CTC 7

Compendium of Therapeutic Choices

Seventh Edition

Published by: Canadian Pharmacists Association, Ottawa, Ontario, Canada

Chair of the Board	Jane Farnham, BScPhm, MBA
Chief Executive Officer	Perry Eisenschmid, BBA, MBA, CDir, HRCCC
Senior Director, Digital Publishing Solutions	James de Gaspé Bonar, PhD
Editor-in-Chief	Barbara Jovaisas, BSc(Pharm), RPh, ELS
Clinical Editors	Lamya Arman, PharmD, RPh Farah Dandachi, BSc(Pharm), MSc Jo-Anne Hutsul, BSc, BSc(Pharm), PhD, RPh Geoff Lewis, BSc(Hons), MSc, RPh Norma Lynn Pearson, BSc(Pharm), RPh Marc Riachi, BSc(Hons), BSc(Pharm), RPh Angela Ross, BScPhm, RPh, ACPR
Scientific Editors	Sonal Acharya, BSc, BA Gustavo Paguaga Anjana Raghuveer, BSc, MSc
Bilingual Pharmacist Editor	Mathilde Vallet, Docteur en pharmacie
Manager, Editorial Processing	Roxanne Bisson
Information Specialist	Laura Léger
Publication Coordinator	Tracy Hume, BA
Product Manager	Marilyn Maynard
Manager, Production Services	Darquise Leblanc
Content Publishing Specialists	Ashley Holmes, BComm(Hons) Kathleen Régimbald
Manager, Graphic Communications	Marilyn Birtwistle
Graphic Designer	Jay Peak

Copyright

Electronic

The content in the *Compendium of Therapeutic Choices (CTC)* is available online and on mobile devices in English and French; to subscribe visit **www.pharmacists.ca**. Licensed content is also available for data integration purposes. For more information on data licensing, please call 1-800-917-9489.

Publisher

Canadian Pharmacists Association / Association des Pharmaciens du Canada

1785 Alta Vista Drive, Ottawa, ON K1G 3Y6 Canada

Comments/Inquiries

Tel: 613-523-7877, 1-800-917-9489 | Fax: 613-523-0445, 1-800-601-1904 | service@pharmacists.ca
Website: www.pharmacists.ca

Printed in Canada

Webcom Inc., 3480 Pharmacy Avenue, Toronto, ON, M1W 2S7 Canada

Website: www.webcomlink.com

Library and Archives Canada Cataloguing in Publication
Compendium of Therapeutic Choices, Seventh Edition (CTC 7)
ISSN: 2368-0210
ISBN: 978-1-894402-89-7

Continues: Therapeutic Choices, Sixth Edition
ISSN: 1495-9208
ISBN: 978-1-894402-75-0

1. Therapeutics – Handbooks, manuals, etc. I. Canadian Pharmacists Association. II. Jovaisas, Barbara.

RM121.5 615.5

Table of Contents

Alterations in Body Temperature

Eye Disorders

Endocrine and Metabolic Disorders

Cardiovascular Disorders

Respiratory Disorders

Gastrointestinal Disorders

Genitourinary Disorders

Sexual Health Disorders

Musculoskeletal Disorders

Skin Disorders

Editor's Message

Welcome to the seventh edition of *Therapeutic Choices*, now titled *Compendium of Therapeutic Choices* (*CTC 7*). This year the Canadian Pharmacists Association (CPhA) has undertaken a strategic rebranding of its products and services, resulting in new titles for many publications. The first edition of this book was published in 1995, a product of the combined vision and creativity of Carmen Krogh and Jean Gray, who recognized the need for reliable, bottom-line information to help healthcare providers make therapeutic decisions at the point of care. Today, the trusted content of this book is available in print, desktop and mobile formats, and is accessed by thousands of physicians, pharmacists and other healthcare providers daily. It has truly become part of the fabric of healthcare delivery in Canada, and CPhA is proud of its growing legacy.

Excerpts from *CTC* chapters form the nucleus of a continuing education offering for physicians and pharmacists. CPhA would like to recognize our 10-year partnership with the McGill Family Practice Research group, in particular Roland Grad and Pierre Pluye, who have worked with us on ground-breaking participatory research that has resulted in several publications. Highlights from *CTC* chapters are linked to McGill's validated information assessment tool, the IAM questionnaire. Data gleaned from thousands of completed questionnaires over the years have provided invaluable feedback, helping us refine the scope and relevance of our content.

CPhA is grateful for the expertise and dedication of the hundreds of authors and reviewers who contribute to this publication. We welcomed many new authors and reviewers into the fold for this edition, and look forward to working together for many to come. The Editorial Advisory Committee provides invaluable strategic guidance on all of CPhA's publications, and their support and counsel are deeply appreciated. A skilled team of clinical and scientific editors contribute significantly to the quality of the content, working with authors and reviewers to ensure that it is current, clearly presented and informed by the best available evidence. The final product would not be possible without the considerable talents of the graphic designers, editorial processing staff, product manager, information technologists and content publishing specialists, who come together from many departments to work magic as a team.

We hope you enjoy the new look of *CTC*. We have made some changes to the seventh edition to optimize the reader experience. The pages are wider, and for the first time we have color in the pages of the chapters. We invite you to tell us how you feel about any aspect of the book, from appearance to usability to the content itself. Feedback helps us provide you with the best possible information, so that you can provide the very best care to your patients.

Barbara Jovaisas, Editor-in-Chief

Editorial Advisory Committee

Authors

Terra Arnason, MD, PhD, FRCP Adult Endocrinology
Clinician Scientist
Division of Endocrinology, Department of Medicine
University of Saskatchewan
Saskatoon, SK

Benoit Bailey, MD, MSc, FRCPC
Division of Emergency Medicine
Department of Pediatrics
Université de Montréal
CHU Sainte-Justine
Montréal, QC

Alan Barkun, MD, CM, FRCPC, FACP, FACG, AGAF, MSc (Clinical Epidemiology)
Professor of Medicine (Gastroenterology)
McGill University
Montreal, QC

Rosemary Basson, MD, FRCP(UK)
University of British Columbia
UBC Hospital, Purdy Pavilion
Vancouver, BC

C. Laird Birmingham, MD, BSc, MHSc, FRCPC, FACP, ABIM, FAED
Professor of Psychiatry
University of British Columbia
Vancouver, BC

David Birnie, MD
Director of the Arrhythmia Service
University of Ottawa Heart Institute
Ottawa, ON

Candice Bjornson, MD, MSc, FRCPC
Pediatric Respirologist
Alberta Children's Hospital
Associate Professor
University of Calgary
Calgary, AB

Edith M. Blondel-Hill, MD, FRCPC
Medical Microbiologist and Infectious Disease Specialist
Medical Director Antimicrobial Stewardship Program
Interior Health Authority
Kelowna General Hospital
Kelowna, BC

Lise Bondy, BSc, MD, FRCPC
Infectious Diseases Resident
University of Toronto
Toronto, ON

Mark Bosma, MD, FRCPC
Assistant Professor of Psychiatry
Associate Postgraduate Program Director
Dalhousie University
Halifax, NS

Susan Bowles, PharmD, MSc, FCCP
Associate Professor
Dalhousie University
Capital District Health Authority
Halifax, NS

Harinderpal Brar, MD, FRCPC
Internal and Critical Care Medicine
Intensivist and General Internist
Surrey Memorial Hospital
Surrey, BC

Marie-Sophie Brochet, BPharm, MSc
Université de Montréal
CHU Sainte-Justine
Montréal, QC

Margaret Burnett , MD, FRCSC, FACOG
Gynecology Section Head
Health Sciences Centre
University of Manitoba
Winnipeg, MB

Vivian P. Bykerk, MD
Associate Professor of Medicine, Weill Cornell Medical College
Director of the Inflammatory Arthritis Center, Division of Rheumatology
Hospital for Special Surgery
New York, NY

Piera Calissi, BSc(Pharm), PharmD, FCSHP
Coordinator Antimicrobial Stewardship Program
Interior Health Authority
Kelowna, BC

Norm R.C. Campbell, MD, FRCPC
Professor of Medicine, Physiology and Pharmacology and Community Health Sciences
University of Calgary
Calgary, AB

Bruce Carleton, BSc, PharmD
Faculty of Medicine
Child & Family Research Institute
University of British Columbia
BC Children's Hospital
Vancouver, BC

George Chami, MD, FRCPC
Gastroenterology and Therapeutic Endoscopy
Pasqua Hospital
Regina, SK

Hugh Chaun, MA, BM, FRCP, FRCP(Ed), FACG, AGAF
University of British Columbia
Vancouver, BC

Victoria Cook, MD, FRCPC
TB Services for Aboriginal Communities
Medical Head, Tuberculosis Services
BC Centre for Disease Control
Vancouver, BC

Robert Côté, MD, FRCPC, FAHA
Senior Neurologist
Montreal General Hospital
Department of Neurology and Neurosurgery
McGill University
Montreal, QC

Amie J. Cullimore, BEd, MD, MSc, FRCSC
Professor of Obstetrics & Gynecology
Associate Chair of Education
McMaster University
Medical Director, Mature Women's Health Program
Staff Obstetrician/Gynecologist
Department of Obstetrics & Gynecology
St. Joseph's Healthcare
Hamilton, ON

Simon de Denus, BPharm, MSc, PhD
Associate Professor
Faculty of Pharmacy
Université de Montréal
Co-director, Heart Failure Research Group
Montreal Heart Institute
Montreal, QC

Virginia Devonshire, MD, FRCPC
Clinical Assistant Professor of Medicine
University of British Columbia
Vancouver, BC

Orna Diav-Citrin, MD
The Israeli Teratology Information Service
Jerusalem, Israel

Simon Dobson, MD, FRCPC
Clinical Associate Professor
Head, Division of Infectious and Immunological Diseases
Department of Pediatrics
BC Children's Hospital
Vancouver, BC

Paul Dorian, MD, MSc, FRCPC
Director, Division of Cardiology
University of Toronto
St. Michael's Hospital
Toronto, ON

David Duperé , MD, FRCPC
Staff Physician, Division of Palliative Medicine
Queen Elizabeth II Health Sciences Centre
Halifax, NS

John M. A. Embil, BSc(Hon), MD, FRCPC, FACP
Winnipeg Regional Health Authority
Diabetic Foot and Complicated Wound Clinic
Health Sciences Centre
University of Manitoba
Winnipeg, MB

Farid Eshghi Esfahani, MD
University of Manitoba
St. Boniface General Hospital
Winnipeg, MB

Karen Ethans, MD, FRCPC, PM&R
Physiatrist
Department of Medicine
University of Manitoba and Health Sciences Centre
Winnipeg, MB

Jean Éthier, MD, FRCPC
Associate professor of Medicine
Centre Hospitalier de l'Université de Montréal
Montreal, QC

Gerald A. Evans, MD, FRCPC
Professor & Chair, Division of Infectious Diseases
Queens' University
Kingston General Hospital
Kingston, ON

Hillel M. Finestone, MDCM, FRCPC
Stroke, Musculoskeletal and Pain Rehabilitation, Electromyography,
Bruyère Continuing Care and The Ottawa Hospital Rehabilitation Centre
Associate Professor of Medicine (Physical Medicine and Rehabilitation)
University of Ottawa
Ottawa, ON

Jonathan Fleming, MB, FRCPC, FABPN, FABSM
Associate Head, Education
Department of Psychiatry
Faculty of Medicine
University of British Columbia
Vancouver, BC

Michael Froeschl, MD, MSc, FRCPC, FACC
Interventional Cardiologist
University of Ottawa Heart Institute
Ottawa, ON

Susan R. Fryters, BScPharm, ACPR
Antimicrobial Utilization/Infectious Diseases Pharmacist
Pharmacy Services
Alberta Health Services
Edmonton, AB

Stan P. George, MD, FRCSC
Department of Ophthalmology and Visual Sciences
Dalhousie University, QEII Health Sciences Centre
Halifax, NS

Paul S. Gibson, MD, FRCPC
Associate Professor of Medicine and Obstetrics & Gynecology
University of Calgary
Calgary, AB

G. Barry Gilliland, MD, FRCPC, FACOG
Clinical Professor of Medicine (Obstetrics, Gynecology and Reproductive Sciences)
College of Medicine
University of Saskatchewan
Saskatoon, SK

Alfred S. Gin, PharmD, FCSHP
Clinical Pharmacist, Infectious Diseases
Department of Pharmaceutical Services
Health Sciences Centre Winnipeg
Assistant Professor of Medicine (Medical Microbiology)
University of Manitoba
Winnipeg, MB

Fabian P. Gorodzinsky, MD, AAPD, FRCPC
Associate Professor (Pediatrics)
University of Western Ontario
London, ON

Michelle M. Graham, MD, FRCPC
Professor of Medicine (Cardiology)
Mazankowski Alberta Heart Institute
University of Alberta Hospital
Edmonton, AB

Gillian Graves, MD, FRCSC
Professor of Obstetrics and Gynecology
Dalhousie University
IWK Health Centre
Halifax, NS

Laurence Green, MD, FRCPC
McGill University
Montreal General Hospital
Montreal, QC

Peter Green, MD, FRCPC
Associate Professor of Dermatology
Dalhousie University
Halifax, NS

S. Grigoriadis, MD, MA, PhD, FRCPC
Head, Women's Mood and Anxiety Clinic: Reproductive Transitions
Associate Professor, Faculty of Medicine, University of Toronto
Toronto, ON

David A. Grimes, MD, FRCPC
Chair and Chief, Division of Neurology
Director, Parkinson's Disease and Movement Disorders Clinic
Associate Professor of Medicine (Neurology)
University of Ottawa
Ottawa, ON

Gord Gubitz, BSc, MD, FRCPC
Assistant Professor of Medicine (Neurology)
Dalhousie University
Director, Neurovascular Clinic
QEII Health Sciences Centre
Halifax, NS

Lyn Guenther, MD, FRCPC
Chair of Dermatology at University of Western Ontario
London, ON

L. Maria Gutschi, BScPhm, PharmD
Canada Chemists
Scientific Consultant, Patented Medicines Prices Review Board
Canadian Forces Health Support Unit
Ottawa, ON

David A. Hanley, MD, FRCPC
Professor of Endocrinology and Metabolism
Departments of Medicine, Community Health Sciences and Oncology
University of Calgary
Calgary, AB

John G. Hanly, MD, MRCPI, FRCPC
Professor of Medicine (Rheumatology)
Dalhousie University
Queen Elizabeth II Health Sciences Centre
Halifax, NS

Marianne Harris, MD, CCFP
AIDS Research Program, St. Paul's Hospital
Clinical Assistant Professor of Medicine (Family Practice)
Associate Member, Division of AIDS, Department of Medicine
University of British Columbia
Vancouver, BC

Glen Hazlewood, MD, FRCPC, PhD(c)
Clinical Scholar
Department of Internal Medicine, Division of Rheumatology
University of Calgary
Calgary, AB

Geralynn Hirsch, MSN, RN-NP
Nurse Practitioner
Medical Services Unit, Division of Gastroenterology
Capital District Health Authority
Halifax, NS

Michael G. Hogan , MD, FRCSC
Orthopaedic Surgeon
Hogan Healthcare Center P.C.
Cumming, GA USA

Shinya Ito, MD, FRCPC
University of Toronto
Clinical Pharmacology & Toxicology
Department of Pediatrics
Hospital for Sick Children
Toronto, ON

W. Bruce Jackson, MD, FRCSC
Professor of Ophthalmology
University of Ottawa Eye Institute
The Ottawa Hospital, General Campus
Ottawa, ON

David Johnson, MD
Professor of Medicine (Pediatrics)
University of Calgary
Calgary, AB

James Johnston, MD, FRCPC
Clinical Assistant Professor
Division of Tuberculosis Control
BC Centre for Disease Control
Vancouver, BC

Gary I. E. Joubert, MD, FRCPC
Associate Professor of Medicine (Pediatrics)
University of Western Ontario
London, ON

Dina Kao, MD, FRCPC
Associate Professor of Medicine (Gastroenterology)
University of Alberta
Edmonton, AB

Suneil Kapur, MD, FRCPC
Assistant Professor of Medicine (Rheumatology)
University of Ottawa
The Ottawa Hospital
Ottawa, ON

Colin A. Kean, BSc
Medical Student
Universita Vita-salute San Raffaele
Milan, Italy

Walter F. Kean, MB, ChB(Glas), MD(Glas), FRCP(Edin, Glas & C)
Clinical Professor of Medicine (Rheumatology)
McMaster University
Hamilton, ON

Paul K. Keith , MD, MSc, FRCPC
Associate Professor of Medicine (Allergy and Clinical Immunology)
McMaster University
Hamilton, ON

James R. Kennedy, MD, FRCPC
Medicine and Pharmacology
University of British Columbia
St Paul's Hospital
Vancouver, BC

Sidney H. Kennedy, MD, FRCPC
Department of Psychiatry
University Health Network and St Michael's Hospital
University of Toronto
Toronto, ON

Tammy M. Keough-Ryan, MD, MSc, FRCPC
Professor of Medicine and Surgery (Nephrology)
Medical Director, Kidney-Pancreas Transplantation, Multi Organ Transplant Program
Dalhousie University, QEII Health Sciences Centre
Halifax, NS

Kathleen J. Kerr, MD, Dip Env Health
Department of Family and Community Medicine, University of Toronto
Environmental Health Clinic, Women's College Hospital
Toronto, ON

Jay Keystone, MD, MSc(CTM), FRCPC
Senior Staff Physician
Department Medicine, Division of Infectious Diseases
University of Toronto
Tropical Disease Unit
Toronto General Hospital
Toronto, ON

Sandra Knowles, BScPhm
Drug Policy Research Specialist
Ontario Drug Policy Research Network (ODPRN)
St. Michael's Hospital
Toronto, ON

Gideon Koren, MD, FRCPC, FACMT, FAACT
Professor of Pediatrics
Director, The Motherisk Program
The Hospital for Sick Children and University of Toronto
University of Toronto
Toronto, ON

Gunnar Kraag, MD, FRCPC
Professor of Medicine (Rheumatology)
University of Ottawa
The Ottawa Hospital
Ottawa, ON

Anne-Louise Lafontaine, MD, MSc, FRCPC
Associate Professor of Medicine (Neurology and Neurosurgery)
Director, McGill Movement Disorder Clinic
McGill University
Montreal, QC

Joanne M. Langley, MD, MSc, FRCPC
Professor of Pediatrics and Community Health and Epidemiology, Dalhousie University
CIHR-GSK Chair in Pediatric Vaccinology
Division of Infectious Diseases, IWK Health Centre
Halifax, NS

Richard Langley, MD, FRCPC
President, Canadian Dermatology Association
Professor of Medicine (Dermatology)
Director of Research
Dalhousie University
Halifax, NS

Richard Lester, MD, FRCPC
Medical Head, STI/HIV Control
Clinical Prevention Services
British Columbia Centre for Disease Control
Vancouver, BC

Mova Leung, BScPhm, PharmD, BCOP
Coordinator - Oncology, Hematology and Immunology
University of Toronto, Faculty of Pharmacy
Toronto, ON

Gisele Li, MD, MSc, FRCSC
Assistant Professor of Medicine (Ophthalmology)
University of Montreal
Montreal, QC

Michael Libman, MDCM, FRCPC
Director, Division of Infectious Diseases
Department of Microbiology
McGill University Health Centre
Associate Professor, McGill University
Montreal, QC

Duane Lichtenwald, MD, FRCPC
Clinical Associate Professor of Medicine
University of Saskatchewan
Saskatoon, SK

Wendy Lim, MD, MSc, FRCPC
Associate Professor of Medicine
McMaster University
St. Joseph's Healthcare
Hamilton, ON

Heather Lochnan, MD, FRCPC
Associate Professor of Medicine (Endocrinology and Metabolism)
University of Ottawa
Ottawa, ON

Mark Loeb, MD, MSc, FRCPC
McMaster University
Hamilton, ON

Timothy P. Lynch, MD, FRCPC
Children's Hospital of Western Ontario
London, ON

Cathy MacLean, MD, FCFP
Professor and Chair of Family Medicine
Memorial University
St John's, NL

Stuart Maddin, MD, FRCPC
Clinical Professor Emeritus of Dermatology and Skin Science
University of British Columbia
Vancouver, BC

Kerry Mansell, BSP, PharmD, CDE
Associate Professor
College of Pharmacy and Nutrition
University of Saskatchewan
Saskatoon, SK

Cindy Marshall, BSc, MD, CCFP, FCFP
Family Health Group
Lower Sackville, NS

David G. McCormack, MD, FRCPC, FCCP
Professor of Medicine (Respirology)
University of Western Ontario
London Health Sciences Centre
London, ON

James McCormack, BSc(Pharm), PharmD
Professor
Faculty of Pharmaceutical Sciences
University of British Columbia
Vancouver, BC

R. Andrew McIvor, MD, MSc, FRCPC
Professory of Medicine
McMaster University
Firestone Institute for Respiratory Health
St. Joseph's Healthcare
Hamilton, ON

Peter J. McLeod, MD, FRCPC, FACP
Professor of Medicine and Pharmacology
McGill University
Montreal, QC

Penny F. Miller, BSc(Pharm), MA(Ed)
Senior Instructor, Clinical Pharmacy Specialist in Family Practice
Faculties of Pharmaceutical Sciences and Medicine
University of British Columbia
Vancouver, BC

Heather I. Milliken, MDCM, FRCPC, CSPQ
Associate Professor of Psychiatry
Director of Continuing Professional Development
Dalhousie University, QEII Health Sciences Centre
Nova Scotia Early Psychosis Program
Halifax, NS

Jeremy Moeller, MD, FRCPC
Assistant Professor of Neurology
Yale University
New Haven, CT USA

Louise Moist, BSc, MSc, MD, FRCPC
Professor of Medicine and Epidemiology and Biostatistics
University of Western Ontario
London, ON

Julio S.G. Montaner, MD, DSc(hon), FRCPC, FCCP, FACP, FRSC, OBC
Professor of Medicine (AIDS)
University of British Columbia
St. Paul's Hospital
BC Centre for Excellence in HIV/AIDS
Vancouver, BC

Val Montessori, MD, FRCPC
Clinical Associate Professor of Medicine (Infectious Diseases)
University of British Columbia
Associate Medical Director, Immunodeficiency Clinic
BC Centre for Excellence in HIV/AIDS
St. Paul's Hospital
Vancouver, BC

Mark Montgomery, MD, FRCPC
Clinical Associate Professor of Pediatrics
University of Calgary
Calgary, AB

Tania Mysak, BSP, PharmD
Clinical Practice Manager North Pharmacy Services
Alberta Health Services
Clinical Academic Colleague
Faculty of Pharmacy and Pharmaceutical Sciences
University of Alberta
Edmonton, AB

Lynne Nakashima, BSc(Pharm), PharmD,
Professional Practice Leader, Pharmacy
BC Cancer Agency
Clinical Professor, Faculty of Pharmaceutical Sciences
University of British Columbia
Vancouver, BC

Mike Namaka, BScPharm, MScPharm, PhD Med
Associate Professor, Faculty of Pharmacy and Medicine
University of Manitoba
President, Manitoba Multiple Sclerosis Research Network Organization
Winnipeg, MB

Pablo B. Nery, MD
Associate Professor of Medicine (Cardiology)
Arrhythmia Service
University of Ottawa Heart Institute
Ottawa, ON

Lindsay E. Nicolle, MD, FRCPC
Professor of Internal Medicine and Medical Microbiology
University of Manitoba
Winnipeg, MB

Richard W. Norman, MD, FRCSC
Chief Urologist
Tantallon Medical Clinics
Upper Tantallon, NS

Mary Noseworthy, MD, FRCPC
Asthma Director
Alberta Children's Hospital
Calgary, AB

Richard I. Ogilvie, MD, FRCPC, FACP
Medicine & Pharmacology
University of Toronto
Hypertension Unit
Toronto Western Hospital
University Health Network
Toronto, ON

Sagar V. Parikh, MD, FRCPC
Professor of Psychiatry
University of Toronto
UHN Toronto Western Hospital
Toronto, ON

Kevork M. Peltekian, MD, FRCPC
Interim Chief and Acting Head, Division of Digestive Care & Endoscopy
Department of Medicine
Dalhousie University and QEII Health Sciences Centre
Halifax, NS

Stephen Phillips, BSc, MBBS, FRCPC
Professor of Medicine (Neurology)
Dalhousie University
Stroke Neurologist
Capital District Health Authority
Halifax, NS

Michael J. Potter, MD, FRCSC
Honorary Professor
Department of Ophthalmology and Visual Sciences
University of British Columbia
Vancouver, BC

William Pryse-Phillips, MD, FRCP, FRCPC, DPM
Emeritus Professor of Medicine (Neurology)
Memorial University of Newfoundland
St. John's, NF

R. Allan Purdy, MD, FRCPC, FACP, FAHS
Professor of Medicine (Neurology)
Dalhousie University, QEII Health Sciences Centre
Department of Medicine
Capital District Health Authority
Halifax, NS

Jeffrey P. Reiss, MD, MSc, FRCPC, DABPN, DFCPA, DFAPA
Professor and Chair, Division of General Adult Psychiatry
Vice-Chair, Department of Psychiatry
Schulich School of Medicine and Dentistry
University of Western Ontario
London, ON

Steven C. Reynolds, MD, FRCPC
Clinical Assistant Professor of Medicine
Infectious Diseases and Critical Care
University of British Columbia
Head and Research Director, Department of Critical Care
Royal Columbian Hospital
Vancouver, BC

Kenneth Rockwood, MD, FRCPC
Geriatric Medicine & Neurology
QEII Health Sciences Centre
Kathryn Allen Weldon Professor of Alzheimer Research
Dalhousie University
Halifax, NS

Ghislaine O. Roederer, MD, PhD
Institut de recherches cliniques de Montréal
Montreal, QC

Alana Rosenthal, MD, FRCPC
Pediatric Infectious Diseases Specialist
Department of Pediatrics
North York General Hospital
North York, ON

Coleman Rotstein, MD, FRCPC, FACP, FIDSA
Professor of Medicine (Infectious Diseases)
Co-director, Immunocompromised Host Infectious Disease
Director, Oncologic Infectious Diseases
University of Toronto,University Health Network
Toronto, ON

André Roussin, MD, FRCPC
Associate Professor of Medecine
University of Montreal
President, Quebec Society of Vascular Sciences
Vice-President Thrombosis Canada
Notre-Dame Hospital (CHUM) and Montreal Heart Institute
Montreal, QC

R. Mark Sadler, MD, FRCPC
Professor of Medicine (Neurology)
Dalhousie University
Co-director, Epilepsy Program
Capital Health Halifax
Halifax, NS

Cheryl A. Sadowski, BSc(Pharm), PharmD, FCSHP
Associate Professor
Faculty of Pharmacy & Pharmaceutical Sciences
University of Alberta
Edmonton, AB

Peter Selby, MBBS, CCFP
Centre for Addiction and Mental Health
Ontario Tobacco Research Unit
University of Toronto
Toronto, ON

Eldon Shaffer, MD, DipABIM, FACP, FRCPC
Professor of Medicine (Gastroenterology)
University of Calgary
Calgary, AB

Arya M. Sharma, MD, FRCPC
Professor and Chair in Obesity Research & Management
Department of Medicine
University of Alberta
Edmonton, AB

Neil H. Shear, MD, FRCPC
Professor of Dermatology and Clinical Pharmacology
Sunnybrook Health Sciences Centre
University of Toronto
Toronto, ON

Robert Sheldon, MD, PhD, FRCPC, FCAHS, FHRS
Professor of Cardiac Sciences
University of Calgary
Calgary, AB

Mathieu Simon, MD, FRCPC, FCCM
Institut Universitaire de Cardiologie et de Pneumologie de Québec
Québec, QC

Kurt Skakum, BSc(Hons), MD, FRCPC
Associate Professor, Medical Director
Consultation-Liaison Psychiatry
Director, Postgraduate Education Department of Psychiatry
University of Manitoba
Assistant Head, Adult Mental Health Program, Winnipeg Regional Health Authority
Winnipeg, MB

C. Douglas Smith, MD, FRCPC
Head, Division of Rheumatology
The Ottawa Hospital and University of Ottawa
Ottawa, ON

Derek Y.F. So, MD, FRCPC, FACC
Associate Professor of Cardiology
Staff Interventional Cardiologist
University of Ottawa Heart Institute
Ottawa, ON

Monica Solbiati, MD
Department of Biomedical and Clinical Sciences
University of Milan
Division of Medicine and Pathophysiology
Luigi Sacco Hospital
Milan, Italy

Paul Stacey, MD, MSc
McMaster University
Hamilton, ON

Andrew Steer, MBBS, BMedSc, MPH, FRACP, PhD
Associate Professor
Principal Research Fellow and Paediatric Infectious Diseases Physician
Centre for International Child Health, Department of Paediatrics, Royal Children's Hospital
University of Melbourne
Royal Children's Hospital
Melbourne, Australia

Robert Strang, MD, MHSc, FRCPC
Chief Medical Officer of Health
Department of Health Wellness
Halifax, NS

Mark G. Swain, MD, MSc, FRCPC
Head, Division of Gastroenterology and Hepatology
Department of Medicine
University of Calgary
Calgary, AB

Richard P. Swinson, MD, FRCPC, FRCPsych
Emeritus Professor and Medical Director of the Anxiety Treatment and Research Centre
Department of Psychiatry and Behavioural Neurosciences
McMaster University and St. Joseph's Hospital
Hamilton, ON

Jerry K.L. Tan, MD, FRCPC
Dermatologist
Windsor, Ontario
Schulich School of Medicine and Dentistry
University of Western Ontario
London, ON

Stephen R. Tan, MD, FRCPC
Associate of the Department of Dermatology
University of Minnesota
St. Paul, MN USA

Laura Targownik, MD, MSHS, FRCPC
Associate Professor of Medicine
Section of Gastroenterology
University of Manitoba
Winnipeg, MB

Taryn Taylor, BKin, MSc, MD, CCFP, Dip Sport & Exercise Medicine
Primary Care Sport Medicine Physician
Carleton Sports Medicine Clinic
Ottawa, ON

Courtney A. Thompson, MD
Physician, Infectious Diseases
University of Toronto
Toronto, ON

W. Grant Thompson, MD, FRCPC, FACG
Emeritus Professor of Medicine
University of Ottawa
Ottawa, ON

Elly Trepman, MD
Department of Medical Microbiology
University of Manitoba
Winnipeg, MB

Ross T. Tsuyuki, PharmD, MSc, FCSHP, FACC
Professor of Medicine (Cardiology)
Faculty of Medicine and Dentistry
University of Alberta
Edmonton, AB

Eldon Tunks, MD, FRCPC
Emeritus Professor of Psychiatry
McMaster University
Department of Physical Medicine and Rehabilitation
Regional Rehabilitation Center, Hamilton General Hospital
Hamilton, ON

Joseph Vayalumkal, MD, FRCPC
Clinical Assistant Professor Pediatrics
Section of Infectious Diseases
University of Calgary
Medical Officer Infection Prevention and Control
Alberta Children's Hospital, Alberta Health Services
Calgary, AB

Adil Virani, BSC(Pharm), PharmD, FCSHP
Director, Lower Mainland Pharmacy Services
Associate Professor
University of British Columbia
Vancouver, BC

Sharon Walmsley, MSc, MD, FRCPC
Professor of Medicine
University of Toronto
Toronto, ON

David Warren, MD, FRCPC
Assistant Director, Pediatric Emergency
Director, Child Protection Program
Children's Hospital, London Health Science Center
Associate Professor
University of Western Ontario
London, ON

Walter Watral, BScPharm, PharmD
Clinical Assistant Professor, Faculty of Pharmacy
University of Manitoba
Clinical Pharmacist, Outpatient Leukemia/BMT Clinic & Clinical Pharmacy Practice Leader
Cancer Care Manitoba
Winnipeg, MB

C. Peter N. Watson, MD, FRCPC
Assistant Professor of Neurology
University of Toronto
Toronto, ON

Lori D. Wazny, BSc(Pharm), PharmD
Clinical Pharmacist, Manitoba Renal Program
Department of Pharmaceutical Services
Health Sciences Centre
Winnipeg, ON

Miriam Weinstein, MD, FRCPC
Associate Professor of Pediatrics and Medicine
University of Toronto
Hospital for Sick Children
Toronto, ON

Philip S. Wells, MD, FRCPC, MSc
Chief/Chair, Department of Medicine
University of Ottawa
The Ottawa Hospital
Ottawa, ON

Michel White, MD, FRCPC, FACC, FESC
Professor of Medicine (Cardiology)
University of Montreal
Montreal Heart Institute
Montreal, QC

Sharon Whiting, MBBS, FRCPC
Children's Hospital of Eastern Ontario
Ottawa, ON

Pearce Wilcox, MD, FRCPC, FACP
Professor of Medicine
University of British Columbia
St. Paul's Hospital
Vancouver, BC

James M. Wright, MD, PhD, FRCPC
Professor, Departments of Medicine,
Anesthesiology, Pharmacology & Therapeutics
University of British Columbia
Vancouver Hospital
Vancouver, BC

Reviewers

David R. Anderson, MD, FRCPC
Professor of Medicine, Pathology and Community Health & Epidemiology
Dalhousie University
Head, Division of Hematology and Deputy Head, Department of Medicine
Capital Health
Halifax, NS

Gary Butterworth, BSc, BSc(Pharm), OD
Optometrist
Winnipeg, MB

Roxane Carr, PharmD, BCPS, FCSHP
Children's & Women's Health Centre of British Columbia
Assistant Professor, Faculty of Pharmaceutical Sciences
University of British Columbia
Vancouver, BC

Alice Yuk-Yan Cheng, MD, FRCPC
Department of Medicine
Trillium Health Partners
Mississauga, ON

Paul J. Daeninck, MD, MSc, FRCPC
Assistant Professor, Internal Medicine and Family Medicine
University of Manitoba
Consultant Medical Oncologist and Coordinator, St. Boniface Hospital Site
Cancer Care Manitoba
Consultant Palliative Medicine Specialist
Regional Palliative Care Program
Winnipeg, MB

Linda Dresser, PharmD, FCSHP
Pharmacotherapy Specialist, Antimicrobial Stewardship
University Health Network, Toronto
Assistant Professor (Status Only), Leslie Dan Faculty of Pharmacy
University of Toronto
Toronto, ON

Barb Evans, BSP, ACPR, MSc, FCSHP
Clinical Manager, Pharmacy Services
Saskatoon Health Region
Clinical Assistant Professor
College of Pharmacy and Nutrition
University of Saskatchewan
Saskatoon, SK

David Gardner, BSCPharm. ACPR, PharmD, MSc
Professor
Department of Psychiatry and College of Pharmacy
Dalhousie University
Halifax, NS

Alfred S. Gin, PharmD, FCSHP
Clinical Pharmacist, Infectious Diseases
Department of Pharmaceutical Services
Health Sciences Centre
Assistant Professor of Medicine (Medical Microbiology)
University of Manitoba
Winnipeg, MB

Helen Grad, MScPhm
Assistant Professor
Faculty of Dentistry and Faculty of Medicine
University of Toronto
Toronto, ON

Anthony J. Ham Pong, MBBS, FRCPC
Consultant, Allergy & Immunology
Assistant Professor (VPT)
Children's Hospital of Eastern Ontario
Ottawa, ON

Brian G. Hardy, BSc, BScPhm, ACPR, PharmD, FCSHP, FCCP
Coordinator, Education and Clinical Programs
Department of Pharmacy
Sunnybrook Health Sciences Centre
Associate Professor, Leslie Dan Faculty of Pharmacy
University of Toronto
Toronto, ON

Lyall Higginson, MD, FRCPC
Internal Medicine, Cardiology
Royal Jubilee Hospital
University of British Columbia
Victoria, BC

Shinya Ito, MD, FRCPC
Professor and Head
Division of Clinical Pharmacology and Toxicology
Department of Pediatrics
Hospital for Sick Children
University of Toronto
Toronto, ON

Derek Jorgenson, BSP, PharmD, FCSHP
Associate Professor
College of Pharmacy and Nutrition
University of Saskatchewan
West Winds Primary Health Centre
Saskatoon, SK

David N. Juurlink, BPhm, MD, PhD, FRCPC, FACMT, FAACT
Professor of Medicine (Pediatrics and Health Policy)
University of Toronto
Divisions of General Internal Medicine and Clinical Pharmacology & Toxicology
Sunnybrook Health Sciences Centre
Institute for Clinical Evaluative Sciences
Ontario Poison Centre
Toronto, ON

Steven Katz, PharmD
Associate Clinical Professor of Medicine (Rheumatology)
University of Alberta
Edmonton, AB

Jamie Kellar, RPh, BScHK, BScPhm, PharmD
Pharmacy Clinician Educator/Advanced Practice Pharmacy
The Centre for Addiction and Mental Health
Assistant Professor
Leslie Dan Faculty of Pharmacy University of Toronto
Toronto, ON

Heather Kertland, PharmD, FCSHP
Clinical Pharmacy Specialist/Leader
St. Michael's Hospital
Assistant Professor
University of Toronto, Leslie Dan Faculty of Pharmacy
Toronto, ON

Sandra Knowles, RPh, ACPR, BScPhm
Drug Safety Pharmacist
Sunnybrook Health Sciences Centre
University of Toronto
Toronto, ON

Michael Libman, MDCM, FRCPC
Director, Division of Infectious Diseases
Department of Microbiology
McGill University Health Centre
Associate Professor, McGill University
Montreal, QC

Mark J. Makowsky, BSP, PharmD, ACPR
Associate Professor
Faculty of Pharmacy and Pharmaceutical Sciences
University of Alberta
Edmonton, AB

Anne Massicotte, BPharm, MSc
Drug Information Pharmacist
The Ottawa Hospital, Civic Campus
Ottawa, ON

Doreen Matsui, MD, FRCPC
Department of Pediatrics
Children's Hospital, London Health Sciences Centre
University of Western Ontario
London, ON

Peter J. McLeod, MD, FRCPC, FACP
Professor, Medicine and Pharmacology
McGill University
Montreal, QC

G.B. Meterissian, MD, FRCPC
Department of Psychiatry
Faculty of Medicine
McGill University
Montreal General Hospital Site
McGill University Health Center
Montreal, QC

Scott Murray, MD, FRCPC
Division of Dermatology
Dalhousie University
Halifax, NS

Tania Mysak, BSP, PharmD
Clinical Practice Manager North Pharmacy Services
Alberta Health Services
Clinical Academic Colleague
Faculty of Pharmacy and Pharmaceutical Sciences
University of Alberta
Edmonton, AB

C. Jane Richardson, BSP, PhD, FCSHP
Consulting Pharmacist
Saskatoon, SK

Stuart J. Rosser, MD, FRCPC, MPH
Assistant Professor of Medicine (Infectious Diseases)
University of Alberta
Edmonton, AB

Robert Siemens, MD, FRCSC
Department of Urology
Kingston General Hospital
Queen's University
Kingston, ON

Jose Silveira, BSc, MD, FRCPC, Dip ABAM
Assistant Professor, Department of Psychiatry
University of Toronto
Director, Mental Health and Addiction
Chief of Psychiatry
St. Joseph's Health Centre
Toronto, ON

Neil Skjodt, MD, MSc, FRCPC, FCCP, DABSM, FAASM
Specialist in Internal, Respiratory Critical Care and Sleep Medicine
Adjunct Associate Professor
Canadian Centre for Behavioural Neuroscience
Lethbridge, AB

Kathryn Slayter, BScPhm, PharmD, FCSHP
Clinical Pharmacy Specialist, Division of Infectious Diseases, Department of Medicine
Clinical Coordinator, Department of Pharmacy
Capital District Health Authority
Canadian Centre for Vaccinology
Adjunct Assistant Professor, Faculties of Medicine and Health Professions
Dalhousie University
Halifax, NS

Penelope Smyth, BSc, MD, FRCPC
Assistant Professor of Medicine
University of Alberta
Neurologist, MS Specialist
WMC Health Sciences Centre
Edmonton, AB

Laura Targownik, MD, MSHS, FRCPC
Associate Professor of Medicine
Section of Gastroenterology
University of Manitoba
Health Sciences Centre
Winnipeg, MB

Peter Thomson, BSc(Pharm), PharmD
Clinical Resource Pharmacist, Medicine Program
Winnipeg Regional Health Authority
Clinical Associate Professor, Faculty of Pharmacy
University of Manitoba
Winnipeg, MB

Deborah L. Thompson, BScPharm, PharmD, BCPP
Clinical Pharmacy Specialist
Fraser Health Mental Health and Substance Use Services
Langley, BC

Nese Yuksel, BScPharm, PharmD, ACPR, FCSHP, NCMP
Associate Professor
Faculty of Pharmacy and Pharmaceutical Sciences
University of Alberta
Edmonton, AB

Editorial Policy

Editorial Process

Chapters and appendices in the *Compendium of Therapeutic Choices* (*CTC*) are written by expert authors and are based on the best available evidence. The Canadian Pharmacists Association (CPhA) employs a rigorous review process to ensure that the information is accurate and unbiased. Content is extensively reviewed and validated by skilled CPhA editors and by at least two reviewers (physicians and pharmacists) who are recognized experts in the relevant clinical area.

CPhA asks authors and reviewers to disclose any potential conflicts of interest, and does not accept funding from pharmaceutical manufacturers for any content that we develop.

Description and Limitations of Information

Although based on the best available evidence, *CTC* also contains selected information representing the experience and opinions of individual authors, particularly if evidence is limited. The authors, editors and publisher have made every attempt to ensure the accuracy of the information at the time of printing. Users should be aware that the text may contain information, statements and dosages for drugs different from those approved by the Therapeutic Products Directorate, Health Canada. Users are advised that the information presented in this text is not intended to be all inclusive. Consequently, health care providers are encouraged to seek additional and confirmatory information to meet their practice requirements and standards as well as the information needs of the patient.

Errata

In spite of CPhA's rigorous review process, should a major error occur it will be corrected immediately on www.e-therapeutics.ca and posted on www.pharmacists.ca. All errors will be corrected in the next print edition.

How to Use the *Compendium of Therapeutic Choices*

The *Compendium of Therapeutic Choices* Seventh Edition (*CTC 7*) includes 128 chapters and 4 appendices. Each chapter presents essential therapeutic information organized in easily readable text, algorithms and tables. Drug tables appear at the end of the chapter. References follow the Suggested Readings section.

Drug therapy is discussed using generic drug names. Brand name inclusion in the chapters is not intended as an endorsement of a product. Many Canadian brand names are listed in the drug tables. These are not all inclusive and are not listed in any order of preference. Within drug tables, classes and drugs are presented in alphabetical order, unless otherwise stated.

A list of common abbreviations can be found in the Glossary of Abbreviated Terms at the back of the book. Microorganism names are spelled out in full the first time they occur in a chapter, and abbreviated thereafter.

The true cost of a specific therapy involves a number of elements including the manufacturer's list price, the mark-up and the dispensing fee, the length of drug therapy and costs related to drug administration. Prices used to determine cost of therapy in this book represent the acquisition cost in Ottawa at the time of writing. Drug costs in the tables do not include any mark-up or dispensing fees. Unless otherwise stated, costs are presented comparatively with the use of the $ symbol. For most conditions, calculations were made with the cost of the lowest priced product at the usual dosage for a given period. The treatment period selected for most chronic conditions is 30 days. However, treatment periods vary, and the legend accompanying each table should be consulted.

Readers of *CTC 7* requiring more detailed information on pediatric therapy should consult specialized texts.

Appendix I addresses dosage adjustment in patients with reduced renal function. Within each chapter's drug table(s), a small icon (❥) appears after the drug name if dosage adjustment should be considered.

The use of drugs during pregnancy is the subject of Appendix II. Appendix III discusses drug use during breastfeeding.

Information on nutritional supplements for adults is found in Appendix IV.

A level of evidence system has been introduced in this edition. Selected text is given a rating of SORT A, B or C based on the Strength of Recommendation Taxonomy system, which was developed to evaluate the body of evidence for primary care interventions.[1]

SORT[1] Code	Definition
A	Based on consistent AND good-quality patient-oriented evidence
B	Based on inconsistent OR limited-quality patient-oriented evidence
C	Based on consensus, disease-oriented evidence, usual practice, expert opinion, or case series for studies of diagnosis, treatment, prevention or screening

1. Ebell MH, Siwek J, Weiss BD et al. Strength of Recommendation Taxonomy (SORT): a patient-centered approach to grading evidence in the medical literature. *Am Fam Physician* 2004;69:549-57. Available from: http://www.aafp.org/afp/2004/0201/p548.html.

Chapter 1
Acute Agitation

Kurt Skakum, MD, FRCPC and
Jeffrey P. Reiss, MD, MSc, FRCPC, DABPN, DFCPA, DFAPA

Acute agitation is a dangerous condition that occurs in 10–20% of hospitalized patients who are acutely ill.[1] For the well-being and safety of patients and caregivers, it is essential that agitated patients are treated quickly, effectively and safely. As a first step, the underlying cause of agitation must be determined and treated whenever possible.

Acute agitation is defined as a "state of anxiety accompanied by motor restlessness."[2] Aggression, defined as a "behaviour leading to self assertion",[2] is often mislabeled as agitation and can occur in association with acute agitation. Agitation can occur in many clinical settings. This chapter will focus on the management of agitation in adults in the emergency room or in-patient units such as psychiatry or medical/surgical wards.

Agitation can be associated with delirium from any cause, including infection, neurologic conditions (e.g., trauma, seizure, stroke or tumor), intoxication, drug withdrawal (see Chapter 12), adverse drug reactions such as toxicity, allergy or akathisia, endocrine disorders, blood sugar irregularities, cardiovascular problems and electrolyte disturbances. Psychiatric conditions that can cause agitation include psychosis, mania, depression, anxiety and personality disorders. Agitation is also frequently associated with dementia.

As practitioners transition to the DSM-5[3] they should be aware of several changes to terminology and diagnostic criteria affecting some of the disorders described in this chapter. Most significantly, the former category of dementia is removed and has been replaced with the wider category of neurocognitive disorders (NCD). This new category now includes delirium as well as mild or major NCDs associated with conditions such as Alzheimer's disease, frontotemporal neurocognitive disorder, Lewy body disease, vascular neurocognitive disorder, traumatic brain injury, substance/medication-induced disorder, HIV infection, prion disease, Parkinson's disease, Huntington's disease, and others.

This chapter still refers to dementia and discusses delirium separately from dementia. Agitation in patients with neurocognitive disorder due to traumatic brain injury deserves separate mention, since significant research is published on this specific condition. Additionally, other psychiatric conditions associated with agitation will be referred to by their generic descriptors (e.g., psychosis, mania, depression, anxiety and personality disorders) rather than a DSM-5 specific diagnosis.

Goals of Therapy

- Create a safe environment for the treatment of the agitated patient and other patients
- Keep the work environment safe for staff
- Ameliorate the agitated state
- Prevent further episodes of agitation/aggression

Investigations

- Obtain history from the patient and descriptions of the patient's behaviour from staff and other collateral sources. Include:
  - triggers for the behaviour
  - previous episodes of agitation
  - description of the nature of the agitation
- Review medications and concomitant medical conditions
- Determine whether the agitation is accompanied by other symptoms such as confusion, clouded consciousness, cognitive impairment or physical symptoms such as fever, hypoxia or pain
- Mental status examination, a complete physical examination and relevant laboratory investigations are essential to the diagnosis

Therapeutic Choices

Figure 1 illustrates an algorithm for the management of acute agitation associated with several conditions.

Nonpharmacologic Choices

Give special attention to safety when encountering an acutely agitated/aggressive patient. This includes safety of the agitated individual, other patients and staff in the environment. Often, both nonpharmacologic and pharmacologic interventions will be necessary. Address patients in a calm, reassuring yet confident tone of voice. There should be no hesitancy to have additional staff nearby. Direct patients to attempt to control their behaviour and reassure them that the environment is safe and that they have no reason to be fearful. Ask what the problem is and how it can be resolved. If necessary, patients can be asked to take medication to help reduce their distress.

Due to safety concerns or adverse reactions in elderly patients with dementing illnesses, use pharmacologic agents sparingly. Employ psychosocial interventions in this population where possible.[4] Consultation with responsive behavioural specialists can be beneficial in these cases.

If verbal approaches are unsuccessful, patients may need to be physically restrained or secluded. Details on the application of restraint and seclusion are not addressed in this chapter.

Pharmacologic Choices

Delirium

Delirium is a condition in which an acute onset of impairment in consciousness and cognition is associated with a medical/physical cause. The impairment typically fluctuates over the course of the day.

The first step is to determine and remove the underlying cause of delirium. If agitation persists because the cause cannot be identified or the patient does not respond, it may be necessary to treat the patient pharmacologically. Antipsychotics (see Table 1) are first-line medications in these instances. **Haloperidol** is the most studied and effective medication for decreasing agitation in delirious patients. It can be given by mouth or by im/iv injection. Small, regularly scheduled doses are preferred over "as needed" dosing. The mid-potency first-generation antipsychotic **loxapine** and second-generation antipsychotics such as **olanzapine**, **risperidone** and **quetiapine** have also been used to treat delirium.[5] Risperidone or olanzapine oral disintegrating tablets may be beneficial for patients who are not willing to swallow tablets.[6] Olanzapine immediate-acting injection may be required for highly agitated or uncooperative patients who cannot or are unwilling to take oral medications.

When used for several weeks to months, antipsychotics have been associated with an increased risk of stroke and death in elderly patients with dementia. To manage acute confusional states with agitation or aggression in the elderly, use antipsychotics (for the briefest possible duration) only when the benefits clearly outweigh the risks.[7,8] See also Dementia, below.

Figure 1: Management of Acute Agitation

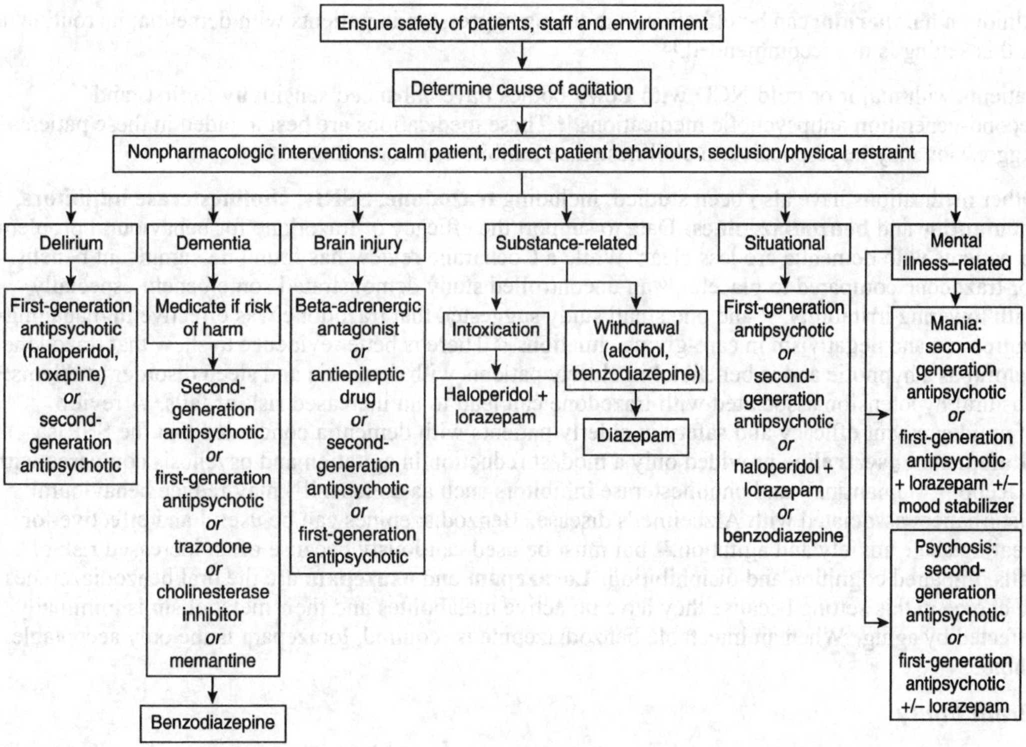

Reserve **benzodiazepines** (preferably those with a longer half-life such as diazepam or chlordiazepoxide) for cases where symptoms are attributed to alcohol or benzodiazepine withdrawal. More information about managing drug withdrawal syndromes can be found in Chapter 12.

Dementia

Patients with various forms of dementia frequently exhibit agitation. Management of behavioural problems in older adults with dementia is also discussed in the Dementia chapter (see Chapter 5).These behaviours can be disruptive to the care environment and are potentially dangerous. Always document the occurrence, frequency and nature of the behavioural disturbance and any recognizable triggers. If medications are necessary they should be prescribed following the “start low, go slow” principle, and reassessed regularly.

Considering the potential increased risks (e.g., stroke, death) and the limited tolerability and benefit in many patients, the decision to use antipsychotic agents for agitation or aggression in patients with dementia needs to be made on an individual basis and with caregiver support and consent (see also Chapter 5).[8,9,10] Because of a more favourable side effect profile, the use of second-generation antipsychotics is increasing over first-generation antipsychotics.[11] **Risperidone** has a favourable effect on agitation and other behavioural symptoms (total behaviour, aggression and psychosis) associated with Alzheimer's disease.[12] Initiate risperidone at a dose of 0.25 mg daily and titrate to a usual effective daily dose of 1 mg, with an upper limit of 2 mg. The higher dosage may offer an efficacy advantage but does so at the risk of increased side effects including falls. **Olanzapine** can be started at 2.5 mg daily and titrated to 5–10 mg per day to reduce aggressiveness, anxiety and euphoria.[12] Olanzapine immediate-acting injection may be helpful for patients who refuse or are unable to take oral medications. There is little evidence on the use of **quetiapine** in the control of agitation and aggression in patients with dementia.

Although **haloperidol** can be effective in reducing aggression in patients with dementia, its routine use in this setting is not recommended.[13]

Patients with major or mild NCD with Lewy bodies have enhanced sensitivity to first- and second-generation antipsychotic medications.[14] These medications are best avoided in these patients. Aggression may be responsive to cholinesterase inhibitors or memantine.[15]

Other medications have also been studied, including **trazodone**, **SSRIs**, **cholinesterase inhibitors**, **memantine** and **benzodiazepines**. Data to support the efficacy of trazodone for behavioural problems in patients with dementia are less clear. While a Cocharane review has found no significant benefit for trazodone compared to placebo,[16] an uncontrolled study demonstrated some benefit especially with lowering irritability, [17] and one small study suggested that trazodone was effective in managing aggression and negativism in care-giving situations.[18] There is better evidence to show that trazodone is helpful as a hypnotic and is beneficial in elderly patients with dementia and sleep disorder problems.[19] Postural hypotension associated with trazodone can lead to an increased risk of falls. A review of antidepressant efficacy and safety in elderly patients with dementia concluded that the SSRIs **citalopram** or **sertraline** provided only a modest reduction in agitation and psychosis compared with placebo.[20] Memantine[21] and cholinesterase inhibitors such as donepezil[22] may reduce behavioural disturbances associated with Alzheimer's disease. Benzodiazepines can be useful and effective for treating acute anxiety and agitation,[23] but must be used cautiously because of an increased risk of falls, impaired cognition and disinhibition. **Lorazepam** and **oxazepam** are the oral benzodiazepines of choice in this setting because they have no active metabolites and their metabolism is minimally affected by aging. When an injectable benzodiazepine is required, lorazepam is the only acceptable choice.

Brain Injury

Give priority to minimizing the potential side effects when choosing a treatment in patients with brain injury. Many medications from different classes have been used in this setting, though conclusive evidence is lacking. A Cochrane review of the treatment of agitation and aggression in patients with acquired brain injury (e.g., anoxic brain injury, encephalitis, trauma; stroke not included)[24] found that the best evidence, though still limited, was for **beta-adrenergic antagonists**. High doses of **propranolol** were effective in reducing the incidence of aggression. Antiepileptic drugs such as **carbamazepine** and **divalproex** are also used. There is concern about paradoxical disinhibition when **benzodiazepines** are used in brain-injured patients. **Antipsychotics** seem to have a generally anti-aggressive effect regardless of the etiology.

Small studies have evaluated several other medications in this patient population. The evidence is not strong enough to recommend the use of **tricyclic antidepressants**, **SSRIs**, **amantadine**, **buspirone**, **stimulants** and **lithium** as first-line agents.

Mental Illness-associated Agitation

Psychosis

With acutely psychotic individuals, short-acting parenteral formulations of **antipsychotics** either alone or in combination with parenteral **lorazepam** are recommended (see also Chapter 11).

Do *not* combine im olanzapine with benzodiazepines because of the associated cardiac and respiratory complications.

Rapidly dissolving or liquid formulations of second-generation antipsychotics with or without benzodiazepines are an effective alternative to im medications,[25,26] but are not practical for uncooperative patients. **Risperidone** is available in liquid and rapidly dissolving tablet preparations. **Olanzapine** is available in a rapidly dissolving wafer form. Several first-generation antipsychotics are also available in oral liquid formulations.

Mania

The acute control of severe agitation in patients with mania involves both short-term treatment and initiation of longer term mood stabilizers. Initially, second-generation antipsychotics (**risperidone**, **olanzapine**, **quetiapine**, **aripiprazole** or **ziprasidone**) are effective in establishing control of agitated behaviour. If oral medications cannot be administered, im injection is an effective alternative; im olanzapine, *alone* or a first-generation antipsychotic with a benzodiazepine can be used. Generally speaking, benzodiazepines should not be used as monotherapy.[27] Initiation of a mood stabilizer should also be undertaken in the acute phase of treatment (see Chapter 4).

Situational Agitation/Aggression

Agitation/aggression that is not attributable to any of the previously discussed causes, but more related to personality factors, is a common occurrence in emergency rooms. There is a relative lack of well-studied interventions in this setting. Nonpharmacologic interventions are essential. The most common medications used are **first-generation antipsychotics** along with a **benzodiazepine**, either by oral administration or im injection (e.g., **haloperidol** 5 mg po/im plus **lorazepam** 2 mg po/im). Emerging evidence supports the use of second-generation antipsychotics in this setting.[28]

Choices during Pregnancy and Breastfeeding

Agitation is usually an acute and short-lived condition. Employ nonpharmacologic methods as a first-line treatment in any patient displaying agitation, especially those who are pregnant or breastfeeding. Use pharmacologic treatments for agitation only in situations where there is significant risk of harm to the patient, infant, staff or other patients on the treatment unit, and with informed consent.

If agitation during pregnancy or postpartum is associated with a chronic mental illness (e.g., due to nonadherence with medication), discuss with the patient and/or their next of kin the risks and benefits of restarting or continuing the specific medication. Information on the use of antipsychotics and antidepressants during pregnancy or breastfeeding can be found in Chapter 6 and Chapter 11.

A discussion of general principles on the use of medications in these special populations, such as obtaining informed consent, can be found in Appendix II and Appendix III. Other specialized reference sources are also provided in these appendices.

Therapeutic Tips

- Implement measures to prevent delirium (and any attendant agitation) in hospitalized patients (e.g., provide aids such as clocks and calendars to keep patients orientated, mobilize patients early following surgery, prevent sleep deprivation, optimize functioning and communication with eyeglasses/hearing aids).
- In elderly patients with dementia, use antipsychotics only when nonpharmacologic measures have failed, and if patients are severely agitated, psychotic and/or a danger to themselves or others.
- Use lower doses of antipsychotics in older patients; re-evaluate the need for continued therapy regularly.

Table 1: Drugs Used for the Management of Acute Agitation

Class	Drug	Dose	Adverse Effects	Drug Interactions	Cost[a]
Antidepressants	*trazodone* generics	Brain injury: 25–50 mg HS po Maximum: 200 mg HS Dementia (for sedation): 25–100 mg/day po	Sedation, nausea, headache, dry mouth, orthostatic hypotension, priapism (rare).	May potentiate effects of other CNS depressants and augment hypotensive effects of antihypertensives.	$
Antiepileptic Drugs	*carbamazepine immediate-release* Tegretol, generics	Mania: 800–1200 mg/day po in 2–4 divided doses Target serum levels (based on data for seizure control): 17–50 µg/L Brain injury: 200–300 mg BID–TID po	Rash, cognitive impairment, sedation, hyponatremia.	Induces cytochrome P450 enzymes; may increase clearance of many other drugs such as oral contraceptives, lovastatin, meperidine, morphine, nifedipine, oxycodone, trazodone.	$
	divalproex sodium Epival, generics	Brain injury: 250–500 mg TID po Target serum level (based on data for seizure control): 400–700 µmol/L	Nausea, tremor, sedation; rarely, edema.	Inhibits glucuronidation; may decrease clearance of other drugs such as lamotrigine and lorazepam.	$
Antipsychotics, First-generation	*haloperidol* generics	Delirium: 0.5–2.5 mg BID po/im Dementia: 0.5–1 mg BID po Psychosis: 5–10 mg/day po/im Mania: 5–10 mg/day po/im	Sedation, parkinsonism, akathisia, acute dystonia, neuroleptic malignant syndrome. Haloperidol: QT_c prolongation.	Additive effects with other CNS depressants, antagonism of dopamine agonists. Haloperidol: Avoid combining with other drugs that increase QT_c interval.	$–$$
	loxapine Xylac, generics	Delirium: 12.5–50 mg/day po Psychosis: 25–50 mg/day po	See haloperidol.	See haloperidol.	$
	zuclopenthixol acetate, intramuscular Clopixol-Acuphase	Psychosis: 50–150 mg im; duration of action 2–3 days	See haloperidol.	See haloperidol.	$$$–$$$$$/ 2–3 days
Antipsychotics, Second-generation	*aripiprazole* Abilify	Mania: 15 mg/day po as acute monotherapy; 10–15 mg/day if used as co-therapy with lithium or valproate Psychosis: 10–15 mg/day po	Akathisia, dizziness, orthostatic hypotension, headache, GI complaints, tremor, sedation.	Carbamazepine (or other strong inducers of CYP2D6 or CYP3A4 such as phenytoin, rifampin) can decrease aripiprazole levels significantly. Ketoconazole, quinidine, fluoxetine or paroxetine (or other strong inhibitors of CYP2D6 or CYP3A4) can increase levels substantially.	$

Class	Drug	Dose	Adverse Effects	Drug Interactions	Cost[a]
	olanzapine, oral Zyprexa, Zyprexa Zydis, generics	Delirium: 5–10 mg/day po Dementia: 2.5–5 mg/day po Psychosis: 10–30 mg/day po Mania: 5–20 mg/day po	Anticholinergic effects, akathisia, dizziness, neuroleptic malignant syndrome.	Additive sedation with CNS depressants; antagonism of dopamine agonists; may potentiate antihypertensive drug effects.	$–$$
	olanzapine, intramuscular Zyprexa Intramuscular	Delirium or mania: 2.5–10 mg im; repeat in 2 h and 6 h PRN to a maximum of 30 mg/24 h Use maximum of 2.5 mg/dose in debilitated patients, 5 mg in elderly patients	See olanzapine, oral.	See olanzapine, oral. Should **not** be administered simultaneously with parenteral benzodiazepines due to reports of cardiac and respiratory problems including deaths.	$$$–$$$$$
	quetiapine Seroquel, generics	Delirium: 25–100 mg/day po Dementia: 12.5–50 mg/day po Psychosis: 300–800 mg/day po Mania: start with 100 mg/day po; increase by 100 mg/day as needed to 300–600 mg/day divided BID	Sedation, dizziness, neuroleptic malignant syndrome.	Additive sedation with CNS depressants; antagonism of dopamine agonists; may potentiate antihypertensive drug effects.	$
	risperidone ❥ Risperdal Preparations, generics	Delirium: 0.5–2 mg/day po Psychosis: 2–8 mg/day po Dementia: 0.25–2 mg/day po Mania: 2–3 mg/day po	Akathisia, dizziness, neuroleptic malignant syndrome.	Additive sedation with CNS depressants; antagonism of dopamine agonists; may potentiate antihypertensive drug effects.	$
	ziprasidone Zeldox	Mania: start with 40 mg BID po; increase as needed up to 80 mg BID po Psychosis: start with 40 mg BID po; increase as needed up to 80 mg BID po	Insomnia, extrapyramidal side effects; consider ECG at baseline and periodically to monitor effect on QT_c interval.	Carbamazepine decreases ziprasidone levels significantly; do not use with other drugs that prolong the QT_c interval.	$
Benzodiazepines	*clonazepam* Rivotril, generics	Mania: 0.25–0.5 mg BID–TID po	Sedation, dizziness, cognitive impairment; rarely, respiratory depression can occur in this setting.	Additive sedation and possibly cardiorespiratory depression with other CNS depressants.	$
	lorazepam Ativan, generics	Dementia: 0.5–1 mg Q6–8H po Mania/psychosis, adjunctively with antipsychotics: 1–2 mg po/im	See clonazepam.	See clonazepam.	$

(cont'd)

Table 1: Drugs Used for the Management of Acute Agitation *(cont'd)*

Class	Drug	Dose	Adverse Effects	Drug Interactions	Cost[a]
	oxazepam generics	Dementia: 10–15 mg TID po	See clonazepam.	See clonazepam.	$
Beta$_1$-adrenergic Antagonists	*propranolol* generics	Brain injury: 20–40 mg daily po; increase by 20 mg/day Maximum: 640 mg/day Monitor heart rate and blood pressure	Bradycardia, hypotension, heart block, sedation.	Additive hypotension with other antihypertensives; additive sedation with other CNS depressants.	$

[a] Cost of 1-day supply unless otherwise specified; includes drug cost only.

Dosage adjustment may be required in renal impairment; see Appendix I.

Legend: $ < $5 $–$$ < $5–15 $$ $5–15 $$$ $15–25 $$$-$$$$$ $15– 45 $$$$ $25–35 $$$$$ $35–45

Suggested Readings

Marder SR. A review of agitation in mental illness: treatment guidelines and current therapies. *J Clin Psychiatry* 2006;67(Suppl 10):13-21.

Nassisi D, Korc B, Hahn S et al. The evaluation and management of the acutely agitated elderly patient. *Mt Sinai J Med* 2006;73(7):976-84.

Stern TA, Rosenbaum JF, Fava M et al. Chapter 18: Delirium. In: *Massachusetts General Hospital comprehensive clinical psychiatry*. 1st ed. Philadelphia (PA): Mosby/Elsevier; 2008. p. 217-29.

References

1. Trzepacz PT. Delirium. Advances in diagnosis, pathophysiology and treatment. *Psychiatr Clin North Am* 1996;19(3):429-48.
2. Dorland WAN. *Dorland's illustrated medical dictionary*. 27th ed. Philadelphia (PA): Saunders; 1988.
3. American Psychiatric Association. *Diagnostic and statistical manual of mental disorders: DSM-5*. 5th ed. Washington (DC): American Psychiatric Publishing; 2013.
4. Richter T, Meyer G, Möhler R et al. Psychosocial interventions for reducing antipsychotic medication in care home residents. *Cochrane Database Syst Rev* 2012;(12):CD008634.
5. Cook IA. *Guideline watch: Practice guideline for the treatment of patients with delirium*. Arlington (VA): American Psychiatric Association; 2004. Available from: psychiatryonline.org/guidelines.aspx. Accessed March 29, 2011.
6. Nordstrom K, Allen MH. Alternative delivery systems for agents to treat acute agitation: progress to date. *Drugs* 2013;(16):1783-92.
7. Caine ED. Clinical perspectives on atypical antipsychotics for the treatment of agitation. *J Clin Psychiatry* 2006;67(Suppl 10):22-31.
8. Herrmann N, Lanctot KL. Atypical antipsychotics for neuropsychiatric symptoms of dementia: malignant or maligned? *Drug Saf* 2006;29(10):833-43.
9. Schneider LS, Tariot PN, Dagerman KS et al. Effectiveness of atypical antipsychotic drugs in patients with Alzheimer's disease. *N Engl J Med* 2006;355(15):1525-38.
10. Schneeweiss S, Setoguchi S, Brookhart A et al. Risk of death associated with the use of conventional versus atypical antipsychotic drugs among elderly patients. *CMAJ* 2007;176(5):627-32.
11. Alexopoulos GS, Jeste DV, Chung H et al. The expert consensus guideline series. Treatment of dementia and its behavioral disturbances. Introduction, methods, commentary, and summary. *Postgrad Med* 2005;Spec No:6-22.
12. Ballard C, Waite J. The effectiveness of atypical antipsychotics for the treatment of aggression and psychosis in Alzheimer's disease. *Cochrane Database Syst Rev* 2006;(1):CD003476.
13. Lonergan E, Luxenberg J, Colford J. Haloperidol for agitation in dementia. *Cochrane Database Syst Rev* 2002;(2):CD002852.
14. McKeith IG, Dickson DW, Lowe J et al. Diagnosis and management of dementia with Lewy bodies: third report of the DLB Consortium. *Neurology* 2005;65(12):1863-72.
15. Zupancic M, Mahajan A, Handa K. Dementia with lewy bodies: diagnosis and management for primary care providers. *Prim Care Companion CNS Disord* 2011;13(5):PCC.11r01190.
16. Martinson-Torres G, Fioravanti M, Grimley EJ. Trazodone for agitation in dementia. *Cochrane Database Syst Rev* 2004;(4):CD004990.
17. Lopez-Pousa S, Garre-Olmo J, Vilalta-Franch J et al. Trazodone for Alzheimer's disease: a naturalistic follow-up study. *Arch Gerontol Geriatr* 2008;47(2):207-15.
18. Kitamura Y, Kudo Y, Imamura T. [Trazodone for the treatment of behavioral and psychological symptoms of dementia (BPSD) in Alzheimer's disease: a retrospective study focused on the aggression and negativism in caregiving situations]. *No To Shinkei* 2006;58(6):483-8. [Japanese].
19. Camargos EF, Pandolfi MB, Freitas MP et al. Trazodone for the treatment of sleep disorders in dementia: an open-label, observational study and review. *Arq Neuropsiquiatr* 2011;69(1):44-9.
20. Seitz DP, Adunuri N, Gill SS et al. Antidepressants for agitation and psychosis in dementia. *Cochrane Database Syst Rev* 2011;(2):CD008191.
21. Cummings JL, Schneider E, Tariot PN et al. Behavioral effects of memantine in Alzheimer disease patients receiving donepezil treatment. *Neurology* 2006;67(1):57-63.
22. Cummings JL, McRae T, Zhang R et al. Effects of donepezil on neuropsychiatric symptoms in patients with dementia and severe behavioral disorders. *Am J Geriatr Psychiatry* 2006;14(7):605-12.
23. American Psychiatric Association. *Practice guideline for the treatment of patients with Alzheimer's disease and other dementias of late life*. Arlington (VA): APA; 2007. Available from: psychiatryonline.org/guidelines.aspx. Accessed March 29, 2011.
24. Fleminger S, Greenwood RJ, Oliver DL. Pharmacological management for agitation and aggression in people with acquired brain injury. *Cochrane Database Syst Rev* 2006;(4):CD003299.
25. American Psychiatric Association. *Practice guideline for the treatment of patients with schizophrenia*. Arlington (VA): APA; 2004. Available from: psychiatryonline.org/guidelines.aspx. Accessed March 29, 2011.
26. Canadian Psychiatric Association. Clinical practice guidelines. Treatment of schizophrenia. *Can J Psychiatry* 2005;50(13 Suppl 1):7S-57S.
27. Yatham LN, Kennedy SH, Parikh SV et al. Canadian Network for Mood and Anxiety treatments (CANMAT) and International Society for Bipoloar Disorders (ISBD) collaborative update of CANMAT guidelines for the management of patients with bipolar disorder: update 2013. *Bipolar Disord* 2013;15(1):1-44.
28. Rund DA, Ewing JD, Mitzel K et al. The use of intramuscular benzodiazepines and antipsychotic agents in the treatment of acute agitation or violence in the emergency department. *J Emerg Med* 2006;31(3):317-24.

Chapter 2
Anxiety Disorders

R. P. Swinson, MD, FRCPsych, FRCPC

The Diagnostic and Statistical Manual of Mental Disorders 5th edition (DSM-5) contains several significant changes to the classification of anxiety disorder:[1]

- Panic disorder and agoraphobia are no longer linked in a single diagnosis. Each has separate criteria and patients with both disorders are now coded with 2 diagnoses.
- Obsessive-compulsive disorder (OCD) and post-traumatic stress disorder (PTSD) are reclassified as separate disorders—obsessive-compulsive and related disorders, and trauma- and stressor-related disorders, respectively. Management of OCD and PTSD are discussed in separate chapters (see Chapter 9 and Chapter 10).
- Two disorders, separation anxiety disorder and selective mutism, have been added to anxiety disorders. Both disorders were previously classified in "disorders usually first diagnosed in infancy, childhood, or adolescence".

Goals of Therapy

- Eliminate or decrease symptomatic anxiety
- Eliminate or decrease anxiety-based disability
- Prevent recurrence
- Treat comorbid conditions

Investigations

- Thorough history with attention to:
  - nature and onset of symptoms
  - nature and extent of disability
  - presence of comorbid medical or psychiatric conditions

Note: Treat comorbid mood disorders, especially depression, as the primary condition.

- Interview questions assist in obtaining an accurate diagnosis (Table 1, Table 2)
- Physical examination to exclude endocrine or cardiac disorders and to look for signs of substance use
- Laboratory tests:
  - CBC, liver function tests, gamma-glutamyl transpeptidase (GGT to screen for alcohol use), thyroid indices (supersensitive TSH), ECG

Note: Treat physical disorders of recent onset before making a definitive diagnosis of an anxiety disorder.

Therapeutic Choices

Relatively mild anxiety states in response to life circumstances are frequently time-limited; many patients will respond to anxiety management strategies without medication. Support, problem-solving and relaxation techniques or mindfulness may be helpful as the environmental crisis resolves.

However, specific anxiety or mood disorders may develop as a consequence of the original stressor. See Figure 1 for an illustration of the management of anxiety disorders.

Table 1: Classification of Anxiety Disorders[1]

Type of Anxiety Disorder	Clinical Features
Separation anxiety disorder	Childhood onset of fear of separation from attachment figures (parents, siblings) that is excessive for the developmental stage.
Selective mutism	Childhood onset of failure to speak in school or other social situations when the individual does speak in other settings. May impede academic progression.
Specific phobia	Severe anxiety triggered by a specific feared object or situation (e.g., spiders, flying, heights) often leading to avoidance behaviour.
Social anxiety disorder (social phobia)	Intense anxiety provoked by social or performance situations in which embarrassment might occur; often leads to avoidance behaviour.
Panic disorder	Recurrent unexpected abrupt panic attacks with persistent anxiety concerning recurrence.
Agoraphobia	Marked fear or anxiety of 2 or more situations: public transportation, open spaces, closed spaces, crowds, being outside of home alone. Leads to avoidance of these situations.
Generalized anxiety disorder	Excessive worry and anxiety about a number of events or activities on more days than not over a period of ≥6 months.
Anxiety disorder due to another medical condition	Anxiety or panic attacks directly caused by a medical condition (e.g., thyroid dysfunction, hypoglycemia, heart failure, arrhythmia, COPD, vitamin B_{12} deficiency, encephalitis).
Substance/medication-induced anxiety disorder	Anxiety or panic attacks directly caused by use or discontinuation of a substance (e.g., alcohol, amphetamines, anticholinergics, caffeine, cannabis, cocaine, corticosteroids, hallucinogens), capable of producing the symptoms of anxiety.
Other specified anxiety disorder	Symptoms of anxiety disorders not meeting full diagnostic criteria, e.g., limited-symptom panic attacks, generalized anxiety not occurring on more days than not.
Unspecified anxiety disorder	Distressing anxiety symptoms that fail to meet diagnostic criteria for specific anxiety disorders.

Table 2: Interview Questions to Establish Specific Anxiety Diagnosis[a]

Questions	Further Inquiry
Do you have sudden episodes of intense anxiety?	Establish nature of attack.
Do you have difficulty going to places to which you used to be able to go?	Inquire about crowded places, line-ups, movies, highways, distance from home.
Do you have difficulty talking to people in authority or speaking in public?	Establish situations (one-on-one or groups).
Are you afraid of blood, small animals or heights?	Establish precise feared situation.
Do you have thoughts that keep going in your mind that you can't stop?	Ask nature of thoughts (illness, harm, sex).
Do you worry a lot of the time?	Ask about worries related to health, family, job and finances.

[a] The order of asking the questions can be varied. The order represented in Table 2 reflects the sequence in the *Diagnostic and statistical manual of mental disorders: DSM-5*[1] in which panic attacks are diagnosed first, followed by phobic disorders, and generalized anxiety disorder. Anxiety disorders that do not fit into the above categories are atypical. Accurate diagnosis is recommended before instituting treatment.

Nonpharmacologic Choices

- Specific *cognitive behavioural therapy* (CBT) tailored to the primary diagnosis may be required. An online resource at McMaster University (www.pter.mcmaster.ca) provides more information about CBT.
- Caffeine or other stimulant use should be reduced and controlled.
- Alcohol use should be minimal; it should not be used to control anxiety.
- Recommend aerobic exercise several times per week. Exercise has been found to reduce some symptoms of panic and agoraphobia but CBT is significantly more effective.[2]
- Educate patient about regular sleep habits and sleep hygiene.
- Stress reduction, including relaxation training and time management, is often helpful initially. Mindfulness meditation is increasingly used in anxiety disorders with good effect.

Figure 1: **Management of Anxiety Disorders**

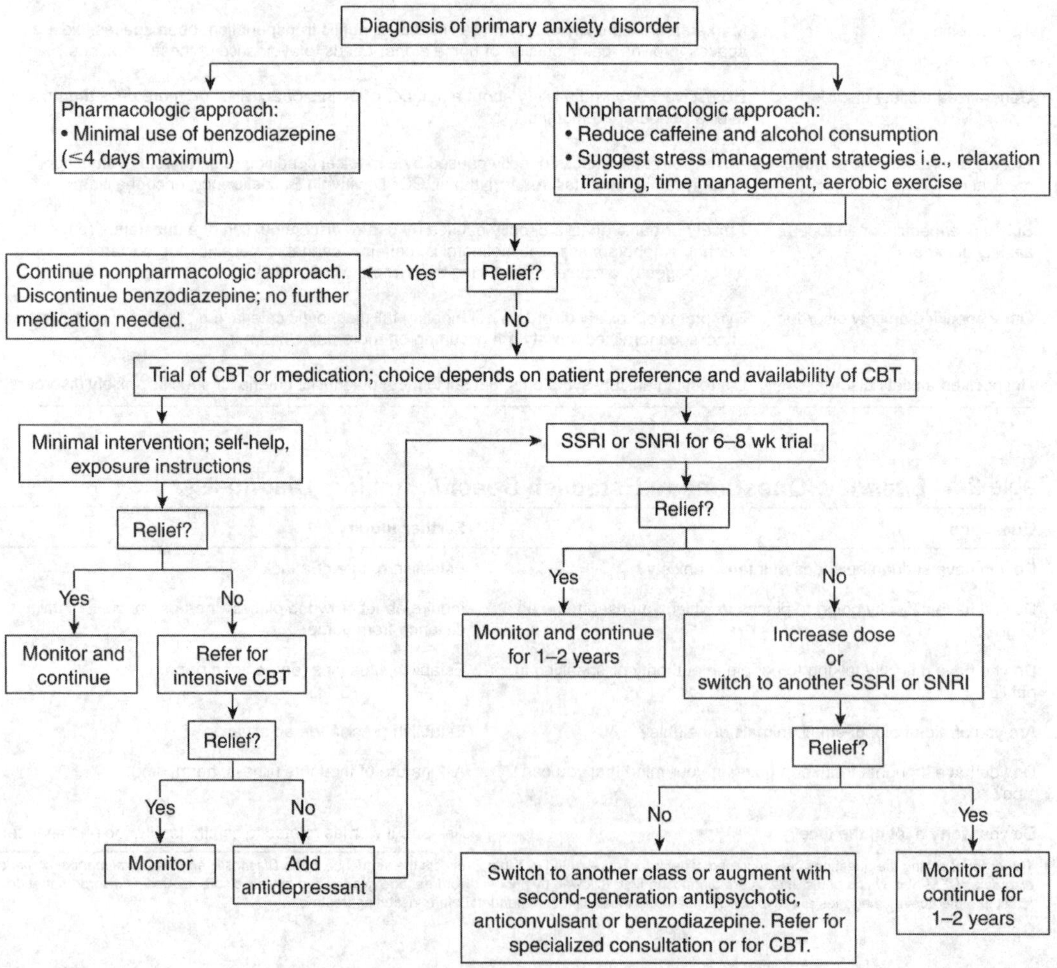

Abbreviations: CBT = cognitive behavioural therapy; SNRI = serotonin-norepinephrine reuptake inhibitor; SSRI = selective serotonin reuptake inhibitor

Pharmacologic Choices

The role of drug therapies varies among anxiety disorders. Drug treatment is rarely required for specific phobias. In the other anxiety disorders, drug therapy is the most common intervention, especially when intensity of symptoms and disability are moderate to severe. A psychiatric consultation is recommended for any patient who does not improve with a trial of 2 separate antidepressants. A list of drug choices is provided in Table 3.

Available information on the treatment of panic disorder, agoraphobia and panic disorder with agoraphobia (PDA) is based on studies that did not separate patients into groups with either panic disorder or agoraphobia.[3] Although DSM-5 makes the distinction between the 2 separate conditions or PDA, studies are needed to determine whether available pharmacologic agents differentially treat each condition.

Panic Disorder

Antidepressants

The SSRIs **citalopram**, **escitalopram**, **fluoxetine**, **fluvoxamine**, **paroxetine** and **sertraline** are all effective in reducing panic attacks. **Venlafaxine**, a serotonin-norepinephrine reuptake inhibitor (SNRI), has also demonstrated efficacy. SSRIs and SNRIs are first-choice agents in treating panic disorder with or without agoraphobia.[4,5] There is usually a delay in response to these agents that may be accompanied by initial agitation. Augmenting the SSRI or SNRI with a brief course of a low-dose benzodiazepine (no longer than 8 weeks, to minimize risk of dependence/withdrawal) can increase adherence to medication and produce a more rapid response than with antidepressants alone.[6]

The tricyclic antidepressants (TCAs) **imipramine**, **desipramine** and **clomipramine** have been shown to reduce the frequency and severity of panic attacks[7] and are inexpensive. The different side effect profiles of TCAs and SSRIs can be used to guide treatment choice. **Mirtazapine** has been effective in open-label trials.[8,9] The older monoamine oxidase inhibitors (MAOIs) **phenelzine** and **tranylcypromine** are also effective but more difficult to use because of the dietary restrictions and potential for serious drug interactions.[10]

The dosage requirements and length of treatment for antidepressants in panic disorder are similar to those for major depression (see Chapter 6). However, the initial dose should be as low as possible (e.g., 10 mg daily for TCAs or fluoxetine), and then increased as tolerated to the usual antidepressant dose range; higher starting doses may cause patients to become agitated and discontinue treatment abruptly. Determining the duration of drug treatment is of great importance; medication is usually required for months or years. Evidence has shown that a majority of patients will suffer relapse after benzodiazepines or antidepressants are discontinued.[11]

Taper doses gradually if antidepressants must be discontinued or dose-reduced. Abrupt dosage changes may cause the patient to experience antidepressant discontinuation syndrome. More information about this syndrome is included in the Depression chapter (see Chapter 6).

Benzodiazepines

Pharmacologic treatment is guided by the acuity of panic disorder at presentation. Low doses of high-potency benzodiazepines can be used to abort initial panic attacks and may control high-frequency attacks later in the development of the disorder. **Clonazepam** 0.25–0.5 mg BID frequently makes panic attacks more manageable. **Lorazepam** and **diazepam** can also be used.

Although there is considerable evidence for the efficacy of benzodiazepines as monotherapy for panic disorder, they are best reserved for those cases where SSRI/SNRI treatment has not been successful or if the antidepressant response needs augmentation.

Short-term use of benzodiazepines is best. For patients who have been maintained on stable low doses for years, the potential benefits of discontinuing benzodiazepines (e.g., decreased risk of sedation/falls or dependence/withdrawal) should be weighed against the potential increase in frequency or severity of panic attacks when benzodiazepines are stopped.[11]

Agoraphobia and Panic Disorder with Agoraphobia

The pharmacologic treatment of agoraphobia with or without panic disorder is the same as for panic disorder. Much of the disability in agoraphobia arises from avoidance behaviour rather than the panic attacks. The degree of avoidance is frequently under-reported by patients; careful questioning or standardized questionnaires may be needed for a complete assessment. The avoidance can be addressed with CBT, even if medication reduces or eliminates accompanying panic attacks. CBT is effective alone or combined with medication.[11,12] Access to specialized CBT is often limited by financial factors.

Social Anxiety Disorder (Social Phobia)

This excessive fear of being criticized or negatively evaluated by others presents as shyness, avoidance of social contact or difficulty dealing with authority figures. The disorder may be present from childhood and often becomes noticeable in adolescence. It is particularly important to rule out comorbid major depression and alcohol use. CBT or other psychotherapy may be necessary to deal with significant social anxiety, even when medication is used.

SSRI and SNRI antidepressants are the mainstay of medical treatment for social anxiety disorder. These agents are effective for generalized social anxiety and for milder cases manifesting as stage fright or fear of public speaking. **Escitalopram**,[13,14] **fluvoxamine**,[15,16] **paroxetine**,[17,18] **sertraline**[19,20] and **venlafaxine**[21] have demonstrated efficacy. Simple stage fright or fear of public speaking may respond to low-dose **propranolol** (10 mg) taken 30 minutes before the event; in generalized social anxiety disorder propranolol is usually ineffective.[22,23]

Results for **moclobemide** vary but it may be effective, particularly in higher doses.[24] When used at doses above 600 mg/day, moclobemide loses its isoenzyme specificity for MAO-A. Caution patients taking higher doses about consumption of tyramine-rich foods such as aged cheeses, smoked meats, beer and red wine.

There is some evidence to support a trial of **gabapentin**[25] or **pregabalin**[26] in patients not responding to first-line measures. Benzodiazepines, particularly **clonazepam**,[27] are effective but should be used with the same restrictions (i.e., short-term use of lowest effective dose) as in other anxiety disorders.

Specific Phobia

Medication is not usually indicated for the treatment of specific fear of heights, animals, injections or other common triggers. As little as 6 hours of CBT is often successful in producing marked, enduring change.

Generalized Anxiety Disorder

Generalized anxiety disorder (GAD) is characterized by excessive and uncontrollable worry related to everyday-life concerns such as safety of family members, financial/job security and health. Patients with GAD frequently exhibit depressed mood and other anxiety symptoms. CBT is the most effective psychosocial treatment but often requires 20 or more sessions to be successful.[28]

SSRIs and SNRIs are established as first-line drug treatment for generalized anxiety disorder. Numerous studies demonstrate the efficacy of **duloxetine**[29], **escitalopram**,[30,31] **paroxetine**,[32] **sertraline** or **venlafaxine**.[33] **Pregabalin** is now an established first-line treatment for GAD with the advantage of providing rapid onset of relief.[34,35,36] While effective in GAD, **imipramine** is limited by its side effect profile and safety concerns in overdose. It is usually reserved for use in patients for whom first-line agents are not effective. **Bupropion** is also an option.[37]

Quetiapine is effective in GAD both as monotherapy and to augment antidepressant medication.[38] At a dose of 150 mg daily, it has been shown to rapidly reduce many symptoms of GAD. Quetiapine is generally regarded as a second-line choice due to its side-effect profile of weight gain and potential effects on metabolic regulation.

Low-dose benzodiazepines (e.g., **bromazepam**, **clonazepam**, **diazepam**, **lorazepam**) can be used for symptom relief for several weeks at a time; caution is advised regarding the risk of dependence and discontinuation symptoms.

Buspirone is an azapirone with a low potential for abuse and less sedation compared to benzodiazepines. Like antidepressants, it has a relatively slow onset of effect. When switching from long-term benzodiazepine therapy to buspirone, it is important that the benzodiazepine is not discontinued abruptly; there is no cross-tolerance between the 2 drug classes and benzodiazepine withdrawal symptoms could be precipitated.

Choices during Pregnancy and Breastfeeding

Anxiety Disorders and Pregnancy

Anxiety disorders have onset early in life, are frequently chronic in nature and their severity waxes and wanes in response to environmental events. Pregnancy may be accompanied by increased or decreased anxiety.

It is important to screen for the presence of anxiety symptoms prior to conception if possible. Screening can be repeated during the pregnancy and in particular postpartum. If a woman is suffering from marked anxiety related to pregnancy and breastfeeding, it is imperative to screen for the presence of mood symptoms and suicidality.

In any circumstances where a woman experiences severe anxiety or mood disorder symptoms during pregnancy or postpartum, referral to a psychiatrist may be necessary. In major centres, women's mental health programs are usually available and are attuned to responding to consultation requests quickly.

Preconceptional treatment can be offered for anxiety disorders that are producing significant distress or interfering with functioning. Panic disorder with agoraphobia may prevent a woman from attending medical appointments.

Management during Pregnancy

There is good evidence that psychological treatments can have beneficial effects for more than half of those who persist with a treatment program. CBT can be administered without restriction throughout pregnancy. Therapies based in meditative or relaxation techniques may be more acceptable than pharmacologic approaches.[39]

If anxiety symptoms are severe and produce significant impairment, medications can be appropriate and effective.[40] The 2 main classes of medications used for anxiety disorders are **SSRI** or **SNRI** antidepressants and **benzodiazepines**.

SSRIs or SNRIs may cause agitation, sweating, nausea, GI distress and weight gain. There have been reports of a slightly higher (but still low) risk of congenital abnormalities involving the heart or cleft lip/palate.[41] When used in the third trimester, these drugs may be associated with neonatal withdrawal symptoms such as tremors, increased muscle tone, feeding or digestive problems or respiratory distress. Whether benzodiazepines confer an increased risk of congenital malformations is controversial. Benzodiazepines administered shortly before delivery can result in floppy infant syndrome or neonatal withdrawal symptoms.

The use of SSRIs, SNRIs or benzodiazepines may be warranted in patients with severe symptoms that could affect fetal or maternal safety or health. In general, the lowest effective dose should be used for the shortest time necessary. General principles for management of depression during pregnancy are applicable to the management of anxiety disorders.[42,43] See also Chapter 6 for information on management of depression during pregnancy and breastfeeding.

Anxiety Disorders and Breastfeeding

In the postpartum period, severe anxiety can impede the mother's sleep and erode her confidence in caring for her child. If a woman refuses to be involved with caring for her child, an urgent psychiatric consultation is needed and treatment considerations should include admitting the mother and child to hospital.

As in pregnancy, nonpharmacologic options should be used whenever possible in the postpartum period, particularly in breastfeeding women. If drug therapy is necessary, consider **paroxetine** or **sertraline**, since both have low concentrations in breast milk.[44] When possible, avoid benzodiazepines due to potential accumulation, sedation and impaired temperature regulation in the infant.

A discussion of general principles on the use of medications in these special populations can be found in Appendix II and Appendix III. Other specialized reference sources are also provided in these appendices.

Therapeutic Tips

- Short-term interventions such as psychological therapies, relaxation techniques and benzodiazepines may be effective.
- Assess a drug's effectiveness after a trial of an adequate dosage taken for a sufficient length of time.
- If the first antidepressant at optimal dosage is not effective or not tolerated, switch to another first-line antidepressant.
- If the second antidepressant is not effective, switch to an agent from a different drug class or augment with an appropriate medication. See Figure 1.
- Restrict benzodiazepines to short-term use (i.e., 6–8 weeks) to assist with SSRI/SNRI-related agitation.
- Limit the "as-needed" use of short-acting benzodiazepines as much as possible; ideally, such use should *not* be continued for longer than 4 days.

Table 3: Drugs Used for the Management of Anxiety Disorders

Class	Drug	Type of Anxiety	Dose	Adverse Effects	Drug Interactions	Comments	Cost[a]
Antidepressants, tricyclic	*clomipramine* Anafranil, generics	PD, AG	75–225 mg/day po	CNS effects (agitation on initiation of therapy, confusion, drowsiness, headache), anticholinergic effects (dry mouth, blurred vision, constipation, etc.), weight gain, nausea, cardiovascular effects (tachycardia, arrhythmias, orthostatic hypotension), anorgasmia, erectile dysfunction.	May increase effect of anticholinergic drugs, CNS depressants, warfarin; do not use MAOIs concurrently.	May take 2–3 months for maximum effect.	$-$$
	desipramine generics	PD, AG, GAD	75–300 mg/day po	See clomipramine.	See clomipramine.	See clomipramine.	$$-$$$$
	imipramine generics	PD, AG, GAD	75–300 mg/day po	See clomipramine.	See clomipramine.	See clomipramine.	$$-$$$$
Antipsychotics, Second-generation	*quetiapine* Seroquel, Seroquel XR, generics	GAD	Initial: 50 mg daily po Titrate to 150 mg daily po, or higher if necessary.[45] Usual maximum: 400 mg daily po	Sedation, dizziness, weight gain, orthostatic hypotension, hepatic aminotransferase elevation, headache, anticholinergic effects, increased risk of diabetes and dyslipidemia, movement disorders; may lower thyroid hormone levels, modest QT_c prolongation.	Additive sedation with CNS depressants; may potentiate antihypertensive drug effects; inhibitors of CYP3A4 such as clarithromycin, erythromycin, grapefruit juice, ketoconazole or prednisone may increase quetiapine levels; inducers of CYP3A4 such as carbamazepine, phenytoin or rifampin may decrease quetiapine levels. Use with caution with drugs known to prolong the QT_c interval.	Used as augmentation therapy with first-line agents in GAD, or as monotherapy after failure of first-line therapies. Advise patients about antipsychotic-associated body temperature dysregulation and prevention of heat stroke (e.g., hydration, sun protection).	$$

(cont'd)

Table 3: **Drugs Used for the Management of Anxiety Disorders** *(cont'd)*

Class	Drug	Type of Anxiety	Dose	Adverse Effects	Drug Interactions	Comments	Cost[a]
Azapirones	*buspirone* generics	GAD	Initial: 5 mg BID–TID po Titrate gradually to effective dose. Maximum: 60 mg/day po	Nausea, headache, dizziness, restlessness/insomnia.	Avoid use with MAOIs.	Onset of effect not as rapid as with benzodiazepines.	$$$-$$$$$
Benzodiazepines	*clonazepam* Rivotril, generics	GAD, PD, AG	0.25–0.5 mg BID po	Drowsiness (tolerance develops with continued therapy), dizziness, reduced concentration, retrograde amnesia, physical dependence; rarely, paradoxical anger or hostility.	Warn patients re: concomitant use of alcohol, other CNS depressants (increased effect).	Discontinue gradually to avoid rebound anxiety; avoid in pregnancy; contraindicated in patients with known history of abuse; dose escalation is rare in patients taking benzodiazepines for chronic anxiety; use lower doses in elderly.	$
Beta$_1$-adrenergic Antagonists	*propranolol* generics	SAD (specific task-related anxiety)	10 mg po 30 min before task PRN	Hypotension.	Caution re: increased bradycardia with amiodarone.	For occasional use in situations such as public speaking, performing; not useful in generalized social anxiety disorder.	$
GABA Derivatives	*gabapentin* ❥ Neurontin, generics	SAD See Comments.	Initial: 300 mg/day po Usual: 900–1800 mg/day po in 2 divided doses	Somnolence, dizziness, ataxia, vision changes.	Magnesium- and aluminum-containing antacids may decrease the absorption of gabapentin.	Not a first-line agent; may be useful in patients not responding to first-line measures. Not an approved indication.	$-$$
	pregabalin ❥ Lyrica, generics	GAD, SAD	Initial: 150 mg/day po in 2–3 divided doses May be increased to 150 mg BID po after 1 wk if necessary	Dizziness, sedation, peripheral edema.	No known significant drug interactions.	First-line agent for GAD. May be useful in patients not responding to or not tolerating other first-line measures.	$$
Monoamine Oxidase Inhibitors	*phenelzine* Nardil	PD, AG	45–90 mg/day po	Insomnia, dizziness, orthostatic hypotension, edema, sexual dysfunction.	Concurrent use with sympathomimetic agents, tyramine or levodopa may result in hypertensive crisis; do not use with serotonergic drugs such as SSRIs, SNRIs, TCAs, meperidine, tryptophan due to high risk for fatal serotonin syndrome).	Stringent dietary restrictions are necessary. Avoid tyramine-containing foods.	$$-$$$

Class	Drug	Type of Anxiety	Dose	Adverse Effects	Drug Interactions	Comments	Cost[a]
	tranylcypromine Parnate	PD, AG	20–60 mg/day po	See phenelzine.	See phenelzine.	See phenelzine.	$$-$$$
Reversible Inhibitors of Monoamine Oxidase-A	*moclobemide* Manerix, generics	SAD	300–600 mg/day po	Nausea, insomnia.	Do not use with meperidine, TCAs, SSRIs.	Dietary restrictions are not required at usual doses.	$
Selective Serotonin Reuptake Inhibitors	*citalopram* Celexa, CTP 30, generics	PD, AG, SAD	20–40 mg/day po Up to 60 mg/day po may be required in appropriately selected patients.	Agitation (on initiation of therapy), nausea, anorgasmia, insomnia, diarrhea, increased risk of GI bleeding; dose-related QT_c prolongation.	Serotonin syndrome with MAOIs (hypertension, tremor, agitation, hypomania); caution with other serotonergic drugs including amphetamine derivatives, dextromethorphan, dihydroergotamine, linezolid, lithium, meperidine, pentazocine, selegiline, St. John's wort, trazodone, triptans, tryptophan (increased risk of serotonin syndrome); increased risk of GI bleeding with NSAIDs, antiplatelet agents. SSRIs are substrates and inhibitors of several cytochrome P450 isoenzymes. This may result in reduced clearance of many drugs (e.g., clozapine, methadone, mexiletine, phenytoin, pimozide, propafenone) or decreased enzymatic conversion of a prodrug to its active form (e.g., clopidogrel, codeine, tamoxifen). Avoid combined use with drugs associated with prolonged QT_c interval/torsades de pointes, such as amiodarone, azithromycin, clarithromycin, domperidone, erythromycin, haloperidol, methadone, pimozide, quinine, sotalol, ziprasidone.	May take 2–3 months for maximum effect. Discontinue gradually.	$

(cont'd)

Table 3: **Drugs Used for the Management of Anxiety Disorders** *(cont'd)*

Class	Drug	Type of Anxiety	Dose	Adverse Effects	Drug Interactions	Comments	Cost[a]
	escitalopram Cipralex, Cipralex MELTZ	PD, AG, GAD	10–20 mg/day po	See citalopram.	See citalopram.	See citalopram.	$$$
	fluoxetine Prozac, generics	PD, AG, SAD	20–80 mg/day po	Agitation (on initiation of therapy), nausea, anorgasmia, insomnia, headache, reduced appetite, diarrhea, increased risk of GI bleeding.	See citalopram.	See citalopram.	$-$$
	fluvoxamine Luvox, generics	PD, AG, SAD	150–300 mg/day po	Agitation (on initiation of therapy), nausea, anorgasmia, anticholinergic effects, sedation, increased risk of GI bleeding.	See citalopram.	See citalopram.	$-$$
	paroxetine immediate-release ❥ Paxil, generics	PD, AG, SAD	20–60 mg/day po	See fluvoxamine.	See citalopram.	See citalopram.	$-$$
	paroxetine controlled-release ❥ Paxil CR	PD, AG, SAD	12.5–37.5 mg/day po	See fluvoxamine.	See citalopram.	See citalopram.	$$$
	sertraline Zoloft, generics	PD, AG, SAD	50–200 mg/day po	Agitation (on initiation of therapy), nausea, anorgasmia, insomnia, diarrhea, increased risk of GI bleeding.	See citalopram.	See citalopram.	$-$$

Class	Drug	Type of Anxiety	Dose	Adverse Effects	Drug Interactions	Comments	Cost[a]
Serotonin-Norepinephrine Reuptake Inhibitors	*duloxetine* Cymbalta	GAD	60–120 mg daily po	Nausea, insomnia, dizziness, asthenia.	Do not use with MAOIs; caution with other serotonergic drugs including amphetamine derivatives, dextromethorphan, dihydroergotamine, linezolid, lithium, meperidine, pentazocine, selegiline, St. John's wort, trazodone, triptans, tryptophan (increased risk of serotonin syndrome). Substrate of CYP1A2 and CYP2D6; caution with inducers or inhibitors of these isoenzymes.	May take 2–3 months for maximum effect. Discontinue gradually. Avoid in severe renal dysfunction.	$125–240
	venlafaxine extended-release Effexor XR, generics	GAD, SAD	37.5–225 mg/day po	See duloxetine.	Do not use with MAOIs. Substrate of CYP2D6 and CYP3A4; caution with inducers or inhibitors of these isoenzymes.	See duloxetine.	$-$$

[a] Cost of 30-day supply, unless otherwise specified; includes drug cost only.

Dosage adjustment may be required in renal impairment; see Appendix I.

Abbreviations: AG = agoraphobia; GAD = generalized anxiety disorder; MAOI = monoamine oxidase inhibitor; PD = panic disorder; SAD = social anxiety disorder; SNRI = serotonin-norepinephrine reuptake inhibitor; SSRI = selective serotonin reuptake inhibitor; TCA = tricyclic antidepressant

Legend: $ < $25 $-$$ < $25–50 $$ $25–50 $$-$$$ $25–75 $$$ $50–75 $$-$$$$ $25–100 $$$$ $75–100 $$$-$$$$$ $50–125 $$$$$ $100–125

Suggested Readings

American Psychiatric Association. *Practice guidelines for the treatment of patients with panic disorder*. 2nd ed. Washington (DC): APA; 2009.

Baldwin DS, Anderson IM, Nutt DJ et al. Evidence-based guidelines for the pharmacological treatment of anxiety disorders: recommendations from the British Association for Psychopharmacology. *J Psychopharmacol* 2005;19(6):567-96.

Bandelow B, Sher L, Bunevicius R et al. Guidelines for the pharmacological treatment of anxiety disorders, obsessive-compulsive disorder and posttraumatic stress disorder in primary care. *Int J Pyschiatry Clin Pract* 2012;16(2):77-84.

Ravindran H, Stein M. The pharmacologic treatment of anxiety disorders: a review of progress. *J Clin Psych* 2010;71(7):839-54.

Swinson R, Anthony M, Bleau P et al. Canadian Psychiatric Association. Clinical practice guidelines. Management of anxiety disorders. *Can J Psychiatry* 2006;51(8 Suppl 2):9S-91S.

U.K. National Institute for Health and Care Excellence. NICE clinical guidelines CG159. *Social anxiety disorder: recognition, assessment and treatment*. May 2013. Available from: publications.nice.org.uk/social-anxiety-disorder-recognition-assessment-and-treatment-cg159.

References

1. American Psychiatric Association. *Diagnostic and statistical manual of mental disorders: DSM-5*. 5th ed. Arlington (VA): APA; 2013.
2. Hovland A, Nordhus IH, Sjøbø T et al. Comparing physical exercise in groups to group cognitive behaviour therapy for the treatment of panic disorder in a randomized controlled trial. *Behav Cogn Psychother* 2013;41(4):408-32.
3. Van Apeldoorn FJ, Van Hout WJ, Timmerman ME et al. Rate of improvement during and across three treatments for panic disorder with or without agoraphobia: cognitive behavioral therapy, selective serotonin reuptake inhibitor or both combined. *J Affect Disord* 2013;150(2):313-9.
4. Swinson R, Anthony M, Bleau P et al. Canadian Psychiatric Association. Clinical practice guidelines. Management of anxiety disorders. *Can J Psychiatry* 2006;51(8 Suppl 2):9S-91S.
5. Boyer W. Serotonin uptake inhibitors are superior to imipramine in alleviating panic attacks: a meta-analysis. In: Darcourt G, ed. *Current therapeutic approaches to panic and other anxiety disorders*. New York (NY): Karger; 1994.
6. Goddard AW, Brouette T, Almai A et al. Early coadministration of clonazepam with sertraline for panic disorder. *Arch Gen Psychiatry* 2001;58(7):681-6.
7. Mavissakalian MR, Perel JM. Long-term maintenance and discontinuation of imipramine therapy in panic disorder with agoraphobia. *Arch Gen Psychiatry* 1999;56(9):821-7.
8. Boshuisen ML, Slaap BR, Vester-Blokland ED et al. The effect of mirtazapine in panic disorder: an open label pilot study with a single-blind placebo run-in period. *Int Clin Psychopharmacol* 2001;16(6):363-8.
9. Sarchiapone M, Amore M, De Risio S et al. Mirtazapine in the treatment of panic disorder: an open-label trial. *Int Clin Psychopharmacol* 2003;18(1):35-8.
10. Buigues J, Vallejo J. Therapeutic response to phenelzine in patients with panic disorder and agoraphobia with panic attacks. *J Clin Psychiatry* 1987;48(2):55-9.
11. Marks IM, Swinson RP, Basoglu M et al. Alprazolam and exposure alone and combined in panic disorder with agoraphobia. A controlled study in London and Toronto. *Br J Psychiatry* 1993;162:776-87.
12. van Apeldoorn FJ, van Hout WJ, Mersch PP et al. Is a combined therapy more effective than either CBT or SSRI alone? Results of a multicenter trial on panic disorder with or without agoraphobia. *Acta Psychiatr Scand* 2008;117(4):260-70.
13. Kasper S, Stein D, Loft H et al. Escitalopram in the treatment of social anxiety disorder: randomised, placebo-controlled, flexible-dosage study. *Br J Psychiatry* 2005;186:222-6.
14. Lader M, Stender K, Burger V et al. Efficacy and tolerability of escitalopram in 12- and 24-week treatment of social anxiety disorder: randomised, double-blind, placebo-controlled, fixed-dose study. *Depress Anxiety* 2004;19(4):241-8.
15. Davidson J, Yaryura-Tobias J, DuPont R et al. Fluvoxamine-controlled release formulation for the treatment of generalized social anxiety disorder. *J Clin Psychopharmacol* 2004;24(2):118-25.
16. Westenberg HG, Stein DJ, Yang H et al. A double-blind placebo-controlled study of controlled release fluvoxamine for the treatment of generalized social anxiety disorder. *J Clin Psychopharmacol* 2004;24(1):49-55.
17. Baldwin D, Bobes J, Stein DJ et al. Paroxetine in social phobia/social anxiety disorder. Randomised, double-blind, placebo-controlled study. Paroxetine Study Group. *Br J Psychiatry* 1999;175:120-6.
18. Liebowitz MR, Stein MB, Tancer M et al. A randomized, double-blind, fixed-dose comparison of paroxetine and placebo in the treatment of generalized social anxiety disorder. *J Clin Psychiatry* 2002;63(1):66-74.
19. Liebowitz MR, DeMartinis NA, Weihs K et al. Efficacy of sertraline in severe generalized social anxiety disorder: results of a double-blind, placebo-controlled study. *J Clin Psychiatry* 2003;64(7):785-92.
20. Van Ameringen MA, Lane RM, Walker JR et al. Sertraline treatment of generalized social phobia: a 20-week, double-blind, placebo-controlled study. *Am J Psychiatry* 2001;158(2):275-81.
21. Rickels K, Mangano R, Khan A. A double-blind, placebo-controlled study of a flexible dose of venlafaxine ER in adult outpatients with generalized social anxiety disorder. *J Clin Psychopharmacol* 2004;24(5):488-96.
22. Falloon IR, Lloyd GG, Harpin RE. The treatment of social phobia. Real-life rehearsal with nonprofessional therapists. *J Nerv Ment Dis* 1981;169(3):180-4.
23. Liebowitz MR, Schneier F, Campeas R et al. Phenelzine vs atenolol in social phobia. A placebo-controlled comparison. *Arch Gen Psychiatry* 1992;49(4):290-300.

24. Stein DJ, Cameron A, Amrein R et al. Moclobemide is effective and well tolerated in the long-term pharmacotherapy of social anxiety disorder with or without comorbid anxiety disorder. *Int Clin Psychopharmacol* 2002;17(4):161-70.
25. Pande AC, Davidson JR, Jefferson JW et al. Treatment of social phobia with gabapentin: a placebo-controlled study. *J Clin Psychopharmacol* 1999;19(4):341-8.
26. Pande AC, Feltner DE, Jefferson JW et al. Efficacy of the novel anxiolytic pregabalin in social anxiety disorder: a placebo-controlled, multicenter study. *J Clin Psychopharmacol* 2004;24(2):141-9.
27. Otto MW, Pollack MH, Gould RA et al. A comparison of the efficacy of clonazepam and cognitive-behavioral group therapy for the treatment of social phobia. *J Anxiety Disord* 2000;14(4):345-58.
28. Borkovec TD, Ruscio AM. Psychotherapy for generalized anxiety disorder. *J Clin Psychiatry* 2001;62(Suppl 11):37-42.
29. Mancini M, Perna G, Rossi A et al. Use of duloxetine in patients with an anxiety disorder, or with comorbid anxiety and major depressive disorder: a review of the literature. *Expert Opin Pharmacother* 2010;11(7):1167-81.
30. Davidson JR, Bose A, Korotzer A et al. Escitalopram in the treatment of generalized anxiety disorder: double-blind, placebo controlled, flexible-dose study. *Depress Anxiety* 2004;19(4):234-40.
31. Goodman WK, Bose A, Wang Q. Treatment of generalized anxiety disorder with escitalopram: pooled results from double-blind, placebo-controlled trials. *J Affect Disord* 2005;87(2-3):161-7.
32. Pollack MH, Zaninelli R, Goddard A et al. Paroxetine in the treatment of generalized anxiety disorder: results of a placebo-controlled, flexible-dosage trial. *J Clin Psychiatry* 2001;62(5):350-7.
33. Davidson JR, DuPont RL, Hedges D et al. Efficacy, safety, and tolerability of venlafaxine extended release and buspirone in outpatients with generalized anxiety disorder. *J Clin Psychiatry* 1999;60(8):528-35.
34. Rickels K, Pollack MH, Feltner DE et al. Pregabalin for treatment of generalized anxiety disorder: a 4-week, multicenter, double-blind, placebo-controlled trial of pregabalin and alprazolam. *Arch Gen Psychiatry* 2005;62(9):1022-30.
35. Feltner DE, Crockatt JG, Dubovsky SJ et al. A randomized, double-blind, placebo-controlled, fixed-dose, multicenter study of pregabalin in patients with generalized anxiety disorder. *J Clin Psychopharmacol* 2003;23(3):240-9.
36. Baldwin S, Ajel K, Masdrakis VG et al. Pregabalin for the treatment of generalized anxiety disorder: an update. *Neuropsychiatr Dis Treat* 2013;9:883-92.
37. Bystritsky A, Kerwin L, Eiduson S et al. A pilot controlled trial of bupropion vs. escitalopram in generalized anxiety disorder (GAD). *Neuropsychopharmacol* 2005;30(Suppl 1):S101.
38. Bandelow B, Chouinard G, Bobes J et al. Extended-release quetiapine fumarate (quetiapine XR): a once-daily monotherapy effective in generalized anxiety disorder. Data from a randomized, double-blind, placebo- and active-controlled study. *Int J Neuropsychopharmacol* 2010;13(3):305-20.
39. Olatunji BO, Cisler JM, Deacon BJ. Efficacy of cognitive behavioral therapy for anxiety disorders: a review of meta-analytic findings. *Psychiatr Clin North Am* 2010;33(3):557-77.
40. ACOG Committee on Practice Bulletins—Obstetrics. ACOG Practice Bulletin: Clinical management guidelines for obstetrician-gynecologists number 92, April 2008 (replaces practice bulletin number 87, November 2007). Use of psychiatric medications during pregnancy and lactation. *Obstet Gynecol* 2008;111(4):1001-20.
41. Tuccori M, Montagnani S, Testi A et al. Use of selective serotonin reuptake inhibitors during pregnancy and risk of major and cardiovascular malformations: an update. *Postgrad Med* 2010;122(4):49-65.
42. Yonkers KA, Wisner KL, Stewart DE et al. The management of depression during pregnancy: a report from the American Psychiatric Association and the American College of Obstetricians and Gynecologists. *Gen Hosp Psychiatry* 2009;31(5):403-13.
43. Academy of Breastfeeding Medicine Protocol Committee. ABM clinical protocol #18: use of antidepressants in nursing mothers. *Breastfeed Med* 2008;3(1):44-52.
44. Weissman AM, Levy BT, Hartz AJ et al. Pooled analysis of antidepressant levels in lactating mothers, breast milk, and nursing infants. *Am J Psychiatry* 2004;161(6):1066-78.
45. Bandelow B, Bobes J, Ahokas A et al. Results from a phase III study of once-daily extended release quetiapine fumarate (quetiapine XR) monotherapy in patients with generalized anxiety disorder. Presented at 7th International Forum of Mood and Anxiety Disorders 5–7 December 2007; Budapest, Hungary.

Chapter 3
Attention-Deficit Hyperactivity Disorder

Adil Virani, BSc(Pharm), Pharm D, FCSHP

Attention-deficit hyperactivity disorder (ADHD) is the most common pediatric neuropsychiatric disorder and affects 4–12% of North American school-aged children.[1] ADHD is characterized by 3 hallmark symptoms—inattention, hyperactivity and impulsivity—the presence and severity of which vary among individuals.[1,2] Symptoms present before the age of 12 and may persist into adulthood.[2,3] It is estimated that ADHD occurs in 3–4% of adults.[3] Symptoms often interfere with normal development, are present in 2 or more settings such as at home, work or school, and have a direct unfavourable impact on social, academic, cognitive or occupational functioning.[3] Individuals affected by ADHD may be diagnosed as primarily inattentive or primarily hyperactive/impulsive or, as is most commonly observed, they may have a majority of both inattentive and hyperactive symptoms as listed in Table 1.[3,4]

Goals of Therapy

- Eliminate or significantly decrease core ADHD symptoms
- Improve behavioural, academic and/or occupational performance
- Improve self-esteem and social functioning
- Minimize adverse effects of medications
- Improve quality of life

Investigations

- Currently there are no objective tests that unequivocally diagnose ADHD
- The diagnosis of ADHD is based on evidence of 6 or more specific behaviours/symptoms for children and at least 5 in those over 17 years of age. These symptoms will have persisted for at least 6 months to a degree that is inconsistent with developmental level and impacted overall functioning.[3] The criteria are listed in Table 1.
- Interview the patient, family/caregivers, teachers/assistants and psychologists (where applicable) to identify:
  - nature and duration of ADHD symptoms
  - impact of symptoms on functioning
  - age of onset
  - social interactions with family and peers
  - situations that exacerbate or ameliorate symptoms
  - symptoms suggestive of other potentially comorbid disorders such as oppositional defiant disorder, conduct disorder, mood/anxiety disorders, tic disorders and/or learning disabilities
- Various assessment/rating scales can be used to collect the above information and assess progress; see the Canadian Attention Deficit Hyperactivity Disorder Resource Alliance (CADDRA) ADHD guidelines at www.caddra.ca to find the most appropriate assessment vehicles and treatment suggestions for individual patients[5]
- Physical examination/medical history to assess hearing, vision, thyroid function, neurologic status, cardiac function, history of dysmorphic disorder (such as Down syndrome) or anemia

- Birth/prenatal history including in utero exposure to substances and premature birth[6]
- Baseline blood pressure, heart rate, height and weight (especially if stimulants are likely to be used)
- According to the CADDRA guideline,[5] baseline ECG is not required for every patient prior to initiating stimulant therapy. However, it is reasonable to consider in some patients, such as those with a personal or family history of cardiac problems or who present with raised blood pressure or heart rate on examination.

Table 1: DSM-5 Criteria for Diagnosing ADHD

A. Either (1) or (2):

(1) Six or more of the following symptoms of *inattention* have persisted for at least 6 months to a degree that is maladaptive and inconsistent with developmental level (if over the age of 17, a minimum of 5 symptoms are needed):

a. Often fails to give close attention to details or makes careless mistakes in schoolwork, at work, or during other activities (e.g., overlooks or misses details, work is inaccurate)
b. Often has difficulty sustaining attention in tasks or play activities (e.g., has difficulty remaining focused during lectures, conversations, or lengthy reading)
c. Often does not seem to listen when spoken to directly (e.g., mind seems elsewhere, even in the absence of any obvious distraction)
d. Often does not follow through on instructions and fails to finish schoolwork, chores, or duties in the workplace (e.g., starts tasks but quickly loses focus and is easily distracted)
e. Often has difficulty organizing tasks and activities (e.g., difficulty managing sequential tasks; difficulty keeping materials and belongings in order; messy, disorganized work; has poor time management; fails to meet deadlines)
f. Often avoids, dislikes, or is reluctant to engage in tasks that require sustained mental effort (e.g., schoolwork or homework; preparing reports, completing forms, reviewing lengthy papers)
g. Often loses things necessary for tasks or activities (e.g., school materials, pencils, books, tools, wallets, keys, paperwork, eyeglasses, mobile phones)
h. Is often easily distracted by extraneous stimuli (for older adolescents and adults, may include unrelated thoughts)
i. Is often forgetful in daily activities (e.g., in doing chores, running errands; for older adolescents and adults, returning calls, paying bills, keeping appointments)

(2) Six or more of the following symptoms of *hyperactivity-impulsivity* have persisted for at least 6 months to a degree that is maladaptive and inconsistent with developmental level (if over the age of 17, a minimum of 5 symptoms are needed):

a. Often fidgets or taps with hands or feet or squirms in seat
b. Often leaves seat in situations when remaining seated is expected (e.g., classroom, office, workplace)
c. Often runs about or climbs excessively in situations where it is inappropriate; in adolescents or adults, may be limited to feeling restless
d. Often unable to play or engage in leisure activities quietly
e. Is often "on the go" acting as if "driven by a motor"
f. Often talks excessively
g. Often blurts out answers before questions have been completed (e.g., completes other people's sentences; cannot wait for turn in conversation)
h. Often has difficulty waiting for his/her turn (e.g., while waiting in line)
i. Often interrupts or intrudes on others (e.g., butts into conversations, games or activities; may start using other peoples things without asking or receiving permission; may intrude into or take over what others are doing)

B. Several hyperactive-impulsive or inattentive symptoms that cause impairment were present *before 12 years of age*

C. Several hyperactive-impulsive or inattentive symptoms are *present in 2 or more settings,* e.g., at school or work *and* at home

D. Clear evidence that the symptoms interfere with, or reduce the quality of, social, academic, or occupational functioning

E. The symptoms do not occur exclusively during the course of schizophrenia, or other psychotic disorder and are not better accounted for by another mental disorder (e.g., mood, anxiety, dissociative or personality disorders or substance intoxication or withdrawal)

Reprinted with permission from the *Diagnostic and Statistical Manual of Mental Disorders, Fifth Edition, (Copyright ©2013). American Psychiatric Association.* All Rights Reserved.

Therapeutic Choices

An algorithm for the management of attention-deficit hyperactivity disorder is presented in Figure 1.

Figure 1: Management of Attention-Deficit Hyperactivity Disorder[9]

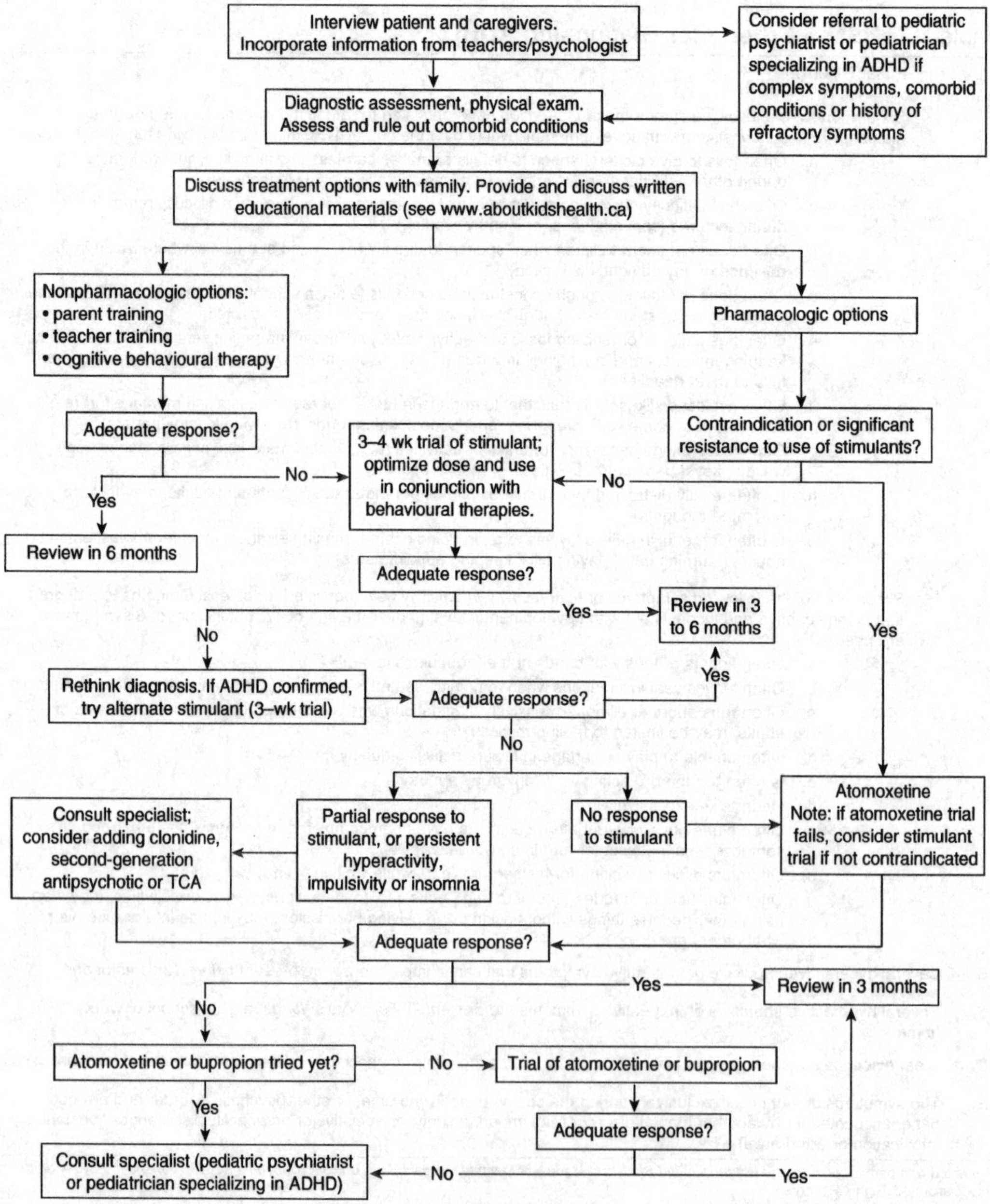

Abbreviations: ADHD = attention-deficit hyperactivity disorder; TCA = tricyclic antidepressant

Evidence suggests that a combination of nonpharmacologic (e.g., behaviour modification programs) and pharmacologic therapies constitutes the best treatment strategy for children with ADHD.[7,8] Stimulant medications and atomoxetine are the most effective treatment for the core symptoms of ADHD (hyperactivity, impulsiveness and inattention).[5,8,9] Behavioural therapies play an important role in improving social interactions, self-esteem and the common behaviours seen in ADHD.[8,10]

Nonpharmacologic Choices

Some clinicians, parents and/or patients may prefer, and require guidance about, approaches such as behaviour management, dietary changes, physical exercise, psychotherapy, neurofeedback (EEG biofeedback) and hypnosis. Evidence for nonpharmacologic therapies alone is lacking while high-quality RCTs have shown that stimulants have the greatest effect on core symptoms.[11,12,13] When compared to stimulants, these nonpharmacologic options are less effective at reducing the core symptoms of ADHD.[4,8,10]

- *Behavioural therapies* are designed to minimize negative behaviours and promote positive ones by teaching parents (and sometimes teachers) techniques to improve a child's behaviours.[2]
  - The Multimodal Treatment Study of ADHD (MTA) is one of the largest (597 children aged 7–9 with the combined subtype of ADHD) and longest RCTs comparing behavioural therapy with pharmacologic therapy and combined behavioural/pharmacologic therapy. This trial found that behavioural therapy alone was inferior to pharmacologic therapy alone at reducing core ADHD symptoms.[8] Combined behavioural/pharmacologic therapy was shown to be more effective at reducing oppositional behaviours and anxiety while improving social interactions and self-esteem when compared to either treatment strategy alone.
  - Another RCT, involving 103 children aged 7–9 years, confirmed the greater benefit of stimulant medications over behavioural strategies on core ADHD symptoms, and demonstrated a sustained benefit over a 2-year period.[10]
  - Parental training may increase confidence and reduce stress for parents.[14]
  - Management of behaviour by way of parent- or teacher-training is considered first-line in preschool-aged children.[15] Addition of stimulant medication is reserved for preschoolers with moderate to severe ADHD who do not respond to behavioural therapy if the benefit outweighs the harm.
- The elimination of certain foods from the *diet* in an effort to minimize ADHD symptoms is not based on evidence from clinical trials, but rather on observations that some children exhibit more severe hyperactive behaviours in association with certain sugars, dyes or preservatives.[11]
- Mind-body therapies such as *neurofeedback* or *hypnosis* are geared toward training the patient's mind (by modifying brainwave activity) to influence physical responses to ADHD symptoms.[13] Though some interesting research has been conducted in this area, well-designed trials are still required to confirm the efficacy of these strategies in reducing core ADHD symptoms.[12,13]

Pharmacologic Choices

Stimulants

Stimulant medications (**dextroamphetamine, lisdexamfetamine, methylphenidate, mixed salts amphetamine**) have been considered first-line agents for treating ADHD for decades.[2,4,5,9] Their efficacy at reducing core ADHD symptoms has been demonstrated in a wide range of patients aged 6 years to adult.[5,9] Controlled trials consistently demonstrate that at least 70% of patients receiving stimulant therapy will have a clinically significant decrease in core ADHD symptoms.[2,4,8,9]

Stimulants have not been adequately studied in terms of important long-term outcomes such as quality of life, employment, school completion and long-term morbidity or mortality.

No clinical predictors of who will benefit from which stimulant have been identified; therefore, the choice of agent will depend on patient and physician preferences.[9] Patients who do not tolerate or respond to one stimulant after 3–4 weeks of therapy should be switched to an alternative stimulant.[9] Currently, there are no RCTs assessing the benefits and harms of using long-term stimulant therapy, e.g., >2 years. Three-year follow up of the participants of the MTA study found that children given stimulants were on average 2 cm shorter and weighed 2.7 kg less than children who were never medicated during the same 3 years.[16]

Though methylphenidate sustained-release tablets, e.g., Ritalin SR and dextroamphetamine sustained-release spansules (Dexedrine) have a longer duration of action (up to 8 hours) than their immediate-release counterparts, they often require more than once-daily dosing.

Long-acting formulations of mixed salts amphetamine (Adderall XR), methylphenidate (Biphentin and Concerta) and lisdexamfetamine (Vyvanse) have a duration of action of 8–14 hours and are as effective as appropriately dosed shorter-acting stimulants.[5,9] Advantages of these long-acting products include single daily dosing, potential for improved adherence, avoidance of the need for medication administration at school, decreased abuse potential and decreased risk of rebound hyperactivity. Given these advantages, it has been recommended that long-acting agents be used first-line for treatment of ADHD.[5]

Health Canada and regulatory agencies in other countries have issued advisories about the possible association of stimulants (and atomoxetine) with cardiovascular risks such as sudden cardiac death in those with underlying cardiac anomalies, and with adverse psychiatric symptoms such as hallucinations and agitation. The FDA has issued a warning that stimulants and atomoxetine may be associated with rare reports of priapism in male children, adolescents and adults taking these medications.[17] Inform patients (and parents/caregivers where appropriate) about the cardiovascular or psychiatric risks, the possibility of prolonged erections (>2 h) and the need to seek medical attention if these risks occur.

Though **modafinil** is a CNS stimulant that promotes wakefulness in the treatment of narcolepsy, it is less effective than other stimulants in ADHD and is not often used. It is not approved for use in ADHD. There is some evidence from double-blind trials in children and adults that modafinil (170–425 mg/day) is superior to placebo in decreasing core symptoms of ADHD.[18,19]

Atomoxetine

Atomoxetine, a norepinephrine reuptake inhibitor, is indicated for the treatment of children ≥6 years of age, adolescents and adults with ADHD. It is not classified as a stimulant and is not a controlled substance. The efficacy and tolerability of atomoxetine have been studied in several well-designed trials.[20,21,22,23,24,25,26] RCTs confirm that after 6–12 weeks of treatment, atomoxetine reduces core ADHD symptoms by at least 25–30% in 60–70% of individuals.[21,24,26] The efficacy of atomoxetine approaches that of stimulants. While some guidelines list it as a first-line option, the available evidence supports a role in therapy for those who have either not responded to or not tolerated an adequate trial of stimulant medications. It should also be considered for those with ADHD and comorbid substance abuse disorder or depression.[9,27]

Antidepressants

In general, antidepressants are considered less effective than stimulants in the management of ADHD in children; hence, they are considered as second- or third-line options or as adjunctive therapy.[2,5,9] Antidepressants may benefit patients with comorbid conditions such as depression, anxiety, enuresis or tic disorders.[20]

Bupropion, a norepinephrine and dopamine reuptake inhibitor, is moderately effective for the treatment of ADHD in both children and adults.[20,28,29,30,31] Although there are insufficient data from RCTs to recommend its use, some evidence suggests **venlafaxine**, a serotonin-norepinephrine reuptake inhibitor, may be helpful in the management of ADHD, particularly in adults.[9,27,32]

Many controlled trials have examined the effects of TCAs such as **desipramine**, **imipramine** and **nortriptyline** in the short-term treatment of ADHD.[33] TCAs are less effective than stimulants at reducing the core symptoms of ADHD. Despite the fact that most TCA studies have significant design flaws such as open label design or lack of randomization, the benefits of TCAs may outweigh their risks in some patients who cannot take stimulants, atomoxetine or bupropion.[6,9,20,33]

Alpha$_2$-Adrenergic Agonists

The alpha$_2$-adrenergic agonists **clonidine** and **guanfacine** are second- or third-line agents for ADHD.[2,9] They primarily reduce symptoms of aggression, impulsivity and hyperactivity and have less pronounced benefits on inattention. When used concurrently with stimulants, clonidine and guanfacine often target sleep disruptions, aggression, impulsivity, comorbid oppositional defiant disorder and tics.[6,20]

Guanfacine was approved by Health Canada in 2013, making it the first selective alpha$_2$-adrenoceptor agonist officially indicated for the treatment of ADHD in children aged 6–12 years. It can be used as monotherapy or as adjunctive therapy with psychostimulants. Compared to clonidine, guanfacine has more selective neuronal activity and a longer duration of action, resulting in less sedation and less hypotension. Several RCTs and open-label studies in children with ADHD have demonstrated that guanfacine 1–4 mg/day had a clinically and statistically superior effect on ADHD symptoms compared with placebo.[34,35,36] There are no adequate head-to-head comparisons of guanfacine with stimulants or the less-expensive clonidine. The most common adverse effects of guanfacine are sedation and headaches. Data comparing guanfacine to other potential ADHD treatments are limited.

Antipsychotics

Some antipsychotics may negatively affect cognition in patients with ADHD. A systematic review of the role of second-generation antipsychotics (primarily risperidone) in ADHD failed to confirm that these agents benefit this patient population.[37]

Low doses of second-generation antipsychotics (SGAs) such as **risperidone** may be moderately effective for the *behavioural symptoms* seen in hyperactive and impulsive children when stimulants alone are ineffective or not tolerated;[5] SGAs have little effect on inattention. Also, SGAs are sometimes used to decrease behaviours seen in children with comorbid conduct disorder, oppositional defiant disorder, autistic disorders, impulse control disorders and Tourette's syndrome.

Natural Health Products

Though evidence from well-designed randomized trials is sparse, various natural health products such as herbs, vitamins and nutritional supplements have been tried on the basis of their traditional uses. For example, agents with possible anxiolytic, sedative or hypnotic effects, e.g., **chamomile**, **valerian**, **melatonin**, have been used in children who are restless, anxious or having sleep difficulties.[11] These herbs may play a role in calming a hyperactive child or promoting sleep in children with ADHD and insomnia. Other agents of interest include antioxidants such as **blue-green algae**, **various B vitamins**, **ginkgo biloba**, **pycnogenol** and **evening primrose oil** (essential fatty acids). In general, concerns regarding efficacy and quality of natural health products make it difficult to support their use in place of existing prescription medications; however, after evaluating potential drug interactions and clinical risks, it may be possible to use some of these products safely in conjunction with approved therapies.

Therapeutic Tips

- When selecting a pharmacologic regimen, consider the child's daily schedule, predominant ADHD symptoms, likelihood of adherence, patient preferences (including medication cost) and risk of adverse effects.
- Cross-over trials of stimulant vs. placebo or other stimulants ("n of 1" trials) can be helpful in assessing the response to medication in a patient for whom therapeutic benefit is uncertain.

- A small portion of patients prescribed long-acting stimulants may require additional afternoon doses of immediate-release stimulants to help with homework and control of early evening symptoms. This is more common with methylphenidate sustained-release products such as Ritalin SR.
- Sustained-release or long-acting stimulant tablets should not be crushed or chewed. In younger children who are unable to swallow certain medications, note that Adderall XR, Dexedrine spansules, Vyvanse and Biphentin capsules can be opened and sprinkled on soft foods such as yogurt or applesauce, and Vyvanse can be mixed with water.
- Monitor children taking stimulants for potential growth suppression—record weight and height at baseline and then monthly. Plot on growth charts and compare measurements with established norms for a given child's age/gender.
- Some clinicians raise concerns about the risk of substance abuse with stimulants. Though this can occur, trials evaluating substance abuse in those with ADHD have found that adequately treated children have a lower risk of substance abuse later in life when compared to those who are untreated.[38] If drug diversion is suspected, consider switching to an agent with less abuse potential.
- A reasonable trial with stimulants is 3–4 weeks although improvement of core ADHD symptoms is often observed in the first week of therapy. If a patient responds adequately with minimal adverse effects, it is reasonable to continue therapy for 6–12 months, depending on patient circumstances.
- While ADHD is a lifelong condition for most individuals, symptoms may dissipate as some patients enter adolescence. Weaning the stimulant for a 2–3 week period (usually in the summer months) once a year may provide an opportunity to reassess behaviours and to confirm whether the stimulant is still required for the next school term.
- Extended “drug holidays” from stimulants, e.g., several months over the summer holidays, are generally not recommended in children with moderate-to-severe ADHD symptoms who are doing well on the stimulant. The return of symptoms and resultant effects on behaviour and self-esteem do not typically outweigh the risks of taking the medication. Drug holidays (at times of low environmental stresses) from stimulants may be useful when adverse effects (such as growth suppression or weight loss >10% of initial body weight) are present or when attempting to assess the continued benefit.
- When switching from stimulant therapy to atomoxetine or an antidepressant, a lower dose of the stimulant can be continued and tapered over approximately 3 weeks while the new drug takes effect.
- An ADHD medication chart available at www.caddra.ca/medical-resources/medication-chart is a useful resource for healthcare professionals.
- Helpful information tips for teachers and parents are available at the US Department of Education website (www2.ed.gov/rschstat/research/pubs/adhd/adhd-teaching_pg3.html).
- Approximately 50% of children and adolescents with *tic disorders* also have ADHD. In general, ADHD symptoms are more disabling than tics in patients with both. Though **stimulants** may exacerbate tics in some individuals, they can be safely used in the majority of patients with both disorders [Evidence: SORT B].[39] **Clonidine** alone or in combination with stimulants is also effective in improving both ADHD and tic symptoms in patients with both conditions [Evidence: SORT A].[39]

SORT (Strength of Recommendation Taxonomy) is a rating system (A, B or C) that addresses the quality of available evidence.
For more information consult **How to Use *Compendium of Therapeutic Choices*** on page xxv.

Table 2: **Drugs Used in Attention-Deficit Hyperactivity Disorder**

Class	Drug	Dose	Adverse Effects	Drug Interactions	Comments	Cost[a]
Alpha$_2$-adrenergic Agonists	*clonidine* Catapres, Dixarit, generics	Initial: 0.05–0.1 mg/day po Usual: 3–10 µg/kg/day po (0.05–0.4 mg/day), once daily or in divided doses To discontinue, reduce dose by 0.1 mg every 3–7 days	Hypotension, sedation and dizziness common initially; dry mouth; could exacerbate depression.	Avoid concurrent use with TCAs. Additive effects with other CNS depressants such as ethanol.	Caution in patients with cardiovascular disease or depression.	$
	guanfacine Intuniv XR	Initial: 1 mg/day po Increase dose in increments of 1 mg/wk to a maximum of 4 mg/day po To discontinue, reduce dose by 1 mg every 3–7 days	Somnolence, fatigue, headache, upper abdominal pain, bradycardia, hypotension (minor).	See clonidine Inhibitors of CYP3A4 such as clarithromycin, ketoconazole will significantly increase guanfacine serum concentrations. Inducers of CYP3A4 such as carbamazepine, systemic dexamethasone, phenobarbital, phenytoin, rifampin, will significantly reduce guanfacine serum concentrations.	Selective alpha$_{2a}$-adrenergic agonists In Canada, indicated only in children 6–12 years. During and after discontinuation, monitor blood pressure and heart rate until they return to normal.	$$$$$
Antidepressants, Dual Action	*bupropion* Wellbutrin SR, generics	Initial: 2–3 mg/kg/day po Usual: 200–300 mg/day po in 2 divided doses. Single doses should not exceed 150 mg	Agitation, dry mouth, insomnia, headache, constipation, nausea, vomiting, nervousness, dizziness, sweating, hypertension and tachycardia. Significant: suicidal ideation, seizures (0.5–1% incidence). Avoid in patients with a history of seizure disorders, eating disorders or significant head injury. Seizure risk increased with doses >300 mg/day.	Inducers of CYP2D6 or CYP3A4 such as carbamazepine, phenytoin or rifampin may decrease plasma level of bupropion and increase level of hydroxybupropion (active metabolite). Plasma concentration of venlafaxine or TCAs such as imipramine, desipramine or nortriptyline may increase due to inhibition of CYP2D6 by bupropion. Avoid use with MAOIs; may cause mania, excitation, hyperpyrexia.	It may take 2–4 wk before effects on ADHD symptoms are seen. Be vigilant for initiation of other medications that can decrease the seizure threshold, such as chloroquine, theophylline, tramadol or ciprofloxacin.	$
Antidepressants, Serotonin-Norepinephrine Reuptake Inhibitors	*venlafaxine* Effexor XR, generics	Adults: Initial: 37.5–75 mg daily po for 1 wk; titrate gradually to 150–300 mg po daily Maximum 450 mg/day po	Nausea, drowsiness, nervousness, dizziness, dry mouth, may increase BP if dose >300 mg/day.	Inhibitors of CYP2D6 or CYP3A4 such as clarithromycin, erythromycin, grapefruit, fluoxetine or paroxetine may decrease venlafaxine clearance; avoid use with MAOIs; caution with other serotonergic drugs (serotonin syndrome).	Make take up to 4 wk for optimal drug effect.	$

(cont'd)

Table 2: **Drugs Used in Attention-Deficit Hyperactivity Disorder** *(cont'd)*

Class	Drug	Dose	Adverse Effects	Drug Interactions	Comments	Cost[a]
Antidepressants, Tricyclic	*desipramine* generics	6–12 y: 10–20 mg/day po in 3–4 divided doses Adolescents: 30–50 mg/day po in 3–4 divided doses Usual maximum 150 mg/day	Postural hypotension, anticholinergic effects (dry mouth, constipation, urinary retention), dizziness, nausea, drowsiness, weakness, tremor, weight gain, asymptomatic ECG changes and tachycardia. Significant: arrhythmias (potential for fatal arrhythmias in overdose). Where possible, avoid in patients with a history of cardiovascular conduction disturbances, urinary retention, seizure disorders, hyperthyroidism.	Avoid with MAOIs—may cause mania, excitation, hyperpyrexia. Inducers of CYP2D6 or CYP3A4 such as carbamazepine, phenytoin or rifampin may decrease effect. Inhibitors of CYP2D6 or CYP3A4 such as clarithromycin, erythromycin, grapefruit juice, fluoxetine or paroxetine may increase effect and toxicity.	May require 3–4 wk to see beneficial effects.	$
	imipramine generics	6–12 y: 10–20 mg/day po in 3–4 divided doses Adolescents: 30–50 mg/day po in 3–4 divided doses Usual maximum 150 mg/day	See desipramine.	See desipramine.	See desipramine.	$
	nortriptyline Aventyl, generics	6–12 y: 10–20 mg/day po in 3–4 divided doses Adolescents: 30–50 mg/day po in 3–4 divided doses Usual maximum 150 mg/day	See desipramine.	See desipramine.	See desipramine.	$
Antipsychotics, Second-generation	*risperidone* Risperdal Preparations, generics	Initial: 0.25–0.5 mg HS po; increase at weekly intervals by 0.5 mg/day po in 2 divided doses as needed Usual maintenance dose 0.75–1.5 mg/day po	Weight gain, drowsiness, headache, orthostatic hypotension, dyspepsia, dose-related extrapyramidal effects; hyperprolactinemia. Advise patients about antipsychotic-associated body temperature dysregulation and prevention of heat stroke (e.g., hydration, sun protection.	Inhibitors of CYP2D6 or CYP3A4 such as clarithromycin, erythromycin, grapefruit, fluoxetine or paroxetine may increase effect and toxicity; inducers of these isoenzymes, such as carbamazepine, phenytoin or rifampin may reduce effect.	Used for behavioural symptoms (hyperactivity, impulsivity) when stimulants alone are ineffective or not tolerated. Oral liquid should not be mixed with cola or tea; may be mixed with water, orange juice or low-fat milk.	$

Class	Drug	Dose	Adverse Effects	Drug Interactions	Comments	Cost[a]
Norepinephrine Reuptake Inhibitors	*atomoxetine* Strattera, generics	Children ≤70 kg: 0.5 mg/kg/day po × 10 days, then 0.8 mg/kg/day po × 10 days, then 1–1.2 mg/kg/day po >70 kg: 40 mg/day po × 10 days, then 60 mg/day po × 10 days, then increase to target of 80 mg/day po if necessary One dose in a.m. or 2 divided doses (a.m. and late afternoon) Maximum 100 mg/day po	Headaches, rhinorrhea, upper abdominal pain, nausea, sedation, vomiting, decreased appetite, dizziness, fatigue, emotional lability and small increases in heart rate and blood pressure. Significant: suicidal ideation, sudden cardiac death, liver toxicity, exacerbation of tics.	Inhibitors of CYP2D6 such as fluoxetine, paroxetine or quinidine can increase plasma levels. "Slow metabolizers" such as some Asian populations may have extended elimination half-lives. Concurrent use of salbutamol may increase heart rate.	Dosing based on patient's weight. Requires 3–4 wk to see beneficial effects.	$$$$
Stimulants	*methylphenidate immediate-release tablets* Ritalin, generics	Initial: 0.3 mg/kg/day po Usual: 0.15–1 mg/kg/day po **or** 10–60 mg/day po in 1–3 divided doses	**Common, usually transient—continue therapeutic trial:** anorexia, insomnia, weight loss, irritability, dizziness, weepiness, headache, abdominal pain. **Transient—stop and re-evaluate:** "zombie-like" effects, psychotic reactions (such as hallucinations), agitation, tachycardia, hypertension, growth failure, rebound hyperactivity, leukopenia, blood dyscrasias. **Overdose symptoms—stop and retitrate:** "glassy eyes," insomnia, hyperactivity. **Significant:** sudden cardiac death reported; neurologic symptoms; exacerbation of tics; avoid in patients with a history of cardiovascular conduction disturbances, hypertension, acute psychotic episodes and hyperthyroidism. If seizures occur, or if frequency increases in patient with controlled epilepsy, stop and re-evaluate.	*Stimulants:* avoid concurrent use with irreversible MAOIs such as phenelzine or tranylcypromine. Other drugs that inhibit MAO, such as moclobemide, can also increase hypertensive effect of stimulant. Concurrent use of theophylline may increase risk of tachycardia, palpitations, dizziness, weakness. *Methylphenidate:* may increase plasma levels of phenytoin, phenobarbital, TCAs. *Carbamazepine:* decreases plasma levels of methylphenidate. *Methylphenidate:* reduces metabolism of warfarin, resulting in increased INR.	Last daily dose should be given before 4 p.m. to avoid insomnia. Doses greater than 60 mg/day usually do not result in additional efficacy in children. Pharmacokinetics reflect wide individual variations; strict weight-based dosing may not be predictive of clinical effect; titrate dose against response. Potential for abuse; use cautiously, especially in adolescents.	$

(cont'd)

Table 2: **Drugs Used in Attention-Deficit Hyperactivity Disorder** *(cont'd)*

Class	Drug	Dose	Adverse Effects	Drug Interactions	Comments	Cost[a]
	methylphenidate sustained-release tablets Ritalin SR, generics	20–60 mg/day po in 1 or 2 divided doses	See methylphenidate immediate-release.	See methylphenidate immediate-release.	See methylphenidate immediate-release. May be used in combination with immediate-release formulation.	$
	methylphenidate controlled-release capsules Biphentin	10–60 mg QAM po	See methylphenidate immediate-release.	See methylphenidate immediate-release.	See methylphenidate immediate-release. Capsule contents can be sprinkled on soft food such as applesauce, ice cream or yogurt.	$$$
	methylphenidate bilayer controlled-release tablets Concerta, generics	18–72 mg QAM po	See methylphenidate immediate-release.	See methylphenidate immediate-release.	See methylphenidate immediate-release. Consult product monograph for dosage conversion from other methylphenidate formulations. Generic product is bioequivalent; clinical equivalence is unknown.	$$
	dextroamphetamine immediate-release tablets Dexedrine	0.15 mg/kg/day po **or** 2.5–40 mg/day po in 1–3 divided doses	See methylphenidate immediate-release.	See methylphenidate immediate-release. *Dextroamphetamine:* Acidifying agents such as fruit juices or ascorbic acid can decrease absorption and increase elimination of dextroamphetamine. Alkalinizing agents such as sodium bicarbonate can increase absorption and decrease elimination of dextroamphetamine.		$$

Class	Drug	Dose	Adverse Effects	Drug Interactions	Comments	Cost[a]
	dextroamphetamine sustained-release spansules Dexedrine	0.15 mg/kg/day po **or** 10–40 mg QAM po	See methylphenidate immediate-release.	See methylphenidate immediate-release. See dextroamphetamine immediate-release.	Capsule contents can be sprinkled on soft food such as applesauce, ice cream or yogurt.	$$$
	lisdexamfetamine Vyvanse	Initial (≥6 y): 30 mg QAM po May increase to 50 mg daily po after 1 wk if necessary	See methylphenidate immediate-release.	See methylphenidate immediate-release.	May be taken with or without food. Capsule contents can be mixed with water or sprinkled on soft food such as applesauce, ice cream or yogurt.	$$$$$
	mixed salts amphetamine extended-release capsules Adderall XR	10–30 mg QAM po	See methylphenidate immediate-release.	See methylphenidate immediate-release.	Capsule contents can be sprinkled on applesauce and eaten immediately without chewing; doses should not be divided or stored.	$$$$

[a] Cost of 30-day supply of mean dosage; based on 35 kg body weight; includes drug cost only.

Dosage adjustment may be required in renal impairment; see Appendix I

Abbreviations: ADHD = attention-deficit hyperactivity disorder; MAOI = monoamine oxidase inhibitor; TCA = tricyclic antidepressant

Legend: $ < $30 $$ $30–60 $$$ $60–90 $$$$ $90–120 $$$$$ $120–150

Suggested Readings

Canadian Attention Deficit Hyperactivity Disorder Resource Alliance (CADDRA). *Canadian ADHD practice guidelines*. 3rd ed. Toronto (ON): CADDRA; 2011. Available from: www.caddra.ca/pdfs/caddraGuidelines2011.pdf.

Jensen PS, Hinshaw SP, Swanson JM et al. Findings from the NIMH Multimodal Treatment Study of ADHD (MTA): implications and applications for primary care providers. *J Dev Behav Pediatr* 2001;22(1):60-73.

National Collaborating Centre for Mental Health. NICE Clinical Guideline 72. *Attention deficit hyperactivity disorder: diagnosis and management of ADHD in children, young people and adults*. September 2008. Available from: www.nice.org.uk/nicemedia/pdf/CG072NiceGuidelineV2.pdf.

Pliszka SR, Crismon ML, Hughes CW et al. The Texas Children's Medication Algorithm Project: revision of the algorithm for pharmacotherapy of attention-deficit/hyperactivity disorder. *J Am Acad Child Adolesc Psychiatry* 2006;45(6):642-57.

Rappley MD. Clinical practice. Attention deficit-hyperactivity disorder. *N Engl J Med* 2005;352(2):165-73.

References

1. Akinbami LJ, Liu X, Pastor PN et al. Attention deficit hyperactivity disorder among children aged 5-17 years in the United States, 1998-2009. *NCHS Data Brief* 2011;(70):1-8.
2. Subcommittee on Attention-Deficit/Hyperactivity Disorder; Steering Committee on Quality Improvement and Management et al. ADHD: clinical practice guideline for the diagnosis, evaluation, and treatment of attention-deficit/hyperactivity disorder in children and adolescents. *Pediatrics* 2011;128(5):1007-22.
3. American Psychiatric Association. *Diagnostic and statistical manual of mental disorders: DSM-5*. 5th ed. Washington (DC): American Psychiatric Publishing; 2013.
4. Rappley MD. Clinical practice. Attention deficit-hyperactivity disorder. *N Engl J Med* 2005;352(2):165-73.
5. Canadian Attention Deficit Hyperactivity Disorder Resource Alliance (CADDRA). *Canadian ADHD practice guidelines*. 3rd ed. Toronto (ON): CADDRA; 2011. Available from: www.caddra.ca/pdfs/caddraGuidelines2011.pdf. Accessed January 21, 2014.
6. Linnet KM, Dalsgaard S, Obel C et al. Maternal lifestyle factors in pregnancy risk of attention deficit hyperactivity disorder and associated behaviors: review of the current evidence. *Am J Psychiatry* 2003;160(6):1028-40.
7. Daley KC. Update on attention-deficit/hyperactivity disorder. *Curr Opin Pediatr* 2004;16(2):217-26.
8. A 14-month randomized clinical trial of treatment strategies for attention-deficit/hyperactivity disorder. The MTA Cooperative Group. Multimodal Treatment Study of Children with ADHD. *Arch Gen Psychiatry* 1999;56(12):1073-86.
9. Pliszka SR, Crismon ML, Hughes CW et al. The Texas Children's Medication Algorithm Project: revision of the algorithm for pharmacotherapy of attention-deficit/hyperactivity disorder. *J Am Acad Child Adolesc Psychiatry* 2006;45(6):642-57.
10. Abikoff H, Hechtman L, Klein RG et al. Symptomatic improvement in children with ADHD treated with long-term methylphenidate and multimodal psychosocial treatment. *J Am Acad Child Adolesc Psychiatry* 2004;43(7):802-11.
11. Chan E. The role of complementary and alternative medicine in attention-deficit hyperactivity disorder. *J Dev Behav Pediatr* 2002;23(1 Suppl):S37-45.
12. The use of alternative therapies in treating children with attention deficit hyperactivity disorder. *Paediatr Child Health* 2002;7(10):710-30.
13. Fox DJ, Tharp DF, Fox LC. Neurofeedback: an alternative and efficacious treatment for attention deficit hyperactivity disorder. *Appl Psychophysiol Biofeedback* 2005;30(4):365-73.
14. Zwi M, Jones H, Thorgaard C et al. Parent training interventions for Attention Deficit Hyperactivity Disorder (ADHD) in children aged 5 to 18 years. *Cochrane Database Syst Rev* 2011;(12):CD003018.
15. Murray, DW. Treatment of preschoolers with attention-deficit/hyperactivity disorder. *Curr Psychiatry Rep* 2010;12(5):374-81.
16. Swanson JM, Elliott GR, Greenhill LL et al. Effects of stimulant medication on growth rates across 3 years in the MTA follow-up. *J Am Acad Child Adolesc Psychiatry* 2007;46(8):1015-27.
17. U.S. Food and Drug Administration. *Methylphenidate ADHD medications: drug safety communication-risk of long-lasting erections*. Available from: www.fda.gov/safety/medwatch/safetyinformation/safetyalertsforhumanmedicalproducts/ucm378876.htm. Accessed May 26, 2014.
18. Biederman J, Swanson JM, Wigal SB et al. Efficacy and safety of modafinil film-coated tablets in children and adolescents with attention-deficit/hyperactivity disorder: results of a randomized, double-blind, placebo-controlled, flexible-dose study. *Pediatrics* 2005;116(6):e777-84.
19. Biederman J, Swanson JM, Wigal SB et al. A comparison of once-daily modafinil in children with attention-deficit/hyperactivity disorder: a randomized, double-blind, and placebo-controlled study. *J Clin Psychiatry* 2006;67(5):727-35.
20. Banaschewski T, Roessner V, Dittman RW et al. Non-stimulant medications in the treatment of ADHD. *Eur Child Adolesc Psychiatry* 2004;13(Suppl 1):102-16.
21. Michelson D, Faries D, Wernicke J et al. Atomoxetine in the treatment of children and adolescents with attention-deficit/hyperactivity disorder: a randomized, placebo-controlled, dose-response study. *Pediatrics* 2001;108(5):e83.
22. Biederman J, Heiligenstein JH, Faries D et al. Efficacy of atomoxetine versus placebo in school-age girls with attention-deficit/hyperactivity disorder. *Pediatrics* 2002;110(6):e75.
23. Michelson D, Allen AJ, Busner J et al. Once-daily atomoxetine treatment for children and adolescents with attention deficit hyperactivity disorder: a randomized, placebo-controlled study. *Am J Psychiatry* 2002;159(11):1896-901.
24. Spencer T, Heiligenstein JH, Biederman J et al. Results from 2 proof-of-concept, placebo-controlled studies of atomoxetine in children with attention-deficit/hyperactivity disorder. *J Clin Psychiatry* 2002;63(12):1140-7.

25. Michelson D, Adler L, Spencer T et al. Atomoxetine in adults with ADHD: two randomized, placebo-controlled studies. *Biol Psychiatry* 2003;53(2):112-20.
26. Kelsey DK, Sumner CR, Casat CD et al. Once-daily atomoxetine treatment for children with attention-deficit/hyperactivity disorder, including an assessment of evening and morning behavior: a double-blind, placebo-controlled trial. *Pediatrics* 2004;114(1):e1-8.
27. Bezchlibnyk-Butler KZ, Virani AS, eds. *Clinical handbook of psychotropic drugs for children and adolescents*. Cambridge (MA): Hogrefe & Huber; 2004.
28. Casat CD, Pleasants DZ, Van Wyck Fleet J. A double-blind trial of bupropion in children with attention deficit disorder. *Psychopharmacol Bull* 1987;23(1):120-2.
29. Barrickman LL, Perry PJ, Allen AJ et al. Bupropion versus methylphenidate in the treatment of attention-deficit hyperactivity disorder. *J Am Acad Child Adolesc Psychiatry* 1995;34(5):649-57.
30. Kuperman S, Perry PJ, Gaffney GR et al. Bupropion SR vs. methylphenidate vs. placebo for attention deficit hyperactivity disorder in adults. *Ann Clin Psychiatry* 2001;13(3):129-34.
31. Wilens TE, Spencer TJ, Biederman J et al. A controlled clinical trial of bupropion for attention deficit hyperactivity disorder in adults. *Am J Psychiatry* 2001;158(2):282-8.
32. Motavalli Mukaddes N, Abali O. Venlafaxine in children and adolescents with attention deficit hyperactivity disorder. *Psychiatry Clin Neurosci* 2004;58(1):92-5.
33. Spencer T, Biederman J, Wilens T et al. Pharmacotherapy of attention-deficit hyperactivity disorder across the life cycle. *J Am Acad Child Adolesc Psychiatry* 1996;35(4):409-32.
34. Biederman J, Melmed RD, Patel A et al. A randomized, double-blind, placebo-controlled study of guanfacine extended release in children and adolescents with attention-deficit/hyperactivity disorder. *Pediatrics* 2008;121(1):e73-84.
35. Sallee FR, McGough J, Wigal T et al. Guanfacine extended release in children and adolescents with attention-deficit/hyperactivity disorder: a placebo-controlled trial. *J Am Acad Child Adolesc Psychiatry* 2009;48(2):155-65.
36. Newcorn JH, Stein MA, Childress AC et al. Randomized, double-blind trial of guanfacine extended release in children with attention-deficit/hyperactivity disorder: morning or evening administration. *J Am Acad Child Adolesc Psychiatry* 2013;52(9):921-30.
37. Einarson TR, Iskedjian M. *Novel antipsychotics for patients with attention-deficit hyperactivity disorder: a systematic review*. Ottawa (ON): Canadian Coordinating Office for Health Technology Assessment (CCOHTA); 2001. Available from: www.cadth.ca/en/products/health-technology-assessment/publication/268.
38. Wilens TE, Faraone SV, Biederman J et al. Does stimulant therapy of attention-deficit/hyperactivity disorder beget later substance abuse? A meta-analytic review of the literature. *Pediatrics* 2003;111(1):179-85.
39. Pringsheim T, Steeves T. Pharmacological treatment for Attention Deficit Hyperactivity Disorder (ADHD) in children with comorbid tic disorders. *Cochrane Database Syst Rev* 2011;(4):CD007990.

Psychiatric Disorders

Chapter 4
Bipolar Disorder

Sagar V. Parikh, MD, FRCPC

Bipolar disorder is a complex, recurrent mood disorder that affects 1–2% of the population.[1] It is defined as having experienced either a manic episode (with or without a history of major depressive episode), or a hypomanic episode (with a current or past history of major depressive episode). DSM-5 criteria also require that mania or hypomania must include abnormally and persistently increased goal-directed activity or energy.[2] See Table 1 and Table 2.

Symptoms of mania include changes in mood, energy, sleep requirements and ability to concentrate, and in some cases psychotic symptoms.

Table 1: Description of Bipolar Disorder Episodes[2]

Type of Episode	Features
Manic episode	**Mood:** Abnormally and persistently elevated, expansive or irritable; must have concomitant increase in activity or energy; psychotic symptoms may occur **Duration:** At least 1 week, causing significant distress/disability, or requiring hospital admission ***Plus:*** If mood is elevated or expansive, 3 or more of the following features must be present. If mood is predominantly irritable, 4 or more are required. • Grandiosity • More talkative • Excessive involvement in pleasurable activities that may have unpleasant consequences • Less need for sleep • Flight of ideas • Distractability • More goal-directed activity
Hypomanic episode	**Mood:** Same symptoms as for mania, but milder and not disabling; *no* psychotic symptoms **Duration:** 4 days or longer
Major depressive episode	**Mood:** Depressed most of the day OR markedly diminished interest or pleasure (anhedonia) **Duration:** At least 2 weeks, with significant change from previous functioning ***Plus:*** Four or more of the following: • Insomnia or hypersomnia • Significant weight loss/gain or change in appetite • Fatigue or loss of energy • Psychomotor retardation or agitation (observable) • Worthlessness or excessive guilt • Impaired thinking, concentrating or making decisions • Recurrent thoughts of death, suicidal ideation or attempt/plan
Manic or hypomanic episode with mixed features	Criteria met *during same time period* for hypomanic episode or manic episode with 3 or more features of depressive episode
Depressive episode with mixed features	Criteria met *during same time period* for a major depressive episode with 3 or more features of manic or hypomanic episode

Table 2: **Classification of Bipolar Disorder**[2]

Disorder	Features
Bipolar I Disorder	Lifetime history of at least one clear-cut manic episode, with or without episodes of hypomania or depression
Bipolar II Disorder	History of hypomanic episode and major depressive episodes, with no history of a full manic episode
Other Specified (or unspecified) Bipolar and Related Disorders	Most diagnostic criteria for bipolar disorder met, but not all; e.g., duration of episode shorter than required for diagnosis, or history of hypomanic episodes but no depressive episodes that meet diagnostic criteria
Cyclothymic Disorder	Recurrent episodes of hypomania and mild (subthreshold) depressive symptoms

Symptoms of depression include oversleeping or profound tiredness (the most common symptom of bipolar depression), pessimism, inability to socialize, decreased cognitive abilities and possibly suicidal or psychotic symptoms.

Bipolar disorder is formally divided into 3 categories: bipolar I disorder, bipolar II disorder and bipolar disorder not otherwise specified (Table 2).[2] Diagnosis of bipolar disorder is often difficult as the illness is perhaps the most complex psychiatric disorder. It has the most variable clinical presentation and is associated with the highest number of episodes, the highest degree of comorbidity and the highest mortality of the major psychiatric conditions. When bipolar disorder is severe and psychotic symptoms are present, it resembles schizophrenia. When accompanied by substance abuse, it mimics a pure substance abuse disorder. In a severe depression phase, it resembles unipolar major depression. When the symptoms are mild and changing rapidly, it resembles borderline personality disorder.

Goals of Therapy

- Control symptoms of acute episode
- Prevent recurrences
- Provide ancillary care for comorbid psychiatric conditions such as anxiety or substance abuse or medical conditions such as endocrine/metabolic disorders

Investigations

- It is estimated that one-third of patients appearing in primary care settings with symptoms suggestive of unipolar major depression are actually experiencing depression in the context of bipolar illness.[3] Ask all depressed patients about possible hypomanic or manic symptoms in their past. While no screening test is ideal, the Mood Disorder Questionnaire (MDQ), available from http://bipolar.stanford.edu/mdq.html, is a helpful, self-completed form that asks systematic yes/no questions about the symptoms of mania;[4] an adolescent version also has been developed.[5] Two or more "yes" answers on the MDQ should prompt a more thorough clinical review of symptoms, including questioning family/friends if possible.
- The diagnosis of bipolar disorder depends not just on the clinical presentation but, very importantly, on a reliable collateral history from a friend or family member who can corroborate episodes of elevated mood, inappropriate behaviour, decreased sleep with increased energy or grandiosity.
- It is critical to determine whether the patient has a *family history* of mood disorders, substance abuse or bipolar disorder itself.
- Laboratory investigations:
  - depend in part on the age and acute presentation of the patient

- for all patients, basic blood tests include CBC, electrolytes, renal function, liver function and thyroid function; bHCG to rule out pregnancy before prescribing drugs contraindicated in pregnant women.
- metabolic parameters including weight, lipid profile and fasting blood sugars at the time of initiation of any treatment
- for patients with any unusual symptoms, neurologic signs or symptoms, or a first manic or hypomanic episode after age 40, include structural imaging of the brain such as CAT or MRI

Therapeutic Choices

Bipolar disorder is a complex illness that can only be partly managed by a sole physician; a team approach is ideal. At a minimum, it is helpful to have access to a nurse who will provide education and coping strategies as well as ongoing monitoring and support. The comprehensive treatment of bipolar disorder is reviewed in detail in the CANMAT treatment guidelines,[1,6,7,8] which are the basis for the recommendations that follow. Key additional resources such as treatment manuals and web sites are also listed in the CANMAT guidelines.

Nonpharmacologic Choices

- Psychoeducation is a recommended intervention consisting of information about the illness as well as training in coping strategies and recognition of episodes early in their genesis [Evidence: SORT B*].[9,10] Structured group psychoeducational programs have been shown to substantially reduce the risk of relapse of manic, mixed and depressive episodes. A recommended source of information on psychoeducation is *Structured Group Psychotherapy for Bipolar Disorder* (see Suggested Readings), which is available in both English and French and provides explicit advice for effective psychoeducation over the course of 6 treatment sessions.
- To prevent an incipient manic or depressive episode from becoming a flagrant episode, conduct a "relapse drill," which trains patients to recognize their unique warning symptoms and respond in a specific treatment fashion which might include:
  - changes in medication strategies
  - rapid contact with the treating physician
  - additional steps to regulate sleep and other behaviours

Pharmacologic Choices

Pharmacologic therapy varies according to the type and stage of the episode being treated. Since treatment for this condition is lifelong, engaging the patient in collaborative decision-making is critical. Except in situations where there is a severe episode or medical emergency, discuss the pros and cons of 2 or 3 pharmacologic options to inform and support the patient's decision.

Manic Episodes

Moderate to severe mania is usually treated in hospital; mild mania, which by psychiatric definition is distinct from hypomania (see Table 1), may be treated on an outpatient basis. The first step in treating mania is to assess for risk of aggressive behaviour or violence to others, suicide, degree of insight and the ability to adhere to treatment (Figure 1).[7] If the patient is taking an antidepressant, it should be discontinued. Complicating issues such as other medical conditions, particularly substance abuse problems, will need attention.

* SORT (Strength of Recommendation Taxonomy) is a rating system (A, B or C) that addresses the quality of available evidence. For more information consult **How to Use *Compendium of Therapeutic Choices*** on page xxv.

Specific medication strategies for mania depend on whether the patient is already on maintenance therapy and is experiencing a breakthrough episode or whether the individual is unmedicated. If the patient is already taking a first-line agent (**lithium** or **divalproex** or a **second-generation ("atypical") antipsychotic**), dosage adjustment may be sufficient after checking blood levels where appropriate. In moderate-to-severe manic episodes, addition of another medication is usually necessary.

In previously unmedicated patients, initiate treatment with a first-line agent (Table 3, Table 6). When the episode is particularly severe, initiate treatment with a 2-drug combination such as lithium or divalproex plus a second-generation antipsychotic. Continue treatment on any particular regimen for 2 weeks at therapeutic doses before assessing whether a change is necessary. Various other treatment options are shown in Figure 1.

Figure 1: Management of Acute Mania in Bipolar Disorder

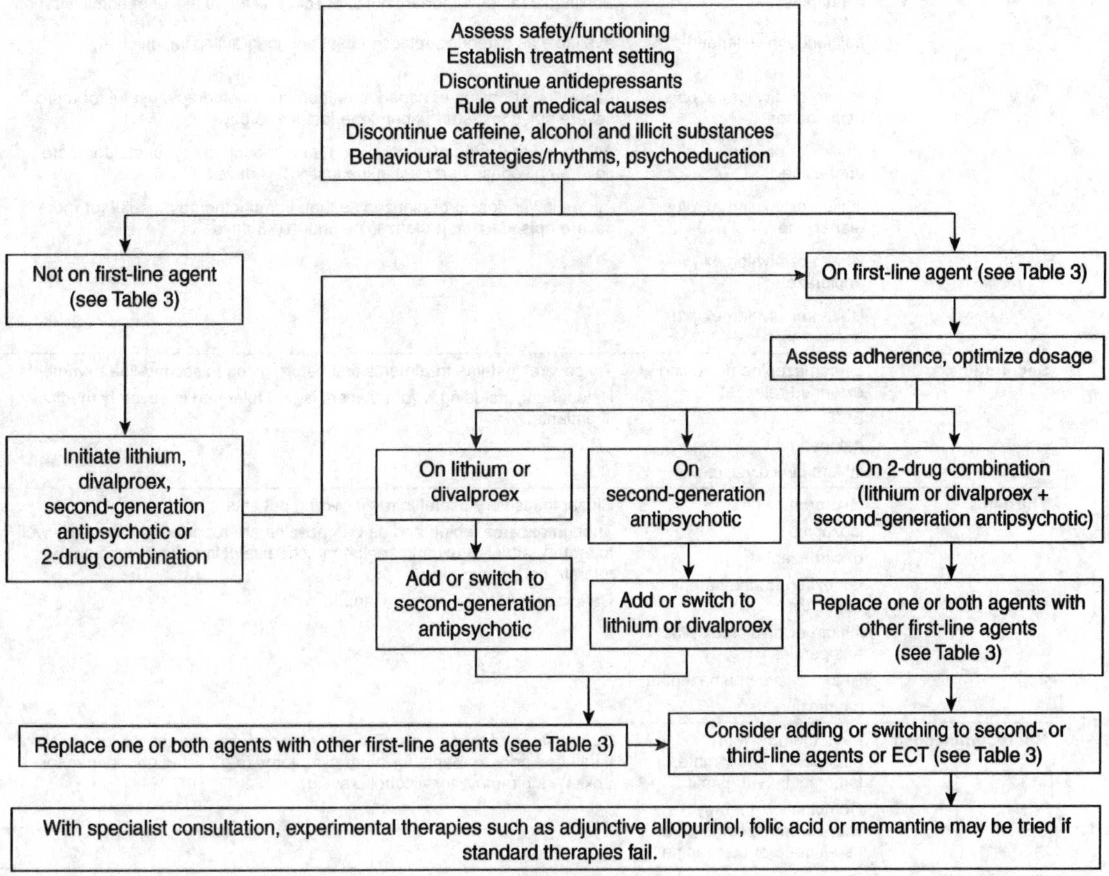

ECT = electroconvulsive therapy
Adapted with permission from Yatham LN, Kennedy SH, Parikh SV et al. Canadian Network for Mood and Anxiety Treatments (CANMAT) and International Society for Bipolar Disorders (ISBD) collaborative update of CANMAT guidelines for the management of patients with bipolar disorder: update 2013. *Bipolar Disord* 2013;15(1):1-44.

Table 3: **Pharmacologic Management of Acute Mania in Bipolar Disorder**

Place in Therapy	Drugs[a,b]	Comments
First-line	lithium	Aim for blood levels near the high end of therapeutic range as tolerated, i.e., 1–1.2 mmol/L (0.5–0.8 mmol/L in elderly patients).
	divalproex	Loading dose is an option (20 mg/kg); aim for blood levels high in therapeutic range.
	olanzapine	May start with therapeutic dose of 15 mg; note peak sedation is 3–4 hours after ingestion, so may dose earlier in evening.
	risperidone	Monitor regularly for orthostatic hypotension and extrapyramidal side effects, e.g., parkinsonism, akathisia.
	quetiapine (including extended-release)	Need to titrate dose rapidly; monitor for sedation, hypotension.
	aripiprazole	
	ziprasidone	Consider pretreatment ECG; usually need ≥120 mg/day.
	asenapine	Sublingual tablet; important not to eat or drink for 10 min after administration.
	paliperidone extended-release	Available as extended-release tablet and long-acting im injection.
	lithium or divalproex *plus* risperidone	Allows lower dosing of risperidone than in monotherapy; useful for more severe episodes; start risperidone first × 1–3 days.
	lithium or divalproex *plus* quetiapine	Allows lower dosing of quetiapine than in monotherapy; useful for more severe episodes; start quetiapine first × 1–3 days.
	lithium or divalproex *plus* olanzapine	Allows lower dosing of olanzapine than in monotherapy; useful for more severe episodes; start olanzapine first × 1–3 days.
	lithium or divalproex *plus* aripiprazole	
	lithium or divalproex *plus* asenapine	
Second-line	carbamazepine (including extended-release) ECT haloperidol lithium *plus* divalproex	Try several first-line treatments first before going to second-line treatments. Haloperidol, including iv formulation, is well tolerated in severely medically ill patients.
Third-line	chlorpromazine clozapine oxcarbazepine tamoxifen (monotherapy or adjunctive) lithium or divalproex *plus* haloperidol lithium *plus* carbamazepine cariprazine	Clozapine is very useful in rapid-cycling patients. Though oxcarbazepine and carbamazepine are reported to be equally well tolerated, a trial of oxcarbazepine may be useful in patients who cannot tolerate carbamazepine. Cariprazine not available in Canada.
Not recommended	Monotherapy with gabapentin, topiramate, lamotrigine, verapamil Combination therapy with carbamazepine plus risperidone or olanzapine	Use of some of these agents as *adjuncts* may be appropriate, especially if initiated prior to mania for other symptoms (e.g., using gabapentin for anxiety, topiramate for alcohol craving).

[a] Pharmacologic treatment of hypomanic episodes in bipolar II disorder is similar.
[b] Treatment trials typically run 2 weeks at therapeutic doses. Adjunctive benzodiazepine use is common, e.g., clonazepam 1–2 mg BID. If patient is not on first-line agent, start first-line agent monotherapy; if more serious, consider dual therapy. If on maintenance therapy, optimize dosing prior to adding new medication.
Abbreviations: ECT = electroconvulsive therapy

Depressive Episodes

As with acute mania, first assess the patient for basic safety issues, including potential suicidality, comorbid medical problems or substance abuse. Next, the strategy depends on whether the patient is on medication and has had a breakthrough episode of major depression, or whether they are medication free (Figure 2).[7] In an unmedicated patient, therapy may begin with **lithium**, **lamotrigine** or **quetiapine**. If the depression is severe, therapy can be initiated with 2 agents, such as lithium plus quetiapine (Table 4, Table 7).

Figure 2: Management of Depressive Episodes in Bipolar Disorder

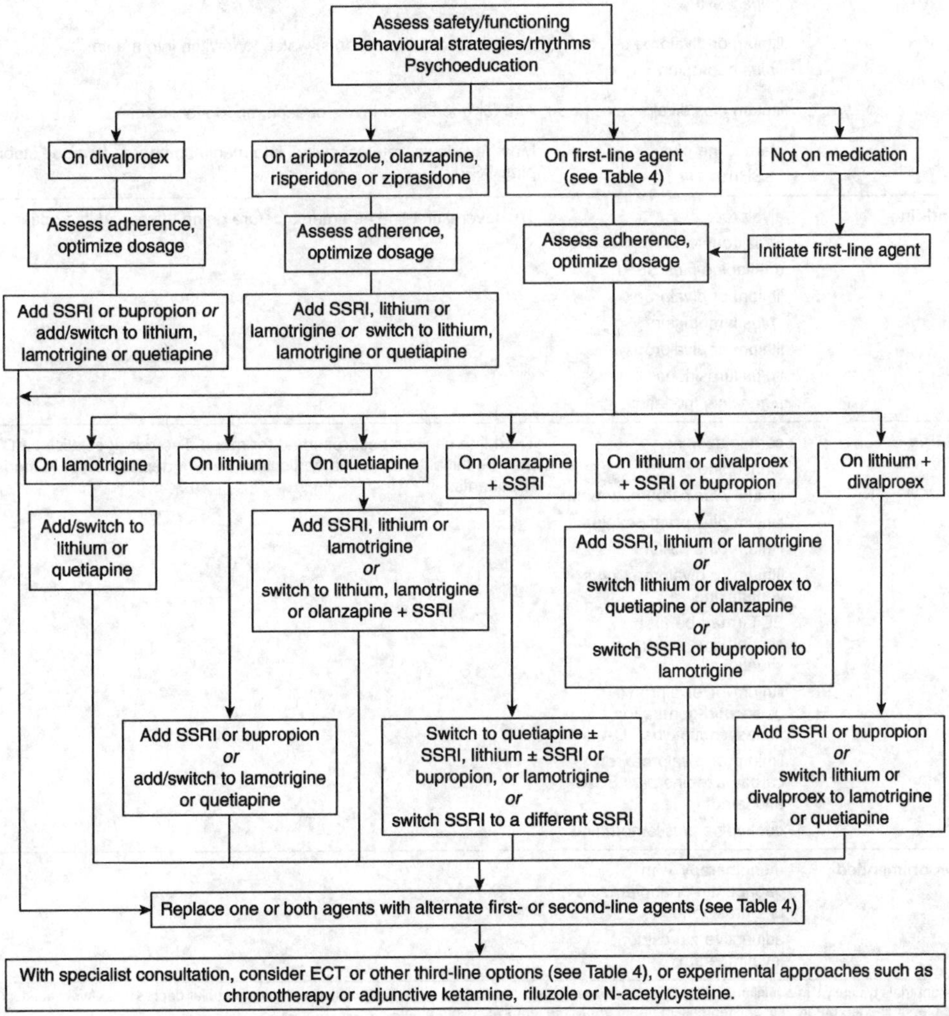

Abbreviations: SSRI = selective serotonin reuptake inhibitor; ECT = electroconvulsive therapy
Adapted with permission from Yatham LN, Kennedy SH, Parikh SV et al. Canadian Network for Mood and Anxiety Treatments (CANMAT) and International Society for Bipolar Disorders (ISBD) collaborative update of CANMAT guidelines for the management of patients with bipolar disorder: update 2013. *Bipolar Disord* 2013;15(1):1-44.

Table 4: **Pharmacologic Management of Acute Depression in Bipolar Disorder**

Place in Therapy	Drugs[a]	Comments
First-line	lithium	Aim for blood levels near the high end of therapeutic range as tolerated, i.e., 1–1.2 mmol/L (0.5–0.8 mmol/L in elderly patients). Measure serum concentration 9–13 hours post-dose. May be useful for those with high risk of suicide or self harm.
	lamotrigine	Slow titration schedule in turn slows response but mitigates risk of adverse effects including rash; useful for milder episodes.
	quetiapine (including extended-release)	Monotherapy studies showed doses of 300 or 600 mg/day to be equally effective; lower dose preferred if patient is medication-naïve.
	lithium or divalproex *plus* SSRI	Prefer shorter half-life SSRIs in case of switch to mania.
	lithium or divalproex *plus* bupropion	As with all antidepressants, watch for switch into mania.
	lithium *plus* divalproex	Aim for good blood levels of each mood stabilizer.
	olanzapine *plus* SSRI	May have lower rates of switch into mania compared to mood stabilizer plus SSRI.
Second-line	divalproex lurasidone[b] quetiapine *plus* SSRI lithium or divalproex *plus* lamotrigine lithium or divalproex *plus* lurasidone *adjunctive* modafinil	Try several first-line treatments before going to second-line options.
Third-line	carbamazepine olanzapine lithium *plus* carbamazepine lithium *plus* pramipexole lithium *plus* MAOI lithium or divalproex *plus* venlafaxine ECT (may be first- or second-line in certain situations) lithium or divalproex or second-generation antipsychotic *plus* TCA lithium or divalproex or carbamazepine *plus* SSRI and lamotrigine quetiapine *plus* lamotrigine	Third-line choices best reserved for mood disorder specialists. ECT may be initial treatment in particularly severe depression or in medically ill patients.
Not recommended	monotherapy with gabapentin or aripiprazole or ziprasidone adjunctive ziprasidone or levetiracetam	

[a] Treatment trials typically run a minimum of 2–4 weeks at therapeutic doses. Response is often slower than in unipolar depression. Avoid antidepressants if possible, or shorten duration of antidepressant treatment to prevent switch into mania.

[b] Though existing guidelines list it as a second-line option, lurasidone was approved by Health Canada in 2014 for treatment of bipolar depressive episodes, either as monotherapy or in conjunction with lithium or valproate.

Abbreviations: ECT = electroconvulsive therapy; MAOI = monoamine oxidase inhibitor; SSRI = selective serotonin reuptake inhibitor; TCA = tricyclic antidepressant

Bipolar depression is difficult to treat; steps to follow if there is an inadequate response after 2–4 weeks of therapy are outlined in Figure 2. Two key emerging observations are that specific psychosocial strategies are potentially valuable for bipolar depression, and that combining 2 traditional mood stabilizers such as **lithium** plus **divalproex** may also be of some value. Although **antidepressants** can be considered in moderate-to-severe cases, there is some potential to destabilize and promote a more rapid-cycling course in susceptible individuals. Thus, the use (with caution) of short courses of antidepressants (e.g., ≤3–4 months), is prudent. Intensive psychosocial interventions for acute bipolar depression also have some efficacy, compared to brief psychosocial intervention, while usual bipolar medications are maintained.[11]

Maintenance Therapy for Bipolar Disorder

When patients recover from an acute episode and remain well for at least 2 months, they are defined as being in the maintenance phase of the illness. Unmedicated, such individuals have an approximately 70% chance of experiencing another episode over the next year and an approximately 95% chance of having a recurrence within 5 years. To prevent relapse, interventions include psychosocial strategies such as psychoeducation, cognitive-behavioural therapy, family therapy and interpersonal and social rhythm therapy. Key characteristics of effective psychosocial therapies that improve medication adherence include education about the disorder (including the likelihood of relapse), training in self-monitoring, education about how to manage side effects, development of strategies to manage stressors and attention to the patient's own belief system and attitude towards the illness.

Give patients the opportunity to discuss the impact of the illness on their life and their beliefs about potential effects of long-term medication use. To facilitate longer-term adherence, repeat a brief version of psychoeducation periodically, e.g., annually.

Table 5 lists a number of effective options for relapse prevention.

Bipolar Disorder in Children and Adolescents

Bipolar disorder typically emerges in adolescence, most often as depression.[12] An initial depressive episode is impossible to distinguish from unipolar depression. The existence of first-degree relatives with bipolar disorder in an adolescent presenting with an initial depression is suggestive of an eventual bipolar diagnosis, but treatment is usually initiated on the assumption that the teenager has unipolar depression. Other key predictors of an eventual shift to a bipolar diagnosis include the presence of particularly severe or psychotic symptoms in a teen who is unmistakably depressed (as opposed to someone who likely has schizophrenia). If the teen does have an initial presentation of hypomania or mania, the presentation is often one of a mixed state, where the mood is predominantly irritable and symptoms of both mania and depression are present in the same week (see Table 1).[13]

Both mania and depression have been documented in pre-teens, therefore bipolar disorder may be reliably diagnosed by a specialist at a very early age. ADHD presents a major differential challenge, with the key distinguishing feature remaining the episodic nature (weeks or months) of the bipolar disorder, while ADHD symptoms are present on a continuous daily basis. Bipolar treatment options are limited by a lack of clinical trials in children and adolescents, but some evidence exists for the efficacy of the usual adult treatments such as **lithium, divalproex**, **quetiapine** and **ziprasidone**.[14] Given the various diagnostic and medication controversies associated with children, refer to a child psychiatrist for treatment.

Bipolar Disorder in the Elderly

When bipolar disorder begins early in life, it is a lifelong illness that, if untreated, continues to manifest with more frequent episodes and shorter periods of recovery over the decades. The illness does *not* typically progress to an extremely rapid-cycling form of illness, and elderly bipolar patients usually will have major periods of euthymia. A small number of individuals experience a first onset of bipolar illness in their sixties or later; symptoms are typical of adult mania but irritability may be prominent.[15] Often these individuals have a history of comorbid neurologic problems and an elevated all-cause mortality rate. Clinical trials are relatively rare in the elderly, so most treatment parameters are extrapolated from the adult literature.[16] All second-generation antipsychotics carry warnings about potential elevated stroke risk and mortality in the elderly, but the significant morbidity and mortality associated with bipolar disorder in this population compels consideration of these agents for treatment.

Choices during Pregnancy and Breastfeeding

Since bipolar disorder often starts early in life, many women will be living with the disorder at the time they are considering having children. Key management principles include careful risk assessment for each woman, namely the risk of pregnancy destabilizing the illness and the possibility of severe episodes resulting in the death of either the patient or child, or both. Untreated women with bipolar disorder are particularly susceptible to postpartum depression, including depression with psychotic features that may result in harm to the child. Despite such cautions, most women with bipolar disorder are able to manage pregnancy successfully. Collaborative management of the pregnancy by a psychiatrist, an obstetrician and a family physician is recommended, including consultation with an agency specializing in information on medications during and following pregnancy, such as Motherisk, available at www.motherisk.org. Because most psychiatric medications pose some teratogenic risk, and many are excreted in breast milk, medication management during and following pregnancy requires extensive consideration and review with the patient.[17] If medication is to be discontinued prior to conception, it should be tapered with medical supervision.[18]

Creation of a "pregnancy contract" is recommended; in consultation with the doctor, a patient creates a 1-page document that summarizes her typical symptoms in mania and in depression, and lists preferred treatment options for each phase of illness. That document is then shared among the treatment team and the patient's family, and serves as a nonbinding but helpful "advance directive" should a new episode of illness arise.

A discussion of general principles on the use of medications in these special populations can be found in Appendix II and Appendix III. Other specialized reference sources are also provided in these appendices.

Therapeutic Tips

- A key feature of bipolar disorder is recurrent nonadherence to medication; including the patient in decision-making, together with psychoeducation, promotes a strong therapeutic alliance and enhances medication adherence.
- Patients taking lithium need to maintain their usual salt and caffeine intake and monitor fluid intake and output, making adjustments in the event of unexpected losses due to vomiting or diarrhea.
- During acute manic episodes, patients may exhibit increased tolerance to lithium.
- Advise patients taking antipsychotics about antipsychotic-associated body temperature dysregulation and strategies to prevent heat stroke (e.g., hydration, sun protection).
- For lithium-associated cognitive impairment, check lithium level and thyroid function. Lowering the dose or using a slow-release formulation may improve cognitive function.
- Patients who experience tremor while taking lithium may benefit from elimination of dietary caffeine, lithium dose reduction or addition of a **beta-blocker** such as propranolol or atenolol.
- Patients who experience diarrhea while taking slow-release lithium preparations may fare better with immediate-release formulations,[19] particularly the oral liquid citrate salt.[20]

Table 5: **Maintenance Treatment Regimens for Bipolar Disorder**[a]

Place in Therapy	Drugs	Comments
First-line	lithium	Blood levels can be individualized—some patients have efficacy at lower end of normal therapeutic range; levels lower than for acute episode
	lamotrigine	Effective only for prophylaxis against depressive relapses
	olanzapine	Equal to lithium overall in relapse prevention, but better at preventing relapse to mixed episodes
	divalproex	RCT support is lacking but clinical observation suggests effective relapse prevention
	quetiapine	Effective in preventing both manic and depressive relapses
	risperidone long-acting injection	Mainly for prevention of mania
	aripiprazole	Mainly for prevention of mania
	lithium or divalproex *plus* quetiapine	Effective in preventing both manic and depressive relapses
	lithium or divalproex *plus* ziprasidone	Mainly for prevention of mania; watch for emergent insomnia.
	lithium or divalproex *plus* risperidone long-acting injection	Mainly for prevention of mania
	lithium or divalproex *plus* aripiprazole	Mainly for prevention of mania
Second-line	carbamazepine paliperidone extended-release lithium *plus* divalproex lithium *plus* carbamazepine lithium or divalproex *plus* olanzapine lithium *plus* lamotrigine olanzapine *plus* fluoxetine lithium *plus* risperidone	Try several first-line treatments before going to second-line treatments. These recommendations are based primarily on open-label studies. May be able to use antidepressants concurrently for a long time in some patients with clear histories of predominantly depressive relapses.
Third-line	asenapine	Third-line choices best reserved for mood disorder specialists
	adjunctive therapy with: phenytoin clozapine ECT topiramate omega-3 fatty acids oxcarbazepine gabapentin asenapine	
Not recommended	adjunctive flupenthixol; monotherapy with gabapentin, topiramate or antidepressants	Patients with bipolar II disorder may rarely benefit from monotherapy with antidepressants

[a] While the goal is ultimately complete relapse prevention, in individuals with severe illness reduction in the frequency, duration and intensity of relapse may be more realistic. Psychosocial interventions are critical to reduce relapse.

Abbreviations: ECT = electroconvulsive therapy; RCT = randomized controlled trial; SSRI = selective serotonin reuptake inhibitor

Table 6: First-line Drug Therapy for Mania in Bipolar Disorder

Class	Drug	Dose	Adverse Effects	Drug Interactions	Cost[a]
Antipsychotics, second-generation	*aripiprazole* Abilify	15 mg/day po Maximum 30 mg/day	Akathisia, dizziness, orthostatic hypotension, headache, GI complaints, tremor, sedation. Advise patients about antipsychotic-associated body temperature dysregulation and prevention of heat stroke (e.g., hydration, sun protection).	Carbamazepine (or other strong inducers of CYP2D6 or CYP3A4 such as phenytoin, rifampin) can reduce aripiprazole levels significantly. Ketoconazole, quinidine, fluoxetine or paroxetine (or other strong inhibitors of CYP2D6 or CYP3A4) can increase levels substantially.	$$$$$
	asenapine Saphris	5 mg BID sl Instruct patients not to eat or drink for 10 minutes after placing tablet under tongue	Sedation, orthostasis, hypotension, dizziness, weight gain, EPS Advise patients about antipsychotic-associated body temperature dysregulation and prevention of heat stroke (e.g., hydration, sun protection).	Decreased asenapine clearance with fluvoxamine.	$$$$
	olanzapine Zyprexa, Zyprexa Zydis, generics	5–20 mg/day po	Weight gain, metabolic disturbances, anticholinergic side effects in elderly, akathisia. Monitor periodically for movement disorders. Advise patients about antipsychotic-associated body temperature dysregulation and prevention of heat stroke (e.g., hydration, sun protection).	Fluvoxamine and ciprofloxacin elevate olanzapine levels.	$$$
	paliperidone extended-release ◗ Invega	3–12 mg/day po	Insomnia, headaches, weight gain, orthostasis, rhinitis, anxiety, dose-related hyperprolactinemia and EPS. Advise patients about antipsychotic-associated body temperature dysregulation and prevention of heat stroke (e.g., hydration, sun protection).	Minimal risk of drug interactions. Carbamazepine may decrease paliperidone concentrations.	$117–350
	quetiapine Seroquel, generics	400–800 mg/day po	Weight gain, sedation, orthostasis, metabolic disturbances. Monitor periodically for movement disorders, including akathisia. Advise patients about antipsychotic-associated body temperature dysregulation and prevention of heat stroke (e.g., hydration, sun protection).	Ketoconazole dramatically increases quetiapine levels. Watch for hypotension with antihypertensives.	$$

Class	Drug	Dose	Adverse Effects	Drug Interactions	Cost[a]
	risperidone Risperdal Preparations, generics	3–6 mg/day po	Weight gain, orthostasis, dose-related EPS, metabolic disturbances. Advise patients about antipsychotic-associated body temperature dysregulation and prevention of heat stroke (e.g., hydration, sun protection).	Avoid combining with carbamazepine.	$$
	ziprasidone Zeldox	120–160 mg/day po in 2 divided doses, with food (≥500 kcal)	Insomnia, EPS; consider ECG at baseline and periodically to monitor effect on QT_c interval. Advise patients about antipsychotic-associated body temperature dysregulation and prevention of heat stroke (e.g., hydration, sun protection).	Carbamazepine decreases levels significantly; do not use with other drugs that prolong the QT_c interval.	$$$$$
Mood Stabilizers	*divalproex sodium* Epival, generics	750–2000 mg/day po, adjusted according to serum levels (target range 350–800 µmol/L)	Weight gain, thrombocytopenia, polycystic ovary syndrome, teratogenic; rarely: hyperammonemia, hepatotoxicity.	Avoid combining with carbamazepine. Use caution if combining with lamotrigine.	$
	lithium carbonate immediate-release Carbolith, Lithane, generics	900–2100 mg/day po, guided by serum concentrations (target 1–1.2 mmol/L, 0.5–0.8 mmol/L in elderly patients) Measure serum concentrations 9–13 h post-dose Single daily dose preferred	Highly toxic in overdose. Measure electrolytes and do 24-h urine for ClCr when starting long-term treatment. Monitor thyroid and renal function at least every 6 months.	Toxic levels may result when adding NSAIDs, ACEIs, ARBs and especially thiazide diuretics. Reduce lithium dose and check serum level if long-term treatment with these agents is required. Avoid large changes in salt or coffee intake. Stop lithium temporarily during acute intermittent illnesses causing fluid and electrolyte losses.	$
	lithium carbonate controlled-release Lithmax	900–2100 mg/day po, guided by serum concentrations (target 1–1.2 mmol/L, 0.5–0.8 mmol/L in elderly patients) Measure serum concentrations 9–13 h post-dose Single daily dose preferred	See lithium carbonate immediate-release.	See lithium carbonate immediate-release.	$$

(cont'd)

Table 6: **First-line Drug Therapy for Mania in Bipolar Disorder** *(cont'd)*

Class	Drug	Dose	Adverse Effects	Drug Interactions	Cost[a]
	lithium citrate syrup ◗ generic (8 mmol/5 mL; approximately equivalent to 300 mg lithium carbonate/5 mL)	900–2100 mg/day po, guided by serum concentrations (target 1–1.2 mmol/L, 0.5–0.8 mmol/L in elderly patients) Measure serum concentrations 9–13 h post-dose Single daily dose preferred	See lithium carbonate immediate-release.	See lithium carbonate immediate-release.	$$
	valproic acid Depakene, Apo-Valproic Capsules, other generics	750–2000 mg/day po, adjusted according to serum levels (target range 350–800 µmol/L)	See divalproex sodium.	See divalproex sodium.	$

[a] Cost of 30-day supply of mean dose (unless specific cost range provided); includes drug cost only.
◗ Dosage adjustment may be required in renal impairment; see Appendix I.
ACEIs = angiotensin converting enzyme inhibitors; ARBs = angiotensin receptor blockers; ClCr = creatinine clearance; EPS = extrapyramidal symptoms; NSAIDs = nonsteroidal anti-inflammatory drugs
Legend: $ < $30 $$ $30–60 $$$ $60–90 $$$$ $90–120 $$$$$ $120–150

Table 7: First-line Drug Therapy for Depression in Bipolar Disorder[a]

Class	Drug	Dose	Adverse Effects	Drug Interactions	Cost[b]
Antipsychotics, second-generation	*quetiapine* Seroquel, Seroquel XR, generics	Usual: 300 mg/day po Maximum: 600 mg/day po	Weight gain, sedation, orthostasis, metabolic disturbances. Advise patients about antipsychotic-associated body temperature dysregulation and prevention of heat stroke (e.g., hydration, sun protection).	Ketoconazole dramatically increases quetiapine levels. Monitor for hypotension with antihypertensives.	$$
Mood Stabilizers	*divalproex sodium* Epival, generics	750–2000 mg/day po, adjusted according to serum levels (target range 350–690 µmol/L)	Weight gain, thrombocytopenia, polycystic ovary syndrome, teratogenic; rarely: hyperammonemia, hepatotoxicity.	Avoid combining with carbamazepine. Use caution if combining with lamotrigine.	$
	lamotrigine Lamictal, generics	100–300 mg/day po	Rash common; severe rash rare.	Divalproex doubles blood level of lamotrigine; always initiate slowly.	$
	lithium carbonate immediate-release (kidney symbol) Carbolith, Lithane, generics	600–1800 mg/day po, adjusted according to serum levels (target 1–1.2 mmol/L, 0.5–0.8 mmol/L in elderly patients) Measure serum concentration 9–13 h post-dose.	Highly toxic in overdose. Measure electrolytes and do 24-h urine for ClCr when starting long-term treatment. Monitor thyroid and renal function at least every 6 months. Inform patients of signs/symptoms of toxicity such as ataxia, tremor, sedation or agitation, diarrhea, vomiting.	Toxic levels may result when adding NSAIDs, ACEIs, ARBs and especially thiazide diuretics. Reduce lithium dose and check serum level if long-term treatment with these agents is required. Avoid large changes in salt or coffee intake. Stop lithium temporarily during acute intermittent illnesses causing fluid and electrolyte losses.	$
	lithium carbonate controlled-release (kidney symbol) Lithmax	600–1800 mg/day po, adjusted according to serum levels (target 1–1.2 mmol/L, 0.5–0.8 mmol/L in elderly patients) Measure serum concentration 9–13 h post-dose.	See lithium carbonate immediate-release.	See lithium carbonate immediate-release.	$$

(cont'd)

Table 7: First-line Drug Therapy for Depression in Bipolar Disorder[a] *(cont'd)*

Class	Drug	Dose	Adverse Effects	Drug Interactions	Cost[b]
	lithium citrate syrup (renal icon) generic (8 mmol/5 mL; approximately equivalent to 300 mg lithium carbonate/5 mL)	600–1800 mg/day po, adjusted according to serum levels (target 1–1.2 mmol/L, 0.5–0.8 mmol/L in elderly patients) Measure serum concentration 9–13 h post-dose.	See lithium carbonate immediate-release.	See lithium carbonate immediate-release.	$$
	valproic acid Depakene, Apo-Valproic Capsules, other generics	750–2000 mg/day po, adjusted according to serum levels (target range 350–690 µmol/L)	See divalproex.	See divalproex.	$

[a] Detailed information on antidepressants can be found in Table 3.
[b] Cost of 30-day supply for mean dose; includes drug cost only.
(renal icon) Dosage adjustment may be required in renal impairment; see Appendix I.
ACEIs = angiotensin converting enzyme inhibitors; ARBs = angiotensin receptor blockers; ClCr = creatinine clearance; NSAIDs = nonsteroidal anti-inflammatory drugs
Legend: $ < $25 $$ $25–50

Table 8: First-line Maintenance Therapy for Bipolar Disorder

Class	Drug	Dose	Adverse Effects	Drug Interactions	Cost[a]
Antipsychotics, second-generation	*aripiprazole* Abilify	15 mg/day po Maximum 30 mg/day	Akathisia, dizziness, orthostatic hypotension, headache, GI complaints, tremor, sedation. Advise patients about antipsychotic-associated body temperature dysregulation and prevention of heat stroke (e.g., hydration, sun protection).	Carbamazepine (or other strong inducers of CYP2D6 or CYP3A4 such as phenytoin, rifampin) can decrease aripiprazole levels significantly. Ketoconazole, quinidine, fluoxetine or paroxetine (or other strong inhibitors of CYP2D6 or CYP3A4) can increase levels substantially.	$$$$$
	olanzapine Zyprexa, Zyprexa Zydis, generics	5–20 mg/day po	Weight gain, metabolic disturbances, anticholinergic side effects in elderly, akathisia. Monitor periodically for movement disorders. Advise patients about antipsychotic-associated body temperature dysregulation and prevention of heat stroke (e.g., hydration, sun protection).	Fluvoxamine and ciprofloxacin increase olanzapine levels.	$$$
	quetiapine Seroquel, Seroquel XR, generics	Usual: 300 mg/day po Maximum: 600 mg/day	Weight gain, sedation, orthostasis, metabolic disturbances. Advise patients about antipsychotic-associated body temperature dysregulation and prevention of heat stroke (e.g., hydration, sun protection).	Ketoconazole dramatically increases quetiapine levels. Monitor for hypotension with antihypertensives.	$
	risperidone long-acting injection Risperdal Consta	25 mg im Q2 wk, by deep gluteal im injection Maximum: 50 mg Q2 wk	Weight gain, orthostasis, dose-related EPS, metabolic disturbances. Advise patients about antipsychotic-associated body temperature dysregulation and prevention of heat stroke (e.g., hydration, sun protection).	Avoid combining with carbamazepine.	$345
	ziprasidone Zeldox	20–80 mg BID po with food (≥500 kcal)	Insomnia, EPS; consider ECG at baseline and periodically to monitor effect on QT_c interval. Advise patients about antipsychotic-associated body temperature dysregulation and prevention of heat stroke (e.g., hydration, sun protection).	Carbamazepine decreases levels significantly; do not use with other drugs that prolong the QT_c interval.	$$$$$

(cont'd)

Table 8: First-line Maintenance Therapy for Bipolar Disorder *(cont'd)*

Class	Drug	Dose	Adverse Effects	Drug Interactions	Cost[a]
Mood Stabilizers	*divalproex sodium* Epival, generics	750–2000 mg/day po, adjusted according to serum levels (target range 350–690 µmol/L)	Weight gain, thrombocytopenia, polycystic ovary syndrome, teratogenic; rarely: hyperammonemia, hepatotoxicity.	Avoid combining with carbamazepine. Use caution if combining with lamotrigine.	$
	lamotrigine Lamictal, generics	100–300 mg/day po	Rash common; severe rash rare.	Divalproex doubles blood level of lamotrigine; always initiate dosing slowly.	$
	lithium carbonate immediate-release (renal symbol) Carbolith, Lithane, generics	600–1800 mg/day po, adjusted according to serum levels (target range 0.6–1 mmol/L, 0.5–0.8 mmol/L in elderly patients) Measure serum concentration 9–13 hours post-dose	Highly toxic in overdose. Measure electrolytes and do 24-h urine for ClCr when starting long-term treatment. Monitor thyroid and renal function at least every 6 months.	Toxic levels may result when adding NSAIDs, ACEIs, ARBs and especially thiazide diuretics. Reduce lithium dose and check serum level if long-term treatment with these agents is required. Avoid large changes in salt or coffee intake. Stop lithium temporarily during acute intermittent illnesses causing fluid and electrolyte losses.	$
	lithium carbonate controlled-release (renal symbol) Lithmax	600–1800 mg/day po, adjusted according to serum levels (target range 0.6–1 mmol/L, 0.5–0.8 mmol/L in elderly patients) Measure serum concentration 9–13 hours post-dose	See lithium carbonate immediate-release.	See lithium carbonate immediate-release.	$$
	lithium citrate syrup (renal symbol) generic (8 mmol/5 mL; approximately equivalent to 300 mg lithium carbonate/5 mL)	600–1800 mg/day po, adjusted according to serum levels (target range 0.6–1 mmol/L, 0.5–0.8 mmol/L in elderly patients) Measure serum concentration 9–13 hours post-dose	See lithium carbonate immediate-release.	See lithium carbonate immediate-release.	$$
	valproic acid Depakene, Apo-Valproic Capsules, other generics	750–2000 mg/day po, adjusted according to serum levels (target range 350–690 µmol/L)	See divalproex.	See divalproex.	$

[a] Cost of 30-day supply for mean dose unless otherwise specified; includes drug cost only.

(renal symbol) Dosage adjustment may be required in renal impairment; see Appendix I.

ACEIs = angiotensin converting enzyme inhibitors; ARBs = angiotensin receptor blockers; ClCr = creatinine clearance; EPS = extrapyramidal symptoms; NSAIDs = nonsteroidal anti-inflammatory drugs

Legend: $ < $30 $$ $30–60 $$$ $60–90 $$$$ $90–120 $$$$$ $120–150

Suggested Readings

Bauer MS, McBride L. *Structured group psychotherapy for bipolar disorder: the life goals program.* 2nd ed. New York (NY): Springer; 2003.

Sharma V. Considerations in the pharmacotherapy of bipolar disorder during and after pregnancy. *Curr Drug Saf* 2011;6(5):318-23.

Yatham LN, Kennedy SH, O'Donovan C et al. Canadian Network for Mood and Anxiety Treatments (CANMAT) guidelines for the management of patients with bipolar disorder: consensus and controversies. *Bipolar Disord* 2005;7(Suppl 3):5-69.

Yatham LN, Kennedy SH, O'Donovan C et al. Canadian Network for Mood and Anxiety Treatments (CANMAT) guidelines for the management of patients with bipolar disorder: update 2007. *Bipolar Disord* 2006;8(6):721-39.

Yatham LN, Kennedy SH, Schaffer A et al. Canadian Network for Mood and Anxiety Treatments (CANMAT) and International Society for Bipolar Disorders (ISBD) collaborative update of CANMAT guidelines for the management of patients with bipolar disorder: update 2009. *Bipolar Disord* 2009;11(3):225-55.

Yatham LN, Kennedy SH, Parikh SV et al. Canadian Network for Mood and Anxiety Treatments (CANMAT) and International Society for Bipolar Disorders (ISBD) collaborative update of CANMAT guidelines for the management of patients with bipolar disorder: update 2013. *Bipolar Disord* 2013;15(1):1-44.

References

1. Yatham LN, Kennedy SH, O'Donovan C et al. Canadian Network for Mood and Anxiety Treatments (CANMAT) guidelines for the management of patients with bipolar disorder: consensus and controversies. *Bipolar Disord* 2005;7(Suppl 3):5-69.
2. American Psychiatric Association. *Diagnostic and statistical manual of mental disorders: DSM-5.* 5th ed. Washington (DC): American Psychiatric Publishing; 2013.
3. Berk M, Dodd S, Berk L. The management of bipolar disorder in primary care: a review of existing and emerging therapies. *Psychiatry Clin Neurosci* 2005;59(3):229-39.
4. Hirschfeld RM, Williams JB, Spitzer RL et al. Development and validation of a screening instrument for bipolar spectrum disorder: the Mood Disorder Questionnaire. *Am J Psychiatry* 2000;157(11):1873-5.
5. Wagner KD, Hirschfeld RM, Emslie GJ et al. Validation of the Mood Disorder Questionnaire for bipolar disorders in adolescents. *J Clin Psychiatry* 2006;67(5):827-30.
6. Yatham LN, Kennedy SH, O'Donovan C et al. Canadian Network for Mood and Anxiety Treatments (CANMAT) guidelines for the management of patients with bipolar disorder: update 2007. *Bipolar Disord* 2006;8(6):721-39.
7. Yatham LN, Kennedy SH, Schaffer A et al. Canadian Network for Mood and Anxiety Treatments (CANMAT) and International Society for Bipolar Disorders (ISBD) collaborative update of CANMAT guidelines for the management of patients with bipolar disorder: update 2009. *Bipolar Disord* 2009;11(3):225-55.
8. Yatham LN, Kennedy SH, Parikh SV et al. Canadian Network for Mood and Anxiety Treatments (CANMAT) and International Society for Bipolar Disorders (ISBD) collaborative update of CANMAT guidelines for the management of patients with bipolar disorder: update 2013. *Bipolar Disord* 2013;15(1):1-44.
9. Parikh SV, Zaretsky A, Beaulieu S et al. A randomized controlled trial of psychoeducation or cognitive behavioural therapy in bipolar disorder: A Canadian network for mood and anxiety treatments (CANMAT) study. *J Clin Psychiatry* 2012;73(6)803-10.
10. Colom F, Vieta E, Sanchez-Moreno R et al. Group psychoeducation for stabilized bipolar disorders: 5-year outcome of a randomized clinical trial. *Br J Psychiatry* 2009;194:260-5.
11. Miklowitz DJ, Otto MW, Frank E et al. Psychosocial treatments for bipolar depression: a 1-year randomized trial from the Systematic Treatment Enhancement Program. *Arch Gen Psychiatry* 2007;64(4):419-26.
12. Schapiro NA. Bipolar disorders in children and adolescents. *J Pediatr Health Care* 2005;19(3):131-41.
13. Kowatch RA, Youngstrom EA, Danielyan A et al. Review and meta-analysis of the phenomenology and clinical characteristics of mania in children and adolescents. *Bipolar Disord* 2005;7(6):483-96.
14. Kowatch RA, DelBello MP. Pediatric bipolar disorder: emerging diagnostic and treatment approaches. *Child Adolesc Psychiatr Clin N Am* 2006;15(1):73-108.
15. Al Jurdi R, Pulakhandam S, Kunik ME et al. Late-life mania: assessment and treatment of late-life manic symptoms. *Geriatrics* 2005;60(10):18-20,22-3.
16. Aziz R, Lorberg B, Tampi RR. Treatments for late-life bipolar disorder. *Am J Geriatr Pharmacother* 2006:4(4):347-64.
17. Yonkers KA, Wisner KL, Stowe Z et al. Management of bipolar disorder during pregnancy and the postpartum period. *Am J Psychiatry* 2004;161(4):608-20.
18. Gentile S. Prophylactic treatment of bipolar disorder in pregnancy and breastfeeding: focus on emerging mood stabilizers. *Bipolar Disord* 2006;8(3):207-20.
19. Vismari L, Pires MLN, Benedito-Silva AA et al. Bioavailability of immediate and controlled release formulations of lithium carbonate. *Rev Bras Psiquitr* 2002;24(2):74-9.
20. Bezchlibnyk-Butler KZ, Jeffries JJ, editors. *Clinical handbook of psychotropic drugs*. 15th ed. [Seattle]: Hogrefe & Huber Publishers; 2005.

Chapter 5
Dementia

Kenneth Rockwood, MD, FRCPC and
Mark Bosma, MD, FRCPC

Dementia is a syndrome of acquired global impairment of cognitive function sufficient to interfere with normal activities. The most common causes are Alzheimer's disease, vascular dementia, a mixture of the two, Lewy body dementia and frontotemporal dementia. Dementia is also recognized as a complication of Parkinson's disease. Dementias are almost always progressive, deteriorating illnesses in which treatment options are different at various stages of the illness (see Table 1).

Table 1: **Stages of Dementia**

Stage	Characteristics	Corresponding FAST Rating[a]
Preclinical	Subjective complaints accompanied by very mild objective cognitive decline; functioning is unimpaired. This stage has considerable overlap with normal aging and may or may not progress to dementia.	3
Mild	Impaired instrumental activities of daily living (IADL), e.g., driving, medication use, finances, use of telephone and housekeeping	4
Moderate	In addition to IADL impairment, personal activities of daily living (PADL) such as bathing, feeding, dressing and toileting can be done only with prompting	5
Severe	PADL cannot be done even with prompting	6
Terminal	Patients must be fed and become immobile and mute	7

[a] Included because many jurisdictions use the Functional Assessment Staging Tool (FAST)[1] in adjudicating reimbursement for dementia medications.

Goals of Therapy

- Alter the natural disease progression to meet patients' and caregivers' goals
- Treat cognitive, behavioural and psychological symptoms
- Alleviate caregiver burden
- Minimize medication side effects

Investigations

Dementia

- Careful history with attention to memory impairment and potentially reversible causes, especially medications. Cognitive impairment can be assessed using the Montreal Cognitive Assessment (MoCA)[2], or Mini-Mental State Examination (MMSE);[3] functional disability is measured with tools such as the Disability Assessment for Dementia[4] or the Functional Assessment Staging Tool (FAST)[1]
- Medication history to rule out drug-induced cognitive impairment, e.g., anticholinergics
- Physical examination to identify the cause, which is rarely reversible[5]
- Laboratory tests: CBC, electrolytes, kidney function, TSH, calcium, blood glucose.

- Neuroimaging (usually CT head scan) if:
  - age <60 years
  - new onset
  - rapid progression
  - post-head injury
  - focal or lateralizing signs
  - history of cancer
  - use of anticoagulants
  - early urinary incontinence and gait disorder
  - unusual cognitive symptoms

Responsive Behaviours in Dementia

A strategy for evaluating and managing behavioural problems in the older adult is illustrated in Figure 1.

Responsive Behaviours in Dementia (RBD) are seen in 3 contexts:

- Part of the *neurocognitive* disorder. These problems usually occur predictably, according to the stage of dementia. In Alzheimer's disease, for example, depression and apathy often occur early, when the dementia is mild. In contrast, psychosis and agitated behaviour tend to occur in the moderate to later stages. If agitation is seen early, more aggressive medical investigation is warranted.
- Related to *psychiatric* problems that predate the dementia, such as depression, anxiety, psychosis and personality issues. Elicit a careful psychiatric history; psychiatric syndromes that occurred earlier in the patient's life may recur (often in slightly different guises, reflecting cognitive impairment) and can guide treatment.

Figure 1: **Evaluation and Management of the Older Adult with Behavioural Problems**

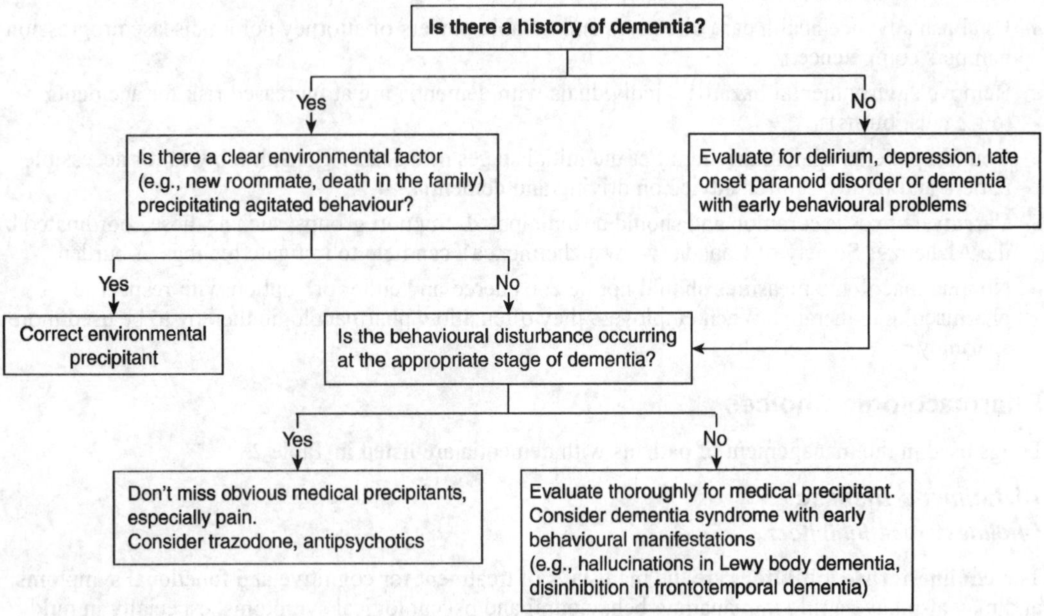

- A *delirium-like* presentation, typically associated with a medical and/or environmental precipitant.[6] (See Figure 1.) The diagnostic approach in the setting of delirium includes:
  - history of concomitant symptoms, environmental precipitants or medication changes
  - examination for focal or lateralizing signs or meningismus; both sets of signs will usually be absent. Evaluate toxic or metabolic causes, as well as signs of infection or heart failure
  - laboratory tests: CBC, electrolytes, urea, creatinine, glucose, urinalysis, chest radiograph

Note: It is unusual for delusions or hallucinations to occur in early dementia. When this happens, it can indicate that the person is suffering from Lewy body dementia, in which case avoid antipsychotics as they can precipitate an antipsychotic sensitivity syndrome. Fluctuation in the level of consciousness, a hallmark of delirium, can also be seen in patients with Lewy body dementia. Increasingly, delirium that either persists or only partly resolves is being recognized.[7] For this reason, there can be significant difficulty in distinguishing delirium from dementia, particularly Lewy body dementia. Therefore, care must be taken to avoid antipsychotics in such patients, in whom a careful trial of a cholinesterase inhibitor is likely warranted.

Therapeutic Choices

Nonpharmacologic Choices

- Nonpharmacologic approaches are first-line therapy for behavioural symptoms of dementia, especially agitation; they are often sufficient to make a noticeable improvement in the target symptoms. Strategies include:
  - clear and respectful communication
  - changes to the physical environment such as ensuring safe places to wander
  - caregiver strategies such as distraction, avoiding confrontation and providing stimulation and structure
  - a multidisciplinary approach with involvement of services such as psychology and recreation therapy to decrease agitation with the use of activity programs and other behavioural interventions
- Involve family and other caregivers in all nonpharmacologic therapy.
- Establish advance health care directives and durable powers of attorney before disease progression hampers competence.
- Remove environmental hazards—individuals with dementia are at increased risk for accidents (e.g., falls, burns).
- Counsel patients against driving after the initial stages of disease. Consult nibw.ca for accessible patient and family-centred advice on driving and dementia.
- Caregiver stress is common and should be anticipated. Support groups, such as those coordinated by the Alzheimer Society of Canada (www.alzheimer.ca), can help to mitigate feelings of burden.
- Nonpharmacologic measures should not be considered an "either/or" option with respect to pharmacologic therapy. When employed, they often allow pharmacologic therapy to be used more sparingly.[8]

Pharmacologic Choices

Drugs used in the management of patients with dementia are listed in Table 2.

Alzheimer's Disease

Cholinesterase Inhibitors

The **cholinesterase inhibitors** are the mainstays of treatment for cognitive and functional symptoms, and may also have a role in managing behavioural and psychological symptoms, especially in mild to moderate dementia. Donepezil, rivastigmine and galantamine have distinct structures and modes of action. However, in the absence of blinded, controlled, head-to-head trials, all 3 agents seem to be of equal efficacy. While clinically detectable, benefits are small to moderate on average,[9] and in many patients can consist mainly of disease stabilization. Treatment response and side effects can vary among individuals; patients who do not respond to one cholinesterase inhibitor might respond to another. In untreated patients with mild to moderate dementia, a decline of 2–4 points per year on the MMSE scale is expected; therefore, an annual decline of less than 2 points while on drug therapy indicates a beneficial effect. For each of the drugs, higher doses have better outcomes. The usual treatment response is that some symptoms improve, others stabilize and still others worsen. Reduction in repetitive questioning is a common treatment goal in patients with mild to moderate Alzheimer's disease and usually corresponds to a generally positive treatment effect.[10]

Define and monitor target symptoms. Effectiveness is considered to be either improvement or no change in target symptoms. A strategy of setting individual goals for treatment and measuring their attainment at regular intervals has been shown to detect a range of beneficial treatment effects.[10,11] Follow-up to detect side effects is advised. Monitor treatment effects 2 weeks after initiating therapy or increasing dosage, then every 3 months.

Very few trials have addressed clinical meaningfulness explicitly, so inferences for practice are needed.[12] Most trials were double-blinded for only 3–6 months, except for two 12-month trials[13,14] and one 24-month[15] trial of **donepezil**. Donepezil was effective in 3- to 6-month trials in patients with *mild to moderate* Alzheimer's disease (MMSE scores 10 to 26).[16] It was also effective in *moderate to severe* Alzheimer's disease (MMSE 0 to 17),[16,17] and is the only cholinesterase inhibitor approved for all disease severities. Donepezil and memantine were evaluated over 52 weeks in an independent trial (not sponsored by a manufacturer) involving 295 community-dwelling patients with moderate or severe Alzheimer's disease who had already received donepezil for at least 3 months.[18] Patients were randomized to continue or discontinue donepezil, discontinue donepezil and start memantine, or continue donepezil and add memantine. Patients who continued taking donepezil showed beneficial effects on both cognition and function. The effect was also seen with memantine alone, but was not greater than with continuing donepezil. The combination of donepezil and memantine provided no significant improvement over donepezil alone. The initial daily dose (5 mg) of donepezil is usually taken at night, but can be taken in the morning if sleep disturbances occur. After 4 weeks try increasing to the target dose of 10 mg/day. There is some evidence for a higher dose (23 mg/day) but the formulation is not available in Canada.[19]

Experience in pure vascular dementia (e.g., post stroke) suggested that a 5 mg dose might offer benefit over 10 mg,[20] but a large trial showed no significant benefit of either dose on both the pre-specified primary outcomes.[21]

Rivastigmine is initiated at 1.5 mg BID and increased to the minimum effective dose of 3 mg BID after 30 days.[22] The maximum dose is 6 mg BID po, although a consistent dose-response relationship has not been demonstrated. For some patients, TID dosing is most effective, with the same maximum total daily dose of 12 mg.[23] Rivastigmine was effective in a double-blind trial in patients with Lewy body dementia,[24] and for patients with dementia associated with Parkinson's disease.[25] A trial of rivastigmine delivered by transcutaneous patch showed evidence of modest benefit compared with placebo, and fewer side effects compared with the oral formulation.[26]

Galantamine has been shown to be effective in several studies,[11,27] including one in patients with mixed Alzheimer's disease and vascular dementia.[28] A Canadian multicentre trial suggested that patients treated with galantamine were more likely to meet clinical treatment goals than those on placebo.[11] Galantamine is available as an extended-release formulation administered once daily.

The cardiac safety of cholinesterase inhibitors has been reviewed in several reports. Although one registry report indicated an increased need for cardiac pacing, a second cohort study suggested that the risk of cardiac events overall is not increased in patients receiving cholinesterase inhibitors, and may even be lower than in patients with dementia who are not receiving the drugs.[29,30] Another registry study suggested that all cholinesterase inhibitors have comparable cardiac safety profiles.[31]

N-methyl-D-aspartate (NMDA) Receptor Antagonists

The proposed mechanism of action of the NMDA receptor antagonist **memantine** is to block glutamate-induced neuronal excitotoxicity, a process that is implicated as a final common pathway in neuronal death. Meta-analyses suggest memantine has a small to moderately beneficial effect on cognition, activities of daily living (ADL) and behaviour in moderate to severe Alzheimer's disease at 6 months.[32,33] The Cochrane review is more guarded.[34] A trial of **memantine with donepezil** suggested the combination added benefit in patients with moderate to severe Alzheimer's disease.[35] The generalizability of this remains unclear, and whether combination therapy has any role in mild disease is not yet known. A more recent study showed no benefit of the combination in patients with moderate to severe Alzheimer's who were already taking donepezil.[18]

If using memantine to elicit a greater response than already achieved with cholinesterase inhibitors, or when cholinesterase inhibitors are contraindicated or poorly tolerated (e.g., GI side effects), the best standard for individualized clinical decision making is to identify target symptoms and monitor carefully. Reduce the dose in patients with mild to moderate renal failure. Dosage reductions may also be necessary in other conditions (e.g., renal tubular acidosis, some urinary tract infections) or concomitant drug therapy (e.g., carbonic anhydrase inhibitors).

Historically, the cost-effectiveness of cholinesterase inhibitors and of memantine has been disparaged. However, this has become more favourable with the introduction of generic alternatives and lower costs plus improved efficacy data.[36]

Other Therapies

Despite many trials, clinically significant beneficial effects of **ergoloid mesylates** in Alzheimer's disease have not been demonstrated.

High-dose **vitamin E** (2000 IU alpha-tocopherol per day), initially appeared to slow the progression of dementia.[37] In light of more recent data suggesting additional adverse effects or no benefit in a range of conditions, use of high-dose vitamin E is not recommended and any supplementation might be questionable.[38]

In the largest study of disease progression to date, **selegiline** proved more effective than placebo, but no more effective than vitamin E alone in delaying death, institutionalization and progression to severe dementia.[37]

Whether extracts of **ginkgo biloba** are beneficial in patients with cognitive impairment and dementia has been the subject of much study. A Cochrane review concluded that while there appears to be little risk of harm, with similar adverse effects in treatment and placebo groups, there was no consistent evidence of beneficial effects on cognition.[39]

Vascular Dementia

With the aim of slowing disease progression, vascular risk factors should be modified, particularly to ensure good control of hypertension (<140/80 mm Hg), and it seems reasonable to use lipid-lowering agents for dyslipidemias (see Chapter 37 and Chapter 39).

Dementia with Lewy Bodies and the Dementia of Parkinson's Disease

Patients with dementia with Lewy bodies often present with hallucinations and early parkinsonism, which can precede cognitive impairment. This psychosis can be worsened by antipsychotics.[40] Patients with dementia with Lewy bodies have severe antipsychotic sensitivity reactions that can precipitate irreversible parkinsonism, further impair consciousness and induce autonomic disturbances. These reactions occur in 40–50% of patients and increase mortality.

Clinical trial data for the use of **rivastigmine**[24] demonstrate that small doses can sometimes be dramatically effective, and leave the potential for subsequent dose titration over time. Prescribing considerations are similar to those for Alzheimer's disease. Similarly, a placebo-controlled trial in the treatment of patients with Parkinson's disease who had been diagnosed with dementia found statistically significant improvement in cognition, function and behaviour in rivastigmine-treated patients.[25] The size of the treatment effect appears to be comparable with that reported for cholinesterase inhibitors in Alzheimer's disease.

Prevention of Dementia

Cardiovascular risk factors increase the chance of all causes of late-life dementia, including Alzheimer's disease. Evidence from the Syst-Eur trial suggests that the incidence of dementia can be halved in elderly patients treated for systolic hypertension.[41] Further, a meta-analysis that included data from the Hypertension in the Very Elderly Trial (indapamide ± perindopril vs. placebo) demonstrated a role for **antihypertensive treatment** in dementia prevention.[42]

Despite the failure of some trials, there is some evidence to show that long-term use of **NSAIDs** might be protective for Alzheimer's disease,[43] although their routine use is not recommended due to their associated adverse effects. One report suggested NSAIDs may even increase the risk of dementia.[44]

Evidence does not support the use of **statins** solely for prevention of dementia.[45] Prior enthusiasm for the use of **estrogen**, based on observational studies, has not been sustained by experimental evidence which on balance suggests net harm.

Physical exercise (30 minutes of exercise more vigorous than a brisk walk, at least 3 times per week) appears to be the minimum required to confer consistent benefit.[46]

Responsive Behaviours in Dementia (RBD)

Nonpharmacologic Approaches

Nonpharmacologic interventions are the preferred method of treatment of RBD, due to the lower risk of adverse effects. Interventions with varying levels of evidence include music therapy, Snoezelen sessions (controlled multisensory stimulation therapy), aromatherapy, bright light therapy, exposure to white noise, massage and touch interventions, and involvement in structured recreational activities.[47]

Antidepressants

Many patients in the early stages of dementia experience depression. Occasionally, depression can manifest with prominent cognitive impairment. Previously known as pseudodementia, it is also referred to as dementia of depression. A significant proportion of these patients will progress to dementia.

Most experienced psychiatrists agree that antidepressants are effective in the treatment of depression in patients with dementia.[48] Current evidence for treatment of depression in dementia using antidepressant medication is inconclusive. A recent placebo-controlled RCT comparing mirtazapine, sertraline and placebo for treatment of depression in dementia failed to show efficacy for treatment with antidepressants.[49] Several recent reviews, including 2 meta-analyses, examined randomized placebo-controlled trials of antidepressants for depression in Alzheimer's disease. Although individual studies showed significant benefit, overall there was a lack of evidence of efficacy.[50,51,52,53] However, there are few controlled studies specifically focused on the antidepressant treatment of these patients.

When choosing an antidepressant, it is important to take several factors into account. SSRIs are less likely than tricyclic antidepressants (TCAs) to cause anticholinergic side effects or to worsen orthostatic hypotension, which are common and problematic in this population. An increased risk of hyponatremia/SIADH, possibly potentiated by concurrent thiazide use, has been reported in elderly patients taking SSRIs.[54,55] Monitoring of electrolytes is recommended in this setting, because of the effect of hyponatremia on cognitive function. If using a TCA (because of lack of response or sensitivity to an SSRI) choose **desipramine** or **nortriptyline**, because of their lower propensity to cause anticholinergic effects. Older adults and those with dementia often require longer exposure to antidepressants; trials can be 2–3 months (see Chapter 6 for dosing information). Although trials should be longer, there are often early indications that the antidepressant is working—there may be improvement in vegetative symptoms such as sleep, appetite and energy before improvement of mood.

Limited evidence suggests that antidepressants improve nondepression-related RBD in dementia,[56] although antidepressants are commonly used for anxiety (including compulsive behaviour), aggression and sexually inappropriate behaviour. A Cochrane review reported that **sertraline** and **citalopram** reduced symptoms of agitation when compared with placebo in two studies.[57] An RCT found that citalopram was as effective as risperidone in treating either agitation or psychotic symptoms in patients with dementia, but further studies are required to confirm this finding.[58]

Antipsychotics

For RBD associated with dementia, especially if psychotic symptoms are evident, the second-generation antipsychotics are considered first-line. Because the elderly demented brain is exquisitely sensitive to antipsychotics, initial doses should be small. **Risperidone** can be started at a daily dose of 0.25 mg, with 1 mg being the optimal dose and 2 mg/day the upper limit.[59,60] **Olanzapine**, started at 2.5 mg and increased to 5–10 mg/day, was effective in a placebo-controlled trial in nursing home patients with Alzheimer's disease.[61] A Cochrane review suggests risperidone and olanzapine are useful in reducing aggression in patients with dementia.[62]

There is less evidence to support the use of **quetiapine**, but an RCT showed that a dose of 200 mg/day was effective for treating agitation associated with dementia.[63] Evidence to support the use of **aripiprazole** is limited, but a few studies showed improvement in aggression and psychosis.[64] To date there have been no published RCTs of **clozapine** in the treatment of RBD of dementia.[56] Individual considerations sometimes dictate the use of these medications, especially if risperidone or olanzapine have proved to be ineffective or have resulted in side effects. A Cochrane review of **haloperidol** for agitation in dementia recommended against its routine use.[65] Periodic reassessment of RBD is essential; even in the absence of therapy, the natural history is gradual diminution of these problems.

Extrapyramidal side effects (EPS) are more commonly seen with the first-generation antipsychotics but can occur with the second-generation agents (especially with doses over 2 mg/day of risperidone). Tardive dyskinesia (TD), a potentially irreversible movement disorder, is also more common with first-generation antipsychotics. In patients over 60 years of age, TD occurs in 29% of patients after 1 year and in up to 63% after 3 years of use.[66] A shorter study found an incidence of TD of 2.6% with risperidone after 9 months.[67] For patients with baseline movement disorders or those who develop EPS with other second-generation antipsychotics, **quetiapine** may be the best option.

The risk of serious adverse events with all antipsychotics is significant. An increased risk of stroke and death has been demonstrated with second-generation antipsychotics compared to placebo, and observational comparisons suggest the risk may be higher with first-generation antipsychotics.[56,68,69] In 2005, Health Canada issued an advisory stating that the use of second-generation antipsychotics in elderly patients with dementia was associated with a 1.6 times greater mortality rate compared with placebo.[70] The Clinical Antipsychotic Trials of Intervention Effectiveness (CATIE) study in Alzheimer's Disease[71] showed that the chance of benefiting from a second-generation antipsychotic (risperidone, olanzapine, quetiapine) was equal to the risk of experiencing an adverse effect such as EPS, parkinsonism, sedation or confusion/mental status changes. A dilemma presented by the data is that psychotic symptoms will improve with antipsychotic therapy in some patients with dementia, but which patients will respond cannot be determined in advance. A trial of second-generation antipsychotic therapy is warranted in patients with severe symptoms, particularly when psychosis is present or there is a risk of harm to self or others, or when nonpharmacologic measures are ineffective in patients with significant distress.

Cholinesterase Inhibitors and Memantine

As mentioned earlier, cholinesterase inhibitors are the mainstay of treatment for cognitive and functional symptoms of dementia. They are now commonly used for the treatment of RBD, with less risk of serious adverse events compared to antipsychotics. Multiple RCTs have shown statistically significant improvement in RBD with cholinesterase inhibitors. However, the overall effect on these behaviours appears to be small, suggesting questionable clinical significance.[56,72,73] Evidence for the use of memantine is similar, with statistically significant improvement that may be undetectable by clinicians.[72,73]

Trazodone for Behavioural and Sleep Disturbances

Trazodone, a serotonergic antidepressant, is often used successfully to manage agitated behaviour, with some RCT evidence to support its use.[74] Trazodone is also used to treat disrupted sleep/wake cycles and "sun downing" (worsening of behaviour as darkness falls). In a systematic review of various medications used to treat sleep disturbances associated with AD, one small study with 30 participants demonstrated that low-dose trazodone was beneficial, no benefit was seen with melatonin and ramelteon (not available in Canada) and evidence was lacking for many other widely prescribed drugs.[75] Trazodone 50 mg QHS administered for 2 weeks increased daily sleeping time by 43 minutes with no serious adverse effects.[76]

Benzodiazepines

Data on the efficacy of benzodiazepines for RBD in dementia are conflicting. Although their use can result in oversedation, falls and worsening cognition, benzodiazepines are sometimes indicated for severe agitation, especially when other agents fail. Low doses of a short-acting agent without active metabolites (e.g., **lorazepam** 0.5–1 mg, **oxazepam** 5–10 mg, **temazepam** 15 mg) may be tried. In an acute situation, to manage severely agitated patients, **lorazepam** 0.5–1 mg can be mixed in the same syringe with **haloperidol** (0.5, 1 or 1.5 mg) and given im every 8 hours for a maximum of 3 days. A double-blind, randomized, controlled comparison of im lorazepam and im olanzapine found them to be equally effective.[77]

Others

Beta-blockers (particularly **pindolol**), **carbamazepine**, **divalproex**, **lithium** and **buspirone** have been used successfully in case reports, but more robust evidence is lacking. These agents seem to work best when the problem behaviour mimics the psychiatric syndrome for which the drug is efficacious (e.g., lithium for cycling and manic features).

Therapeutic Tips

- Tips for *monitoring treatment effects* on target symptoms:
  - in certain provinces, reimbursement of drug costs by the provincial drug plan is predicated on monitoring degrees of improvement/worsening of target symptoms. Symptoms should be described precisely, e.g., instead of "impaired function," state "cannot carry on a conversation; will call only 1 or 2 well-known numbers; cannot remember how often he has called." For many symptoms, it is important to quantify how often they occur, e.g., asks the same question up to 20 times per day
  - the most common target symptoms include repetitive questioning, decreased initiative (especially for social and leisure activities and for instrumental activities of daily living), irritability, impaired recent memory and disorientation. A web site with the most common symptoms of dementia is available (www.dementiaguide.com). Subscribers to the site can use a symptom tracking option to aid in communicating with their physicians about the effects of treatment

- Tips for using **antidepressants** in dementia include:
  - start at low doses
  - monitor patient for side effects
  - increase dosage until the recommended range is reached
  - continue to increase the dose as side effects permit until the patient benefits or the maximum dose has been reached; effective doses will be similar to those used to treat younger adults
  - maintain therapy for 4–6 weeks after the first indication of symptomatic improvement (e.g., improved mood, appetite, sleep or energy) *before* evaluating the success of treatment; symptoms like sleep, appetite and energy may improve earlier in treatment but it may take 6–8 weeks for improvement in psychological symptoms such as depressed mood or anhedonia
- Tips for using **antipsychotics** in dementia include:
  - reserve for patients with severe behavioural symptoms, particularly with psychosis or risk of harm to self or others, or if nonpharmacologic measures are ineffective. Use a second-generation agent first, with caregiver support and consent
  - start low, go slow; keep the dose as low as possible
  - treat to a designated endpoint, usually an improvement in symptoms rather than their complete resolution
  - evaluate therapy at 1, 3 and 6 months, then every 6 months. Symptoms may subside naturally and the antipsychotic can then be tapered
  - antipsychotic-induced akathisia (increased motor restlessness) may be misinterpreted as lack of drug effect. This can initiate a cycle of increased antipsychotic use and worsening akathisia; the escalating dose of antipsychotic can then result in extrapyramidal rigidity to the point of immobility. Beware the elderly patient with dementia who requires large or increasing doses of antipsychotics, especially if the patient seems even worse after their administration
  - beware of antipsychotic sensitivity, manifested as rigidity, autonomic dysregulation, cognitive deterioration (including delirium, and even coma). This can be a hallmark of Lewy body dementia, and antipsychotics are best avoided in these patients

Table 2: **Drugs Used for the Treatment of Dementia**

Class	Drug	Dose	Adverse Effects	Drug Interactions	Cost[a]
Antipsychotics	*olanzapine* Zyprexa, Zyprexa Zydis, generics	Initial: 2.5 mg/day po Usual: 5–10 mg/day po	Extrapyramidal symptoms, sedation, constipation, GI upset, weight gain, metabolic dysregulation (type 2 diabetes); Increased risk of stroke and death.	Toxicity may be increased by inhibitors of CYP1A2 such as ciprofloxacin, fluvoxamine, ketoconazole. Effectiveness may be decreased by inducers of CYP1A2 such as carbamazepine, cigarette smoking, phenobarbital, primidone, rifampin.	$$
	quetiapine Seroquel, generics	Initial: 12.5 mg/day po Usual: 25–50 mg/day po Maximum: 200 mg/day po	See olanzapine.	Toxicity may be increased by inhibitors of CYP3A4 such as clarithromycin, erythromycin, grapefruit juice, ketoconazole. Effectiveness may be decreased by inducers of CYP3A4 such as carbamazepine, phenytoin, rifampin.	$
	risperidone ❥ Risperdal preparations, generics	Initial: 0.25 mg/day po Usual: 1 mg/day po Maximum: 2 mg/day po	See olanzapine.	Toxicity may be increased by inhibitors of CYP2D6 or CYP3A4 such as erythromycin, grapefruit juice, paroxetine, prednisone. Effectiveness may be decreased by inducers of CYP2D6 or CYP3A4 such as carbamazepine, phenytoin, rifampin.	$
Cholinesterase Inhibitors	*donepezil* Aricept, Aricept RDT, generics	Initial: 5 mg/day po Target: 10 mg/day po Adjust dose after 4 wk	*Cholinesterase inhibitors:* Theoretically, these agents may lower seizure threshold, increase the risk of GI ulceration or bleeding or exacerbate COPD or asthma. *Donepezil:* >10%: headache, nausea, diarrhea. <10%: vomiting, anorexia, fatigue, sleep disturbance, syncope, muscle cramps, urinary frequency. Uncommon: bradycardia, heart block.	*Cholinesterase inhibitors:* Theoretical concern regarding antagonistic effect of combined therapy with cholinesterase inhibitors and drugs with anticholinergic activity, or additive bradycardic effects when combined with beta-blockers or calcium channel blockers; few reports of actual interactions. *Donepezil:* Toxicity may be increased by inhibitors of CYP2D6 or CYP3A4 such as paroxetine, erythromycin, prednisone, grapefruit juice. Effectiveness may be reduced by inducers of CYP2D6 or CYP3A4 such as carbamazepine, phenytoin, rifampin.	$$

(cont'd)

Table 2: **Drugs Used for the Treatment of Dementia** *(cont'd)*

Class	Drug	Dose	Adverse Effects	Drug Interactions	Cost[a]
	galantamine extended-release Reminyl ER, generics	Initial: 8 mg daily po Target: 16–24 mg daily po Adjust dose at 4-wk intervals	See cholinesterase inhibitors. *Galantamine:* >10%: nausea, vomiting, diarrhea. <10%: bradycardia, syncope, dizziness, headache, sleep disturbance, fatigue, abdominal pain, weight loss, UTI, urinary incontinence, rhinitis. Rare: heart block, seizures, delirium.	See cholinesterase inhibitors. *Galantamine:* Toxicity may be increased by inhibitors of CYP2D6 or CYP3A4 such as paroxetine, erythromycin, prednisone, grapefruit juice. Effectiveness may be decreased by inducers of CYP2D6 or CYP3A4 such as carbamazepine, phenytoin, rifampin.	$$
	rivastigmine oral Exelon, generics	Initial: 1.5 mg BID po Target: 6–12 mg/day po Adjust dose monthly; take with breakfast and dinner	See cholinesterase inhibitors. *Rivastigmine:* >10%: headache, dizziness, nausea/vomiting, diarrhea, abdominal pain, anorexia. <10%: fatigue, insomnia, syncope, dyspepsia, weight loss, UTI, rhinitis. Rare: heart block, delirium, seizures.	See cholinesterase inhibitors. *Rivastigmine:* None reported; not metabolized by cytochrome P450 system.	$$
	rivastigmine transdermal patch Exelon Patch	Initial: Apply 1 Exelon 5 transdermal patch daily; if well tolerated, increase to Exelon 10 patch after at least 4 weeks If switching from oral rivastigmine, use Exelon 5 for patients taking <3 mg BID po, and Exelon 10 for patients taking 3–6 mg BID po	See rivastigmine oral.	See rivastigmine oral.	$$$$$
N-methyl-D-aspartate Receptor Antagonists	*memantine* Ebixa, generics	Initial: 5 mg daily; po increase by 5 mg daily, at weekly intervals, to 10 mg BID starting at week 4	Generally well tolerated; dizziness (7%), headache (6%), confusion (6%), constipation (5%), nausea/vomiting (3%).	None reported; not affected by cytochrome P450 system. Theoretically, urinary alkalizers such as carbonic anhydrase inhibitors may decrease the clearance of memantine.	$$$$

Class	Drug	Dose	Adverse Effects	Drug Interactions	Cost[a]
Serotonergic Antidepressants	*trazodone* generics	Initial: 25–50 mg QHS po Usual: Insomnia: 50 mg QHS po Other responsive behaviours: 100–200 mg/day po in divided doses Maximum: 400 mg/day in divided doses	Drowsiness, orthostatic hypotension, nausea, vomiting, headache, dry mouth, priapism (rare).	Toxicity may be increased by inhibitors of CYP3A4 such as clarithromycin, erythromycin, grapefruit juice, ketoconazole). Effectiveness may be reduced by inducers of CYP3A4 such as carbamazepine, phenytoin, rifampin).	$

[a] Cost of 30-day supply of target or usual dose; includes drug cost only.

Dosage adjustment may be required in renal impairment; see Appendix I

Legend: $ < $30 $$ $30–60 $$$ $60–90 $$$$ $90–120 $$$$$ $120–150

Suggested Readings

Gauthier S, ed. *Clinical diagnosis and management of Alzheimer's disease.* 3rd ed. Boca Raton (FL): Taylor & Francis; 2006.

Gauthier S, Patterson C, Chertkow H et al. Recommendations of the 4th Canadian Consensus Conference on the Diagnosis and Treatment of Dementia (CCCDTD4). *Can Geriatr J* 2012;15(4):120-6.

Herrmann N, Lanctôt K, Hogan DB. Pharmacological recommendations for the symptomatic treatment of dementia: the Canadian Consensus Conference on the Diagnosis and Treatment of Dementia 2012. *Alzheimers Res Ther* 2013;5(Suppl 1):S5.

References

1. Reisberg B. Functional assessment staging (FAST). *Psychopharmacol Bull* 1988;24(4):653-9.
2. Nasreddine ZS, Phillips NA, Bedirian V et al. The Montreal Cognitive Assessment, MoCA: a brief screening tool for mild cognitive impairment. *J Am Geriatr Soc* 2005;53(4):695-9.
3. Folstein MF, Folstein SE, McHugh PR. "Mini-mental state". A practical method for grading the cognitive state of patients for the clinician. *J Psychiatr Res* 1975;12(3):189-98.
4. Gelinas I, Gauthier L, McIntyre M et al. Development of a functional measure for persons with Alzheimer's disease: the disability assessment for dementia. *Am J Occup Ther* 1999;53(5):471-81.
5. Clarfield AM. The decreasing prevalence of reversible dementias: an updated meta-analysis. *Arch Intern Med* 2003;163(18):2219-29.
6. Fick DM, Agostini JV, Inouye SK. Delirium superimposed on dementia: a systematic review. *J Am Geriatr Soc* 2002;50(10):1723-32.
7. Cole MG, Ciampi A, Belzile E et al. Persistent delirium in older hospital patients: a systematic review of frequency and prognosis. *Age Ageing* 2009;38(1):19-26.
8. Ballard C, Corbett A. Management of neuropsychiatric symptoms in people with dementia. *CNS Drugs* 2010;24(9):729-39.
9. Rockwood K. Size of the treatment effect on cognition of cholinesterase inhibition in Alzheimer's disease. *J Neurol Neurosurg Psychiatry* 2004;75(5):677-85.
10. Rockwood K, Fay S, Jarrett P et al. Effect of galantamine on verbal repetition in AD: a secondary analysis of the VISTA trial. *Neurology* 2007;68(14):1116-21.
11. Rockwood K, Fay S, Song X et al. Attainment of treatment goals by people with Alzheimer's disease receiving galantamine: a randomized controlled trial. *CMAJ* 2006;174(8):1099-105.
12. Molnar FJ, Man-Son-Hing M, Fergusson D. Systematic review of measures of clinical significance employed in randomized controlled trials of drugs for dementia. *J Am Geriatr Soc* 2009;57(3):536-46.
13. Mohs RC, Doody RS, Morris JC et al. A 1-year, placebo-controlled preservation of function survival study of donepezil in AD patients. *Neurology* 2001;57(3):481-8.
14. Winblad B, Engedal K, Soininen H et al. A 1-year, randomized, placebo-controlled study of donepezil in patients with mild to moderate AD. *Neurology* 2001;57(3):489-95.
15. Courtney C, Farrell, Gray R et al. Long-term donepezil treatment in 565 patients with Alzheimer's disease (AD2000): randomised double-blind trial. *Lancet* 2004;363(9427):2105-15.
16. Birks J, Harvey RJ. Donepezil for dementia due to Alzheimer's disease. *Cochrane Database Syst Rev* 2006;(1):CD001190.
17. Winblad B, Kilander L, Eriksson S et al. Donepezil in patients with severe Alzheimer's disease: double-blind, parallel-group, placebo-controlled study. *Lancet* 2006;367(9516):1057-65.
18. Howard R, McShane R, Lindesay J et al. Donepezil and memantine for moderate-to-severe Alzheimer's disease. *N Engl J Med* 2012;366(10):893-903.
19. Farlow MR, Salloway S, Tariot PN et al. Effectiveness and tolerability of high-dose (23 mg/d) versus standard-dose (10 mg/d) donepezil in moderate to severe Alzheimer's disease: a 24-week, randomized, double-blind study. *Clin Ther* 2010;32(7):1234-51.
20. Roman GC, Wilkinson DG, Doody RS et al. Donepezil in vascular dementia: combined analysis of two large-scale clinical trials. *Dement Geriatr Cogn Disord* 2005;20(6):338-44.
21. Roman GC, Salloway S, Black SE et al. Randomized, placebo-controlled, clinical trial of donepezil in vascular dementia: differential effects by hippocampal size. *Stroke* 2010;41(6):1213-21.
22. Birks J. Cholinesterase inhibitors for Alzheimer's disease. *Cochrane Database Syst Rev* 2006;(1):CD005593.
23. Feldman HH, Lane R; Study 304 Group. Rivastigmine: a placebo controlled trial of twice daily and three times daily regimens in patients with Alzheimer's disease. *J Neurol Neurosurg Psychiatry* 2007;78(10):1056-63.
24. McKeith I, Del Ser T, Spano P et al. Efficacy of rivastigmine in dementia with Lewy bodies: a randomised, double-blind, placebo-controlled international study. *Lancet* 2000;356(9247):2031-6.
25. Emre M, Aarsland D, Albanese A et al. Rivastigmine for dementia associated with Parkinson's disease. *N Engl J Med* 2004;351(24):2509-18.
26. Winblad B, Cummings J, Andreasen N et al. A six-month double-blind, randomized, placebo-controlled study of a transdermal patch in Alzheimer's disease—rivastigmine patch versus capsule. *Int J Geriatr Psychiatry* 2007;22(5):456-67.
27. Loy C, Schneider L. Galantamine for Alzheimer's disease and mild cognitive impairment. *Cochrane Database Syst Rev* 2006;(1):CD001747.
28. Erkinjuntti T, Kurz A, Gauthier S et al. Efficacy of galantamine in probable vascular dementia and Alzheimer's disease combined with cerebrovascular disease: a randomised trial. *Lancet* 2002;359(9314):1283-90.
29. Gill SS, Anderson GM, Fischer HD et al. Syncope and its consequences in patients with dementia receiving cholinesterase inhibitors: a population-based cohort study. *Arch Intern Med* 2009;169(9):867-73.
30. Nordström P, Religa D, Wimo A et al. The use of cholinesterase inhibitors and the risk of myocardial infarction and death: a nationwide cohort study in subjects with Alzheimer's disease. *Eur Heart J* 2013;34(33):2585-91.
31. Fosbøl EL, Peterson ED, Holm E et al. Comparative cardiovascular safety of dementia medications: a cross-national study. *J Am Geriatr Soc* 2012;60(12):2283-9.

32. Smith M, Wells J, Borrie M. Treatment effect size of memantine therapy in Alzheimer disease and vascular dementia. *Alzheimer Dis Assoc Disord* 2006;20(3):133-7.
33. Winblad B, Jones RW, Wirth Y et al. Memantine in moderate to severe Alzheimer's disease: a meta-analysis of randomised clinical trials. *Dement Geriatr Cogn Disord* 2007;24(1):20-7.
34. McShane R, Areosa Sastre A, Minakaran N. Memantine for dementia. *Cochrane Database Syst Rev* 2006;(2):CD003154.
35. Tariot PN, Farlow MR, Grossberg GT et al. Memantine treatment in patients with moderate to severe Alzheimer disease already receiving donepezil: a randomized controlled trial. *JAMA* 2004;291(3):317-24.
36. Hyde C, Peters J, Bond M et al. Evolution of the evidence on the effectiveness and cost-effectiveness of acetylcholinesterase inhibitors and memantine for Alzheimer's disease: systematic review and economic model. *Age Ageing* 2013;42(1):14-20.
37. Sano M, Ernesto C, Thomas RG et al. A controlled trial of selegiline, alpha-tocopherol, or both as treatment for Alzheimer's disease. The Alzheimer's Disease Cooperative Study. *N Engl J Med* 1997;336(17):1216-22.
38. Bjelakovic G , Nikolova D, Gluud LL et al. Mortality in randomized trials of antioxidant supplements for primary and secondary prevention: systematic review and meta-analysis. *JAMA* 2007;297(8):842-57.
39. Birks J, Grimley Evans J. Ginkgo biloba for cognitive impairment and dementia. *Cochrane Database Syst Rev* 2009;(1):CD003120.
40. McKeith IG , Galasko D, Kosaka K et al. Consensus guidelines for the clinical and pathologic diagnosis of dementia with Lewy bodies (DLB): report of the consortium on DLB international workshop. *Neurology* 1996;47(5):1113-24.
41. Forette F, Seux ML, Staessen JA et al. The prevention of dementia with antihypertensive treatment: new evidence from the Systolic Hypertension in Europe (Syst-Eur) study. *Arch Intern Med* 2002;162(18):2046-52.
42. Peters R, Beckett N, Forette F et al. Incident dementia and blood pressure lowering in the Hypertension in the Very Elderly Trial cognitive function assessment (HYVET-COG): a double-blind, placebo controlled trial. *Lancet Neurol* 2008;7(8):683-9.
43. Etminan M, Gill S, Samii A. Effect of non-steroidal anti-inflammatory drugs on risk of Alzheimer's disease: systematic review and meta-analysis of observational studies. *BMJ* 2003;327(7407):128.
44. Breitner JC, Haneuse SJ, Walker R et al. Risk of dementia and AD with prior exposure to NSAIDs in an elderly community-based cohort. *Neurology* 2009;72(22):1899-905.
45. McGuinness B, O'Hare J, Craig D et al. Statins for the treatment of dementia. *Cochrane Database Syst Rev* 2010;(8):CD007514.
46. Middleton LE, Yaffe K. Promising strategies for the prevention of dementia. *Arch Neurol* 2009;66(10):1210-5.
47. Conn D, Gibson M, Feldman S et al. *National guidelines for seniors' mental health: the assessment and treatment of mental health issues in long term care homes*. Toronto (ON): Canadian Coalition for Seniors' Mental Health; 2006.
48. Swartz M, Barak Y, Mirecki I et al. Treating depression in Alzheimer's disease: integration of differing guidelines. *Int Psychogeriatr* 2000;12(3):353-8.
49. Banerjee S, Hellier J, Dewey M et al. Sertraline or mirtazapine for depression in dementia (HTA-SADD): a randomized, multicentre, double-blind, placebo-controlled trial. *Lancet* 2011;378(9789):403-11.
50. Enache D, Winblad B, Aarsland D. Depression in dementia: epidemiology, mechanisms, and treatment. *Curr Opin Psychiatry* 2011;24(6):461-72.
51. Modrego PJ. Depression in Alzheimer's disease. Pathophysiology, diagnosis, and treatment. *J Alzheimers Dis* 2010;21(4):1077-87.
52. Nelson JC, Devanand DP. A systematic review and meta-analysis of placebo-controlled antidepressant studies in people with depression and dementia. *J Am Geriatr Soc* 2011;59(4):577-85.
53. Sepehry AA, Lee PE, Hsiung GY et al. Effect of selective serotonin reuptake inhibitors in Alzheimer's disease with comorbid depression: a meta-analysis of depression and cognitive outcomes. *Drugs Aging* 2012;29(10):793-806.
54. Rosner MH. Severe hyponatremia associated with the combined use of thiazide diuretics and selective serotonin reuptake inhibitors. *Am J Med Sci* 2004;327(2):109-11.
55. Kirby D, Harrigan S, Ames D. Hyponatraemia in elderly psychiatric patients treated with Selective Serotonin Reuptake Inhibitors and venlafaxine: a retrospective controlled study in an inpatient unit. *Int J Geriatr Psychiatry* 2002;17(3):231-7.
56. Sink KM, Holden KF, Yaffe K. Pharmacological treatment of neuropsychiatric symptoms of dementia: a review of the evidence. *JAMA* 2005;293(5):596-608.
57. Seitz DP, Adunuri N, Gill SS et al. Antidepressants for agitation and psychosis in dementia. *Cochrane Database Syst Rev* 2011;(2):CD008191.
58. Pollock BG, Mulsant BH, Rosen J et al. A double-blind comparison of citalopram and risperidone for the treatment of behavioral and psychotic symptoms associated with dementia. *Am J Geriatr Psychiatry* 2007;15(11):942-52.
59. Katz IR, Jeste DV, Mintzer JE et al. Comparison of risperidone and placebo for psychosis and behavioral disturbances associated with dementia: a randomized, double-blind trial. Risperidone Study Group. *J Clin Psychiatry* 1999;60(2):107-15.
60. De Deyn PP, Rabheru K, Rasmussen A et al. A randomized trial of risperidone, placebo, and haloperidol for behavioral symptoms of dementia. *Neurology* 1999;53(5):946-55.
61. Street JS, Clark WS, Gannon KS et al. Olanzapine treatment of psychotic and behavioral symptoms in patients with Alzheimer disease in nursing care facilities: a double-blind, randomized, placebo-controlled trial. The HGEU Study Group. *Arch Gen Psychiatry* 2000;57(10):968-76.
62. Ballard C, Waite J. The effectiveness of atypical antipsychotics for the treatment of aggression and psychosis in Alzheimer's disease. *Cochrane Database Syst Rev* 2006;(1):CD003476.
63. Zhong KX, Tariot PN, Mintzer J et al. Quetiapine to treat agitation in dementia: a randomized, double-blind, placebo-controlled study. *Curr Alzheimer Res* 2007;4(1):81-93.
64. Ballard C, Corbett A. Management of neuropsychiatric symptoms in people with dementia. *CNS Drugs* 2010;24(9):729-39.
65. Lonergan E, Luxenberg J, Colford J. Haloperidol for agitation in dementia. *Cochrane Database Syst Rev* 2002;(2):CD002852.
66. Jeste DV. Tardive dyskinesia in older patients. *J Clin Psychiatry* 2000;61(Suppl 4):27-32.
67. Jeste DV, Lacro JP, Bailey A et al. Lower incidence of tardive dyskinesia with risperidone compared with haloperidol in older patients. *J Am Geriatr Soc* 1999;47(6):716-9.
68. Gill SS, Rochon PA, Herrmann N et al. Atypical antipsychotic drugs and risk of ischaemic stroke: population based retrospective cohort study. *BMJ* 2005;330(7489):445.
69. Schneeweiss S, Setoguchi S, Brookhart A et al. Risk of death associated with the use of conventional versus atypical antipsychotic drugs among elderly patients. *CMAJ* 2007;176(5):627-32.
70. Health Canada. *Health Canada advises consumers about the important safety information on atypical antipsychotic drugs and dementia*. Available from: www.healthycanadians.gc.ca/recall-alert-rappel-avis/hc-sc/2005/13696a-eng.php.
71. Schneider LS, Tariot PN, Dagerman KS et al. Effectiveness of atypical antipsychotic drugs in patients with Alzheimer's disease. *N Engl J Med* 2006;355(15):1525-38.

72. Passmore MJ, Gardner DM, Polak Y et al. Alternatives to atypical antipsychotics for the management of dementia-related agitation. *Drugs Aging* 2008;25(5):381-98.
73. Raina P, Santaguida P, Ismaila A et al. Effectiveness of cholinesterase inhibitors and memantine for treating dementia: evidence review for a clinical practice guideline. *Ann Intern Med* 2008;148(5):379-97.
74. Henry G, Williamson D, Tampi RR. Efficacy and tolerability of antidepressants in the treatment of behavioral and psychological symptoms of dementia, a literature review of evidence. *Am J Alzheimers Dis Other Demen* 2011;26(3):169-83.
75. McCleery J, Cohen DA, Sharpley AL. Pharmacotherapies for sleep disturbances in Alzheimer's disease. *Cochrane Database Syst Rev* 2014;3:CD009178.
76. Camargos EF, Louzada LL, Quintas JL et al. Trazodone improves sleep parameters in Alzheimer disease patients: a randomized, double-blind, and placebo-controlled study. *Am J Geriatr Psychiatry* 2014 Jan 4. pii:S1064-7481(14)00003-7.
77. Meehan KM, Wang H, David SR et al. Comparison of rapidly acting intramuscular olanzapine, lorazepam, and placebo: a double-blind, randomized study in acutely agitated patients with dementia. *Neuropsychopharmacology* 2002;26(4):494-504.

Chapter 6
Depression

Sidney H. Kennedy, MD, FRCPC
Sagar V. Parikh, MD, FRCPC and
Sophie Grigoriadis, MD, PhD, FRCPC

In the Diagnostic and Statistical Manual of Mental Disorders 5th edition (DSM-5), depressive disorders (Table 1) include the specific illnesses of major depressive disorder (MDD) and persistent depressive disorder.[1] Major depressive episodes may be single or, more often, recurrent. Persistent depressive disorder, or dysthymia, is a consolidation of dysthymic disorder and chronic major depressive disorder.

Other disorders in this category are disruptive mood dysregulation disorder, premenstrual dysphoric disorder, substance-induced mood disorder (caused by substances such as alcohol or medications), mood disorder due to a general medical condition (when the depression is thought to be a direct physiological consequence of the medical disorder), other specified depressive disorder (depressive episodes deviating from the precise criteria for MDD) and unspecified depressive disorder.

Table 1: Clinical Features of Major Depressive Episode and Persistent Depressive Disorder[1]

Syndrome	Essential Features[a,b]
Major Depressive Episode	Five or more of the following on most days for at least 2 weeks. At least 1 symptom must be depressed mood or loss of interest/pleasure: • Depressed mood, e.g., felling sad, empty, hopeless • Markedly diminished interest or pleasure • Significant weight loss or weight gain • Insomnia or hypersomnia • Psychomotor agitation or retardation • Fatigue or loss of energy • Feelings of worthlessness or excessive guilt • Diminished ability to think or concentrate, or indecisiveness • Recurrent thoughts of death/suicide or suicide attempt
Persistent Depressive Disorder (Dysthymia)	Depressed mood for most of the day, more days than not, for at least 2 years, plus at least 2 of the following[c]: • Poor appetite or overeating • Insomnia or hypersomnia • Low energy or fatigue • Low self-esteem • Poor concentration or difficulty making decisions • Feelings of hopelessness

[a] Not due to medically or drug-induced conditions or normal bereavement.
[b] Symptoms must be associated with impairment in social, occupational or other areas of functioning.
[c] In children and adolescents, mood can be irritable and the duration must be at least 1 year.
Reprinted with permission from the *Diagnostic and Statistical Manual of Mental Disorders, Fifth Edition, (Copyright ©2013). American Psychiatric Association.* All Rights Reserved.

Goals of Therapy

- Achieve remission of depressive symptoms
- Prevent suicide
- Restore optimal functioning
- Prevent recurrence

Investigations

The following screening questions/assessment tools are recommended for use by primary care physicians:

- The Patient Health Questionnaire (PHQ-9)[2] is a self-reported version of the DSM-IV criteria for a major depressive episode. (At the time of writing, the DSM-5 version was not available.) The first 2 questions from the PHQ-9 serve as a useful and rapid screening tool:[3]
  - "During the past month, how often have you been bothered by feeling down, depressed or hopeless?"
  - "During the past month, how often have you been bothered by little interest or pleasure in doing things?"
- The seven-item Hamilton Depression Rating Scale (HAM-D-7)[4] is a validated, brief, physician assessment designed to assess severity and remission.
- The Mood Disorder Questionnaire (MDQ)[5] is a useful screening instrument for manic or hypomanic symptoms.
- The Edinburgh Postnatal Depression Scale (EPDS)[6] (available at www.cfp.ca/content/suppl/2011/07/07/57.7.777.DC1/MotheRisk.pdf) is the most widely used and well-validated tool to screen for depressive symptoms during pregnancy and the postpartum.

Therapeutic Choices

The most impressive evidence for the success of pharmacologic and depression-specific psychological therapies, in terms of both clinical efficacy and restoration of occupational functioning, comes from controlled trials involving multifaceted health system interventions.[7,8] These interventions, tested mostly in primary care settings, involve physicians working in conjunction with another healthcare provider (e.g., nurses, psychologists, psychiatrists); the physician prescribes the antidepressants while the other practitioner educates the patient about depression and monitors the progress during treatment.[9,10] Multifaceted interventions can substantially reduce long-term expense and increase the likelihood of the patient returning to work for only a modest cost.[11,12,13] Unfortunately not all clinicians and patients have access to these resources.

Nonpharmacologic Choices

The efficacy of both *cognitive behavioural therapy* (CBT) and a specific model of *interpersonal therapy* (IPT) in treating depression has been shown over decades of research and summarized in numerous meta-analyses. While pharmacotherapy is preferable in severe depression and also when comorbid personality disorders are present, psychotherapies are as effective as medication for depression of mild to moderate severity.

Each type of intervention has subtle advantages in specific circumstances and patient preferences are important to consider. IPT may be preferable when major interpersonal issues are present. Newer versions of CBT and IPT have evolved and show particular promise. *Mindfulness-based CBT* (mCBT) is particularly effective in preventing relapse into depression,[14] and *acceptance and commitment therapy* (ACT) has some efficacy in acute depression.[15] CBT is also available on the Internet, in some cases at no charge (e.g., www.moodgym.anu.edu.au/welcome and www.llttf.com). One meta-analysis has shown web-based CBT to be equivalent to therapist-delivered CBT.[16] Patients should be encouraged to complete the modules and simple homework exercises on these sites, in tandem with attending routine clinical care visits.

Motivational interviewing is a type of psychotherapy that is strikingly effective for treatment of substance abuse when depression is also present.[17] Its effects are primarily on the substance abuse, not on the depressive symptoms.

In addition to psychotherapy, measures to enhance adherence to antidepressant therapy are useful. Psychoeducation with the following 5 simple messages is effective:[18]

- Take medication daily
- Call this number for questions about side effects or other issues
- Remember that it may take 2–4 weeks to see a noticeable effect from antidepressants
- Continue to take medication even if you are feeling better
- Do not stop taking your antidepressant without checking with your physician

There is some evidence for the benefit of regular *physical exercise* as an adjunct to pharmacotherapy and/or psychotherapy in mild-to-moderate depression, but not as monotherapy.[19]

Pharmacologic Choices

Figure 1 illustrates an algorithm for the pharmacologic management of depression with or without a remission of symptoms.

Figure 1: Pharmacologic Treatment of Depression[20]

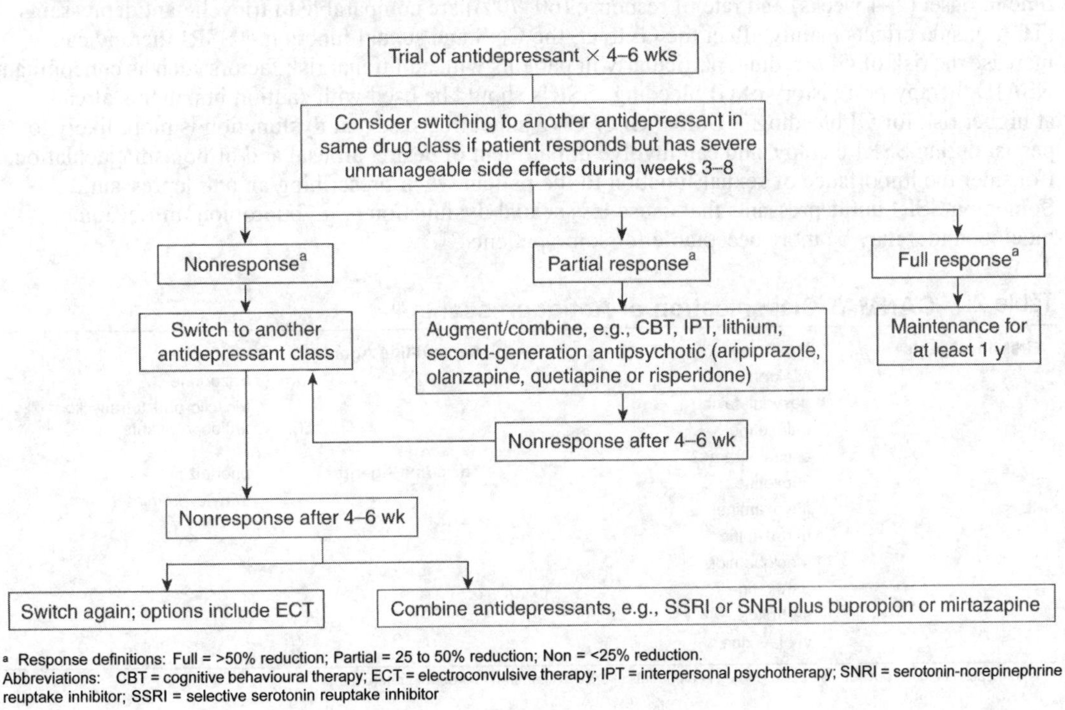

[a] Response definitions: Full = >50% reduction; Partial = 25 to 50% reduction; Non = <25% reduction.

Abbreviations: CBT = cognitive behavioural therapy; ECT = electroconvulsive therapy; IPT = interpersonal psychotherapy; SNRI = serotonin-norepinephrine reuptake inhibitor; SSRI = selective serotonin reuptake inhibitor

Although diagnostic criteria for MDD and persistent depressive disorder (see Table 1) differ , recommendations for the use of antidepressants are the same in both conditions. Table 2 lists first-, second- and third-line antidepressants according to the 2009 CANMAT guidelines.[20] Table 3 provides more details about the drugs used to treat depression. A minimum therapeutic dose should be achieved in the first 2 weeks of treatment, and increased if necessary over the next 4–6 weeks. Patients need to be informed of common side effects and that some of these unwanted effects usually subside within 2 weeks. Consider switching within the same class during weeks 3–8 if a favourable response is overshadowed by persistent and troublesome side effects that do not respond to measures such as adjusting the dose or time of administration.

A meta-analysis of head-to-head comparisons among 12 antidepressants identified 4 agents with superior efficacy: escitalopram, mirtazapine, sertraline and venlafaxine.[21] When acceptability (based on drop-out rates) was considered, the leading 4 agents were escitalopram, sertraline, bupropion and citalopram. Based on this systematic review, escitalopram and sertraline appear to be 2 of the most effective and well-tolerated options.

Regulatory authorities have issued cautions that highlight the potential of antidepressants to increase suicidal ideation, particularly in children and young adults. Clinicians are faced with complex decisions about when to use CBT and/or pharmacotherapy to treat depression in younger age groups, and are advised to monitor patients carefully for any emergent suicidal ideation or acts, particularly during the early phase of treatment. The risk of emergent or worsening suicidal ideation must be weighed against the risks associated with untreated depression (suicide, increased duration and severity of illness, higher incidence of relapse).

Selective Serotonin Reuptake Inhibitors (SSRIs)

Greater tolerability and ease of dosing are key reasons SSRIs are first-choice antidepressants. Both time to onset (2–4 weeks) and rate of response (60–70%) are comparable to tricyclic antidepressants (TCAs); side effects mainly affect the GI tract, the CNS and sexual function.[20] SSRI therapy can increase the risk of GI bleeding, particularly in patients with additional risk factors such as concomitant NSAID therapy or a history of GI bleeding. SSRIs should be used with caution in patients already at higher risk for GI bleeding.[22] Unlike GI or CNS side effects, sexual dysfunction is more likely to persist during SSRI therapy, and can involve impairment of desire, arousal and/or orgasm/ejaculation. Consider the importance of sexual function to the patient when prescribing an antidepressant. Some non-SSRI antidepressants that cause less sexual dysfunction (e.g., bupropion, mirtazapine, moclobemide) may be more acceptable for some patients.[20]

Table 2: CANMAT Classification of Antidepressants[20]

First-line Agents[a]	bupropion citalopram desvenlafaxine duloxetine escitalopram fluoxetine fluvoxamine mirtazapine moclobemide paroxetine sertraline venlafaxine	**Second-line Agents**[a]	quetiapine trazodone tricyclic and tetracyclic antidepressants
		Third-line Agents[a]	phenelzine tranylcypromine

[a] Within each category, antidepressants are listed in alphabetical order rather than in order of preference.

Six SSRIs are currently available in Canada (**citalopram**, **escitalopram**, **fluoxetine**, **fluvoxamine**, **paroxetine** and **sertraline**). Escitalopram, the stereoisomer of citalopram, has a similar side effect profile but superior efficacy to citalopram,[23] and is at least as effective as venlafaxine.[24] With the exception of fluoxetine, all SSRIs are commonly associated with discontinuation effects when stopping therapy. See Antidepressant Discontinuation Syndrome for more information. These effects can be severe and protracted in a small proportion of patients. Patients should be assessed regularly during and after treatment discontinuation for withdrawal symptoms and relapse.

Dual Action Antidepressants

Bupropion is thought to exert antidepressant effects through norepinephrine and dopamine reuptake inhibition.[25] It is a first-line agent for MDD and is also indicated for smoking cessation under a different brand name.[26] Bupropion is contraindicated in patients with a seizure disorder or recent history of anorexia or bulimia nervosa, and should be used with extreme caution where there is a history of head trauma or prior seizure. Treatment-emergent GI disturbance occurs less frequently with bupropion compared to SSRIs. Bupropion provides patients with the best treatment option regarding sexual side effects.[27]

Trazodone is a potent postsynaptic serotonin ($5HT_2$) receptor antagonist with weak serotonin reuptake inhibitory effects.[28] Because of severe daytime sedation, trazodone is rarely prescribed at therapeutic antidepressant doses (300–400 mg daily) but is often prescribed at lower doses (50–100 mg) as a hypnotic in combination with other antidepressants.[29] Tolerance, as seen with benzodiazepines, does not develop with trazodone and there is the potential for trazodone to enhance antidepressant effects.

Mirtazapine acts on both the noradrenergic and serotonergic systems. It has a lower rate of GI and sexual side effects but is associated with sedation and weight gain.[30]

Serotonin-Norepinephrine Reuptake Inhibitors (SNRIs)

Venlafaxine is a serotonin-norepinephrine reuptake inhibitor (SNRI) that has inhibitory effects on serotonin reuptake at any therapeutic dose. At doses of >150 mg daily it also inhibits norepinephrine reuptake. Compared to SSRIs, rates of remission have been reported to be 6–10 % higher with venlafaxine, although these results are mainly due to venlafaxine's superiority over fluoxetine.[31,32] Dose-related hypertension occurs rarely, and is more likely to be seen at doses ≥225 mg. Monitor blood pressure and avoid use in patients with uncontrolled hypertension.

Duloxetine is an SNRI that appears to exert effects on both serotonin and norepinephrine systems at the starting dose of 60 mg daily, and has comparable efficacy to venlafaxine.[33] In addition to depression, duloxetine is indicated for neuropathic pain and for pain associated with fibromyalgia. Isolated cases of hepatic injury have been reported but there is no requirement for routine monitoring of liver enzymes.

Desvenlafaxine, an SNRI, is the active metabolite of venlafaxine. The recommended dose is 50 mg daily, although safety data are available for 100 mg daily. In the treatment of depression, the response and remission rates at 8 weeks are 51–63% and 31–45%, respectively. Common adverse effects include insomnia, somnolence, dizziness and nausea.[34,35]

Tricyclic Antidepressants (TCAs)

TCAs are generally reserved as second-line medications. **Amitriptyline** is the most frequently prescribed TCA, often at considerably lower doses of 25–50 mg per day for nighttime sedation or analgesia. **Nortriptyline**, a metabolite of amitriptyline and a secondary amine, has been used to treat depression in older populations for many years. **Clomipramine**, the most serotonergic TCA, is still favoured in the treatment of obsessive compulsive disorder. In all cases, TCA use is limited by tolerability and safety concerns, especially cardiotoxicity following overdose.

Monoamine Oxidase Inhibitors (MAOIs)

Prescribing of the *irreversible* monoamine oxidase inhibitors (MAOIs) **phenelzine** and **tranylcypromine** is generally reserved for specialized mood disorder clinics because these agents are associated with potentially fatal food and drug interactions (serotonin syndrome, hypertensive crisis). Nevertheless, all prescribers and pharmacists should be aware of these risks and how they can avoided when faced with a patient taking an irreversible MAOI. Despite the potential risks, under careful conditions phenelzine 30–90 mg daily or tranylcypromine 20–60 mg daily may prove effective where other antidepressants have failed.

Moclobemide is a *reversible* and selective MAO-A inhibitor that does not require the same dietary restrictions as irreversible MAOIs. Moclobemide is a well-tolerated alternative to SSRI or SNRI agents, particularly in patients with a significant anxiety component to their depressive episode. Although it is often perceived as being less effective than irreversible MAOIs, this has not been substantiated in clinical trials.

Antipsychotics

Extended-release **quetiapine**, a second-generation or "atypical" antipsychotic agent, has been approved in Canada for the treatment of depression and is considered to be a second-line option.[20,36]

Aripiprazole is approved as an adjunct to antidepressants in adults with MDD who have not had an adequate response to antidepressants alone during the current episode.

See Treatment-Resistant Depression for information regarding the role of antipsychotics in the treatment of depression.

Natural Health Products

Several natural health products have been evaluated for the treatment of depression. It is important to consider potential drug interactions with these products since many should not be used in combination with prescription antidepressants.

There is evidence to show that **St. John's wort** is effective and a potential first-line monotherapy option for patients with MDD of mild to moderate severity.[19] As an inducer of CYP3A4 and intestinal P-glycoprotein, St. John's wort can decrease the bioavailability of many drugs. When combined with other serotonergic medications, there is an increased risk of serotonin syndrome. Consider potential interactions before recommending this agent.

S-adenosyl-L-methionine (SAMe), a synthetic form of a dietary amino acid, may be an effective second-line monotherapy option for the treatment of mild to moderate depression.[19] SAMe is well tolerated with few adverse effects, but may be associated with an increased risk of serotonin syndrome when combined with other serotonergic drugs.

Available evidence supports the use of **omega-3 fatty acids**, either alone or adjunctively, as second-line treatment of mild to moderate depression.[19]

Folic acid and **vitamin D** supplementation may have a beneficial effect on depression. Adjunctive L-methylfolate 15 mg/day showed significantly greater efficacy compared with continued SSRI therapy plus placebo.[37] More study is needed to clarify the potential role for these 2 supplements.

Duration of Treatment—Relapse Prevention

Evidence supports the use of maintenance antidepressant therapies for a minimum period of 1 year, particularly when the intervals between depressive episodes become shorter and the disability associated with each depressive episode worsens. After achieving remission in a first episode, treat for 1 year. For recurrent episodes, treat for at least 2 years. CBT and IPT may also be effective in reducing the risk of relapse.[38]

In general, taper antidepressants slowly to minimize the risk of discontinuation-emergent symptoms. Among newer antidepressants, paroxetine and venlafaxine are most likely to produce discontinuation symptoms such as insomnia, dizziness, nausea and diarrhea. See Antidepressant Discontinuation Syndrome for more information.

Treatment-Resistant Depression

Antidepressants can be switched either within a medication class or to a different class. Most physicians switch out of class, e.g., from SSRI to SNRI or TCA, when there has been no response to the first drug. Consider switching within class in the presence of a favourable clinical response hampered by persistent, unmanageable side effects. Generally there is no need for a *washout period*; a *crossover technique* can be applied whereby the dose of the first agent is tapered while the dose of the new antidepressant is gradually increased. Exceptions include: switching to an irreversible MAOI from another antidepressant where a washout period of 5 half-lives is recommended; switching from an irreversible MAOI (phenelzine or tranylcypromine) to any other antidepressant, where a 2-week washout is required; switching from moclobemide, where a 5-day washout is recommended; and switching from fluoxetine to an irreversible MAOI, where a 5-week washout is recommended. Similarly, due to its long half-life, exercise caution when starting other antidepressants after fluoxetine discontinuation.

Augmentation or *combination* therapy is recommended when a patient tolerates the first antidepressant but has only a partial response.[20] **Lithium carbonate** at a dose of 600–900 mg daily has been most evaluated, although triiodothyronine 25–50 µg daily was equally effective in the large Sequenced Treatment Alternatives to Relieve Depression (STAR*D) trial.[39] Several second-generation antipsychotics including **aripiprazole**, **olanzapine**, **quetiapine** and **risperidone** have also proved effective in augmenting antidepressant response, particularly where insomnia and anxiety symptoms persist.[40] Antipsychotic augmentation is not recommended for long-term use, and close monitoring for movement disorders, weight gain and cardiometabolic effects is indicated. The combination of **bupropion** with SSRIs is also an option.[41,42] Psychostimulant agents including modafinil and methylphenidate have enhanced motivation and energy but not overall symptoms of depression.[43]

A combination of pharmacotherapy and psychotherapy (specifically IPT or CBT) is superior to either modality alone. In mild to moderate cases, combination therapy provides little synergy to either treatment alone, but does provide protection against early relapse compared to either treatment alone. Pharmacotherapy typically facilitates more rapid relief of symptoms, but does not prevent relapse if the medication is stopped; both IPT and CBT reduce relapse for up to 3 years after completion of a course of psychotherapy. For moderate to severe depression, or refractory depression, combination therapy should be strongly considered, particularly in individuals with a history of more than 3 previous depressions.[44]

Neurostimulation Therapies

Electroconvulsive therapy (ECT) is efficacious in 80–90% of depressed patients, a response rate that is superior to any single antidepressant drug, although relapse and recurrence rates are high in the absence of other prophylactic treatments.[45,46]

Other neurostimulation therapies, including *repetitive transcranial magnetic stimulation* (rTMS), *vagus nerve stimulation* (VNS) and *deep brain stimulation* (DBS) are emerging alternatives.[47]

Bipolar Disorder

Although bipolar disorder has a lower prevalence (1–2%) than MDD, individuals with bipolar disorder experience more depressive episodes than those with MDD.[48] Patients presenting with depression should be questioned about past manic or hypomanic episodes, since many have difficulty recalling such episodes, and treatment of bipolar disorder differs significantly. The primary pharmacotherapy for bipolar disorder is a mood stabilizer with other medications as needed (see Chapter 4).

Antidepressant Discontinuation Syndrome

If antidepressants are abruptly discontinued or dose-reduced, patients are at risk of experiencing discontinuation syndrome.[49] This syndrome is often reported with SSRIs, most likely because these drugs are first-line agents, but patients are at risk if they have been taking any antidepressant for 6 weeks or more. Patients taking agents with a shorter half-life, e.g., paroxetine, are at greatest risk.

Patients experience somatic, neurologic and psychological symptoms attributed to a rapid decrease in the availability of 5-HT,[50] within 1–7 days of stopping the drug. If untreated, symptoms will subside within 3 weeks.

As prevention, inform patients that discontinuation syndrome may occur if they abruptly stop or reduce the dose of their medication. Taper antidepressant doses gradually by approximately 25% per week and monitor for a re-emergence of depressive symptoms.[49] Fluoxetine has a long half-life and can be tapered more rapidly than other SSRIs.

Reassure patients who experience discontinuation syndrome that the condition is not serious or life-threatening and severe symptoms will usually resolve in 3 days or less. The syndrome can be reversed by restarting the antidepressant and tapering the dose more slowly. Alternatively, if a slow taper is poorly tolerated, substitute with one dose of fluoxetine 10–20 mg po. Patients can experience side effects such as nausea and imbalance. Consider a herbal product containing ginger if drug interactions or adverse effects limit use of other possible antinausea medications[51] (see Chapter 64).

Choices during Pregnancy and Breastfeeding

Depression during Pregnancy

During pregnancy, symptoms of depression are common and can be difficult to disentangle from symptoms frequently reported during pregnancy (fatigue, sleeplessness, appetite changes). Symptoms are highly predictive of subsequent postpartum depression. The decision to initiate or continue treatment during pregnancy should be based on a risk-benefit analysis that considers both the fetus and mother. Untreated maternal depression is associated with untoward effects for the fetus/neonate, the mother and her partner.[52,53,54]

Management

If symptoms are mild or if criteria for a mild depressive episode are met, psychotherapy such as IPT is the first treatment option. For episodes of moderate severity, antidepressant medication should be considered, especially in women with a past history of depression. Evidence suggests that these medications are not major teratogens, although a statistical association may exist between cardiovascular malformations, such as ventricular or atrial septal defects, and fetal exposure to antidepressants, and specifically **paroxetine**.[55,56,57] Adverse delivery outcomes such as preterm birth have also been statistically associated with antenatal antidepressant use although the clinical relevance is not certain.[58] Third-trimester **SSRI** exposure may be associated with an increased risk of persistent pulmonary hypertension in the newborn.[59,60,61] Other potential postbirth adverse effects include transient neonatal withdrawal or discontinuation symptoms such as tremors, shivering, increased muscle tone, feeding or digestive problems or respiratory distress.[62,63] If antidepressants are prescribed during pregnancy, use the lowest effective dose. Counsel the mother about the possibility that the newborn may experience transient withdrawal symptoms and may require monitoring by a pediatrician, especially when higher doses are needed.

Postpartum Depression

Rates of postpartum depression vary according to the severity of the episode. Postpartum "blues" affects up to 80% of women.[64] Postpartum major depression occurs in up to 16% of new mothers in Canada and postpartum psychosis in ≤0.1%.[65,66,67]

"The blues" is not a disorder per se, given that it is so common and symptoms are self-limiting, requiring only monitoring and supportive care. However, women with postpartum blues are at risk of developing a depressive episode.

Management

Psychotherapy, preferably IPT and CBT, should be considered first for the treatment of postpartum depression, particularly if the mother is breast-feeding. When the illness is more severe, psychotherapy may be inadequate or inappropriate, in which case antidepressant treatment should be initiated. For breastfeeding patients, consider **paroxetine**, **sertraline** and **nortriptyline**,[68] due to their low concentrations in breast milk.

A discussion of general principles on the use of medications in these special populations can be found in Appendix II and Appendix III. Other specialized reference sources are also provided in these appendices.

Therapeutic Tips

- Choose 1 or 2 agents from several antidepressant classes and use them consistently.
- Provide structured psychoeducation with the initial prescription. Reinforce and add to this during regular follow-up visits.
- Reinforce the importance of maintenance therapy beyond the acute phase.
- Serum drug concentrations are not useful with SSRIs, MAOIs and newer antidepressants. There is a limited role for monitoring serum levels with some TCAs such as amitriptyline, desipramine, imipramine and nortriptyline.
- Provide patients with reliable information on drug interactions and dietary restrictions. Some patient-friendly Internet resources are available at medicationinfoshare.com/tools/, including pamphlets about serotonin syndrome (medicationinfoshare.com/wp-content/uploads/2013/01/MIS-Serotonin-Syndrome-Jan-2013.pdf) and food and drug interaction information for patients taking irreversible MAOI therapy, e.g., MAO Inhibitors—Food and Drug Interactions—What You Should Know, developed by Dr. David Gardner and Anne Marentette at Dalhousie University; available at medicationinfoshare.com/wp-content/uploads/2012/02/MAOI-restrictions-pamphlet.pdf.
- In nonresponders, review alcohol and drug abuse history, assess medication adherence and confirm diagnosis.
- Refer for psychiatric consultation if the patient has psychotic symptoms or acute suicidal ideation, or after failure of 3 treatment trials.
- When discontinuing antidepressants, taper slowly over 4–6 weeks. This is particularly important for paroxetine and venlafaxine. A patient information pamphlet about stopping antidepressants is available at medicationinfoshare.com/wp-content/uploads/2014/03/MIS-Stopping-Antidepressants-Feb-20141.pdf.
- For patient education, consider recommending web sites such as www.canmat.org or moodgym.anu.edu.au, or self-help books such as *Mind Over Mood*[69] or *Feeling Good*[70].

Table 3: Drug Therapy for Depression

Class	Drug	Oral Dose	Adverse Effects	Drug Interactions	Cost[a]
Antipsychotics, Second-generation	*aripiprazole* Abilify	2 mg daily Augmentation of first-line antidepressants	EPS (akathisia, parkinsonism), dizziness, orthostatic hypotension, headache, GI complaints, nasopharyngitis, tremor, sedation, insomnia. Advise patients about antipsychotic-associated body temperature dysregulation and prevention of heat stroke (e.g., hydration, sun protection).	Strong inducers of CYP2D6 or CYP3A4 (e.g., carbamazepine, phenytoin, rifampin) can decrease aripiprazole levels substantially. Strong inhibitors of CYP2D6 or CYP3A4 (e.g., ketoconazole, quinidine, fluoxetine, paroxetine) can increase levels substantially.	$$$$
	olanzapine Zyprexa, Zyprexa Zydis, generics	2.5–10 mg daily Augmentation of SSRIs	Weight gain, dizziness, sedation, anticholinergic effects, hepatic aminotransferase elevation, orthostatic hypotension, increased risk of diabetes and dyslipidemia, EPS (especially akathisia). Advise patients about antipsychotic-associated body temperature dysregulation and prevention of heat stroke (e.g., hydration, sun protection).	Sedation with CNS depressants; may potentiate antihypertensive drug effects; inhibitors of CYP1A2 or CYP2D6 (e.g., diltiazem, fluvoxamine, paroxetine) may increase olanzapine levels; inducers CYP1A2 or CYP2D6 (e.g., barbiturates, carbamazepine, phenytoin, rifampin or cigarette smoking) may decrease olanzapine levels.	$$
	quetiapine extended-release Seroquel XR, generics	Initial: 50 mg daily for 2 days, then 150 mg daily; if necessary can increase to 300 mg on or after day 4 Usual: 150 mg/day High: 300 mg/day Low doses can be used to augment SSRIs	Sedation, dizziness, weight gain, orthostatic hypotension, hepatic transaminase elevation, headache, anticholinergic effects, increased risk of diabetes and dyslipidemia, possible increased risk of cataracts; may reduce thyroid hormone levels.	Additive sedation with CNS depressants; may potentiate antihypertensive drug effects; inhibitors of CYP3A4 such as clarithromycin, erythromycin, grapefruit juice, ketoconazole or prednisone may increase quetiapine levels; inducers of CYP3A4 such as carbamazepine, phenytoin or rifampin may reduce quetiapine levels.	$
	risperidone Risperdal Preparations, generics	0.5–2 mg daily Augmentation of SSRIs	Sedation, headaches, weight gain, orthostatic hypotension, rhinitis, anxiety, dose-related hyperprolactinemia and EPS. Risk of intraoperative floppy iris syndrome in patients undergoing cataract surgery who have been exposed to risperidone.	Additive sedation with CNS depressants; may potentiate antihypertensive drug effects; inhibitors of CYP3A4 (e.g., clarithromycin, erythromycin, grapefruit juice, ketoconazole, prednisone) may increase risperidone levels; induces of CYP3A3 (e.g., carbamazepine, phenytoin, rifampin) may decrease risperidone levels.	$

Class	Drug	Oral Dose	Adverse Effects	Drug Interactions	Cost[a]
Dual Action Antidepressants	*bupropion* Wellbutrin SR, Wellbutrin XL, generics	SR formulation (doses >150 mg/day should be given in divided doses; maximum single dose = 150 mg): Initial:[b] 150 mg/day Usual: 150–300 mg/day High:[c] 375–450 mg/day XL formulation (given once daily): Initial:[b] 150 mg/day Usual: 150–300 mg/day High:[c] 450 mg/day	Agitation, insomnia, anorexia; contraindicated in anorexia or bulimia nervosa and seizure disorders.	Use with MAOIs may lead to potentially fatal reaction initially presenting with tremor, agitation, hypomania, hyperthermia and/or hypertension. May increase levels of cyclophosphamide, ifosfamide and orphenadrine.	$
	mirtazapine Remeron, Remeron RD, generics	Initial:[b] 15–30 mg/day Usual: 30–45 mg/day High:[c] 60 mg/day	Weight gain, sedation.	Use with MAOIs may lead to potentially fatal reaction initially presenting with tremor, agitation, hypomania, hyperthermia and/or hypertension. Sedative effects may be potentiated by alcohol or diazepam. Orally disintegrating tablets can be taken without water.	$
	trazodone generics	Initial:[b] 150–200 mg/day Usual: 300–400 mg/day High:[c] 600 mg/day	Drowsiness, orthostatic hypotension, nausea, headache, dry mouth, priapism.	May potentiate effects of other CNS depressants and augment hypotensive effects of antihypertensives. Avoid use with MAOIs.	$
Irreversible MAOIs	*phenelzine* Nardil	Initial:[b] 15–30 mg/day Usual: 30–75 mg/day High:[c] 90–120 mg/day	Edema, postural hypotension, insomnia, sexual dysfunction.	Concurrent sympathomimetics may increase BP; use with meperidine causes agitation, hyperpyrexia, circulatory collapse and death; SSRIs, TCAs, levodopa may increase effects and side effects; tyramine-containing food may cause hypertensive crisis (see Therapeutic Tips).	$$
	tranylcypromine Parnate	Initial:[b] 10–20 mg/day Usual: 20–60 mg/day High:[c] 60–80 mg/day	See phenelzine.	See phenelzine.	$$

(cont'd)

Table 3: **Drug Therapy for Depression** *(cont'd)*

Class	Drug	Oral Dose	Adverse Effects	Drug Interactions	Cost[a]
Reversible Inhibitors of Monoamine Oxidase-A	*moclobemide* Manerix, generics	Initial:[b] 200–300 mg/day Usual: 450–600 mg/day High:[c] 900 mg/day	Nausea, insomnia, dizziness.	Use with irreversible MAOIs may lead to potentially fatal reaction initially presenting with tremor, agitation, hypomania, hyperthermia and/or hypertension. Avoid sympathomimetics, meperidine; caution with opioids, antihypertensives, antipsychotics, SSRIs, selegiline, excessive tyramine, alcohol; reduce dose with cimetidine.	$
Selective Serotonin Reuptake Inhibitors	*citalopram* Celexa, CTP 30, generics	Initial:[b] 10–20 mg/day Usual:[d] 20–40 mg/day High:[c] 40 mg/day	Nausea, dry mouth, sleep disturbance, somnolence, sweating, sexual dysfunction, increased risk of GI bleeding, SIADH, dose-dependent QT_c prolongation, discontinuation syndrome.	SSRIs: Use with MAOIs leads to potentially fatal reaction initially presenting with tremor, agitation, hypomania, hyperthermia and/or hypertension. Increased risk of GI bleeding with NSAIDs, antiplatelet agents. Inhibitors of cytochrome P450 enzymes such as cimetidine, clarithromycin, erythromycin, fluconazole, indinavir, isoniazid, itraconazole, ketoconazole, quinidine or ritonavir may increase SSRI levels. All SSRIs inhibit certain cytochrome P450 isoenzymes and can reduce the clearance of many drugs such as clozapine, methadone, mexiletine, phenytoin, pimozide or propafenone, or decrease the enzymatic conversion of a prodrug such as clopidogrel, codeine or tamoxifen to its active form. Inducers of cytochrome P450 enzymes (e.g., carbamazepine, phenobarbital, phenytoin, rifampin) can increase the clearance of SSRIs. Avoid combined use with drugs associated with prolonged QT_c interval/torsades de pointes, such as amiodarone, azithromycin, clarithromycin, domperidone, erythromycin, haloperidol, methadone, pimozide, quinine, sotalol, ziprasidone.	$

Class	Drug	Oral Dose	Adverse Effects	Drug Interactions	Cost[a]
	escitalopram Cipralex, Cipralex MELTZ	Initial:[b] 10 mg/day Usual:[d] 10–20 mg/day High:[c] 20 mg/day	See citalopram.	See citalopram.	$$
	fluoxetine Prozac, generics	Initial:[b] 10–20 mg/day Usual:[d] 20–40 mg/day High:[c] 60–80 mg/day	Nausea, nervousness, anorexia, insomnia, sexual dysfunction, increased risk of GI bleeding.	See citalopram.	$$
	fluvoxamine Luvox, generics	Initial:[b] 50–100 mg/day Usual:[d] 150–200 mg/day High:[c] 400 mg/day	Nausea, drowsiness, sweating, anorexia, sexual dysfunction, increased risk of GI bleeding. Discontinuation syndrome.	See citalopram.	$
	paroxetine, immediate-release Paxil, generics	Initial:[b] 10–20 mg/day Usual:[d] 20–40 mg/day High:[c] 60 mg/day	Nausea, drowsiness, fatigue, sweating, constipation, dry mouth, dizziness, sexual dysfunction, increased risk of GI bleeding. Discontinuation syndrome.	See citalopram.	$
	paroxetine, controlled-release Paxil CR	Initial:[b] 12.5–25 mg/day Usual:[d] 25–50 mg/day High:[c] 75 mg/day	See paroxetine immediate-release.	See citalopram.	$$$
	sertraline Zoloft, generics	Initial:[b] 25–50 mg/day Usual:[d] 50–100 mg/day High:[c] 150–200 mg/day	Nausea, tremors, diarrhea, dry mouth, sexual dysfunction, increased risk of GI bleeding. Discontinuation syndrome.	See citalopram.	$
Serotonin-Norepinephrine Reuptake Inhibitors	*desvenlafaxine* ❥ Pristiq	Initial: 50 mg daily Usual: 50 mg daily High: 100 mg daily	See venlafaxine.	Use with MAOIs may lead to potentially fatal reaction initially presenting with tremor, agitation, hypomania, hyperthermia and/or hypertension. Potent inhibitors of CYP3A4 may increase desvenlafaxine levels.	$$$
	duloxetine Cymbalta	Initial/Usual: 60 mg/day If necessary for tolerability may start with 30 mg/day and increase to 60 mg in 1–2 wk High: 120 mg/day	Nausea, drowsiness, insomnia, dizziness, dry mouth.	Use with MAOIs may lead to potentially fatal reaction initially presenting with tremor, agitation, hypomania, hyperthermia and/or hypertension. Do not use with potent inhibitors of CYP1A2 such as ciprofloxacin, fluvoxamine, ketoconazole.	$$$$

(cont'd)

Table 3: **Drug Therapy for Depression** *(cont'd)*

Class	Drug	Oral Dose	Adverse Effects	Drug Interactions	Cost[a]
	venlafaxine ◗ Effexor XR, generics	Initial:[b] 37.5–75 mg/day Usual: 112.5–225 mg/day High:[c] 300–375 mg/day	Nausea, sleep disturbance, drowsiness, nervousness, dizziness, dry mouth. Dose-related hypertension occurs rarely, particularly at doses ≥225 mg/day.	Use with MAOIs may lead to potentially fatal reaction initially presenting with tremor, agitation, hypomania, hyperthermia and/or hypertension. Inhibitors of CYP2D6 or CYP3A4 may increase venlafaxine levels.	$
Tetracyclic Antidepressants	*maprotiline* generics	Initial:[b] 75 mg/day Usual: 75–150 mg/day High:[c] 200 mg/day	Anticholinergic (dry mouth, blurred vision, constipation, urinary hesitancy, tachycardia, delirium), antihistaminergic (sedation, weight gain), orthostatic hypotension, lowered seizure threshold; sexual dysfunction.	Use with MAOIs may lead to potentially fatal reaction initially presenting with tremor, agitation, hypomania, hyperthermia and/or hypertension. Barbiturates, carbamazepine and rifampin may decrease effect; cimetidine and antipsychotics may increase effect and toxicity; possible interaction with antiarrhythmics (may lead to increased effect of either drug); may reduce antihypertensive effect of clonidine; may augment hypotensive effect of thiazides.	$$$
Tricyclic Antidepressants	*amitriptyline* generics	Initial:[b] 25–50 mg/day Usual: 75–200 mg/day High:[c] 250–300 mg/day	Anticholinergic (dry mouth, blurred vision, constipation, urinary hesitancy, tachycardia, delirium), antihistaminergic (sedation, weight gain), orthostatic hypotension, lowered seizure threshold; sexual dysfunction.	Use with MAOIs may lead to potentially fatal reaction initially presenting with tremor, agitation, hypomania, hyperthermia and/or hypertension. Barbiturates, carbamazepine and rifampin may decrease effect; cimetidine and antipsychotics may increase effect and toxicity; possible interaction with antiarrhythmics (may lead to increased effect of either drug); may reduce antihypertensive effect of clonidine; may augment hypotensive effect of thiazides.	$
	clomipramine Anafranil, generics	Initial:[b] 25–50 mg/day Usual: 75–200 mg/day High:[c] 250–300 mg/day	See amitriptyline.	See amitriptyline.	$
	desipramine generics	Initial:[b] 25–50 mg/day Usual: 75–200 mg/day High:[c] 250–300 mg/day	See amitriptyline.	See amitriptyline.	$$
	doxepin Sinequan, generics	Initial:[b] 25–50 mg/day Usual: 75–200 mg/day High:[c] 250–300 mg/day	See amitriptyline.	See amitriptyline.	$

Class	Drug	Oral Dose	Adverse Effects	Drug Interactions	Cost[a]
	imipramine generics	Initial:[b] 25–50 mg/day Usual: 75–200 mg/day High:[c] 250–300 mg/day	See amitriptyline.	See amitriptyline.	$$
	nortriptyline Aventyl, generics	Initial:[b] 25–50 mg/day Usual: 75–150 mg/day High:[c] 200 mg/day	See amitriptyline.	See amitriptyline.	$
	trimipramine generics	Initial:[b] 25–50 mg/day Usual: 75–200 mg/day High:[c] 250–300 mg/day	See amitriptyline.	See amitriptyline.	$$
Natural Health Products	*omega-3 fatty acids*	1–2 g per day of an EPA-DHA mixture	Mild GI upset, fishy aftertaste; risk of bleeding documented (minimal with doses <3 g/day).	Potential additive bleeding risk with drugs such as warfarin, ASA, other antiplatelet agents.	$
	SAMe (S-adenosyl-L-methionine)	400–1600 mg/day, in 2–3 divided doses	Mild insomnia, constipation, dizziness, nausea, dry mouth, sweating; case reports of increased anxiety, mania or hypomania in patients with bipolar disorder.	Avoid concurrent use with other serotonergic drugs such as antidepressants (possible serotonin syndrome).	$$
	St. John's wort (Hypericum perforatum)	Usual: 300 mg TID Range: 300–1800 mg/day, in 2–3 divided doses	Photosensitivity (rare), GI upset, dizziness, insomnia, restlessness, agitation; cases of mania or hypomania reported. Avoid during pregnancy and lactation.	Avoid concurrent use with MAOIs (possible hypertensive crisis). Avoid concurrent use with SSRIs (possible serotonin syndrome). May decrease bioavailability of many drugs including cyclosporine, digoxin, indinavir, oral contraceptives, theophylline, warfarin.	$

[a] Cost of 30-day supply for mean usual dose; includes drug cost only.
[b] Lower starting dose indicated where previous side effect experience or polypharmacy; often applies to elderly patients.
[c] Higher doses often exceed upper doses in manufacturers' product monographs and are usually associated with increased risk of adverse effects. These doses should be used with caution in appropriately selected patients.
[d] For SSRIs, upper starting dose may be usual dose, e.g., fluoxetine 20 mg or sertraline 50 mg; otherwise, increments every 5–7 days.
Dosage adjustment may be required in renal impairment; see Appendix I.
Abbreviations: EPA-DHA = eicosapentaenoic acid-docosahexaenoic acid; GI = gastrointestinal; MAOI = monoamine oxidase inhibitor; RIMA = reversible inhibitor of monoamine oxidase A; SIADH = syndrome of inappropriate antidiuretic hormone ; SNRI = serotonin-norepinephrine reuptake inhibitor; SSRI = selective serotonin reuptake inhibitor; TCA = tricyclic antidepressant
Legend: $ < $30 $$ $30–60 $$$ $60–90 $$$$ $90–120

Suggested Readings

Australia. Beyondblue. *Perinatal mental health.* Available from: www.beyondblue.org.au/resources/health-professionals/perinatal-mental-health. Accessed June 3, 2014.

Bilsker D, Paterson R. *Antidepressant skills workbook.* 2nd ed. Burnaby (BC): Simon Fraser University; BC Mental Health & Addiction Services; 2005. Available from: www.comh.ca/antidepressant-skills/adult/. Accessed June 3, 2014.

Hollon SD, Jarrett RB, Nierenberg AA et al. Psychotherapy and medication in the treatment of adult and geriatric depression: which monotherapy or combined treatment? *J Clin Psychiatry* 2005;66(4):455-68.

Kennedy SH. Lam RW, Nutt DJ et al. *Treating depression effectively: applying clinical guidelines.* 2nd ed. London (GB): Informa Healthcare; 2007.

Lam RW, Kennedy SH, Grigoriadis S et al. Canadian Network for Mood and Anxiety Treatments (CANMAT) clinical guidelines for the management of major depressive disorder in adults. III. Pharmacotherapy. *J Affect Disord* 2009;117(Suppl 1):S26-43.

Lam RW, Wan DD, Cohen NL et al. Combining antidepressants for treatment-resistant depression: a review. *J Clin Psychiatry* 2002;63(8):685-93.

Yatham LN, Kennedy SH, Schaffer A et al. Canadian Network for Mood and Anxiety Treatments (CANMAT) and International Society for Bipolar Disorders (ISBD) collaborative update of CANMAT guidelines for the management of patients with bipolar disorder: update 2009. *Bipolar Disord* 2009;11(3):225-55.

References

1. American Psychiatric Association. *Diagnostic and statistical manual of mental disorders: DSM-5.* 5th ed. Washington (DC): American Psychiatric Association; 2013.
2. Kroenke K, Spitzer RL, Williams JB. The PHQ-9: validity of a brief depression severity measure. *J Gen Intern Med* 2001;16(9):606-13.
3. Arroll B, Khin N, Kerse N. Screening for depression in primary care with two verbally asked questions: cross sectional study. *BMJ* 2003;327(7424):1144-6.
4. McIntyre RS, Konarski JZ, Mancini DA et al. Measuring the severity of depression and remission in primary care: validation of the HAMD-7 scale. *CMAJ* 2005;173(11):1327-34.
5. Hirschfeld RM. The mood disorder questionnaire: a simple, patient-rated screening instrument for bipolar disorder. *Prim Care Companion J Clin Psychiatry* 2002;4(1):9-11.
6. Cox JL, Holden JM, Sagovsky R. Detection of postnatal depression. Development of the 10-item Edinburgh Postnatal Depression Scale. *Br J Psychiatry* 1987;150:782-6.
7. Wells KB, Sherbourne C, Schoenbaum M et al. Impact of disseminating quality improvement programs for depression in managed primary care: a randomized controlled trial. *JAMA* 2000;283(2):212-20.
8. Von Korff M, Goldberg D. Improving outcomes in depression. *BMJ* 2001;323(7319):948-9.
9. Rost K, Nutting P, Smith JL et al. Managing depression as a chronic disease: a randomised trial of ongoing treatment in primary care. *BMJ* 2002;325(7370):934-7.
10. Katon W, Von Korff M, Lin E et al. Collaborative management to achieve depression treatment guidelines. *J Clin Psychiatry* 1997;58(Suppl 1):20-3.
11. Simon GE, Von Korff M, Ludman EJ et al. Cost-effectiveness of a program to prevent depression relapse in primary care. *Med Care* 2002;40(10):941-50.
12. Schoenbaum M, Unutzer J, McCaffrey D et al. The effects of primary care depression treatment on patients' clinical status and employment. *Health Serv Res* 2002;37(5):1145-58.
13. Lave JR, Frank RG, Schulberg HC et al. Cost-effectiveness of treatments for major depression in primary care practice. *Arch Gen Psychiatry* 1998;55(7):645-51.
14. Kuyken W, Byford S, Taylor RS et al. Mindfulness-based cognitive therapy to prevent relapse in recurrent depression. *J Consult Clin Psychol* 2008;76(6):966-78.
15. Powers MB, Zum Vorde Sive Vording MB, Emmelkamp PM. Acceptance and commitment therapy: a meta-analytic review. *Psychother Psychosom* 2009;78(2):73-80.
16. Spek V, Cuijpers P, Nyklicek I et al. Internet-based cognitive behaviour therapy for symptoms of depression and anxiety: a meta-analysis. *Psychol Med* 2007;37(3):319-28.
17. Parikh SV, Segal ZV, Grigoriadis S et al. Canadian Network for Mood and Anxiety Treatments (CANMAT) clinical guidelines for the management of major depressive disorder in adults. II. Psychotherapy alone or in combination with antidepressant medication. *J Affect Disord* 2009;117(Suppl 1):S15-25.
18. Lin EH, Von Korff M, Katon W et al. The role of the primary care physician in patients' adherence to antidepressant therapy. *Med Care* 1995;33(1):67-74.
19. Ravindran AV, Lam RW, Filteau MJ et al. Canadian Network for Mood and Anxiety Treatments (CANMAT) clinical guidelines for the management of major depressive disorder in adults. V. Complementary and alternative medicine treatments. *J Affect Disord* 2009;117(Suppl 1):S54-64.
20. Lam RW, Kennedy SH, Grigoriadis S et al. Canadian Network for Mood and Anxiety Treatments (CANMAT) clinical guidelines for the management of major depressive disorder in adults. III . Pharmacotherapy. *J Affect Disord* 2009;117(Suppl 1):S26-43.

21. Cipriani A, Furukawa TA, Salanti G et al. Comparative efficacy and acceptability of 12 new-generation antidepressants: a multiple-treatments meta-analysis. *Lancet* 2009;373(9665):746-58.
22. Loke YK, Trivedi AN, Singh S. Meta-analysis: gastrointestinal bleeding due to interaction between selective serotonin uptake inhibitors and non-steroidal anti-inflammatory drugs. *Aliment Pharmacol Ther* 2008;27(1):31-40.
23. Montgomery S, Hansen T, Kasper S. Efficacy of escitalopram compared to citalopram: a meta-analysis. *Int J Neuropsychopharmacol* 2011;14(2):261-8.
24. Bielski RJ, Ventura D, Chang CC. A double-blind comparison of escitalopram and venlafaxine extended release in the treatment of major depressive disorder. *J Clin Psychiatry* 2004;65(9):1190-6.
25. Stahl SM. Basic psychopharmacology of antidepressants, part 1: Antidepressants have seven distinct mechanisms of action. *J Clin Psychiatry* 1998;59(Suppl 4):5-14.
26. Jorenby D. Clinical efficacy of bupropion in the management of smoking cessation. *Drugs* 2002;62(Suppl 2):25-35.
27. Clayton AH, Pradko JF, Croft HA et al. Prevalence of sexual dysfunction among newer antidepressants. *J Clin Psychiatry* 2002;63(4):357-66.
28. Kent JM. SNaRIs, NaSSAs, and NaRIs: new agents for the treatment of depression. *Lancet* 2000;355(9207):911-8.
29. Bossini L, Casolaro I, Koukouna D et al. Off-label uses of trazodone: a review. *Expert Opin Pharmacother* 2012;13(12):1707-17.
30. Thase ME, Nierenberg AA, Keller MB et al. Efficacy of mirtazapine for prevention of depressive relapse: a placebo-controlled double-blind trial of recently remitted high-risk patients. *J Clin Psychiatry* 2001;62(10):782-8.
31. Smith D, Dempster C, Glanville J. Efficacy and tolerability of venlafaxine compared with selective serotonin reuptake inhibitors and other antidepressants: a meta-analysis. *Br J Psychiatry* 2002;180:396-404.
32. Nemeroff CB, Entsuah R, Benattia I et al. Comprehensive analysis of remission (COMPARE) with venlafaxine versus SSRIs. *Biol Psychiatry* 2008;63(4):424-34.
33. Perahia DG, Pritchett YL, Kajdasz DK et al. A randomized, double-blind comparison of duloxetine and venlafaxine in the treatment of patients with major depressive disorder. *J Psychiatr Res* 2008;42(1):22-34.
34. Sopko MA, Ehret MJ, Grgas M. Desvenlafaxine: another "me too" drug? *Ann Pharmacother* 2008;42(10):1439-46.
35. Lourenco MT, Kennedy SH. Desvenlafaxine in the treatment of major depressive disorder. *Neuropsychiatr Dis Treat* 2009;5:127-36.
36. Cutler AJ, Montgomery SA, Feifel D et al. Extended release quetiapine fumarate monotherapy in major depressive disorder: a placebo- and duloxetine-controlled study. *J Clin Psychiatry* 2009;70(4):526-39.
37. Papakostas GI, Shelton RC, Zajecka JM et al. L-methylfolate as adjunctive therapy for SSRI-resistant major depression: results of two randomized, double-blind, parallel-sequential trials. *Am J Psychiatry* 2012;169(12):1267-74.
38. Parikh S, Segal ZV, Grigoriadis S et al. Canadian Network for Mood and Anxiety Treatments (CANMAT) clinical guidelines for the management of major depressive disorder in adults. II. Psychotherapy alone or in combination with antidepressant medication. *J Affect Disord* 2009;117(Suppl 1):S15-25.
39. Fava M, Rush AJ, Trivedi MH et al. Background and rationale for the sequenced treatment alternatives to relieve depression (STAR*D) study. *Psychiatr Clin North Am* 2003;26(2):457-94.
40. Kennedy SH, Lam RW. Enhancing outcomes in the management of treatment resistant depression: a focus on atypical antipsychotics. *Bipolar Disord* 2003;5(Suppl 2):36-47.
41. Kennedy SH, McCann SM, Masellis M et al. Combining bupropion SR with venlafaxine, paroxetine, or fluoxetine: a preliminary report on pharmacokinetic, therapeutic, and sexual dysfunction effects. *J Clin Psychiatry* 2002;63(3):181-6.
42. Zisook S, Rush AJ, Haight BR et al. Use of bupropion in combination with serotonin reuptake inhibitors. *Biol Psychiatry* 2006;59(3):203-10.
43. Ravindran AV, Kennedy SH, O'Donovan MC et al. Osmotic-release oral system methylphenidate augmentation of antidepressant monotherapy in major depressive disorder: results of a double-blind, randomized, placebo-controlled trial. *J Clin Psychiatry* 2008;69(1):87-94.
44. Hollon SD, Jarrett RB, Nierenberg AA et al. Psychotherapy and medication in the treatment of adult and geriatric depression: which monotherapy or combined treatment? *J Clin Psychiatry* 2005;66(4):455-68.
45. Sackeim HA, Haskett RF, Mulsant BH et al. Continuation pharmacotherapy in the prevention of relapse following electroconvulsive therapy: a randomized controlled trial. *JAMA* 2001;285(10):1299-307.
46. UK ECT Review Group. Efficacy and safety of electroconvulsive therapy in depressive disorders: a systematic review and meta-analysis. *Lancet* 2003;361(9360):799-808.
47. Kennedy SH, Giacobbe P. Treatment resistant depression–advances in somatic therapies. *Ann Clin Psychiatry* 2007;19(4):279-87.
48. Kusumakar V. Antidepressants and antipsychotics in the long-term treatment of bipolar disorder. *J Clin Psychiatry* 2002;63(Suppl 10):23-8.
49. Warner CH, Bobo W, Warner C et al. Antidepressant discontinuation syndrome. *Am Fam Physician* 2006;74(3):449-56.
50. Renoir T. Selective serotonin reuptake inhibitor antidepressant treatment discontinuation syndrome: a review of the clinical evidence and the possible mechanisms involved. *Front Pharmacol* 2013;4:45.
51. Natural Medicines Comprehensive Database. *Ginger*. Available from: naturaldatabase.therapeuticresearch.com. Accessed May 14, 2014. Subscription required.
52. Bonari L, Pinto N, Ahn E et al. Perinatal risks of untreated depression during pregnancy. *Can J Psychiatry* 2004;49(11):726-35.
53. Grote NK, Bridge JA, Gavin AR et al. A meta-analysis of depression during pregnancy and the risk of preterm birth, low birth weight, and intrauterine growth restriction. *Arch Gen Psychiatry* 2010;67(10):1012-24.
54. Grigoriadis S, VonderPorten EH, Mamisashvili L et al. The impact of maternal depression during pregnancy on perinatal outcomes: a systematic review and meta-analysis. *J Clin Psychiatry* 2013;74(4):e321-41.
55. Tuccori M, Montagnani S, Testi A et al. Use of selective serotonin reuptake inhibitors during pregnancy and risk of major and cardiovascular malformations: an update. *Postgrad Med* 2010;122(4):49-65.
56. Wurst KE, Poole C, Ephross SA et al. First trimester paroxetine use and the prevalence of congenital, specifically cardiac, defects: a meta-analysis of epidemiological studies. *Birth Defects Res A Clin Mol Teratol* 2010;88(3):159-70.
57. Grigoriadis S, VonderPorten EH, Mamisashvili L et al. Antidepressant exposure during pregnancy and congenital malformations: is there an association? a systematic review and meta-analysis of the best evidence. *J Clin Psychiatry* 2013;74(4):e293-308.
58. Ross LE, Grigoriadis S, Mamisashvili L et al. Selected pregnancy and delivery outcomes after exposure to antidepressant medication: a systematic review and meta-analysis. *JAMA Psychiatry* 2013;70(4):436-43.
59. Chambers CD, Hernandez-Diaz S, Van Marter LJ et al. Selective serotonin-reuptake inhibitors and risk of persistent pulmonary hypertension of the newborn. *N Engl J Med* 2006;354(6):579-87.
60. Kieler H, Artama M, Engeland A et al. Selective serotonin reuptake inhibitors during pregnancy and risk of persistent pulmonary hypertension in the newborn: population based cohort study from the five Nordic countries. *BMJ* 2012;344:d8012.

61. Grigoriadis S, Vonderporten EH, Mamisashvili L et al. Prenatal exposure to antidepressants and persistent pulmonary hypertension of the newborn: systematic review and meta-analysis. *BMJ* 2014;348:f6932.
62. Lattimore KA, Donn SM, Kaciroti N et al. Selective serotonin reuptake inhibitor (SSRI) use during pregnancy and effects on the fetus and newborn: a meta-analysis. *J Perinatol* 2005;25(9):595-604.
63. Grigoriadis S, VonderPorten EH, Mamisashvili L et al. The effect of prenatal antidepressant exposure on neonatal adaptation: a systematic review and meta-analysis. *J Clin Psychiatry* 2013;74(4):e309-20.
64. O'Hara MW, Schlechte JA, Lewis DA et al. Prospective study of postpartum blues. Biologic and psychosocial factors. *Arch Gen Psychiatry* 1991;48(9):801-6.
65. O'Hara MW, Swain AM. Rates and risk of postpartum depression–a meta-analysis. *Int Rev Psychiatry* 1996;8(1):37-54.
66. Sword W, Watt S, Gafni A et al. *The Ontario mother and infant survey postpartum health and social service utilization: a five-site Ontario study*. Ottawa (ON): Canadian Health Services Research Foundation; 2001.
67. Kendell RE, Chalmers JC, Platz C. Epidemiology of puerperal psychoses. *Br J Psychiatry* 1987;150:662-73.
68. Weissman AM, Levy BT, Hartz AJ et al. Pooled analysis of antidepressant levels in lactating mothers, breast milk, and nursing infants. *Am J Psychiatry* 2004;161(6):1066-78.
69. Greenberger D, Padesky CA. *Mind over mood: change how you feel by changing the way you think*. New York (NY): Guilford Press; 1996.
70. Burns DD. *Feeling good: the new mood therapy*. New York (NY): HarperCollins; 1999.

Chapter 7
Eating Disorders

C. Laird Birmingham, MD, MHSc, FRCPC, FACP, ABIM, FAED

The Diagnostic and Statistical Manual of Mental Disorders, 5th edition (DSM-5) published in 2013 provides new definitions for eating disorders.[1]

Anorexia nervosa primarily affects adolescent girls and young women. It is characterized by a distorted body image and excessive dieting that leads to severe weight loss and a pathological fear of becoming fat. Diagnostic criteria for anorexia nervosa *no longer require* the "refusal" to maintain a normal body weight, amenorrhea or the absence of at least 3 menstrual cycles.

Bulimia nervosa is characterized by frequent episodes of binge-eating followed by inappropriate behaviours such as self-induced vomiting to avoid weight gain. In DSM-5 the frequency of binge-eating and compensatory behaviours diagnostic criteria has been reduced to weekly (from twice weekly).

Goals of Therapy

- Assess and treat coexistent nutritional deficiencies
- Assess and treat the effects of malnutrition, e.g., osteoporosis, hypoglycemia, dehydration
- Improve cognitive and emotional function
- Identify and treat psychiatric comorbidity, e.g., anxiety, depression, family dysfunction, self-injurious behaviour, suicidal ideation
- Reduce or eliminate binge and purge behaviour
- Develop healthy eating habits
- For anorexia nervosa, achieve and maintain a healthy weight and body mass index (BMI)
- Prevent relapse

Investigations

- A thorough history with special attention to:
  - weight, eating habits, binge and purge behaviour, menstruation (in females), body image, use of vomiting, laxatives (oral formulations or rectal suppositories), diuretics, ipecac, products marketed as weight loss supplements, fasting and excessive exercising
  - developmental and psychological history
  - depression, anxiety, suicidal ideation, family dysfunction and sexual abuse
  - symptoms of malnutrition including chest wall pain, palpitations, loss of consciousness, hematemesis, seizures, abdominal pain, muscle weakness or cramping, episodes of confusion
  - dietary history
- Physical examination for parotid hypertrophy, jugular venous pressure, edema, abnormal dentition, Russell's sign (scarring over the knuckles caused by using the hand to induce vomiting); for anorexia nervosa, look also for postural hypotension, tachycardia, lanugo hair, hypercarotenemia, height, weight, measurements of body fat, proximal myopathy, neuromuscular hyperirritability (Chvostek's and Trousseau's signs)[2]
- Laboratory tests:

  - sodium, potassium, chloride, bicarbonate, creatinine, magnesium, calcium, phosphorus, zinc, vitamin B_{12}, ferritin; for anorexia nervosa, add ECG, hemoglobin, WBC count, urinalysis, RBC, folate and blood glucose (fasting and 2 hours after eating)
- For anorexia nervosa, a psychiatric and nutritional assessment if symptoms continue and weight does not normalize with 1–2 months of weekly follow-up and counselling[3]

Anorexia Nervosa

Therapeutic Choices

Figure 1 is an algorithm illustrating the management of anorexia nervosa.

Nonpharmacologic Choices

- Develop and maintain a rapport and therapeutic alliance.
- Consider the need for and role of family intervention and treatment (especially for children and adolescents).
- Set step-wise nutritional goals.
- Use nutritional supplements (e.g., Ensure, Boost) to achieve weight gain if not possible with food. Supportive nursing care at mealtime may improve success.[4] Tube feeding may be necessary if oral feeding fails.
- Exercise should be limited. A supervised graded exercise plan (such as nonexercise yoga) can reduce anxiety while not interfering with the rate of weight gain.[5]
- Warming by means of a warm room or warming vest may reduce anxiety, hasten recovery and improve the chances of long-term recovery.[6]
- Monitor binge and purge behaviour and set goals for normalization, e.g., a gradual tapering of laxatives.

Figure 1: **Management of Anorexia Nervosa**

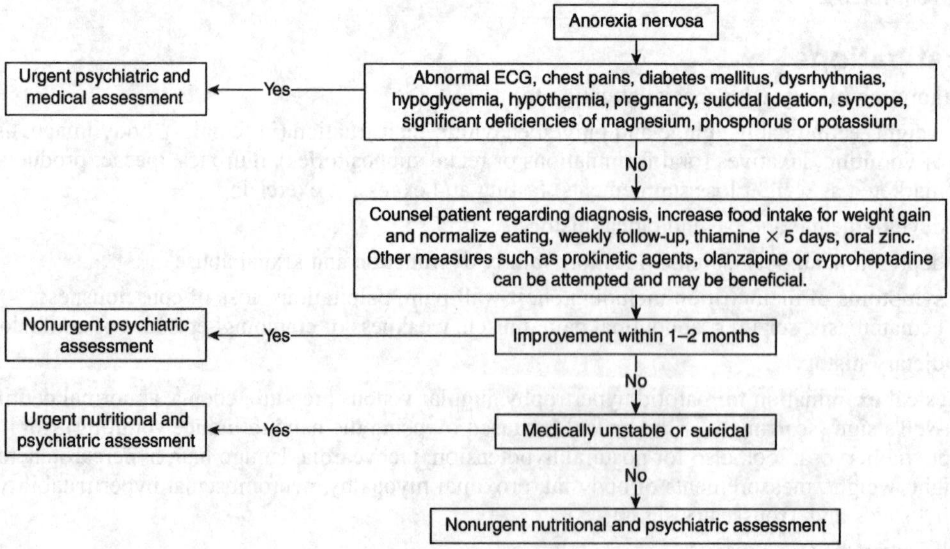

Pharmacologic Choices[7,8]

Table 1 lists drugs used in the management of anorexia nervosa.

Prokinetic Agents

The prokinetic agents **domperidone** and **metoclopramide** can reduce the feeling of fullness caused by decreased intestinal motility during the early stages of feeding.[9]

Unless the antinauseant effect of metoclopramide is needed, domperidone is the preferred agent because it has a lower incidence of extrapyramidal side effects. On rare occasions when the feeling of fullness is limiting a patient's treatment and domperidone or metoclopramide are not effective, consider adding **erythromycin**.[10,11]

Prokinetic agents have the potential to cause QT_c prolongation, especially in patients with other risk factors such as hypokalemia or hypoglycemia. Cisapride, the only prokinetic agent to be studied in this patient group, was withdrawn from the market because of its association with an increased rate of dysrhythmia and death.

Prucalopride is a newer 5-HT_4 receptor agonist that can help to normalize colonic function and treat constipation in patients with anorexia nervosa.[12] Unlike previously marketed 5-HT_4 agonists, prucalopride does not act at other receptors and does not cause cardiac complications associated with a prolonged QT_c interval. Prucalopride should be initiated at 2 mg daily po and should be decreased if possible to 1 mg daily po after 1–2 months.

Other Therapies

In patients with anorexia nervosa, **zinc gluconate** (100 mg daily po for 2 months) can increase the rate of weight gain (average 0.15 kg per day compared to 0.08 kg per day for placebo), irrespective of the serum zinc measurement.[13] Nausea affects about 2% of patients who take oral zinc; take with food to reduce this adverse effect.[8]

Olanzapine, a second-generation antipsychotic, decreases anorexic rumination resulting in improved motivation and may thereby promote weight gain, even in chronic anorexia nervosa.[14,15] A randomized controlled trial supported these findings and demonstrated that the rate of weight gain was not increased in patients with anorexia nervosa (beyond the weight gain olanzapine would be expected to cause in a person without anorexia).[16] This is important because anorexia nervosa sufferers would not use the medication if weight gain were rapid. Doses of 2.5–5 mg per day have been effective, with a maximum dose of 20 mg per day. Do not use olanzapine long term unless the benefits outweigh the risk of developing a movement disorder as an adverse effect. Duration of therapy is usually around 3 months—until it is no longer needed for weight gain and to a maximum BMI of 17 kg/m^2. If continued beyond this, olanzapine can cause a rapid increase in appetite and weight gain. Olanzapine can cause metabolic effects such as dyslipidemia. Diabetes due to reduced insulin sensitivity is also a potential adverse effect, but has not been observed in this patient group to date.

Cyproheptadine 4–16 mg at bedtime may be useful, particularly in chronic anorexia nervosa. It may cause a modest weight gain and can be used as a hypnotic.[17,18]

Benzodiazepines (e.g., **clonazepam**) can be used to treat severe anxiety. Take care to avoid dependence. Begin with clonazepam at 0.25–0.5 mg BID and cautiously titrate if necessary, no faster than every 3 days. The second-generation antipsychotic **quetiapine** is often used to manage anxiety in this setting because it is more effective than benzodiazepines and is not associated with dependence.[19,20]

SSRI antidepressants such as **fluoxetine** should be used only for coexistent depression, purge behaviour or anxiety disorders including obsessive-compulsive disorder, and if cardiac status is stable (e.g., QT_c less than 450 milliseconds; see Bulimia Nervosa, Antidepressants).[21]

Give **thiamine** 100 mg daily for 5 days at the beginning of feeding to prevent the development of Wernicke-Korsakoff syndrome (encephalopathy).

Ondansetron is not effective in controlling nausea or vomiting associated with eating disorders.[22]

Therapeutic Tips

- Realistic targets for weight gain are 0.9–1.4 kg per week in hospitalized patients and 0.2–0.5 kg per week for patients in outpatient programs.[23]
- Hypoglycemia can occur when the patient starts eating because liver glycogen stores are depleted. Measure blood glucose 2 hours after meals for the first 1–2 days of feeding and if confusion occurs.[24]
- Treat chronic laxative abuse by slowly tapering laxatives over months to years.[25] Prucalopride is effective in normalizing bowel movements in many patients with chronic laxative abuse.
- Body fat must be normalized for psychological treatment to be effective and for cure. Normal body fat[26] will allow normal cognitive and physiologic function.
- Refeeding syndrome is a serious complication that can occur when patients are treated for eating disorders.[27] Serious electrolyte disturbances, the hallmark of which is hypophosphatemia, can occur when patients are fed after a prolonged period of minimal caloric intake or starvation. Careful management by experienced clinicians is required.
- Women with anorexia nervosa can become pregnant when amenorrheic.[28]
- Refusal of treatment is common. Carefully reassess the treatment plan if this occurs.[29] Family therapy is particularly important for the treatment of children and adolescents.
- Suicidality, worsening depression and/or an inability to gain weight are indicators for referral to an eating disorders specialist. Outpatient, residential or inpatient eating disorder treatment may be required.[30]

Bulimia Nervosa

Therapeutic Choices

Figure 2 is an algorithm illustrating the management of bulimia nervosa.

Nonpharmacologic Choices

- Cognitive behavioural therapy and interpersonal therapy are helpful in addressing cognitive and emotional issues and reinforcing normal eating behaviour. Monitor the patient's progress.[3]
- Assess for suicidal ideation and depression and treat if present.
- Psychoeducational groups addressing nutritional and psychological issues can enhance individual therapy.[31,32]
- Various forms of guided self-help therapy (including Internet-based therapy) may be effective for patients with no coexistent psychiatric conditions, especially early in the course of the disease.[33,34,35,36,37]

Pharmacologic Choices

Table 2 lists drugs used in the management of bulimia nervosa.

Antidepressants

Antidepressants are effective in reducing binge-eating episodes by ≥50% in two-thirds of patients. There is no correlation between the presence of comorbid depression and antibulimic effects of the antidepressant, nor is there any evidence that one antidepressant is more effective than another.[38]

SSRIs, **venlafaxine** or **trazodone** can be used; **fluoxetine** is supported by the most evidence.[39,40,41] Trazodone can be useful in patients with insomnia associated with bulimia nervosa. Due to toxicity and poor adherence, do not prescribe tricyclic antidepressants, MAOIs, or bupropion. Bupropion has been associated with an increased risk of seizures in patients with eating disorders.

If symptoms persist after a trial of counselling and a trial of an antidepressant, treatment by a multidisciplinary team may be necessary. If therapy is effective, continue for at least 6 months, and preferably 1 year.

Therapeutic Tips

- Purging can reduce or prevent drug absorption. When pharmacotherapy is not effective, ask the patient about the timing of both purging behaviour and dose administration.
- A temporary worsening of binge and purge behaviour often occurs during psychological treatment, e.g., when a long-suppressed traumatic event such as sexual abuse is uncovered and addressed, or with significant life stress. This does not indicate a worsening in the patient's overall condition.
- Treatment with more than 1 antidepressant at the same time is not recommended—there are no proven advantages and there is a potential to increase adverse effects and cost.
- Response to medication will vary from patient to patient—a trial of several agents may be needed to find one that is effective.
- When an antidepressant is effective, continue for 6–12 months.
- When discontinuing antidepressants, taper the dose gradually to prevent the development of antidepressant discontinuation syndrome. For more information see Antidepressant Discontinuation Syndrome in Chapter 6.
- Treatment of psychiatric comorbidity is necessary for long-term cure.

Figure 2: **Management of Bulimia Nervosa**

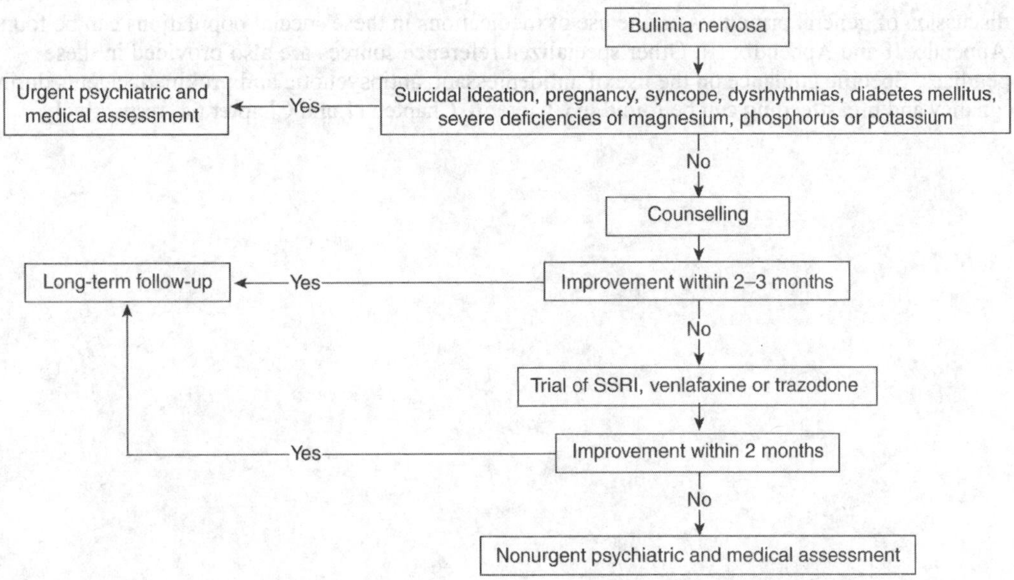

Choices during Pregnancy and Breastfeeding

Eating Disorders and Pregnancy

Amenorrheic patients with anorexia nervosa may ovulate and unless effective contraception is used, pregnancy can occur in these patients.[42,43,44,45,46] Medications, including oral contraceptives, may be missed, vomited or not absorbed.[47]

Eating disorder symptoms improve during pregnancy in two-thirds of women, but worsen in one-third.[48,49,50] In patients with eating disorders, the delivery is usually normal and the newborn is almost always healthy.[51,52] Nutrient deficiencies in the mother may affect the fetus.

Management

- Assess for depression or suicidality.[53,54]
- Reassess all medications regarding their risk in pregnancy, and discontinue or change drug therapy as required. An individual risk-benefit assessment should guide decision making.[55,56] As with any medical condition during pregnancy, use nonpharmacologic measures preferentially when possible.
- Biochemistry must be measured (see Investigations).
- Follow as a high-risk pregnancy, unless the eating disorder is mild.
- A dietitian should make recommendations for diet and nutrient supplements.
- Children are often aware of their mother's eating disorder and may take on a caregiver's role within the first few years of life. They also have an increased likelihood of developing disordered eating and body image.[57]

Eating Disorders and Breastfeeding

If the symptoms of eating disorders (particularly anorexia nervosa) are severe, breast milk production can be affected. Nevertheless most patients with eating disorders can successfully breastfeed their babies. Refer lactating women with eating disorders to a dietitian to optimize maternal and infant nutrition.

A discussion of general principles on the use of medications in these special populations can be found in Appendix II and Appendix III. Other specialized reference sources are also provided in these appendices. Specific guidance on the use of antidepressant, antipsychotic and prokinetic agents during pregnancy and breastfeeding can be found in Chapter 6, Chapter 11 and Chapter 64, respectively.

Table 1: **Drugs Used in Anorexia Nervosa**

Class	Drug	Dose	Adverse Effects	Drug Interactions	Cost[a]
Antipsychotics, Second-generation	*olanzapine* Zyprexa, Zyprexa Zydis, generics	2.5–20 mg/day po	Drowsiness, akathisia, dyslipidemia.	Fluvoxamine may increase olanzapine serum concentrations; other SSRIs are less likely to exhibit this interaction. Inducers of CYP1A2 such as carbamazepine, rifampin or cigarette smoking may decrease olanzapine serum concentrations; conversely, quitting smoking may necessitate a dose reduction to avoid toxicity. Inhibitors of CYP1A2 such as ciprofloxacin or ketoconazole may increase effects and toxicity of olanzapine. Caution re: other drugs with potential EPS such as metoclopramide; avoid concurrent use.	$$$
	quetiapine Seroquel, generics	12.5–50 mg before meals and at bedtime po Used to manage severe anxiety in this setting	Drowsiness, EPS effects, QT_c prolongation.	Increased hypotension with antihypertensives; additive sedation with CNS depressants, including alcohol; inhibitors of CYP3A4 such as erythromycin, clarithromycin, fluoxetine or ketoconazole can increase the effects and toxicity of quetiapine. Caution with other drugs that prolong the QT_c interval.	$
Benzodiazepines	*clonazepam* Rivotril, generics	Initial: 0.25–0.5 mg BID po May titrate cautiously at 3-day intervals if needed Usual maximum: 2–5 mg/day	Sedation, ataxia, weakness, dependence.	Potentiates effects of other CNS depressants, including alcohol.	$
$5\text{-}HT_4$ Receptor Agonists	*prucalopride* Resotran	1–2 mg daily po	Abdominal pain, diarrhea, headache, nausea.	Monitor therapy if combined with p-glycoprotein inhibitors such as erythromycin, ketoconazole, verapamil, cyclosporine. May increase prucalopride serum concentration and adverse effects. Prucalopride-induced diarrhea may affect the absorption of oral contraceptives.	$$$$
Prokinetic Agents	*domperidone* generics	10–20 mg 30 min before meals po May also be given at bedtime to deal with residual food ingested in evening	Diarrhea, abdominal discomfort, hyperprolactinemia, drowsiness; can prolong QT_c interval.	Opioids and antimuscarinics may antagonize action of domperidone in the gut. Caution with other drugs that prolong the QT_c interval.	$

(cont'd)

Table 1: **Drugs Used in Anorexia Nervosa** *(cont'd)*

Class	Drug	Dose	Adverse Effects	Drug Interactions	Cost[a]
	erythromycin generics	125 mg BID po	Diarrhea, abdominal discomfort, prolonged QT_c interval, dysrhythmias.	Inhibitor of CYP1A2 and potent inhibitor of CYP3A4; may increase effect and toxicity of substrates of these isoenzymes such as isotretinoin, mirtazapine, morphine, oxycodone, quetiapine, theophylline, trazodone, tricyclic antidepressants, venlafaxine. Caution with other drugs that prolong the QT_c interval.	$
	metoclopramide Metonia, generics	5–20 mg 30 min before meals po	Diarrhea, abdominal discomfort, hyperprolactinemia, drowsiness, restlessness; can prolong QT_c interval. Rarely, can cause EPS.	Avoid alcohol and other CNS depressants (additive sedative effects). Caution with other drugs that prolong the QT_c interval. Additive risk of EPS with antipsychotics; avoid concurrent use.	$
Supplements, mineral	*zinc gluconate* generics	100 mg daily po with meals for 2 months	Nausea; can cause a copper deficiency if taken in excess for months.	Zinc may reduce the serum concentration and efficacy of tetracycline; tetracycline doses should be taken 2–3 h before zinc.	$
Supplements, vitamin	*thiamine* generics	100 mg daily po × 5 days at start of refeeding	None expected.	None known.	$

[a] Cost of 30-day supply of mean dose; includes drug cost only.
Dosage adjustment may be required in renal impairment; see Appendix I.
Abbreviations: EPS = extrapyramidal symptoms
Legend: $ < $15 $$ $15–40 $$$ $40–65 $$$$ $65–100

Table 2: Drugs Used in Bulimia Nervosa

Class	Drug	Dose	Adverse Effects	Drug Interactions	Cost[a]
Selective Serotonin Reuptake Inhibitors[b]	*fluoxetine* Prozac, generics	20–60 mg daily po	Anxiety, GI discomfort (common), sexual dysfunction, increased risk of GI bleeding.	Do not use with MAOIs; inhibits CYP2D6—may increase effects and toxicity of many drugs including atomoxetine, dextromethorphan, mirtazapine, risperidone, TCAs; increased risk of GI bleeding with NSAIDs, antiplatelet agents.	$$
Serotonin Agonists	*trazodone* generics	100–500 mg daily po in single or divided doses	Sedation (common), anticholinergic adverse effects less common than with other TCAs.	Avoid use with MAOIs; caution with other serotonergic drugs such as SSRIs, SNRIs; inhibitors of CYP3A4 such as erythromycin, clarithromycin or ketoconazole can increase effects and toxicity of trazodone.	$
Serotonin-Norepinephrine Reuptake Inhibitors	*venlafaxine* (renal symbol) Effexor XR, generics	75–150 mg daily po	Nausea, drowsiness, nervousness, dizziness, dry mouth, hypertension at doses >300 mg.	Inhibitors of CYP2D6 or CYP3A4 such as erythromycin, clarithromycin, fluphenazine or ketoconazole can increase effects and toxicity of venlafaxine; do not use with MAOIs; caution with trazodone (serotonin syndrome).	$

[a] Cost of 30-day supply; includes drug cost only.
[b] For other SSRIs, see Chapter 6.
(renal symbol) Dosage adjustment may be required in renal impairment; see Appendix I.
Abbreviations: SNRI = serotonin-norepinephrine reuptake inhibitor; TCA = tricyclic antidepressant; XR = extended-release
Legend: $ < $15 $$ $15-45

Suggested Readings

Aigner M, Treasure J, Kaye W et al. World Federation of Societies of Biological Psychiatry (WFSBP) guidelines for the pharmacological treatment of eating disorders. *World J Biol Psychiatry* 2011;12(6):400-43.

American Dietetic Association. Position of the American Dietetic Association: nutrition intervention in the treatment of anorexia nervosa, bulimia nervosa, and other eating disorders. *J Am Diet Assoc* 2006;106(12):2073-82.

American Psychiatric Association. Treatment of patients with eating disorders, third edition. *Am J Psychiatry* 2006;163(7 Suppl):4-54.

Bacaltchuk J, Hay P. Antidepressants versus placebo for people with bulimia nervosa. *Cochrane Database Syst Rev* 2003;(4):CD003391.

Beumont P, Hay P, Beumont D et al. Australian and New Zealand clinical practice guidelines for the treatment of anorexia nervosa. *Aust N Z J Psychiatry* 2004;38(9):659-70.

Birmingham CL, Treasure J. *The medical management of eating disorders*. 2nd ed. Cambridge (GB): Cambridge University Press; 2010.

National Collaborating Centre for Mental Health; National Institute of Clinical Excellence. *Eating disorders: core interventions in the treatment and management of anorexia nervosa, bulimia nervosa and related eating disorders*. London (GB): NICE; 2004. Available from: www.nice.org.uk/nicemedia/live/10932/29218/29218.pdf.

References

1. American Psychiatric Association. *Diagnostic and statistical manual of mental disorders: DSM-5*. 5th ed. Washington (DC): American Psychiatric Publishing; 2013.
2. Tyler I, Birmingham CL. The interrater reliability of physical signs in patients with eating disorders. *Int J Eat Disord* 2001;30(3):343-5.
3. American Dietetic Association. Position of the American Dietetic Association: nutrition intervention in the treatment of anorexia nervosa, bulimia nervosa, and other eating disorders. *J Am Diet Assoc* 2006;106(12):2073-82.
4. Leichner P, Hall D, Calderon R. Meal support training for friends and families of patients with eating disorders. *Eat Disord* 2005;13(4):407-11.
5. Thien V, Thomas A, Markin D et al. Pilot study of a graded exercise program for the treatment of anorexia nervosa. *Int J Eat Disord* 2000;28(1):101-6.
6. Bergh C, Brodin U, Lindberg G et al. Randomized controlled trial of a treatment for anorexia and bulimia nervosa. *Proc Natl Acad Sci U S A* 2002;99(14):9486-91.
7. Zhu AJ, Walsh BT. Pharmacologic treatment of eating disorders. *Can J Psychiatry* 2002;47(3):227-34.
8. Aigner M, Treasure J, Kaye W et al. World Federation of Societies of Biological Psychiatry (WFSBP) guidelines for the pharmacological treatment of eating disorders. *World J Biol Psychiatry* 2011;12(6):400-43.
9. Leung M, Birmingham CL. Food fight: the management of anorexia nervosa and bulimia nervosa. *Pharmacy Practice* 1997;13(10):62-72.
10. Stacher G, Peeters TL, Bergmann H et al. Erythromycin effects on gastric emptying, antral motility and plasma motilin and pancreatic polypeptide concentrations in anorexia nervosa. *Gut* 1993;34(2):166-72.
11. Ray WA, Murray KT, Meredith S et al. Oral erythromycin and the risk of sudden death from cardiac causes. *N Engl J Med* 2004;351(11):1089-96.
12. Tack J, Stanghellini V, Dubois D et al. Effect of prucalopride on symptoms of chronic constipation. *Neurogastroenterol Motil* 2014;26(1):21-7.
13. Su JC, Birmingham CL. Zinc supplementation in the treatment of anorexia nervosa. *Eat Weight Disord* 2002;7(1):20-2.
14. La Via MC, Gray N, Kaye WH. Case reports of olanzapine treatment of anorexia nervosa. *Int J Eat Disord* 2000;27(3):363-6.
15. Mehler C, Wewetzer C, Schulze U et al. Olanzapine in children and adolescents with chronic anorexia nervosa. A study of five cases. *Eur Child Adolesc Psychiatry* 2001;10(2):151-7.
16. Mondraty N, Birmingham CL, Touyz S et al. Randomized controlled trial of olanzapine in the treatment of cognitions in anorexia nervosa. *Australas Psychiatry* 2005;13(1):72-5.
17. Halmi KA, Eckert E, LaDu TJ et al. Anorexia nervosa. Treatment efficacy of cyproheptadine and amitriptyline. *Arch Gen Psychiatry* 1986;43(2):177-81.
18. Halmi KA, Eckert E, Falk JR. Cyproheptadine for anorexia nervosa. *Lancet* 1982;1(8285):1357-8.
19. Powers PS, Bannon Y, Eubanks R et al. Quetiapine in anorexia nervosa patients: an open label outpatient pilot study. *Int J Eat Disord* 2007;40(1):21-6.
20. Sattar SP, Bhatia SC, Petty F. Potential benefits of quetiapine in the treatment of substance dependence disorders. *J Psychiatry Neurosci* 2004;29(6):452-7.
21. Walsh BT, Kaplan AS, Attia E et al. Fluoxetine after weight restoration in anorexia nervosa: a randomized controlled trial. *JAMA* 2006;295(22):2605-12.
22. Fung SM, Ferrill MJ. Treatment of bulimia nervosa with ondansetron. *Ann Pharmacother* 2001;35(10):1270-3.
23. American Psychiatric Association. Treatment of patients with eating disorders, third edition. *Am J Psychiatry* 2006;163(7 Suppl):4-54.
24. Puddicombe DM, Birmingham CL. Using the glucagon test to predict hypoglycemia in anorexia nervosa. *Eat Weight Disord* 2006;11(2):e72-4.
25. Harper J, Leung M, Birmingham CL. A blinded laxative taper for patients with eating disorders. *Eat Weight Disord* 2004;9(2):147-50.
26. Lear SA, Humphries KH, Kohli S et al. The use of BMI and waist circumference as surrogates of body fat differs by ethnicity. *Obesity (Silver Spring)* 2007;15(11):2817-24.
27. Birmingham CL, Treasure J. *The medical management of eating disorders*. 2nd ed. Cambridge (GB): Cambridge University Press; 2010.
28. Mehler PS. Diagnosis and care of patients with anorexia nervosa in primary care settings. *Ann Intern Med* 2001;134(11):1048-59.

29. Geller J, Cockell SJ, Drab DL. Assessing readiness for change in the eating disorders: the psychometric properties of the readiness and motivation interview. *Psychol Assess* 2001;13(2):189-98.
30. Kaplan AS. Psychological treatments for anorexia nervosa: a review of published studies and promising new directions. *Can J Psychiatry* 2002;47(3):235-42.
31. Davis R, McVey G, Heinmaa M et al. Sequencing of cognitive-behavioral treatments for bulimia nervosa. *Int J Eat Disord* 1999;25(4):361-74.
32. Hay PJ, Bacaltchuk J, Stefano S. Psychotherapy for bulimia nervosa and binging. *Cochrane Database Syst Rev* 2004;(3):CD000562.
33. Dolemeyer R, Tietjen A, Kersting A et al. Internet-based interventions for eating disorders in adults: a systematic review. *BMC Psychiatry* 2013;13:207.
34. Wagner G, Wagner G, Penelo E et al. Is technology assisted guided self-help successful in treating female adolescents with bulimia nervosa? *Neuropsychiatr* 2013;27(2):66-73.
35. Högdahl L, Birgegård A, Björck C. How effective is bibliotherapy-based self-help cognitive behavioral therapy with Internet support in clinical settings? Results from a pilot study. *Eat Weight Disord* 2013;18(1):37-44.
36. Fairburn CG. *Overcoming binge eating: the proven program to learn why you binge and how you can stop*. 2nd ed. New York (NY): Guilford; 2013.
37. Perkins SJ, Murphy R, Schmidt U et al. Self-help and guided self-help for eating disorders. *Cochrane Database Syst Rev* 2006;(3):CD004191.
38. Bacaltchuk J, Hay P. Antidepressants versus placebo for people with bulimia nervosa. *Cochrane Database Syst Rev* 2003;(4):CD003391.
39. Goldstein DJ, Wilson MG, Thompson VL et al. Long-term fluoxetine treatment of bulimia nervosa: Fluoxetine Bulimia Nervosa Research Group. *Br J Psychiatry* 1995;166(5):660-6.
40. Romano SJ, Halmi KA, Sarkar NP et al. A placebo-controlled study of fluoxetine in continued treatment of bulimia nervosa after successful acute fluoxetine treatment. *Am J Psychiatry* 2002;159(1):96-102.
41. Fluoxetine in the treatment of bulimia nervosa. A multicenter, placebo-controlled, double-blind trial. Fluoxetine Bulimia Nervosa Collaborative Study Group. *Arch Gen Psychiatry* 1992;49(2):139-47.
42. Beumont P, Tam P. Anorexia nervosa, infertility and pregnancy. *Med J Aust* 2001;174(3):155-6.
43. Crow SJ, Thuras P, Keel PK et al. Long-term menstrual and reproductive function in patients with bulimia nervosa. *Am J Psychiatry* 2002;159(6):1048-50.
44. Kye SL. Pregnancy in women with eating disorders. *Am J Psychiatry* 2002;159(7):1249-50.
45. Moschos S, Chan JL, Mantzoros CS. Leptin and reproduction: a review. *Fertil Steril* 2002;77(3):433-44.
46. Beumont PJ. Anorexia, LHRH and ovulation. *Med J Aust* 1985;142(1):77-8.
47. Abraham S, Taylor A, Conti J. Postnatal depression, eating, exercise, and vomiting before and during pregnancy. *Int J Eat Disord* 2001;29(4):482-7.
48. Crow SJ, Agras WS, Crosby R et al. Eating disorder symptoms in pregnancy: a prospective study. *Int J Eat Disord* 2008;41(3):277-9.
49. Micali N, Treasure J, Simonoff E. Eating disorders symptoms in pregnancy: a longitudinal study of women with recent and past eating disorders and obesity. *J Psychosom Res* 2007;63(3):297-303.
50. Ward VB. Eating disorders in pregnancy. *BMJ* 2008;336(7635):93-6.
51. Franko DL, Blais MA, Becker AE et al. Pregnancy complications and neonatal outcomes in women with eating disorders. *Am J Psychiatry* 2001;158(9):1461-6.
52. Micali N, Simonoff E, Treasure J. Risk of major adverse perinatal outcomes in women with eating disorders. *Br J Psychiatry* 2007;190:255-9.
53. Morgan JF, Lacey JH, Chung E. Risk of postnatal depression, miscarriage, and preterm birth in bulimia nervosa: retrospective controlled study. *Psychosom Med* 2006;68(3):487-92.
54. Bodnar LM, Sunder KR, Wisner KL. Treatment with selective serotonin reuptake inhibitors during pregnancy: deceleration of weight gain because of depression or drug? *Am J Psychiatry* 2006;163(6):986-91.
55. Norre J, Vandereycken W, Gordts S. The management of eating disorders in a fertility clinic: clinical guidelines. *J Psychosom Obstet Gynaecol* 2001;22(2):77-81.
56. Franko DL, Spurrell EB. Detection and management of eating disorders during pregnancy. *Obstet Gynecol* 2000;95(6 Pt 1):942-6.
57. Stein A, Woolley H, Senior R et al. Treating disturbances in the relationship between mothers with bulimic eating disorders and their infants: a randomized, controlled trial of video feedback. *Am J Psychiatry* 2006;163(5):899-906.

Chapter 8
Insomnia

Jonathan A.E. Fleming, MB, FRCPC, FABPN, FABSM

Insomnia is defined as dissatisfaction with sleep quality or quantity that is associated with one or more of the following features: difficulty falling asleep, difficulty staying asleep or early morning awakening without being able to return to sleep. The diagnosis requires that the sleep disturbance causes distress or impairment in functioning, occurs at least 3 nights per week for at least 3 months, and is not substance related.[1] Insomnia is a common symptom of a number of psychiatric and medical conditions including depression, anxiety and pain.

Goals of Therapy

- Promote subjectively sound and restorative sleep when external (e.g., stress, noise, jet lag) or internal (e.g., pain, anxiety) factors disrupt natural sleep
- Reduce subjective daytime impairment (e.g., dysphoria, fatigue, decreased alertness) associated with sleep loss
- Potentiate the effectiveness of behavioural interventions in managing patients with chronic insomnia[2]

Investigations

- A complete sleep history (Table 1) is *essential:*
  - to quantify current sleep performance and daytime impairment
  - to determine the outcome of previous interventions
  - to rule out other sleep pathologies including those for which hypnotics are contraindicated and potentially lethal, e.g., obstructive sleep apnea
- Completion of a sleep diary (Table 3) for one week, to quantify sleep performance and variability
- Psychiatric workup to rule out associated mental disorders (especially mood and anxiety disorders, drug and alcohol use)
- Medical workup to rule out associated medical disorders (especially those associated with nocturnal discomfort or pain such as arthritis, Parkinson's disease)
- Thorough drug history including prescription and nonprescription medications, herbal or other natural remedies, caffeine, nicotine, alcohol and recreational drugs
- Self-rating scales for depression and anxiety symptoms (such as the PHQ-9 available from www.ncbi.nlm.nih.gov/pmc/articles/PMC1495268/#app1 or the GAD-7 available from www.mpho.org/resource/d/34008/GAD708.19.08Cartwright.pdf) are useful screening tools for identifying depressive or anxiety disorders causing insomnia

  Note: Insomnia can be both an early symptom and a cause of depression.

Therapeutic Choices

Nonpharmacologic Choices

- Instruct patient in sleep hygiene, emphasizing the importance of rising at the same time 7 days a week, even when taking hypnotics (Figure 1, Table 2); monitor and encourage adherence throughout treatment and follow-up (important to success of *any* intervention).

- Suggest relaxation exercises (available as free downloads for home use, e.g., www.allaboutdepression.com/relax).
- Consider sleep restriction, stimulus control (avoidance of sensory arousal) or other behavioural approaches such as cognitive behavioural therapy (CBT-I),[3] either alone or in conjunction with pharmacologic interventions. Online CBT-I self-help programs are available for a fee from www.sleepio.com or cbtforinsomnia.com.
- Aerobic exercise, a useful modifier of stress and dysphoric moods, also promotes deeper and more restful sleep; encourage patients with insomnia to eliminate daytime rest periods and increase exercise, just as brisk walking (Table 2).

Pharmacologic Choices

Short courses of hypnotics (Figure 1, Table 4) are useful combined with good sleep hygiene (Table 2). A comprehensive evaluation, education stressing the importance of sleep hygiene (especially preventing extended sleeping such as naps or nocturnal sleep periods of more than 8 hours) and careful monitoring of progress are important. With these measures, use of the preferred agents (short-acting benzodiazepines or benzodiazepine receptor agonists) is usually straightforward in patients with insomnia.

It is inappropriate to use the sedative side effect of another medication (e.g., antidepressants, antihistamines, antipsychotics such as quetiapine[4]) to avoid using a benzodiazepine or benzodiazepine receptor agonist, in cases where the latter agents are the treatment of choice.

Generally, self-medication with nonprescription agents such as diphenhydramine is not recommended. For distressing insomnia lasting more than a few days, patients should see their physician for an accurate diagnosis of symptoms and monitoring of the treatment plan.

Table 1: The Sleep History

1. Time data (can also be collected as part of a sleep diary—Table 3)
Did you nap or lie down to rest today? If yes, when and for how long?
What time did you go to bed last night?
What time did you put out the lights?
How long did it take you to fall asleep?
How many times did you awaken last night?
How long was your longest awake period; when was it? What time did you finally awaken?
What time did you get out of bed?
How many hours of sleep did you get last night?
2. Questions about the sleep period
Do physical symptoms, such as pain, prevent you from falling asleep?
Do mental or emotional symptoms (e.g., worry or anxiety) prevent you from falling asleep?
When you awaken during the night, what awakens you? (Snoring? Gasping for air? Dreams/nightmares? Noise?)
When you get up for the day, do you have any symptoms? (Headache? Confusion? Sleepiness?)
3. Questions for the patient's bed partner
Does your partner snore, gasp or make choking sounds during the night?
Does your partner stop breathing during the night?
Do your partner's legs twitch, jerk or kick during the night?
Has your partner's use of alcohol, nicotine, caffeine or other drugs changed recently?
Has your partner's mood or emotional state changed recently?
What do you think is the cause of your partner's sleep problem?

Benzodiazepines

All benzodiazepines have sedative and hypnotic properties, but differ significantly in potency and pharmacokinetics. All may cause confusion and ataxia, especially in the elderly and the medically ill. Benzodiazepines also confer a significant risk of dependence and withdrawal symptoms with long-term use, and judicious therapeutic trials for insomnia involve use for up to 2 weeks.

Benzodiazepines that have been studied in sleep-disturbed patients are generally preferred over other agents. When insomnia is secondary to prominent anxiety symptoms, a long-acting benzodiazepine (such as **clonazepam**) given at night may promote sleep and also manage daytime anxiety. It is inappropriate to use one benzodiazepine to manage anxiety during the day and a different one as a bedtime hypnotic agent, in the same patient.

Figure 1: **Management of Insomnia**

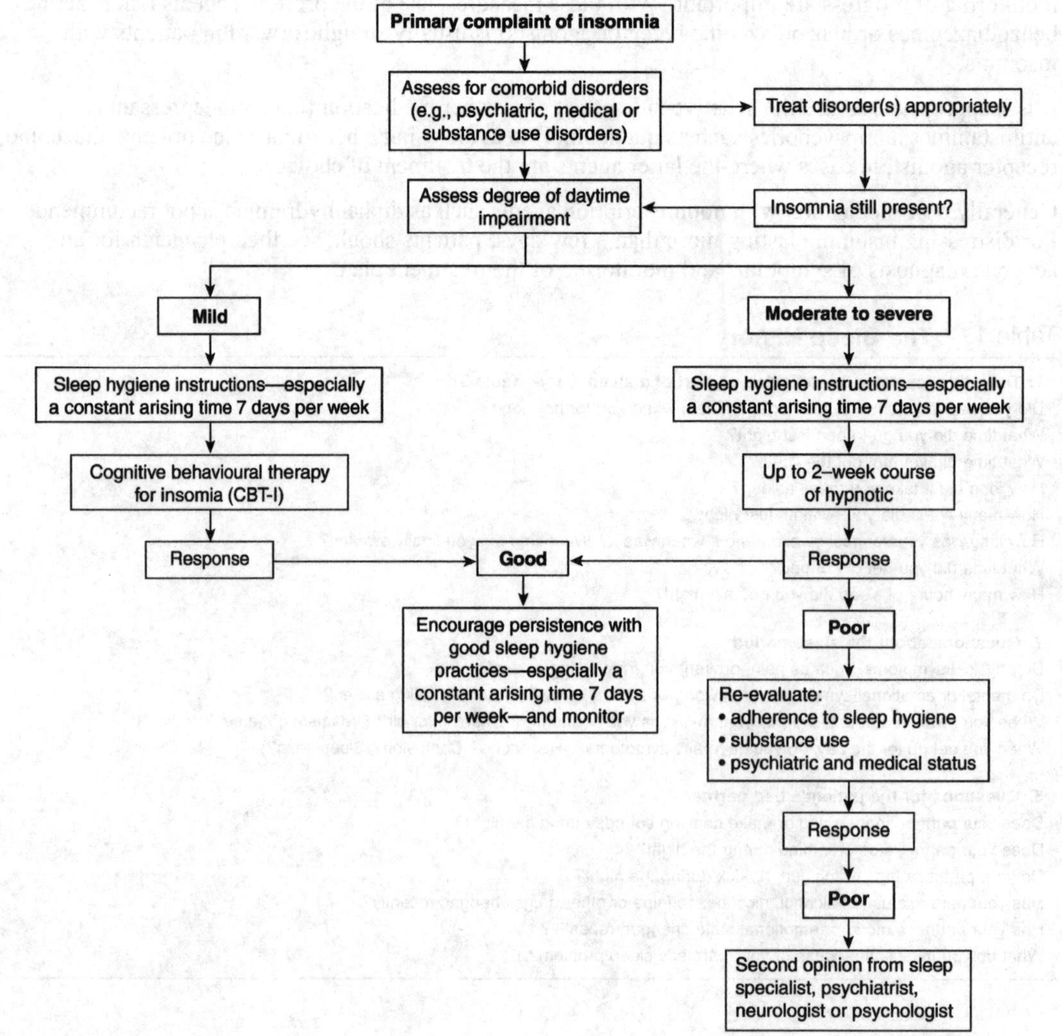

Table 2: **Sleep Hygiene Guidelines**

1. Keep a regular sleep-wake schedule, with a consistent arising time 7 days per week.
2. Restrict the sleep period to the average sleep time you have obtained each night over the preceding week.
3. Avoid sleeping in, extensive periods of horizontal rest or daytime napping; these activities usually affect the subsequent night's sleep.
4. Get regular exercise every day: about 40 minutes of an activity with sufficient intensity to cause sweating. If evening exercise prevents sleep, schedule the exercise earlier in the day.
5. Avoid caffeine, nicotine, alcohol and other recreational drugs, all of which disturb sleep. If you must smoke do not do so after 7:00 p.m.
6. Plan a quiet period before lights out; a warm bath may be helpful.
7. Avoid large meals late in the evening; a light carbohydrate snack (e.g., crackers and warm milk) before bedtime can be helpful.
8. Turn the clock face away and always use the alarm. Looking at the clock time on awakening can cause emotional arousal (performance anxiety or anger) that prevents return to sleep.
9. As much as possible, keep the bedroom dark and soundproofed. If you live in a noisy area, consider ear plugs.
10. Use the bedroom only for sleep and intimacy; using the bed as a reading place, office or media centre conditions you to be alert in a place that should be associated with quiet and sleep. If you awaken during the night and are wide awake, get up, leave the bedroom and do something quiet until you feel drowsy-tired, then return to bed.

Note: Pharmacologic (or any) interventions will be less effective if these guidelines are not followed. In mild cases of insomnia, sleep hygiene strategies, practised consistently and together, may be sufficient to reinstate a normal sleep pattern.

In Canada, 4 benzodiazepines (flurazepam, nitrazepam, temazepam and triazolam) are officially indicated for insomnia. However, **flurazepam** and **nitrazepam** are not recommended, particularly in the elderly.[5] Because of their longer half-lives, flurazepam and nitrazepam accumulate with repeated dosing and are associated with more hangover effects than shorter-acting agents. In the elderly, they cause higher cortical impairment resulting in confusion and falls.

Temazepam is a good all-purpose hypnotic with a half-life sufficient to cover the sleep period without causing hangover effects. However, few hypnotics have proven tolerability in the elderly, and temazepam may be associated with falls in this population.[6] It causes less rebound insomnia than more potent agents such as lorazepam.

Triazolam has a fast onset and short duration of action, which makes it more suited to use in *initial insomnia* (first third of the night) than *maintenance insomnia* (last third of the night). Because these pharmacokinetic properties may confer a higher risk of abuse and dependence, a shorter treatment course (5–7 days) is recommended for triazolam. In addition to causing rebound insomnia, triazolam has a unique, dose-related adverse effect profile (confusion, agitation and amnesia) making it unsuitable for use in the elderly.[7] Some experts recommend against use of triazolam in any patient.

Although the number of comparative studies is relatively small, **oxazepam** is as effective as the benzodiazepines that are officially indicated for insomnia.[8,9] In patients with initial insomnia, oxazepam should be given 60–90 minutes before bedtime because of its slow absorption, although patients should be aware that some sedation/impairment could occur before this time. Conversely, patients who have no difficulty falling asleep but experience maintenance insomnia can take oxazepam when getting into bed.

There are few trials studying the effects of **lorazepam** on insomnia. Lorazepam may cause significant rebound effects such as anxiety and tension.[10]

Table 3: **Sleep Diary**

Date							
Daytime							
Caffeine intake (what, when)							
Alcohol intake (what, when)							
Nicotine use (what, when)							
Naps (start time, end time)							
Exercise (what, when)							
Overall daytime functioning, on a scale of 1 to 5 (1 = alert, energetic; 5 = fatigued, sleepy)							
Nighttime							
What time did you go to bed?							
Did you watch television in bed?							
Did you read in bed?							
How long did it take to fall asleep?							
For each time you woke up during the night, record the following: 1. Time you were awake (e.g., 1:10–2:30 a.m.) 2. What woke you up (e.g., snoring, gasping for air, bad dreams, pet, noise)?							
What time did you *wake up* for the day?							
What time did you *get out of bed* for the day?							
How many hours of sleep did you get?							
How did you feel when you woke up this morning, on a scale of 1 to 5? (1 = refreshed, alert; 5 = fatigued, sleepy)							

Benzodiazepine Receptor Agonists

Although not a benzodiazepine, the cyclopyrrolone **zopiclone** acts at the benzodiazepine receptor and so has similar therapeutic and side effects. Although psychomotor impairment associated with combined use of zopiclone and small amounts of alcohol has been shown to be minor, zopiclone can have residual or hangover effects that could impair morning driving, when used with or without alcohol.[11] Compared with benzodiazepines, tolerance to zopiclone's hypnotic effect may be delayed and rebound insomnia may be reduced.[12] **Eszopiclone**, the active (S+) isomer of zopiclone, shares similar pharmacologic properties to the racemic compound but is more potent.[13] Several studies have demonstrated efficacy in transient and chronic insomnia. One study showed continued efficacy over 12 months of use with no evidence of tolerance or a withdrawal syndrome or rebound insomnia on discontinuation.[14] Eszopiclone in not available in Canada.

Zolpidem is an imidazopyrine with preferential affinity to benzodiazepine type I receptors. Memory disturbances and complex sleep behaviours (night eating, somnambulism) have been reported in patients using zolpidem. Gender and age-based differences in metabolic clearance of zolpidem and incidence of complex sleep behaviours have led to lower dosing recommendations for women and elderly patients.[15,16] As with all hypnotics, zolpidem must not be combined with alcohol.

Other Hypnotics

The toxicity and drug interaction profile of **chloral hydrate** make it less safe than benzodiazepines. Tolerance to its hypnotic effect typically develops within 2 weeks. Its use is not recommended.[17] **Barbiturates** are contraindicated in the management of insomnia due to their unacceptable safety profile.[18]

In high dosages (>1 g), **L-tryptophan** has a hypnotic effect, but it is not as predictable as that seen with traditional hypnotics.[19] It may be useful when one wishes to avoid benzodiazepines.

Use of **melatonin** (1–5 mg) in the management of insomnia remains controversial.[20] A meta-analysis of nineteen studies on the effects of melatonin on insomnia showed a decrease in the time to onset of sleep (weighted mean difference 7.06 minutes), an increase in total sleep time (weighted mean difference 8.25 minutes) and an improvement in overall sleep quality.[21] Improvement increased with dose and treatment duration; trials with higher dosages and longer duration had greater effects on shortening sleep onset latency and increasing total sleep time. Though the effect size is smaller than for other pharmacologic treatments for insomnia, melatonin may have a role in the management of insomnia given its relatively benign side effect profile.

Ramelteon, a novel compound with chronohypnotic properties (causing phase shifts in circadian rhythm) and high selectivity for MT_1 and MT_2 melatonin receptors, is available in the US but not in Canada. In various animal models, ramelteon has demonstrated hypnotic properties[22] with no effect on learning, memory or motor coordination. Human studies in young adults and elderly patients show it is effective and well tolerated.[23]

Choices during Pregnancy and Breastfeeding

Insomnia and Pregnancy

Disrupted sleep is one of the most frequently reported complaints of pregnant women, and tends to worsen as the pregnancy progresses.[24] Multiple endogenous factors, such as endocrine changes, physical discomfort and bladder distention, contribute to this common complaint. In the postpartum period, exogenous factors, e.g., the child's sleep-wake and feeding schedules, further disrupt sleep. Additionally, psychological factors, e.g., anxiety, or the emergence of psychiatric disorders during the pregnancy or after the birth can add to the insomnia burden with persistent sleep complaints increasing the risk of postpartum mood disorders.[25] Two sleep disorders, sleep apnea[26] and restless legs syndrome (see Chapter 24),[27] are known to worsen during pregnancy and may present as insomnia in the pregnant patient.

There has been little research on the effects of insomnia during pregnancy on maternal functioning and no randomized controlled studies of any intervention in this population. Regardless of cause, it is likely that significantly disrupted sleep during pregnancy and in the postpartum period will impair the mother's quality of life by causing similar daytime impairments to those seen in the nonpregnant population,[28] and that this impairment may adversely affect the mother-child bond.

When insomnia is severe, carefully consider the risk-benefit ratio to both the mother and developing fetus when using a pharmacologic intervention.[29] Although lacking empirical evidence, intermittent dosing using the safest medication, at the lowest effective dose, combined with behavioural strategies is reasonable.

Management of Insomnia during Pregnancy and Postpartum Period

Although not well studied, clinical experience suggests that behavioural techniques are effective in pregnant patients with insomnia and are the treatments of choice when distress and impairment are mild to moderate.

Evidence for the safety of psychotropics in human pregnancy is derived from patients who have been inadvertently exposed to these medications at conception. Orofacial malformations were the most feared consequence of **benzodiazepine** exposure but the risk appears small (0.1% vs. 0.06%) and in some studies, nonexistent.[30]

Benzodiazepines are associated with more prenatal and perinatal risks than **zopiclone**.[31] Neonatal flaccidity, hypothermia, respiratory depression and feeding difficulties have been reported in infants whose mothers received benzodiazepines late in pregnancy; these infants may also be at risk of experiencing withdrawal symptoms during the postnatal period. **Zolpidem** has been associated with a higher risk of preterm deliveries, delivery of small-for-gestational-age infants and cesarean delivery, and is not recommended in pregnancy.[32]

Although derived from limited data, available evidence suggests the preferred hypnotic for use in pregnancy is zopiclone.[33,34]

Diphenhydramine, an antihistamine commonly used as a nonprescription hypnotic (though not recommended), may cause neonatal depression if used during labour, and whether it enters breast milk is unknown.[35]

Insomnia and Breastfeeding

A review of hypnotic drug use during breastfeeding suggests that with respect to **benzodiazepines**,[36] **zolpidem**[37] and **zopiclone**,[36] the amount of active drug excreted in breast milk is generally quite low, and they can be used safely with appropriate monitoring. Behavioural interventions to manage insomnia are preferred, but should medications be required, low doses of short-acting benzodiazepines or benzodiazepine receptor agonists (used intermittently or for short periods) appear relatively safe.

When long-acting benzodiazepines are used during pregnancy, they should be switched to short-acting agents before delivery, to minimize effects on the fetus. There is a risk of inducing a withdrawal syndrome, particularly if high-potency benzodiazepines (such as **alprazolam**) are withdrawn abruptly. When there is marked functional impairment in the mother, supportive assistance from a relative, nanny or nurse, may improve coping. Regulating the sleep period as much as possible and ensuring regular exercise (such as walking) will help both mood and sleep performance. Monitor the baby for signs of sedation (e.g., lethargy, drowsiness, poor suckling, weight loss) or other adverse effects, and to ensure appropriate thriving.

A discussion of general principles on the use of medications in these special populations can be found in Appendix II and Appendix III. Other specialized reference sources are also provided in these appendices.

Therapeutic Tips

- Sleep diaries (Table 3) are often helpful in delineating the initial complaint, monitoring progress and facilitating withdrawal.
- The degree of daytime impairment directs the intervention: if there is an acute change in daytime functioning, a short course of hypnotics may be indicated; if the daytime impairment is mild or chronic, try a behavioural intervention (e.g., sleep restriction) first.
- Always start hypnotics at the lowest dose and use them for the shortest possible time.
- Set realistic treatment goals with the patient, mainly to minimize daytime impairment; a chronic poor sleeper will not be turned into a good sleeper overnight.
- Warn patients about combined effects when hypnotics are used with other CNS depressants. They should never be combined with alcohol.
- If a short course of a hypnotic has been used, plan to withdraw it at a low-stress time, e.g., a weekend. Two nights before the planned withdrawal, the patient should shorten the sleep time (while staying on the medication) by 20 minutes. This modest degree of sleep deprivation will promote physiological sleepiness, which should counterbalance any sleep disruption associated with withdrawal. This shortened sleep period should be maintained for one week.
- Insomnia often occurs as a symptom, comorbid condition or prodrome of other psychiatric conditions such as depression and/or anxiety disorders.[38,39] Chronic sleep disturbance of at least 1 year in duration increases the risk of a mood disorder in subsequent years.[40,41] Vigilance is required for the emergence of a mood disorder, which should be managed with appropriate specific therapy. Short-term use of adjunctive hypnotic agents such as benzodiazepines or benzodiazepine receptor agonists may be appropriate and beneficial in select patients with depression [Evidence: SORT B*].[42,43]

---

* SORT (Strength of Recommendation Taxonomy) is a rating system (A, B or C) that addresses the quality of available evidence. For more information consult **How to Use *Compendium of Therapeutic Choices*** on page xxv.

Table 4: Drugs Used to Manage Insomnia

Class	Drug	Dose (bedtime PRN)	Adverse Effects	Drug Interactions	Comments	Cost[a]
Benzodiazepines	*lorazepam* Ativan, generics	Initial: 0.5 mg po Maximum: 1 mg po	*Benzodiazepines:* dose-dependent ataxia, dizziness; dependence/withdrawal symptoms. *Lorazepam:* may cause more rebound insomnia on withdrawal than temazepam or oxazepam; may cause amnesia with higher dosages.	Additive sedation with CNS depressants such as alcohol.	Widely used as a hypnotic although not officially indicated.	$
	oxazepam generics	Initial: 10–15 mg po Maximum: 30 mg po	See benzodiazepines.	See lorazepam.	Slowly absorbed; should be taken 60–90 min before bedtime for *initial* insomnia, but some sedation/impairment may occur earlier; no hangover effects. Not officially indicated as a hypnotic.	$
	temazepam Restoril, generics	Initial: 15 mg po Maximum: 30 mg po	See benzodiazepines.	Substrate of CYP3A4; metabolism could be increased by inducers (e.g., carbamazepine, phenytoin) or decreased by inhibitors (e.g., cimetidine, clarithromycin, efavirenz, erythromycin, grapefruit juice, itraconazole, ketoconazole, ritonavir) of the enzyme.	Good all-purpose hypnotic; does not accumulate.	$
	triazolam generics	Initial: 0.125 mg po Maximum: 0.25 mg po	See benzodiazepines. *Triazolam:* anterograde amnesia (especially with higher dosages, concurrent use of alcohol) and other potency and dose-related side effects (rebound insomnia, daytime anxiety) have limited its use; useful for *initiating* sleep.	See temazepam.	Absence of hangover effects is an advantage (does not affect daytime alertness). Higher risk of abuse/dependence than other benzodiazepines. Avoid in elderly patients, especially in doses >0.125 mg.	$$

Class	Drug	Dose (bedtime PRN)	Adverse Effects	Drug Interactions	Comments	Cost[a]
Benzodiazepine Receptor Agonists	*zolpidem* Sublinox	Men (<65 y): 5–10 mg po Women: 5 mg po Elderly patients (≥65 y): 5 mg po	Complex sleep behaviours such as night eating, somnambulism, with no recollection of such activities. Discontinue immediately if such reactions occur.	Do not combine with alcohol. Additive sedation with other CNS depressants. Increased risk of complex sleep behaviours in combination with other CNS-active drugs. Avoid zolpidem in patients taking moderate to strong inhibitors of CYP3A4 such as clarithromycin, erythromycin, grapefruit juice, itraconazole, ketoconazole, metronidazole, sertraline, verapamil, due to risk of decreased zolpidem clearance.	Use only when there is a period of at least 7–8 h before planned awakening. Avoid in patients with a history of somnambulism.	$$$
	zopiclone Imovane, Rhovane, generics	Initial: 3.75 mg po (geriatric) Usual adult dose: 7.5 mg po Maximum: 7.5 mg po	Major adverse effect is bitter/metallic taste.	Minimal additive effects with low doses of alcohol.	Does not accumulate; minimal cognitive effects;[44] may cause less rebound on withdrawal.	$$
Serotonin Precursors	*L-tryptophan* Tryptan, generics	1–3 g 20 min before bedtime po	May cause serotonin syndrome (shivering, diaphoresis, hypomanic behaviour and ataxia) alone (rarely) or when combined with other serotonergic drugs.	Combined therapy with serotonergic drugs such as triptans, SSRIs, SNRIs or MAOIs can increase the risk of serotonin syndrome.	Alternative to benzodiazepines and benzodiazepine receptoragonists; erratic response.	$$$

[a] Cost of 14-day supply; includes drug cost only.

Abbreviations: MAOI = monamine oxidase inhibitor; SNRI = serotonin-norepinephrine reuptake inhibitor; SSRI = selective serotonin reuptake inhibitor

Legend: $ < $2 $$ $2–15 $$$ $15–30

Suggested Readings

McMillan JM, Aitken E, Holroyd-Leduc JM. Management of insomnia and long-term use of sedative-hypnotic drugs in older patients. *CMAJ* 2013;185(17):1499-505.

National Institute for Health and Care Excellence. *Antenatal and postnatal mental health: clinical management and service guidance*. Issued February 2007. Available from: www.nice.org.uk/CG045.

Roehrs T, Roth T. Insomnia pharmacotherapy. *Neurotherapeutics* 2012;9(4):728-38.

Wilson SJ, Nutt DJ, Alford C et al. British Association for the Psychopharmacology consensus statement on evidence-based treatment of insomnia, parasomnias and circadian rhythm disorders. *J Psychopharmacol* 2010;24(11):1577-601.

References

1. American Psychiatric Association. *Diagnostic and statistical manual of mental disorders: DSM-5*. 5th ed. Washington (DC): American Psychiatric Publishing; 2013.
2. Vallieres A, Morin CM, Guay B. Sequential combinations of drug and cognitive behavioral therapy for chronic insomnia: an exploratory study. *Behav Res Ther* 2005;43(12):1611-30.
3. Edinger JD, Means MK. Cognitive-behavioral therapy for primary insomnia. *Clin Psychol Rev* 2005;25(5):539-58.
4. Anderson SL, Vande Griend JP. Quetiapine for insomnia: a review of the literature. *Am J Health Syst Pharm* 2014;71(5):394-402.
5. Reynolds CF et al. Treatment of insomnia in the elderly. In: Salzman C, ed. *Clinical geriatric psychopharmacology*. 3rd ed. Baltimore (MD): Williams & Wilkins; 1998.
6. Frels C, Williams P, Narayanan S et al. Iatrogenic causes of falls in hospitalised elderly patients: a case-control study. *Postgrad Med J* 2002;78(922):487-9.
7. Schneider DL. Insomnia. Safe and effective therapy for sleep problems in the older patient. *Geriatrics* 2002;57(5):24-6, 29, 32.
8. Bliwise D, Seidel W, Greenblatt DJ et al. Nighttime and daytime efficacy of flurazepam and oxazepam in chronic insomnia. *Am J Psychiatry* 1984;141(2):191-5.
9. Feldmeier C, Kapp W. Comparative clinical studies with midazolam, oxazepam and placebo. *Br J Clin Pharmacol* 1983;16(Suppl 1):151S-155S.
10. Kales A, Bixler EO, Soldatos CR et al. Lorazepam: effects on sleep and withdrawal phenomena. *Pharmacology* 1986;32(3):121-30.
11. Vermeeren A. Residual effects of hypnotics: epidemiology and clinical implications. *CNS Drugs* 2004;18(5):297-328.
12. Voderholzer U, Riemann D, Hornyak M et al. A double-blind, randomized and placebo-controlled study on the polysomnographic withdrawal effects of zopiclone, zolpidem and triazolam in healthy subjects. *Eur Arch Psychiatry Clin Neurosci* 2001;251(3):117-23.
13. Melton ST, Wood JM, Kirkwood CK. Eszopiclone for insomnia. *Ann Pharmacother* 2005;39(10):1659-66.
14. Roth T, Walsh JK, Krystal A et al. An evaluation of the efficacy and safety of eszopiclone over 12 months in patients with chronic primary insomnia. *Sleep Med* 2005;6(6):487-95.
15. Greenblatt DJ, Harmatz JS, von Moltke LL et al. Comparative kinetics and response to the benzodiazepine agonists triazolam and zolpidem: evaluation of sex-dependent differences. *J Pharmacol Exp Ther* 2000;293(2):435-43.
16. Health Canada. *Sublinox (zolpidem tartrate)—new dosage recommendations to minimize risk of next-day impairment in both women and men—for health professionals*. 2014. Available from: healthycanadians.gc.ca/recall-alert-rappel-avis/hc-sc/2014/37415a-eng.php.
17. Frankland A, Robinson MJ. Fatal chloral hydrate overdoses: unnecessary tragedies. *Can J Psychiatry* 2001;46(8):763-4.
18. Morgan WW. Abuse liability of barbiturates and other sedative-hypnotics. *Adv Alcohol Subst Abuse* 1990;9(1-2):67-82.
19. Schneider-Helmert D, Spinweber CL. Evaluation of L-tryptophan for treatment of insomnia: a review. *Psychopharmacology (Berl)* 1986;89(1):1-7.
20. Olde Rikkert MG, Rigaud AS. Melatonin in elderly patients with insomnia. A systematic review. *Z Gerontol Geriatr* 2001;34(6):491-7.
21. Ferracioli-Oda E, Qawasmi A, Bloch MH. Meta-analysis: melatonin for the treatment of primary sleep disorders. *PLoS One* 2013;8(5):e63773.
22. Erman M, Seiden D, Zammit G et al. An efficacy, safety, and dose-response study of Ramelteon in patients with chronic primary insomnia. *Sleep Med* 2006;7(1):17-24.
23. Pandi-Perumal SR, Srinivasan V, Spence DW et al. Ramelteon: a review of its therapeutic potential in sleep disorders. *Adv Ther* 2009;26(6):613-26.
24. Facco FL, Kramer J, Ho KH et al. Sleep disturbances in pregnancy. *Obstet Gynecol* 2010;115(1):77-83.
25. Goyal D, Gay CL, Lee KA. Patterns of sleep disruption and depressive symptoms in new mothers. *J Perinat Neonatal Nurs* 2007;21(2):123-9.
26. Maasilta P, Bachour A, Teramo K et al. Sleep-related disordered breathing during pregnancy in obese women. *Chest* 2001;120(5):1448-54.
27. Kranick SM, Mowry EM, Colcher A et al. Movement disorders and pregnancy: a review of the literature. *Mov Disord* 2010;25(6):665-71.
28. Kyle SD, Morgan K, Espie CA. Insomnia and health-related quality of life. *Sleep Med Rev* 2010;14(1):69-82.
29. Einarson A, Selby P, Koren G. Abrupt discontinuation of psychotropic drugs during pregnancy: fear of teratogenic risk and impact of counselling. *J Psychiatry Neurosci* 2001;26(1):44-8.
30. Addis A, Dolovich LR, Einarson TR et al. Can we use anxiolytics during pregnancy without anxiety? *Can Fam Physician* 2000;46:549-51.
31. Wikner BN, Stiller CO, Bergman U et al. Use of benzodiazepines and benzodiazepine receptor agonists during pregnancy: neonatal outcome and congenital malformations. *Pharmacoepidemiol Drug Saf* 2007;16(11):1203-10.
32. Wang LH, Lin HC, Lin CC et al. Increased risk of adverse pregnancy outcomes in women receiving zolpidem during pregnancy. *Clin Pharmacol Ther* 2010;88(3):369-74.
33. Wilson SJ, Nutt DJ, Alford C et al. British Association for Psychopharmacology consensus statement on evidence-based treatment of insomnia, parasomnias and circadian rhythm disorders. *J Psychopharmacol* 2010;24(11):1577-601.
34. Diav-Citrin O, Okotore B, Lucarelli K et al. Pregnancy outcome following first-trimester exposure to zopiclone: a prospective controlled cohort study. *Am J Perinatol* 1999;16(4):157-60.
35. Buhimschi CS, Weiner CP. Medications in pregnancy and lactation: Part 2. Drugs with minimal or unknown human teratogenic effect. *Obstet Gynecol* 2009;113(2 Pt 1):417-32.

36. Fortinguerra F, Clavenna A, Bonati M. Psychotropic drug use during breastfeeding: a review of the evidence. *Pediatrics* 2009;124(4):e547-56.
37. Pons G, Francoual C, Guillet P et al. Zolpidem excretion in breast milk. *Eur J Clin Pharmacol* 1989;37(3):245-8.
38. Alvaro PK, Roberts RM, Harris JK. A systematic review assessing bidirectionality between sleep disturbances, anxiety, and depression. *Sleep* 2013;36(7):1059-68.
39. Sivertsen B, Salo P, Mykletun A et al. The bidirectional association between depression and insomnia: the HUNT study. *Psychosom Med* 2012;74(7):758-65.
40. Ford DE, Kamerow DB. Epidemiologic study of sleep disturbances and psychiatric disorders. An opportunity for prevention? *JAMA* 1989;262(11):1479-84.
41. Baglioni C, Battagliese G, Feige B et al. Insomnia as a predictor of depression: a meta-analytic evaluation of longitudinal epidemiological studies. *J Affect Disord* 2011;135(1-3):10-9.
42. Lam RW, Kennedy SH, Grigoriadis S et al. Canadian Network for Mood and Anxiety Treatments (CANMAT) clinical guidelines for the management of major depressive disorder in adults. III. Pharmacotherapy. *J Affect Disord* 2009;117(Suppl 1):S26-43.
43. Furukawa TA, Streiner DL, Young LT. Antidepressants plus benzodiazepines for major depression. *Cochrane Database Syst Rev* 2005;(1):CD001026.
44. Silva A, Collao A, Orellana M et al. Zopiclone, but not brotizolam, impairs memory storage during sleep. *Neurosci Res* 2003;47(2):241-3.

Psychiatric Disorders

Chapter 9
Obsessive-Compulsive Disorder

R. P. Swinson, MD, FRCPsych, FRCPC

Obsessive-compulsive disorder (OCD) is now classified separately from anxiety disorders in the Diagnostic and Statistical Manual of Mental Disorders 5th edition (DSM-5).[1] Related conditions in the same classification include body dysmorphic disorder, hoarding disorder, trichotillomania (hair-pulling disorder), excoriation disorder, and OCD that is substance/medication-induced or related to another medical condition.

OCD frequently starts early in life and often becomes a chronic condition. The mean age of onset is about 20 years with 25% of cases beginning by age 14. On average the onset is earlier in males. The defining symptoms are obsessions and compulsions. Obsessions are thoughts, images or urges that provoke anxiety and are unwanted, repetitive and difficult to control. Compulsions consist of repetitive behaviours that may be visible, such as washing or turning a light switch on and off, or may be mental actions such as counting or repeating a phrase in a precise manner. In severe OCD these ritualistic behaviours may occupy hours each day and can be extremely disabling.

Goals of Therapy

- Eliminate or decrease symptoms of OCD
- Eliminate or decrease OCD-associated disability
- Prevent recurrence
- Treat comorbid conditions

Investigations

- Thorough history with attention to:
  - nature and onset of symptoms
  - nature and extent of disability
  - presence of comorbid medical or psychiatric conditions

Note: Treat comorbid mood disorders, especially depression, as the primary condition.

- Criteria and interview questions assist in obtaining an accurate diagnosis (Table 1, Table 2)
- Physical examination to exclude endocrine or cardiac disorders and to look for signs of substance use
- Laboratory tests:
  - CBC, liver function tests, gamma-glutamyl transpeptidase (GGT to screen for alcohol use), thyroid indices (supersensitive TSH), ECG

Note: Treat physical disorders of recent onset before making a definitive diagnosis of an OCD.

Therapeutic Choices

Cognitive behavioural therapy (CBT) and pharmacotherapy with SSRIs or SNRIs are considered to be first-line treatments for OCD. The efficacy for both modalities is supported by a significant number of high-quality studies. A combination of these 2 modalities may help to increase the clinical response or reduce the risk of relapse when medication is discontinued.

Table 1: **Diagnosis Criteria**[2]

- Presence of obsessions (persistent, disturbing thoughts that cannot be reasoned away) or compulsions (uncontrollable impulses to do something against one's conscious will)
- Patient has recognized that the obsessions or compulsions are excessive or unreasonable
- Obsessions/compulsions cause distress, are time consuming or interfere with patient's routine, occupation, or academic or social functioning
- Obsessions/compulsions are not due to substance abuse or another medical or mental disorder

Table 2: **Interview Questions to Identify Presence of Obsessions or Compulsions**[2]

Obsessions	Is patient experiencing disturbing thoughts, images or urges that recur or are difficult to ignore? For example, "Do troubling thoughts or images come into your mind without you wanting to have them and are they difficult to get rid of?"
Compulsions	Does patient feel compelled to do something that doesn't make sense to them or that they don't want to do? For example, "Do you feel that you have to count, wash, clean or check things repeatedly when you know that it isn't really necessary?"

Nonpharmacologic Choices

Two psychological treatments for OCD, *exposure and response prevention* (ERP) and *cognitive therapy* (CT), have been shown repeatedly to be more effective than no treatment or supportive therapies.[3,4] Some studies have found that ERP is more effective than medication.[5] In one randomized trial in an outpatient setting, ERP, clomipramine, and a combination of both were found to be significantly more effective than placebo in 122 adults with OCD. ERP and ERP plus clomipramine were superior to clomipramine alone. ERP reduced the Yale Brown Obsessive Compulsive scale (YBOCS) score by 55% and the Clinical Global Impression improvement scale (CGI-I) by 32%. The ERP in this study was intensive and may be difficult to replicate in regular clinical practice.

Brain stimulation therapies have recently been investigated in the treatment of OCD. *Transcranial magnetic stimulation* (TMS) and *deep brain stimulation* (DBS) have been used to treat OCD that has not responded to the usual first-line therapies. TMS consists of the application of magnetic stimulation to targeted areas of the brain.[6,7,8]

In a small study of 17 patients, DBS reduced YBOCS scores by 25% after 12 months of stimulation in the ventral capsule/ventral striatum area.[9] A review of 90 patients receiving DBS in the internal capsule/ventral striatum showed a 50% decrease in YBOCS scores in the first 3 months of treatment. The limited number and low quality of available clinical trials keeps this technique from being recognized as a standard treatment. However, DBS is available as an alternative prior to selecting an ablative technique.[10]

Pharmacologic Choices

Drug therapy is indicated for many patients and is often more readily available than CBT. First-, second- and third-line options are listed in Figure 1, Table 3 and Table 4.

The SSRIs **citalopram, escitalopram, fluoxetine, fluvoxamine, paroxetine** and **sertraline**, in usual antidepressant doses, are recommended as first-line treatment for OCD.[2,11] It may take up to 12 weeks of therapy to produce a significant change in symptoms;[12] a trial at full dosage for at least 6 weeks is required to assess the potential benefit of each SSRI. A recent study demonstrated that a 20% reduction in baseline YBOCS score at week 4 predicted response at week 12. Subjects who had less than 20% improvement had only a 20% chance of response at week 12 compared to 55% for those with greater improvement.[13] There is no strong evidence to suggest that SSRIs vary in efficacy, but patients may respond to or tolerate one drug better than others in the same class. Second-line options include **clomipramine**, **venlafaxine** and **mirtazapine**. Clomipramine and venlafaxine are effective, but use is limited by their respective side effect profiles; mirtazapine is less effective and causes significant weight gain. Although SSRIs and SNRIs are better tolerated than clomipramine, some patients may experience agitation early in therapy leading to discontinuation of these drugs. To minimize early adverse effects, initiate SSRIs or SNRIs with lower doses and titrate slowly to an effective dose.

If successful, treatment should continue for a minimum of 6 months in acute therapy and may continue for years. When stopping any antidepressant, taper gradually to minimize discontinuation effects and warn patients to report any early signs of relapse.[2] For more information about antidepressant discontinuation syndrome, see Chapter 6.

It is estimated that 40–60% of patients do not respond adequately to SSRIs. In these instances consider increasing the dose or augmentation with another mode of therapy. If available, CBT can be used to augment pharmacologic treatment response.[14,15] First- (i.e., haloperidol) and second-generation (i.e., olanzapine, quetiapine, risperidone, aripiprazole) antipsychotics have been studied in this setting. A systematic review and a meta-analysis have concluded that antipsychotic augmentation of SSRI treatment will benefit about 30% of patients.[16,17] While olanzapine was not shown to be better than placebo, limited data support the addition of **quetiapine** or **risperidone** to SSRIs to increase the response in OCD. There is insufficient evidence to guide the use of one over the other. Adverse effects (e.g., sedation) will affect the tolerability of this group of drugs and must be weighed carefully against the limited benefits they provide.

In a 12-week placebo-controlled study, **topiramate** plus an SSRI improved patient compulsion scores, but not obsessions.[18] Some other agents such as **riluzole**, **tramadol**, **gabapentin** and **pindolol** have shown some benefit as augmentation therapy in patients who were refractory to other treatments.[2] The efficacy of other agents affecting glutamatergic systems, such as **ketamine** and **memantine**, are being investigated for their ability to reduce OCD symptoms when combined with an SSRI.[19,20]

Benzodiazepines alone are not usually helpful in treating OCD.

In DSM-5, hoarding disorder and body dysmorphic disorder (BDD) have been separated from OCD and now have their own diagnostic category. Standard treatment for hoarding disorder consists of CBT and serotonergic medications; for nonresponders augmentation with second-generation antipsychotics or haloperidol may be beneficial.[21] BDD also responds to the same treatment regimens as OCD and hoarding disorder.[22,23]

Figure 1: Drug Therapy for Obsessive-Compulsive Disorder

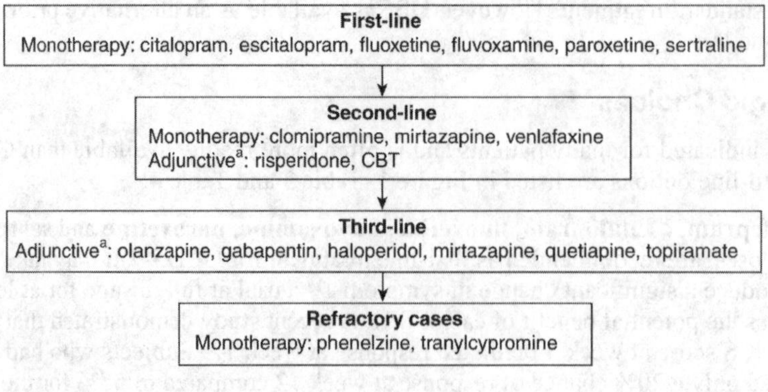

[a] Add on to first- or second-line monotherapy.
Abbreviations: CBT = cognitive behavioural therapy

Choices during Pregnancy and Breastfeeding

OCD and Pregnancy

During pregnancy, obsessive-compulsive symptoms, particularly obsessional ideas about causing harm to the baby, may worsen and can be extremely disturbing. These ideas are often accompanied by marked guilt and depression. Many people with psychiatric disorders do not bring their distress to the attention of healthcare providers.

Whenever possible, it is important to screen for the presence of OCD or other psychiatric symptoms before conception occurs. Screening can be repeated during the pregnancy and particularly postpartum. If a woman is suffering from marked psychological distress related to pregnancy and breastfeeding, it is imperative to screen for the presence of mood symptoms and suicidality.

When a woman experiences severe psychiatric symptoms during pregnancy or postpartum, referral to a psychiatrist may be necessary. In major centres, women's mental health programs are usually available and are attuned to responding to consultation requests quickly.

Preconceptional treatment can be offered for disorders that are producing significant distress or are interfering with functioning. Obsessive-compulsive disorder with high fear of contamination may prevent a woman from entering settings where there is a perceived high risk of coming into contact with infections.

Management during Pregnancy

There is good evidence to show that psychological treatments can have beneficial effects for more than half of those who persist with a treatment program. CBT can be administered without restriction throughout pregnancy. Therapies based in meditative or relaxation techniques may be more acceptable than pharmacologic approaches.[24]

If symptoms are severe and producing significant impairment, medications can be appropriate and effective.[25] **SSRIs**, **SNRIs** and **TCAs** are initial treatment options for OCD in the pregnant patient.

SSRIs and SNRIs may cause agitation, sweating, nausea, GI distress and weight gain. There have been reports of a slightly higher (but still low) risk of congenital abnormalities involving the heart or cleft lip/palate.[26] Use of these drugs in the 3rd trimester may be associated with neonatal withdrawal symptoms such as tremors, increased muscle tone, feeding or digestive problems or respiratory distress.

The use of SSRIs and SNRIs may be warranted in patients with severe symptoms that could affect fetal or maternal safety or health. In general, the lowest effective dose should be used for the shortest time necessary. General principles for management of depression during pregnancy are applicable to the management of OCD disorders.[26,27] See also Chapter 6 for information on management of depression during pregnancy and breastfeeding.

OCD and Breastfeeding

In the postpartum period, severe anxiety can impede the mother's sleep and erode her confidence in caring for her child. A woman with severe OCD can be so tormented by thoughts of potentially harming her child that she may refuse to be involved with caring for it. In such cases a psychiatric consultation is urgently required, and treatment consideration should include admitting the mother and child to hospital.

As in pregnancy, nonpharmacologic options should be used whenever possible in the postpartum period, particularly in breastfeeding women. If drug therapy is necessary, consider **paroxetine** and **sertraline**, since both have low concentrations in breast milk.[28]

A discussion of general principles on the use of medications in these special populations can be found in Appendix II and Appendix III. Other specialized reference sources are also provided in these appendices.

Therapeutic Tips

- If response to initial therapy is not adequate, optimize the dose and assess adherence before switching agents.
- If the first antidepressant at optimal dosage is not effective or not tolerated, switch to another first-line antidepressant.
- If the second antidepressant is not effective consider switching to clomipramine or add risperidone as adjunctive therapy.

Table 3: Drugs for First-line Management of Obsessive-Compulsive Disorder[2]

Class	Drug	Dose	Adverse Effects	Drug Interactions	Comments	Cost[a]
Selective Serotonin Reuptake Inhibitors	*citalopram* Celexa, CTP 30, generics	Initial: 10–20 mg/day po Target: 20–40 mg/day po Maximum: 40 mg/day	Agitation (on initiation of therapy), nausea, anorgasmia, insomnia, headache, increased appetite, diarrhea, increased risk of GI bleeding. Dose-related QT_c prolongation.	Serotonin syndrome with MAOIs (hypertension, tremor, agitation, hypomania); caution with other serotonergic drugs including amphetamine derivatives, dextromethorphan, dihydroergotamine, linezolid, lithium, meperidine, pentazocine, selegiline, St. John's wort, trazodone, triptans, tryptophan (increased risk of serotonin syndrome); increased risk of GI bleeding with NSAIDs, antiplatelet agents. SSRIs are substrates and inhibitors of several cytochrome P450 isoenzymes. This may result in decreased clearance of many drugs (e.g., clozapine, methadone, mexiletine, phenytoin, pimozide, propafenone) or reduced enzymatic conversion of a prodrug to its active form (e.g., clopidogrel, codeine, tamoxifen). Avoid combined use with drugs associated with prolonged QT_c interval/torsades de pointes, such as amiodarone, azithromycin, clarithromycin, domperidone, erythromycin, haloperidol, methadone, pimozide, quinine, sotalol, ziprasidone.	May take 2–3 months for maximum effect. Discontinue gradually.	$
	escitalopram Cipralex, Cipralex MELTZ	Initial: 10–20 mg/day po Target: 20–40 mg/day po Maximum: 40 mg/day po	See citalopram.	See citalopram.	See citalopram.	$$$
	fluoxetine Prozac, generics	Initial: 10–20 mg/day po Target: 40–80 mg/day po Maximum: 80 mg/day po	Agitation (on initiation of therapy), nausea, anorgasmia, insomnia, headache, increased appetite, diarrhea, increased risk of GI bleeding.	See citalopram.	See citalopram.	$$

(cont'd)

Table 3: **Drugs for First-line Management of Obsessive-Compulsive Disorder[2]** *(cont'd)*

Class	Drug	Dose	Adverse Effects	Drug Interactions	Comments	Cost[a]
	fluvoxamine Luvox, generics	Initial: 50–100 mg/day po Target: 200–300 mg/day po Maximum: 300 mg/day po	See fluoxetine.	See citalopram.	See citalopram.	$$
	paroxetine immediate-release Paxil, generics	Initial: 10–20 mg/day po Target: 40–60 mg/day po Maximum: 60 mg/day po	See fluoxetine.	See citalopram.	See citalopram.	$
	paroxetine controlled-release Paxil CR	25–50 mg/day po	See fluoxetine.	See citalopram.	See citalopram.	$$$$
	sertraline Zoloft, generics	Initial: 50–100 mg/day po Target: 200 mg/day po Maximum: 200 mg/day po	See fluoxetine.	See citalopram.	See citalopram.	$

[a] Cost of 30-day supply of mean dosage; includes drug cost only.
Dosage adjustment may be required in renal impairment; see Appendix I.
Abbreviations: MAOI = monoamine oxidase inhibitor; NSAID = nonsteroidal anti-inflammatory drug; SSRI = selective serotonin reuptake inhibitor
Legend: $ < $30 $$ $30–60 $$$ $60–90 $$$$ $90–120

Table 4: **Drugs for Second- and Third-line Management of Obsessive-Compulsive Disorder**[2]

Class	Drug	Dose	Adverse Effects	Drug Interactions	Comments	Cost[a]
Antidepressants, noradrenergic and specific serotonergic	*mirtazapine* Remeron, Remeron RD, generics	30–60 mg QHS po	Somnolence, increased appetite/weight gain, dizziness.	Do not use with MAOIs. Additive sedation with other CNS depressants such as alcohol, benzodiazepines; substrate of CYP1A2, 2D6 and 3A4—caution with inhibitors or inducers of these isoenzymes.	**Second-line** monotherapy when SSRIs fail. Orally disintegrating tablets can be taken without water.	$
Antidepressants, serotonin-norepinephrine reuptake inhibitors	*venlafaxine* Effexor XR, generics	Initial: 37.5–75 mg/day po Usual: 112.5–225 mg/day po High: 300–375 mg/day po	Nausea, sleep disturbance, drowsiness, nervousness, dizziness, dry mouth. Dose-related hypertension occurs rarely, particularly at doses ≥225 mg/day.	Use with MAOIs may lead to potentially fatal reaction initially presenting with tremor, agitation, hypomania, hyperthermia and/or hypertension. Inhibitors of CYP2D6 or CYP3A4 may increase venlafaxine levels.	**Second-line** monotherapy when SSRIs fail.	$$
Antidepressants, tricyclic	*clomipramine* Anafranil, generics	100–250 mg/day po Adjunctive: 10–50 mg/day po	CNS effects (agitation on initiation of therapy, confusion, drowsiness, headache), anticholinergic effects (dry mouth, blurred vision, constipation, etc.), weight gain, nausea, cardiovascular effects (tachycardia, arrhythmias, orthostatic hypotension), anorgasmia, erectile dysfunction.	May increase effect of anticholinergic drugs, CNS depressants, warfarin; do not use MAOIs concurrently.	**Second-line** monotherapy when SSRIs fail. **Third-line** augmentation therapy with SSRI or SNRI. May take 2–3 months for maximum effect.	$$$
Antipsychotics, First-generation	*haloperidol*, generics	5–10 mg daily po	Sedation, parkinsonism, akathisia, EPS, neuroleptic malignant syndrome, QT_c prolongation.	Additive effects with other CNS depressants, antagonism of dopamine agonists.	**Third-line** augmentation of SSRI or SNRI. Use only if second-generation antipsychotics not effective or not tolerated.	$$

(cont'd)

Table 4: Drugs for Second- and Third-line Management of Obsessive-Compulsive Disorder[2] *(cont'd)*

Class	Drug	Dose	Adverse Effects	Drug Interactions	Comments	Cost[a]
Antipsychotics, Second-generation	*olanzapine* Zyprexa, Zyprexa Zydis, generics	Initial: 2.5 mg daily po Titrate gradually to desired effect, usually 2.5–5 mg daily po. May need to increase to a maximum of 10 mg per day po	Weight gain, dizziness, sedation, anticholinergic effects, hepatic aminotransferase elevation, orthostatic hypotension, increased risk of diabetes and dyslipidemia, EPS (especially akathisia), QT_c prolongation.	Sedation with CNS depressants; may potentiate antihypertensive drug effects; inhibitors of CYP1A2 or CYP2D6 such as diltiazem, fluvoxamine or paroxetine may increase olanzapine levels; inducers of CYP1A2 or CYP3A4 such as barbiturates, carbamazepine, phenytoin or rifampin may decrease olanzapine levels.	**Third-line** augmentation of SSRI or SNRI. Advise patients about antipsychotic-associated body temperature dysregulation and prevention of heat stroke (e.g., hydration, sun protection).	$$
	quetiapine Seroquel, Seroquel XR, generics	Initial: 50 mg daily po Titrate to 150 mg daily po, or higher if necessary. Usual maximum: 400 mg daily po	Sedation, dizziness, weight gain, orthostatic hypotension, hepatic aminotransferase elevation, headache, anticholinergic effects, increased risk of diabetes and dyslipidemia, possible increased risk of cataracts; may decrease thyroid hormone levels, QT_c prolongation.	Additive sedation with CNS depressants; may potentiate antihypertensive drug effects; inhibitors of CYP3A4 such as clarithromycin, erythromycin, grapefruit juice, ketoconazole or prednisone may increase quetiapine levels; inducers of CYP3A4 such as carbamazepine, phenytoin or rifampin may decrease quetiapine levels.	**Third-line** augmentation of SSRI or SNRI. Advise patients about antipsychotic-associated body temperature dysregulation and prevention of heat stroke (e.g., hydration, sun protection).	$$
	risperidone ➊ Risperdal preparations, generics	0.5–3 mg daily po	Insomnia, headaches, weight gain, lipid and glucose dysregulation, orthostatic hypotension, rhinitis, anxiety, dose-related hyperprolactinemia, EPS and QT_c prolongation. Risk of intraoperative floppy iris syndrome in patients undergoing cataract surgery who have been exposed to risperidone.	Additive sedation with CNS depressants; may potentiate antihypertensive drug effects; inhibitors of CYP3A4 such as clarithromycin, erythromycin, grapefruit juice, ketoconazole or prednisone) may increase risperidone levels; inducers of CYP3A4 such as carbamazepine, phenytoin or rifampin may decrease risperidone levels.	**Second-line** augmentation of SSRI or SNRI or clomipramine. Advise patients about antipsychotic-associated body temperature dysregulation and prevention of heat stroke (e.g., hydration, sun protection).	$$
GABA Derivatives	*gabapentin* ➊ Neurontin, generics	Initial: 300 mg/day po Usual: 900–1800 mg/day po in 2 divided doses	Somnolence, dizziness, ataxia, vision changes.	Magnesium- and aluminum-containing antacids may decrease the absorption of gabapentin.	**Third-line** augmentation of SSRI or SNRI.	$$$

Class	Drug	Dose	Adverse Effects	Drug Interactions	Comments	Cost[a]
Monoamine Oxidase Inhibitors	*phenelzine* Nardil	45–90 mg/day po	Insomnia, dizziness, orthostatic hypotension, edema, sexual dysfunction.	Concurrent use with sympathomimetic agents, tyramine or levodopa may result in hypertensive crisis; do not use with serotonergic drugs such as SSRIs, SNRIs, TCAs, meperidine, tryptophan (increased risk of serotonin syndrome).	Only for **refractory cases**. Stringent dietary restrictions (tyramine-containing foods) are necessary.	$$$$
	tranylcypromine Parnate	20–60 mg/day po	See phenelzine.	See phenelzine.	See phenelzine.	$$$$
Other Antiepileptic Drugs	*topiramate* Topamax, generics	Initial: 15–25 mg daily po Increase by 15 mg/day at weekly intervals or 25 mg/day every 1–2 wk Range: 50–400 mg/day in 2 divided doses po[18]	CNS effects (e.g., dizziness, ataxia, tremor, sedation, cognitive impairment), GI symptoms (e.g., nausea, dyspepsia, constipation), weight loss (can be beneficial in some patients). Possible increased risk of oral clefts if used during the first trimester; avoid topiramate for migraine prophylaxis during pregnancy.	Additive depressant effects with other CNS depressants. May decrease effectiveness of oral contraceptives; use oral contraceptives containing at least 35 µg estrogen and add barrier contraceptive protection (condoms). Inhibitors of CYP2C19 may increase topiramate levels (e.g., SSRIs, isoniazid, omeprazole, moclobemide). Phenytoin and carbamazepine can decrease topiramate levels.	**Third-line** augmentation of SSRI or SNRI. May raise risk of nephrolithiasis; maintain adequate hydration during therapy; avoid in patients with renal stones. May cause acute myopia, with consequent angle closure glaucoma that responds to drug discontinuation; advise patients to consult an ophthalmologist or emergency room *immediately* if they have acute painful/red eyes or decreased/blurred vision. Warn patients about CNS depressant effects; possible risk associated with driving, other hazardous activities.	$$$

[a] Cost of 30-day supply of mean dosage; includes drug cost only.
Dosage adjustment required in renal impairment; see Appendix I.
Abbreviations: EPS = extrapyramidal symptoms; GABA = gamma-aminobutyric acid; MAOI = monoamine oxidase inhibitor; SNRI = serotonin-norepinephrine reuptake inhibitor; SSRI = selective serotonin reuptake inhibitor; TCA = tricyclic antidepressant
Legend: $ < $15 $$ $15–30 $$$ $30–45 $$$$ $45–60

Suggested Readings

Antony MM, Norton PJ. *The anti-anxiety workbook: proven strategies to overcome worry, phobias, panic, and obsessions*. New York (NY): Guilford Press; 2009.

Baldwin DS, Anderson IM, Nutt DJ et al. Evidence-based guidelines for the pharmacological treatment of anxiety disorders: recommendations from the British Association for Psychopharmacology. *J Psychopharmacol* 2005;19(6):567-96.

Canadian Psychiatric Association. Clinical practice guidelines. Management of anxiety disorders. *Can J Psychiatry* 2006;51(8 Suppl 2):9S-91S.

Ravindran LN, Stein MB. The pharmacologic treatment of anxiety disorders: a review of progress. *J Clin Psych* 2010;71(7):839-54.

References

1. American Psychiatric Association. *Diagnostic and statistical manual of mental disorders: DSM-5*. 5th ed. Washington (DC): American Psychiatric Publishing; 2013.
2. Canadian Psychiatric Association. Clinical practice guidelines. Management of anxiety disorders. *Can J Psychiatry* 2006;51(8 Suppl 2):9S-91S.
3. Shafran R, Radomsky AS, Coughtrey AE et al. Advances in the cognitive behavioural treatment of obsessive compulsive disorder. *Cogn Behav Ther* 2013;42(2):265-74.
4. Foa EB, Wilson R. *Stop obsessing: how to overcome your obsessions and compulsions*. Rev. ed. New York (NY): Bantam; 2001.
5. Foa EB, Liebowitz MR, Kozak MJ et al. Randomized, placebo-controlled trial of exposure and ritual prevention, clomipramine, and their combination in the treatment of obsessive-compulsive disorder. *Am J Psychiatry* 2005;162(1):151-61.
6. Richter MA, de Jesus DR, Hoppenbrouwers S et al. Evidence for cortical inhibitory and excitatory dysfunction in obsessive compulsive disorder. *Neuropsychopharmacology* 2012;37(5):1144-51.
7. B lom RM, Figee M, Vulink N et al. Update on repetitive transcranial magnetic stimulation in obsessive-compulsive disorder: different targets. *Curr Psychiatry Rep* 2011;13(4):289-94.
8. Jaafari N, Rachid F, Rotge JY et al. Safety and efficacy of repetitive transcranial magnetic stimulation in the treatment of obsessive-compulsive disorder: a review. *World J Biol Psychiatry* 2012;13(3):164-77.
9. Greenberg BD, Gabriels LA, Malone DA et al. Deep brain stimulation of the ventral internal capsule/ventral striatum for obsessive-compulsive disorder: worldwide experience. *Mol Psychiatry* 2010;15(1):64-79.
10. Blomstedt P, Sjoberg RL, Hansson M et al. Deep brain stimulation in the treatment of obsessive-compulsive disorder. *World Neurosurg* 2013;80(6):e245-53.
11. Soomro GM, Altman D, Rajagopal S et al. Selective serotonin re-uptake inhibitors (SSRIs) versus placebo for obsessive compulsive disorder (OCD). *Cochrane Database Syst Rev* 2008;(1):CD001765.
12. McDougle CJ, Epperson CN, Pelton GH et al. A double-blind, placebo-controlled study of risperidone addition in serotonin reuptake inhibitor-refractory obsessive-compulsive disorder. *Arch Gen Psychiatry* 2000;57(8):794-801.
13. da Conceicao Costa DL, Shavitt RG, Castro Cesar RC et al. Can early improvement be an indicator of treatment response in obsessive-compulsive disorder? Implications for early-treatment decision-making. *J Psychiatr Res* 2013;47(11):1700-7.
14. Olatunji BO, Cisler JM, Deacon BJ. Efficacy of cognitive behavioral therapy for anxiety disorders: a review of meta-analytic findings. *Psychiatr Clin North Am* 2010;33(3):557-77.
15. Simpson HB, Foa EB, Liebowitz MR et al. Cognitive behavioral therapy vs risperidone for augmenting serotonin reuptake inhibitors in obsessive compulsive disorder. *JAMA Psychiatry* 2013;70(11):1190-9.
16. Dold M, Aigner M, Lanzenberger et al. Antipsychotic augmentation of serotonin reuptake inhibitors in treatment-resistant obsessive-compulsive disorder: a meta-analysis of double-blind, randomized, placebo-controlled trials. *Int J Neuropsychopharmacol* 2013;16(3):557-74.
17. Komossa K, Depping AM, Meyer M et al. Second-generation antipsychotics for obsessive compulsive disorder. *Cochrane Database Syst Rev* 2010;(12):CD008141.
18. Berlin HA, Koran LM, Jenike MA et al. Double-blind, placebo-controlled trail of topiramate augmentation in treatment-resistant obsessive-compulsive disorder. *J Clin Psychiatry* 2011;72(5):716-21.
19. Rodriguez CI, Kegeles LS, Levinson A et al. Randomized controlled crossover trial of ketamine in obsessive-compulsive disorder: proof-of-concept. *Neuropsychopharmacology* 2013;38(12):2475-83.
20. Kariuki-Nyuthe C, Gomez-Mancilla B, Stein DJ. Obsessive compulsive disorder and the glutamatergic system. *Curr Opin Psychiatry* 2014;27(1):32-7.
21. Saxena S. Pharmacotherapy of compulsive hoarding. *J Clin Psychol* 2011;67(5):477-84.
22. Hadley SJ, Greenberg J, Hollander E. Diagnosis and treatment of body dysmorphic disorder in adolescents. *Curr Psychiatry Rep* 2002;4(2):108-13.
23. Ipser JC, Sander C, Stein DJ. Pharmacotherapy and psychotherapy for body dysmorphic disorder. *Cochrane Database Syst Rev* 2009;(1):CD005332.
24. ACOG Committee on Practice Bulletins–Obstetrics. ACOG Practice Bulletin: Clinical management guidelines for obstetrician-gynecologists number 92, April 2008 (replaces practice bulletin number 87, November 2007). Use of psychiatric medications during pregnancy and lactation. *Obstet Gynecol* 2008;111(4):1001-20.
25. Tuccori M, Montagnani S, Testi A et al. Use of selective serotonin reuptake inhibitors during pregnancy and risk of major and cardiovascular malformations: an update. *Postgrad Med* 2010;122(4):49-65.
26. Yonkers KA, Wisner KL, Stewart DE et al. The management of depression during pregnancy: a report from the American Psychiatric Association and the American College of Obstetricians and Gynecologists. *Gen Hosp Psychiatry* 2009;31(5):403-13.
27. Academy of Breastfeeding Medicine Protocol Committee. ABM clinical protocol #18: use of antidepressants in nursing mothers. *Breastfeed Med* 2008;3(1):44-52.
28. Weissman AM, Levy BT, Hartz AJ et al. Pooled analysis of antidepressant levels in lactating mothers, breast milk, and nursing infants. *Am J Psychiatry* 2004;161(6):1066-78.

Chapter 10
Post-traumatic Stress Disorder

R. P. Swinson, MD, FRCPsych, FRCPC

In the Diagnostic and Statistical Manual of Mental Disorders 5th edition (DSM-5), *post-traumatic stress disorder* (PTSD) is classified with other trauma- and stressor-related disorders that are diagnosed as occurring due to exposure to a traumatic or stressful event.[1] Other conditions in this classification include reactive attachment disorder, acute stress disorder and adjustment disorders. Previously PTSD was listed as an anxiety disorder.

PTSD is characterized by significant distress or impairment in functioning of at least 1 month's duration in response to a traumatic event described as exposure to actual or threatened death, serious injury or sexual violence. Symptoms have been divided into 4 main categories and are included in Table 1. Children 6 years of age or younger with the disorder are now diagnosed using a separate set of criteria.

Goals of Therapy

- Eliminate or decrease symptoms of PTSD
- Eliminate or decrease PTSD-based disability
- Prevent recurrence
- Treat comorbid conditions

Investigations

The assessment for PTSD requires a detailed exploration of the nature and circumstances of the traumatic event and its affect on the patient. It is important to be sensitive to the person's potential inability to recall these details without becoming overwhelmed. It may take a number of sessions to allow for a complete understanding of the circumstances of the traumatic experience(s).

- Thorough history with attention to:
  - nature of symptoms and onset
  - nature and extent of disability
  - presence of comorbid medical or psychiatric conditions (see Initial Management)
- Criteria to assist in obtaining an accurate diagnosis (Table 1)
- Physical examination to exclude endocrine or cardiac disorders and to look for signs of substance use
- Laboratory tests:
  - CBC, liver function tests, gamma-glutamyl transpeptidase (GGT; to screen for alcohol use), thyroid indices (supersensitive TSH), ECG

Note: Treat physical disorders of recent onset before making a definitive diagnosis of PTSD.

Therapeutic Choices

An illustration of the management of post-traumatic stress disorder is provided in Figure 1.

Table 1: Diagnosis Criteria for PTSD[1]

Symptoms	Examples
Repeated intrusion symptoms after the traumatic event	Intrusive memories, distressing dreams, dissociative symptoms such as flashbacks, intense distress cued by aspects of the trauma
Avoidance	Attempts to avoid memories, thoughts, feelings or external reminders associated with the triggering event
Negative cognition and mood	A broad category that may include a distorted sense of blame of self or others, inability to recall aspects of the traumatic event, loss of interest in activities
Arousal	Hypervigilance, sleep disturbances, self-destructive behaviour, irritability, verbal or physical aggression, recklessness

Figure 1: Management of Post-traumatic Stress Disorder

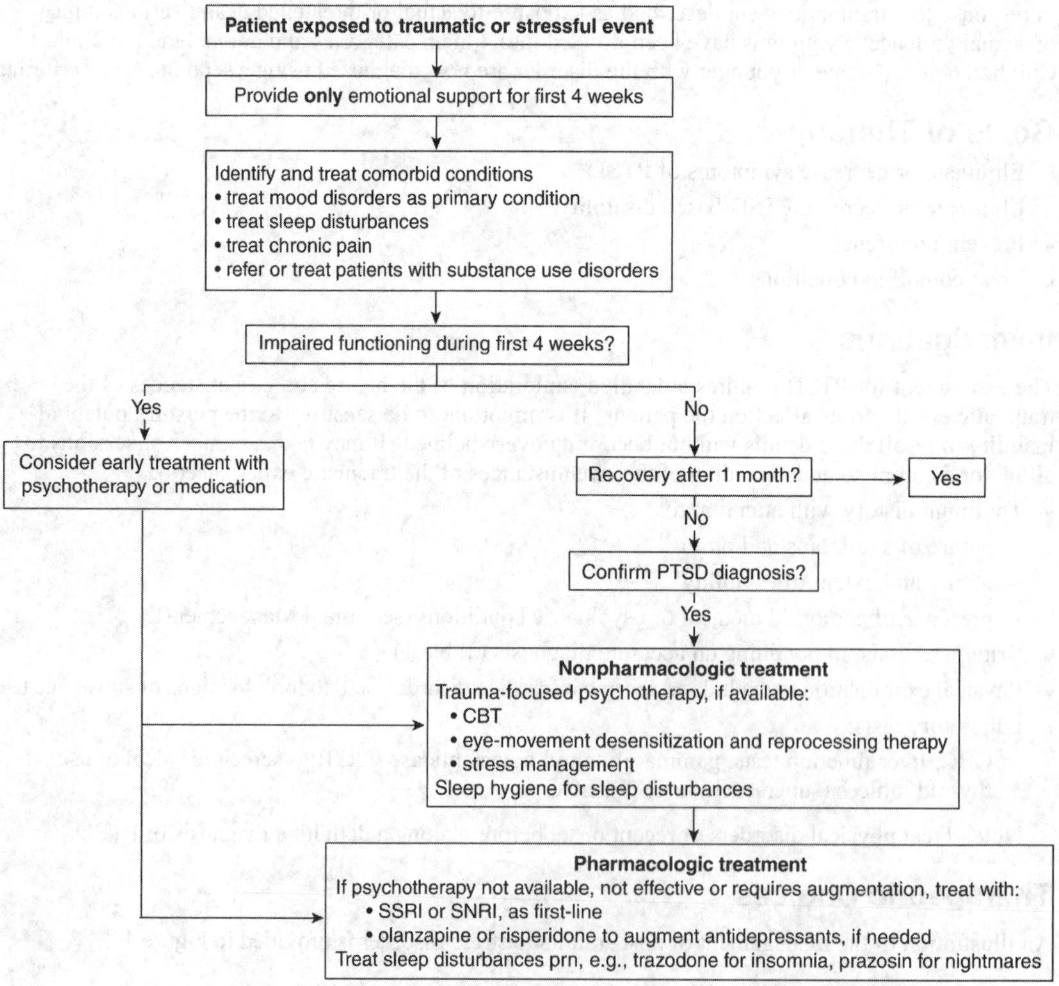

Abbreviations: CBT = cognitive behavioural therapy; PTSD = post-traumatic stress disorder; SNRI = serotonin-norepinephrine reuptake inhibitor; SSRI = selective serotonin reuptake inhibitor

Initial Management

Most people who experience trauma do not go on to develop either acute stress disorder or PTSD. In the first 4 weeks following a traumatic event, psychotherapy or pharmacotherapy, including benzodiazepines, should not be started. During this initial phase, help patients to understand that acute responses to trauma are common and often short term. Allow them to use their natural resilience and usual emotional supports to recover. Psychological debriefing, a short intervention delivered in group settings during the first 2 weeks following a traumatic event, may hamper natural recovery and is not usually recommended.[2] There is little evidence to show that medication taken immediately after a traumatic event can prevent the onset of PTSD.[3] In one small study, **propranolol** administered within a few hours of the trauma showed some promise.[4] Newer agents are being investigated.[5]

For those individuals who are overwhelmed and have impaired functioning, psychotherapy or medication may need to be instituted within the first 4 weeks following the traumatic event.

Treat comorbid mood disorders, especially depression, as the primary condition. It is important to manage comorbid chronic pain and sleep disturbances in patients with PTSD. Patients with PTSD often attempt to self-treat and can have substance use disorders; referral to a specialized program may be necessary.

Nonpharmacologic Choices

Whenever possible, trauma-focused psychotherapy is recommended before initiating pharmacotherapy. Several psychological approaches have been investigated in the treatment of PTSD and acute stress disorder.

Cognitive behavioural therapy (CBT) that is initiated at least 1 month after the trauma occurs is very effective in reducing symptoms of PTSD.[2] Evidence shows that therapies focused on the trauma, such as trauma-focused CBT, eye movement desensitization and reprocessing therapy or stress management, are more effective than more general approaches.[6] Support that does not deal with the trauma directly is no more effective than being on a waiting list.[7]

Pharmacologic Choices

The management of PTSD depends on the nature, severity and frequency of the trauma and requires a multimodal treatment program. Short-term treatment with medication may benefit patients who do not have access to CBT. See Table 2 for a list of these drugs.

SSRI and SNRI antidepressants have been shown to reduce the severity of all the component symptoms of PTSD. **Fluoxetine**, **paroxetine**,[8] **sertraline**[9] and **venlafaxine**[10] are first-line options. Other antidepressants with evidence of efficacy include **fluvoxamine**,[11] **mirtazapine**,[12,13] **moclobemide**[14] and **phenelzine**[15,16] and are considered second-line choices. Second-generation antipsychotics such as **risperidone** and **olanzapine** may be effective in augmenting the effects of antidepressants in some patients who do not respond to first-line PTSD treatment.[17,18]

Monotherapy with benzodiazepines is not recommended due to the effects on disinhibition and the high rates of substance use disorders in patients with PTSD.

Sleep disturbances are common in patients with PTSD. Although evidence from clinical trials is limited in this patient population, several PTSD practice guidelines support the use of **trazodone**[19] in the management of insomnia that has not responded to nonpharmacologic therapy (e.g., sleep hygiene) or treatment for comorbid conditions. **Prazosin** is an $alpha_1$-adrenergic antagonist that reduces sympathetic outflow in the brain. A systematic review based on a small but positive evidence base concluded that prazosin is an important pharmacologic option in reducing the frequency and intensity of nightmares and improving sleep in patients with PTSD [Evidence: SORT B].[20]

Choices during Pregnancy and Breastfeeding

PTSD and Pregnancy

Women who have encountered trauma during their lives may experience a worsening or relapse of PTSD symptoms during pregnancy.

Many people with PTSD do not bring their distress to the attention of their caregivers. If possible, screen patients for the presence of PTSD or anxiety symptoms prior to conception. Screening can usefully be repeated during the pregnancy and particularly postpartum. It is imperative to screen for the presence of mood symptoms and suicidality in a woman who is suffering from marked psychological distress related to pregnancy and breastfeeding.

It may be necessary to refer women experiencing severe PTSD symptoms during pregnancy or postpartum to a psychiatrist. Women's mental health programs are usually available in major centres and these programs customarily respond quickly to consultation requests.

Treatment for PTSD or other psychiatric disorders that are producing significant distress or interfering with functioning can be offered to women before conception.

Management during Pregnancy

Evidence-based psychotherapies such as CBT can be administered without restriction throughout pregnancy. There is good evidence to show that psychological treatments can have beneficial effects for more than half of the patients who remain with a treatment program. Therapies based in meditative or relaxation techniques may be more acceptable to the patient than pharmacologic approaches.[21]

If PTSD symptoms are severe and producing significant impairment, medications can be appropriate and effective.[22] **SSRI/SNRI antidepressants** are the mainstay of pharmacologic therapy for PTSD during pregnancy.

SSRIs/SNRIs may cause agitation, sweating, nausea, gastrointestinal distress and weight gain. There have been reports of a slightly higher (but still low) risk of congenital abnormalities involving the heart or cleft lip/palate.[23] Use of these drugs in the third trimester may be associated with neonatal withdrawal symptoms such as tremors, increased muscle tone, feeding or digestive problems or respiratory distress. Whether benzodiazepines confer an increased risk of congenital malformations is controversial.

The use of SSRIs or SNRIs may be warranted in patients with severe symptoms that could affect fetal or maternal safety or health. In general, use the lowest effective dose for the shortest time necessary. General principles for management of depression during pregnancy are applicable to the management of PTSD.[24,25]

PTSD and Breastfeeding

In the postpartum period, severe distress can impede the mother's sleep and erode her confidence in caring for her child.

As in pregnancy, nonpharmacologic options should be used whenever possible in the postpartum period, particularly in breastfeeding women. If drug therapy is necessary, consider **paroxetine** and sertraline, since both drugs appear in low concentrations in breast milk.[26]

---

* SORT (Strength of Recommendation Taxonomy) is a rating system (A, B or C) that addresses the quality of available evidence. For more information consult **How to Use *Compendium of Therapeutic Choices*** on page xxv.

A discussion of general principles on the use of medications in these special populations can be found in Appendix II and Appendix III. Other specialized reference sources are also provided in these appendices.

Therapeutic Tips

- Trauma-focused psychotherapy is recommended as first-line treatment for PTSD whenever possible.
- Assess a drug's effectiveness after a trial of an adequate dosage taken for an adequate length of time.
- If one antidepressant is not effective, switch to a second agent from the same or different drug class.
- If a second antidepressant is not effective, switch to an agent from a different drug class.
- Families of persons with PTSD can be significantly affected; refer spouses, children or other family members to marital or family counselors when indicated.

Table 2: **Drugs Used in the Management of Post-traumatic Stress Disorder**

Class	Drug	Dose	Adverse Effects	Drug Interactions	Comments	Cost[a]
Alpha$_1$-adrenergic Antagonists	*prazosin* Minipress, generics	Initial: 1 mg QHS po Increase by 1–2 mg QHS po until effective dose reached (range 3–15 mg QHS po)	Orthostatic hypotension (particularly following first dose), dizziness.	Increased risk of orthostatic hypotension with other antihypertensives or PDE-5 inhibitors (sildenafil, tadalafil, vardenafil). As a p-glyoprotein inducer, prazosin may reduce the efficacy of dabigatran or linagliptin, though interactions with these drugs have not been reported clinically.	Used to improve sleep and/or reduce nightmares in patients with PTSD. Current or past use of alpha$_1$-adrenergic antagonists increases the risk of intraoperative floppy iris syndrome during cataract surgery; discontinuing the drug preoperatively does not eliminate the risk. Inform the ophthalmologist if prazosin has been used at any time prior to cataract surgery.	$
Antipsychotics, Second-generation	*olanzapine* Zyprexa, Zyprexa Zydis, generics	Initial: 2.5 mg daily po Titrate gradually to desired effect, usually 2.5–5 mg daily po. May need to increase to a maximum of 10 mg per day po.	Weight gain, dizziness, sedation, anticholinergic effects, hepatic aminotransferase elevation, orthostatic hypotension, increased risk of diabetes and dyslipidemia, extrapyramidal effects (especially akathisia).	Sedation with CNS depressants; may potentiate antihypertensive drug effects; inhibitors of CYP1A2 or CYP2D6 such as diltiazem, fluvoxamine or paroxetine may increase olanzapine levels; inducers of CYP1A2 or CYP3A4 such as barbiturates, carbamazepine, phenytoin or rifampin may decrease olanzapine levels.	Used as augmentation therapy with first-line agents in PTSD. Advise patients about antipsychotic-associated body temperature dysregulation and prevention of heat stroke (e.g., hydration, sun protection).	$-$$
	risperidone Risperdal Preparations, generics	Initial: 1 mg daily po Titrate gradually to desired effect, usually 1–2 mg daily po. May need to increase to a maximum of 4 mg daily po	Insomnia, headaches, weight gain, orthostatic hypotension, rhinitis, anxiety, dose-related hyperprolactinemia and extrapyramidal effects.	Additive sedation with CNS depressants; may potentiate antihypertensive drug effects; inhibitors of CYP3A4 such as clarithromycin, erythromycin, grapefruit juice, ketoconazole or prednisone) may increase risperidone levels; inducers of CYP3A4 such as carbamazepine, phenytoin or rifampin may decrease risperidone levels.	Used as augmentation therapy with first-line agents in PTSD. Advise patients about antipsychotic-associated body temperature dysregulation and prevention of heat stroke (e.g., hydration, sun protection).	$

Class	Drug	Dose	Adverse Effects	Drug Interactions	Comments	Cost[a]
Monoamine Oxidase Inhibitors	*phenelzine* Nardil	45-90 mg/day po	Insomnia, dizziness, orthostatic hypotension, edema, sexual dysfunction.	Concurrent use with sympathomimetic agents, tyramine or levodopa may result in hypertensive crisis; do not use with serotonergic drugs such as SSRIs, SNRIs, TCAs, meperidine, tryptophan (increased risk of serotonin syndrome).	Stringent dietary restrictions (tyramine-containing foods) are necessary.	$$$
Noradrenergic and Specific Serotonergic Antidepressants	*mirtazapine* Remeron, Remeron RD, generics	15-45 mg QHS po	Somnolence, increased appetite/weight gain, dizziness.	Do not use with MAOIs; additive sedation with other CNS depressants such as alcohol, benzodiazepines; substrate of CYP1A2, 2D6 and 3A4—caution with inhibitors or inducers of these isoenzymes.		$
Reversible Inhibitors of Monoamine Oxidase-A	*moclobemide* Manerix, generics (RIMAs)	300–600 mg/day po	Nausea, insomnia.	Do not use with meperidine, TCAs, SSRIs.	Dietary restrictions are not required at usual doses.	$
Selective Serotonin Reuptake Inhibitors	*fluvoxamine* Luvox, generics	150–300 mg/day po	Agitation (on initiation of therapy), nausea, anorgasmia, anticholinergic effects, sedation, increased risk of GI bleeding.	Serotonin syndrome with MAOIs (hypertension, tremor, agitation, hypomania); caution with other serotonergic drugs including amphetamine derivatives, dextromethorphan, dihydroergotamine, linezolid, lithium, meperidine, pentazocine, selegiline, St. John's wort, trazodone, triptans, tryptophan (increased risk of serotonin syndrome); increased risk of GI bleeding with NSAIDs, antiplatelet agents. SSRIs are substrates and inhibitors of several cytochrome P450 isoenzymes. This may result in decreased clearance of many drugs (e.g., clozapine, methadone, mexiletine, phenytoin, pimozide,	May take 2–3 months to achieve maximum effect. Discontinue gradually.	$$

(cont'd)

Table 2: **Drugs Used in the Management of Post-traumatic Stress Disorder** *(cont'd)*

Class	Drug	Dose	Adverse Effects	Drug Interactions	Comments	Cost[a]
				propafenone) or decreased enzymatic conversion of a prodrug to its active form (e.g., clopidogrel, codeine, tamoxifen). Avoid combined use with drugs associated with prolonged QT_c interval/torsades de pointes, such as amiodarone, azithromycin, clarithromycin, domperidone, erythromycin, haloperidol, methadone, pimozide, quinine, sotalol, ziprasidone.		
	paroxetine immediate-release Paxil, generics	Usual dose: 20–40 mg/day po Maximum dose: 60 mg/day po	Agitation (on initiation of therapy), nausea, anorgasmia, anticholinergic effects, sedation, increased risk of GI bleeding.	See fluvoxamine.	May take 2–3 months for maximum effect. Discontinue gradually.	$
	paroxetine controlled-release Paxil CR	12.5–37.5 mg/day po	Agitation (on initiation of therapy), nausea, anorgasmia, anticholinergic effects, sedation, increased risk of GI bleeding.	See fluvoxamine.	May take 2–3 months for maximum effect. Discontinue gradually.	$$$-$$$$$
	sertraline Zoloft, generics	50–200 mg/day po	Agitation (on initiation of therapy), nausea, anorgasmia, insomnia, diarrhea, increased risk of GI bleeding.	See fluvoxamine.	May take 2–3 months for maximum effect. Discontinue gradually.	$

Class	Drug	Dose	Adverse Effects	Drug Interactions	Comments	Cost[a]
Serotonergic Antidepressants	*trazodone* generics	Initial: 25–50 mg QHS po May increase gradually up to 100 mg QHS po as needed/tolerated	Drowsiness, orthostatic hypotension, nausea, vomiting, headache, dry mouth, priapism (rare).	Toxicity may be increased by inhibitors of CYP3A4 such as clarithromycin, erythromycin, grapefruit juice, ketoconazole). Effectiveness may be decreased by inducers of CYP3A4 such as carbamazepine, phenytoin, rifampin).	For management of insomnia. Not a Health Canada-approved indication.	$
Serotonin-Norepinephrine Reuptake Inhibitors	*venlafaxine extended-release* (kidney symbol) Effexor XR, generics	37.5–225 mg/day po	Nausea, insomnia, dizziness, asthenia.	Do not use with MAOIs. Substrate of CYP2D6 and CYP3A4; caution with inducers or inhibitors of these isoenzymes.	May take 2–3 months for maximum effect. Discontinue gradually. Avoid in severe renal dysfunction.	$

[a] Cost of 30-day supply; includes drug cost only.

(kidney symbol) Dosage adjustment may be required in renal impairment; see Appendix I.

Abbreviations: MAOI = monoamine oxidase inhibitor; NSAID = nonsteroidal anti-inflammatory drug; PTSD = post-traumatic stress disorder; SNRI = serotonin-norepinephrine reuptake inhibitor; SSRI = selective serotonin reuptake inhibitor; TCA = tricyclic antidepressant

Legend: $ < $25 $-$$ < $25–50 $$ $25–50 $$$ $50–75 $$$$ $75–100 $$$-$$$$$ $50–125 $$$$$ $100–125

Suggested Readings

Baldwin DS, Anderson IM, Nutt DJ et al. Evidence-based guidelines for the pharmacological treatment of anxiety disorders: recommendations from the British Association for Psychopharmacology. *J Psychopharmacol* 2005;19(6):567-96.

Bandelow B, Sher L, Bunevicius R et al. Guidelines for the pharmacological treatment of anxiety disorders, obsessive-compulsive disorder and posttraumatic stress disorder in primary care. *Int J Psych Clin Pract* 2012;16(2):77-84.

Bisson JI, Roberts NP, Andrew M et al. Psychological therapies for post-traumatic stress disorder (PTSD) in adults. *Cochrane Database Syst Rev* 2013;12:CD003388.

Canadian Psychiatric Association. Clinical practice guidelines. Management of anxiety disorders. *Can J Psychiatry* 2006;51(8 Suppl 2):9S-91S.

Ravindran LN, Stein MB. The pharmacologic treatment of anxiety disorders: a review of progress. *J Clin Psych* 2010;71(7):839-54.

References

1. American Psychiatric Association. *Diagnostic and statistical manual of mental disorders: DSM-5*. 5th ed. Washington (DC): American Psychiatric Association; 2013.
2. Kavan MG, Elsasser GN, Barone EJ. The physician's role in managing acute stress disorder. *Am Fam Physician* 2012;86(7):643-9.
3. Bandelow B, Sher L, Bunevicius R et al. Guidelines for the pharmacological treatment of anxiety disorders, obsessive-compulsive disorder and posttraumatic stress disorder in primary care. *Int J Psych Clin Pract* 2012;16(2):77-84.
4. Pitman RK, Sanders KM, Zusman RM et al. Pilot study of secondary prevention of posttraumatic stress disorder with propranolol. *Biol Psychiatry* 2002;51(2):189-92.
5. Steckler T, Risbrough V. Pharmacological treatment of PTSD—established and new approaches. *Neuropharmacology* 2012;62(2):617-27.
6. Canadian Psychiatric Association. Clinical practice guidelines. Management of anxiety disorders. *Can J Psychiatry* 2006;51(8 Suppl 2):9S-91S.
7. Bisson JI, Roberts NP, Andrew M et al. Psychological therapies for post-traumatic stress disorder (PTSD) in adults. *Cochrane Database Syst Rev* 2013;12:CD003388.
8. Marshall RD, Beebe KL, Oldham M et al. Efficacy and safety of paroxetine treatment for chronic PTSD: a fixed-dose, placebo-controlled study. *Am J Psychiatry* 2001;158(12):1982-8.
9. Brady K, Pearlstein T, Asnis GM et al. Efficacy and safety of sertraline treatment of posttraumatic stress disorder: a randomized controlled trial. *JAMA* 2000;283(14):1837-44.
10. Seedat S, Stein DJ, Ziervogel C et al. Comparison of response to a selective serotonin reuptake inhibitor in children, adolescents, and adults with posttraumatic stress disorder. *J Child Adolesc Psychopharmacol* 2002;12(1):37-46.
11. Escalona R, Canive JM, Calais LA et al. Fluvoxamine treatment in veterans with combat-related post-traumatic stress disorder. *Depress Anxiety* 2002;15(1):29-33.
12. Connor KM, Davidson JR, Weisler RH et al. A pilot study of mirtazapine in post-traumatic stress disorder. *Int Clin Psychopharmacol* 1999;14(1):29-31.
13. Davidson JR,Weisler RH, Butterfield MI et al. Mirtazapine vs. placebo in posttraumatic stress disorder: a pilot trial. *Biol Psychiatry* 2003;53(2):188-91.
14. Neal LA, Shapland W, Fox C. An open trial of moclobemide in the treatment of post-traumatic stress disorder. *Int Clin Psychopharmacol* 1997;12(4):231-7.
15. Frank JB, Kosten TR, Giller EL et al. A randomized clinical trial of phenelzine and imipramine for posttraumatic stress disorder. *Am J Psychiatry* 1988;145(10):1289-91.
16. Kosten TR, Frank JB, Dan E et al. Pharmacotherapy for posttraumatic stress disorder using phenelzine or imipramine. *J Nerv Ment Dis* 1991;179(6):366-70.
17. Wang HR, Woo YS, Bahk WM. Atypical antipsychotics in the treatment of posttraumatic stress disorder. *Clin Neuropharm* 2013;36(6):216-22.
18. Krystal JH, Rosenheck RA, Cramer JA et al. Adjunctive risperidone treatment for antidepressant-resistant symptoms of chronic military service-related PTSD: a randomized trial. *JAMA* 2011;306(5):493-502.
19. Bossini L, Casolaro I, Koukouna D et al. Off-label uses of trazodone: a review. *Expert Opin Pharmacother* 2012:13(12):1707-17.
20. Kung S, Zelde E, Lapid MI. Treatment of nightmares with prazosin: a systematic review. *Mayo Clin Proc* 2012;87(9):890-900.
21. Olatunji BO, Cisler JM, Deacon BJ. Efficacy of cognitive behavioral therapy for anxiety disorders: a review of meta-analytic findings. *Psychiatr Clin North Am* 2010;33(3):557-77.
22. ACOG Committee on Practice Bulletins—Obstetrics. ACOG Practice Bulletin: Clinical management guidelines for obstetrician-gynecologists number 92, April 2008 (replaces practice bulletin number 87, November 2007). Use of psychiatric medications during pregnancy and lactation. *Obstet Gynecol* 2008;111(4):1001-20.
23. Tuccori M, Montagnani S, Testi A et al. Use of selective serotonin reuptake inhibitors during pregnancy and risk of major and cardiovascular malformations: an update. *Postgrad Med* 2010;122(4):49-65.
24. Yonkers KA, Wisner KL, Stewart DE et al. The management of depression during pregnancy: a report from the American Psychiatric Association and the American College of Obstetricians and Gynecologists. *Gen Hosp Psychiatry* 2009;31(5):403-13.
25. Academy of Breastfeeding Medicine Protocol Committee. ABM clinical protocol #18: use of antidepressants in nursing mothers. *Breastfeed Med* 2008;3(1):44-52.
26. Weissman AM, Levy BT, Hartz AJ et al. Pooled analysis of antidepressant levels in lactating mothers, breast milk, and nursing infants. *Am J Psychiatry* 2004;161(6):1066-78.

Chapter 11
Psychoses

Heather Milliken, MDCM, FRCPC, CSPQ

Psychoses are brain disorders that cause a distortion of, or loss of contact with, reality and affect a patient's ability to think, feel, perceive and act. Psychotic symptoms include delusions, hallucinations, disorganized thinking and bizarre or disorganized behaviour. Approximately 3% of people worldwide will experience at least one psychotic episode during their lifetime. See Table 1 for a list of differential diagnoses.

The age of onset of schizophrenia spectrum psychotic disorders is usually late adolescence/early adulthood. There is increased emphasis on earlier detection and intervention[1,2,3] because the duration of untreated psychosis correlates to poorer outcomes in both the short- and long-term.[4,5]

Common prodromal psychosis symptoms (in order of decreasing frequency) include:

- reduced concentration and attention
- reduced drive and motivation; lack of energy
- depressed mood
- sleep disturbance
- anxiety
- social withdrawal
- deterioration in functioning
- irritability

Increasingly research has focused on the identification and treatment of individuals who are at “clinical high-risk” of developing a psychotic disorder or may be in the prodromal phase.[6,7,8]

A number of tools including structured interviews and rating scales have been developed to identify individuals who may meet criteria for being at “clinical high-risk” of progressing to a psychotic disorder.[9] Some studies evaluating the effectiveness of psychosocial and pharmacologic options to prevent the onset of a psychotic disorder in “at-risk” individuals are encouraging but these measures are considered experimental and not recommended for routine clinical use.

Family physicians can play an important role in early detection.[10,11] If a person is suspected of having “prodromal psychosis” symptoms, referral to a specialized early psychosis program (if available), psychiatrist or community mental health team is recommended.

Goals of Therapy

- Reduce psychotic agitation in acute episodes
- Achieve remission of:
  - positive symptoms such as delusions, hallucinations, disordered thinking and disorganized behaviour
  - negative symptoms such as apathy, anhedonia, social withdrawal
  - mood symptoms such as dysphoria, anxiety, emotional lability
  - cognitive symptoms such as impaired attention, concentration and memory

Table 1: **Differential Diagnosis of Psychotic Episodes**[12]

Disorder	Characteristics
Schizophrenia	Signs of illness for ≥6 months; psychotic symptoms (delusions and/or hallucinations and/or disorganized speech) for ≥1 month; social/occupational dysfunction
Schizophreniform psychosis	Similar to schizophrenia except duration of illness of <6 months
Schizoaffective disorder	Uninterrupted period of illness in which symptoms of schizophrenia and mood disorder occur concurrently; during lifetime duration of illness, ≥2 weeks of delusions or hallucinations in absence of major mood episode; major mood episode is present >50% of total duration of illness
Delusional disorder	Nonbizarre delusions for ≥1 month and does not meet criteria for schizophrenia
Brief psychotic disorder	Psychotic symptoms for ≥1 day but <1 month; may or may not be related to marked stressor; eventual full return to premorbid level of functioning
Substance-induced psychotic disorder	Delusions or hallucinations develop during or within 1 month of substance intoxication or withdrawal or are etiologically related to medication use and are not better accounted for by another psychotic disorder
Psychotic disorder associated with another medical condition	Delusions or hallucinations are direct physiological consequence of a medical condition and occur in absence of delirium
Psychotic disorder not elsewhere classified	Psychotic symptoms present but criteria for specific disorder not met or there is insufficient or contradictory information
Major depression with psychotic features	Major depressive episode with concurrent mood-congruent (most common) or mood-incongruent psychotic symptoms
Bipolar disorder	Manic episode with concurrent mood-congruent (most common) or mood-incongruent psychotic symptoms

- Reduce risk of psychiatric comorbidity, particularly suicide and depression
- Reduce risk of substance abuse
- Facilitate recovery of functioning and healthy development
- Reduce risk of social isolation due to alienation from family, friends and social supports
- Reduce risk of physical comorbidity including metabolic syndrome and cardiovascular disease
- Prevent recurrence of psychotic episodes

Investigations

- Family physicians are often the initial contact for a person experiencing a first psychotic episode. They should have a high index of suspicion in any young individual who is experiencing persistent changes in behaviour, mood and functioning, especially in the presence of other risk factors such as substance abuse or a family history of mental illness, particularly history of psychotic disorders.
- In addition to the common prodromal symptoms, signs and symptoms of possible first-episode psychosis include:[1]
  - rapid fluctuations in mood (emotional lability) or showing very little emotion or facial expression
  - unreasonable suspiciousness
  - insomnia; restlessness and pacing at night

  - unusual or bizarre behaviour
  - unusual perceptual experiences including hypersensitivity, illusions and/or brief intermittent hallucinations
  - difficulties in thinking such as organizing and/or expressing thoughts
- Substance use (particularly cannabis) is common in first-episode psychosis. Individuals may therefore be misdiagnosed with a substance-induced psychosis and not receive appropriate ongoing treatment. Cannabis use can trigger the onset of a schizophrenia spectrum disorder in genetically vulnerable individuals[13]
- Even in the presence of substance use, have a high index of suspicion of a functional psychosis if:
  - symptoms precede the onset of substance use
  - symptoms are bizarre or there is marked thought disorder
  - symptoms persist beyond the period of intoxication or withdrawal
- Individuals with a suspected first episode of psychosis require urgent services. If available, refer to a psychiatrist, community mental health clinic or specialized early psychosis program[14]
- Appropriate investigations, based on both the phase of the psychotic disorder and individual patient characteristics, are listed in Table 2
- In an acute psychotic episode, assess the nature and extent of psychopathology:
  - thorough history of presenting problems with special attention to onset and course of prodromal symptoms
  - onset, characteristics and severity of psychotic symptoms
  - changes in behaviour and functioning
  - history of any suicidal ideation or behaviour and/or aggressive/violent ideation or behaviour
  - history of substance use/abuse in relation to onset and course of psychotic symptoms
- A thorough mental status examination is essential. Competency to consent to treatment needs to be assessed in all acutely psychotic individuals
- Obtain information from as many sources as possible since individuals with psychotic disorders are often poor historians:
  - interview family members whenever possible with the consent of the individual. If a patient is unwilling to give consent to interview family members, a clinician may still accept collateral information provided by a family member (e.g., in a phone call) but cannot divulge any information that would constitute a breach of patient confidentiality. If a patient is judged unable to give informed consent then legally a substitute decision maker (usually a family member) has to be contacted in order to provide informed consent on behalf of the patient
- A variety of clinical rating scales can be used at baseline and repeated periodically to monitor for symptomatic and functional recovery following an acute psychotic episode:
  - the Clinical Global Impression Scales for Severity (CGI-S)[15] and for Change (CGI-C)[15] and Global Assessment of Functioning (GAF)[14] for documenting changes over time are easy to use
  - training is required in order to reliably use the Brief Psychiatric Rating Scale (BPRS, available at www.priory.com/psych/bprs.htm) and the Positive and Negative Syndrome Scale (PANSS). Alternatively, the semistructured interview guide SCI-PANSS[16] takes approximately 30–40 minutes to complete and can be helpful in eliciting signs and symptoms of psychopathology
- Patients with only partial symptomatic and/or functional recovery following an acute psychotic episode require diagnostic reassessment by a psychiatrist

Table 2: **Investigations and Monitoring of Psychoses**

Parameter	Phase of Illness, Recommended Monitoring/Frequency[14,17]
Psychopathology	**First episode:** baseline then weekly for first 4–8 weeks; more often if clinically indicated **Recurrent acute episode:** baseline then weekly for first 4–8 weeks; more often if clinically indicated **Stabilization phase:** monthly for first 6 months following first or recurrent acute episode; more often if clinically indicated **Stable phase:** every 3 months for individuals with good symptomatic and functional recovery and medication adherence; more often for individuals with poor medication adherence; residual symptoms; poor functioning; substance abuse
Substance use	**First episode:** baseline **Recurrent acute episode:** baseline **Stabilization phase:** at every patient visit or as clinically indicated **Stable phase:** at every patient visit or as clinically indicated
Level of functioning (activities of daily living; social and occupational functioning)	**First episode:** premorbid level of functioning; baseline assessment of current functioning **Recurrent acute episode:** baseline assessment of current functioning **Stabilization phase:** monthly for first 6 months following first or acute episode **Stable phase:** every 3 months
Past psychiatric history	**First episode:** baseline **Recurrent acute episode:** baseline with focus on past antipsychotic treatment including type of medication, dose, side effects, response, duration of treatment and medication adherence **Stabilization/Stable phases:** N/A
Family psychiatric history	**First episode:** baseline **Recurrent acute episode:** baseline **Stabilization/Stable phases:** N/A
Developmental history (mother's obstetrical history including pre- and perinatal complications); developmental milestones; history of learning disabilities	**First episode:** baseline **Recurrent acute episode:** N/A **Stabilization/Stable phases:** N/A
Medical history (past and current conditions including treatment)	**First episode:** baseline **Recurrent acute episode:** baseline **Stable phase:** yearly
Extrapyramidal signs and symptoms (parkinsonism, dystonia, akathisia, dyskinesia)	**First episode:** baseline; when dosage of antipsychotic is changed or new antipsychotic is started, then weekly for 2–4 weeks **Recurrent acute episode:** baseline; when dosage of antipsychotic is changed or new antipsychotic is started, then weekly for 2–4 weeks **Stabilization phase:** as clinically indicated **Stable phase:** every 6 months or more often for individuals at higher risk
Cognitive functions (estimates of premorbid IQ, current IQ, attention and concentration, working memory, verbal and visual learning and memory, executive functions such as abstract thinking, reasoning, problem solving, judgment)	**First episode:** referral to a psychologist is recommended for neurocognitive testing within 3 months after psychotic symptoms have remitted **Recurrent acute episode:** N/A **Stabilization phase:** N/A **Stable phase:** referral to a psychologist for neurocognitive testing as clinically indicated (clinical evidence of ongoing cognitive impairment that affects functioning)

(cont'd)

Table 2: **Investigations and Monitoring of Psychoses** *(cont'd)*

Parameter	Phase of Illness, Recommended Monitoring/Frequency[14,17]
Functional enquiry and physical examination with focus on current complaints, endocrine and sexual function, vital signs, weight, body mass index (BMI)	**First episode:** baseline and then as clinically indicated; weight and BMI monthly for 6 months; baseline waist circumference; blood pressure at baseline and 12 weeks or more often if clinically indicated **Recurrent acute episode:** baseline and then as clinically indicated; weight and BMI monthly for 6 months after initiation of a new antipsychotic; baseline waist circumference; blood pressure at baseline and 12 weeks or more often if clinically indicated **Stabilization phase:** as clinically indicated **Stable phase:** as clinically indicated; weight and BMI every 3 months when on stable antipsychotic dosage: waist circumference annually; blood pressure annually or more often if clinically indicated; functional enquiry (including endocrine and sexual function) and physical exam at least yearly
Laboratory investigations (including CBC and differential, electrolytes, kidney and liver function, fasting glucose and lipid profile, TSH, baseline prolactin, routine urinalysis, urine drug screen if clinically indicated, tests for STIs, HIV and hepatitis if clinically indicated)	**First episode:** baseline; fasting glucose at baseline and repeat at 12 weeks or more often as clinically indicated; fasting lipid profile at baseline and 12 weeks, and repeat as clinically indicated **Recurrent acute episode:** baseline; fasting glucose at baseline and repeat at 12 weeks or more often as clinically indicated; fasting lipid profile at baseline and 12 weeks and repeat as clinically indicated **Stabilization phase:** as clinically indicated **Stable phase:** fasting glucose annually or more frequently if gaining weight or symptomatic; fasting lipid profile annually or every 6 months if LDL or triglyceride levels above normal range; other tests as clinically indicated
CT brain	**First episode:** recommended **Recurrent acute episode:** as clinically indicated

Abbreviations: N/A = not applicable

Therapeutic Choices

- Antipsychotic medications are the most effective treatment of schizophrenia and related psychotic disorders[18,19] but need to be integrated with psychosocial interventions to optimize outcome.[14]
- Both pharmacologic and psychosocial interventions should be tailored to the individual, based on phase of illness, severity of symptoms, past history of treatment response (if applicable), degree of insight and acceptance of treatment, presence of comorbid psychiatric/physical disorders and family medical/psychiatric history.

Nonpharmacologic Choices

First Episode/Recurrent Acute Episode

- Determine appropriate treatment setting (least restrictive setting possible), ensure safety and reduce environmental stressors and stimuli.
- Acutely agitated patients and those at imminent risk of harm to self or others will require hospitalization, if necessary on an involuntary basis. Criteria for involuntary psychiatric assessment and/or admission are determined by each province's mental health legislation.
- See patient frequently (for outpatients at least weekly for first 4–6 weeks) in order to:
  - build rapport
  - provide support, practical advice and psychoeducation
  - promote medication adherence
  - monitor treatment response (both adverse effects and improvement in symptoms)
- Foster a collaborative therapeutic relationship between the patient, family/caregivers and treatment team.

Stabilization/Stable Phases

- In schizophrenia and related psychotic disorders, recovery (stabilization phase) from an acute psychotic episode usually occurs over 6 months but may take longer and may be incomplete.
  - focus on medication adherence, stress management, assessment of signs and symptoms of postpsychotic depression and suicidality, assessment of substance use and education about early warning signs of relapse
- Psychosocial interventions such as individual psychoeducation, family psychoeducation, cognitive-behavioural therapies (CBT), motivational interviewing, social and vocational skills training and peer support groups have been shown to improve functional outcome and community reintegration, promote treatment adherence and help prevent relapse.[14]
- Maintain continuity of care with an individual clinician or multidisciplinary treatment team.
- Individuals with serious ongoing illness and functional disability or comorbid problems such as substance abuse may benefit from referral to an Assertive Community Treatment (ACT) team if available.[14]

Pharmacologic Choices

Choice of Antipsychotic

Two major classes of antipsychotics are currently available in Canada:

- **First-generation** antipsychotics (FGAs), also known as "typical" or "conventional" antipsychotics, can be classified according to their chemical structure (e.g., phenothiazines such as **fluphenazine** or butyrophenones such as **haloperidol**) or potency (low, intermediate, high) as determined by dopamine D_2-receptor binding affinity (see Table 6).
- **Second-generation** antipsychotics (SGAs) or "atypical" antipsychotics (**aripiprazole**, **asenapine**, **clozapine**, **lurasidone**, **olanzapine**, **paliperidone**, **quetiapine**, **risperidone** and **ziprasidone**) have greater 5HT affinity relative to D_2 affinity. The duration of binding to D_2 receptors and differences in binding affinity to other neurotransmitters (serotonergic, muscarinic, histaminic, alpha-adrenergic) may account for clinical differences in dosing requirements and side effect profiles among SGAs (see Table 7).[20] Aripiprazole, asenapine, lurasidone and ziprasidone have slightly different binding affinities compared to other SGAs:
  - **aripiprazole** has partial agonist activity at D_2 and $5HT_{1A}$ receptors and potent antagonism activity at $5HT_{2A}$ receptors (potential efficacy in treating negative and depressive symptoms). It can be given once daily with or without food, and is usually given in the morning because it can be activating and cause insomnia. Changes in dosage should be made no more frequently than every 14 days due to its uniquely long half-life. Aripiprazole is also available in a long acting injectable formulation that is administered once a month.
  - **asenapine** is derived from the antidepressant mirtazapine and is a potent multireceptor antagonist with strong affinity for a number of serotonergic and dopaminergic receptors.[21] Asenapine dissolves rapidly after being administered sublingually and is given twice daily due to its short half-life. Oral hypoesthesia and paresthesia may occur directly after administration and usually resolves within 1 hour. Hypersensitivity reactions including anaphylaxis and angioedema have occurred in patients treated with asenapine, often after the first dose.[22] Inform patients of the signs and symptoms of a serious allergic reaction and advise them to seek immediate medical attention if they occur. The initial and target dose for the treatment of schizophrenia and related psychotic disorders is 5 mg twice daily. An increase in dose to 10 mg twice daily is recommended only after clinical assessment.
  - **lurasidone** has high affinity for D_2, $5\text{-}HT_{2A}$ and $5\text{-}HT_7$ receptors, moderate affinity for alpha-adrenergic receptors and little or none for muscarinic and histaminic receptors. Lurasidone is given once daily with food (minimum of 350 calories, irrespective of fat content) to maximize

bioavailability, usually with the supper meal or a bedtime snack. The initial and target dose is 40 mg daily, with most patients responding to 40–80 mg daily. Doses higher than 80 mg daily may be required by some patients. Consultation with a psychiatrist is recommended prior to increasing the dose above 80 mg daily. Lurasidone is generally well tolerated with minimal effect on weight, glucose, cholesterol or triglycerides.[23] The most common side effects are nausea, somnolence, akathisia and dose-related EPS.[22] Nausea is related to initiation of therapy and increases in dosage, and can be persistent and distressing to patients. It is often worst 2–3 hours post dose (time of peak plasma levels) and does not appear to be related to the presence or absence of food. Nausea can be managed by lowering or splitting the dose (e.g., 40 mg twice daily rather than 80 mg once daily) or giving the dose at bedtime. Ginger or peppermint remedies may also be helpful.

- **paliperidone** is the active metabolite of risperidone. It is not metabolized by the liver and therefore has minimal risk of drug-drug interactions compared to other oral antipsychotics. The oral extended-release formulation is intended for once-daily dosing with or without food. Morning administration is recommended as it can cause insomnia. Paliperidone palmitate is available as a prolonged-release injectable suspension. In contrast to long-acting injectable risperidone, initiation of treatment involves a loading dose strategy with 2 initial injections in the deltoid muscle 7 days apart followed by monthly maintenance injections in either the deltoid or gluteal muscles. Supplementation with oral antipsychotics during the first 3 weeks after initiation of treatment is not required (see Table 7). Patient acceptance may be improved with monthly maintenance doses of paliperidone palmitate compared to risperidone long-acting injections given every 2 weeks.
- **ziprasidone** has agonist activity at $5HT_{1A}$ receptors and, unlike other SGAs, has antagonist activity at $5HT_{1D}$ receptors and moderate inhibition of synaptic reuptake of serotonin and norepinephrine. Though once-daily dosing may be appropriate for some patients, ziprasidone usually requires twice-daily administration due to its short half-life (6.6 hours), and must be taken with food (at least 500 calories) to ensure optimal absorption and therapeutic serum concentrations. Bioavailability of ziprasidone is reduced by 50% if taken on an empty stomach. It is important to educate patients and family members/caregivers regarding adequate caloric intake and to monitor patients' food intake for several weeks following initiation of treatment.

- All FGAs and SGAs, with the exception of clozapine, have similar efficacy in treating the positive (psychotic) symptoms of schizophrenia and related disorders. While some studies have found that SGAs may have advantages in first-episode psychosis[24,25] i.e., in improving negative symptoms, mood and cognitive deficits[26,27] and in preventing relapse[28] and rehospitalization, overall the results have been mixed and greater efficacy for SGAs has not been consistently demonstrated.[29] **Clozapine** is the only antipsychotic with proven efficacy in treatment-resistant schizophrenia,[18] in reducing hostility and aggression,[30,31] persistent suicidality[32] and all-cause mortality.[33]
- With the exception of clozapine, SGAs are now considered a first-line treatment choice.[26,27,34] Clozapine is reserved for treatment-resistant schizophrenia due to the risk of agranulocytosis and the need for regular blood monitoring. The major differences between the FGAs and SGAs (and among individual SGAs), are in side effect profiles, safety and tolerability (see Table 5).

Dosing and Duration of Treatment

Tailor treatment to the specific phase of the disorder, and to the patient's signs and symptoms.[14,34]

Acute Phase

An algorithm in Figure 1 illustrates the management of patients in the acute phase of a psychotic episode.

Figure 1: Management of Acute Psychotic Episodes

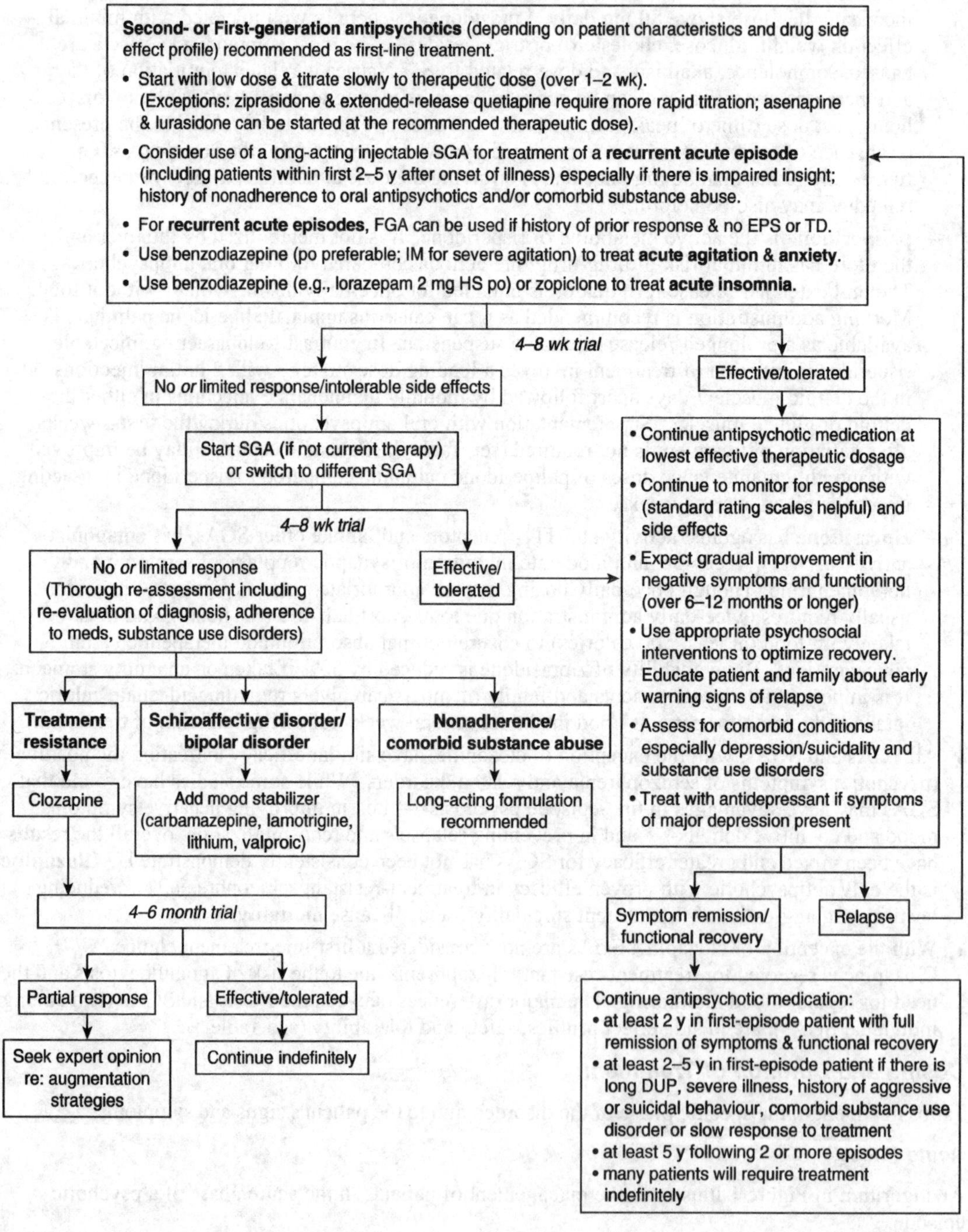

Abbreviations: DUP = duration of untreated psychosis; EPS = extrapyramidal symptoms; FGA = first-generation antipsychotic; SGA = second-generation antipsychotic; TD = tardive dyskinesia

- **Haloperidol** im has been the most widely used treatment for psychotic agitation. Haloperidol 5 mg im combined with **lorazepam** 2 mg im has been shown to be more effective than haloperidol alone.[35]
- While only studied in mildly to moderately agitated patients, **olanzapine** 2.5–10 mg im appears to have efficacy similar to haloperidol and causes less EPS.[36,37] Do not use the parenteral formulations of benzodiazepines and olanzapine in combination as there have been reports of cardiac and respiratory problems including deaths.
- Rapid-dissolving oral formulations of olanzapine and risperidone are as effective as haloperidol im[38] if the patient is able and willing to take oral medications.
- **Zuclopenthixol acetate** is an injectable FGA with a pharmacokinetic profile (peak serum level in 24–48 hours, declining to one-third of peak concentration in 72 hours) that may reduce the number of injections required in severe acute agitation and/or aggression. It should not be used in antipsychotic-naïve patients.
- Patients with *first-episode psychosis* are more responsive to lower doses of antipsychotics,[39,40] have a greater rate of recovery[39] and are more prone to side effects.
  - starting doses for asenapine (5 mg twice daily) and lurasidone (40 mg daily) are also the target therapeutic doses.
  - when initiating SGAs (with the exception of ziprasidone and extended-release quetiapine), begin with a low dose and titrate gradually over 1–2 weeks up to the usual therapeutic range (see Table 7). Aripiprazole, lurasidone, olanzapine, paliperidone, extended-release quetiapine and risperidone are usually administered once daily. Although twice-daily dosing is recommended for immediate-release quetiapine, many patients can be maintained on a single daily dose at bedtime.[41] Twice-daily dosing with meals (of at least 500 calories) is recommended for ziprasidone.
  - optimal dosing for **ziprasidone** is 80–160 mg daily for first-episode psychosis and 120–160 mg daily for chronic schizophrenia. Rapid titration to the target dose is required; slow titration is associated with poorer outcomes and the development of restlessness, agitation and insomnia (ziprasidone-induced activation syndrome) that occurs at the lower end of the dose range (20–40 mg BID). Advise patients that they may experience some initial restlessness or agitation that should subside with rapid titration to the target dose. The recommended titration schedule for an early psychosis outpatient is:[42]

Day 1:	20 mg AM, 40 mg PM
Day 2:	40 mg AM, 60 mg PM
Day 3:	60 mg AM, 60 mg PM
Day 4:	Reassess

  - extended-release **quetiapine** is usually administered once daily, preferably in the evening. The recommended initial dose is 300 mg daily. Dosage increases can be made rapidly at intervals as short as 1 day and in increments of up to 300 mg/day, to a range of 400–800 mg daily
  - if an FGA is used, consider an intermediate-potency agent such as **loxapine** or **perphenazine**
  - benzodiazepines can be used to treat anxiety and agitation while titrating the dose of antipsychotic
- With the exception of ziprasidone and extended-release quetiapine (both are quickly titrated to avoid adverse reactions), rapid titration and high doses of antipsychotics do not accelerate or enhance response and are rarely indicated. Even in patients with a chronic course, doses in the range of 2–5 mg of haloperidol are as effective as 10–40 mg and associated with fewer side effects and greater tolerability.[43] Only a very small subgroup of patients appears to benefit from high-dose therapy.[44] Doses exceeding the recommended daily maximum (e.g., olanzapine >20 mg/day or quetiapine >800 mg/day) are sometimes required but should be used under the care of a psychiatrist.

- An adequate trial of antipsychotic therapy is 4–8 weeks at a dose within the usual therapeutic range.[14,27,34] Patients who fail to demonstrate even minimal response by that time are unlikely to benefit from a longer trial; consider switching to a different antipsychotic and consulting a psychiatrist.
- There is no good evidence to guide switching from one antipsychotic medication to another. *Crossover medication strategies*, over 2 weeks to 3 months,[45] are preferred. It is important to complete the crossover; combination therapy with more than 1 antipsychotic medication is not supported by evidence and should be used only in exceptional circumstances under the care of a psychiatrist. Patients successfully stabilized on **clozapine** have not been shown to benefit from switching to any other antipsychotic medication, or from the addition of a second antipsychotic.[14] SwitchRx (www.switchrx.ca) is a Canadian online tool that provides clinicians with guidance on how to transition patients from one antipsychotic to another.

Stabilization/Stable Phases

- During the stabilization (recovery) phase patients are vulnerable to relapse. Avoid changes in antipsychotic medication unless there are intolerable side effects or persistent residual symptoms that are distressing and/or disabling to the patient.
- *Maintenance* therapy is essential to prevent relapse. First-episode psychosis is associated with a 70–90% risk of relapse within 5 years. A significant percentage of patients relapse as early as the second year following discontinuation of antipsychotic therapy for first-episode psychosis.[46]
  - continue maintenance pharmacotherapy for at least 1–2 years for first-episode patients who achieve symptom remission and functional recovery.[14,34] Longer treatment (2–5 years) may be required for individuals with a long duration of untreated psychosis, more severe illness, slower response, substance abuse and history of suicidal or aggressive behaviour.[14,34] For patients with a history of 2 or more episodes, continue maintenance pharmacotherapy until the patient has been stable and relapse-free for at least 5 years.[14]
  - many patients will require antipsychotic treatment indefinitely.
  - in general, the lowest effective antipsychotic dose used during the acute phase should also be used in maintenance treatment.[14,18]
- Poor medication adherence is common in patients with schizophrenia and related psychotic disorders. Adherence rates of <70–80% are associated with a significantly increased risk of relapse and hospitalization.[47,48] Patients who discontinue medications are 5 times more likely to relapse.[19] Recovery from recurrent acute psychotic episodes (relapses) may take longer with each subsequent episode and the degree of recovery may not be as great, resulting in persistent residual symptoms and functional disability.[19]
- Long-acting injectable antipsychotics (LAIs) are as effective as oral antipsychotics. In addition to promoting adherence, LAIs may improve rates of remission and decrease the risk of relapse and rehospitalization.[49] LAI usage rates in Canada are low (6.3%) compared to the rest of the world (15–80%).[49] Canadian qualitative studies of physician and patient attitudes toward LAIs indicate that physicians' lack of knowledge and training in the use of LAIs, negative biases toward LAIs (treatment of "last resort") and unfounded beliefs regarding patients' rejection of LAIs due to fear of needles may contribute to the low rates of use.[50,51]
- Consider LAIs (e.g., aripiprazole, paliperidone palmitate or risperidone) in all phases of illness but especially in the first 2–5 years after onset of illness when patients are most vulnerable ("critical period").[52]
- When discontinuing medication, gradually reduce the dose by ≤20% every 2–4 weeks. Reduce over a period of 6–12 months for first episode patients and 6–24 months if patients have experienced 2 or more episodes.[14,18] Monitor closely and if the patient experiences early signs of relapse, restabilize them on the previously effective dose of antipsychotic as quickly as possible.

Treatment of Comorbid Conditions

Depression and Suicidality

- Depressive symptoms are common in the prodromal phase preceding the onset of a first episode of psychosis. In the acute phase, particularly in multiple-episode patients, depressive symptoms usually remit along with the positive psychotic symptoms.
  - SGAs may be more effective than FGAs in treating depressive symptoms[53] in the acute phase. There is no evidence to support the use of an antidepressant in the acute phase.[14]
- Major depressive episodes occur as often in individuals diagnosed with schizophrenia as in those with either schizoaffective disorder or nonpsychotic major depression.[54]
  - patients with first-episode psychosis have a greater risk of depression compared to multiple-episode patients, particularly in the stabilization phase (postpsychotic depression),[55] and depressive symptoms tend to increase for the first 3 months following a first episode of psychosis[56]
- It can be difficult to differentiate between depression and ongoing negative symptoms or antipsychotic-induced emotional blunting, and rating scales such as the HAM-D and Beck Depression Inventory have not been validated in individuals with schizophrenia. The Calgary Depression Scale for Schizophrenia[57] can be used to differentiate between negative symptoms and symptoms of major depression.
- Antidepressant medication may be useful in the treatment of major depression in the stabilization or stable phases.[56] Although there have been few studies, there is limited support for CBT.

Substance Abuse

- Higher rates of substance abuse/dependence disorders are found in individuals with schizophrenia (lifetime prevalence of 47–50%) compared to the general population. Persistent substance abuse is associated with poor treatment adherence, greater risk of suicidality and aggression and significantly poorer outcomes.
- Rates of smoking in individuals with schizophrenia and related psychotic disorders are extremely high (70% in Canada),[58] compared to a rate of approximately 20% in the general population (www.smoke-free.ca). Patients with psychotic disorders are more likely to be heavy smokers and are 2–3 times more likely than nonsmokers to abuse other substances.[59]
  - it is estimated that patients with schizophrenia have a life expectancy that is 20% lower than the general population. This is mostly attributable to increased rates of cardiovascular disease and metabolic syndrome, for which smoking is a significant risk factor.[60]
  - smoking induces the metabolism of some antipsychotics (e.g., clozapine and olanzapine). Consequently smokers require higher doses of these antipsychotics, leading to increased side effects and adverse events.[61,62]
  - actively encourage smoking cessation even though success rates are low in patients with psychotic disorders (in patients with psychoses, only 9% are former smokers compared to 14–49% in the general population).[58] **Nicotine replacement therapies** may be helpful. Use caution with **bupropion** due to the risk of exacerbation of psychosis. **Varenicline** can be considered for patients with psychotic disorders when other smoking cessation options have failed.[63] Inform the patient of the risks and benefits associated with this medication and monitor diligently for new or worsening neuropsychiatric symptoms. For patients with a psychotic disorder and a history of depressed mood, suicidal ideation, behaviours of self-harm, suicide attempts, agitation or hostility, consider a consultation with a psychiatrist.
- The prevalence of cannabis use in individuals with psychotic disorders is higher than in the general population, particularly in early psychosis where rates of use are as high as 86% and rates of DSM IV cannabis abuse/dependence range from 14–28%.[64] Cannabis use is associated with poor

antipsychotic adherence, greater severity and chronicity of symptoms and 4 times the risk of relapse.[65]

- In patients (and particularly in those with first-episode psychosis) who appear to have been using substances as a form of "self-medication," substance abuse may remit spontaneously with recovery from the acute episode.
- A "harm reduction" approach that incorporates motivational interviewing is recommended for individuals with comorbid substance abuse problems. Refer patients with persistent substance abuse to a mental health program that can provide a comprehensive, integrated approach.[66]

Side Effects of Antipsychotics

Table 4 compares the side effect profile of second-generation antipsychotics. Table 5 provides guidance on the assessment and management of antipsychotic-induced side effects.

- Closely monitor and manage side effects since they are the leading cause of nonadherence to medication.
- Patients taking antipsychotics long-term ranked the most burdensome and function impairing side effects as follows: sedation/tiredness, weight gain, difficulty thinking/concentrating and restlessness.[67]

Neuroleptic Malignant Syndrome (NMS)

- Neuroleptic malignant syndrome is a medical emergency with a high mortality rate. It is a rare but serious side effect characterized by muscle rigidity, fever, autonomic disturbance, labile blood pressure, fluctuating levels of consciousness, and elevated levels of creatine kinase (CK) and WBC.
- NMS has been reported with all antipsychotics and can occur at any dosage and at any time. Dehydration is a risk factor (see also Table 5).

Table 4: Comparative Side Effects of Second-generation Antipsychotics

Drug	Sedation	Insomnia	Extra-pyramidal Side Effects[a]	Weight Gain	Metabolic Abnormalities[b]	Hyperpro-lactinemia	Cardiovascular Effects[c]
aripiprazole	+/–	++	++	+	+/–	+/–	+
asenapine	+/–	+/–	+	+/–	+/–	+/–	+
clozapine	++++	–	–	++++	++++	–	++
lurasidone	+	+/–	+	+/–	+/–	+/–	+
olanzapine	+++/++	–	+/–	++++	++++	+/–	+
paliperidone	+/–	++	+++/++	++/+	+/–	+++/++	+
quetiapine	+++	–	–	+++	++	–	+
risperidone	+	+	+++	++	+/–	+++	+
ziprasidone	+	+	+	+/–	+/–	+	++

Legend: ++++ = high; +++ = moderate; ++ = low; + = very low; +/– = minimal or none; – = equivalent to placebo

[a] Includes akathisia.

[b] Includes glucose abnormalities and dyslipidemias.

[c] Includes orthostatic hypotension and/or QT_c prolongation.

Table 5: **Antipsychotic-induced Side Effects: Assessment, Monitoring and Management**[14,89,90]

Side Effect	Assessment, Monitoring and Management
Neuroleptic malignant syndrome	**Assessment:** physical exam with focus on level of consciousness; vital signs (fever, tachycardia, fluctuations in BP); look for evidence of muscle rigidity **Monitoring:** rare, but can occur with any antipsychotic at any dose and at any time; risk factors include young age, male gender, neurologic disabilities, dehydration, agitation, exhaustion, rapid or parenteral administration of antipsychotic **Management:** medical emergency; discontinue antipsychotic and provide supportive care (hydration and cooling); other measures may include **dantrolene** 2–3 mg/kg TID to QID iv (maximum 10 mg/kg daily) and/or **bromocriptine** 2.5–5 mg TID po, increasing by 2.5 mg TID Q24H (maximum 60 mg daily)[45]
Sedation and cognitive effects	**Assessment:** ask patient about daytime drowsiness, excessive sleep, cognitive "dulling"; obtain collateral information from caregivers and family **Monitoring:** see outpatients at least weekly for first 4–6 wk after initiating new antipsychotic **Management:** use SGAs as first-line treatment to reduce risk of cognitive side effects; low initial dose and gradual titration based on degree of sedation, especially with clozapine and first-episode psychosis (exceptions include quetiapine XR and ziprasidone for which rapid titration is recommended). Give entire daily dose at HS if possible to reduce daytime drowsiness; do not use anticholinergic antiparkinsonian agents prophylactically and avoid prolonged use when treating acute EPS
Extrapyramidal side effects (EPS; dystonia, parkinsonism, akathisia, tardive dyskinesia, tardive dystonia, tardive akathisia)	**Assessment:** rating scales such as Simpson Angus Scale, Barnes Akathisia Scale or Extrapyramidal Syndrome Rating Scale (ESRS)[91] are useful to assess EPS and the Abnormal Involuntary Movement Scale or the ESRS is used to assess tardive dyskinesia (TD) **Monitoring:** baseline assessment in antipsychotic-naïve first-episode patients, in multiple-episode patients when initiating a new antipsychotic, and in first-episode and multiple-episode patients whenever dosage of antipsychotic is changed; assess weekly for 2–4 wk or until EPS resolves; in stable patients assess for TD every 6 months or more often in patients at higher risk (on FGAs, erratic medication adherence or intermittent treatment, female, age >55, diagnosis of an affective disorder, substance abuse, diabetes) **Management:** prevention is key—use SGAs first-line; if EPS occurs, first reduce dose; consider switch to SGA if on FGA; prophylactic use of anticholinergics such as benztropine, procyclidine and trihexyphenidyl is not recommended even with FGAs, and should usually be used only on a short-term basis to treat parkinsonism associated with FGAs;[92] anticholinergics are generally not recommended with SGAs[93] For *akathisia*, if dose reduction is not effective, beta-blockers (e.g., **propranolol** 10–120 mg/day) are the treatment of choice with monitoring for hypotension; benzodiazepines also provide symptom relief; anticholinergics are ineffective IM **benztropine** or **diphenhydramine** can be used to treat *acute dystonia* (acute torticollis or oculogyric crisis), followed by reduction in dose or switch to SGA There is no evidence-based treatment for TD—prevention is key—use SGAs first-line; antiparkinsonian medications are not effective and may worsen symptoms; if TD occurs suggest consultation with a psychiatrist; consider switching to an SGA; consider clozapine trial for persistent, severe TD
Weight gain	**Assessment:** baseline weight, body mass index (BMI) and waist circumference **Monitoring:** weight and BMI monthly for 6 months with new antipsychotic then every 3 months when on a stable dosage; waist circumference annually **Management:** prevention is critical as weight reduction is especially difficult in individuals with mental illness; educate about risk of weight gain and provide dietary and exercise counselling; if weight increases >7% over baseline, implement behavioural weight reduction program; if unsuccessful assess risks/benefits of continuing current antipsychotic vs. switching; no consistent evidence of efficacy of adjunctive weight loss pharmacotherapy

(cont'd)

Table 5: **Antipsychotic-induced Side Effects: Assessment, Monitoring and Management[14,89,90]** *(cont'd)*

Side Effect	Assessment, Monitoring and Management
Glucose abnormalities	**Assessment:** baseline fasting plasma glucose; HbA_{1c} if difficult to obtain fasting plasma glucose; oral glucose tolerance test (OGTT) if evidence of impaired glucose tolerance; obtain family history and medical history **Monitoring:** inquire about signs and symptoms of emergent diabetes; fasting plasma glucose 12 wk after initiating new antipsychotic, then yearly; more frequent monitoring required if significant weight gain or if symptomatic; OGTT if evidence of impaired glucose tolerance **Management:** educate about signs and symptoms of emergent diabetes; if diabetes is diagnosed, follow the Canadian Diabetes Association guidelines for diabetes and mental health (guidelines.diabetes.ca/Browse/Chapter18); consider switching to another antipsychotic
Dyslipidemias	**Assessment:** baseline fasting lipid profile (total cholesterol, LDL, HDL, triglycerides) **Monitoring:** fasting lipid profile at 12 wk after initiation of a new antipsychotic, then annually; more frequent monitoring if significant weight gain, and every 6 months if LDL and/or triglycerides above the normal range **Management:** change in diet; consider switching to ziprasidone;[77,94] consult Canadian Cardiovascular Society guidelines for management of dyslipidemia at www.onlinecjc.ca/article/S0828-282X(12)01510-3/fulltext
Cardiovascular side effects	**Assessment:** baseline vital signs; obtain family history and medical history; ECG in individuals >40 y and as clinically indicated **Monitoring:** blood pressure at 12 wk then annually (monitor more frequently when initiating clozapine, until stable dose reached); vital signs and ECG as clinically indicated and with changes in medication; monitor QT_c when affected by multiple medications **Management:** educate about risks and prevention of orthostatic hypotension; if symptoms persist, decrease dose of antipsychotic if possible or switch to another antipsychotic
Endocrine and sexual side effects	**Assessment:** baseline functional inquiry including menstrual history and libido in women and libido, erectile and ejaculatory function in men; baseline prolactin level in first episode psychosis, before initiating antipsychotic associated with hyperprolactinemia and when clinically indicated **Monitoring:** monitor monthly for 3 months after initiating a new antipsychotic, then yearly. **Management:** determine underlying cause of endocrine or sexual dysfunction and treat accordingly; consider drugs for erectile dysfunction For clinically significant hyperprolactinemia, first reduce dose of antipsychotic; if dose reduction not tolerated (emergence of or increase in psychotic symptoms) consider switching to an antipsychotic not associated with risk of hyperprolactinemia

Sedation, Insomnia and Cognitive Side Effects

- Sedation is a very common side effect, especially after starting a new antipsychotic or increasing the dose. It can be very disabling and distressing. Sedation occurs most frequently with low-potency FGAs, clozapine, olanzapine[14] or quetiapine; and to a lesser extent with asenapine[22] and lurasidone.[22] Several antipsychotics (aripiprazole, risperidone [mild], ziprasidone) have the potential to cause sedation or insomnia. Adjust the dose to provide the greatest amount of the total daily dosage at the time of day (i.e., morning or evening) to help manage these side effects.[68] Aripiprazole can cause dose-related somnolence but can also be activating and cause insomnia. Paliperidone is associated with insomnia. Both are usually administered in the morning.
- FGAs can cause a subjective cognitive "dulling" effect and do not improve cognitive deficits, whereas SGAs have shown statistically significant improvement on a variety of cognitive measures[69,70] but clinical significance has not been demonstrated.
- Concomitant medications such as anticholinergics (used to treat EPS) and antiepileptic drugs (used as mood stabilizers) can worsen cognitive deficits[71,72] and may add to the sedative effect.
- Cognitive deficits are correlated with poorer functional outcomes such as social and occupational functioning and activities of daily living.[73]

Extrapyramidal Side Effects

- The major advantage of the SGAs is the significantly reduced risk of EPS (acute dystonia, parkinsonism, akathisia) and tardive dyskinesia (TD) compared to FGAs.[18,26,27,74,75] However, higher doses of risperidone, paliperidone and ziprasidone can cause parkinsonism and akathisia, and higher doses of olanzapine can cause akathisia. Although risk increases with higher doses, aripiprazole, asenapine and lurasidone can cause akathisia at any dose. Risk of parkinsonism is low with asenapine and lurasidone but can occur at higher doses.
- *Parkinsonism* can be associated with dysphoria, decreased concentration and slowing of cognition.
- *Akathisia* (subjective and objective restlessness) is often misidentified as psychotic agitation which can result in an increase in dose of the offending antipsychotic.
- *Tardive dyskinesia* consists of repetitive, involuntary choreoathetoid movements usually involving the buccal-oral-lingual musculature, face, trunk, extremities or respiratory muscles and can be permanent and disabling.
  - the incidence is 5% per year with FGAs and the cumulative risk is up to 50% even if low doses of FGAs are used.[14] The incidence is significantly less with aripiprazole, asenapine, lurasidone, olanzapine, paliperidone, risperidone and ziprasidone. Quetiapine and clozapine have rates of TD equivalent to placebo. Clozapine may improve existing TD.[14]
  - inform patients of the risk of TD when initiating treatment with any antipsychotic medication, especially an FGA.

Weight Gain, Diabetes and Dyslipidemia

- Antipsychotic-induced weight gain and metabolic side effects are serious, given that individuals with schizophrenia and bipolar disorder are already at higher risk of metabolic syndrome compared to the general population.
- For FGAs, the risk of weight gain is greatest with low-potency agents.
- For many SGAs, there is a higher risk of weight gain compared to FGAs. Among SGAs, clozapine and olanzapine are associated with the greatest weight gain followed by quetiapine, risperidone, paliperidone and aripiprazole.[76] Asenapine, lurasidone and ziprasidone are associated with minimal or no weight gain. In the CATIE schizophrenia trial, ziprasidone was the only agent to show improvement in weight and metabolic parameters following a switch from another SGA.[77]
- In studies of 1 year or longer, weight gain did not correlate to dosage therefore dose reductions are unlikely to result in weight loss. In some individuals weight gain may be rapid. Weight usually plateaus over time, although it can continue to increase for over a year. Weight gain often leads to treatment nonadherence and requests to stop or switch antipsychotic medication.
- Compared to FGAs, SGAs are associated with greater risk of glucose abnormalities including hyperglycemia, insulin resistance, new onset type 2 diabetes, exacerbation of type 1 diabetes and diabetic ketoacidosis.[78] Type 2 diabetes is 2–4 times more prevalent in individuals with schizophrenia compared to the general population, and abnormal glucose tolerance and insulin resistance are also more common.[79]
- Independent of risks for weight gain, there are different degrees of risk for glucose abnormalities among SGAs. Clozapine and olanzapine have the highest risk. Aripiprazole, asenapine, lurasidone, paliperidone, risperidone, and ziprasidone have minimal risk of glucose abnormalities.
- Hyperlipidemia has been associated with clozapine and olanzapine. Increased triglycerides have been reported with quetiapine. Aripiprazole, asenapine, lurasidone, paliperidone, risperidone and ziprasidone have not been associated with dyslipidemia.[80,81] Switching to ziprasidone from other agents such as olanzapine or quetiapine has demonstrated improvements in dyslipidemia.[76]
- In first-episode psychosis, treatment with an SGA with less risk of weight gain and metabolic side effects is recommended.

- Consider switching patients with antipsychotic-induced weight gain and metabolic side effects to an SGA with a lower risk of these side effects (considering risks vs. benefits of switch).
  - the Canadian Diabetes Association recommends use of an SGA that is associated with less risk of weight gain, glucose abnormalities and dyslipidemia in individuals with high-risk of weight gain, diabetes, metabolic syndrome and cardiovascular disease.[82]

Cardiovascular Side Effects

- Orthostatic hypotension is the most common antipsychotic-induced cardiovascular side effect, particularly in elderly patients or those with heart disease or diabetes. It is more common with low-potency first-generation antipsychotics and with clozapine, but can occur with aripiprazole, asenapine, lurasidone, olanzapine, quetiapine or risperidone.
- Prolongation of the QT_c interval is associated with torsades de pointes, and can cause recurrent syncope, ventricular fibrillation and sudden cardiac death. Clinically, a QT_c interval of >450 msec is concerning.[83]
  - QT_c prolongation occurs with chlorpromazine, pimozide (particularly at doses >8 mg/day) and haloperidol, although the incidence is low. The SGAs olanzapine, quetiapine and risperidone cause modest QT_c prolongation (mean <30 msec).[84] Minimal QT_c prolongation has been reported with aripiprazole, asenapine, clozapine and lurasidone.[22,85]
  - **ziprasidone** has a greater (though modest) capacity for QT_c interval prolongation compared to other antipsychotics. It is contraindicated in individuals with a known history of QT_c interval prolongation, including congenital long QT_c syndrome or individuals with recent acute myocardial infarction or uncompensated heart failure. Baseline ECGs are not required unless clinically indicated. Before initiating therapy in individuals at risk for electrolyte disturbance, particularly hypokalemia and/or hypomagnesemia (e.g., history of kidney disease, diuretic therapy, water intoxication, eating disorders, prolonged vomiting/diarrhea, alcoholism), measure baseline electrolytes and correct abnormalities.
  - to date there has been no significant increase in morbidity or mortality associated with SGA-induced QT_c interval prolongation. Nevertheless, all antipsychotics that prolong the QT_c interval should not be combined with any other drug that is known to prolong QT_c.[22,42] Consult the ziprasidone product monograph and other references such as www.azcert.org for an extensive list of drugs that may prolong the QT_c interval. Advise patients taking ziprasidone to consult their physician and/or pharmacist before taking any concomitant medications.
- Antipsychotic drugs confer a dose-related increase in the risk of sudden cardiac death.[86] This risk is increased when more than one antipsychotic is used concurrently.
- **Clozapine** is associated with an increased risk of myocarditis (especially in but not limited to the first month of therapy), pericarditis, pericardial effusion, cardiomyopathy, heart failure, myocardial infarction and mitral insufficiency. If signs and symptoms of any of these disorders appear, seek urgent assessment by a cardiologist.

Endocrine and Sexual Side Effects

- Hyperprolactinemia is a common side effect of FGAs (especially high-potency agents such as haloperidol), risperidone and paliperidone (especially at higher doses). Transient hyperprolactinemia can occur with olanzapine and ziprasidone. No differences in prolactin levels have been found with aripiprazole, asenapine, clozapine, lurasidone or quetiapine compared to placebo.[22,87,88]
  - hyperprolactinemia often causes no clinically significant effects but can be associated with menstrual irregularities and galactorrhea in women, galactorrhea and gynecomastia in men and sexual dysfunction in both men and women. Sexual dysfunction, however, is associated with all antipsychotics and is not necessarily related to elevated prolactin levels alone.
  - reducing the antipsychotic dose is the first approach to managing clinically significant side effects associated with hyperprolactinemia.

Choices during Pregnancy and Breastfeeding

Prenatal and Perinatal Risk Factors for Schizophrenia

A number of prenatal and perinatal factors have been associated with an increased risk of schizophrenia in the offspring to varying degrees. These include malnutrition, viral illnesses such as influenza, obesity, x-ray radiation, exposure to cats infected with toxoplasmosis gondii protozoa, use of analgesics (ASA), season of birth (lack of sunlight exposure/vitamin D deficiency), maternal-fetal Rh incompatibility, low birth weight and obstetric complications (hypoxia).

Psychosis and Pregnancy

The onset of a first episode of psychosis during pregnancy is uncommon but if it occurs it is considered a psychiatric emergency and requires treatment because of the potential adverse effects of psychosis on both mother and fetus. Women who experience a psychotic episode during pregnancy have twice the rate of adverse outcomes including stillbirth, infant death, prematurity and small for gestational age even when controlling for other variables including age, education, smoking, marital status, parity and pregnancy-induced hypertension.[95]

Although women with schizophrenia may have lower fertility rates compared to the general population, their relative fertility has increased since deinstitutionalization, possibly due to a change in drug selection. High potency antipsychotics are prescribed less often or at lower doses, resulting in less effect on prolactin levels and ovulation inhibition. More recent studies have found similar numbers of pregnancies in women with schizophrenia compared to the general population.[96,97] Women with schizophrenia also have higher rates of unplanned and unwanted pregnancies, less social support, poorer antenatal care, poorer nutrition, greater use of tobacco, alcohol and illicit substances and the majority experience intermittent loss of custody.[98]

Women with schizophrenia and related psychotic disorders should receive counselling about contraception and pregnancy early in the course of their illness. If a pregnancy is planned, a consultation with a psychiatrist is recommended to evaluate the risks/benefits of maintenance antipsychotics during pregnancy. Pregnancy in a woman being treated for schizophrenia is considered high-risk; referrals to a mental health clinic and obstetrician are recommended, and if possible, the pregnancy should be managed through a high-risk clinic.

Psychosis and the Postpartum Period

Postpartum psychosis usually occurs within 2–4 weeks after delivery. The rate of postpartum psychosis is 1–2/1000 births. This is a psychiatric emergency because of the rare but serious risk of suicide and infanticide. If hospitalization is required and the mother's condition does not pose a risk to the newborn, the mother and baby should be kept together, ideally in a specialized unit.

In the postpartum period the risk of relapse of schizophrenia and related psychosis is high (~24%) and is greatest during the first 3 months. Women with schizoaffective disorder are particularly at risk.[99]

Antipsychotics and Pregnancy

There have been no randomized controlled trials of FGAs or SGAs in pregnant patients. Teratogenic effects have not been demonstrated with the use of antipsychotics during pregnancy but data are limited, particularly for the newer SGAs (aripiprazole, asenapine, lurasidone, paliperidone, ziprasidone). Hypertonia in neonates has been noted following prepartum use of high-potency FGAs.

While minimizing exposure to all medications is advisable, especially during the first trimester, the risks/benefits of antipsychotic use and the choice of medication must be carefully weighed for each patient, considering factors such as severity of past psychotic episodes, vulnerability to relapse, remission versus ongoing residual symptoms, current substance use, level of functioning, availability of social supports and history of prior response including side effects (EPS, weight gain, diabetes).

For many women with schizophrenia and related psychotic disorders, maintenance antipsychotics during pregnancy at the lowest dose possible to prevent relapse will be recommended, as maintenance therapy may ultimately reduce risks to the fetus associated with an acute psychotic relapse, such as exposure to higher maternal doses of medication.[98]

Antipsychotics and the Postpartum Period

Because of the high-risk of relapse in the postpartum period, re-start antipsychotics immediately after the delivery if they were discontinued during pregnancy. Closely monitor women maintained on low-dose maintenance antipsychotics during pregnancy for early signs of relapse, as an increase of dose may be needed in the postpartum period.

Antipsychotics and Breastfeeding

All antipsychotics pass into breast milk. The American Academy of Pediatrics considers excretion of less than 10% of a drug into breast milk to be compatible with breastfeeding.[100] Less than 3% of a dose of FGAs is excreted into breast milk.[100] Drowsiness and lethargy have been reported, although many studies cite no adverse events.[100] Less than 5% of quetiapine is excreted into breast milk and no adverse effects of any other SGAs on breastfeeding infants have been reported, but data are very limited.

There is no consensus regarding breastfeeding in women being treated with antipsychotics; some experts recommend against breastfeeding until further data are available.[98] The potential benefits of breastfeeding must be weighed against potential adverse effects, and discussed with each individual patient.

A discussion of general principles on the use of medications in these special populations can be found in Appendix II and Appendix III. Other specialized reference sources are also provided in these appendices.

Therapeutic Tips

- Initiate treatment before the development of a crisis such as self-harm, aggression or violence.[14,34]
- Provide treatment in the least restrictive setting, considering safety issues, availability of community resources (including both caregiver and mental health supports), the patient's insight and competency to consent to treatment and ability to cooperate with treatment.[14,34]
- Integrate psychosocial interventions such as patient and family psychoeducation, supportive therapy, motivational interviewing and stress management with the use of antipsychotic medications in order to promote adherence to treatment and optimize outcomes.[14,34]
- Conduct baseline and regular ongoing assessments of signs and symptoms, possible comorbid conditions, level of functioning, response to treatment, side effects and medication adherence during all phases of the disorder. A variety of standardized scales and semi-structured interviews facilitate these assessments.[14]
- To ensure continuity of care, longitudinal follow-up by the same clinician or multidisciplinary team is optimal.[14,34]

Table 6: **First-generation Antipsychotics**

Class	Drug	Dose	Adverse Effects	Drug Interactions	Comments	Cost[a]
Antipsychotics, First-generation, low potency	*chlorpromazine* generics	Initial: 50–100 mg/day po Usual: 200–400 mg/day po Maximum: 1000–2000 mg/day po Divided in 1–3 doses/day	More common with low-potency agents: sedation, cardiovascular effects, anticholinergic effects, weight gain, lower seizure threshold, photosensitivity. More common with high-potency agents: increased prolactin, EPS, NMS, tardive movement disorders. Liver function abnormalities.	Additive effects with other CNS depressants, anticholinergics, alpha-adrenergic antagonists; inhibitors of cytochrome P450 enzymes (e.g., TCAs, fluoxetine, fluvoxamine, paroxetine) may increase serum levels; inducers of cytochrome P450 enzymes (e.g., carbamazepine, phenytoin) may decrease serum levels; effects of levodopa may be inhibited.	Advise patients about antipsychotic-associated body temperature dysregulation and prevention of heat stroke (e.g., hydration, sun protection).	$$
	methotrimeprazine, generics	Initial: 25–75 mg/day po Usual: 100–200 mg/day po Maximum: 1000 mg/day po Divided in 1–3 doses/day	See chlorpromazine.	See chlorpromazine.	See chlorpromazine.	$$
Antipsychotics, First-generation, intermediate potency	*loxapine* Xylac, generics	Initial: 10–20 mg/day po Usual: 20–100 mg/day po Maximum: 250 mg/day po Divided in 2–3 doses/day	See chlorpromazine.	See chlorpromazine.	See chlorpromazine.	$
	perphenazine generics	Initial: 4–12 mg/day po Usual: 12–48 mg/day po Maximum: 48–64 mg/day po Divided in 2–3 doses/day	See chlorpromazine.	See chlorpromazine.	See chlorpromazine.	$
	zuclopenthixol Clopixol	Initial: 10–20 mg/day po Usual: 20–60 mg/day po Maximum: 100 mg/day po Divided in 1–3 doses/day	See chlorpromazine.	See chlorpromazine.	See chlorpromazine.	$$$

(cont'd)

Table 6: **First-generation Antipsychotics** *(cont'd)*

Class	Drug	Dose	Adverse Effects	Drug Interactions	Comments	Cost[a]
	zuclopenthixol acetate injection Clopixol Acuphase	50-150 mg im Q2–3 days. Maximum: cumulative dose of 400 mg or 4 injections	See chlorpromazine.	See chlorpromazine.	See chlorpromazine. Not to be used in antipsychotic-naïve patients with first-episode psychosis. Intended for use in acute psychosis, for up to 2 wk.	$ /50 mg dose
	zuclopenthixol decanoate long-acting injection Clopixol Depot	Range: 100–400 mg im Q2–4 wk Usual dose: 150–300 mg im Q2–4 wk	See chlorpromazine.	See chlorpromazine.	See chlorpromazine.	$$
Antipsychotics, First-generation, high potency	*flupentixol* Fluanxol	Initial: 3–6 mg/day po Usual: 9–24 mg/day po Maximum: 24 mg/day po Divided in 2 doses/day	See chlorpromazine.	See chlorpromazine.	See chlorpromazine.	$$$$
	flupentixol decanoate long-acting injection Fluanxol Depot	Range: 20–100 mg im Q2–3 wk Usual dose: 20–40 mg im Q2–3 wk	See chlorpromazine.	See chlorpromazine.	See chlorpromazine.	$$
	fluphenazine generics	Initial: 2–5 mg/day po Usual: 2.5–10 mg/day po Maximum: 20 mg/day po Divided in 1–2 doses/day	See chlorpromazine.	See chlorpromazine.	See chlorpromazine.	$
	fluphenazine decanoate long-acting injection Modecate	Range: 12.5–100 mg im Q2–3 wk Usual dose: 25–50 mg im Q2–3 wk	See chlorpromazine.	See chlorpromazine.	See chlorpromazine. Preferred route is im; can be given sc.	$$
	haloperidol generics	Initial: 1.5–3 mg/day po Usual: 4–12 mg/day po Maximum: 20 mg/day po Divided in 1–3 doses/day	See chlorpromazine.	See chlorpromazine.	See chlorpromazine.	$
	haloperidol decanoate long-acting injection generics	Range/usual dose: 50–300 mg im Q4 wk	See chlorpromazine.	See chlorpromazine.	See chlorpromazine. Dose is approximately 10–15 × daily oral dose.	$$

Class	Drug	Dose	Adverse Effects	Drug Interactions	Comments	Cost[a]
	pimozide Orap, generics	Initial: 2–4 mg/day po Usual: 2–12 mg/day po Maximum: 12 mg/day po Divided in 1–2 doses/day	See chlorpromazine. Pimozide: QT_c prolongation with doses >8 mg/day.	See chlorpromazine. Pimozide: avoid use with sertraline due to increased risk of QT_c prolongation.	See chlorpromazine.	$
	pipotiazine decanoate long-acting injection Piportil L4	Range: 25–250 mg im Q4 wk Usual dose: 75–150 mg im Q4 wk	See chlorpromazine.	See chlorpromazine.	See chlorpromazine.	$$$
	thiothixene Navane	Initial: 5–10 mg/day po Usual: 15–30 mg/day po Maximum: 60 mg/day po Divided in 1–2 doses/day	See chlorpromazine.	See chlorpromazine.	See chlorpromazine.	$$$
	trifluoperazine generics	Initial: 2–10 mg/day po Usual: 6–20 mg/day po Maximum: 40 mg/day po Divided in 1–2 doses/day	See chlorpromazine.	See chlorpromazine.	See chlorpromazine.	$

[a] Cost of 30-day supply of mean usual dose unless otherwise specified; includes drug cost only.
Legend: $ < $25 $$ $25–50 $$$ $50–75 $$$$ $75–100
Abbreviations: CV = cardiovascular; EPS = extrapyramidal symptoms; NMS = neuroleptic malignant syndrome; TCA = tricyclic antidepressant

Table 7: **Second-generation Antipsychotics**

Class	Drug	Dose	Adverse Effects	Drug Interactions	Comments	Cost[a]
Antipsychotics, Second-generation	*aripiprazole* Abilify	Initial: 10–15 mg/day po In first-episode psychosis: 2–5 mg then gradually titrate to 10–15 mg/day Titration: If necessary increase dose after 2 wk Maximum: 30 mg/day	EPS (akathisia, parkinsonism), dizziness, orthostatic hypotension, headache, GI complaints, nasopharyngitis, tremor, sedation, insomnia.	Carbamazepine (or other strong inducers of CYP2D6 or CYP3A4 such as phenytoin, rifampin) can decrease aripiprazole levels significantly. Ketoconazole, quinidine, fluoxetine or paroxetine (or other strong inhibitors of CYP2D6 or CYP3A4) can increase levels substantially.	Advise patients about antipsychotic-associated body temperature dysregulation and prevention of heat stroke (e.g., hydration, sun protection).	$
	aripiprazole prolonged release injectable suspension Abilify Maintena	Ensure patient tolerates aripiprazole oral doses before initiating im dose. Initial: 400 mg im one dose. Continue aripiprazole 10–20 mg daily po × 14 days Maintenance: 400 mg monthly im In first-episode psychosis: 300 mg monthly im	See aripiprazole. Consider dose reduction to 300 mg monthly im if adverse reactions with higher dose.	See aripiprazole. Concomitant administration of CYP3A4 inducers for more than 14 days may cause lower aripiprazole levels and reduce efficacy. Increased sedation when combined with alcohol or other CNS drugs.	See aripiprazole. Dose adjustments recommended when patients are adding or discontinuing concomitant strong inhibitors of CYP3A4 or CYP2D6.	$$$
	asenapine Saphris	Initial: 5 mg BID sl Titration: Target therapeutic dose same as initial dose (5 mg BID sl) Maximum: 10 mg BID sl	Hypersensitivity reactions, oral hypoesthesia and paresthesia, orthostatic hypotension, sedation, insomnia, akathisia, EPS, constipation. Minimal effect on weight, glucose, lipids.	May potentiate antihypertensive drug effects. Strong inhibitors of CYP1A2 (such as fluvoxamine) increase asenapine levels. Other CYP1A2 inducers or inhibitors may affect asenapine levels.	See aripiprazole. Instruct patients to handle the tablet with dry hands, to place it immediately under the tongue, to allow it to dissolve completely (do not chew or swallow) and to not drink or eat for 10 minutes afterward. If asenapine is taken in combination with other oral medications it should be taken last.	$

Class	Drug	Dose	Adverse Effects	Drug Interactions	Comments	Cost[a]
	clozapine Clozaril, Gen-Clozapine, generics	Initial: 12.5–25 mg/day po Titration: Increase by 12.5–25 mg on 2nd day and then by 25–50 mg daily po depending on tolerance Usual: 300–600 mg/day po Maximum: 900 mg/day Divided in 1–3 doses/day	Agranulocytosis (<1%), seizures (1–5%; dose-related), sedation, orthostatic hypotension, tachycardia, fever, nausea, weight gain, hypersalivation (30–50%), urinary incontinence; increased risk of diabetes and hyperlipidemia; myocarditis and other cardiac effects (see Pharmacologic Choices).	Additive sedation with CNS depressants; may potentiate antihypertensive drug effects; inhibitors of CYP1A2, such as diltiazem, fluvoxamine or propranolol, or of CYP3A4, such as clarithromycin, erythromycin, grapefruit juice or prednisone, may increase clozapine levels; inducers of CYP1A2 or CYP3A4 such as carbamazepine, phenytoin, rifampin or cigarette smoking may reduce clozapine levels; respiratory depression with higher doses of benzodiazepines; avoid use with bone marrow suppressants and drugs that lower the seizure threshold.	See aripiprazole.	$$
	lurasidone Latuda	Initial: 40 mg daily po (with food) Titration: Target therapeutic dose same as initial dose (40 mg daily po) Usual: 40–80 mg daily po Maximum: 160 mg daily po	Nausea and vomiting, sedation, akathisia, EPS, orthostatic hypotension, insomnia.	May potentiate antihypertensive drug effects; do not use in combination with strong inhibitors of CYP3A4 such as ketoconazole; do not exceed doses of 40 mg daily po in combination with other inhibitors of CYP3A4 such as diltiazem, clarithromycin, erythromycin, prednisone, grapefruit, grapefruit juice (increased lurasidone levels); do not use in combination with strong inducers of CYP3A4 such as carbamazepine, phenytoin (decreased lurasidone levels).	See aripiprazole. Administer with meals of >350 kcal to maximize absorption and therapeutic effect.	$
	olanzapine Zyprexa, Zyprexa Zydis (rapid-dissolving oral tablets), generics	Initial: 5–10 mg/day po Titration: Increase by 2.5–5 mg every 3–4 days Usual: 10–20 mg/day Maximum: 20 mg/day (product monograph). Doses of up to 40 mg/day are used in clinical practice under care of a psychiatrist Frequency: 1 dose/day; higher doses may be given in 2 divided doses	Weight gain, dizziness, sedation, anticholinergic effects, hepatic aminotransferase elevation, orthostatic hypotension, increased risk of diabetes and dyslipidemia, EPS (especially akathisia).	Sedation with CNS depressants; may potentiate antihypertensive drug effects; inhibitors of CYP1A2 or CYP2D6 such as diltiazem, fluvoxamine, or paroxetine may increase olanzapine levels; inducers of CYP1A2 or CYP3A4 such as barbiturates, carbamazepine, phenytoin, rifampin or cigarette smoking may decrease olanzapine levels.	See aripiprazole.	$

(cont'd)

Table 7: Second-generation Antipsychotics *(cont'd)*

Class	Drug	Dose	Adverse Effects	Drug Interactions	Comments	Cost[a]
	olanzapine injection Zyprexa Intramuscular	Initial: 5–10 mg im Usual: 10 mg im. If necessary 2nd dose of 5–10 mg im may be given 2 h after first injection Maximum: 20 mg/day (oral and im) with no more than 3 injections in 24 h	See oral olanzapine.	See oral olanzapine. Should not be administered simultaneously with parenteral benzodiazepines due to reports of cardiac and respiratory problems including deaths.	See aripiprazole.	$ /10 mg dose
	paliperidone Invega	Initial: 3–6 mg daily po Titration: If necessary increase by 3 mg per day at 5-day intervals Maximum: 12 mg daily	Insomnia, headaches, weight gain, orthostatic hypotension, rhinitis, anxiety, dose-related hyperprolactinemia and EPS. Risk of intraoperative floppy iris syndrome in patients undergoing cataract surgery who have been exposed to paliperidone.	Minimal risk of drug interactions. Carbamazepine may decrease paliperidone serum concentrations.	See aripiprazole. Less orthostatic hypotension and weight gain and more insomnia compared to risperidone.	$$
	paliperidone palmitate long-acting injectable Invega Sustenna	Initial: 150 mg im (deltoid muscle) and 100 mg im (deltoid muscle) 7 days later. No oral supplementation required Usual: 100 mg im monthly in either deltoid or gluteal muscle Range: 25–150 mg im monthly	See paliperidone.	See paliperidone.	See aripiprazole. Less orthostatic hypotension and weight gain and more insomnia compared to risperidone.	$$$
	quetiapine immediate-release Seroquel, generics	Initial: 50–100 mg/day po Titration: Increase by 100 mg/day Usual: 600 mg/day Maximum: 800 mg/day (product monograph). Doses of up to 1200 mg/day used in clinical practice under care of a psychiatrist Divided in 1–3 doses/day	Sedation, dizziness, weight gain, orthostatic hypotension, hepatic aminotransferase elevation, headache, anticholinergic effects, increased risk of diabetes and dyslipidemia, possible increased risk of cataracts; may reduce thyroid hormone levels.	Additive sedation with CNS depressants; may potentiate antihypertensive drug effects; inhibitors of CYP3A4 (e.g., clarithromycin, erythromycin, grapefruit juice, ketoconazole, prednisone) may increase quetiapine levels; inducers of CYP3A4 (e.g., carbamazepine, phenytoin, rifampin) may decrease quetiapine levels.	See aripiprazole.	$

Class	Drug	Dose	Adverse Effects	Drug Interactions	Comments	Cost[a]
	quetiapine extended-release Seroquel XR, generics	Initial: 300 mg QHS po (200 mg for first-episode psychosis) Titration: May increase dose in increments of ≤300 mg/day at intervals ≥1 day Usual: 400–800 mg/day Given as a once-daily dose, generally in the evening	See quetiapine immediate-release.	See quetiapine immediate-release.	See aripiprazole.	$
	risperidone Risperdal Preparations, generics	Initial: 0.5–1 mg/day po Titration: Increase by 0.5–1 mg po every 3–4 days Usual: 2–6 mg/day po Maximum: 6 mg/day po Frequency: 1 dose/day, preferably QHS	Sedation, headaches, weight gain, orthostatic hypotension, rhinitis, anxiety, dose-related hyperprolactinemia and EPS. Risk of intraoperative floppy iris syndrome in patients undergoing cataract surgery who have been exposed to risperidone.	Additive sedation with CNS depressants; may potentiate antihypertensive drug effects; inhibitors of CYP3A4 (e.g., clarithromycin, erythromycin, grapefruit juice, ketoconazole, prednisone) may increase risperidone levels; inducers of CYP3A4 (e.g., carbamazepine, phenytoin, rifampin) may decrease risperidone levels.	See aripiprazole.	$
	risperidone long-acting injection Risperdal Consta	Initial: 25 mg im every 2 wk (oral supplementation with current antipsychotic required for first 3 wk) Titration: Depending on response, increase by 12.5 mg every 4–8 wk Usual: 25–37.5 mg im every 2 wk. Some patients can be maintained on a dose of 12.5 mg every 2 wk Maximum: 50 mg im every 2 wk	See oral risperidone. Adverse effects may be less severe compared to oral risperidone due to decreased peak to trough serum fluctuations.	See oral risperidone.	See aripiprazole.	$$$
	ziprasidone Zeldox	Start with 40 mg BID po (20 mg BID for antipsychotic-naïve first-episode patients) and rapidly titrate in the first wk up to 120–160 mg/day Administer doses with food (see Comments)	Orthostatic hypotension, EPS, sedation, insomnia. Prolonged QT-interval; contraindicated in patients with history of QT_c prolongation, recent MI, uncompensated heart failure or with concomitant use of any other drug that prolongs the QT_c interval.	Contraindicated with any other drug that prolongs the QT_c interval such as: commonly used antibiotics such as azithromycin, clarithromycin and erythromycin; antiarrhythmics such as amiodarone, ibutilide, procainamide, quinidine and sotalol; lithium, methadone and venlafaxine.	Administer with meals of ≥500 kcal to maximize absorption and therapeutic effect. See aripiprazole.	$

(cont'd)

Table 7: **Second-generation Antipsychotics** *(cont'd)*

Class	Drug	Dose	Adverse Effects	Drug Interactions	Comments	Cost[a]
			Rapid titration is recommended to avoid ziprasidone-induced "activation" syndrome consisting of anxiety, restlessness, insomnia, increased energy and hypomanic-like symptoms which develop soon after treatment initiation and occur at the lower end of the dosage range (20–40 mg BID po).	May potentiate antihypertensive drug effects.		

[a] Cost of 30-day supply of mean usual dose unless otherwise specified; includes drug cost only.

Dosage adjustment may be required in renal impairment; see Appendix I

Abbreviations: EPS = extrapyramidal symptoms

Legend: $ < $150 $$ $150–350 $$$ $350–550

Suggested Readings

Canadian Psychiatric Association. Clinical practice guidelines. Treatment of schizophrenia. *Can J Psychiatry* 2005;50(13 Suppl 1):7S-57S.

Faulkner G, Cohn TA. Pharmacologic and nonpharmacologic strategies for weight gain and metabolic disturbance in patients treated with antipsychotic medications. *Can J Psychiatry* 2006;51(8):502-11.

Gardner DM, Baldessarini RJ, Waraich P. Modern antipsychotic drugs: a critical overview. *CMAJ* 2005;172(13):1703-11.

Gardner DM, Murphy AL, Kutcher S et al. Evidence review and clinical guidance for the use of ziprasidone in Canada. *Ann Gen Psychiatry* 2013;12(1):1.

Gardner DM, Teehan MD. *Antipsychotics and their side effects*. Cambridge (GB): Cambridge University Press; 2011.

Long-acting injectable antipsychotics: recommendations for clinicians. *Can J Psychiatry* 2013;58(5 Suppl 1):1S-36S. Available from: publications.cpa-apc.org/browse/documents/593.

References

1. Nova Scotia Early Psychosis Program, Capital Health Mental Health Program, Capital Health and the Department of Psychiatry, Dalhousie University. *The sooner the better: get help early for psychosis. Information guide*. Halifax (NS): Nova Scotia Early Psychosis Program; 2003. Available from: earlypsychosis.medicine.dal.ca/resources/FinalBooklet_July14_2008.pdf. Accessed January 27, 2014.
2. McGorry PD, Killackey EJ. Early intervention in psychosis: a new evidence based paradigm. *Epidemiol Psychiatr Soc* 2002;11(4):237-47.
3. McGorry PD, Killackey EJ, Yung A. Early intervention in psychosis: concepts, evidence and future directions. *World Psychiatry* 2008;7(3):148-56.
4. Perkins D, Gu H, Boteva K et al. Relationship between untreated psychosis and outcome in first-episode schizophrenia: a critical review and meta-analysis. *Am J Psychiatry* 2005;162(10):1785-804.
5. Craig TJ, Bromet EJ, Fennig S et al. Is there an association between duration of untreated psychosis and 24-month clinical outcome in a first-admission series? *Am J Psychiatry* 2000;157(1):60-6.
6. Preti A, Cella M. Randomized-controlled trials in people at ultra high risk of psychosis: a review of treatment effectiveness. *Schizophr Res* 2010;123(1):30-6.
7. Yung AR, Phillips LJ, Yuen et al. Psychosis prediction: 12-month follow up of a high-risk ("prodromal") group. *Schizophr Res* 2003;60(10):21-32.
8. Amminger GP, Shafer MR, Papageorgiou K et al. Long-chain omega-3 fatty acids for indicated prevention of psychotic disorders: a randomized, placebo-controlled trial. *Arch Gen Psychiatry* 2010;67(2):146-54.
9. Miller TJ, McGlashan TH, Rosen JL et al. Prodromal assessment with the structured interview for prodromal syndromes and the scale of prodromal symptoms: predictive validity, interrater reliability, and training to reliability. *Schizophr Bull* 2003;29(4):703-15.
10. Stowkowy J, Colijn MA, Addington J. Pathways to care for those at clinical high risk of developing psychosis. *Early Interv Psychiatry* 2013;7(1):80-3.
11. Addington J, Van Mastrigt S, Hutchinson J et al. Pathways to care: help seeking behaviour in first episode psychosis. *Acta Psych Scand* 2002;106(5):285-64.
12. American Psychiatric Association. Task Force on DSM-V. *Diagnostic and statistical manual of mental disorders: DSM-V*. 5th ed. Washington (DC): American Psychiatric Publishing; 2013.
13. Caspi A, Moffitt TE, Cannon M et al. Moderation of the effect of adolescent-onset cannabis use on adult psychosis by a functional polymorphism in the catechol-O-methyltransferase gene: longitudinal evidence of a gene X environment interaction. *Biol Psychiatry* 2005;57(10):1117-27.
14. Canadian Psychiatric Association. Clinical practice guidelines. Treatment of schizophrenia. *Can J Psychiatry* 2005;50(13 Suppl 1):7S-57S.
15. Guy W; National Institute of Mental Health. Psychopharmacology Research Branch; Early Clinical Drug Evaluation Program. *ECDEU assessment manual for psychopharmacology*. Rockville (MD): U.S. Dept. of Health, Education, and Welfare, Public Health Service, Alcohol, Drug Abuse, and Mental Health Administration, National Institute of Mental Health, Psychopharmacology Research Branch, Division of Extramural Research Programs; 1976. p. 217-22.
16. Kay SR, Fiszbein A, Opler LA. The positive and negative syndrome scale (PANSS) for schizophrenia. *Schizophr Bull* 1987;13(2):261-76.
17. American Diabetes Association; American Psychiatric Association; American Association of Clinical Endocrinologists et al. Consensus development conference on antipsychotic drugs and obesity and diabetes. *Diabetes Care* 2004;27(2):596-601.
18. Siegfried SI, Fleischhacker W, Lieberman JA. Pharmacological treatment of schizophrenia. In: Lieberman JA, Murray RM, eds. *Comprehensive care of schizophrenia: a textbook of clinical management*. London (GB): Martin Dunitz; 2001. p. 59-94.
19. Zipursky RB. Optimal pharmacologic management of the first episode of schizophrenia. In: Zipursky RB, Schulz SC, eds. *The early stages of schizophrenia*. 1st ed. Washington (DC): American Psychiatric Pub; 2002.
20. Seeman P. Atypical antipsychotics: mechanism of action. *Can J Psychiatry* 2002;47(1):27-38.
21. Shahid M, Walker GB, Zorn SH et al. Asenapine: a novel psychopharmacologic agent with a unique human receptor signature. *J Psychopharmacol* 2009;23(1):65-73.
22. Canadian Pharmacists Association. *CPS: Compendium of pharmaceuticals and specialties*. Ottawa (ON): CPhA; 2013.
23. Meltzer HY, Cuchiarro J, Silva R et al. Lurasidone in the treatment of schizophrenia: a randomized, double-blind, placebo- and olanzapine-controlled study. *Am J Psychiatry* 2011;168(9):957-67.
24. Emsley RA. Risperidone in the treatment of first-episode psychotic patients: a double-blind multicenter study. Risperidone Working Group. *Schizophr Bull* 1999;25(4):721-9.
25. Sanger TM, Lieberman JA, Tohen M et al. Olanzapine versus haloperidol treatment in first-episode psychosis. *Am J Psychiatry* 1999;156(1):79-87.
26. Canadian Psychiatric Association. *Practical guide for schizophrenia management*. Ottawa (ON): CPA; 2000.

27. Marder SR, Essock SM, Miller AL et al. The Mount Sinai conference on the pharmacotherapy of schizophrenia. *Schizophr Bull* 2002;28(1):5-16.
28. Csernansky JG, Mahmoud R, Brenner R et al. A comparison of risperidone and haloperidol for the prevention of relapse in patients with schizophrenia. *N Engl J Med* 2002;346(1):16-22.
29. Conley RR, Love RC, Kelly DL et al. Rehospitalization rates of patients recently discharged on a regimen of risperidone or clozapine. *Am J Psychiatry* 1999;156(6):863-8.
30. Citrome L, Volavka J, Czobor P et al. Effects of clozapine, olanzapine, risperidone, and haloperidol on hostility among patients with schizophrenia. *Psychiatr Serv* 2001;52(11):1510-4.
31. Kane JM, Marder SR, Schooler NR et al. Clozapine and haloperidol in moderately refractory schizophrenia: a 6-month randomized and double-blind comparison. *Arch Gen Psychiatry* 2001;58(10):965-72.
32. Meltzer HY, Okayli G. Reduction of suicidality during clozapine treatment of neuroleptic-resistant schizophrenia: impact on risk-benefit assessment. *Am J Psychiatry* 1995;152(2):183-90.
33. Tiihonen J, Lonnqvist J, Wahlbeck K et al. 11-year follow-up of mortality in patients with schizophrenia: a population-based cohort study (FIN11 study). *Lancet* 2009;374(9690):620-7.
34. International Early Psychosis Association. *Draft consensus statement—principles and practice in early psychosis*. Victoria (AU): IEPA; 2003.
35. Battaglia J, Moss S, Rush J et al. Haloperidol, lorazepam, or both for psychotic agitation? A multicenter, prospective, double-blind, emergency department study. *Am J Emerg Med* 1997;15(4):335-40.
36. Breier A, Meehan K, Birkett M et al. A double-blind, placebo-controlled dose-response comparison of intramuscular olanzapine and haloperidol in the treatment of acute agitation in schizophrenia. *Arch Gen Psychiatry* 2002;59(5):441-8.
37. Wright P, Birkett M, David SR et al. Double-blind, placebo-controlled comparison of intramuscular olanzapine and intramuscular haloperidol in the treatment of acute agitation in schizophrenia. *Am J Psychiatry* 2001;158(7):1149-51.
38. Currier GW, Chou JC, Feifel D et al. Acute treatment of psychotic agitation: a randomized comparison of oral treatment with risperidone and lorazepam versus intramuscular treatment with haloperidol and lorazepam. *J Clin Psychiatry* 2004;65(3):386-94.
39. Lieberman J, Jody D, Geisler S et al. Time course and biologic correlates of treatment response in first-episode schizophrenia. *Arch Gen Psychiatry* 1993;50(5):369-76.
40. Lieberman JA, Koreen AR, Chakos M et al. Factors influencing treatment response and outcome of first-episode schizophrenia: implications for understanding the pathophysiology of schizophrenia. *J Clin Psychiatry* 1996;57(Suppl 9):5-9.
41. Chengappa KN, Parepally H, Brar JS et al. A random-assignment, double-blind, clinical trial of once- vs twice-daily administration of quetiapine fumarate in patients with schizophrenia or schizoaffective disorder: a pilot study. *Can J Psychiatry* 2003;48(3):187-94.
42. Gardner DM, Murphy AL, Kutcher S et al. Evidence review and clinical guidance for the use of ziprasidone in Canada. *Ann Gen Psychiatry* 2013;12(1):1.
43. Stone CK, Garve DL, Griffith J et al. Further evidence of a dose-response threshold for haloperidol in psychosis. *Am J Psychiatry* 1995;152(8):1210-2.
44. Thompson C. The use of high-dose antipsychotic medication. *Br J Psychiatry* 1994;164(4):448-58.
45. Weiden PJ et al. *Breakthroughs in antipsychotic medications: a guide for consumers, families, and clinicians*. New York (NY): Norton; 1999.
46. Robinson D, Woerner MG, Alvir JM et al. Predictors of relapse following response from a first episode of schizophrenia or schizoaffective disorder. *Arch Gen Psychiatry* 1999;56(3):241-7.
47. Kane JM. Problems of compliance in the outpatient treatment of schizophrenia. *J Clin Psychiatry* 1983;44(6 Pt 2):3-6.
48. Valenstein M, Copeland LA, Blow FC et al. Pharmacy data identify poorly adherent patients with schizophrenia at increased risk for admission. *Med Care* 2002;40(8):630-9.
49. Manchanda R, Chue P, Malla A et al. Long-acting injectable antipsychotics: evidence of effectiveness and use. *Can J Psychiatry* 2013;58(5 Suppl 1):5S-13S.
50. Iver S, Banks N, Roy MA et al. A qualitative study of experiences with and perceptions regarding long-acting injectable antipsychotics: Part I—patient perspectives. *Can J Psychiatry* 2013;58(5 Suppl 1):14S-22S.
51. Iver S, Banks N, Roy MA et al. A qualitative study of experiences with and perceptions regarding long-acting injectable antipsychotics: Part II—physician perspectives. *Can J Psychiatry* 2013;58(5 Suppl 1):23S-9S.
52. Malla A, Tibbo P, Chue P et al. Long-acting injectable antipsychotics: recommendations for clinicians *Can J Psychiatry* 2013;58(5 Suppl 1):30S-5S.
53. Davis JM, Chen N, Glick ID. A meta-analysis of the efficacy of second-generation antipsychotics. *Arch Gen Psychiatry* 2003;60(6):553-64.
54. Sands JR, Harrow M. Depression during the longitudinal course of schizophrenia. *Schizophr Bull* 1999;25(1):157-71.
55. Koreen AR, Siris SG, Chakos M et al. Depression in first-episode schizophrenia. *Am J Psychiatry* 1993;150(11):1643-8.
56. Addington D, Addington J, Patten S. Depression in people with first-episode schizophrenia. *Br J Psychiatry Suppl* 1998;172(33):90-2.
57. Addington D, Addington J, Schissel B. A depression rating scale for schizophrenics. *Schizophr Res* 1990;3(4):247-51.
58. de Leon J, Diaz FJ. A meta-analysis of worldwide studies demonstrates an association between schizophrenia and tobacco smoking behaviors. *Schizophr Res* 2005;76(2-3):135-57.
59. Ziedonis DM, Kosten TR, Glazer WM et al. Nicotine dependence and schizophrenia. *Hosp Community Psychiatry* 1994;45(3):204-6.
60. Goff DC, Cather C, Evins AE et al. Medical morbidity and mortality in schizophrenia: guidelines for psychiatrists. *J Clin Psychiatry* 2005;66(2):183-94.
61. Dalack GW, Meador-Woodruff JH. Smoking, smoking withdrawal and schizophrenia: case reports and a review of the literature. *Schizophr Res* 1996;22(2):133-41.
62. Haustein KO, Haffner S, Woodcock BG. A review of the pharmacological and psychopharmacological aspects of smoking and smoking cessation in psychiatric patients. *Int J Clin Pharmacol Ther* 2002;40(9):404-18.
63. Williams JM, Anthenelli RM, Morris CD et al. A randomized, double-blind, placebo-controlled study evaluating the safety and efficacy of varenicline for smoking cessation in patients with schizophrenia or schizoaffective disorder. *J Clin Psychiatry* 2012;73(5):654-60.
64. Edwards J, Elkins K, Hinton M et al. Randomized controlled trial of a cannabis-focused intervention for young people with first-episode psychosis. *Acta Psychiatr Scand* 2006;114(2):109-17.
65. Linszen DH, Dingemans PM, Nugter MA et al. Patient attributes and expressed emotion as risk factors for psychotic relapse. *Schizophr Bull* 1997;23(1):119-30.
66. Drake RE, Mueser KT, Brunette MF et al. A review of treatments for people with severe mental illnesses and co-occurring substance use disorders. *Psychiatr Rehabil J* 2004;27(4):360-74.

67. Meehan T, Stedman T, Wallace J. Consumer strategies for coping with antipsychotic medication side effects. *Autralas Psychiatry* 2011;19(1):74-7.
68. Harvey PD, Meltzer H, Simpson GM et al. Improvement in cognitive function following a switch to ziprasidone from conventional antipsychotics, olanzapine, or risperidone in outpatients with schizophrenia. *Schizophr Res* 2004;66(2-3):101-13.
69. Bilder RM, Goldman RS, Volavka J et al. Neurocognitive effects of clozapine, olanzapine, risperidone, and haloperidol in patients with chronic schizophrenia or schizoaffective disorder. *Am J Psychiatry* 2002;159(6):1018-28.
70. Velligan DI, Miller AL. Cognitive dysfunction in schizophrenia and its importance to outcome: the place of atypical antipsychotics in treatment. *J Clin Psychiatry* 1999;60(Suppl 23):25-8.
71. Chakos M, Lieberman J, Hoffman E et al. Effectiveness of second-generation antipsychotics in patients with treatment-resistant schizophrenia: a review and meta-analysis of randomized trials. *Am J Psychiatry* 2001;158(4):518-26.
72. Raggi MA, Mandrioli R, Sabbioni C et al. Atypical antipsychotics: pharmacokinetics, therapeutic drug monitoring and pharmacological interactions. *Curr Med Chem* 2004;11(3):279-96.
73. Velligan DI, Mahurin RK, Diamond PL et al. The functional significance of symptomatology and cognitive function in schizophrenia. *Schizophr Res* 1997;25(1):21-31.
74. Casey DE. Tardive dyskinesia and atypical antipsychotic drugs. *Schizophr Res* 1999;35(Suppl):S61-6.
75. Leucht S, Pitschel-Walz G, Abraham D et al. Efficacy and extrapyramidal side-effects of the new antipsychotics olanzapine, quetiapine, risperidone, and sertindole compared to conventional antipsychotics and placebo. A meta-analysis of randomized controlled trials. *Schizophr Res* 1999;35(1):51-68.
76. Shriqui CL. Atypical antipsychotics. *Can J CME* 2002;65-80. Available from: www.stacommunications.com/journals/pdfs/cme/julycme/g.pdf. Accessed January 27, 2014.
77. Lieberman JA, Stroup TS, McEvoy JP et al. Effectiveness of antipsychotic drugs in patients with chronic schizophrenia. *N Engl J Med* 2005;353(12):1209-23.
78. Sernyak MJ, Leslie DL, Alarcon RD et al. Association of diabetes mellitus with use of atypical neuroleptics in the treatment of schizophrenia. *Am J Psychiatry* 2002;159(4):561-6.
79. Buse JB. Metabolic side effects of antipsychotics: focus on hyperglycemia and diabetes. *J Clin Psychiatry* 2002;63(Suppl 4):37-41.
80. Casey DE. Dyslipidemia and atypical antipsychotic drugs. *J Clin Psychiatry* 2004;65(Suppl 18):27-35.
81. Marder SR, Essock SM, Miller AL et al. Physical health monitoring of patients with schizophrenia. *Am J Psychiatry* 2004;161(8):1334-49.
82. Woo V, Harris SB, Houlden RI. Canadian Diabetes Association position paper: Antipsychotic medications and associated risks of weight gain and diabetes. *Can J Diabetes* 2005;29:111-2.
83. Vieweg WV. Mechanisms and risks of electrocardiographic QT interval prolongation when using antipsychotic drugs. *J Clin Psychiatry* 2002;63(Suppl 9):18-24.
84. U.S. Food and Drug Administration. FDA Psychopharmacological Drugs Advisory Committee. *Briefing document for Zeldox capsules (Ziprasidone HCl)*. Rockville (MD): FDA, Pfizer; 2000. Available from: www.fda.gov/ohrms/dockets/ac/00/backgrd/3619b1a.pdf. Accessed January 27, 2014.
85. Feinstein RE, Khawaja IS, Nurenberg JR et al. Cardiovascular effects of psychotropic drugs. *Curr Probl Cardiol* 2002;27(5):190-240.
86. Ray WA, Chung CP, Murray KT et al. Atypical antipsychotic drugs and the risk of sudden cardiac death. *N Engl J Med* 2009;360(3):225-35.
87. Atmaca M, Kuloglu M, Tezcan E et al. Quetiapine is not associated with increase in prolactin secretion in contrast to haloperidol. *Arch Med Res* 2002;33(6):562-5.
88. Knegtering H, van der Moolen AE, Castelein S et al. What are the effects of antipsychotics on sexual dysfunctions and endocrine functioning? *Psychoneuroendocrinology* 2003;28(Suppl 2):109-23.
89. Cohn TA, Sernyak MJ. Metabolic monitoring for patients treated with antipsychotic medications. *Can J Psychiatry* 2006;51(8):492-501.
90. Gardner DM, Teehan MD. *Antipsychotics and their side effects*. Cambridge (GB): Cambridge University Press; 2011.
91. De Deyn PP, Wirshing WC. Scales to assess efficacy and safety of pharmacologic agents in the treatment of behavioral and psychological symptoms of dementia. *J Clin Psychiatry* 2001;62(Suppl 21):19-22.
92. Stahl SM, Grady MM. A critical review of atypical antipsychotic utilization: comparing monotherapy with polypharmacy and augmentation. *Curr Med Chem* 2004;11(3):313-27.
93. Serretti A, De Ronchi D, Lorenzi C et al. New antipsychotics and schizophrenia: a review on efficacy and side effects. *Curr Med Chem* 2004;11(3):343-58.
94. Weiden PJ. Switching antipsychotics as a treatment strategy for antipsychotic-induced weight gain and dyslipidemia. *J Clin Psychiatry* 2007;68(Suppl 4):34-9.
95. Nilsson E, Lichtenstein P, Cnattingius S et al. Women with schizophrenia: pregnancy outcome and infant death among their offsprings. *Schizophr Res* 2002;58(2-3):221-9.
96. Odegard O. Fertility of psychiatric first admissions in Norway 1936-1975. *Acta Psychiatr Scand* 1980;62(3):212-20.
97. Howard LM, Kumar R, Thornicroft G. Psychosocial characteristics and needs of mothers with psychotic disorders. *Br J Psychiatry* 2001;178:427-32.
98. Yaeger D, Smith HG, Altshuler LL. Atypical antipsychotics in the treatment of schizophrenia during pregnancy and the postpartum. *Am J Psychiatry* 2006;163(12):2064-70.
99. McNeil TF. A prospective study of postpartum psychoses in a high-risk group. 1. Clinical characteristics of the current postpartum episodes. *Acta Psychiatr Scand* 1986;74(2):205-16.
100. Centre for Addiction and Mental Health. *Exposure to psychotropic medications and other substances during pregnancy and lactation: a handbook for health care providers*. Toronto (ON): CAMH; 2007. Available from: www.camh.ca/en/education/about/camh_publications/Pages/exposure_psychotropic_meds_pregnancy.aspx. Accessed January 27, 2014.

Chapter 12
Drug Withdrawal Syndromes

James R. Kennedy, MD, FRCPC

Treatment of drug withdrawal syndromes requires attention to both the biological (medical) model and the behavioural (psychosocial) model. Alcohol and benzodiazepine withdrawal can result in medically important sequelae such as seizures and autonomic instability. Opioid withdrawal results in markedly unpleasant symptoms without important medical sequelae. Stimulant withdrawal is almost exclusively behavioural with the most important risks being suicidality and, less commonly, hallucinosis with amphetamines.

Withdrawal syndrome diagnosis requires:[1]

- The development of a substance-specific syndrome due to cessation or reduction of prolonged substance use
- Clinically significant distress or impairment of functioning
- The absence of a medical or other psychiatric disorder that can cause the syndrome

Goals of Therapy

- Anticipate, prevent and treat complications
- Relieve symptoms
- Assess for and treat comorbidities (medical and psychiatric)
- Facilitate definitive psychosocial/behavioural treatment
- Prevent relapse

Investigations

- Detailed history and physical examination to evaluate severity of abuse of the substance (amount, frequency, duration) and comorbid medical and psychiatric conditions
- Specific assessment tools such as the Clinical Institute Withdrawal Assessment for Alcohol (CIWA-Ar)[2] or CIWA-Benzo[3]
- Laboratory tests and/or imaging to assess comorbidities/complications revealed in history and physical (complete blood count, renal/liver function, electrolytes, magnesium, phosphorus, chest x-ray, CT of head)
- Drug screening: blood alcohol or urine screen for benzodiazepines may be helpful in the trauma or emergency patient where history is inadequate

Therapeutic Choices

Figure 1 illustrates a process for managing patients experiencing drug withdrawal.

Nonpharmacologic Choices

- Nonjudgmental approach to explain process, reassure and support.
- Psychosocial treatment program (cognitive behavioural therapy, motivational enhancement therapy, interpersonal therapy, 12-step, group and family therapies).[4]

Figure 1: **Management of Drug Withdrawal Syndromes**

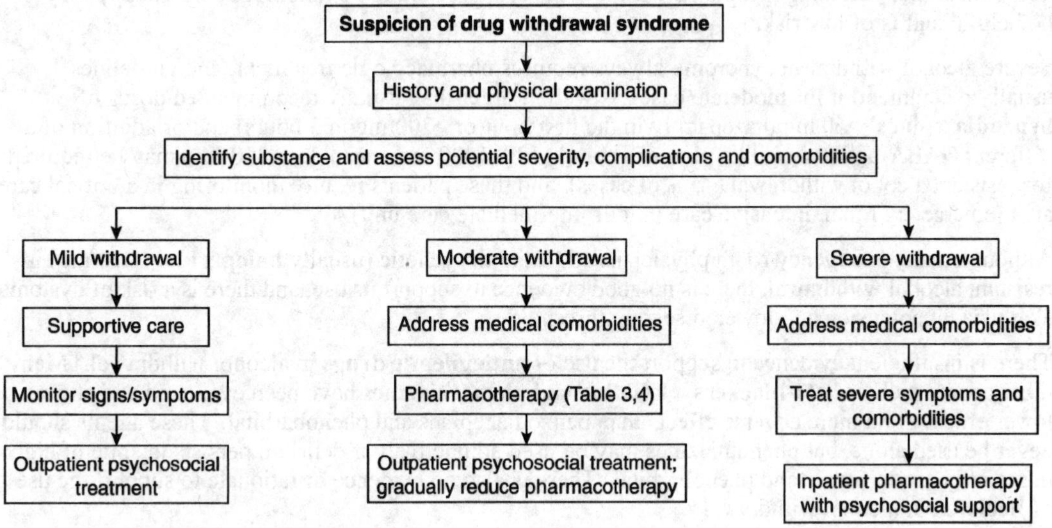

Pharmacologic Choices

General principles:

- Monitor signs and symptoms.
- Treat specific symptoms of withdrawal and associated complications and comorbidities (medical and psychiatric).
- Substitute abused drug with one of same or similar class (a cross-tolerant agonist that is less likely to be abused, usually with longer half-life).
- Substitute abused drug with one that blocks its reinforcing effects (antagonist).

Alcohol Withdrawal Syndrome

Assessment

Diagnostic criteria for the withdrawal syndromes associated with alcohol, benzodiazepines, opioids and stimulants is provided in Table 1.

The severity of the alcohol withdrawal syndrome and its complications correlate directly but inconsistently with the intensity and duration of alcohol use. These complications can include undernutrition (thiamine deficiency), low potassium, magnesium and phosphorus, liver disease and bleeding diathesis (increased INR, impaired platelet function/thrombocytopenia), CNS disorders (seizures, Wernicke encephalopathy, trauma) autonomic dysfunction (hypertension, dehydration, pyrexia), infections (pneumonia, aspiration, cellulitis) and psychosis (hallucinations, delusions). Mild withdrawal symptoms include tremor, irritability and insomnia, usually lasting 48–72 hours. A minority of patients experience more severe symptoms with onset around 48 hours and lasting up to about 5 days, which may include autonomic instability, seizures, hallucinations, delusions and hyperthermia. In the small proportion of fatalities following acute alcohol withdrawal (approximately 0.25%), cardiac complications such as arrhythmias are the most common cause. The CIWA-Ar is an effective assessment tool.[2]

Management

Medications used in the management of alcohol withdrawal are listed in Table 3.

Approximately two-thirds of patients with mild to moderate withdrawal symptoms can be managed with supportive treatment and monitoring, although comparison with pharmacotherapy is not described in the literature.[5] Blunting symptoms with low-dose, short-duration **benzodiazepine** therapy may be helpful and is of low risk.

Severe alcohol withdrawal syndrome always requires pharmacologic treatment, and guidelines usually recommend it for moderate cases as well. Larger than usually recommended doses of **benzodiazepines** (>50 mg diazepam iv in the first hour or >200 mg in 3 hours) and/or addition of a different GABA-active drug like **phenobarbital** (130–1430 mg, mean dose 390 mg) may be required for resistant alcohol withdrawal (<5% of cases), and these patients require monitoring in a critical care area (emergency room, intensive care unit or intermediate care unit).[6,7]

Although many emergency room physicians add an antipsychotic (usually **haloperidol** 5–10 mg) in resistant alcohol withdrawal, there is no good evidence to support its use, and there is a risk of dystonia, akathisia, hypotension and lowered seizure threshold.

There is insufficient evidence to support the use of **antiepileptic drugs** in alcohol withdrawal.[8] Many other agents such as **beta-blockers**, **clonidine** and **phenothiazines** have been evaluated and show lower efficacy and more adverse effects than benzodiazepines and phenobarbital. These agents should never be used alone, but phenothiazines may be used adjunctively if delirium persists in spite of high doses of benzodiazepine and phenobarbital. There is also no evidence or rationale to support the use of **baclofen** in alcohol withdrawal.[9]

Patients admitted to hospital for surgical illness may have occult alcohol dependence, and appropriate prophylaxis and management of alcohol withdrawal syndromes with benzodiazepines can prevent complications.[10]

Table 1: **Diagnostic Criteria for Substance-specific Withdrawal Syndromes**[1]

Alcohol	**Stimulants (Cocaine and Amphetamines)**
Two or more of:	Dysphoric mood, plus 2 or more of:
Autonomic hyperactivity (e.g., sweating, pulse >100 bpm)	Fatigue
Increased hand tremor	Vivid, unpleasant dreams
Insomnia	Insomnia or hypersomnia
Nausea/vomiting	Increased appetite
Transient visual, tactile or auditory hallucinations	Psychomotor retardation or agitation
Psychomotor agitation	**Benzodiazepines**
Anxiety	Two or more of:
Grand mal seizures	Autonomic hyperactivity
Opioids	(e.g., sweating, pulse >100 bpm)
Three or more of:	Increased hand tremor
Dysphoric mood	Insomnia
Nausea/vomiting	Nausea/vomiting
Muscle aches	Transient visual, tactile or auditory hallucinations
Lacrimation, rhinorrhea	Psychomotor agitation
Pupillary dilation, piloerection, sweating	Anxiety
Diarrhea	Grand mal seizures (only after abrupt cessation of high doses)
Yawning	
Fever	
Insomnia	

Rehabilitation

Cognitive behavioural therapy, group therapy and self-help groups such as Alcoholics Anonymous form the mainstay of long-term rehabilitation and maintenance of abstinence; there is conflicting evidence to support the use of pharmacotherapy (**acamprosate**, **naltrexone**) in this setting.[11] Results from clinical trials of acamprosate have been mixed.[12,13,14] A Cochrane review reported a modest effect of naltrexone on reducing the quantity of alcohol intake.[15] There is a risk of precipitating withdrawal in opioid-dependent patients.

Stimulant (Cocaine and Amphetamine) Withdrawal Syndrome

Assessment

Symptoms of cocaine withdrawal include mostly psychosocial, subtle and medically unimportant symptoms and signs, except for the risk of acute severe depression and suicidality in a small percentage of patients. See Table 1 for diagnostic criteria. The toxic state is manifested by agitation, tachycardia and anorexia, and conversely the withdrawal state is characterized by somnolence and increased appetite. Depression, anxiety, anhedonia and sleep disturbance may also occur, resolving over several weeks. Suicidality is uncommon and requires direct assessment.

Amphetamine withdrawal shares most of the characteristics of cocaine withdrawal, but may include psychotic features or a more severe depressed mood and may last longer. Drug craving replaces the withdrawal syndrome and may last several months. After withdrawal from methamphetamine ("crystal meth"), a persistent psychosis may occur and become permanent (uncommon) or last several weeks, usually responding well to low-dose antipsychotics (for dosing information, see Chapter 11).[16] Look for medical complications of stimulant use such as cardiomyopathy, local or systemic abscess, endocarditis, HIV and hepatitis B and C.

Management

Evaluation of a variety of pharmacotherapy approaches both for treatment of stimulant withdrawal syndrome and for relapse prevention has yielded inconsistent results, reflecting lack of efficacy. Dopamine agonists, such as **amantadine**[17] or **bromocriptine**[18] have demonstrated no significant benefit. **Desipramine** and other antidepressants have little or no effectiveness for withdrawal or relapse prevention, but may have a role in comorbid depression or anxiety. Agonist replacement therapy with sustained-release **amphetamine** or **methylphenidate** has shown benefit in relapse prevention, but regulatory concerns may limit their use, unless underlying attention deficit disorder co-exists.[19] Making this diagnosis requires psychiatric expertise.

Rehabilitation

Although **buprenorphine** and **methadone** may offer benefit to patients with mixed opioid and stimulant dependence, no drug therapy is consistently effective for treating pure stimulant dependence. Intensive outpatient, abstinence-oriented psychosocial treatment, especially *cognitive behavioural therapy*, is the most effective treatment, in addition to addressing the psychiatric comorbidities.

Opioid Withdrawal Syndrome

Assessment

Symptoms of opioid withdrawal are not medically serious, with muscle aches, restlessness and insomnia predominating. See Table 1 for diagnostic criteria. The acute withdrawal syndrome usually lasts about 1 week, except for withdrawal from methadone, with drug craving often persisting for several months.

Management

Drugs used in the management of opioid withdrawal are listed in Table 4.

Abstinence-based treatment may be desirable, but the most effective treatment by far continues to be replacement therapy with a long-acting agonist like **methadone** or the partial agonist **buprenorphine**, available as a sublingual combination product with **naloxone**, an opioid antagonist that is not sufficiently absorbed orally/sublingually to cause opioid withdrawal, but is included to discourage injection use. Methadone and buprenorphine can be initiated with the first withdrawal symptoms. Higher *maintenance* doses (methadone 60–100 mg or buprenorphine 8–24 mg/day) are more effective than lower doses. Because of methadone's long half-life of about 30 hours, the risk of narcosis (opioid-induced stupor or unconsciousness) in patients with an unknown degree of opioid tolerance is high in the first few days, and requires expertise and vigilance. Buprenorphine is a partial opiate agonist with a long half-life (36 hours) and generally does not cause narcosis in overdose.[20]

Clonidine, an alpha-2 agonist that decreases the neuronal output of norepinephrine, can be used to blunt the neuradrenergic signs/symptoms of withdrawal such as chills and flushing, but muscle aches and cravings usually persist. **Naltrexone**, a long-acting opioid antagonist, is ineffective in decreasing long-term opioid use, even with psychosocial support.[21] In addition, naltrexone-based withdrawal, alone or with anesthesia, results in no benefit compared to other detoxification treatments, and anesthesia or heavy sedation carries unacceptable risks.[22]

When there is a need to withdraw prescribed opioid therapy, a gradual reduction of the drug by approximately 10% weekly is safe, avoids withdrawal symptoms and is best done as an outpatient.

Rehabilitation

The best long-term results are obtained with replacement therapy (methadone or buprenorphine) combined with cognitive behavioural or group therapy, counselling and 12-step support. If methadone or buprenorphine discontinuation is considered, the best outcomes occur with slow tapering over many weeks.[4]

Benzodiazepine Withdrawal Syndrome

Assessment

Assessing benzodiazepine withdrawal syndrome is associated with 3 challenges:

- distinguishing recurrence of anxiety, panic or insomnia from the onset of withdrawal symptoms
- assessing risk of seizures and autonomic hyperactivity
- selecting the best treatment for any underlying psychiatric condition.

The withdrawal syndrome begins within 1–2 days of abrupt discontinuation (up to 5–10 days for benzodiazepines with longer half-lives) and can be severe, with hypertension, tachycardia and hyperreflexia progressing to seizures if there was long-term, high-dose use. See Table 1 for diagnostic criteria. In chronic anxiety and panic disorders, chronic dosing may be very high (even >100 mg diazepam per day) and may be associated with alcohol overuse, i.e., sedative self-treatment. A number of factors correlate with severity of the benzodiazepine withdrawal syndrome: high daily dose, use of agents with short half-life, long duration of use, diagnosis of panic disorder, presence of severe disorders personality disorders and concomitant alcohol or substance abuse.

Management

The only effective treatment for prolonged high-dose benzodiazepine dependence involves switching to a benzodiazepine with a long half-life (if not already taking one) and prolonged tapering of daily dose, combined with supportive therapy and eventually cognitive therapy for the underlying condition. Most Canadian experts use **diazepam** or **clonazepam** for replacement therapy (Table 2). Initial tapering of the daily dose of diazepam or clonazepam to 50% of the starting dose can usually occur over a 2- to 4-week period. The last 50% frequently takes many weeks, sometimes with periods of several weeks with no dosage change.[24]

Because patients with personality disorders tolerate distress poorly, they often drop out early; an intensive supportive and cognitive behavioural program should coincide with benzodiazepine tapering and may include periods of maintenance. Patients can be managed in an intensive outpatient program. Few patients (those with comorbid cardiovascular disease, severe alcoholism or previous seizures) require a short hospitalization.

Rehabilitation

For patients being treated for benzodiazepine dependence, the best strategy for managing an underlying psychiatric condition such as insomnia, generalized anxiety, panic disorder or mood disorder is *cognitive behavioural therapy*.[4,25] Pharmacotherapy should be directed to the specific underlying condition and should have a low risk of dependence; options for managing insomnia include **trazodone** (25–100 mg at bedtime). **Buspirone** can be used for generalized anxiety, and has low abuse potential and reasonable but not dramatic efficacy. See also Chapter 2, Chapter 6 and Chapter 8.

Neonatal Withdrawal Syndrome

Neonates may suffer withdrawal symptoms due to in utero exposure to drugs such as alcohol, benzodiazepines, opioids, barbiturates, nicotine, cannabinoids, cocaine, amphetamines and SSRI antidepressants. Neonatal abstinence syndrome usually refers specifically to neonatal opioid withdrawal.

For management of irritability, tachycardia, insomnia and for prevention of seizures associated with neonatal alcohol or benzodiazepine withdrawal, benzodiazepines and phenobarbital are effective and safe. Phenobarbital withdrawal usually does not require pharmacotherapy due to its long half-life. Neonatal withdrawal from cannabinoids, nicotine, SSRI antidepressants, cocaine or amphetamines is treated with supportive care only. Nicotine-associated small-for-dates babies and fetal alcohol spectrum disorder are potential long-term sequelae associated with use of those substances during pregnancy.

Table 2: **Dosage Equivalents of Benzodiazepines**

Benzodiazepine	Elimination Half-life[a]	Approximate Equivalent Oral Dosage[23] (mg)
Clorazepate	Long	10
Chlordiazepoxide	Long	25
Diazepam	Long	5
Flurazepam	Long	15
Alprazolam	Intermediate	0.5
Bromazepam	Intermediate	3
Clonazepam	Intermediate	0.25
Lorazepam	Intermediate	1
Nitrazepam	Intermediate	2.5
Oxazepam	Intermediate	15
Temazepam	Intermediate	10
Triazolam	Short	0.25

[a] Short = ≤5 h; Intermediate = 5–60 h; Long = ≥100 h.

Neonatal Abstinence Syndrome

Assessment

Neonatal abstinence syndrome (NAS) refers specifically to neonatal withdrawal from maternal opioid use, usually methadone or heroin. The onset of symptoms is usually 48–72 hours after birth for most opioids, but about 4–14 days for methadone. Expression of NAS is widely variable and is unrelated to the maternal daily dose of methadone.[26] Clinical manifestations relate to the central/autonomic nervous systems and the gastrointestinal tract. Affected infants display a characteristic high-pitched cry, as well as irritability, insomnia, hypertonia, hyperreflexia, tremor and convulsions. They often experience vomiting, diarrhea, feeding problems, sweating, yawning, tachypnea, congestion/sneezing and fever. It is important to evaluate for potential differential diagnoses including neonatal sepsis, meningitis, hypoglycemia, hypocalcemia, hypomagnesemia or colic.

There are several scoring systems for assessment and guiding treatment of NAS; the modified Finnegan Neonatal Abstinence Scoring System (31 items) is the most widely used for both research and treatment.[26] The Finnegan score is assessed every 2–4 hours.

Management

Nonpharmacologic treatment is the standard of care for babies with NAS, and includes swaddling, holding, gentle rocking, pacifier use, frequent small feeds with hypercaloric formula, frequent diaper changes with barrier ointment, and most importantly an environment that is quiet, has low light and white noise. Use of **methadone** in a breastfeeding mother may ameliorate withdrawal symptoms in the infant through transfer of approximately 2.8% of the maternal dose to breast milk. The American Academy of Pediatrics considers any maternal dose of methadone to be compatible with breastfeeding.[27] For infants with moderate to severe withdrawal, pharmacotherapy may provide additional benefits. A Cochrane review compared opioid treatment to supportive care alone, phenobarbital or diazepam.[28] Compared to supportive care alone, opioid treatment resulted in reduction in time to regain birth weight and shorter duration of supportive care, but longer hospital stay (possibly due to a policy-based requirement for hospitalization to receive opioids). Opioid therapy reduced seizure incidence and special care nursery admissions compared to phenobarbital, and reduced treatment failure (inadequate control of symptoms, requirement for additional pharmacotherapy, seizures, mortality) compared to diazepam.

The best studied opioid treatment regimen uses *diluted* **tincture of opium** (equivalent to morphine 0.4 mg/mL), with or without **phenobarbital** (added when there was polydrug withdrawal or maximum doses of opioid had been achieved).[29] This treatment regimen was safe and effective, with many of the infants sent home on phenobarbital which was weaned by the pediatrician. There was a 48% decrease in the length of hospitalization, less time with severe withdrawal scores and markedly decreased cost. It is important to be aware of the neonatal half-life of phenobarbital of 200–400 hours (around 100 hours in adults).

Clonidine should not be used alone, but when used adjunctively with opioids can reduce length of hospital stay, decrease seizures and decrease treatment failures, in doses of 1 μg/kg every 4 hours.[30]

Table 3: **Pharmacologic Management of Alcohol Withdrawal**

Class	Drug	Indication/Symptom	Dose	Comments	Cost[a]
Barbiturates	*phenobarbital*[6,7] Phenobarb, generics	Severe withdrawal refractory to benzodiazepine therapy (>50 mg diazepam given in 1 h or >200 mg in 3 h).	60 mg Q20–30 min po or iv	High dose may be required (up to total of 1000 mg). Should be used in a critical care area.	po: $ iv: $$
Benzodiazepines	*chlordiazepoxide* generics	Autonomic hyperactivity, agitation/tremor, hallucinations, seizures.	10–50 mg Q10–20 min po	Goal is suppression of symptoms with no more than mild sedation. Onset of action 1–2 h for chlordiazepoxide po.	$
	diazepam Diazemuls, Valium, generics	See chlordiazepoxide.	5–10 mg po or iv Q10–20 min; see Comments.	Goal is suppression of symptoms with no more than mild sedation. Mild withdrawal: give Q1H. Moderate withdrawal: give Q20–60 min. Severe withdrawal: give Q10–20 min. Onset of action 1 min for diazepam iv.	po: $ iv: $$
	lorazepam Ativan, generics	See chlordiazepoxide.	1–2 mg Q20–60 min po or iv	Goal is suppression of symptoms with no more than mild sedation. Onset of action 5–15 min for lorazepam iv.	po: $ iv: $$
Vitamins	*thiamine* (vitamin B_1) Thiamiject, generics	Treatment/prevention of Wernicke's encephalopathy.	50–100 mg daily iv or po for duration of withdrawal	Best practice is to administer thiamine to all patients with alcohol withdrawal. Should be administered prior to iv dextrose, to avoid precipitation of Wernicke's encephalopathy.	$

[a] Cost of a single administration; includes drug cost only.
Legend: $ < $1 $$ $1–5

Table 4: Pharmacologic Management of Opioid Withdrawal in Adults

Class	Drug	Dose	Comments	Cost[a]
Alpha$_2$-adrenergic Agonists	*clonidine* Catapres, Dixarit, generics	0.1–0.5 mg/day Q8H po for 7 days, then taper over 3–5 days	Blunts some withdrawal symptoms. Use only for acute detoxification and when patient prefers over methadone. Maintain fluid intake and monitor for hypotensive effects; hold next dose if blood pressure <85/55 mm Hg.	$
Opioid Agonists	*methadone* Metadol, Methadose	Acute withdrawal symptoms in new patients: 10–20 mg Q2–4H po until stable (usually 20–60 mg). If not to be continued as maintenance, taper by 5 mg/day over 1–2 wk Maintenance: 40–100 mg/day po	High relapse rate without maintenance therapy. Long half-life (24–36 h). Higher maintenance doses (60–100 mg) associated with better outcomes.	$$
Partial Opioid Agonists	*buprenorphine/naloxone* Suboxone	Long-term maintenance : 8–24 mg (buprenorphine) daily sl. Dose is usually initiated at 4 mg (1 or 2 doses the first day) and titrated to the lowest effective maintenance dose	Start with first signs of withdrawal (if switching from methadone, start at least 24 h after last dose). Prescribed and dispensed in accordance with Suboxone Education Program (www.suboxonecme.ca)	$$$

[a] Cost of 7-day supply of mean dose; includes drug cost only.
Legend: $ < $25 $$ $25–50 $$$ $50–75

Suggested Readings

Kleber HD, Weiss RD, Anton RF et al. Treatment of patients with substance use disorders, second edition. American Psychiatric Association. *Am J Psychiatry* 2007;164(4 Suppl):5-123.

National Institute for Health and Care Excellence. *Alcohol dependence and harmful alcohol use.* London (GB): NICE; 2011. Available from: guidance.nice.org.uk/CG115.

Spies CD, Rommelspacher H. Alcohol withdrawal in the surgical patients: prevention and treatment. *Anesth Analg* 1999;88(4):946-54.

Voshaar RC, Couvee JE, van Balkom AJ et al. Strategies for discontinuing long-term benzodiazepine use: meta-analysis. *Br J Psychiatry* 2006;189:213-20.

References

1. American Psychiatric Association. *Diagnostic and statistical manual of mental disorders: DSM-5*. 5th ed. Washington (DC): American Psychiatric Association; 2013.
2. Sullivan JT, Sykora K, Schneiderman J et al. Assessment of alcohol withdrawal: the revised clinical institute withdrawal assessment for alcohol scale (CIWA-Ar). *Br J Addict* 1989;84(11):1353-7.
3. Busto UE, Sykora K, Sellers EM. A clinical scale to assess benzodiazepine withdrawal. *J Clin Psychopharmacol* 1989;9(6):412-6.
4. Kleber HD, Weiss RD, Anton RF et al. Treatment of patients with substance use disorders, second edition. American Psychiatric Association. *Am J Psychiatry* 2007;164(4 Suppl):5-123.
5. Naranjo CA, Sellers EM, Chater K et al. Nonpharmacologic intervention in acute alcohol withdrawal. *Clin Pharmacol Ther* 1983;34(2):214-9.
6. Hack JB, Hoffman RS, Nelson LS. Resistant alcohol withdrawal: does an unexpectedly large sedative requirement identify these patient early? *J Med Toxicol* 2006;2(2):55-60.
7. Gold JA, Rimal B, Nolan A et al. A strategy of escalating doses of benzodiazepines and phenobarbital administration reduce the need for mechanical ventilation in delirium tremens. *Crit Care Med* 2007;35(3):724-30.
8. Minozzi S, Amato L, Vecchi S et al. Anticonvulsants for alcohol withdrawal. *Cochrane Database Syst Rev* 2010;(3):CD005064.
9. Liu J, Wang L. Baclofen for alcohol withdrawal. *Cochrane Database Syst Rev* 2011;(1):CD008502.
10. Spies CD, Dubisz N, Funk W et al. Prophylaxis of alcohol withdrawal syndrome in alcohol dependent patients admitted to the intensive care unit following tumour resection. *Br J Anaesth* 1995;75(6):734-9.
11. Krystal JH, Cramer JA, Krol WF et al. Naltrexone in the treatment of alcohol dependence. *N Engl J Med* 2001;345(24):1734-9.
12. Anton RF, O'Malley SS, Ciraulo DA et al. Combined pharmacotherapies and behavioral interventions for alcohol dependence: the COMBINE study: a randomized controlled trial. *JAMA* 2006;295(17):2003-17.
13. Umhau JC, Schwandt ML, Usala J et al. Pharmacologically induced alcohol craving in treatment seeking alcoholics correlates with alcoholism severity, but is insensitive to acamprosate. *Neuropsychopharmacology* 2011;36(6):1178-86.
14. McNeely J, Sherman S. ACP Journal Club. Review: Acamprosate increases abstinence in patients with alcohol dependence. *Ann Intern Med* 2011;154(2):JC1-10.
15. Rosner S, Hackl-Herrwerth A, Leucht S et al. Opioid antagonists for alcohol dependence. *Cochrane Database Syst Rev* 2010;(12):CD001867.
16. Curran C, Byrappa N, McBride A. Stimulant psychosis: systematic review. *Br J Psychiatry* 2004;185:196-204.
17. Weddington WW, Brown BS, Haertzen CA et al. Changes in mood, craving, and sleep during short-term abstinence reported by male cocaine addicts: a controlled, residential study. *Arch Gen Psychiatry* 1990;47(9):861-8.
18. Moscovitz H, Brookoff D, Nelson L. A randomized trial of bromocriptine for cocaine users presenting to the emergency department. *J Gen Intern Med* 1993;8(1):1-4.
19. Grabowski J, Shearer J, Merril J et al. Agonist-like, replacement pharmacotherapy for stimulant abuse and dependence. *Addict Behav* 2004;29(7):1439-64.
20. Petry NM, Bickel WK, Badger GJ. A comparison of four buprenorphine dosing regimens in the treatment of opioid dependence. *Clin Pharmacol Ther* 1999;66(3):306-14.
21. Minozzi S, Amato L, Vecchi S et al. Oral naltrexone maintenance treatment for opioid dependence. *Cochrane Database Syst Rev* 2011;(2):CD001333.
22. Gowing LT, Ali RL. The place of detoxification in treatment of opioid dependence. *Curr Opin Psychiatry* 2006;19(3):266-70.
23. Bezchlibnyk-Butler KZ, Jeffries JJ, eds. *Clinical handbook of psychotropic drugs*. 20th ed. Ashland (OH): Hogrefe & Huber Publishers; 2014.
24. Rickels K, DeMartinis N, Rynn M et al. Pharmacologic strategies for discontinuing benzodiazepine treatment. *J Clin Psychopharmacol* 1999;19(6 Suppl 2):12S-16S.
25. Spiegel DA. Psychological strategies for discontinuation in benzodiazepine treatment. *J Clin Psychopharmacol* 1999;19(6 Suppl 2):17S-22S.
26. Finnegan LP, Connaughton JF, Kron RE et al. Neonatal abstinence syndrome: assessment and management. *Addict Dis* 1975;2(1-2):141-58.
27. American Academy of Pediatrics Committee on Drugs. Transfer of drugs and other chemical into human milk. *Pediatrics* 2001;108(3):776-89.
28. Osborn DA, Jeffery HE, Cole MJ. Opiate treatment for opiate withdrawal in newborn infants. *Cochrane Database Syst Rev* 2010;(10):CD002059.
29. Coyle MG, Ferguson A, Lagasse L et al. Diluted tincture of opium (DTO) and phenobarbital versus DTO alone for neonatal opiate withdrawal in term infants. *J Pediatr* 2002;140(5):561-4.
30. Agthe AG, Kim GR, Mathias KB et al. Clonidine as an adjunct therapy to opioids for neonatal abstinence syndrome: a randomized, controlled trial. *Pediatrics* 2009;123(5):e849-56.

Substance-related Disorders

Chapter 13
Smoking Cessation

Peter Selby, MBBS, FCFP

Tobacco use kills approximately 37 000 Canadians annually, primarily from cardiac disease, lung cancer and respiratory diseases such as COPD.[1] The toxicity of cigarette smoke is due to the inhalation of about 7000 chemicals including 70 carcinogens.[2] Cigarettes are highly addictive because of the rapid delivery of nicotine to the mesolimbic reward pathways, combined with activity in the motivational and learning circuitry of the brain.[3] The short half-life of nicotine (60–90 minutes) forces repeated administration to maintain nicotine levels.[4] Other psychoactive compounds in smoke include MAO-A and MAO-B inhibitors.[5] The polyaromatic hydrocarbons (PAHs) are inducers of CYP1A1, 1A2 and 2E1 enzymes that have clinical implications when smokers quit.[6]

Goals of Therapy[7]

- The ultimate goal is to help smokers achieve complete and sustained remission from tobacco use disorder
- An intermediate goal is to help them achieve complete and sustained remission from cigarette smoking and/or other forms of tobacco products such as chewing tobacco
- To help smokers understand that:
  - smoking cessation is a process not a singular event; helping smokers stay engaged in the process of behaviour change is a major objective of therapy
  - the best odds of quitting are achieved when behavioural and pharmacologic interventions are used to complement each other
  - reduction in smoking by 50% in those unable or unwilling to quit is controversial because there is no long-term health benefit.[8] However, reduction is associated with subsequent successful quitting[9]

Investigations

- Figure 1 provides a general assessment questionnaire
- Measures of physical dependence include the Fagerström Test of Nicotine Dependence.[10] A shorter version is the Heaviness of Smoking Index, which assesses the level of tobacco dependence based on questions such as: "How early in the day do you smoke your first cigarette?" and "How many cigarettes do you smoke per day?"[11] The earlier a person smokes the first cigarette of the day and the more cigarettes smoked per day, the higher the level of dependence.
- Motivation can be assessed along a continuum by asking the following 2 questions:
  - "Given everything going on in your life right now, on a scale of 1 to 10, where 10 is the most important thing to do right now, how important is it for you to quit smoking altogether?"
  - "Given everything going on in your life right now, on a scale of 1 to 10, where 10 is the most confident you have felt about anything, how confident do you feel you will be able to quit smoking altogether?"

Figure 1: **Tobacco-smoking History Questionnaire**

1. Tobacco use history

a. Current (past year):

i. Quantity: number of cigarettes smoked per day_____

ii. Frequency/pattern:

a. weekday ________

b. weekend ________

iii. Time to first cigarette after waking up (in minutes): ________

iv. Type(s): cigarettes: ☐ yes ☐ no;
cigars: ☐ yes ☐ no;
cigarellos: ☐ yes ☐ no;
others (☐ bidis, ☐ kretek)

b. Past history:

i. Age of onset of smoking (years) ________

ii. Maximum smoked per day (lifetime) ________

iii. Number of past quit attempts (24 hours or more of intentional cessation) ________

iv. Past methods used to quit:
____

v. Utility of method used to quit:
____

vi. What led to a relapse? (check all that apply)
withdrawal: ☐ yes ☐ no;
negative mood: ☐ yes ☐ no;
habit: ☐ yes ☐ no;
being with other smokers: ☐ yes ☐ no;
stress: ☐ yes ☐ no;
other________________

2. Other drug use

a. Caffeine: ☐ yes ☐ no: cups per day _____

b. Alcohol: ☐ yes ☐ no: drinks per day _____

c. Marijuana: (especially if smoked)
☐ yes ☐ no: joints per day _____

3. Concurrent mental health problems

a. Depression: ☐ yes ☐ no

b. Anxiety: ☐ yes ☐ no

c. Eating disorders: ☐ yes ☐ no

d. Bipolar disease: ☐ yes ☐ no

e. Schizophrenia: ☐ yes ☐ no

4. Environmental assessment

a. Living with smokers: ☐ yes ☐ no

b. Workplace smoking: ☐ yes ☐ no

5. Consequences of smoking

a. Health — cardiac: ☐ yes ☐ no
respiratory: ☐ yes ☐ no
cancer: ☐ yes ☐ no
others: ☐ yes ☐ no

b. Social/Family — feeling ostracized, advice to stop from friends/family

c. Financial: costs of cigarettes _______ per pack of 20 (small pack)

6. Concurrent medications

a. Benzodiazepines: ☐ yes ☐ no

b. Antipsychotics: ☐ yes ☐ no

c. Antidepressants: ☐ yes ☐ no

d. Others: ________________

7. Allergies and intolerances especially to smoking cessation medications

☐ yes ☐ no

8. A rapid assessment of motivation

a. High importance and confidence, ready to quit in the next 30 days

b. High importance low confidence, wants to quit but needs help

c. Low importance, low confidence, doesn't want to quit

d. Low importance, high confidence, discounts the importance of quitting but has high self efficacy

9. Physical examination

a. Blood pressure ______ mm Hg

b. Height ______ metres

c. Weight ______ kg

c. Waist circumference ______ cm

Treatment plan for those who want to quit within 30 days:

10. Quit date

a. ☐ yes__________; If yes offer self-help material and follow up

b. ☐ no: If no, within 6 months?
Advise to quit and follow up as needed

11. Counselling

a. In person: ☐ yes ☐ no

b. Telephone: ☐ yes ☐ no

c. Internet: ☐ yes ☐ no

12. Pharmacotherapy

Drug	Start date
Nicotine replacement therapy:	
a. Patch ☐ 21 mg ☐ 14 mg ☐ 7 mg ☐ 15 mg ☐ 10 mg ☐ 5 mg	
b. Gum ☐ 2 mg ☐ 4 mg	
c. Inhaler ☐ 4 mg	
d. Lozenge ☐ 2 mg ☐ 4 mg	
Bupropion: dose ________	
Varenicline: dose ________	
Nortriptyline: dose ________	
Clonidine: dose ________	

____
Signature

____
Date

To provide optimal support for smoking cessation, health care professionals need proper training.[12,13] The "5 As Approach" is a universally adopted tool clinicians may utilize as part of a smoking cessation program. The 5 As consist of the following steps:

- *Ask* about tobacco use.
- *Advise* your patient to quit.
- *Assess* readiness to quit. Employ motivational interviewing and reflective listening if patient is not ready.
- *Assist* in smoking cessation via behavioural plan and/or pharmacotherapy.
- *Arrange* follow up 4 weeks post quit date.

Clinicians can be trained in this approach via several programs including QUIT[14] and TEACH.[15] For more information view the algorithm for tailoring pharmacotherapy in primary care setting.[16]

Therapeutic Choices

This chapter will focus on smokers who want to quit in the next 30 days. Figure 2 provides an algorithm for smoking cessation strategies based on readiness to quit and level of tobacco use dependence.

Nonpharmacologic Choices

Tobacco use disorder is a chronic relapsing condition for which multiple courses of therapy might be required. Current interventions including behavioural therapy for 8–24 weeks have shown to be effective at follow up 6 months post-treatment. Only a small number of patients achieve long-term remission of >1 year following a single course of therapy. Long-term clinical trials are needed to establish the effects of prolonged pharmacotherapy in preventing relapse.[7] Though widely promoted, there is no evidence for the efficacy of hypnosis or acupuncture.

The 5 evidence-based steps required to successfully quit include the following:[7]

- setting a target quit date
- getting professional help
- enlisting social support
- using medication to quit smoking
- using problem-solving methods of counselling to quit and remain smoke free.

It should be noted that abrupt stopping on the quit day and gradual reduction to stop are associated with comparable quit rates [Evidence: SORT A*].[17] Patients can be given an option as to how they wish to quit . Gradual smoking reduction interventions include reducing smoking by a predetermined percentage from baseline, increasing the interval between cigarettes, and increasing the time from waking to the first cigarette of the day. All gradual reduction methods should culminate in a quit day.

There is a dose-response relationship between counselling and quit success.[7] Estimated abstinence rates increase from 13.4% with minimal counselling contact time (<3 minutes) to an average of 22% with contact time >10 minutes. Optimal total contact time is 91–300 minutes, yielding abstinence rates of approximately 28%.[7] Smokers who are attempting to quit should be counselled at least once prior to their quit date, the week following their quit date and weekly thereafter as necessary to optimize therapy and to identify and manage early relapse.[7] Formats that have been shown to be effective include face-to-face (individual or group) counselling as well as contact by telephone, mobile text messages and Internet sites.[18,19,20,21] Examples include www.smokershelpline.ca, www.stopsmokingcentre.net and www.pregnets.ca for pregnant smokers.

* SORT (Strength of Recommendation Taxonomy) is a rating system (A, B or C) that addresses the quality of available evidence. For more information consult **How to Use *Compendium of Therapeutic Choices*** on page xxv.

Figure 2: **Management of Smoking Cessation**

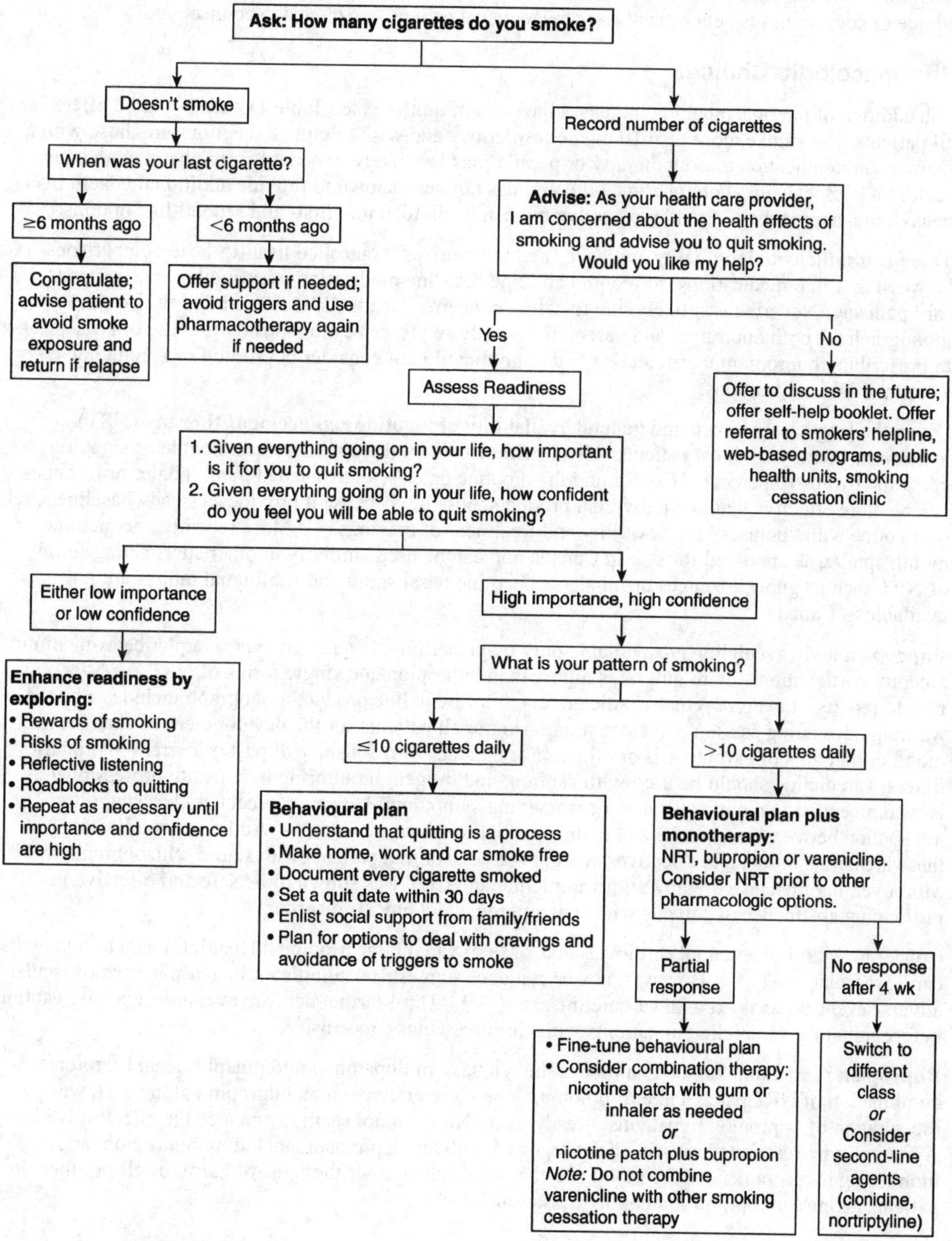

Abbreviations: NRT = nicotine replacement therapy

Increasing the amount of counseling sessions for smokers receiving pharmacotherapy is likely to increase the efficacy of pharmacotherapy by about 10–25%, with at least 4 sessions in person or by telephone showing added benefit.[22] A combination of pharmacotherapy and behavioural support (brief advice or counseling) is better than brief advice, usual care or less intensive counseling.[23]

Pharmacologic Choices

The addition of pharmacotherapy increases the odds of quitting (see Table 1) and should be offered to all patients who smoke more than 10 cigarettes per day and wish to quit. Exceptions are those with a known contraindication to drug therapy or populations less likely to benefit from pharmacotherapy such as adolescents in whom pharmacotherapy has not been shown to provide additional benefit over behavioural approaches.[7,24,25] Pharmacotherapy can be divided into first- and second-line options.[7]

There is insufficient high-quality evidence (i.e., randomized, controlled head-to-head comparisons between first-line medications) to recommend one first-line medication over another in a stepped care pathway. Nevertheless, likely due to safety concerns, Health Canada modified the product monograph for both bupropion and varenicline to advise prescribers to consider the use of NRT prior to prescribing bupropion or varenicline,[26] though they do not consider bupropion or varenicline as second-line medications.

Given the long safety record and general availability of **nicotine replacement therapy** (NRT), it is first-line therapy for most patients. Nicotine replacement therapy increases the rate of smoking cessation by 50–70 percent.[27] Combining the nicotine patch with as-needed gum, inhaler or lozenges can be more effective than the individual products, possibly because it provides a steady baseline level of nicotine with "boluses" for flexibility and treatment of cravings.[27,28] More recently, the nicotine mouth spray was approved for sale in Canada and can be used similarly to other short-acting forms of NRT such as gums, lozenges or inhalers. Nicotine nasal spray and sublingual tablets are not available in Canada.

Bupropion and **varenicline** are available only by prescription. Varenicline is an $alpha_4beta_2$-nicotinic receptor partial agonist with quit rates higher than bupropion and single forms of NRT.[28,29,30,31,32,33] Due to reports of neuropsychiatric side effects, the varenicline product monograph includes a boxed warning advocating caution and close monitoring in all patients for the development of changes in mood or thoughts of harm to self or others. For patients with a history of past or current psychiatric illness, varenicline should be used with caution, and diligent monitoring by a health professional is recommended to monitor for new or worsening symptoms. However, recent studies suggest no association between varenicline and neuropsychiatric adverse events.[34,35] Additional studies suggest that varenicline is safe and effective for smoking cessation in patients with stable schizophrenia.[36,37,38] Moreover, maintenance therapy with varenicline and CBT was shown to be safe and effective in prolonging abstinence in patients with schizophrenia and bipolar disorder.[39]

Concerns regarding potential cardiovascular risks of varenicline prompted Health Canada to review its cardiovascular safety.[40,41] However, newer evidence suggests no significant increase in cardiovascular adverse events associated with varenicline use.[42,43,44,45] Until further data are available, exercise caution before initiating varenicline in patients with cardiovascular concerns.

Bupropion is an aminoketone that blocks the reuptake of dopamine, norepinephrine and serotonin. A combination of NRT patch and bupropion may be more effective than bupropion alone.[27] However, the addition of bupropion in patients already using NRT did not seem to enhance the effect of NRT.[27] Agitation-type reactions have also been reported with antidepressants including bupropion, and monitoring is recommended for mood or behavioural changes or thoughts of harm to self or others in patients taking bupropion for smoking cessation.

Table 1: **Odds Ratios of Selected Pharmacotherapies**[28]

Intervention	Odds Ratio (95% CI)[a]	No. of Studies
Placebo	1	267
Nicotine gum	1.68 (1.51–1.88)	56
Nicotine patch	1.91 (1.71–2.14)	43
Nicotine inhaler, lozenge or spray	2.04 (1.75–2.38)	16
Bupropion	1.85 (1.63–2.1)	6
Nicotine patch plus as-needed inhaler, gum or spray	2.73 (2.07–3.65)	2
Varenicline	2.89 (2.4–3.48)	15

[a] Odds ratios were derived from comparisons with placebo.

Second-line pharmacotherapies such as **clonidine**[46,47] and **nortriptyline**[48,49] have evidence of efficacy but are not officially indicated for smoking cessation. Nortriptyline can be used in otherwise healthy individuals with minimal risk of cardiac disease or overdose when first-line therapies are either unaffordable or have not worked. Clonidine may be used in those with coexisting hypertension, where appropriate. However, postural hypotension can be problematic and the drug must be tapered to prevent rebound hypertension.

Cytisine, natural product derived from the seeds of *Laburnum anagyroides* (also known as Cytisus Laburnum, Golden Rain or Golden Chain acacia), is a partial nicotine agonist that demonstrated efficacy over placebo in an RCT.[50] Its limitations include multiple daily doses and lack of availability in Canada.

Choice of medication should depend on patient preference and absence of contraindications (such as recent MI or stroke for nicotine replacement therapy). Initially, monotherapy is preferred. Combination therapy such as the nicotine patch combined with either as-needed nicotine dosage forms (gum, inhaler or lozenge) or bupropion is associated with higher 6-month abstinence rates than monotherapy.[7,51] However, cost may be a limiting factor and combination therapy should be reserved for those in whom monotherapy was unsuccessful or those with severe nicotine addiction. Varenicline in combination with bupropion showed promise in an open label trial.[52] However, varenicline is contraindicated in combination with NRT. Table 2 lists pharmacotherapy for smoking cessation.

Special Considerations

Electronic Delivery Systems (EDS)

It is important to note that only those electronic delivery systems (EDS, electronic cigarettes or e-cigarettes) *without* nicotine or health claims can be legally imported and sold in Canada.[53]

EDS look and behave like cigarettes, but they contain a battery-powered mechanism to heat and vapourize a liquid chemical mixture composed of varying amounts of nicotine, propylene glycol, other chemicals and/or impurities. The vapour produced and glowing tip resemble the smoke and burning tip of an actual cigarette which may satisfy the behaviors associated with smoking (handling of cigarette, and inhaling of smoke).

Health Canada does not recommend using EDS due to lack of safety information regarding exposure to vapourized propylene glycol (among other chemicals used in the products) and their unknown long term effects.[53] Legally, EDS currently marketed and sold in Canada cannot contain nicotine. However, nicotine-containing cartridges or "e-juice" is easily available via the Internet. EDS are not regulated; some products contain nicotine while others contain varying levels of other chemicals. Over 400 brands of electronic cigarettes are available.[54] Despite widespread availability and use, the efficacy of EDS for smoking cessation is unproven. The first RCT to examine the efficacy of nicotine-containing EDS showed similar abstinence rates between EDS and nicotine patches and no significant differences in adverse events.[55] There is worldwide debate concerning EDS, since their potential benefits may or may not outweigh their potential risks.[56]

Post-smoking Cessation Weight Gain

From a health perspective, the risks from continuing to smoke outweigh the risks of weight gain.[57,58] Address potential weight gain associated with smoking cessation, since quitting smoking with or without pharmacotherapy is associated with changes in body weight.[59,60] Pharmacotherapy for smoking cessation (NRT, bupropion and varenicline) are associated with less weight gain than quitting using behavioral methods alone.[61] Bupropion is associated with the least weight gain due to its anorexiant properties.

Most changes occur in the first 3 months of quitting with an average increase of 4–5 kg at 12 months. It should be noted that 16% of quitters lose weight and only 13% gain more than 10 kg.[62] Advise patients to focus on quitting smoking and to manage food cravings by eating low-calorie snacks such as carrots, celery sticks and/or use sugar-free candy and gum. Encourage physical activity as well.

Drug Interactions with Smoking Cessation

Be aware of the effect of smoking on hepatic metabolism. Induction of CYP1A2 by cigarette smoking can increase the clearance and potentially necessitate higher doses of drugs such as caffeine, clozapine, diazepam, estrogens, fluvoxamine, methadone, nifedipine, olanzapine, rasagiline, theophylline, trifluoperazine or warfarin. Conversely, a reduction of the dose may be required if the patient quits smoking. Patients should be made aware of the potentially increased effects (and side effects) of caffeine when they quit smoking.

Choices during Pregnancy and Breastfeeding

Smoking and Pregnancy

Smoking before, during and after pregnancy is associated with negative outcomes for both mother and baby.[63,64,65,66,67,68] Nicotine readily crosses the placenta and is concentrated on the fetal side. Moreover, carbon monoxide and other teratogens and carcinogens in cigarette smoke also cross the placenta. Adverse effects such as intrauterine growth retardation, increased risk of sudden infant death syndrome (SIDS) and potential behavioural and metabolic effects manifesting in childhood make tobacco smoke one of the most damaging teratogens, with permanent and significant morbidity and mortality. Smoking is also associated with a reduction in the amount of breast milk.

Most women who smoke will attempt to quit when they discover they are pregnant, but the majority will ultimately continue to smoke. Factors associated with successful quit attempts include first pregnancy, first trimester, low level of tobacco dependence, sharing a household with nonsmokers, higher education and not suffering from depression. The relapse rate postpartum is about 60% at 6 months, and reflects the chronic relapsing nature of tobacco addiction.

Pregnancy is seen as a "teachable moment" in terms of smoking cessation. Quitting at anytime during pregnancy is associated with improved birth outcomes. Routine screening for tobacco use is recommended for all pregnant women, as well as interventions to help smokers quit. There are no known risks to stopping "cold turkey" while pregnant, and quitting should not be delayed until the postpartum period because the motivation to stop smoking diminishes once the pregnancy is completed. There is reluctance to use pharmacotherapy in pregnancy due to the known and unknown adverse effects of available treatment.[69] The risk/benefit equation for smoking cessation pharmacotherapy in pregnancy depends on whether there is additional benefit over behavioural measures. With NRT it is unlikely there is any additional risk incurred from using the lowest effective dose of nicotine, considering it will be delivered via less dangerous routes. Any potential harm from using NRT must be weighed against that caused by continued smoking.

Management Prior to Conception

Reduction in smoking prevalence in women of childbearing age can potentially improve maternal and fetal health.[70] Whenever feasible, both potential parents should be given assistance to quit smoking, as women whose partners smoke are less likely to quit.

Sperm cells are rendered abnormal (altered morphology, number and motility) by tobacco smoke.[70] DNA-adducts and benzopyrene (a carcinogen from tobacco smoke) are incorporated into the gamete, with the major contribution from sperm. Men should quit smoking for at least 3 months prior to attempted conception, to allow sufficient time for replacement of the abnormal sperm. Since smoking is a major reversible cause of infertility, all couples should be given assistance to quit smoking prior to undergoing fertility treatment. Smoking cessation pharmacotherapy can be used during this period without concern for teratogenic effects.

Management during Pregnancy and Postpartum Period

Screen all pregnant women for smoking status and exposure to second-hand smoke at the first appointment and periodically during the pregnancy. All should be advised and assisted to stop smoking completely as soon as possible.[71,72] Behavioural treatment, either in person (individual/group) or telephone-based, is recommended. The combination of multiple components (e.g., peer support and counselling) may have the best likelihood of success.[73] Avoid pharmacotherapy unless the woman is unable to quit using behavioural measures alone. There is no good evidence for the efficacy or safety of NRT, bupropion or varenicline in pregnancy.[74,75] Recent studies comparing the efficacy of the nicotine patch to placebo in pregnant smokers found no difference in quit rates by the end of pregnancy and inconsistent findings on increased birth weight in the offspring.[76,77,78]

It is also possible that women who find it hard to quit while pregnant might also have other substance use disorders, and be involved in the criminal justice system.[79] Mental illnesses such as depression were not associated with failure to stop smoking when pregnant.[80]

Given the teratogenic nature of tobacco, the practitioner and the pregnant patient face a dilemma when she is unable to quit smoking. When possible, such women should be referred to an expert in smoking cessation in pregnancy, and a teratology information centre such as Motherisk should be consulted. Offer the lowest effective dose of short-acting nicotine (gum), to eliminate exposure to smoke and minimize the amount of nicotine exposure to the fetus.[81] This may be continued for 8–12 weeks with the goal of maintaining abstinence. There is no agreement on the maximum number of pieces per day. Reserve the transdermal patch for heavily dependent smokers and those who do not respond to the gum, and recommend removal after 16 hours, e.g., at bedtime, to reduce fetal nicotine exposure.[7,82] Bupropion may be used, especially in those women with an additional diagnosis of depression, as long as there are no contraindications. Use of bupropion during pregnancy has not been associated with a higher risk of congenital malformations.[83] Data regarding the safety of varenicline during pregnancy are still very limited.

Smoking and Breastfeeding

Smoking reduces the production and quality of breast milk.[84] However, the amount of nicotine exposure is minimal and overall the benefits of breastfeeding outweigh the risks of continued smoking. NRT and bupropion may be used if the benefits outweigh the potential risks. There are no published data on the safety of varenicline or its transmission to breast milk.

Continued breastfeeding is associated with delayed relapse in women who have quit smoking.[85] If women smoke and also breastfeed, educate them about the risks to the baby from second-hand smoke, and advise them to smoke outdoors and not to smoke just before or during breastfeeding. Changing clothes and hand-washing also reduce the “off-gassing” of toxins after smoking a cigarette.

A discussion of general principles on the use of medications in these special populations can be found in Appendix II and Appendix III. Other specialized reference sources are also provided in these appendices.

Therapeutic Tips

- Encourage smokers who have slips while on medication to continue medication for at least 4 weeks and use behavioural interventions to help them to stop smoking.[86]
- If smokers using the patch complain of unmanageable cravings and smoke cigarettes, add nicotine gum, lozenge or inhaler as a breakthrough medication.[7]
- Although smoking cessation may have a positive effect on mental health after 6 weeks of quitting in the general population as well as in patients suffering from psychiatric disorders,[87] it is important to monitor for low mood and emergence of depression in smokers who quit, regardless of the method used to quit.[88]
- Create a therapeutic relationship in which the patient can report back at the first signs of a relapse to abort it as soon as possible.
- For adolescents, school-based programs that provide complex interventions with elements of cognitive behavioural therapy (CBT) matched to stages of change show promise.[89,90] Additionally, behavioral counseling interventions may prevent tobacco smoking among school-aged children and adolescents.[91]

Table 2: Pharmacologic Agents Used for Smoking Cessation

Class	Drug	Dose	Adverse Effects	Drug Interactions[a]	Comments	Cost[b]
Alpha$_2$-adrenergic Receptor Agonists	*clonidine* Catapres, generics	0.1 mg BID po starting up to 3 days before or on the quit date. Titrate up by 0.1 mg/day po once per week as tolerated to a maximum of 0.4 mg/day. Duration of therapy ranges from 3–10 weeks	Common: sedation, dizziness, hypotension, dry mouth. Less common: anxiety, irritability, memory problems.	Avoid concurrent use with tricyclic antidepressants. Additive effects with other CNS depressants such as ethanol. Additive hypotensive effect when combined with antihypertensive drugs.	Monitor blood pressure and heart rate during treatment initiation. Taper gradually to avoid rebound hypertension when stopping treatment.	$
Antidepressants	*bupropion* Zyban	150 mg daily po × 3 days then 150 mg BID po × 7–12 weeks. Begin 1–2 weeks before the selected quit date	Usual: insomnia, dry mouth, dizziness, restlessness, difficulty concentrating. Unusual: hypersensitivity reactions, increased risk of seizures at higher dosages; agitation-type reactions involving mood/behavioural changes.	Inhibits CYP2D6; may decrease clearance of atomoxetine, duloxetine, fluoxetine, fluvoxamine, paroxetine, risperidone, sertraline, venlafaxine; may decrease effectiveness of codeine and tamoxifen. Do not use with MAO inhibitors (possible mania, excitation, hyperpyrexia). May be safely combined with NRT (monitor for treatment-emergent hypertension).	Not recommended in patients with conditions predisposing to seizures, history of seizures, current eating disorder or severe hepatic impairment. Least expensive of oral medications officially indicated for smoking cessation.	$$
	nortriptyline Aventyl, generics	25 mg/day po titrated to 75–100 mg/day po. Quit day is usually set between 1 and 4 weeks; medication is continued for 12 weeks	Common: dry mouth, blurred vision, constipation, dizziness, sedation. Less common: confusion, arrhythmias, urinary retention.	Do not use with MAO inhibitors (may cause mania, excitation, hyperpyrexia). Inducers of CYP2D6 or CYP3A4 such as carbamazepine, phenytoin or rifampin may decrease effect. Inhibitors of CYP2D6 or CYP3A4 such as clarithromycin, erythromycin, grapefruit juice, fluoxetine or paroxetine may increase effect and toxicity.	Caution in patients with cardiovascular disease or arrhythmias. Consider measuring serum levels to reach therapeutic dose (based on efficacy data for depression).	$

(cont'd)

Table 2: **Pharmacologic Agents Used for Smoking Cessation** *(cont'd)*

Class	Drug	Dose	Adverse Effects	Drug Interactions[a]	Comments	Cost[b]
Nicotine Receptor Partial Agonists	*varenicline* Champix	0.5 mg daily po for 3 days then BID for 4 days then 0.5–1 mg BID po for 12 weeks. Patient should quit smoking 1–2 weeks after starting varenicline. If patient is still smoking 4 weeks after starting, reassess therapy; can be continued for an additional 12 weeks if patient has benefited. If 1 mg BID not tolerated, can reduce to 0.5 mg BID. No tapering necessary when discontinuing	Nausea (30%); may be mitigated by taking on a full stomach, increasing water intake or reducing dose. May cause insomnia; take second daily dose at suppertime. Neuropsychiatric side effects such as suicidal/homicidal ideation have been reported; monitor closely for changes in mood/behaviour. Close monitoring by health professional for those with pre-existing psychiatric disorders.	Should not be combined with nicotine replacement therapy due to increased risk of adverse effects.	Does not induce cytochrome P450 enzymes; excreted renally unchanged. Efficacy is dose related.	$$$$$
Nicotine Replacement, immediate-release	*nicotine bitartrate dihydrate lozenge* Thrive	Initial strength: 1 mg if <20 cigarettes per day, 2 mg if ≥20 cigarettes per day. Dosing frequency: see nicotine polacrilex lozenges; maximum 15/day for 2 mg strength, 25/day for 1 mg strength	Hiccups, GI disturbances, jaw pain and orodental problems.	Avoid use of acidic beverages and foods (coffee, fruit juices, soft drinks, alcohol) while chewing and 15 min before (decreases absorption).	Lozenges should be allowed to slowly dissolve and moved from one side of the mouth to the other periodically.	$
	nicotine inhaler Nicorette Inhaler	1 cartridge, as needed first 6–12 weeks: Encourage patient to use at least 6 cartridges/day for the first 3–6 weeks. Maximum 12/day. Tapering: gradual reduction in use over next 6–12 weeks, stopping when reduced to 1–2/day	Mild local irritation (cough, throat irritation, stomatitis, rhinitis) that may decline with continued use; headache, nausea, dyspepsia.	No known significant drug interactions.	Not a true inhaler—each cartridge lasts for about 20 min of puffing and delivers 4 mg of nicotine, of which approximately 2 mg is absorbed buccally. "Hand-mouth" activity from using the inhaler is preferred by some quitters while others find it to be a trigger. Useful in those with poor oral health or dentures and in those who cannot chew gum. Cold temperatures can decrease the absorption rate. If spending time in cold environments, store inhaler in a warm place such as an inner clothing pocket.	$$

Class	Drug	Dose	Adverse Effects	Drug Interactions[a]	Comments	Cost[b]
	nicotine mouthspray Nicorette QuickMist	Use 1–2 sprays every 30–60 min Maximum dose: 2 sprays/episode, 4 sprays/h, 64 sprays/day Spray must be primed with first use or after 2 days of not using	Altered sense of taste, headache, hiccups, nausea and vomiting, dyspepsia, oral soft tissue pain, stomatitis, salivary hypersecretion, burning lips, dry mouth.	No known significant drug interactions.	Each spray delivers 1 mg of nicotine. Mouthspray absorbed through buccal mucosa. Avoid acidic beverages and foods (coffee, fruit juices, soft drinks, alcohol) during use and 15 min before use as this may decrease absorption.	$$
	nicotine polacrilex gum Nicorette Gum, Thrive, generics	**Stopping abruptly:** 10–12 pieces/day (initial dose of 2 mg for lighter smokers, 4 mg for heavier smokers—consult individual product insert) Maximum 20 pieces/day, for up to 6 months **Stopping gradually in those not ready to quit:** use lowest effective dose of gum to relieve acute cravings, to prolong interval between cigarettes. Goal is to reduce smoking by 50% within 4 months, and quit within 6 months. Maximum 20 pieces/day, for no more than 12 months **Tapering:** 1 piece/day each week, as withdrawal symptoms allow	See nicotine bitartrate dihydrate lozenge.	See nicotine bitartrate dihydrate lozenge.	Instruct patient to bite down once or twice then park gum between the teeth and gums for about 1 min. Use 4 mg in heavily dependent smokers. May be used for temporary abstinence, e.g., to comply with smoking restrictions on airplanes.	$

(cont'd)

Table 2: **Pharmacologic Agents Used for Smoking Cessation** *(cont'd)*

Class	Drug	Dose	Adverse Effects	Drug Interactions[a]	Comments	Cost[b]
	nicotine polacrilex lozenge Nicorette Lozenge	Nicotine: use initial strength of 2 mg if first cigarette of the day >30 min after waking, 4 mg if ≤30 min Weeks 1–6: 1 lozenge Q1–2H PRN (maximum 15/day) Weeks 7–9: 1 lozenge Q2–4H PRN Weeks 10–12: 1 lozenge Q4–8H PRN Discontinue when dose has been reduced to 1–2 lozenges/day Use beyond 6 months generally not recommended	See nicotine bitartrate dihydrate lozenge.	See nicotine bitartrate dihydrate lozenge.	See nicotine bitartrate dihydrate lozenge.	$$
Nicotine Replacement, sustained-release	*nicotine transdermal patch* Habitrol, Nicoderm, generics	**Habitrol:** >20 cigarettes/day: 1 patch (21 mg/24 h) daily × 3–4 weeks ≤20 cigarettes/day: 1 patch (14 mg/24 h) daily × 3–4 weeks Total daily doses of nicotine may be increased up to 35 mg per day for smokers previously using 21–40 cigarettes a day, and up to 40 mg per day for smokers previously using more than 40 cigarettes a day.[92,93] This may be achieved by using additional patches or chewing pieces or the combination of both. Using more than 1 patch or doses >21 mg/day requires physician supervision. **Tapering:** reduce strength of patch (i.e., from 21 to 14 to 7 mg/24 h) every 3–4 weeks **Nicoderm:** 21 mg/24 h × 6 weeks then 14 mg/24 h × 2 weeks then 7 mg/24 h × 2 weeks If patient has cardiovascular disease, weighs less than 45 kg or smokes <½ pack/day begin	Skin sensitivity and irritation (most common); abnormal dreams; insomnia; nausea, dyspepsia.	No known significant drug interactions.	Start patch on the quit date. Advise not to smoke cigarettes while using the patch, though this is generally safe and does not indicate treatment failure. Educate users on the signs and symptoms of nicotine toxicity. **Habitrol:** Takes longer to reach peak levels than Nicoderm; should not use while exercising; major supplier of the generic/store brands. **Nicoderm:** More rapid onset and shorter time to peak effects; may be worn while exercising; although not recommended by the manufacturer, can be cut without damaging the delivery device. **Nicorette:** Better dosing flexibility and outcomes with gum/patch combination therapy.	$$$$

Class	Drug	Dose	Adverse Effects	Drug Interactions[a]	Comments	Cost[b]
		with 14 mg/24 h × 6 weeks then decrease to 7 mg/24 h × 2 weeks **Nicorette:** 15 mg patch daily × 6 weeks. If desired, decrease to 10 mg daily × 2 weeks then 5 mg daily × 2 weeks before discontinuing. Maximum 10 weeks				

[a] Cigarette smoking can increase the clearance of many drugs through mechanisms such as induction of cytochrome P450 enzymes CYP1A1, 1A2 or 2E1. Patients taking drugs such as caffeine, clozapine, diazepam, estrogens, fluvoxamine, methadone, nifedipine, olanzapine, rasagiline, theophylline, trifluoperazine or warfarin may require dosage reduction when they quit smoking.

[b] Cost of 100 pieces of gum or lozenges, 42 cartridges, 150 sprays, 28 patches or 30-day supply of tablets; includes drug cost only.

Dosage adjustment may be required in renal impairment; see Appendix I.

Abbreviations: CVS = cardiovascular; NRT = nicotine replacement therapy

Legend: $ < $25 $$ $25–50 $$$ $50–75 $$$$ $75–100 $$$$$ $100–125

Suggested Readings

Cahill K, Stevens S, Perera R et al. Pharmacological interventions for smoking cessation: an overview and network meta-analysis. *Cochrane Database Syst Rev* 2013;5:CD009329.

CAN-ADAPTT: The Canadian Action Network for the Advancement, Dissemination and Adoption of Practice-informed Tobacco Treatment. *Smoking cessation knowledge exchange network & clinical practice guidelines*. Available from: www.nicotinedependenceclinic.com.

Els C, Kunyk D, Selby P. *Disease interrupted: tobacco reduction and cessation.* CreateSpace, a DBA of On-Demand Publishing; 2012.

Fiore MC, Jaen CR, Baker TB et al. Clinical practice guideline. *Treating tobacco use and dependence: 2008 update.* Washington (DC): Public Health Service, U.S. Department of Health and Human Services; 2008.

George TP, ed. *Medication treatments for nicotine dependence.* Boca Raton (FL): CRC/Taylor & Francis; 2007.

Marcano Belisario JS, Bruggeling MN, Gunn LH et al. Interventions for recruiting smokers into cessation programmes. *Cochrane Database Syst Rev* 2012;12:CD009187.

Treatobacco.net. Independent, authoritative information on the treatment of tobacco dependence. Available from: www.treatobacco.net.

References

1. Health Canada. Canadian Tobacco Use Monitoring Survey (CTUMS). *Summary of annual results for 2011.* Available from: www.hc-sc.gc.ca/hc-ps/tobac-tabac/research-recherche/stat/_ctums-esutc_2011/ann_summary-sommaire-eng.php. Accessed February 25, 2013.
2. U.S. Department of Health & Human. Report of the Surgeon General. *How tobacco smoke causes disease: the biology and behavioral basis for smoking-attributable disease.* 2010. Available from: www.surgeongeneral.gov/library/reports/tobaccosmoke/index.html.
3. Picciotto MR, Mineur YS. Molecules and circuits involved in nicotine addiction: the many faces of smoking. *Neuropharmacology* 2014;76(Pt B):545-53.
4. Le Houezec J. Role of nicotine pharmacokinetics in nicotine addiction and nicotine replacement therapy: a review. *Int J Tuberc Lung Dis* 2003;7(9):811-9.
5. Fowler JS, Logan J, Wang GJ et al. Monoamine oxidase and cigarette smoking. *Neurotoxicology* 2003;24(1):75-82.
6. Desai HD, Seabolt J, Jann MW. Smoking in patients receiving psychotropic medications: a pharmacokinetic perspective. *CNS Drugs* 2001;15(6):469-94.
7. Fiore MC, Jaen CR, Baker TB et al. *Clinical practice guideline. Treating tobacco use and dependence: 2008 update.* Washington (DC): Public Health Service, U.S. Department of Health and Human Services; 2008. Available from: http://bphc.hrsa.gov/buckets/treatingtobacco.pdf
8. Tverdal A, Bjartveit K. Health consequences of reduced daily cigarette consumption. *Tob Control* 2006;15(6):472-80.
9. Hyland A, Levy DT, Rezaishiraz H et al. Reduction in amount smoked predicts future cessation. *Psychol Addict Behav* 2005;19(2):221-5.
10. Heatherton TF, Kozlowski LT, Frecker RC et al. The Fagerstrom Test for Nicotine Dependence: a revision of the Fagerstrom Tolerance Questionnaire. *Br J Addict* 1991;86(9):1119-27.
11. Kozlowski LT, Porter CQ, Orleans CT et al. Predicting smoking cessation with self-reported measures of nicotine dependence: FTQ, FTND, and HSI. *Drug Alcohol Depend* 1994;34(3):211-6.
12. Prokhorov AV, Hudmon KS, Marani S et al. Engaging physicians and pharmacists in providing smoking cessation counseling. *Arch Intern Med* 2010;170(18):1640-6.
13. Carson KV, Verbiest ME, Crone MR et al. Training health professionals in smoking cessation. *Cochrane Database Syst Rev* 2012;5:CD000214.
14. Canadian Pharmacists Association. *QUIT (Quit Using and Inhaling Tobacco) smoking cessation program.* Available from: www.pharmacists.ca/index.cfm/education-practice-resources/professional-development/quit/.
15. Centre for Addiction and Mental Health. *TEACH certificate program in intensive tobacco cessation counselling.* Available from: www.camh.ca/en/education/about/AZCourses/Pages/Sample-Course_9.aspx.
16. Centre for Addiction and Mental Health. *Algorithm for tailoring pharmacotherapy in primary care setting.* Available from: https://www.nicotinedependenceclinic.com/English/teach/resources/Visual%20Aids/Tobacco%20Algorithm%20updated%20Nov%202013.pdf
17. Lindson-Hawley N, Aveyard P, Hughes JR. Reduction versus abrupt cessation in smokers who want to quit. *Cochrane Database Syst Rev* 2012;11:CD008033.
18. Chen YF, Madan J, Welton N et al. Effectiveness and cost-effectiveness of computer and other electronic aids for smoking cessation: a systematic review and network meta-analysis. *Health Technol Assess* 2012;16(38):1-205.
19. Whittaker R, McRobbie H, Bullen C et al. Mobile phone-based interventions for smoking cessation. *Cochrane Database Syst Rev* 2012;11:CD006611.
20. Civljak, Stead LF, Hartmann-Boyce J et al. Internet-based interventions for smoking cessation. *Cochrane Database Syst Rev* 2013;7:CD007078.
21. Ramon JM, Nerin I, Comino A et al. A multicentre randomized trial of combined individual and telephone counselling for smoking cessation. *Prev Med* 2013;57(3):183-8.
22. Stead LF, Lancaster T. Behavioural interventions as adjuncts to pharmacotherapy for smoking cessation. *Cochrane Database Syst Rev* 2012;12:CD009670.
23. Stead LF, Lancaster T. Combined pharmacotherapy and behavioural interventions for smoking cessation. *Cochrane Database Syst Rev* 2012;10:CD008286.
24. Patnode CD, O'Connor E, Whitlock EP et al. Primary care-relevant interventions for tobacco use prevention and cessation in children and adolescents: a systematic evidence review for the U.S. Preventative Services Task Force. *Ann Intern Med* 2013;158(4):253-60.

25. Johnston V, Liberato S, Thomas D. Incentives for prevention smoking in children and adolescents. *Cochrane Database Syst Rev* 2012;10:CD008645.

26. Health Canada. *Champix (varenicline tartrate) and Zyban (bupropion hydrochloride)—Revision to the Consumer information of non-nicotine smoking cessation aids—For health professionals*. Available from: healthycanadians.gc.ca/recall-alert-rappel-avis/hc-sc/2013/33621a-eng.php.

27. Stead LF, Perera R, Bullen C et al. Nicotine replacement therapy for smoking cessation. *Cochrane Database Syst Rev* 2012;11:CD000146.

28. Cahill K, Stevens S, Perera R et al. Pharmacological interventions for smoking cessation: an overview and network meta-analysis. *Cochrane Databse Syst Rev* 2013;5:CD009329.

29. Cahill K, Stead LF, Lancaster T. Nicotine receptor partial agonists for smoking cessation. *Cochrane Database Syst Rev* 2012;4:CD006103.

30. Cinciripini PM, Robinson JD, Karam-Hage M et al. Effects of varenicline and bupropion sustained-release use plus intensive smoking cessation counseling on prolonged abstinence from smoking and on depression, negative affect, and other symptoms of nicotine withdrawal. *JAMA Psychiatry* 2013;70(5):522-33.

31. Keating GM, Siddiqui MA. Varenicline: a review of its use as an aid to smoking cessation therapy. *CNS Drugs* 2006;20(11):945-60.

32. Oncken C, Gonzales D, Nides M et al. Efficacy and safety of the novel selective nicotinic acetylcholine receptor partial agonist, varenicline, for smoking cessation. *Arch Intern Med* 2006;166(15):1571-7.

33. Tonstad S, Tonnesen P, Hajek P et al. Effect of maintenance therapy with varenicline on smoking cessation: a randomized controlled trial. *JAMA* 2006;296(1):64-71.

34. Cinciripini PM, Robinson JD, Karam-Hage M et al. Effects of varenicline and bupropion sustained-release use plus intensive smoking cessation counseling on prolonged abstinence from smoking and on depression, negative affect, and other symptoms of nicotine withdrawal. *JAMA Psychiatry* 2013;70(5):522-33.

35. Gibbons RD, Mann JJ. Varenicline, smoking cessation, and neuropsychiatric adverse events. *Am J Psychiatry* 2013;170(12):1460-7.

36. Pachas GN, Cather C, Pratt SA et al. Varenicline for smoking cessation in schizophrenia: safety and effectiveness in a 12-week, open-label trial. *J Dual Diagn* 2012;8(2):117-25.

37. Williams JM, Anthenelli RM, Morris CD et al. A randomized, double-blind, placebo-controlled study evaluating the safety and efficacy of varenicline for smoking cessation in patients with schizophrenia or schizoaffective disorder. *J Clin Psychiatry* 2012;73(5):654-60.

38. Weiner E, Buchholz A, Coffay A et al. Varenicline for smoking cessation in people with schizophrenia: a double blind randomized pilot study. *Schizophr Res* 2011;129(1):94-5.

39. Evins AE, Cather C, Pratt SA et al. Maintenance treatment with varenicline for smoking cessation in patients with schizophrenia and bipolar disorder: a randomized clinical trial. *JAMA* 2014;311(2):145-54.

40. Singh S, Loke YK, Spangler JG et al. Risk of serious adverse cardiovascular events associated with varenicline: a systemic review and meta-analysis. *CMAJ* 2011;183(12):1359-66.

41. Health Canada. *Health Canada reviewing stop-smoking drug Champix (varenicline tartrate) and potential risk of heart problems in patients with heart disease*. Available from: www.healthycanadians.gc.ca/recall-alert-rappel-avis/hc-sc/2011/13619a-eng.php. Accessed February 5, 2014.

42. Rigotti NA, Pipe AL, Benowitz NL et al. Efficacy and safety of varenicline for smoking cessation in patients with cardiovascular disease: a randomized trial. *Circulation* 2010;121(2):221-9.

43. Prochaska JJ, Hilton JF. Risk of cardiovascular serious adverse events associated with varenicline use for tobacco cessation: systematic review and meta-analysis. *BMJ* 2012;344:e2856.

44. Svanstrom HS, Pasternak B, Hviid A. Use of varenicline for smoking cessation and risk of serious cardiovascular events: nationwide cohort study. *BMJ* 2012;345:e7176.

45. Mills EJ, Thorlund K, Eapen S et al. Cardiovascular events associated with smoking cessation pharmacotherapies: a network meta-analysis. *Circulation* 2014;129(1):28-41.

46. Gourlay S, Forbes A, Marriner T et al. A placebo-controlled study of three clonidine doses for smoking cessation. *Clin Pharmacol Ther* 1994;55(1):64-9.

47. Glassman AH, Stetner F, Walsh BT et al. Heavy smokers, smoking cessation, and clonidine. Results of a double-blind, randomized trial. *JAMA* 1988;259(19):2863-6.

48. Hughes JR, Stead LF, Lancaster T. Antidepressants for smoking cessation. *Cochrane Database Syst Rev* 2007;(1):CD000031.

49. Frishman WH, Mitta W, Kupersmith A et al. Nicotine and non-nicotine smoking cessation pharmacotherapies. *Cardiol Rev* 2006;14(2):57-73.

50. West R, Zatonski W, Cedzynska M et al. Placebo-controlled trial of cytisine for smoking cessation. *N Engl J Med* 2011;365(13):1193-200.

51. Smith SS, McCarthy DE, Japuntich SJ et al. Comparative effectiveness of 5 smoking cessation pharmacotherapies in primary care clinics. *Arch Intern Med* 2009;169(22):2148-55.

52. Ebbert JO, Croghan IT, Sood A et al. Varenicline and bupropion sustained-release combination therapy for smoking cessation. *Nicotine Tob Res* 2009;11(3):234-9.

53. Health Canada. *Health Canada advises Canadians not to use electronic cigarettes*. Available from: www.healthycanadians.gc.ca/recall-alert-rappel-avis/hc-sc/2009/13373a-eng.php.

54. U.S. Food and Drug Administration (FDA). *Summary of results: laboratory analysis of electronic cigarettes conducted by FDA*. Available from: www.fda.gov/newsevents/publichealthfocus/ucm173146.htm.

55. Bullen C, Howe C, Laugesen M et al. Electronic cigarettes for smoking cessation: a randomised controlled trial. *Lancet* 2013;382(9905):1629-37.

56. Caponnetto P, Campagna D, Cibella F et al. EffiCiency and safety of an eLectronic cigAreTte (ECLAT) as tobacco cigarettes substitute: a Prospective 12-month randomized control design study. *PLoS One* 2013;8(6):e66317.

57. Peto R, Whitlock G, Jha P. Effects of obesity and smoking on U.S. life expectancy. *N Engl J Med* 2010;362(9):855-6.

58. Clair C, Rigotti NA, Porneala B et al. Association of smoking cessation and weight change with cardiovascular disease among adults with and without diabetes. *JAMA* 2013;309(10):1014-21.

59. O'Hara P, Connett JE, Lee WW et al. Early and late weight gain following smoking cessation in the Lung Health Study. *Am J Epidemiol* 1998;148(9):821-30.

60. Fagerstrom K, Balfour DJ. Neuropharmacology and potential efficacy of new treatments for tobacco dependence. *Expert Opin Investig Drugs* 2006;15(2):107-16.

61. Farley AC, Hajek P, Lycett D et al. Interventions for preventing weight gain after smoking cessation. *Cochrane Database Syst Rev* 2012;1:CD006219.

62. Aubin HJ, Farley A, Lycett D et al. Weight gain in smokers after quitting cigarettes: meta-analysis. *BMJ* 2012;345:e4439.

63. Al-Sahab B, Saqib M, Hauser G et al. Prevalence of smoking during pregnancy and associated risk factors among Canadian women: a national survey. *BMC Pregnancy Childbirth* 2010;10:24.

64. Agrawal A, Scherrer JF, Grant JD et al. The effects of maternal smoking during pregnancy on offspring outcomes. *Prev Med* 2010;50(1-2):13-8.
65. Andres RL, Day MC. Perinatal complications associated with maternal tobacco use. *Semin Neonatol* 2000;5(3):231-41.
66. Public Health Agency of Canada. *What mothers say: the Canadian maternity experiences survey*. Ottawa (ON): PHAC; 2009. Available from: www.phac-aspc.gc.ca/rhs-ssg/survey-eng.php. Accessed May 31, 2013.
67. Cnattingius S. The epidemiology of smoking during pregnancy: smoking prevalence, maternal characteristics, and pregnancy outcomes. *Nicotine Tob Res* 2004;6(Suppl 2):S125-40.
68. Crawford JT, Tolosa JE, Goldenberg RL. Smoking cessation in pregnancy: why, how, and what next. *Clin Obstet Gynecol* 2008;51(2):419-35.
69. Coleman T, Chamberlain C, Davey MA et al. Pharmacological interventions for promoting smoking cessation during pregnancy. *Cochrane Database Syst Rev* 2012;9:CD010078.
70. Practice Committee of the American Society for Reproductive Medicine. Smoking and infertility. *Fertil Steril* 2006;86(5 Suppl 1):S172-7.
71. Lumley J, Chamberlain C, Dowswell T et al. Interventions for promoting smoking cessation during pregnancy. *Cochrane Database Syst Rev* 2009;(3):CD001055.
72. Fang WL, Goldstein AO, Butzen AY et al. Smoking cessation in pregnancy: a review of postpartum relapse prevention strategies. *J Am Board Fam Pract* 2004;17(4):264-75.
73. Likis FE, Andrews JC, Fonnesbeck CJ et al. Smoking cessation interventions in pregnancy and postpartum care. *Evidence Report/Technology Assessment* No.214. AHRQ Publication No. 14-E001-EF. Rockville (MD): Agency for Healthcare Research and Quality; February 2014. Available from: effectivehealthcare.ahrq.gov/ehc/products/517/1871/smoking-pregnancy-infants-report-140226.pdf.
74. Kapur B, Hackman R, Selby P et al. Randomized, double-blind, placebo-controlled trial of nicotine replacement therapy in pregnancy. *Curr Ther Res* 2001;62(4):274-8.
75. Pollak KI, Oncken CA, Lipkus IM et al. Nicotine replacement and behavioral therapy for smoking cessation in pregnancy. *Am J Prev Med* 2007;33(4):297-305.
76. Wisborg K, Henriksen TB, Jespersen LB et al. Nicotine patches for pregnant smokers: a randomized controlled study. *Obstet Gynecol* 2000;96(6):967-71.
77. Coleman T, Cooper S, Thornton JG et al. A randomized trial of nicotine-replacement therapy patches in pregnancy. *N Engl J Med* 2012;366(9):808-18.
78. Berlin I, Grangé G, Jacob N et al. Nicotine patches in pregnant smokers: randomised placebo controlled, multicentre trial of efficacy. *BMJ* 2014;348:g1622.
79. Masho SW, Bishop DL, Keyser-Marcus L et al. Least explored factors associated with prenatal smoking. *Matern Child Health J* 2013;17(7):1167-74.
80. Massey SH, Compton MT. Psychological differences between smokers who spontaneously quit during pregnancy and those who do not: a review of observational studies and directions for future research. *Nicotine Tob Res* 2013;15(2):307-19.
81. Oncken C, Dornelas E, Greene J et al. Nicotine gum for pregnant smokers: a randomized controlled trial. *Obstet Gynecol* 2008;112(4):859-67.
82. Osadchy A, Kazmin A, Koren G. Nicotine replacement during pregnancy: recommended or not recommended? *J Obstet Gynaecol Can* 2009;31(8):744-7.
83. Einarson A, Choi J, Einarson TR et al. Incidence of major malformations in infants following antidepressant exposure in pregnancy: results of a large prospective cohort study. *Can J Psychiatry* 2009;54(4):242-6.
84. American Academy of Pediatrics Committee on Drugs. Transfer of drugs and other chemicals into human milk. *Pediatrics* 2001;108(3):776-89.
85. Kendzor DE, Businelle MS, Costello TJ et al. Breast feeding is associated with postpartum smoking abstinence among women who quit smoking due to pregnancy. *Nicotine Tob Res* 2010;12(10):983-8.
86. Mallin R. Smoking cessation: integration of behavioral and drug therapies. *Am Fam Physician* 2002;65(6):1107-14.
87. Taylor G, McNeill A, Girling A et al. Change in mental health after smoking cessation: systematic review and meta-analysis. *BMJ* 2014;348:g1151.
88. Smith SS, Jorenby DE, Leischow SJ et al. Targeting smokers at increased risk for relapse: treating women and those with a history of depression. *Nicotine Tob Res* 2003;5(1):99-109.
89. Sussman S, Sun P, Dent CW. A meta-analysis of teen cigarette smoking cessation. *Health Psychol* 2006;25(5):549-57.
90. Grimshaw GM, Stanton A. Tobacco cessation interventions for young people. *Cochrane Database Syst Rev* 2006;(4):CD003289.
91. Moyer VA; U.S. Preventive Services Task Force. Primary care interventions to prevent tobacco use in children and adolescents: U.S. Preventive Services Task Force recommendation statement. *Pediatrics* 2013;132(3):560-5.
92. Dale LC, Hurt RD, Offord KP et al. High-dose nicotine patch therapy. Percentage of replacement and smoking cessation. *JAMA* 1995;274(17):1353-8.
93. Dale LC, Hurt RD, Hays JT. Drug therapy to aid in smoking cessation. Tips on maximizing patients' chances for success. *Postgrad Med* 1998;104(6):75-8, 83-4.

Chapter 14
Acute Pain

Benoit Bailey, MD, MSc, FRCPC

Pain is one of the most common symptoms experienced by patients. Acute pain is temporary and may last for minutes or up to several weeks. It needs to be recognized, assessed for cause and treated appropriately as soon as possible. The absence of treatment can lead to physiological and psychological adverse effects. Treatment should be tailored to the level and type of pain. The absence of a diagnosis, including for patients with abdominal pain, should not delay measures to relieve pain.

Goals of Therapy

- Recognize that the patient is experiencing pain
- Relieve the pain until the cause is treated
- Identify and treat the cause of pain

Investigations

- Observe the patient for behavioural signs of pain, e.g., agitation, anxiety, crying, gritting of teeth, withdrawal from activities
- Solicit self-reports of the pain
- Inquire about the medical history and perform a physical examination to determine the cause and severity of the pain
- Inquire about medication self-treatment history and possible allergy or adverse reactions to analgesics
- Use laboratory investigations as appropriate to determine the cause of the pain
- Use a *pain scale* to measure and assess pain
- Frequently evaluate response to treatment

Note: The use of a pain scale can help reduce oligoanalgesia (undertreatment of pain).[1] Record the results of this assessment as for a vital sign, and use it to judge the efficacy of interventions. The easy-to-use verbal numeric scale, also known as the numeric rating scale, asks the patient to grade pain from 0 (no pain) to 10 (worst pain) and is validated in adults and children ≥8 years.[2] Other pain scales such as the standardized colour analogue scale or the Wong-Baker Faces Pain Rating Scale can be used in children as young as 4–5 years or 3–6 years, respectively.[3] The PAINAD tool was developed to assess pain in adults with cognitive impairment.[4]

Therapeutic Choices

Nonpharmacologic Choices

Assess patients presenting with acute pain quickly, calmly and with empathy. Provide reassurance and encourage patients to verbalize their pain at all stages of treatment. Initiate immediate measures to decrease pain (e.g., immobilize a fracture, apply dressings to burns, employ cold or heat or other techniques such as relaxation, imagery and distraction) until pharmacologic treatment is started and takes effect. Do not wait until a full assessment is made to start pharmacologic treatment.

Pharmacologic Choices

Table 3 provides a list of opioid and non-opioid medications for the treatment of acute pain.

Oral Analgesics

As a first step for mild to moderate pain, initiate treatment with a nonopioid analgesic (i.e., acetaminophen or nonsteroidal anti-inflammatory drug [NSAID]), either alone or in combination with an oral opioid depending on the nature/severity of the pain and the patient's medical and medication history. If pain persists and is still moderate or worsening, consider adding an oral opioid to the"first-step" drug if not already tried. For patients with severe acute pain, starting a parenteral opioid is usually more appropriate (Figure 1).

Nonopioid Analgesics

Acetaminophen can be used for mild to moderate pain. Compared to full-dose NSAIDs, acetaminophen has fewer adverse effects and drug interactions but is less effective and has no anti-inflammatory action.[5] Acetaminophen can be used with oral opioids for additive analgesic effect.

Nonsteroidal anti-inflammatory drugs (NSAIDs) are a heterogeneous group of medications with analgesic, antipyretic and anti-inflammatory properties. Medications from all 5 classes of nonselective NSAIDs (i.e., salicylates, fenamates, propionic acid derivatives, oxicams, acetic acid derivatives) are effective for mild to moderate pain. Prescribing information for all classes of NSAIDs can be found in Chapter 82. Full single doses of most NSAIDs provide more effective analgesia than full doses of ASA or acetaminophen.[5] Choosing an NSAID can be difficult; some patients respond well to a certain class but not to others and cost can be an important factor.

Adverse effects associated with single (or a few) doses of nonselective NSAIDs are limited and are qualitatively similar to those of ASA. Chronic use is associated with GI effects (ulceration, bleeding and perforation) and renal failure. Combining a proton-pump inhibitor (PPI) once daily or misoprostol 200 µg QID po with an NSAID effectively provides protection from GI toxicity.[6] Some combinations are commercially available in Canada (e.g., naproxen/esomeprazole, Vimovo; diclofenac/misoprostol, Arthrotec). Unlike other NSAIDs, ASA irreversibly inhibits platelet function for the lifetime of the platelet (8–10 days) even after a single therapeutic dose. In contrast, platelet function returns to normal when other NSAIDs have been eliminated from the body (within approximately 24 hours for most NSAIDs). NSAIDs can precipitate asthma in ASA-sensitive patients. Avoid NSAIDs in patients with a history of peptic ulcer disease, renal failure or heart failure.

COX-2 selective NSAIDs such as celecoxib may cause less severe GI toxicity than nonselective NSAIDs, but are more expensive and have a poorly-defined role and unstudied adverse effect profile in the treatment of acute pain.

ASA can be given with opioids for additive analgesic effect. Avoid using ASA in children less than 18 years of age if they have a fever or viral illness such as flu or chickenpox or any unidentified infection, because of a possible increased risk of Reye's syndrome—a rare but serious condition that causes brain and liver damage. ASA can also precipitate asthma in ASA-sensitive patients.

Ibuprofen 200 mg provides equivalent analgesia to ASA 650 mg or acetaminophen 650 mg; a dose of 400 mg is superior and longer acting, and provides comparable analgesia to the combination of acetaminophen/codeine.[5,7] A 10 mg/kg dose of ibuprofen is as safe as a 15 mg/kg dose of acetaminophen, although GI bleeding has been reported with ibuprofen.[8]

Naproxen has a longer duration of action than ASA.[5] Compared to ASA 650 mg, naproxen 250 mg is equally effective and naproxen 500 mg is superior.[9] Naproxen is available as oral tablets or rectal suppositories. Naproxen sodium 220 mg (equivalent to naproxen 200 mg) is available as an oral nonprescription analgesic.

Figure 1: **Management of Acute Pain**

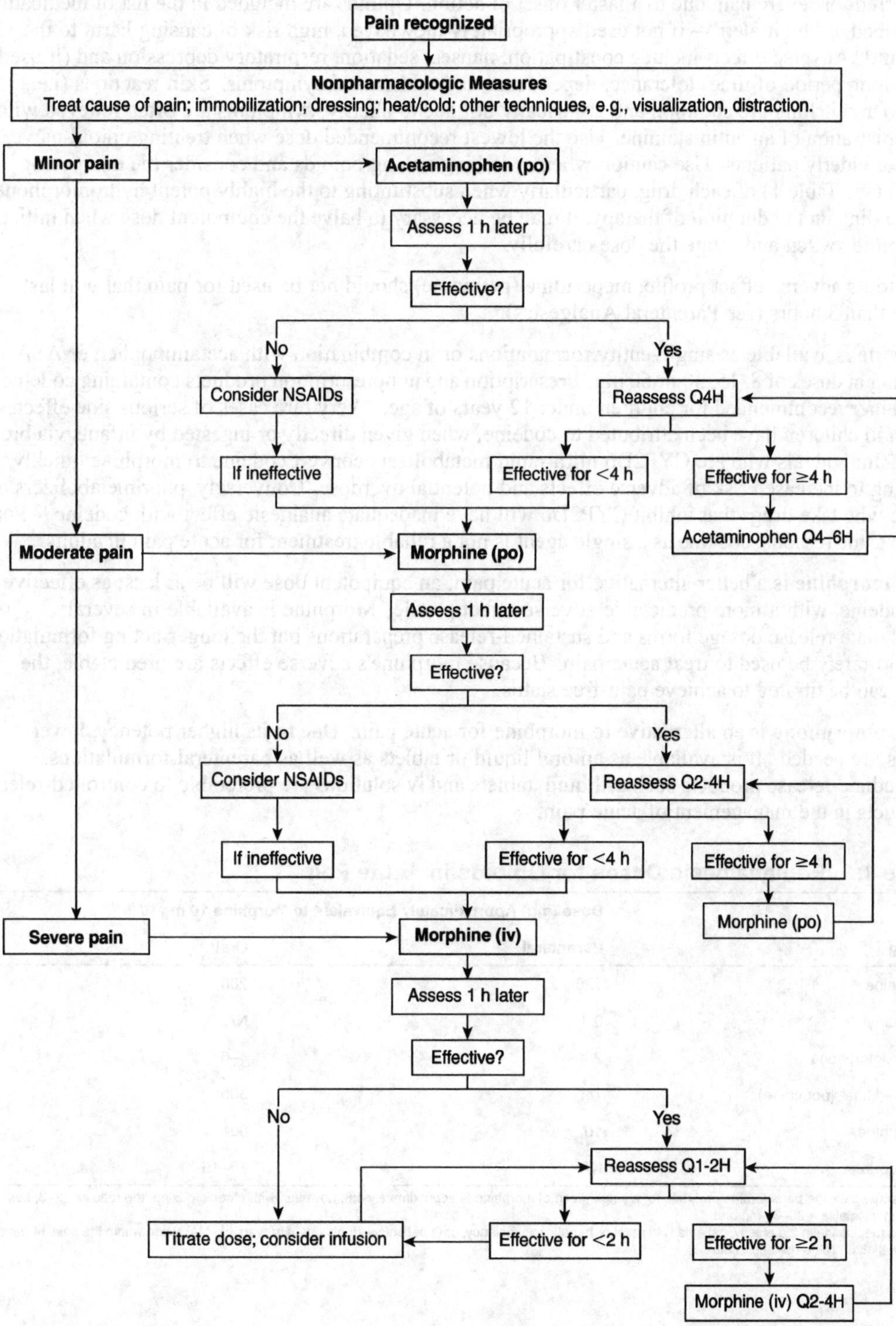

Opioids

Oral opioids can be used for the treatment of moderate to severe pain. The parenteral route may be preferred for severe pain due to a faster onset of action. Opioids are included in the list of medications described as "high-alert"—if not used appropriately they have a high risk of causing harm to the patient.[10] Adverse effects include constipation, nausea, sedation, respiratory depression and (if used for a long period of time) tolerance, dependence and withdrawal symptoms. Skin reactions (i.e., hives) and itching are common and are usually not due to allergy; symptoms are often relieved with administration of an antihistamine. Use the lowest recommended dose when treating opioid-naïve, frail or elderly patients. Use caution when switching among opioids and consider the equipotent doses (see Table 1) of each drug, particularly when substituting to the highly potent hydromorphone. Depending on the duration of therapy, it may be necessary to halve the equipotent dose when initiating an opioid switch and titrate the dose carefully.

Due to its adverse effect profile, meperidine (pethidine) should not be used for pain that will last more than 3 hours (see Parenteral Analgesics).

Codeine is available as single-entity formulations or in combination with acetaminophen or ASA 325 mg at doses of 8, 15, 30 or 60 mg. Prescription and nonprescription products containing codeine are no longer recommended for children under 12 years of age.[11] Very rare cases of serious side effects and death in children have been attributed to codeine, when given directly or ingested by infants via breast milk. Individuals who are CYP2D6 ultra-rapid metabolizers convert codeine to morphine quickly, leading to increased risk of adverse effects and potential overdose. Conversely, poor metabolizers or those who take drugs that inhibit CYP2D6 will have inadequate analgesic effect with codeine.[12] For these same reasons, codeine as a single agent is not a reliable treatment for acute pain in adults.

Oral **morphine** is a better alternative for acute pain; an equipotent dose will be at least as effective as codeine, with a more predictable adverse effect profile. Morphine is available in several immediate-release dosage forms and sustained-release preparations but the longer-acting formulations should rarely be used to treat acute pain. Because morphine's adverse effects are predictable, the dose can be titrated to achieve pain-free status.

Hydromorphone is an alternative to morphine for acute pain. Due to its higher potency, lower doses are needed. It is available as an oral liquid or tablets as well as parenteral formulations. Immediate-release products such as liquid, tablets and iv solutions are preferable to controlled-release products in the management of acute pain.

Table 1: **Equianalgesic Doses for Opioids in Acute Pain**

	Dose (mg) Approximately Equivalent to Morphine 10 mg IV	
Drug	**Parenteral**	**Oral**
Codeine	120	200
Fentanyl	0.1	NA
Hydromorphone	2	4–6
Meperidine[b] (pethidine)	75	300
Morphine	10	60[a]
Oxycodone	NA	10–15

[a] For acute pain, the parenteral-to-oral ratio for a single dose of morphine is approximately 1:6; however, with chronic dosing, the ratio is 1:2–3, i.e., 10 mg injectable ≈ 20–30 mg oral.

[b] Avoid meperidine in the elderly, patients with renal or hepatic insufficiency, or in patients with history of irreversible MAOI use within the past 14 days.

Abbreviations: NA = not applicable

Oxycodone is available in single-entity immediate-release or controlled-release formulations and in combination with acetaminophen. Immediate-release formulations with or without acetaminophen are an effective alternative for acute pain management; use with caution since oxycodone is often a drug of choice for patients with drug seeking behaviour or substance abuse disorders.

Tramadol is a unique analgesic. It is structurally related to morphine and codeine and acts through opioid and nonopioid mechanisms. Although it appears to have less abuse potential and minimal effect on respiratory function, tramadol causes more nausea compared to other opioids and may not be as effective unless combined with another analgesic such as acetaminophen.[13,14] Tramadol should not be used as a first-line analgesic for acute pain [Evidence: SORT B*].[14,15,16]

Parenteral Analgesics

IV administration is less painful and has a more rapid and predictable onset of action compared with the sc and im routes. The intranasal route is sometimes used with fentanyl.[17]

In case overdosage occurs, keep **naloxone** (Table 2) on hand when administering opioids parenterally. Respiratory depression rarely occurs as long as the opioid is titrated to the level of pain.

NSAIDs

Ketorolac is an NSAID that can be given im or iv for the treatment of moderate to severe pain. A dose of 30 mg is comparable to approximately 12 mg of morphine.[5] Ketorolac has the same adverse effect profile as the oral nonselective NSAIDs. The pharmacologic effect cannot be titrated but the drug can be used when opioids are contraindicated. Limit its use to 5 days' duration to minimize adverse effects. Ketorolac is effective for the treatment of pain associated with renal colic.

Ibuprofen, at a dose of 400 mg or 800 mg administered as an iv infusion every 6 hours, significantly decreased pain at rest and with movement when used adjunctively with iv opioids, for short-term management of postoperative pain.[18] The 800 mg dose, but not 400 mg, significantly reduced opioid requirements.

Opioids

Morphine is the gold standard to which other opioids are compared. Its advantages (i.e., over meperidine) include a longer duration of action, and metabolism that is not affected by liver and renal disease. It can be administered as continuous infusion or as patient-controlled analgesia (PCA), a pump programmed to deliver a preset amount of drug by continuous infusion or repeated boluses, as well as smaller bolus doses for breakthrough pain.

Table 2: **Treatment of Opioid-induced Respiratory Depression**

Class	Drug	Dose
Opioid Antagonists	*naloxone* generics	Adults and children >5 y or >20 kg weight: 0.4–2 mg Q2–3 min iv, depending on response Children ≤5 y or 20 kg weight: 0.1 mg/kg Q2–3 min iv, depending on response Maximum dose: 10 mg. **Note:** May need to repeat in 1–2 h, depending on half-life of opioid. Continuous infusion may be used for overdoses of long-acting opiates. Starting dose is 2/3 of the initial dose that was effective for the patient, administered per hour by infusion *or* 0.4–0.8 mg/h in adults and 0.05–0.15 mg/kg/h in children. Titrate to effect.

* SORT (Strength of Recommendation Taxonomy) is a rating system (A, B or C) that addresses the quality of available evidence. For more information consult **How to Use *Compendium of Therapeutic Choices*** on page xxv.

Fentanyl is a synthetic opioid with a duration of action of only 30–60 minutes, making it an ideal analgesic for brief procedures. It can be administered by infusion, but this offers no advantage over morphine in terms of efficacy, and is much more costly. Fentanyl has almost no hemodynamic effects and does not induce histamine release, unlike morphine and meperidine. Rapid iv administration can lead to chest wall rigidity that could interfere with ventilation. A single dose of intranasal fentanyl can be used to rapidly treat acute pain when there is no iv access (such as on arrival to the emergency department).[17] This requires an atomizer device as well as established policy and procedures for administration. The intranasal dose should be followed by administration of an iv opioid in all cases, where required.

Meperidine is not considered a first-line option in the treatment of acute pain and should not be given for pain that is expected to last more than 3 hours where morphine is a better choice. Limit its use to short-term (i.e., 24–48 hours) due to the accumulation of normeperidine, a neurotoxic metabolite that can cause seizures in some patients and CNS effects such as tremors, hyperreflexia, hallucinations. Avoid using meperidine in patients with renal failure or liver disease and in those who have received MAOIs in the past 14 days. In some hospitals, meperidine has been removed from the formulary because of these concerns.

Topical and Local Anesthesia

Topical NSAIDs can be used to treat acute musculoskeletal conditions.[19] They provide local pain relief with fewer systemic effects compared to oral NSAIDs. See Chapter 82 for information on topical NSAIDs availability.

Infiltrative techniques using **lidocaine** are frequently used for minor procedures. A dose of 3–5 mg/kg (maximum 300 mg) can be used for direct infiltration or regional nerve block. Coadministration of **epinephrine** allows an increase of lidocaine dose to 5–7 mg/kg, unless epinephrine is contraindicated (e.g., if tissue vascularity is poor or if distal vasculature is involved). If allergy to amide-type local anesthetics (e.g., lidocaine, bupivacaine) is suspected, an ester (e.g., procaine, tetracaine, benzocaine) can be used because of the absence of cross-reactivity.

For small facial lacerations, a mixture of **tetracaine** 0.5–1%, **epinephrine** (adrenaline) 0.25–0.5% and **cocaine** 1–4% (**TAC**) can be applied topically (volume 3 mL; maximum topical cocaine dose 6 mg/kg). The restricted status of cocaine limits its usefulness. A mixture of lidocaine 0.4%, epinephrine 0.1% and tetracaine 0.05% (**LET**), in a dose of 2 mL topically, is as effective as TAC.

Topical anesthetics such as eutectic mixture of local anesthetics (**EMLA**), **amethocaine** (tetracaine; Ametop) or **liposomal lidocaine** (Maxilene) can be used to reduce pain associated with minor procedures such as needle insertion on intact skin. EMLA, containing **prilocaine** and **lidocaine**, causes vasoconstriction potentially making cannulation difficult. To be effective, a large amount should be applied and covered with an occlusive dressing for at least 45–60 minutes.

Amethocaine is superior to EMLA in preventing pain associated with needle insertion in children.[20] It requires a shorter application time (30 minutes) than EMLA (45–60 minutes). Amethocaine causes vasodilation and may induce hypersensitivity with repeated use. Liposomal lidocaine is as effective as EMLA in decreasing pain associated with venipuncture or iv cannulation. It has minimal vasoactive properties and requires an application time of 30 minutes. An occlusive dressing is not required, but it is recommended in young children.

Inhalation Pain Management

Inhaled **nitrous oxide** (N_20) 30–50% can be used as an analgesic.[21] Advantages include rapid onset and short duration of action. Contraindications include altered level of consciousness, severe maxillofacial injuries, chronic obstructive pulmonary disease, acute pulmonary edema, pneumothorax, shock, decompression sickness, bowel obstruction and major chest injury. It can produce lightheadedness, drowsiness, nausea, vomiting and excitement.

Choices during Pregnancy and Breastfeeding

Acute pain is a common occurrence during pregnancy and in breastfeeding mothers. These conditions need not preclude the use of analgesics. However, prescribing the safest alternative for the fetus or newborn is paramount.

Pregnancy

For mild pain, the drug of choice is usually **acetaminophen**. During pregnancy, the use of **NSAIDs** should be restricted to the first or second trimester; even short-term NSAID use after 32 weeks is associated with a substantial increase in the risk of premature closure of the ductus arteriosus, and is not recommended.[22] For more severe pain, **opioids** can be used at all stages of pregnancy. If opioids are used during the late stage of labour, the newborn should be monitored for signs of respiratory depression. When opioids are used at high doses or more than sporadically in late pregnancy, monitor the newborn for signs of withdrawal. Neonatal withdrawal can occur when therapeutic doses of opioids are used in late pregnancy.[23]

Breastfeeding

For mild pain, the drug of choice is **acetaminophen**. **NSAIDs** can be used safely during breastfeeding. Generally, most immediate-release **opioids** taken while breastfeeding are safe if limited to therapeutic doses and relatively short-term use. Because of potential toxicity, **codeine**[12,24] or **meperidine** are not recommended if safer alternatives are available. When possible, it is advisable to wait at least 2 hours after taking an opioid before breastfeeding.[25] With exposure to more than a few doses of any opioid, particularly high doses, the breastfed child needs to be monitored for signs of respiratory depression.

A discussion of general principles on the use of medications during pregnancy and breastfeeding can be found in Appendix II and Appendix III. Other specialized reference sources are also provided in these appendices.

Therapeutic Tips

- Choose the medication and route of administration according to the severity of the pain and the desired onset and duration of action.
- Opioid analgesics can be safely given before full assessment and diagnosis in acute abdominal pain, without increasing the risk of errors in diagnosis or treatment.[26,27]
- Consider adding sedatives to analgesics, particularly for painful procedures. However, sedative use should not replace analgesics.
- Choose the most appropriate analgesic for elderly patients, considering hepatic and renal function and concurrent medications.
- Allow an adequate amount of time (according to the analgesic's onset of action), before performing a painful procedure or assessing whether an analgesic is effective.
- Monitor the patient's level of consciousness and for the presence of adverse effects after administering an analgesic.
- Reassess the need for analgesics frequently, using a pain scale.
- Avoid administering opioids on an "as-needed" basis. A regular schedule of administration is more effective.
- Consult specialized acute pain services as needed.

Table 3: Analgesics for the Treatment of Acute Pain

Class	Drug	Dose	Adverse Effects	Drug Interactions	Cost[a]
Analgesics, nonopioid	*acetaminophen* Atasol Preparations, Tempra, Tylenol, generics	**Children:** 10–15 mg/kg/dose Q4H po; oral suspension available 15–20 mg/kg/dose Q4H pr Maximum: 5 doses/day **Adults:** 325–650 mg Q4H po or pr Maximum: 4 g/day	Hepatotoxicity in overdose or supratherapeutic dosing.	Enhanced anticoagulant effect of warfarin with regular use of >2 g/day of acetaminophen.	$
	ASA Aspirin, Coated Aspirin, generics	**Children:** 10–15 mg/kg/dose Q4H po Maximum: 5 doses/day **Adults:** 325–650 mg Q4H po Maximum: 4 g/day	GI upset. Avoid in patients with renal failure, peptic ulcer disease, heart failure and ASA-sensitive asthma.	Warfarin: increased anticoagulant effect. Antihypertensives (diuretics, beta-blockers, ACE inhibitors, alpha-blockers): possible reduction in antihypertensive effect; may require additional antihypertensive therapy. Lithium may interfere with sodium/water balance. Monitor lithium levels when NSAID added. Increased risk of GI bleeding with SSRIs.	$
	ibuprofen, oral Advil, Motrin, Motrin (Children's), generics	**Children:** 10 mg/kg/dose Q6–8H po; oral suspension available Maximum: 40 mg/kg/day, not to exceed adult dose **Adults:** 200–400 mg Q6–8H po Maximum: 1.2 g/day	See ASA.	See ASA.	$
	ibuprofen, parenteral Caldolor	**Adults:** For postoperative pain in conjunction with iv opioids, in patients undergoing general anesthesia: 400–800 mg Q6H iv Dilute each dose in 250 mL compatible fluid and administer over 30 min **Usual maximum:** 2400 mg/24 h × 1 day; do not exceed 3200 mg in 24 h	See ASA.	See ASA.	$$$$$/ 800 mg vial
	ketorolac, parenteral ❾ Toradol, generics	**Children:** 0.2–1 mg/kg/dose Q4–6H im or iv Maximum: 30 mg/dose **Adults:** 10–30 mg Q4–6H im or iv Maximum: 120 mg/day	See ASA.	See ASA.	$$

Class	Drug	Dose	Adverse Effects	Drug Interactions	Cost[a]
	naproxen Naprosyn, generics	**Children:** 5–7 mg/kg/dose Q8–12H po; oral suspension available Maximum: 1000 mg/day **Adults:** 500 mg initially, then 250 mg Q6–8H po Maximum: 1250 mg/day	See ASA.	See ASA.	$
	naproxen sodium Aleve (220 mg), Anaprox (275 mg; 550 mg), generics	**Adults:** 220–550 mg Q8–12H po Maximum: 1375 mg/day (maximum dose for nonprescription use is 440 mg/day)	See ASA.	See ASA.	$
Analgesics, opioid	*fentanyl* generics	**Children:** 0.5–3 µg/kg/dose Q1–2H iv **Adults:** 50–100 µg Q1–2H iv Titrate to effect	*All opioids:* sedation, constipation.	*All opioids:* additive sedation with other CNS depressants, e.g., alcohol; potential enhancement of opioid effects with lidocaine. *Fentanyl:* inhibitors of CYP3A4 (e.g., cimetidine, efavirenz, erythromycin, itraconazole, ketoconazole, ritonavir) may potentiate fentanyl's opioid effects.	$$
	hydromorphone ❩ Dilaudid, Dilaudid-HP, generics	**Adults:** 1–2 mg Q4H po 0.25–0.5 mg Q1H iv	See fentanyl.	See fentanyl.	po: $ iv: $$
	morphine ❩ M.O.S., MS-IR, Statex, generics	Titrate to effect. **Immediate-release oral:** **Children:** 0.2–0.5 mg/kg/dose Q4–6H **Adults:** 10–30 mg Q4–6H **IV: Children:** Intermittent: 0.1–0.2 mg/kg/dose Q2–4H Continuous infusion: 0.01–0.05 mg/kg/h Breakthrough pain during infusion: 0.01–0.05 mg/kg/dose **Adults:** Intermittent: 2.5–10 mg Q2–4H iv Continuous infusion: 1–10 mg/h Breakthrough pain during infusion: 2.5–5 mg/dose	See fentanyl.	See fentanyl.	$

(cont'd)

Table 3: **Analgesics for the Treatment of Acute Pain** *(cont'd)*

Class	Drug	Dose	Adverse Effects	Drug Interactions	Cost[a]
	meperidine (pethidine) ❥ generics	**Parenteral:** **Children:** 1–1.5 mg/kg/dose Q3–4H iv Maximum: 100 mg/dose; not recommended for ongoing use **Adults:** 50–100 mg Q3–4H iv Maximum: 100 mg/dose; not recommended for ongoing use	See fentanyl. Seizures can occur when used in renal failure. May cause tremors, hyperreflexia, hallucinations. Avoid in liver disease and those who have received MAOIs within the last 14 days.	See fentanyl. *Meperidine:* potentially life-threatening serotonin syndrome with nonselective MAOIs.	$$
	oxycodone ❥ Oxy-IR, generics	**Adults:** 2.5–5 mg Q4H po	See fentanyl.	See fentanyl.	$

[a] Cost per dose (based on body weights of 20 kg for children and 70 kg for adults); includes drug cost only.
❥ Dosage adjustment may be required in renal impairment; see Appendix I.
Legend: $ <$1 $$ $1–3 $$$ $3–6 $$$$ $6–9 $$$$$ $9–12

Suggested Readings

Drugs for pain. *Treat Guidel Med Lett* 2013;11(128):31-42.

Macintyre PE, Scott DA, Schug SA et al. *Acute pain management: scientific evidence*. 3rd ed. Melbourne (AU): Australian and New Zealand College of Anaesthetists and Faculty of Pain Medicine; 2010. p. 491. Available from: www.anzca.edu.au/resources/books-and-publications/acutepain.pdf.

Moore ND. In search of an ideal analgesic for common acute pain. *Acute Pain* 2009;11(3):129-37.

References

1. Drendel AL, Brousseau DC, Gorelick MH. Pain assessment for pediatric patients in the emergency department. *Pediatrics* 2006;117(5):1511-8.
2. Bailey B, Daoust R, Doyon-Trottier E et al. Validation and properties of the verbal numeric scale in children with acute pain. *Pain* 2010;149(2):216-21.
3. Stinson JN, Kavanagh T, Yamada J et al. Systematic review of the psychometric properties, interpretability and feasibility of self-report pain intensity measures for use in clinical trials in children and adolescents. *Pain* 2006;125(1-2):143-57.
4. Warden V, Hurley AC, Volicer L. Development and psychometric evaluation of the pain assessment in advanced dementia (PAINAD) scale. *J Am Med Dir Assoc* 2003;4(1):9-15.
5. Drugs for pain. *Treat Guidel Med Lett* 2013;11(128):31-42.
6. Rostom A, Dubé C, Jolicoeur E et al. Gastroduodenal ulcers associated with the use of non-steroidal anti-inflammatory drugs: a systematic review of preventative pharmacological interventions. Ottawa (ON): Canadian Coordinating Office for Health Technology Assessment. *Technology Overview* March 2004;12:1-20. Available from: www.cadth.ca/media/pdf/261_gastro_ov_e.pdf. Accessed May 5, 2014.
7. Lesko SM, Mitchell AA. An assessment of the safety of pediatric ibuprofen. A practitioner-based randomized clinical trial. *JAMA* 1995;273(12):929-33.
8. Pierce CA, Voss B. Efficacy and safety of ibuprofen and acetaminophen in children and adults: a meta-analysis and qualitative review. *Ann Pharmacother* 2010;44(3):489-506.
9. Isomaki H, Martio J, Kaarela K et al. Comparison of the analgesic effect of ten nonsteroidal anti-inflammatory drugs. *Br J Rheumatol* 1984;23(1):61-5.
10. Institute for Safe Medications. *ISMP's list of high-alert medications*. Available from: www.ismp.org/tools/highalertmedications.pdf. Accessed May 5, 2014.
11. Health Canada. *Health Canada's review recommends codeine only be used in patients aged 12 and over*. Available from: www.healthycanadians.gc.ca/recall-alert-rappel-avis/hc-sc/2013/33915a-eng.php. Accessed May 2, 2014.
12. MacDonald N, MacLeod SM. Has the time come to phase out codeine? *CMAJ* 2010;182(17):1825.
13. Grond S, Sablotzki A. Clinical pharmacology of tramadol. *Clin Pharmacokinet* 2004;43(13):879-923.
14. Sachs CJ. Oral analgesics for acute nonspecific pain. *Am Fam Physician* 2005;71(5):913-8.
15. Turturro MA, Paris PM, Larkin GL. Tramadol versus hydrocodone-acetaminophen in acute musculoskeletal pain: a randomized, double-blind clinical trial. *Ann Emerg Med* 1998;32(2):139-43.
16. Stubhaug A, Grimstad J, Breivik H. Lack of analgesic effect of 50 and 100 mg oral tramadol after orthopaedic surgery: a randomized, double-blind, placebo and standard active drug comparison. *Pain* 1995;62(1):111-8.
17. Prommer E, Thompson L. Intranasal fentanyl for pain control: current status with a focus on patient considerations. *Patient Prefer Adherence* 2011;5:157-64.
18. Southworth S, Peters J, Rock A et al. A multicenter, randomized, double-blind, placebo-controlled trial of intravenous ibuprofen 400 and 800 mg every 6 hours in the management of postoperative pain. *Clin Ther* 2009;31(9):1922-35.
19. Massey T, Derry S, Moore RA et al. Topical NSAIDs for acute pain in adults. *Cochrane Database Syst Rev* 2010;(6):CD007402.
20. Lander JA, Weltman BJ, So SS. EMLA and amethocaine for reduction of children's pain associated with needle insertion. *Cochrane Database Syst Rev* 2006;(3):CD004236.
21. Pedersen RS, Bayat A, Steen NP et al. Nitrous oxide provides safe and effective analgesia for minor paediatric procedures–a systematic review. *Dan Med J* 2013;60(6):A4627.
22. Koren G, Florescu A, Costei AM et al. Nonsteroidal antiinflammatory drugs during third trimester and the risk of premature closure of the ductus arteriosus: a meta-analysis. *Ann Pharmacother* 2006;40(5):824-9.
23. Babb M, Koren G, Einarson A. Treating pain during pregnancy. *Can Fam Physician* 2010;56(1):25, 27.
24. Madadi P, Ross CJ, Hayden MR et al. Pharmacogenetics of neonatal opioid toxicity following maternal use of codeine during breastfeeding: a case-control study. *Clin Pharmacol Ther* 2009;85(1):31-5.
25. Bennett PN. *Drugs and human lactation: a comprehensive guide to the content and consequences of drugs, micronutrients, radiopharmaceuticals, and environmental and occupational chemicals in human milk*. 2nd ed. New York (NY): Elsevier; 1996. p. 712.
26. Ranji SR, Dolman LE, Simel DL et al. Do opiates affect the clinical evaluation of patients with acute abdominal pain? *JAMA* 2006;296(14):1764-74.
27. Manterola C, Vial M, Moraga J et al. Analgesia in patients with acute abdominal pain. *Cochrane Database Syst Rev* 2011;(1):CD005660.

Chapter 15
Bell's Palsy

William Pryse-Phillips, MD, FRCP, FRCPC, DPM

Bell's palsy is a lower motor neuron paralysis of the facial nerve, often due to herpes simplex virus-1 infection, causing inflammation and edema.[1] It affects about 20 persons per 100 000 per year without gender predominance.[2] The incidence increases until age 40 and remains static until late adult life, when it again increases. Bell's palsy occurs more frequently in pregnant women and in patients with diabetes or hypertension.

Up to 85% of patients achieve spontaneous complete recovery without treatment. Those who will not recover cannot be identified by clinical features,[3] although incomplete paralysis carries a better prognosis. In <10% of cases the palsy recurs on either side.

Goals of Therapy

- Promote complete recovery of function through prevention of denervation
- Protect the eye from corneal abrasion
- Alleviate pain

Investigations

The classic presentation of Bell's palsy includes abrupt onset of facial weakness affecting the upper and lower face, ear pain and altered taste. Involvement of other cranial nerves, remote CNS signs and systemic features would indicate further inquiry for the conditions listed in Table 1.

Investigations are seldom needed after a complete history and physical examination have excluded other causes of peripheral facial palsy.

- EMG and facial nerve conduction studies may help with prognosis but only after 8–10 days
- Computed tomography (CT) scan is appropriate if trauma is a likely cause
- Cranial magnetic resonance imaging (MRI) may be indicated in the presence of atypical features such as fever, the immunocompromised state or other focal neurological symptoms or signs
- No laboratory tests are useful

Table 1: **Differential Diagnosis of Unilateral Bell's Palsy**

- Ramsay Hunt syndrome (herpes zoster infection; vesicles in the ear or throat)
- Facial nerve tumors (usually painless; examine for neurofibromatosis)
- Cerebellopontine angle tumors (added neurologic signs)
- Parotid tumors (clinical examination)
- Mastoiditis (clinical examination; deafness, discharge)
- Lyme disease (skin and joint signs)
- Neurosarcoidosis (chest x-ray)
- Brainstem lesions such as multiple sclerosis (other neurologic signs)
- Rarely, diabetic ischemic cranial neuropathies, HIV and TB

Bilateral facial palsy is a feature of Guillain-Barré syndrome, Lyme disease, sarcoid and Wegener's granulomatosis, and of other even more rare conditions.

Therapeutic Choices

Nonpharmacologic Choices

See also Eye Care.

No high quality trials have been published that would allow any conclusion about the efficacy of acupuncture, although one study suggested that strong (i.e., painful) stimulation did have a better therapeutic effect than painless acupuncture.[4] The value of physical therapy is also unproven.[5]

Pharmacologic Choices

Figure 1 illustrates clinical management of Bell's Palsy. See Table 2 for detailed drug therapy choices.

Eye Care

To prevent corneal abrasions in any eye that cannot be closed voluntarily:

- lubricate with ophthalmic drops or ointment
- tape the eyelid closed at night and protect with glasses during the day

Analgesics

Ibuprofen or **acetaminophen** with or without **codeine** is occasionally required for the first day or two. More potent opioids such as morphine are rarely needed.

Corticosteroids

Corticosteroids have been shown to improve rates of full recovery as well as time to complete recovery.[6,7] Early treatment (initiated within 72 hours of symptom onset) provides maximal benefit.[7,8] Theoretically, the anti-inflammatory action of corticosteroids minimizes nerve damage, thus improving outcomes. In addition, there is good anecdotal evidence that early corticosteroid therapy reduces pain while clinical experience suggests that corticosteroid-treated patients are less likely to develop denervation. The following basic regimen is recommended: **prednisone** 1 mg/kg po daily for 5 days, then taper over another 5 days (see Figure 1 and Table 2).[8]

In the case of *complete* facial paralysis, corticosteroid treatment showed clinically and statistically significant improvement in recovery of function,[9] a report not cited in the American Academy of Neurology guideline.[10] A systematic review of the use of corticosteroids in children with Bell's palsy concluded that in cases of complete facial paralysis, corticosteroid therapy is not advisable.[11]

Antivirals

Antiviral therapy (**acyclovir**, **famciclovir** or **valacyclovir**) *alone* provides no significant benefit over placebo in the treatment of Bell's palsy [Evidence: SORT A*].[6,7] Whether antivirals confer any additional benefit over corticosteroids alone is controversial.[12,13] Some studies have demonstrated no additional benefit[6,7] while others show possible benefit, particularly in patients with more severe facial paralysis at presentation.[14,15,16] Because adverse effects are minimal, antiviral therapy may be offered in conjunction with corticosteroids, particularly in patients with more severe paralysis at presentation, though evidence of significant additional benefit is not clearly established [Evidence: SORT C*].[10]

In Ramsay Hunt syndrome (herpes zoster infection of the VII cranial nerve, typically with a visible skin eruption), antiviral therapy seems appropriate.

* SORT (Strength of Recommendation Taxonomy) is a rating system (A, B or C) that addresses the quality of available evidence. For more information consult **How to Use *Compendium of Therapeutic Choices*** on page xxv.

Figure 1: Management of Bell's Palsy

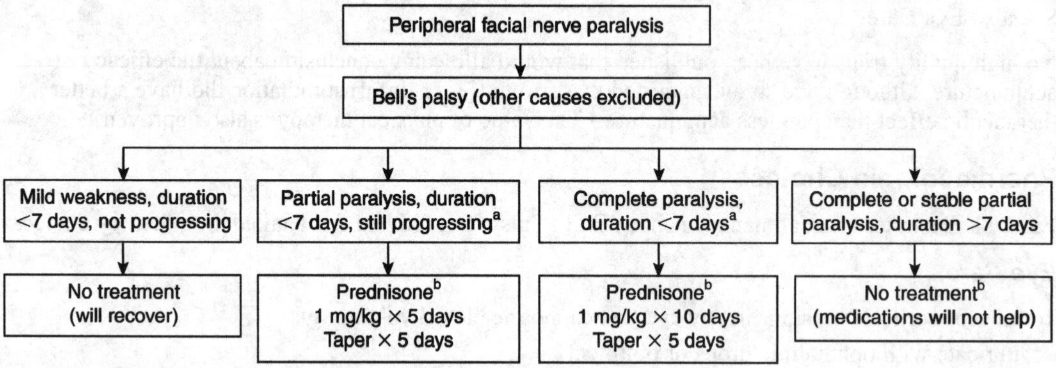

a Greatest benefit is seen when treatment is initiated up to 72 hours after symptom onset; evidence of benefit is less clear for treatment initiated 4–7 days after onset.[8]
b The addition of antiviral therapy is not routinely warranted based on current evidence.

Table 2: Drug Therapy for Bell's Palsy

Class	Drug	Dose	Adverse Effects	Cost[a]
Antivirals	*acyclovir* Zovirax Oral, generics	400 mg 5 times daily po × 10 days	Headache, nausea.	$$$
	famciclovir Famvir, generics	500 mg TID po × 1 wk	See acyclovir.	$$$
	valacyclovir Valtrex, generics	1000 mg TID po × 1 wk	See acyclovir.	$$$
Corticosteroids	*prednisone* Winpred, generics	1 mg/kg daily po × 5 days,[b] then taper over another 5 days	GI upset, hyperglycemia, sodium and fluid retention, hypokalemia, hypocalcemia.	$

a Cost of 1 course of treatment, based on 70 kg weight; includes drug cost only.
b In cases of complete facial paralysis, treat for 10 days then taper over another 5 days.
Dosage adjustment may be required in renal impairment; see Appendix I.
Legend: $ < $5 $$ $5–25 $$$ $25–50

Surgical Procedures

A systematic review judged the quality of evidence to be low and insufficient to determine the benefit or harm of surgical interventions for nerve decompression in patients with Bell's palsy.[17]

Choices during Pregnancy and Breastfeeding

While Bell's Palsy occurs 2–4 times more often in women of childbearing age than men of the same age, it is not clear if the incidence is greater in pregnant versus nonpregnant women.[18,19,20,21]

Most cases of Bell's palsy in pregnant women occur in the third trimester of pregnancy or during the first few postpartum weeks.[21] In a retrospective population-based analysis of 242 000 deliveries over 20 years, the onset of Bell's palsy during pregnancy and the puerperium was shown to be significantly associated with obesity, chronic hypertension, severe preeclampsia and associated Caesarian deliveries.[22] This study did not find a link between Bell's palsy and adverse perinatal outcomes such as low Apgar scores, perinatal mortality or congenital malformations.

Unfortunately, the prognosis for a satisfactory recovery for women who develop a complete facial paralysis with Bell's palsy while pregnant is significantly worse than for the general population.[23] Whether this is due to differing etiologies or to a reluctance to prescribe corticosteroids during pregnancy has not been ascertained.

Supportive care is appropriate for most pregnant patients since the majority of patients will recover spontaneously. The decision to use **corticosteroids** for Bell's palsy in pregnant patients should be made on an individual basis after discussing the risks and benefits with the patient. The effect of these drugs on the fetus is unclear and varies depending on the trimester; pregnant patients were excluded from studies evaluating corticosteroids for Bell's palsy.

A discussion of general principles on the use of medications in these special populations can be found in Appendix II and Appendix III. Other specialized reference sources are also provided in these appendices.

Therapeutic Tips

- No treatment is needed for mild weakness that is no longer evolving.
- Use **prednisone** as soon as possible in all cases of Bell's palsy involving paralysis unless there is a potential contraindication to steroid use, such as diabetes or peptic ulcer disease.
- There is no good evidence for benefit from prednisone that is started more than 7 days after the onset of symptoms.
- No evidence supports the use of antiviral therapy alone.
- Based on available evidence, routine use of antiviral agents with prednisone for Bell's palsy cannot be recommended. There may be some benefit of this drug combination in severe cases.

Suggested Readings

Baringer JR. Herpes simplex virus and Bell palsy. *Ann Intern Med* 1996;124(1 Pt 1):63-5.

Baugh RF, Basura GJ, Ishii LE et al. Clinical practice guidelines: Bell's palsy. *Otolaryngol Head Neck Surg* 2013;149(3 Suppl):S1-27.

Roob G, Fazekas F, Hartung HP. Peripheral facial palsy: etiology, diagnosis and treatment. *Eur Neurol* 1999;41(1):3-9.

Salinas RA, Alvarez G, Daly F et al. Corticosteroids for Bell's palsy (idiopathic facial paralysis). *Cochrane Database Syst Rev* 2010;(3):CD001942.

References

1. Morrow MJ. Bell's palsy and herpes zoster oticus. *Curr Treat Options Neurol* 2000;2(5):407-16.
2. Rowlands S, Hooper R, Hughes R et al. The epidemiology and treatment of Bell's palsy in the UK. *Eur J Neurol* 2002;9(1):63-7.
3. Jabor MA, Gianoli G. Management of Bell's palsy. *J La State Med Soc* 1996;148(7):279-83.
4. Xu SB, Huang B, Zhang CY et al. Effectiveness of strengthened stimulation during acupuncture for the treatment of Bell palsy: a randomized controlled trial. *CMAJ* 2013;185(6):473-9.
5. Teixeira LJ, Valbuza JS, Prado GF. Physical therapy for Bell's palsy (idiopathic facial paralysis). *Cochrane Database Syst Rev* 2011;(12):CD006283.
6. Sullivan FM, Swan IR, Donnan PT et al. Early treatment with prednisolone or acyclovir in Bell's palsy. *N Engl J Med* 2007;357(16):1598-607.
7. Engstrom M, Berg T, Stjenquist-Desatnik A et al. Prednisolone and valaciclovir in Bell's palsy: a randomised, double-blind, placebo-controlled, multicentre trial. *Lancet Neurol* 2008;7(11):993-1000.
8. Baugh RF, Basura GJ, Ishii LE et al. Clinical practice guidelines: Bell's palsy. *Otolaryngol Head Neck Surg* 2013;149(3 Suppl):S1-27.
9. Ramsey MJ, DerSimonian R, Holtel MR et al. Corticosteroid treatment for idiopathic facial nerve paralysis: a meta-analysis. *Laryngoscope* 2000;110(3 Pt 1):335-41.
10. Gronseth GS, Paduga R; American Academy of Neurology. Evidence-based guideline update: steroids and antivirals for Bell Palsy: report of the Guideline Development Subcommittee of the American Academy of Neurology. *Neurology* 2012;79(22):2209-13.
11. Salman MS, MacGregor DL. Should children with Bell's palsy be treated with corticosteroids? A systematic review. *J Child Neurol* 2001;16(8):565-8.
12. Quant EC, Jeste SS, Muni RH et al. The benefits of steroids versus steroids plus antivirals for treatment of Bell's palsy: a meta-analysis. *BMJ* 2009;339:b3354.
13. de Almeida JR, Al Khabori M, Guyatt GH et al. Combined corticosteroid and antiviral treatment for Bell palsy: a systematic review and meta-analysis. *JAMA* 2009;302(9):985-93.
14. Hato N, Murakami S, Gyo K. Steroid and antiviral treatment for Bell's palsy. *Lancet* 2008;371(9627):1818-20.

15. Minnerop M, Herbst M, Fimmers R et al. Bell's palsy: combined treatment of famciclovir and prednisone is superior to prednisone alone. *J Neurol* 2008;255(11):1726-30.
16. Lee HY, Byun JY, Park MS et al. Steroid-antiviral treatment improves the recovery rate in patients with severe Bell's palsy. *Am J Med* 2013;126(4):336-41.
17. McAllister K, Walker D, Donnan PT et al. Surgical interventions for the early management of Bell's palsy. *Cochrane Database Syst Rev* 2013;(10):CD007468. Available from: onlinelibrary.wiley.com/doi/10.1002/14651858.CD007468.pub3/abstract.
18. Vrabec JT, Isaacson B, Van Hook JW. Bell's palsy and pregnancy. *Otolaryngol Head Neck Surg* 2007;137(6):858-61.
19. Cohen Y, Lavie O, Granovsky-Grisaru S et al. Bell palsy complicating pregnancy: a review. *Obstet Gynecol Surv* 2000;55(3):184-8.
20. Peitersen E. Bell's palsy: the spontaneous course of 2,500 peripheral facial nerve palsies of different etiologies. *Acta Otolaryngol Suppl* 2002;(549):4-30.
21. Shmorgun D, Chan WS, Ray JG. Association between Bell's palsy in pregnancy and pre-eclampsia. *QJM* 2002;95(6):359-62.
22. Katz A, Sergienko R, Dior U et al. Bell's palsy during pregnancy: is it associated with adverse perinatal outcome? *Laryngoscope* 2011;121(7)1395-8.
23. Gillman GS, Schaitkin BM, May M et al. Bell's palsy in pregnancy: a study of recovery outcomes. *Otolaryngol Head Neck Surg* 2002;126(1):26-30.

Chapter 16
Chronic Spasticity

Virginia Devonshire, MD, FRCPC

Spasticity is an involuntary velocity-dependent increase in muscle tone resulting from injury to the motor pathways in the brain or spinal cord. It is common in spinal cord injury, multiple sclerosis, stroke and cerebral palsy. Spasticity usually occurs as part of the upper motor neuron (UMN) complex and consists of weakness, hyper-reflexia, Babinski's sign and slow coordination.

Spasticity can impair feeding, dressing, bowel/bladder function, hygiene and gait. It can also reduce joint range of movement, cause contractures (shortening of muscles that leads to joint dysfunction) and result in significant pain and skin breakdown. However, spasticity is not always impairing and can facilitate some movements by providing posture and tone in what would otherwise be a flaccid limb. It can allow weight bearing in a plegic limb by essentially "bracing" that limb. Further, treatment of spasticity can sometimes worsen ambulation by unmasking limb weakness. Thus, spasticity should only be treated when it interferes with function and care, or results in pain.

Goals of Therapy

- Improve functional movements and gait
- Improve range of movement and limit contracture formation
- Reduce pain and spasms
- Improve seating and positioning; reduce skin breakdown
- Improve care, e.g., perineal care and catheterization

Investigations

- No investigations needed if seen as part of a UMN complex already diagnosed.
- Spasticity in isolation needs investigation for the underlying pathology.

Therapeutic Choices

An algorithm for the management of chronic spasticity is shown in Figure 1.

Nonpharmacologic Choices

Search for aggravating factors if spasticity has increased in a stable patient. This can include pressure areas, infections (bladder, toenail, etc.), bladder stones, constipation and DVTs.

Always recommend physical measures including daily stretching and range-of-movement exercises. Braces may be used to maintain a spastic limb in a reflex-inhibiting posture and prevent contractures.

Surgical treatment of spasticity tends to be reserved for the most refractory cases and is rarely considered. Orthopedic procedures, such as lengthening, releasing or transferring a tendon, do not treat the underlying spasticity but may help optimize function and prevent contractures.

Figure 1: **Management of Chronic Spasticity**

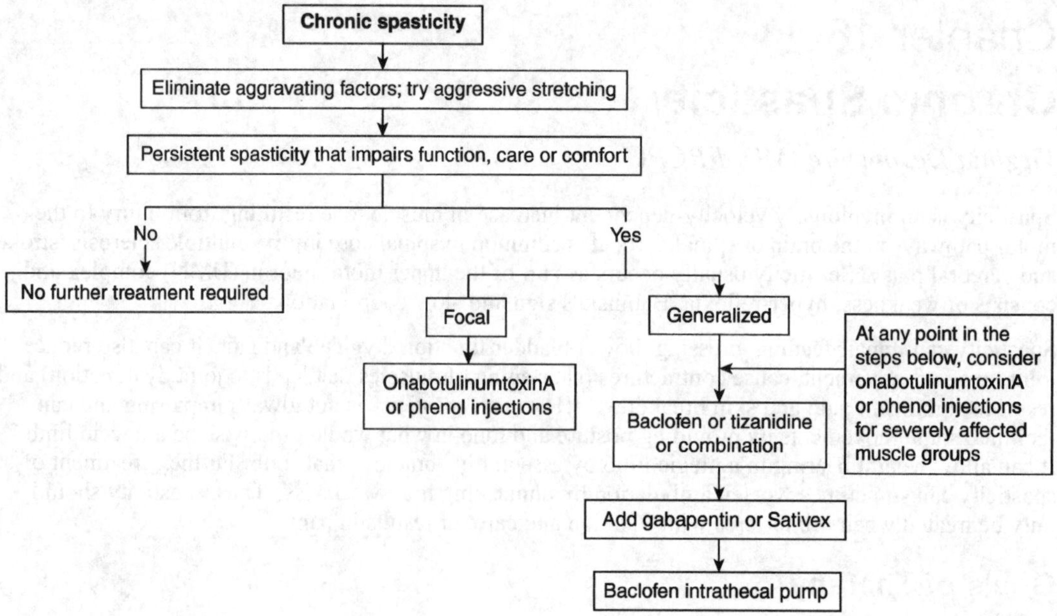

Pharmacologic Choices

The treatment for *focal* spasticity that occurs in a limited number of muscle groups differs from that which occurs in a more *generalized* pattern.

Oral medications (Table 1) remain important in the treatment of generalized spasticity. Most drugs recommended for management of spasticity have a central mode of action. A number of randomized clinical trials have demonstrated efficacy of antispasticity medications, although systematic reviews have found that the studies were limited.[1,2] Clinical experience has shown that efficacy is better in spasticity of spinal origin (multiple sclerosis, spinal cord injury) than of cerebral origin (brain injury and stroke).

Baclofen is the standard initial medication for spasticity. It must be titrated gradually to an effective dose typically in the range of 30–80 mg/day. Adverse effects such as sedation can limit its use in patients who are brain-injured. Abrupt discontinuation can result in confusion, seizures and hallucinations.

Tizanidine monotherapy is a another good first-line choice;[3] it can also be combined with baclofen as the 2 agents have different sites of action. It is best to start with a low dose of 2 mg at night and increase gradually. Side effects of dry mouth and drowsiness can limit the use of tizanidine, particularly in brain-injured patients.

Benzodiazepines such as **diazepam** and **clonazepam** can be useful for treating spasms especially if these are problematic at night. Daytime use of these drugs is limited by their sedating effects.

Gabapentin may be a useful alternative or addition in managing spasticity especially if there is concurrent neuropathic pain.[4]

Sativex, a cannabis extract delivered by buccal spray, has shown modest efficacy in phase 3 clinical trials and is officially indicated for the treatment of spasticity in patients with multiple sclerosis.

Compared with placebo, significantly more patients experienced improvement in neuropathic pain, spasticity and sleep disturbance.[5,6] It may also be beneficial as add-on therapy.[7]

Although it is officially indicated in the management of spasticity and widely used, there is insufficient evidence to recommend dantrolene.[8,9]

Focal treatment of spastic muscles involves chemodenervation using local agents such as onabotulinumtoxinA or phenol injections to reduce spasticity selectively, leaving some muscle groups with tone that is functional. Local treatment is more effective for focal spasticity, avoids the significant CNS side effects associated with systemic therapy and may also benefit patients with spasticity of cerebral origin when other drug therapies are less effective. **Phenol** injections block nerves going to specific spastic muscle groups; treatment is repeated every 6 months as required. Injections can be uncomfortable with adverse effects that include pain, dysesthesias and infection. **Onabotulinumtoxin type A** injections may be better tolerated than phenol.[10] The toxin blocks the release of acetylcholine at the neuromuscular junction, causing weakness (reduced tone) in the treated muscle. The effect lasts 3 months, after which collateral sprouting occurs. It is a relatively safe medication with few serious side effects.

Intrathecal delivery of medication is usually indicated when oral medications fail to control spasticity or side effects are intolerable. A programmable pump, usually implanted in the anterior abdominal wall, delivers small continuous or bolus amounts of drug (usually **baclofen**) into the spinal fluid. Cognitive side effects are minimal because the drug is acting locally at the level of the spinal cord. The effect on spasticity can be profound, although it is more effective for lower limb tone due to a concentration gradient from lumbar to cervical levels.[11]

Therapeutic Tips

- Treat the patient, not the spasticity. The goal is improved comfort or function.
- Titrate medications slowly to a maximum tolerated dose before switching or adding agents.
- Consider earlier referral to a neurologist/physiatrist for focal treatment if the spasticity is limited to a focal area and/or is of cerebral origin (therefore less likely to respond to oral agents).
- Muscle spasms occurring during the night can interrupt sleep. Diazepam or clonazepam can be very helpful in reducing these nocturnal spasms.
- Sativex may be helpful if pain is also present.

Table 1: Drug Therapy for Chronic Spasticity

Class	Drug	Dose	Adverse Effects	Drug Interactions	Cost[a]
Alpha$_2$-Adrenergic Agonists	*tizanidine* ❥ Zanaflex, generics	Adults: Start with 2 mg QHS po; titrate by 2 mg per day Q3–5 days to a maximum of 36 mg/day in 3–4 divided doses	Dry mouth, sedation, dizziness, hypotension, weakness, hallucinations, hepatotoxicity (monitor liver function tests).	Increased hypotensive effect with antihypertensives. Decreased clearance with oral contraceptives or TCAs. Decreased clearance with CYP1A2 inhibitors such as cimetidine, ciprofloxacin, fluvoxamine, ketoconazole. May increase phenytoin levels.	$$$$$
Benzodi-azepines	*clonazepam* Rivotril, generics	Adults: 0.5–2 mg QHS po	Sedation, ataxia, weakness, dependence.	Potentiates effects of other CNS depressants including alcohol.	$
	diazepam Valium, generics	Adults: Start with 2.5 mg QHS po; titrate by 2.5 mg Q3–7 days to a maximum of 60 mg/day in 3–4 divided doses For nocturnal spasms: 5–10 mg QHS po Children: 0.1–0.8 mg/kg/day po in 2–3 divided doses	See clonazepam.	See clonazepam.	$
Botulinum Toxins	*onabotulinumtoxinA* Botox	Dosage ranges vary for focal spasticity and depend on site of administration: 10–50 units (total) in 1–2 injection sites up to 100–200 units (total) in 1–4 sites im Q12–16 wk Maximum dose 360 units per treatment	Hypertonia, ecchymosis, muscular weakness, injection site pain, fever, headache, paresthesia, hot flush, nausea, hyperhidrosis, skin odor abnormal, pruritus, alopecia.	Drugs interfering with neuromuscular transmission may potentiate the effect of onabotulinumtoxinA. Caution with aminoglycoside antibiotics (amikacin, gentamicin, neomycin, streptomycin, tobramycin) and neuromuscular blocking agents (anticholinesterases, lincosamides, magnesium, polymyxins, quinidine, succinylcholine, tubocurarine)	$375/ 100-unit vial
Cannabinoids	*delta-9-tetrahydro-cannabinol/ cannabidiol* Sativex	4–12 buccal sprays daily, titrated to lowest effective maintenance dose	Fatigue, nausea, vertigo, diarrhea, dry mouth.	Additive effects with CNS depressants such as alcohol, opioids. Potent inhibitors of CYP3A4 such as ketoconazole may lead to higher Sativex concentrations.	$230/unit

Class	Drug	Dose	Adverse Effects	Drug Interactions	Cost[a]
GABA Derivatives	*baclofen* (kidney symbol) Lioresal, generics	Adults:Start with 5 mg BID to TID po; increase by 5–15 mg/day Q3–5 days to a maximum of 120 mg/day in 3–4 divided doses Children: Same titration as for adults, but with a maximum of 60 mg/day	Sedation, weakness, nausea, dizziness, lowered seizure threshold.	Potential additive CNS depression with tricyclic antidepressants, opioids, benzodiazepines and antihypertensives.	$$
	gabapentin (kidney symbol) Neurontin, generics	Adults: Start with 100 mg TID po; increase by 100 mg per dose Q3 days to a maximum of 800 mg QID Not a Health Canada–approved indication.	Sedation, dizziness, fatigue, weight gain.	Antacids may decrease absorption of gabapentin; separate doses by at least 2 h.	$$$

[a] Cost of tablets is per 30-day supply at the maximum adult dose unless otherwise specified; includes drug cost only.

(kidney symbol) Dosage adjustment may be required in renal impairment; see Appendix I.

Legend: $ < $30 $$ $30–60 $$$ $60–90 $$$$ $90–120 $$$$$ $120–150

Suggested Readings

Baker JA, Pereira G. The efficacy of Botulinum Toxin A for spasticity and pain in adults: a systematic review and meta-analysis using the grades of recommendation, assessment, development and evaluation approach. *Clin Rehabil* 2013;27(12):1084-96.

Gracies JM, Nance P, Elovic E et al. Traditional pharmacologic treatments for spasticity. Part II: General and regional treatments. *Muscle Nerve Suppl* 1997;6:S92-120.

Thompson AJ, Jarrett L, Lockley L et al. Clinical management of spasticity. *J Neurol Neurosurg Psychiatry* 2005;76(4):459-63.

References

1. Shakespeare DT, Boggild M, Young C. Anti-spasticity agents for multiple sclerosis. *Cochrane Database Syst Rev* 2003;(4):CD001332.
2. Taricco M, Pagliacci MC, Telaro E et al. Pharmacological interventions for spasticity following spinal cord injury: results of a Cochrane systematic review. *Eura Medicophys* 2006;42(1):5-15.
3. Nance PW, Bugaresti J, Shellenberger K et al. Efficacy and safety of tizanidine in the treatment of spasticity in patients with spinal cord injury. North American Tizanidine Study Group. *Neurology* 1994;44(11 Suppl 9):S44-51.
4. Cutter NC, Scott DD, Johnson JC et al. Gabapentin effect on spasticity in multiple sclerosis: a placebo-controlled, randomized trial. *Arch Phys Med Rehabil* 2000;81(2):164-9.
5. Collin C, Ehler E, Waberzinek G et al. A double-blind, randomized, placebo-controlled, parallel-group study of Sativex, in subjects with symptoms of spasticity due to multiple sclerosis. *Neurol Res* 2010;32(5):451-9.
6. Wade DT, Makela P, Robson P et al. Do cannabis-based medicinal extracts have general or specific effects on symptoms of multiple sclerosis? A double-blind, randomized, placebo-controlled study on 160 participants. *Mult Scler* 2004;10(4):434-41.
7. Novotna A, Mares J, Ratcliffe S et al. A randomized, double-blind, placebo-controlled, parallel-group, enriched-design study of nabiximols (Sativex®), as add-on therapy, in subjects with refractory spasticity caused by multiple sclerosis. *Eur J Neurol* 2011;18(9):1122-31.
8. Yelnik AP, Simon O, Bensmail D et al. Drug treatments for spasticity. *Ann Phys Rehabil Med* 2009;52(10):746-56.
9. Simon O, Yelnik AP. Managing spasticity with drugs. *Eur J Phys Rehabil Med* 2010;46(3):401-10.
10. Simpson DM. Clinical trials of botulinum toxin in the treatment of spasticity. *Muscle Nerve Suppl* 1997;6:S169-75.
11. Coffey JR, Cahill D, Steers W et al. Intrathecal baclofen for intractable spasticity of spinal origin: results of a long-term multicenter study. *J Neurosurg* 1993;78(2):226-32.

Chapter 17
Headache in Adults

R. Allan Purdy, MD, FRCPC, FACP, FAHS

Goals of Therapy

- Relieve or abolish pain and associated symptoms such as nausea/vomiting
- Prevent recurrent symptoms in primary headache disorders, e.g., migraine, tension-type and cluster
- Diagnose and manage serious causes of headache, e.g., tumor, arteritis, infection, hemorrhage
- Prevent complications of medication usage

Investigations

Figure 1 illustrates a diagnostic algorithm for headache.

- A thorough history and physical examination are most important for a correct diagnosis.[1] Note characteristics of the headache:
  - onset: sudden versus gradual
  - temporal profile: progressive versus self-limited
  - frequency/pattern of recurrence: e.g., during menses (menstrual migraine), strictly unilateral (always on the same side) and occurring in clusters separated by months or years (episodic cluster headache)
  - associated symptoms: nausea, vomiting, sensitivity to light, noise or odours, systemic or other neurologic signs or symptoms
  - degree of interference with activities of daily life caused by migraine
- The physical examination should be normal; if any abnormalities are found (especially visual, motor, reflex, sensory, speech or cognitive), investigation is warranted
- CT/MR scans are not routine but must be done if any organic etiology is suspected (see Table 1)
- Lumbar puncture if subarachnoid hemorrhage, encephalitis, high- or low-pressure headache syndromes or meningitis is suspected
- Laboratory tests (on an individual basis)
  - ESR for suspected temporal arteritis
  - endocrine, biochemical, infection work-up
  - search for malignancy if indicated
- Facial pain may need a thorough assessment by a dental specialist familiar with headaches and facial pain and/or an ENT specialist if sinus or other ENT disorders are suspected

Therapeutic Choices

If serious structural CNS causes for headache and facial pain have been ruled out, the primary headache disorders can be managed as follows.[2,3]

Figure 1: Diagnosis and Initial Assessment of Headache

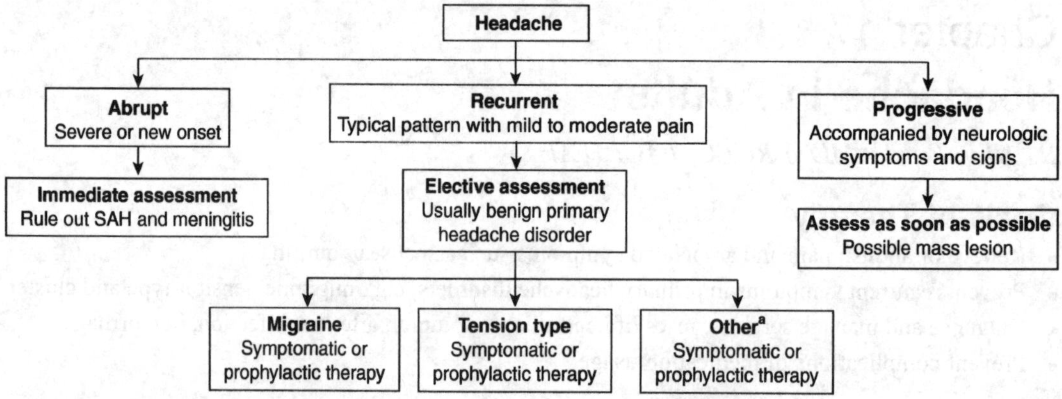

[a] Any headache not recognized as migraine, tension headache or known cause is in the "other" group. Investigate if no response to usual treatments.
Abbreviations: SAH = subarachnoid hemorrhage

Table 1: Red Flags for Serious Headache

Patient Factors	Red Flags
Age of onset	Child, or middle-aged to elderly patient
Type of onset	Severe and abrupt
Temporal sequence	Progressive severity or increased frequency
Pattern	Significant change in headache pattern
Neurologic signs	Stiff neck, focal signs, reduced consciousness
Systemic signs	Fever, appears sick, abnormal examination

Caution: If headache does not fit typical pattern, a serious diagnosis can be missed.

Nonpharmacologic Choices

- The management of headache is as much art as science; the science is improving, but the art remains important:
  - after serious causes are excluded, the interaction with the patient is the first and most important therapeutic choice
  - communicate with patients to let them know their headache is real, and that they have a specific diagnosis
  - determine patients' expectations and explain management options
- Advise patients to:
  - avoid triggers, especially in migraine, e.g., too much or too little sleep, irregular meals, lack of regular exercise, extremes of stress or relaxation, known dietary triggers
  - apply ice; sleep or rest in a dark, noise-free room
- Try informal psychotherapy (family physician); refer to a psychologist or psychiatrist if psychiatric comorbidity present
- Try biofeedback, relaxation therapy, cognitive-behavioural therapy, psychotherapy, acupuncture and/or nerve blocks, individualized to each patient[3]

- Refer to neurologist and/or specialized headache or pain management unit if problems too complex, such as chronic daily headache, or require multidisciplinary approach

Pharmacologic Choices

Evidence-based guidelines for symptomatic and prophylactic therapies have been published.[4,5,6] Drugs used for treatment of acute headache are presented in Table 2.

Symptomatic Treatment

For acute treatment of migraine headache, see Figure 2.

Analgesics

Acetaminophen, ASA, diclofenac, ibuprofen and **naproxen** are effective for mild to moderate headache pain.[6] *Medication-overuse headache* can result from overuse of analgesics, which limits their long-term potential. To avoid medication-overuse headache, nonopioid analgesics should be used less than 15 days per month; opioids and analgesic-opioid combination products should be used less than 10 days per month. **Codeine** and **tramadol** have limited use in benign headache disorders because there is no evidence of superior effectiveness, yet there is potential for dependency, medication-induced headache and withdrawal syndrome. **Butalbital** compounds and **butorphanol** nasal spray should generally be avoided for these reasons.

Ergot Derivatives

Dihydroergotamine mesylate (DHE) has similar actions to the triptans but also interacts centrally with dopamine and adrenergic receptors, accounting for some of its side effects. It can be used to treat acute intractable headache or withdrawal from analgesics. DHE produces no dependence. Ergot derivatives may produce rebound headaches if used 10 days per month or more.

Figure 2: **Management of Acute Migraine**[44]

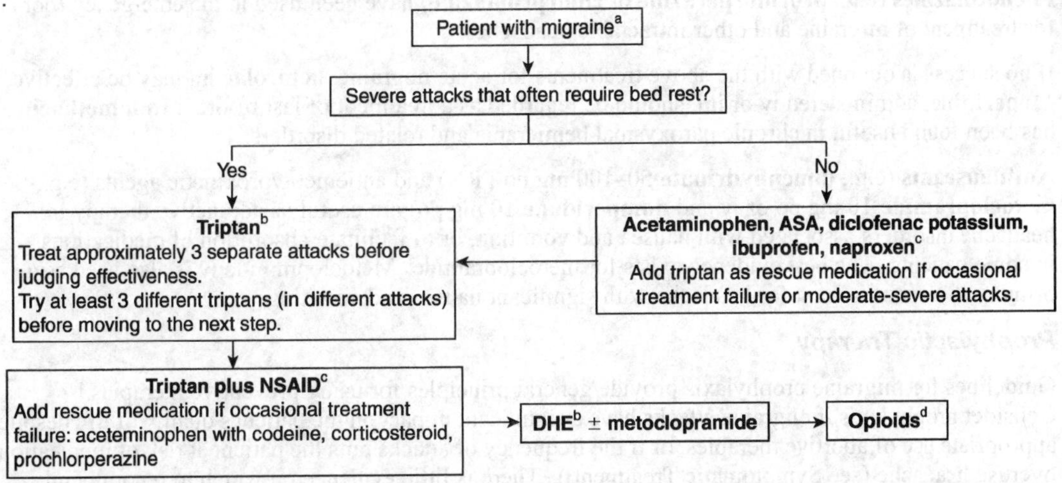

a Treatment is stepped up for the next attack if the patient is not pain free (or almost pain free) 2 hours post-dose with no significant side effects and is able to resume usual activities.
b Do *not* use 2 different triptans in the same 24-hour period. Do *not* use a triptan and dihydroergotamine (DHE) in the same 24-hour period.
c Use NSAIDs with caution in patients with GI or cardiovascular risk factors.
d Not recommended for routine use. Monitor frequency of use carefully.

Triptans

The triptans currently available to abort migraine include **almotriptan, eletriptan, frovatriptan, naratriptan, rizatriptan, sumatriptan** and **zolmitriptan**. All act on serotonin (5-HT) subclass 1B and 1D receptors, on extracerebral blood vessels and neurons respectively. The supposed mechanism of action is prevention of neurogenically sterile inflammatory responses around vessels and vasoconstriction. The newer agents may alter pain transmission centrally at the level of the trigeminal nucleus of the medulla, an action that may or may not have clinical benefits.

Overall, there is now good evidence that the available triptans are efficacious, generally well tolerated and safe.[7] Meta-analyses reveal that differences among the triptans are relatively small, but may be clinically meaningful to patients.[8,9,10] However, the benefits in individual patients may vary, as may patient preference for specific formulations (injection, nasal spray, tablets or fast-melt tablets).[11]

Subcutaneous sumatriptan has the fastest onset of action and remains the most efficacious triptan for a severe migraine attack. It is also useful in an acute cluster headache. There are few trials comparing triptans to each other. Rizatriptan may provide faster relief than a number of other oral triptans.[6] Almotriptan may have fewer adverse effects.[6] Naratriptan has a slow onset of action with maximal efficacy at 4 hours, lower headache recurrence rate and near placebo rates of side effects. Naratriptan may be best for moderately severe migraine attacks and for individuals who have low tolerance for side effects or high pain recurrence rates.

All triptans are contraindicated in patients with cardiac disorders, sustained hypertension, basilar and hemiplegic migraine.

To avoid medication-overuse headache, triptans should be used less than 10 days per month.

Others

Corticosteroids can be useful in many headache disorders, including status migrainosus, cluster headache and cerebral neoplasms with edema (especially metastatic lesions). Corticosteroids in temporal arteritis relieve headache and may prevent blindness.

Phenothiazines (e.g., **prochlorperazine** or **chlorpromazine**) have been used in the emergency room for treatment of migraine and other intractable headaches.

If no success is obtained with the above treatments for acute migraine, **ketorolac** im may be effective. **Meperidine**, administered iv or im, should be regarded as a treatment of last resort.[12] **Indomethacin** has been found useful in chronic paroxysmal hemicrania and related disorders.

Antinauseants (e.g., **dimenhydrinate** 50–100 mg po PRN) and antiemetic/prokinetic agents (e.g., **metoclopramide** 10 mg po or iv and **domperidone** 10 mg po) are useful as adjunctive therapy in headache disorders associated with nausea and vomiting, or to facilitate absorption of medications in some patients. The best evidence exists for metoclopramide. Metoclopramide iv is also used as a primary therapeutic agent for headache with significant nausea and vomiting.

Prophylactic Therapy

Guidelines for migraine prophylaxis provide general principles for using preventive therapies.[13,14] Consider prophylaxis if migraine attacks have a significant impact on the patient's quality of life despite appropriate use of abortive therapies, or if the frequency of attacks puts the patient at risk of medication overuse headache (see Symptomatic Treatment). There is little evidence on which to recommend an optimal duration of prophylaxis. Guidelines suggest a trial of at least 2 months, following dose titration, before assessing benefit. Advise patients to maintain a headache diary to monitor headache triggers, frequency and intensity, menstrual cycle, use of preventive and abortive medications and side effects. Successful prophylaxis is usually defined as a ≥50% reduction in headache frequency or days with headache, though some patients may report improved response to abortive therapy or decreased headache severity or duration. If no benefit after a 2-month trial at the target/optimal dose, try a different medication. If prophylaxis is deemed beneficial, continue for 6–12 months then consider tapering the dose to assess ongoing need. If headache intensity and frequency increase, the dose can be increased to previously effective levels.[13]

Clinical guidelines include recommendations for the following medications for migraine prophylaxis. Consider efficacy, adverse effects, comorbid conditions (such as hypertension, depression, obesity), migraine severity and patient preference when deciding which prophylactic agents to try.[13,14] For information on drugs used in the prevention of migraine, see Table 3.

Beta-blockers

Beta-blockers are commonly used and efficacious in migraine prophylaxis; their mechanism of action is uncertain. Effective agents lack partial agonist activity, but CNS penetration, membrane stabilization and cardioselectivity do not influence efficacy. **Propranolol**, **metoprolol** and **nadolol** are good initial choices.[13] Propranolol has been studied more than other beta-blockers for migraine prophylaxis.[15] **Atenolol** is also effective, though supported by less evidence.[13] Atenolol and nadolol may have fewer CNS side effects due to comparatively lower blood brain barrier penetration.

Tricyclic Analgesics

Amitriptyline and **nortriptyline** are effective for migraine, especially in patients who also have tension-type headache. Analgesic doses are lower than those required for affective disorders.[13] They do not produce dependence and are relatively safe medications in this setting. Nortriptyline may be better tolerated, particularly in older patients, because of fewer anticholinergic side effects.

Serotonin-norepinephrine Reuptake Inhibitors

Venlafaxine reduces the number of headache days in patients with migraine,[16] and may be useful in some patients with comorbid depression or anxiety.[13]

Calcium Channel Blockers

These drugs may work by modulating neurotransmitter function rather than producing vasodilation or protecting against hypoxia. **Verapamil** is useful in migraine prophylaxis,[13] but evidence for verapamil is more robust for cluster headache prophylaxis.[17] **Flunarizine** is a selective calcium entry blocker and has good efficacy in migraine, but can precipitate depression and should be avoided in patients with a history of depression.[13,14]

ACE Inhibitors

Limited evidence suggests **lisinopril** (10 mg po daily initially, increasing to 20 mg po daily after 1 week) may be effective in reducing headache frequency.[13,14,18] Proposed mechanisms for efficacy include altered sympathetic activity, decreased free radical activity, increased prostacyclin synthesis and reduced degradation of bradykinin, encephalin and substance P.

Angiotensin Receptor Blockers

Moderate quality evidence supports the efficacy of **candesartan** (8 mg po daily initially, increasing to 16 mg po daily after 1 week) in the prevention of migraine, with minimal side effects.[13,14,19] Efficacy in migraine prophylaxis may be due to direct vasoconstriction, increased sympathetic discharge and/or adrenal medullary catecholamine release.

Antiepileptic Drugs

Valproic acid and **divalproex sodium** are effective in migraine prophylaxis and may work by modulating gamma aminobutyric acid (GABA) receptors in the peripheral trigeminovascular system.[13,14] Guidelines for use have been published.[20] Because of an increased risk of neural tube defects, avoid these agents for migraine prophylaxis during pregnancy. See Choices during Pregnancy and Breastfeeding for more information.

Topiramate can reduce migraine frequency in doses up to 100 mg per day or occasionally higher. Avoid in patients with renal stones. Topiramate can cause increased intraocular pressure that responds to drug discontinuation. Weight loss is a side effect that can be beneficial in some patients. Start topiramate at a very low dose of 15–25 mg and increase very slowly to avoid cognitive side effects.[13,14,21,22] Avoid topiramate for migraine prophylaxis during pregnancy.

There is insufficient evidence to recommend the use of **gabapentin** for migraine prophylaxis.[23]

Serotonin Antagonists

Pizotifen (pizotyline) is helpful in migraine at maximal dosage if tolerated.[13,14]

Triptans

Efficacy has been demonstrated for the short-term use (5–7 days, starting 2 days before menses) of **frovatriptan** 2.5 mg po once to twice daily, to prevent *menstrually associated migraine*.[25] Perimenstrual use of **naratriptan** 1 mg po BID or **zolmitriptan** 2.5 mg po BID-TID may also be effective in this setting.[14,26,27]

Natural Health Products

Evidence suggests modest efficacy for 4 natural health products for prevention of migraine. **Butterbur** (75 mg po BID) is supported by the best evidence.[28,29] Use only formulations that are free of hepatotoxic pyrrolizidine alkaloids ("PAs"). **Magnesium citrate** (300 mg elemental magnesium po BID), **riboflavin** (400 mg po daily) and **coenzyme Q10** (100 mg po TID) may also be helpful.[13,14]

Others

Lithium 300 mg TID is useful in the prophylactic management of chronic cluster headache.[30]

Evidence of efficacy of **botulinum toxin type A** in preventing episodic migraine is lacking;[13,31] however, it may be effective in the management of chronic migraine.[32]

Choices during Pregnancy and Breastfeeding

Migraine and Pregnancy/Postpartum Period

Migraine often improves during pregnancy but in roughly 30–40% it either worsens or does not change. Postpartum migraine flares are common. The occurrence of migraine during pregnancy does not appear to increase the risk of preterm labour, low birth weight or congenital abnormalities. However, migraine may be associated with a higher risk of maternal complications of pregnancy such as gestational hypertension, pre-eclampsia and pregnancy-related stroke. When treating headache during pregnancy and the postpartum period, a high degree of suspicion is prudent to avoid missing serious causes such as cerebral venous thrombosis, pre-eclampsia/eclampsia, intracranial hemorrhage or headaches associated with epidural anesthesia.[38,39,40]

Pre-pregnancy Considerations

Women with migraine should use effective contraception if pregnancy is not desired, particularly if they are taking medications that are contraindicated during pregnancy. **Folic acid** supplementation (0.4–1 mg daily) is recommended, beginning at least 2–3 months prior to conception and continuing postpartum for at least 4–6 weeks, or as long as breastfeeding is continued. Women taking medications that can interfere with folate function (e.g., barbiturates, valproate) should take folic acid 5 mg daily beginning at least 3 months prior to conception and continuing until 10–12 weeks postconception, at which time they can switch to a dose of 0.4–1 mg daily. When possible, preventive and acute headache medications should be discontinued before attempting to conceive; this is also a logical time to begin training in nonpharmacologic measures such as biofeedback.[38,39,40,41]

Management during Pregnancy and Postpartum Period[38,39,40]

Nonpharmacologic approaches (see Nonpharmacologic Choices) should be used first-line; for the majority of women whose migraine improves during pregnancy, nonpharmacologic measures supplemented with occasional use of **acetaminophen** may suffice. For women with frequent disabling headaches or who experience severe nausea and vomiting leading to dehydration, the benefits of further drug treatment may outweigh the risks. **Ibuprofen** and **naproxen** can be used during the first or second trimester but should be avoided in the latter stages of pregnancy because they may cause constriction of the fetal ductus arteriosis. ASA, indomethacin and barbiturates should generally be avoided during pregnancy. Opioids such as meperidine or acetaminophen/codeine are occasionally used for severe headache, but should be avoided near term because of the risk of respiratory depression of the fetus. Severe nausea can be managed with **metoclopramide** or **prochlorperazine**.

Ergot derivatives restrict uterine blood flow and should not be used during pregnancy. **Triptans** are generally avoided as well, although evidence is beginning to support a lack of additional risk to the mother or fetus, particularly with sumatriptan. Also avoid vasoconstricting agents such as ergots and triptans in the postpartum period because of a possible increased risk of postpartum stroke or angiopathy.

When prophylactic medication is deemed necessary during pregnancy due to frequent, severe migraine or associated severe nausea and vomiting, **propranolol** is the preferred agent. Beta-blockers have been associated with intrauterine growth retardation and reduced placental weight. Discontinue beta blockers a few days before delivery if possible; monitor neonates exposed to beta-blockers near term for symptoms such as bradycardia, hypoglycemia and other potential effects of beta-blockade.[38,42] **Magnesium** may also be reasonable considering its efficacy when given iv for pre-eclampsia.[43] Other preventive medications are generally avoided.

When possible, refer patients with severe migraine during pregnancy to a specialist in gynecologic endocrinology or to a high-risk pregnancy clinic.

Migraine and Breastfeeding[38,39,40]

Lactation may have a positive effect on migraine activity, and breastfeeding should be encouraged. As in pregnancy, use nonpharmacologic measures first-line during breastfeeding. When medication is required, **acetaminophen** is the preferred abortive agent. **Ibuprofen** is considered the NSAID of choice in breastfeeding. Avoid ergot derivatives, barbiturates and opioids. **Sumatriptan** has been studied more than other triptans in lactation and is considered compatible with breastfeeding, although it is prudent to avoid vasoconstricting agents in the initial postpartum period; other triptans should be used with caution. **Metoclopramide**, **domperidone**, **dimenhydrinate**, and **prochlorperazine** are all considered safe in breastfeeding.

For prophylaxis, **propranolol** and **magnesium** are the preferred options.**Valproic acid/divalproex sodium** is considered compatible with breastfeeding. Other prophylactic agents should be avoided or used with appropriate caution and monitoring of the infant.

For a discussion of general principles of drug use during pregnancy and breastfeeding see Appendix II and Appendix III. Other specialized reference sources are included in these appendices.

Chronic Daily Headache and Medication-overuse Headache

Chronic headache occurs daily or almost daily for 15 days per month, for 6 months or longer. The most common causes of these headaches are *chronic migraine* and *chronic tension-type headache*.

In the former there is history of migraine attacks and over several years the migraine attacks become more frequent. Soon the migraine characteristics give way to chronic daily headache with a daily or near-daily background headache that often resembles a typical "tension-type headache." People with chronic tension-type headache may have no history of distinct migraine.

Patients with these disorders frequently use excessive amounts of abortive agents, including ergots, acetaminophen, ASA and opioid analgesics. They can have rebound headaches as a result of *medication-overuse headache*, while some may have symptoms of depression or other psychological comorbidities. Medication-overuse headache can also occur with the overuse of triptans.[33] Most will improve in days or a few weeks with the discontinuation of these medications, especially mixed analgesics.

Generally, simple analgesics should be used less than 15 days per month in primary headache disorders such as migraine or tension-type headache or they will lead to the development of medication-overuse headache and chronic daily headache.[34] Further, if chronic daily headache develops, other useful abortive and prophylactic medications usually have less efficacy.

Management includes recognition of these disorders, tapering and stopping the offending agent(s), and starting a prophylactic medication such as **amitriptyline** or another agent listed in Table 3. During withdrawal, particularly in patients with transformed migraine, use abortive agents such as **DHE** or a **triptan** for treatment of the migraine headaches that emerge. Short-term admission to hospital may be required to use the Raskin protocol (using DHE)[35,37] and give support. If psychological comorbidities such as depression are present, they must be managed and treated. Consider referral to a multidisciplinary pain management clinic for cases failing to respond to therapy.

Therapeutic Tips

- Give abortive treatment, without exceeding recommended dosages, as soon as possible after headache onset.
- To avoid medication overuse headache, use simple analgesics less than 15 days per month, and ergots, triptans, opioids or analgesic combinations less than 10 days per month.
- A calendar or diary of headaches is useful in follow-up assessment.[36]
- Keep a record of medications (usefulness, dosage and side effects).
- Different medications may need to be tried, including different members of the same class, such as triptans.
- Follow-up is most important in managing chronic headache.
- Reassurance and explanation are most important to the patient in the long term.
- Always offer hope to patients with chronic headache even if no cure is available; most primary headaches can be controlled.

Table 2: **Medications for Symptomatic Treatment of Headache**

Class	Drug	Dose (per attack)	Adverse Effects	Drug Interactions	Comments	Cost[a]
Analgesics	*acetaminophen* Atasol Preparations, Tylenol, generics	650–1300 mg Q4H po × 1–2 doses	Potential hepatotoxicity with chronic use of high doses (particularly in heavy drinkers) or in acute overdose.	Alcohol: See Adverse Effects May enhance anticoagulant effect of warfarin, particularly at doses >1.3 g/day for >1 wk	Use less than 15 days/month for headache; great risk of rebound headache; for symptomatic treatment only.	$
	ASA Aspirin, Coated Aspirin, generics	650–1300 mg Q4H po × 1–2 doses	GI upset (usually the only more common adverse effect when single doses are used to treat acute headache). For a detailed description of adverse effects associated with continuous or frequent NSAID use see Chapter 82, Table 2.	Warfarin: increased anticoagulant effect. Antihypertensives (diuretics, beta-blockers, ACE inhibitors, alpha-blockers): possible reduction in antihypertensive effect; may require additional antihypertensive therapy. Lithium may interfere with sodium/water balance. Monitor lithium levels when NSAID added. Increased risk of GI bleeding with SSRIs.	See acetaminophen.	$
	diclofenac potassium Voltaren Rapide, generics	50 mg Q6–8H po × 1–2 doses	See ASA.	See ASA.	See acetaminophen.	$
	diclofenac potassium powder Cambia	50 mg single dose Dissolve contents of one sachet in 30–60 mL water	See ASA.	See ASA.	Powder for oral solution has faster onset of action.	$$$

(cont'd)

Table 2: Medications for Symptomatic Treatment of Headache *(cont'd)*

Class	Drug	Dose (per attack)	Adverse Effects	Drug Interactions	Comments	Cost[a]
	ibuprofen Advil, Motrin, Motrin Liquid Gels, Motrin IB Super Strength generics	400–800 mg Q6H po × 1–2 doses	See ASA.	See ASA.	See acetaminophen. Liquid-containing capsules may have faster onset of action.	$
	ketorolac Toradol IM, generics	30–60 mg im; maximum 120 mg/24 h	Pain at the injection site, sweating, GI upset.	See ASA.		$
	naproxen Naprosyn, generics	**Acute migraine:** 500–750 mg po; after at least 30 minutes, an additional dose of 250–500 mg may be given to a maximum daily dose of 1250 mg **Mild to moderate headache pain:** 500 mg Q12H or 250 mg Q6–8H po; maximum 1000 mg/day	See ASA.	See ASA.	Use less than 15 days/month for symptomatic treatment of headache.	$
	naproxen sodium Aleve, Anaprox, generics	**Acute migraine:** 550–825 mg po; after at least 30 minutes, an additional dose of 375–550 mg may be given to a maximum daily dose of 1375 mg **Mild to moderate headache pain:** 550 mg Q12H or 275 mg Q6–8H po; maximum 1100 mg/day **Nonprescription use**: 220 mg Q12H po	See ASA.	See ASA.	See naproxen. Useful in preventing premenstrual migraine attacks when taken BID perimenstrually for 2 wk, starting 7 days before menses.[45]	$
Ergot Derivatives	*dihydroergotamine injection* generics	0.5–1 mg sc, im or iv; may repeat at 1 h; maximum 4 doses/24 h Administration of dihydroergotamine is preceded by metoclopramide 10 mg iv or prochlorperazine 5 mg iv[35,37] Administer iv meds *slowly*	Chest pain, tingling, nausea, vomiting, parasthesias, cramps and/or vasoconstriction occur infrequently and are of short-duration; watch for hypotension (rare).	Contraindicated in patients taking potent inhibitors of CYP3A4 (e.g., cimetidine, clarithromycin, efavirenz, erythromycin, itraconazole, ketoconazole, ritonavir).	Not as potent a vasoconstrictor as ergotamine; mainly venoconstrictor; contraindicated in pregnancy, cardiac disorders, hypertension, sepsis, PVD, PUD, renal or liver disease; no risk of dependence; good for attacks beginning in emergency room and for treating medication-overuse headaches.	$
	dihydroergotamine nasal spray Migranal	1 spray (0.5 mg) in each nostril; may repeat in 15 min if no effect with first dose; maximum 2 mg (4 sprays) per day	Rhinitis, nausea, taste disturbance.	See dihydroergotamine injection.	Convenient, bypasses GI tract. See dihydroergotamine injection.	$

Class	Drug	Dose (per attack)	Adverse Effects	Drug Interactions	Comments	Cost[a]
Triptans	*almotriptan* Axert, generics	Oral: 6.25–12.5 mg; if headache returns after initial relief, may repeat in 2 h; maximum 2 doses/24 h	*All triptans:* chest discomfort, fatigue, dizziness, paresthesias, drowsiness, nausea, throat symptoms.	See Comments. *Almotriptan:* inhibitors of CYP3A4 (e.g., cimetidine, clarithromycin, efavirenz, erythromycin, grapefruit juice, itraconazole, ketoconazole and ritonavir) may increase bioavailability of almotriptan.	*All triptans:* do not use if *any* cardiac-like symptoms; contraindicated in ischemic heart disease, sustained hypertension, pregnancy, basilar or hemiplegic migraine, ergotamine-containing products or with MAOIs (except eletriptan, frovatriptan and naratriptan); caution with SSRIs or SNRIs (increased risk of serotonin syndrome); do not use a triptan within 24 h after another triptan; use less than 10 days/month to avoid medication-overuse headache. Second dose not likely to be effective if first dose provided no relief.	$$
	eletriptan Relpax, generics	Oral: 20–40 mg; if headache returns after initial relief from 20 mg dose, may take an additional 20 mg in 2 h; maximum 40 mg/24 h	See almotriptan.	See Comments. *Eletriptan*: contraindicated within 72 h of the following inhibitors of CYP3A4: clarithromycin, itraconazole, ketoconazole, nelfinavir and ritonavir, or any potent inhibitor of CYP3A4.	See almotriptan.	$$
	frovatriptan Frova	Oral: 2.5 mg; if headache recurs after initial relief, may repeat in 4–24 h; maximum 5 mg/24 h	See almotriptan.	See Comments. *Frovatriptan*: oral contraceptives and propranolol may increase frovatriptan serum concentrations by 30–60%.	See almotriptan.	$$$
	naratriptan Amerge, generics	Oral: 1–2.5 mg; if headache returns after initial relief, may repeat dose in 4 h; maximum 5 mg/24 h	See almotriptan. Naratriptan may have a lower incidence of side effects than other triptans.	See Comments.	See almotriptan.	$$

(cont'd)

Table 2: **Medications for Symptomatic Treatment of Headache** *(cont'd)*

Class	Drug	Dose (per attack)	Adverse Effects	Drug Interactions	Comments	Cost[a]
	rizatriptan Maxalt, Maxalt RPD, generics	Oral: 5–10 mg; if headache returns after initial relief, may repeat dose in 2 h; maximum 20 mg/24 h	See almotriptan.	See Comments. *Rizatriptan:* use with caution in patients taking propranolol (increased bioavailability of rizatriptan).	See almotriptan. *Rizatriptan:* fastmelt wafers can be taken without water.	$$
	sumatriptan Imitrex, Imitrex DF, generics	Oral: 25–100 mg; if headache returns after initial relief, may repeat in 2 h; maximum 200 mg/24 h Injectable: 6 mg sc; may repeat in 1 h; maximum 2 injections/24 h Nasal spray: 5–20 mg intranasally; may repeat in 2 h; maximum 40 mg/24 h	See almotriptan. Nasal spray: taste disturbance, nausea.	See Comments.	See almotriptan. *Sumatriptan nasal spray:* faster onset than with oral formulations.	Oral: $$ SC: $$$$$ Nasal: $$$
	zolmitriptan Zomig, Zomig Rapimelt, Zomig Nasal Spray, generics	Oral: 2.5–5 mg; may repeat in 2 h; maximum 10 mg/24 h Nasal Spray: 2.5 mg or 5 mg; may repeat in 2 h; maximum 10 mg/24 h	See almotriptan.	See Comments. Maximum dose of zolmitriptan 5 mg/24 h if also on fluvoxamine or cimetidine.	See almotriptan. *Zolmitriptan:* orally dispersible tablets can be taken without water; nasal spray available as 2.5 mg or 5 mg per dose.	$$

[a] Cost per dose; includes drug cost only.

Dosage adjustment may be required in renal impairment; see Appendix I.

Abbreviations: PUD = peptic ulcer disease; PVD = peripheral vascular disease

Legend: $ < $5 $$ $5–10 $$$ $10–20 $$$$ $20–30 $$$$$ $30–40

Table 3: **Medications for Migraine Prophylaxis**

Class	Drug	Dose	Adverse Effects	Drug Interactions	Comments	Cost[a]
Antiepileptic Drugs	*divalproex sodium* Epival, generics	Initial: 250–500 mg/day po; increase by 250 mg/day at weekly intervals as needed/tolerated (usual range 500–1500 mg/day po in 2 divided doses	See valproic acid.	Inhibits CYP2C9 and may decrease the clearance of substrates (e.g., fluoxetine, fluvastatin, sertraline, verapamil, warfarin); avoid ASA or warfarin; carbamazepine, phenytoin and phenobarbital can significantly increase clearance; may increase depressant effect of alcohol.	Do liver function tests prior to initiation of therapy and periodically, especially in the first 6 months of therapy and if symptoms of hepatic dysfunction occur.	$$
	topiramate ◗ Topamax, generics	Initial: 15–25 mg daily po; increase by 15 mg/day at weekly intervals or 25 mg/day every 1–2 wk (usual range 25–50 mg BID po)	CNS effects (e.g., dizziness, ataxia, tremor, sedation, cognitive impairment), GI symptoms (e.g., nausea, dyspepsia, constipation), weight loss (can be beneficial in some patients). Possible increased risk of oral clefts if used during the 1st trimester; avoid topiramate for migraine prophylaxis during pregnancy.	Additive depressant effects with other CNS depressants. May decrease effectiveness of oral contraceptives; use oral contraceptives containing at least 35 μg estrogen and add barrier contraceptive protection (condoms). Inhibitors of CYP2C19 may increase topiramate levels (e.g., SSRIs, isoniazid, omeprazole, moclobemide). Phenytoin and carbamazepine can decrease topiramate levels.	May increase risk of nephrolithiasis; maintain adequate hydration during therapy; avoid in patients with renal stones. May cause acute myopia, with consequent angle closure glaucoma that responds to drug discontinuation; advise patients to consult an ophthalmologist or emergency room *immediately* if they have acute painful/red eyes or decreased/blurred vision. Warn patients about CNS depressant effects; possible risk associated with driving, other hazardous activities.	$$
	valproic acid, (valproate) Depakene, Apo-Valproic, other generics	Initial: 250–500 mg/day po; increase by 250 mg daily at weekly intervals as needed/tolerated (usual range 500–1500 mg/day po in 2 divided doses	Nausea, alopecia, tremor, weight gain, increased hepatic enzymes; neural tube defects can occur if used during pregnancy.	See divalproex sodium.	See divalproex sodium.	$$

(cont'd)

Table 3: **Medications for Migraine Prophylaxis** *(cont'd)*

Class	Drug	Dose	Adverse Effects	Drug Interactions	Comments	Cost[a]
Beta$_1$-adrenergic Antagonists	*atenolol* Tenormin, generics	Initial: 50 mg daily po; increase by 50 mg daily every 1–2 wk as needed/tolerated (usual range 100–150 mg daily po)	Fatigue, impotence, bradycardia and hypotension, GI symptoms, bronchospasm, heart failure, depression.	Possible bradycardia with dipyridamole; antacids may decrease absorption.	Contraindicated in asthma, insulin-dependent diabetes or heart block; avoid abrupt withdrawal; consider long-acting formulations. Atenolol and nadolol may have fewer CNS side effects. If beta-blocker therapy is deemed necessary during pregnancy, propranolol is the preferred agent.	$
	metoprolol Lopresor, Betaloc, generics	Initial: 50 mg BID po; increase by 25 mg BID every 1–2 wk as needed/tolerated (usual range 100– 200 mg/day po)	See atenolol.	See atenolol.	See atenolol.	$
	nadolol generics	Initial: 20–40 mg daily po; increase by 20–40 mg daily every 1–2 wk as needed/tolerated (usual range 80–160 mg/day po)	See atenolol.	See atenolol.	See atenolol. Nadolol and atenolol may have fewer CNS side effects.	$$
	propranolol generics	Initial: 20–40 mg BID po; increase by 20 mg BID every 1–2 wk as needed/tolerated (usual range 80–160 mg/day po)	See atenolol.	See atenolol.	See atenolol.	$
Calcium Channel Blockers	*flunarizine* generics	Initial: 5 mg QHS po; increase to 10 mg QHS po after 1–2 wk	Weight gain, extrapyramidal effects, drowsiness, depression.	Additive sedation with other CNS depressants, such as alcohol, benzodiazepines, opioids.	Long latency to onset; many patients have side effects; contraindicated in hypotension, heart failure and arrhythmia; avoid if severe constipation. Do not use flunarizine in depressed patients or those with extrapyramidal disorders.	$$
	verapamil Isoptin SR, generics	Initial: 40 mg TID po or 160 mg once daily po (long-acting formulation); increase to 240–320 mg/day po over 1–2 wk	Bradycardia, hypotension, constipation.	Inhibits CYP3A4 and may decrease the clearance of CYP3A4 substrates (e.g., lovastatin, sildenafil).	See flunarizine.	$$

Class	Drug	Dose	Adverse Effects	Drug Interactions	Comments	Cost[a]
Others	*lithium* Carbolith, Lithane, Lithmax, generics	300 mg TID po	GI upset, tremor, polyuria, hypothyroidism.	ACE inhibitors, angiotensin II receptor blockers, NSAIDs and thiazide diuretics increase lithium serum levels; a potential effect on lithium levels should be considered whenever other drugs are started or discontinued; significant dosage adjustment may be required.	Used in chronic cluster headache; contraindicated in renal dysfunction, dehydration, heart failure.	$
Serotonin Antagonists	*pizotifen* Sandomigran, Sandomigran DS	Start with 0.5 mg QHS po; gradually increase to TID; if needed/tolerated may increase to 4 mg/day po	Drowsiness, weight gain.	Additive sedation with other CNS depressants (e.g., alcohol).	Consider QHS dosing at higher doses.	$$$
Serotonin-norepinephrine Reuptake Inhibitors	*venlafaxine* Effexor XR, generics	Initial: 37.5 mg daily po; increase by 37.5 mg/day at weekly intervals as needed/tolerated to 150 mg daily po	Nausea, sleep disturbance, drowsiness, nervousness, dizziness, dry mouth. Dose-related hypertension occurs rarely, particularly at doses ≥225 mg/day.	Use with MAOIs may lead to potentially fatal reaction initially presenting with tremor, agitation, hypomania, hyperthermia and/or hypertension. Inhibitors of CYP2D6 or CYP3A4 (such as bupropion, clarithromycin, erythromycin, itraconazole, ketoconazole, quinidine, ritonavir) may increase venlafaxine levels.	May be useful for some patients with comorbid anxiety or depression.	$
Tricyclic Analgesics (TCAs)	*amitriptyline* Elavil	Initial: 10 mg QHS po; increase by 10 mg/day po every 1–2 wk as needed/tolerated (usual range 20–40 mg QHS po; may increase up to 150 mg/day po if needed/tolerated)	All TCAs: weight gain, drowsiness, anticholinergic symptoms (e.g., dry mouth, constipation), lower seizure threshold, confusion.	All TCAs: increased sedation with other CNS depressants (e.g., alcohol). *Amitriptyline*: metabolized by many cytochrome P450 enzymes—clearance may be affected by inhibitors (e.g., cimetidine, ciprofloxacin, clarithromycin, diltiazem, erythromycin, fluoxetine, fluvoxamine, isoniazid, itraconazole, ketoconazole, paroxetine, valproic acid), inducers (e.g., phenobarbital, carbamazepine, phenytoin, rifampin, smoking) or other substrates of these enzymes.	All TCAs: dose can be cumulative, adjustments needed; contraindicated if significant cardiac disease, glaucoma, prostate disease or hypotension; start with low dosage in elderly or in patients sensitive to these agents.	$

(cont'd)

Table 3: **Medications for Migraine Prophylaxis** *(cont'd)*

Class	Drug	Dose	Adverse Effects	Drug Interactions	Comments	Cost[a]
	doxepin Sinequan, generics	Initial: 25 mg QHS po; increase by 25 mg/day every 1–2 wk as needed/tolerated (usual range 25–100 mg QHS po)	See amitriptyline.	All TCAs: increased sedation with other CNS depressants (e.g., alcohol). *Doxepin*: metabolized by CYP2D6; clearance may be altered by inducers (e.g., carbamazepine, phenobarbital, phenytoin, rifampin), inhibitors (e.g., celecoxib, fluoxetine, imatinib, paroxetine, quinidine) or other substrates of the enzyme.	See amitriptyline.	$
	nortriptyline Aventyl, generics	Initial: 10 mg QHS po; increase by 10 mg/day every 1–2 wk as needed/tolerated (usual range 20–40 mg QHS po; may increase to 150 mg/day po if needed tolerated)	See amitriptyline.	All TCAs: increased sedation with other CNS depressants (e.g., alcohol). *Nortriptyline*: metabolized by CYP1A2 and CYP2D6. Clearance may be affected by inducers (e.g., carbamazepine, phenobarbital, primidone, phenytoin, rifampin, smoking), inhibitors (e.g., celecoxib, cimetidine, ciprofloxacin, clarithromycin, diltiazem, erythromycin, ethinyl estradiol, fluvoxamine, isoniazid, ketoconazole, fluoxetine, imatinib, paroxetine, quinidine) or other substrates of either enzyme.	See amitriptyline.	$

[a] Cost of 30-day supply; includes drug cost only.

Dosage adjustment may be required in renal impairment; see Appendix I.

Legend: $ < $15 $$ $15–30 $$$ $45–60

Suggested Readings

Pringsheim T, Davenport W, Mackie G et al. Canadian Headache Society guideline for migraine prophylaxis. *Can J Neurol Sci* 2012;39(2 Suppl 2):S1-59.

Worthington I, Pringsheim T, Gawel MJ et al. Canadian Headache Society guideline: acute drug therapy for migraine headache. *Can J Neurol Sci* 2013;40(5 Suppl 3):S1-80.

References

1. Purdy RA. Clinical evaluation of a patient presenting with headache. *Med Clin North Am* 2001;85(4):847-63.
2. Pryse-Phillips WE, Dodick DW, Edmeads JG et al. Guidelines for the diagnosis and management of migraine in clinical practice. Canadian Headache Society. *CMAJ* 1997;156(9):1273-87.
3. Pryse-Phillips WE, Dodick DW, Edmeads JG et al. Guidelines for the nonpharmacologic management of migraine in clinical practice. Canadian Headache Society. *CMAJ* 1998;159(1):47-54.
4. Silberstein SD. Practice parameter: evidence-based guidelines for migraine headache (an evidence-based review): report of the Quality Standards Subcommittee of the American Academy of Neurology. *Neurology* 2000;55(6):754-62.
5. Snow V, Weiss K, Wall EM et al. Pharmacologic management of acute attacks of migraine and prevention of migraine headache. *Ann Intern Med* 2002;137(10):840-9.
6. Worthington I, Pringsheim T, Gawel MJ et al. Canadian Headache Society guideline: acute drug therapy for migraine headache. *Can J Neurol Sci* 2013;40(5 Suppl 3):S1-80.
7. Dodick D, Lipton RB, Martin V et al. Consensus statement: cardiovascular safety profile of triptans (5-HT agonists) in the acute treatment of migraine. *Headache* 2004;44(5):414-25.
8. Ferrari MD, Goadsby PJ, Roon KI et al. Triptans (serotonin, 5-HT1B/1D agonists) in migraine: detailed results and methods of a meta-analysis of 53 trials. *Cephalalgia* 2002;22(8):633-58.
9. Ferrari MD, Roon KI, Lipton RB et al. Oral triptans (serotonin 5-HT(1B/1D) agonists) in acute migraine treatment: a meta-analysis of 53 trials. *Lancet* 2001;358(9294):1668-75.
10. Pascual J, Mateos V, Roig C et al. Marketed oral triptans in the acute treatment of migraine: a systematic review on efficacy and tolerability. *Headache* 2007;47(8):1152-68.
11. Dodick DW, Silberstein S, Dahlof CG. Is there a preferred triptan? *Headache* 2002;42(1):1-7.
12. Friedman BW, Kapoor A, Friedman MS et al. The relative efficacy of meperidine for the treatment of acute migraine: a meta-analysis of randomized controlled trials. *Ann Emerg Med* 2008;52(6):705-13.
13. Pringsheim T, Davenport W, Mackie G et al. Canadian Headache Society guideline for migraine prophylaxis. *Can J Neurol Sci* 2012;39(2 Suppl 2):S1-59.
14. Holland S, Silberstein SD, Freitag F et al. Evidence-based guideline update: NSAIDs and other complementary treatments for episodic migraine prevention in adults: report of the Quality Standards Subcommittee of the American Academy of Neurology and the American Headache Society. *Neurology* 2012;78(17):1346-53.
15. Linde K, Rossnagel K. Propranolol for migraine prophylaxis. *Cochrane Database Syst Rev* 2004;(2):CD003225.
16. Ozyalcin SN, Talu GK, Kiziltan E et al. The efficacy and safety of venlafaxine in the prophylaxis of migraine. *Headache* 2005;45(2):144-52.
17. Leone M, D'Amico D, Frediani F et al. Verapamil in the prophylaxis of episodic cluster headache: a double-blind study versus placebo. *Neurology* 2000;54(6):1382-5.
18. Schrader H, Stovner LJ, Helde G et al. Prophylactic treatment of migraine with angiotensin converting enzyme inhibitor (lisinopril): randomised, placebo controlled, crossover study. *BMJ* 2001;322(7277):19-22.
19. Tronvik E, Stovner LJ, Helde G et al. Prophylactic treatment of migraine with an angiotensin II receptor blocker: a randomized controlled trial. *JAMA* 2003;289(1):65-9.
20. Silberstein SD. Divalproex sodium in headache: literature review and clinical guidelines. *Headache* 1996;36(9):547-55.
21. Brandes JL, Saper JR, Diamond M et al. Topiramate for migraine prevention: a randomized controlled trial. *JAMA* 2004;291(8):965-73.
22. Young WB, Hopkins MM, Shechter AL et al. Topiramate: a case series study in migraine prophylaxis. *Cephalalgia* 2002;22(8):659-63.
23. Linde M, Mulleners WM, Chronicle EP et al. Gabapentin or pregabalin for the prophylaxis of episodic migraine in adults. *Cochrane Database Syst Rev* 2013;(6):CD010609.
24. Silberstein SD, Goadsby PJ. Migraine: preventive treatment. *Cephalalgia* 2002;22(7):491-512.
25. Brandes JL, Poole A, Kallela M et al. Short-term frovatriptan for the prevention of difficult-to-treat menstrual migraine attacks. *Cephalalgia* 2009;29(11):1133-48.
26. Newman L, Mannix LK, Landy S et al. Naratriptan as short-term prophylaxis of menstrually associated migraine: a randomized, double-blind, placebo-controlled study. *Headache* 2001;41(3):248-56.
27. Tuchman MM, Hee A, Emeribe U et al. Oral zolmitriptan in the short-term prevention of menstrual migraine: a randomized, placebo-controlled study. *CNS Drugs* 2008;22(10):877-86.
28. Lipton RB, Gobel K, Einhaupl KM et al. Petasites hybridus root (butterbur) is an effective preventative treatment for migraine. *Neurology* 2004;63(12):2240-4.
29. Diener HC, Rahlfs VW, Danesch U. The first placebo-controlled trial of a special butterbur root extract for the prevention of migraine: reanalysis of efficacy criteria. *Eur Neurol* 2004;51(2):89-97.
30. Bussone G, Leone M, Peccarisi G et al. Double blind comparison of lithium and verapamil in cluster headache prophylaxis. *Headache* 1990;30(7):411-7.
31. Shuhendler AJ, Lee S, Siu M et al. Efficacy of botulinum toxin type A for the prophylaxis of episodic migraine headaches: a meta-analysis of randomized double-blind, placebo-controlled trials. *Pharmacotherapy* 2009;29(7):784-91.
32. Jackson JL, Kuriyama A, Hayashino Y. Botulinum toxin A for prophylactic treatment of migraine and tension headaches in adults: a meta-analysis. *JAMA* 2012;307(16):1736-45.
33. Limmroth V, Katsarava Z, Fritsche G et al. Features of medication overuse headache following overuse of different acute headache drugs. *Neurology* 2002;59(7):1011-4.
34. Silberstein SD, Welch KM. Painkiller headache. *Neurology* 2002;59(7):972-4.
35. Raskin NH. Repetitive intravenous dihydroergotamine as therapy for intractable migraine. *Neurology* 1986;36(7):995-7.

36. Becker WJ, Worthington I. Diary completion instructions. *Can J Neurol Sci* 2013;40(5 Suppl 3):S79-80.
37. Raskin NH. Modern pharmacotherapy of migraine. *Neurol Clin* 1990;8(4):857-65.
38. Loder E. Migraine in pregnancy. *Semin Neurol* 2007;27(5):425-33.
39. Menon R, Bushnell CD. Headache and pregnancy. *Neurologist* 2008;14(2):108-18.
40. Loder E, Silberstein SD. Headaches in women. In: Silberstein SD, Lipton RB, Dodick DW, eds. *Wolff's headache and other head pain*. 8th ed. Oxford (GB): Oxford University Press; 2008.
41. Wilson RD, Johnson JA, Wyatt P et al. Pre-conceptional vitamin/folic acid supplementation 2007: the use of folic acid in combination with a multivitamin supplement for the prevention of neural tube defects and other congenital anomalies. *J Obstet Gynaecol Can* 2007;29(12):1003-26.
42. Briggs GG, Freeman RK, Yaffe, SJ. *Drugs in pregnancy and lactation: a reference guide to fetal and neonatal risk*. 9th ed. Philadelphia (PA): Wolters Kluwer Health; Lippincott Williams & Wilkins; 2011.
43. Drugs and Lactation Database (LactMed). Bethesda (MD): U.S. National Library of Medicine. Available from: toxnet.nlm.nih.gov/cgi-bin/sis/htmlgen?LACT. Accessed October 21, 2009.
44. Werner JB, Worthington I. Guideline summary for primary care physicians. *Can J Neurol Sci* 2013;40(3):S63-68.
45. Sances G, Martignoni E, Fioroni L et al. Naproxen sodium in menstrual migraine prophylaxis: a double-blind placebo controlled study. *Headache* 1990;30(11):705-9.

Neurologic Disorders

Chapter 18
Headache in Children

Sharon Whiting, MBBS, FRCPC

Headaches occur commonly in children and adolescents. They may occur as a primary disorder such as migraine, or accompany systemic disorders or infectious diseases. In Canada, more than 25% of 12- to 13-year-olds experience headache at least weekly.[1] The prevalence of migraine shows an increase with age, i.e., 2.4% in 12- to 14-year-olds and 5% in 15- to 19-year-olds.[2]

Migraine in children is usually associated with at least one of the following: vomiting, photophobia, family history of migraine.

Goals of Therapy

- Make an accurate diagnosis of headache[3]
- Relieve or abort pain and associated symptoms
- Prevent further headaches

Investigations

- The history is the key to the diagnosis of headache and should be obtained from both parent and child with attention to:
  - specific questions such as where pain began, progress, duration, frequency, relieving and aggravating factors (especially sleep loss, excitement, certain foods, relief with activity) and associated symptoms such as vomiting and photophobia
  - specific neurologic symptoms such as seizures, visual disturbances, difficulty with balance, personality change, weakness
  - symptoms suggestive of renal, cardiac, dental or infectious disease
  - degree of interference with school and social life, e.g., pedMIDAS questionnaire[4]
  - analgesic use
  - child's growth and development, behaviour, academic function

Note: During the interview, observe interaction between parent and child.

- Physical examination:
  - blood pressure, vital signs, palpation of sinuses, examination of teeth, neck stiffness, examination of optic fundi
  - height, weight, head circumference
  - thorough neurologic examination including cranial nerves, muscle tone, power and reflexes and coordination tests
- Investigations:
  - sinus x-rays if sinusitis suspected
  - CT followed by lumbar puncture with measurement of opening pressure if pseudotumor cerebri suspected based on history of raised intracranial pressure with a negative CT
  - lumbar puncture if infectious process suspected

- CT and/or MRI if abnormal neurologic examination, decreased visual acuity, recent behaviour change, increasing severity and frequency of headaches, or if headache does not fit a known pattern

- The routine use of any diagnostic study is not indicated when the clinical history has no associated risk factors and the child's examination is normal[5]
- Investigations based on headache profile can be found in Figure 1.

Tension-type Headache

Therapeutic Choices

Nonpharmacologic Choices

- Psychological evaluation
- Relaxation therapy
- Biofeedback

Pharmacologic Choices

- Simple analgesics (**acetaminophen**, **ASA**) and NSAIDs, such as **ibuprofen** or **naproxen**, are effective for the treatment of acute tension-type headache (Table 1). Because of the possible association with Reye's syndrome, avoid ASA in children and adolescents for headache or fever associated with viral illness such as influenza or chickenpox.[6]
- **Amitriptyline** (Table 2) is effective in reducing headache frequency and severity.[7,8] Preventive therapy may be appropriate when headaches are frequent and significantly disabling and disruptive.

Medication-overuse Headache

The occurrence of headache induced by chronic use of analgesics, such as acetaminophen and NSAIDs, is now recognized in pediatric patients. Treatment involves education and gradual withdrawal of analgesic drugs. Consider use of a prophylactic agent (Table 2).[9]

Figure 1: **Investigations Based on Headache Profile**

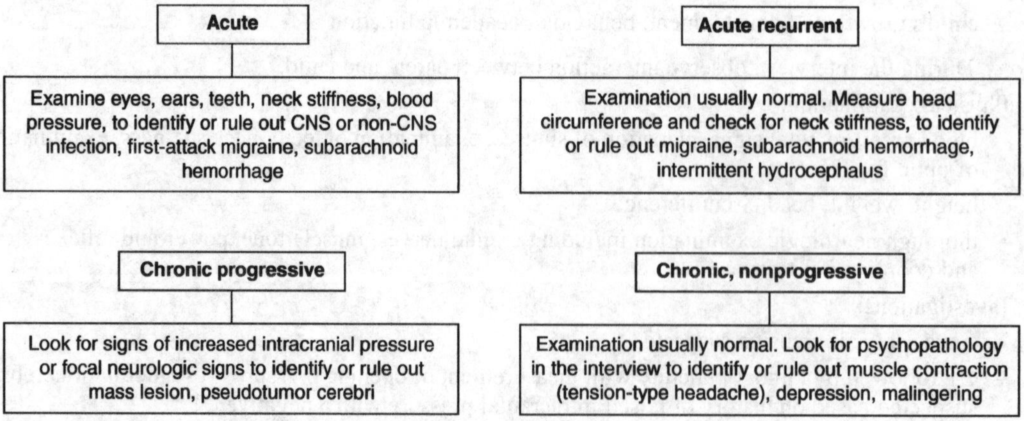
Acute
Examine eyes, ears, teeth, neck stiffness, blood pressure, to identify or rule out CNS or non-CNS infection, first-attack migraine, subarachnoid hemorrhage
Acute recurrent
Examination usually normal. Measure head circumference and check for neck stiffness, to identify or rule out migraine, subarachnoid hemorrhage, intermittent hydrocephalus
Chronic progressive
Look for signs of increased intracranial pressure or focal neurologic signs to identify or rule out mass lesion, pseudotumor cerebri
Chronic, nonprogressive
Examination usually normal. Look for psychopathology in the interview to identify or rule out muscle contraction (tension-type headache), depression, malingering

Migraine

Therapeutic Choices

Nonpharmacologic Choices

After exclusion of mass lesion or other causes:

- Provide reassurance and information about the headache condition.
- Discuss triggers of migraine, e.g., lack of sleep, too much sleep, excitement, foods, stress, menstruation.
- Encourage sleep at the time of headache and medication early in the course of the headache.
- Biofeedback and relaxation therapy are effective.

Pharmacologic Choices

These can be divided into medication given at the time of the headache (symptomatic) and medication to prevent headache (prophylactic).[10]

Symptomatic Treatments (Table 1)

Analgesics

Intermittent oral analgesics, given as early in the course of the headache as feasible, are the mainstay of pharmacologic management of childhood migraine. **Acetaminophen**, **ibuprofen** and **ASA** are effective at appropriate doses.[11] As for tension-type headache, avoid ASA in children and adolescents for fever or headache associated with viral illness such as varicella or influenza. Two evaluations of the evidence for treatment of migraine in children concluded that ibuprofen and acetaminophen are effective.[10,12,13]

Combination products containing ASA, caffeine and butalbital ± codeine (e.g., Fiorinal) should generally be avoided, but may be appropriate in exceptional circumstances when initial agents fail. These sedating drugs have abuse potential and should be reserved for adolescents (12–18 years) for brief periods only. Take care to avoid unnecessary opioids.

Antiemetics

Nausea and vomiting occur in up to 90% of young migraine sufferers and besides being disabling, inhibit oral administration of analgesics. Antiemetics alone (e.g., **chlorpromazine**,[14] **prochlorperazine**, **metoclopramide**) are surprisingly effective in relieving all symptoms including the headache.[15]

Ergot Derivatives

Ergotamine compounds have very limited use in pediatrics for the following reasons:

- Auras are uncommon and inconsistent; therefore, warning indicators that trigger the time to treat with ergot are often unreliable.
- Ergots can exacerbate gastrointestinal upset.
- Ergots are contraindicated in complicated migraine syndromes because of the risk of increasing vasospasm.

Oral dihydroergotamine showed no significant difference in headache improvement in a study comparing it with placebo.[16] In severe intractable headache, dihydroergotamine can be used iv in combination with an antiemetic in the emergency department.[17]

Triptans

Of the 7 agents available in Canada (**almotriptan, eletriptan, frovatriptan, naratriptan, rizatriptan, sumatriptan** and **zolmitriptan**), only almotriptan is specifically approved for use in children aged

12–18 years, though several triptans have been shown to be safe in this age group.[13,18,19] The best evidence exists for nasal sumatriptan, shown to be safe and effective for acute migraine pain in adolescents 12 years and older.[20,21,22] Consider triptans for use in adolescents with moderate to severe migraine that is unresponsive to conventional analgesics [Evidence: SORT B*].[13,18,19] Unpleasant taste is a common side effect.

Prophylactic Agents (Table 2)

A practice parameter on the pharmacologic treatment of childhood migraine examined the evidence for efficacy of several medications.[10] Although many are in current use and may be effective, only **flunarizine** was deemed probably effective based on evidence. Flunarizine has been shown to significantly reduce headache frequency and severity in children.[23,24]

Although evidence of its efficacy is lacking, **pizotifen** (pizotyline) may be helpful.

Evidence for **propranolol** is conflicting, although it is commonly used and is effective in some cases.[25] Propranolol is contraindicated in reactive airway disease, diabetes mellitus and bradyarrhythmias. Symptoms of depression are an under-reported but common side effect in adolescents.

Despite a lack of evidence of efficacy, **cyproheptadine,** an antihistamine with antiserotonergic and calcium channel blocking properties, is widely used as a prophylactic agent. Its use in older children and adolescents is limited by sedation and increased appetite/weight gain.

Amitriptyline has shown efficacy in adults; studies in children are limited.[8,26]

NSAIDs reduce headache frequency and severity in adults, presumably through prostaglandin inhibition. Although evidence of efficacy in children is lacking, **naproxen sodium** can be tried in adolescents as prophylaxis (see Therapeutic Tips).

Valproic acid has been studied in children;[27,28] however, there is insufficient evidence to recommend its use.[10] Phenobarbital and phenytoin are no longer used.

Topiramate is approved for migraine prophylaxis in adults. While not specifically approved for use in children it is used in adolescents.[8,29,30]

Riboflavin 200 mg/day may be effective in reducing migraine frequency and intensity of migraine.[31]

Therapeutic Tips

- There are very few controlled trials of pharmacologic management of childhood migraine; hence, anecdotal experience prevails. Most young patients with migraine do not require daily medication but need access to reliable analgesia at home and at school.
- Children are debilitated by nausea and vomiting and benefit greatly from antiemetics. Rest and sleep are usually very helpful.
- Consider prophylactic agents for children who cycle through periods of time when they experience such frequency of headache that their lifestyle is disrupted, or when isolated or infrequent events are severe and complex.
- For prophylaxis, consider medications with the fewest side effects first. Cyproheptadine is usually used in *younger children*. For *adolescents*, consider using propranolol, amitriptyline, naproxen sodium or flunarizine.
- A period of 6–12 months is a reasonable trial of prophylactic medication, followed by very gradual tapering and discontinuation to assess ongoing need.

* SORT (Strength of Recommendation Taxonomy) is a rating system (A, B or C) that addresses the quality of available evidence. For more information consult **How to Use *Compendium of Therapeutic Choices*** on page xxv.

- Calendars/diaries are helpful in identifying triggers, headache patterns, frequency and severity and are invaluable for management and evaluation of response to therapy.
- The prognosis for children with migraine is favourable with 50% of patients reporting improvement within 6 months after medical intervention, regardless of treatment methods used.
- Most children respond to reassurance, general advice and simple remedies for attacks when they occur.

Table 1: Drug Treatment of Headache in Children

Class	Drug	Dose[a]	Adverse Effects	Drug Interactions	Comments	Cost[b]
Analgesics	*acetaminophen* Atasol Preparations, Tempra, Tylenol, generics	10–15 mg/kg/dose Q4H prn	GI upset; liver toxicity in overdose.	May enhance anticoagulant effect of warfarin, particularly with doses of >1.3 g/day for >1 wk.	Analgesics are the most commonly used abortive medications for headache. Limit use to <15 days per month to avoid medication-overuse headache.	$
	ASA Aspirin, Coated Aspirin, generics	Age ≥12 y: single dose of 500–650 mg per headache	GI upset (usually the only more common adverse effect when single doses are used to treat acute headache). For a detailed description of adverse effects associated with continuous or frequent NSAID use, see Chapter 82, Table 2.	Warfarin: increased anticoagulant effect.	Because of the concern of Reye's syndrome, ASA should *not* be used in the context of headache or fever associated with a viral illness; do not use more frequently than Q4–6H.	$
	ibuprofen Advil, Motrin, Motrin Children's, generics	5–10 mg/kg/dose, up to 4 times daily	See ASA.	See ASA.		$
	naproxen sodium Aleve, Anaprox, Maxidol, generics	Age >2 y: 5–7 mg/kg/dose Q8–12H prn	See ASA.	See ASA.		$
Analgesics, combination	*butalbital* ❥ + *ASA + caffeine ± codeine* Fiorinal, Fiorinal C1/4, C1/2, generics	Adolescents: 50–100 mg (1–2 tablets) up to 4 times daily	GI upset; dependence and tolerance to barbiturates and opioids.	Possible additive sedation with other CNS depressants, e.g., alcohol.	Should generally be avoided. May be appropriate in exceptional circumstances. Limit use to adolescents, no more than 2 days/wk, 7 days/month. Risk of tolerance, addiction and misuse.	$$
Antiemetics	*chlorpromazine* generics	Oral/IM: 1 mg/kg to a maximum of 25 mg Q8H IV: 0.1 mg/kg Q10–15 min prn to a maximum of 30 mg	Hypotension.	Possible additive sedation with other CNS depressants, e.g., alcohol.	Can cause hypotension when given iv; used in the emergency department.	$

Class	Drug	Dose[a]	Adverse Effects	Drug Interactions	Comments	Cost[b]
	metoclopramide Metonia, other generics	IV: Adolescents: 0.1– 0.2 mg/kg (≤10 mg) single dose May repeat once if necessary; maximum 20 mg	Extrapyramidal dysfunction.	Possible enhanced sedative effect of alcohol.	Use iv in adolescents in the emergency department. See also dihydroergotamine.	$
	prochlorperazine generics	Oral: 2.5–5 mg BID prn IV: Adolescents: 10 mg	Extrapyramidal dysfunction.	Possible additive sedation with other CNS depressants, e.g., alcohol.	Used iv in adolescents in the emergency department.	$
Ergot Derivatives	*dihydroergo-tamine injection* generics	>6 years: 0.1–0.25 mg/dose iv May repeat Q20 min × 3 Give metoclopramide 0.2 mg/kg/dose (maximum 20 mg) 30 min prior to iv dihydroergotamine	Flushed feeling, tingling in extremities, nausea and vomiting.	Do not use with potent inhibitors of CYP3A4 such as cimetidine, clarithromycin, efavirenz, erythromycin, itraconazole, ketoconazole and ritonavir.	Useful in patients with severe and prolonged migraine headache; protocol to take place in hospital; contraindicated in complicated migraine, coronary heart disease, abnormal blood pressure, abnormal ECG.	$$
	dihydroergo-tamine nasal spray Migranal	>6 years: 1 spray into each nostril May repeat in 15 min if required	Nausea, taste disturbance, rhinitis.	See dihydroergotamine injection.	Contraindicated in complicated migraine, coronary heart disease, abnormal blood pressure, abnormal ECG.	$$
Triptans	*almotriptan* Axert, generics	≥12 y: Oral: 6.25 mg at start of headache; if headache returns, dose may be repeated after 2 h; no more than 2 doses in a 24-h period	Chest discomfort, fatigue, dizziness, paresthesias, drowsiness, nausea, throat symptoms.	All triptans: Do not use with ergotamine-containing products. Caution with SSRIs. Do not use a triptan within 24 h after another triptan. Almotriptan: Do not use with MAOIs. Inhibitors of CYP3A4 (e.g., cimetidine, clarithromycin, efavirenz, erythromycin, grapefruit juice, itraconazole, ketoconazole and ritonavir) may increase bioavailability of almotriptan.	Consider for adolescents 12–18 y who are unresponsive to conventional analgesics; do not use if *any* cardiac-like symptoms; contraindicated in ischemic heart disease, sustained hypertension, pregnancy, basilar or hemiplegic migraine; use less than 10 days/month to avoid medication-overuse headache.	$$$
	eletriptan Relpax, generics	≥12 y: Oral: 20–40 mg as soon after headache onset as possible; if initial dose is 20 mg and headache returns after ≥2 h, may repeat 20 mg dose; maximum 40 mg in a 24-h period	See almotriptan.	See almotriptan. Eletriptan: Contraindicated within 72 h of the following inhibitors of CYP3A4: clarithromycin, itraconazole, ketoconazole, nelfinavir and ritonavir, or any potent inhibitor of CYP3A4.	See almotriptan.	$$$

(cont'd)

Table 1: **Drug Treatment of Headache in Children** *(cont'd)*

Class	Drug	Dose[a]	Adverse Effects	Drug Interactions	Comments	Cost[b]
	frovatriptan Frova	≥12 y: Oral: 2.5 mg; if headache recurs after initial relief, may repeat in 4–24 h; maximum 5 mg/24 h	See almotriptan.	See almotriptan. Frovatriptan: Oral contraceptives and propranolol may increase frovatriptan serum concentrations by 30–60%.	See almotriptan.	$$$$
	naratriptan ◗ Amerge, generics	≥12 y: Oral: 1 mg at start of headache; if partial response or headache returns, dose may be repeated once after 4 h; maximum dose of 5 mg in a 24-h period	See almotriptan. Naratriptan may be associated with fewer side effects than the other triptans.	See almotriptan.	See almotriptan.	$$$
	rizatriptan Maxalt, Maxalt RPD, generics	≥12 y: Oral: 5–10 mg (tablet or wafer) at start of headache Do not repeat if no relief from first dose; if headache returns 2 h or more after partial or complete relief from an initial 5 mg dose, may repeat 5 mg dose (daily maximum 10 mg)	See almotriptan.	See almotriptan. Rizatriptan: Do not use with MAOIs. Use with caution in patients taking propranolol (increased bioavailability of rizatriptan).	See almotriptan. Fastmelt wafers can be taken without water.	$$$$
	sumatriptan Imitrex Nasal Spray, Imitrex DF, generics	≥12 y: 25 mg tablet or 20 mg nasal spray at start of headache Do not repeat if no relief from first dose; if headache returns 2 h or more after first dose, may repeat dose (daily maximum 2 doses)	See almotriptan. Nasal spray may cause taste disturbance.	See almotriptan. Sumatriptan: Do not use with MAOIs.	See almotriptan. Faster onset with nasal spray than with oral formulations.	$$$
	zolmitriptan Zomig, Zomig Rapimelt, Zomig Nasal Spray, generics	≥12 y: 2.5–5 mg (tablet, orally dispersible tablet or nasal spray) at start of headache Do not repeat if no relief from first dose; if headache returns 2 h or more after first dose, may repeat dose (daily maximum 2 doses)	See almotriptan. Nasal spray may cause taste disturbance.	See almotriptan. Zolmitriptan: Do not use with MAOIs. Maximum dose of 5 mg/24 h if also taking fluvoxamine or cimetidine.	See almotriptan. Zolmitriptan orally dispersible tablets can be taken without water.	$$$

[a] Not to exceed maximum adult dose.
[b] Cost per dose, based on 20 kg body weight; includes drug cost only.
◗ Dosage adjustment may be required in renal impairment; see Appendix I.
Legend: $ < $1 $$ $1–5 $$$ $5–10 $$$$ $10–15

Table 2: **Drugs Used for Prophylaxis of Headache in Children**

Class	Drug[a]	Dose	Adverse Effects	Drug Interactions	Comments	Cost[b]
Antiepileptic Drugs	*topiramate* Topamax, generics	Adolescents: Start at 25 mg daily, increase by 25 mg daily at weekly intervals to 100 mg/day in 1 or 2 divided doses	Most common: somnolence, anorexia, weight loss, paresthesias. Less common: psychomotor slowing, metabolic acidosis.	Avoid use with alcohol or other CNS depressants.	Used in adolescents.	$$$
Antihistamines	*cyproheptadine* generics	Age 2–6 y: 2 mg Q8–12H (maximum 12 mg/day) Age 7–14 y: 4 mg Q8–12H (maximum 16 mg/day)	Drowsiness, weight gain.	Possible additive sedation with other CNS depressants, e.g., alcohol.	More useful in younger children; use in older children and adolescents limited by sedation and increased appetite/weight gain.	$$
Beta$_1$-adrenergic Antagonists	*propranolol* generics	Oral: 0.6–1.5 mg/kg/day in 2–3 divided doses	Fatigue, bradycardia, hypotension, depression.	Antacids may decrease absorption.	Contraindicated in asthma, diabetes, heart block, bradyarrhythmias, pregnancy; avoid abrupt withdrawal.	$
Calcium Channel Blockers	*flunarizine* generics	Oral: 5 mg/day	Bradycardia, hypotension, depression, drowsiness.	Additive sedation with other CNS depressants.	May take several weeks to be effective; do not use in depressed patients or those with extrapyramidal disorders.	$$
NSAIDs	*naproxen sodium* Aleve, Anaprox, Maxidolgenerics	Adolescents: 220–550 mg twice daily	For a detailed description of adverse effects associated with continuous NSAID use, see Chapter 82, Table 2.	Warfarin: increased anticoagulant effect. Antihypertensives (diuretics, beta-blockers, ACE inhibitors, alpha-blockers): possible reduction in antihypertensive effect; may require additional antihypertensive therapy. Lithium may interfere with sodium/water balance. Monitor lithium levels when NSAID added.	Used in adolescents.	Aleve NonRx: $$ Rx: $$

(cont'd)

Table 2: Drugs Used for Prophylaxis of Headache in Children *(cont'd)*

Class	Drug[a]	Dose	Adverse Effects	Drug Interactions	Comments	Cost[b]
Tricyclic Analgesics (TCAs)	*amitriptyline* Elavil	10–150 mg/day	Weight gain, drowsiness; anticholinergic symptoms such as dry mouth and constipation.	Possible additive sedation with other CNS depressants, e.g., alcohol; metabolized by cytochrome P450 enzyme system—clearance may be affected by inhibitors (e.g., erythromycin, fluoxetine, fluvoxamine, isoniazid, itraconazole, ketoconazole, paroxetine, valproic acid), inducers (e.g., phenobarbital, carbamazepine, phenytoin, rifampin) or other substrates of these enzymes.	Contraindicated in significant cardiac disease or hypotension.	$
Serotonin Antagonists	*pizotifen* Sandomigran/ Sandomigran DS	Oral: 0.5–1.5 mg/day in divided doses	Sedation and weight gain.	Possible additive sedation with other CNS depressants including alcohol.	Start medication slowly and increase over 1–3 wk.	$$-$$$

[a] Not to exceed maximum adult dose.
[b] Cost of 30-day supply based on 20 kg body weight; includes drug cost only.
Dosage adjustment may be required in renal impairment; see Appendix I.
Abbreviations: NonRx = nonprescription product; Rx = prescription product
Legend: $ < $10 $$ $10–20 $$-$$$ $10–30 $$$ $20–30

Suggested Readings

Brna PM, Dooley JM. Headaches in the pediatric population. *Semin Pediatr Neurol* 2006;13(4):222-30.
Friedman G. Advances in paediatric migraine. *Paediatr Child Health* 2002;7(4):239-43.
Hershey AD. Recent developments in pediatric headache. *Curr Opin Neurol* 2010;23(3):249-53.
Lewis DW. Headaches in children and adolescents. *Am Fam Physician* 2002;65(4):625-32.
Lewis DW. Toward the definition of childhood migraine. *Curr Opin Pediatr* 2004;16(6):628-36.
Winner P. Pediatric headache.*Curr Opin Neurol* 2008;21(3):316-22.

References

1. Dooley JM, Gordon KE, Wood EP. Frequent headaches in Canadian adolescents: prevalence and associated features. *Eur J Paediatr Neurol* 2003;7:357-8.
2. Gordon KE, Dooley JM, Wood EP. Prevalence of reported migraine headaches in Canadian adolescents. *Can J Neurol Sci* 2004;31(3):324-7.
3. Overview of diagnosis and management of paediatric headache. Part I: diagnosis. *J Headache Pain* 2011(1):13-23.
4. Hershey AD, Powers SW, Vockell AL et al. PedMIDAS: development of a questionnaire to assess disability of migraines in children. *Neurology* 2001;57(11):2034-9.
5. Lewis DW, Ashwal S, Dahl G et al. Practice parameter: evaluation of children and adolescents with recurrent headaches: report of the Quality Standards Subcommittee of the American Academy of Neurology and the Practice Committee of the Child Neurology Society. *Neurology* 2002;59(4):490-8.
6. Steiner TJ, Lange R, Voelker M. Aspirin in episodic tension-type headache: placebo-controlled dose-ranging comparison with paracetamol. *Cephalalgia* 2003;23(1):59-66.
7. Hershey AD, Powers SW, Bentti AL et al. Effectiveness of amitriptyline in the prophylactic management of childhood headaches. *Headache* 2000;40(7):539-49.
8. Sezer T, Kandemir H, Alehan F. A randomized trial comparing amitriptyline versus topiramate for the prophylaxis of chronic daily headache in pediatric patients. *Int J Neurosci* 2013;123(8):553-6.
9. Mathew NT, Kurman R, Perez F. Drug induced refractory headache--clinical features and management. *Headache* 1990;30(10):634-8.
10. Lewis D, Ashwal S, Hershey A et al. Practice parameter: pharmacological treatment of migraine headache in children and adolescents: report of the American Academy of Neurology Quality Standards Subcommittee and the Practice Committee of the Child Neurology Society. *Neurology* 2004;63(12):2215-24.
11. Hamalainen ML, Hoppu K, Valkeila E et al. Ibuprofen or acetaminophen for the acute treatment of migraine in children: a double-blind, randomized, placebo-controlled, crossover study. *Neurology* 1997;48(1):103-7.
12. Damen L, Bruijn JK, Verhagen AP et al. Symptomatic treatment of migraine in children: a systematic review of medication trials. *Pediatrics* 2005;116(2):e295-302.
13. Termine C, Ozge A, Antonaci F et al. Overview of the diagnosis and management of pediatric headache. Part II: therapeutic management. *J Headache Pain* 2011;12(1):25-34.
14. Logan P, Lewis D. Towards evidence based emergency medicine: best BETs from the Manchester Royal Infirmary. Chlorpromazine in migraine. *Emerg Med J* 2007;24(4):297-300.
15. Iserson KV. Parenteral chlorpromazine treatment of migraine. *Ann Emerg Med* 1983;12(12):756-8.
16. Hamalainen ML, Hoppu K, Santavuori PR. Oral dihydroergotamine for therapy-resistant migraine attacks in children. *Pediatr Neurol* 1997;16(2):114-7.
17. Linder SL. Treatment of childhood headache with dihydroergotamine mesylate. *Headache* 1994;34(10):578-80.
18. Eiland LS, Hunt MO. The use of triptans for pediatric migraines. *Paediatr Drugs* 2010;12(6):379-89.
19. Wöber-Bingöl Ç. Pharmacological treatment of acute migraine in adolescents and children. *Paediatr Drugs* 2013;15(3):235-46.
20. Winner P, Rothner AD, Wooten JD et al. Sumatriptan nasal spray in adolescent migraineurs: a randomized, double-blind, placebo-controlled, acute study. *Headache* 2006;46(2):212-22.
21. Winner P, Rothner AD, Saper J et al. A randomized, double-blind, placebo-controlled study of sumatriptan nasal spray in the treatment of acute migraine in adolescents. *Pediatrics* 2000;106(5):989-97.
22. Ahonen K, Hamalainen ML, Rantala H et al. Nasal sumatriptan is effective in treatment of migraine attacks in children: a randomized trial. *Neurology* 2004;62(6):883-7.
23. Sorge F, De Simone R, Marano E et al. Flunarizine in prophylaxis of childhood migraine. A double-blind, placebo-controlled, crossover study. *Cephalalgia* 1988;8(1):1-6.
24. Martinez-Lage JM. Flunarizine (Sibelium) in the prophylaxis of migraine. An open, long-term, multicenter trial. *Cephalalgia* 1988;8(Suppl 8):15-20.
25. Ludvigsson J. Propranolol used in prophylaxis of migraine in children. *Acta Neurol Scand* 1974;50(1):109-15.
26. Hershey AD, Powers SW, Bentti AL et al. Effectiveness of amitriptyline in the prophylactic management of childhood headaches. *Headache* 2000;40(7):539-49.
27. Caruso JM, Brown WD, Exil G et al. The efficacy of divalproex sodium in the prophylactic treatment of children with migraine. *Headache* 2000;40(8):672-6.
28. Serdaroglu G, Erhan E, Tekgul H et al. Sodium valproate prophylaxis in childhood migraine. *Headache* 2001;42(8):819-22.
29. Winner P, Gendolla A, Stayer C et al. Topiramate for prevention of migraine in adolescents: a pooled analysis of efficacy and safety. *Headache* 2006;46(10):1503-10.
30. Lakshmi CV, Singhi P, Malhi P et al. Topiramate in the prophylaxis of pediatric migraine: a double-blind placebo-controlled trial. *J Child Neurol* 2007;22(7):829-35.
31. Condo M, Posar A, Arbizzani A et al. Riboflavin prophylaxis in pediatric and adolescent migraine. *J Headache Pain* 2009;10(5):361-5.

Neurologic Disorders

Chapter 19
Multiple Sclerosis

Michael Namaka, BSc Pharm, MSc Pharm, PhD
Karen Ethans, MD, FRCPC, PM&R and
Farid Esfahani, MD

Pathophysiology

Multiple sclerosis (MS) is a chronic neurologic disorder characterized by targeted destruction of central nervous system (CNS) myelin, as well as axonal degeneration and loss. The precise pathogenic mechanisms are not clearly understood, but in the early stages neural damage is thought to result from immune-mediated destruction of myelin.[1] The most widely accepted theory of what triggers MS involves an autoimmune response to a foreign molecule with a structure similar to a component of CNS myelin.[2] MS is now proposed to be a biphasic disease consisting of an initial focal inflammatory phase, followed later by a primarily degenerative phase, with inflammation that is more diffuse.[3]

As a result of demyelination, the propagation of electrical nerve signals is interrupted, leading to a vast array of clinical symptoms including numbness, weakness, fatigue, cognitive difficulties, ataxia, optic neuritis, bowel/bladder abnormalities and neuropathic pain.[4] The areas of eroded myelin along CNS axonal tracts are referred to as lesions or plaques. Though early acute lesions often have the ability to remyelinate, repeated insult or severe initial insult leads to chronic lesions.[5,6,7] The ultimate failure to repair demyelinated lesions and the axonal loss result in the neurologic deficits characteristic of MS.

Prevalence

The global prevalence of MS is an estimated 2–2.5 million cases, distributed unevenly throughout the world. Prevalence ranges from 5 cases per 100 000 in tropical areas such as Asia, to 100–200 cases per 100 000 in temperate areas such as Northern Europe, United States, Canada, New Zealand and parts of Australia. Canada has the fifth highest prevalence of MS in the world. The prairie and the Atlantic provinces have higher rates compared to other provinces. Women are more than twice as likely to develop MS, though men generally have a worse prognosis, owing to their greater tendency to develop the primary progressive form of MS.[8] Childhood exposure to various environmental factors may also play a role in the development of MS later in life. For example, it has been shown that people who emigrate to a new country/region before age 15 acquire the new region's susceptibility to MS; conversely, if emigration takes place after age 15, susceptibility to MS is retained from the country/region of origin.[9]

Etiology

No specific gene has been directly linked to MS; however, first-degree relatives of people with MS are at an approximately 5% increased risk of developing the disease.[10] Some research scientists postulate that MS develops because of a genetic predisposition to mount an immune response to an environmental stimulus. The environmental factor most likely to be associated with MS susceptibility is low sunlight exposure/vitamin D synthesis,[11] which may explain the greater incidence of MS at higher latitudes.[12] Viral infections such as measles, canine distemper virus, human herpesvirus and Epstein-Barr virus (EBV) are also potential risk factors for MS.[13] Other factors such as dietary fat, antioxidants, nutrition and hormones have also been implicated.[14]

Disease Course

The clinical presentation of MS is highly individualized. Four basic types of MS are identified: i) relapsing remitting (RRMS); ii) primary progressive (PPMS); iii) secondary progressive (SPMS); and iv) progressive relapsing (PRMS). Most patients (80%) present with an initial acute episode known as a clinically isolated syndrome. Various sets of criteria have been proposed for making an accurate diagnosis of MS, differing slightly in with respect to the timing and location of recurrent episodes.[15,16] The most widely accepted are the McDonald criteria, most recently revised in 2010.[15] In about 10–20% of cases, the disease is progressive from the outset. PPMS may involve temporary minor improvements but is steadily progressive. PRMS is characterized by a progressive course from the outset with clear, superimposed, acute relapses but continued progression between relapses. The vast majority of cases (85–90%) follow a relapsing remitting course at onset. Approximately 65% of patients with RRMS develop secondary progressive MS beginning around 15–20 years from the onset of their disease, usually around the age of 40.[17]

Goals of Therapy

- Reduce the number, severity and duration of MS attacks with demonstrated improvements on MRI and brain atrophy measures
- Slow relapse-related disease progression and delay time to permanent disability
- Improve quality of life

Investigations

Investigations are guided by clinical presentation and may be more extensive or limited depending on how clearly the history, physical examination and MRI indicate multiple sclerosis.

- Complete blood count with differential
- Liver function tests (ALT, AST)
- Antinuclear antibody, rheumatoid factor and C-reactive protein
- Thyroid-stimulating hormone
- Vitamin D levels
- Vitamin B_{12} (deficiency can mimic MS symptoms)
- MRI ± gadolinium to identify and quantify lesions in brain and/or spinal cord
- Cerebrospinal fluid exam for oligoclonal banding and visual evoked potential, to support the diagnosis
- Complete neurologic exam

Therapeutic Choices

Nonpharmacologic Choices

There are currently no nonpharmacologic treatment strategies that affect the disease course of RRMS, but some symptoms may be improved through the use of nonpharmacologic measures.[18] For example: physiotherapy and stretching are used to help manage spasticity and gait disturbances; fluid intake restriction and pelvic floor exercises can be helpful for bladder symptoms; surgical interventions such as stereotactic thalamotomy or deep brain stimulation may benefit patients with localized tremor; respiratory training may improve inspiratory and expiratory muscle strength in patients with mild to moderate dysfunction.

The potential role of chronic cerebrospinal venous insufficiency (CCSVI) as a causative factor for MS has generated interest in the news media. CCSVI is a state of chronically impaired venous drainage from the CNS. Work done by a group in Italy indicated that a procedure involving endovascular balloon angioplasty or stent placement provided significant relief for patients with MS.[19,20] Significant limitations to this study (lack of investigator blinding or proper control groups) and negative outcomes associated with vascular stents put the validity of this therapy into question.[21] Subsequent studies (including one large Canadian study)[22] have indicated that CCSVI is not associated with MS, revealing no significant difference in the cerebral and cervical venous drainage between patients with MS and healthy subjects.[23,22] Further, MS patients who do have CCSVI do not appear to have more severe symptoms than MS patients without CCSVI.[24]

Pharmacologic Choices

Although there is no known cure for MS, several disease-modifying therapies have been shown to reduce the rate of relapses in RRMS, which may ultimately reduce/delay disease progression. Disease-modifying therapies have little or no effect on primary or secondary progressive MS, except in cases of progressive disease where frequent relapses continue to occur.

Short courses of high-dose **corticosteroids**, e.g., **methylprednisolone** 1 g iv daily for 3–5 days possibly followed by tapering doses of oral prednisone for several days,[25] are sometimes used to reduce the severity and duration of acute relapses but do not alter the disease course. The optimal dose and route of administration have not been established, and varied protocols are in use across the spectrum of care delivery centres.[26]

This discussion will focus on disease-modifying therapies for MS (Table 2, Figure 1). Information on management of various MS-related symptoms or associated conditions can be found in Chapter 4, Chapter 6, Chapter 11, Chapter 16, Chapter 21, Chapter 68 and Chapter 74.

First-line Disease-modifying Therapies

Glatiramer

Glatiramer acetate is an immunomodulator with effects similar to interferon beta on reduction in relapse rates and MRI-detectable lesion burden in RRMS.[4,27] Its proposed mechanism of action involves inhibition of myelin reactive T cells, decreased T cell proliferation and decreased interferon-γ secretion.[28,29,30] Glatiramer has also demonstrated neuroprotective effects linked to increased brain-derived neurotrophic factor (BDNF) expression, though the exact mechanism remains unclear.[31,32] A review by the Cochrane Multiple Sclerosis group concluded that glatiramer reduces relapse rates in patients with RRMS but fails to prevent disease progression.[33] Glatiramer has no effect on primary or secondary progressive MS. Overall, glatiramer is well tolerated with few side effects, most notably a rare, acute, transient, postinjection reaction with flushing, chest tightness, palpitations and dyspnea.[34]

Interferons

Interferon beta is a standard first-line therapy option in the treatment of MS. Interferon therapy reduces the frequency of relapses and the size/number of lesions detectable on MRI,[35,36] and reduces the rate of conversion to clinically definite MS following an initial clinically isolated syndrome from 45–50% to 28–35% over 2–3 years.[37,38,39] Whether interferon therapy delays onset of the progressive phase of the disease or slows progression of disability in patients with secondary progressive MS is uncertain.[40,41]

Studies suggest several potential mechanisms of action in MS.[28,29,42,43] The most common side effects associated with interferon treatment include local injection site reactions and flu-like symptoms.[44] The development of neutralizing antibodies can diminish the clinical response to interferon therapy.[35,36] Serious hepatotoxicity occurs rarely.

Figure 1: **Management of Multiple Sclerosis**

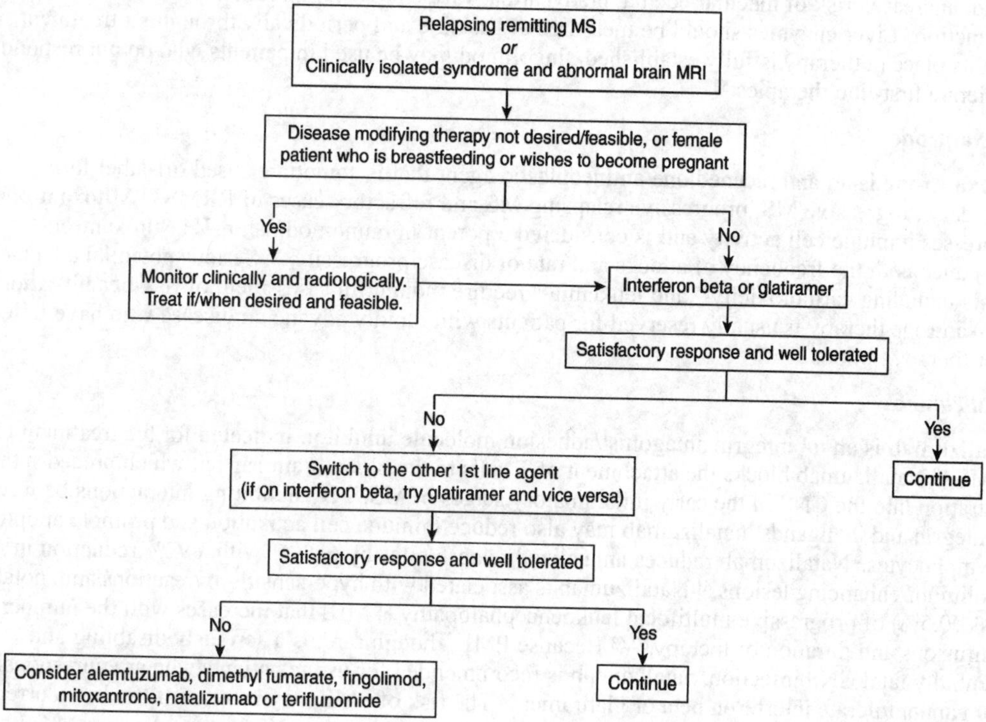

Abbreviations: MS = multiple sclerosis

Alternative Disease-modifying Therapies

Alemtuzumab

Alemtuzumab is a monoclonal antibody that binds to CD52 on activated lymphocytes and targets their destruction, leading to a reduction in relapse rates and sustained accumulation of disability in patients with RRMS. Alemtuzumab was associated with a 50% greater reduction in relapse rates compared to interferon beta.[45,46] Adverse effects include infusion reactions, infection and emergent autoimmunity, mainly affecting the thyroid gland.

Dimethyl Fumarate

Dimethyl fumarate is an oral agent for management of RRMS. Though its exact mechanism of action is unknown, dimethyl fumarate activates the nuclear factor (erythroid-derived 2)-like 2 (Nrf2) pathway, which is involved in the cellular response to oxidative stress. Dimethyl fumarate has been shown to decrease the proportion of patients who had relapsed at 2 years by around 40%, reduce the annualized relapse rate by 53% and decrease the number of new or enlarging brain lesions.[47,48] An exploratory comparison showed no significant differences between dimethyl fumarate and glatiramer.[47] Common side effects include flushing, nausea, vomiting, diarrhea, and abdominal pain. Decreased lymphocytes, proteinuria and increased liver enzymes can also occur.

Fingolimod

Fingolimod is a sphingosine-1-phosphate receptor agonist that blocks the egress of activated, presumably autoimmune lymphocytes into the circulating bloodstream from lymphoid tissues.[49] Phase

III clinical trials showed oral fingolimod was well tolerated and effective in reducing annualized relapse rates by ~50% and MRI-detected inflammatory activity in patients with RRMS.[50,51] Precautions include increased risk of macular edema, bradycardia, varicella-zoster infection and reversible hepatic dysfunction. Liver enzymes should be measured at baseline and periodically throughout treatment. Until its place in therapy is fully established, fingolimod may be used in patients who do not respond to or tolerate first-line therapies.[52]

Mitoxantrone

Mitoxantrone is an anthracenedione antineoplastic agent that is sometimes used off-label for secondary progressive MS, progressive relapsing MS and refractory cases of RRMS.[53] Mitoxantrone suppresses immune cell activity and is considered a potent immunomodulator.[53,54] Mitoxantrone can reduce both the frequency of attacks and rate of disease progression.[53] Serious potential adverse effects including cardiotoxicity[55] and leukemia[56] require thoughtful assessment of risk-benefit ratio. Mitoxantrone therapy is usually reserved for patients with rapidly advancing disease who have failed other therapy options.[57]

Natalizumab

Natalizumab is an α4 integrin antagonist/adhesion molecule inhibitor, indicated for the treatment of RRMS.[58] Natalizumab blocks the attachment of T cells to the blood brain barrier, which precedes their infiltration into the CNS in the early inflammatory stages of MS.[59] By inhibiting interactions between α4 integrin and its ligands, natalizumab may also reduce immune cell activation and promote apoptosis of lymphocytes. Natalizumab reduces annualized relapse rates by 68%,[60] with a 92% reduction in gadolinium-enhancing lesions.[61] Natalizumab is associated with hypersensitivity reactions and, notably, a risk (0.5%) of progressive multifocal leukoencephalopathy (PML) that increases with the number of infusions and duration of therapy.[62,63] Because PML, though rare, is a seriously disabling and potentially fatal CNS infection, natalizumab is recommended for use in patients who are unresponsive to or cannot tolerate interferon beta or glatiramer.[64] The risk of PML may increase if used concurrently with or subsequent to interferon beta or other immunomodulating drugs.[63]

Teriflunomide

Teriflunomide is an oral immune modulator that reduces T- and B-cell activity through inhibition of dihydroorotate dehydrogenase-mediated pyrimidine synthesis. Teriflunomide has been shown to reduce the annualized relapse rate by approximately 50% and the proportion of patients with confirmed disease progression by about 25% in clinical trials.[65,66,67]

Adjunctive Therapies

Fampridine

Fampridine (4-aminopyridine) is approved in Canada to improve walking ability in patients with MS. As a selective blocker of a subset of voltage-activated potassium channels with little or no effect on sodium or calcium channels, fampridine directly targets the nervous system, apparently by increasing the ability of action potentials to traverse demyelinated areas of the axon without losing strength.[68] A phase III study using sustained-release oral fampridine showed significantly greater improvement in walking speed compared to placebo (35% vs. 8%).[69]

Choices during Pregnancy and Breastfeeding

Multiple Sclerosis and Pregnancy

Women diagnosed with MS who become pregnant have been reported to have a period of decreased disease activity during the course of their pregnancy.[70,71] This phenomenon has been observed in other immune-mediated disease states such as rheumatoid arthritis, and is believed to result from changes in the immune system that are necessary to prevent an immune response to the non-self tissue of the fetus.[72] However, following delivery of the baby, patients are more likely to experience a relapse, particularly if relapse rate prior to pregnancy was high.[73] Although several studies have attempted to pharmacologically mimic the hormonal fluctuations believed to be responsible for the quiescence of MS during pregnancy, results have been inconclusive.[74] One series of clinical trials showed a beneficial effect of sex hormone therapy in female patients with clinically definite MS. An equal number of patients with relapsing remitting and secondary progressive disease were recruited, with a mean age of 44 years and a mean expanded disability status scale (EDSS)[75] score of 3.3. The study showed a significant reduction in both T helper cells and inflammatory markers of disease activity in patients treated with estradiol.[76]

Management of Multiple Sclerosis during Pregnancy

The use of immunosuppressive or immunomodulator agents in pregnancy is not routinely advised.[77] **Teriflunomide**, the active metabolite of leflunomide, is contraindicated in pregnancy and in women of childbearing potential who are not using reliable birth control. Women who become pregnant while taking teriflunomide are advised to undergo a drug washout regimen using **cholestyramine** to enhance elimination. Details of this procedure may be found in Chapter 87.

Though there are no definitive guidelines recommending the discontinuation of other immunomodulators prior to conception, clinical experience and anecdotal reports generally support stopping therapy 2–3 months prior to conception.[78] This precautionary recommendation applies to both men and women with MS who are considering starting a family. Though studies of small numbers of pregnant women have suggested the use of **interferon beta** or **glatiramer** during pregnancy is not linked to an increased risk of birth defects,[79,80,81] the treating physician and patient must always weigh the potential risks and benefits associated with treatment during pregnancy.

Multiple Sclerosis and Breastfeeding

Though infants can be exposed to immunomodulating agents via breast milk, a significant risk associated with breastfeeding during immunomodulator therapy has not been reported.[78] Because breastfeeding during the postpartum period may actually have a protective effect to the mother in terms of relapse,[82] most clinicians favour the cessation of immunomodulator treatment during breastfeeding to avoid possible adverse effects on the developing infant.[83] Corticosteroids can be used for acute relapses if necessary.[84]

A discussion of general principles on the use of medications in these special populations can be found in Appendix II and Appendix III. Other specialized reference sources are also provided in these appendices.

Therapeutic Tips

- RRMS is the most common form of MS and is most likely to respond to immunomodulator therapy.
- Though there is no cure for the disease, the decision to treat early with immunomodulator therapy is associated with improved long-term neurologic outcomes and quality of life when compared to no treatment.[39]
- All MS patients able to tolerate vitamin D should commence therapy with a supplement (at least 1000 IU per day), especially if their levels are low. While there is little evidence of benefit from vitamin D supplementation for MS, there are other potential benefits and no known risk of harm.
- Start treatment with the endpoint in mind, understanding the strengths and limitations of each therapy. For example, disease-modifying therapies are not effective for progressive patients without relapse, and MS-specific therapy may not be required for patients with a history of clinically or radiologically isolated syndrome who remain stable clinically and radiographically.

Table 1: First-line Disease-modifying Therapies for Multiple Sclerosis

Class	Drug	Dose	Adverse Effects	Drug Interactions	Cost[a]
Immune Modulators	*glatiramer* Copaxone	20 mg daily sc	Injection site pain, post-injection reaction, flushing, chest pain, anxiety, hypertonia, joint pain, weakness, nausea, palpitations.	No serious interactions reported.	$1402
	interferon beta-1a Avonex, Rebif	Rebif: 8.8 μg 3 times weekly × 2 wk sc, then 22 μg 3 times weekly × 2 wk sc, then 44 μg 3 times weekly sc Avonex: 30 μg weekly im	Flu-like symptoms such as fever, chills, myalgias; injection site reactions; depression, fatigue, headache; neutralizing antibodies. Elevated liver enzymes (serious hepatotoxicity rare), decreased platelets, pancytopenia, hypertension, tachycardia.	May lessen immune response to live vaccines.	Avonex: $1655 Rebif (44 μg 3 times/wk): $1976
	interferon beta-1b Betaseron, Extavia	0.25 mg (8×10^6 IU) every second day sc	See interferon beta-1a.		Betaseron: $1976 Extavia: $1565

[a] Cost of 4-week (28-day) supply at usual dose. Prices reflect acquisition cost in Ottawa at time of publishing and include no mark-ups or fees. Costs may vary among provinces.

Table 2: **Alternative Disease-modifying Therapies for Multiple Sclerosis**

Class	Drug	Dose	Adverse Effects	Drug Interactions	Cost[a]
Adhesion Molecule Inhibitors	*natalizumab* Tysabri	300 mg Q4 wk iv	Headache, fatigue, arthralgias, infection, depression, increased liver enzymes. Progressive multifocal leukoencephalopathy (rare but potentially fatal).	Combined therapy with interferon beta-1a (Avonex) has increased natalizumab levels by 30%.	$3235
Antiproliferative Agents	*mitoxantrone* generics	12 mg/m^2 Q3 months iv Maximum: cumulative dose of 100–140 mg/m^2 or treatment duration of 2–3 y	Nausea, anxiety, fatigue, menstrual disturbances, alopecia, infection, blue-green discoloration of urine, sclera for 24 h post treatment. Cardiac toxicity (systolic dysfunction, heart failure; risk increases with higher cumulative dose).	Decreased immune response to vaccines.	$350[b]
Anti-CD52 Monoclonal Antibodies	*alemtuzumab* Lemtrada	Initial course: 12 mg daily iv × 5 days Second course, 12 months after first: 12 mg daily iv × 3 days	Infusion reactions (headache, rash, fever, nausea, urticaria, pruritus), autoimmunity (e.g., (thrombocytopenic purpura, anti-glomerular basement membrane disease, Grave's hyperthyroidism), infection (potentially serious). Antiviral prophylaxis recommended. Progressive multifocal leukoencephalopathy (rare but potentially fatal).	Avoid live vaccines.	$10500/ 12 mg vial
Immune Modulators	*dimethyl fumarate* Tecfidera	Initial dose: 120 mg bid po × 7 days Usual dose: 240 mg bid po	Gastrointestinal (nausea, vomiting, diarrhea, abdominal pain), flushing, decreased lymphocytes, decreased liver enzymes, proteinuria. Monitor CBC, liver function, urinalysis.	Avoid live vaccines.	$1854

(cont'd)

Table 2: **Alternative Disease-modifying Therapies for Multiple Sclerosis** *(cont'd)*

Class	Drug	Dose	Adverse Effects	Drug Interactions	Cost[a]
	fingolimod Gilenya	0.5 mg daily po	Bradyarrhythmias (baseline ECG if not available from previous 6 months; monitor patient for at least 6 h following first dose; first-dose monitoring should be repeated if treatment is interrupted for ≥1 day within the first 2 wk, for ≥7 days during weeks 3 and 4, or for >2 wk after the first month of therapy); QT_c interval prolongation; infection (baseline CBC if not available from previous 6 mo); increased liver enzymes; macular edema; decreased blood pressure following first dose, increased blood pressure with ongoing therapy.	Avoid live vaccines during fingolimod therapy and for 2 months after. Caution with strong inhibitors of CYP3A4 or CYP4F2 such as ketoconazole (increased fingolimod exposure). Caution with other drugs that can prolong the QTc interval such as amiodarone, azithromycin, chlorpromazine, clarithromycin, erythromycin, fluoxetine, haloperidol, lithium, methadone, quinidine, tricyclic antidepressants, venlafaxine.	$2504
Pyrimidine Synthesis Inhibitors	*teriflunomide* Aubagio	14 mg once daily po	Elevated hepatic enzymes, potential for more serious liver toxicity. Monitor hepatic enzymes at baseline and monthly for at least 6 months after initiating teriflunomide. Animal date suggest potential teratogenic risk; contraindicated in pregnancy. Wash-out protocol using cholestyramine to enhance elimination can be used to minimize exposure in patients with suspected liver damage or women who become pregnant while taking teriflunomide. See Chapter 87 for details. Alopecia, diarrhea, hypertension, neutropenia, paresthesias, rash.	BRCP efflux transporter inhibitors such as cyclosporine, eltombopag or gefitinib may increase teriflunomide exposure. Decreased INR in patients taking warfarin; monitor closely. Avoid live vaccines. Do not use with leflunomide, pimecrolimus, tacrolimus.	$1571

[a] Cost of 4-week (28-day) supply at usual dose unless otherwise specified. Prices reflect acquisition cost in Ottawa at time of publishing and include no mark-ups or fees. Costs may vary among provinces.
[b] Based on 3 months' therapy in a person with body surface area of 1.73 m².

Table 3: Adjunctive Therapy for Multiple Sclerosis

Class	Drug	Dose	Adverse Effects	Drug Interactions	Cost[a]
Potassium Channel Blockers	*fampridine* ◗ Fampyra	10 mg Q12H po Swallow whole with glass of water; do not take with food Assess improvement in walking ability after 4 wk; discontinue if no benefit Advise patients not to take doses less than 12 h apart; missed doses should not be taken late; omit the missed dose, and resume with the next scheduled dose	Dose-related increased risk of seizures; avoid in patients with renal impairment or history of seizures; do not exceed usual dose. Urinary tract infection; insomnia; dizziness; headache; nausea; balance disorder; paresthesia; weakness.	Decreased fampridine clearance/increased risk of seizures may result from concurrent use of organic cation transporter (OCT2) inhibitors such as cimetidine or quinidine, or OCT2 substrates such as carvedilol, metformin, pindolol, procainamide, propranolol, ranitidine, varenicline.	$550

[a] Cost of 4-week (28-day) supply at usual dose; includes drug cost only. Prices reflect acquisition cost in Ottawa at time of publishing and include no mark-ups or fees. Costs may vary among provinces.

◗ Dosage adjustment may be required in renal impairment; see Appendix I.

Suggested Readings

Houtchens MK. Pregnancy and multiple sclerosis. *Semin Neurol* 2007;27(5):434-41.

Kappos L, Bates D, Hartung HP et al. Natalizumab treatment for multiple sclerosis: recommendations for patient selection and monitoring. *Lancet Neurol* 2007;6(5):431-41.

Namaka M, Turcotte D, Leong C et al. Multiple sclerosis: etiology and treatment strategies. *Consult Pharm* 2008;23(11):886-96.

Ozenci V, Kouwenhoven M, Link H. Cytokines in multiple sclerosis: methodological aspects and pathogenic implications. *Mult Scler* 2002;8(5):396-404.

Thompson AJ, Toosy AT, Ciccarelli O. Pharmacological management of symptoms in multiple sclerosis: current approaches and future directions. *Lancet Neurol* 2010;9(12):1182-99.

References

1. Korn T. Pathophysiology of multiple sclerosis. *J Neurol* 2008;255(Suppl 6):2-6.
2. Alto M, Kapoor S, Simms L et al. Molecular mimicry and multiple sclerosis. *Neural Regen Res*, 2011;6(17):1322-33.
3. Ludwin SK. The pathogenesis of multiple sclerosis: relating human pathology to experimental studies. *J Neuropathol Exp Neurol* 2006;65(4):305-18.
4. Namaka M, Turcotte D, Leong C et al. Multiple sclerosis: etiology and treatment strategies. *Consult Pharm* 2008;23(11):886-96.
5. Frost EE, Nielsen JA, Le TQ et al. PDGF and FGF2 regulate oligodendrocyte progenitor responses to demyelination. *J Neurobiol* 2003;54(3):457-72.
6. Albert M, Antel J, Bruck W et al. Extensive cortical remyelination in patients with chronic multiple sclerosis. *Brain Pathol* 2007;17(2):129-38.
7. Patani R, Balaratnam M, Vora A et al. Remyelination can be extensive in multiple sclerosis despite a long disease course. *Neuropathol Appl Neurobiol* 2007;33(3):277-87.
8. Kantarci O, Wingerchuk D. Epidemiology and natural history of multiple sclerosis: new insights. *Curr Opin Neurol* 2006;19(3):248-54.
9. Compston A, Coles A. Multiple sclerosis. *Lancet* 2008;372(9648):1502-17.
10. Compston A. The genetic epidemiology of multiple sclerosis. *Philos Trans R Soc Lond B Biol Sci* 1999;354(1390):1623-34.
11. Solomon AJ, Whitham RH. Multiple sclerosis and vitamin D: a review and recommendations. *Curr Neurol Neurosci Rep* 2010;10(5):389-96.
12. Milo R, Kahana E. Multiple sclerosis: geoepidemiology, genetics and the environment. *Autoimmun Rev* 2010;9(5):A387-94.
13. Salvetti M, Giovannoni G, Aloisi F. Epstein-Barr virus and multiple sclerosis. *Curr Opin Neurol* 2009;22(3):201-6.
14. Ascherio A, Munger KL. Environmental risk factors for multiple sclerosis. Part I: the role of infection. *Ann Neurol* 2007;61(4):288-99.
15. Polman CH, Reingold SC, Banwell B et al. Diagnostic criteria for multiple sclerosis: 2010 revisions to the McDonald criteria. *Ann Neurol* 2011;69(2):292-302.
16. Montalban X, Tintore M, Swanton J et al. MRI criteria for MS in patients with clinically isolated syndromes. *Neurology* 2010;74(5):427-34.
17. Confavreux C, Vujusic S. Age at disability milestones in multiple sclerosis. *Brain* 2006;129(Pt 3):595-605.
18. Thompson AJ, Toosy AT, Ciccarelli O. Pharmacological management of symptoms in multiple sclerosis: current approaches and future directions. *Lancet Neurol* 2010;9(12):1182-99.
19. Zamboni P, Galeotti R. The chronic cerebrospinal venous insufficiency syndrome. *Phlebology* 2010;25(6):269-79.
20. Zamboni P, Galeotti R, Menegatti E et al. A prospective open label study of endovascular treatment of chronic cerebrospinal venous insufficiency. *J Vasc Surg* 2009;50(6):1348-58.e1-3.
21. Doepp F, Paul F, Valdueza JM et al. No cerebrocervical venous congestion in patients with multiple sclerosis. *Ann Neurol* 2010;68(2):173-83.
22. Traboulsee AL, Knox KB, Machan L et al. Prevalence of extracranial venous narrowing on catheter venography in people with multiple sclerosis, their siblings, and unrelated healthy controls: a blinded, case-control study. *Lancet* 2014;383(9912):138-45.
23. Experimental multiple sclerosis vascular shunting procedure halted at Stanford. *Ann Neurol* 2010;67(1):A13-5.
24. Leone C, D'Amico E, Cilia S et al. Cognitive impairment and "invisible symptoms" are not associated with CCSVI in MS. *BMC Neurol* 2013;13(1):97.
25. Shaygannejad V, Ashtari F, Alinaghian M et al. Short-term safety of pulse steroid therapy in multiple sclerosis relapses. *Clin Neuropharm* 2013;36(1):1-3.
26. Goodin DS. Glucocorticoid treatment of multiple sclerosis. *Handb Clin Neurol* 2014;122:455-64.
27. O'Connor P, Filippi M, Arnason B et al. 250 microg or 500 microg interferon beta-1b versus 20 mg glatiramer acetate in relapsing-remitting multiple sclerosis: a prospective, randomised, multicentre study. *Lancet Neurol* 2009;8(10):889-97.
28. Dhib-Jalbut S. Mechanisms of action of interferons and glatiramer acetate in multiple sclerosis. *Neurology* 2002;58(8 Suppl 4):S3-9.
29. Yong VW. Differential mechanisms of action of interferon-beta and glatiramer aetate in MS. *Neurology* 2002;59(6):802-8.
30. Greenstein JI. Current concepts of the cellular and molecular pathophysiology of multiple sclerosis. *Dev Neurobiol* 2007;67(9):1248-65.
31. Arnon R, Aharoni R. Neuroprotection and neurogeneration in MS and its animal model EAE effected by glatiramer acetate. *J Neural Transm* 2009;116(11):1443-9.
32. Aharoni R, Eilam R, Domev H et al. The immunomodulator glatiramer acetate augments the expression of neurotrophic factors in brains of experimental autoimmune encephalomyelitis mice. *Proc Natl Acad Sci U S A* 2005;102(52):19045-50.
33. La Mantia L, Munari LM, Lovati R. Glatiramer acetate for multiple sclerosis. *Cochrane Database Syst Rev* 2010;(5):CD004678.
34. Ziemssen T, Neuhaus O, Hohlfeld R. Risk-benefit assessment of glatiramer acetate in multiple sclerosis. *Drug Saf* 2001;24(13):979-90.
35. Interferon beta-1b is effective in relapsing-remitting multiple sclerosis. I. Clinical results of a multicenter, randomized, double-blind, placebo-controlled trial. The IFNB Multiple Sclerosis Study Group. *Neurology* 1993;43(4):655-61.
36. Paty DW, Li DK. Interferon beta-1b is effective in relapsing-remitting multiple sclerosis. II. MRI analysis results of a multicenter, randomized, double-blind, placebo-controlled trial. UBC MS/MRI Study Group and the IFNB Multiple Sclerosis Study Group. *Neurology* 1993;43(4):662-7.
37. Jacobs LD, Beck RW, Simon JH et al. Intramuscular interferon beta-1a initiated during a first demyelinating event in multiple sclerosis. CHAMPS Study Group. *N Engl J Med* 2000;343(13):898-904.
38. Comi G, Filippi M, Barkhof F et al. Effect of early interferon treatment on conversion to definite multiple sclerosis: a randomised study. *Lancet* 2001;357(9268):1576-82.

39. Kappos L, Freedman MS, Polman CH et al. Effect of early versus delayed interferon beta-1b treatment on disability after a first clinical event suggestive of multiple sclerosis: a 3-year follow-up analysis of the BENEFIT study. *Lancet* 2007;370(9585):389-97.
40. Kappos L, Polman C, Pozzilli C et al. Final analysis of the European multicenter trial on IFNbeta-1b in secondary-progressive MS. *Neurology* 2001;57(11):1969-75.
41. Panitch H, Miller A, Paty D et al. Interferon beta-1b in secondary progressive MS: results from a 3-year controlled study. *Neurology* 2004;63(10):1788-95.
42. Airas L, Niemela J, Yegutkin G et al. Mechanism of action of IFN-beta in the treatment of multiple sclerosis: a special reference to CD73 and adenosine. *Ann N Y Acad Sci* 2007;1110:641-8
43. Kraus J, Voigt K, Schuller AM et al. Interferon-beta stabilizes barrier characteristics of the blood-brain barrier in four different species in vitro. *Mult Scler* 2008;14(6):843-52.
44. Melanson M, Grossberndt A, Klowak M et al. Fatigue and cognition in patients with relapsing multiple sclerosis treated with interferon beta. *Int J Neurosci* 2010;120(10):631-40.
45. Cohen JA, Coles AJ, Arnold DL et al. Alemtuzumab versus interferon beta 1a as first-line treatment for patients with relapsing-remitting multiple sclerosis: a randomised controlled phase 3 trial. *Lancet* 2012;380(9856):1819-28.
46. Coles AJ, Twyman CL, Arnold DL et al. Alemtuzumab for patients with relapsing multiple sclerosis after disease-modifying therapy: a randomised controlled phase 3 trial. *Lancet* 2012;380(9856):1829-39.
47. Fox RJ, Miller DH, Phillips JT et al. Placebo-controlled phase 3 study of oral BG-12 or glatiramer in multiple sclerosis. *N Engl J Med* 2012;367(12):1087-97.
48. Gold R, Kappos L, Arnold DL et al. Placebo-controlled phase 3 study of oral BG-12 for relapsing multiple sclerosis. *N Engl J Med* 2012;367(12):1098-107.
49. Horga A, Montalban X. FTY720 (fingolimod) for relapsing multiple sclerosis. *Expert Rev Neurother* 2008;8(5):699-714.
50. Kappos L, Radue EW, O'Connor P et al. A placebo-controlled trial of oral fingolimod in relapsing multiple sclerosis. *N Engl J Med* 2010;362(5):387-401.
51. Cohen JA, Barkhof F, Comi G et al. Oral fingolimod or intramuscular interferon for relapsing multiple sclerosis. *N Engl J Med* 2010;362(5):402-15.
52. Brinkmann V, Billich A, Baumruker T et al. Fingolimod (FTY720): discovery and development of an oral drug to treat multiple sclerosis. *Nat Rev Drug Discov* 2010;9(11):883-97.
53. Fox EJ. Management of worsening multiple sclerosis with mitoxantrone: a review. *Clin Ther* 2006;28(4):461-74.
54. Martinelli Boneschi F, Rovaris M, Capra R et al. Mitoxantrone for multiple sclerosis. *Cochrane Database Syst Rev* 2005;(4):CD002127.
55. Namaka MP, Turcotte DA, Klowak M et al. Early mitoxantrone-induced cardiotoxicity detected in secondary progressive multiple sclerosis. *Clin Med Insights Ther* 2011;3:449-58.
56. Marriott JJ, Miyasaki JM, Gronseth G et al. Evidence report: the efficacy and safety of mitoxantrone (Novantrone) in the treatment of multiple sclerosis: report of the Therapeutics and Technology Assessment Subcommittee of the American Academy of Neurology. *Neurology* 2010;74(18):1463-70.
57. Goodin DS, Arnason BG, Coyle PK et al. The use of mitoxantrone (Novantrone) for the treatment of multiple sclerosis: report of the Therapeutics and Technology Assessment Subcommittee of the American Academy of Neurology. *Neurology* 2003;61(10):1332-8.
58. Polman CH, O'Connor PW, Havrdova E et al. A randomized, placebo-controlled trial of natalizumab for relapsing multiple sclerosis. *N Engl J Med* 2006;354(9):899-910.
59. Correale J, Villa A. The blood-brain-barrier in multiple sclerosis: functional roles and therapeutic targeting. *Autoimmunity* 2007;40(2):148-60.
60. Polman CH, O'Connor PW, Havrdova E et al. A randomized, placebo-controlled trial of natalizumab for relapsing multiple sclerosis. *N Engl J Med* 2006;354(9):899-910.
61. Miller DH, Khan OA, Sheremata WA et al. A controlled trial of natalizumab for relapsing multiple sclerosis. *N Engl J Med* 2003;348(1):15-23.
62. Aksamit AJ. Review of progressive multifocal leukoencephalopathy and natalizumab. *Neurologist* 2006;12(6):293-8.
63. Clifford DB, De Luca A, Simpson DM et al. Natalizumab-associated progressive multifocal leukoencephalopathy in patients with multiple sclerosis: lessons from 28 cases. *Lancet Neurol* 2010;9(4):438-46.
64. Kappos L, Bates D, Hartung HP et al. Natalizumab treatment for multiple sclerosis: recommendations for patient selection and monitoring. *Lancet Neurol* 2007;6(5):431-41.
65. Freedman MS, Wolinsky JS, Wamil B et al. Teriflunomide added to interferon-beta in relapsing multiple sclerosis: a randomized phase II trial. *Neurology* 2012;78(23):1877-85.
66. O'Connor P, Wolinsky JS, Confavreux C et al. Randomized trial of oral teriflunomide for relapsing multiple sclerosis. *N Engl J Med* 2011;365(14):1293-303.
67. He D, Xu Z, Dong S et al. Teriflunomide for multiple sclerosis. *Cochrane Database Syst Rev* 2012;12:CD009882.
68. Judge SI, Bever CT. Potassium channel blockers in multiple sclerosis: neuronal Kv channels and effects of symptomatic treatment. *Pharmacol Ther* 2006;111(1):224-59.
69. Goodman AD, Brown TR, Krupp LB et al. Sustained-release oral fampridine in multiple sclerosis: a randomised, double-blind, controlled trial. *Lancet* 2009;373(9665):732-8.
70. Rinta S, Airas L, Elovaara I. Is the modulatory effect of pregnancy in multiple sclerosis associated with changes in blood apoptotic molecules? *Acta Neurol Scand* 2010;122(3):168-74.
71. Nicot A. Gender and sex hormones in multiple sclerosis pathology and therapy. *Front Biosci (Landmark Ed)* 2009;14:4477-515.
72. Chaouat G. Placental immunoregulatory factors. *J Reprod Immunol* 1987;10(3):179-88.
73. Hellwig K, Brune N, Haghikia A et al. Reproductive counselling, treatment and course of pregnancy in 73 German MS patients. *Acta Neurol Scand* 2008;118(1):24-8.
74. Vukusic S, Confavreux C. [Multiple sclerosis and pregnancy]. *Rev Neurol (Paris)* 2006;162(3):299-309. [French].
75. Kurtzke JF. Rating neurologic impairment in multiple sclerosis: an expanded disability status scale (EDSS). *Neurology* 1983;33(11):1444-52.
76. Sicotte NL, Liva SM, Klutch R et al. Treatment of multiple sclerosis with the pregnancy hormone estriol. *Ann Neurol* 2002;52(4):421-8.
77. Houtchens MK. Pregnancy and multiple sclerosis. *Semin Neurol* 2007;27(5):434-41.
78. Moreau T, Brunot S, Couvreur G et al. [Pregnancy and multiple sclerosis]. *Presse Med* 2010;39(3):389-94. [French].
79. Amato MP, Portaccio E, Ghezzi A et al. Pregnancy and fetal outcomes after interferon-β exposure in multiple sclerosis. *Neurology* 2010;75(20):1794-802.
80. Fragoso YD, Finkelsztejn A, Kaimen-Maciel DR et al. Long-term use of glatiramer acetate by 11 pregnant women with multiple sclerosis: a retrospective, multicentre case series. *CNS Drugs* 2010;24(11):969-76.

81. De Las Heras V, De Andres C, Tellez N et al. Pregnancy in multiple sclerosis patients treated with immunomodulators prior to or during part of the pregnancy: a descriptive study in the Spanish population. *Mult Scler* 2007;13(8):981-4.
82. Hellwig K, Haghikia A, Agne H et al. Protective effect of breastfeeding in postpartum relapse rate of mothers with multiple sclerosis. *Arch Neurol* 2009;66(12):1580-1.
83. Gulick EE, Johnson S. Infant health of mothers with multiple sclerosis. *West J Nurs Res* 2004;26(6):632-49.
84. Houtchens MK, Kolb CM. Multiple sclerosis and pregnancy: therapeutic considerations. *J Neurol* 2013;260(5):1202-14.

Chapter 20
Muscle Cramps

Virginia Devonshire, MD, FRCPC

Muscle cramps are sudden, involuntary contractions of one or more muscle groups that are caused by hyperexcitability of the anterior horn cells or peripheral nerves that subserve them. A common condition that occurs more frequently in older patients, cramps are typically painful in nature and can last up to a quarter of an hour. In many cases, cramps recur multiple times and leave residual pain. Common cramps often occur at rest (usually at night, involving the calf or foot) or after overuse of a muscle. The cause is usually unknown but muscle cramps have been associated with acute extracellular volume depletion (diarrhea, vomiting, excessive sweating; "heat cramps"), medications, metabolic disorders including hormonal changes (pregnancy, hypothyroidism, uremia, liver disease), hereditary disorders and rarely, autoimmune conditions (antibodies against voltage-gated potassium channels).

Goals of Therapy

- Prevent and relieve cramps
- Avoid or minimize side effects of pharmacologic therapy

Investigations

- Check for contributing factors such as excessive muscle use, acute volume depletion.
- Perform laboratory tests for BUN, creatinine, sodium, potassium, magnesium, phosphorus, calcium, thyroid, glucose and CK.
- Check for iatrogenic causes[1] such as diuretics, angiotensin receptor blockers, lithium, cyclosporine, nifedipine, cholesterol-lowering agents, salbutamol, donepezil, phenothiazines, raloxifene and alcohol.
- Consider a possible underlying pathology if cramps occur in unusual muscle groups or during activities, or if they occur in the setting of weakness, muscular atrophy/fasciculations or sensory symptoms, though some (i.e., cramp-fasciculation syndrome) may still be benign.
  - electromyography to rule out motor neuron disease or peripheral neuropathy
- Differentiate from spasms, spasticity, dystonia (co-contraction of agonist/antagonist muscles during a movement or posture), restless legs, tetany or myalgias. Assess for peripheral vascular disease as it can have symptoms that present as leg cramps.

Therapeutic Choices

Nonpharmacologic Choices

Reassure patients of the benign nature of cramps. Nonpharmacologic approaches should be the mainstay of treatment. Most cramps can be relieved by stretching the affected muscle. For calf cramps, the patient stands two feet from a wall and leans into the wall, stretching the Achilles tendon. Fluid imbalances can be corrected, and regular stretching may be of benefit in preventing cramps.

Pharmacologic Choices

For decades **quinine sulfate** has been used "off-label" to manage nocturnal leg cramps (see Table 1). Its proposed mechanism of action involves decreasing the responsiveness of the motor endplate to nerve stimulation and increasing the muscle refractory period. The American Academy of Neurology reported that there is good evidence to show that quinine is modestly effective in the treatment of muscle cramps.[2] However, health regulators worldwide, including Health Canada, have received numerous reports of adverse reactions even at lower doses.[3] Many of the cases reported were for serious or life-threatening side effects such as thrombocytopenia, Stevens-Johnson syndrome, vasculitis and cardiac arrhythmias. Severe thrombocytopenia has occurred within days or after months of use. Other adverse effects such as tinnitus, headache, nausea, visual or gait disturbances and abdominal pain were also reported. Quinine is not recommended for the routine management of nocturnal leg cramps [Evidence: SORT C*].[2] When other measures have failed in patients with severe symptoms, a trial of quinine (200–300 mg QHS for 4–6 weeks) may be reasonable provided that the patient is properly monitored and informed of the risks [Evidence: SORT B*].[4] Treatment should be interrupted every 3 months to assess further need.[5]

There is minimal evidence for other therapies for leg cramps. A crossover trial of **vitamin E** failed to show any benefit.[6] Results for **magnesium** therapy (300–900 mg per day) have been mixed.[7,8] Small, randomized, double-blind or cross-over studies have shown potential benefit of **diltiazem** 30 mg daily[9] or **vitamin B complex**.[10] Open-labelled trials of **gabapentin**[11] and **verapamil**[12] showed some potential benefit. These studies are of insufficient sample size to allow for recommendation of the respective therapies; therefore, risk-benefit analysis must guide therapy for individual patients.

Therapeutic Tips

- Nocturnal leg cramps (almost exclusively calf cramps) are common in the later stages of pregnancy. Generally these are best managed with stretching, but vitamin B complex supplementation could be considered.
- Check patient's medication history carefully to rule out drug-related causes before treating cramps.
- Use **quinine** cautiously, only if cramps are frequent and severe and nonpharmacologic measures have failed.
- Advise patients to report any signs of unusual bleeding (e.g., nosebleeds, bleeding gums, blood in the urine/stool, easy bruising or petechiae) to a healthcare professional immediately.
- Regularly reassess use of **quinine**, as cramps can resolve spontaneously or after a short duration of therapy.
- Cramps rarely need referral unless associated with other neurologic complaints or signs.

---

* SORT (Strength of Recommendation Taxonomy) is a rating system (A, B or C) that addresses the quality of available evidence. For more information consult **How to Use *Compendium of Therapeutic Choices*** on page xxv.

Table 1: Drugs Used in the Management of Nocturnal Leg Cramps

Class	Drug	Dose	Adverse Effects	Drug Interactions	Comments	Cost[a]
Cinchona Alkaloids	*quinine sulfate* generics	For patients with severe symptoms in whom other measures have failed: trial of 200–300 mg QHS po × 4–6 wk May continue if beneficial and well tolerated	Headache, dizziness, tinnitus, gait disturbances, visual impairment, cardiac arrhythmias, potentially fatal thrombocytopenia.	May potentiate effect of warfarin; monitor INR. May decrease digoxin clearance. Ketoconazole may reduce quinine clearance and increase toxicity. Rifampin may increase quinine clearance.	Advise patients of potential risks and monitor for serious side effects. With ongoing use, withdraw therapy every 3 months to reassess need.	$

[a] Cost of 30-day supply; includes drug cost only.
Legend: $ $5–15

Suggested Readings

Butler JV, Mulkerrin EC, O'Keeffe ST. Nocturnal leg cramps in older people. *Postgrad Med J* 2002;78(924):596-8.

Katzberg HD, Khan AH, So YT. Assessment: symptomatic treatment for muscle cramps (an evidence-based review): report of the Therapeutics and Technology Assessment Subcommittee of the American Academy of Neurology. *Neurology* 2010;74(8):691-6.

MedicineNet.com. *Muscle cramps facts*. San Clemente (CA): MedicineNet; reviewed 2012. Available from: www.medicinenet.com/muscle_cramps/article.htm. Accessed Jan 27, 2014.

References

1. Conforti A, Chiamulera C, Moretti U et al. Musculoskeletal adverse drug reactions: a review of literature and data from ADR spontaneous reporting databases. *Curr Drug Saf* 2007;2(1):47-63.
2. Katzberg HD, Khan AH, So YT. Assessment: symptomatic treatment for muscle cramps (an evidence-based review): report of the therapeutics and technology assessment subcommittee of the American academy of neurology. *Neurology* 2010;74(8):691-6.
3. Younger-Lewis C. Quinine sulfate and serious adverse reactions. *Can Adverse React Newsl* 2011;21(2):5. Available from: hc-sc.gc.ca/dhp-mps/medeff/bulletin/carn-bcei_v21n2-eng.php.
4. El-Tawil S, Al Musa T, Valli H et al. Quinine for muscle cramps. *Cochrane Database Syst Rev* 2010;(12):CD005044.
5. Coppin RJ, Wicke DM, Little PS. Managing nocturnal leg cramps–calf-stretching exercises and cessation of quinine treatment: a factorial randomized controlled trial. *Br J Gen Pract* 2005;55(512):186-91.
6. Connolly PS, Shirley EA, Wasson JH et al. Treatment of nocturnal leg cramps. A crossover trial of quinine vs vitamin E. *Arch Intern Med* 1992;152(9):1877-80.
7. Frusso R, Zarate M, Augustovski F et al. Magnesium for the treatment of nocturnal leg cramps: a crossover randomized trial. *J Fam Pract* 1999;48(11):868-71.
8. Roffe C, Sills S, Crome P et al. Randomised, cross-over, placebo controlled trial of magnesium citrate in the treatment of chronic persistent leg cramps. *Med Sci Monit* 2002;8(5):CR326-30.
9. Voon WC, Sheu SH. Diltiazem for nocturnal leg cramps. *Age Ageing* 2001;30(1):91-2.
10. Chan P, Huang TY, Chen YJ et al. Randomized, double-blind, placebo-controlled study of the safety and efficacy of vitamin B complex in the treatment of nocturnal leg cramps in elderly patients with hypertension. *J Clin Pharmacol* 1998;38(12):1151-4.
11. Serrao M, Rossi P, Cardinali P et al. Gabapentin treatment for muscle cramps: an open-label trial. *Clin Neuropharmacol* 2000;23(1):45-9.
12. Baltodano N, Gallo BV, Weidler DJ. Verapamil vs quinine in recumbent nocturnal leg cramps in the elderly. *Arch Intern Med* 1988;148(9):1969-70.

Chapter 21
Neuropathic Pain

C. Peter N. Watson, MD, FRCPC

Pain described as neuropathic is initiated or caused by a primary lesion or dysfunction in the nervous system. The terms "peripheral" or "central" are used to differentiate lesions that are located in the peripheral and central nervous systems, respectively (see Table 1). This chapter focuses on peripheral neuropathic pain, but the same principles may be applied to central pain. "Neuralgia" is a historical term for neuropathic pain that suggests pain with a paroxysmal, brief, lancinating quality.

Goals of Therapy

- Reduce severe or moderate pain to mild and tolerable. Both patient and physician should understand that total pain relief is not realistic for most of these difficult problems
- Find a balance between pain relief and acceptable side effects
- Restore quality of life to the extent possible

Investigations

- History with attention to:
  - temporal profile and characteristics of the pain
  - functional status, mood, quality of life, insomnia, sexual function, previous and current treatments, especially concurrent medications (chemotherapy, isoniazid, antiretrovirals and others)[1]
  - present or past chemical dependency, especially if opioids are considered
- Physical examination:
  - determine areas of sensory loss (hypoesthesia) and skin sensitivity characteristic of neuropathic pain (Table 2)
  - determine other neurologic findings that might indicate a progressive lesion requiring imaging and surgery
  - determine concurrent conditions that contribute to the pain problem, e.g., concomitant muscular pain and psychological factors
- Other investigations:
  - imaging with CT or MR scanning if a space-occupying lesion is suspected
  - electromyography
  - diagnostic sympathetic blockade if complex regional pain syndrome is suspected

Therapeutic Choices

Nonpharmacologic Choices

Neuropathic pain is often severe and debilitating. Always consider combining pharmacotherapy with appropriate psychological and physical measures. Although evidence is lacking, many nonpharmacologic strategies can be used to provide benefit in some patients. Reduce sleep deprivation and improve physical conditioning to rehabilitate patients and improve their quality of life. Patients can minimize chronic neuropathic pain by getting adequate rest and avoiding further aggravation. Continued medical visits provide important psychological support and hope for desperate patients who have failed standard therapy and are being treated with medication using a trial and error approach.

Surgery may be helpful for patients with trigeminal neuralgia who do not respond to pharmacotherapy. Some patients with nerve root compression who do not respond to conservative management may benefit from surgical options, see Nerve Root Compression: Cervical and Lumbar Radiculopathy. Surgical treatment has no role in postherpetic neuralgia and other types of neuropathic pain in the majority of patients.

Pharmacologic Choices

In recent years, the therapeutic armamentarium for neuropathic pain has grown with the addition of serotonin-norepinephrine reuptake inhibitor (SNRI) antidepressants, tramadol and cannabinoids. The Canadian Pain Society provides recommendations for the treatment of neuropathic pain (Figure 1) based on randomized controlled trials.[2,3] The recommended therapies can be used in many types of chronic neuropathic pain; the acute pain of herpes zoster and the unique condition of trigeminal neuralgia are considered separately. Certain types of neuropathic pain are much more intractable to treatment (e.g., central post-stroke pain) and drug combinations may be needed for optimal relief. Some individual patients with the more easily treated types of neuropathic pain may also fail to respond to usual treatment options.

Acute Neuropathic Pain—Herpes Zoster[4]

A live attenuated **varicella zoster vaccine** to prevent herpes zoster and postherpetic neuralgia[5] is available in Canada. More information on this vaccine and its efficacy can be found in Chapter 112.

Table 1: **Types of Neuropathic Pain**

Peripheral Neuropathic Pain	Central Neuropathic Pain
Nerve root pain	Central poststroke pain
Carpal tunnel syndrome	Spinal cord injury pain
Trigeminal neuralgia	Brain injury
Postherpetic neuralgia	Multiple sclerosis
Incisional neuralgia	Syringomyelia
Nerve trauma (causalgia)	
Phantom limb pain	

Table 2: **Definitions Related to Neuropathic Pain**

Allodynia	Pain resulting from a non-noxious stimulus to normal skin, such as touch
Causalgia (CRPS II)	Burning pain due to traumatic injury of a peripheral nerve
Hyperalgesia	Abnormally painful response to a stimulus, especially a repetitive stimulus, as well as a decreased pain threshold
Hyperpathia	Abnormally exaggerated subjective response to painful stimuli

Abbreviations: CRPS II = complex regional pain syndrome type II

The varicella-zoster virus lies dormant in dorsal root ganglia following initial infection; risk factors for reactivation include age (>50 years) and decreased immunologic competence. Severe or stabbing pain and dysesthesia are soon followed by vesicular eruption in the affected dermatomes—thoracic and cranial dermatomes are affected in about 50% and 15% of cases, respectively. Pain may precede the rash by days or radicular (nerve root) pain may occur with no rash (zoster sine herpete), making diagnosis difficult. Motor deficits occur in more severe cases. When herpes zoster affects the forehead, observe for eye complications and refer to an ophthalmologist when necessary.

Early treatment of herpes zoster can reduce the severity of the infection; however, there is no evidence that antivirals will prevent postherpetic neuralgia.[6] Oral antivirals (**acyclovir**, **famciclovir**, **valacyclovir**) are most effective if started within 72 hours of the onset of the rash. Even if the rash has not appeared, the sudden occurrence of severe, acute neuropathic pain unilaterally in the forehead or thoracic area in an individual over age 60 is reasonable cause to initiate antiviral drug therapy, since these agents are safe and well tolerated. For prescribing information see Chapter 112.

In addition to instituting an antiviral agent, it is important to relieve the acute pain. This may be accomplished with early treatment with **amitriptyline** and/or **gabapentin** and if necessary **opioids** or *nerve blocks*. Corticosteroid therapy may improve quality of life (resolution of acute neuritis, uninterrupted sleep and return to normal activity)[7] but does not accelerate healing or reduce the incidence of postherpetic neuralgia.[8] Limit use of corticosteroids to healthy patients with moderate to severe pain. Corticosteroids increase the risk of immunosuppression and are not appropriate for high-risk patients (e.g., immunosuppressed, elderly, patients with diabetes, hypertension, GI ulcers).

The risk of *chronic postherpetic neuralgia* increases with age and with severity of the eruption. Management of postherpetic neuralgia is described in Chronic Peripheral Neuropathic Pain, below.

Trigeminal Neuralgia

Trigeminal neuralgia, also known as *tic douloureux*, is different from other neuropathic pain and therapy is both pharmacologic (Table 4) and surgical. Trigeminal neuralgia is confined to the face, shows a predilection for the second or third trigeminal divisions, is brought on by tactile stimuli in trigger areas such as the nasolabial region and gingiva, and is electric shock-like in quality. Almost always unilateral, it generally afflicts persons over the age of 50 and often follows a remitting course. Trigeminal neuralgia usually responds to **carbamazepine**, a treatment that is generally not effective for other types of neuropathic pain unless there is a shock-like component.[2] The sustained-release formulation is given every 8–12 hours and may improve adherence, lessen untoward effects and provide a more sustained effect. Measuring serum levels is not necessary unless there is a need to assess adherence or concerns regarding toxicity. **Oxcarbazepine** may have advantages over carbamazepine, from which it is derived, in that it is given twice daily and has fewer side effects and drug interactions.[9] Randomized controlled trials comparing the efficacy of these 2 agents are lacking; oxcarbazepine appears to have a higher propensity to cause hyponatremia, particularly in the young.

Clinical experience has shown that other pharmacologic approaches are inferior to carbamazepine, but may be helpful as adjunctive therapy. If some relief is achieved with carbamazepine but side effects are unacceptable, a good strategy is to switch to oxcarbazepine or reduce the dose of carbamazepine to tolerability and add **baclofen**.[10] If adequate relief is not achieved, add **phenytoin** or replace baclofen with phenytoin. **Gabapentin**, **pregabalin**, **clonazepam** and **valproic acid** may be tried if other strategies fail.

If medical therapy is insufficient, a variety of *neurosurgical options* have a high success rate in experienced hands. Procedures include potentially curative microvascular decompression, ablative procedures such as glycerol instillation or balloon compression of the gasserian ganglion, and the gamma knife. MRI can help identify candidates for microvascular decompression by ruling out other causes of nerve compression. There is a risk of recurrence with all ablative surgeries and a <10% risk of anesthesia dolorosa (nerve injury pain caused by surgery) with all procedures.

Figure 1: **Management of Chronic Peripheral Neuropathic Pain**[3]

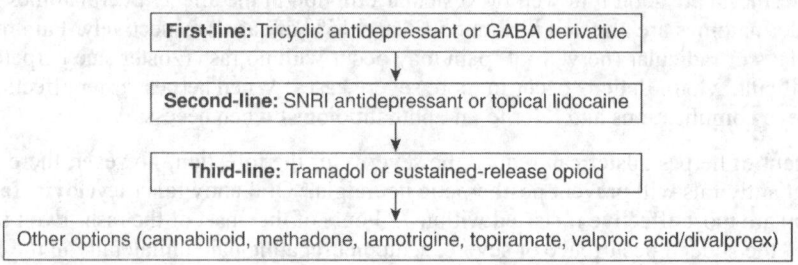

First-line: Tricyclic antidepressant or GABA derivative

↓

Second-line: SNRI antidepressant or topical lidocaine

↓

Third-line: Tramadol or sustained-release opioid

↓

Other options (cannabinoid, methadone, lamotrigine, topiramate, valproic acid/divalproex)

Chronic Neuropathic Pain

Nerve Root Compression: Cervical and Lumbar Radiculopathy

The commonest form of neuropathic pain involves nerve root compression in the cervical and lumbar areas (usually C5 or C6 and L5 or S1) associated with degenerative change and disc herniation or scar tissue. In the acute phase, **NSAIDs** or **acetaminophen/codeine** may be effective. Where necessary, additional pain relief can be achieved with stronger **opioids**, an appropriate regimen of rest and avoidance of further aggravation.

This pain often settles with conservative management. Consider surgical treatment if medical treatment fails over 6–12 weeks and if neuroimaging with CT or MR shows a surgically treatable lesion, if acute pain is excruciating and intractable, or if a neurologic deficit and a correctable lesion are present. Signs of a progressive neurologic deficit such as weakness or muscle wasting should prompt urgent surgical consultation as early as possible. Investigate if pain does not resolve within a reasonable time frame, or if this is the first episode in an elderly person (because of possible malignancy or other serious illness).

Complex Regional Pain Syndrome Type I (CRPS I)[11]

CRPS I, formerly known as reflex sympathetic dystrophy or sympathetically maintained pain, is thought to be neuropathic pain with neurovascular and dystrophic changes. It may result from penetrating or crush injuries to nerves but sometimes occurs after stroke or MI. Characteristics include burning pain, hyperalgesia, hyperpathia and allodynia, sweating, rubor and coldness of the affected limb. When clearly associated with nerve injury, it is referred to as CRPS II, known historically as causalgia and treated as for chronic peripheral neuropathic pain (see Chronic Peripheral Neuropathic Pain).

If CRPS I symptoms persist for a few months, the patient may experience a widening of the painful area, cool cyanotic skin, a glossy appearance to the skin, altered hair growth and progressive loss of function. Some patients will progress to dystrophic changes, osteoporosis, nail changes, subcutaneous thinning with pointed digits, and further loss of function with contractures or frozen shoulder and continued severe pain.

While CRPS I was thought to be due to sympathetic overactivity, evidence now points to a disorder involving upregulation of adrenergic receptors. Although sympathetic blocks often provide temporary relief, sympathectomy does not necessarily result in permanent resolution. Bier blocks using guanethidine are ineffective. Physical therapy, corticosteroids, sympathectomies and repeated sympathetic blocks have limited success. At follow up, two-thirds of patients are likely to have continued pain, and only about 25% return to fully normal activity. Manage these patients with the same agents used to treat neuropathic pain; some may require chronic opioid therapy.

Chronic Peripheral Neuropathic Pain

This category of neuropathic pain conditions includes *postherpetic neuralgia, diabetic neuropathy, causalgia* (CRPS II), *incisional neuralgias* following mastectomy, thoracotomy or bypass surgery, *phantom limb pain* and other neuropathies. Guidelines for the treatment of chronic peripheral neuropathic pain have been developed by the Canadian Pain Society and others.[2,3] **Tricyclic antidepressants** (TCAs) and GABA derivatives such as **gabapentin** and **pregabalin** are considered first-line agents (Figure 1, Table 5). SNRI antidepressants (**duloxetine**, **venlafaxine**) and topical **lidocaine** can be considered second-line. Lidocaine 5% topical formulations may be helpful in postherpetic neuralgia;[12] a transdermal patch is available in the United States but not yet in Canada. Other topical treatments, such as topical **ASA**, **diclofenac**, **menthol** and **capsaicin** are unproven or of modest efficacy. They may be helpful as adjunctive therapy combined with an oral analgesic, or as monotherapy for elderly patients if oral agents are not tolerated. Caution patients that capsaicin may cause a nonharmful burning sensation on the skin, mucous membranes and conjunctiva.

Opioids such as **morphine**, **hydromorphone**, **oxycodone**, **transdermal fentanyl** and **tramadol** can be used third-line. Guidance for the use of opioids in this setting is presented in Table 3. If pain persists, use a trial and error approach with a variety of drugs including **cannabinoids** (e.g., dronabinol, tetrahydrocannabinol/cannabidiol), **methadone**, **lamotrigine** and **topiramate**. Cannabinoids have been studied mainly in pain associated with multiple sclerosis. Methadone may be useful when refractory chronic neuropathic pain co-exists with opioid dependency; it requires prescribing authorization and specialized knowledge and should be used only by experienced clinicians. Avoid **meperidine** as chronic use can lead to an accumulation of the metabolite normeperidine and cause excitotoxicity. When used alone or combined with **acetaminophen**, codeine is a poor choice for severe pain of any kind. Conversion of **codeine** to morphine in the liver is unreliable in individuals who are rapid or slow CYP2D6 metabolizers, leading to increased risk of adverse effects or poor pain control, respectively.

Although the evidence for the recommended therapeutic approaches is mainly from studies of patients with postherpetic neuralgia and diabetic neuropathy, patients with phantom limb pain or other chronic peripheral neuropathic pain may derive benefit.

Table 3: Guidelines for Use of Opioids in Chronic Nonmalignant Pain

- Consider after other reasonable therapies have failed.
- Perform a complete pain and psychosocial history, physical examination and appropriate diagnostic tests. A history of substance abuse, tension-type headaches, frequent migraine headache, muscular pain (myofascial pain, fibromyalgia) or pain that appears to be largely determined by psychologic factors is a *relative* contraindication to the use of opioid therapy.
- A single physician/prescriber/pharmacy is optimal. The prescriber may choose to set up a contract with the patient. The agreement should specify the drug regimen, possible side effects, the functional restoration program and that violations may result in termination of opioid therapy.
- The opioid analgesic of choice should be administered around the clock and may include a provision of "rescue doses" for breakthrough pain. Controlled-release preparations include morphine, oxycodone, hydromorphone, tramadol and transdermal fentanyl. Avoid meperidine primarily because of accumulation of its excitotoxic metabolite normeperidine. Codeine is a poor analgesic for moderate to severe pain because it has to be metabolized to morphine. Drug administration should include a titration phase to minimize side effects. If a graded analgesic response to incremental doses is not observed, the patient may not be opioid-responsive, and opioid treatment should probably be terminated.
- The patient should be seen monthly or more often for the first few months and every 2–3 months thereafter. At each visit assess pain relief (0–10 scale), mood, side effects, quality of life, adherence to functional goals and presence of drug-related behaviour. Optimally, affix a copy of the prescription and drug therapy flow sheet to the medical record.
- The goal of opioid therapy is to make the pain tolerable. For some patients with chronic noncancer pain (e.g., postherpetic neuralgia), the administration of an opioid analgesic can mean the difference between bearable and unbearable pain.

Choices during Pregnancy and Breastfeeding[13,14,15]

When possible, use nonpharmacologic measures and avoid any pharmacologic options mentioned above during pregnancy. If drug therapy is deemed necessary, consider the risks and benefits of each drug to ensure an informed decision is made. Of the antidepressants, tricyclics such as **amitriptyline** appear relatively safe and are probably preferred but its effect on lactation and breastfeeding is unknown and may be of concern. SNRIs such as **venlafaxine** and **duloxetine**, while not associated with an increased risk of congenital malformations, are less effective than tricyclics for neuropathic pain and have been associated with short-term neurobehavioural symptoms in the neonate such as agitation, jitteriness and poor feeding.

There are limited data regarding **baclofen** in pregnancy but it is thought to be compatible with breastfeeding.

Carbamazepine is associated with an increased risk of major and minor malformations including neural tube defects. If carbamazepine is to be used during pregnancy, folate supplementation (5 mg/day) is recommended, beginning prior to conception and continued in pregnancy.[16] Less is known about the safety of **oxcarbazepine** during pregnancy, but as with carbamazepine, folate supplementation 5 mg/day is considered prudent. Both carbamazepine and oxcarbazepine are thought to be compatible with breastfeeding.

Clonazepam is probably safe in pregnancy after the first trimester but because of its low molecular weight may cause sedation in the breastfed infant. **Valproate** is not recommended for neuropathic pain during pregnancy because of the increased risk of neural tube defects, but is considered compatible with breastfeeding. Until more is known about the safety of **gabapentin** or **pregabalin**, avoid these agents for the treatment of neuropathic pain during pregnancy and breastfeeding.

Morphine and **oxycodone** have not been associated with an increased risk of major malformations but, as with all **opioids**, may depress respiratory and GI function and cause sedation and/or withdrawal syndromes in the newborn. Keep in mind that many patients with chronic noncancer pain require high doses of opioids, and the safety data regarding malformations with morphine and oxycodone may not apply in these cases. When infants are exposed to opioids through breast milk, monitor for possible GI or CNS depressant effects.

A discussion of general principles on the use of medications in these special populations can be found in Appendix II and Appendix III. Other specialized reference sources are also provided in these appendices.

Therapeutic Tips

- Two to 3 months constitutes a reasonable trial of medication for neuropathic pain.
- While patients frequently report poor response to previous treatment with amitriptyline, carbamazepine or other agents, these drugs have often been used at a dose that is too high or too low and for a duration that is too short. It is useful to re-institute these drugs and evaluate their effectiveness when used appropriately: start low, go slow, increase dose until relief of symptoms or side effects occur and treat side effects when possible.
- Be sure the patient understands the goals of therapy: reduction in pain from moderate or severe to mild, at the price of some side effects that may be tolerable or treatable.
- Use a pain assessment tool, such as a scale of 0–10 where 0 is no pain and 10 the worst pain imaginable, to evaluate pain with and without activity, and before and after medication.
- As a matter of course, prescribe an **artificial saliva mouth spray** with TCAs and a **bowel regimen** with TCAs or opioids.
- Use controlled-release formulations of carbamazepine and opioids (see Table 3).
- It may be possible to reduce or gradually withdraw medication after initial control of pain and a period of relief of 1–3 months (pain such as postherpetic neuralgia may resolve spontaneously and trigeminal neuralgia may go into remission). Gradually reduce dosage to avoid withdrawal symptoms.

- If a drug is not effective, try different drugs within the same class (e.g., TCAs or GABA derivatives), drugs of different classes or a combination of drugs for a possible additive or synergistic effect. Do not combine TCAs with SNRIs.
- If opioids are used, guidelines (see Table 3) are important and should be worked through with the patient.
- A trial and error approach of scientifically unproven treatments is reasonable if standard therapy fails.
- If chronic neuropathic pain is being managed in general practice, semi-annual or annual visits to a pain specialist (where available) help provide support to the family practitioner for contentious approaches such as opioids, and offer the chance to provide a novel therapy for the patient.

Table 4: Drug Therapy for Trigeminal Neuralgia

Class	Drug	Dose	Adverse Effects	Drug Interactions	Comments	Cost[a]
Antiepileptic Drugs	*carbamazepine immediate-release* Tegretol, generics	Initial: 100 mg BID to QID po Increase by 100 mg daily at weekly intervals to 400–1200 mg/day or more, in 2–4 divided doses, until good pain control or intolerable side effects Give doses before meals	Drowsiness, ataxia, dizziness, nausea, hyponatremia; allergic reactions, e.g., rash; rarely, hepatitis or bone marrow suppression.	Induces several cytochrome P450 isoenzymes, potentially increases the clearance of many drugs, such as OCs, warfarin, risperidone or TCAs; clearance may be reduced by CYP3A4 inhibitors such as erythromycin, grapefruit juice, itraconazole or ketoconazole.	To improve detection of rare idiosyncratic reactions that usually occur in the first 3 months, complete blood count, electrolytes and liver function tests are suggested every 1–2 wk during that time.	$
	carbamazepine controlled-release Tegretol CR, generics	Initial: 100 mg Q8–12H po Increase at weekly intervals as needed to 400–1200 mg daily in 2 divided doses	See carbamazepine immediate-release.	See carbamazepine immediate-release.	See carbamazepine immediate-release.	$
	clonazepam Rivotril, generics	Initial: 1.5 mg/day po Maximum: 20 mg/day	Sedation.	Additive sedation with CNS depressants such as alcohol; serum levels potentially increased by CYP3A4 inhibitors, such as cimetidine, clarithromycin, erythromycin, grapefruit juice, ketoconazole, lamotrigine, ritonavir or verapamil, or reduced by inducers of CYP3A4, such as carbamazepine, phenytoin or rifampin.	Important to discontinue gradually to avoid withdrawal symptoms.	$

Class	Drug	Dose	Adverse Effects	Drug Interactions	Comments	Cost[a]
	divalproex sodium Epival, generics	Initial: 250 mg BID po; increase by 250 mg/day every 3–4 days as necessary Usual maintenance: 750–1000 mg/day in 2–4 divided doses	Nausea, alopecia, tremor, weight gain, increased hepatic enzymes; neural tube defects can occur if used during pregnancy; do liver function tests prior to initiation of therapy and periodically, especially in first 6 months of therapy and if symptoms of hepatic dysfunction occur.	Inhibits CYP2C9 and may reduce clearance of its substrates, such as fluoxetine, fluvastatin, sertraline, verapamil or warfarin; avoid with ASA or warfarin; carbamazepine, phenytoin and phenobarbital can significantly increase clearance of valproic acid; may increase depressant effect of alcohol.	Do not use for neuropathic pain in pregnancy due to increased risk of neural tube defects.	$
	oxcarbazepine Trileptal, generics	Initial: 75–150 mg BID po Maximum: 1200 mg/day	See carbamazepine immediate-release. Hyponatremia may be more common than with carbamazepine, especially in younger patients.	May have lower propensity for drug interactions than carbamazepine, but comparative trials are lacking.	Possible alternative to carbamazepine in terms of efficacy; generally fewer side effects.	$$$
	phenytoin Dilantin Capsules, Dilantin Infatabs, generics	100–300 mg QHS po, depending on age	Ataxia, drowsiness, nausea; gingival hyperplasia; skin rash 5–10%, rarely very serious; increased liver enzymes; blood dyscrasias; dose-related encephalopathy; coarse facial features with long-term use.	Induces several cytochrome P450 isoenzymes, potentially increasing the clearance of many drugs, such as OCs, warfarin, risperidone and TCAs.	Dosage increases should be small and gradual because of saturation kinetics. Serum concentrations can help guide dosage and assess adherence.	$
	valproic acid Depakene, Apo-Valproic, other generics	Initial: 125 mg BID po; increase by 250 mg/day every 1–2 wk as necessary Usual maintenance: 750–1000 mg/day in 2–4 divided doses	See divalproex sodium.	See divalproex sodium.	See divalproex sodium.	$
GABA Derivatives	*gabapentin* Neurontin, generics	Initial: 300–400 mg/day po in divided doses May increase at weekly intervals to BID then TID Maximum: 3600 mg/day	Sedation, ataxia, tremor; less commonly, GI upset, peripheral edema, vision changes, weight gain.	Administration with aluminum/magnesium-containing antacids may decrease bioavailability.	Not a Health Canada–approved indication.	$$

(cont'd)

Table 4: Drug Therapy for Trigeminal Neuralgia *(cont'd)*

Class	Drug	Dose	Adverse Effects	Drug Interactions	Comments	Cost[a]
	pregabalin (kidney symbol) Lyrica, generics	Initial: 50–150 mg per day po in 2 divided doses Increase dose weekly by 50–150 mg/day Usual effective dose: 300–600 mg/day Maximum: 600 mg/day	Sedation, ataxia, edema, diplopia, weight gain, dry mouth.	No known significant drug interactions.	BID dosing is an advantage over gabapentin.	$$
Muscle Relaxants	*baclofen* (kidney symbol) Lioresal Oral, generics	Initial: 10 mg BID po Maximum: 20 mg TID	Sedation, muscle weakness, nausea, dizziness.	Potential additive CNS depression with benzodiazepines, opioids, TCAs and some antihypertensive agents.	Gradual withdrawal is important to minimize the potential for seizures. May be useful add-on to carbamazepine.	$

[a] Cost of 30-day supply of usual dose; includes drug cost only.
(kidney symbol) Dosage adjustment may be required in renal impairment; see Appendix I.
Abbreviations: OC = oral contraceptive; TCA = tricyclic antidepressant
Legend: $ < $25 $$ $25–50 $$$ $50–75 $$$$ $75–100 $$$$$ $100–125

Table 5: Drug Therapy for Chronic Peripheral Neuropathic Pain

Class	Drug	Dose	Adverse Effects	Drug Interactions	Comments	Cost[a]
Anesthetics, Topical	*lidocaine 5%* Lidodan, Maxilene, Xylocaine Ointment	Apply to painful areas TID–QID PRN	No significant side effects when used appropriately (e.g., on intact skin). Excessive use, application to abraded skin or use of occlusive covering may result in systemic effects such as bradycardia, hypotension.	No known significant drug interactions.	Not to be used with occlusive covering. Most effective in postherpetic neuralgia.	$/30 g tube
Antidepressants, Tricyclic	*amitriptyline* Elavil	Initial: 10–25 mg QHS po Increase by 10–25 mg daily at weekly intervals, until pain relief or side effects	All TCAs: dry mouth, constipation, drowsiness, blurred vision, urinary retention, weight gain, confusion, tachycardia.	All TCAs: metabolized by cytochrome P450; potential interactions with other substrates, inhibitors (e.g., erythromycin, fluoxetine, fluvoxamine, isoniazid, itraconazole, ketoconazole, paroxetine, valproic acid), or inducers (e.g., carbamazepine, phenobarbital, phenytoin, rifampin); increased sedation with other CNS depressants such as alcohol; increased anticholinergic effects with other anticholinergic agents.	Avoid in patients with prostatic hyperplasia (because TCAs may cause/exacerbate urinary retention) and in significant heart disease because of cardiac toxicity (e.g., arrhythmias).	$
	desipramine generics	Initial: 10–25 mg QHS po Increase by 10–25 mg daily at weekly intervals, until pain relief or side effects	See amitriptyline.	See amitriptyline.	See amitriptyline.	$
	nortriptyline Aventyl, generics	Initial: 10–25 mg QHS po Increase by 10–25 mg daily at weekly intervals, until pain relief or side effects	See amitriptyline.	See amitriptyline.	See amitriptyline.	$

(cont'd)

Table 5: Drug Therapy for Chronic Peripheral Neuropathic Pain *(cont'd)*

Class	Drug	Dose	Adverse Effects	Drug Interactions	Comments	Cost[a]
Antiepileptic Drugs	*divalproex sodium* Epival, generics	Initial: 250 mg BID po; increase by 250 mg/day every 3–4 days as necessary Usual maintenance: 750–1000 mg/day in 2–4 divided doses	Nausea, alopecia, tremor, weight gain, increased hepatic enzymes; neural tube defects can occur if used during pregnancy; do liver function tests prior to initiation of therapy and periodically, especially in 1st 6 months of therapy and if symptoms of hepatic dysfunction occur.	Inhibits CYP2C9 and may reduce clearance of its substrates, such as fluoxetine, fluvastatin, sertraline, verapamil or warfarin; avoid with ASA or warfarin; carbamazepine, phenytoin and phenobarbital can significantly increase clearance of valproic acid; may increase depressant effect of alcohol.	Do not use to treat neuropathic pain during pregnancy due to increased risk of neural tube defects.	$
	valproic acid Depakene, Apo-Valproic, other generics	Initial: 125 mg BID po; increase by 250 mg/day every 1–2 wk as necessary Usual maintenance: 750–1000 mg/day in 2–4 divided doses	See divalproex sodium.	See divalproex sodium.	See divalproex sodium.	$
GABA Derivatives	*gabapentin* ❥ Neurontin, generics	Initial: 300–400 mg/day po in divided doses May increase at weekly intervals to BID then TID Maximum: 3600 mg/day	Sedation, ataxia, tremor; less commonly, GI upset, peripheral edema, vision changes, weight gain.	Administration with aluminum/magnesium-containing antacids may decrease bioavailability.	Not a Health Canada–approved indication.	$$
	pregabalin ❥ Lyrica, generics	Initial: 50–150 mg daily po in 2 divided doses Increase dose weekly by 50–150 mg/day Usual effective dose: 300–600 mg/day Maximum: 600 mg/day	Sedation, ataxia, edema, diplopia, weight gain, dry mouth.	No known significant drug interactions.	BID dosing is an advantage.	$$

Class	Drug	Dose	Adverse Effects	Drug Interactions	Comments	Cost[a]
Opioids	*fentanyl transdermal* Duragesic MAT, generics	Initial: apply one 12 μg/h transdermal patch Q72H Start low and go slow; increase until relief of symptoms or unacceptable side effects	All opioids: nausea, constipation, drowsiness, risk of addiction; allergic reactions, e.g., rash, itch.	All opioids: additive sedation with other CNS depressants such as alcohol; potential enhancement of opioid effects with lidocaine. Fentanyl: inhibitors of CYP3A4, such as cimetidine, efavirenz, erythromycin, itraconazole, ketoconazole or ritonavir, may potentiate fentanyl's pharmacologic effects.	Follow dosing conversion in product monograph when switching from other opioids; do not use in children or opioid-naïve individuals because of the risk of respiratory depression.	$$$
	hydromorphone immediate-release Dilaudid, generics	Initial: 1–2 mg Q4H PRN po Start low and go slow; increase until relief of symptoms or unacceptable side effects	See fentanyl.	See fentanyl.		$
	hydromorphone controlled-release Hydromorph Contin, Jurnista	Initial: Hydromorph Contin: 3 mg Q8–12H po Jurnista: 4 mg once daily Start low and go slow; increase until relief of symptoms or unacceptable side effects	See fentanyl.	See fentanyl.		$$
	morphine immediate-release ❥ MS-IR, Statex, generics	Initial: 5–15 mg Q4–6H PRN po Start low and go slow; increase until relief of symptoms or unacceptable side effects	See fentanyl.	See fentanyl. Morphine: decreased analgesic effect with somatostatin, rifampin.	After 1–2 wk, convert to equivalent daily dose of controlled-release formulation.	$
	morphine controlled-release ❥ Kadian, M-Eslon, MS Contin, generics	Initial: 20–30 mg/day po Kadian: once daily or in divided doses Q12H M-Eslon, MS Contin: divided doses Q8–12H Titrate slowly as needed until relief of symptoms or unacceptable side effects	See fentanyl.	See fentanyl. Morphine: decreased analgesic effect with somatostatin, rifampin.		$
	oxycodone immediate-release Oxy-IR, Supeudol, generics	Initial: 5–10 mg Q4–6H po Start low and go slow; increase until relief of symptoms or unacceptable side effects	See fentanyl.	See fentanyl.		$

(cont'd)

Table 5: **Drug Therapy for Chronic Peripheral Neuropathic Pain** *(cont'd)*

Class	Drug	Dose	Adverse Effects	Drug Interactions	Comments	Cost[a]
	oxycodone controlled-release OxyNEO, generics	Initial: 10–20 mg Q12H po Start low and go slow; increase until relief of symptoms or unacceptable side effects	See fentanyl.	See fentanyl.		$$
	oxycodone/naloxone controlled-release Targin	Initial: 1 tablet (oxycodone 10 mg/naloxone 5 mg) Q12H po Start low and go slow; increase until relief of symptoms or unacceptable side effects Maximum: oxycodone 40 mg/naloxone 20 mg Q12H	See fentanyl.	See fentanyl.	The role of naloxone in this preparation is for the relief of opioid-induced constipation. Single doses should not exceed oxycodone 40 mg/naloxone 20 mg. If higher doses are needed to achieve adequate pain relief, supplementation with a single-entity controlled-release oxycodone formulation is an option, though this may reduce the beneficial effect of the naloxone.	$$$$$
	tramadol controlled-release ❥ Durela, Ralivia, Tridural, Zytram XL	Durela, Ralivia or Tridural: start with 100 mg once daily po; may increase gradually to maximum 300 mg daily Zytram XL: start with 150 mg once daily; may increase at weekly intervals to maximum 400 mg daily	Respiratory depression, sedation, ataxia, constipation, seizures, nausea, orthostatic hypotension.	Do not use if MAOIs taken within past 14 days. Caution with drugs that lower seizure threshold, e.g., SSRIs, TCAs, bupropion. Increased sedation with other CNS depressants. Carbamazepine may decrease analgesic effect of tramadol. Clearance of tramadol (and conversion to its active M1 metobolite) may be decreased by inhibitors of CYP2D6 such as fluoxetine, paroxetine or quinidine, increasing the risk of seizures or serotonin syndrome. Clearance may also be reduced by inhibitors of CYP3A4 such as erythromycin, itraconazole or ketoconazole.	Do not break, crush or chew sustained-release tramadol tablets. They must be swallowed whole to prevent the rapid release and absorption of excessive doses of tramadol.	$$$$

Class	Drug	Dose	Adverse Effects	Drug Interactions	Comments	Cost[a]
Serotonin-Norepinephrine Reuptake Inhibitors	*duloxetine* Cymbalta	60 mg daily to BID po	Nausea, drowsiness, insomnia, dizziness, dry mouth.	Do not use with potent inhibitors of CYP1A2 (e.g., fluvoxamine) or MAOIs.	Second-line choice after TCAs or GABA derivatives.	$$$$$
	venlafaxine Effexor XR, generics	Initial: 37.5 mg daily po Increase weekly by 37.5 mg/day Usual effective dose: 150–225 mg/day Maximum: 375 mg/day	Hypertension, ataxia, sedation, insomnia, nausea, hyperhidrosis, dry mouth, constipation, anxiety, anorexia.	Clearance may be reduced by inhibitors of CYP2D6 such as cannabidiol, fluoxetine, paroxetine or quinidine, or by inhibitors of CYP3A4 such as erythromycin, itraconazole, ketoconazole or grapefruit juice. Contraindicated with MAOIs.	Less effective than TCAs for neuropathic pain.	$

[a] Cost of 30-day supply of usual dose; includes drug cost only.

Dosage adjustment may be required in renal impairment; see Appendix I.

Abbreviations: MAOI = monoamine oxidase inhibitor; SNRI = serotonin-norepinephrine reuptake inhibitor; SSRI = selective serotonine reuptake inhibitor; TCA = tricyclic antidepressant

Legend: $ < $25 $$ $25–50 $$$ $50–75 $$$$ $75–100 $$$$$ $100–125

Suggested Readings

Gilron I, Watson CP, Cahill CM et al. Neuropathic pain: a practical guideline for the clinician. *CMAJ* 2006;175(3):265-75.

Harden RN, Baron R, Janig W, eds. *Complex regional pain syndrome*. Seattle (WA): IASP Press; 2001.

Oxman MN, Levin MJ, Johnson GR et al. A vaccine to prevent herpes zoster and postherpetic neuralgia in older adults. *N Eng J Med* 2005;352(22):2271-84.

Toth C, Moulin DE. *Neuropathic pain: causes, management and understanding*. Cambridge (GB): Cambridge University Press; 2013.

Watson CP, Gershon AA, eds. *Herpes zoster and postherpetic neuralgia*. 2nd ed. New York (NY): Elsevier; 2001.

References

1. Drug-induced peripheral neuropathies. *Prescrire Int* 2013;22(141):208-12.
2. Gilron I, Watson CP, Cahill CM et al. Neuropathic pain: a practical guideline for the clinician. *CMAJ* 2006;175(3):265-75.
3. Moulin DE, Clark AJ, Gilron I et al. Pharmacological management of chronic neuropathic pain - consensus statement and guidelines from the Canadian Pain Society. *Pain Res Manag* 2007;12(1):13-21.
4. Watson CP, Gershon AA, eds. *Herpes zoster and postherpetic neuralgia*. 2nd ed. New York (NY): Elsevier; 2001.
5. Oxman MN, Levin MJ, Johnson GR et al. A vaccine to prevent herpes zoster and postherpetic neuralgia in older adults. *N Eng J Med* 2005;352(22):2271-84.
6. Chen N, Li Q, Yang J et al. Antiviral treatment for preventing postherpetic neuralgia. *Cochrane Database Syst Rev* 2014;2:CD006866.
7. Whitley RJ, Weiss H, Gnann JW et al. Acyclovir with and without prednisone for the treatment of herpes zoster. A randomized, placebo-controlled trial. The National Institute of Allergy and Infections Diseases Collaborative Antiviral Study Group. *Ann Intern Med* 1996;125(5):376-83.
8. Han Y, Zhang J, Chen N et al. Corticosteroids for preventing postherpetic neuralgia. *Cochrane Database Syst Rev* 2013;3:CD005582.
9. Zhou M, Chen N, He L et al. Oxcarbazepine for neuropathic pain. *Cochrane Database Syst Rev* 2013;3:CD007963.
10. Fromm GH, Terrence CF, Chattha AS. Baclofen in the treatment of trigeminal neuralgia: double-blind study and long-term follow-up. *Ann Neurol* 1984;15(3):240-4.
11. Harden RN, Baron R, Janig W, eds. *Complex regional pain syndrome*. Seattle (WA): IASP Press; 2001.
12. Hansson PT, Fields HL, Hill RG et al., eds. *Neuropathic pain: pathophysiology and treatment*. Seattle (WA): IASP Press; 2001.
13. Briggs GG, Freeman RK, Yaffe SJ, eds. *Drugs in pregnancy and lactation: a reference guide to fetal and neonatal risk*. 9th ed. Philadephia (PA): Wolters Kluwer Health; Lippincott Williams & Wilkins; 2011.
14. Schaefer C, Peters P, Miller RK, eds. *Drugs during pregnancy and lactation*. 2nd ed. London (GB): Elsevier; 2007.
15. Drugs and Lactation Database (LactMed). Bethesda (MD): U.S. National Library of Medicine. Available from: toxnet.nlm.nih.gov/cgi-bin/sis/htmlgen?LACT. Accessed April 4, 2011.
16. Wilson RD, Johnson JA, Wyatt P et al. Pre-conceptional vitamin/folic acid supplementation 2007: the use of folic acid in combination with a multivitamin supplement for the prevention of neural tube defects and other congenital anomalies. *J Obstet Gynaecol Can* 2007;29(12):1003-26.

Chapter 22
Parkinson's Disease

D.A. Grimes, MD, FRCPC

Parkinson's disease (PD) is a chronic, progressive, neurodegenerative disease whose cardinal features are tremor, bradykinesia and rigidity. Nonmotor features such as dementia, psychosis and autonomic dysfunction (excessive sweating, bladder frequency/urgency, orthostasis) often become the more disabling features as the disease progresses. Currently available treatments significantly decrease morbidity and mortality; however, no treatment to date has been definitively shown to impact the underlying disease process.[1] Medications providing the most benefit are directed at replenishing dopamine within the brain.

Goals of Therapy

- Improve functioning and quality of life
- Minimize acute and long-term side effects of medications
- Instill a positive outlook, despite the chronic, progressive nature of PD

Investigations

- The clinical diagnosis of PD can be made with confidence if the classic features of a unilateral or asymmetric resting tremor plus bradykinesia and rigidity are present. The patient's earliest complaints may include fatigue, loss of smell, sleep disorders, general slowness, poor handwriting and a tremulous feeling in one arm, without obvious tremor.
- Early postural instability, autonomic dysfunction, early and prominent dementia, impaired eye movements, rapid progression and poor response to dopaminergic therapy are not features of early PD, and if present suggest a different diagnosis.
- Perform imaging studies in young patients or those with atypical features. Exclude Wilson's disease in young patients by performing a serum ceruloplasmin, a slit-lamp examination and a 24-hour urine for copper.
- Exclude drug-induced parkinsonism. The most common drug causes include first- and second-generation antipsychotic agents and central dopamine-blocking antiemetics, e.g., metoclopramide and prochlorperazine.

Therapeutic Choices

Nonpharmacologic Choices

- Patient education via books, websites and local and national Parkinson societies (all available through the Parkinson Society Canada, www.parkinson.ca).
- Stress importance of staying active and having a regular exercise routine.
- Encourage awareness of the important roles of allied health professionals such as speech, physical and occupational therapists, and home care as the disease becomes more advanced.
- Some patients may benefit from surgery. See Surgery, below.

Pharmacologic Choices

Drug therapy choices for PD are listed in Table 1. An algorithm in Figure 1 provides a guide to the initial management of PD.

Levodopa

Levodopa is converted to dopamine within presynaptic dopaminergic neurons. Although used alone when first discovered, today it is combined with a DOPA decarboxylase inhibitor, **carbidopa** or **benserazide**, to enhance distribution to the brain and minimize acute side effects such as nausea and vomiting.

There is theoretical concern that levodopa could be toxic to already damaged dopaminergic neurons through a mechanism involving excess oxidative stress.[2] There is little evidence for this from in vitro studies, in vivo animal models or human studies.[3]

Over time, many PD patients develop symptoms such as dysarthria, gait disorders, postural instability and cognitive dysfunction that are poorly responsive to levodopa therapy. The cause is mainly disease-related degeneration of nondopaminergic neuronal systems, and not that levodopa has become ineffective for the initial symptoms for which it was started.[2,3]

Though initially effective, in many patients levodopa therapy is eventually complicated by motor fluctuations and dyskinesia; these complications develop in up to 50% of patients after 5 years.[4,5] In the early stages of PD, patients enjoy a long-lasting response following a single dose of levodopa. With disease progression and longer-term treatment, patients begin to experience motor fluctuations, such as end-of-dose "wearing off" of effectiveness or periods of fluctuating response known as "on-off" phenomena, and a variety of patterns of dyskinesia such as peak-dose dyskinesia (occurring during the peak effect of the dose), diphasic dyskinesia (occurring at the beginning and/or end of a dosing interval) and off-period dystonia (painful spasms, usually of the feet, occurring upon morning rising or when a dose is wearing off). There is also increasing recognition that nonmotor symptoms such as excessive perspiration, anxiety, cognitive changes and shortness of breath do occur and can fluctuate with the motor features of the disease.

Figure 1: Initial Pharmacologic Management of Parkinson's Disease

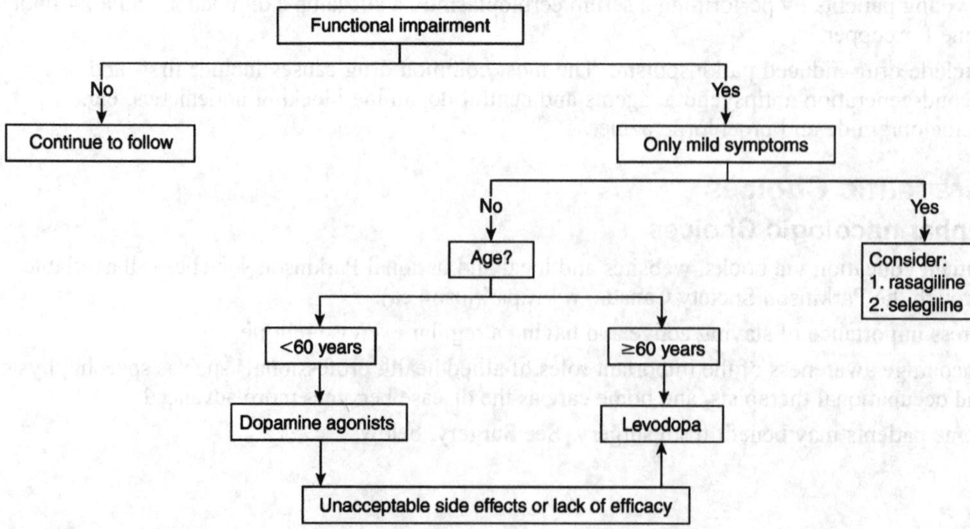

The pathophysiology of motor complications is not completely understood, but the leading theory suggests they are related to pulsatile stimulation of dopamine receptors resulting from intermittent dosing and levodopa's short plasma half-life.[5]

Factors shown to increase the risk of levodopa-induced dyskinesia include higher doses of levodopa, longer duration of treatment, severity of the underlying nigral degeneration and a younger age of disease onset.[5] Delaying the use of levodopa to preserve its effectiveness and minimize adverse effects, especially in young-onset patients, has been the standard of practice in many movement disorder centres; however, this approach is being questioned as the risks and benefits of delayed versus earlier treatment appears to be less clear,[6] and the use of levodopa in younger patients is increasing.[1] Slow-release preparations of levodopa benefit patients having difficulty with "wearing-off," although good randomized trials are lacking;[7] there is no evidence that initiating treatment with controlled-release levodopa provides an advantage over immediate-release formulations.[8] Other strategies to minimize pulsatile stimulation of dopamine, such as combining levodopa with a COMT inhibitor, have not delayed onset of motor fluctuations, and may actually increase the risk of dyskinesia.[9]

A variety of strategies can be used to help treat patients who have developed "wearing off" or dyskinesia (Figure 2).

Dopamine Agonists

Bromocriptine, **pramipexole** and **ropinirole** are effective as monotherapy in the early stages of the disease, and as adjunctive therapy with levodopa for more advanced patients with motor complications.[7,8] **Pergolide** was withdrawn from the Canadian market in 2007 because of its association with cardiac valvulopathy;[10,11] it is now available through Health Canada's Special Access Programme for patients who meet specific criteria. **Rotigotine**, available as a transdermal patch formulation, has been shown to be effective in reducing Parkinson's disease symptoms [Evidence: SORT A*].[12] Transdermal delivery results in stable plasma concentrations (which avoids pulsatile stimulation of dopamine receptors), offers an alternative for patients wishing to reduce oral medications, and may result in improved adherence.

Compared to levodopa, dopamine agonists are associated with fewer motor complications in the first 5 years of the disease, but it is unclear whether this translates into benefits in the long term, when these problems become more significant.[7,8] Although all clinical trials demonstrate a lower efficacy compared to levodopa, this difference does not seem to affect quality-of-life scores in early disease.[8,13] Because of the lower incidence of motor complications, dopamine agonists are typically used as initial therapy in younger patients, then levodopa is added in the case of poor tolerance or inadequate benefit, or later because of waning efficacy of the dopamine agonist; however, this strategy is being re-examined[6] and the use of levodopa in younger patients is rising.[1]

Because bromocriptine can cause pulmonary fibrosis, the newer, non-ergot dopamine agonists (pramipexole and ropinirole) are better choices. Daytime sleepiness or sudden irresistible attacks of sleep can occur with all of the dopamine replacement medications, including levodopa, but occur more frequently with dopamine agonists compared to levodopa.[14] Impulse control disorders such as hypersexual behaviour and pathologic gambling occur in up to 15% of patients taking dopamine agonists. It is important to discuss these significant side effects with your patient.[15] Additional difficulties with dopamine agonists, compared to levodopa, include more GI upset, orthostatic hypotension and psychiatric reactions (hallucinations and confusion); in addition, supplementary levodopa is almost always required for supervening disability after varying periods of time. For these reasons, there has been a shift away from using dopamine agonists.

---

* SORT (Strength of Recommendation Taxonomy) is a rating system (A, B or C) that addresses the quality of available evidence. For more information consult **How to Use *Compendium of Therapeutic Choices*** on page xxv.

Figure 2: **Management of Levodopa-associated Motor Complications**

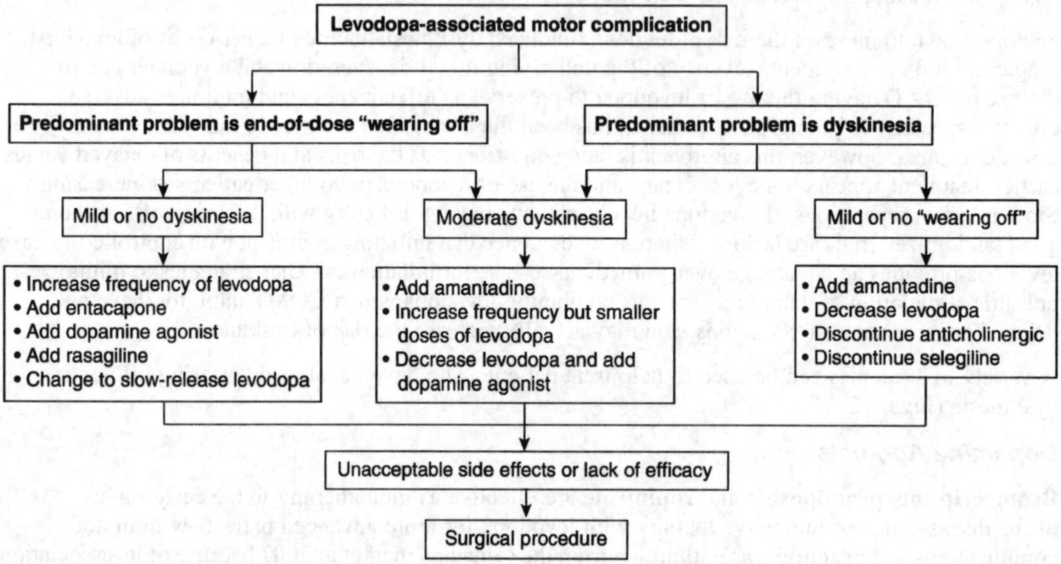

MAO-B Inhibitors

Early clinical evaluations of **selegiline**, an irreversible inhibitor of monoamine oxidase B (MAO-B), suggested that it might slow the progression of PD. Evidence now indicates that it does not have a substantial neuroprotective effect, and most of the apparent benefit during the first year of treatment is likely due to its very mild effects on symptoms.[8] In addition, it does not delay the development of dyskinesia or fluctuations associated with chronic levodopa therapy. A second, more potent, MAO-B inhibitor **rasagiline** is now available as initial treatment to improve motor symptoms and for patients with more advanced disease to help with "wearing off." Studies have suggested it may slow disease progression but this remains controversial.[16]

Amantadine

Amantadine provides mild-to-modest improvement in about two-thirds of early PD patients and improves levodopa-induced dyskinesia in the later stages of the disease.[7] Its exact mechanism of action is unclear but it may release dopamine from the presynaptic terminals or block its reuptake. Amantadine is an N-methyl-D-aspartate (NMDA) antagonist, which may account for some of its antiparkinsonian efficacy. NMDA receptor blockade confers a neuroprotective effect in some animal models of parkinsonism, and it has been suggested that amantadine improves survival in PD patients; however, this is unproven. Amantadine is not recommended as a drug of first choice in the early management of Parkinson's disease.[1] It is easy to use and usually well tolerated; leg edema, erythema and livedo reticularis (a reversible condition characterized by bluish, mottled appearance of the skin, mainly of the lower extremities) are the most common adverse events. In patients with cognitive deficits, amantadine can increase confusion and should not be used.

Anticholinergics

Anticholinergic drugs such as **benztropine**, **ethopropazine**, **procyclidine** and **trihexyphenidyl** have been used in the treatment of PD for decades, since before the availability of levodopa. Their major putative effect is on tremor, with little or no effect on bradykinesia; however, this has not been well studied.[2] They can be used as monotherapy or as adjuncts to dopaminergic therapy. Their many side effects (e.g., dry mouth, urinary retention, constipation) limit their use, especially in the elderly, and they are not recommended as drugs of first choice.[1]

COMT Inhibitors

COMT (catechol-O-methyl transferase), an enzyme that helps metabolize levodopa, is found in both the brain and in the peripheral nervous system. COMT inhibitors such as **entacapone** help prevent peripheral metabolism of levodopa, which increases its availability to the brain, and have no effect if not used in conjunction with levodopa. Despite some studies showing additional improvement in activities of daily living, in nonfluctuating patients their use should be limited to patients with wearing off.[7] Most of their side effects relate to increased dopaminergic activity in the brain, e.g., dyskinesia and, less often, confusion/hallucinations. Because of this, levodopa dosage may have to be reduced by up to 30% when a COMT inhibitor is initiated. **Tolcapone** was the first COMT inhibitor to be approved, but because of associated hepatotoxicity it is now available only through Health Canada's Special Access Programme, for use in exceptional cases. Entacapone is not associated with liver toxicity, but 2 other potential side effects are diarrhea (often weeks to months after initiation) and a harmless discolouration of the urine that patients need to be warned about.

Surgery

Recognition that there is a limit to the medical management of PD brought about a resurgence of surgical treatments. Two main surgical procedures have been shown to be effective: lesioning procedures and deep brain stimulation (DBS). Surgical treatment of PD mainly targets the thalamus (improves tremor), globus pallidum (improves dyskinesias and bradykinesia) and the subthalamic nucleus (improves bradykinesia, tremor and dyskinesias).[1] Lesioning procedures such as pallidotomy and thalamotomy are performed rarely. DBS is the surgical treatment of choice in patients with advanced disease in whom medications can no longer control motor symptoms,[1] though use of subthalamic DBS in patients with early motor complications has shown promise.[17] It is important for patients to understand that these surgeries are not a cure; functioning will increase only to the level of their best "on" times, and postural instability does not improve. Poor cognition is a contraindication to these procedures.

Complications: Depression, Psychosis, Dementia

Depression is common in PD, but keep in mind that a lack of facial expression in a patient with PD does not necessarily indicate sadness or depression. Selective serotonin reuptake inhibitors (SSRIs) and tricyclic antidepressants (TCAs) have been the mainstay of therapy for depression in patients with PD, yet there is a surprising lack of evidence to guide the choice of antidepressant.[18] TCAs should be used cautiously because their anticholinergic effects are more likely to induce delirium, especially in memory-impaired patients; they may also aggravate orthostatic hypotension, which can increase the risk of falls.

Psychosis and *dementia* are also very common in PD, typically in patients with more advanced disease. All medications used to treat the motor symptoms can contribute to psychosis in a dose-related fashion. As the disease progresses, PD medications often need to be reduced or withdrawn because of worsening of the patient's cognitive status. Usually, anticholinergics are withdrawn first, then selegiline, rasagiline, amantadine, dopamine agonists and COMT inhibitors, until only levodopa remains. At that point, reducing the dose of levodopa is an option. Review other (non-PD) medications carefully to ensure they are not also contributing to the psychosis. For patients in whom an optimum balance cannot be found by adjusting PD medications, antipsychotics are sometimes used. All antipsychotics have some potential to reduce control of movement disorders. The second-generation (atypical) antipsychotic **clozapine** appears to have the lowest risk and has shown clear benefit in randomized controlled trials for management of psychotic symptoms in patients with PD.[1,18] **Quetiapine** has not shown consistent benefit in clinical trials yet is often tried first to avoid the blood monitoring requirements with clozapine use.[1] Avoid **olanzapine** as it has not been shown to be effective and is poorly tolerated.[1]

Cholinesterase inhibitors (e.g., **donepezil**, **rivastigmine**) have a modest impact on improving dementia, but careful observation for deterioration in motor function is required.[18]

Therapeutic Tips

- Symptomatic treatment is not necessary in the early stage of PD when symptoms are noticed but not troublesome. All drugs have the potential to cause side effects that would outweigh their benefits at this stage in the disease.
- Start medication at low doses and titrate slowly, especially in the elderly, to minimize the acute side effects of medications.
- When levodopa or a dopamine agonist are initiated, **domperidone** (10–20 mg ½ hour prior to each dose) can be helpful to minimize gastric upset or orthostatic hypotension.
- Individualize patient management based on the severity of disease, level of disability, cost, patient preference and patient's age.
- Nonmotor difficulties such as dysarthria, sleep disturbance, depression, dementia and postural instability are common, especially as the disease progresses. Managing these effectively with the assistance of allied health professionals is important for maximizing a patient's quality of life.[1]
- Parkinsonism-hyperpyrexia syndrome (similar to neuroleptic malignant syndrome) is a potentially fatal complication of Parkinson's disease treatment, usually associated with abrupt reduction or discontinuation of dopaminergic drugs. Hyponatremia is also a risk factor. Medications should be reduced or withdrawn slowly. "Drug holidays" to reduce motor complications are not a recommended practice.[1]
- Pregnancy and breastfeeding are uncommon considerations among patients with Parkinson's disease. Expert consultation should be sought where possible; amantadine should be avoided.

Table 1: **Drugs Used in the Treatment of Parkinson's Disease**

Class	Drug	Dose	Adverse Effects	Drug Interactions	Cost[a]
Anticholinergic Agents	*benztropine* Benztropine, other generics	1–2 mg BID po	Dry mouth, blurred vision, constipation, urinary retention, aggravation of glaucoma, confusion, memory impairment. Avoid in elderly. Risk of parkinsonism-hyperpyrexia syndrome with abrupt discontinuation; taper gradually. Drug holidays not recommended.	Amantadine may increase anticholinergic effects.	$
	ethopropazine Parsitan	25 mg BID–50 mg TID po	See benztropine.	See benztropine.	$
	procyclidine generics	5 mg TID po	See benztropine.	See benztropine.	$
	trihexyphenidyl generics	Initial: 1 mg BID po Usual: 2 mg TID po	See benztropine.	See benztropine.	$
COMT Inhibitors	*entacapone* Comtan, generics	200 mg po with each dose of levodopa; maximum 8 × daily	Dyskinesia, nausea, sleep disorder, anorexia, diarrhea, hallucinations; urine discolouration. Risk of parkinsonism-hyperpyrexia syndrome with abrupt discontinuation; taper gradually. Drug holidays not recommended.	Potentiates levodopa; increased dyskinesia, psychosis. Avoid dobutamine, dopamine, epinephrine, isoproterenol, nonselective MAOIs.	$
Dopamine Agonists	*bromocriptine* generics	Initial: 1.25 mg BID po Usual: 5–10 mg TID po	Nausea, vomiting, orthostatic hypotension, hallucinations, psychosis, erythromelalgia (burning pain, warmth and redness of the extremities), pleural fibrosis (obtain a baseline chest x-ray before initiating therapy). Risk of parkinsonism-hyperpyrexia syndrome with abrupt discontinuation; taper gradually. Drug holidays not recommended.	Antihypertensives, diuretics, tricyclic antidepressants may increase hypotensive action.	$$$–$$$$

(cont'd)

Table 1: **Drugs Used in the Treatment of Parkinson's Disease** *(cont'd)*

Class	Drug	Dose	Adverse Effects	Drug Interactions	Cost[a]
	pramipexole ❥ Mirapex, generics	Initial: 0.125 mg TID po Usual: 0.5–1 mg TID po	Orthostatic hypotension, somnolence, confusion, hallucinations, nausea, vomiting, sudden sleep attacks; caution patients about potential compulsive behaviours such as pathologic gambling or hypersexual behaviour; caution patients about driving or operating dangerous machinery. Risk of parkinsonism-hyperpyrexia syndrome with abrupt discontinuation; taper gradually. Drug holidays not recommended.	See bromocriptine.	$
	ropinirole ReQuip, generics	Initial: 0.25 mg TID po Usual: 3–6 mg TID po	See pramipexole.	See bromocriptine. Ciprofloxacin increases levels of ropinirole.	$$
	rotigotine Neupro	Initial: 2 mg/24 h transdermal patch once daily Increase at weekly intervals as needed, to a maximum of 16 mg/24 h Usual: 6–8 mg/24 h Apply to clean, dry, intact skin on abdomen, thigh, hip, flank, shoulder or upper arm. Avoid using same site twice within 14 days.	See pramipexole. Application site reactions can occur.	See bromocriptine.	$$$$$
Levodopa Preparations	*levodopa/carbidopa, immediate-release* Sinemet, generics	Initial: 50/12.5 mg BID po Usual: 100/25 mg–150/37.5 mg TID–QID po	Nausea, vomiting, orthostatic hypotension, dyskinesias, hallucinations, confusion. Risk of parkinsonism-hyperpyrexia syndrome with abrupt discontinuation; taper gradually. Drug holidays not recommended.	Antihypertensives, diuretics, tricyclic antidepressants may increase hypotensive action.	$
	levodopa/carbidopa, controlled-release Sinemet CR, generics	Initial: 100/25 mg[b] BID po Usual: 200/50 mg[b] QID po	See levodopa/carbidopa, immediate-release. Decreased "kick" compared to Sinemet immediate-release; patterns of dyskinesia may be more complex.	See levodopa/carbidopa, immediate-release.	$$$

Class	Drug	Dose	Adverse Effects	Drug Interactions	Cost[a]
	levodopa/ benserazide Prolopa	Initial: 50/12.5 mg BID po Usual: 100/25 mg–150/37.5 mg TID–QID po	See levodopa/carbidopa, immediate-release.	See levodopa/carbidopa, immediate-release.	$$
Levodopa/COMT Inhibitor Combinations	*levodopa/carbidopa/ entacapone* Stalevo	50/12.5/200 mg, 100/25/200 mg or 150/37.5/200 mg TID–QID po, depending on previous levodopa/carbidopa and/or entacapone dose	See levodopa/carbidopa. See entacapone.	See levodopa/carbidopa. See entacapone.	$$$–$$$$
MAO-B Inhibitors	*rasagiline* Azilect	Monotherapy: 1 mg daily po Adjunctive therapy: 0.5–1 mg daily po Mild hepatic impairment: 0.5 mg daily maximum; avoid in patients with severe impairment	Insomnia, confusion, hallucinations, increased dyskinesia, autonomic dysfunction. Risk of parkinsonism-hyperpyrexia syndrome with abrupt discontinuation; taper gradually. Drug holidays not recommended.	Avoid use with dextromethorphan, meperidine, pseudoephedrine, TCAs, MAO-A inhibitors, SNRIs, SSRIs. Use lower dose of 0.5 mg daily in patients taking ciprofloxacin or other CYP1A2 inhibitors.	$$$$$
	selegiline (deprenyl) generics	2.5 mg daily–5 mg BID po Give before 1 p.m.	See rasagiline.	Avoid use with atomoxetine, bupropion, dextroamphetamine, dextromethorphan, meperidine, pseudoephedrine, TCAs, MAO-A inhibitors, SSRIs. May need to reduce dose in women taking oral contraceptives.	$
N-methyl-D-aspartate (NMDA) Receptor Antagonists	*amantadine* ➊ generics	Usual: 100 mg BID po	Nausea, constipation, dry mouth, insomnia, anxiety, impaired concentration, livedo reticularis, orthostatic hypotension, ankle edema. Use with caution in elderly; avoid in pregnancy and in patients with cognitive deficits. Risk of parkinsonism-hyperpyrexia syndrome with abrupt discontinuation; taper gradually. Drug holidays not recommended.	Anticholinergic agents may increase effects.	$

[a] Cost of 30-day supply of usual dose; includes drug cost only.
[b] Compared to Sinemet immediate-release formulation, bioavailability of Sinemet CR is 25–30% lower and duration of action 25–30% longer.
➊ Dosage adjustment is required in renal impairment; see Appendix I.
Abbreviations: MAOI = monoamine oxidase inhibitor; SNRI = serotonin-norepinephrine reuptake inhibitor; SSRI = selective serotonin reuptake inhibitor; TCA = tricyclic antidepressant
Legend: $ < $50 $$ $50–100 $$$ $100–150 $$$-$$$$ $100–200 $$$$ $150–200 $$$$$ $200–250

Suggested Readings

Grimes D, Gordon J, Snelgrove B et al. Canadian guidelines on Parkinson's disease. *Can J Neurol Sci* 2012;39(Suppl 4):S1-30.

Miyasaki JM, Martin W, Suchowersky O et al. Practice parameter: initiation of treatment for Parkinson's disease: an evidence-based review: report of the Quality Standards Subcommittee of the American Academy of Neurology. *Neurology* 2002;58(1):11-7.

National Collaborating Centre for Chronic Conditions. *Parkinson's disease: national clinical guideline for diagnosis and management in primary and secondary care.* London (GB): Royal College of Physicians; 2006. Available from: www.nice.org.uk/nicemedia/live/10984/30087/30087.pdf.

Pahwa R, Factor SA, Lyons KE et al. Practice parameter: treatment of Parkinson disease with motor fluctuations and dyskinesia (an evidence-based review): report of the Quality Standards Subcommittee of the American Academy of Neurology. *Neurology* 2006;66(7):983-95.

Suchowersky O, Gronseth G, Perlmutter J et al. Practice parameter: neuroprotective strategies and alternative therapies for Parkinson disease (an evidence-based review): report of the Quality Standards Subcommittee of the American Academy of Neurology. *Neurology* 2006;66(7):976-82.

References

1. Grimes D, Gordon J, Snelgrove B et al. Canadian guidelines on Parkinson's disease. *Can J Neurol Sci* 2012;39(Suppl 4):S1-30.
2. Grimes DA, Lang AE. Treatment of early Parkinson's disease. *Can J Neurol Sci* 1999;26(Suppl 2):S39-44.
3. Fahn S. Does levodopa slow or hasten the rate of progression of Parkinson's disease? *J Neurol* 2005;252(Suppl 4):IV37-IV42.
4. Lang AE, Lozano AM. Parkinson's disease. Second of two parts. *N Engl J Med* 1998;339(16):1130-43.
5. Olanow CW, Obeso JA, Stocchi F. Drug insight: continuous dopaminergic stimulation in the treatment of Parkinson's disease. *Nat Clin Pract Neurol* 2006;2(7):382-92.
6. Schapria AH, Obeso J. Timing of treatment initiation in Parkinson's disease: a need for reappraisal? *Ann Neurol* 2006;59(3):559-62.
7. Stowe R, Ives N, Clarke CE et al. Meta-analysis of the comparative efficacy and safety of adjuvant treatment to levodopa in later Parkinson's disease. *Mov Disord* 2011;26(4):587-98.
8. Miyasaki JM, Martin W, Suchowersky O et al. Practice parameter: initiation of treatment for Parkinson's disease: an evidence-based review: report of the Quality Standards Subcommittee of the American Academy of Neurology. *Neurology* 2002;58(1):11-7.
9. Stocchi F, Rascol O, Kieburtz K et al. Initiating levodopa/carbidopa therapy with and without entacapone in early Parkinson disease: the STRIDE-PD study. *Ann Neurol* 2010;68(1):18-27.
10. Baseman DG, O'Suilleabhain PE, Reimold SC et al. Pergolide use in Parkinson disease is associated with cardiac valve regurgitation. *Neurology* 2004;63(2):301-4.
11. Van Camp G, Flamez A, Cosyns B et al. Treatment of Parkinson's disease with pergolide and relation to restrictive valvular heart disease. *Lancet* 2004;363(9416):1179-83.
12. Zhou, CQ, Li SS, Chen ZM et al. Rotigotine transdermal patch in Parkinson's disease: a systematic review and meta-analysis. *PLoS ONE* 2013;8(7):e69738.
13. Holloway RG, Shoulson I, Fahn S et al. Pramipexole vs levodopa as initial treatment for Parkinson disease: a 4-year randomized controlled trial. *Arch Neurol* 2004;61(7):1044-53.
14. Hobson DE, Lang AE, Martin WR et al. Excessive daytime sleepiness and sudden-onset sleep in Parkinson disease: a survey by the Canadian Movement Disorders Group. *JAMA* 2002;287(4):455-63.
15. Weintraub D, Koester J, Potenza MN et al. Impulse control disorders in Parkinson disease: a cross-sectional study of 3090 patients. *Arch Neurol* 2010;67(5):589-95.
16. Olanow CW, Rascol O, Hauser R et al. A double-blind, delayed-start trial of rasagiline in Parkinson's disease. *N Engl J Med* 2009;361(13):1268-78.
17. Schuepbach WM, Rau J, Knudsen K et al. Neurostimulation for Parkinson's disease with early motor complications. *N Engl J Med* 2013;368(7):610-22.
18. Miyasaki JM, Shannon K, Voon V et al. Practice parameter: evaluation and treatment of depression, psychosis, and dementia in Parkinson disease (an evidence-based review): report of the Quality Standards Subcommittee of the American Academy of Neurology. *Neurology* 2006;66(7):996-1002.

Neurologic Disorders

Chapter 23
Persistent Hiccups

James M. Wright, MD, PhD, CRCPC

Persistent (2–30 days) or intractable (>1 month) hiccups are unusual but distressing. They may cause insomnia, weight loss or depression and are associated with metabolic causes and abnormalities of the CNS, ear, throat, diaphragm, thorax and abdomen.

Goals of Therapy

- Stop or decrease frequency or intensity of hiccups
- Prevent recurrence

Investigations

- Complete history (including medication and alcohol use) and physical examination to provide clues for further investigations. If no abnormalities are identified, it is reasonable to do a CBC, electrolytes, creatinine and chest x-ray
  - drug-induced persistent hiccups are uncommon; alcohol, corticosteroids and benzodiazepines are the drugs most frequently implicated[1]
- Further investigations depend on findings from the history, physical and baseline investigations, e.g., upper GI tract endoscopy, CT brain, abdominal ultrasound

If all investigations are negative or etiologic treatment is impossible, a therapeutic trial to stop the hiccups is warranted.

Therapeutic Choices

Nonpharmacologic Choices

- Vagal stimulation (e.g., posterior pharyngeal wall stimulation with a finger, forced expiration against a closed glottis for 10 seconds in the sitting position) is worth trying.
- If gastric distention is identified as the cause, gastric aspiration is effective.
- Poor-quality studies have reported temporary or permanent relief of intractable hiccups with acupuncture, but no randomized, placebo-controlled trials testing this approach have been published.[2]
- Phrenic nerve disruption is reserved for cases where all else has failed.

Pharmacologic Choices

Table 1 details the medications used in the management of persistent or intractable hiccups

One randomized controlled cross-over trial comparing baclofen with placebo was identified (see Baclofen, below).[3] Most treatment recommendations are based on case reports or open trials in small numbers of patients.

Dopamine Antagonists

Chlorpromazine historically has been the drug of choice.[4] It has been used iv (25–50 mg over 0.5–1 hour) in the emergency room. A trial of 25–50 mg TID–QID po for 2–3 days is also reasonable but experience suggests that oral therapy may be less effective than the iv route. **Haloperidol** 2–5 mg im or 2–10 mg po has also been effective in some cases.[5] **Metoclopramide**, 10 mg iv or im followed by 5–10 mg TID–QID po, has been successful.[6] It may act as a dopamine antagonist or by enhancing gastric emptying. Adverse effects of dopamine antagonists include acute dystonia and postural hypotension. If chronic therapy is required, use back-titration to find the lowest effective dose taken once daily.

Baclofen

Baclofen has been effective in intractable hiccups, with maintenance therapy required in at least 50% of cases.[7] A randomized double-blind cross-over trial in 4 patients with intractable hiccups demonstrated that baclofen did not eliminate the hiccups, but did increase hiccup-free periods and decrease hiccup severity.[3] Starting with 5 mg BID, the dose is increased gradually every 2–3 days to a maximum daily dose of 80 mg. If effective, baclofen should not be discontinued suddenly. The minimum maintenance dose can be determined by gradually reducing the dose over time. Since baclofen is excreted by the kidney, much lower doses are required in the presence of renal failure (e.g., 2.5 mg BID). Side effects (drowsiness, weakness, nausea and fatigue) are relatively frequent.

Other Drugs

In case reports or case series, many other drugs such as **amantadine**,[8] **amitriptyline**,[9] **carbamazepine**,[10] **gabapentin**,[11] **nifedipine**[12] and **valproic acid**[13] have been found to be effective.

Duration of Treatment

When a drug is effective in aborting the hiccups, taper the dose downwards after 3 days. If hiccups return, find the lowest dose that will suppress them. If they do not return, the drug can be tapered and stopped.

Therapeutic Tips

- When a drug is effective, hiccups generally stop abruptly within a few hours; in some cases, the frequency and severity may slowly decrease.
- Attempt to withdraw treatments gradually; maintenance therapy may be required in some cases.
- Avoid benzodiazepines, as worsening of hiccups has been reported.
- When a drug is ineffective, there is no need to continue treatment for more than 3 days.

Table 1: Drugs Used in Persistent or Intractable Hiccups

Class	Drug	Dose	Adverse Effects	Drug Interactions	Cost[a]
Dopamine Antagonists[b]	*chlorpromazine* generics	ER: 25–50 mg iv over 30–60 min Oral: 25–50 mg TID–QID × 2–3 days	Anticholinergic effects, extrapyramidal effects, hypotension, sedation.	Additive sedative effects with CNS depressants, including alcohol.	$
	haloperidol generics	ER: 2–5 mg im Oral: 2–10 mg once daily × 2–3 days	Sedation, extrapyramidal effects.	See chlorpromazine.	im: $$ po: $
	metoclopramide (renal) Metonia, other generics	ER: 10 mg iv or im Oral: 5–10 mg TID–QID × 2–3 days	Diarrhea, abdominal cramps, hyperprolactinemia, sedation, extrapyramidal effects, headache.	See chlorpromazine.	im/iv: $$ po: $
Muscle Relaxants[b]	*baclofen* (renal) Lioresal Oral, generics	Start with 5 mg BID po; increase gradually every 2–3 days to a maximum of 80 mg per day	Sedation, muscle weakness, nausea, dizziness, lowered seizure threshold.	Additive sedative effects with CNS depressants, including alcohol.	$

[a] Cost per day for oral therapy, unless otherwise specified; includes drug cost only.
[b] If chronic therapy required, establish lowest effective dose using gradual back-titration.
(renal) Dosage adjustment may be required in renal impairment; see Appendix I.
Abbreviations: CNS = central nervous system; ER = emergency room
Legend: $ <$2 $$ $2–5

Suggested Readings

Friedman NL. Hiccups: a treatment review. *Pharmacotherapy* 1996;16(6):986-95.
Woelk CJ. Managing hiccups. *Can Fam Physician* 2011;57(6):672-5, e198-201.

References

1. Drug-induced hiccups. *Prescrire Int* 1999;8(39):23.
2. Moretto EN, Wee B, Wiffen PJ et al. Interventions for treating persistent and intractable hiccups in adults. *Cochrane Database Syst Rev* 2013;1:CD008768.
3. Ramirez FC, Graham DY. Treatment of intractable hiccup with baclofen: results of a double-blind randomized, controlled, cross-over study. *Am J Gastroenterol* 1992;87(12):1789-91.
4. Friedgood CE, Ripstein CB. Chlorpromazine (thorazine) in the treatment of intractable hiccups. *J Am Med Assoc* 1955;157(4):309-10.
5. Ives TJ, Fleming MF, Weart CW et al. Treatment of intractable hiccups with intramuscular haloperidol. *Am J Psychiatry* 1985;142(11):1368-9.
6. Madanagopolan N. Metoclopramide in hiccup. *Curr Med Res Opin* 1975;3(6):371-4.
7. Guelaud C, Similowski T, Bizec JL et al. Baclofen therapy for chronic hiccup. *Eur Respir J* 1995;8(2):235-7.
8. Wilcox SK, Garry A, Johnson MJ. Novel use of amantadine: to treat hiccups. *J Pain Symptom Manage* 2009;38(3):460-5.
9. Peabody CA, Dewitt J, Herrin S et al. Intractable hiccups treated with amitriptyline. *Am J Psychiatry* 1988;145(8):1036-7.
10. McFarling DA, Susac JO. Letter: Carbamazepine for hiccoughs. *JAMA* 1974;230(7):962.
11. Porzio G, Aielli F, Verna L et al. Gabapentin in the treatment of hiccups in patients with advanced cancer: a 5-year experience. *Clin Neuropharmacol* 2010;33(4):179-80.
12. Lipps DC, Jabbari B, Mitchell MH et al. Nifedipine for intractable hiccups. *Neurology* 1990;40(3 Pt 1):531-2.
13. Jacobson PL, Messenheimer JA, Farmer TW. Treatment of intractable hiccups with valproic acid. *Neurology* 1981;31(11):1458-60.

Chapter 24
Restless Legs Syndrome

Anne-Louise Lafontaine, MD, MSc, FRCPC

Restless legs syndrome (RLS), also known as Willis-Ekbom disorder, is a neurologic disorder characterized by an unpleasant sensation in the legs accompanied by an urge to move the legs, especially at bedtime.[1] The cause of primary RLS is not definitively known but is believed to involve a genetic component as well as dysfunctional dopaminergic transmission and low brain iron stores. Secondary RLS is associated with many conditions such as diabetes mellitus, end-stage renal disease (anemia may play a role), iron deficiency, multiple sclerosis, Parkinson's disease, pregnancy and venous insufficiency. Drugs such as alcohol, antidepressants, antipsychotics, caffeine, metoclopramide and nicotine can aggravate symptoms.

Symptoms of RLS occur when the limbs are at rest, and are relieved by movement. In severe cases, symptoms may extend to the arms and trunk. Symptoms are commonly bilateral and symmetrical, but on occasion can be unilateral. The prevalence of RLS is estimated to be 5–15% in the general population,[1,2] is higher in women and increases with age. Patients often use the following terms to describe the symptoms of RLS: a "creepy-crawly", "burning", "nagging", "aching", "painful", "itching-bones" or "electric-current" sensation. These unpleasant sensations may last hours and may persist throughout the night causing sleep disturbance in some patients.

All of the following 4 criteria are required for a diagnosis of RLS:[3]

- An urge to move the legs, usually accompanied or caused by unpleasant sensations in the legs.
- Symptoms begin or worsen during periods of rest or inactivity such as lying or sitting.
- Symptoms are partially or totally relieved by movement, such as walking or stretching, for at least as long as the activity continues.
- Symptoms are worse in the evening or at night, or may occur only in the evening or at night.

Supportive clinical features include a positive family history, response to dopaminergic therapy and periodic limb movements during wakefulness (PLM) or during sleep (PLMS).[3]

Intermittent RLS is defined as symptoms that occur on average less than twice a week but are troublesome enough to require treatment less often than daily. In *chronic persistent* RLS, symptoms cause moderate to severe distress and are frequent and bothersome enough to require daily therapy.[4] Symptoms occur on average at least twice a week. Patients with *refractory* RLS are those who experience inadequate response and/or intolerable side effects and/or "augmentation" (see Goals of Therapy) not responding to more frequent dosing, while receiving first-line therapy for daily symptoms.

Goals of Therapy

- Improve the symptoms of motor restlessness and discomfort
- Improve sleep
- Improve function in patients experiencing daytime symptoms
- Reduce the PLMS, if disruptive
- Reduce the potential for "rebound" or "augmentation" with drug therapy
  - "rebound" is the recurrence of symptoms during the night or early morning coinciding with the end-of-dose wearing off of effectiveness.[5]

- "augmentation" is the occurrence of symptoms earlier in the day than they occurred prior to treatment, a shorter latency time to symptom onset when at rest, an increase in the severity of symptoms with shorter treatment effect and/or spread of symptoms to involve the upper extremities and trunk.[6]

Investigations

- History from patient and partner regarding sleep and PLMS
- CBC, electrolytes, BUN, creatinine, fasting glucose, serum iron, ferritin and iron saturation
- Nerve conduction studies can be performed if peripheral neuropathy is suspected
- Polysomnography should be performed if there is a clinical suspicion of sleep apnea or concurrent sleep disorder
- Consider vascular insufficiency, e.g., varicose veins, as potential contributing factor

Therapeutic Choices

Nonpharmacologic Choices

While pharmacologic therapy is needed for moderate to severe symptoms, nonpharmacologic measures may be useful in milder cases:

- Engage in mental alertness activities (playing cards, video games or doing crossword puzzles) to reduce symptoms during times of boredom.[7]
- Abstain from alcohol, caffeine and nicotine.[7]
- Take hot baths, stretch and exercise moderately.[8]
- Discontinue medications that may be contributing to symptoms, e.g., antidepressants, antipsychotics, dopamine-blocking antiemetics and sedating antihistamines.[7]
- Minimize aggravating factors such as sleep deprivation.
- In patients with RLS and varicose veins, consider sclerotherapy to improve RLS symptoms.[9]

In patients who do not respond to pharmacotherapy or experience intolerable side effects, consider a trial of pneumatic compression devices (PCDs), garments that are intermittently inflated and deflated with compressed air using an electrical pneumatic pump. In a small randomized sham-controlled study of one month's duration, patients who wore PCDs on their legs for at least 1 hour daily prior to the usual onset time of moderate to severe RLS symptoms had improvement in quality of life scores and clinically significant improvement in RLS symptoms.[10]

Pharmacologic Choices

Studies have shown that 25–30% of patients with RLS are iron deficient.[11] The incidence of secondary RLS is increased in patients with conditions associated with iron deficiency such as pregnancy and end-stage renal disease. Furthermore, RLS may be the only clinical indicator of iron deficiency and can be more severe in patients with serum ferritin less than 50 µg/L (normal range is 40–200 µg/L).[4] When patients present with RLS symptoms, investigate for the possible presence and cause of iron deficiency. Although a systematic review concluded there was insufficient evidence to determine whether iron would benefit any or all patients with RLS,[12] a trial of **oral iron therapy** should be considered for patients in whom a deficiency is detected [Evidence: SORT C*].[13] For more information about treatment of iron deficiency anemia, see Chapter 99.

* SORT (Strength of Recommendation Taxonomy) is a rating system (A, B or C) that addresses the quality of available evidence. For more information consult **How to Use *Compendium of Therapeutic Choices*** on page xxv.

The choice of pharmacologic agent depends on the severity of RLS symptoms. See Table 1 for a list of drug therapy options for RLS.

Levodopa preparations, benzodiazepines or low-potency opioids are good options for treatment of intermittent RLS.[4] In chronic persistent RLS, dopamine agonists or GABA derivatives are the preferred agents. Both are associated with a lower risk of augmentation compared to levodopa.[4,14] Figure 1 illustrates the clinical management of intermittent and chronic persistent RLS.

In patients with refractory RLS, lower doses of single-agent therapy are not effective. Consider combining treatment from different drug classes, i.e., dopamine agonists, GABA derivatives, benzodiazepines or opioids.[4,14] Figure 2 illustrates clinical management of refractory RLS.

Pharmacotherapy for Intermittent RLS

Levodopa Preparations

Many clinical trials have shown **levodopa/carbidopa** to be effective for the treatment of RLS.[15] While levodopa may be suitable for patients with intermittent symptoms, its short half-life increases the potential for rebound and/or augmentation and makes it a poor choice for patients with daily symptoms.

Figure 1: **Management of Intermittent and Chronic Persistent Restless Legs Syndrome[4]**

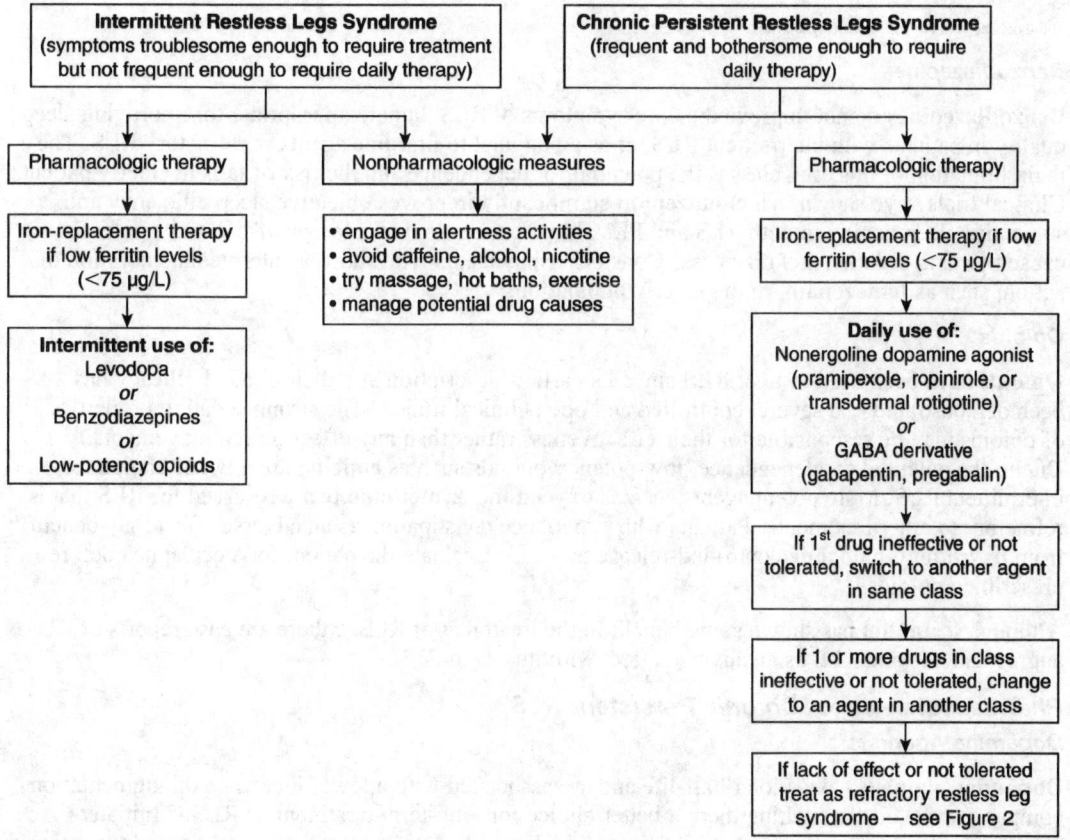

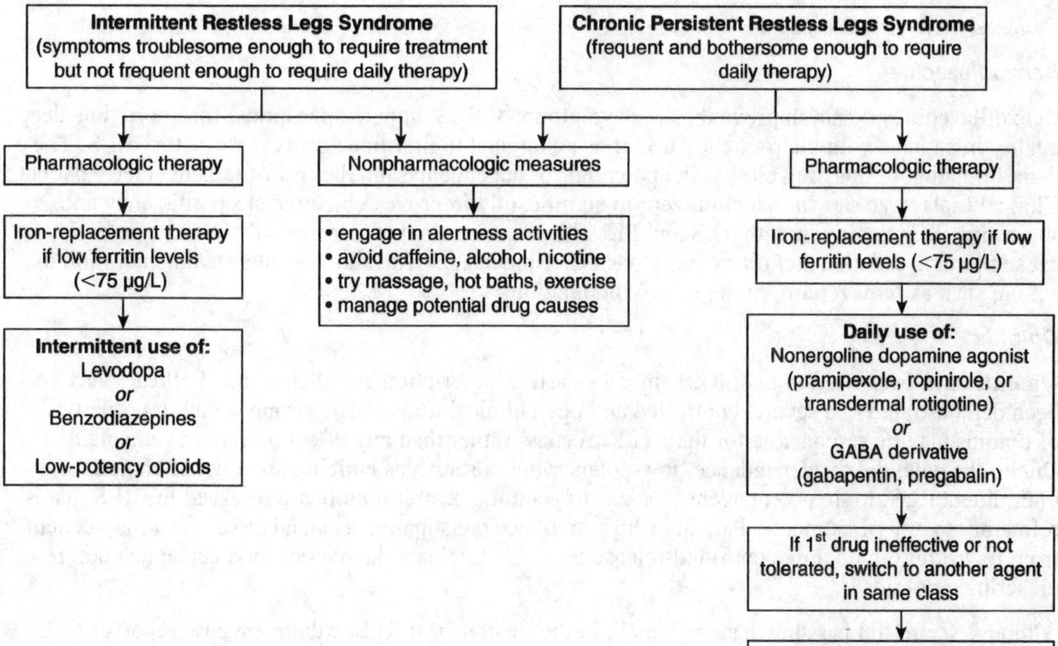

Figure 2: **Management of Refractory Restless Legs Syndrome**[4]

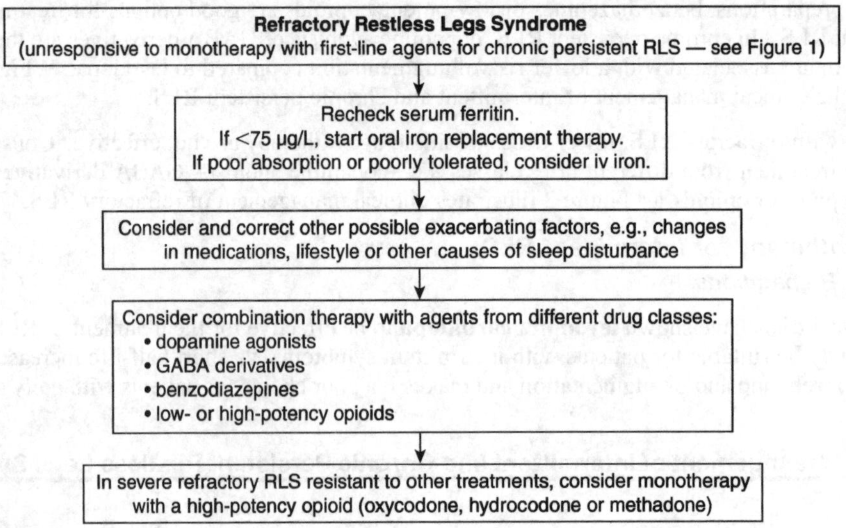

Abbreviations: RLS=restless legs syndrome

Benzodiazepines

Benzodiazepines do not improve the core symptoms of RLS, but are appropriate for improving sleep quality in patients with intermittent RLS, or as an adjunct to first-line agents in refractory RLS. The main limitation of this drug class is the potential for dependence and the risk of falls in elderly patients. Clinical trials have shown that **clonazepam** significantly improves objective sleep efficiency and subjective sleep quality in both RLS and PLMS.[16] Clonazepam has a long half-life and a potential to cause morning sedation and dizziness. Consider using agents with short or intermediate duration of action, such as **temazepam**, in the elderly population.

Opioids

Opioids have been used to treat RLS since its earliest description and their clinical efficacy has been demonstrated in a several controlled and open clinical trials.[17] The strong sedating properties of opioids may be responsible for their effectiveness rather than any effect on leg movements. Due to the potential for dependence, low-potency opioids such as **codeine** are a better choice for intermittent RLS. More potent agents such as **oxycodone** or **methadone** are reserved for RLS that is refractory to other treatments. Patients who experience constipation as an adverse effect may benefit from **oxycodone-naloxone** controlled-release tablets.[18] Evaluate the patient for sleep apnea before prescribing opioids.[19]

Although **tramadol** has shown some benefit in the treatment of RLS[20], there are case reports of RLS augmentation[21] and RLS as an adverse effect with this agent.[22]

Pharmacotherapy for Chronic Persistent RLS

Dopamine Agonists

Dopamine agonists have a long-half-life and are associated with a lower incidence of augmentation compared to levodopa, making them a better choice for long-term treatment of RLS.[19] Initiate treatment with a dopamine agonist in patients who have severe symptoms, excessive weight, comorbid depression, cognitive impairment or are at increased risk for falling.[19] The efficacy of bromocriptine,[23] pergolide,[24,25] pramipexole,[26] ropinirole[27] and rotigotine[28] in the treatment of RLS has been established in controlled clinical trials. These agents improve sleep efficiency and decrease the frequency of periodic limb movements during sleep. Side effects of dopamine agonists include nausea, sedation and lightheadedness and these generally decrease after the first few months of therapy.[19] Clinicians should inform patients that dopamine agonists are associated with a high risk (6–17%) of developing a compulsive behaviour such as pathological gambling and hypersexuality.[19,29] These disorders may occur more frequently in women and may be associated with higher doses of drugs. Monitor for these behaviours at each patient visit and discontinue or decrease the dosage of the dopamine agonist if the adverse effect is significant.[19] When discontinuing dopamine agonist treatment, taper the dose gradually to minimize withdrawal symptoms.[19]

Bromocriptine and **pergolide** are ergoline derivatives that are associated with a higher frequency of adverse effects. Pergolide is no longer available in Canada. It was withdrawn from the market in 2007 due to reports of cardiac valvulopathy.[30]

Pramipexole and **ropinirole** are nonergoline derivatives and have a more favourable side effect profile in patients with RLS. When used at higher doses in the treatment of Parkinson's disease they have been associated with a higher incidence of sudden sleep attacks. For RLS, pramipexole is started at 0.125 mg po taken 2 hours before the onset of symptoms and the dose is increased every 4–5 days until it is effective.[19] The average dose is 0.5 mg but some patients may require up to 2 mg daily. The starting dose of ropinirole is 0.25 mg/day with an average effective dose being in the 1–4 mg/day range. Some patients may require an additional dose given in the late afternoon if symptoms arise earlier in the day.

Rotigotine is a nonergolinic dopamine agonist that is officially approved to treat symptoms of moderate to severe idiopathic RLS in patients 18 years or older. The transdermal system is formulated to deliver rotigotine over a 24-hour period. To minimize skin irritation, advise patients to apply the patch only on intact, undamaged skin and not to use the same application site for at least 14 days. The patches should not be cut. Avoid the use of external heat to the area where the patch is applied as this would increase the release of the drug from the patch.

GABA Derivatives

GABA derivatives are alternatives to dopamine agonists in the treatment of chronic persistent RLS. Consider these agents first in patients who have severe sleep disturbance, comorbid insomnia or anxiety, painful RLS, or a history of compulsive behaviour or anxiety.[19] **Gabapentin** and **pregabalin** are administered once or twice daily later in the day (afternoon, evening or before sleep). Gabapentin was shown to be effective in open[31] and double-blind, randomized controlled trials.[32] Initiate gabapentin at 300 mg po daily and titrate to effect; typical doses range from 900–1800 mg/day.[4] Consider pregabalin in patients who develop augmentation (see Goals of Therapy) with a dopamine agonist. In a year-long double-blind trial, 719 patients with RLS were randomized to once daily doses of pregabalin 300 mg, pramipexole 0.25 mg, pramipexole 0.5 mg or 12 weeks of placebo followed by 40 weeks of one of the active treatments.[33] Pregabalin was shown to significantly improve RLS symptom scores compared to placebo, and significantly lower augmentation rates compared to pramipexole 0.5 mg. To minimize adverse effects, start pregabalin at 100 mg po daily and increase every 2–3 days to an effective dose usually in the range of 150–450 mg/day.[4] Major side effects of these agents include drowsiness and unsteady gait, especially in the elderly. Suicide-related events have been reported with GABA derivatives; monitor patients for signs of suicidal ideation and behaviours.

Gabapentin enacarbil is a novel prodrug of gabapentin that is not currently available in Canada. This agent was developed to address the pharmacokinetic limitations of gabapentin and can be administered once daily. Its effectiveness in the treatment of RLS has been shown in several randomized, controlled trials.[34]

Other Agents

Antiepileptic drugs such as carbamazepine and valproic acid have not been as rigorously studied as the GABA derivatives.[35,36] There is some evidence for improved RLS symptoms with other agents such as amantadine,[37] baclofen[38] and clonidine.[39] These drugs should be reserved for patients who develop tolerance to recommended first-line agents.

Choices during Pregnancy and Breastfeeding

RLS and Pregnancy

RLS symptoms are common during pregnancy with an estimated prevalence of 10–20%.[40] The exact cause is not known but deficiency of iron and vitamins may be involved. Symptoms of RLS are most often a feature of the third trimester and are usually temporary, with most symptoms disappearing soon after childbirth.

None of the drugs used to treat RLS are known to be safe in pregnancy. Nonpharmacologic choices are therefore the safest treatments for women who experience RLS during pregnancy. It is important to rule out iron, magnesium or folate deficiency, as appropriate supplementation may be helpful. RLS typically becomes more severe as the pregnancy progresses. If pharmacologic therapy is deemed necessary, waiting until the third trimester will reduce the risk of adverse pregnancy outcomes. **Dopamine agonists** are not recommended. **Opioids** can be used but should be avoided near term because of the risk of respiratory depression in the newborn. For most pregnant women, RLS is temporary and the symptoms will typically resolve postpartum. Educating pregnant women about the self-limiting nature of symptoms may allay fears.

RLS and Breastfeeding

As in pregnancy, nonpharmacologic choices are the safest option for women experiencing RLS when breastfeeding. There is no available information on the use of **pramipexole**, **ropinirole** and **rotigotine** in breastfeeding women, but these drugs suppress serum prolactin and may interfere with lactation.[41] Limited information indicates that maternal doses of **gabapentin** and **pregabalin** may produce relatively low levels in infant serum.[41] Limited data indicate that **levodopa** is poorly excreted into breast milk and that sustained-release formulations may result in a smaller amount of drug transferred to the breastfed infant than immediate-release products.[42] Several studies indicate that levodopa can decrease serum prolactin during lactation, but a reduced prolactin level may not affect breastfeeding in a mother with established lactation.[43,44] The effect of long-term use of levodopa on breastfeeding has not been adequately evaluated.

A discussion of general principles on the use of medications in these special populations can be found in Appendix II and Appendix III. Other specialized reference sources are also provided in these appendices.

Therapeutic Tips

- Always consider nonpharmacologic management.
- When possible, discontinue drugs that may be contributing to symptoms.
- Drugs should be started at the lowest dose, administered 1–2 hours before bedtime, and gradually titrated to the lowest effective dose.
- Optimizing long-term therapy may be difficult; if one drug loses its effectiveness, switching to another drug in the same or a different class may be effective.
- For symptoms beginning earlier in the day, a second daily dose can be prescribed in the afternoon, and if needed, in the morning.
- Intractable RLS may require the use of polytherapy.

- Levodopa is associated with a higher incidence of rebound. Restrict its use to the treatment of intermittent RLS.
- Augmentation occurs less frequently with dopamine agonists than with levodopa. Manage augmentation by alternating medications, i.e., switch between drug classes every few months as needed.
- For patients taking dopamine agonists, monitor at each visit for the emergence of compulsive behaviours.
- The Willis-Ekbom Disease Foundation website (www.willis-ekbom.org) is a good resource for healthcare providers and patients.

Table 1: Drug Therapy for Restless Legs Syndrome

Class	Drug	Dose	Adverse Effects	Drug Interactions	Cost[a]
Benzodiazepines	*clonazepam* Rivotril, generics	0.25–2 mg QHS po	Sedation, dizziness, dependence.	Additive sedation with other CNS depressants such as alcohol.	$
	temazepam Restoril, generics	15–30 mg QHS po	See clonazepam.	See clonazepam.	$
	triazolam generics	0.125–0.25 mg QHS po	See clonazepam.	See clonazepam.	$
Dopamine Agonists	*bromocriptine* generics	7.5 mg QHS po	Nausea, vomiting, lightheadedness, hallucinations, psychosis, erythromelalgia (burning pain, warmth and redness of the extremities), pleural fibrosis. Risk of parkinsonism-hyperpyrexia syndrome with abrupt discontinuation; taper gradually. Drug holidays not recommended.	First-generation antipsychotics decrease effect of dopamine agonists.	$$$
	pramipexole Mirapex, generics	0.125–0.75 mg/day po; at least 2 hours before usual time of symptom onset May need up to 2 mg/day.	Orthostatic hypotension, somnolence, confusion, hallucinations, nausea, vomiting, insomnia, sudden sleep attacks. Caution patients about potential compulsive behaviours such as pathologic gambling or hypersexual behaviour. Caution patients about driving or operating dangerous machinery. Risk of parkinsonism-hyperpyrexia syndrome with abrupt discontinuation; taper gradually. Drug holidays not recommended.	See bromocriptine.	$
	ropinirole ReQuip, generics	0.25–4 mg/day po May be given in 2–3 divided doses if needed.	See pramipexole.	See bromocriptine.	$

Class	Drug	Dose	Adverse Effects	Drug Interactions	Cost[a]
	rotigotine Neupro	1–3 mg/24 h transdermal patch once daily Apply to clean, dry intact skin on abdomen, thigh, hip, flank, shoulder or upper arm. Avoid using the same site twice within 14 days.	Lightheadedness, confusion, hallucinations, nausea, vomiting, sedation, fatigue, headache. Caution patients about potential compulsive behaviours such as pathologic gambling or hypersexual behaviour. Risk of parkinsonism-hyperpyrexia syndrome with abrupt discontinuation; taper gradually. Drug holidays not recommended. Application site reactions can occur.	First-generation antipsychotics decrease effect of dopamine agonists.	$100–200
GABA Derivatives	*gabapentin* ◗ Neurontin, generics	300–2400 mg daily po May be given in 2–3 divided doses if needed. Not a Health Canada-approved indication.	Sedation, dizziness, ataxia, tremor, vision changes, weight gain.	May enhance CNS depressant effects when coadministered with other CNS depressants. May cause peripheral edema/weight gain when coadministered with thiazolidinediones (pioglitazone, rosiglitazone).	$$$$
	pregabalin ◗ Lyrica, generics	100–450 mg/day po May be given in 2 divided doses if needed. Not a Health Canada-approved indication.	Sedation, dizziness, ataxia, tremor, vision changes, weight gain.	See gabapentin.	$$$
Levodopa Preparations	*levodopa/carbidopa* Sinemet, Sinemet CR, generics	50/12.5–200/50 mg QHS po	Nausea, vomiting, lightheadedness, dry mouth, "rebound" and "augmentation".	First-generation antipsychotics decrease effect of levodopa. Antihypertensives, diuretics, tricyclic antidepressants may increase hypotensive action. Reduced absorption with high-protein meals.	$
Opioids	*codeine immediate-release* ◗ generics	30–180 mg/day po May be given in 2–3 divided doses if needed.	Sedation, constipation, dependence.	Additive sedation with other CNS depressants such as alcohol.	$
	codeine sustained-release ◗ Codeine Contin	50–150 mg daily po divided Q12H	See codeine immediate-release.	See codeine immediate-release.	$$

(cont'd)

Table 1: Drug Therapy for Restless Legs Syndrome *(cont'd)*

Class	Drug	Dose	Adverse Effects	Drug Interactions	Cost[a]
	methadone Metadol, generics	5–40 mg/day po May be given in 2 divided doses if needed.	See codeine immediate-release. May prolong QT_c interval.	See codeine immediate-release. Caution with other drugs that can cause QT_c interval prolongation such as amiodarone, erythromycin, quinidine.	$$$
	oxycodone immediate-release Oxy-IR, Supeudol, generics	5–30 mg daily po May be given in 2–3 divided doses if needed.	See codeine immediate-release.	See codeine immediate-release.	$$
	oxycodone sustained-release OxyNEO, generics	10–20 mg HS po	See codeine immediate-release.	See codeine immediate-release.	$$
	oxycodone/naloxone controlled-release Targin	10–20 mg (oxycodone component) HS po	See codeine immediate-release. Role of naloxone is to relieve opioid-induced constipation.	See codeine immediate-release.	$$$

[a] Cost of 30-day supply of mean dose; includes drug cost only.
Dosage adjustment may be required in renal impairment; see Appendix I.
Legend: $ < $15 $$ $15–30 $$$ $30–45 $$$$ $45–60

Suggested Readings

Aurora RN, Kristo DA, Bista SR et al. The treatment of restless legs syndrome and periodic limb movement disorder in adults–an update for 2012: practice parameters with an evidence-based systematic review and meta-analyses: an American Academy of Sleep Medicine Clinical Practice Guideline. *Sleep* 2012;35(8):1039-62.

Ekbom K, Ulfberg J. Restless legs syndrome. *J Intern Med* 2009;266(5):419-31.

Silber MH, Becker PM, Earley C et al. Willis-Ekbom Disease Foundation revised consensus statement on the management of restless legs syndrome. *Mayo Clin Proc* 2013;88(9):977-86.

References

1. Ekbom KA. Restless legs syndrome. *Neurology* 1960;10:868-73.
2. Lavigne GJ, Montplaisir JY. Restless legs syndrome and sleep bruxism: prevalence and associations among Canadians. *Sleep* 1994;17(8):739-43.
3. Allen RP, Picchietti D, Hening WA et al. Restless legs syndrome: diagnostic criteria, special considerations, and epidemiology. A report from the restless legs syndrome diagnosis and epidemiology workshop at the National Institutes of Health. *Sleep Med* 2003;4(2):101-19.
4. Silber MH, Becker PM, Earley C et al. Willis-Ekbom Disease Foundation revised consensus statement on the management of restless legs syndrome. *Mayo Clin Proc* 2013;88(9):977-86.
5. Guilleminault C, Cetel M, Philip P. Dopaminergic treatment of restless legs and rebound phenomenon. *Neurology* 1993;43(2):445.
6. Allen RP, Earley CJ. Augmentation of the restless legs syndrome with carbidopa/levodopa. *Sleep* 1996;19(3):205-13.
7. Silber MH, Ehrenberg BL, Allen RP et al. An algorithm for the management of restless legs syndrome. *Mayo Clin Proc* 2004;79(7):916-22.
8. Ryan M, Slevin JT. Restless legs syndrome. *Am J Health Syst Pharm* 2006;63(17):1599-612.
9. Kanter AH. The effect of sclerotherapy on restless legs syndrome. *Dermatol Surg* 1995;21(4):328-32.
10. Lettieri CJ, Eliasson AH. Pneumatic compression devices are an effective therapy for restless legs syndrome: a prospective, randomized, double-blind, sham-controlled trial. *Chest* 2009;135(1):74-80.
11. Allen RP, Auerbach S, Bahrain H et al. The prevalence and impact of restless legs syndrome on patients with iron deficiency anemia. *Am J Hematol* 2013;88(4):261-4.
12. Trotti LM, Bhadriraju S, Becker LA. Iron for restless legs syndrome. *Cochrane Database Syst Rev* 2012;5:CD007834.
13. Wang J, O'Reilly B, Venkataraman R et al. Efficacy of oral iron in patients with restless legs syndrome and low-normal ferritin: a randomized, double-blind, placebo-controlled study. *Sleep Med* 2009;10(9):973-5.
14. Garcia-Borreguero D, Grunstein R, Sridhar G et al. A 52-week open-label study of the long-term safety of ropinirole in patients with restless legs syndrome. *Sleep Med* 2007;8(7-8):742-52.
15. Montplaisir J, Lapierre O, Warnes H et al. The treatment of the restless legs syndrome with or without periodic leg movements in sleep. *Sleep* 1992;15(5):391-5.
16. Saletu M, Anderer P, Saletu-Zyhlarz G et al. Restless legs syndrome (RLS) and periodic limb movement disorder (PLMD): acute placebo-controlled sleep laboratory studies with clonazepam. *Eur Neuropsychopharmacol* 2001;11(2):153-61.
17. Ondo WG. Methadone for refractory restless legs syndrome. *Mov Disord* 2005;20(3):345-8.
18. Trenkwalder C, Benes H, Grote L et al. Prolonged release oxycodone-naloxone for treatment of severe restless legs syndrome after failure of previous treatment: a double-blind, randomized, placebo-controlled trial with an open-label extension. *Lancet Neurol* 2013;12(12):1141-50.
19. Garcia-Borreguero D, Kohnen R, Silber MH et al. The long-term treatment of restless legs syndrome/Willis-Ekbom disease: evidence-based guidelines and clinical consensus best practice guidance: a report from the International Restless Legs Syndrome Study Group. *Sleep Med* 2013;14(7):675-84.
20. Lauerma H, Markkula J. Treatment of restless legs syndrome and tramadol: an open study. *J Clin Psychiatry* 1999;60(4):241-4.
21. Vetrugno R, La Morgia C, D'Angelo R et al. Augmentation of restless legs syndrome with long-term tramadol treatment. *Mov Disord* 2007;22(3):424-7.
22. Perez-Lloret S, Rey MV, Bondon-Guitton E et al. Drugs associated with restless legs syndrome: a case/noncase study in the French Pharmacovigilance Database. *J Clin Psychopharmacol* 2012;32(6):824-7.
23. Walters AS, Hening WA, Kavey N et al. A double-blind randomized crossover trial of bromocriptine and placebo in restless legs syndrome. *Ann Neurol* 1988;24(3):455-8.
24. Wetter TC, Stiasny K, Winkelmann J et al. A randomized controlled study of pergolide in patients with restless legs syndrome. *Neurology* 1999;52(5):944-50.
25. Trenkwalder C, Hundemer HP, Lledo A et al. Efficacy of pergolide in treatment of restless legs syndrome: the PEARLS Study. *Neurology* 2004;62(8):1391-7.
26. Montplaisir J, Nicolas A, Denesle R et al. Restless legs syndrome improved by pramipexole: a double-blind randomized trial. *Neurology* 1999;52(5):938-43.
27. Adler CH, Hauser RA, Sethi K et al. Ropinirole for restless legs syndrome: a placebo-controlled crossover trial. *Neurology* 2004;62(8):1405-7.
28. Trenkwalder C, Benes H, Poewe W et al. Efficacy of rotigotine for treatment of moderate-to-severe restless legs syndrome: a randomised, double-blind, placebo-controlled trial. *Lancet Neurol* 2008;7(7):595-604.
29. Tippman-Peikert M, Park JG, Boeve BF et al. Pathologic gambling in patients with restless legs syndrome treated with dopaminergic agonists. *Neurology* 2007;68(4):301-3.
30. Van Camp G, Flamez A, Cosyns B et al. Treatment of Parkinson's disease with pergolide and relation to restrictive valvular heart disease. *Lancet* 2004;363(9416):1179-83.
31. Happe S, Klosch G, Saletu B et al. Treatment of idiopathic restless legs syndrome (RLS) with gabapentin. *Neurology* 2001;57(9):1717-19.
32. Garcia-Borreguero D, Larrosa O, de la Llave Y et al. Treatment of restless legs syndrome with gabapentin: a double-blind, cross-over study. *Neurology* 2002;59(10):1573-9.
33. Allen RP, Chen C, Garcia-Borrequero D et al. Comparison of pregabalin with pramipexole for restless legs syndrome. *N Engl J Med* 2014;370(7):621-31.
34. Yaltho TC, Ondo WG. The use of gabapentin enacarbil in the treatment of restless legs syndrome. *Ther Adv Neurol Disord* 2010;3(5):269-75.

35. Eisensehr I, Ehrenberg BL, Rogge Solti S et al. Treatment of idiopathic restless legs syndrome with slow-release valproic acid compared with slow-release levodopa/benserazid. *J Neurol* 2004;251(5):579-83.
36. Hornyak M, Scholz H, Kohnen R et al. What treatment works best for restless legs syndrome? Meta-analyses of dopaminergic and non-dopaminergic medications. *Sleep Med Rev* 2014;18(2):153-64.
37. Evidente VG, Adler CH, Caviness HN et al. Amantadine is beneficial in restless legs syndrome. *Mov Disord* 2000;15(2):324-7.
38. Guilleminault C, Flagg W. Effect of baclofen on sleep-related periodic leg movements. *Ann Neurol* 1984;15(3):234-9.
39. Handwerker JV, Palmer RF. Clonidine in the treatment of "restless leg" syndrome. *N Engl J Med* 1985;313(19):1228-9.
40. Manconi M, Govoni V, De Vito A et al. Restless legs syndrome and pregnancy. *Neurology* 2004;63(6):1065-9.
41. Drugs and Lactation Database (LactMed). Bethesda (MD): U.S. National Library of Medicine. Available from: toxnet.nlm.nih.gov/cgi-bin/sis/htmlgen?LACT.
42. Thulin PC, Woodward WR, Carter JH et al. Levodopa in human breast milk: clinical implications. *Neurology* 1998;50(6):1920-1.
43. Kaulhausen H, Oney T, Leyendecker G. Inhibition of the renin-aldosterone axis and of prolactin secretion during pregnancy by L-dopa. *Br J Obstet Gynaecol* 1982;89(6):483-8.
44. Rao R, Scommegna A, Frohman LA. Integrity of central dopaminergic system in women with postpartum hyperprolactinemia. *Am J Obstet Gynecol* 1982;143(8):883-7.

Chapter 25
Seizures and Epilepsy

Jeremy J. Moeller, MD, FRCPC and
R. Mark Sadler, MD, FRCPC

Epilepsy is a neurological disorder characterized by a predisposition to unprovoked seizures. Treatment of epilepsy entails not only prevention of seizures but also the management of biological, cognitive, psychological and social consequences of this disorder. This chapter focuses mainly on the role of antiepileptic drugs (AEDs) in adults with epilepsy, but also outlines some other important considerations in the pharmacologic management of this complex disease.

The International League Against Epilepsy (ILAE) provides a practical definition of epilepsy as a brain disease defined by either 2 unprovoked seizures occurring more than 24 hours apart or one unprovoked seizure and a high (>60%) probability of further seizures over the next 10 years.[1] There are many seizure types and epilepsy syndromes, and the classification system for seizures and epileptic disorders can be intimidating to new learners.[2] Since traditional terminology is still used by most practising clinicians, for the purposes of clarity both traditional and newer terminology for epileptic seizure types are provided.

Goals of Therapy

- Appropriately manage patients presenting with a first seizure (see Pharmacologic Choices, The First Seizure)
- Prevent seizure recurrence in patients with an established diagnosis of epilepsy, i.e., recurrent seizures
- Prevent or minimize adverse effects of antiepileptic drugs (AEDs)
- Optimize quality of life, e.g., employment, psychosocial interactions, driving

Investigations

Figure 1 illustrates an algorithm for the management of seizures and epilepsy.

History

- The most important factor in making a diagnosis is a detailed history of the patient's "spells" obtained from both the patient and a witness (see Clinical Features).
- Is there an aura (rising abdominal sensation, sudden fear or anxiety, feeling of déjà-vu)? An aura indicates the onset of a focal seizure, and its features provide valuable clues to the anatomic site of the seizure onset. Lack of an aura may be due to focal (partial) seizures that spread very rapidly, or generalized seizures.
- Inquire about history of recurrent or prolonged seizures in childhood, intracranial infection, head trauma, stroke, any systemic disorders that may affect the CNS (such as malignancies, fluid and electrolyte disorders), family history of seizures or other neurologic diseases.
- Determine whether there are concerns such as use of drugs (prescribed or recreational) and alcohol, sleep deprivation, or symptoms of raised intracranial pressure.

Figure 1: **Management of Seizures and Epilepsy**

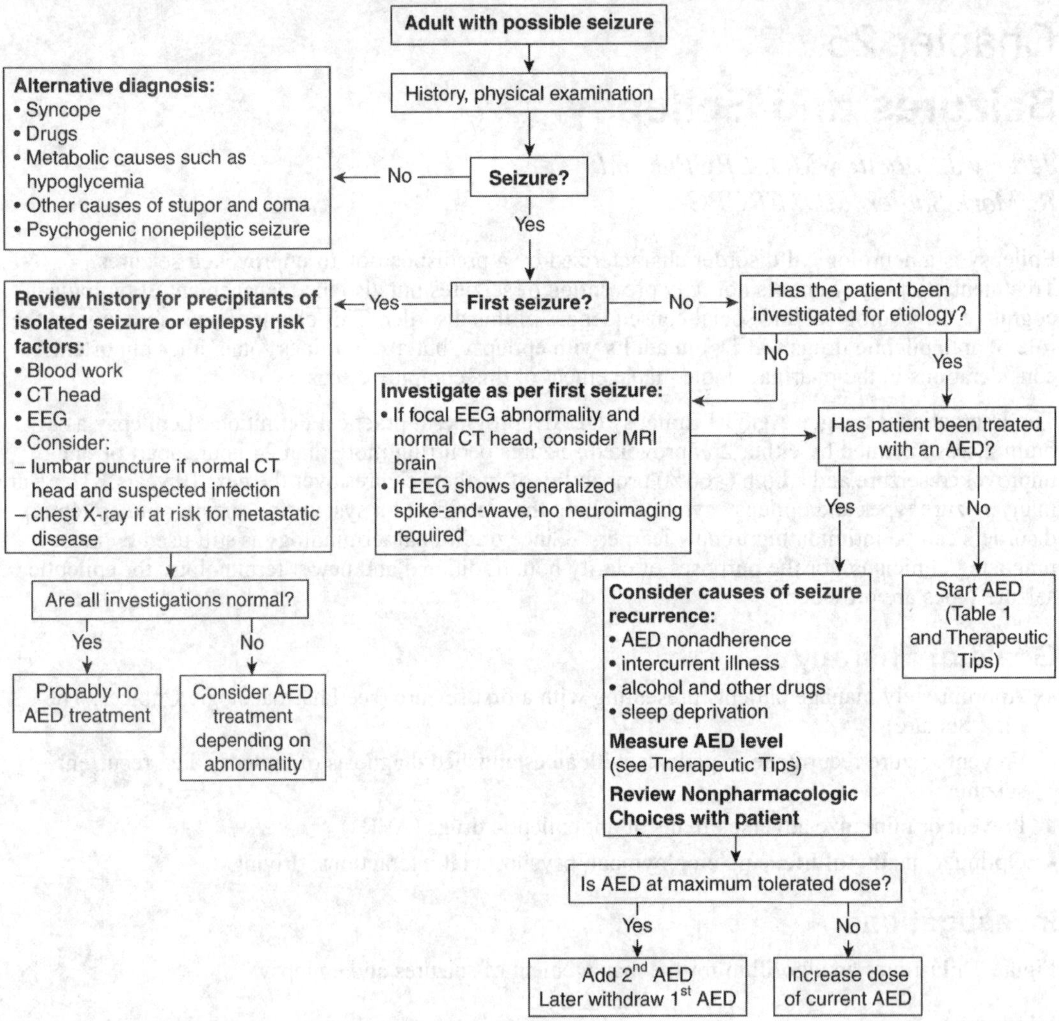

Abbreviations: AED = antiepileptic drug; CT = computed tomography; EEG = electroencephalogram; MRI = magnetic resonance imaging

Clinical Features[3,4]

- Focal seizures (partial seizures)
  - Focal seizures without impairment of awareness (simple partial seizures):
    - motor, sensory, autonomic or cognitive features
    - usually brief (<60 seconds)
  - Focal seizures with impairment of awareness (complex partial seizures):
    - focally originating seizures characterized by behavioral arrest, often manifested as a blank stare
    - usual duration of 1–2 minutes
    - frequently accompanied by motor automatisms, e.g., lip smacking and chewing movements

    - brief postictal confusion is common
    - can begin without impairment of awareness before progressing, or can have impairment of awareness at onset
    - commonly misdiagnosed as absence seizures
- Generalized seizures
  - Absence ("petit mal"):
    - last only seconds (usually 5–10)
    - recur daily (often in clusters) in the untreated patient
    - no warning signs or postictal confusion
    - onset in childhood or adolescence (almost never *begin* in adulthood)
  - Generalized tonic-clonic ("grand mal"):
    - can begin as a focal seizure (secondarily generalized) or can involved the entire brain at onset (primarily generalized)
    - a careful history may help identify focal/partial features at onset, thereby distinguishing secondarily generalized from primarily generalized tonic-clonic seizures
    - fairly uniform sequence of motor features (tonic and clonic phases)
    - impaired consciousness
    - duration of 1–2 minutes
    - postictal stupor, confusion and headache
  - Atonic seizures:
    - abrupt loss of consciousness and muscle tone
    - no other motor features
    - return to awareness within seconds
    - occur as part of a clinical syndrome in patients with childhood-onset epilepsy, significant intellectual disability and other seizure types
    - virtually never occur in otherwise intellectually and physically normal adults
  - Myoclonic seizures:
    - a generalized seizure type consisting of brief, bilateral "shock-like" jerks
    - multifocal asynchronous myoclonic jerks most commonly occur in the setting of a metabolic encephalopathy
- Consider whether the clinical features suggest one of the entities commonly mistaken for epileptic seizures, such as syncope or psychogenic nonepileptic spells, migraine or transient ischemic attack (TIA).

Physical Examination

- Look for evidence of any systemic disorder that can affect the central nervous system, such as malignancy, infection or autoimmune disorder
- Look for focal or lateralizing findings in the neurologic examination (hemianopia, motor weakness, hemisensory disturbance, reflex asymmetry, language dysfunction)
- Assess potential injuries sustained during a generalized tonic-clonic seizure, e.g., tongue laceration, shoulder dislocation or vertebral compression fracture or a focal seizure with alteration of awareness (complex partial seizure), e.g., burns, lacerations or contusions

Laboratory Investigations[5]

- For the patient presenting with a *first seizure*, consider:
  - CBC, glucose, electrolytes, calcium, renal and hepatic function
  - alcohol levels, toxicology screen, infection screen such as urinalysis and urine cultures (especially in elderly or developmentally-challenged population).
  - chest x-ray if metastatic disease is a consideration
  - electroencephalogram (EEG) to support the clinical impression of seizures and to determine whether the seizure is focal or primarily generalized. The interictal EEG may show focal spikes in patients with focal (partial) seizures or generalized spike-waves in the primarily generalized epilepsies. The EEG may also be helpful in determining the likelihood of seizure recurrence. A normal EEG does not rule out epilepsy or the possibility of future seizures.
  - computed tomography (CT) head scan. Adults should have a CT scan unless they are otherwise well and their EEG demonstrates generalized spike-and-wave discharges, which indicate one of the primarily generalized seizure syndromes that are not accompanied by gross structural brain abnormalities. Patients should have a CT scan before any clinically warranted lumbar puncture.
  - lumbar puncture if the presenting clinical features suggest intracranial infection (meningitis, encephalitis) or a CT-negative subarachnoid hemorrhage
  - magnetic resonance imaging (MRI) if the patient has focal (partial) seizures of unknown etiology and negative CT scan
- For the patient with known epilepsy treated with AEDs who is presenting with a seizure recurrence, assess:
  - factors that may precipitate loss of seizure control (medication nonadherence, intercurrent illness with fever and vomiting, sleep deprivation, alcohol, nonprescription drug use)
  - the addition of a drug that may promote seizures or interact with AEDs
  - sudden withdrawal from alcohol, benzodiazepines, barbiturates
  - AED serum levels (phenytoin, phenobarbital, primidone, carbamazepine, valproic acid). Serum levels for other AEDs may be difficult to obtain and are of limited clinical value. (Nonadherence with AED therapy is the most common cause of seizure breakthrough in patients with known epilepsy.)

Therapeutic Choices

Nonpharmacologic Choices

- Avoid sleep deprivation.
- Keep alcohol consumption to a minimum. Cocaine and amphetamines must be avoided because of their proconvulsant properties. The evidence for marijuana as a "pro-" or "anti-" seizure drug is inconclusive.
- Ask patients about their use of herbal remedies and dietary supplements. Many will try natural health products without the knowledge of their physicians. Some of these products may have proconvulsant properties or important pharmacologic interactions with AEDs.[6]
- Discuss seizure precautions with patient and family members.
- Advise patients about the requirement for driving restrictions. Regulations regarding seizures and driving vary by province and can be obtained through provincial departments of transportation.
- Certain types of diets, including the ketogenic diet and the Modified Atkins Diet, may reduce seizure frequency in some patients. However, these treatments require strict adherence to a high-fat, low-carbohydrate diet and are not practical for most adults with epilepsy.[7]

- Consider epilepsy surgery for patients with medically refractory focal (partial) seizures resistant to multiple AEDs.[8]
- Other complementary practices (yoga, meditation, relaxation training and acupuncture) have limited evidence supporting their efficacy in epilepsy. However, these practices should not necessarily be discouraged; they may benefit the overall physical and psychological health of the patient, and are often associated with a low risk of harm.

Pharmacologic Choices

Deciding whether AED treatment is indicated following a first seizure is an important consideration (see The First Seizure, below).

The choice of an AED depends on the seizure type (Table 1), potential for drug interactions and side effects (Table 3), cost (Table 3) and physician familiarity with the drug.[9,10]

There is some evidence for a drug of first choice in both *focal (partial)* and *generalized* epilepsy syndromes. In a large, multicentre trial of "new" AEDs for patients with a partial epilepsy syndrome, **lamotrigine** was better tolerated than **carbamazepine**, and was similarly effective in obtaining long-term seizure freedom.[11] The other AEDs used in the trial, gabapentin and topiramate, were not superior to carbamazepine.

Table 1: **Suggested Therapeutic Options for Antiepileptic Drugs**[9,10]

Seizure Type	First Choice Monotherapy[a,b]	Alternative Monotherapy or Add-on[a]
Generalized tonic-clonic	carbamazepine lamotrigine phenytoin valproic acid/divalproex	clobazam levetiracetam topiramate
Absence	ethosuximide	clobazam lamotrigine levetiracetam topiramate valproic acid/divalproex
Myoclonic and atonic	valproic acid/divalproex	clobazam lamotrigine levetiracetam rufinamide topiramate
Focal (partial) seizures with or without 2° generalization	carbamazepine lamotrigine levetiracetam phenytoin	clobazam gabapentin lacosamide oxcarbazepine perampanel phenobarbital primidone topiramate valproic acid/divalproex vigabatrin

[a] AEDs are listed alphabetically; the order does not reflect a preference ranking.
[b] See Pharmacologic Choices for further discussion of first-choice monotherapy.

A parallel trial for patients with generalized epilepsy syndromes showed that **valproic acid** was superior to lamotrigine and topiramate.[12] Valproic acid was particularly effective in maintaining long-term seizure freedom in patients with idiopathic generalized epilepsy. However, the trial was not designed to measure pregnancy outcomes, and there is evidence that among the commonly used AEDs valproic acid may pose the highest risk to the fetus in pregnant women with epilepsy.

Levetiracetam monotherapy was not superior to the "older" AEDs in a large, open-label study comparing levetiracetam to controlled-release carbamazepine (in patients with focal seizures) and valproic acid (in patients with generalized epilepsy syndromes).[13] There is no strong evidence comparing other newer agents such as oxcarbazepine and lacosamide to the older AEDs.

For childhood absence epilepsy, **ethosuximide** and **valproic acid** are similarly effective in preventing seizures, and both medications are superior to lamotrigine.[14] Ethosuximide is associated with lower rates of attention difficulties than valproic acid, and is usually the drug of first choice in childhood absence epilepsy. However, ethosuximide is not effective in preventing other seizure types such as generalized tonic-clonic seizures, and should not be used as monotherapy in children with multiple seizure types.

Basic principles for initiating AED therapy:

- Select a single AED (Table 1).
- Start the AED at a fraction of the initial target dose (Table 3) to minimize the risk of dose-dependent adverse effects (exceptions are phenytoin and phenobarbital).
- Inform patient of potential risks of treatment (especially life-threatening hypersensitivity reactions).
- Evaluate the patient after the initial target dose has been achieved. Make a small dosage reduction if dose-related adverse effects are problematic. Slowly increase the dose if seizures have recurred.
- Add a second AED if the maximum tolerated dose of the first AED has failed to achieve satisfactory seizure control. Gradually withdraw the first AED after the maintenance dose of the second drug has been achieved. Polytherapy is usually reserved until monotherapy with 2–3 drugs has failed.

The First Seizure

- Whether to treat with AEDs after the first seizure can be a difficult decision for the patient and physician and must be individualized.[15,16] Many patients will not require AED treatment after a single seizure. The decision should be guided by clinical factors as outlined above and a careful conversation with the patient in which the risks associated with recurrent seizures (e.g., driving restrictions, injury) are weighed against the risks of long-term AED therapy.
- Most patients come to medical attention with a primarily or secondarily generalized tonic-clonic seizure. At least one-third of these patients have experienced prior unrecognized nocturnal tonic-clonic seizures and/or nonconvulsive seizures. It is important to determine if the event was *truly* the first seizure. Generally, patients whose history indicates potentially unrecognized or misdiagnosed prior seizures should be treated, as the risk for seizure recurrence is high.
- Not all patients with a single tonic-clonic seizure will have a recurrence. The overall risk of recurrence after a single unprovoked seizure is 40% within 2 years, but the degree of risk can be stratified based on other factors. For example, the recurrence risk in a patient with a normal EEG >2 years after a single unprovoked seizure is approximately 25%, compared to a risk of approximately 50% in a patient with epileptiform discharges on EEG.
- An increased risk of recurrence is suggested if one or more of the following features is present:[5,15,16]
  - identifiable remote cause of increased seizure risk, such as severe head injury
  - focally originating seizure
  - abnormal neurologic examination
  - epileptiform discharges on EEG

Status Epilepticus (SE)

- "Convulsive" SE was traditionally defined as recurrent primarily or secondarily generalized tonic-clonic seizures lasting >30 minutes, or intermittent seizures lasting >30 minutes, without return to baseline consciousness between events. However, almost all "isolated" tonic-clonic seizures last <2 minutes;[17] a tonic-clonic seizure lasting >5 minutes most likely suggests "impending SE" and should be treated aggressively.[18]
- Any seizure type (absence, focal [partial]) can evolve to nonconvulsive status epilepticus and this diagnosis should be considered in any patient with unexplained coma.
- Predisposing factors include subtherapeutic AED serum levels (often related to nonadherence), drug withdrawal (alcohol, benzodiazepines), acute or chronic structural brain injury or tumour.
- Psychogenic nonepileptic seizures (psychiatrically-based behaviours that are not associated with abnormal EEG rhythms) can be confused with convulsive SE because of some similarities on clinical presentation. There are clinical and EEG features that help to differentiate psychogenic nonepileptic events from epileptic seizures. Conversely, absence or partial complex SE is often misdiagnosed as a psychiatric condition.
- Convulsive SE is associated with high morbidity and mortality, related to underlying cause and the effects of seizures on the brain. Brain injury begins at 30–45 minutes after onset of SE; aggressive treatment of seizures is important to optimize outcome. With convulsions lasting longer than 5 minutes, early treatment with an adequate dose of benzodiazepine showed a trend toward lower rates of respiratory complications than no treatment;[19] do not withhold initial benzodiazepine treatment because of concerns about respiratory suppression. Table 2 outlines a suggested treatment protocol.

Table 2: **Initial Management of Convulsive Status Epilepticus in Adults**[17,18,20]

Time	Management
0–5 min	History, physical examination. Oral airway, oxygen. Consider intubation. Venous blood (glucose, blood counts, electrolytes, calcium, renal and liver function, AED blood levels, consider drug screen). Arterial blood gases. Monitor ECG, pulse oximetry, blood pressure.
6–10 min	Start 2 large-bore iv saline infusions. 50 mL dextrose 50% iv. Thiamine 100 mg im or iv. Lorazepam 2 mg iv; repeat once if seizures persist ***or*** if no iv access: midazolam 5 mg im; repeat once if seizures persist ***or*** diazepam 20 mg pr; can use rectal gel formulation or iv solution.
11–30 min	Phenytoin 20 mg/kg iv (maximum rate = 50 mg/min) ***or*** phenobarbital 20 mg/kg iv (50–75 mg/min) ***or*** midazolam 10 mg iv bolus, then 0.05–0.4 mg/kg/h ***or*** propofol 2–5 mg/kg iv bolus followed by infusion at 2–10 mg/kg/h.
31–60 min	Obtain neuroimaging (CT, MRI) if etiology of SE not known; consider lumbar puncture if a possibility of meningitis-encephalitis. Admit to intensive care unit, obtain expert advice, arrange EEG.

Abbreviations: AED = antiepileptic drug; CT = computed tomography; ECG = electrocardiogram; EEG = electroencephalogram; MRI = magnetic resonance imaging; SE = status epilepticus

General Safety Measures and Seizure Precautions

- To reduce the risk of burns during seizures:
  - discourage smoking
  - encourage patients to use microwave ovens and place pots and pans on the rear burners of stoves
- Avoid heights and ladders.
- Avoid use of power tools.
- Showers are preferable to tub baths because of the risk of drowning.
- Assess recreational activities as well as current and planned employment, and counsel accordingly.
- Patients with active epilepsy who are caregivers for young children should not bathe them without assistance and should not use change tables for clothing or diaper changes.
- Assess driving status. Physicians should be aware of their legal obligations to local departments of transportation (mandatory vs. discretional reporting).
- Some patients may benefit from membership in an epilepsy support group.

Choices during Pregnancy and Breastfeeding

Because seizure disorders often affect female patients during their childbearing years, it is important to consider the interaction between pregnancy/breastfeeding and the patient with epilepsy in a positive and proactive manner.[21,22,23] Approximately 90% of women with epilepsy who are seizure-free for at least 9 months prior to pregnancy will remain seizure-free during pregnancy.

Prepregnancy Considerations

- Contraception:
  - there is an increased risk of combined oral contraceptive (COC) failure in women taking enzyme-inducing AEDs (carbamazepine, oxcarbazepine, phenobarbital, phenytoin, primidone, topiramate). Ideally the COC should contain ≥50 µg ethinyl estradiol; however, no COC products currently available in Canada contain >35 µg. In addition to hormonal methods, the use of a barrier method (condoms) is recommended for increased contraceptive effect and to reduce the risk of sexually transmitted infections. However, barrier methods should not replace more effective methods of contraception such as COCs.
  - other contraceptive methods (intrauterine devices, progestin depot injection formulations) may be reasonable alternatives for women with epilepsy. Encourage use of condoms with these methods as well.
- Discuss pregnancy plans prior to conception:
  - is AED treatment still required?
  - AED polytherapy probably increases the risk of congenital malformations compared to monotherapy. Consider withdrawing the least helpful AEDs if the patient is treated with AED polytherapy. The least helpful AED is the drug that had the smallest effect on seizure frequency when added.
  - if possible, avoid valproic acid in women of childbearing age, particularly those who are planning to become pregnant, because of increased risk of major congenital malformations and poor cognitive outcome. However, the risk of teratogenesis with valproic acid must be balanced against potential risk associated with uncontrolled seizures.
  - women of childbearing potential who take AEDs should receive continuous **folic acid** supplementation (at least 1 mg/day; some experts recommend 5 mg/day) to potentially reduce the risk of teratogenic effects associated with AEDs.

Choices during Pregnancy

- AEDs during pregnancy:[24]
  - available evidence does not allow selection of one or more AEDs that are "best" for preventing teratogenesis or negative perinatal outcomes
  - over 90% of women with epilepsy treated with AEDs have successful pregnancies and outcomes
  - follow AED levels as they may drop significantly during pregnancy due to increased clearance
  - do not switch AEDs during pregnancy to avoid teratogenesis. The risk of major congenital malformations is highest in the first trimester, before many women have discovered that they are pregnant. A change of AED therapy during pregnancy exposes the fetus to risks associated with polytherapy and exposes the mother to the risks of serious adverse effects (including hypersensitivity reaction) and uncontrolled seizures and/or status epilepticus.
- Obtain expert obstetrical advice on timing and type of ultrasound to detect fetal malformations.
- Vitamin K is routinely given to all newborns at delivery to prevent hemorrhagic disease of the newborn. It is unclear whether prenatal oral vitamin K supplementation in women taking AEDs provides any additional benefit.[25]

Choices during Breastfeeding

- Breastfeeding should not be discouraged. Many AEDs transfer into breast milk, but the clinical significance of this is uncertain. Infants whose mothers are taking **barbiturates** may be sedated; infants exposed to barbiturates prepartum who are not breastfed may have barbiturate withdrawal symptoms in the first week after delivery.
- Follow AED levels as they may rise precipitously in the first weeks post-delivery.

A discussion of general principles on the use of medications in these special populations can be found in Appendix II and Appendix III. Other specialized reference sources are also provided in these appendices.

Therapeutic Tips

- Obtain a baseline CBC and serum liver aminotransferases if treating with an AED that may cause a hypersensitivity syndrome involving blood or liver; repeat in 4–6 weeks. Mild elevations (<2–3 times the upper limit of normal) in liver enzymes and/or modest reductions in blood counts (e.g., neutropenia with carbamazepine, thrombocytopenia with valproic acid) are relatively common. These minor changes do not require discontinuation of treatment; follow such abnormalities with serial blood tests. If CBC and liver enzymes remain stable, the frequency of repeat blood work can be gradually decreased. Yearly blood work is appropriate in stable patients.
- Do not rely on serum AED levels alone to guide therapy. Some patients will have satisfactory seizure control at low AED levels, while others have dose-related toxicity with AED levels in the "therapeutic" range. Obtain a serum AED level when the patient is seizure-free and has no dose-related toxicity; this AED level may serve as a reference point for the future if seizures or drug toxicity occur. A useful adage is "treat the patient, not the serum level."
- With many AEDs, drug interactions are potential problems. Drugs with hepatic enzyme-inducing properties (carbamazepine, oxcarbazepine, phenobarbital, phenytoin, primidone, topiramate) may reduce the levels of concomitant medications. Consider the presence (or absence) of other medications when selecting an AED.
- It is reasonable to refer any patient with uncontrolled seizures despite adequate trials of 2–3 AEDs to a tertiary-care epilepsy centre for further evaluation.

Table 3: **Antiepileptic Drugs**

Class	Drug	Dose	Adverse Effects[a]	Advantages	Disadvantages	Cost[b]
Barbiturates	*phenobarbital* Phenobarb, other generics	90–120 mg/day HS po	Sedation prominent, rash 5%, depression, diminished libido.	Long half-life; daily dosing; inexpensive.	Potent inducer of cytochrome P450, therefore many potential drug interactions; may decrease efficacy of hormonal contraceptives; metabolism inhibited by valproic acid; declining use because of adverse effect profile.	$
	primidone generics	Initial: 125 mg HS po × 3 days, 125 mg BID po × 3 days, 125 mg TID po × 3 days Usual maintenance: 500–1000 mg/day in 3–4 divided doses	See phenobarbital. Some patients intolerant of low-dose primidone.	Primidone metabolized to phenobarbital but parent compound has significant antiseizure properties.	Potent inducer of cytochrome P450, therefore many potential drug interactions; may decrease efficacy of hormonal contraceptives; metabolism inhibited by valproic acid; declining use because of adverse effect profile; requires QID dosing (to maintain high primidone/phenobarb ratio); slow dose titration.	$
Benzodiazepines	*clobazam* Frisium, generics	Initial: 5–15 mg/day po, preferably at HS Usual maintenance: 20–40 mg/day in 1 or 2 divided doses	Irritability, depression.	Very safe; daily or BID dosing; broad spectrum; rapid onset; few drug interactions; can be useful as "add-on" for patients "nearly" seizure free.	Tolerance (initial good response followed by loss of seizure control).	$
Carboxylic Acid Derivatives	*valproic acid* Depakene, Apo-Valproic, generics	Initial: 250 mg BID po; increase by 250 mg/day Q3–4 days as necessary. Usual maintenance: 750–1000 mg/day in 2–4 divided doses	Nausea, weight gain, tremor, hair loss, blood dyscrasias, hepatotoxicity rarely; edema rarely; menstrual irregularities; teratogenicity.	Often may use BID dosing; broad spectrum; no hepatic enzyme induction; very low incidence of rash; cognitive effects generally less than with other older AEDs; drug of first choice for patients with mixed 1° generalized seizures (generalized tonic-clonic, myoclonus, absence).	Inhibits hepatic enzymes, therefore many potential drug interactions; least desirable option for women of childbearing potential.	$

Class	Drug	Dose	Adverse Effects[a]	Advantages	Disadvantages	Cost[b]
	divalproex sodium Epival, generics	Initial: 250 mg BID po; increase by 250 mg/day Q3–4 days Usual maintenance: 750–1000 mg/day in 2 divided doses	See valproic acid.	Often may use BID dosing; broad spectrum; no hepatic enzyme induction; very low incidence of rash; cognitive effects generally less than other older AEDs; drug of first choice for patients with mixed 1° generalized seizures (generalized tonic-clonic, myoclonus, absence); GI tolerability may be better than with valproic acid.	Inhibits hepatic enzymes, therefore many potential drug interactions; least desirable option for women of childbearing potential.	$
Gamma Aminobutyric Acid (GABA) Derivatives	*gabapentin* Neurontin, generics	Initial: 300 mg once daily po; increase by 300 mg/day Q5–7 days up to 300 mg TID, then titrate TID dose. Usual maintenance: 900–3600 mg/day divided Q6–8H	Tremor, vision changes.	No known significant drug interactions; well tolerated; safe; not metabolized; can use in liver failure.	TID dosing; not for 1° generalized seizures; expensive at high doses; best used as add-on drug.	$$
	vigabatrin Sabril	Initial: 1000 mg/day po in 1–2 divided doses Usual maintenance: 2000–4000 mg/day in 1–2 divided doses	Low incidence of psychosis, depression; irreversible visual field problems.	BID dosing; well tolerated; few drug interactions; easy to use; linear pharmacokinetics; does not exhibit dermatologic, hepatic or hematologic adverse effects.	**Reports of visual field defects have severely limited use of this drug**. May worsen absence seizures, myoclonus; expensive at high doses.	$$$
Hydantoin Derivatives	*phenytoin* Dilantin, generics	Usual maintenance: 300–400 mg/day po If used, loading doses should be administered carefully	Gingival hyperplasia; rash 5–10%, which rarely can be very serious; increased liver enzymes; blood dyscrasias; dose-related encephalopathy; coarse facial features with long-term use.	Daily or BID dosing; parenteral form available; inexpensive.	Inducer of cytochrome P450, therefore many potential drug interactions; may decrease efficacy of hormonal contraceptives; long-term cosmetic adverse effects; dosing complicated by saturation kinetics.	$

(cont'd)

Table 3: **Antiepileptic Drugs** *(cont'd)*

Class	Drug	Dose	Adverse Effects[a]	Advantages	Disadvantages	Cost[b]
Iminostilbene Derivatives	*carbamazepine immediate-release* Tegretol, generics	Initial: 100 mg BID po; increase by 200 mg/day Q3–4 days Usual maintenance: 800–1200 mg/day in 2–4 divided doses, with meals when possible	Rash 5–10%, which rarely can be very serious; increased liver enzymes; transient neutropenia (common); aplastic anemia (extremely rare); hyponatremia.	Linear pharmacokinetics.	Substrate of CYP3A4 and inducer of CYP1A2, 3A4, 2C9, 2C19, 2D6, 3A4 and 2C8, therefore many potential drug interactions; may decrease efficacy of hormonal contraceptives; available only as oral formulations; may worsen absence seizures; may produce or exacerbate myoclonus.	$
	carbamazepine controlled-release Tegretol CR, generics	Initial: 100 mg BID po; increase by 200 mg/day Q3–4 days Usual maintenance: 800–1200 mg/day in 2 divided doses with meals	See carbamazepine immediate-release.	BID dosing; linear pharmacokinetics; CR preparation may be better tolerated and improve compliance.	See carbamazepine immediate-release.	$
	oxcarbazepine Trileptal, generics	Initial: 300 mg BID po; increase by ≤600 mg/day at weekly intervals Usual maintenance: 1200–2400 mg/day in 2 divided doses	Similar to carbamazepine but slightly higher risk of hyponatremia; skin rash cross-reaction with carbamazepine.	BID dosing; efficacy may be similar to carbamazepine but better tolerated; no autoinduction of liver enzymes.	May decrease efficacy of hormonal contraceptives; available only as oral formulation.	$$$–$$$$
Succinimide Derivatives	*ethosuximide* Zarontin	Initial: 500 mg/day po in 1 or 2 divided doses; increase by 250 mg/day Q4–7 days Usual maintenance: 750–1000 mg/day	GI upset.	Few drug interactions.	For absence seizures only; confers no protection for generalized tonic-clonic seizures.	$
Other Antiepileptic Drugs	*lacosamide* Vimpat	Initial: 50–100 mg/day po in 2 divided doses; increase by 50 mg/day at 1 to 2-wk intervals Usual maintenance: 200–400 mg/day in 2 divided doses	Dizziness, ataxia, sedation (more common with faster rates of titration). PR interval prolongation; caution in patients with conduction abnormalities.	BID dosing; no known significant drug interactions.	Cost; limited postmarketing clinical data compared to older AEDs.	$$$–$$$$

Class	Drug	Dose	Adverse Effects[a]	Advantages	Disadvantages	Cost[b]
	lamotrigine Lamictal, generics	Initial: 25 mg Q2 days po to 50 mg/day, depending on concurrent AED therapy; after 2 wk give same dose BID × 2 wk, then increase by 100 mg/day at 1 to 2-wk intervals Usual maintenance: 300–400 mg/day in 2 divided doses	Rash 5–10%, which rarely can be very serious; insomnia.	BID dosing; broad spectrum; no enzyme induction (few interactions); some patients report feeling more "alert"; increasing evidence for monotherapy; increasing use for 1° generalized seizures.	Very slow dose titration; metabolism markedly inhibited by valproic acid/divalproex sodium and increased by enzyme-inducing AEDs (carbamazepine, phenytoin, phenobarbital, primidone); available only as oral formulation; expensive at high doses; addition of hormonal contraceptives may reduce lamotrigine serum levels by up to 50%.	$$
	levetiracetam Keppra, generics	Initial: 1000 mg/day po in 2 divided doses; increase by 1000 mg/day at weekly intervals Usual maintenance: 1000–3000 mg/day in 2 divided doses	Sleepiness, decreased energy, headache, irritability, depression.	BID dosing; broad spectrum; no drug interactions; rapid titration.	Cost; psychiatric side effects (see Adverse Effects).	$$–$$$
	perampanel Fycompa	Initial: 2 mg/day HS po; increase by 2 mg at 2-wk intervals as tolerated Patients taking enzyme-inducing AEDs (carbamazepine, phenytoin, oxcarbazepine) can start at 4 mg/day. Usual maintenance: 8–12 mg/day HS	Serious psychiatric reactions, such as aggression, irritability and homicidal ideation, in patients with and without prior psychiatric history; increase monitoring during titration and at high doses; avoid alcohol. Dizziness, sleepiness, fatigue, unsteadiness.	Daily dosing.	Cost; decreased efficacy of hormonal contraceptives; limited postmarketing data compared to older AEDs.	$$$$
	rufinamide Banzel	Initial: 400 mg/day po in 2 divided doses; increase by 5 mg/kg/day at 2-wk intervals as tolerated Usual maintenance: 1800–3200 mg/day in 2 divided doses	Headache, sleepiness, dizziness, nausea/vomiting; rash, which rarely can be very serious; shortening of QT_c interval.	Indicated for adjunctive treatment of generalized seizures in Lennox-Gastaut syndrome.		$400–800

(cont'd)

Table 3: **Antiepileptic Drugs** *(cont'd)*

Class	Drug	Dose	Adverse Effects[a]	Advantages	Disadvantages	Cost[b]
	stiripentol Diacomit	Increase dose gradually over 3 days to recommended dose of 50 mg/kg/day po in 2–3 divided doses. Discontinuation: gradually reduce dosage over 1 month to reduce risk of seizures.	Neurological (drowsiness, sleepiness) or GI (loss of appetite, nausea, weight loss).	Adjunctive therapy for refractory generalized tonic-clonic seizures in severe myoclonic epilepsy in infancy or Dravet syndrome not responding to clobazam and valproate alone.		~$2800
	topiramate ❥ Topamax, generics	Initial: 100 mg/day po in 2 divided doses Usual maintenance: 200–400 mg/day	Cognitive problems common; kidney stones; weight loss; headache; fingers/toes paresthesias.	BID dosing; broad spectrum; safe; few drug interactions; potent AED with broad spectrum of activity.	Slow titration; decreased efficacy of hormonal contraceptives; cost; cognitive effects commonly limit use.	$

[a] Virtually all AEDs can produce sedation, fatigue, cognitive impairment, dizziness and ataxia in a dose-dependent fashion.
[b] Cost of 30-day supply for usual maintenance dose, based on 70 kg body weight, unless otherwise specified; includes drug cost only.
❥ Dosage adjustment may be required in renal impairment; see Appendix I.
Abbreviations: AED = antiepileptic drug; CR = controlled-release; GI = gastrointestinal
Legend: $ < $50 $$ $50–150 $$-$$$ $50–250 $$$ $150–250 $$$-$$$$ $150–350 $$$$ $250–350

Suggested Readings

Chen JW, Wasterlain CG. Status epilepticus: pathophysiology and management in adults. *Lancet Neurol* 2006;5(3):246-56.

Duncan JS, Sander JW, Sisodiya SM et al. Adult epilepsy. *Lancet* 2006;367(9516):1087-100.

French JA, Pedley TA. Initial management of epilepsy. *N Engl J Med* 2008;359(2):166-76.

Perucca E, Tomson T. The pharmacological treatment of epilepsy in adults. *Lancet Neurol* 2011;10(5):446-56.

Tomson T, Hiilesmaa V. Epilepsy in pregnancy. *BMJ* 2007;335(7623):769-73.

References

1. Fisher RS, Acevedo C, Arzimanoglou A et al. ILAE Official Report: a practical clinical definition of epilepsy. *Epilepsia* 2014;55(4):475-82.
2. Berg AT, Berkovic SF, Brodie MJ et al. Revised terminology and concepts for organization of seizures and epilepsies: report of the ILAE Commission on Classification and Terminology, 2005-2009. *Epilepsia* 2010;51(4):676-85.
3. French JA, Pedley TA. Initial management of epilepsy. *N Engl J Med* 2008;359(2):166-76.
4. Duncan JS, Sander JW, Sisodiya SM et al. Adult epilepsy. *Lancet* 2006;367(9516):1087-100.
5. Krumholz A, Wiebe S, Gronseth G et al. Practice Parameter: evaluating an apparent unprovoked first seizure in adults (an evidence-based review): report of the Quality Standards Subcommittee of the American Academy of Neurology and the American Epilepsy Society. *Neurology* 2007;69(21):1996-2007.
6. Schachter SC. Complementary and alternative medical therapies. *Curr Opin Neurol* 2008;21(2):184-9.
7. Neal EG, Chaffe H, Schwartz RH et al. The ketogenic diet for the treatment of childhood epilepsy: a randomised controlled trial. *Lancet Neurol* 2008;7(6):500-6.
8. Spencer S, Huh L. Outcomes of epilepsy surgery in adults and children. *Lancet Neurol* 2008;7(6):525-37.
9. Perucca E, Tomson T. The pharmacological management of epilepsy in adults. *Lancet Neurol* 2011;10(5):446-56.
10. Glauser T, Ben-Menachem E, Bourgeois B et al. Updated ILAE evidence review of antiepileptic drug efficacy and effectiveness as initial monotherapy for epileptic seizures and syndromes. *Epilepsia* 2013;54(3):551-63.
11. Marson AG, Al-Kharusi AM, Alwaidh M et al. The SANAD study of effectiveness of carbamazepine, gabapentin, lamotrigine, oxcarbazepine, or topiramate for treatment of partial epilepsy: an unblinded randomised controlled trial. *Lancet* 2007;369(9566):1000-15.
12. Marson AG, Al-Kharusi AM, Alwaidh M et al. The SANAD study of effectiveness of valproate, lamotrigine, or topiramate for generalised and unclassifiable epilepsy: an unblinded randomised controlled trial. *Lancet* 2007;369(9566):1016-26.
13. Trinka E, Marson AG, Van Paesschen W et al. KOMET: an unblinded, randomised, two parallel-group, stratified trial comparing the effectiveness of levetiracetam with controlled-release carbamazepine and extended-release sodium valproate as monotherapy in patients with newly diagnosed epilepsy. *J Neurol Neurosurg Psychiatry* 2013;84(10):1138-47.
14. Glauser TA, Cnaan A, Shinnar S et al. Ethosuximide, valproic acid, and lamotrigine in childhood absence epilepsy. *N Engl J Med* 2010;362(9):790-9.
15. Marson A, Jacoby A, Johnson A et al. Immediate versus deferred antiepileptic drug treatment for early epilepsy and single seizures: a randomised controlled trial. *Lancet* 2005;365(9476):2007-13.
16. Pohlman-Eden B, Behgi E, Camfield C et al. The first seizure and its management in adults and children. *BMJ* 2006;332(7537):339-42.
17. Chen JW, Wasterlain CG. Status epilepticus: pathophysiology and management in adults. *Lancet Neurol* 2006;5(3):246-56.
18. Arif H, Hirsch LJ. Treatment of status epilepticus. *Semin Neurol* 2008;28(3):342-54.
19. Alldredge BK, Gelb AM, Isaacs SM et al. A comparison of lorazepam, diazepam, and placebo for the treatment of our-of-hospital status epilepticus. *N Engl J Med* 2001;345(9):631-7.
20. Silbergleit R, Durkalski V, Lowenstein D et al. Intramuscular versus intravenous therapy for prehospital status epilepticus. *N Engl J Med* 2012;366(7):591-600.
21. Harden CL, Hopp J, Ting TY et al. Practice parameter update: management issues for women with epilepsy—focus on pregnancy (an evidence-based review): obstetrical complications and change in seizure frequency: report of the Quality Standards Subcommittee and Therapeutics and Technology Assessment Subcommittee of the American Academy of Neurology and American Epilepsy Society. *Neurology* 2009;73(2):126-32.
22. Harden CL, Meador KJ, Pennell PB et al. Practice parameter update: management issues for women with epilepsy—focus on pregnancy (an evidence-based review): teratogenesis and perinatal outcomes: report of the Quality Standards Subcommittee and Therapeutics and Technology Assessment Subcommittee of the American Academy of Neurology and American Epilepsy Society. *Neurology* 2009;73(2):133-41.
23. Harden CL, Pennell PB, Koppel BS et al. Practice parameter update: management issues for women with epilepsy—focus on pregnancy (an evidence-based review): vitamin K, folic acid, blood levels, and breastfeeding: report of the Quality Standards Subcommittee and Therapeutics and Technology Assessment Subcommittee of the American Academy of Neurology and American Epilepsy Society. *Neurology* 2009;73(2):142-9.
24. Hernández-Diaz S, Smith CR, Shen A et al. Comparative safety of antiepileptic drugs during pregnancy. *Neurology* 2012;78(21):1692-9.
25. Kazmin A, Wong RC, Sermer M et al. Antiepileptic drugs in pregnancy and hemorrhagic disease of the newborn: an update. *Can Fam Physician* 2010;56(12):1291-2.

Chapter 26
Fever in Children

Joanne M. Langley, MD, MSc, FRCPC

Fever is a regulated physiologic response in which a new thermal balance point (set-point) for body temperature is established by the hypothalamus. In response, the body establishes a new equilibrium of heat loss and production to maintain homeostasis at the higher temperature.[1] Fever is distinguished from disorders of temperature regulation, such as hyperthermia, where heat production exceeds heat loss without an increase in the thermoregulatory set-point (see Chapter 27). Normal body temperature varies by 0.5°C throughout the day. A common definition of fever is a temperature consistently over 38°C (rectal or rectal equivalent).[2] The febrile response rarely exceeds 41–42°C.[1] The most frequent cause of fever in children is infection and is part of a beneficial host response to control and eliminate pathogens.[3] Fever itself is not harmful.

Temperature measurement from the rectum, mouth or tympanic membrane reflects core temperature. Although measurement error can occur with any method, *rectal* thermometry is recommended in Canada as the gold standard for definitive measurement of temperature in children ≤5 years.[2] *Oral* thermometry is recommended for confirmation of fever in children >5 years. *Axillary* temperature can be used for screening low-risk children of all ages while *tympanic* temperature measurement can be used as a screening tool for low-risk children ≥2 years.[2]

Goals of Therapy

- Provide patient comfort
- Relieve parental anxiety
- Balance the benefit of symptomatic treatment with possible adverse effects and cost of medication

There is no evidence that reduction of temperature via antipyretic therapy is beneficial to the child.[3,4] Available antipyretics also have analgesic effects, which can decrease discomfort if present. Most guidelines recommend consideration of antipyretics only for febrile children who appear distressed or unwell.[3,5] Evidence suggests that antipyretic therapy does not prevent febrile seizures.[3,6,7]

Investigations

Fever is a symptom/sign, not a diagnosis, and most commonly is an adaptive response to an infection. Fever may also occur in malignancy, rheumatologic or immunologic diseases.

- History and physical examination to ascertain associated symptoms and source of the fever
- Clinical judgment determines whether the underlying process is benign (e.g., viral upper respiratory tract infection) or life-threatening (e.g., bacterial meningitis)
- Bacteremia is more likely present if the temperature is >41.1°C in young children;[8] therefore, blood cultures may be warranted
- Aggressiveness of the laboratory and diagnostic imaging evaluation depends on the clinical assessment of the severity of illness, symptoms pointing to a focus of infection, the child's age (especially if <3 months) and immune status[5,8]
  - may include culture of suspected sources of infection (e.g., urine, blood, cerebrospinal fluid) or imaging studies (e.g., chest radiograph)

– nonspecific tests such as C-reactive protein or WBC ± differential are not sufficiently sensitive or specific to replace clinical assessment of the severity of illness of a febrile child

Therapeutic Choices

Nonpharmacologic Choices

Physical methods for heat reduction use convection, evaporation or conduction to counteract the body's attempt to maintain a higher temperature set-point (fever). The body opposes physical cooling by attempting to re-establish a high temperature through shivering and vasoconstriction.[9] Pharmacologic methods are preferred because they lower the hypothalamic set-point—an effect analogous to setting a thermostat in the home.

In the rare instance where core temperatures exceed 41–42°C, physical methods may be used in addition to pharmacologic methods. There is little evidence that these are of additional benefit to antipyretic medication, and they are associated with patient discomfort:[9]

- Sponging with tepid or cold water uses evaporation to dissipate body heat. Alcohol is not recommended for sponging as it may be absorbed through the skin, inhaled or accidentally ingested by the child.
- Ice packs or cooling (hypothermia) blankets may be applied to the skin to lower body temperature by conduction.
- Circulating fans, sometimes directed over ice before reaching the patient, use convection to transfer heat away from the skin surface.

Pharmacologic Choices

Acetaminophen and **ibuprofen** are the therapeutic choices available for managing fever in children. They have been studied in large populations and are considered safe in therapeutic doses.[3] National guidelines in the United States[3] and the United Kingdom[5] recommend use of antipyretics only for the treatment goal of patient comfort.

The dose, frequency of administration and adverse effects associated with acetaminophen and ibuprofen differ (Table 1). With regard to efficacy in temperature reduction, one systematic review of randomized trials showed comparable efficacy of a single dose of either drug in terms of pain relief, with about 15% more children in the ibuprofen group having temperature reduction at 4 and 6 hours.[10] The clinical significance of these marginal benefits is unclear.

ASA is not recommended in children under 15 years of age because of the potentially increased risk of Reye's syndrome.

Naproxen sodium has not been studied in children for the treatment of fever and therefore is not recommended in children under 12 years of age.

A response to antipyretic therapy does not exclude the possibility that serious underlying illness is present. Clinical decision-making should not be based on response to fever treatment.

Some clinicians recommend alternating acetaminophen and ibuprofen administration to reduce fever. However, there is insufficient evidence to support this as a routine practice and it is not recommended [Evidence: SORT C*].[3,5,11] While alternating or combining acetaminophen and ibuprofen may result in a greater period of time without fever, the clinical benefit of this difference is uncertain. It has not been shown to be either safe or more effective in improving discomfort than a single antipyretic. In

* SORT (Strength of Recommendation Taxonomy) is a rating system (A, B or C) that addresses the quality of available evidence. For more information consult **How to Use *Compendium of Therapeutic Choices*** on page xxv.

addition, potential risks of prescribing 2 antipyretics may include parental confusion and dosing errors with associated toxicity.

Therapeutic Tips

- Use doses of acetaminophen or ibuprofen based on the child's weight, not on age. Maximum dose per day should be specified.
- Concentrations of liquid acetaminophen and ibuprofen preparations vary according to product. Remind caregivers to check the concentration of a product each time medication is given.
- Acetaminophen is the drug most frequently involved in analgesic overdose in children under 6 years old. Store antipyretics in locked cabinets to prevent inappropriate access. Instruct parents to use a calibrated measuring device, and educate them about the many formulations available and the potential for error with substitution or combination of products.

Table 1: Antipyretic Medications for Children

Class	Drug	Dose	Adverse Effects	Comments	Cost[a]
NSAIDs	*ibuprofen* Advil, Motrin (Children's), Motrin, generics	5–10 mg/kg Q6–8H po as needed for symptom management; maximum 40 mg/kg/day or 2400 mg/day	Uncommon with infrequent use and recommended dose. GI intolerance and bleeding, allergic reactions, tinnitus, visual disturbances, nephropathy. Dehydration enhances risk of renal toxicity.	Limited data exist for the use of ibuprofen in children <2 months. Do not give if dehydration is present; ensure child has adequate intake of fluids. Avoid in the presence of renal dysfunction. Available as tablets and suspension. Some nonprescription products contain ibuprofen in combination with other drugs. Advise parents and caregivers to check labels carefully to avoid inadvertent administration of excessive doses.	$
Para-aminophenol Derivatives	*acetaminophen* Atasol Preparations, Tempra, Tylenol, generics	10–15 mg/kg/dose Q4–6H po as needed for symptom management; maximum 75 mg/kg/day or 4 g/day, whichever is less	Uncommon with infrequent use and recommended dose. Hypersensitivity, agranulocytosis and anemia (rare). Chronic use and overdose associated with hepatotoxicity, nephropathy. Potential for toxicity enhanced if concurrent dehydration, prolonged fasting, diabetes mellitus, obesity, concomitant viral infection or family history of hepatotoxic reaction.	Rectal administration results in erratic absorption and should be used under health care provider supervision. Available as oral drops, tablets, chewtabs, suppositories and suspension. Many nonprescription products contain acetaminophen in combination with other drugs. Advise parents and caregivers to check labels carefully to avoid inadvertent administration of excessive doses.	$

[a] Cost of 1-day supply; available without prescription.
Legend: $ < $2

Suggested Readings

Canadian Paediatric Society. Caring for Kids. *Fever and temperature taking*. Available from: www.caringforkids.cps.ca/handouts/fever_and_temperature_taking.

National Institute for Health and Clinical Excellence. CG160. *Feverish illness in children: assessment and initial management in children younger than 5 years*. London (GB): NICE; 2013. Available from: guidance.nice.org.uk/CG160.

Section on Clinical Pharmacology and Therapeutics; Committee on Drugs, Sullivan JE et al. Fever and antipyretic use in children. *Pediatrics* 2011;127(3):580-7.

References

1. Mackowiak PA, Wasserman SS, Levine MM. A critical appraisal of 98.6 degrees F, the upper limit of the normal body temperature, and other legacies of Carl Reinhold August Wunderlich. *JAMA* 1992;268(12):1578-80.
2. Leduc D, Woods S; Community Pediatrics Committee. *Temperature measurement in paediatrics*. Ottawa (ON): Canadian Paediatric Society; reaffirmed January 2013. Available from: www.cps.ca/en/documents/position/temperature-measurement. Accessed December 19, 2013.
3. Section on Clinical Pharmacology and Therapeutics; Committee on Drugs, Sullivan JE et al. Fever and antipyretic use in children. *Pediatrics* 2011;127(3):580-7.
4. Russell FM, Shann F, Curtis N et al. Evidence on the use of paracetamol in febrile children. *Bull World Health Organ* 2003;81(5):367-72.
5. National Institute for Health and Clinical Excellence. CG160. *Feverish illness in children: assessment and initial management in children younger than 5 years*. London (GB): NICE; 2013. Available from: guidance.nice.org.uk/CG160. Accessed December 19, 2013.
6. Meremikwu M, Oyo-Ita A. Paracetamol for treating fever in children. *Cochrane Database Syst Rev* 2002;(2):CD003676.
7. Offringa M, Newton R. Prophylactic drug management for febrile seizures in children. *Cochrane Database Syst Rev* 2012;4:CD003031.
8. Hui C, Neto G, Tsertsvadze A et al. *Diagnosis and management of febrile infants (0-3 months). Evidence report/technology assessment, No. 205*. Rockville (MD): Agency for Healthcare Research and Quality; March 2012. Available from: www.ncbi.nlm.nih.gov/books/NBK92690.
9. Meremikwu M, Oyo-Ita A. Physical methods for treating fever in children. *Cochrane Database Syst Rev* 2003;(2):CD004264.
10. Perrott DA, Piira T, Goodenough B et al. Efficacy and safety of acetaminophen vs ibuprofen for treating children's pain or fever: a meta-analysis. *Arch Pediatr Adolesc Med* 2004;158(6):521-6.
11. Wong T, Stang AS, Ganshorn H et al. Combined and alternating paracetamol and ibuprofen therapy for febrile children. *Cochrane Database Syst Rev* 2013;10:CD009572.

Alterations in Body Temperature

Chapter 27
Thermoregulatory Disorders in Adults

Mathieu Simon, MD, FRCPC, FCCM

Body temperature is normally maintained within a very narrow range to allow for normal metabolism. Disorders of thermoregulation can therefore produce a wide variety of symptoms ranging from minor discomfort to life-threatening emergencies.

Hyperthermia refers to a symptomatic increase in core body temperature >38.2°C.[1] Hyperthermia may occur in vulnerable populations (extreme of ages, chronic diseases), with illicit or prescription drugs (e.g., anticholinergics, antipsychotics, beta-lactams, salicylates, succinylcholine, sympathomimetics, tricyclic antidepressants) that interfere with normal heat dissipation mechanisms or in healthy individuals exercising or working in extreme heat conditions. Clinical manifestations represent the adverse effects of increased body temperature and the secondary activation of inflammatory and coagulation cascades on various organ systems.[2]

While *hyperthermia* is the result of a failure of the heat-regulating mechanisms to deal with exposure to the environment, *fever* is most often the sign of an underlying infectious or inflammatory process and is mediated by the hypothalamus (see Chapter 26). The distinction between fever and hyperthermia relies on findings from medical history such as hyperthermia resulting from environmental or toxic exposures and fever accompanying infectious, inflammatory or cancerous diseases. *Hyperpyrexia*, a fever of >41.5°C, results from impairment of both heat loss mechanisms and the hypothalamic thermostat set point. It is most often a sign of an overwhelming infection.

Hypothermia, a common but often unrecognized problem, is defined as a core body temperature <35°C.[3] Core temperature <32°C predisposes patients to ventricular fibrillation, which could be preceded by ECG changes such as QT-interval prolongation, T-wave inversion and atrial fibrillation.[4] Hypothermia may develop when exposed to a cold environment but may also occur in vulnerable populations (e.g., elderly, those with alcoholism, hypothalamic dysfunction, hypothyroidism, prolonged immobilization, malnutrition) even at normal environmental temperatures.[5] Drugs such as clonidine[6] and second-generation ("atypical") antipsychotics[7] may also increase the risk of accidental hypothermia.

In treating thermoregulatory disorders, it is important to focus on the cause of the temperature variance rather than the absolute thermometer reading. There is limited evidence to support the optimal treatment of patients with either hyperthermia or hypothermia.

Goals of Therapy

- Treat underlying cause
- Restore normal body temperature by cooling in hyperthermia and warming in hypothermia
- Prevent, diagnose and treat uncommon but lethal complications
- Avoid unnecessary, ineffective or dangerous interventions

Investigations

Hyperthermia and hypothermia are more commonly signs of an underlying illness rather than primary problems. To establish the appropriate diagnosis and institute definitive therapy consider the following:

- History and physical exam:
  - environmental exposure and the context in which the symptoms developed, e.g., activities, exposure to different types of medications (see Table 1), immobilization, medical conditions
  - neurologic status, e.g., headache, confusion, seizure
  - hyperthermia: exclude infection, assess hydration status. Inquire about the use of medications (anticholinergics, antipsychotics, serotonergics, volatile anesthetics), recreational drugs (amphetamines, cocaine, phencyclidine) and consider intoxication (ASA, organophosphates, tricyclic antidepressant overdose). Endocrinopathies (pheochromocytoma, thyrotoxicosis) may also present with hyperthermia
- Objective measurements:
  - accurate measurement of core body temperature
    - Use electronic devices. Standard glass/mercury thermometers will not record temperature below 32°C or above 42°C. Frequent calibration of electronic instruments is mandatory. Tympanic thermometers are not recommended in extreme temperature disorders as they may provide inaccurate readings[20]
  - assess vital signs: pulse, respiration
  - order tests according to the clinical setting:
    - Blood glucose, electrolytes (sodium, calcium, potassium), renal profile, CBC, creatine kinase (CK), coagulation panel (INR, PTT), blood gases, ECG, blood or urine cultures, liver enzymes, urine myoglobin (only helpful if positive), thyroid function tests, toxicology screen

Table 1: **Clinical Characteristics of Hyperthermia Syndromes**

Diagnosis	Characteristics
Heat cramps	Core body temperature is normal, skin is moist and cool Occurs in muscles following vigorous exercise in the heat Caused by salt depletion from excess sweating combined with hypotonic fluid replacement, resulting in dilutional hyponatremia[8]
Heat exhaustion	Core body temperature is minimally increased and is between 37°C and 40°C[3] Consequence of salt and water losses Symptoms: muscle cramps, diaphoresis, headache, nausea, vomiting, orthostatic syncope[3]
Heat stroke	Core body temperature ≥40.6°C[3] *Classic:* develops over several days during heat waves and affects primarily the elderly or those suffering from chronic illness[9] *Exertional:* occurs acutely with workers, endurance athletes or soldiers submitted to conditions of high heat and humidity without appropriate access to salt and water[10,11,12] Signs and symptoms: dehydration, central nervous system dysfunction (delirium, seizure, coma) and hot, dry skin[3,13] Complications such as disseminated intravascular coagulation, rhabdomyolysis, renal failure, seizures and permanent neurologic damage can result[14,15]
Malignant hyperthermia	Drug-induced reaction characterized by genetic susceptibility to generalized and sustained skeletal muscle contraction after exposure to depolarizing muscle relaxants such as succinylcholine or volatile anesthetic agents, such as halothane or isoflurane[16,17] Sustained muscle contraction and increased metabolism result in hyperthermia, metabolic acidosis, increased serum creatine kinase (CK) Duchenne disease and myotonic muscular dystrophy have been associated with an increased incidence of malignant hyperthermia[18]
Neuroleptic malignant syndrome (NMS)	Drug-induced idiosyncratic reaction characterized by hyperthermia, altered mentation, muscle rigidity[19] and autonomic instability, e.g., cardiac arrhythmias Drugs implicated are most often phenothiazines (e.g., chlorpromazine) and butyrophenones (e.g., haloperidol) or withdrawal of a dopaminergic agent (e.g., levodopa) resulting in reduced central dopamine neurotransmission

Hyperthermia

Therapeutic Choices

Nonpharmacologic Choices

Therapy is directed toward reducing heat production and increasing thermal dissipation (Table 2).

- Ensure adequate airway, breathing and circulation (ABC).
- Rest, cooling (icepacks, cooling blankets) and rehydration (iv electrolytes) is the mainstay of treatment.
- Monitor core body temperature continuously.[24] Discontinue cooling when core body temperature normalizes to prevent risk of iatrogenic hypothermia.

Pharmacologic Choices

Antipyretics are ineffective in treating hyperthermia since the hypothalamic thermostat set point is normal.[25] Malignant hyperthermia and neuroleptic malignant syndrome require prompt pharmacologic therapy and demand special attention. Clinical characteristics of both conditions are listed in Table 1.

Malignant Hyperthermia

To reverse this potentially lethal condition, prompt recognition of malignant hyperthermia is imperative, as well as interruption of the surgery, cessation of the offending drug, external cooling and administration of a muscle relaxant (**dantrolene** 2.5 mg/kg every 5 minutes iv up to 10 mg/kg cumulative dose, although rarely up to 30 mg/kg may be needed).[24,26,27] This can be followed by further administration of dantrolene 1 mg/kg Q4–6H for 24 hours to prevent recurrence of symptoms. Some experts suggest continuing dantrolene in a dosing regimen of 4–8 mg/kg/day po divided into 4 doses for 2–3 days after an episode of malignant hyperthermia.[28] The Malignant Hyperthermia Association of the United States (MHAUS) provides 24-hour crisis support and a management protocol is available on their website at www.mhaus.org/healthcare-professionals/managing-a-crisis.

Table 2: **Nonpharmacologic Management of Heat Cramps, Heat Exhaustion and Heat Stroke**

Cause	Treatment
Heat cramps	Rest and oral rehydration with a salt-containing solution, e.g., 1 teaspoonful (5 mL) of salt in 500 mL of water Normal saline iv (e.g., 2–3 L over 4–6 hours) is infrequently indicated[21]
Heat exhaustion	Rest in a cool environment External cooling with fan and rehydration Avoid strenuous exercise for 2–3 days[14]
Heat stroke	Primary objective: rapid lowering of core temperature below 39.4°C Rehydration and immediate cooling; ideal approach is tepid (20°C) water misting enhanced by fan evaporation. Definitive studies on the optimal cooling method are lacking and optimal management is controversial. Despite this, cooling should not be delayed.[22] Icepacks (wrapped in towels to avoid skin injury) and tepid water sponging are alternative approaches. Cooling should not be too intense since it could trigger shivering and increase heat generation In the hospital setting, cold-water immersion is not recommended because it induces peripheral vasoconstriction, which is counterproductive, and does not permit close monitoring of the patient. In the field, however, priority should be given to rapidly reducing body temperature, and cold-water immersion remains a valid and possibly life-saving option in this setting[23]

Neuroleptic Malignant Syndrome

Treatment of neuroleptic malignant syndrome involves prompt cessation of the offending agent and nonspecific supportive therapy (hydration, cooling). Limited evidence exists to support administration of dopaminergic agonists (**bromocriptine** 2.5–20 mg TID po or through a nasogastric tube), and possibly the use of a **muscle relaxant** (**nondepolarizing neuromuscular blockers** or **dantrolene**).[24,26,29] Experience in the treatment of this uncommon condition remains limited.

Hypothermia

Therapeutic Choices

Nonpharmacologic Choices

Resuscitation and rewarming are the mainstay of treatment of hypothermia. In resuscitating a patient, ensure adequate airway, breathing and circulation. Resuscitate patient until temperature is between 32°C and 35°C. Assess vital signs carefully as severe hypothermia may result in barely perceptible pulse and respiration as well as unstable cardiac arrhythmias with high risk of cardiac arrest. Rewarming takes precedence once initial resuscitation has been initiated. The 3 progressive modalities of rewarming are *passive external rewarming*, *active external rewarming* and *active core rewarming* (Table 3). Monitor core body temperature continuously through a rectal or esophageal probe. Discontinue warming when core body temperature normalizes to prevent risk of iatrogenic hyperthermia.

Table 3: Hypothermia: Rewarming Modalities

Rewarming Modality	Characteristics
Passive external rewarming	Minimize heat loss by removing wet or frozen clothing and keep the patient dry and covered with warm blankets. Relies on the patient's ability to shiver, which is lost below 32°C. It is an essential first-line intervention but additional steps should be taken in more severe hypothermia.
Active external rewarming	Refers to the use of warming blankets or warm water immersion. Use in stable patients with minimal metabolic abnormalities, since paradoxical acidosis and worsening of core hypothermia may result due to peripheral vasodilatation induced by external rewarming while thoracic and abdominal organs remain cold. If used, active external rewarming should be limited to the trunk.[30]
Active core rewarming	Favoured approach in severe hypothermia. Heated iv normal saline (40–43°C) should be administered through a peripheral line. Using a central line allows for faster rewarming, but insertion may be complicated by malignant arrhythmia and significant bleeding secondary to coagulopathy. If a blood warmer is not available, iv solutions could be heated in a microwave oven but only if they do not contain dextrose and the temperature is monitored before administration.[31] Blood cannot be heated in a microwave because of its high cellular and protein content. Mechanical ventilation using heated gases (40–45°C) is another simple and effective technique.[32] Heated peritoneal lavage through a temporary dialysis catheter using 2000 mL of dialysate at 44°C exchanged every 20 minutes can increase core temperature by up to 2°C/hour. Disseminated intravascular coagulation, intra-abdominal bleeding and electrolyte imbalance are the most common complications.[33] Heated enemas, nasogastric lavage, bladder irrigation[33,34] and open and closed thoracic lavage[35] have all been attempted with mixed results. Heated cardiopulmonary bypass provides the fastest and most physiologic means of active core rewarming. This technique is usually limited to the management of patients suffering cardiac arrest or those with unstable hemodynamics and arrhythmias.[5,34] Transfer of severely hypothermic patients to a hospital where the technique is available should be considered but is often impossible considering the extreme risks involved in the transport of these patients.

Electrical defibrillation for ventricular fibrillation is less effective at core temperatures <30°C but should be attempted if a patient is in ventricular fibrillation or unstable ventricular tachycardia. If one shock (120–200 J and 360 J respectively for biphasic and monophasic defibrillators) is unsuccessful in restoring normal sinus rhythm, attention should be switched to aggressive rewarming while continuing advanced cardiac life support (ACLS) until body temperature reaches 30°C, when defibrillation attempts are more likely to be successful (see Figure 1).[5,36] Manoeuvres such as endotracheal intubation or simply moving the patient could be sufficient triggers for ventricular fibrillation[37] but this should not discourage initial in-field stabilization and evacuation.

Favourable outcomes following prolonged resuscitation in the hypothermic patient are well described, especially in children. Hypothermia victims should not be pronounced dead until rewarmed to a near normal core temperature.[3,36] This is especially true of near-drowning victims because immersion in cold water results in rapid cooling of the entire body that may provide some survival advantages such as protecting the brain and organs.

Controversies still exist about the utility of temperature-corrected arterial pH and blood gases relative to the hypothermia. Most literature suggests that uncorrected pH, pO_2 and pCO_2 values are more physiologic and more valuable to the clinician in guiding the therapeutic interventions.[38]

Pharmacologic Choices

Since hypothermia is often associated with alcohol intoxication, **thiamine** supplementation is part of the supportive therapy. Administer **glucose** and **naloxone** if opioid overdose is suspected. Consider other sources of intoxication and their specific treatments.

Prophylactic antibiotics are controversial. Some advocate wide-spectrum antibiotic coverage for the first 3 days but there are no clinical trial data to support this recommendation. Routine use of barbiturates or corticosteroids is discouraged.

Hypothermic patients will usually require fluid resuscitation with warm isotonic solutions. Monitoring of electrolytes is imperative, especially serum K^+. In the past, vasopressors were avoided because they were considered ineffective and possibly arrhythmogenic.[39] However, research in animal models suggests that vasopressor use may increase rates of return of spontaneous circulation in hypothermic cardiac arrest.[40] Based on this information the American Heart Association ACLS guidelines suggest it may be reasonable to consider administration of a vasopressor in hypothermic cardiac arrest.[36]

Pharmacologic management of cardiac arrest in hypothermic patients is difficult and clinical experience is scarce. Most studies focus on case reports or animal models. Antiarrhythmic agents have long been considered ineffective until after rewarming. Evidence derived from animal models of hypothermic arrest now suggests that the ACLS algorithms could be used safely and effectively in hypothermic patients while rewarming, including those with severe hypothermia.[40] Below a core body temperature of 30°C, at least one sequence of medications should be tried in accordance with ACLS guidelines used for normothermic patients.[5,36] Once core temperature reaches 30°C, standard ACLS guidelines may be applied. Avoid bretylium and procainamide in hypothermic cardiac arrest.[40,41]

Therapeutic Hypothermia

Controlled hypothermia has been studied in an attempt to improve survival and neurologic outcomes in cardiac arrest survivors. Initially indicated only for comatose survivors of out-of-hospital ventricular fibrillation, the practice is now considered a standard of care in comatose post-cardiac arrest patients irrespective of the initial rhythm. Mild hypothermia reaching 32–34°C and extending for 12–24 hours from the time of the arrest, is generally advocated in otherwise hemodynamically stable survivors.[42,43,44,45] Therapeutic hypothermia (also called targeted temperature management) is being investigated in emerging indications ranging from neurotrauma and spinal injuries to multiple trauma in the battlefield, with varying results. More recently, a randomized trial showed similar rates of death and neurologic outcome whether temperature was targeted to 33°C or 36°C.[46]

The first step in reducing core temperature is to expose the patient by removing clothing and protective coverings and reduce room temperature. Fans and water may be used to increase convective heat loss. Icepacks or cooling blankets are also useful in maintaining hypothermia. To quickly reach the desired core temperature, infusion of 1–2 L of normal saline refrigerated to 4°C is often necessary.

Without muscle relaxation, shivering would prevent induction of therapeutic hypothermia and would be very uncomfortable to the patient. Furthermore, shivering increases both cardiac output and oxygen consumption, two undesirable situations following cardiac resuscitation. Prevention of shivering is accomplished with sedation and muscle relaxation. Although any muscle relaxants could be used (with the exception of succinylcholine whose depolarizing effect is ill suited for this indication), **cisatracurium** is often considered the agent of choice. Its short duration of action requires that it be used as a continuous iv infusion, but also makes early assessment of any neurologic sequelae easier once discontinued.[47]

Therapeutic Tips

- Nonpharmacologic management is the basis of therapy for true thermoregulation disorders.
- Hypothermic patients are prone to cardiac arrhythmia. ECG monitoring is mandatory. Aggressive resuscitation and rewarming are warranted.
- While the effectiveness of most medications used in cardiac resuscitation is probably temperature dependent, the old suggestion to avoid them until a minimal degree of rewarming is achieved finds little scientific support. Although overmedication of the hypothermic patient could cause toxicity during rewarming, one complete pharmacologic sequence based on the rhythm-appropriate ACLS guidelines is probably advisable at this time.
- Hypothermia results in reduced activity of many hepatic enzymes, notably cytochrome P450. Drugs that are metabolized by the liver may require dosage modification during therapeutic hypothermia.[44]
- Consider thermoregulation disorders in the differential diagnosis of confusion and coma
- While treating severe hypothermia, close monitoring of serum K^+ is important. Rapid rewarming may induce severe hyperkalemia.
- Avoid **alpha-adrenergic agonists** in hyperthermia as they may decrease heat dissipation through vasoconstriction.
- **Dantrolene** is not effective in heat stroke.[48]

Figure 1: **Hypothermia Treatment**[36]

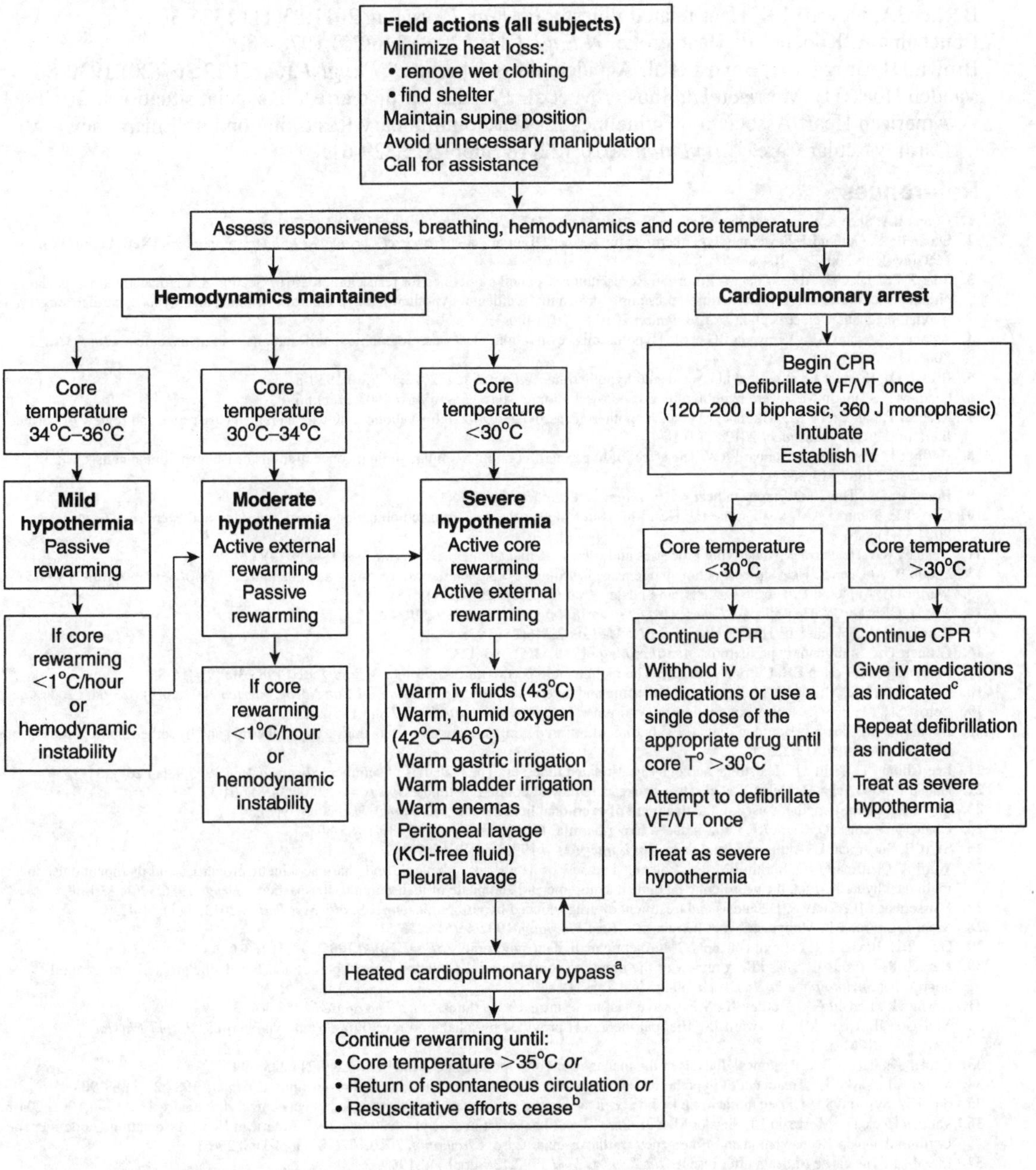

[a] Cardiac arrest and hemodynamic collapse are seen as the two usual indications for cardiopulmonary bypass in the setting of severe hypothermia.
[b] Successful resuscitations after prolonged ACLS, although unusual, have been reported, most of them in the pediatric literature. ACLS and active rewarming should, in most cases, be continued until the core temperature reaches 35°C.
[c] Use longer than standard intervals between doses.
Abbreviations: CPR = cardiopulmonary resuscitation; VF = ventricular fibrillation; VT = ventricular tachycardia

Suggested Readings

Atha WF. Heat-related illness. *Emerg Med Clin North Am* 2013;31(4):1097-108.

Becker JA, Stewart LK. Heat-related illness. *Am Fam Physician* 2011;83(11):1325-30.

Bouchama A, Knochel JP. Heat stroke. *N Engl J Med* 2002;346(25):1978-88.

Brown DJ, Brugger H, Boyd J et al. Accidental hypothermia. *N Engl J Med* 2012;367(20):1930-8.

Vanden Hoek TL, Morrison LJ, Shuster M et al. Part 12: cardiac arrest in special situations: 2010 American Heart Association Guidelines for Cardiopulmonary Resuscitation and Emergency Cardiovascular Care. *Circulation* 2010;122(18 Suppl 3):S829-61.

References

1. Cunha BA, Shea KW. Fever in the intensive care unit. *Infect Dis Clin North Am* 1996;10(1):185-209.
2. Dinarello C, Gelfand J. Fever and hyperthermia. In: Kasper DL et al., eds. *Harrison's principles of internal medicine.* New York (NY): McGraw-Hill; 2005. p. 104-8.
3. Soar J, Perkins GD, Abbas G et al. European Resuscitation Council guidelines for resuscitation 2010. Section 8. Cardiac arrest in special circumstances: electrolyte abnormalities, poisoning, drowning, accidental hypothermia, hyperthermia, asthma, anaphylaxis, cardiac surgery, trauma, pregnancy, electrocution. *Resuscitation* 2010;81(10):1400-33.
4. Aslam AF, Aslam AK, Vasavada BC et al. Hypothermia: evaluation, electrocardiographic manifestations, and management. *Am J Med* 2006;119(4):297-301.
5. Brown DJ, Brugger H, Boyd J et al. Accidental hypothermia. *N Engl J Med* 2012;367(20):1930-8.
6. Quail MT, Shannon M. Severe hypothermia caused by clonidine. *Am J Emerg Med* 2003;21(1):86.
7. Kreuzer P, Landgrebe M, Wittmann M et al. Hypothermia associated with antipsychotic drug use: a clinical case series and review of current literature. *J Clin Pharmacol* 2012;52(7):1090-7.
8. Gaffin SL, Koratich M, Hubbard RW. The effect of hyperthermia on intracellular sodium concentrations of isolated human cells. *Ann N Y Acad Sci* 1997;813:637-9.
9. Bouchama A. The 2003 European heat wave. *Intensive Care Med* 2004;30(1):1-3.
10. Coris EE, Ramirez AM, Van Durme DJ. Heat illness in athletes: the dangerous combination of heat, humidity and exercise. *Sports Med* 2004;34(1):9-16.
11. Delaney KA. Heatstroke. Underlying processes and lifesaving management. *Postgrad Med* 1992;91(4):379-88.
12. Yaqub B, Al Deeb S. Heat strokes: aetiopathogenesis, neurological characteristics, treatment and outcome. *J Neurol Sci* 1998;156(2):144-51.
13. Waruiru C, Appleton R. Febrile seizures: an update. *Arch Dis Child* 2004;89(8):751-6.
14. Tek D, Olshaker JS. Heat illness. *Emerg Med Clin North Am* 1992;10(2):299-310.
15. Bouchama A, Knochel JP. Heat stroke. *N Engl J Med* 2002;346(25):1978-88.
16. Gronert GA. Malignant hyperthermia. *Anesthesiology* 1980;53(5):395-423.
17. Nelson TE, Flewellen EH. Current concepts. The malignant hyperthermia syndrome. *N Engl J Med* 1983;309(7):416-8.
18. Rosenbaum HK, Miller JD. Malignant hyperthermia and myotonic disorders. *Anesthesiol Clin North America* 2002;20(3):623-64.
19. Caroff SN, Mann SC. Neuroleptic malignant syndrome. *Med Clin North Am* 1993;77(1):185-202.
20. Ducharme MB, Frim J, Bourdon L et al. Evaluation of infrared tympanic thermometers during normothermia and hypothermia in humans. *Ann N Y Acad Sci* 1997;813:225-9.
21. Lee-Chiong TL, Stitt JT. Heatstroke and other heat-related illnesses. The maladies of summer. *Postgrad Med* 1995;98(1):26-8, 31-3, 36.
22. Hadad E, Rav-Acha M, Heled Y et al. Heat stroke: a review of cooling methods. *Sports Med* 2004;34(8):501-11.
23. Smith JE. Cooling methods used in the treatment of exertional heat illness. *Br J Sports Med* 2005;39(8):503-7.
24. Chan TC, Evans SD, Clark RF. Drug-induced hyperthermia. *Crit Care Clin* 1997;13(4):785-808.
25. Styrt B, Sugarman B. Antipyresis and fever. *Arch Intern Med* 1990;150(8):1589-97.
26. Ward A, Chaffman MO, Sorkin EM. Dantrolene. A review of its pharmacodynamic and pharmacokinetic properties and therapeutic use in malignant hyperthermia, the neuroleptic malignant syndrome and an update of its use in muscle spasticity. *Drugs* 1986;32(2):130-68.
27. Musselman ME, Saely S. Diagnosis and treatment of drug-induced hyperthermia. *Am J Health Syst Pharm* 2013;70(1):34-42.
28. Moore JL, Rice EL. Malignant hyperthermia. *Am Fam Physician* 1992;45(5):2245-51.
29. Guze BH, Baxter LR. Current concepts. Neuroleptic malignant syndrome. *N Engl J Med* 1985;313(3):163-6.
30. Harnett RM, Pruitt JR, Sias FR. A review of the literature concerning resuscitation from hypothermia: Part I--the problem and general approaches. *Aviat Space Environ Med* 1983;54(5):425-34.
31. Anshus JS, Endahl GL, Mottley JL. Microwave heating of intravenous fluids. *Am J Emerg Med* 1985;3(4):316-9.
32. Morrison JB, Conn ML, Hayward JS. Thermal increment provided by inhalation rewarming from hypothermia. *J Appl Physiol* 1979;46(6):1061-5.
33. Reuler JB, Parker RA. Peritoneal dialysis in the management of hypothermia. *JAMA* 1978;240(21):2289-90.
34. Maresca L, Vasko JS. Treatment of hypothermia by extracorporeal circulation and internal rewarming. *J Trauma* 1987;27(1):89-90.
35. Hall KN, Syverud SA. Closed thoracic cavity lavage in the treatment of severe hypothermia in human beings. *Ann Emerg Med* 1990;19(2):204-6.
36. Vanden Hoek TL, Morrison LJ, Shuster M et al. Part 12: cardiac arrest in special situations: 2010 American Heart Association Guidelines for Cardiopulmonary Resuscitation and Emergency Cardiovascular Care. *Circulation* 2010;122(18 Suppl 3):S829-61.
37. Lloyd EL. The cause of death after rescue. *Int J Sports Med* 1992;13(Suppl 1):S196-9.
38. Danzl DF, Pozos RS, Auerbach PS et al. Multicenter hypothermia survey. *Ann Emerg Med* 1987;16(9):1042-55.
39. Rankin AC, Rae AP. Cardiac arrhythmias during rewarming of patients with accidental hypothermia. *Br Med J (Clin Res Ed)* 1984;289(6449):874-7.
40. Wira CR, Becker JU, Martin G et al. Anti-arrhythmic and vasopressor medications for the treatment of ventricular fibrillation in severe hypothermia: a systematic review of the literature. *Resuscitation* 2008;78(1):21-9.
41. Danzl DF, Sowers MB, Vicario SJ et al. Chemical ventricular defibrillation in severe accidental hypothermia. *Ann Emerg Med* 1982;11(12):698-9.

42. Peberdy MA, Callaway CW, Neumar RW et al. Part 9: post-cardiac arrest care: 2010 American Heart Association Guidelines for Cardiopulmonary Resuscitation and Emergency Cardiovascular Care. *Circulation* 2010;122(18 Suppl 3):S768-86.
43. Hypothermia after Cardiac Arrest Study Group. Mild therapeutic hypothermia to improve the neurologic outcome after cardiac arrest. *N Engl J Med* 2002;346(8):549-56.
44. Delhaye C, Mahmoudi M, Waksman R. Hypothermia therapy: neurological and cardiac benefits. *J Am Coll Cardiol* 2012;59(3):197-210.
45. Arrich J, Holzer M, Havel C et al. Hypothermia for neuroprotection in adults after cardiopulmonary resuscitation. *Cochrane Database Syst Rev* 2012;9:CD004128.
46. Nielsen N, Wetterslev J, Cronberg T et al. Targeted temperature management at 33°C versus 36°C after cardiac arrest. *N Engl J Med* 2013;369(23):2197-206.
47. Chamorro C, Borallo JM, Romera MA et al. Anesthesia and analgesia protocol during therapeutic hypothermia after cardiac arrest: a systematic review. *Anesth Analg* 2010;110(5):1328-35.
48. Bouchama A, Cafege A, Devol EB et al. Ineffectiveness of dantrolene sodium in the treatment of heatstroke. *Crit Care Med* 1991;19(2):176-80.

Chapter 28
Age-related Macular Degeneration

Michael J. Potter, MD, FRCSC

Age-related macular degeneration (AMD) is classified as *dry* or *wet* (*exudative*) AMD. The dry form is characterized by drusen (white to yellow spots in the central retina) and may or may not be associated with gradual deterioration in central vision. Wet AMD is responsible for the vast majority of severe vision loss, and always occurs in the setting of pre-existing dry AMD. The wet form is caused by the presence of a choroidal neovascular membrane (CNV). There are a number of similar conditions causing central visual loss, the most common of which is pathologic myopia.

In the Western world, almost a third of people over the age of 75 develop the dry form of AMD.[1] About 90% of severe vision loss, however, is seen in the 5% of these individuals who go on to develop the wet form of the disease.

Up to 30% of the risk of vision loss in AMD is attributable to smoking.[2] Hypertension[2,3,4] and family history[2] of AMD are also risk factors. Vision loss from wet AMD in 1 eye is associated with a 50% risk of vision loss in the fellow eye over 5 years.[5,6,7] At this time, nutrition (aside from eating a balanced diet) and the wearing of sunglasses do not appear to have a significant impact on visual outcomes in AMD.

Goals of Therapy

- Minimize loss of vision
- Improve vision if possible
- Minimize enlargement of central scotomas
- Optimize function and quality of life

Investigations

- Thorough history with attention to:
  - vision loss
    - recent changes
    - central visual changes such as a central scotoma (central blur in centre of visual field)
    - metamorphopsia (distortion such that straight lines appear curved or crooked)
  - AMD in patient or first-degree relatives
- Physical examination with attention to:
  - visual acuity
  - Amsler grid (see Figure 1)
  - funduscopy (dilated fundus exam with slit-lamp biomicroscopy

  Note: The retinal exam alone may be inadequate to exclude the presence of a treatable lesion in wet AMD.
- Fluorescein angiography:
  - available only at large centres and interpreted by retinal specialists

  - involves intravenous injection of fluorescein sodium, followed by photography of the ocular fundus
  - considered the gold standard for investigating AMD

Note: Some patients have allergic reactions to fluorescein sodium, which is chemically unrelated to x-ray contrast and contains no iodine. Severe reactions are rare.

- Optical coherence tomography:
  - widely available
  - noninvasive
  - uses infrared light to generate a cross-sectional view of the macula
  - considered the gold standard for treatment decisions using vascular endothelial growth factor inhibitors

Figure 1: Amsler Grid

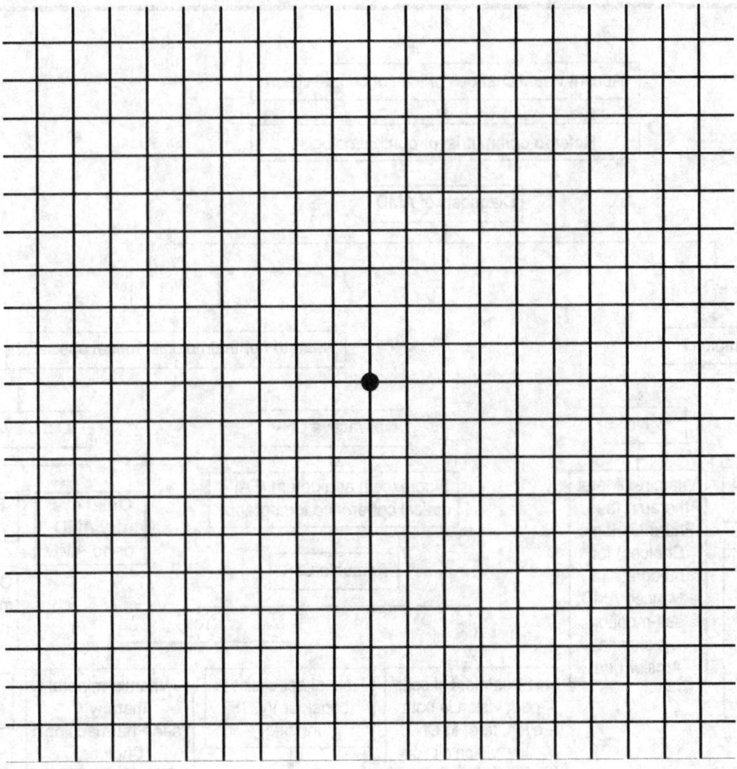

Instructions for the patient:

- Use adequate lighting, and wear the glasses you would normally use to read.
- Cover 1 at eye at a time and test the other.
- With the open eye, stare at the centre dot while considering the following questions:
  - Is any corner or border of the grid not visible?
  - Are there any broken or missing lines?
  - Are any of the lines blurry, curved or wavy?
- Repeat the test 2–3 times per week. Tell your eye care professional if you answer yes to any of the questions.

Source: St. Luke's Cataract & Laser Institute. Eye-Q. *Amlser grid.* Available from: www.stlukeseye.com/eyeq/amsler.html.

Therapeutic Choices

An algorithm for the management of age-related macular degeneration is presented in Figure 2.

Nonpharmacologic Choices

Smoking is a major risk factor for AMD. Advise patients to quit smoking and to maintain a balanced diet. See also Prevention.

The *Amsler grid* (Figure 1) is useful for self-monitoring by patients. A central blur or distortion in either eye can indicate the onset of the wet form of AMD. The test must be performed with 1 eye closed, then repeated with the other eye. Reading glasses must be used for the test, if the patient customarily requires them. The grid should be placed 33 cm from the eyes.

Visual aids such as magnifiers, high-power glasses and reading machines can enable many visually handicapped persons to read enough to perform common household tasks. Low vision clinics sponsored by the Canadian National Institute for the Blind are widely available in Canada.

Figure 2: **Management of Age-related Macular Degeneration**

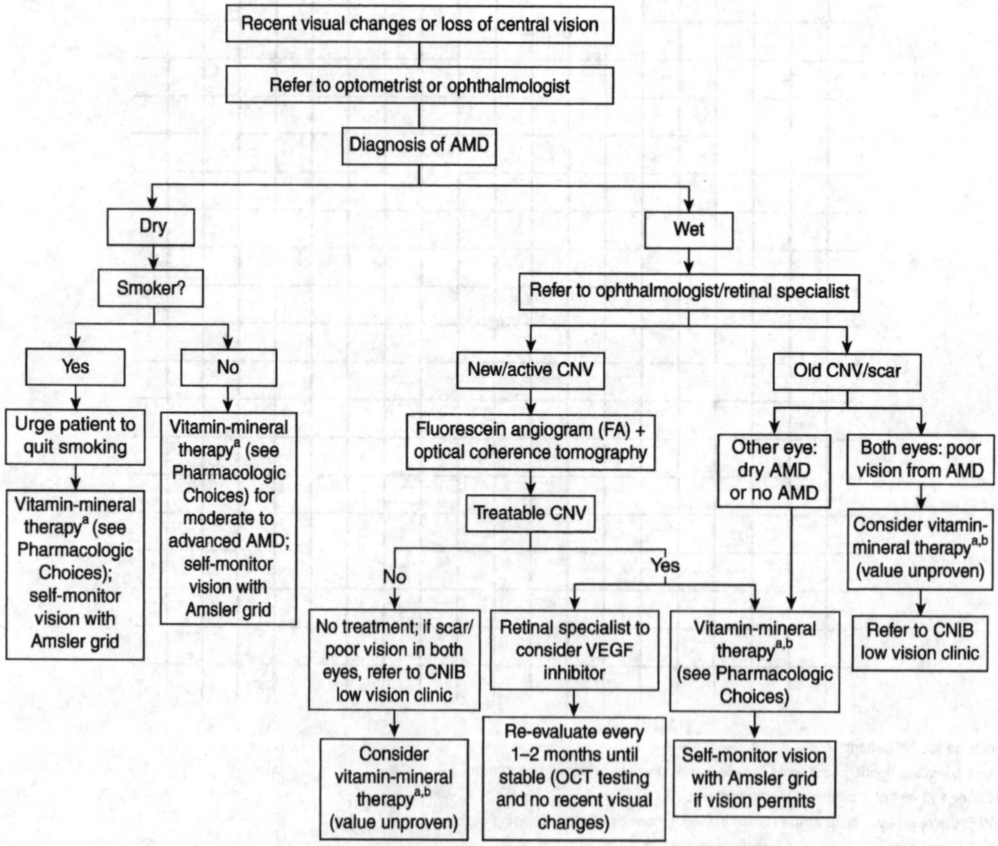

[a] Vitamin-mineral formulations containing beta-carotene are no longer recommended; see Table 2.
[b] If patient smokes, encourage smoking cessation.
Abbreviations: AMD = age-related macular degeneration; CNIB = Canadian National Institute for the Blind; CNV = choroidal neovascular membrane; OCT = optical coherence tomography; VEGF = vascular endothelial growth factor

Pharmacologic Choices

Drug treatment options for AMD are listed in Table 1.

Vascular Endothelial Growth Factor (VEGF) Inhibitors

Studies have proven that the vascular endothelial growth factor (VEGF) inhibitors are effective in decreasing vision loss in wet AMD.[8,9,10,11] By decreasing VEGF levels in the extracellular space, these drugs inhibit growth and cause regression of new blood vessels in CNV membranes. They also stabilize the blood-retinal barrier, thereby reducing macular edema and restoring normal anatomy. All VEGF inhibitors are injected directly into the vitreous cavity of the eye following application of topical anesthesia and antiseptic eye drops, usually povidone-iodine. Patients with a known allergy to iodine should alert their treating physician. Alternatives such as chlorhexidine topical solution are currently available in Canada.

Four VEGF inhibitors are available in Canada: bevacizumab, ranibizumab, aflibercept and pegaptanib. There is excellent evidence supporting the use of **ranibizumab**, a monoclonal antibody fragment derived from bevacizumab that demonstrates a higher VEGF binding affinity than its antecedent.[10,11] Ninety percent of patients receiving ranibizumab lost less than 3 lines on a specialized vision chart and 40% of patients showed improvement at 2 years.[10] The monoclonal antibody **bevacizumab** has been in widespread use since 2005 when it was approved for the treatment of colon cancer. It is frequently used off-label for several retinal diseases, including wet AMD. Large-scale multicenter controlled clinical trials have shown no statistically significant differences between bevacizumab and ranibizumab for visual outcomes of patients with wet AMD.[12,13,14,15,16] Minor differences in other outcome measures, such as intraretinal edema and atrophy were reported, however. There are also small differences in the half-lives of the 2 drugs, and tachyphylaxis has been reported with both, with improvements upon switching to the other drug. Because of the very large difference in cost and minimal evidence to show that one is superior to the other, most physicians will initiate treatment with bevacizumab.

Aflibercept is the most recent addition to the anti-VEGF group of drugs. It is a fusion protein of binding domains from human VEGF receptors 1 and 2 with the constant region (Fc) of human immunoglobulin G. Recent studies including 2 large scale multicenter controlled clinical trials showed equivalent efficacy at 96 weeks for aflibercept and ranibizumab in the treatment of wet AMD.[17]

In large multicenter randomized controlled clinical trials, **pegaptanib** was shown to reduce vision loss at a rate similar to that of photodynamic therapy (see Photodynamic Therapy below)[8,9] but, unlike bevacizumab, ranibizumab and aflibercept, has not shown actual improvement in vision. It is rarely used today.

The frequency of administration varies with the drug. Aflibercept may be used at monthly or bimonthly intervals; ranibizumab is generally used monthly and bevacizumab is administered every 6 weeks. While the endpoints of treatment with AMD have not been fully established, most patients will require 6–8 injections during the first year of therapy, and fewer afterwards. As patients stabilize or improve (based on the results of ocular coherence tomography testing, clinical examination and visual acuity), physicians may elect to increase the dosing interval, or treat on an "as needed" (prn) basis, with any of these drugs.

Side effects of these drugs are uncommon. The most worrisome is due to the injection procedure—bacterial endophthalmitis occurs at a frequency of 1 in 1000 procedures or less. Severe loss of vision is the hallmark of endophthalmitis. Pain and redness of the eye may also be present. Because irreversible blindness may occur, endophthalmitis is considered a medical emergency that requires immediate treatment by an ophthalmologist; management includes biopsy for bacterial culture followed by intravitreal injection of antibiotics. Often surgery is necessary, and outcomes vary widely depending on the duration and nature of the infection. Patients receiving intravitreal VEGF inhibitors are warned to seek medical attention immediately if they develop symptoms of endophthalmitis. Many patients will have mild pain from the drug injection procedure, which does not necessarily indicate a problem. Subconjunctival hemorrhage is also common and generally resolves within 2 weeks. A large fraction of patients undergoing intraocular injection will have a subconjuntival hemorrhage, usually manifested as a small red spot at the injection site on the white of the eye. Generally the spot will go away within a few days and has no effect on the inside of the eye or on any macular disease. Patients may shower or bathe normally afterward. Subconjunctival blood is more common in patients taking ASA or warfarin, and patients with a propensity for bleeding should discuss this issue with their doctor prior to treatment.

The recurrence rate of AMD following successful treatment has not been firmly established, but appears to be very high. Lifelong vigilance for recurrence is likely necessary, including self-monitoring with the Amsler grid (Figure 1).

Anti-VEGF therapy has also become the standard treatment of diabetic macular edema, branch and central retinal vein occlusion with macular edema, and various other retinal diseases.

Photodynamic Therapy

Photodynamic therapy (PDT) is no longer used as primary therapy for most forms of AMD. PDT[18,19,20,21] with **verteporfin** may be indicated in patients with a suitable CNV lesion from rare forms of wet AMD or related conditions. Today it is most commonly used for the treatment of central serous retinopathy, also known as central serous chorioretinopathy. This condition usually presents in young men, is not caused by macular degeneration and has a more benign course. PDT may also be used for polypoidal choroidal vasculopathy, a form of macular degeneration that is more common in East Asia, particularly Japan. Indocyanine green angiography, a procedure similar to fluorescein angiography, may be necessary to make this diagnosis.

Verteporfin is a porphyrin derivative that, when activated by light in the presence of oxygen, generates free radicals that damage the neovascular endothelium and occlude the vessels. Verteporfin is contraindicated in patients with porphyria; severe liver disease is a relative contraindication.

PDT has been shown to significantly reduce vision loss compared to placebo.[19,20,21] Patients usually do not recover lost vision, and indeed often lose further vision after the initiation of therapy before plateauing at levels higher than untreated patients. Individual patient response may vary from the averages in the large studies.

Treatment decisions require the interpretation of fluorescein angiograms together with clinical evaluation by a retinal specialist. PDT involves administration of intravenous verteporfin followed by a low-level (nonthermal) laser light that is aimed at the CNV lesion through a magnifying contact lens using a slit-lamp. The 10-minute infusion is followed by a 5-minute waiting period. The laser light is then applied for 83 seconds.

Patients must be in semi-darkness for the treatment, and remain so for 48 hours afterward. Skin is photosensitive during this time, and a severe burn may result if sunlight or bright lights strike the patient anywhere on the body. This warning includes tanning salons, halogen examination lights used in emergency wards, surgical lights and lighting used for dental procedures. Ultraviolet sunscreens provide no protection from this photosensitivity reaction.

Inadvertent subcutaneous extravasation of verteporfin can cause pain and prolonged photosensitivity of the overlying skin until the drug has been metabolized.

Prevention

Advise patients to quit smoking to reduce their risk of AMD. Encourage a balanced diet.

Numerous vitamins and mineral supplements are marketed to help reduce the risk of AMD. Choosing a product with safe ingredients in effective strengths requires careful assessment of the most recent evidence.

In the large multicentred Age-Related Eye Disease Study (AREDS), a daily treatment (given in 2 divided doses) with a combination of **beta-carotene** 25 000 IU, **vitamin C** 500 mg, **vitamin E** 400 IU, **zinc** 80 mg and **copper** 2 mg reduced patients' AMD-associated vision loss by 25% over 7 years.[22] The increased risk of lung cancer in smokers taking beta-carotene supplements reported in earlier studies[23,24] and in AREDS prompted the recommendation to avoid beta-carotene in smokers and former smokers and led to the marketing of a supplement formulation without beta-carotene. The more recent AREDS2 was a large multicenter clinical trial that concluded there was no additional reduction in vision loss when lutein plus zeaxanthin, **omega-3** plus **omega-6 long chain fatty acids** or all 4 were added to the original AREDS formula.[25] In a subgroup of study patients who were randomized to one of 4 AREDS formulations (the original, no beta-carotene, lower-dose zinc, or no beta-carotene plus lower-dose zinc) the progression of AMD was not affected when beta-carotene was removed and zinc doses were lowered. A small but worrisome increased risk of lung cancer was observed in AREDS2 patients (and on re-examination, AREDS patients) who took formulations containing beta-carotene. This increased risk was observed in nonsmokers (some former smokers and some not) but was not fully quantified. Because of these concerns, beta-carotene–containing formulations are no longer recommended for the prevention of progression to AMD (see Table 2).[25]

Many vitamin products containing lutein, zeaxanthin and omega-3 fatty acids are now marketed for improving eye health. Omega supplements were shown not to be of value in AMD.[25] Formulations with a lower dose of zinc (total of 25 mg daily) may be as effective and cause less nausea.[25] **Lutein** and **zeaxanthin** are structurally and functionally related to beta-carotene and vitamin A, occur naturally in foods and are concentrated in the macula. The AREDS researchers have proposed that the lutein and zeaxanthin combination may be an effective and safer alternative than beta-carotene for future formulations, however, more research is required.

Other contraindications to beta-carotene include severe liver disease, renal insufficiency, renal dialysis and pregnancy. While beta-carotene appears to be less teratogenic than vitamin A, no definitive data on risk are available. Women of child-bearing potential are below the age for which vitamins have been proven effective. High-dose vitamin C and E supplementation is contraindicated in renal disease, and high-dose vitamin C has been noted to cause oxalosis, resulting in kidney stones. High-dose zinc may cause gastric disturbances as well as the rare, severe sideroblastic form of anemia. Fish liver oils may contain high doses of vitamins A and E, and toxicity could result from taking multiple supplements with overlapping constituents. Because it is known to exacerbate retinitis pigmentosa, vitamin E is contraindicated in certain non-AMD inherited retinal degenerations.[26] Patients with such retinal conditions should not take AREDS vitamin formulations containing vitamin E. Copper was included in the AREDS formula to reduce the likelihood of anemia in patients taking large amounts of zinc.

Table 1: Drug Therapy for Wet Age-related Macular Degeneration

Class	Drug	Dose	Comments	Cost[a]
Photodynamic Therapy	*verteporfin* Visudyne	6 mg/m² diluted to a total volume of 30 mL and given iv over 10 min; may need to be repeated at 3-month intervals	Use only in **rare** forms of wet AMD. IV infusion is followed by laser light delivery, i.e., 50 J/cm² at a fluence of 600 mW/cm² (standard fluence); 25 J/cm² at a fluence of 300 mW/cm² (low fluence) is also in use. Patients must avoid exposure of skin or eyes to sunlight or bright indoor light for 2 days. Severe back pain, which occurs rarely during verteporfin infusions, remits when the infusion is stopped. Severe and potentially irreversible vision loss occurs rarely following therapy.	~$1900/15 mg single-dose vial
Vascular Endothelial Growth Factor Inhibitors	*aflibercept* Eylea	2 mg intravitreal injection every 4 wk × 3 months; then 2 mg every 8 wk	VEGF Inhibitors: Mild eye pain is common; does not necessarily indicate a problem. Subconjunctival hemorrhage is also common and resolves spontaneously. Endophthalmitis occurs rarely but is a medical emergency requiring immediate treatment by an ophthalmologist.	~$1500/2 mg vial
	bevacizumab Avastin	1.25 mg intravitreal injection every 1–2 months	See aflibercept. Bevacizumab: Widely used off-label.	~$550/ 100 mg vial
	ranibizumab Lucentis	0.5 mg intravitreal injection every 1–2 months	See aflibercept.	~$1700 /2.3 mg single-dose vial

[a] Includes drug cost only.
Abbreviations: AMD = age-related macular degeneration; VEGF = vascular endothelial growth factor

Table 2: Vitamin-Mineral Supplements for Age-related Macular Degeneration

Class	Drug[a]	Dose	Comments	Cost[b]
Combination Vitamin/Mineral Supplements	*vitamin C 250 mg + vitamin E 200 IU + copper 1 mg + zinc 40 mg + lutein 5 mg* Vitalux-S, generics	1 caplet BID po	Formulated to match the doses in the AREDS2 trial.[25] Take with food to reduce nausea that may be associated with zinc dose. Note: contains no beta-carotene. Formulas containing beta-carotene may increase the risk of lung cancer. Lutein 5 mg content yields zeaxanthin 250 µg. Caution with other vitamin-mineral supplements containing overlapping ingredients.	$$

[a] Because of an increased risk of lung cancer, mainly in smokers[23,24] but also in former smokers and nonsmokers,[25] formulations containing beta-carotene are not recommended.
[b] Cost of 30-day supply; includes drug cost only.
Legend: $ < $10 $$ $10–15

Suggested Readings

Age-Related Eye Disease Study 2 Research Group. Lutein + zeaxanthin and omega-3 fatty acids for age-related macular degeneration: the Age-Related Eye Disease Study 2 (AREDS2) randomized clinical trial. *JAMA* 2013;309(19):2005-15.

CATT Research Group, Martin DF, Maguire MG et al. Ranibizumab and bevacizumab for neovascular age-related macular degeneration. *N Engl J Med* 2011;364(20):1897-908.

Klein R, Klein BE, Tomany SC et al. Ten-year incidence and progression of age-related maculopathy: the Beaver Dam eye study. *Ophthalmology* 2002;109(10):1767-79.

References

1. Leibowitz HM, Krueger DE, Maunder LR et al. The Framingham Eye Study monograph: an ophthalmological and epidemiological study of cataract, glaucoma, diabetic retinopathy, macular degeneration, and visual acuity in a general population of 2631 adults, 1973-1975. *Surv Ophthalmol* 1980;24(Suppl):335-610.
2. Hyman LG, Lilienfeld AM, Ferris FL et al. Senile macular degeneration: a case-control study. *Am J Epidemiol* 1983;118(2):213-27.
3. Kahn HA, Leibowitz HM, Ganley JP et al. The Framingham Eye Study. II. Association of ophthalmic pathology with single variables previously measured in the Framingham Heart Study. *Am J Epidemiol* 1977;106(1):33-41.
4. Klein BE, Klein R. Cataracts and macular degeneration in older Americans. *Arch Ophthalmol* 1982;100(4):571-3.
5. Bressler SB, Bressler NM, Fine SL et al. Natural course of choroidal neovascular membranes within the foveal avascular zone in senile macular degeneration. *Am J Ophthalmol* 1982;93(2):157-63.
6. Chandra SR, Gragoudas ES, Friedman E et al. Natural history of disciform degeneration of the macula. *Am J Ophthalmol* 1974;78(4):579-82.
7. Gass JD. Drusen and disciform macular detachment and degeneration. *Arch Ophthalmol* 1973;90(3):206-17.
8. Gragoudas ES, Adamis AP, Cunningham ET et al. Pegaptanib for neovascular age-related macular degeneration. *N Engl J Med* 2004;351(27):2805-16.
9. VEGF Inhibition Study in Ocular Neovascularization (V.I.S.I.O.N.) Clinical Trial Group; Chakravarthy U, Adamis AP et al. Year 2 efficacy results of 2 randomized controlled clinical trials of pegaptanib for neovascular age-related macular degeneration. *Ophthalmology* 2006;113(9):1508.e1-25.
10. Rosenfeld PJ, Brown DM, Heier JS et al. Ranibizumab for neovascular age-related macular degeneration. *N Engl J Med* 2006;355(14):1419-31.
11. Brown DM, Kaiser PK, Michels M et al. Ranibizumab versus verteporfin for neovascular age-related macular degeneration. *N Engl J Med* 2006;355(14):1432-44.
12. Avery RL, Pieramici DJ, Rabena MD et al. Intravitreal bevacizumab (Avastin) for neovascular age-related macular degeneration. *Ophthalmology* 2006;113(3):363-372.e5.
13. Lazic R, Gabric N. Intravitreally administered bevacizumab (Avastin) in minimally classic and occult choroidal neovascularization secondary to age-related macular degeneration. *Graefes Arch Clin Exp Ophthalmol* 2007;245(1):68-73.
14. Rich RM, Rosenfeld PJ, Puliafito CA et al. Short-term safety and efficacy of intravitreal bevacizumab (Avastin) for neovascular age-related macular degeneration. *Retina* 2006;26(5):495-511.
15. Yoganathan P, Deramo VA, Lai JC et al. Visual improvement following intravitreal bevacizumab (Avastin) in exudative age-related macular degeneration. *Retina* 2006;26(9):994-8.
16. CATT Research Group, Martin DF, Maguire MG et al. Ranibizumab and bevacizumab for neovascular age-related macular degeneration. *N Engl J Med* 2011;364(20):1897-908.
17. Schmidt-Erfurth U, Kaiser PK, Korobelnik JF et al. Intravitreal aflibercept injection for neovascular age-related macular degeneration: ninety-six–week results of the VIEW studies. *Ophthalmology* 2014;121(1):193-201.
18. Verteporfin Roundtable Participants. Guidelines for using verteporfin (Visudyne) in photodynamic therapy for choroidal neovascularization due to age-related macular degeneration and other causes: update. *Retina* 2005;25(2):119-34.
19. Verteporfin Roundtable 2000 and 2001 Participants; Treatment of age-related macular degeneration with photodynamic therapy (TAP) study group principal investigators; Verteporfin in photodynamic therapy (VIP) study group principal investigators. Guidelines for using verteporfin (Visudyne) in photodynamic therapy to treat choroidal neovascularization due to age-related macular degeneration and other causes. *Retina* 2002;22(1):6-18.
20. Verteporfin In Photodynamic Therapy Study Group. Verteporfin therapy of subfoveal choroidal neovascularization in age-related macular degeneration: two-year results of a randomized clinical trial including lesions with occult with no classic choroidal neovascularization—Verteporfin in Photodynamic Therapy Report 2. *Am J Ophthalmol* 2001;131(5):541-60.
21. Bressler NM; Treatment of Age-Related Macular Degeneration with Photodynamic Therapy (TAP) Study Group. Photodynamic therapy of subfoveal choroidal neovascularization in age-related macular degeneration with verteporfin: two-year results of 2 randomized clinical trials-TAP Report 2. *Arch Ophthalmol* 2001;119(2):198-207.
22. Age-Related Eye Disease Study Research Group. A randomized, placebo-controlled, clinical trial of high-dose supplementation with vitamins C and E, beta carotene, and zinc for age-related macular degeneration and vision loss: AREDS report no. 8. *Arch Ophthalmol* 2001;119(10):1417-36.
23. Albanes D, Heinonen OP, Huttunen JK et al. Effects of alpha-tocopherol and beta-carotene supplements on cancer incidence in the Alpha-Tocopherol Beta-Carotene Cancer Prevention Study. *Am J Clin Nutr* 1995;62(6 Suppl):1427S-1430S.
24. Omenn GS, Goodman GE, Thornquist MD et al. Risk factors for lung cancer and for intervention effects in CARET, the Beta-Carotene and Retinol Efficacy Trial. *J Natl Cancer Inst* 1996;88(21):1550-9.
25. Age-Related Eye Disease Study 2 Research Group. Lutein + zeaxanthin and omega-3 fatty acids for age-related macular degeneration: the Age-Related Eye Disease Study 2 (AREDS2) randomized clinical trial. *JAMA* 2013;309(19):2005-15.
26. Berson EL, Rosner B, Sandberg MA et al. A randomized trial of vitamin A and vitamin E supplementation for retinitis pigmentosa. *Arch Ophthalmol* 1993;111(6):761-72.

Chapter 29
Cataract Surgery Postoperative Care

Stan P. George, MD, FRCSC

It is difficult for a primary care practitioner to manage and diagnose the complications of a postoperative cataract patient without the benefit of a slit lamp or indirect ophthalmoscope; frequently even a Snellen acuity chart is unavailable. The goal of this chapter is to review symptoms and signs that would allow a primary care practitioner to identify cases that should be urgently referred to the ophthalmologist.

Goals of Therapy

- Control inflammation
- Prevent infection
- Maintain eye comfort
- Promote early visual rehabilitation

The goals of the *postoperative assessment* are to:

- Detect intraocular infection in its early stages
- Detect postoperative uveitis or intraocular pressure (IOP) elevation
- Detect other abnormalities in the postoperative course such as a retinal detachment, iris prolapse, wound leak, flat anterior chamber, excessive corneal edema or intraocular hemorrhage

Investigations

Figure 1 illustrates an assessment process for the postoperative cataract patient.

Figure 1: **Evaluation of the Postoperative Cataract Patient by the Primary Care Practitioner**

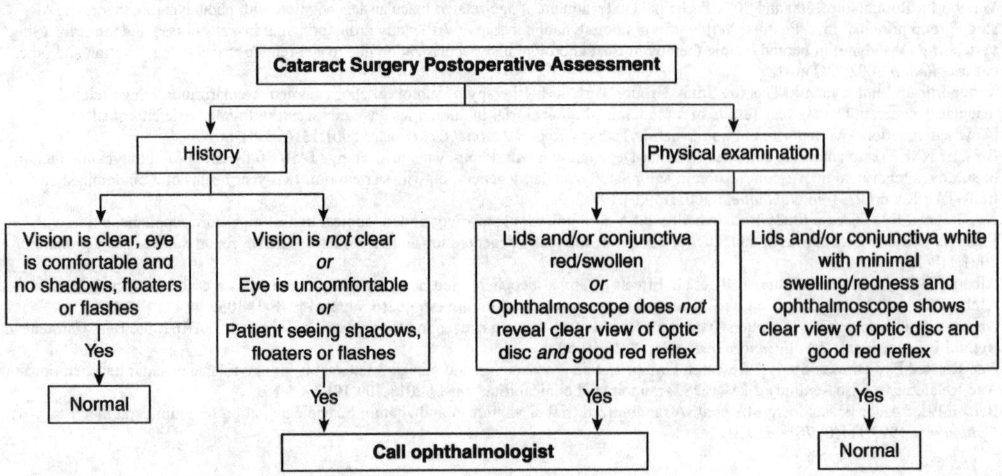

- Pain:
  - the postoperative eye should be comfortable. At worst, the patient may have a mild foreign-body sensation
  - more intense pain suggests increased IOP, increased inflammation and/or infection (not uncommon in the first 24 hours)
- History of recent trauma:
  - any trauma to the eye in the early postoperative phase requires thorough reassessment with a slit lamp
- Change in vision (worsening, darkening, loss of detail or peripheral visual loss):
  - any significant change could indicate infection, hemorrhage, retinal detachment or other acute intraocular pathology requiring immediate attention
- Visual phenomena (flashing lights, dark shadows or floaters):
  - worsening of floaters requires thorough reassessment to rule out infection, retinal tear or detachment, or uveitis
  - in the first few days or weeks after implantation of an intraocular lens, many patients notice a glare or shadow in the peripheral vision (dysphotopsia); in this time frame it is usually not a cause for concern provided that confrontation visual field testing (finger counting using peripheral vision) is normal
  - using a pinhole to test visual acuity will eliminate the effect of refractive error if the patient has apparent reduced acuity
- Itching of the eye (as predominant symptom):
  - suggests allergy to medications
- Examination of eye:
  - swelling of lids and/or conjunctiva suggests drug allergy or infection
  - pupil(s) should react normally to light unless a mydriatic agent has been used. Photophobia (glare sensitivity and pain from light exposure) can indicate anterior uveitis or corneal haze (from infection, inflammation or increased IOP)
  - the cornea should be clear of any clouding or infiltrates (to rule out corneal or anterior segment infection, inflammation or intraocular pressure elevation); the cornea should reflect a clear, well-demarcated image when the direct ophthalmoscope or pupil light is shined on it
  - use the ophthalmoscope to see if the disc is clearly viewed and a red reflex is present (to rule out vitreous clouding, inflammation or infection)
- Review of ocular medications:
  - reinforce proper use
  - clarify any confusion
  - discuss with family member
- Verify follow-up visits with surgeon

Therapeutic Choices

Pharmacologic Choices

Postoperative ophthalmic medications may include:

- **Antibacterials** (Table 1)
  - a broad-spectrum antibacterial is used perioperatively to reduce the risk of endophthalmitis. Although there is some evidence that prophylactic antibacterials are beneficial,[1] the evidence is

weak.[2] Nonetheless, not using perioperative topical antibacterials could be problematic from a medical-legal point of view as they have become a standard of care.

- one study demonstrated the efficacy of preoperative topical **povidone iodine** in reducing the rate of endophthalmitis.[3] The use of perioperative fourth-generation topical fluoroquinolones (**besifloxacin, gatifloxacin, moxifloxacin**)[4,5] is very common; however, many surgeons still prefer a formulation that combines an antibacterial with a corticosteroid in the same bottle, e.g., tobramycin/dexamethasone (Tobradex), for ease of use and to improve adherence to therapy.

- **Glaucoma medications** (Table 2)
  - used to lower the intraocular pressure after eye surgery. In patients with pre-existing glaucoma, medication regimen may be modified in postoperative period to protect against early postoperative rise in intraocular pressure.
- **Anti-inflammatory agents** (Table 3)
  - used during the first few postoperative weeks to reduce inflammation and the risk of developing cystoid macular edema.
- **Dilators** and **cycloplegics** (Table 4)
  - used to keep iris away from implant during early healing period and to improve comfort by decreasing ciliary muscle spasm.
- A mild analgesic may be required (e.g., **acetaminophen** 500 mg every 4–6 hours).
- Sedation is rarely needed.
- Other systemic medications should be continued.

Therapeutic Tips

- Any changes to postoperative ophthalmic medications should be discussed with the treating ophthalmologist.
- Initiate topical antibacterials immediately following surgery rather than waiting until the first postoperative day.[6,7,8]
- Advise patients to separate the administration of different eye drops by a period of at least 5 minutes. Counsel them to close the eye and put pressure on the inner canthus after instilling drops in order to reduce the transfer of ophthalmic medication to the nasal and/or oral mucosa where it can be absorbed systemically.
- Any worsening of vision, floaters or eye redness, especially in the first postoperative week, should be considered endophthalmitis until proven otherwise and requires urgent assessment by an ophthalmologist.
- Treatment with many medications in this setting is for a limited course, therefore any remaining ophthalmic medication should be disposed of properly.
- Patients having clear corneal cataract surgery should take all their usual medications, including anticoagulants and antiplatelet agents, on the day of surgery.

Table 1: Antibacterials for Cataract Surgery Postoperative Care

Class	Drug	Duration of Use	Adverse Effects	Comments	Cost[b]
Aminoglycosides	*neomycin combinations, ophthalmic* Maxitrol	7–10 days	Extended use may cause conjunctivitis or epitheliopathy reactions to the eye.	High concentrations on and in the eye lead to broader bacterial coverage than traditional in vitro testing suggests.	$
	tobramycin, ophthalmic Tobrex, generics	7–10 days	See neomycin combinations, ophthalmic.	See neomycin combinations, ophthalmic.	$
Antibiotic Combinations	*bacitracin ± polymyxin B ± gramicidin, ophthalmic* Polysporin, generics	7–10 days	Allergic/hypersensitivity reactions.	Good broad-spectrum coverage but hypersensitivity reactions in some patients, especially with longer use.	$
Fluoroquinolones	*besifloxacin, ophthalmic* Besivance	7–10 days	Blurred vision, local irritation or discomfort.	4th generation fluoroquinolone; improved broad-spectrum activity, especially against gram-positive organisms.	$$
	ciprofloxacin, ophthalmic Ciloxan, generics	7–10 days	Formation of white crystalline precipitate on a corneal defect after administration.	Excellent broad-spectrum profile and minimal ocular surface toxicity; very commonly used; may be used orally if lens capsule ruptured during cataract surgery.	$
	ciprofloxacin, oral ➔ Cipro, generics	500 mg Q12H po × 7–10 days	Abdominal pain, headache, dizziness, photosensitivity, hepatitis, pseudomembranous colitis, cartilage toxicity.	Used orally if lens capsule ruptured during cataract surgery.	$$
	gatifloxacin, ophthalmic Zymar	7–10 days	Well tolerated and minimal eye toxicity with topical administration. Allergic reactions uncommon. Blurred vision, local irritation or discomfort.	See besifloxacin.	$$
	moxifloxacin, ophthalmic Vigamox	7–10 days	See gatifloxacin, ophthalmic.	See besifloxacin.	$$
	ofloxacin, ophthalmic Ocuflox, generics	7–10 days	See gatifloxacin, ophthalmic.	See ciprofloxacin, ophthalmic.	$
	ofloxacin, oral ➔ generics	400 mg Q12H po × 7–10 days	See ciprofloxacin, oral.	Used orally if lens capsule ruptured during cataract surgery.	$$$

[a] Cost of smallest available pack size or 10-day supply for oral treatment; includes drug cost only.
➔ Dosage adjustment may be required in renal impairment; see Appendix I.
Legend: $ < $10 $$ $10–20 $$$ $20–30

Table 2: Glaucoma Medications for Cataract Surgery Postoperative Care

Class	Drug	Duration of Use	Adverse Effects	Comments	Cost[a]
Alpha$_2$-adrenergic Agonists	*apraclonidine* Iopidine	Used as long as intraocular pressure is elevated, or permanently in patients with pre-existing glaucoma	Common ocular reactions include hyperemia and a burning sensation.	Potent in controlling postoperative pressure spikes; avoid in patients with severe cardiovascular disease in light of alpha-adrenergic effects; use with caution in patients taking tricyclic antidepressants.	$$$
	brimonidine 0.2% Alphagan, generics	Used as long as intraocular pressure is elevated, or permanently in patients with pre-existing glaucoma	See apraclonidine.	See apraclonidine.	$
	brimonidine 0.15% Alphagan P, generics	Used as long as intraocular pressure is elevated, or permanently in patients with pre-existing glaucoma	See apraclonidine.	See apraclonidine. Contains purite as preservative rather than benzalkonium chloride; may have slightly lower incidence of ocular allergy than brimonidine 0.2%.	$
Beta-adrenergic Antagonists	*betaxolol* Betoptic S, generics	Used as long as intraocular pressure is elevated, or permanently in patients with pre-existing glaucoma	Symptoms of systemic beta blockade can be precipitated or aggravated with beta-blocking eye drops (e.g., bradycardia, arrhythmia, hypotension, bronchospasm); potentially serious systemic effects in patients with asthma, obstructive lung disease or borderline cardiac function.	Efficacious and cost effective with minimal ocular toxicity; avoid in asthmatics or patients with obstructive lung disease or borderline cardiac function.	$
	levobunolol Betagan, generics	Used as long as intraocular pressure is elevated, or permanently in patients with pre-existing glaucoma	See betaxolol.	See betaxolol.	$
	timolol Timoptic, generics	Used as long as intraocular pressure is elevated, or permanently in patients with pre-existing glaucoma	See betaxolol.	See betaxolol.	$
	timolol gel-forming solution Timoptic XE, generics	Used as long as intraocular pressure is elevated, or permanently in patients with pre-existing glaucoma	See betaxolol.	See betaxolol. Once-daily formulation improves adherence.	$

Class	Drug	Duration of Use	Adverse Effects	Comments	Cost[a]
Carbonic Anhydrase Inhibitors	*acetazolamide, oral* ❥ generics	250 mg up to QID; used for very high intraocular pressure on a short-term basis	Should not be used in patients with sulfonamide allergy; systemic hypersensitivity reactions may develop. See also Chapter 30.	Carbonic anhydrase inhibitors more commonly used *topically* as adjunctive agents to reduce intraocular pressure. Oral formulation usually used short-term for severe rises in pressure or treatment failure with topical formulations.	$
	brinzolamide Azopt	Topical use may be long-term	See acetazolamide. Conjunctivitis and blepharitis are not uncommon side effects with topical carbonic anhydrase inhibitors.	See acetazolamide.	$$
	dorzolamide Trusopt, generics	Topical use may be long-term	See acetazolamide. Conjunctivitis and blepharitis are not uncommon side effects with topical carbonic anhydrase inhibitors.	See acetazolamide.	$
	methazolamide, oral generics	50–100 mg BID–TID; used for very high intraocular pressure on a short-term basis	See acetazolamide.	See acetazolamide.	$$$$
Prostaglandins	*bimatoprost* Lumigan RC	Used as long as intraocular pressure is elevated, or permanently in patients with pre-existing glaucoma	Brown pigmentation of the iris; darkening of the periocular skin; thickening and elongation of eye lashes. Hyperemia not uncommon in first month of use.	Very potent pressure-lowering agents with once-daily application.	$$$$
	latanoprost Xalatan, generics	Used as long as intraocular pressure is elevated, or permanently in patients with pre-existing glaucoma	See bimatoprost.	See bimatoprost.	$$
	travoprost Travatan Z	Used as long as intraocular pressure is elevated, or permanently in patients with pre-existing glaucoma	See bimatoprost.	See bimatoprost.	$$$

[a] Cost of smallest available pack size or 30-day supply of oral therapy; includes drug cost only.

❥ Dosage adjustment may be required in renal impairment; see Appendix I.

Legend: $ < $10 $$ $10–20 $$$ $20–30 $$$$ $30–40

Table 3: Ophthalmic Anti-inflammatories for Cataract Surgery Postoperative Care

Class	Drug	Duration of Use	Adverse Effects	Comments	Cost[a]
Corticosteroids	*dexamethasone* Maxidex	3–4 wk; longer if evidence of cystoid macular edema	Elevated intraocular pressure; anti-inflammatory effects can mask signs of infection.	Commonly used after all types of eye surgery.	$
	difluprednate 0.05% Durezol	Start 24 h after surgery, continue for 2 wk then taper. 1 drop into conjunctival sac of affected eye QID	See dexamethasone.	Preservative is sorbic acid.	$$$
	fluorometholone Flarex, FML, generics	3–4 wk; longer if evidence of cystoid macular edema	See dexamethasone.	See dexamethasone. Less elevation of intraocular pressure compared to dexamethasone or prednisolone, but less potent.	$
	loteprednol 0.5% Lotemax	3–4 wk; longer if evidence of cystoid macular edema	See dexamethasone.	See dexamethasone. Less elevation of intraocular pressure compared to dexamethasone or prednisolone.	$$$
	prednisolone Pred Mild, Pred Forte, Minims Prednisolone, generics	3–4 wk; longer if evidence of cystoid macular edema	See dexamethasone.	See dexamethasone. Minims prednisolone are preservative-free.	$
	rimexolone Vexol	3–4 wk; longer if evidence of cystoid macular edema	See dexamethasone.	See dexamethasone. Less elevation of intraocular pressure compared to dexamethasone or prednisolone.	$$
NSAIDs	*diclofenac* Voltaren Ophtha	3–4 wk; longer if evidence of cystoid macular edema	Mild to moderate burning on instillation; epitheliopathy and possible ulceration with prolonged and frequent use.	Used as a substitute for steroids to decrease inflammation without the risk of elevating intraocular pressure; reduces risk of developing cystoid macular edema; should not be used in patients with asthma or allergies to ASA or NSAIDs.	$
	ketorolac Acular, Acuvail, generics	3–4 wk; longer if evidence of cystoid macular edema	See diclofenac.	See diclofenac.	$
	nepafenac Nevanac	3–4 wk; longer if evidence of cystoid macular edema	See diclofenac.	See diclofenac.	$$

[a] Cost of smallest available pack size; includes drug cost only.
Legend: $ < $10 $$ $10–20 $$$ $20–30

Table 4: Ophthalmic Dilators and Cycloplegics for Cataract Surgery Postoperative Care

Class	Drug	Duration of Use	Adverse Effects	Comments	Cost[a]
Dilators and Cycloplegics	*cyclopentolate* Cyclogyl, generics	First few weeks after surgery	Uncommonly, systemic anticholinergic side effects (e.g., flushing, tachycardia, urinary retention).	Less commonly used with modern cataract surgery in light of smaller incisions and less postoperative inflammation.	$$
	phenylephrine Mydfrin, generics	First few weeks after surgery	Rarely, tachycardia and hypertension.	See cyclopentolate.	$
	tropicamide Mydriacil, generics	First few weeks after surgery	See cyclopentolate.	See cyclopentolate.	$$

[a] Cost of smallest available pack size; includes drug cost only.
Legend: $ < $10 $$ $10–20

Suggested Readings

American Academy of Ophthalmology. Cataract and Anterior Segment Panel. *Preferred practice pattern: cataract in the adult eye*. San Francisco (CA): American Academy of Ophthalmology; 2011. Available from: one.aao.org/preferred-practice-pattern/cataract-in-adult-eye-ppp--october-2011.

Fintelmann RE, Naseri A. Prophylaxis of postoperative endophthalmitis following cataract surgery: current status and future directions. *Drugs* 2010;70(11):1395-409.

Gerstenblith AT, Rabinowitz MP. *The Wills eye manual: office and emergency room diagnosis and treatment of eye disease*. 6th ed. Philadelphia (PA): Lippincott Williams & Wilkins; 2012.

Harper RA, ed. *Basic ophthalmology*. 9th ed. San Francisco (CA): American Academy of Ophthalmology; 2010.

Tasman W, Jaeger EA, eds. *Duane's ophthalmology on DVD-ROM*. 2013 ed. Philadelphia (PA): Lippincott Williams & Wilkins; 2012.

References

1. Allen HF, Mangiaracine AB. Bacterial endophthalmitis after cataract extraction. II. Incidence in 36,000 consecutive operations with special reference to preoperative topical antibiotics. *Arch Ophthalmol* 1974;91(1):3-7.
2. Ciulla TA, Starr MB, Masket S. Bacterial endophthalmitis prophylaxis for cataract surgery: an evidence-based update. *Ophthalmology* 2002;109(1):13-24.
3. Speaker MG, Menikoff JA. Prophylaxis of endophthalmitis with topical povidone-iodine. *Ophthalmology* 1991;98(12):1769-75.
4. Callegan MC, Ramirez R, Kane ST et al. Antibacterial activity of the fourth generation flouroquinolones gatifloxacin and moxifloxacin against ocular pathogens. *Adv Ther* 2003;20(5):246-52.
5. Deramo VA, Lai JC, Fastenberg DM et al. Acute endophthalmitis in eyes treated prophylactically with gatifloxacin and moxifloxacin. *Am J Ophthmol* 2006;142(5):721-5.
6. Jensen MK, Fiscella RG, Crandall AS et al. A retrospective study of endophthalmitis rates comparing fluoroquinolone antibiotics. *Am J Ophthalmol* 2005;139(1):141-8.
7. Jensen MK, Fiscella RG, Moshifar M et al. Third- and fourth-generation fluoroquinolones: retrospective comparison of endophthalmitis after cataract surgery performed over ten years. *J Cataract Refract Surg* 2008;34(9):1460-7.
8. Lloyd JC, Braga-Mele R. Incidence of postoperative endophthalmitis in a high-volume cataract surgicentre in Canada. *Can J Ophthalmol* 2009;44(3):288-92.

Chapter 30

Glaucoma

Gisèle Li, MSc, MD, FRCSC

Glaucoma is the term used to describe a group of ocular diseases that have optic neuropathy leading to vision loss in common. Characteristically, the optic disc is cupped, and peripheral field loss precedes deterioration of visual acuity. Elevated intraocular pressure (IOP) is the most important, and only modifiable, risk factor for glaucoma.[1] Other risk factors (Table 1) are likely important in the pathogenesis of this neurodegenerative condition.[2]

Goals of Therapy

- Prevent, halt or slow progressive visual loss
- Preserve the structure and function of the optic nerve
- Eliminate pain and improve vision in acute forms

Investigations

- Thorough history with special attention to:
  - nature of any ocular disturbances, e.g., loss of peripheral vision, halos around lights, decreased visual acuity
  - quality of any pain, e.g., deep orbital, brow or headache
  - associated systemic symptoms, e.g., abdominal pain, nausea and vomiting

  Note: The most common varieties of glaucoma are chronic. Generally, symptoms are associated only with *acute* types of glaucoma and warrant an urgent referral to an ophthalmologist or emergency room. Most patients with chronic glaucoma are asymptomatic until they reach the advanced stages of the disease.

Table 1: **Risk Factors for the Development of Glaucoma**

Type of Glaucoma	Open-angle Glaucoma	Angle-closure Glaucoma Acute	Chronic
Acquired, Primary	Elevated IOP Advanced age[7] Black ethnicity[8] Hispanic ethnicity (Mexican ancestry)[9] Positive family history Myopia[10] Vascular diseases such as migraine,[11] hypertension[12] or nocturnal hypotension[13]	Female gender Advanced age[7] Positive family history Hyperopia White ethnicity	Advanced age[7] Positive family history Hyperopia
Acquired, Secondary	Blunt or penetrating trauma Previous intraocular surgery Previous intraocular inflammation Corticosteroid use (ophthalmic, systemic, nasal or inhaled)	Proliferative diabetic retinopathy and central retinal vein occlusion (neovascular angle-closure glaucoma)	
Congenital	Positive family history		

- Careful assessment of risk factors (Table 1)
- History of drug use that can cause or worsen glaucoma:
  - corticosteroids (common)
  - drugs with antimuscarinic activity (rare), e.g., antihistamines, decongestants, antidepressants, antispasmodics
  - the anticonvulsant topiramate has been associated with acute angle-closure glaucoma[3]
- Physical examination:
  - positive findings include constricted visual field, optic disc cupping and elevated IOP

  Note: Screening for elevated IOP *alone* lacks adequate sensitivity and specificity for the detection of glaucoma. Up to 50% of people with glaucoma have IOP in the normal range (<21 mm Hg).[4] Furthermore, about 90% of people with elevated IOP do *not* have glaucoma, although their risk of developing it are increased.[5]
- Comprehensive eye examination by an ophthalmologist or optometrist
- Laboratory tests:
  - automated perimetry
  - optic disc photography
  - optic disc and retinal imaging[6]

Therapeutic Choices

To achieve therapeutic goals (see Goals of Therapy) the IOP is lowered through the use of medications, laser and/or surgical procedures. This is true even in patients with glaucoma whose pressures are in the normal range.

An algorithm for the management of open-angle glaucoma is presented in Figure 1.

Nonpharmacologic Choices

- Lifestyle modifications have not been shown to alter the outcome of the disease. Aerobic exercise can lower IOP modestly in some patients with glaucoma.[14]
- Laser or surgical procedures are treatment options if drug therapy is unsuccessful (Figure 1, Table 2).

Pharmacologic Choices

- Treat any reversible cause of glaucoma (see Table 1).

  Note: The definitive treatment for *acute angle-closure* glaucoma is a *laser iridotomy or surgical iridectomy*. Aggressive medical treatment is required to ameliorate the damaging effects of extreme IOP elevation until the iridectomy is performed.
- Treat excessive IOP, the only modifiable risk factor in chronic primary *open-angle* glaucoma (the most prevalent form). All treatments listed in Figure 1 and Table 3 exert their therapeutic effect by lowering IOP.
- Some patients with risk factors in addition to elevated IOP may require treatment even in the absence of glaucomatous optic disc and visual field damage.[5]
- Patients with open-angle glaucoma at normal pressures will benefit from further lowering of their IOP.[15]
- Target IOPs for a specific patient are set on the basis of:
  - the extent of glaucomatous damage
  - the IOP range believed to have been associated with that damage

– the burden of therapy to achieve the desired IOP.

- Target pressure is adjusted downward if progressive damage to the optic disc or visual field occurs at the target IOP.[16]
- In some cases, clinicians may want to consider the potential neuroprotective effects or improvement in ocular blood flow afforded by some of the existing ocular hypotensive agents.[17]

Figure 1: Management of Open-angle Glaucoma

Treatment is stepped up if optic disc cupping progresses, the visual field deteriorates or intraocular pressure control is inadequate.

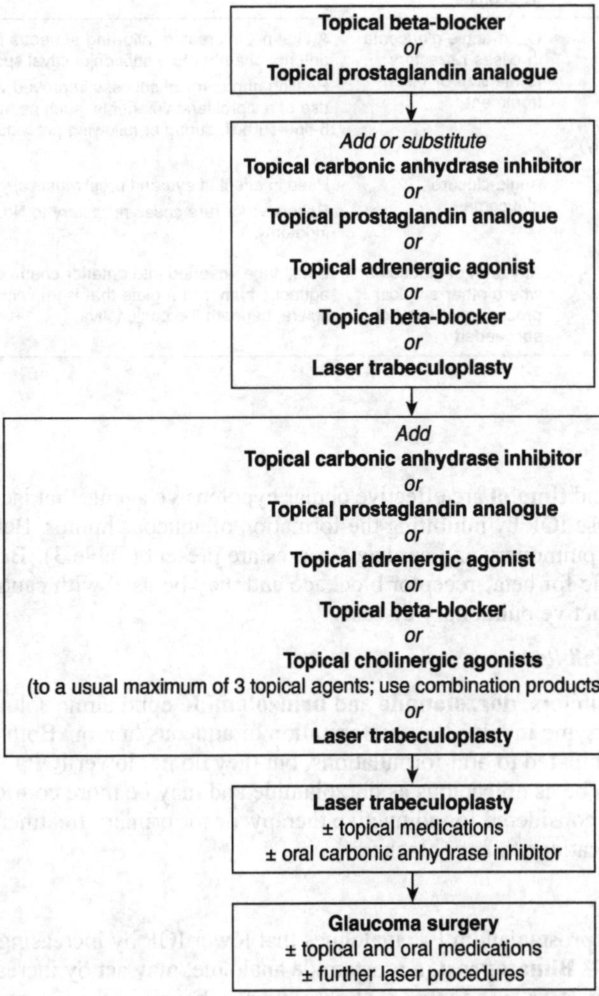
Topical beta-blocker
or
Topical prostaglandin analogue
Add or substitute
Topical carbonic anhydrase inhibitor
or
Topical prostaglandin analogue
or
Topical adrenergic agonist
or
Topical beta-blocker
or
Laser trabeculoplasty
Add
Topical carbonic anhydrase inhibitor
or
Topical prostaglandin analogue
or
Topical adrenergic agonist
or
Topical beta-blocker
or
Topical cholinergic agonists
(to a usual maximum of 3 topical agents; use combination products to improve adherence)
or
Laser trabeculoplasty
Laser trabeculoplasty
± topical medications
± oral carbonic anhydrase inhibitor
Glaucoma surgery
± topical and oral medications
± further laser procedures

Table 2: **Laser and Surgical Treatment of Glaucoma**

Type of Treatment	Procedure	Indication	Description
Laser	Laser trabeculoplasty (argon or selective laser)	Open-angle glaucoma	Laser applications to trabecular meshwork (drainage system). Effect is short-term, e.g., 2 y; most suitable for elderly patients.
	Laser iridotomy	Angle-closure glaucoma	A neodymium:yttrium-aluminum-garnet (Nd:YAG) laser cuts holes in iris to permit flow of aqueous humor directly from posterior to anterior chamber; can be done without incising eyeball. Simple office procedure.
	Laser ciliary body ablation	Advanced refractory glaucomas	Used where other options are limited.
Surgical	Filtration procedures (e.g., trabeculectomy, nonpenetrating deep sclerotomy, viscocanalostomy)	Open-angle glaucoma, in cases refractory to medical or laser treatment	A channel is created, allowing aqueous flow from anterior chamber to a subconjunctival space. Healing and surgical success improved with topical use of antiproliferative agents, such as mitomycin C or 5-fluorouracil, during or following procedure.
	Iridectomy	Angle-closure glaucoma	Used in affected eye and prophylactically in other eye. Reserved for rare cases refractory to Nd:YAG laser iridotomy.
	Drainage tube insertion	Any form of glaucoma, where other surgical procedures have not succeeded	Small tube, inserted into anterior chamber, drains aqueous humor to a plate that is implanted on the sclera, beneath the conjunctiva.

Open-angle Glaucoma

Beta-blockers

Topical **betaxolol**, **levobunolol** and **timolol** are effective ocular hypotensive agents that lack significant ocular side effects.[18] They decrease IOP by inhibiting the formation of aqueous humor. Beta-blockers are contraindicated when certain pulmonary and cardiac diseases are present (Table 3). Betaxolol hydrochloride is relatively specific for beta$_1$-receptor blockade and may be used with caution in selected patients with mild obstructive pulmonary disease.[19]

Topical Carbonic Anhydrase Inhibitors

Like oral carbonic anhydrase inhibitors, **dorzolamide** and **brinzolamide** ophthalmic solutions decrease IOP by inhibiting an enzyme involved in the formation of aqueous humor. Both have limited systemic effects when compared to oral formulations, but they do not lower IOP to the same extent.[20] Brinzolamide appears to be as efficacious as dorzolamide and may be more comfortable on instillation.[21] These drugs can be considered for adjunctive therapy, or for primary treatment in patients with cardiopulmonary contraindications to beta-blockers.

Prostaglandin Analogues

Latanoprost and **travoprost** are prostaglandin $F_{2\alpha}$ analogues that lower IOP by increasing outflow through the uveoscleral pathway.[22] **Bimatoprost**, a prostamide analogue, may act by increasing both uveoscleral and trabecular outflow.[23] These agents are slightly more efficacious than nonselective beta-blockers. Clinical experience with this class has not revealed any significant systemic adverse effects, but a few ocular effects have been noted, including darkening of some brown-coloured irides, lengthening of the eyelashes and mild conjunctival hyperemia.[24] Any of these agents may be considered first-line therapy because of their potencies and excellent safety profiles.

Alpha$_2$-Adrenergic Agonists

Topical epinephrine, the prototype in this class, has not been available in Canada for some time because of unacceptable adverse ocular effects. The epinephrine prodrug dipivefrin has also been discontinued. **Apraclonidine** was the first alpha$_2$-specific agonist introduced, but local allergic reactions have limited its use to the management of acute IOP spikes.[25] Also demonstrating a significant incidence of allergy, **brimonidine** has a higher specificity for the alpha$_2$-receptor and is associated with a less severe conjunctival hyperemia.[26] A formulation of brimonidine (0.15%, preserved with purite rather than benzalkonium chloride) may have a slightly lower rate of ocular allergy than brimonidine 0.2%. Like apraclonidine, brimonidine suppresses the formation of aqueous humor and can be used for a variety of open-angle and angle-closure glaucomas.[27] Brimonidine may also increase uveoscleral outflow.

Cholinergic Agonists

The topical cholinergic agonists **pilocarpine** and **carbachol** directly stimulate muscarinic receptors to contract the ciliary muscle and increase trabecular outflow.[28] These drugs are characterized by ocular side effects, including miosis (with reduced night vision), accommodative spasm (including myopia) and brow ache, and rarely, in predisposed patients, retinal detachment. Rarely is sufficient drug absorbed systemically to cause abdominal cramping or diarrhea. These drugs are poorly tolerated in children and young adults. Carbachol is no longer available in Canada.

Fixed-combination Preparations

There are currently 5 fixed-combination topical glaucoma therapies, each containing timolol, available in Canada. **Brimonidine/timolol**,[29] **brinzolamide/timolol**,[30] **dorzolamide/timolol**,[31] **latanoprost/timolol**[32] and **travoprost/timolol**[33] are all more effective than the individual agents. All combined formulations have similar ocular hypotensive effects. Dorzolamide/timolol has the longest track record. The advantage of the combined agents is improved adherence to therapy.

Oral Carbonic Anhydrase Inhibitors

Acetazolamide and **methazolamide** lower IOP by decreasing the production of aqueous humor. Their use is normally reserved for emergencies because of significant side effects. Approximately 50% of patients are unable to use these agents long term because of GI or CNS difficulties, paresthesias or renal lithiasis.[34] Oral and topical carbonic anhydrase inhibitors can show cross-reactivity in patients allergic to sulfonamides.

Preservatives

Benzalkonium chloride, the most common preservative in eye drops, works by denaturing proteins and causing lysis of cytoplasmic membranes.[35] Unfortunately, as many as 6% of glaucoma patients are allergic to benzalkonium chloride.[36] Prolonged exposure to this preservative can result in superficial damage to the ocular surface[37] and cause symptoms such as irritation, dryness, itchiness and burning. To increase tolerability of glaucoma drops, alternative preservatives have been developed. Travoprost is available with an ionic buffer preservative (see Table 3).[38] Brimonidine is also available with a non-benzalkonium chloride preservative called purite. Some ophthalmic drops are available in preservative-free, single-dose units.

Therapeutic Tips

- Topical glaucoma medications are highly concentrated to allow adequate intraocular penetration. Systemic absorption through the nasal mucosa can be reduced through digital occlusion of the nasolacrimal drainage system for several minutes following instillation of the drops[39] or through eyelid closure for 3–5 minutes.
- Allow 5 minutes between the instillation of different eye drops to avoid a washout of the previously administered medication.

- Nonprescription **antihistamine** products include a caution against use in patients with glaucoma due to potential anticholinergic side effects. Intermittent use of medications with anticholinergic effects will rarely cause a problem in open-angle glaucoma. The caution is included primarily to warn that, in rare instances, drugs with anticholinergic activity can precipitate angle-closure glaucoma in predisposed individuals[40] (e.g., elderly white or Asian females who are significantly hyperopic, have a positive family history and have not yet had a therapeutic or prophylactic iridectomy; see Table 1).
- The Canadian Ophthalmological Society does not support the use of **cannabis** (marijuana) for the treatment of glaucoma due to the short duration of action and the undesirable psychotropic and other systemic side effects.[41] Other more effective and less harmful treatments exist.

Table 3: Drug Therapy for Glaucoma

Class	Drug	Dose[a]	Adverse Effects	Comments	Cost[b]
Alpha$_2$-adrenergic Agonists, ophthalmic	*apraclonidine 0.5%, 1%* Iopidine	1–2 drops Q12H or Q8H	Local allergic reaction, tachycardia, hypotension, headache, tremor.	Contraindicated with MAO inhibitors. Can rarely be used chronically due to more than 40% incidence of marked blepharoconjunctivitis. 1% solution used perioperatively for anterior segment laser treatment.	$$$
	brimonidine 0.2% Alphagan, generics	1 drop Q12H	See apraclonidine.	Contraindicated with MAO inhibitors; not recommended in pediatric patients. Lower incidence of allergy than apraclonidine when used chronically.	$
	brimonidine 0.15% Alphagan P, generics	1 drop Q8H	See apraclonidine.	See brimonidine 0.2%. Contains purite as preservative rather than benzalkonium chloride; may have slightly lower incidence of ocular allergy than brimonidine 0.2%.	$
Alpha$_2$-adrenergic Agonist/Beta-blocker Combinations, ophthalmic	*brimonidine 0.2%/timolol 0.5%* Combigan	1 drop Q12H	See apraclonidine. See betaxolol.	See brimonidine 0.2%. See betaxolol.	$$$$$
Beta-adrenergic Antagonists, ophthalmic	*betaxolol 0.25%* Betoptic S	1 drop QAM or Q12H	Local adverse effects usually minimal: stinging, dry eyes, rarely conjunctivitis. Systemic effects can include bronchospasm, exacerbation of CHF, bradycardia, syncope, depression, impotence, altered response to hypoglycemia, reduction of high-density lipoproteins.	Avoid in patients with bronchial asthma; caution in patients with a history of syncope or bradycardia.	$$
	levobunolol 0.25%, 0.5% Betagan, generics	1 drop QAM or Q12H	See betaxolol.	See betaxolol.	$
	timolol 0.25%, 0.5% Timoptic, generics	1 drop QAM or Q12H	See betaxolol.	See betaxolol.	$
	timolol gel-forming solution 0.25%, 0.5% Timoptic-XE, generics	1 drop once daily	See betaxolol.	See betaxolol. Shake container once before each use.	$

(cont'd)

Table 3: Drug Therapy for Glaucoma *(cont'd)*

Class	Drug	Dose[a]	Adverse Effects	Comments	Cost[b]
Carbonic Anhydrase Inhibitors, ophthalmic	*brinzolamide 1%* Azopt	1 drop Q12H	Bitter, sour or unusual taste, stinging, local allergic reaction.	Dose can be increased to Q8H after 4 wk if inadequate response. Cross-reactivity in patients allergic to sulfonamides.	$$
	dorzolamide 2% Trusopt, generics	Monotherapy: 1 drop Q8H; Adjunctive therapy: 1 drop Q12H	See brinzolamide.	Cross-reactivity in patients allergic to sulfonamides.	$
	dorzolamide 2% preservative-free Trusopt	Monotherapy: 1 drop Q8H; Adjunctive therapy: 1 drop Q12H	See brinzolamide.	Advantageous for patients with allergies to benzalkonium chloride. Ensure tip or fins of the pipette container do not touch the eye; align fins side-to-side to the corners of the eye when administering drops.[42] Cross-reactivity in patients allergic to sulfonamides.	$$$$$
Carbonic Anhydrase Inhibitors, oral	*acetazolamide* generics	250 mg up to QID po	Paresthesias of the extremities, metabolic acidosis, hypokalemia, GI upset, urolithiasis, lethargy and depression, aplastic anemia (rare), Stevens-Johnson syndrome (rare).	Cross-reactivity in patients allergic to sulfonamides.	$$
	methazolamide generics	50–100 mg BID–TID po	See acetazolamide. Side effects are less severe than with acetazolamide.	See acetazolamide.	$$$$$
Carbonic Anhydrase Inhibitor/Beta-blocker Combinations, ophthalmic	*brinzolamide 1%/timolol 0.5%* Azarga	1 drop Q12H	See brinzolamide. See betaxolol.	See brinzolamide. See betaxolol. Shake well before using.	$$$
	dorzolamide 2%/timolol 0.5% Cosopt, generics	1 drop Q12H	See brinzolamide. See betaxolol.	Cross-reactivity in patients allergic to sulfonamides.	$$$
	dorzolamide 2%/timolol 0.5%, preservative-free Preservative-free Cosopt	1 drop Q12H	See brinzolamide. See betaxolol.	Advantageous for patients with allergies to benzalkonium chloride. Cross-reactivity in patients allergic to sulfonamides.	$$$

Class	Drug	Dose[a]	Adverse Effects	Comments	Cost[b]
Cholinergic Agonists, ophthalmic	*pilocarpine 1%, 2%, 4%,* Isopto Carpine drops	1 drop QID	Reduced vision in patients with cataracts, blurred vision due to refractive shift, brow ache, GI upset (rare).	Poorly tolerated in children and younger adults.	$
Prostaglandin Analogues, ophthalmic	*bimatoprost 0.01%* Lumigan RC	1 drop once daily in evening	Conjunctival hyperemia, foreign body sensation, burning, stinging, itching, increased iris pigmentation, increased eyelash length.	Once-daily dosing should not be exceeded; more frequent administration may reduce effectiveness.	$$$$
	latanoprost 0.005% Xalatan, generics	1 drop once daily in evening	Foreign body sensation, burning, stinging, itching, increased iris pigmentation, increased eyelash length.	See bimatoprost.	$$
	travoprost 0.004% Travatan Z	1 drop once daily in evening	See bimatoprost.	See bimatoprost. Formulated with a non-benzalkonium chloride preservative.	$$$
Prostaglandin Analogue/Beta-blocker Combinations, ophthalmic	*latanoprost 0.005%/timolol 0.5%* Xalacom, generics	1 drop once daily	See bimatoprost. See betaxolol.	See bimatoprost. See betaxolol.	$$
	travoprost 0.004%/timolol 0.5% DuoTrav PQ	1 drop once daily Administer in morning or evening	See bimatoprost. See betaxolol.	See bimatoprost. See betaxolol. Formulated with a non-benzalkonium chloride preservative.	$$$$

[a] Ophthalmic solutions are applied in affected eye(s)
[b] Cost of smallest available pack size or 30-day supply for oral medications; includes drug cost only.
Dosage adjustment may be required in renal impairment; see Appendix I.
Legend: $ < $10 $$ $10–20 $$$ $20–30 $$$$ $30–40 $$$$$ $40–50

Suggested Readings

American Academy of Ophthalmology. Glaucoma Panel. *Primary angle closure PPP—2010.* San Francisco (CA): AAO; 2010. Available from: one.aao.org/preferred-practice-pattern/primary-angle-closure-ppp--october-2010.

American Academy of Ophthalmology. Glaucoma Panel. *Primary open-angle glaucoma PPP—2010.* San Francisco (CA): AAO; 2010. Available from: one.aao.org/preferred-practice-pattern/primary-openangle-glaucoma-ppp--october-2010.

American Academy of Ophthalmology. Glaucoma Panel. *Primary open-angle glaucoma suspect PPP—2010.* San Francisco (CA): AAO; 2010. Available from: one.aao.org/preferred-practice-pattern/primary-openangle-glaucoma-suspect-ppp--october-20.

Canadian Ophthalmological Society evidence-based clinical practice guidelines for the management of glaucoma in the adult eye. *Can J Ophthalmol* 2009;44(Suppl 1):1-93.

Morrison JC, Pollack IP, eds. *Glaucoma: science and practice.* New York (NY): Thieme; 2003.

References

1. Sommer A, Tielsch JM, Katz J et al. Relationship between intraocular pressure and primary open angle glaucoma among white and black Americans. The Baltimore Eye Survey. *Arch Ophthalmol* 1991;109(8):1090-5.
2. Drance SM. Bowman Lecture. Glaucoma--changing concepts. *Eye* 1992;6(Pt 4):337-45.
3. Fraunfelder FW, Fraunfelder FT, Keates EU. Topiramate-associated acute, bilateral, secondary angle-closure glaucoma. *Ophthalmology* 2004;111(1):109-11.
4. Grodum K, Heijl A, Bengtsson B. A comparison of glaucoma patients identified through mass screening and in routine clinical practice. *Acta Ophthalmol Scand* 2002;80(6):627-31.
5. Kass MA, Heuer DK, Higginbotham EJ et al. The Ocular Hypertension Treatment Study: a randomized trial determines that topical ocular hypotensive medication delays or prevents the onset of primary open-angle glaucoma. *Arch Ophthalmol* 2002;120(6):701-13.
6. Greenfield DS, Weinreb RN. Role of optic nerve imaging in glaucoma clinical practice and clinical trials. *Am J Ophthalmol* 2008;145(4):598-603.
7. Quigley HA, Vitale S. Models of open-angle glaucoma prevalence and incidence in the United States. *Invest Ophthalmol Vis Sci* 1997;38(1):83-91.
8. Tielsch JM, Sommer A, Katz J et al. Racial variations in the prevalence of primary open angle glaucoma. The Baltimore Eye Survey. *JAMA* 1991;266(3):369-74.
9. Varma R Ying-Lai M, Francis BA et al. Prevalence of open-angle glaucoma and ocular hypertension in Latinos: the Los Angeles Latino Eye Study. *Ophthalmology* 2004;111(8):1439-48.
10. Hitchings R. Normal-tension glaucoma. In: Yanoff M, Duker JS, eds. *Ophthalmology*. London (GB): Mosby; 1999. p. 1-4.
11. Phelps CD, Corbett JJ. Migraine and low-tension glaucoma. A case-control study. *Invest Ophthalmol Vis Sci* 1985;26(8):1105-8.
12. Tielsch JM, Katz J, Sommer A et al. Hypertension, perfusion pressure, and primary open-angle glaucoma. A population-based assessment. *Arch Ophthalmol* 1995;113(2):216-21.
13. Graham SL, Drance SM, Wijsman K et al. Ambulatory blood pressure monitoring in glaucoma. The nocturnal dip. *Ophthalmology* 1995;102(1):61-9.
14. Passo MS, Goldberg L, Elliot DL et al. Exercise training reduces intraocular pressure among subjects suspected of having glaucoma. *Arch Ophthalmol* 1991;109(8):1096-8.
15. Comparison of glaucomatous progression between untreated patients with normal-tension glaucoma and patients with therapeutically reduced intraocular pressures. Collaborative Normal-Tension Glaucoma Study Group. *Am J Ophthalmol* 1998;126(4):487-97.
16. Damji KF, Behki R, Wang L et al. Canadian perspectives in glaucoma management: setting target intraocular pressure range. *Can J Ophthalmol* 2003;38(3):189-97.
17. Lesk MR, Lachaine J. Medical therapy of glaucoma: focus on newer agents. *Ophthalmic Practice* 2003;21(2):46-52.
18. Rafuse PE. Adrenergic antagonists. In: Morrison JC, Pollack IP, eds. *Glaucoma: science and practice*. New York (NY): Thieme; 2003.
19. Berry DP, Van Buskirk EM, Shields MB. Betaxolol and timolol. A comparison of efficacy and side effects. *Arch Ophthalmol* 1984;102(1):42-5.
20. Goldberg I. Carbonic anhydrase inhibitors. In: Morrison JC, Pollack IP, eds. *Glaucoma: science and practice*. New York (NY): Thieme; 2003.
21. Seong GJ, Lee SC, Lee JH et al. Comparisons of intraocular-pressure-lowering efficacy and side effects of 2% dorzolamide and 1% brinzolamide. *Ophthalmologica* 2001;215(3):188-91.
22. Lawlor D et al. Prostaglandin analogs. In: Morrison JC, Pollack IP, eds. *Glaucoma: science and practice*. New York (NY): Thieme; 2003.
23. Brubaker RF, Schoff EO, Nau CB et al. Effects of AGN 192024, a new ocular hypotensive agent, on aqueous dynamics. *Am J Ophthalmol* 2001;131(1):19-24.
24. Johnstone MA. Hypertrichosis and increased pigmentation of eyelashes and adjacent hair in the region of the ipsilateral eyelids of patients treated with unilateral topical latanoprost. *Am J Ophthalmol* 1997;124(4):544-7.
25. Butler P, Mannschreck M, Lin S et al. Clinical experience with the long-term use of 1% apraclonidine. Incidence of allergic reactions. *Arch Ophthalmol* 1995;113(3):293-6.
26. Blondeau P, Rousseau JA. Allergic reactions to brimonidine in patients treated for glaucoma. *Can J Ophthalmol* 2002;37(1):21-6.
27. Serle JB et al. Adrenergic agonists. In: Morrison JC, Pollack IP, eds. *Glaucoma: science and practice*. New York (NY): Thieme; 2003.
28. Derick RJ. Cholinergic agonists. In: Morrison JC, Pollack IP, eds. *Glaucoma: science and practice*. New York (NY): Thieme; 2003.
29. Craven ER, Walters TR, Williams R et al. Brimonidine and timolol fixed-combination therapy versus monotherapy: a 3-month randomized trial in patients with glaucoma or ocular hypertension. *J Ocul Pharmacol Ther* 2005;21(4):337-48.
30. Januleviciene I. Brinzolamide 1%/timolol 0.5%: safety and efficacy of a new fixed-combination IOP-lowering product for glaucoma. *Curr Med Res Opin* 2010;26(11):2575-8.

31. Strohmaier K, Snyder E, DuBiner H et al. The efficacy and safety of the dorzolamide-timolol combination versus the concomitant administration of its components. Dorzolamide-Timolol Study Group. *Ophthalmology* 1998;105(10):1936-44.
32. Higginbotham EJ, Feldman R, Stiles M et al. Latanoprost and timolol combination therapy vs monotherapy: one-year randomized trial. *Arch Ophthalmol* 2002;120(7):915-22.
33. Schuman JS, Katz GJ, Lewis RA et al. Efficacy and safety of a fixed combination of travoprost 0.004%/timolol 0.5% ophthalmic solution once daily for open-angle glaucoma or ocular hypertension. *Am J Ophthalmol* 2005;140(2):242-50.
34. Stamper RL et al. Carbonic anhydrase inhibitors. In: *Becker-Shaffer's diagnosis and therapy of the glaucomas*. 7th ed. St. Louis (MO): Mosby; 1999.
35. Tripathi BJ, Tripathi RC, Kolli SP. Cytotoxicity of ophthalmic preservatives on human corneal epithelium. *Lens Eye Toxic Res* 1992;9(3-4):361-75.
36. van Beek LM, de Keizer RJ, Polak BC et al. Incidence of ocular side effects of topical beta blockers in the Netherlands. *Br J Ophthalmol* 2000;84(8):856-9.
37. Baudouin C. Detrimental effect of preservatives in eyedrops: implications for the treatment of glaucoma. *Acta Ophthalmol* 2008;86(7):716-26.
38. Uusitalo H, Chen E, Pfeiffer N et al. Switching from a preserved to a preservative-free prostaglandin preparation in topical glaucoma medication. *Acta Ophthalmol* 2010;88(3):329-36.
39. Zimmerman TJ, Kooner KS, Kandarakis AS et al. Improving the therapeutic index of topically applied ocular drugs. *Arch Ophthalmol* 1984;102(4):551-3.
40. Abelson MB et al. Antiallergic therapies. In: Zimmerman TJ et al., eds. *Textbook of ocular pharmacology*. Philadelphia (PA): Lippincott-Raven; 1997.
41. Canadian Ophthalmological Society. Position & Policy Statements. *Medical use of marijuana for glaucoma*. Available from: www.cos-sco.ca/advocacy-news/position-policy-statements/medical-use-of-marijuana-for-glaucoma/. Accessed September 23, 2013.
42. Health Canada. *Cosopt (dorzolamide hydrochloride/timolol maleate) preservative-free ophthalmic solution—Risk of eye injury*. Available from: www.healthycanadians.gc.ca/recall-alert-rappel-avis/hc-sc/2014/37909a-eng.php. Accessed February 19, 2014.

Eye Disorders

Chapter 31
Red Eye

W. Bruce Jackson, MD, FRCSC

CPhA acknowledges the contribution of Dr. Sueda Akkor as the previous author of this chapter.

Red eye is common in a wide variety of ocular conditions and signals inflammation. The majority of these conditions are benign but some can have serious consequences. Table 1 lists minor and major/serious causes of red eye. The presence of one or more warning signs (see Table 2) requires immediate referral to an ophthalmologist.

Conjunctivitis is the most common cause of red eye.[1] The majority of infectious (caused by viruses or bacteria) or noninfectious (due to an allergic reaction) cases of conjunctivitis can be treated in primary care but certain cases require referral to a specialist (see Table 3).

Goals of Therapy

- Preserve eyesight
- Prevent structural damage to the eye
- Control and prevent spread of infection
- Control inflammation
- Provide symptomatic relief

Table 1: **Etiology of Red Eye**

Cause	Examples
Infection	Conjunctivitis/keratitis (bacterial, viral, other), lacrimal system infection
Allergy	
Dry eyes (keratoconjunctivitis sicca)	Sjögren's syndrome, vitamin A deficiency, meibomian gland dysfunction (MGD)/ocular rosacea (see Chapter 96), other
Eyelid condition	Blepharitis with secondary conjunctivitis/keratitis; blepharitis and MGD can also be a manifestation of rosacea (see Chapter 96)
Toxic/chemical/other irritants	Ophthalmic medications, contact lens solutions, acids/alkalis, smoke, wind, UV light (e.g., tanning bed, welder's arc)
Traumatic injury	Corneal abrasions, foreign bodies, hyphema (bleeding into the anterior chamber), heat exposure
Ocular inflammation	Iritis, episcleritis, scleritis
Glaucoma	Acute angle-closure glaucoma (see Chapter 30)
Ocular manifestations of skin condition	Rosacea (blepharitis, dry eye; see Chapter 96), herpes simplex, herpes zoster
Other	Subconjunctival hemorrhage, pterygium

Investigations

An algorithm for assessment and management of red eye is presented in Figure 1.

Thorough history to determine:

- unilateral or bilateral eye involvement
- duration and type of symptoms
- allergies
- contact lens wear
- trauma
- previous eye diseases and treatment
- history of previous dermatologic and rheumatologic conditions
- type of discharge
- visual changes
- pain and photophobia

Physical examination:

- pinhole visual acuity if glasses are not available
- pupil size and reaction to light
- inspection of face, eyelids, conjunctiva (to determine type and extent of hyperemia), sclera, cornea (staining with fluorescein)
- globe tenderness by digital pressure through the lids
- preauricular adenopathy
- intraocular pressure if acute glaucoma is suspected

Rule out serious ophthalmic conditions (e.g., corneal ulcer, acute angle closure glaucoma, iritis, scleritis):

- trauma (e.g., chemical, foreign body)
- contact lens wearer
  - possible corneal ulcer
- pain and/or severe photophobia
  - possible acute angle-closure glaucoma (more common in older adults), corneal ulcer, iritis or scleritis
- significant vision changes
  - possible glaucoma, iritis, corneal ulcer
- history of prior ocular disease (e.g., scleritis, iritis)

Danger signs include:

- decreased visual acuity
- irregular pupil(s), e.g., fixed, small or large
- ocular tenderness—pain could indicate iritis, scleritis or glaucoma
- white corneal opacity or corneal haze (with or without fluorescein staining)
- increased intraocular pressure

Table 2: Warning Signs for Ophthalmologist Referral

- Limbal/ciliary injection (redness dominant at the corneoscleral junction), especially unilateral involvement
- Pain *not* relieved by test dose of topical anesthetic drop (proparacaine, tetracaine)
- Pupil abnormalities (miotic or mid-dilated and fixed, irregular, sluggish to light)
- Signs and symptoms of acute angle-closure glaucoma such as red, painful eye with raised intraocular pressure, blurred vision, headache, vomiting or coloured halos around lights
- History of iritis/scleritis/angle-closure glaucoma
- Recent trauma to eye including contact lens wear

Table 3: Diagnosing Conjunctivitis

History	Exposure to person with red eye Upper respiratory tract infection Past history of conjunctivitis Discharge with morning crusting Exposure to ophthalmic medications, chemicals
Signs	Normal pupillary reaction Discharge and/or excessive tearing Lid and conjunctival edema Conjunctival redness
Refer to ophthalmologist	Chlamydia—preauricular node and purulent conjunctivitis plus history of sexual contact Gonococcal—hyperacute conjunctivitis Herpes simplex—usually unilateral, watery discharge and preauricular node (differential diagnosis is viral, i.e., adenovirus), eyelid vesicles Herpes zoster—ocular involvement (usually eyelids, conjunctiva), facial vesicles, corneal complication, uveitis

Therapeutic Choices

Nonpharmacologic Choices

Treatment of red eye depends on the history and symptom presentation as shown in Figure 1.

Instruct patient to:

- Stop wearing contact lenses until the problem is resolved
- Avoid makeup, smoke, wind and other irritants
- Apply cold compresses for allergic or viral conjunctivitis
- Apply warm compresses for blepharitis/styes
- Practise lid hygiene for blepharitis:
  - warm compresses applied to closed eyelids for 10–15 minutes, followed by gentle rubbing of lid margins with warm water; a commercial eyelid wipe followed by rinsing with warm water can also be used for lid hygiene
  - repeat daily at bedtime

Pharmacologic Choices

Once major/serious conditions are ruled out, treatment can be initiated. The choice of treatment depends on the underlying cause (see Table 4, Table 5, Table 6, Table 7 and Table 8).

Figure 1: Management of Red Eye

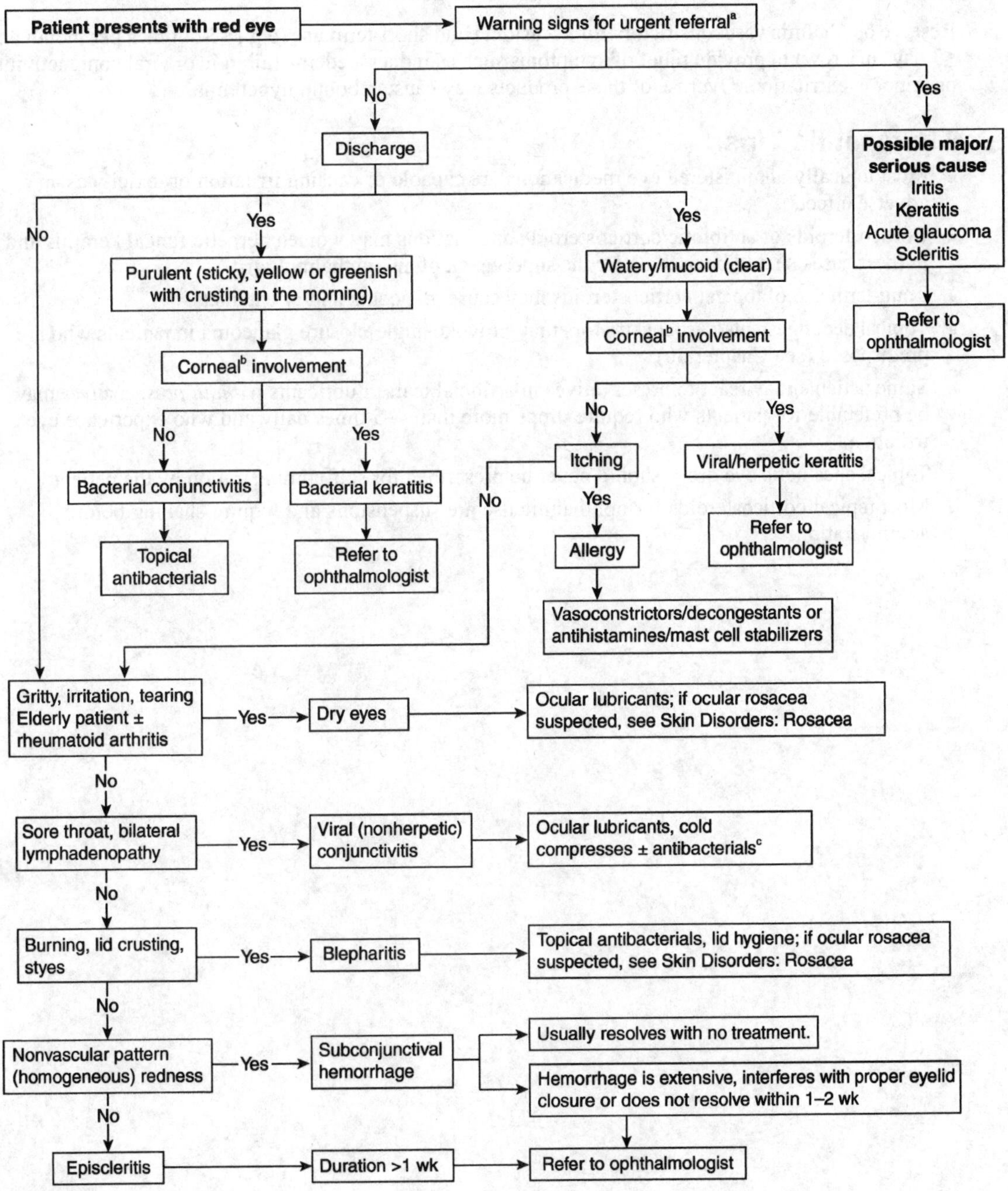

a See Table 2.
b Corneal staining with fluorescein strip indicates corneal involvement.
c Used rarely to prevent secondary bacterial infection.

Viral conjunctivitis does not usually require treatment. Although acute bacterial conjunctivitis is self-limiting, broad-spectrum antibiotic eye drops can shorten recovery time.[2,3] If no improvement is seen after 3–5 days, refer the patient to an ophthalmologist.

Reserve ophthalmic vasoconstrictors for occasional and short-term use (e.g., ≤3–4 times per month and ≤3 days in a row) to provide relief of symptoms such as redness, edema (allergic or viral conjunctivitis) or minor eye irritation. Overuse of these products may cause rebound hyperemia.

Therapeutic Tips

- Most topically administered eye medications are capable of causing irritation or toxicity as an adverse effect.
- Corticosteroids or antibiotic/corticosteroid combinations may worsen herpetic/fungal keratitis and in these cases should be used under the supervision of an ophthalmologist.
- Long-term use of topical corticosteroids may cause glaucoma and/or cataracts.
- Topical decongestants/vasoconstrictors may provoke angle-closure glaucoma in patients who are predisposed (see Chapter 30).
- Some patients may react to preservatives in artificial tears. Lubricants *without preservatives* may be preferable for patients who require drops more than 4–5 times daily and who experience eye irritation.
- Topical anesthetic eye drops should never be prescribed for self-administration by the patient.
- Most topical corticosteroids for ophthalmic use are suspensions and require shaking before administration.

Table 4: Anti-infectives for Red Eye

Class	Drug	Indications	Dose	Adverse Effects	Comments	Cost[a]
Antibacterials, ophthalmic	*besifloxacin* Besivance	Bacterial conjunctivitis.	1 drop in affected eye(s) TID for 7 days	*Antibacterials:* Chronic use may cause corneal epithelial toxicity, allergy and bacterial resistance.		$$
	ciprofloxacin Ciloxan, generics	Bacterial conjunctivitis and corneal ulcers. Fluoroquinolones should be reserved for serious corneal infections.	Drops: 1–2 drops Q2H while awake × 2 days then 2 drops Q4H while awake × 5 days Ointment: 1.25 cm TID × 2 days then BID × 5 days	See besifloxacin.		$
	erythromycin generics	Superficial bacterial infections of the conjunctiva or cornea. Dry eye.	Ointment: 1.25 cm 2–6 times/day	See besifloxacin.		$
	fusidic acid Fucithalmic	External bacterial infection of the eye. Dry eye. Due to its broad-spectrum and BID dosing, fusidic acid is especially useful in children and elderly patients. Enterobacteriaciae and pseudomonas are resistant to fusidic acid.	1 drop Q12H × 7 days	See besifloxacin.	Unit-dose droppers do not contain preservative and may be preferable in patients with atopic dermatitis.	$
	gatifloxacin Zymar	Bacterial conjunctivitis. Fluoroquinolones should be reserved for serious infections.	First 2 days: 1 drop in affected eye(s) Q2H while awake, up to 8 times daily Days 3 to 7: 1 drop QID	See besifloxacin.		$$
	moxifloxacin Vigamox	Bacterial conjunctivitis.	1 drop TID × 7 days	See besifloxacin.	Preservative-free.	$$
	ofloxacin Ocuflox, generics	Bacterial conjunctivitis Fluoroquinolones should be reserved for serious corneal infections.	1–2 drops Q2–4H × 2 days then QID × 5 days	See besifloxacin.		$

(cont'd)

Table 4: Anti-infectives for Red Eye *(cont'd)*

Class	Drug	Indications	Dose	Adverse Effects	Comments	Cost[a]
	polymyxin B/ trimethoprim Polytrim, generics	Acute bacterial conjunctivitis, blepharitis, blepharoconjunctivitis.	Initially 1–3 drops Q1H, gradually decreasing to 1–2 drops 4–6 times daily	See besifloxacin.		$$$
	polymyxin B ± bacitracin ± gramicidin Polysporin Eye/Ear Drops, Polysporin Ophthalmic Ointment, generics	Bacterial conjunctivitis/keratitis; blepharitis/styes. Choose broad-spectrum agent first, guided by patient allergies.	Drops: initially 1–3 drops Q1H, gradually decreasing to 1–2 drops 4–6 times daily Ointment: apply 2–5 times daily	See besifloxacin.	Limit use to 4–5 days.	$
	tobramycin Tobrex, generics	External bacterial infections of the eye.	Drops: 1–2 drops Q4H Ointment: 1.25 cm BID–TID	See besifloxacin.		$
Antivirals, ophthalmic	*trifluridine* Viroptic	Herpes simplex; *not* for herpes zoster infections.	1 drop Q2H while awake to a maximum of 9 drops per day, until lesion re-epithelialized; then 1 drop Q4H, maximum 5 drops per day × 7 days	Chronic use may cause corneal epithelial toxicity, conjunctival scarring and punctal stenosis.		$$$
Antivirals, systemic	*acyclovir* Zovirax Oral, generics	Herpes zoster, herpes simplex.	Herpes zoster: 800 mg 5 times/day po × 7 days Herpes simplex: 400 mg QID po × 14 days	GI upset (uncommon); well tolerated.		$$$$–$$$$$
	famciclovir Famvir, generics	Herpes zoster, herpes simplex.	Herpes zoster: 500 mg TID po × 7 days Herpes simplex: 250 mg TID po × 7 days	GI upset (uncommon); well tolerated.		$$–$$$$
	valacyclovir Valtrex, generics	Herpes zoster, herpes simplex.	Herpes zoster: 1 g TID po × 7 days Herpes simplex: 500 mg TID po × 7 days	GI upset (uncommon); well tolerated.		$$–$$$$

[a] Cost of smallest available pack size; includes drug cost only.

Dosage adjustment may be required in renal impairment; see Appendix I.

Legend: $ < $10 $$ $10–20 $$$ $20–30 $$-$$$$ $20–40 $$$$ $30–40 $$$$-$$$$$ $30–50 $$$$$ $40–50

Table 5: Ocular Lubricants for Red Eye

Class	Drug	Indications	Dose	Adverse Effects	Comments	Cost[a]
Ocular Lubricants	*carboxymethylcellulose* Refresh Celluvisc, Refresh Liquigel, Refresh Plus, Refresh Tears, Refresh Optive Advanced, Refresh Endura	Dry eyes, exposure, lid malpositions, blepharitis, minor irritations.	1–2 drops TID–QID	Preservative toxicity, gels cause filmy/blurry vision.	Refresh Plus and Endura do not contain preservatives.	$
	dextran 70/hypromellose (hydroxypropyl methylcellulose) Bion Tears, Tears Naturale, Tears Naturale Free, Tears Naturale II	See carboxymethylcellulose.	1–2 drops TID–QID	See carboxymethylcellulose.	Bion is preservative-free.	$
	hypromellose (hydroxypropyl methylcellulose) Genteal, Isopto Tears	See carboxymethylcellulose.	1–2 drops TID–QID	See carboxymethylcellulose.		$
	mineral oil/petrolatum Duolube, Hypotears Eye Ointment, Lacri-Lube S.O.P., generics	See carboxymethylcellulose.	Ointment: 0.6 cm to inside of lower lid as needed	See carboxymethylcellulose.		$
	polyvinyl alcohol Hypotears Ophthalmic Solution, Refresh, generics	See carboxymethylcellulose.	1–2 drops TID–QID	See carboxymethylcellulose.		$
	propylene glycol/polyethylene glycol-400 Systane, Systane Balance, Systane Ultra	See carboxymethylcellulose.	1–2 drops as needed	See carboxymethylcellulose.	Systane Ultra is preservative-free.	$
	sodium hyaluronate i-drop, Hylo, Blink	See carboxymethylcellulose.	With preservative: 1 drop up to QID; preservative-free drops can be used more frequently as needed	See carboxymethylcellulose.	i-drop and Hylo are preservative-free.	$

[a] Cost of smallest available pack size; includes drug cost only.
Legend: $ < $10

Table 6: Ophthalmic Anti-allergy Agents for Red Eye

Class	Drug	Indications	Dose	Adverse Effects	Comments	Cost[a]
Antihistamines/ Mast Cell Stabilizers, ophthalmic	*sodium cromoglycate* Cromolyn Eye Drops, Opticrom, generics	Ocular allergies; contact lens wear-related giant papillary conjunctivitis (a hypersensitivity disorder seen in patients with contact lenses or artificial eyes; family practitioners may suspect it in patients complaining of itch and ropy whitish discharge, but diagnosis requires slit lamp exam by an ophthalmologist).	1–2 drops 4–6 times/day	Minor stinging on instillation.	Mast cell stabilizer—does not provide immediate relief. May take 2–3 days to see symptom improvement.	$
	ketotifen fumarate Zaditor, generics	Ocular allergies.	1 drop Q8–12H	See sodium cromoglycate.		$$
	lodoxamide Alomide	Ocular allergies.	1–2 drops QID	See sodium cromoglycate.		$$
	nedocromil Alocril	Ocular allergies.	1–2 drops BID	See sodium cromoglycate.		$$$
	olopatadine 0.1% Patanol, generics	Ocular allergies.	1–2 drops Q6–8H	See sodium cromoglycate.		$$$
	olopatadine 0.2% Pataday, generics	Ocular allergies.	1 drop daily	See sodium cromoglycate.		$$$
	antazoline/naphazoline Refresh Eye Allergy Relief, generics	Ocular allergies.	1–2 drops Q3–4H	See sodium cromoglycate.		$
	pheniramine/naphazoline Naphcon-A, Opcon-A, Visine Advance Allergy	Ocular allergies.	1–2 drops up to QID	See sodium cromoglycate.		$

[a] Cost of smallest available pack size; includes drug cost only.
Legend: $ < $10 $$ $10–20 $$$ $20–30

Table 7: Ophthalmic Anti-inflammatories for Red Eye

Class	Drug	Indications	Dose	Adverse Effects	Comments	Cost[a]
Corticosteroids, ophthalmic	*dexamethasone* Maxidex	Episcleritis, iritis, scleritis, some keratitis, ocular allergy.	Drops: 2 drops Q1H during the day and Q2H during the night; gradually decrease to Q3–4H then to TID–QID Ointment: small amount to conjunctival sac TID–QID	Minor stinging on instillation; may worsen herpetic/fungal keratitis; long-term use may cause glaucoma, cataracts.		$
	difluprednate 0.05% Durezol	Endogenous anterior uveitis	1 drop QID in conjunctival sac of affected eye for 14 days, then taper	See dexamethasone.	Preservative is sorbic acid.	$$$
	fluorometholone FML, FML Forte, Flarex, generics	See dexamethasone.	1–2 drops BID–QID; may be used more frequently during initial 48 h if needed	See dexamethasone.		$
	loteprednol 0.2% Alrex	Seasonal allergic conjunctivitis.	1 drop in affected eye(s) QID for up to 14 days	Minor stinging on instillation; may worsen herpetic/fungal keratitis; rare cases of glaucoma reported with long-term use.		$$$
	prednisolone Pred Mild/Forte, Minims Prednisolone, generics	See dexamethasone.	1–2 drops Q1H during the day and Q2H at night until favourable response, then 1 drop Q4H	See dexamethasone.	Minims Prednisolone is preservative-free.	$$
	rimexolone Vexol	Inflammation following ocular surgery; anterior uveitis.	Postoperative inflammation: 1–2 drops QID × 2 wk, beginning 24 h post-op Uveitis: 1–2 drops Q1H while awake × 1 wk, then Q2H while awake × 1 wk, then QID × 1 wk, then TID × 4 days, then BID × 3 days	See dexamethasone.		$$
NSAIDs, ophthalmic	*diclofenac* Voltaren Ophtha	Episcleritis, minor corneal abrasions; as an adjunct to topical corticosteroids in scleritis, iritis.	1 drop 4–5 times daily	Minor stinging on instillation.		$$

(cont'd)

Table 7: **Ophthalmic Anti-inflammatories for Red Eye** *(cont'd)*

Class	Drug	Indications	Dose	Adverse Effects	Comments	Cost[a]
	ketorolac Acular, Acuvail, generics	Episcleritis, minor corneal abrasions; as an adjunct to topical corticosteroids in scleritis, iritis.	1 drop QID	See diclofenac.		$
	nepafenac Nevanac	Management of pain and inflammation associated with cataract surgery.	1 drop TID beginning 1 day prior to cataract surgery, continued on the day of surgery and × 2 wk postoperatively.	Eyelid margin crusting, eye pain, punctate keratitis, blurred vision, dry eye, pruritis, headache.		$$

[a] Cost of smallest available pack size; includes drug cost only.
Legend: $ < $10 $$ $10–20 $$$ $20–30

Table 8: Ophthalmic Vasoconstrictors/Decongestants for Red Eye

Class	Drug	Indications	Dose	Adverse Effects	Cost[a]
Vasoconstrictors/ Decongestants, ophthalmic	*naphazoline* Clear Eyes, Naphcon Forte, Refresh Redness Relief, generics	Alleviation of redness and/or eyelid edema in allergic or viral conjunctivitis, minor irritation (smoke, dust, wind, chlorinated pool).	1–2 drops Q3–4H PRN × 3–4 days	Minor stinging on instillation; pupillary dilation and angle-closure glaucoma in predisposed persons, e.g., elderly white or Asian females who are significantly hyperopic, have a positive family history and have not had a therapeutic or prophylactic iridotomy. Ophthalmic vasoconstrictors are meant for occasional and short-term use. Overuse may cause rebound hyperemia.	$
	oxymetazoline Visine Workplace, others	See naphazoline.	1–2 drops Q6H PRN × 3–4 days	See naphazoline.	$
	phenylephrine Mydfrin, generics	See naphazoline.	1–2 drops QID PRN × ≤3 days	See naphazoline.	$
	tetrahydrozoline Visine, others	See naphazoline.	1–2 drops BID–QID	See naphazoline.	$

[a] Cost of smallest available pack size; includes drug cost only.
Legend: $ < $10

Suggested Readings

Abnormal eye appearances. In: Frith P. *The eye in clinical practice*. 2nd ed. Oxford (GB): Blackwell Science; 2001. p. 57-84.

Chern Kenneth C, ed. *Emergency ophthalmology: a rapid treatment guide*. New York (NY): McGraw-Hill; 2002. p. 85-128.

Cronau H, Kankanala RR, Mauger T. Diagnosis and management of red eye in primary care. *Am Fam Physician* 2010;81(2):137-44.

Du Toit N, Van Zyl L. The red eye. *S Afr Fam Pract* 2013;55(1):33-40.

Maclean Hunter. *The eye in primary care : a symptom-based approach*. Oxford (GB): Butterworth-Heinemann; 2001. p. 96-114.

Mahmood AR, Narang AT. Diagnosis and management of the acute red eye. *Emerg Med Clin North Am* 2008;26(1):35-55.

Noble J, Lloyd JC. The red eye. *CMAJ* 2011;183(1):81.

Trobe Jonathan D; American Academy of Family Physicians. *The physician's guide to eye care*. 2nd ed. San Francisco (CA): American Academy of Ophthalmology; 2001. p. 41-67.

References

1. Azari AA, Barney NP. Conjunctivitis: a systematic review of diagnosis and treatment. *JAMA* 2013;310(16):1721-9.
2. Sheikh A, Hurwitz B, van Schayck CP et al. Antibiotics versus placebo for acute bacterial conjunctivitis. *Cochrane Database Syst Rev* 2012;9:CD001211.
3. Epling J. Bacterial conjunctivitis. *Clin Evid (Online)* 2012;2012. pii: 0704.

Chapter 32
Diabetes Mellitus

Kerry Mansell, BSP, PharmD, CDE and
Terra Arnason, MD, PhD, FRCPC

Diabetes mellitus is a chronic metabolic disturbance characterized by fasting and/or postprandial hyperglycemia. Rather than a single disease entity, diabetes mellitus is a heterogeneous syndrome that is caused by an absolute or relative lack of insulin, resistance to the action of insulin, or both. Dysglycemia is a term that describes abnormal blood glucose levels without a definite threshold. The term reflects current evidence that minor degrees of blood glucose abnormalities, even those that do not meet the diagnostic threshold for diabetes mellitus, are still associated with increased cardiovascular risk.[1]

Long-term diabetes mellitus may lead to complications that involve the small blood vessels (microangiopathy), large blood vessels (macroangiopathy) and nerves (neuropathy) of multiple organs and systems. Because diabetes is associated with significant dysfunction of numerous metabolic pathways, clinicians must pay close attention to factors such as hypertension and dyslipidemia in addition to blood glucose. Heart disease is the most common cause of death in patients with diabetes.[2]

Classification

Type 1 diabetes mellitus (T1DM) is due to autoimmune beta cell destruction resulting in an absolute deficiency of insulin. T1DM usually presents as acute metabolic symptoms of relatively short duration in a child, adolescent or young adult. If untreated, ketoacidosis may occur. Although onset of T1DM is not common after 30 years of age, some older individuals with type 2 diabetes mellitus may develop markers of autoimmunity and progress quickly to an insulin-dependent state. In North America, T1DM accounts for 5–10% of all patients with diabetes.

Type 2 diabetes mellitus (T2DM) manifests primarily as insulin resistance along with some degree of insulin deficiency. Over time insulin deficiency worsens, resulting in more prominent hyperglycemia. T2DM is commonly discovered incidentally, or is diagnosed in adults who are often obese and have nonspecific symptoms. T2DM makes up 90% of all cases of diabetes mellitus and the prevalence is rising rapidly, particularly in certain ethnic groups, both in Canada and worldwide. It is also being diagnosed more frequently and earlier in obese children and adolescents.

Gestational diabetes is defined as onset or recognition of glucose intolerance in pregnancy.

Other specific causes of diabetes mellitus include genetic syndromes such as maturity-onset diabetes of the young (MODY), or as a result of pancreatic diseases, infectious agents, drugs or other diseases leading to carbohydrate intolerance. Drugs that can perturb blood glucose levels and interfere with glycemic control in patients with diabetes are presented in Table 1.

Goals of Therapy

- Control symptoms
- Establish and maintain glycemic control, while avoiding hypoglycemia
- Prevent or minimize the risk of complications
- Achieve optimal control of associated risk factors such as hypertension, obesity and dyslipidemia

Table 1: **Drugs That Can Cause Dysglycemia**

- Beta-blockers, e.g., atenolol, metoprolol, propranolol[a]
- Corticosteroids, e.g., prednisone
- Diazoxide
- Immunosuppressive agents, e.g., sirolimus, tacrolimus, temsirolimus
- Interferon alfa
- Isoniazid
- Niacin
- Pentamidine
- Protease inhibitors (amprenavir, atazanavir, darunavir, fosamprenavir, indinavir, lopinavir, nelfinavir, ritonavir, saquinavir, tipranavir)
- Second-generation antipsychotic agents, e.g., clozapine, olanzapine, paliperidone, quetiapine, risperidone
- Thiazide or loop diuretics, e.g., chlorthalidone, furosemide, hydrochlorothiazide

[a] Medication-induced dysglycemia should not preclude the use of these medications if clinically indicated.

Investigations

- Diabetes mellitus may present in a variety of settings:
  - asymptomatic; incidental discovery through routine laboratory screening (Figure 1)
  - nonspecific signs and symptoms such as fatigue, lassitude, weight changes
  - presence of diabetic complications such as macrovascular or microvascular changes, neuropathy, kidney disease, erectile dysfunction
  - acute metabolic symptoms such as polyuria, polydipsia, weight loss
  - diabetic ketoacidosis
- The diagnosis of diabetes is established by:[4]
  - a random plasma glucose ≥11.1 mmol/L (random is defined as any time of day without regard to the interval since the last meal) *or*
  - a fasting plasma glucose (FPG) ≥7 mmol/L (fasting is defined as no caloric intake for ≥8 hours) *or*
  - a plasma glucose level ≥11.1 mmol/L 2 hours after a 75 g oral glucose load (oral glucose tolerance test; OGTT) *or*
  - an HbA_{1c} ≥6.5% (in nonpregnant adults) using a standardized, validated assay, in the absence of conditions that affect the accuracy of the HbA_{1c} (not to be used for suspected T1DM)[5]
  - in the absence of clinical symptoms of hyperglycemia, confirming the diagnosis with a repeat test performed on another day.[4] With the exception of a random plasma glucose, the same test should be used to confirm the initial result.

Screening

Screening for T1DM is not recommended. Although research continues there are no interventions proven to prevent or delay its onset.

The Canadian Diabetes Association recommends screening for T2DM every 3 years in individuals over 40 years of age using a fasting plasma glucose (FPG) or HbA_{1c} level. Earlier and more frequent testing should be considered in individuals at a higher risk (Table 2).[6] Alternatively, the Canadian Task Force on Preventive Health Care recommends stratifying adults by risk factor to determine if screening is warranted.[5] A validated tool such as CANRISK is recommended to determine who may benefit from screening for diabetes.[3,5,7]

Figure 1: **Screening and Diagnosis of Diabetes Mellitus[3]**

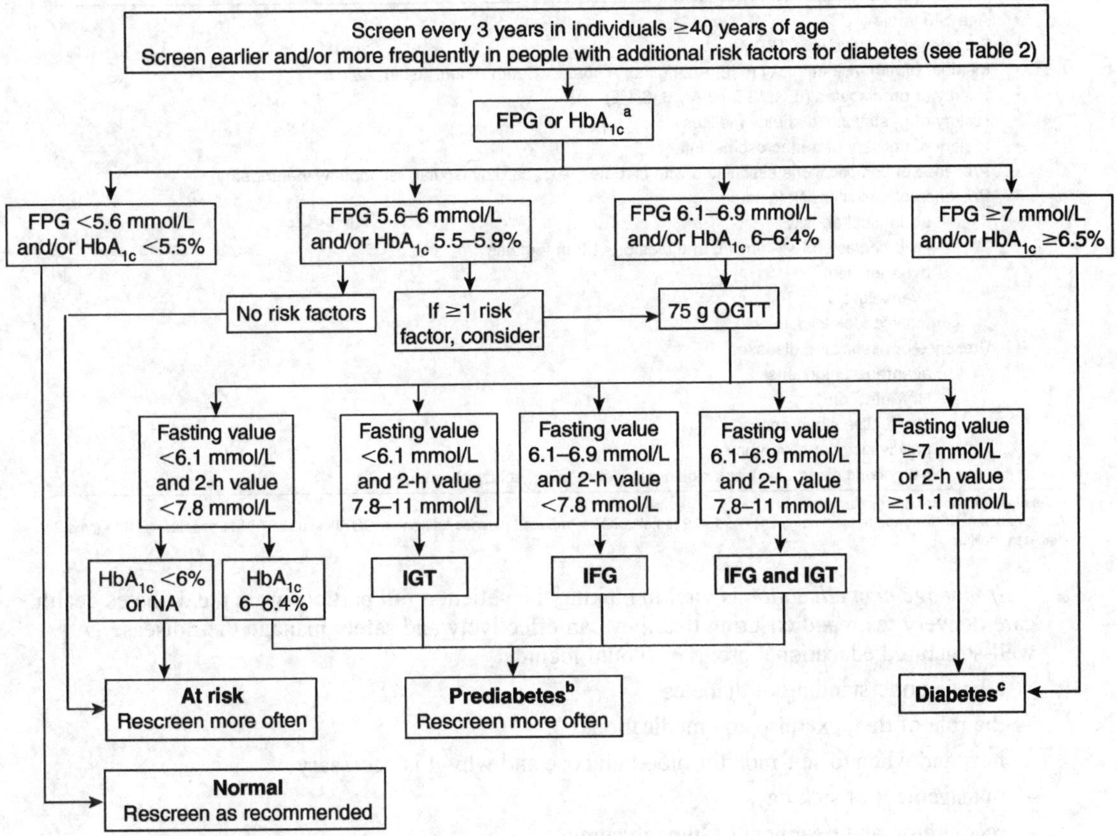

a If both FPG and HbA_{1c} are available, but discordant, use the test that appears furthest to the right side of the algorithm.
b Prediabetes = IFG, IGT or HbA_{1c} 6–6.4%.
c A confirmatory laboratory glucose test (either an FPG, a casual PG or a 2hPG in a 75 g OGTT) must be done on another day in all cases in the absence of unequivocal hyperglycemia accompanied by acute metabolic decompensation.

Abbreviations: 2hPG = 2-hour plasma glucose; HbA_{1c} = glycosylated hemoglobin; FPG = fasting plasma glucose; IFG = impaired fasting glucose; IGT = impaired glucose tolerance; OGTT = oral glucose tolerance test; PG = plasma glucose

Adapted with the permission of the Canadian Diabetes Association.

Type 1 and Type 2 Diabetes Mellitus

Therapeutic Choices

Insulin must be initiated in patients with T1DM at the time of diagnosis and considered in those with T2DM who present with marked hyperglycemia (HbA_{1c} ≥8.5%). In newly diagnosed T2DM with HbA_{1c} <8.5%, lifestyle modifications alone may be appropriate as a first step. However, if glycemic goals are not reached within 2–3 months, initiate therapy with pharmacologic agents.

Nonpharmacologic Choices

Nonpharmacologic therapy plays a pivotal role in the treatment of both type 1 and type 2 diabetes. The use of a flow chart may be helpful to ensure interventions are not overlooked (see www.diabetes.ca for an example).

Table 2: **Risk Factors for Diabetes Mellitus**[3]

- Age ≥40 years
- First-degree relative with T2DM
- Member of high-risk ethnicity (e.g., Aboriginal, Hispanic, South Asian, Asian, African)
- History of prediabetes (IFG, IGT, HbA_{1c} 6–6.4%)
- History of gestational diabetes mellitus
- History of delivery of a macrosomic infant
- Presence of complications associated with diabetes (e.g. cardiovascular, retinopathy, neuropathy)
- Presence of vascular risk factors:[a]
  - abdominal obesity
  - HDL cholesterol <1 mmol/L in males or <1.3 in females
  - hypertension
  - overweight
  - triglycerides ≥1.7 mmol/L
- Presence of associated diseases:
  - acanthosis nigricans[a]
  - HIV infection
  - obstructive sleep apnea
  - polycystic ovary syndrome[a]
  - psychiatric disorders (bipolar disorder, depression, schizophrenia)

[a] Associated with insulin resistance.
Abbreviations: IFG = impaired fasting glucose: 6.1–6.9 mmol/L; IGT = impaired glucose tolerance: OGTT result of 7.8–11 mmol/L; T2DM = type 2 diabetes mellitus

- *Self-management education* is vital in making the patient a full participant in the diabetes health care delivery team and ensuring that they can effectively and safely manage their disease. A well-structured educational program should include:
  - a basic understanding of diabetes
  - the role of diet, exercise and medications
  - how and when to self-monitor blood glucose and why it is necessary
  - management of sick days
  - recognition and treatment of hypoglycemia
  - knowledge of the major side effects of medications and possible medication adjustments in response to changes in diet and activity
  - care of the feet
  - awareness of risk of heart disease and importance of risk factor control including body weight
- Individualize *nutritional management*. Provide counselling by a registered dietitian and include information on nutrients from all the basic food groups. If overweight, reduce total caloric consumption in patients with T2DM to decrease weight and improve metabolic control. For patients on insulin, tailor the distribution of food intake into meals and snacks according to the individual's preference, lifestyle and medications. In patients with T1DM, carbohydrate intake and insulin dose must be linked. Options include advising patients to fix carbohydrate consumption or count the amount of carbohydrate ingested and adjust the insulin dose accordingly.
- *Self-monitoring of blood glucose* (SMBG) is an essential component of normalizing blood glucose for the majority of patients with diabetes mellitus. It allows appropriate recognition of low blood glucose levels and provides immediate feedback about the effects of therapy. SMBG is especially important for patients treated with insulin. In these patients, individualize self-monitoring strategies and take both pre- and postprandial measurements. A minimum of 3 blood sugar measurements per day should be performed for those on basal-bolus insulin regimens.[8] In contrast, the benefits and optimal timing and frequency of SMBG has not yet been established for those who are being managed on oral antihyperglycemics or lifestyle alone. The frequency and duration of blood glucose

monitoring in patients on oral therapy must be individualized, and should be based on factors such as type of oral antihyperglycemic agent, risk of hypoglycemia, presence of concurrent illness, as well as the need to evaluate the effectiveness of new medications or dosage changes. For example, in stable patients receiving metformin alone, who are at low risk of hypoglycemia and meeting their glycemic targets, SMBG may not be necessary. For medications that carry a higher risk of hypoglycemia (e.g., glyburide or insulin), or in patients with risk factors for hypoglycemia (e.g., advanced age, renal dysfunction, multiple comorbidities, hypoglycemia unawareness) SMBG is useful to ensure safety.

- *Physical activity* will improve cardiovascular function, enhance insulin sensitivity and lower blood pressure and lipid levels. Physical activity also helps improve glycemic control in people with T2DM. Patients engaging in physical activity more vigorous than walking should undergo a thorough physical examination to ensure safety prior to commencing the exercise program. Encourage aerobic exercise totaling ≥150 minutes per week along with resistance training at least twice a week.[9] It is imperative to educate patients treated with insulin about the effect of exercise on blood glucose and how to adjust the insulin dosage accordingly. Predictable intensity and duration allows individuals to understand how blood glucose levels will change immediately following the exercise. Typically, blood glucose levels will decrease after moderate intensity exercise but may increase after intense activity (likely a stress response). Teach patients how to time their meals and/or regulate food consumption to ensure the safety of the prescribed exercise regimen.
- *Ongoing monitoring* including directed histories and physical examinations are intended to detect comorbidities and complications; assessments should include:
  - blood pressure measurements at all appropriate visits[10]
  - foot examinations annually. Refer patients at high risk of foot ulceration or amputation and those with existing ulcers to a health care provider trained in foot care management[11]
  - HbA_{1c} measurements every 3 months for patients who have not achieved target values. Testing every 6 months may be acceptable in stable patients who consistently meet glycemic targets[8]
  - assessment of the accuracy of blood glucose meters by comparing blood glucose readings from the glucose meter and a simultaneous phlebotomy draw at least once per year; reading should be within 20%[8]
  - serum creatinine and random urine albumin-creatinine ratio once a year to screen for chronic kidney disease[12]
  - fasting lipid profile, at the time of diagnosis and then annually if results are normal initially.[13] More frequent testing (every 3–6 months) should occur if treatment is initiated.[14]
  - refer to a specialist (ophthalmologist or optometrist) for an eye examination using dilated funduscopy or wide-angle stereoscopic retinal photography at the time of diagnosis in patients with T2DM, and 5 years after diagnosis or at puberty in patients with T1DM; repeat every 1–2 years if initially normal[15]
  - reinforcing skills learned in education and dietary counselling
- *Immunize* patients with diabetes to reduce the risk of complications and hospitalization. In adults, annual influenza immunization and a one-time pneumococcal vaccination is recommended. A second pneumococcal vaccination is recommended for patients over 65 who received their original immunization >5 years earlier at an age <65.[16]

Pharmacologic Choices

Type 1 Diabetes

Insulin may be administered by syringe, pen or continuous subcutaneous insulin infusion (CSII or insulin pump). Although insulins from animal sources are still marketed in Canada, most patients use human insulin and insulin analogues since these agents cause less antibody generation and related adverse reactions (e.g., hypersensitivity, insulin resistance). Human insulins are produced by recombinant DNA technology and have an amino acid sequence identical to endogenous human insulin. Insulin analogues are slightly modified human insulin molecules (Table 7). Rapid-acting insulin analogues (**insulin aspart**, **insulin glulisine**, **insulin lispro**) allow for more flexibility to control postprandial glucose because of their faster onset of action compared with short-acting insulins. The long-acting insulin analogues (**insulin detemir** and **insulin glargine**) appear to produce more predictable effects than intermediate-acting human insulin (NPH) and may be associated with fewer episodes of hypoglycemia, particularly nocturnal hypoglycemia.[17,18,19] However, these long-acting insulin analogues are more expensive than traditional insulins and have not accumulated as much long-term safety and efficacy data.

Insulin degludec is an ultra-long-acting basal insulin recently marketed in other countries but not yet available in Canada. Degludec has a long duration of action in the range of 42 hours.[20] Compared with insulin glargine, it was shown to be as effective at glucose control, with less nocturnal hypoglycemia.[21]

Insulin Regimens (Table 3)

Although an in-depth discussion about the different types of insulin regimens is beyond the scope of this chapter, the Diabetes Control and Complications Trial (DCCT) showed that intensive treatment regimens control blood glucose more effectively than conventional regimens and reduce the risk of long-term diabetic microvascular complications (retinopathy, nephropathy, neuropathy).[22] Follow-up data from the trial demonstrate a long-term benefit of intensive therapy on the risk of cardiovascular events.[23] Newly diagnosed patients and those with poor glycemic control on conventional regimens should be offered the option of intensive diabetes management consisting of basal-bolus insulin regimens. It is essential to assess each patient to determine if an intensive regimens is a suitable option. Less intensive regimens may be a better choice in the frail elderly, unmotivated patients, or those who lack awareness of severe hypoglycemia. In clinical practice, rapid-acting insulin in combination with long-acting insulin is preferred over regular insulin in order to minimize risk of hypoglycemia and improve HbA_{1c} and postprandial glucose levels.[24,25]

Table 3: **Insulin Regimens in Type 1 and Type 2 Diabetes Mellitus**

Rapid- or Short-acting (Bolus)	Intermediate- or Long-acting (Basal)	Comments
Intensive: Multiple-dose Insulin Regimens (Basal-Bolus)		
Regular human insulin, insulin aspart, glulisine or lispro before each meal	NPH (once or twice daily), insulin detemir or glargine at supper *or* bedtime	Flexible. Usually good BG control.
Intensive: Continuous Subcutaneous Insulin Infusion		
Single insulin type delivered by an electronic infusion set: insulin aspart or lispro recommended; basal and boluses delivered according to programmable settings	None	Most flexible but also most expensive. Rapid analogues preferred. May have advantages over multiple dose regimens. DKA may occur quickly after discontinuation, tubing block, or pump failure.
Conventional (not appropriate in type 1 diabetes mellitus)		
None	NPH at breakfast *and* supper	Moderate to poor control of a.m. and overnight BG levels. Minimal control of postprandial glucose.
Regular human insulin, insulin aspart, glulisine or lispro at breakfast and supper	NPH at breakfast *and* supper	Better postprandial control than regimen above.
Regular human insulin, insulin aspart, glulisine or lispro at breakfast and supper	NPH at breakfast *and* bedtime	More likely to be effective until morning.

Abbreviations: BG = blood glucose; DKA = diabetic ketoacidosis

Most lean patients with T1DM require approximately 0.5 units of insulin per kilogram of body mass. In the first few months following a T1DM diagnosis, patients may experience periods where the requirement for insulin is decreased or transiently eliminated. This phenomenon is known as the honeymoon phase. Initiate insulin therapy judiciously in order to minimize the risk of hypoglycemia and adjust the dose every 2–3 days according to blood glucose results. Regular home monitoring allows patients to adjust the dose of insulin in response to abnormal blood glucose levels, effects of diet and exercise and changing blood glucose patterns. Optimal blood glucose control is achieved by matching the timing of insulin injections with caloric intake: regular insulin is given 20–30 minutes before meals and rapid-acting insulin analogues are administered shortly before or within 20 minutes of starting a meal.

The use of insulin pumps and regimens involving multiple doses of rapid-acting insulin (versus regular human insulin) improves the stability of postprandial glucose levels and may also diminish the frequency and severity of hypoglycemia, especially early nocturnal hypoglycemia. In addition, insulin pumps can achieve a tighter and more reproducible degree of glycemic control, particularly in those with a high initial HbA_{1c}, but at a significantly increased expense for the patient.

Adverse Effects of Insulin Therapy

- *Hypoglycemia* is the most common adverse effect of insulin therapy and occurs more frequently in patients aiming for tight control of blood glucose.
  - the only way to completely avoid hypoglycemia is through unacceptably poor glycemic control. Hypoglycemia is most commonly the result of either a missed meal or an unusual amount of exercise. Frequent hypoglycemic events may lead to hypoglycemia unawareness. Teach patients to account for diet and physical activity when planning insulin treatment regimens.
  - *mild* to *moderate* hypoglycemia is manifested by autonomic symptoms: sweating, tremors, tachycardia, hunger, nausea and a general sensation of weakness. It can easily be treated with an oral source of sugar. Fifteen grams of glucose (e.g., 3/4 cup of juice or regular soft drink, 6 Lifesavers) will usually raise the blood glucose approximately 2 mmol/L within 20 minutes.
  - *severe* hypoglycemia requires assistance in its recognition and/or treatment. Neuroglycopenic symptoms such as confusion, altered behavior, difficulty speaking and disorientation can progress to seizures and coma and prevent the patient from appropriately treating the hypoglycemic episode. If the patient is conscious, an **oral glucose** preparation consisting of 20 grams of carbohydrate should be used, preferably as glucose tablets or equivalent. Glucose gel is not a preferred treatment option. It must be swallowed for significant effect and it's effect on blood glucose is very slow.
  - in *unconscious* patients with no iv access, 1 mg of **glucagon** im or sc temporarily increases blood glucose, allowing for the intake of oral carbohydrate. Glucagon is *not* effective in malnourished patients or in alcohol-induced hypoglycemia. If iv access is available, the treatment of choice is 20–50 mL of 50% dextrose iv over 1–3 minutes.
  - assess specifically for *hypoglycemia unawareness* and use strategies to recover awareness, such as relaxing glycemic targets for up to 3 months and increasing patient self-monitoring of BG.[26,27]
- *Localized fat hypertrophy* is most often the result of frequent use of the same injection site. This results in low or unpredictable absorption of insulin from that site.
- *Allergic reactions*, such as urticaria, angioedema, rashes and local erythema, are rare with human insulin. If they do occur, switching to a different insulin manufacturer may help.
- Immune-mediated *insulin resistance*, due to the production of anti-insulin antibodies, is also rare with human insulin. Patients who have developed immune-mediated resistance to animal insulins should be switched to human insulin. Reduce the dose substantially at the initiation of the switch. Concentrated regular insulin, 500 units/mL, may be useful in the treatment of patients requiring very large doses of insulin.

- Concern was raised about a possible association between *breast cancer* and use of insulin glargine.[28] However, a focused look at breast cancer incidence with the use of any type of insulin, including glargine, did not reveal increased rates of cancer.[29]

Type 2 Diabetes Mellitus

Initial management of patients with T2DM generally depends on the HbA_{1c}, as described below:[30]

In patients with an HbA_{1c} <8.5% it is acceptable to initiate nonpharmacologic therapy alone (e.g., diet and exercise); however, medications must be initiated without delay if glycemic targets are not met within 2–3 months [Evidence: SORT B*].[31] Upon starting medication therapy in these patients, monotherapy with **metformin** is usually recommended; however, initial treatment may include a combination of oral agents and/or insulin if the patient is exhibiting hyperglycemic symptoms or if it is unreasonable to expect excellent control with this approach. The patient populations in whom metformin use is contraindicated or cautioned will be discussed in further detail below.

In patients with an HbA_{1c} ≥8.5% at presentation, medication therapy should be initiated immediately (along with diet and exercise). In these patients, combination therapy with 2 medications from different classes is usually required. Bedtime insulin can be considered as an appropriate second agent at this point. Also a conventional/intensive insulin regimen may be appropriate in patients who exhibit extremely high levels at presentation, or for those who are very symptomatic.

In all patients who have been started on antihyperglycemic medications, aim to reach the desired HbA_{1c} target within 3–6 months through dosage titration or addition of other agents (Figure 2).[30] The Canadian Agency for Drugs and Technology in Health (CADTH) has recommended that if the HbA_{1c} target is not met with lifestyle changes, antihyperglycemic medications are to be used in the following order: metformin, metformin *plus* sulfonylurea, then metformin *plus* sulfonylurea *plus* NPH insulin. If patients are unable to use insulin as a third-line option, a DPP-4 inhibitor may be added.[32] These recommendations were made primarily on the basis of the cost-effectiveness of available agents and are reasonable for patients who do not have difficulties using insulin, have no additional risk factors for hypoglycemia and tolerate the suggested medications.

Antihyperglycemic agents (Table 8) can be divided into several broad categories: insulin secretagogues (**sulfonylureas** and **meglitinides**); drugs that decrease hepatic glucose production and/or increase tissue sensitivity to insulin (**thiazolidinediones** and **metformin**); drugs that mimic or enhance incretin hormones (**dipeptidyl peptidase-4 inhibitors** and **glucagon-like peptide-1 receptor agonists**); and drugs that delay or prevent the digestion of complex carbohydrates (the alpha-glucosidase inhibitor **acarbose**). Some data suggest the antiobesity drug, **orlistat**, may prevent the onset of T2DM in obese subjects; however, it has no role in the management of diabetes or blood glucose per se. The mean decrease in HbA_{1c} achieved with metformin, sulfonylureas, repaglinide, liraglutide and the thiazolidinediones has generally ranged from 1–1.5% in clinical trials.[33,34] In contrast, the mean decrease in HbA_{1c} achieved with acarbose, the dipeptidyl peptidase-4 inhibitors and nateglinide is generally lower (≤1%).[34] Typically, the higher the baseline HbA_{1c}, the greater the reduction in HbA_{1c} that can be achieved with treatment.[34]

Dipeptidyl peptidase-4 inhibitors (DPP-4 inhibitors) augment, and glucagon-like peptide-1 (GLP-1) agonists mimic, the actions of GLP-1, an endogenous "incretin" hormone. GLP-1 is secreted in response to food ingestion by endocrine cells found in the gastrointestinal tract.[35] Once released into the circulation, GLP-1 increases insulin secretion, suppresses glucagon secretion during the postprandial period, slows gastric emptying and increases satiety,[36] resulting in better control of postprandial glucose levels.

* SORT (Strength of Recommendation Taxonomy) is a rating system (A, B or C) that addresses the quality of available evidence. For more information consult **How to Use *Compendium of Therapeutic Choices*** on page xxv.

Figure 2: **Stepwise Approach to Type 2 Diabetes**[30]

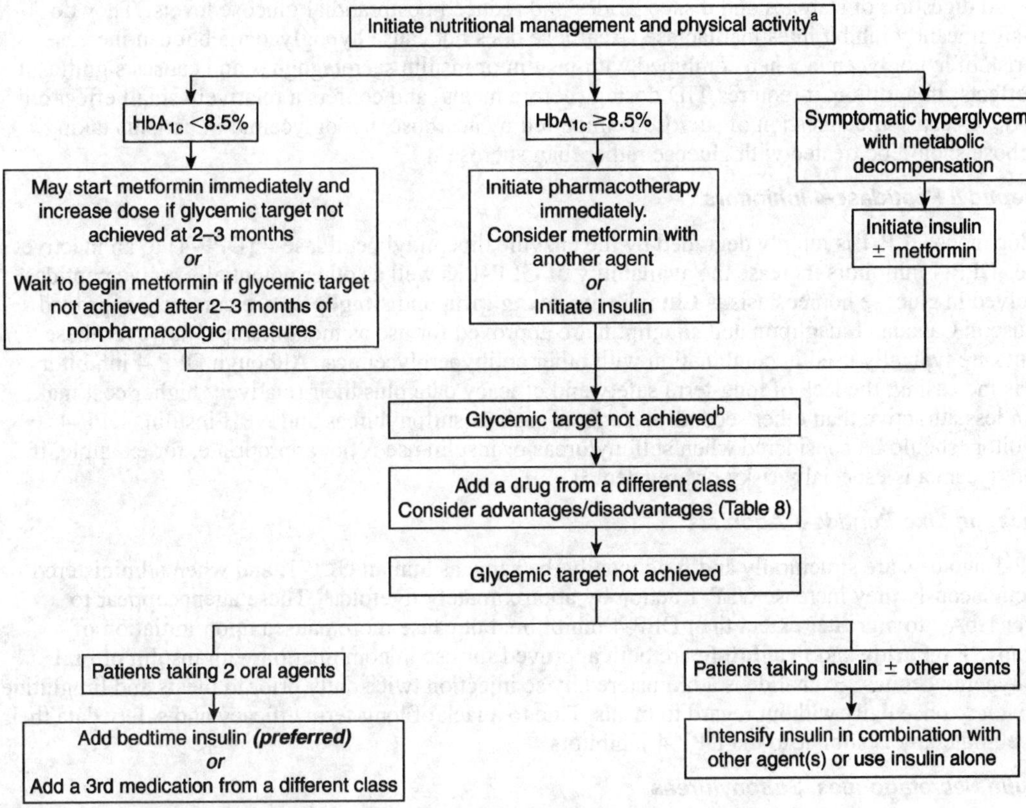

a Reinforce the need to continue lifestyle interventions at every opportunity.
b Drug regimens should be adjusted in a timely fashion so as to achieve the target HbA_{1c} level within 3–6 months.
Abbreviations: HbA_{1c} = glycosylated hemoglobin

Biguanides

Metformin is generally considered the first choice for uncomplicated patients with a new diagnosis of T2DM. It decreases hepatic glucose production and may lower glucose absorption and enhance insulin-mediated glucose uptake. It is not associated with weight gain and the risk of hypoglycemia is low when it is used as monotherapy. Compared with all other available antihyperglycemic medications, it has the strongest evidence suggesting it reduces macrovascular endpoints and mortality based on the UKPDS study in overweight patients.[37] However, it can potentiate the hypoglycemic effects of insulin and sulfonylureas. Although the use of metformin has traditionally been discouraged in patients with heart failure, renal or hepatic disease or hypoxemic states due to the perceived risk of lactic acidosis, a Cochrane review of 347 studies comparing over 70 000 subjects found no increase in the rate of lactic acidosis among patients receiving metformin compared with controls receiving other antihyperglycemic agents.[38] In addition, data primarily from observational studies suggest metformin use might even be beneficial in patients with heart failure, [39] and the risk of lactic acidosis may be primarily related to comorbidity rather than drug use.[40] However, further studies on the effects of metformin in these high-risk populations are needed before routine use could be recommended. Metformin is also routinely held preoperatively and when imaging contrast agents are being given to avoid the possibilities of acute renal failure that may increase the risk of lactic acidosis.

Alpha-glucosidase Inhibitors

Acarbose and **miglitol** (not available in Canada) inhibit intestinal alpha-glucosidases, resulting in delayed digestion of starches and disaccharides and reduced postprandial glucose levels. They do not significantly inhibit intestinal lactase. Acarbose does not cause hypoglycemia but can increase the risk of hypoglycemia when combined with insulin or insulin secretagogues and causes significant GI effects. In addition, it requires TID dosing (before meals) and confers a relatively small effect on HbA_{1c}. Because the digestion of sucrose is impaired by acarbose, hypoglycemia in patients taking acarbose should be treated with glucose rather than sucrose.

Dipeptidyl Peptidase-4 Inhibitors

Endogenous GLP-1 is rapidly degraded by the enzyme dipeptidyl peptidase-4 (DPP-4) to an inactive state. DPP-4 inhibitors increase the availability of GLP-1 as well as other potentially active peptides involved in glucose homeostasis.[36] **Linagliptin**, **saxagliptin** and **sitagliptin** are currently approved for use in Canada. Linagliptin and sitagliptin are approved for use as monotherapy, however these agents are typically used in combination with other antihyperglycemics. Although DPP-4 inhibitor use is increasing, the lack of long-term safety and efficacy data plus their relatively higher cost make them less attractive than other second-line agents such as sulfonylureas and NPH insulin. DPP-4 inhibitors should be considered when sulfonylureas or insulin use is not appropriate, for example, if hypoglycemia is especially risky or prevalent.[41]

Glucagon Like Peptide-1 Agonists

GLP-1 agonists are structurally and functionally the same as human GLP-1, and when administered subcutaneously they increase GLP-1 action by approximately fivefold.[42] These agents appear to lower HbA_{1c} to a greater extent than DPP-4 inhibitors but cause more nausea upon initiation of therapy. **Exenatide** and **liraglutide** are both approved for use in combination with insulin or oral antihyperglycemics. Exenatide is administered by sc injection twice daily prior to meals and liraglutide is given sc once daily without regard to meals. Due to a lack of long-term efficacy and safety data their place in therapy is similar to the DPP-4 inhibitors.

Insulin Secretagogues, Sulfonylureas

The sulfonylureas (SUs) **chlorpropamide**, **gliclazide**, **glimepiride**, **glyburide** and **tolbutamide** stimulate both basal and meal-stimulated insulin release. Significant differences exist between agents. First-generation SUs (chlorpropamide and tolbutamide) are typically not used due to their pharmacokinetic profile and higher affinity for drug interactions. Glyburide is an inexpensive second-generation SU. Compared with other agents in this group, glyburide is associated with a greater risk of hypoglycemia,[43] especially in elderly patients or those with renal impairment. Though more common with glyburide, hypoglycemia and weight gain can occur with any of these agents to varying degrees. Glyburide is included in the BEERS list of medications considered potentially inappropriate for use in the elderly.[44] Additionally, evidence relating to their influence on cardiovascular events is conflicting. SUs are considered as second-line agents for T2DM, either as add-on therapy, or as monotherapy when metformin is contraindicated.

Insulin Secretagogues, Meglitinides

Nateglinide and **repaglinide** promote insulin release, but their actions are much shorter compared with SUs. As a result, these medications need to be taken just prior to meals to reduce postprandial glucose elevations and should be omitted if the meal is missed. Although repaglinide is expected to lower HbA_{1c} to a similar extent as SUs, it is also considered to confer a lower risk of hypoglycemia in the context of missed meals (patients who skip meals could omit the associated repaglinide dose). Nateglinide is similar to repaglinide except it has a weaker effect on HbA_{1c}. FPG usually drops after about 1 month of regular use.[45] It has been theorized that the greater effect on postprandial glucose compared with SUs would translate into a more favourable effect on cardiovascular outcomes;

however, available data suggest their effects are very similar to SUs.[43] Further study is needed to determine if these agents influence clinical outcomes differently than SUs.

Sodium-Glucose Cotransporter 2 Inhibitors

The sodium-glucose cotransporter 2 (SGLT2) inhibitors belong to the most recent drug class being developed for the treatment of T2DM . These agents prevent glucose reabsorption in the kidneys, leading to increased excretion of urinary glucose.[46] Some weight loss is associated with SGLT-2 inhibitors, and their glucose-lowering ability is similar to that of other antihyperglycemic agents.[47,48] **Canagliflozin** has recently been approved for use in Canada. **Dapagliflozin** is available the United States and Europe and other SGLT2 inhibitors are still in development. These agents provide another option for lowering blood glucose, but their role in the management of T2DM is still to be determined.

Thiazolidinediones (TZDs)

Pioglitazone and **rosiglitazone** are agonists at PPARγ receptors located on the cell nucleus. These medications influence gene expression in the cell leading to enhanced insulin sensitivity and lower levels of blood glucose and circulating insulin. The precise mechanism underlying these effects remains unclear.[49] The TZDs also exhibit increased peripheral glucose uptake, enhanced fat cell sensitivity to insulin and decreased hepatic glucose output. The risk of hypoglycemia with TZDs is very low when taken as monotherapy; however, they may enhance the hypoglycemic effects of insulin and SUs. Individual TZDs may differ in their effects on serum lipids.[50] Both agents are associated with weight gain due to increased subcutaneous fat deposition, fluid retention and edema, which is likely the cause of the increased incidence of heart failure in patients receiving TZDs.[49,51] Other reported adverse effects include worsening macular edema[52] and an increased risk of fractures, particularly of the hip and wrist.[53,54]

The cardiovascular safety of thiazolidinediones is in question. Some analyses have reported an increase in the risk of ischemic events such as MI in patients receiving rosiglitazone[55,56] while other research suggests that rosiglitazone confers a protective effect from ischemic events.[57] Studies of pioglitazone have more consistently lacked any signal of increased risk of ischemic events.[57] To ensure that the risks and benefits of this medication have been clearly communicated, Health Canada requires that physicians counsel patients and obtain their written consent for all new and renewed rosiglitazone prescriptions. The FDA has recently removed its prescribing restrictions for rosiglitazone-containing products (Avandia, Avandamet, Avandaryl and generics), after a re-evaluation of the RECORD trial did not show an increased risk of MI.[58]

Concerns have emerged about the increased risk of bladder cancer with pioglitazone.[59] This TZD is now contraindicated in patients with active or previous bladder cancer. Various countries have suspended the sale of both TZDs due to cardiovascular or bladder cancer concerns.

Insulin Regimens for Type 2 Diabetes Mellitus

Due to the progressive nature of T2DM, noninsulin antihyperglycemic agents gradually lose their effectiveness over time. Insulin remains an important option for patients because of its powerful effects on lowering HbA_{1c}. Although it is appropriate to consider insulin initiation at any point in the management of T2DM, it is commonly reserved for the following situations:

- maximum tolerated dose of noninsulin antihyperglycemic agents yet HbA_{1c} still not at target
- end-organ damage (e.g., kidney failure) when some antihyperglycemics are inappropriate
- at initial diagnosis when $HbA_{1c} \geq 8.5\%$
- with metabolic decompensation
- in pregnancy and in women planning pregnancy

The use of insulin is often delayed because of the perceived complexity of self-injections. Also, insulin is associated with weight gain and carries a risk of hypoglycemia; thus, self-monitoring is critical to its safe and effective use. Insulin is eventually required, either alone, or in combination with other agents.[41] Many patients with T2DM require high doses of insulin (≥1 unit/kg) to overcome their significant insulin resistance. There are several commonly used insulin regimens:

- Generally, insulin is added to existing antihyperglycemic therapy when targets are not being met. Daily bedtime injection of basal insulin is prescribed at a dose of 0.1–0.2 units/kg of NPH insulin or long-acting analogue.[41,60] Alternatively, an empiric dose of 5–10 units of intermediate (NPH) or long-acting insulin (glargine or detemir) may be initially chosen depending on whether the patient is lean or obese. Subsequently, the dose is adjusted (~2 units every 3 days) to achieve a fasting glucose <7 mmol/L. Other agents may need to be reduced once glycemic control is achieved; metformin is often continued because it has proven to lower insulin requirements, ameliorate weight gain and reduce the risk of hypoglycemia.[61]
- If glycemic targets are not being met with bedtime insulin in combination with a daytime antihyperglycemic regimen, an intensified insulin regimen can be initiated with the introduction of mealtime insulin(s) depending upon blood glucose patterns. Generally, oral antihyperglycemic medications are discontinued when mealtime insulin injections are added with the exception of metformin, which can help minimize weight gain and reduce the amount of insulin required.
- If glycemic values are extremely high upon initial presentation, then intensive insulin therapy may be started immediately, rather than introducing oral agents. To initiate insulin, start with 40% of the total daily dose (0.5 units/kg total insulin units divided over the 24-hour day) administered as a basal insulin (NPH or long-acting analogue) and 20% of the daily dose administered before meals 3 times daily (regular or rapid-acting analogues). The dose is then adjusted to achieve glycemic targets; fasting and premeal glucose <7 mmol and 2 hour postprandial glucose <10 mmol.
- Insulin may be administered in twice-daily injections of a premixed insulin with two-thirds of the daily dose (0.5 units/kg) administered in the morning before breakfast and the remaining one-third of the daily dose administered before the evening meal (usually 30/70 [30% regular, 70% basal mix] in the a.m. and p.m.). These regimens provide convenience at the expense of flexibility and the ability to correct for abnormal results. However, this approach is a reasonable alternative for patients with diabetes who: have little variation in exercise or food intake from day to day, require home care for insulin injections, or do not have the cognitive ability to adjust insulin doses. In order to achieve glycemic targets with this regimen, both the dose and type of mixture may need to be modified.

Targets for Control

The 2013 Canadian Diabetes Association Clinical Practice Guidelines emphasize that glycemic targets should be individualized based on patient-specific factors. (Table 4). This is similar to recommendations from the American Diabetes Association.[62] The target of HbA_{1c} ≤7% for most patients with T1DM and T2DM is based on grade "A" evidence supporting the relationship between tight glucose control and a reduction in microvascular and neuropathic complications.[63] In contrast, it remains unclear if macrovascular (ischemic) events are influenced by tight glucose control.[64,65,66] A more aggressive HbA_{1c} of ≤6.5% may be targeted in patients with T2DM if the benefits are thought to outweigh the risk of hypoglycemia. Conversely, a higher HbA_{1c} of up to 8.5% may be more appropriate if the risk of hypoglycemia outweighs the benefits of tight control, e.g., in frail elderly patients, those with limited life expectancy or patients with a history of recurrent severe hypoglycemia.[63]

Vascular protection is a critical component of the management strategy for patients with diabetes. In addition to glycemic control, it is essential to simultaneously achieve blood pressure (see Chapter 39) and serum lipid targets (see Chapter 37), promote weight loss to a normal BMI, encourage smoking cessation (see Chapter 13) and prescribe antiplatelet therapy as indicated.[68]

Table 4: **Recommended Targets for Blood Glucose Control**[63,67]

Age (years)	Diabetes Type	HbA_{1c} (%)	FPG/Preprandial Glucose (mmol/L)	2-hour PPG (mmol/L)
>18	T1,T2	≤7[a,b]	4–7	5–10 5–8 if goal HbA_{1c} not reached
0–18	T2	≤7	4–7	No recommendation
13–18	T1	≤7	4–7	5–10 (appropriate for most)
6–12	T1	≤7.5	4–10	No recommendation
<6	T1	≤8	6–10	No recommendation

[a] Consider HbA_{1c} ≤6.5% in some T2DM patients to reduce risk of nephropathy and retinopathy.
[b] Consider HbA_{1c} 7.1–8.5% in T1DM and T2DM for whom the benefit of lower targets do not outweigh the risk of hypoglycemia.
Abbreviations: HbA_{1c} = glycosylated hemoglobin; FPG = fasting plasma glucose; PPG = postprandial plasma glucose; T1 = Type 1 diabetes mellitus; T2 = Type 2 diabetes mellitus

- *Antiplatelet therapy:* Low-dose **ASA** (75–162 mg/day) is recommended in patients with diabetes for secondary prevention in those with established cardiovascular disease.[68] Evidence supporting its use in primary prevention is much less substantial in people with diabetes. Due to the uncertainty of benefit and the risks associated with ASA, routine use is not recommended for primary prevention of cardiovascular events in patients with diabetes.[69] If antiplatelet therapy is deemed necessary and patients are unable to tolerate ASA, **clopidogrel** 75 mg daily may be considered.[69]
- *Cholesterol:* Consider statin treatment for any patient ≥40 years of age with type 1 or type 2 diabetes mellitus, for younger patients with diabetes of more than 15 years' duration and age >30 years, or for patients with documented silent or clinically apparent CVD or microvascular complications of diabetes.[13] The treatment goal is LDL ≤2 mmol/L or a 50% reduction from baseline.[13] Because **fibrates** have limited evidence for further reducing the risk of ischemic events, they should be reserved for specific situations where triglycerides are especially problematic (see Chapter 37). **Niacin** can increase blood glucose levels; thus antihyperglycemic therapy may require adjustment if this agent is used to manage dyslipidemia. Although recent evidence suggests that statin therapy may slightly increase the incidence of new-onset diabetes,[70,71] the beneficial effects of statins outweigh this risk. Statins remain as preferred agents to reduce LDL-C when indicated.[14,72]
- *Blood pressure:* Control of blood pressure (<130/80 mm Hg) is an additional goal of therapy. Diabetes, particularly type 2, is frequently associated with hypertension, and multiple antihypertensive agents are often required to meet this target. Monitor blood pressure regularly and control hypertension if it occurs (see Chapter 39).
- It has been shown that a coordinated, multifactorial intervention involving behaviour modification and pharmacologic therapy targeting hyperglycemia, hypertension, dyslipidemia, body weight, microalbuminuria and platelet activation can significantly reduce the risk of major cardiovascular and microvascular outcomes.[73] These findings illustrate the importance of targeting all associated risk factors in addition to achieving glycemic control.

Choices during Pregnancy and Breastfeeding

Carbohydrate intolerance during pregnancy can occur in patients with diabetes prior to pregnancy and in those who develop diabetes during pregnancy.

Diabetes and Pregnancy

Both type 1 and type 2 diabetes mellitus can occur in women of childbearing age, while *gestational diabetes mellitus* (GDM) is a condition that develops during pregnancy, primarily due to insulin resistance that results from the high levels of gestational hormones (see Figure 3).[74] Regardless of the specific diagnosis type, the existence of diabetes in pregnancy significantly increases the risk of negative outcomes in both the mother and fetus/infant.[75] Pre-existing diabetes (type 1 or 2) increases the risk of miscarriage, perinatal mortality, fetal macrosomia, and congenital malformations, the latter being due to hyperglycemia in the first weeks of gestation.[76] Similarly, GDM increases the risk of fetal hyperinsulinemia, heavier birth weight, higher rates of cesarian deliveries and neonatal hypoglycemia.[74] Children born to mothers with diabetes and mothers with a history of GDM also appear to have an increased risk of developing diabetes in the future.[77]

When diabetes is pre-existing, pre-pregnancy counselling is essential and a target HbA_{1c} of <7 % (or lower if tolerated) should be achieved even before conception. Although the benefits of treating women with pre-existing diabetes have been clearly demonstrated,[74] the benefits of treating GDM are less clear.[78,79] Diabetes treatments confer a risk of hypoglycemia and some may exhibit teratogenic effects, thus careful monitoring and therapeutic selection is required. Fortunately, hypoglycemia may not pose substantial risks to the developing fetus,[76] but instances of diabetic ketoacidosis are very dangerous and can occur in cases such as unrecognized failure of an insulin pump.

Management during Pregnancy

Counsel women of childbearing age with diabetes about the need to plan and prepare for any pregnancy in order to minimize the risks to the fetus and the mother. In the months preceding conception, women should undertake the following risk reduction activities:[74]

Figure 3: **Diagnosis of Gestational Diabetes**[a,74]

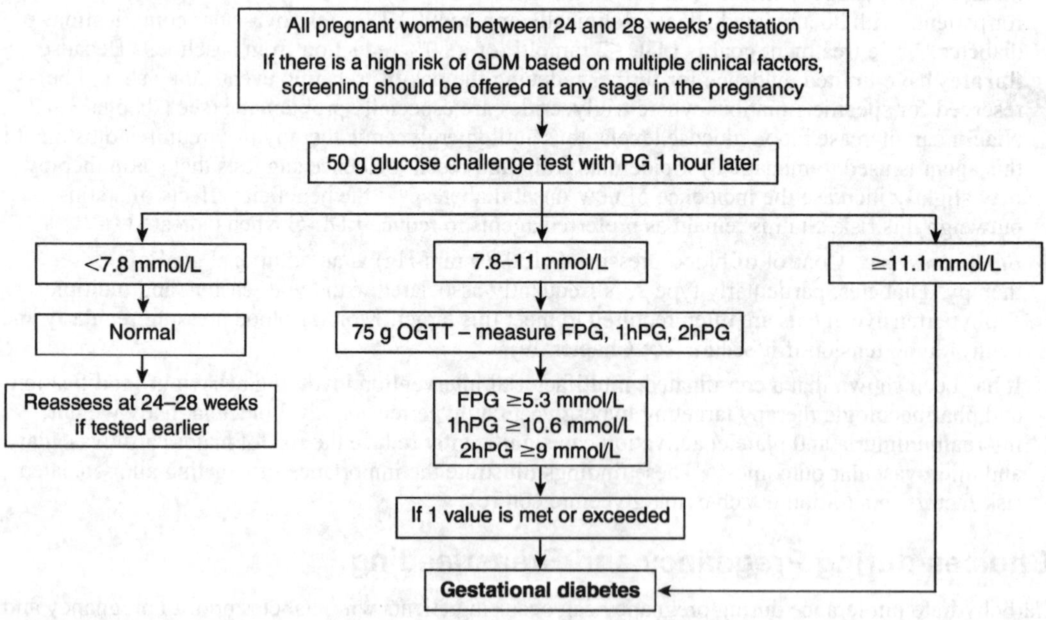

[a] In view of the controversies about diagnostic tests, other accepted methods may be used.
Abbreviations: 1hPG = 1-hour plasma glucose; 2hPG = 2-hour plasma glucose; FPG = fasting plasma glucose; GDM = gestational diabetes mellitus; OGTT = oral glucose tolerance test
Reproduced with permission of the Canadian Diabetes Association.

- Begin **folic acid** supplementation at least 3 months prior to conception. The initial dose should be 5 mg daily and is continued into the pregnancy. After 3 months' gestation, the dose is reduced to 0.4–1 mg daily and continued throughout the pregnancy and for a minimum of 6 months postpartum or until breastfeeding is completed.
- Undergo an *eye exam* because pregnancy can accelerate retinopathy resulting from poor glycemic control. A baseline exam should occur prior to conception and subsequent exams should be scheduled periodically during the pregnancy and for 1 year postpartum.
- Switch to an **insulin regimen** from oral hypoglycemic agents (if not taking already) and aim to achieve an HbA_{1c} level of <7% (<6% if safely achievable).
- Undergo *screening for cardiovascular disease* (or risk factors) and *chronic kidney disease* (CKD). Clinicians should be especially vigilant about CKD and hypertension prior to and throughout pregnancy, given the risk of an additive effect with pregnancy.
- Discontinue any *teratogenic medications* such as ACE inhibitors, angiotensin receptor blockers or statins. The fast-acting insulin analogues lispro and aspart are safe in pregnancy and may provide a decreased risk of hypoglycemia compared with regular insulin.[80,81,82] In women with pre-existing diabetes, NPH insulin or long-acting insulin analogues (detemir and glargine) can be used throughout pregnancy.[83,84]

In women with diabetes who successfully become pregnant, strict glycemic control is recommended, along with frequent self-monitoring of blood glucose. Both pre- and postprandial testing is suggested in order to facilitate the achievement of both targets outlined in Table 5. In addition, ketone testing (urine or blood) may be considered to ensure that the diet is adequate to prevent starvation ketosis.[74] Although it is acceptable to initiate nonpharmacologic therapy (strict diet and exercise) in women who are newly diagnosed with GDM, it is recommended to start multiple daily injections of rapid-acting or regular **insulin** if fasting and postprandial targets have not been met within 2 weeks of adjusting these lifestyle measures.[85,86] In women (excluding type 1 diabetics) who cannot take insulin, it may be reasonable to consider **glyburide** or **metformin**, recognizing that use of either agent is off-label.[79,87]

Table 5: **Recommended Glycemic Targets during Pregnancy**[74]

FPG/Preprandial Glucose (mmol/L)	1-hour Postprandial Glucose (mmol/L)	2-hour Postprandial Glucose (mmol/L)
<5.3	<7.8	<6.7

Abbreviations: FPG = fasting plasma glucose

Diabetes and Breastfeeding

Mothers with diabetes are encouraged to breastfeed to reduce the risk of childhood obesity.[74] Although **insulin** is excreted into breast milk, it poses little risk to the infant because the hormone is degraded in the gastrointestinal tract before reaching the systemic circulation.[87] As a result, breastfeeding mothers receiving insulin do not need to alter their regimen unless it is in response to their individual glycemic levels. Frequent monitoring of blood glucose is extremely important after delivery because insulin requirements may change quickly, and the increased caloric output during breastfeeding theoretically puts the mother at increased risk of hypoglycemia.

Management during Breastfeeding

After delivery, most woman will remain in-hospital for at least 24 hours. During this time, glycemic monitoring should be performed frequently to assess for changes in blood glucose levels. In many cases of GDM, hyperglycemia will resolve completely during this time and antihyperglycemic medications may be discontinued altogether. In addition, all postpartum women with GDM should have their glycemic status assessed by their primary care provider sometime in the months following delivery. All patients diagnosed with GDM should have a 75 g OGTT between 6 weeks and 6 months following delivery to detect persistent hyperglycemia.

In women who require ongoing antihyperglycemic medication, insulin remains the first choice for reasons stated above. However, both **glyburide** and **metformin** have also been used in breastfeeding women with T2DM. Limited data suggest glyburide does not pass into breast milk and metformin appears to have little penetration.[87] Although these agents can be considered for use in breastfeeding mothers, long-term studies have not been done to rule out any unanticipated adverse effects.

A discussion of general principles on the use of medications in these special populations can be found in Appendix II and Appendix III. Other specialized reference sources are also provided in these appendices.

Therapeutic Tips

- Assess all patients every 3–6 months. Study their home monitoring records (if available) and note the occurrence, frequency and trends of hypoglycemia. Hypoglycemia should be addressed before hyperglycemia to ensure patient safety in the short term.
- Review home blood glucose records, looking for predictable glucose trends that can be improved on. Whether glucose readings are printed out, tabulated in a logbook or in the glucometer memory, they must be brought to follow-up appointments, reviewed and discussed.
- Inadequate control is frequently related to poor adherence to diet and/or medications. Chronic infections can also negatively impact glucose control.
- The use of snacks is important in patients on conventional insulin therapy and may be important in those treated with a SU because these regimens are minimally flexible to daily variations in carbohydrate intake. Those treated with acarbose, metformin, thiazolidinedione, meglitinide or a multidose rapid-acting insulin regimen may not require snacks.
- Monitor blood sugar, blood pressure, serum lipids, body weight and for the presence of complications. Foot examination is an integral part of such monitoring.
- Encourage all patients to wear a MedicAlert ID bracelet or the equivalent.

Preventing Type 2 Diabetes Mellitus

The prevalence of T2DM has been rising for decades and is expected to afflict over 2.4 million Canadians by the year 2016.[88] As a result, many studies have focused on preventative strategies aimed at individuals who exhibit risk factors for the development of this disease. Although family history, sedentary lifestyle, obesity and poor diets are risk factors for T2DM, individuals with slightly elevated blood glucose levels are likely at the greatest short-term risk of reaching the diagnostic threshold. Individuals who exhibit elevated blood glucose concentrations (yet below the threshold for diabetes) can be described as having *impaired fasting glucose* (FPG 6.1–6.9 mmol/L), *impaired glucose tolerance* (plasma glucose of 7.8–11 mmol/L 2 hours after a 75 g oral glucose load), or both. Generally, individuals exhibiting slight elevations in blood glucose concentrations have been insulin-resistant for years, but glucose levels were likely maintained by increased insulin secretion.[89] Frequently, insulin resistance is accompanied by other metabolic disruptions that are probably linked by one or more common biologic pathways. Clustering of metabolic risk factors such as central obesity, hypertension, dyslipidemia, insulin resistance and glucose abnormalities is termed the *metabolic syndrome*. It confers a significant short-term risk of overt diabetes and a long-term risk of cardiovascular disease.[90]

Several large studies have examined nonpharmacologic (diet, exercise and weight loss) and pharmacologic strategies aimed at preventing the onset of T2DM in high-risk individuals.

The Finnish Diabetes Prevention Study (DPS)[91] and the Diabetes Prevention Program (DPP)[92] showed that *calorie restriction* along with a supervised *exercise program* of moderate intensity (about 150 minutes/week) significantly reduced the relative risk of progression from prediabetes to diabetes by 58% at 4 years. In the DPS, diabetes was diagnosed in 11% of those randomized to lifestyle intervention versus 23% in the control group. In the DPP study, diabetes developed in 4.8%, 7.8% and 11% of those randomized to lifestyle intervention, metformin and placebo, respectively. The weight loss associated with lifestyle interventions was about 5–6% of initial body weight in these studies. Interestingly, the benefits of the lifestyle changes persisted long after these trials were completed.[93,94] These findings prove the success of lifestyle interventions and the significance for all people at high-risk of developing diabetes.

Other studies have evaluated the impact of pharmacologic interventions on the incidence of T2DM. It has been shown that **metformin**,[92,94] **acarbose**,[95] **TZDs**,[96,97,98,99] and **orlistat**[100] can also reduce the incidence of T2DM in at-risk patients. In one study, rosiglitazone significantly reduced the risk of progression to diabetes from 26% to 11.6% over 3 years compared with placebo; a similar benefit to that reported in the lifestyle intervention trials above. The benefit was offset to some extent by a significantly higher incidence of heart failure relative to placebo (0.5% vs. 0.1%).[96] In contrast, **ramipril** did not prevent the progression from prediabetes to diabetes in this same study.[101] **Nateglinide** was also unsuccessful in preventing diabetes among individuals at risk in a prospective randomized trial.[102]

There are no known safe and effective measures to prevent T1DM although recent advances in immunomodulatory therapies have reached human trials. Time and controlled trials are still needed to review and assess the efficacy and safety of these interventions.[103]

Diabetic Ketoacidosis

Diabetic ketoacidosis is a potentially fatal complication of severe insulin deficiency seen in T1DM that presents as metabolic decompensation. It is characterized by variable hyperglycemia, volume depletion, acidosis, depressed levels of consciousness and detectable ketones in the urine or blood.[104] Upon presentation, patients are depleted in sodium, potassium, chloride and water. Despite body wide potassium depletion, serum potassium is frequently elevated at the time of presentation due to lack of insulin and an inability of potassium to efficiently enter cells. Pre-renal failure may be present secondary to severe dehydration. Hyperglycemia, as well as high triglycerides and free fatty acids, may result in pseudohyponatremia, or falsely low sodium measurements.

Diabetic ketoacidosis is found almost exclusively in T1DM and may be seen at first presentation in newly diagnosed patients, or when insulin use is non-compliant. It is also often associated with the onset of a severe or stressful illness (e.g., severe infection), surgery, trauma or MI in patients who were previously stable. Patients with diabetic ketoacidosis are generally hospitalized. A detailed patient care flow sheet is published in the 2013 Canadian Diabetes Association clinical practice guidelines and is available on-line[105] (guidelines.diabetes.ca/). Management of diabetic ketoacidosis is outlined in Table 6.

Table 6: Management of Diabetic Ketoacidosis (DKA)

Fluids: Patients are always significantly volume depleted. Give iv NS 500 mL for 4 h, then 250 mL for 4 h (faster if in shock), then individualize. Good urinary output is reassuring that volume is being replaced.

Potassium: Potassium chloride is the preparation of choice. Do not give unless urine is being produced; may need to wait for iv fluids to improve volume status. If serum K^+ is <3.5 mmol/L, add 40 mmol/L of fluid; if 3.5–5.5 mmol/L, add 20 mmol/L; if >5.5 mmol/L, do not add K^+, but monitor hourly. Rehydration and insulin will drive K^+ levels down.

Insulin: Do not give insulin if K^+ is <3.3, as insulin will drive K^+ into cells and drop levels further. Once K^+ >3.3, then insulin can be infused at 0.1 units/kg/h using a second iv line. One protocol is as follows: mix 25 units R insulin in 250 mL NS and adjust rate to drop glucose to <14 mmol/L. Continue iv insulin until the anion gap resolves and patient eating without nausea. NEVER stop or hold insulin in DKA. Rather, if the glucose drops below 14 mmol/L, continue the insulin infusion but also switch the saline iv to D5½NS and adjust the iv rate to maintain glucose between 12–14 mmol/L. When anion gap closed and patient eating, overlap iv insulin with subcutaneous insulin by 2 hours before stopping iv. DKA can rapidly reoccur if waiting for subcutaneous insulin to peak.

Bicarbonate: Not first-line therapy and infrequently used. Consider giving 1 ampoule of sodium bicarbonate in 200 mL D5W over 1 h if acidosis is severe and ICU is being considered (e.g., pH <7, lowered LOC).

Laboratory tests: Latest recommendations include bed-side testing for beta-hydroxybutyrate, a ketone that is not detected with standard ketone testing.[106,107] Initial CBC, glucose, electrolytes, urea, creatinine and ABG. Request blood or urine cultures to look for infection as indicated. Radiology looking for infection/trigger as indicated. Repeat electrolyte and glucose hourly, ABG only if severe acidosis persists. Capillary glucose (with bedside glucometer) hourly for trends, but require repeated blood draws for confirmation.

Supportive care: Keep the patient warm and rested. Insert an NG tube if vomiting, and a urinary catheter if anuric (urinary retention may be significant).

Pitfalls:

- Children with DKA are at higher risk of cerebral edema due to treatment of DKA, with associated sodium, pH and glucose shifts. It is essential that a specialized team and monitored setting be used in pediatric cases. A diagnosis of DKA does not initially require detection of ketones. Routine detection of ketones may require both urine and blood testing over time.
- For urinary ketones, Ketostix strips detect aceto-acetate but not hydroxybutyrate; beware of false negatives. Acetone smell may be absent, undetected or unrecognized by some. Where available, use rapid beta-hydroxybutyrate testing.
- Temperature may be low initially—absence of fever does not rule out infection.
- Leukocytosis is usually present and does not necessarily mean infection.
- Low serum sodium may be due to pseudohyponatremia from high glucose or TG.
- High serum potassium is caused by acidosis and may be seen in spite of severe total body potassium depletion.
- Dehydration may mask a respiratory infection; reassess after rehydration and stabilization.
- Severe abdominal pain or signs of an acute abdomen need to be reassessed after stabilization—they often disappear.
- A premature switch to sc insulin and/or discharge results in high recurrence and readmission rates.

Abbreviations: D5½NS = dextrose 5% with ½ normal saline; DKA = diabetic ketoacidosis; K^+ = potassium; LOC = level of consciousness; NS = normal saline; R = regular; TG = triglycerides

Table 7: **Insulin and Analogues**[a]

Class	Drug	Onset	Peak	Duration	Comments	Cost[b]
Very Rapid-acting Insulin Analogues	*insulin aspart* NovoRapid	10–15 min	60–90 min	4–5 h	Appearance: clear.	$$$
	insulin glulisine Apidra	10–15 min	60–90 min	4–5 h	Appearance: clear.	$$$
	insulin lispro Humalog	10–15 min	60–90 min	4–5 h	Appearance: clear.	$$$
Rapid-acting Insulin	*insulin, regular* Humulin R, Novolin ge Toronto	30–60 min	2–4 h	5–8 h	Appearance: clear.	$$
	pork insulin Hypurin Regular	30 min	2–4 h	5–7 h	Appearance: clear. Used only if human insulin or analogues not tolerated.	$$$$/10 ml vial
Intermediate-acting Insulin	*insulin, NPH* Humulin N, Novolin ge NPH	1–2 h	5–8 h	14–18 h	Appearance: cloudy.	$$
	pork insulin, NPH Hypurin NPH	1–3 h	6–12 h	24–28 h	Appearance: cloudy. Used only if human insulin or analogues not tolerated.	$$$$/10 ml vial
Long-acting Insulin Analogues	*insulin detemir* Levemir	1.5 h	Flat, no discernible peak	6–24 h	Appearance: clear. Do not mix with other insulins. Contains a C14 fatty acid chain and is highly bound (98%) to serum albumin. At low doses, duration of action is shorter and may require BID administration to maintain fasting glucose targets.	$$$$$
	insulin glargine Lantus	1.5 h	Flat, no discernible peak	24 h	Appearance: clear. Do not mix with other insulins. An acidic solution (pH 4). After injection the solution is neutralized, and microprecipitates form, from which the drug is slowly released. Do not inject im or iv.	$$$$

(cont'd)

Table 7: **Insulin and Analogues**[a] *(cont'd)*

Class	Drug	Onset	Peak	Duration	Comments	Cost[b]
Mixed (regular/NPH) Human Insulin	*insulin, regular/insulin, NPH* Humulin 30/70, Novolin ge 30/70, 40/60, 50/50	Combination of individual components			Appearance: cloudy.	$$
Mixed Insulin Analogues	*insulin lispro/lispro protamine* Humalog Mix25, Humalog Mix50	10–15 min	Not available	Not available	Appearance: cloudy.	$$$
	insulin aspart/aspart protamine NovoMix 30	10–15 min	60–90 min	15–18 h	Appearance: cloudy.	$$$

[a] Insulin products are shown in order of onset of action, with the very rapid-acting insulin analogues at the top. Mixed insulin products are grouped at the end of the table.
[b] Cost of 5 × 3 mL cartridges unless otherwise specified; drug cost only.
Legend: $ < $25 $$ $25–50 $$$ $50–75 $$$$ $75–100 $$$$$ $100–125

Table 8: Antihyperglycemic Agents

Class	Drug[a]	Dose	Adverse Effects	Drug Interactions	Comments	Cost[b]
Alpha-glucosidase Inhibitors	*acarbose* Glucobay	50–100 mg TID po with each meal; start low and go slow	Flatulence, diarrhea, abdominal pain, cramps, nausea.	Potentiates other antihyperglycemic agents; may reduce metformin bioavailability.	No weight gain; not absorbed; contraindicated in irritable bowel syndrome or inflammatory bowel disease. Use glucose to treat hypoglycemia.	$
Biguanides	*metformin* Glucophage, Glumetza, generics	500–2500 mg/day po divided BID or TID; start low and go slow to minimize GI side effects; little additional benefit above 1500 mg/day	Nausea, diarrhea, abdominal discomfort, anorexia, metallic taste, lactic acidosis if hepatic or renal disease.	Potentiates other oral antihyperglycemic agents; alcohol potentiates hypoglycemic effect.	No weight gain. Contraindicated in hepatic impairment, renal impairment, previous lactic acidosis.	$
Dipeptidyl Peptidase-4 Inhibitors (DPP4Is)	*linagliptin* Trajenta	5 mg once daily po	Nasopharyngitis, hypersensitivity reactions. Rare: pancreatitis.	Clearance of linagliptin is enhanced by strong CYP3A4 inducers, e.g., rifampin.	May be taken with or without food.	$$$
	saxagliptin Onglyza	5 mg once daily po	See linagliptin.	Clearance of saxagliptin is reduced by strong CYP3A4/5 inhibitors, e.g., imidazole antifungals, macrolides. Clearance of saxagliptin is enhanced by strong CYP3A4/5 inducers, e.g., rifampin.	See linagliptin.	$$$
	sitagliptin Januvia	100 mg once daily po	See linagliptin.	Does not inhibit cytochrome P450 isozymes. Low potential for drug interactions.	See linagliptin.	$$$

(cont'd)

Table 8: **Antihyperglycemic Agents** *(cont'd)*

Class	Drug[a]	Dose	Adverse Effects	Drug Interactions	Comments	Cost[b]
Glucagon-Like-Peptide 1 (GLP-1) Agonists	*exenatide* ➔ Byetta	Initial: 5 µg BID sc Increase to 10 µg BID sc after 1 month if required	Nausea, vomiting, diarrhea. Rare: acute pancreatitis.	May reduce rate of absorption of some oral medications.	Causes weight loss. Caution in patients with heart rhythm disturbances and severe renal impairment. Contraindicated in pregnancy and those with personal or family history of medullary thyroid carcinoma or multiple endocrine neoplasia syndrome type 2.	$$$$$
	liraglutide Victoza	Initial: 0.6 mg once daily sc Increase to 1.2–1.8 mg once daily sc	See exenatide.	No significant interactions.	See exenatide.	$$$$$
Insulin Secretagogues, Sulfonylureas	*chlorpropamide* ➔ generics	100–500 mg daily po in 1 dose	Sulfonylureas: prolonged hypoglycemia; weight gain. Chlorpropamide: alcohol-associated flushing; hyponatremia.	Hypoglycemic effect potentiated by salicylates, sulfonamides and monoamine oxidase inhibitors; beta-blockers may mask hypoglycemic symptoms.	Contraindicated in type 1 diabetes, pregnancy.	$
	gliclazide Diamicron, generics	40–320 mg/day po; administer in 2 divided doses if daily dose ≥160 mg	Prolonged hypoglycemia; weight gain.	See chlorpropamide.	See chlorpropamide.	$
	gliclazide, long-acting Diamicron MR, generics	30–120 mg once daily po	Prolonged hypoglycemia; weight gain.	See chlorpropamide.	See chlorpropamide.	$
	glimepiride ➔ Amaryl, generics	1–4 mg once daily po	Prolonged hypoglycemia; weight gain.	See chlorpropamide.	See chlorpropamide.	$
	glyburide ➔ Diabeta, generics	2.5–20 mg/day po; administer in 2 divided doses if daily dose >10 mg	Weight gain; prolonged hypoglycemia. Risk of hypoglycemia may be greater compared with gliclazide and glimepiride, especially in elderly or patients with renal impairment.	See chlorpropamide.	Contraindicated in type 1 diabetes.	$

Class	Drug[a]	Dose	Adverse Effects	Drug Interactions	Comments	Cost[b]
	tolbutamide generics	500 mg BID–TID po Maximum: 3 g/day	Prolonged hypoglycemia; weight gain. GI upset, skin rash, hemolytic anemia, jaundice.	See chlorpropamide. Alcohol and rifampin may accelerate clearance.	See chlorpropamide.	$
Insulin Secretagogues, Meglitinides	*nateglinide* Starlix	60–180 mg po 0–30 min before meals	Hypoglycemia, especially if meal not taken.	Clearance of meglitinides is reduced by strong CYP3A4 inhibitors, e.g., imidazole antifungals, macrolides, protease inhibitors. Clearance of meglitinides is enhanced by strong CYP3A4 inducers, e.g., rifampin, carbamazepine.	Contraindicated in type 1 diabetes, pregnancy.	$$$
	repaglinide GlucoNorm, Apo-Repaglinide, other generics	0.5–4 mg po 0–30 min before meals	Hypoglycemia, especially if meal not taken; weight gain.	See nateglinide. Strong inhibitors of CYP2C8 have the potential to reduce metabolism of repaglinide, e.g., atazanavir, ritonavir, gemfibrozil. Enhanced and prolonged hypoglycemia occurs when taken with gemfibrozil (avoid combined use). Cyclosporine increases plasma concentrations of repaglinide.	Contraindicated in type 1 diabetes, pregnancy.	$
Sodium-Glucose Cotransporter 2 Inhibitors	*canagliflozin* Invokana	100–300 mg once daily po	Increased risk of genitourinary infections; reduced intravascular volume resulting in hypotension; hyperkalemia.	Strong enzyme inducers e.g., rifampin, phenytoin, carbamazepine will reduce plasma levels. Loop diuretics increase risk of hypotension.	Less effective in moderate and ineffective in severe renal impairment.	$$$
Thiazolidinediones (TZDs)	*pioglitazone* Actos, generics	15–45 mg once daily po	Weight gain, fluid retention and hemodilution; worsening heart failure; macular degeneration; increased risk of fractures and possibly bladder cancer.	Potentiates the effect of other antihyperglycemic agents. Gemfibrozil inhibits metabolism and increases plasma levels.	Avoid in patients with heart failure. Effects on CV outcomes being evaluated. Ovulation resumes in previously anovulatory women, e.g., polycystic ovarian syndrome; Increased risk of pregnancy if adequate contraception not used.	$$

(cont'd)

Table 8: **Antihyperglycemic Agents** *(cont'd)*

Class	Drug[a]	Dose	Adverse Effects	Drug Interactions	Comments	Cost[b]
	rosiglitazone Avandia	4–8 mg daily po in 1–2 doses	See pioglitazone.	See pioglitazone.	See pioglitazone. Patient consent required.	$$$$
Combination Products	*rosiglitazone/metformin* Avandamet	If on metformin monotherapy: start with rosiglitazone 2 mg BID po. If on rosiglitazone monotherapy start with metformin 500 mg BID po Maximum: 8 mg/1000 mg BID	See pioglitazone. See metformin.	See pioglitazone. See metformin.	See pioglitazone. See rosiglitazone. See metformin.	$$$$
	sitagliptin/metformin Janumet	If on metformin monotherapy: continue metformin dose, add sitagliptin 50 mg BID po. If on both agents already: continue current doses. Maximum: 50 mg/1000 mg BID	See linagliptin. See metformin.	See sitagliptin. See metformin.	See metformin.	$$$
	sitagliptin/metformin Janumet XR	50/500, 50/1000 or 100/1000 mg once daily po Maximum: 100 mg/2000 mg once daily	See linagliptin. See metformin.	See sitagliptin. See metformin.	See metformin.	$$$

Class	Drug[a]	Dose	Adverse Effects	Drug Interactions	Comments	Cost[b]
	linagliptin/metformin (kidney symbol) Jentadueto	If on metformin monotherapy: continue metformin dose, add linagliptin 2.5 mg BID po. If on both agents already: continue current doses. Maximum: 2.5 mg/1000 mg BID	See linagliptin. See metformin.	See linagliptin See metformin.	See metformin.	$$$
	saxagliptin/metformin (kidney symbol) Komboglyze	If on metformin monotherapy: continue metformin dose, add saxagliptin 2.5 mg BID po. If on both agents already: continue current doses. Maximum: 2.5 mg/1000 mg BID	See linagliptin. See metformin.	See saxagliptin. See metformin.	See metformin.	$$$

[a] Combination therapy: always use agents from different classes; combinations can be used as initial therapy if hyperglycemia is not expected to be controlled by a single agent.
[b] Cost of 30-day supply; includes drug cost only.
(kidney symbol) Dosage adjustment may be required in renal impairment; see Appendix I.
Legend: $ < $30 $$ $30–60 $$$ $60–90 $$$$ $90–120 $$$$$ $120–150

Suggested Readings

American Diabetes Association. ADA clinical practice recommendations—2013. *Diabetes Care* 2013;36(1):S1-108.

Canadian Agency for Drugs and Technologies in Health (CADTH). Optimal Use. *Second- and third-line therapy for patients with type 2 diabetes*. Ottawa (ON): CADTH; July 2013. Available from: www.cadth.ca/en/products/optimal-use/second-line-therapies.

Canadian Diabetes Association Clinical Practice Guidelines Expert Committee. Canadian Diabetes Association 2013 Clinical Practice Guidelines for the Prevention and Management of Diabetes in Canada. *Can J Diabetes* 2013;37(Suppl 1):S1-S212. Available from: guidelines.diabetes.ca/App_Themes/CDACPG/resources/cpg_2013_full_en.pdf.

Canadian Optimal Medication Prescribing and Utilization Service (COMPUS). Optimal therapy recommendations for the prescribing and use of blood glucose test strips. *COMPUS* 2009;3(6):1-50. Available from: www.cadth.ca/media/pdf/compus_BGTS_OT_Rec_e.pdf.

Holman RR, Farmer AJ, Davies MJ et al. Three-year efficacy of complex insulin regimens in type 2 diabetes. *N Engl J Med* 2009;361(18):1736-47.

Kaul S, Bolger AF, Herrington D et al. Thiazolidinedione drugs and cardiovascular risks: a science advisory from the American Heart Association and American College of Cardiology Foundation. *Circulation* 2010;121(16):1868-77.

Skyler JS, Bergenstal R, Bonow RO et al. Intensive glycemic control and the prevention of cardiovascular events: implications of the ACCORD, ADVANCE, and VA diabetes trials: a position statement of the American Diabetes Association and a scientific statement of the American College of Cardiology Foundation and the American Heart Association. *Diabetes Care* 2009;32(1):187-92.

References

1. Emerging Risk Factors Collaboration, Sarwar N, Gao P et al. Diabetes mellitus, fasting blood glucose concentration, and risk of vascular disease: a collaborative meta-analysis of 102 prospective studies. *Lancet* 2010;375(9733):2215-22.
2. Poirier P, Dufour R, Carpentier A et al. Canadian Diabetes Association 2013 Clinical Practice Guidelines for the Prevention and Management of Diabetes in Canada: Screening for the presence of coronary artery disease. *Can J Diabetes* 2013;37(Suppl 1):S105-9. Available from: guidelines.diabetes.ca/App_Themes/CDACPG/resources/cpg_2013_full_en.pdf. Accessed November 22, 2013.
3. Ekoé JM, Punthakee Z, Ransom T et al. Canadian Diabetes Association 2013 Clinical Practice Guidelines for the Prevention and Management of Diabetes in Canada: Screening for type 1 and type 2 diabetes. *Can J Diabetes* 2013;37(Suppl 1):S12-5. Available from: guidelines.diabetes.ca/App_Themes/CDACPG/resources/cpg_2013_full_en.pdf. Accessed September 3, 2013.
4. Goldenberg R, Punthakee Z. Canadian Diabetes Association 2013 Clinical Practice Guidelines for the Prevention and Management of Diabetes in Canada: Definition, classification and diagnosis of diabetes, prediabetes and metabolic syndrome. *Can J Diabetes* 2013;37(Suppl 1):S8-11. Available from: guidelines.diabetes.ca/App_Themes/CDACPG/resources/cpg_2013_full_en.pdf. Accessed September 3, 2013.
5. Canadian Task Force on Preventive Health Care, Pottie K, Jaramillo A et al. Recommendations on screening for type 2 diabetes in adults. *CMAJ* 2012;184(15):1687-96.
6. Charles MA, Fontbonne A, Thibult N et al. Risk factors for NIDDM in white population. Paris prospective study. *Diabetes* 1991;40(7):796-9.
7. Robinson CA, Agarwal G, Nerenberg K. Validating the CANRISK prognostic model for assessing diabetes risk in Canada's multi-ethnic population. *Chron Dis Inj Can* 2011;32(1):19-31.
8. Berard LD, Blumer I, Houlden R et al. Canadian Diabetes Association 2013 Clinical Practice Guidelines for the Prevention and Management of Diabetes in Canada: Monitoring glycemic control. *Can J Diabetes* 2013;37(Suppl 1):S35-9. Available from: guidelines.diabetes.ca/App_Themes/CDACPG/resources/cpg_2013_full_en.pdf. Accessed September 3, 2013.
9. Sigal RJ, Armstrong MJ, Colby P et al. Canadian Diabetes Association 2013 Clinical Practice Guidelines for the Prevention and Management of Diabetes in Canada: Physical activity and diabetes. *Can J Diabetes* 2013;37(Suppl 1):S40-4. Available from: guidelines.diabetes.ca/App_Themes/CDACPG/resources/cpg_2013_full_en.pdf. Accessed September 3, 2013.
10. Gilbert RE, Rabi D, LaRochelle P et al. Canadian Diabetes Association 2013 Clinical Practice Guidelines for the Prevention and Management of Diabetes in Canada: Treatment of hypertension. *Can J Diabetes* 2013;37(Suppl 1):S117-8. Available from: guidelines.diabetes.ca/App_Themes/CDACPG/resources/cpg_2013_full_en.pdf. Accessed September 3, 2013.
11. Bowering K, Embil J. Canadian Diabetes Association 2013 Clinical Practice Guidelines for the Prevention and Management of Diabetes in Canada: Foot care. *Can J Diabetes* 2013;37(Suppl 1):S145-9. Available from: guidelines.diabetes.ca/App_Themes/CDACPG/resources/cpg_2013_full_en.pdf.
12. McFarlane P, Gilbert R, MacCallum L et al. Canadian Diabetes Association 2013 Clinical Practice Guidelines for the Prevention and Management of Diabetes in Canada: Chronic kidney disease in diabetes. *Can J Diabetes* 2013;37(Suppl 1):S129-36. Available from: guidelines.diabetes.ca/App_Themes/CDACPG/resources/cpg_2013_full_en.pdf.
13. Anderson T, Gregoire J, Hegele R et al. 2012 Update of the Canadian Cardiovascular Society guidelines for the diagnosis and treatment of dyslipidemia for the prevention of cardiovascular disease in the adult. *Can J Cardiol* 2013;29(2):151-67.
14. Mancini G, Hegele R, Leiter L. Canadian Diabetes Association 2013 Clinical Practice Guidelines for the Prevention and Management of Diabetes in Canada: Dyslipidemia. *Can J Diabetes* 2013;37(Suppl 1):S110-6. Available from: guidelines.diabetes.ca/App_Themes/CDACPG/resources/cpg_2013_full_en.pdf.

15. Boyd S, Advani A, Altomare F et al. Canadian Diabetes Association 2013 Clinical Practice Guidelines for the Prevention and Management of Diabetes in Canada: Retinopathy. *Can J Diabetes* 2013;37(Suppl 1):S137-41. Available from: guidelines.diabetes.ca/App_Themes/CDACPG/resources/cpg_2013_full_en.pdf.
16. Husein N, Woo V. Canadian Diabetes Association 2013 Clinical Practice Guidelines for the Prevention and Management of Diabetes in Canada: Influenza and pneumococcal immunization. *Can J Diabetes* 2013;37(Suppl 1):S93. Available from: guidelines.diabetes.ca/App_Themes/CDACPG/resources/cpg_2013_full_en.pdf. Accessed September 3, 2013.
17. Ratner RE, Hirsch IB, Neifing JL et al. Less hypoglycemia with insulin glargine in intensive insulin therapy for type 1 diabetes. U.S. Study Group of Insulin Glargine in Type 1 Diabetes. *Diabetes Care* 2000;23(5):639-43.
18. Home P, Bartley P, Russell-Jones D et al. Insulin detemir offers improved glycemic control compared with NPH insulin in people with type 1 diabetes: a randomized clinical trial. *Diabetes Care* 2004;27(5):1081-7.
19. Vague P, Selam JL, Skeie S et al. Insulin detemir is associated with more predictable glycemic control and reduced risk of hypoglycemia than NPH insulin in patients with type 1 diabetes on a basal-bolus regimen with premeal insulin aspart. *Diabetes Care* 2003;26(3):590-6.
20. Freemantle N, Meneghini L, Christensen T et al. Insulin degludec improves health-related quality of life (SF-36®) compared with insulin glargine in people with Type 2 diabetes starting on basal insulin: a meta-analysis of phase 3a trials. *Diabet Med* 2013;30(2):226-32.
21. Ratner RE, Gough SC, Mathieu C et al. Hypoglycaemia risk with insulin degludec compared with insulin glargine in type 2 and type 1 diabetes: a pre-planned meta-analysis of phase 3 trials. *Diabetes Obes Metab* 2013;15(2):175-84.
22. The effect of intensive treatment of diabetes on the development and progression of long-term complications in insulin-dependent diabetes mellitus. The Diabetes Control and Complications Trial Research Group. *N Engl J Med* 1993;329(14):977-86.
23. Nathan DM, Cleary PA, Backlund JY et al. Intensive diabetes treatment and cardiovascular disease in patients with type 1 diabetes. *N Engl J Med* 2005;353(25):2643-53.
24. Siebenhofer A, Plank J, Berghold A et al. Short acting insulin analogues versus regular human insulin in patients with diabetes mellitus. *Cochrane Database Syst Rev* 2006;(2):CD003287.
25. Plank J, Siebenhofer A, Berghold A et al. Systematic review and meta-analysis of short-acting insulin analogues in patients with diabetes mellitus. *Arch Intern Med* 2005;165(12):1337-44.
26. Cryer PE. Banting Lecture. Hypoglycemia: the limiting factor in the management of IDDM. *Diabetes* 1994;43(11):1378-89.
27. Epidemiology of severe hypoglycemia in the Diabetes Control and Complications Trial. The DCCT Research Group. *Am J Med* 1991;90(4):450-9.
28. Mayer D, Shukla A, Enzmann H. Proliferative effects of insulin analogues on mammary epithelial cells. *Arch Physiol Biochem* 2008;114(1):38-44.
29. Grimaldi-Bensouda L, Cameron D, Marty M et al. Risk of breast cancer by individual insulin use: an international multicenter study. *Diabetes Care* 2014;37(1):134-43.
30. Harper W, Clement M, Goldenberg R et al. Canadian Diabetes Association 2013 Clinical Practice Guidelines for the Prevention and Management of Diabetes in Canada: Pharmacologic management of type 2 diabetes. *Can J Diabetes* 2013;37(Suppl 1):S61-8. Available from: guidelines.diabetes.ca/App_Themes/CDACPG/resources/cpg_2013_full_en.pdf. Accessed September 3, 2013.
31. Intensive blood-glucose control with sulphonylureas or insulin compared with conventional treatment and risk of complications in patients with type 2 diabetes (UKPDS 33). UK Prospective Diabetes Study (UKPDS) Group. *Lancet* 1998;352:(9131)837-53.
32. Canadian Agency for Drugs and Technologies in Health (CADTH). Optimal Use. *Second- and third-line therapy for patients with type 2 diabetes*. Ottawa (ON): CADTH; June 2011. Available from: www.cadth.ca/en/products/optimal-use/second-line-therapies. Accessed September 27, 2011.
33. Russell-Jones D, Vaag A, Schmitz O et al. Liraglutide vs insulin glargine and placebo in combination with metformin and sulfonylurea therapy in type 2 diabetes mellitus (LEAD-5 met+SU): a randomised controlled trial. *Diabetologia* 2009;52(10):2046-55.
34. Sherifali D, Nerenberg K, Pullenayegum E et al. The effect of oral antidiabetic agents on A1C levels: a systematic review and meta-analysis. *Diabetes Care* 2010;33(8):1859-64.
35. Brubaker PL. Minireview: update on incretin biology: focus on glucagon-like peptide-1. *Endocrinology* 2010;151(5):1984-9.
36. Peters A. Incretin-based therapies: review of current clinical trial data. *Am J Med* 2010;123(3 Suppl):S28-S37.
37. UK Prospective Diabetes Study (UKPDS) Group. Effect of intensive blood-glucose control with metformin on complications in overweight patients with type 2 diabetes (UKPDS 34). *Lancet* 1998;352(9131):854-65.
38. Salpeter S, Greyber E, Pasternak G et al. Risk of fatal and nonfatal lactic acidosis with metformin use in type 2 diabetes mellitus. *Cochrane Database Syst Rev* 2010;(4):CD002967.
39. Eurich DT, McAlister FA, Blackburn DF et al. Benefits and harms of antidiabetic agents in patients with diabetes and heart failure: systematic review. *BMJ* 2007;335(7618):497.
40. Bodmer M, Meier C, Krahenbauhl S et al. Metformin, sulfonylureas, or other antidiabetes drugs and the risk of lactic acidosis or hypoglycemia: a nested case-control analysis. *Diabetes Care* 2008;31(11):2086-91.
41. Nathan DM, Buse JB, Davidson MB et al. Medical management of hyperglycemia in type 2 diabetes: a consensus algorithm for the initiation and adjustment of therapy: a consensus statement of the American Diabetes Association and the European Association for the Study of Diabetes. *Diabetes Care* 2009;32(1):193-203.
42. Elbrond B, Jakobsen G, Larsen S et al. Pharmacokinetics, pharmacodynamics, safety, and tolerability of a single-dose of NN2211, a long-acting glucagon-like peptide 1 derivative, in healthy male subjects. *Diabetes Care* 2002;25(8):1398-404.
43. Bolen S, Feldman L, Vassy J et al. Systematic review: comparative effectiveness and safety of oral medications for type 2 diabetes mellitus. *Ann Intern Med* 2007;147(6):386-99.
44. American Geriatrics Society 2012 Beers Criteria Expert Panel. American Geriatrics Society updated Beers Criteria for potentially inappropriate medication use in older adults. *J Am Geriatr Soc* 2012;60(4):616-31.
45. Lebovitz HE. Oral therapies for diabetic hyperglycemia. *Endocrinol Metab Clin North Am* 2001;30(4):909-33.
46. Neumiller JJ, White JR, Campbell RK. Sodium-glucose co-transport inhibitors: progress and therapeutic potential in type 2 diabetes mellitus. *Drugs* 2010;70(4):377-85.
47. Cefalu WT, Leiter LA, Yoon KH. Efficacy and safety of canagliflozin versus glimepiride in patients with type 2 diabetes inadequately controlled with metformin (CANTATA-SU): 52 week results from a randomised, double-blind, phase 3 non-inferiority trial. *Lancet* 2013;382(9896):941-50.
48. List JF, Woo V, Morales E et al. Sodium-glucose cotransport inhibition with dapagliflozin in type 2 diabetes. *Diabetes Care* 2009;32(4):650-7.
49. Yki-Jarvinen H. Thiazolidinediones. *N Engl J Med* 2004;351(11):1106-18.

50. Chiquette E, Ramirez G, Defronzo R. A meta-analysis comparing the effect of thiazolidinediones on cardiovascular risk factors. *Arch Intern Med* 2004;164(19):2097-104.
51. Dormandy JA, Charbonnel B, Eckland DJ et al. Secondary prevention of macrovascular events in patients with type 2 diabetes in the PROactive Study (PROspective pioglitAzone Clinical Trial In macroVascular Events): a randomised controlled trial. *Lancet* 2005;366(9493):1279-89.
52. Ryan EH, Han DP, Ramsay RC et al. Diabetic macular edema associated with glitazone use. *Retina* 2006;26(5):562-70.
53. Meier C, Kraenzlin ME, Bodmer M et al. Use of thiazolidinediones and fracture risk. *Arch Intern Med* 2008;168(8):820-5.
54. Bilik D, McEwen LN, Brown MB et al. Thiazolidinediones and fractures: evidence from translating research into action for diabetes. *J Clin Endocrinol Metab* 2010;95(10):4560-5.
55. Diamond GA, Bax L, Kaul S. Uncertain effects of rosiglitazone on the risk for myocardial infarction and cardiovascular death. *Ann Intern Med* 2007;147(8):578-81.
56. Nissen SE, Wolski K. Effect of rosiglitazone on the risk of myocardial infarction and death from cardiovascular causes. *N Engl J Med* 2007;356(24):2457-71.
57. Kaul S, Bolger AF, Herrington D et al. Thiazolidinedione drugs and cardiovascular risks: a science advisory from the American Heart Association and American College of Cardiology Foundation. *Circulation* 2010;121(16):1868-77.
58. Mahaffey KW, Hafley G, Dickerson S et al. Results of a reevaluation of cardiovascular outcomes in the RECORD trial *Am Heart J* 2013;166(2):240-9.
59. Colmers IN, Bowker SL, Majumdar SR et al. Use of thiazolidinediones and the risk of bladder cancer among people with type 2 diabetes: a meta-analysis. *CMAJ* 2012;184(12):E675-83.
60. Holman RR, Farmer AJ, Davies MJ et al. Three-year efficacy of complex insulin regimens in type 2 diabetes. *N Engl J Med* 2009;361(18):1736-47.
61. Douek IF, Allen SE, Ewings P et al. Continuing metformin when starting insulin in patients with Type 2 diabetes: a double-blind randomized placebo-controlled trial. *Diabet Med* 2005;22(5):634-40.
62. American Diabetes Association. Standards of medical care in diabetes—2013. *Diabetes Care* 2013;36(Suppl 1):S11-66.
63. Imran SA, Rabasa-Lhoret R, Ross S. Canadian Diabetes Association 2013 Clinical Practice Guidelines for the Prevention and Management of Diabetes in Canada: Targets for glycemic control. *Can J Diabetes* 2013;37(Suppl 1):S31-4. Available from: guidelines.diabetes.ca/App_Themes/CDACPG/resources/cpg_2013_full_en.pdf. Accessed September 3, 2013.
64. Action to Control Cardiovascular Risk in Diabetes Study Group, Gerstein HC, Miller ME et al. Effects of intensive glucose lowering in type 2 diabetes. *N Engl J Med* 2008;358(24):2545-59.
65. ADVANCE Collaborative Group, Patel A, MacMahon S et al. Intensive blood glucose control and vascular outcomes in patients with type 2 diabetes. *N Engl J Med* 2008;358(24):2560-72.
66. Duckworth W, Abraira C, Moritz T et al. Glucose control and vascular complications in veterans with type 2 diabetes. *N Engl J Med* 2009;360(2):129-39.
67. Wherrett D, Huot C, Mitchell B et al. Canadian Diabetes Association 2013 Clinical Practice Guidelines for the Prevention and Management of Diabetes in Canada: Type 1 diabetes in children and adolescents. *Can J Diabetes* 2013;37(Suppl 1):S153-62. Available from: guidelines.diabetes.ca/App_Themes/CDACPG/resources/cpg_2013_full_en.pdf. Accessed September 3, 2013.
68. Bell AD, Roussin A, Cartier R et al. The use of antiplatelet therapy in the outpatient setting: Canadian Cardiovascular Society guidelines. *Can J Cardiol* 2011;27(Suppl A):S1-59.
69. Stone JA, Fitchett D, Grover S et al. Canadian Diabetes Association 2013 Clinical Practice Guidelines for the Prevention and Management of Diabetes in Canada: Vascular protection in people with diabetes. *Can J Diabetes* 2013;37(Suppl 1):S100-4. Available from: guidelines.diabetes.ca/App_Themes/CDACPG/resources/cpg_2013_full_en.pdf. Accessed September 3, 2013.
70. Ridker PM, Danielson E, Fonseca FA et al. Rosuvastatin to prevent vascular events in men and women with elevated C-reactive protein. *N Engl J Med* 2008;359(21):2195-207.
71. Preiss D, Seshasai SR, Welsh P et al. Risk of incident diabetes with intensive-dose compared with moderate-dose statin therapy: a meta-analysis. *JAMA* 2011;305(24):2556-64.
72. Colbert JD, Stone JA. Statin use and the risk of incident diabetes mellitus: a review of the literature. *Can J Cardiol* 2012;28(5):581-9.
73. Gaede P, Vedel P, Larsen N et al. Multifactorial intervention and cardiovascular disease in patients with type 2 diabetes. *N Engl J Med* 2003;348(5):383-93.
74. Thompson D, Berger H, Feig D et al. Canadian Diabetes Association 2013 Clinical Practice Guidelines for the Prevention and Management of Diabetes in Canada: Diabetes and pregnancy. *Can J Diabetes* 2013;37(Suppl 1):S168-83. Available from: guidelines.diabetes.ca/App_Themes/CDACPG/resources/cpg_2013_full_en.pdf. Accessed September 3, 2013.
75. Balsells M, Garcia-Patterson A, Gich I et al. Maternal and fetal outcome in women with type 2 versus type 1 diabetes mellitus: a systematic review and metaanalysis. *J Clin Endocrinol Metab* 2009;94(11):4284-91.
76. Middleton P, Crowther CA, Simmonds L et al. Different intensities of glycaemic control for pregnant women with pre-existing diabetes. *Cochrane Database Syst Rev* 2010;(9):CD008540.
77. Dabelea D, Knowler WC, Pettitt DJ. Effect of diabetes in pregnancy on offspring: follow-up research in the Pima Indians. *J Matern Fetal Med* 2000;9(1):83-8.
78. Crowther CA, Hiller JE, Moss JR et al. Effect of treatment of gestational diabetes mellitus on pregnancy outcomes. *N Engl J Med* 2005;352(24):2477-86.
79. Alwan N, Tuffnell DJ, West J. Treatments for gestational diabetes. *Cochrane Database Syst Rev* 2009;(3):CD003395.
80. Mathiesen ER, Kinsley B, Amiel SA et al. Maternal glycemic control and hypoglycemia in type 1 diabetic pregnancy: a randomized trial of insulin aspart versus human insulin in 322 pregnant women. *Diabetes Care* 2007;30(4):771-6.
81. Chico A, Saigi I, Garcia-Patterson A et al. Glycemic control and perinatal outcomes of pregnancies complicated by type 1 diabetes: influence of continuous subcutaneous insulin and lispro insulin. *Diabetes Tech Ther* 2010;12(12):937-45.
82. Durnwald CP, Landon MB. A comparison of lispro and regular insulin for the management of type 1 and type 2 diabetes in pregnancy. *J Matern Fetal Neonatal Med* 2008;21(5):309-13.
83. Mathiesen ER, Hod M, Ivanisevic M et al. Maternal efficacy and safety outcomes in a randomized, controlled trial comparing insulin detemir with NPH insulin in 310 pregnant women with type 1 diabetes. *Diabetes Care* 2012;35(10):2012-7.
84. Pollex E, Moreti ME, Koren G et al. Safety of insulin glargine use in pregnancy: a systematic review and meta-analysis. *Ann Pharmacother* 2011;45(1):9-16.
85. Mecacci F, Carignani L, Cioni R et al. Maternal metabolic control and perinatal outcome in women with gestational diabetes treated with regular or lispro insulin: comparison with non-diabetic pregnant women. *Eur J Obstet Gynecol Reprod Biol* 2003;111(1):19-24.

86. Pettitt DJ, Ospina P, Kolaczynski JW et al. Comparison of an insulin analog, insulin aspart, and regular human insulin with no insulin in gestational diabetes mellitus. *Diabetes Care* 2003;26(1):183-6.

87. Briggs GG, Freeman RK, Yaffe SJ. *Drugs in pregnancy and lactation: a reference guide to fetal and neonatal risk.* 9th ed. Philadelphia (PA): Wolters Kluwer Health; Lippincott Williams & Wilkins; 2011.

88. Ohinmaa A, Jacobs P, Simpson S et al. The projection of prevalence and cost of diabetes in Canada: 2000 to 2016. *Can J Diabetes* 2004;28(2):1-8. Available from: www.diabetes.ca/files/johnsonCJDjune2004.pdf. Accessed September 27, 2011.

89. American Diabetes Association. Diagnosis and classification of diabetes mellitus. *Diabetes Care* 2010;33(Suppl 1):S62-69.

90. Eckel RH, Grundy SM, Zimmet PZ. The metabolic syndrome. *Lancet* 2005;365(9468):1415-28.

91. Tuomilehto J, Lindstrom J, Eriksson JG et al. Prevention of type 2 diabetes mellitus by changes in lifestyle among subjects with impaired glucose tolerance. *N Engl J Med* 2001;344(18):1343-50.

92. Knowler WC, Barrett-Connor E, Fowler SE et al. Reduction in the incidence of type 2 diabetes with lifestyle intervention or metformin. *N Engl J Med* 2002;346(6):393-403.

93. Lindstrom J, Ilanne-Parikka P, Peltonen M et al. Sustained reduction in the incidence of type 2 diabetes by lifestyle intervention: follow-up of the Finnish Diabetes Prevention Study. *Lancet* 2006;368(9548):1673-9.

94. Diabetes Prevention Program Research Group, Knowler WC, Fowler SE et al. 10-year follow-up of diabetes incidence and weight loss in the Diabetes Prevention Program Outcomes Study. *Lancet* 2009;374(9702):1677-86.

95. Van de Laar FA, Lucassen PL, Akkermans RP et al. Alpha-glucosidase inhibitors for people with impaired glucose tolerance or impaired fasting blood glucose. *Cochrane Database Syst Rev* 2006;(4):CD005061.

96. Gerstein HC, Yusuf S, Bosch J et al. Effect of rosiglitazone on the frequency of diabetes in patients with impaired glucose tolerance or impaired fasting glucose: a randomised controlled trial. *Lancet* 2006;368(9541):1096-105.

97. Buchanan TA, Xiang AH, Peters RK et al. Preservation of pancreatic beta-cell function and prevention of type 2 diabetes by pharmacological treatment of insulin resistance in high-risk Hispanic women. *Diabetes* 2002;51(9):2796-803.

98. Knowler WC, Hamman RF, Edelstein SL et al. Prevention of type 2 diabetes with troglitazone in the Diabetes Prevention Program. *Diabetes* 2005;54(4):1150-6.

99. Zinman B, Harris SB, Neuman J et al. Low-dose combination therapy with rosiglitazone and metformin to prevent type 2 diabetes mellitus (CANOE trial): a double-blind randomised controlled study. *Lancet* 2010;376(9735):103-11.

100. Torgerson JS, Hauptman J, Boldrin MN et al. XENical in the prevention of diabetes in obese subjects (XENDOS) study: a randomized study of orlistat as an adjunct to lifestyle changes for the prevention of type 2 diabetes in obese patients. *Diabetes Care* 2004;27(1):155-61.

101. Bosch J, Yusuf S, Gerstein HC et al. Effect of ramipril on the incidence of diabetes. *N Engl J Med* 2006;355(15):1551-62.

102. NAVIGATOR Study Group, Holman RR, Haffner SM et al. Effect of nateglinide on the incidence of diabetes and cardiovascular events. *N Engl J Med* 2010;362(16):1463-76.

103. Skyler JS. Prediction and prevention of type 1 diabetes: progress, problems, and prospects. *Clin Pharmacol Ther* 2007;81(5):768-71.

104. Kitabchi AE, Umpierrez GE, Murphy MB et al. Hyperglycemic crises in adult patients with diabetes: a consensus statement from the American Diabetes Association. *Diabetes Care* 2006;29(12):2739-48.

105. Goguen J, Gilbert J. Canadian Diabetes Association 2013 Clinical Practice Guidelines for the Prevention and Management of Diabetes in Canada: Hyperglycemic emergencies in adults. *Can J Diabetes* 2013;37(Suppl 1):S72-6. Available from: guidelines.diabetes.ca/App_Themes/CDACPG/resources/cpg_2013_full_en.pdf. Accessed September 3, 2013.

106. Charles RA, Bee YM, Eng PH et al. Point-of-care blood ketone testing: screening for diabetic ketoacidosis at the emergency department. *Singapore Med J* 2007;48(11):986-9.

107. Naunheim R, Jang TJ, Banet G et al. Point-of-care test identifies diabetic ketoacidosis at triage. *Acad Emerg Med* 2006;13(6):683-5.

Endocrine and Metabolic Disorders

Chapter 33
Obesity

Arya M. Sharma, MD

Obesity is a complex heterogeneous disorder that places individuals at increased risk for adverse mental and/or physical health consequences from excess body fat. The current definition of obesity is based on body mass index (BMI), calculated as weight (kg)/height $(m)^2$; see Table 1. In 2004, 23.1% of Canadians aged 18 or older—an estimated 5.5 million adults—had a BMI of 30 kg/m^2 or more; the prevalence of class II and III obesity was 5.1% and 2.7%, respectively.[1] Childhood obesity is likewise on the rise, affecting more than 500 000 children in Canada.[1]

These figures likely underestimate the impact of excess body weight on health, as weight distribution (central versus peripheral) and ectopic adiposity (hepatic steatosis, increased intramyocellular fat) may increase health risks, even at BMI levels well below the conventional BMI cut-offs.[2] Thus, measures of abdominal obesity, such as waist circumference values exceeding 102 cm (40 inches) in men and 88 cm (35 inches) in women, have been suggested as markers of increased cardiometabolic risk. The BMI and waist circumference classification system is less accurate with respect to young adults who have not yet reached full growth, lean or muscular adults, adults over age 65, and some racial and ethnic groups such as Asian, Black and Canadian First Nations, including Inuit.

More comprehensive staging tools are needed to estimate mortality risk based on adiposity. The Edmonton Obesity Staging System ranks mortality risk in overweight individuals based on obesity-related comorbidities and functional status.[3] This tool is meant to complement anthropometric measures and requires further validation.

Table 1: WHO Classification of Overweight and Obesity in Adults According to Body Mass Index

		Risk of Comorbidities[b]	
Classification	**BMI[a]**	**Waist Circumference Men: ≤40 in (≤102 cm) Women: ≤35 in (≤88 cm)**	**Waist Circumference Men: >40 in (>102 cm) Women: >35 in (>88 cm)**
Underweight	<18.5		
Normal	18.5–24.9	Least	Increased
Overweight	25–29.9	Increased	High
Obese	≥30		
Class I	30–34.9	High	Very high
Class II	35–39.9	Very high	Very high
Class III	≥40	Extremely high	Extremely high

[a] Values are age and gender independent.
[b] Both BMI and a measure of fat distribution (e.g., waist circumference) are important in estimating the risk of comorbidities (type 2 diabetes, hypertension, dyslipidemia).
Adapted with permission from the National Heart, Lung and Blood Institute. Preventing and Managing the Global Epidemic of Obesity. *Report of the World Health Organization Consultation of Obesity*. Geneva (SZ): WHO; June 1997.

Goals of Therapy

- The overall aim is to reduce excess body fat for health and not for cosmetic reasons; reducing weight by 5–10% can result in important health benefits
- Minimum goal: stabilize and prevent further weight gain
- Prevent weight regain
- Prevent and treat obesity-related comorbidities and complications

Strategies for Treatment of Obesity

Obesity is a heterogeneous condition and no single management strategy works for every patient. Psychosocial, emotional or physical barriers may make it difficult for patients to adhere to management strategies. There is currently no cure for obesity; successful management involves a long-term "coping" strategy that allows the patient to reduce their body weight and prevent weight regain. Typically, treatment is characterized by intermittent periods of remission and relapse, commonly referred to as "weight cycling." The health risks of weight cycling versus maintaining a long-term stable weight remain controversial.

The Canadian Obesity Network has developed a set of tools based on the 5As framework for obesity management:

Table 2: **Canadian Obesity Network 5As of Obesity Management**[4]

	Definition	Rationale
Ask	Ask permission to discuss weight; be non-judgmental; explore readiness for change.	Weight is a sensitive issue; avoid verbal or nonverbal cues that imply judgment; indication of readiness may predict outcomes.
Assess	Assess BMI, waist circumference, obesity class (see Table 1); explore root causes of obesity.	BMI alone should not serve as an indicator for obesity interventions.
Advise	Advise on health risks of obesity; benefits of modest weight loss; need for long-term strategy; treatment options.	Health risk of excess weight can vary; avoidance of weight gain and/or modest weight loss can have health benefits; treatment options should consider risk.
Agree	Agree on realistic weight loss expectations and targets; specifics of treatment plan.	Most patients have unrealistic expectations; interventions should focus on changing behavior; providers should seek patient's desire for proposed treatment.
Assist	Assist in identifying and addressing barriers; provide resources and assist in identifying and consulting with appropriate providers; arrange regular follow up.	Most patients have significant barriers to weight management; patients are confused and cannot identify credible from non-credible sources of information; follow up is an essential principle of chronic disease management.

Adapted with permission from the Canadian Obesity Network, 5As of Obesity Management at www.obesitynetwork.ca/5As.

Treatment strategies should acknowledge 2 distinct phases in obesity management:[5]

Phase 1: Induction of weight loss

Weight loss requires caloric restriction. A negative energy balance of about 500 kcal/day results in weight loss of about 1–2 kg (2–4 lb) per month. A kilogram of fat is equivalent to 7780 kcal (3500 kcal/lb). A challenge in this phase is to prevent the concomitant loss of lean body mass, which can be minimized by ensuring the intake of high-quality protein and participation in resistance training. This phase lasts until the patient achieves the weight-loss plateau (usually 3–6 months into the weight-loss phase), at which time the focus of treatment changes to phase 2.

Phase 2: Prevention of weight regain

The induction of weight loss results in complex hormonal and neurobehavioural changes that seek to restore body weight to its original level. There is no evidence that these responses diminish over time. The patient will thus have to continue restricting energy intake indefinitely to the same level as was consumed at the time of the weight-loss plateau. Any increase in energy intake will result in weight regain. Deep-rooted lifestyle changes, intense physical activity, medication and surgery can significantly reduce the likelihood of weight regain.

Setting Treatment Goals

- Treatment goals should focus on improving health status and/or quality of life rather than on just reducing numbers on the scale.
- Significant health benefits can be achieved with a 5–10% weight loss; further weight loss in class I and II obesity may be difficult to achieve and maintain.
- In phase 2 of treatment, the principal goal is to prevent weight regain.
- Increased physical activity in phase 2 can help maintain weight loss and result in further improvements in health and quality of life.

Investigations

- Thorough history including:
  - weight history, including previous attempts at weight loss, precipitating events (e.g., pregnancy, injury) and contributing factors (e.g., corticosteroids, antihyperglycemic agents, antiepileptic drugs or antipsychotics)
  - lifestyle (diet and activity), readiness for change, psychosocial, emotional and physical barriers to lifestyle change, smoking, alcohol, substance abuse
  - reasons for willingness to change and possible health and quality-of-life goals
  - family history of obesity and comorbidities
  - support system and insurance coverage for obesity treatment
  - assess as indicated for anxiety (see Chapter 2), attention deficit (see Chapter 3), depression (see Chapter 6), eating disorders (see Chapter 7) and insomnia (see Chapter 8)
- Physical examination:
  - weight, height, waist circumference, visual impression of weight distribution; calculate BMI
  - vital signs
  - target organ damage, including hepatomegaly, abdominal wall hernias, acanthosis nigricans, intertrigo
  - identify genetic and associated conditions
  - assess for low back pain (see Chapter 80) and osteoarthritis (see Chapter 82) as indicated
  - assess for chronic fatigue syndrome (see Chapter 77) and fibromyalgia (see Chapter 78) as indicated
- Laboratory and diagnostic procedures:
  - screen for diabetes mellitus (see Chapter 32), dyslipidemia (see Chapter 37), hypertension (see Chapter 39) and gout (see Chapter 79)
  - liver function tests—liver ultrasound where indicated
  - discourage routine TSH testing
  - pulmonary functions and sleep studies where indicated

- ECG, exercise test and echocardiography where indicated
- assess for gastroesophageal reflux and gallbladder disease where indicated

Therapeutic Choices (Figure 1)

Nonpharmacologic Choices

Nutrition Planning and Diet Composition

- Regular eating (3 meals, 3 snacks) is an important measure for weight control. Discourage prolonged fasting and skipping of meals—people who eat breakfast are less likely to be obese than people who do not.
- Weight-management strategies include grocery shopping after meals, using smaller dishes and glasses and avoiding energy-dense foods, empty calories in soda pop and snacking in front of the TV.
- All weight-loss diets must be nutritionally adequate to ensure optimal health, and well balanced with respect to macronutrient composition. Discourage extreme diets.
- Ensure an adequate carbohydrate intake of ≥100 g/day (400 kcal/day) to avoid protein breakdown and muscle wasting, and to avoid large shifts in fluid balance. Complex carbohydrates that are high in fibre (e.g., kidney beans) and have a low glycemic index require more time to eat and digest and are associated with greater satiety.
- Ensure a protein intake of ≥1 g/kg/day of high quality mixed proteins to maintain lean body mass and other essential body functions. When energy intake falls below that needed to maintain energy balance, protein requirements increase by 1.75 g for every 100 kcal deficit.
- Fat intake should not exceed 30–35% of total calories consumed, with ≤10% from trans and saturated fat. Low-fat diets are not more effective in weight loss than other hypocaloric diets, but they do reduce cardiovascular risk.
- Use of commercial meal replacements can provide a simple and sustainable adjunct to weight management. A comparison of adult nutrition products, including meal replacement products, is available in the current edition of *Compendium of Products for Minor Ailments* published by the Canadian Pharmacists Association.
- All popular diets result in weight loss and some programs (Jenny Craig, Weight Watchers) may help patients maintain the loss while they remain in the program.[6,7] The long-term efficacy and safety of all diets have not been established in randomized controlled trials.

Physical Activity

Increased physical activity and fitness are clearly associated with a reduction in cardiometabolic risk.[8] Regular physical activity also enhances the patient's sense of well-being, promotes weight maintenance, reduces insulin resistance and the loss of bone mineral density that is associated with weight loss.[9] However, exercise alone is not an effective strategy for weight loss.

Individual patients should be assessed to determine the level of fitness before starting an exercise program. A treadmill stress test should be considered for individuals with elevated cardiovascular risk.

- Exercise coupled with a judicious caloric-deficit meal plan accelerates fat loss while maintaining lean body mass, and helps sustain weight loss over the long term.
- Encourage all patients to spend ≥30 minutes doing continuous or intermittent (minimum of 10-minute bouts accumulated throughout the day) physical activity at least 5 days each week. Initially, physical activity could begin with 5–10 minute bouts, with increasing frequency, duration and intensity over time.
- The initial goal is to increase energy expenditure by 700–1000 kcal/week or about 100–130 kcal daily (Table 3).

- Walking 10 000 steps per day (measured by a pedometer) is associated with increased weight maintenance.
- Promote a daily energy expenditure of about 300 kcal. Recommend a variety of activities that are enjoyable and can be continued for life.
- Resistance training to build lean body mass sustains weight loss in the long term.

Figure 1: **Management of Obesity**

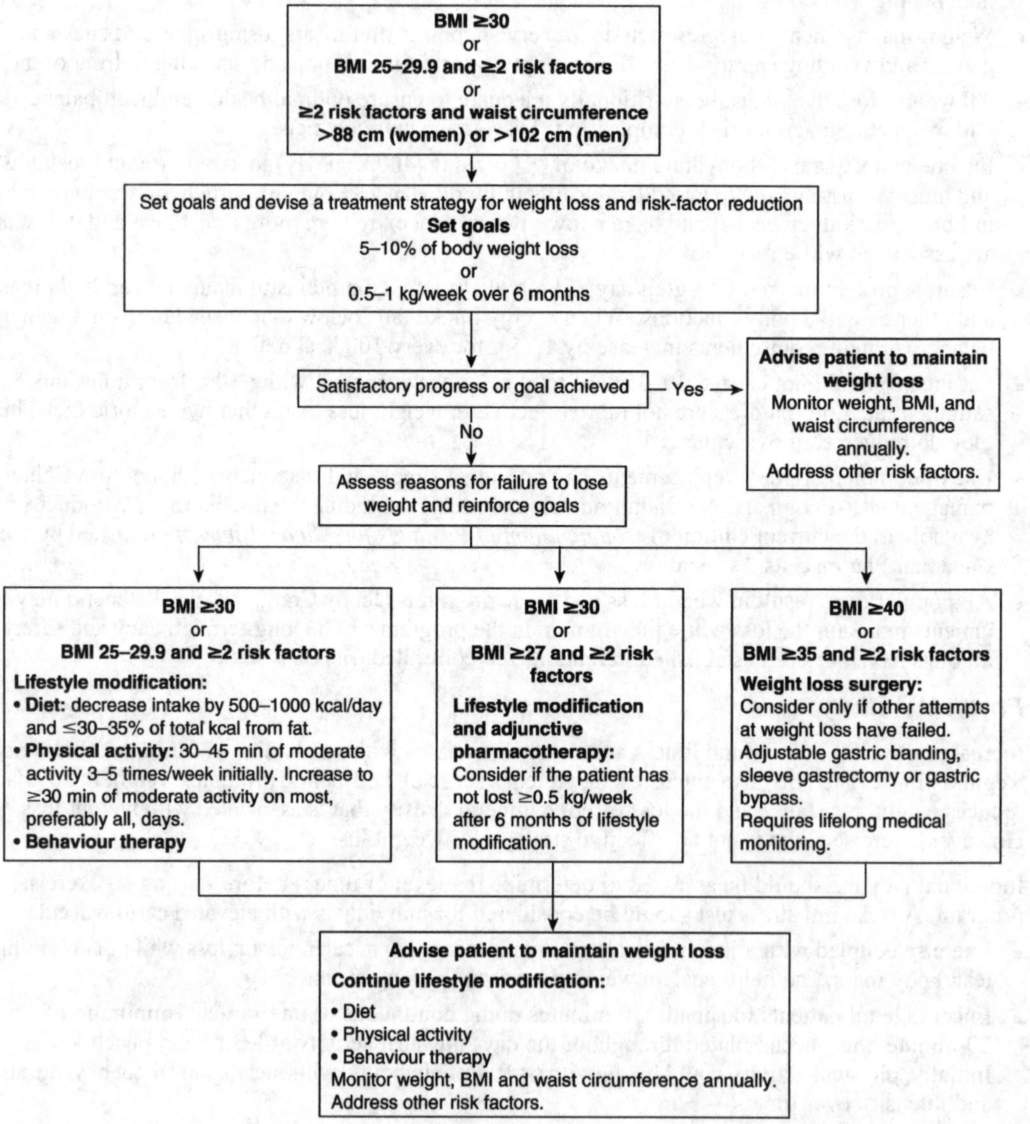

Table 3: **Average Energy Consumption Per Hour of Low-intensity Forms of Physical Activity**

Activity	Average Energy Cost[a] Kilocalories	Kilojoules
Shopping	150	630
Light housework (cleaning, vacuuming)	220	920
Dancing	250	1050
Walking		
4 km/h or 2.5 mph	200	840
6 km/h or 4 mph	300	1260

[a] 1 kilocalorie is approximately 4.2 kilojoules. The calories consumed per hour depend on the intensity of the activity and can range from 150 calories for shopping to just over 300 calories for brisk walking at 6 km/h. An example of low-intensity endurance exercise activity is walking at a brisk pace (6 km/h) for 60 minutes daily (about 50% of maximal oxygen consumption, VO_{2max}).

Pharmacologic Choices

- The combination of lifestyle modification and anti-obesity drug therapy is superior to lifestyle modification alone in achieving a target weight loss of 5–10% over the long term, and may improve health status.
- Discontinuation of anti-obesity medication generally results in weight regain and should therefore be continued as long as there is benefit.
- No anti-obesity drugs have yet shown an effect on mortality.
- **Sibutramine**, a serotonin and norepinephrine reuptake inhibitor (SNRI), was voluntarily withdrawn from the Canadian market in 2010 due to concerns about heart-related adverse events.
- There is no indication that currently available anti-obesity medications are associated with pulmonary hypertension, valvular dysfunction or other cardiovascular abnormalities associated with earlier anti-obesity medications.

Appetite Suppressants

Bupropion is a sympathomimetic drug that has a mild appetite-suppressant effect. Bupropion sustained-release, at a dose of 300 or 400 mg per day for 24 weeks, was well tolerated by obese adults and was associated with weight loss of 7.2% and 10.1%; weight loss was maintained at 48 weeks.[10]

Lorcaserin, an orally active 5-HTc receptor agonist, is available in the United States for the treatment of obesity. In a 1-year randomized controlled trial in obese patients, weight loss with lorcaserin 10 mg twice daily or once daily was 5.8% and 4.7%, respectively, compared with 2.8% with placebo.[11] A similar degree of weight loss with significant improvements in glycemic control was also seen in patients with type 2 diabetes.[12] Common adverse events were headache, back pain, dizziness, nasopharyngitis and nausea. Lorcaserin is currently not available in Canada.

Topiramate/phentermine (controlled release) is approved in the United States for the treatment of obesity. In a 1-year study, change in bodyweight was −1.4 kg, −8.1 kg and −10.2 kg in the patients assigned to placebo, topiramate 46 mg plus phentermine 7.5 mg, and topiramate 92 mg plus phentermine 15 mg, respectively.[13] A similar degree of weight loss was noted in patients with severe obesity.[14] Common adverse events included paresthesia, dry mouth, constipation, dysgeusia and insomnia. This combination is currently not available in Canada.

Lipase Inhibitors

Orlistat is a pancreatic and gastric lipase inhibitor that reduces dietary fat absorption by 30%, resulting in an effective reduction in caloric intake of around 180 kcal/day on a diet containing 60 g of fat.[15]

A high fat intake is poorly tolerated during orlistat therapy because of an increased incidence of GI adverse effects, including bloating, steatorrhea and oily discharge. Orlistat is less effective in patients on low-fat diets and is difficult to take for individuals with irregular eating patterns. In randomized, double-blind long-term trials, patients lost on average 2.9% more weight over 1 year than those on placebo.[16] Orlistat is approved for use in obese patients with type 2 diabetes mellitus, in whom it improves glycemic and metabolic control.

Incretins

Liraglutide is a glucagon-like peptide-1 (GLP-1) agonist currently approved for the treatment of type 2 diabetes mellitus (T2DM). Preliminary evidence suggests that liraglutide 3 mg daily subcutaneously, a dose higher than currently recommended for managing T2DM, may also promote[17] and maintain weight loss.[18] Liraglutide is currently under investigation for the treatment of obesity.

Bariatric Surgery

Evidence suggests that bariatric surgery provides significant psychosocial and health benefits in patients with severe obesity,[19] including reduction in both cardiovascular and all-cause mortality.[20,21,22] Maintenance of weight loss for up to 15 years has also been demonstrated.[23] As a result, bariatric surgery should be considered in patients with severe obesity (Class II or III) [Evidence: SORT B*].[19,20,21,22,24] Furthermore, the superiority of bariatric surgery to conventional treatment in preventing and controlling diabetes in obese patients has been demonstrated.[25,26,27,28,29]

Risks and long-term complications of bariatric surgery vary depending on baseline patient characteristics and type of surgery performed. One year mortality rates postsurgery range from 0.3%–4.6%; long-term mortality data are not available.[30,31,32] Postoperative complications occur in 17% of patients and the re-operation rate is 7%.[32] Complications most commonly include GI obstruction, surgical site infections and incisional hernia.[33]

Eligibility for Bariatric Surgery

Bariatric surgery should be considered in individuals with BMI ≥40 kg/m², or BMI ≥35 kg/m² if they have comorbidities.[34] Relative contraindications for bariatric surgery include severe heart failure, unstable coronary artery disease, end-stage lung disease, active cancer diagnosis/treatment, cirrhosis with portal hypertension, Crohn's disease, uncontrolled drug or alcohol dependency, severely impaired intellectual capacity. Laparoscopic surgery may be difficult or impossible in patients with giant ventral hernias, severe intra-abdominal adhesions, large liver, high BMI with central obesity or physiological intolerance of pneumoperitoneum.

A team approach to perioperative care is mandatory with special attention to nutritional and metabolic issues.[35] The best outcomes are achieved by interdisciplinary teams working in high-volume centres and are largely dependent on appropriate patient selection and follow up. Patients with underlying psychiatric or emotional issues should be carefully evaluated. Counsel on the need for lifelong nutritional changes to avoid nutritional complications.

Nutritional Counseling

Postoperative nutritional therapy following bariatric surgery depends on the type of bariatric procedure performed.[35] All post-bariatric surgery patients should have routine screening for nutritional deficiencies. See Table 4 below for specific recommendations. Drugs to avoid after bariatric surgery include GI irritants, such as oral bisphosphonates and NSAIDs.

* SORT (Strength of Recommendation Taxonomy) is a rating system (A, B or C) that addresses the quality of available evidence. For more information consult **How to Use *Compendium of Therapeutic Choices*** on page xxv.

Table 4: **Postoperative Follow Up for Bariatric Surgery**

Follow up	LAGB	LSG	RYGB	BPD/BPD-DS
Visits: initial, interval until stable, once stable (months)	1, 1–2, 12	1, 3–6, 12	1, 3, 6–12	1, 3, 6
CBC, chemistry panel with each visit (iron at baseline and when needed)	Y	Y	Y	Y
Lipid evaluation every 6–12 months	Y	Y	Y	Y
Bone densitometry every 2 years	Y	Y	Y	Y
24-hour urinary excretion yearly (initial at 6 months)	Y	Y	Y	Y
Vitamin B_{12} yearly (3–6 months if supplemented)	Y	Y	Y	Y
Folic acid, iron, vitamin D, iPTH	N	N	Y	Y
Vitamin A every 6–12 months	N	N	Optional	Y
Copper, zinc, selenium	N	N	Y	Y
Thiamine	Y	Y	Y	Y
Assess need for antihypertensives, gout therapy and gallstone prophylaxis with each visit	Y	Y	Y	Y

Abbreviations: BPD/BPD-DS = laparoscopic biliopancreatic diversion/BPD-duodenal switch; CBC = complete blood count; DXA = dual energy x-ray absorptiometry; iPTH = intact parathyroid hormone; LAGB = laparoscopic adjustable gastric banding ; LSG = laparoscopic sleeve gastrectomy; RYGB = laparascopic Roux-en-Y gastric bypass

Choices during Pregnancy and Breastfeeding

Obesity and Pregnancy

Obesity during pregnancy has been associated with gestational diabetes, gestational hypertension, pre-eclampsia, birth defects, Cesarean delivery, fetal macrosomia, perinatal deaths, postpartum anemia and childhood obesity in offspring.[36]

Recent guidelines recommend that preconceptional and interconceptional counselling be made available to all women of reproductive age, to raise awareness of possible pregnancy complications associated with obesity and how to prevent them.[37,38]

Pre-pregnancy Considerations

Adipose tissue is critical in controlling the regulation of estrogen production and the concentration of sex hormone-binding globulin in the blood. Body weight and composition play an important role in pubertal maturation, whereby excessive weight gain at younger ages is associated with earlier menarche and menstrual problems including amenorrhea, oligomenorrhea and long menstrual cycles.[39] Obesity is a strong risk factor for polycystic ovarian syndrome, which results in menstrual irregularities and chronic anovulation. In the United States, 25% of ovulatory infertility may be attributable to overweight and obesity.[40]

Menstrual functioning, ovulation and fertility improve with weight loss. In women with polycystic ovarian syndrome, as little as a 5% reduction in weight has been associated with improved fertility.[41] Maintaining this weight loss may prove challenging for women of childbearing age. Restrained eating, dieting or weight cycling prior to pregnancy have been associated with gaining more weight during pregnancy.

Bariatric surgery for morbidly obese women has been associated with better outcomes in mother and child.[42] However, due to the possibility of nutritional deficiencies, women becoming pregnant after bariatric surgery are advised to seek care from an obstetrician specializing in high-risk pregnancies.

Management during Pregnancy and Postpartum Period

Maternal Complications during Pregnancy

During pregnancy, obese women are at increased risk for gestational diabetes mellitus (GDM) and preeclampsia[37] and should be screened for glucose intolerance early in prenatal care. Tight glucose control in women with GDM seems to reduce the risk for preeclampsia.

Maternal Complications in the Peripartum Period

Cesarean deliveries and associated morbidities are more common among obese women.[37] Overweight or obese women have more postoperative complications following cesarean delivery.[37] These include: wound infection/breakdown, excessive blood loss, deep venous thrombophlebitis and postpartum endometritis. Labour is also longer in overweight and obese women.

Birth Outcomes

Congenital anomalies are more common in infants born to obese mothers. Neural tube defects (NTDs) are approximately twice as frequent, with spina bifida being more common than anencephaly. Other birth defects that can occur more frequently include: oral clefts, heart anomalies, hydrocephaly and abdominal wall abnormalities. Maternal obesity has been found to be a risk factor for intrauterine fetal death and stillbirth.[43]

Management

During pregnancy all overweight and obese women should be informed about current gestational weight gain target goals, but also advised to not lose weight during pregnancy. They should be counselled about eating healthy diets and be encouraged to be physically active. Because of the potential effect on vitamin absorption, **orlistat** is not recommended during pregnancy. Information regarding the safety of **bupropion** during pregnancy is conflicting; the risks are likely small and bupropion should not necessarily be withheld during pregnancy.[44] The potential benefits and risks of continuing bupropion should be discussed with the patient.

Obesity and Breastfeeding

Maternal overweight or obesity may be associated with decreased rates of breastfeeding.[38] This is concerning, as breastfeeding has been associated with reduced development of obesity later in life. A high BMI before conception has been shown to be inversely related to the successful initiation of breastfeeding, the duration of lactation and the amount of milk produced. Overweight and obesity adversely affect lactation performance in a variety of ways.[38] There are mechanical difficulties associated with latching on and proper positioning of the infant. The high cesarean section rates among this subpopulation delays the onset of first suckling. If first suckling occurs ≥48 hours after delivery, prolactin response will be lower, which may compromise milk production and over time lead to early cessation of lactation.

Overweight and obese mothers should be encouraged to breastfeed as well as eat a healthy diet and engage in regular exercise. It is unlikely that **orlistat** is excreted in breast milk since only traces are absorbed orally.[45] However, the drug can cause vitamin deficiencies, which may be undesirable in breastfeeding women. Its use is therefore not recommended. Limited evidence suggests that **bupropion** is excreted in breast milk in very small amounts and unlikely to cause side effects in breastfed infants.[46] However there are two case reports of possible seizure in breastfed infants.

A discussion of general principles on the use of medications in these special populations can be found in Appendix II and Appendix III. Other specialized reference sources are also provided in these appendices.

Therapeutic Tips

- Obesity is a chronic disease—focus on long-term strategies rather than short-term interventions.
- Identify psychosocial, emotional and physical barriers—addressing these may be required before obesity treatment is initiated.
- Focus on improvements in health and quality of life, not on changes in body weight. Weight loss of only 3% can achieve health benefits; reaching a BMI $\leq 25\ kg/m^2$ is not necessary to achieve health benefits.
- Correct disordered eating; encourage 3 meals and 3 snacks. Avoid hunger because it leads to binge eating.
- Meal replacements are an easy, efficient and inexpensive way to facilitate portion control. Recommend meal replacements that do not contain trans fats, have a low glycemic load and are high in fibre.
- Exercise is not the best way to lose weight, but can reduce visceral fat, increase cardiovascular fitness and help with weight maintenance.
- Prepare the patient for the weight-loss plateau; managing expectations is an important part of obesity management.

Table 5: Drugs Used for the Management of Obesity

Class	Drug	Dose	Adverse Effects	Drug Interactions	Comments	Cost[a]
Lipase Inhibitors	*orlistat* Xenical	120 mg daily to TID po with each meal containing fat	Oily spotting, flatus with discharge, fecal urgency.	Decreased absorption of soluble vitamins. Administer cyclosporine at least 2 h apart from orlistat.	Contraindicated in patients with chronic malabsorption syndrome or cholestasis. Minimal systemic absorption. Advise patients to take a multivitamin daily ≥2 h before or after orlistat or at bedtime.	$$$
Noradrenergic Appetite Suppressants	*bupropion* ❥ Wellbutrin SR, generics	Initial: 150 mg daily po Maximum: 150 mg BID	Dry mouth, constipation, agitation, insomnia and anxiety. Seizures occur rarely (risk increases with dose).	Avoid concurrent use of drugs that lower the seizure threshold.	Not approved for obesity. To minimize seizure risk, single doses should not exceed 150 mg and the total daily dose should not exceed 300 mg. Caution in patients with hepatic impairment.	$

[a] Cost of 30-day supply; includes drug cost only.
Legend: $ <$20 $$ $75–100 $$$ $125–150

Suggested Readings

Dietz WH, Robinson TN. Clinical practice. Overweight children and adolescents. *N Engl J Med* 2005;352(20):2100-9.

Freedhoff Y, Sharma AM. *Best weight: a practical guide to office-based obesity management.* Edmonton (AB): Canadian Obesity Network; 2010.

Haslam DW, James WP. Obesity. *Lancet* 2005;366(9492):1197-209.

Jensen MD, Ryan DH, Apovian CM et al. 2013 AHA/ACC/TOS guideline for the management of overweight and obesity in adults: a report of the American College of Cardiology/American Heart Association Task Force on Practice Guidelines and The Obesity Society. *J Am Coll Cardiol* 2013 Nov 7. [Epub ahead of print].

Lau DC, Douketis JD, Morrison KM et al. 2006 Canadian clinical practice guidelines on the management and prevention of obesity in adults and children [summary]. *CMAJ* 2007;176(8):S1-13.

O'Mara NB. Bariatric surgery and medication use. *Canadian Pharmacist's Letter* 2013;20(12):291228.

Strychar I. Diet in the management of weight loss. *CMAJ* 2006;174(1):56-63.

Yanovski SZ, Yanovski JA. Long-term drug treatment for obesity: a systematic and clinical review. *JAMA* 2014;311(1):74-86.

References

1. Tjepkema M. *Measured obesity. Adult obesity in Canada: measured height and weight.* In: Nutrition: findings from the Canadian Community Health Survey 2004;(1). Available from: www.statcan.gc.ca/pub/82-620-m/2005001/pdf/4224906-eng.pdf. Accessed January 11, 2012.
2. Franzosi MG. Should we continue to use BMI as a cardiovascular risk factor? *Lancet* 2006;368(9536):624-5.
3. Padwal RS, Pajewski NM, Allison DB et al. Using the Edmonton obesity staging system to predict mortality in a population-representative cohort of people with overweight and obesity. *CMAJ* 2011;183(14):E1059-66.
4. Vallis M, Piccinini-Vallis H, Sharma AM et al. Clinical review: modified 5 As: minimal intervention for obesity counseling in primary care. *Can Fam Physician* 2013;59(1):27-31.
5. Merchant A, Yusuf S, Sharma AM. A cardiologist's guide to waist management. *Heart* 2006;92(7):865-6.
6. Rock CL, Flatt SW, Sherwood NE et al. Effect of a free prepared meal and incentivized weight loss program on weight loss and weight loss maintenance in obese and overweight women: a randomized controlled trial. *JAMA* 2010;304(16):1803-10.
7. Jebb SA, Ahern AL, Olson AD et al. Primary care referral to a commercial provider for weight loss treatment versus standard care: a randomised controlled trial. *Lancet* 2011;378(9801):1485-92.
8. Shaw K, Gennat H, O'Rourke P et al. Exercise for overweight or obesity. *Cochrane Database Syst Rev* 2006;(4):CD003817.
9. Villareal DT, Fontana L, Weiss EP et al. Bone mineral density response to caloric restriction-induced weight loss or exercise-induced weight loss: a randomized controlled trial. *Arch Intern Med* 2006;166(22):2502-10.
10. Anderson JW, Greenway FL, Fujioka K et al. Bupropion SR enhances weight loss: a 48-week double-blind, placebo-controlled trial. *Obes Res* 2002;10(7):633-41.
11. Fidler MC, Sanchez M, Raether B et al. A one-year randomized trial of lorcaserin for weight loss in obese and overweight adults: the Blossom trial. *J Clin Endocrinol Metab* 2011;96(10):3067-77.
12. O'Neil PM, Smith SR, Weissman NJ et al. Randomized placebo-controlled clinical trial of lorcaserin for weight loss in type 2 diabetes mellitus: the BLOOM-DM study. *Obesity* 2012;20(7):1426-36.
13. Gadde KM, Allison DB, Ryan DH et al. Effects of low-dose, controlled-release, phentermine plus topiramate combination on weight and associated comorbidities in overweight and obese adults (CONQUER): a randomised, placebo-controlled, phase 3 trial. *Lancet* 2011;377(9774):1341-52.
14. Allison DB, Gadde KM, Garvey WT et al. Controlled-release phentermine/topiramate in severely obese adults: a randomized controlled trial (EQUIP). *Obesity* 2012;20(2):330-42.
15. Hutton B, Fergusson D. Changes in body weight and serum lipid profile in obese patients treated with orlistat in addition to a hypocaloric diet: a systematic review of randomized clinical trials. *Am J Clin Nutr* 2004;80(6):1461-8.
16. Rucker D, Padwal R, Li SK et al. Long term pharmacotherapy for obesity and overweight: updated meta-analysis. *BMJ* 2007;335(7631):1194-9.
17. Astrup A, Rossner S, Van Gaal L et al. Effects of liraglutide in the treatment of obesity: a randomized, double-blind, placebo-controlled study. *Lancet* 2009;374(9701):1606-16.
18. Wadden TA, Hollander P, Klein S et al. Weight maintenance and additional weight loss with liraglutide after low-calorie-diet induced weight loss: the SCALE Maintenance randomized study. *Int J Obes (Lond)* 2013;37(11):1443-51.
19. Buchwald H, Avidor Y, Braunwald E et al. Bariatric surgery: a systematic review and meta-analysis. *JAMA* 2004;292(14):1724-37.
20. Sjöström L, Peltonen M, Jacobson P et al. Bariatric surgery and long-term cardiovascular events. *JAMA* 2012;307(1):56-65.
21. Adams TD, Gress RE, Smith SC et al. Long-term mortality after gastric bypass surgery. *N Engl J Med* 2007;357(8):753-61.
22. Sjöström L, Narbro K, Sjöström CD et al. Effects of bariatric surgery on mortality in Swedish subjects. *N Engl J Med* 2007;357(8):741-52.
23. O'Brien PE, MacDonald L, Anderson M et al. Long-term outcomes after bariatric surgery: fifteen-year follow-up of adjustable gastric banding and a systematic review of the bariatric surgical literature. *Ann Surg* 2013;257(1):87-94.
24. Lau DC, Douketis JD, Morrison KM et al. 2006 Canadian clinical practice guidelines on the management and prevention of obesity in adults and children [summary]. *CMAJ* 2007;176(8):S1-13.
25. Gloy VL, Briel M, Bhatt DL et al. Bariatric surgery versus non-surgical treatment for obesity: a systematic review and meta-analysis of randomized controlled trials. *BMJ* 2013;347:f5934.
26. Carlsson LM, Peltonen M, Ahlin S et al. Bariatric surgery and prevention of type 2 diabetes in Swedish obese subjects. *N Engl J Med* 2012;367(6):695-704.

27. Schauer PR, Kashyap SR, Wolski K et al. Bariatric surgery versus intensive medical therapy in obese patients with diabetes. *N Engl J Med* 2012;366(17):1567-76.
28. Mingrone G, Panunzi S, De Gaetano C et al. Bariatric surgery versus conventional medical therapy for type 2 diabetes. *N Engl J Med* 2012;366(17):1577-85.
29. Schauer PR, Bhatt DL, Kirwan JP et al. Bariatric surgery versus intensive medical therapy for diabetes—3-year outcomes. *N Engl J Med* 2014 Mar 31. [Epub ahead of print].
30. Flum DR, Salem L, Elrod JA et al. Early mortality among Medicare beneficiaries undergoing bariatric surgical procedures. *JAMA* 2005;294(15):1903-8.
31. Shikora SA, Kim JJ, Tarnoff ME et al. Laparoscopic Roux-en-Y gastric bypass: results and learning curve of a high-volume academic program. *Arch Surg* 2005;140(4):362-7.
32. Chang SH, Stoll CR, Song J et al. The effectiveness and risks of bariatric surgery: an updated systematic review and meta-analysis, 2003-2012. *JAMA Surg* 2014;149(3):275-87.
33. Encinosa WE, Bernard DM, Chen CC et al. Healthcare utilization and outcomes after bariatric surgery. *Med Care* 2006;44(8):706-12.
34. Jensen MD, Ryan DH, Apovian CM et al. 2013 AHA/ACC/TOS guideline for the management of overweight and obesity in adults: a report of the American College of Cardiology/American Heart Association Task Force on Practice Guidelines and The Obesity Society. *J Am Coll Cardiol* 2013 Nov 7. [Epub ahead of print].
35. Mechanick JI, Youdim A, Jones DB et al. Clinical practice guidelines for the perioperative nutritional, metabolic, and nonsurgical support of the bariatric surgery patient—2013 updates: cosponsored by American Association of Clinical Endocrinologists, The Obesity Society, and American Society for Metabolic & Bariatric Surgery. *Objesity (Silver Spring)* 2013;21(Suppl 1):S1-27.
36. Waller DK, Shaw GM, Rasmussen SA et al. Prepregnancy obesity as a risk factor for structural birth defects. *Arch Pediatr Adolesc Med* 2007;161(8):745-50.
37. Davies GA, Maxwell C, McLeod L et al. SOCG clinical practice guidelines: obesity in pregnancy. No. 239, February 2010. *Int J Gynaecol Obstet* 2010;110(2):165-73.
38. Siega-Riz AM, King JC. Position of the American Dietetic Association and American Society for Nutrition: obesity, reproduction, and pregnancy outcomes. *J Am Diet Assoc* 2009;109(5):918-27.
39. Pasquali R, Pelusi C, Genghini S et al. Obesity and reproductive disorders in women. *Hum Reprod Update* 2003;9(4):359-72.
40. Rich-Edwards JW, Goldman MB, Willett WC et al. Adolescent body mass index and infertility caused by ovulatory disorder. *Am J Obstet Gynecol* 1994;171(1):171-7.
41. Sarwer DB, Allison KC, Gibbons LM et al. Pregnancy and obesity: a review and agenda for future research. *J Womens Health (Larchmt)* 2006;15(6):720-33.
42. Lesko J, Peaceman A. Pregnancy outcomes in women after bariatric surgery compared with obese and morbidly obese controls. *Obstet Gynecol* 2012;119(3):547-54.
43. King JC. Maternal obesity, metabolism, and pregnancy outcomes. *Annu Rev Nutr* 2006;26:271-91.
44. Briggs GG, Freeman RK, Yaffe SJ. *Drugs in pregnancy and lactation: a reference guide to fetal and neonatal risk.* 9th ed. Philadelphia: Wolters Kluwer Health; Lippincott Williams & Wilkins; 2011.
45. Orlistat. In: Drugs and Lactation Database (LactMed). Besthesda (MD): U.S. National Library of Medicine. Available from: toxnet.nlm.nih.gov/.
46. Bupropion. In: Drugs and Lactation Database (LactMed). Besthesda (MD): U.S. National Library of Medicine. Available from: toxnet.nlm.nih.gov/.

Chapter 34
Thyroid Disorders

Heather Lochnan, MD, FRCPC

Thyroid disease is extremely common, with women more frequently affected than men. The symptoms associated with thyroid disease are often nonspecific. A high index of suspicion coupled with a low threshold for screening for thyroid disease will capture most affected patients.

This chapter addresses hypothyroidism, hyperthyroidism and thyroid nodules and goitre.

Goals of Therapy

- Achieve a euthyroid state in patients with hyperthyroidism or hypothyroidism
- Recognize which patients with goitre or thyroid nodules require treatment
- Manage patients with thyroid disease during all stages of life, including pregnancy

Hypothyroidism

Hypothyroidism is a clinical syndrome that usually results from a deficiency of thyroid hormone or, in areas with sufficient iodine supply, autoimmune thyroid disease (Table 1). Rarely, it can be due to resistance to thyroid hormone. An elevated thyroid-stimulating hormone (TSH) measurement is a very sensitive indicator of hypothyroidism but may be low or normal in pituitary or hypothalamic disease. *Subclinical hypothyroidism* is defined by an elevated TSH with normal thyroid hormone levels.[1] If subclinical hypothyroidism is confirmed, consider treatment, especially in patients with TSH >10 mU/L (normally 0.3–6 mU/L, depending on the laboratory), an abnormal lipid profile, symptoms of hypothyroidism and in patients who are antithyroid peroxidase (anti-TPO)-positive or who are planning a pregnancy.[2,3]

Table 1: **Causes of Hypothyroidism**

Cause	Comments
Hashimoto's thyroiditis	Most common cause; anti-TPO levels very high
Iatrogenic	Causes include: surgical removal of thyroid; ^{131}I therapy; drugs such as amiodarone, iodinated contrast agents, lithium, sulfonylureas
Hypothyroid phase of subacute thyroiditis	Usually transient
Congenital	Aplasia of thyroid; dyshormonogenesis
Iodine deficiency	Rare in North America
Recovering phase of nonthyroidal illness	Transiently elevated TSH
Pituitary disorder	*Secondary* hypothyroidism; TSH low or normal; fT_4 usually low
Hypothalamic disorder	*Tertiary* hypothyroidism; TSH low or normal; fT_4 usually low
Resistance to thyroid hormone	High TSH, fT_3 and fT_4

Abbreviations: anti-TPO = antithyroid peroxidase; fT_3 = free triiodothyronine; fT_4 = free thyroxine

Investigations

- Thorough history with attention to:
  - symptoms such as fatigue, impaired memory, constipation, cold intolerance and changes in skin or hair
- Physical examination with attention to:
  - appearance, e.g., coarse features, dry skin and hair
  - hypertension, bradycardia
  - delayed relaxation phase of reflexes
  - extreme cases may present with myxedema coma (hypotension, coma, hypothermia)
- Laboratory investigations:
  - TSH
  - free triiodothyronine (fT_3)
  - free thyroxine (fT_4)
  - antithyroid peroxidase (anti-TPO)

Therapeutic Choices

Pharmacologic Choices

Levothyroxine (L-T_4)

Replacement therapy with L-T_4 alone is the treatment of choice[4] (see Table 4). The goal is to normalize the TSH level. Replacement dosages average 1.6 µg/kg/day in adults and 10–16 µg/kg/day in newborns. Dosage adjustment is made every 4–6 weeks as needed. Generally, it takes 6 weeks to attain a new steady state after dosage adjustments. In the elderly, or in patients with coronary artery disease, start with a dose as low as 12.5 µg/day as tolerated, and titrate every 4 weeks. High doses may be associated with an increased risk of fracture in elderly patients.[5]

Liothyronine (Triiodothyronine, T_3)

T_3 is used for short-term management of patients with thyroid cancer undergoing withdrawal of L-T_4, when recombinant TSH is not an option, in order to prepare for radioactive iodine therapy. The combination of L-T_4 and T_3 is occasionally used for replacement therapy, though recent studies have shown little or no benefit of combination therapy and there is concern of causing adverse effects with T_3.[6,7] Dessicated thyroid comes from animal thyroid, may not provide reliable dosing, and presents no clear therapeutic advantage.

Choices during Pregnancy and Breastfeeding

Hypothyroidism and Pregnancy

Hypothyroidism can be associated with infertility and miscarriage as well as with lower intelligence scores in children of women who had elevated TSH at the time of conception.[8,9] Women who are on thyroid hormone replacement or who are at risk of hypothyroidism should have a preconception TSH measurement and ensure it is normalized. In the first trimester TSH levels are usually low due to high beta HCG levels. If a woman's first-trimester TSH is not suppressed, this may indicate under-treatment with thyroxine or a new diagnosis of hypothyroidism; follow with a repeat TSH or adjust the dose of thyroxine.

Management

Women who are known to be hypothyroid and are taking thyroid hormone replacement should be advised to increase their thyroid hormone dose by 2 extra tablets per week immediately following a positive pregnancy test. Further dose adjustment should be based on TSH levels.[10] Thyroid binding globulins increase during pregnancy so requirements for L-T_4 replacement may increase by up to 50% during pregnancy to maintain TSH at around 2–5 mU/L.[11] Throughout pregnancy, women on thyroid hormone replacement should have a TSH level every 6 weeks or 4 weeks after a dosage adjustment. Remember the TSH level may be low in the first trimester, and no reduction in dosage is required if the fT_4 and fT_3 levels are normal.

An ideal TSH level is less than 2.5 mU/L in the first trimester, less than 3 mU/L in the second and third trimesters.[8,12]

Postpartum, thyroid hormone requirements return to prepregnancy values. Iron supplements, which can lead to decreased absorption of thyroxine, are frequently used in pregnant women. Separate administration times by at least 6 hours (see Table 4).

Reassure women that their thyroid hormone therapy is safe during pregnancy and breastfeeding and that thyroid hormone replacement is important to ensure a healthy pregnancy and normal fetal development.

Referral to an endocrinologist is indicated if, despite dosage adjustment, the patient continues to have TSH out of target range.

Hypothyroidism and Breastfeeding

Untreated or inadequately treated hypothyroidism in the breastfeeding mother will augment symptoms of fatigue, cold intolerance and constipation but is not likely to have effects on the baby.

Management

Manage hypothyroidism just as in the nonbreastfeeding woman; avoid over-replacement with thyroid hormone.

A discussion of general principles on the use of medications in these special populations can be found in Appendix II and Appendix III. Other specialized reference sources are also provided in these appendices.

Therapeutic Tips

- One way to make a quick dosage adjustment and allow the patient to use the thyroxine tablets they have on hand is to ask the patient to take one extra pill per week (if TSH is slightly above target) or one less per week (if TSH is slightly below target).
- Numerous drugs can interfere with the absorption and metabolism of L-T_4 (Table 4). Iron supplementation frequently decreases L-T_4 absorption.
- If symptoms are serious, consider a patient's fitness to drive.
- *Myxedema coma* is a medical emergency associated with severe hypothyroidism. Typical symptoms include hypotension and decreased level of consciousness. Patients are treated with **levothyroxine** 300–500 µg iv initially, followed by 100 µg iv daily, and concomitant corticosteroids such as hydrocortisone 100 mg Q8H iv. Supportive therapy and passive rewarming are indicated as required.

Hyperthyroidism

Hyperthyroidism (thyrotoxicosis) is defined as the syndrome of excessive thyroid hormone production and its effects (Table 2). *Subclinical hyperthyroidism* is common and can be a risk factor for atrial fibrillation.[13,14] In subclinical hyperthyroidism, TSH is suppressed while thyroid hormone levels are normal. Treatment is indicated if the patient is frail and/or elderly, has other risk factors for atrial fibrillation, has osteoporosis or has symptoms of hyperthyroidism.

Table 2: **Causes of Hyperthyroidism**

Cause	Comments
Graves' disease	Due to thyroid-stimulating immunoglobulins activating the TSH receptor; most common cause of hyperthyroidism; patients frequently have eye disease and possibly pretibial myxedema;[15] RAIU is elevated and thyroid scan with pertechnetate or ^{123}I shows a diffuse pattern
Subacute thyroiditis	Scan poorly defines the gland; RAIU is very low
Postpartum thyroiditis	Scan poorly defines the gland; RAIU is very low (not recommended if patient is lactating)
Toxic nodule	Thyroid scan shows hot area
Toxic multinodular goitre	Scan shows multiple hot areas; RAIU is slightly elevated
Iodine excess	Usually in setting of multinodular goitre; RAIU is low
Iatrogenic	Due to over-treatment with thyroid hormones; scan shows no thyroid; 0% RAIU
Struma ovarii	Very rare; thyroid hormone production in ectopic sites; RAIU is 0%; body scan will show thyroid tissue in ovary
Metastatic thyroid cancer	With large tumor burden
TSH-producing pituitary adenoma	TSH elevated
Stimulation of TSH receptor by excessive human chorionic gonadotropin	Examples are hydatidiform mole, hyperemesis gravidarum, other tumors; TSH is low or undetectable

Abbreviations: RAIU = radioactive iodine uptake; TSH = thyroid-stimulating hormone

Thyroid storm is a life-threatening medical emergency characterized by severe thyrotoxicosis as well as other signs and symptoms. It has many causes including radioactive iodine, infection, trauma, surgery or withdrawal from antithyroid drugs.

Investigations

- A thorough history with attention to:
  - symptoms such as weight loss, palpitations, diarrhea, heat intolerance and anxiety
- Physical examination with attention to:
  - signs such as eyelid lag, stare and the ophthalmopathy associated with Graves' disease; tachycardia; hyperreflexia; warm, moist skin; goitre or nodules
- Laboratory tests, nuclear medicine and imaging:
  - TSH, fT_3, fT_4
  - thyroid scan (scintigraphy); contraindicated in pregnancy
  - radioactive iodine uptake (RAIU); contraindicated in pregnancy

Note: Suppression of TSH can be seen in nonthyroidal illness, depression or treatment with corticosteroids and some centrally acting medications (e.g., domperidone, metoclopramide, dopamine).

Therapeutic Choices

Nonpharmacologic Choices

Consider thyroid surgery in patients with thyroid nodules, large goitre (see Thyroid Nodules and Goitre) and occasionally in patients with Graves' disease. Surgery is part of the management of thyroid cancer and ectopic production of thyroid hormone. Medical therapy with antithyroid drugs is frequently initiated prior to surgery to make the patient euthyroid if possible. Follow closely postoperatively to determine if thyroid replacement is required; avoid hypothyroidism in patients with Graves' ophthalmopathy.

Pharmacologic Choices

Use **radioactive iodine (^{131}I)** to ablate thyroid tissue in patients with Graves' disease, toxic autonomous nodules and toxic multinodular goitres. Inducing hypothyroidism is the main risk associated with its use. RAI is contraindicated in pregnancy. In patients with significant ophthalmopathy, use with caution, or use **corticosteroids** concomitantly.[16]

Methimazole and **propylthiouracil** decrease the production of thyroid hormones; Propylthiouracil can also block the conversion of L-T_4 to T_3. Both drugs must be stopped about 5 days prior to a thyroid scan (scintigraphy), radioactive iodine uptake or treatment with ^{131}I. Propylthiouracil may make the thyroid more resistant to ^{131}I.[17] Side effects of these agents include allergy, rash, agranulocytosis and, rarely, hepatotoxicity and nephrotoxicity. Methimazole is the preferred drug due to a lower incidence of serious (sometimes fatal) hepatotoxicity. Propylthiouracil should be avoided in children.[18] For dosing information see Table 5.

Beta-adrenergic blockers ameliorate the symptoms of adrenergic excess and are usually used adjunctively in the management of Graves' disease or toxic nodules. Propranolol and nadolol can decrease the conversion of L-T_4 to T_3. Use beta-blockers with caution in patients with asthma, obstructive respiratory disorders or Raynaud's phenomenon.

Iodine, in the form of oral **Lugol's solution** (6.3 mg iodide per drop), blocks thyroid hormone production. Iodine can be used in the acute management of severe hyperthyroidism. It should be given 1 hour after administration of an antithyroid drug.

Consider **corticosteroids** as adjuvant therapy in treatment-resistant cases.

Patients may inquire about whether to take selenium. **Selenium** 100 µg twice daily may help prevent worsening of mild Graves' ophthalmopathy and could be considered as supplemental therapy.[19] Patients should discuss this option with their eye care specialist.

The management of *thyroid storm* involves supportive therapy in conjunction with aggressive treatment with antithyroid medications, beta-blockers and corticosteroids. Use acetaminophen for hyperthermia, and avoid ASA and other NSAIDs.[20] Plasmapheresis can be considered in unresponsive cases.

Choices during Pregnancy and Breastfeeding

Hyperthyroidism and Pregnancy

During pregnancy, hyperthyroidism due to Graves' disease is the most likely scenario to be encountered. Hyperthyroidism due to subacute thyroiditis or other causes is possible though less common.[21] In general hyperthyroidism in pregnancy is well tolerated but should be treated to target the level of fT_3 and fT_4 near the upper limits of normal. Women with hyperthyroidism should achieve good control prior to conception and if treated with radioactive iodine should consult with a physician prior to planning a pregnancy to ensure thyroid levels are normal.[22,23] In general a woman should wait at least 6 months after receiving radioactive iodine before conceiving due to radiation precautions. Hypothyroidism is a frequent outcome of radioactive iodine therapy and thyroid replacement may be necessary.[8]

Untreated hyperthyroidism could increase the risk of fetal loss. Women with Graves' disease and their doctors should be aware that those treated with surgery or radioactive iodine may have a significant titre of stimulating thyroid receptor antibodies that could result in hyperthyroidism in the fetus or newborn. Treatment with antithyroid drugs could also affect the fetus and baby so the lowest doses necessary to achieve the treatment goals should be used during pregnancy and lactation.

In most women with Graves' disease hyperthyroidism may ameliorate during the second and third trimester and treatment may not be required. Unfortunately, like other autoimmune disorders, it may flare again in the postpartum period.

Management

Prior to conception, ensure that thyroid levels are well controlled. **Propylthiouracil** remains preferable to **methimazole** during the first trimester of pregnancy due to increased risk of congenital abnormalities with methimazole. Switch women using methimazole to propylthiouracil. Methimazole is an acceptable second choice if propylthiouracil is contraindicated and drug therapy is necessary. Propylthiouracil confers a risk of serious hepatotoxicity; consider switching back to methimazole after the first trimester if feasible without disrupting control.[8,25]

During pregnancy, women typically require lower doses of antithyroid medication and often go into remission. Monitoring is best done by measuring TSH, fT_3 and fT_4 every 6–8 weeks, and more often if a change in clinical status or dose is made. Aim for free hormone levels at or near the upper limit of normal to avoid overtreatment. The TSH is not the best guide and it is anticipated the TSH level will remain low.

At approximately 22 weeks' gestation, the titre of TSH receptor antibodies (TRAb) should be measured; a high titre may mean higher risk of hyperthyroidism for the fetus or newborn and specific monitoring by a neonatologist should be considered in those cases. Alternatively, if the titre is low in the first trimester, risks to the fetus are very low.[8,25]

To screen for potential side effects of antithyroid medication, a CBC with differential and ALT should be done simultaneously. Remind patients to stop the drug and contact their physician if they have fever, rash or jaundice. Blood work should be drawn to ensure the neutrophil count and ALT are normal before restarting the medication.

Avoid overtreatment of hyperthyroidism to avoid inducing hypothyroidism in the fetus or newborn. Ensure the mother's and baby's physicians are aware of the diagnosis of Graves' disease and any treatments given, even if the mother's disease is in remission.

Graves' disease may reactivate in the postpartum period. Women should be reminded of the symptoms of hyperthyroidism (e.g., rapid unexpected weight loss, heat intolerance, palpitations and tremor) and urged to have their thyroid levels checked if they suspect a problem.

Referral to an endocrinologist is reasonable for any patient who requires antithyroid medication during pregnancy; if not feasible the physician may choose to discuss the case by telephone with a specialist. Women with high titres of TRAb should have their case reviewed by an endocrinologist, and require intensive fetal assessment.

Hyperthyroidism and Breastfeeding

Hyperthyroidism during breastfeeding should be treated or could have detrimental effects on the mother (atrial fibrillation, bone loss and psychological effects in the short term; myopathy and cardiomyopathy long term). The goal is to ensure the fT_3 and fT_4 levels are near the upper limit of normal and not to overtreat. Hyperthyroidism may obviously be Graves' disease in someone with a prior history or could be the result of postpartum thyroiditis. Other causes are possible but less likely. In all cases, if the cause is not clear refer to an endocrinologist. Avoid the use of radioactive scans or radioactive iodine treatment during breastfeeding.

Management

Methimazole is now the preferred antithyroid drug during breastfeeding due to concerns of serious hepatotoxicity associated with propythiouracil, though **propylthiouracil** can be used if methimazole is contraindicated or not tolerated, or if warranted to facilitate care of the patient.

The baby's physician should be aware the mother is using antithyroid medication and may decide to check the baby's TSH level, especially if the mother is on a high dose (to ensure the baby is not made hypothyroid). **Beta-blockers** can be used for short-term management of symptomatic hyperthyroidism until control is achieved with antithyroid drugs. **Radioactive iodine** therapy should be postponed until breastfeeding is stopped. Thyroid hormone levels should be checked every 4–6 weeks until control is stable and then every 3 months.

To screen for potential side effects of antithyroid medication, a CBC with differential and ALT should be done simultaneously. Remind patients to stop the drug and contact their physician if they have fever, rash or jaundice. Blood work should be drawn to ensure the neutrophil count and ALT are normal before restarting the medication.

Women can be reassured that hyperthyroidism can be successfully managed in pregnant and breastfeeding women to ensure good health for the mother and baby. Management is a team approach and women must ensure their physicians are aware of their thyroid condition and medications.

A discussion of general principles on the use of medications in these special populations can be found in Appendix II and Appendix III. Other specialized reference sources are also provided in these appendices.

Therapeutic Tips

- Patients with Graves' disease may have prolonged suppression of TSH, despite normalization or decreased levels of thyroid hormones. Follow TSH, fT_3 and fT_4 levels.
- Patients on **propylthiouracil** or **methimazole** can develop a gradual neutropenia which may be detected by regular measurement of white blood cell counts with a differential. In many cases it occurs suddenly, and patients should be advised to contact their physician immediately if symptoms of infection occur.
- Warn patients who decline treatment of the risks of untreated hyperthyroidism, which include myopathy, cardiac arrhythmias, cardiomyopathy and osteoporosis.
- If symptoms are serious or remain uncontrolled, consider a patient's fitness to drive.

Thyroid Nodules and Goitre

Individuals with goitre may be at higher risk for disorders of thyroid function and should be screened with a TSH level. Goitres in euthyroid patients can be problematic if growing or causing compressive symptoms. The usual treatment is surgery. Thyroid suppression with **levothyroxine** can be considered in some cases, including pediatric cases, as it may help prevent further growth and in some cases shrink the gland.

Thyroid nodules are very common. They may be identified incidentally by ultrasound, CT or MRI of the neck.[24] Solitary nodules are concerning, but large or growing nodules within a multinodular goitre should be investigated similarly to a solitary nodule. Clinical history and high-quality ultrasound assessment for presence or absence of concerning features in each nodule with comparison to previous scans is useful to determine when to proceed to fine needle aspiration biopsy (see Figure 1).

Figure 1: **Management of Thyroid Nodules**

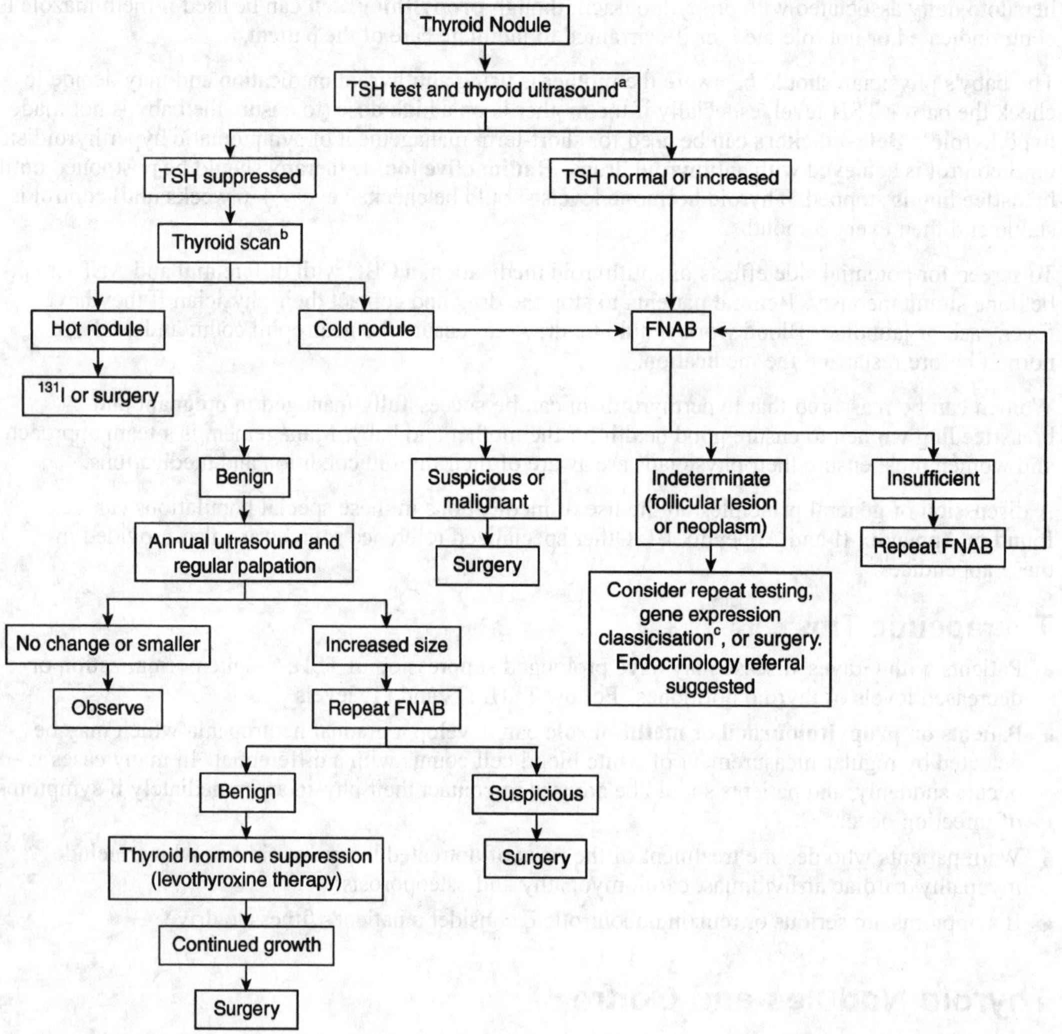

a The ultrasound report should note the size and characteristics of each nodule. Hypoechoic nodules ≥1.5cm, or nodules with concerning clinical history, features or growth should have FNAB.

b Nodules with intense activity of radioisotope are considered "hot" and are almost always benign. Those with less intense activity of radioisotope are considered "cold" and may be cancerous (3–15%).

c Not widely available at this time

Abbreviations: FNAB = fine needle aspiration biopsy; TSH = thyroid-stimulating hormone

Therapeutic Choices

Nonpharmacologic Choices

Surgery is the definitive therapy. Surgical pathology will confirm or exclude malignancy and reduce compressive symptoms. The risks associated with surgery include hypothyroidism, hypoparathyroidism and vocal cord paralysis. Consider surgery if 2 or more risk factors for malignancy (Table 3) are present.

Table 3: **Risk Factors for Thyroid Cancer**[27]

<20 or >60 years of age	Male gender
Family history of thyroid cancer	Previous malignancy
Lymphadenopathy	Prior radiation exposure
Nodule >4 cm in size or rapidly growing	Vocal cord paralysis
Nodule fixed to soft tissue	

Pharmacologic Choices

Radioactive iodine therapy can be used to treat a multinodular goitre or a *hot* nodule, with an associated risk of hypothyroidism (see Table 4).

Thyroid suppression therapy is no longer routinely used for nodules.[26] **Levothyroxine** can be considered to prevent further growth of a *benign* nodule.[28] The goal is to keep TSH below 1 mU/L, and above the lower limit of the normal range. In this setting, the risk of inducing hyperthyroidism is minimal.

Therapeutic Tips

- Ultrasound can be helpful to document the size of a goitre or nodule and whether it is changing in size. Some features on ultrasound may raise suspicion of malignancy.
- A thyroid scan is rarely needed if the TSH is normal.
- Repeat fine needle aspiration biopsy (FNAB) if a nodule is growing.

Table 4: Drugs Used in the Management of Hypothyroidism

Class	Drug	Dose	Adverse Effects	Drug Interactions	Comments	Cost[a]
Thyroid Hormones	*levothyroxine* (*L-T₄*) Eltroxin, Synthroid	Average adult replacement: 1.6 μg/kg/day po; elderly patients may need less Start with 12.5–25 μg/day po in those at risk of angina	Symptoms of hyperthyroidism if over-treated; possible exacerbation of angina.	Absorption may be reduced by iron salts, calcium salts, cholestyramine (separate administration by 6 h), colestipol and sucralfate. Response to warfarin may vary. Glycemic control may decline with initiation of levothyroxine, potentially necessitating dosage adjustment of antihyperglycemic agents.	Monitor TSH levels to adjust initial dosage after 6–8 wk, then as required or annually; adrenal insufficiency may be uncovered; dosage may have to be increased during pregnancy to maintain TSH in desired range; check TSH Q4 wk in first trimester, Q6 wk until ~32 weeks' gestation, and 4–6 wk after any dosage adjustment.	$
	liothyronine (T_3) (triiodothyronine) Cytomel	Up to 25 μg BID po for short-term management in patients with thyroid cancer after stopping levothyroxine	See levothyroxine.	See levothyroxine. T_3 is not reported to interact with iron salts.		$$$

[a] Cost of 30-day supply; includes drug cost only.
Legend: $ < $5 $$ $5–25 $$$ $25–50

Table 5: **Drugs Used in the Management of Hyperthyroidism**

Class	Drug	Dose	Adverse Effects	Drug Interactions	Comments	Cost[a]
Antithyroid Agents	*methimazole* (MMI) Tapazole	10–30 mg daily po in 2–3 divided doses; higher doses are sometimes necessary Thyroid storm: up to 40 mg BID may be required	Risk of skin rash, allergic reaction, agranulocytosis, rarely hepatotoxicity.	Thyroid status influences response to warfarin. Monitor INR when antithyroid medication dose altered.	Warn patient to stop medication if rash, fever, sore throat or jaundice develop. MMI preferred first-line agent, especially in children, *except* during the first trimester of pregnancy when PTU is preferred. MMI first choice when breastfeeding.	$$–$$$
	propylthiouracil (PTU) Propyl-Thyracil	Initially 50–100 mg TID po in most cases; reduce dose in renal failure Thyroid storm: up to 1200 mg daily in divided doses	Risk of skin rash; allergic reaction; agranulocytosis; rarely, severe hepatotoxicity that may be fatal.	See methimazole.	See methimazole. In pregnancy, use the lowest PTU dose necessary to maintain thyroid hormone in the upper normal range. Avoid PTU in children.	$$$
$Beta_1$-adrenergic Antagonists, nonselective	*propranolol* generics	Hyperthyroidism: 10–40 mg QID po Thyroid storm: 40–120 mg Q6H po or 0.5–2 mg iv slowly Q4–6H, if no evidence of cardiac decompensation	Bradycardia, dizziness, fatigue, headache, hypotension.	Bradycardia with digoxin or nondihydropyridine CCBs Cardiodepressant effects with nondihydropyridine CCBs and amiodarone	Avoid in patients with asthma or conditions associated with bradycardia; taper once thyrotoxicosis improved. Controls tachycardia.	$
$Beta_1$-adrenergic Antagonists, selective	*atenolol* Tenormin, generics	Initial dose: 25–50 mg daily po, may increase to 200 mg daily	See propranolol.	See propranolol.	See propranolol. May have faster onset of action compared to propranolol. Controls tachycardia.	$
	metoprolol Betaloc, Lopresor, generics	50 mg QID po, may increase to 100 mg QID	See propranolol.	See propranolol.	See propranolol. May have faster onset of action compared to propranolol. Controls tachycardia.	$

(cont'd)

Table 5: **Drugs Used in the Management of Hyperthyroidism** *(cont'd)*

Class	Drug	Dose	Adverse Effects	Drug Interactions	Comments	Cost[a]
Corticosteroids, systemic	*dexamethasone* generics	Thyroid storm: 2 mg Q6H po or iv; continue until free T_3 level controlled	Numerous effects especially if prolonged use; acutely: elevated blood glucose, risk of avascular necrosis, altered mood.	Effects can be diminished with concomitant medications such as phenytoin.	Reserved for emergency adjunctive management of hyperthyroidism or myxedema coma, in conjunction with specific management of thyroid disorder.	$ for 3 days' oral therapy
	hydrocortisone sodium succinate Solu-Cortef, generics	Myxedema coma: 100 mg Q8H iv; taper when stable	See dexamethasone.	See dexamethasone.	See dexamethasone.	$$ for 3 days' iv therapy
Iodine	*iodine*	Thyroid storm: Lugol's solution, 3–5 drops Q6H po, 1 h after antithyroid drug Prior to thyroidectomy: if hyperthyroidism reasonably controlled, use Lugol's solution 2–6 drops TID po × 7 days preceding operation	Allergy, hypersensitivity.		Administer 1 h after PTU or MMI; blocks radioactive iodine uptake.	$
Iodine, radioactive	*sodium iodide* ^{131}I Draximage Sodium Iodide I131	Graves' disease: ~370 MBq (10 mCi) po; more might be used for a toxic nodule or nodular goitre, or less if uptake is very high	High risk of hypothyroidism; possible worsening of Graves' ophthalmopathy; risk of radiation thyroiditis.		Given as single oral dose; usually only one dose required.	~$175/ per dose

[a] Cost of 30-day supply unless otherwise specified; includes drug cost only.

Dosage adjustment may be required in renal impairment; see Appendix I

Abbreviations: CCB = calcium channel blocker; MBq = megabecquerels; mCi = megacurie; MMI = methimazole; PTU = propylthiouracil; T_3 = triiodothyronine; TSH = thyroid-stimulating hormone

Legend: $ < $10 $$ $10–20 $$–$$$ $10–30 $$$ $20–30

Suggested Readings

American Thyroid Association. *Professional guidelines*. Available from: thyroidguidelines.org.

Cooper DS. Antithyroid drugs. *N Engl J Med* 2005;352(9):905-17.

De Groot L, Abalovich M, Alexander EK et al. Management of thyroid dysfunction during pregnancy and postpartum: an Endocrine Society clinical practice guideline. *J Clin Endocrinol Metab* 2012;97(8):2543-65.

Gharib H, Papini E, Paschke R et al. American Association of Clinical Endocrinologists, Associazione Medici Endocrinologi and European Thyroid Association medical guidelines for clinical practice for the diagnosis and management of thyroid nodules. *Endocr Pract* 2010;16(Suppl 1):1-43.

Klein I, Ojamaa K. Thyroid hormone and the cardiovascular system. *N Engl J Med* 2001;344(7):501-9.

Thyroid Disease Manager. South Dartmouth (MA): Endocrine Education. Available from: www.thyroidmanager.org.

References

1. Cooper DS. Clinical practice. Subclinical hypothyroidism. *N Engl J Med* 2001;345(4):260-5.
2. Surks MI, Ortiz E, Daniels GH et al. Subclinical thyroid disease: scientific review and guidelines for diagnosis and management. *JAMA* 2004;291(2):228-38.
3. Rodondi N, den Elzen WP, Bauer DC et al. Subclinical hypothyroidism and the risk of coronary heart disease and mortality. *JAMA* 2010;304(12):1365-74.
4. American Thyroid Association. *Professional guidelines*. Available from: thyroidguidelines.org. Accessed July 7, 2011.
5. Turner MR, Camacho X, Fischer HD et al. Levothyroxine dose and risk of fractures in older adults: nested case-control study. *BMJ* 2011;342:d2238.
6. Escobar-Morreale HF, Botella-Carretero JI, Escobar del Rey F et al. Review: Treatment of hypothyroidism with combinations of levothyroxine plus liothyronine. *J Clin Endocrinol Metab* 2005;90(8):4946-54.
7. Bunevicius R, Kazanavicius G, Zalinkevicius R et al. Effects of thyroxine as compared with thyroxine plus triiodothyronine in patients with hypothyroidism. *N Engl J Med* 1999;340(6):424-9.
8. De Groot L, Abalovich M, Alexander EK et al. Management of thyroid dysfunction during pregnancy and postpartum: an Endocrine Society clinical practice guideline. *J Clin Endocrinol Metab* 2012;97(8):2543-65.
9. Rosene-Montella K. *Medical care of the pregnant patient*. 2nd ed. Philadelphia (PA): ACP Press/American College of Physicians; 2008.
10. Yassa L, Marqusee E, Fawcett R et al. Thyroid hormone early adjustment in pregnancy (the THERAPY) trial. *J Clin Endocrinol Metab* 2010;95(7):3234-41.
11. Alexander EK, Marqusee E, Lawrence J et al. Timing and magnitude of increases in levothyroxine requirements during pregnancy in women with hypothyroidism. *N Engl J Med* 2004;351(3):241-9.
12. Garber JR, Cobin RH, Gharib H et al. Clinical practice guidelines for hypothyroidism in adults: cosponsored by the American Association of Clinical Endocrinologists and the American Thyroid Association. *Endocr Pract* 2012;18(6):988-1028.
13. Weetman AP. Graves' disease. *N Engl J Med* 2000;343(17):1236-48.
14. Toft AD. Clinical practice. Subclinical hyperthyroidism. *N Engl J Med* 2001;345(7):512-6.
15. Sawin CT, Geller A, Wolf PA et al. Low serum thyrotropin concentrations as a risk factor for atrial fibrillation in older persons. *N Engl J Med* 1994;331(19):1249-52.
16. Bartalena L, Marcocci C, Bogazzi F et al. Relation between therapy for hyperthyroidism and the course of Graves' ophthalmopathy. *N Engl J Med* 1998;338(2):73-8.
17. Imseis RE, Vanmiddlesworth L, Massie JD et al. Pretreatment with propylthiouracil but not methimazole reduces the therapeutic efficacy of iodine-131 in hyperthyroidism. *J Clin Endocrinol Metab* 1998;83(2):685-7.
18. Rivkees SA, Mattison DR. Propylthiouracil (PTU) hepatoxicity in children and recommendations for discontinuation of use. *Int J Pediatr Endocrinol* 2009;2009:132041.
19. Marcocci C, Kahaly GJ, Krassas GE et al. Selenium and the course of mild Graves' orbitopathy. *N Engl J Med* 2011;364(20):1920-31.
20. Larsen PR. Salicylate-induced increases in free triiodothyronine in human serum. Evidence of inhibition of triiodothyronine binding to thyroxine-binding globulin and thyroxine-binding prealbumin. *J Clin Invest* 1972;51(5):1125-34.
21. Mestman JH. Hyperthyroidism in pregnancy. *Best Pract Res Clin Endocrinol Metab* 2004;18(2):267-88.
22. Millar LK, Wing DA, Leung AS et al. Low birth weight and preeclampsia in pregnancies complicated by hyperthyroidism. *Obstet Gynecol* 1994;84(6):946-9.
23. Patil-Sisodia K, Mestman JH. Graves hyperthyroidism and pregnancy: a clinical update. *Endocr Pract* 2010;16(1):118-29.
24. Tan GH, Gharib H. Thyroid incidentalomas: management approaches to nonpalpable nodules discovered incidentally on thyroid imaging. *Ann Intern Med* 1997;126(3):226-31.
25. Stagnaro-Green A, Abalovich M, Alexander E et al. Guidelines of the American Thyroid Association for the diagnosis and management of thyroid disease during pregnancy and postpartum. *Thyroid* 2011;21(10):1081-125.
26. Gharib H, Mazzaferri EL. Thyroxine suppressive therapy in patients with nodular thyroid disease. *Ann Intern Med* 1998;128(5):386-94.
27. Mazzaferri EL, Kloos RT. Clinical review 128: current approaches to primary therapy for papillary and follicular thyroid cancer. *J Clin Endocrinol Metab* 2001;86(4):1447-63.
28. Ridgway EC. Medical treatment of benign thyroid nodules: have we defined a benefit? *Ann Intern Med* 1998;128(5):403-5.

Chapter 35
Acute Coronary Syndromes

Michelle Graham, MD, FRCPC

The term "acute coronary syndrome" (ACS) refers to any clinical symptoms compatible with acute myocardial ischemia, from ST segment elevation myocardial infarction (STEMI) to non-ST segment elevation myocardial infarction (NSTEMI) and unstable angina. Treatment centres should have a standardized approach to patients with ACS to ensure the most rapid assessment and initiation of treatment possible.

The following discussion relates to any ACS that is associated with primary coronary events caused by plaque erosion and/or rupture, fissuring or dissection.

Unstable Angina (UA) and Non-ST Segment Elevation Myocardial Infarction (NSTEMI)

Goals of Therapy

- Decrease mortality and complications
- Reduce the severity or eliminate episodes of ischemia
- Prevent further myocardial injury

Investigations

- Careful history with special attention to pain (quality, severity, location, radiation, precipitating and relieving factors), duration of symptoms, previous cardiac history, cardiac risk factors (smoking status, diabetes mellitus, hyperlipidemia, hypertension, family history of first-degree relative with MI before age 55 if male or 65 if female) and effect of nitroglycerin
- Physical examination, with attention to the presence of hypertension, heart failure or valvular heart disease
- Laboratory tests:
  - ECG, CBC, electrolytes, glucose, creatinine and lipid profile (within 24 hours of presentation)
  - troponin, a highly accurate, sensitive and specific indicator of myocardial injury.[1] Measurement allows reliable stratification of risk and prediction of outcomes in individual patients.[2,3] Elevation of cardiac troponin levels may result from pulmonary embolus or nonischemic mechanisms of myocardial injury, such as myocarditis, severe heart failure or cardiac trauma. Additionally, troponins are elevated in 30–50% of patients with pericarditis as a result of epicardial inflammation, and have also been reported in critical illness, sepsis, neurologic events, hypothyroidism, chemotherapy-induced myocardial toxicity and renal insufficiency.
- A careful search for secondary causes of ischemia, e.g., anemia, fever, infection, arrhythmia, thyroid disease
- Echocardiography can be used early when clinical history and ECG are nondiagnostic—the presence of regional wall motion abnormalities with chest pain is suggestive of underlying ischemia

Table 1: **Clinical Features Used to Calculate TIMI Risk Score**[4]

One point is assigned for each of the following clinical features:
• age >65 y
• ≥3 cardiac risk factors (hypercholesterolemia, hypertension, diabetes mellitus, current smoker, family history of coronary artery disease)
• ≥50% coronary artery stenosis
• any ASA use within the past 7 days
• ≥2 episodes of angina within the last 24 hours
• elevation in cardiac markers (troponin or creatine kinase-myocardial band)
• ST segment deviation ≥0.5 mm on ECG

The TIMI (Thrombolysis in Myocardial Infarction) Risk Score is a risk stratification tool for patients with unstable angina or NSTEMI (UA/NSTEMI), using clinical features present at the time of initial assessment in the emergency department (Table 1). It predicts the risk of both death and early recurrent ischemic events and is used to tailor different evidence-based therapies to appropriate patients. As the risk score increases, so too do adverse outcomes; for example, there is a 5% risk of major adverse cardiac events in patients with a risk score of 0 or 1, and a 41% risk in those with a risk score of 6 or 7.[4]

The Global Registry of Acute Coronary Events (GRACE) score is a more comprehensive risk stratification tool (www.outcomes-umassmed.org/grace/acs_risk/acs_risk_content.html). While more complicated, it is a web-based tool that can be easily used to improve risk calculation. When compared to the TIMI Risk Score, this model has been found to better discriminate risk of 1-month and 1-year mortality in patients with ACS.[5]

Therapeutic Choices

The management of patients with UA/NSTEMI has evolved significantly (see Figure 1). Evidence from randomized clinical trials now strongly supports the use of the "invasive strategy": early, urgent coronary angiography followed if possible by revascularization with percutaneous coronary intervention (PCI) or bypass surgery in all high-risk patients. Patients are at high risk if they have one or more of the following features: positive cardiac enzymes, ST segment changes, TIMI Risk Score ≥3, recurrent ischemic symptoms, heart failure, hemodynamic instability, sustained ventricular tachycardia or a prior revascularization procedure such as a coronary artery bypass graft (CABG) or PCI.[6]

Nonpharmacologic Choices

All patients admitted with UA/NSTEMI should be placed on bedrest while ischemia is ongoing, then gradually mobilized when symptoms have stabilized. Use supplemental oxygen in patients with inadequate arterial oxygen saturation to keep SaO_2 above 90%. Continuous ECG monitoring for potentially lethal arrhythmias and ST segment shifts (if available) is indicated in all high-risk patients.

Pharmacologic Choices

Table 2 provides details on the medications used in UA/NSTEMI.

Nitrates

Initial attempts at symptom relief should involve the use of **nitroglycerin**, first with sublingual tablets or spray. Intravenous nitroglycerin is indicated in patients whose symptoms are not relieved promptly (within 15–20 minutes). Longer-acting oral or topical nitrates can be used when patients are symptom free to prevent recurrent episodes of ischemia. The use of sildenafil, tadalafil or vardenafil in the previous 24 hours or the presence of significant hypotension is a contraindication to the use of nitrates.

Figure 1: **Early Management of UA/NSTEMI**

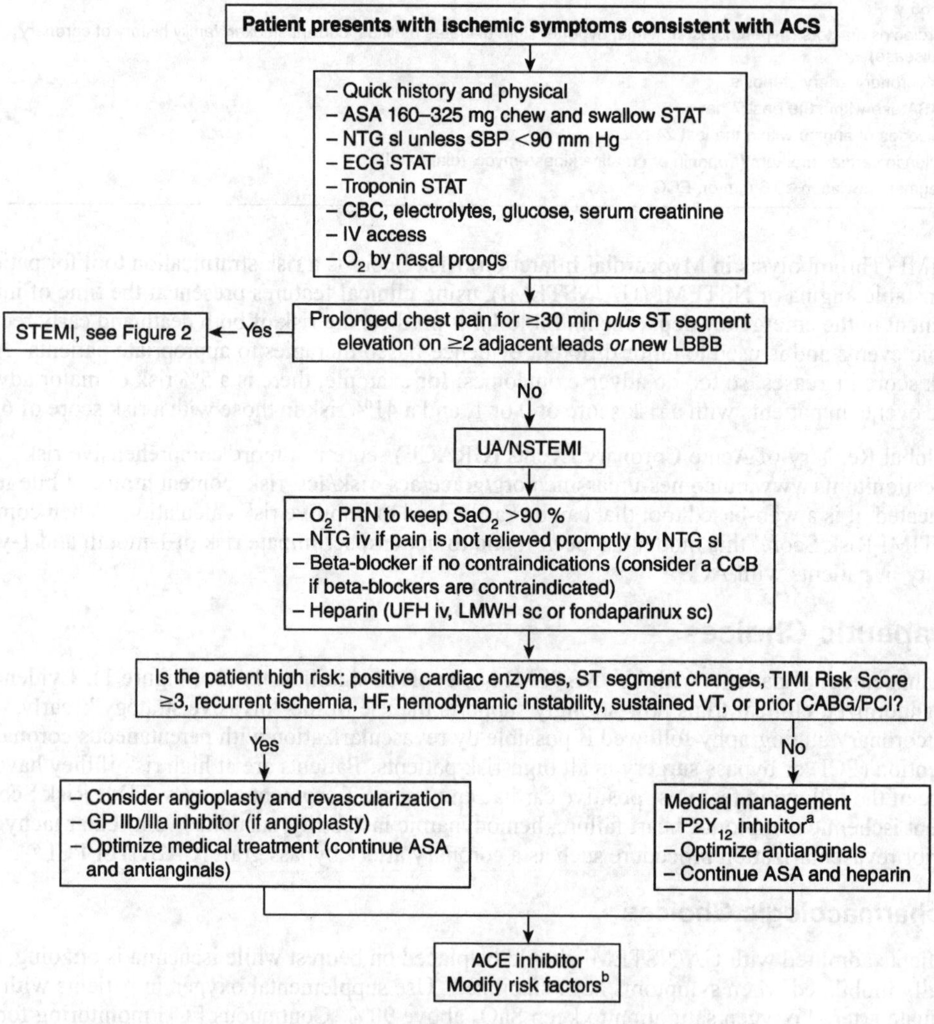
Patient presents with ischemic symptoms consistent with ACS
– Quick history and physical
– ASA 160–325 mg chew and swallow STAT
– NTG sl unless SBP <90 mm Hg
– ECG STAT
– Troponin STAT
– CBC, electrolytes, glucose, serum creatinine
– IV access
– O2 by nasal prongs
Prolonged chest pain for ≥30 min plus ST segment elevation on ≥2 adjacent leads or new LBBB
Yes
STEMI, see Figure 2
No
UA/NSTEMI
– O2 PRN to keep SaO2 >90 %
– NTG iv if pain is not relieved promptly by NTG sl
– Beta-blocker if no contraindications (consider a CCB if beta-blockers are contraindicated)
– Heparin (UFH iv, LMWH sc or fondaparinux sc)
Is the patient high risk: positive cardiac enzymes, ST segment changes, TIMI Risk Score ≥3, recurrent ischemia, HF, hemodynamic instability, sustained VT, or prior CABG/PCI?
Yes
No
– Consider angioplasty and revascularization
– GP IIb/IIIa inhibitor (if angioplasty)
– Optimize medical treatment (continue ASA and antianginals)
Medical management
– P2Y12 inhibitor a
– Optimize antianginals
– Continue ASA and heparin
ACE inhibitor
Modify risk factors b

[a] The recommended $P2Y_{12}$ inhibitors are: clopidogrel, prasugrel and ticagrelor.
[b] See Chapter 41.

Abbreviations: ACE = angiotensin converting enzyme; ACS = acute coronary syndrome; CABG = coronary artery bypass graft; CBC = complete blood count; CCB = calcium channel blocker; DVT = deep vein thrombosis; GP = glycoprotein; HF = heart failure; LBBB = left bundle branch block; LMWH = low-molecular-weight heparin; NTG = nitroglycerin; PCI = percutaneous coronary intervention; SaO_2 = oxygen saturation; SBP = systolic blood pressure; STEMI = ST segment elevation myocardial infarction; TIMI = Thrombolysis in Myocardial Infarction; UA/NSTEMI = unstable angina or non-ST segment elevation myocardial infarction; UFH = unfractionated heparin; VT = ventricular tachycardia

$Beta_1$-adrenergic Antagonists (Beta-blockers) and Calcium Channel Blockers

Start beta-blockers as soon as possible in all patients without contraindications: reactive airway disease; bradycardia (heart rate ≤50 beats per minute); second- or third-degree heart block without a functioning pacemaker; hypotension (SBP <100 mm Hg). The dose should be titrated as tolerated to achieve target doses. If anginal pain is ongoing at presentation, beta-blockers can be initially administered intravenously, followed by oral therapy.

Calcium channel blockers can be used to control ongoing symptoms of ischemia in patients who are receiving maximum tolerated doses of beta-blockers and adequate doses of nitrates. In addition, these agents are used in patients who cannot tolerate beta-blockers and in those with variant angina (coronary spasm). Nondihydropyridine calcium channel blockers should be used with caution when administered with beta-blockers to avoid left ventricular (LV) dysfunction, severe bradycardia or increasing atrioventricular (AV) nodal block. Avoid immediate-release nifedipine because of potential adverse outcomes such as stroke.[7]

Angiotensin Converting Enzyme (ACE) Inhibitors

ACE inhibitors reduce mortality in patients with LV systolic dysfunction or clinical heart failure, diabetes or recent MI, and in a broad spectrum of patients with high-risk chronic coronary artery disease.[8,9] Therefore, use these agents (ideally initiated within 24 hours of presentation) in all of these patient groups and in patients with hypertension not controlled with beta-blockers and nitrates.

Anticoagulation Therapy

Heparins and Fondaparinux

Heparin is a key component in the successful management of patients with ACS. Studies of ASA with either unfractionated heparin (UFH) or low-molecular-weight heparins (LMWH) have shown a 3–3.5% absolute reduction (50–60% relative reduction) in the rate of death or MI in the first week.[10,11] UFH has important limitations due to significant variability in anticoagulant response. LMWHs have the advantage of ease of administration, predictable anticoagulant response and no need for monitoring. Clinical trials have demonstrated the superiority of **enoxaparin** over UFH, but have shown neutral or unfavourable trends with other LMWHs (**dalteparin** and **nadroparin**).[12,13,14,15] A direct comparison favoured enoxaparin over **tinzaparin**.[16] Enoxaparin is therefore the preferred agent in patients with UA/NSTEMI who do not have significant renal dysfunction (estimated ClCr >30 mL/min). In those with an estimated ClCr ≤30 mL/min, UFH is appropriate. The optimal duration of heparin therapy is unknown but generally is 2–5 days. Heparin is usually not administered following successful PCI.

Fondaparinux, a direct inhibitor of factor Xa, is as effective as enoxaparin in patients with NSTEMI ACS, so it can be considered as an alternative anticoagulant in this setting. It is associated with a lower incidence of major bleeding according to the results of a large randomized trial.[17]

Direct Thrombin Inhibitors

Bivalirudin, a reversible direct thrombin inhibitor with a quick onset of action and short half-life, has a predictable antithrombotic response. Clinical studies demonstrate positive outcomes in patients with ACS.[18] Bivalirudin use is considered a reasonable strategy in patients with ACS undergoing PCI with concomitant thienopyridine and/or glycoprotein IIb/IIIa inhibitor use.

Antiplatelet Therapy

ASA

ASA provides a significant benefit in patients with acute coronary syndromes.[18] If patients with suspected UA/NSTEMI are not already receiving ASA, it should be initiated promptly and continued long term.

Thienopyridines

Thienopyridine antiplatelet agents block the $P2Y_{12}$ platelet receptor. In the CURE (Clopidogrel in Unstable angina to prevent Recurrent ischemic Events) trial, **clopidogrel** (plus **ASA**) significantly reduced the incidence of major adverse cardiac events in patients with ACS compared with ASA alone, and reduced the incidence of recurrent ischemia, an effect which was evident within a few hours.[19] The benefit of clopidogrel was consistent among patients, regardless of their TIMI Risk Score.[20] The major benefits were noted at 30 days, with small additional benefits observed over the subsequent treatment period (average 8 months). There was an excess of both major and minor bleeding in the clopidogrel group during the trial, with an insignificant trend towards an increase in life-threatening bleeding. Bleeding risks increase with higher ASA doses.[21] Because of this risk, many hospitals with cardiac catheterization facilities do not initiate clopidogrel until it is clear that bypass surgery is not needed for appropriate revascularization. Clopidogrel should be held for a minimum of 5 days in patients scheduled for bypass surgery.[19,20]

Regulatory authorities have noted the diminished effectiveness of clopidogrel in patients who are unable to convert it to its active form. Patients with diminished CYP2C19 function due to genetic polymorphisms activate clopidogrel poorly and have higher cardiovascular event rates, both following an ACS and after PCI. Tests are available to identify these individuals. However, there is little evidence that increasing the dose of clopidogrel or changing to another agent improves outcomes overall. For this reason, routine genetic testing is not recommended at this time [Evidence: SORT C*].[22]

Prasugrel is a more potent platelet inhibitor than clopidogrel. In a large clinical trial of patients with ACS who were undergoing PCI, it was associated with lower ischemic event rates, including stent thrombosis. However, there was a significant increase in bleeding events, particularly in those over age 75, those with body weight <60 kg and in patients with a history of stroke or transient ischemic attack.[23] The use of prasugrel should be considered in those patients with ACS undergoing stent implantation who are at higher risk for stent thrombosis (previous stent thrombosis, STEMI, history of diabetes mellitus). A recent study (TRILOGY-ACS) did not demonstrate superiority of prasugrel over clopidogrel in patients with ACS who are managed medically.[24] Prasugrel is not recommended as first-line therapy unless coronary anatomy has been defined. However, when it has been started and CABG is considered optimal therapy, it should be held for a minimum of 7 days prior to surgery.

Ticlopidine is rarely used due to the better safety profile of other antiplatelet agents.

Cyclopentyltriazolopyrimidines

Cyclopentyltriazolopyrimidines also block the $P2Y_{12}$ receptor. **Ticagrelor** has similar potency and speed of onset to prasugrel, but does not require metabolic activation. In a large clinical trial of patients with ACS, the use of ticagrelor was associated with both lower mortality and ischemic events compared to clopidogrel, but with an increase in non-CABG–related bleeding.[25] Ticagrelor is recommended as first-line therapy in patients with ACS, but may not be available on all formularies. Ticagrelor should be held for a minimum of 5 days prior to CABG. Dyspnea and ventricular pauses are side effects that may be associated with ticagrelor therapy but rarely result in its discontinuation.

Glycoprotein IIb/IIIa Inhibitors

Numerous trials have demonstrated the efficacy of these agents in the treatment of high-risk patients with UA/NSTEMI undergoing coronary angiography and subsequent PCI. Clinical trials support the use of **eptifibatide** and **tirofiban** at the time of admission or immediately before PCI.[26,27,28,29,30] **Abciximab** is also effective, but cost limits its use to the cardiac catheterization laboratory. The benefit of these agents is less clear in patients for whom an initial conservative management approach is planned. Patients receiving any of these agents must be carefully monitored for bleeding. However, the combined use of glycoprotein IIb/IIIa inhibitors and heparin appears to be safe.[18] Thrombocytopenia is a complication of treatment with these agents so platelet counts should be monitored.

Therapeutic Tips

- The standard dose of **ASA** is 81 mg daily.
- Discontinue **clopidogrel** or **ticagrelor** 5 days prior to bypass surgery to decrease the risk of bleeding.

* SORT (Strength of Recommendation Taxonomy) is a rating system (A, B or C) that addresses the quality of available evidence. For more information consult **How to Use *Compendium of Therapeutic Choices*** on page xxv.

ST Segment Elevation Myocardial Infarction (STEMI)

STEMI represents the extreme of the ACS spectrum and is considered to be a medical emergency, and therefore requires urgent assessment and treatment.

Goals of Therapy

- Decrease mortality and complications
- Reduce or contain infarct size
- Salvage functioning myocardium and prevent remodelling
- Re-establish patency of the infarct-related artery

Investigations

- Rapid, targeted history and physical examination, with particular attention to onset of symptoms, contraindications to use of thrombolytic agents (see Table 2) and evidence of high-risk features (tachycardia, hypotension, heart failure)
- ECG STAT, then every 8 hours for the first 24 hours, then daily for 3 days. In addition, repeat the ECG with each recurrence of chest pain
- Baseline troponin STAT, and then every 8 hours until enzymatic confirmation of the diagnosis (see Unstable Angina (UA) and Non-ST Segment Elevation Myocardial Infarction (NSTEMI), Investigations for further discussion of troponin)
- CBC to rule out the presence of anemia and establish baseline platelet count, baseline electrolytes, creatinine, fasting lipid profile (within 24 hours of presentation) and liver enzyme tests
- Portable chest x-ray (CXR) STAT
- Echocardiography to assess LV function after stabilization and treatment. Echocardiography is also used emergently when there is suspicion of acute mechanical complications post-MI

Therapeutic Choices

The care of patients with STEMI is summarized in Figure 2.

Nonpharmacologic Choices

Place all patients on bedrest with supplemental oxygen and continuous ECG monitoring. Begin gradual mobilization after stabilization, provided there is no evidence of complications.

Primary Percutaneous Coronary Intervention (PCI)

Urgent coronary angiography with PCI is considered first-line therapy for all patients who can access appropriate high-volume cardiac catheterization facilities.[31] Primary PCI is indicated in patients with contraindications to thrombolytic therapy or cardiogenic shock, and is preferred in patients over the age of 75 because of a higher risk of intracranial hemorrhage and higher overall early mortality seen with thrombolytic agents in this age group.[32,33,34] For all patients who cannot access PCI within 2 hours, a pharmacoinvasive strategy (involving administration of thrombolytic therapy followed by either immediate or more routine transfer to a cardiac catheterization centre) is now recommended as a first-line approach.[31] Heparin agents are used post-PCI at the discretion of the treating physician.

Pharmacologic Choices

Table 2 provides details on the medications used in STEMI.

Figure 2: **Early Management of STEMI**

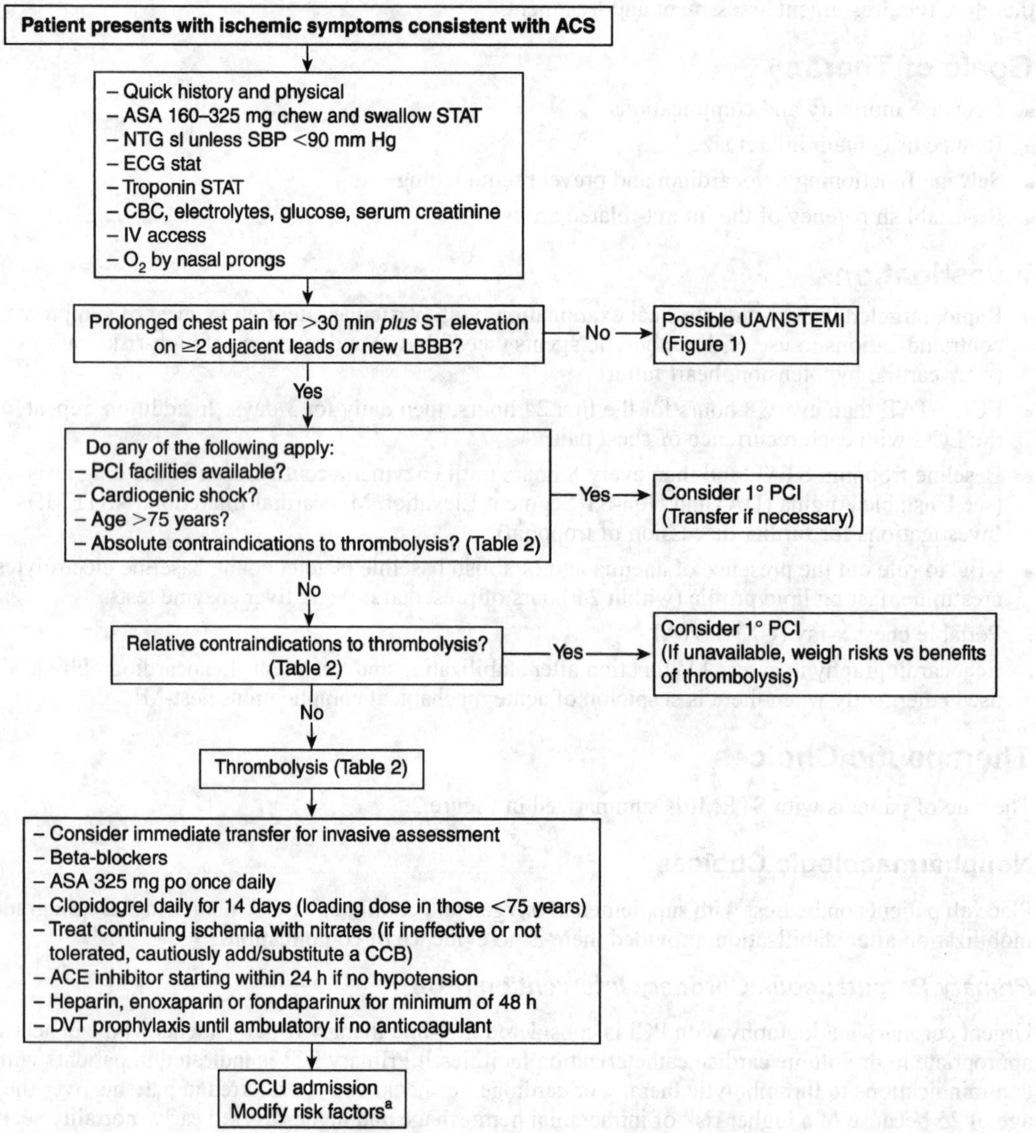
Patient presents with ischemic symptoms consistent with ACS
– Quick history and physical
– ASA 160–325 mg chew and swallow STAT
– NTG sl unless SBP <90 mm Hg
– ECG stat
– Troponin STAT
– CBC, electrolytes, glucose, serum creatinine
– IV access
– O_2 by nasal prongs
Prolonged chest pain for >30 min *plus* ST elevation on ≥2 adjacent leads *or* new LBBB?
No
Possible UA/NSTEMI (Figure 1)
Yes
Do any of the following apply:
– PCI facilities available?
– Cardiogenic shock?
– Age >75 years?
– Absolute contraindications to thrombolysis? (Table 2)
Yes
Consider 1° PCI (Transfer if necessary)
No
Relative contraindications to thrombolysis? (Table 2)
Yes
Consider 1° PCI (If unavailable, weigh risks vs benefits of thrombolysis)
No
Thrombolysis (Table 2)
– Consider immediate transfer for invasive assessment
– Beta-blockers
– ASA 325 mg po once daily
– Clopidogrel daily for 14 days (loading dose in those <75 years)
– Treat continuing ischemia with nitrates (if ineffective or not tolerated, cautiously add/substitute a CCB)
– ACE inhibitor starting within 24 h if no hypotension
– Heparin, enoxaparin or fondaparinux for minimum of 48 h
– DVT prophylaxis until ambulatory if no anticoagulant
CCU admission
Modify risk factors[a]

[a] See Chapter 41.

Abbreviations: ACE = angiotensin converting enzyme; ACS = acute coronary syndrome; CCB = calcium channel blocker; CCU = cardiac care unit; DVT = deep vein thrombosis; LBBB = left bundle branch block; NTG = nitroglycerin; PCI = percutaneous coronary intervention; UA/NSTEMI = unstable angina or non-ST segment elevation myocardial infarction

Thrombolytic Therapy

Thrombolytic therapy administered early in the course of STEMI substantially reduces morbidity and mortality, particularly if the patient presents within 6 hours of symptom onset.[31] The benefit is reduced for patients who present 6–12 hours after the onset of symptoms, and evidence of benefit is much less clear for those who present more than 12 hours after the onset of symptoms. The greatest absolute benefit is seen where the risk of mortality is highest (anterior MI, previous MI).

Heparins

Administer intravenous **unfractionated heparin** to all STEMI patients receiving alteplase or tenecteplase. **Enoxaparin** is an alternative, and has been shown to be superior to UFH in patients treated with tenecteplase. It must be used with caution in patients older than 75 (dosage adjustment required) or those with renal insufficiency (estimated ClCr <30 mL/min) because of an increased risk of bleeding.[35] Heparins should be continued for a minimum of 48 hours and use can be extended in patients with high-risk features.

ASA

ASA significantly reduces mortality in patients with STEMI. If patients are not already receiving ASA, it should be initiated promptly and continued long term.[31]

Beta$_1$-adrenergic Antagonists (Beta-blockers)

These agents are recommended to reduce the risk of recurrent MI in all STEMI patients without contraindications, and are particularly useful when sinus tachycardia and hypertension are present. They should be initiated once hemodynamic stability is achieved. Titrate doses to a resting heart rate of 50–60 bpm.

Calcium Channel Blockers

Calcium channel blockers increase morbidity and mortality in patients with STEMI and are not recommended.[36] They may be used *cautiously* to relieve ischemia or to achieve rate control in patients with atrial fibrillation if beta-blockers are contraindicated. Consider low-dose **diltiazem**, e.g., 90–120 mg daily in divided doses, with heart rate monitored closely.

Nitrates

Unlike UA/NSTEMI, iv, oral or topical nitrates should be used in patients with STEMI only if ischemia is persistent or recurrent, or if the patient has a large anterior MI, hypertension or heart failure.[37]

ACE Inhibitors and Angiotensin Receptor Blockers

ACE inhibitors are routinely recommended, unless contraindicated, in all patients post-STEMI and should ideally be started within 24 hours of the event unless the patient is hypotensive (SBP <100 mm Hg).[31] Doses should be increased every 24 hours as tolerated for inpatients and at 1- to 2-week intervals for outpatients. Based on the results of the HOPE trial, it is reasonable to continue an ACE inhibitor indefinitely, even in patients with preserved LV function.[9] An angiotensin receptor blocker should be used in STEMI patients who cannot tolerate an ACE inhibitor and have either clinical or radiological signs of heart failure or documented LV dysfunction.

Aldosterone Antagonists

Long-term use of an aldosterone antagonist such as **spironolactone** or **eplerenone** reduces morbidity and mortality in STEMI patients with clinical evidence of heart failure, LV ejection fraction <40% or both, based on the results of 2 randomized trials.[38,39] Caution must be used in patients with renal insufficiency or pre-existing hyperkalemia, and in those receiving ACE inhibitors concomitantly.[38,39]

Clopidogrel

In patients with STEMI treated with fibrinolysis, clopidogrel increases patency of the infarct-related artery and decreases ischemic complications according to the results of 2 randomized trials;[40,41] therefore, routine use should be considered in these patients. Recent recommendations suggest an increased dose (150 mg/day) for the first 6 days of treatment.[42]

Complications of STEMI

Recurrent or Ongoing Ischemia

Optimize antianginal therapy, and consider urgent coronary angiography and possible revascularization for all patients with recurrent or ongoing ischemia.

Heart Failure

Treat heart failure aggressively (see Chapter 38). In addition, consider angiography and possible revascularization in patients with LV ejection fraction <40% after MI.

Arrhythmias

Asymptomatic premature ventricular contractions (PVCs) do not require therapy. Symptomatic ectopy may require therapy, usually with a beta-blocker. Class IC agents are contraindicated. Patients with sustained ventricular arrhythmias require investigation to rule out recurrent ischemia and may require subsequent electrophysiologic assessment.[43] Consider urgent electrical or pharmacologic cardioversion in patients with atrial fibrillation causing ischemia or heart failure. Treat all patients with atrial fibrillation to control ventricular rate (usually with a beta-blocker or digoxin if there is concomitant heart failure) and consider oral anticoagulant therapy.

Patients with an ejection fraction <30% 1 month post-MI or 3 months post-revascularization should be referred for automatic implantable cardioverter-defibrillator therapy (AICD) for prevention of sudden cardiac death.[44]

Pericarditis

Pericarditis, although uncommon, usually presents within 72 hours post-MI, and symptoms usually resolve within 3–4 days. Symptomatic pericarditis can be treated by increasing the dose of **ASA** to 650 mg QID for 1–2 weeks. If ASA is ineffective, an **NSAID** or **corticosteroid** can be added. Discontinuation of anticoagulants is unnecessary if pericarditis occurs early postinfarction, but caution is required if a patient presents with pericarditis weeks or months after MI (Dressler's syndrome) because of the risk of pericardial bleeding and tamponade.[45]

Mechanical Complications

Ruptured papillary muscle (and severe mitral regurgitation), ventricular septal defects or ventricular free wall rupture are infrequent but devastating problems that can present with acute cardiac arrest or cardiogenic shock. Patients should be considered for emergency angiography and surgical intervention, but even with urgent treatment, the mortality rate associated with these conditions is very high.

Therapeutic Tips

- The goal for thrombolytic treatment is a door-to-needle time of 30 minutes or less.
- The goal for primary PCI is a door-to-dilatation time of 90 minutes or less.
- Careful attention to maximum pain relief is important.
- In patients with right ventricular infarcts:
  - avoid nitrates and diuretics
  - use fluids and inotropes to treat hypotension
- Administer beta-blockers in the first 24 hours to all patients without contraindications. Increase the dose every 12 hours (every 24 hours for once-daily beta-blockers), if tolerated (monitor blood pressure and heart rate), until the patient has reached adequate beta-blockade (HR ≤55–65 bpm).

- Start ACE inhibitors within 24 hours post-MI. The choice of agent can depend on practitioner preference, hospital formulary or financial constraints for the individual patient.
- In smokers, reinforce early (within 24 hours) and frequently the need to quit smoking.
- Stool softeners may be used in the immediate post-MI period to prevent straining with bowel movements.
- Anxiolytics may be used on an as-needed basis in the immediate post-MI period.

Table 2: Drugs Used in Acute Coronary Syndromes

Class	Drug	Dose	Adverse Effects	Drug Interactions	Cost[a]
ACE Inhibitors	*captopril* generics	Initial: 6.25 mg Q8H po Target: 50 mg Q8H po	Proteinuria (1%), neutropenia (rare), rash, angioedema, hypotension, alterations in taste, nausea, anorexia, dizziness, hyperkalemia, dry cough (common). Caution in patients with renovascular hypertension, renal insufficiency, bilateral renal artery stenosis or single kidney with renal artery stenosis.	Increased risk of neutropenia with allopurinol, antiarrhythmics, corticosteroids. Hyperkalemia with amiloride, spironolactone, triamterene. Hypotension with diuretics. Avoid concurrent therapy with lithium.	$$
	cilazapril Inhibace, generics	Initial: 0.5 mg daily po Target: 2.5 mg daily po	See captopril.	See captopril.	$
	enalapril Vasotec, generics	Initial: 2.5 mg BID po Target: 10 mg BID po	See captopril.	See captopril.	$
	fosinopril generics	Initial: 5 mg daily po Target: 20 mg daily po	See captopril.	See captopril.	$
	lisinopril Zestril, Prinivil, generics	Initial: 2.5 mg daily po Target: 20 mg daily po	See captopril.	See captopril.	$
	quinapril Accupril, generics	Initial: 5 mg daily po Target: 20 mg daily po	See captopril.	See captopril.	$
	ramipril Altace, generics	Initial: 1.25–2.5 mg BID po Target: 5 mg BID or 10 mg daily po	See captopril.	See captopril.	$
Aldosterone Antagonists	*eplerenone* Inspra	Initial: 25 mg daily po Target: 50 mg daily po	Hyperkalemia, dehydration, dizziness, diarrhea, nausea.	Hyperkalemia with ACE inhibitors, ARBs. NSAIDs. Strong inhibitors/inducers of CYP3A4.	$$$$
	spironolactone Aldactone, generics	Initial: 12.5 mg daily po Target: 25–50 mg daily po	Rash, urticaria, gynecomastia, nausea, vomiting, diarrhea, confusion, hyperkalemia, agranulocytosis, SLE.	Hyperkalemia with ACE inhibitors, digoxin, NSAIDs.	$
Antiplatelet Agents	*ASA* Aspirin, Coated Aspirin, Entrophen, generics	80–325 mg/day po	Gastritis, gastric/duodenal ulceration (rarely bronchospasm). Nausea, vomiting, GI hemorrhage, tinnitus, vertigo, hypersensitivity.	Bleeding increased with heparin (low risk) and warfarin; other NSAIDs.	$

Class	Drug	Dose	Adverse Effects	Drug Interactions	Cost[a]
	clopidogrel Plavix, generics	Loading dose: pre-PCI or STEMI: 300–600 mg UA/NSTEMI: 300 mg (omit if risk of bleeding high) Maintenance: 75 mg daily po	Bleeding, rash, purpura. Similar tolerability to ASA.	Caution with NSAIDs. PPI use may reduce clopidogrel efficacy.	$
	prasugrel Effient	Loading dose: 60 mg, then 10 mg daily po	Increased risk of bleeding. Caution in patients >75 y, body weight <60 kg. Contraindicated if history of ischemic stroke.	Caution with NSAIDs.	$$$$
	ticagrelor Brilinta	Loading dose: 180 mg, then 90 mg BID po	Increased risk of bleeding, bradycardia, headache, nausea, transient dyspnea. Increased serum creatinine, uric acid.	Caution with NSAIDs. Avoid strong CYP3A4 inhibitors (e.g., clarithromycin). May increase digoxin levels.	$$$$
Beta$_1$-adrenergic Antagonists, selective with ISA	*acebutolol* Sectral, generics	Initial: 100–200 mg BID po Target: 400 mg BID po	Bronchospasm, HF, hypotension, sleep disturbance, dizziness, fatigue, anorexia, nausea, AV block, bradycardia, claudication, Raynaud's phenomenon, lethargy, drowsiness.	Enhanced cardiodepressant effect with calcium channel blockers, antiarrhythmics, anesthetics. Increased bradycardia with digoxin. Hypertension with alpha-agonists.	$
Beta$_1$-adrenergic Antagonists, selective without ISA	*atenolol* Tenormin, generics	Initial: 50 mg/day po Target: 100 mg/day po	See acebutolol.	See acebutolol.	$
	metoprolol Lopresor, generics	IV: 5 mg over 1–2 min, repeat Q5min (maximum 15 mg) Initial: 25–50 mg QID po Target: 100 mg BID po po can be started 15 min after iv	See acebutolol.	See acebutolol.	$
Beta$_1$-adrenergic Antagonists, nonselective without ISA	*nadolol* generics	Initial: 40–80 mg/day po Target: 160 mg/day po	See acebutolol.	See acebutolol.	$
	propranolol generics	Initial: 40 mg BID–TID po Target: 60 mg QID po	See acebutolol.	See acebutolol.	$
	timolol generics	Initial: 5–10 mg BID po Target: 10 mg BID po	See acebutolol.	See acebutolol.	$
Calcium Channel Blockers	*amlodipine* Norvasc, generics	5–10 mg/day po	Hypotension, flushing, marked peripheral edema.		$

(cont'd)

Table 2: **Drugs Used in Acute Coronary Syndromes** *(cont'd)*

Class	Drug	Dose	Adverse Effects	Drug Interactions	Cost[a]
	diltiazem Cardizem CD, Tiazac, Tiazac XC, generics	120–360 mg/day po Give IR formulations TID or QID; CD and XC once daily	Bradycardia, heart block, edema, hypotension.	Additive effect with β-blockers, digoxin, amiodarone. Monitor for excessive bradycardia.	\$–\$\$\$
	verapamil Isoptin SR, generics	180–480 mg/day po Give IR formulations TID; SR BID	Bradycardia, heart block, hypotension, constipation, flushing, edema.	See diltiazem.	\$\$
Direct Thrombin Inhibitors	*bivalirudin* Angiomax	Bolus: 0.75 mg/kg iv, then 1.75 mg/kg/h	Bleeding, allergic reactions (rare).	Use caution with other drugs that affect hemostasis.	\$465 (250 mg vial)[b]
Glycoprotein IIb/IIIa Inhibitors	*eptifibatide* Integrilin, generics	Bolus: 180 μg/kg iv over 1–2 min, then 2 μg/kg/min Maximum: 15 mg/h ClCr <50 mL/min: infuse at 1 μg/kg/min	Bleeding (risk of serious bleeding appears to be low), primarily at puncture sites. Thrombocytopenia. Allergic reactions.	Use caution with other drugs that affect hemostasis.	\$250[b]
	tirofiban Aggrastat	0.4 μg/kg/min iv × 30 min then 0.1 μg/kg/min × 48–72 h ClCr <30 mL/min: 0.2 μg/kg/min iv × 30 min then 0.05 μg/kg/min × 72 h	See eptifibatide.	See eptifibatide.	\$345[b]
Low Molecular Weight Heparins	*dalteparin* Fragmin	120 IU/kg BID sc Maximum: 10 000 IU/dose	Hematoma at injection site, bleeding, thrombocytopenia; caution if ClCr <30 mL/min.	Bleeding increased with ASA (low risk) and warfarin.	\$\$[b]
	enoxaparin Lovenox	1 mg/kg BID sc Maximum: 100 mg for the first 2 doses Post-thrombolytic: 30 mg iv bolus in addition to first sc dose If ≥75 y, omit bolus and reduce dose to 0.75 mg/kg BID (75 mg maximum for first 2 doses)	See dalteparin. Caution in elderly patients and those with renal insufficiency. **Preferred LMWH in ACS.**	See dalteparin.	\$\$[b]
Nitrates	*isosorbide dinitrate* generics	Initial: 30–90 mg/day po Divide dose TID (allow a 12 h nitrate-free period)	Headache (up to 50%; tolerance may develop), tachycardia, palpitation, hypotension, syncope (rare), dizziness, nausea, flushing, weakness.	Potential hypotensive effect with vasodilators. Contraindicated with recent (<24 h) use of sildenafil, tadalafil or vardenafil; use with caution when hypotension present.	\$

Class	Drug	Dose	Adverse Effects	Drug Interactions	Cost[a]
	isosorbide-5-mononitrate Imdur, generics	30–60 mg daily po	See isosorbide dinitrate	See isosorbide dinitrate	$
	nitroglycerin, intravenous generics	Initial: 10–150 µg/min iv (titrate to symptoms and blood pressure)	Frequent BP monitoring is required for iv nitroglycerin. See isosorbide dinitrate	See isosorbide dinitrate	$[b]
	nitroglycerin, sublingual Nitrostat, Nitrolingual Pumpspray, generics	Tablet: 0.3–0.6 mg sl PRN Q5 min Spray: 0.4 mg sl PRN Q5 min	See isosorbide dinitrate	See isosorbide dinitrate	$/ container
	nitroglycerin, transdermal Minitran, Nitro-Dur, Transderm-Nitro, Trinipatch, generics	0.2–0.8 mg/h patch applied daily for 10–12 h	See isosorbide dinitrate Contact dermatitis.	See isosorbide dinitrate	$$
Specific Factor Xa Inhibitors	*fondaparinux* Arixtra, generics	2.5 mg daily sc First dose iv if STEMI	Bleeding, allergic reactions (rare). Not recommended as sole agent in patients undergoing PCI due to risk of catheter thrombosis.	Use caution with other drugs that affect hemostasis.	$[b]
Thrombolytics	*alteplase* Activase rt-PA	Bolus: 15 mg iv, then 0.75 mg/kg × 30 min (maximum 50 mg), then 0.5 mg/kg × 60 min (maximum 35 mg) Maximum dose: 100 mg Start heparin with infusion	Bleeding (can be fatal). Absolute contraindications: pericarditis, previous intracranial hemorrhage; known malignant intracranial neoplasm, known cerebral vascular lesion, ischemic stroke within 3 months **except** acute stroke within 3 h; suspected aortic dissection; active bleeding or bleeding diathesis (excluding menses); significant closed head or facial trauma within 3 months. Relative contraindications: history of chronic severe, poorly controlled HTN, severe uncontrolled HTN (BP >180/110 mm Hg)[c]; prior CVA greater than 3 months or known intracerebral pathology not covered above; traumatic or prolonged (>10 min) CPR or major surgery (<3 wk); noncompressible venous punctures; recent (2–4 wk) internal bleeding; pregnancy; active peptic ulcer; current use of anticoagulants.		$2746 (100 mg vial)[b]

(cont'd)

Table 2: **Drugs Used in Acute Coronary Syndromes** *(cont'd)*

Class	Drug	Dose	Adverse Effects	Drug Interactions	Cost[a]
	tenecteplase TNKase	<60 kg: 30 mg iv × 1 60–69 kg: 35 mg iv × 1 70–79 kg: 40 mg iv × 1 80–89 kg: 45 mg iv × 1 ≥90 kg: 50 mg iv × 1 Given as iv bolus over 5 s	See alteplase.		$2835 (50 mg vial)[b]
Unfractionated Heparin	*heparin, unfractionated* Heparin LEO, generics	60–70 U/kg iv bolus Maximum: 5000 U then 12–15 U/kg/h Adjust to maintain aPTT at 1.5–2 × control. First aPTT 4 h after bolus Post-thrombolytic: bolus 60 U/kg iv Maximum: 4000 U then 12 U/kg/h Adjust to maintain aPTT at 1.5–2 × control. First aPTT 6 h after bolus	Bleeding, thrombocytopenia.	Bleeding increased with ASA (low risk) and warfarin; aPTT response may be blunted with concurrent iv nitroglycerin (controversial).	$[b]

[a] Cost of 30-day supply unless otherwise specified; includes drug cost only except where noted.
[b] Cost of average 1-day supply.
[c] Could be an absolute contraindication in low-risk patients with STEMI.
Dosage adjustment may be required in renal impairment; see Appendix I.
Abbreviations: aPTT = activated partial thromboplastin time; AV = atrioventricular; BP = blood pressure; CPR = cardiopulmonary resuscitation; CVA = cerebrovascular accident; GI = gastrointestinal; GU = genitourinary; HF = heart failure; HTN = hypertension; ISA = intrinsic sympathomimetic activity; LMWH = low-molecular-weight heparin; NSAID = nonsteroidal anti-inflammatory drug; NTG = nitroglycerin; PCI = percutaneous coronary intervention; PPI = proton pump inhibitor; s = seconds; SCr = serum creatinine; SL = sublingual; SLE = systemic lupus erythematosus; SR = sustained release; STEMI = ST segment elevation myocardial infarction; U = units; UA/NSTEMI = unstable angina or non-ST segment elevation myocardial infarction
Legend: $ < $25 $$ $25–50 $-$$$ < $25–75 $$$ $50–75 $$$$ $75–100

Suggested Readings

2012 Writing Committee Members, Jneid H, Anderson JL et al. 2012 ACCF/AHA focused update of the guideline for the management of patients with unstable angina/non-ST-segment elevation myocardial infarction (updating the 2007 guideline and replacing the 2011 focused update): a report of the American College of Cardiology Foundation/American Heart Association Task Force on Practice Guidelines. *Circulation* 2012;126(7):875-910.

Boersma E, Harrington RA, Moliterno DJ et al. Platelet glycoprotein IIb/IIIa inhibitors in acute coronary syndromes: a meta-analysis of all major randomised clinical trials. *Lancet* 2002;359(9302):189-98.

O'Gara PT, Kushner FG, Ascheim DD et al. 2013 ACCF/AHA guideline for the management of ST-elevation myocardial infarction: executive summary: a report of the American College of Cardiology Foundation/American Heart Association Task Force on Practice Guidelines. *Circulation* 2013;127(4):529-55.

References

1. Alpert JS, Thygesen K, Antman E et al. Myocardial infarction redefined—a consensus document of The Joint European Society of Cardiology/American College of Cardiology Committee for the redefinition of myocardial infarction. *J Am Coll Cardiol* 2000;36(3):959-69.
2. Heidenreich PA, Alloggiamento T, Melsop K et al. The prognostic value of troponin in patients with non-ST elevation acute coronary syndromes: a meta-analysis. *J Am Coll Cardiol* 2001;38(2):478-85.
3. Ottani F, Galvani M, Nicolini FA et al. Elevated cardiac troponin levels predict the risk of adverse outcome in patients with acute coronary syndromes. *Am Heart J* 2000;140(6):917-27.
4. Antman EM, Cohen M, Bernink PJ et al. The TIMI risk score for unstable angina/non-ST elevation MI: a method for prognostication and therapeutic decision making. *JAMA* 2000;284(7):835-42.
5. Yan AT, Yan RT, Tan M et al. Risk scores for risk stratification in acute coronary syndromes: useful but simpler is not necessarily better. *Eur Heart J* 2007;28(9):1072-8.
6. Cannon CP, Weintraub WS, Demopoulos LA et al. Comparison of early invasive and conservative strategies in patients with unstable coronary syndromes treated with the glycoprotein IIb/IIIa inhibitor tirofiban. *N Engl J Med* 2001;344(25):1879-87.
7. Grossman E, Messerli FH, Grodzicki T et al. Should a moratorium be placed on sublingual nifedipine capsules given for hypertensive emergencies and pseudoemergencies? *JAMA* 1996;276(16):1328-31.
8. Indications for ACE inhibitors in the early treatment of acute myocardial infarction: systematic overview of individual data from 100,000 patients in randomized trials. ACE Inhibitor Myocardial Infarction Collaborative Group. *Circulation* 1998;97(22):2202-12.
9. Yusuf S, Sleight P, Pogue J et al. Effects of an angiotensin-converting-enzyme inhibitor, ramipril, on cardiovascular events in high-risk patients. The Heart Outcomes Prevention Evaluation Study Investigators. *N Engl J Med* 2000;342(3):145-53.
10. Holdright D, Patel D, Cunningham D et al. Comparison of the effect of heparin and aspirin versus aspirin alone on transient myocardial ischemia and in-hospital prognosis in patients with unstable angina. *J Am Coll Cardiol* 1994;24(1):39-45.
11. Theroux P, Ouimet H, McCans J et al. Aspirin, heparin, or both to treat acute unstable angina. *N Engl J Med* 1988;319(17):1105-11.
12. Comparison of two treatment durations (6 days and 14 days) of a low molecular weight heparin with a 6-day treatment of unfractionated heparin in the initial management of unstable angina or non-Q wave myocardial infarction: FRAX.I.S. (FRAxiparine in Ischaemic Syndrome). *Eur Heart J* 1999;20(21):1553-62.
13. Antman EM, McCabe CH, Gurfinkel EP et al. Enoxaparin prevents death and cardiac ischemic events in unstable angina/non-Q-wave myocardial infarction. Results of the thrombolysis in myocardial infarction (TIMI) 11B trial. *Circulation* 1999;100(15):1593-601.
14. Cohen M, Demers C, Gurfinkel EP et al. A comparison of low-molecular-weight heparin with unfractionated heparin for unstable coronary artery disease. Efficacy and Safety of Subcutaneous Enoxaparin in Non-Q-Wave Coronary Events Study Group. *N Engl J Med* 1997;337(7):447-52.
15. Klein W, Buchwald A, Hillis SE et al. Comparison of low-molecular-weight heparin with unfractionated heparin acutely and with placebo for 6 weeks in the management of unstable coronary artery disease. Fragmin in unstable coronary artery disease study (FRIC). *Circulation* 1997;96(1):61-8.
16. Michalis LK, Katsouras CS, Papamichael N et al. Enoxaparin versus tinzaparin in non-ST-segment elevation acute coronary syndromes: the EVET trial. *Am Heart J* 2003;146(2):304-10.
17. Yusuf S, Mehta SR, Chrolavicius S et al. Comparison of fondaparinux and enoxaparin in acute coronary syndromes. *N Engl J Med* 2006;354(14):1464-76.
18. Anderson JL, Adams CD, Antman EM et al. ACC/AHA 2007 guidelines for the management of patients with unstable angina/non-ST-elevation myocardial infarction: a report of the American College of Cardiology/American Heart Association Task Force on Practice Guidelines (Writing Committee to revise the 2002 guidelines for the management of patients with unstable angina/non-ST-elevation myocardial infarction): developed in collaboration with the American College of Emergency Physicians, the Society for Cardiovascular Angiography and Interventions and the Society of Thoracic Surgeons: endorsed by the American Association of Cardiovascular and Pulmonary Rehabilitation and the Society for Academic Emergency Medicine. *Circulation* 2007;116(7):e148-304.
19. Yusuf S, Zhao F, Mehta SR et al. Effects of clopidogrel in addition to aspirin in patients with acute coronary syndromes without ST-segment elevation. *N Engl J Med* 2001;345(7):494-502.
20. Budaj A, Yusuf S, Mehta SR et al. Benefit of clopidogrel in patients with acute coronary syndromes without ST-segment elevation in various risk groups. *Circulation* 2002;106(13):1622-6.
21. Mehta SR, Yusuf S, Peters RJ et al. Effects of pretreatment with clopidogrel and aspirin followed by long-term therapy in patients undergoing percutaneous coronary intervention: the PCI-CURE study. *Lancet* 2001;358(9281):527-33.
22. ACCF/AHA clopidogrel clinical alert: approaches to the FDA "boxed warning": a report of the American College of Cardiology Foundation Task Force on Clinical Expert Consensus Documents and the American Heart Association. *Circulation* 2010;122(5):537-57.

23. Wiviott SD, Braunwald E, McCabe CH et al. Prasugrel versus clopidogrel in patients with acute coronary syndromes. *N Engl J Med* 2007;357(2):2001-15.
24. Roe MT, Armstrong PW, Fox KA et al. Prasugrel versus clopidogrel for acute coronary syndromes without revascularization. *N Eng J Med* 2012;367(14):1297-309.
25. Wallentin L, Becker RC, Budaj A et al. Ticagrelor versus clopidogrel in patients with acute coronary syndromes. *N Engl J Med* 2009;361(11):1045-57.
26. A comparison of aspirin plus tirofiban with aspirin plus heparin for unstable angina. Platelet Receptor Inhibition in Ischemic Syndrome Management (PRISM) Study Investigators. *N Engl J Med* 1998;338(21):1498-505.
27. Inhibition of the platelet glycoprotein IIb/IIIa receptor with tirofiban in unstable angina and non-Q-wave myocardial infarction. Platelet Receptor Inhibition in Ischemic Syndrome Management in Patients Limited by Unstable Signs and Symptoms (PRISM-PLUS) Study Investigators. *N Engl J Med* 1998;338(21):1488-97.
28. Labinaz M, Kilaru R, Pieper K et al. Outcomes of patients with acute coronary syndromes and prior coronary artery bypass grafting: results from the platelet glycoprotein IIb/IIIa in unstable angina: receptor suppression using integrilin therapy (PURSUIT) trial. *Circulation* 2002;105(3):322-7.
29. Moliterno DJ, Yakubov SJ, DiBattiste PM et al. Outcomes at 6 months for the direct comparison of tirofiban and abciximab during percutaneous coronary revascularisation with stent placement: the TARGET follow-up study. *Lancet* 2002;360(9330):355-60.
30. O'Shea JC, Hafley GE, Greenberg S et al. Platelet glycoprotein IIb/IIIa integrin blockade with eptifibatide in coronary stent intervention: the ESPRIT trial: a randomized controlled trial. *JAMA* 2001;285(19):2468-73.
31. O'Gara PT, Kushner FG, Ascheim DD et al. 2013 ACCF/AHA guideline for the management of ST-elevation myocardial infarction: a report of the American College of Cardiology Foundation/American Heart Association Task Force on Practice Guidelines. *Circulation* 2013;127(4):e362-425.
32. Grines CL, Browne KF, Marco J et al. A comparison of immediate angioplasty with thrombolytic therapy for acute myocardial infarction. The Primary Angioplasty in Myocardial Infarction Study Group. *N Engl J Med* 1993;328(10):673-9.
33. Hochman JS, Sleeper LA, White HD et al. One-year survival following early revascularization for cardiogenic shock. *JAMA* 2001;285(2):190-2.
34. Thiemann DR, Coresh J, Schulman SP et al. Lack of benefit for intravenous thrombolysis in patients with myocardial infarction who are older than 75 years. *Circulation* 2000;101(19):2239-46.
35. Antman EM, Morrow DA, McCabe CH et al. Enoxaparin versus unfractionated heparin with fibrinolysis for ST-elevation myocardial infarction. *N Engl J Med* 2006;354(14):1477-88.
36. Yusuf S, Held P, Furberg C. Update of effects of calcium antagonists in myocardial infarction or angina in light of the second Danish Verapamil Infarction Trial (DAVIT-II) and other recent studies. *Am J Cardiol* 1991;67(15):1295-7.
37. Yusuf S, Collins R, MacMahon S et al. Effect of intravenous nitrates on mortality in acute myocardial infarction: an overview of the randomised trials. *Lancet* 1988;1(8594):1088-92.
38. Pitt B, Zannad F, Remme WJ et al. The effect of spironolactone on morbidity and mortality in patients with severe heart failure. Randomized Aldactone Evaluation Study Investigators. *N Engl J Med* 1999;341(10):709-17.
39. Pitt B, Remme W, Zannad F et al. Eplerenone, a selective aldosterone blocker, in patients with left ventricular dysfunction after myocardial infarction. *N Engl J Med* 2003;348(14):1309-21.
40. Chen ZM, Jiang LX, Chen YP et al. Addition of clopidogrel to aspirin in 45,852 patients with acute myocardial infarction: randomised placebo-controlled trial. *Lancet* 2005;366(9497):1607-21.
41. Sabatine MS, Cannon CP, Gibson CM et al. Addition of clopidogrel to aspirin and fibrinolytic therapy for myocardial infarction with ST-segment elevation. *N Engl J Med* 2005;352(12):1179-89.
42. Tanguay JF, Bell AD Ackman ML et al. Canadian Cardiovascular Society. *2012 CCS antiplatelet therapy guidelines*. Available from: www.ccsguidelineprograms.ca/index.php?option=com_content&=article&=141&=82#AP.
43. Moss AJ, Zareba W, Hall WJ et al. Prophylactic implantation of a defibrillator in patients with myocardial infarction and reduced ejection fraction. *N Engl J Med* 2002;346(12):877-83.
44. Gregoratos G, Abrams J, Epstein AE et al. ACC/AHA/NASPE 2002 guideline update for implantation of cardiac pacemakers and antiarrhythmia devices: summary article: a report of the American College of Cardiology/American Heart Association Task Force on Practice Guidelines (ACC/AHA/NASPE Committee to Update the 1998 Pacemaker Guidelines). *Circulation* 2002;106(16):2145-61.
45. Berman J, Haffajee CI, Alpert JS. Therapy of symptomatic pericarditis after myocardial infarction: retrospective and prospective studies of aspirin, indomethacin, prednisone, and spontaneous resolution. *Am Heart J* 1981;101(6):750-3.

Cardiovascular Disorders

Chapter 36
Acute Stroke

Stephen J. Phillips, BSc, MBBS, FRCPC and
Gord Gubitz, BSc, MD, FRCPC (Edin)

Stroke, recognized clinically as the sudden onset of a focal disturbance of central nervous system function, may be caused by cerebral infarction (ischemic stroke, responsible for about 85% of all strokes) or intracerebral hemorrhage.[1] The third main stroke subtype, subarachnoid hemorrhage, more often causes sudden onset of severe headache with or without impaired consciousness. The Heart and Stroke Foundation promotes awareness of the warning signs of possible stroke, which are presented in Table 1.

There is no acute-phase intervention of proven value for intracerebral hemorrhage. Post-acute treatment of primary intracerebral hemorrhage is similar to that of ischemic stroke except that antithrombotic drugs are avoided. Treatment of subarachnoid hemorrhage is primarily nonpharmacologic (ablation of the bleeding source). Refer patients with suspected subarachnoid hemorrhage to a neurosurgical centre immediately.

Goals of Therapy

- Minimize brain damage
- Prevent complications
- Reduce risk of recurrence
- Restore function of the individual

Investigations

The evaluation of patients with suspected stroke is highly time dependent. Specific stroke treatments (alteplase) can be provided only within the first 4.5 hours of symptom onset in patients with ischemic stroke (see Figure 1).

Table 1: **Warning Signs of Stroke**

Weakness	Sudden loss of strength or numbness in the face, arm or leg
Difficulty with speech	Sudden confusion or trouble speaking
Vision problems	Sudden trouble with vision
Headache	Sudden severe and unusual headache
Dizziness	Loss of balance, especially with any of the above signs

Figure 1: **Emergency Department Management of Patients with Suspected Stroke**

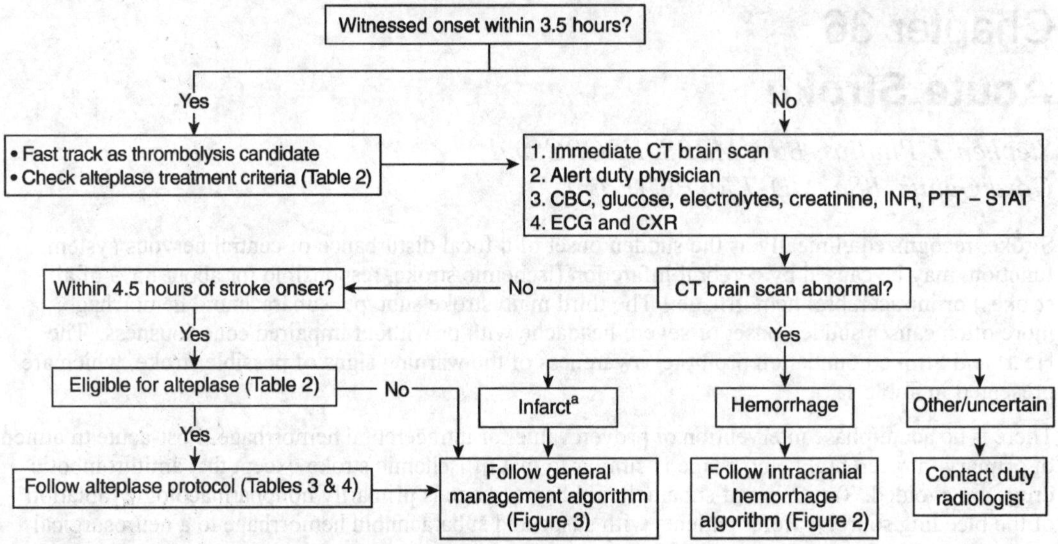

[a] Notify neurosurgeon if cerebellar infarct with mass effect on 4th ventricle (see Neurosurgical Intervention text).
Abbreviations: CBC = complete blood count; CT = computed tomography; CXR = chest x-ray; ECG = electrocardiogram; PTT = partial thromboplastin time; STAT = immediately/urgently
Adapted with permission from *Nova Scotia guidelines for stroke care*. Halifax (NS): Cardiovascular Health Nova Scotia; 2008.

Use the clinical history, physical examination, imaging studies and other ancillary investigations to confirm the diagnosis and exclude stroke mimics such as subdural hematoma, Todd's paresis (post seizure), brain abscess, herpes simplex encephalitis, hypoglycemia, brain tumour (primary or secondary), multiple sclerosis, migraine and conversion disorder.

- History:
  - time of onset, symptoms at onset, course of symptoms since onset
  - antecedent trauma or illness, previous neurovascular events
  - vascular comorbidity (angina, MI, heart failure, atrial fibrillation, peripheral and renal vascular disease)
  - vascular disease risk factors (hypertension, smoking, diabetes mellitus, dyslipidemia, excessive alcohol intake, body mass index, exercise, family history of vascular disease or hemostatic disorders)
  - other health problems (particularly peptic ulcer disease or other disorders that predispose to bleeding)
  - pre-stroke cognitive and functional status
  - place of residence and social supports
  - medications (particularly anticoagulant and antiplatelet drugs)
- Physical examination:
  - to localize the lesion by brain region and vascular territory
  - to determine stroke syndrome, severity and cause
  - to assess comorbid conditions

- Laboratory and radiological tests:
  - CBC, INR, PTT, glucose (to rule out hypoglycemia as a stroke mimic), electrolytes, urea, creatinine, liver function tests, albumin
  - fasting glucose, hemoglobin A_{1c}, cholesterol panel (for risk factor modification)
  - ECG (to look for atrial fibrillation, MI and left ventricular hypertrophy)
  - chest x-ray (to look for heart disease, lung cancer)
  - CT (or MR) brain scan is required immediately[2] for all patients to rule out intracerebral hemorrhage and stroke mimics. For patients who are found to have intracranial hemorrhage, the *location* of the hemorrhage determines subsequent treatment (see Figure 2)
  - if CT scan is negative for blood but subarachnoid hemorrhage is still suspected, lumbar puncture is indicated
  - urgent (same or next day) vascular imaging (duplex carotid ultrasonography, CT angiography or MR angiography) to determine the degree of carotid stenosis in patients with nondisabling carotid territory strokes who are fit for carotid endarterectomy[2]
  - 24-hour ECG (Holter) monitor and echocardiography (transthoracic ± transesophageal) to search for a cardiac source of emboli in patients with a recent history of MI or cardiac surgery, and patients with a large-vessel territory (nonlacunar) stroke and neurovascular imaging studies showing no large-vessel disease, provided anticoagulation is not contraindicated
  - other investigations if indicated:
    - antiphospholipid antibodies, protein C, protein S, antithrombin, factor V Leiden and prothrombin gene mutation if hypercoagulable state suspected
    - blood cultures and urgent echocardiogram if infectious endocarditis suspected
    - inflammatory markers (ESR, CRP, ANA) as a screen for vasculitis
    - lumbar puncture if suspected vasculitis, syphilis or other CNS infections
    - malignancy work-up (CT chest, abdomen, pelvis)
    - syphilis serology

Figure 2: Approach to a Finding of Intracranial Hemorrhage on CT Scan

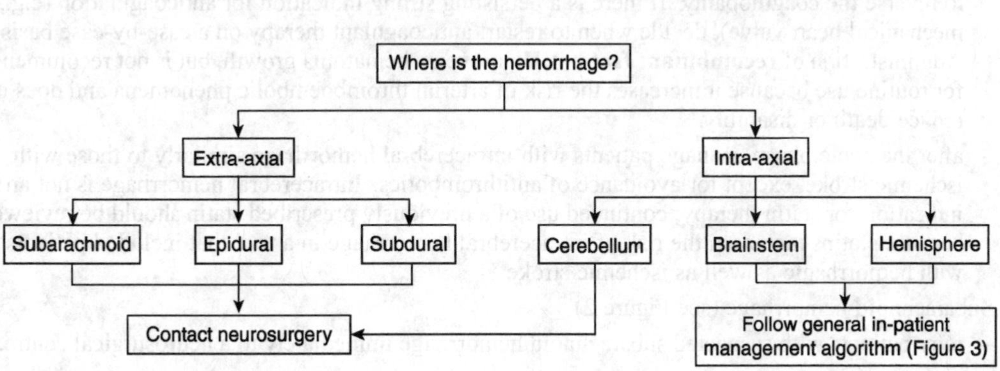

Abbreviations: CT = computed tomography
Adapted with permission from *Nova Scotia guidelines for stroke care*. Halifax (NS): Cardiovascular Health Nova Scotia; 2008.

Therapeutic Choices

Nonpharmacologic Choices

Aneurysmal Subarachnoid Hemorrhage

Ablation of the aneurysm reduces the risk of rebleeding. Endovascular coiling is superior to neurosurgical clipping for ruptured intracranial aneurysm anatomically suitable for either procedure.[3]

Carotid Endarterectomy

Patients with carotid territory transient ischemic attack (TIA) or nondisabling stroke and ipsilateral 70–95% internal carotid artery stenosis (measured on a catheter angiogram or by 2 concordant noninvasive imaging modalities) should be offered carotid endarterectomy (CEA) within 2 weeks of the incident TIA or stroke unless contraindicated.[2] CEA is also appropriate for *selected* patients with moderate (50–69%) symptomatic stenosis. These patients should be evaluated by a physician with expertise in stroke management. Carotid stenting may be considered for patients who are not CEA candidates for technical, anatomical or medical reasons.[4]

Neurosurgical Intervention

- Ischemic stroke
  - *decompressive hemicraniectomy* may be performed on patients with massive hemispheric infarcts whose level of consciousness is declining. Evidence from a pooled analysis of 3 smaller randomized trials found an increase in survival for these patients when treated with craniectomy. However, survivors did incur significant amounts of disability.[5] Consensus opinion is that patients with large cerebellar infarcts may benefit from surgical decompression.
- Intracerebral hemorrhage (see Figure 2)
  - patients with cerebellar hemorrhage should have an urgent neurosurgical consultation for consideration of *posterior fossa craniotomy* and evacuation of the hemorrhage.[2] The place of neurosurgical intervention for supratentorial intracerebral hemorrhage is unclear and the subject of ongoing research.[6] Patients with supratentorial intracerebral hemorrhage should be cared for on a stroke unit.[2]
  - treat patients with acute intracerebral hemorrhage and an established coagulopathy or a history of warfarin use with **prothrombin complex concentrate**, **vitamin K** or fresh-frozen plasma to reverse the coagulopathy. If there is a persisting strong indication for anticoagulation (e.g., mechanical heart valve), decide when to restart anticoagulant therapy on a case-by-case basis. Administration of **recombinant factor VIIa** prevents hematoma growth, but is not recommended for routine use because it increases the risk of arterial thromboembolic phenomena and does not reduce death or disability.[7]
  - after the acute phase, manage patients with intracerebral hemorrhage similarly to those with ischemic stroke, except for avoidance of antithrombotics. Intracerebral hemorrhage is not an indication for statin therapy; continued use of a previously prescribed statin should be reviewed because statins increased the risk of intracerebral hemorrhage in a trial that included patients with hemorrhagic as well as ischemic stroke.[8]
- Subarachnoid hemorrhage (see Figure 2)
  - refer patients with suspected subarachnoid hemorrhage immediately to a neurosurgical centre.[2]

General Supportive Care

- Outcomes are optimized by care on a stroke unit provided by a coordinated interdisciplinary team (see Figure 3).
- Start rehabilitation as soon as the patient is medically stable.
- Family and community supports are important for social reintegration.

- Expert nursing care and early mobilization are the mainstays of treatment.
- Use oxygen if pulse oximetry shows desaturation (SaO_2 <90%).[12]
- Elevated body temperature is associated with poor outcome after stroke.[13,14,15] Symptomatic treatment of pyrexia (and investigation of its cause) is recommended.[16]
- Hyperglycemia is associated with poor outcome after stroke and should be treated,[2] but there is no definitive clinical trial data to support the use of intravenous insulin.[17]

Aspiration Pneumonia and Malnutrition[16]

- Review the nutritional status (prealbumin, weight) on admission to identify patients who were malnourished before their stroke.
- Give *nothing by mouth* if any of the following are present: reduced level of consciousness, severe dysarthria, wet voice, weak cough, impaired palatal sensation, inability to sit, suspected aspiration.
- Monitor recovery from dysphagia using serial bedside swallowing assessments, best performed by an experienced dysphagia team.
- A videofluoroscopic examination (modified barium swallow) may be required to exclude significant aspiration when the results of the bedside examination are ambiguous.
- Tube feeding may be required if significant aspiration is demonstrated or suspected. Initially, this is usually done via a nasogastric tube. If swallowing does not improve, tube feeding via percutaneous endoscopic gastrostomy (PEG) may be necessary. The FOOD trial did not support early initiation of PEG feeding in dysphagic stroke patients.[18]
- Parenteral nutrition is required only in exceptional circumstances.
- Give a texture-modified diet for dysphagic patients at lower risk of aspiration. Additional iv fluids are often necessary for these patients.

Figure 3: **General Management of the Stroke Patient**

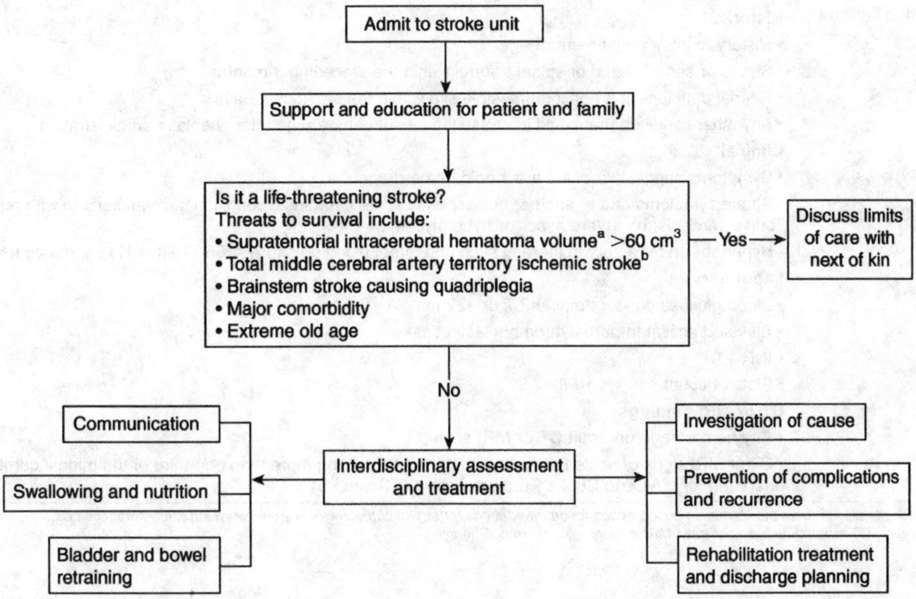

[a] Hematoma volume (cm^3) = A×B×C/2 where A = largest diameter (cm) on CT scan, B = diameter (cm) perpendicular to A, C = number of 1 cm scan slices showing hematoma.[9,10]
[b] Hemiparesis and hemianopia with either aphasia or visuospatial deficit.[11]

Venous Thromboembolism[16]

- Early mobilization (even if only up in a chair) is recommended (as soon as possible after admission to hospital).
- Maintain adequate hydration.
- The use of graduated compression stockings is not recommended.[19,20]
- Pneumatic compression stockings reduce the risk of deep vein thrombosis and increase the likelihood of survival after stroke, and because they do not cause bleeding they can be used in patients who have had an intracerebral hemorrhage.[21]

Pharmacologic Choices

Ischemic Stroke

Thrombolytics

Alteplase (rt-PA) should be administered iv as soon as possible following stroke onset in patients who meet strict eligibility criteria [Evidence: SORT A*].[2,12] See Figure 1, Table 2, Table 3 and Table 4. A meta-analysis concluded that thrombolysis within 3 hours significantly increased the chance (from 317 to 407 per 1000 patients treated) of being alive and independent 1–6 months after ischemic stroke.[22] This overall benefit was found despite an increase in early intracranial hemorrhage. Health Canada currently approves administration within 3 hours of stroke onset, though evidence from randomized trials demonstrates benefit up to at least 4.5 hours.[2,22]

Intra-arterial administration of thrombolytic agents and nonpharmacologic methods of achieving recanalization are presently of limited clinical application, except in highly specialized centres where randomized trials are ongoing.

Table 2: **Alteplase in Acute Ischemic Stroke: Treatment Criteria**

Treatment Criteria	• Ischemic stroke causing measurable neurologic deficit in a patient ≥18 years • Stroke onset >1 h and ≤4.5 h before alteplase administration
Exclusion Criteria	**Historical** • History of intracranial hemorrhage • Stroke or serious head or spinal trauma within the preceding 3 months • Arterial puncture at a noncompressible site within the previous 7 days • Any other condition that could increase the risk of hemorrhage after alteplase administration **Clinical** • Symptoms suggestive of subarachnoid hemorrhage • Stroke symptoms due to another nonischemic acute neurologic condition such as seizure with postictal Todd's paralysis, or severe hypo- or hyperglycemia • Hypertension refractory to therapy such that target blood pressure <185/110 mm Hg cannot be reached **Laboratory** • Blood glucose concentration <2.7 or >22 mmol/L • Elevated activated partial thromboplastin time • INR >1.7 • Platelet count <100 × 10^9/L **CT or MRI Findings** • Any hemorrhage on brain CT or MRI scan • CT or MRI signs of acute hemispheric infarction involving more than one-third of the middle cerebral artery territory (Alberta Stroke Program Early CT Score <5)

Adapted with permission from the *Canadian best practice recommendations for stroke care*, available from: www.strokebestpractices.ca.
Abbreviations: CT = computed tomography; MRI = magnetic resonance imaging

* SORT (Strength of Recommendation Taxonomy) is a rating system (A, B or C) that addresses the quality of available evidence. For more information consult **How to Use *Compendium of Therapeutic Choices*** on page xxv.

Table 3: Alteplase in Acute Ischemic Stroke: Monitoring[12]

Blood Pressure and Neurologic Signs
• Baseline, then Q15 min × 2 h after starting alteplase, then Q30 min × 6 h, then Q1H until 24 h after starting alteplase
• Call MD if the systolic BP is >180 mm Hg or if the diastolic BP is >110 mm Hg on 2 or more occasions taken 5–10 min apart
• Stop the infusion, obtain emergency CT scan and notify MD if there is neurologic deterioration, severe headache, or new onset of nausea or vomiting
Blood Glucose
• Call MD if glucose >12 mmol/L
Lines and Tubes
• Delay placement of nasogastric tubes, indwelling catheters or intra-arterial pressure catheters
Medications
• No anticoagulant or antiplatelet drug for 24 h
• Acetaminophen 650 mg po or pr Q4H if body temperature is ≥38°C, or for analgesia
• O_2 via nasal prongs or face mask to keep O_2 saturation >90%
• After the alteplase infusion is completed, continue iv normal saline (with or without KCl)
Investigations
• CT brain scan after 24 h

Abbreviations: CT = computed tomography; MD = medical doctor

Venous Thromboembolism[16]

- In the absence of contraindications, use **low molecular weight heparin** (LMWH) or **unfractionated heparin** (UH) in prophylactic doses (see Chapter 48) for patients with acute *ischemic stroke* who cannot move one or both lower limbs or mobilize independently.
- **ASA** (80–325 mg daily) reduces the risk of thromboembolism.[23]
- In patients with *hemorrhagic stroke* use of LMWH or UH is controversial.

Antithrombotic Drug Treatment

- Avoid in patients with hemorrhagic stroke.

Antiplatelet Therapy[2]

- If intracranial hemorrhage is excluded by CT scan, but alteplase is not indicated, give **ASA** 160 mg immediately. Follow with ASA 80–325 mg daily.
- When alteplase is used, wait until intracranial hemorrhage is excluded by CT scan 24 hours later and give **ASA** 160 mg once. Follow with ASA 80–325 mg daily.
- Administer **ASA** as a suppository or via nasogastric tube to dysphagic patients. Use enteric-coated formulation for patients who can swallow. No evidence supports the use of ASA doses greater than 325 mg/day for secondary stroke prevention. The GI side effects of ASA are dose related.
- For patients who were taking ASA prior to their stroke, consider other antiplatelet agents, such as **clopidogrel** 75 mg daily or a **ASA/dipyridamole** 25/200 mg twice daily; these regimens have not been adequately tested in acute stroke, but in longer term secondary prevention trials they were superior to ASA and equivalent to each other.[2] ASA-dipyridamole capsules should not be administered via nasogastric tube.
- The use of combined **ASA** and **clopidogrel** in the first month after a nondisabling stroke (or TIA) reduces the risk of major stroke recurrence at 3 months without increasing the likelihood of serious bleeding.[24,25]
- The combination of **ASA** and **clopidogrel** is not recommended for long-term secondary stroke prevention.

Anticoagulant Therapy

- Immediate systemic anticoagulation with treatment doses of UH, LMWH, heparinoids or specific thrombin inhibitors is not recommended in the setting of acute ischemic stroke, not even for patients in atrial fibrillation (AF), because there is no evidence of short- or long-term benefit. Specifically, reduction in early recurrent ischemic stroke is completely offset by an increase in major intracranial and extracranial bleeding.[26] For patients with AF and ischemic stroke, most physicians use ASA until an oral anticoagulant is started.
- ASA is as effective as warfarin for secondary stroke prevention in patients in normal sinus rhythm, and does not require laboratory monitoring.
- For patients in AF without contraindications to anticoagulation, use **apixaban**, **dabigatran**, **rivaroxaban** or **warfarin** at a dose to maintain the INR in the range of 2–3.[2] For patients who cannot be anticoagulated, use enteric-coated **ASA** 80–325 mg daily.
- The choice of oral anticoagulant should be based on patient factors including age, renal function, additional health factors, likelihood of adherence and patient preferences. Dabigatran and rivaroxaban are contraindicated if ClCr <30 mL/min; apixaban is contraindicated if ClCr <15mL/min.
- The best time to initiate anticoagulant therapy is unclear. For patients with minor stroke, it is common practice to start warfarin as soon as brain imaging has excluded intracranial hemorrhage. In patients with more severe strokes, it is common practice to repeat brain imaging after 2–14 days to exclude asymptomatic intracranial hemorrhage before starting warfarin. The RELY trial[27] of dabigatran did not enroll patients within the first 14 days after stroke, or patients with severe stroke within the previous 6 months. The ROCKET AF trial[28] of rivaroxaban did not enroll patients with a history of TIA within 3 days prior to the event, stroke within 14 days, and severely disabling strokes within 3 months. The ARISTOTLE trial[29] of apixaban did not enrol patients within the first 7 days after stroke.

For information on postacute antithrombotic treatment, carotid endarterectomy and risk factor modification, see Chapter 42.

Blood Pressure Lowering Treatment[2]

Randomized controlled trials have not defined the optimal time to initiate blood pressure lowering therapy after stroke.[30] Oral blood pressure lowering treatment should be initiated (or modified) prior to discharge from hospital in patients whose blood pressure is ≥140/90 mm Hg.

Subarachnoid Hemorrhage

Nimodipine 60 mg po Q4H for 3 weeks reduces the risk of secondary vasospasm and cerebral infarction.[31] Consider a dose of 30 mg po Q2H in patients who are very sensitive to the blood pressure lowering effects (Table 5).

Therapeutic Tips

- Formal acute stroke protocols help reduce logistical delays.
- The effectiveness of thrombolytic therapy with **alteplase** is exquisitely time dependent; delays of any sort *should not be tolerated.* A minority of patients present to hospital within the first 90 minutes of stroke onset, leaving limited time to act. Immediate contact with the patient, rapid triage, and (most importantly) *staying with the patient* continuously during the clinical assessment, CT scan, blood tests and consent procedures are vital in ensuring that the appropriate steps are being taken as rapidly as possible prior to alteplase administration.
- Determining the time of stroke onset is critical in deciding to use alteplase, but checking the clock is not a natural reaction in the setting of an acute stroke. Encourage patients and families to think of

"time anchors" (e.g., what was on the radio or TV at the time, or at what point in the patient's daily routine the symptoms first occurred).

- Patients with acute stroke are often unable to communicate. When possible, the next-of-kin should travel with the patient to hospital (or between hospitals if the patient is transferred) to provide collateral history and consent for treatment before the time window for intervention closes.
- If the patient is referred to a tertiary care hospital, have the STAT blood work (CBC, INR) drawn at the community hospital and the results faxed to the referral centre as soon as possible.
- Point-of-care INR testing , if available, can provide results quickly.
- Signs of infarction on a CT scan done within 4.5 hours of stroke onset are usually subtle. If the CT scan of a patient being considered for treatment with alteplase shows a very definite infarct in a location that explains the presenting clinical symptoms and signs, recheck the time of onset.

Suggested Readings

Heart and Stroke Foundation. *Canadian best practice recommendations for stroke care*. Available from: www.strokebestpractices.ca

Donnan GA, Fisher M, Macleod M et al. Stroke. *Lancet* 2008;371(9624):1612-23.

Internet Stroke Center. *Stroke trials registry*. Available from: www.strokecenter.org/trials.

Stroke Unit Trialists' Collaboration. Organised inpatient (stroke unit) care for stroke. *Cochrane Database Syst Rev* 2013;(9):CD000197.

Wardlaw JM, Murray V, Berge E et al. Recombinant tissue plasminogen activator for acute ischemic stroke: an updated systematic review and meta-analysis. *Lancet* 2012;379(9834):2364-72.

Table 4: Drugs Used to Treat Acute Ischemic Stroke

Class	Drug	Dose	Adverse Effects	Comments	Cost[a]
Antiplatelet Agents	*ASA* Aspirin, Coated Aspirin, generics	Initial: 160 mg Maintenance: 80–325 mg daily	Nausea, vomiting, hemorrhage, hypersensitivity reactions (rarely bronchospasm).	If alteplase is to be administered, wait 24 h before initiating ASA. If alteplase is not used, start ASA as soon as intracranial hemorrhage is excluded by CT scan. Use enteric-coated formulations for patients who can swallow. Give via nasogastric tube or as a suppository to dysphagic patients.	<$1
Thrombolytics	*alteplase* Activase rt-PA	0.9 mg/kg (maximum 90 mg) iv over 60 min. Give 10% of the total dose as an initial bolus over 1 min	Superficial bleeding, internal bleeding (i.e., gastrointestinal, genitourinary, respiratory tract, retroperitoneal), intracranial hemorrhage. Cerebral edema, cerebral herniation, seizures and new onset ischemic stroke may occur and be life threatening.	Review inclusion and exclusion criteria before administering (Table 2). No anticoagulant or antiplatelet drugs for 24 h after administration.	$2746/100 mg vial

[a] Cost of a 1-day supply; includes drug cost only.

Table 5: Drugs Used to Treat Subarachnoid Hemorrhage

Class	Drug	Dose	Adverse Effects	Comments	Cost[a]
Calcium Channel Blockers	*nimodipine* Nimotop	60 mg Q4H po for 21 days 30 mg Q2H po may be used if hypotension significant	Hypotension (5%), nausea, bradycardia and rash.	Crushing tablets for nasogastric administration is not recommended since bioavailability reduces with time. If necessary, crush and administer immediately.	$2670

[a] Cost of 21-day supply; includes drug cost only.

References

1. Warlow C, Sudlow S, Dennis M et al. Stroke. *Lancet* 2003;362(9391):1211-24.
2. Casaubon LK, Suddes M. Hyperacute stroke care. Lindsay MP, Gubitz G, Baylet M et al., eds. In: *Canadian best practice recommendations for stroke care*. 4th ed. Available from: www.strokebestpractices.ca/wp-content/uploads/2010/10/Ch3_SBP2013_Hyper-Acute-_23MAY13_EN_-FINAL5.pdf. Accessed April 2, 2014.
3. Molyneux A, Kerr R, Stratton I et al. International Subarachnoid Aneurysm Trial (ISAT) of neurosurgical clipping versus endovascular coiling in 2143 patients with ruptured intracranial aneurysms: a randomised trial. *Lancet* 2002;360(9342):1267-74.
4. Brott TG, Hobson RW, Howard G et al. Stenting versus endarterectomy for treatment of carotid-artery stenosis. *N Engl J Med* 2010;363(1):11-23.
5. Vahedi K, Hofmeijer J, Juettler E et al. Early decompressive surgery in malignant infarction of the middle cerebral artery: a pooled analysis of three randomised controlled trials. *Lancet Neurol* 2007;6(3):215-22.
6. Prasad K, Mendelow AD, Gregson B. Surgery for primary supratentorial intracerebral haemorrhage. *Cochrane Database Syst Rev* 2008;(4):CD000200.
7. Diringer MN, Skolnick BE, Mayer SA et al. Thromboembolic events with recombinant activated factor VII in spontaneous intracerebral hemorrhage: results from the Factor Seven for Acute Hemorrhagic Stroke (FAST) trial. *Stroke* 2010;41(1):48-53.
8. Goldstein LB, Amarenco P, Szarek M et al. Hemorrhagic stroke in the Stroke Prevention by Aggressive Reduction in Cholesterol Levels study. *Neurology* 2008;70(24 Pt 2):2364-70.
9. Broderick JP, Brott TG, Duldner JE et al. Volume of intracerebral hemorrhage. A powerful and easy-to-use predictor of 30-day mortality. *Stroke* 1993;24(7):987-93.
10. Broderick JP, Brott TG, Grotta JC. Intracerebral hemorrhage volume measurement. *Stroke* 1994;25(5):1081.
11. Bamford J, Sandercock P, Dennis M et al. Classification and natural history of clinically identifiable subtypes of cerebral infarction. *Lancet* 1991;337(8756):1521-6.
12. Adams HP, del Zoppo G, Alberts MJ et al. Guidelines for the early management of adults with ischemic stroke: a guideline from the American Heart Association/American Stroke Association Stroke Council, Clinical Cardiology Council, Cardiovascular Radiology and Intervention Council, and the Atherosclerotic Peripheral Vascular Disease and Quality of Care Outcomes in Research Interdisciplinary Working Groups: The American Academy of Neurology affirms the value of this guideline as an educational tool for neurologists. *Circulation* 2007;115(20):e478-534.
13. Jorgensen HS, Reith J, Pedersen PM et al. Body temperature and outcome in stroke patients. *Lancet* 1996;348(9021):193.
14. Jorgensen HS, Reith J, Nakayama H et al. What determines good recovery in patients with the most severe strokes? The Copenhagen Stroke Study. *Stroke* 1999;30(10):2008-12.
15. Reith J, Jorgensen HS, Pedersen PM et al. Body temperature in acute stroke: relation to stroke severity, infarct size, mortality and outcome. *Lancet* 1996;347(8999):422-5.
16. Casaubon LK, Suddes M. Acute inpatient stroke care. Lindsay MP, Gubitz G, Baylet M et al., eds. In: *Canadian best practice recommendations for stroke care*. 4th ed. Available from: www.strokebestpractices.ca/wp-content/uploads/2010/10/Ch4_SBP2013_Acute-Inpatient-Care_22MAY13_EN_FINAL4.pdf. Accessed April 2, 2014.
17. Gray CS, Hildreth AJ, Sandercock PA et al. Glucose-potassium-insulin infusions in the management of post-stroke hyperglycaemia: the UK Glucose Insulin in Stroke Trial (GIST-UK). *Lancet Neurol* 2007;6(5):397-406.
18. Dennis MS, Lewis SC, Warlow C et al. Effect of timing and method of enteral tube feeding for dysphagic stroke patients (FOOD): a multicentre randomised controlled trial. *Lancet* 2005;365(9461):764-72.
19. CLOTS Trials Collaboration, Dennis M, Sandercock PA et al. Effectiveness of thigh-length graduated compression stockings to reduce the risk of deep vein thrombosis after stroke (CLOTS trial 1): a multicentre, randomised controlled trial. *Lancet* 2009;373(9679):1958-65.
20. CLOTS Trials Collaboration, Dennis M, Sandercock P et al. The effect of graduated compression stockings on long-term outcomes after stroke: the CLOTS trials 1 and 2. *Stroke* 2013;44(4):1075-9.
21. CLOTS (Clots in Legs Or sTockings after Stroke) Trials Collaboration, Dennis M, Sandercock P et al. Effectiveness of intermittent pneumatic compression in reduction of risk of deep vein thrombosis in patients who have had a stroke (CLOTS 3): a multicentre randomised controlled trial. *Lancet* 2013;382(9891):516-24.
22. Wardlaw JM, Murray V, Berge E et al. Recombinant tissue plasminogen activator for acute ischemic stroke: an updated systematic review and meta-analysis. *Lancet* 2012;379(9834):2364-72.
23. Antithrombotic Trialists' Collaboration. Collaborative meta-analysis of randomised trials of antiplatelet therapy for prevention of death, myocardial infarction, and stroke in high risk patients. *BMJ* 2002;324(7329):71-86.
24. Wang Y, Wang Y, Zhao X et al. Clopidogrel with aspirin in acute minor stroke or transient ischemic attack. *N Engl J Med* 2013;369(1):11-9.
25. Wong KS, Wang Y, Leng X et al. Early dual versus mono antiplatelet therapy for acute non-cardioembolic ischemic stroke or transient ischemic attack: an updated systematic review and meta-analysis. *Circulation* 2013;128(15):1656-66.
26. Sandercock PA, Counsell C, Kamal AK. Anticoagulants for acute ischemic stroke. *Cochrane Database Syst Rev* 2008;(4):CD000024.
27. Connolly SJ, Ezekowitz MD, Yusuf S et al. Dabigatran versus warfarin in patients with atrial fibrillation. *N Engl J Med* 2009;361(12):1139-51.
28. Patel MR, Mahaffey KW, Garg J et al. Rivaroxaban versus warfarin in nonvalvular atrial fibrillation. *N Engl J Med* 2011;365(10):883-91.
29. Granger CB, Alexander JH, McMurray JJ et al. Apixaban versus warfarin in patients with atrial fibrillation. *N Engl J Med* 2011;365(11):981-92.
30. Sare GM, Geeganage C, Bath PM. High blood pressure in acute stroke: to treat or not to treat? *Int J Stroke* 2007;2(3):172-3.
31. Rinkel GJ. Medical management of patients with aneurysmal subarachnoid hemorrhage. *Int J Stroke* 2008;3(3):193-204.

Chapter 37
Dyslipidemias

Ghislaine O. Roederer, MD, PhD

The majority of dyslipidemias result from interaction between environmental and genetic factors. Understanding the contribution of each factor in the dyslipidemic patient is beyond the scope of this chapter. Nevertheless, it is essential to rule out secondary causes of dyslipidemia that, when identified and potentially eliminated, can prevent unnecessary treatment. In addition, the use of lipid-lowering agents in the management of cardiovascular (CV) disease is increasingly emphasized.

Screening of the lipid profile is recommended in children with a family history of hypercholesterolemia or chylomicronemia, men ≥40 years, women who are ≥50 years or postmenopausal. Individuals of at-risk ethnicities (South Asian, First Nation) may be screened at an earlier age.[1] Screen all patients with the following risk factors irrespective of age:[1]

- abdominal aneurysm
- chronic obstructive pulmonary disease
- chronic kidney disease (eGFR <60 mL/min/1.73 m^2)
- clinical manifestations of hyperlipidemias (xanthomas, xanthelasmas, premature arcus cornealis)
- current cigarette smoking
- diabetes
- erectile dysfunction
- evidence of atherosclerosis
- family history of premature coronary artery disease
- HIV infection treated with HAART
- hypertension
- inflammatory diseases (inflammatory bowel disease, systemic lupus erythematosus, rheumatoid arthritis, psoriasis)
- BMI >27 kg/m^2

Goals of Therapy

- Reduce risk of CV and cerebrovascular disease
- Prevent pancreatitis from severe hypertriglyceridemia

Investigations

Clinical evaluation should focus on:

- Medical history:
  - Past or present CV disease: angina, aortic aneurysm, claudication, erectile dysfunction, MI, stroke or TIA
  - possible causes of secondary dyslipidemia (Table 1)
  - major CV risk factors (Figure 1, Figure 2)

- Family history:
  - premature CVD (<55 years in males, <65 in females) in first-degree relatives
  - dyslipidemia
- Physical examination:
  - waist circumference
  - bilateral brachial blood pressure
  - funduscopy (lipemia retinalis, retinopathies)
  - cardiovascular evaluation (bruits, peripheral pulses)
  - hepatosplenomegaly
  - lipid deposits (premature arcus cornealis, xanthomas, xanthelasmas)
- Laboratory tests:
  - lipid and lipoprotein levels

  Note that the Friedewald equation, LDL-C=Total-C − (HDL-C+TG/2.2) cannot be used if triglyceride levels are >4.52 mmol/L, if type III dysbetalipoproteinemia or if chylomicrons are present.

  - use the same laboratory for repeated measurements
  - a 12-hour fast is required for triglyceride levels
  - obtain 2 or 3 measurements at 4- to 6-week intervals to establish a baseline before initial diagnosis of a dyslipidemic phenotype. At least one measurement should include a lipoprotein profile, i.e., high-density lipoprotein cholesterol (HDL-C) and low-density lipoprotein cholesterol (LDL-C)
  - other lab investigations to rule out frequent causes of secondary dyslipidemias (Table 1) and establish baseline levels for CK and liver transaminases

Figure 1: **Management of Dyslipidemia**[1]

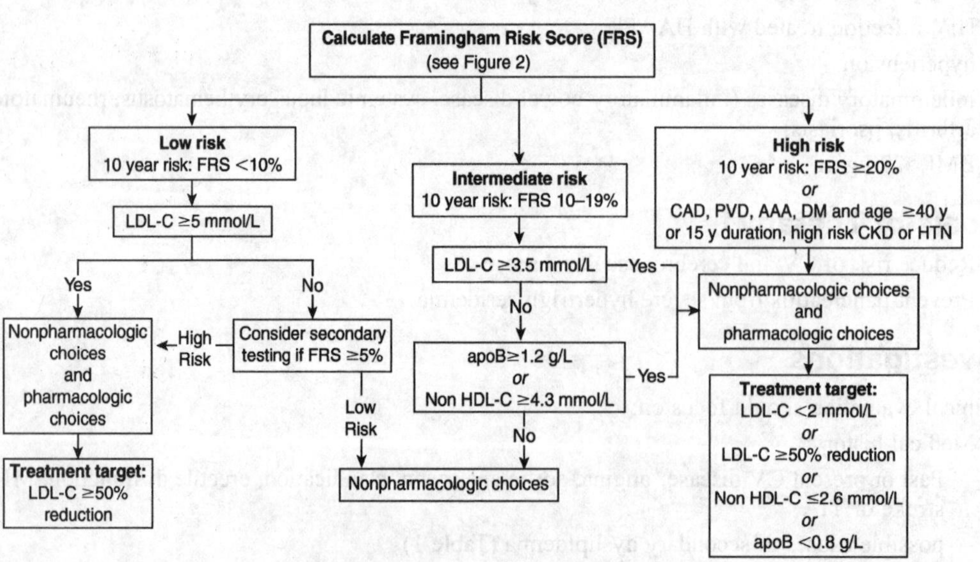

Abbreviations: AAA = abdominal aortic aneurysm; apoB = apolipoprotein B; CAD = coronary artery disease; CKD = chronic kidney disease; DM = diabetes mellitus; HDL-C = high-density lipoprotein cholesterol; hsCRP = high sensitivity C-reactive protein; HTN = hypertension; LDL-C = low-density lipoprotein cholesterol; PVD = peripheral vascular disease; TC = total cholesterol
Legend: Non HDL-C = TC − HDL-C

Figure 2: **Estimating the 10-year Risk of Total Cardiovascular Disease (Framingham Heart Study)[30]**

MEN

Age group, yr	Risk Points
30–34	0
35–39	2
40–44	5
45–49	7
50–54	8
55–59	10
60–64	11
65–69	13
70–74	14
≥75	15

Smoker	Risk Points
No	0
Yes	4

Diabetic	Risk Points
No	0
Yes	3

Total cholesterol level, mmol/L	Risk Points
<4.1	0
4.1–5.19	1
5.2–6.19	2
6.2–7.2	3
>7.2	4

Systolic Blood Pressure, mm Hg	Risk Points Untreated	Risk Points Treated
<120	−2	0
120–129	0	2
130–139	1	3
140–159	2	4
≥160	3	5

HDL-C Level, mmol/L	Risk Points
>1.6	−2
1.3–1.6	−1
1.2–1.29	0
0.9–1.19	1
<0.9	2

Total Risk Points	10-year Risk, %
≤−3	<1
−2	1.1
−1	1.4
0	1.6
1	1.9
2	2.3
3	2.8
4	3.3
5	3.9
6	4.7
7	5.6
8	6.7
9	7.9
10	9.4
11	11.2
12	13.3
13	15.6
14	18.4
15	21.6
16	25.3
17	29.4
≥18	>30

Total Risk Points [ ] 10-Year Risk % [ ]

WOMEN

Age group, yr	Risk Points
30–34	0
35–39	2
40–44	4
45–49	5
50–54	7
55–59	8
60–64	9
65–69	10
70–74	11
≥75	12

Smoker	Risk Points
No	0
Yes	3

Diabetic	Risk Points
No	0
Yes	4

Total cholesterol level, mmol/L	Risk Points
<4.1	0
4.1–5.19	1
5.2–6.19	3
6.2–7.2	4
>7.2	5

Systolic Blood Pressure, mm Hg	Risk Points Untreated	Risk Points Treated
<120	−3	−1
120–129	0	2
130–139	1	3
140–149	2	5
150–159	4	6
≥160	5	7

HDL-C Level, mmol/L	Risk Points
>1.6	−2
1.3–1.6	−1
1.2–1.29	0
0.9–1.19	1
<0.9	2

Total Risk Points	10-year Risk, %
≤−2	<1
−1	1.0
0	1.2
1	1.5
2	1.7
3	2.0
4	2.4
5	2.8
6	3.3
7	3.9
8	4.5
9	5.3
10	6.3
11	7.3
12	8.6
13	10.0
14	11.7
15	13.7
16	15.9
17	18.5
18	21.5
19	24.8
20	27.5
≥21	>30

Total Risk Points [ ] 10-Year Risk % [ ]

Instructions: Add risk points for each of the risk factors shown on the left for either men or women. Determine the 10-Year risk estimate from the chart on the right.

Adapted with permission from D'Agostino RB, Vasan RS, Pencina MJ et al. General cardiovascular risk profile for use in primary care: the Framingham Heart Study. *Circulation* 2008;117(6):743-53.

Table 1: **Common Causes of Secondary Hyperlipidemia**

Conditions	Medications[a]
Alcohol excess	Beta-blockers without intrinsic sympathomimetic or alpha-blocking activity
Chronic renal failure	Corticosteroids
Diabetes/Metabolic syndrome	Highly active antiretroviral therapy (HAART)
Excess weight	Hormone replacement therapy (HRT)
Hypothyroidism	Oral contraceptives
Nephrotic syndrome	Thiazide diuretics
Obstructive liver disease	
Pregnancy	

[a] Medication-induced dyslipidemia should not preclude the use of these medications if clinically indicated.

Criteria for Intervention

Global CV risk assessment described in the recommendations from the Canadian Cardiovascular Society[1] stratifies patients into 1 of 3 categories of CV risk, using the Framingham Risk Score (FRS). It is recommended to double the Framingham score when there is a family history of premature CV disease. Based on the risk score, the target lipid levels are shown in Figure 1.

Optional targets, after reaching LDL-C goals may be:[1]

- Non-HDL-C <2.6 mmol/L
- Apolipoprotein B <0.8 g/L

These particular tests have shown a stronger correlation with CV events than LDL-C. While apolipoprotein B testing may not be widely available, non-HDL-C can be calculated from routine tests (non-HDL-C = total-C − HDL-C).

Some individuals with an intermediate FRS and moderately elevated lipid values may still benefit from pharmacologic therapy. These individuals can be identified using testing of specific biomarkers (lipoprotein(a), hsCRP, HbA_{1c} or urine albumin:creatinine ratio), or by using certain noninvasive tests (graded exercise stress test, carotid imaging, ankle-brachial index or coronary artery calcium).[1] Consider referring these individuals for specialist assessment.

Metabolic syndrome is an association of metabolic abnormalities. The classification used by the International Diabetes Federation is suggested to reflect the ethnic make-up of Canada (Table 2). Management includes weight reduction, increased physical activity and treatment of lipid and nonlipid risk factors.

Renal transplant patients and those with diabetes or end-stage renal disease are considered to be at very high risk. High triglyceride levels (2.3–11.3 mmol/L) are an additional CV risk factor when associated with atherogenic dyslipidemias, e.g., familial combined hyperlipidemia, insulin resistance, diabetes, chronic kidney disease. Very high triglyceride levels (>10 mmol/L) are a risk factor for pancreatitis.

Therapeutic Choices

Nonpharmacologic Choices

- *Diet*, aimed at reducing blood lipid levels and weight (if needed), should always be part of the treatment. For secondary prevention and high-risk individuals, medication is introduced simultaneously. For primary prevention, a 3-month dietary trial (Table 3) is recommended before considering medication; during this time, take 2 (ideally 3) lipid and lipoprotein measurements. The Mediterranean, Portfolio or DASH diets can also be recommended.[1]

Plant sterols have been reported to reduce LDL-cholesterol levels by 5–15%.[3] The benefit is observed after taking 2 g daily for 3 weeks, preferably on a regular twice-daily schedule. Natural sources are unable to provide such an intake, so specific sterol-enriched foods must be used (e.g., yogurt, margarine, fruit juice).

- Other lifestyle changes are important to further modify lipoprotein profile and reduce the risk of CVD, e.g., stress management, weight loss, physical activity and smoking cessation. Smoking cessation can help raise HDL-C.

Pharmacologic Choices

Table 4 summarizes the effects of lipid-lowering drugs on lipoproteins. See Table 6 for prescribing information on drugs used in the management of dyslipidemias.

Resins

The bile acid-sequestering resins **cholestyramine**, **colesevelam** and **colestipol** reduce plasma LDL and can slightly increase HDL levels. They have a strong safety record. Resins are appropriate lipid-lowering agents in children and in pregnant or breastfeeding women.

Table 2: **International Diabetes Federation Classification of the Metabolic Syndrome**[2]

Risk Factor	Defining Level
Central obesity[a]	Waist circumference:
• Caucasian	Men ≥94 cm; Women ≥80 cm
• South Asians	Men ≥90 cm; Women ≥80 cm
• Chinese	Men ≥90 cm; Women ≥80 cm
• Japanese	Men ≥90 cm; Women ≥80 cm
• Ethnic South and Central Americans, First Nations	Use South Asian recommendations until more specific data are available
• Eastern Mediterranean and Middle East (Arabic) populations, Sub-Saharan Africans	Use Caucasian data until more specific data are available
Triglyceride level	≥1.7 mmol/L
HDL-C level	
• Men • Women	<1.03 mmol/L <1.29 mmol/L
Blood pressure	≥130/85 mm Hg
Fasting glucose level	≥5.6 mmol/L

[a] Criteria: central obesity required, plus 2 or more other risk factors.
Abbreviations: HDL-C = high-density lipoprotein cholesterol
Adapted with permission from the International Diabetes Federation.

Table 3: **Dietary Interventions**

Step I **Primary Prevention** **(patients with no previous CVD)**	**Step II** **Secondary Prevention[a]** **(patients with prior CVD/atherosclerotic disease and/or at high risk)**
Reduce dietary cholesterol intake to <300 mg/day Restrict fat intake to 30% of calories Increase proportion of mono- and polyunsaturated fats in diet Restrict saturated and trans-fatty acids in diet Encourage fruit and vegetable intake Set plant sterol intake to 1 g bid, using sterol-enriched foods Increase omega-3 fatty acids from fish and plant sources Encourage high-fibre intake (>30 g/day) Limit simple sugars to 8% of total calories Limit alcohol consumption to 5% of total calories	Same as Step I, but further reduce dietary cholesterol intake to <200 mg/day Restrict fat intake to 20% of calories and less than 7% of daily calories as saturated fat and trans-fatty acids

[a] A dietitian's help is usually required to reach and maintain these goals.

Table 4: **Lipid-lowering Agents—Effect on Lipoproteins[4,5]**

	LDL	HDL	TG
Resins	↓ 10–30%	↑ 3–10%	↑ 10–25%
HMG-CoA Reductase Inhibitors	↓ 20–60%	↑ 5–15%	↓ 7–30%[a]
Niacin	↓ 5–25%	↑ 15–35%	↓ 20–50%
Fibrates	↓ 5–20%	↑ 10–35%	↓ 20–50%
Ezetimibe	↓ 14–25%	↑ 1%	↓ 7–9%

[a] Atorvastatin and rosuvastatin have the greatest TG-lowering effect.

HMG-CoA Reductase Inhibitors (Statins)

HMG-CoA reductase inhibitors, the most potent LDL-lowering agents, interfere with the atherosclerotic disease process. Effect on HDL is modest. Significant reductions in CVD morbidity, CVD mortality and total deaths have been associated with their use and they are recommended as first-line lipid-lowering agents.[1] Statins should be initiated at the recommended starting doses and titrated to reach targets. In secondary prevention of CVD all patients should receive statin therapy [Evidence: SORT A*].[6] For primary prevention of CVD in patients at high risk of coronary artery disease statins are also recommended [Evidence: SORT A*].[7] Statins may be considered in patients in lower risk groups based on the individual's global cardiovascular risk (Figure 1, Figure 2)[Evidence: SORT A*].[1,8]

To avoid myotoxic effects, consider statin- and patient-related factors (Table 5).[9] The management of myotoxic effects is presented in Figure 3. Other concerns are the risk of new-onset diabetes[11] and anecdotal reports of memory loss. Although the potential increased risk of diabetes appears to be related to high doses of statins, there are as yet no recommendations against use of high-dose statins.

Some statins are indicated for use in children >10 years old with heterozygous and homozygous familial hypercholesterolemia.[12,13] Refer these patients for care by a specialist.

* SORT (Strength of Recommendation Taxonomy) is a rating system (A, B or C) that addresses the quality of available evidence. For more information consult **How to Use *Compendium of Therapeutic Choices*** on page xxv.

Figure 3: **Diagnosis and Management of Statin-induced Myopathy**[9,10]

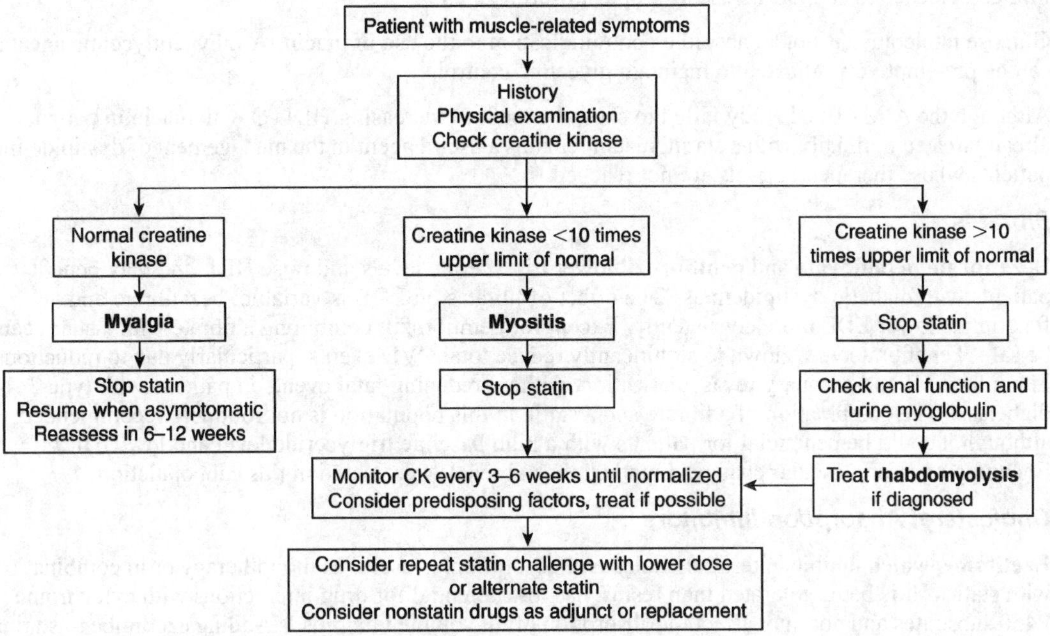

Table 5: **Patient- and Statin-related Factors That May Potentiate Myotoxic Effects**

Patient Factors	Concomitant Medications	Statin Properties
Advanced age (>80 y)	Amiodarone	High statin dose
Alcohol abuse	Azole antifungals (itraconazole, ketoconazole)	High bioavailability
Chronic renal insufficiency	Calcium channel blockers (nondihydropyridines)	Limited protein binding
Excessive grapefruit juice intake	Cyclosporine	High lipophilicity
Frailty, small body frame	Fibrates (particularly gemfibrozil)	Potential for drug-drug interactions metabolized by cytochrome P450 pathways, especially 3A4 and 2C9 (Table 6)
Gender (women are more affected than men)	HIV protease inhibitors	
Hepatic dysfunction	Macrolide antibiotics (clarithromycin, erythromycin)	
Hypothyroidism (untreated)	Nicotinic acid (rarely)	
Inherited myopathies		
Intercurrent infections		
Perioperative periods		
Vigorous exercise		
Vitamin D deficiency		

Nicotinic Acid (Niacin)

Niacin is a B vitamin that at high doses lowers triglycerides and LDL and raises HDL more than any other lipid-lowering agent. It lowers lipoprotein(a), although the clinical significance of this effect is not yet known. The unpleasant side effects of niacin make patient adherence difficult, limiting its usefulness.

Slow-release formulations appear to be more hepatotoxic than immediate-release products.[14] A "no-flush" formulation combining inositol and niacin purports to reduce this adverse effect, but there is limited evidence to support its use as a lipid-lowering agent.

Glucose intolerance is not an absolute contraindication to the use of niacin. Antihyperglycemic agents can be pre-emptively adjusted to maintain glycemic control.

Although the AIM-HIGH study failed to show a benefit in increasing HDL-C with niacin in patients already treated optimally with a statin, niacin remains a useful agent in the management of dyslipidemic patients whose therapeutic goals are not reached.[15]

Fibrates

Bezafibrate, **fenofibrate** and **gemfibrozil** lower triglyceride levels and raise HDL and may benefit patients with diabetic dyslipidemias. The effect of fibrates on LDL is variable; bezafibrate and fenofibrate lower LDL more consistently. Except for gemfibrozil, combining a fibrate with a statin can be safe. Fenofibrate was shown to significantly reduce total CVD events, particularly due to reductions in nonfatal MI and coronary revascularization, without reducing fatal events in patients with type 2 diabetes.[16] The combination of a fibrate and a statin in this population is not routinely recommended, although it could be beneficial for patients with a high baseline triglyceride level and low HDL.[17] Encouraging microvascular changes (ophthalmic and renal) were noted in this subpopulation.[16]

Cholesterol Absorption Inhibitors

Ezetimibe, which inhibits intestinal cholesterol absorption, is useful as monotherapy or in combination with statins. It is better tolerated than resins, has low potential for drug interactions with cytochrome P450 substrates and does not affect the absorption of fat-soluble vitamins.[18] Adding ezetimibe to statins as a complementary LDL-C-lowering agent have been disappointing.[19,20] However, in chronic kidney disease, the combination of simvastatin and ezetimibe significantly and safely reduced the risk of major atherosclerotic and vascular events compared to monotherapy.[21]

Combination Therapy

Agents from different classes can be combined to reach maximal efficacy with an acceptable level of safety, especially if a single drug fails to achieve targets. However, since some combination therapies (such as fibrates and statins) carry an increased risk of drug toxicity, consider referral for such patients.[22]

Microsomal Triglyceride Transfer Protein Inhibitor

Lomitapide has recently received Health Canada approval as adjunctive therapy in adult homozygous familial hypercholesterolemia. It has the potential for significant hepatic toxicity. Referral to a specialized lipid clinic for management is recommended.

Nonprescription Agents

Daily consumption of 10 g **psyllium** may result in a 7% reduction in LDL.[1] The American Heart Association recommends patients with documented coronary heart disease consume about 1 g of **omega-3 fatty acids** daily, though accumulating evidence does not suggest improved cardiovascular outcomes.[23,24] In patients with hypertriglyceridemia, omega-3 fatty acids 2–4 g daily will reduce triglycerides by 25–30%.[1] Patients taking more than 3 g daily of omega-3 fatty acids from supplements should do so only under a physician's care. High intakes could cause excessive bleeding in some people.

Choices during Pregnancy and Breastfeeding

Due to hormonal changes, plasma lipids increase throughout the duration of pregnancy. Total cholesterol concentrations increase 25–50% and total triglycerides by two to fourfold. By midgestation, there is a 50% increase in LDL-C and a 30% rise in HDL-C, followed at term by a slight decrease in HDL-C.[25]

Risk factors for hyperlipidemia also apply to pregnancy and include obesity, weight gain, hypothyroidism, gestational and nongestational diabetes, alcohol consumption, medications and genetic predisposition.[26] Very severe forms of hypertriglyceridemia may increase the risk of pancreatitis.[27]

Prepregnancy Considerations

Risk factor control is recommended throughout the pregnancy. The teratogenicity of lipid-lowering drugs in humans is not well established but appears to be small (if present at all) with statins, and termination of pregnancy is not warranted should fetal exposure occur. However, in order to reduce the risks as much as possible, it is advisable to discontinue all lipid-lowering drugs with the exception of resins.[28]

Management during Pregnancy

Reassure patients that interrupting treatment for the duration of the childbearing period has little impact on the overall cardiovascular risk. Although **resins** may be continued, their GI effects may limit their use. If tolerated, lipid-soluble vitamin supplementation should be implemented. In the very severe cases of pregnancy-induced hyperlipoproteinemia, nonpharmacologic measures can be used.[29]

Management during Postpartum/Breastfeeding

Treatment may be resumed unless breastfeeding is considered. Lipid-lowering drugs are currently not recommended during breastfeeding.

A discussion of general principles on the use of medications in these special populations can be found in Appendix II and Appendix III. Other specialized reference sources are also provided in these appendices.

Therapeutic Tips

- Global cardiovascular management initially involves modification of health behaviours (smoking cessation, diet, weight reduction and maintenance, exercise, stress management) in addition to lipid-lowering medication.
- Lipid-lowering drugs must always be an adjunct to, not a substitution for, diet therapy.
- Treat to reach the target levels.
- Try different agents within the same class in cases of intolerance or insufficient efficacy.
- Long-term clinical and laboratory follow up is essential to monitor lipid-lowering efficacy and safety of therapy. Based on the author's experience, follow-up is suggested every 4 months for the first year, every 6 months for the second year and yearly thereafter, unless some other condition requires closer monitoring.
- Allow 3 months for a stabilized and representative plasma lipid profile after a major medical event. Acute coronary syndromes require immediate statin therapy regardless of the lipid profile.
- Doubling the dose of a statin will further reduce the LDL-C level by only 6% (Figure 1, Figure 2).
- It appears safe to lower target LDL-C levels to 1.8 mmol/L (<70 mg/dL) in individuals with overt coronary heart disease and multiple risk factors.

Table 6: Drugs Used in the Management of Dyslipidemias

Class	Drug	Dose	Adverse Effects	Drug Interactions	Comments	Cost[a]
Cholesterol Absorption Inhibitor	*ezetimibe* Ezetrol	10 mg once daily po at any time of day	Well tolerated. Common: back pain, arthralgia, diarrhea, abdominal pain, fatigue, dizziness, headache. Rare: myopathy, rhabdomyolysis, hepatitis, acute pancreatitis, thrombocytopenia.	Low potential for drug interactions. Potential pharmacokinetic interaction with cyclosporine. Caution when initiating ezetimibe in patients receiving cyclosporine, especially if severe renal insufficiency.	Monitor liver function and CK. In general, can use in children ≥12 y. Not recommended in moderate to severe hepatic impairment.	$$
Fibrates	*bezafibrate* Bezalip SR	400 mg once daily po with evening meal	Upper GI disturbances (nausea, abdominal pain, flatulence), myalgias Increased bile lithogenicity, Increased CK, Increased creatinine (not representative of renal function deterioration).	Caution when combining with statins. Monitor INR with concomitant warfarin use. Increased ezetimibe levels. Monitor for signs of cholelithiasis.	Renal function should be checked at 3, 6 and 12 months, then yearly. Liver function (ALT) checked at least once at 3 months. Check CK if myalgia develops. Useful in diabetic dyslipidemias. Contraindications: hepatic impairment, renal dysfunction, pre-existing gallbladder disease.	$$
	fenofibrate generics	100 mg BID–QID po with meals	See bezafibrate.	See bezafibrate. Monitor renal function with concomitant cyclosporine use.	See bezafibrate.	$$
	fenofibrate microcoated Lipidil Supra, generics	160 mg once daily po with largest meal of the day	See bezafibrate.	See bezafibrate. Monitor renal function with concomitant cyclosporine use.	See bezafibrate.	$
	fenofibrate micronized Lipidil Micro, generics	200 mg once daily po with largest meal of the day	See bezafibrate.	See bezafibrate. Monitor renal function with concomitant cyclosporine use.	See bezafibrate.	$

Class	Drug	Dose	Adverse Effects	Drug Interactions	Comments	Cost[a]
	fenofibrate nanocrystals ❥ Lipidil EZ, generics	145 mg once daily po with or without food Recommended starting dose for patients with renal impairment and in the elderly is 48 mg daily	See bezafibrate.	See bezafibrate. Monitor renal function with concomitant cyclosporine use.	See bezafibrate.	$$
	gemfibrozil ❥ generics	300–1200 mg/day po divided BID 30 min prior to meals	See bezafibrate.	Not to be used in combination with statins. May increase repaglinide and rosiglitazone levels; metabolized by CYP2C8. Monitor INR with concomitant warfarin use.	See bezafibrate.	$
HMG-CoA Reductase Inhibitors	*atorvastatin* Lipitor, generics	Adults: 10–80 mg daily po at any time of day Children:[b] 10–20 mg daily po	Common: Increased CK, Increased transaminases (reversible), mild upper GI disturbances, myalgias (with and without CK elevation), sleep disturbances, headache, rash. Rare: myopathy, rhabdomyolysis, peripheral neuropathy, lupus-like symptoms, impotence.	Avoid with CYP3A4 inhibitors: amiodarone, azoles, cyclosporine, gemfibrozil, grapefruit juice, macrolide antibiotics, nondihydropyridine calcium channel blockers, e.g., verapamil, protease inhibitors.	Start with low doses and titrate up to reach targets while monitoring biochemical markers. Liver function (ALT) should be checked at least once at 3 months. Check CK if myalgia develops. Use caution in patients with moderate to severe renal impairment (<60 mL/min). Contraindications: active liver disease, high alcohol consumption, pregnancy.	$
	fluvastatin Lescol, Lescol XL, generics	Adults and Children:[b] 20–80 mg po daily in 1 or 2 divided doses Give XL formulation once daily anytime	See atorvastatin.	Avoid with CYP2C9 inhibitors: amiodarone, fluconazole, fluoxetine, fluvoxamine.	See atorvastatin.	$
	lovastatin Mevacor, generics	Adults: 20–80 mg daily po with evening meal. May be given in 2 divided doses	See atorvastatin.	See atorvastatin.	See atorvastatin.	$$

(cont'd)

Table 6: **Drugs Used in the Management of Dyslipidemias** *(cont'd)*

Class	Drug	Dose	Adverse Effects	Drug Interactions	Comments	Cost[a]
	pravastatin Pravachol, generics	Adults: 10–40 mg QHS po	See atorvastatin.	Not metabolized through CYP P450 pathway, thus low potential for drug interactions.	See atorvastatin.	$
	rosuvastatin Crestor, generics	Adults: 10–40 mg daily po Initial dose 10 mg/day po except in Asian patients and those receiving cyclosporine (initial dose 5 mg/day po) Children:[b] 5–10 mg daily po	See atorvastatin.	See fluvastatin. Reduced levels with concomitant use of magnesium/aluminum hydroxide-containing antacids.	See atorvastatin. Administer antacids 2 h after rosuvastatin.	$
	simvastatin Zocor, generics	Adults: 10–80 mg po with evening meal Children:[b] 10–40 mg po with evening meal	See atorvastatin.	See atorvastatin.	See atorvastatin.	$
Niacin (Nicotinic Acid) Derivatives	*niacin, immediate-release* Niacin, generics	Start with 50 mg TID po; double dose Q5 days to 1.5–2 g/day Usual dose if tolerated: 1.5–4 g/day divided TID po after meals	Common: hot flushes and pruritus, dry skin, acanthosis nigricans (reversible), reactivation of peptic ulcer, GI disturbances, increased blood glucose, glucose intolerance. Rare: torsades de pointes, severe hepatotoxicity (more frequent with slow-release formulation), increased uric acid, transaminases.	Use caution if using with statins because of potential hepatotoxicity and myopathy.	Greatest HDL-raising effect. Monitor blood glucose, uric acid, transaminases at 3, 6 and 12 months, then yearly. Contraindications: severe peptic ulcer disease, uncontrolled hyperglycemia, severe gout, hepatic disease. Flushing: Reassure patients that symptoms abate with time. Avoid hot drinks, hot showers, spicy food, alcohol for 1–2 h after a dose. Uncoated ASA 325 mg daily may be helpful in the first few weeks of treatment or when increasing the dose. Tolerance develops within several weeks. Avoid missing a dose.	$

Class	Drug	Dose	Adverse Effects	Drug Interactions	Comments	Cost[a]
	niacin, extended-release Niaspan, Niaspan-FCT	Titrate the dose: 0.5 g QHS po after a low-fat snack × 1 month then 1 g QHS ×1 month, then 1.5 g QHS. May increase to 2 g QHS if required	Similar adverse effects to niacin immediate release, although less severe. See niacin, immediate release.	See niacin, immediate release.	Less flushing because taken at bedtime.	$$
Resins	*cholestyramine* Olestyr	Adults: 4 g BID–TID ac po. Maximum 24 g/day divided in 3 doses Children: 240 mg/kg/day po Maximum 16 g/day divided in 3 doses	Common: constipation (>10%), bloating, abdominal fullness, flatulence, increased triglycerides, increased transaminases (reversible). Rare: hyperchloremic acidosis, cholecystitis, cholelithiasis, pancreatitis, malabsorption syndrome, GI bleeding, peptic ulceration.	Administer 1 h before or 4–6 h after concurrent medications due to possible reduced absorption of other drugs in the GI tract.	Start with daily dosing to improve tolerability. Recommend high-fibre diet and high water intake to minimize constipation. May be mixed with juice, soups and applesauce. Add granules to at least 90 mL of fluid. Long-term and high-dose use can prevent the absorption of fat-soluble vitamins and folic acid. Can be used to lower cholesterol and LDL in pregnancy and in children. Some formulations contain phenylalanine; caution in patients with phenylketonuria. Contraindications: biliary obstruction, dysbetalipoproteinemia, TG >3.4 mmol/L.	$$$
	colesevelam Lodalis	1250 mg BID po Maximum 3.75 g/day	See cholestyramine.	See cholestyramine.	See cholestyramine.	$$$$
	colestipol Colestid	Granules: 5 g BID–TID ac po Maximum 30 g/day Tablets: 2 g once daily–BID po Maximum 16 g/day	See cholestyramine.	See cholestyramine.	See cholestyramine.	Granules: $$ Tablets: $

[a] Cost of 30-day supply; includes drug cost only.
[b] Children aged 10 to 17 years (boys and postmenarchal girls).
Dosage adjustment may be required in renal impairment; see Appendix I.
Abbreviations: ALT = alanine transaminase; AST = aspartate transaminase; CK = creatine kinase; LFT = liver function test; SR = slow release; TG = triglycerides
Legend: $ <$25 $$ $25–75 $$$ $75–125 $$$$ $125–175

Suggested Readings

Anderson TJ, Gregoire J, Hegele RA et al. 2012 Update of the Canadian Cardiovascular Society guidelines for the diagnosis and treatment of dyslipidemia for the prevention of cardiovascular disease in the adult. *Can J Cardiol* 2013;29(2):151-67.

Grundy SM, Cleeman JI, Merz CN et al. Implications of recent clinical trials for the National Cholesterol Education Program Adult Treatment Panel III guidelines. *Circulation* 2004;110(2):227-39.

Jialal I. A practical approach to the laboratory diagnosis of dyslipidemia. *Am J Clin Pathol* 1996;106(1):128-38.

Kuoppala J, Lamminpaa A, Pukkala E. Statins and cancer: a systematic review and meta-analysis. *Eur J Cancer* 2008;44(15):2122-32.

Mattar M, Obeid O. Fish oil and the management of hypertriglyceridemia. *Nutr Health* 2009;20(1):41-9.

NACB LMPG Committee Members, Myers GL, Christenson RH et al. NACB LMPG Committee Members, National Academy of Clinical Biochemistry Laboratory Medicine Practice guidelines: emerging biomarkers for primary prevention of cardiovascular disease. *Clin Chem* 2009;55(2):378-84.

Sathasivam S, Lecky B. Statin induced myopathy. *BMJ* 2008;337:a2286.

Seth Loomba R, Arora R. Fibrates: where are we now? *Ther Adv Cardiovasc Dis* 2009;3(1):91-6.

References

1. Anderson TJ, Gregoire J, Hegele RA et al. 2012 update of the Canadian Cardiovascular Society guidelines for the diagnosis and treatment of dyslipidemia for the prevention of cardiovascular disease in the adult. *Can J Cardiol* 2013;29(2):151-67.
2. International Diabetes Federation. *The IDF consensus worldwide definition of the metabolic syndrome.* Brussels (BE); [2006]. Available from: www.idf.org/webdata/docs/MetSyndrome_FINAL.pdf. Accessed January 3, 2014.
3. Abumweis SS, Barake R, Jones PJ. Plant sterols/stanols as cholesterol lowering agents: a meta-analysis of randomized controlled trials. *Food Nut Res* 2008:52.
4. Third Report of the National Cholesterol Education Program (NCEP) Expert Panel on Detection, Evaluation, and Treatment of High Blood Cholesterol in Adults (Adult Treatment Panel III) final report *Circulation* 2002;106(25):3143-421.
5. Hou R, Goldberg AC. Lowering low-density lipoprotein cholesterol: statins, ezetimibe, bile acid sequestrants and combinations: comparative efficacy and safety. *Endocrinol Metab Clin North Am* 2009;38(1):79-97.
6. Baigent C, Keech A, Kearney PM et al. Efficacy and safety of cholesterol-lowering treatment: prospective meta-analysis of data from 90,056 participants in 14 randomised trials of statins. *Lancet* 2005;366(9493):1267-78.
7. Brugts JJ, Yetgin T, Hoeks SE et al. The benefits of statins in people without established cardiovascular disease but with cardiovascular risk factors: meta-analysis of randomised controlled trials. *BMJ* 2009;338:b2376.
8. Taylor F, Huffman MD, Macedo AF et al. Statins for the primary prevention of cardiovascular disease. *Cochrane Database Syst Rev* 2013;1:CD004816.
9. Sathasivam S, Lecky B. Statin induced myopathy. *BMJ* 2008;337:a2286.
10. Mancini GB, Baker S, Bergeron J et al. Diagnosis, prevention, and management of statin adverse effects and intolerance: proceedings of a Canadian Working Group Consensus Conference. *Can J Cardiol* 2011;27(5):635-62.
11. Sattar N, Preiss D, Murray HM et al. Statins and risk of incident diabetes: a collaborative meta-analysis of randomised statin trials. *Lancet* 2010;375(9716):735-42.
12. Kavey RE, Allada V, Daniels SR et al. Cardiovascular risk reduction in high-risk pediatric patients: a scientific statement from the American Heart Association Expert Panel on Population and Prevention Science et al. *Circulation* 2006;114(24):2710-38.
13. Daniels SR, Greer FR; Committee on Nutrition. Lipid screening and cardiovascular health in childhood. *Pediatrics* 2008;122(1):198-208.
14. Guyton JR, Bays HE. Safety considerations with niacin therapy. *Am J Cardiol* 2007;99(6A):22C-31C.
15. AIM-HIGH Investigators, Boden WE, Probstfield JL et al. Niacin in patients with low HDL cholesterol levels receiving intensive statin therapy. *N Eng J Med* 2011;365(24):2255-67.
16. Keech A, Simes RJ, Barter P et al. Effects of long-term fenofibrate therapy on cardiovascular events in 9795 people with type 2 diabetes mellitus (the FIELD study): randomised controlled trial. *Lancet* 2005;366(9500):1849-61.
17. ACCORD Study Group, Ginsberg HN, Elam MB et al. Effects of combination lipid therapy in type 2 diabetes mellitus. *N Engl J Med* 2010;362(17):1563-74.
18. Cannon CP, Giugliano RP, Blazing MA et al. Rationale and design of IMPROVE-IT (IMProved Reduction of Outcomes: Vytorin Efficacy International Trial): comparison of ezetimibe/simvastatin versus simvastatin monotherapy on cardiovascular outcomes in patients with acute coronary syndromes. *Am Heart J* 2008;156(5):826-32.
19. Kastelein JJ, Akdim F, Stroes ES et al. Simvastatin with or without ezetimibe in familial hypercholesterolemia. *N Eng J Med* 2008;358(14):1431-43.
20. Taylor AJ, Villines TC, Stanek EJ et al. Extended-release niacin or ezetimibe and carotid intima-media thickness. *N Engl J Med* 2009;361(22):2113-22.
21. Baigent C, Landray MJ, Reith C et al. The effects of lowering LDL cholesterol with simvastatin plus ezetimibe in patients with chronic kidney disease (Study of Heart and Renal Protection): a randomised placebo-controlled trial. *Lancet* 2011;377(9784):2181-92.
22. Tenenbaum A, Fisman EZ, Motro M et al. Optimal management of combined dyslipidemia: what have we behind statins monotherapy? *Adv Cardiol* 2008;45:127-53.

23. Kris-Etherton PM, Harris WS, Appel LJ. Fish consumption, fish oil, omega-3 fatty acids, and cardiovascular disease. *Circulation* 2002;106(21):2747-57.
24. Rizos EC, Ntzani EE, Bika E et al. Association between omega-3 fatty acid supplementation and risk of major cardiovascular disease events: a systematic review and meta-analysis. *JAMA* 2012;308(10):1024-33.
25. Lain KY, Catalano PM. Metabolic changes in pregnancy. *Clin Obstet Gynecol* 2007;50(4):938-48.
26. Basaran A. Pregnancy-induced hyperlipoproteinemia: review of the literature. *Reprod Sci* 2009;16(5):431-7.
27. Glueck CJ, Christopher C, Mishkel MA et al. Pancreatitis, familial hypertriglyceridemia, and pregnancy. *Am J Obstet Gynecol* 1980;136(6):755-61.
28. Kazmin A, Garcia-Bournissen F, Koren G. Risks of statin use during pregnancy: a systematic review. *J Obstet Gynaecol Can* 2007;29(11):906-8.
29. Klingel R, Gohlen B, Schwarting A et al. Differential indication of lipoprotein apheresis during pregnancy. *Ther Apher Dial* 2003;7(3):359-64.
30. D'Agostino RB, Vasan RS, Pencina MJ et al. General cardiovascular risk profile for use in primary care: the Framingham Heart Study. *Circulation* 2008;117(6):743-53.

Cardiovascular Disorders

Chapter 38
Heart Failure

Simon de Denus, B. Pharm, MSc, PhD and
Michel White, MD, FRCPC, FACC, FESC

Heart failure (HF) is associated with a 5-year mortality rate of 5–50% depending on the severity of symptoms and left ventricular (LV) dysfunction.[1] Patients with HF may require frequent hospitalizations and experience significantly reduced quality of life and exercise tolerance.[1] Typical symptoms of HF include dyspnea, fatigue and fluid retention.[1]

HF is characterized by impaired LV function and reduced LV reserve. HF is generally categorized as systolic HF or HF with preserved ejection fraction (PEF).[2] Less common types of HF, such as restrictive, infiltrative or hypertrophic cardiomyopathy, will not be discussed. Systolic HF is characterized by decreased pump function, dilatation of the left ventricle and decreased LV ejection fraction (LVEF ≤40%). Most clinical trials have been conducted in patients with systolic HF. There is no strong consensus on the definition of HF with PEF or its treatment.[1,2,3,4,5] It is variably defined as the presence of signs and symptoms of HF with LVEF >40% or >50%. HF with PEF can be associated with many conditions (hypertension, arterial stiffness, diabetes mellitus), although abnormal myocardial relaxation, hypertrophy and/or fibrosis are generally present.[1,2,3,4,5]

Goals of Therapy

- Treat modifiable risk factors
- Avoid exacerbating factors (Table 1)
- Prevent disease progression
- Improve symptoms, exercise tolerance and quality of life
- Reduce morbidity and mortality

Investigations

- Perform a history, physical examination and select laboratory tests to establish the diagnosis (Figure 1, Table 2)
- Determine ventricular size and function with transthoracic echocardiography or isotopic ventriculography in all patients with suspected HF. Echocardiography identifies valvular abnormalities and other myocardial problems
- Additional tests should be performed in select individuals to identify the etiology of HF and to guide specific treatment when appropriate
- The New York Heart Association functional classification is commonly used to describe patients with HF (Table 3)

Table 1: **Factors That Can Exacerbate Heart Failure**

Patient-specific Factors	Nonadherence to drug therapy or dietary restrictions
	Anemia
	Arrhythmias
	Infections
	Myocardial ischemia
	Pulmonary embolism
	Renal dysfunction
	Thyroid dysfunction
	Uncontrolled hypertension
	Valvular heart disease
Drugs	**Drugs that cause sodium and fluid retention:**
	Androgens
	Corticosteroids
	Drugs with high sodium content
	Licorice-containing products
	Minoxidil
	NSAIDs including selective COX-2 inhibitors and high-dose salicylates
	Thiazolidinediones (pioglitazone, rosiglitazone)
	Negative inotropes:
	Antiarrhythmic agents except amiodarone and dofetilide
	Beta-blockers at maintenance doses
	Calcium channel blockers: diltiazem, nifedipine, verapamil, but not amlodipine or felodipine
	Itraconazole
	Cardiotoxic drugs:
	Alcohol
	Alkylating agents (cyclophosphamide, ifosfamide)
	Anthracyclines (doxorubicin, epirubicin, mitoxantrone)
	Bevacizumab
	Clozapine
	Cocaine
	Trastuzumab
	Tyrosine kinase inhibitors (imatinib, sunitinib)

Therapeutic Choices

Nonpharmacologic Choices[1,3,4,5]

- Control HF risk factors (hypertension, obesity, diabetes mellitus, supraventricular arrhythmia, dyslipidemia, coronary artery disease and other vascular diseases).
- Avoid exacerbating risk factors.
- Recommend moderate regular physical activity in stable patients.
- Recommend no more than one alcoholic drink per day in all patients. Avoid completely in alcoholic cardiomyopathy.
- Restrict sodium intake in all patients (<2–3 g/day; 1–2 g/day in those with severe HF).
- Restrict fluid intake (<1.5–2 L/day) in patients with fluid retention that is not easily controlled with diuretics, or in patients with hyponatremia.
- Annual influenza vaccination in all patients.
- Pneumococcal vaccination in all patients.
- Daily weight. Advise patients who gain 0.5 kg/day on several consecutive days or 2 kg in 3 days to alert their team or physician.

Figure 1: Evaluation of Patients with Heart Failure

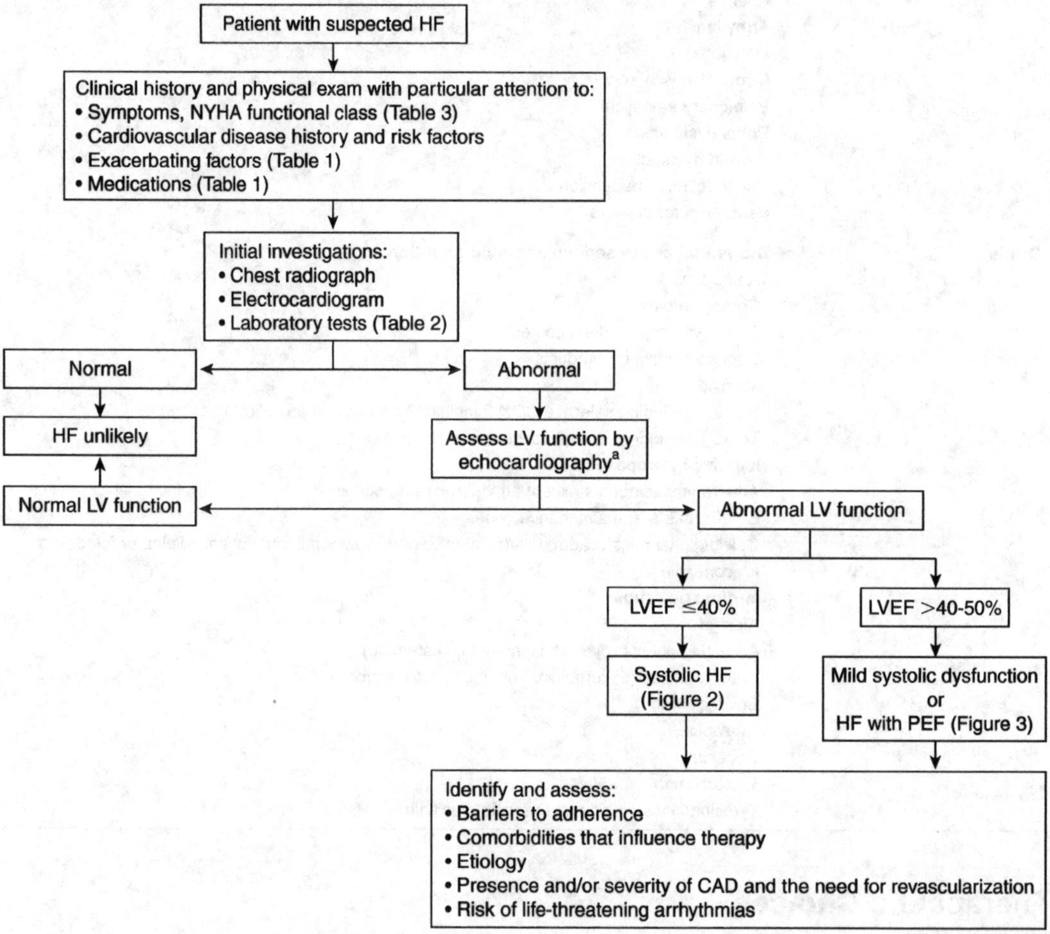

[a] Echocardiography (two-dimensional or transthoracic) is used to determine LVEF, chamber size, wall thickness, valve function and presence of pericardial disease. Consider other diagnostic investigations if inconclusive (e.g., magnetic resonance imaging or cardiac catheterization).

Abbreviations: HF = heart failure; LV = left ventricular; LVEF = LV ejection fraction; PEF = preserved ejection fraction

Table 2: Laboratory Investigations for Evaluation of Patients with Heart Failure

All patients	Complete blood count
	Serum creatinine, electrolytes, urea, albumin, uric acid and transaminase levels
	Fasting plasma glucose and serum lipids
	Thyroid function tests
	Urinalysis
Select patients	Brain natriuretic peptide (BNP) or N-terminal proBNP (NT-proBNP)[a]
	Iron studies, ferritin and transferrin
	HIV test

[a] BNP or NT-proBNP is particularly useful in the emergency care setting. Value in primary care is not definitive, but it can be used to aid diagnosis and treatment of patients with suspected LV dysfunction. Natriuretic peptides should not be used to screen for LV dysfunction.

Table 3: **New York Heart Association (NYHA) Functional Classification**

Class	Characteristics
I	No symptoms with ordinary activity
II	Symptoms occur with ordinary activity
III	Symptoms occur with less than ordinary activity
IV	Symptoms occur at rest or with minimal activity

Device Therapy

Given their cost, the following devices should generally be reserved for patients who do not have significant comorbidities that are expected to significantly limit survival.

- *Implantable cardioverter defibrillators* (ICDs) are recommended for stable patients with a history of sudden cardiac arrest, ventricular fibrillation (VF) or hemodynamically unstable sustained ventricular tachycardia (VT) in the absence of reversible factors (secondary prevention). Primary ICD placement should be considered in patients with ischemic cardiomyopathy with either:
  - NYHA class II-III and LVEF ≤35%
  - NYHA class I and LVEF ≤30%, where the LVEF is measured at least 1 month post-MI and at least 3 months after a coronary revascularization procedure

  In patients with nonischemic cardiomyopathy, primary ICD therapy should be considered in patients with NYHA class II-III and LVEF ≤35% measured after at least 9 months of optimal medical therapy.
- *Cardiac resynchronization therapy* (CRT) should be considered in patients with NYHA class III and ambulatory NYHA class IV despite optimal medical therapy who are in sinus rhythm with QRS interval ≥130 msec, left bundle branch block QRS morphology and LVEF ≤35%.[1,7] For NYHA class II patients in sinus rhythm receiving optimal medical therapy, CRT is recommended if the QRS duration is ≥130 msec with LBBB QRS morphology and an LVEF ≤30%. Patients with a QRS >150 msec may derive the most benefit from CRT.
- *Left ventricular assist devices* (LVAD) should be used as a bridge to transplantation. Use of LVADs as a bridge to recovery is controversial.[8]
- *Continuous positive airway pressure* (CPAP) should be considered in patients with obstructive sleep apnea.[4]

Reperfusion and Surgery

- *Revascularization*, either by percutaneous coronary intervention or coronary artery bypass surgery, should be performed in select patients with symptomatic ischemia or if reperfusion may improve dysfunctional myocardium.[1]
- *Cardiac transplantation* should be considered in patients with severe refractory HF, despite optimal therapy, who would otherwise have a good life expectancy.[1]

Pharmacologic Choices

Systolic Heart Failure

In the absence of contraindications, the cornerstone of therapy for systolic HF in all patients with an LVEF ≤40% (NYHA class I–IV) is long-term treatment with the combination of an angiotensin converting enzyme (ACE) inhibitor and a beta-blocker (Figure 2). Diuretics are used to control signs and symptoms of hypervolemia. Digoxin, angiotensin II receptor blockers (ARBs), aldosterone antagonists or the combination of isosorbide dinitrate/hydralazine are used in select individuals.[5]

Figure 2: **Drug Therapy of Systolic Heart Failure**[3]

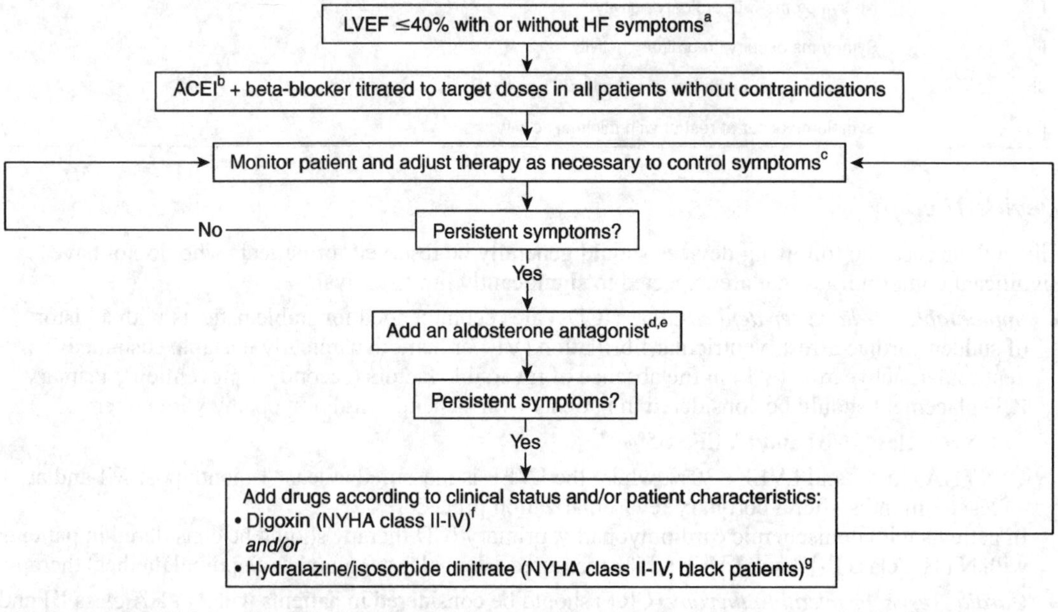

a Identify and manage risk factors, educate all patients about their disease and implement nonpharmacologic treatment. Consider ICD and resynchronization therapy in select patients.
b Use an ARB in patients with ACEI-induced cough that is intolerable or angioedema (although there is a low risk of angioedema with ARBs). Alternatively, substitute hydralazine/isosorbide dinitrate combination therapy for ACEI and/or ARB-induced hyperkalemia, renal dysfunction or angioedema.
c Use diuretics to minimize fluid retention. Consider combination diuretic therapy in patients with severe symptoms.
d Avoid the combination of an ACEI plus an ARB and an aldosterone antagonist because of the risk of hyperkalemia.
e If an aldosterone antagonist is not tolerated, consider adding an ARB to ACEI therapy.
f Digoxin may be used earlier to control the ventricular rate in patients with atrial fibrillation, usually in combination with a beta-blocker.
g Consider hydralazine/isosorbide dinitrate therapy in the patient who cannot tolerate an ACEI or ARB.
Abbreviations: ACEI = angiotensin converting enzyme inhibitor; ARB = angiotensin II receptor blocker; LVEF = left ventricular ejection fraction; NYHA = New York Heart Association

Preference should be given to the use of agents for which mortality and morbidity benefits have been established in large randomized clinical trials (Table 4). Drugs used in the treatment of HF are presented in Table 5. Target doses are those used in such trials.

Consider a patient's comorbid conditions, such as renal failure, when contemplating the use of a particular class of medication, a specific agent and the target dosage.

ACE Inhibitors

ACE inhibitors are recommended in all patients because they improve symptoms and reduce the risk of hospitalization, MI and death in patients with systolic HF.[9,10,11] Start with a low dose and titrate at 7- to 14-day intervals to the target dose, or maximum tolerated dose if the target dose cannot be reached. Treatment with target doses is more effective than low doses.[12] Measure serum creatinine, potassium and blood pressure before initiating an ACE inhibitor or increasing the dose and 7–14 days after any increase in dosage.[5] An increase in serum creatinine of up to 30% is expected and acceptable after initiation of an ACE inhibitor.[1] If the increase in serum creatinine is greater than 30%, other causes of worsening renal function should first be excluded. In particular, assess volume status, as an increase in serum creatinine often appears in patients who are hypovolemic because of excessive diuresis. If no other cause for the worsening renal function can be identified, reduce the dose or discontinue the ACE inhibitor. Although data are limited, the authors recommend periodically reassessing the potential of restarting ACE inhibitors or increasing the dose if the patient's condition improves. Patients at greatest risk of hyperkalemia are those with moderate to severe renal dysfunction, high baseline potassium, diabetes mellitus and those receiving potassium-sparing diuretics.[13]

Beta-blockers

Beta-blockers improve symptoms and reduce the risk of hospitalization and death in patients with systolic HF.[14,15,16,17] They are recommended in all patients with an LVEF ≤40%.[5] Prescribe only the beta-blockers that have been shown to reduce mortality: **bisoprolol**, **carvedilol** and **metoprolol succinate** (not available in Canada).[5] **Metoprolol tartrate** is available in Canada, but has not been shown to reduce mortality in patients with HF. In fact, mortality and hospital admissions were significantly more frequent in patients treated with metoprolol tartrate (target dose 50 mg BID) than with carvedilol (25 mg BID) in a large randomized trial.[18] The target dose of metoprolol tartrate used in this trial was lower than the target dose of controlled-release metoprolol succinate that significantly decreased mortality in a large placebo-controlled trial.[14]

In HF patients, initiate beta-blockers at a very low dose and slowly titrate the dose at 2- to 4-week intervals.[5] Beta-blockers should not be initiated, or their doses increased, while patients are acutely decompensated. Nevertheless, once the hypervolemia has resolved, beta-blockers should be carefully initiated with close monitoring before the end of the hospitalization.[19] Monitor blood pressure and heart rate before initiating a beta-blocker and before any increase in dose. Watch for the signs and symptoms of HF decompensation when initiating or increasing the dose of a beta-blocker, paying particular attention to the daily morning weight.[5] Beta-blockers should not be stopped abruptly.[1] Refer patients with severe HF (NYHA class III–IV) to an HF specialist for initiation of a beta-blocker.[1]

Diuretics

Diuretics are recommended to control signs and symptoms of volume overload. **Thiazide diuretics** can be used in patients with minimal fluid retention, but **loop diuretics**, usually **furosemide**, are required in most patients.[1,3,4,5] Use of **ethacrynic acid** is limited to patients with an allergy to furosemide. Thiazides have poor efficacy as monotherapy in patients with creatinine clearance <50 mL/min.[20] Higher doses of furosemide are required in patients with renal dysfunction.[20] Use the lowest effective dose.[5] Measure serum creatinine and electrolytes before and 3–7 days after initiation of a diuretic and then as indicated (until serum potassium and renal function are stable) after increasing the dose. It is important to highlight that although diuretics are extremely effective in reducing symptoms, they do not modify the natural course of HF and do not decrease mortality. Hence, following the resolution of symptoms, focus on optimizing agents shown to reduce cardiovascular events and on minimizing diuretic dosage. Finally, it is important to periodically reassess the doses of diuretics. Although dosage increases are frequently required in individuals whose condition deteriorates, diuretic doses can sometimes be reduced or stopped in select individuals, particularly those who demonstrate long-term improvements in cardiac function.

Thiazide and loop diuretics deplete potassium and magnesium. Serum potassium should be maintained at ≥4 mmol/L because hypokalemia increases the risk of fatal ventricular arrhythmias and digoxin toxicity.[1] In patients with refractory volume overload, consider the addition of a low-dose thiazide intermittently (e.g., a few times/week) to a loop diuretic.[1,3,4,5] This strategy should be used only by experienced clinicians with close monitoring of weight, renal function and serum potassium because of the risk of severe and potentially fatal dehydration and electrolyte imbalances.[1,3,4,5] When prescribed once daily, diuretics should generally be taken in the morning. When prescribed twice daily or more, the last dose should be taken before 4:00 p.m. to avoid diuresis during the night.

Potassium-sparing diuretics may be used to prevent hypokalemia and hypomagnesemia in patients treated with thiazides or loop diuretics.[3] Eplerenone and spironolactone (see Aldosterone Antagonists) should be preferred given their cardiovascular benefits.

Angiotensin II Receptor Blockers

Angiotensin II receptor blockers (ARBs) are an alternative to ACE inhibitors in patients with ACE inhibitor-induced cough or angioedema. Patient education and follow-up are essential because ARB-induced angioedema has been reported.[4,21] In patients who are intolerant of ACE inhibitors, **candesartan** has reduced the combined endpoint of cardiovascular death or hospitalizations for HF.[21] Data suggest that **valsartan** has a comparable effect on mortality and morbidity to captopril in patients with HF complicating an acute MI.[22] **Losartan** titrated to a dose of 150 mg daily is also a reasonable alternative.[23] Similar to ACE inhibitors, ARBs are associated with renal dysfunction and hyperkalemia; thus, ARBs should not be substituted for ACE inhibitors specifically for these adverse events.[22] Considerations for initiation, dosage titration and monitoring for ARBs are the same as for ACE inhibitors.

Addition of an ARB may be considered in patients with persistent symptoms despite optimal therapy with an ACE inhibitor and a beta-blocker who do not tolerate an aldosterone antagonist.[1,24] Although no large randomized trial has compared aldosterone antagonists to ARBs, the addition of an aldosterone antagonist is generally preferred to an ARB in patients who remain symptomatic despite the use of a beta-blocker and an ACE inhibitor, because clinical studies with these agents have produced greater benefit.[3] **Candesartan** has reduced cardiovascular mortality and hospitalizations for HF.[24] **Valsartan** has reduced morbidity but not mortality.[25] Limited data suggest that an ARB may be a valuable addition to an ACE inhibitor in patients not receiving a beta-blocker.[1] Close monitoring of vital signs, serum creatinine and potassium is essential when combining an ACE inhibitor and an ARB. The combination of an ACE inhibitor, an ARB and an aldosterone antagonist is not recommended because of the uncertainty regarding the benefit and safety of this combination.[1]

Aldosterone Antagonists

In patients with chronic HF who remain symptomatic despite optimal use of ACE inhibitors and beta-blockers, an aldosterone antagonist (**eplerenone** or **spironolactone**) should be used to reduce mortality and morbidity [Evidence: SORT B*].[26,27]

Canadian guidelines recommend their use in high-risk patients with NYHA class II symptoms, specifically individuals aged >55 years with LVEF ≤30% (or ≤35% if QRS interval >130 msec) and recent (within 6 months) hospitalization for CV disease or with elevated BNP or NT-proBNP levels. They are also recommended as additional therapy in NYHA class III-IV patients with LVEF <30% (Figure 2).

Aldosterone antagonists should not be used in patients with a baseline potassium >5 mmol/L, serum creatinine >221 µmol/L or creatinine clearance <30 mL/min.[4] Monitor vital signs, serum creatinine and potassium 3 days and 7 days after initiating or titrating the dose of aldosterone antagonists and repeat as necessary until the potassium level and renal function are stable.[5] Monitoring should then be performed monthly for 3 months and then every 3 months.[5]

Eplerenone, unlike spironolactone, does not produce gynecomastia and is therefore the agent of choice in individuals who have experienced this adverse effect.[5] Eplerenone appears to have a similar risk of hyperkalemia and renal dysfunction as spironolactone, so should not be used as a substitute in these situations. Prospective comparative data between these agents is limited. The choice is left to the discretion of the clinician and will likely be influenced by reimbursement considerations.

Digoxin

Digoxin improves symptoms and reduces the risk of hospitalization for HF, but does not reduce mortality in patients with moderate to severe persistent symptoms (NYHA class II–IV) receiving an

* SORT (Strength of Recommendation Taxonomy) is a rating system (A, B or C) that addresses the quality of available evidence. For more information consult **How to Use *Compendium of Therapeutic Choices*** on page xxv.

ACE inhibitor.[4,28] Digoxin may be considered in patients with persisting symptoms despite the use of a beta-blocker, an ACE inhibitor (or an ARB) and an aldosterone antagonist (or an ARB). It may also be considered for control of the ventricular rate in patients with atrial fibrillation that cannot be controlled by beta-blockers, or in patients who cannot tolerate beta-blockers.[5] Individualize the dosage based on the patient's age, weight, renal function and concomitant drugs; the usual range is from 0.0625–0.25 mg daily. Lower doses may be appropriate in select patients. Given the narrow therapeutic index of digoxin, pay particular attention to identifying and preventing potential drug interactions. Check digoxin serum concentrations when renal function changes significantly, an interacting drug is added or discontinued or when digoxin toxicity is suspected. Serum concentrations may also be verified after steady state is achieved, particularly in elderly patients and those with renal dysfunction.[4,29] Measure trough serum concentrations at least 8 hours after administration and adjust the dose to maintain the serum concentration between 0.6 and 1 nmol/L, which is associated with greater reductions in hospitalization and, possibly, a reduction in all cause and HF-associated mortality.[30,31]

Nitrates/Hydralazine

The combination of isosorbide dinitrate plus hydralazine reduces mortality and morbidity in black patients with NYHA class III–IV HF and is recommended in addition to standard therapy in this setting.[32] Use of this combination may also be considered in black patients with NYHA class II HF[1,4,32] and in other HF patients who do not tolerate ACE inhibitors and ARBs.[1]

Nitrate monotherapy is valuable in treating symptoms of exercise-induced dyspnea or angina, paroxysmal nocturnal dyspnea and orthopnea. Nitrates have not been shown to reduce mortality in the absence of hydralazine.[1]

Omega-3 Polyunsaturated Fatty Acid Supplementation

Based on a trial that suggested a modest reduction of cardiovascular events with low-dose omega-3 polyunsaturated fatty acid (n-3 PUFA),[33] some guidelines suggest that low-dose n-3 PUFA (1 g/day) may be considered in patients with mild to moderate HF.[4,34] Whether higher doses of n-3 PUFA are more effective is unknown, but doses of more than 3 g/day have been associated with excessive bleeding.[34] Monitor the INR in patients receiving warfarin following n-3 PUFA initiation.[34] Because n-3 PUFA are food supplements, patients should consult their pharmacist to help in the selection of a reliable n-3 PUFA brand that most closely matches the formulation studied in HF (850–882 mg eicosapentaenoic acid and docosahexaenoic acid as ethyl esters in an average ratio of 1:1.2).

Calcium Channel Blockers

Felodipine and **amlodipine** are safe, but do not reduce mortality or morbidity in patients with systolic HF.[35,36] They may be useful in select patients with persistent angina despite the use of beta-blockers and nitrates or in patients with uncontrolled hypertension despite the use of an ACEI, aldosterone antagonist, beta-blocker and a diuretic.[3]

Avoid diltiazem and verapamil in patients with systolic HF because of their negative inotropic effects[1,3,4,5] and nifedipine because of the lack of data.

Antiarrhythmics

Consider **amiodarone** to maintain sinus rhythm in select patients with atrial fibrillation.[4] Amiodarone also reduces the frequency of repetitive ICD discharges.

Avoid all other antiarrhythmic drugs.[3,37] Antiarrhythmics are not recommended for prevention of sudden cardiac death because they do not reduce mortality. It should be emphasized that a strategy of maintaining sinus rhythm in patients with HF is not superior to ventricular rate control in patients with a history of atrial fibrillation.[38]

HMG-CoA Reductase Inhibitors (Statins)

Although the benefit of statins in the primary and secondary prevention of coronary artery disease is well established, 2 trials have suggested that the benefits of statins in patients with HF may be limited, even if they have coronary artery disease.[39,40] Nevertheless, patients included in these trials were relatively older (mean age at baseline of 69 and 73 years) and presented with a baseline LDL cholesterol of only 3.2 mmol/L and 3.5 mmol/L, respectively. Consequently, it is reasonable to continue treating younger patients and/or patients who are at high risk of cardiovascular events (recent MI, diabetes and known vascular disease). Because these trials did not study the impact of statin discontinuation, it is reasonable to continue the use of these agents in patients who are receiving them.

Heart Failure with Preserved Ejection Fraction

In patients with HF with PEF, focus treatment on control of risk factors (hypertension, diabetes mellitus, ventricular rate in patients with supraventricular arrhythmias), volume status and decreasing heart rate to optimize filling time.[1,4] Trials have suggested that the chronic use of **renin-angiotensin system modulators** does not significantly reduce the risk of mortality in patients with HF with PEF.[41,42,43] Nevertheless, these agents should be used to treat hypertension, particularly in patients with diabetes, left ventricular hypertrophy, nephropathy or coronary artery disease because of their established efficacy and end-organ protection in these patient populations. **Beta-blockers** are recommended in patients with CAD, prior MI, hypertension or atrial fibrillation to control ventricular rate (Figure 3).[4] **Diuretics** should be used to optimize volume status.[1] **Verapamil** or **diltiazem** may be considered to control the ventricular rate in patients with supraventricular arrhythmias[1,4] or angina, in those who cannot tolerate a beta-blocker.[4] Calcium channel blockers may also be considered in patients with hypertension.[4]

Decompensated Heart Failure

Few large, randomized trials have been performed in patients with decompensated or acute HF. Intravenous **loop diuretics** are recommended in patients with signs and symptoms of fluid retention (e.g., **furosemide** 40–200 mg 2–3 times daily based on renal function or the patient's usual dose of furosemide).[1,4,20]

Figure 3: **Management of Heart Failure with Preserved Ejection Fraction (HF with PEF)**

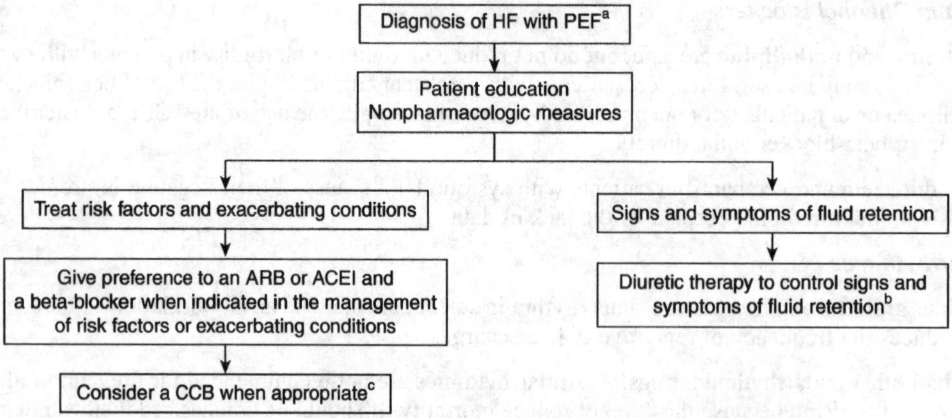

[a] There is no strong consensus on the definition of HF with PEF or its treatment.
[b] Diuretics should be used with care because excessive diuresis may decrease cardiac output and compromise renal function in HF with PEF.
[c] CCBs may improve symptoms by decreasing heart rate and increasing diastolic filling time.
Abbreviations: ACEI = angiotensin converting enzyme inhibitor; ARB = angiotensin II receptor blocker; CCB = calcium channel blocker

Use combinations of diuretics, or add a vasodilator such as **nitroglycerin** or **nitroprusside** for hospitalized patients who do not respond to intravenous furosemide.[1,4] Although clinical guidelines recommend the use of **nesiritide**, this drug is no longer available in Canada. Intravenous vasodilators with a loop diuretic can be used initially in patients with moderate to severe symptoms of pulmonary congestion or those with severe hypertension.[1,4] Sublingual nitroglycerin can be given before intravenous nitroglycerin. Invasive monitoring is recommended when administering nitroprusside.[4] Take care to prevent cyanide and thiocyanide toxicity with nitroprusside; avoid in patients with hepatic or renal failure.[3]

In patients with low cardiac output, **milrinone** or **dobutamine** is indicated if the systolic blood pressure is >90 mm Hg,[1] and dobutamine if the systolic blood pressure is <90 mm Hg.[1] Limit the use of vasopressors (**dopamine** or **norepinephrine**) to patients with significant hypotension.[1] Dosages of these agents are based on vital signs, clinical status, comorbidities and the treatment regimen of the patient. In select patients, invasive monitoring of hemodynamic parameters may be used to adjust the dose.

Choices during Pregnancy and Breastfeeding

Heart Failure and Pregnancy

Pregnancy is accompanied by important cardiovascular hemodynamic alterations including increases in blood volume, heart rate and cardiac output, as well as a reduction in peripheral vascular resistance and blood pressure.[44] In women with existing HF, pregnancy may be associated with significant risk for the mother depending on the severity of the HF and comorbid conditions.[44] Most experts agree that HF with an LVEF <35–40%, or NYHA functional class III or IV, are contraindications to pregnancy because of the high risk of cardiovascular events and mortality.[45] This risk is further increased in the presence of other cardiovascular pathologies.[45] Because many of the pharmacologic agents used in HF are teratogenic, pharmacologic treatments should be selected and optimized based on their cardiovascular benefits for the mother and risks to the fetus.[45]

Peripartum cardiomyopathy (PPCM), defined as HF with LVEF <45% in the last month of the pregnancy or within 5 months of the delivery in the absence of pre-existing cardiac disease,[45] has an incidence of 1 in 3000–4000 live births.[44]

Management during Pregnancy

The 2010 Canadian Cardiovascular Society guidelines recommend that women with pre-existing HF be evaluated and counselled by an expert in HF and pregnancy before becoming pregnant.[45] The risk of the pregnancy and of the transmission of inheritable cardiac diseases, if applicable, should be addressed.[45]

Women should be monitored closely during the pregnancy, at the time of delivery and in the postpartum period.[45] Should worsening of new onset HF be suspected in a pregnant woman, cardiac testing should include an echocardiogram.[45] Radiation should be minimized.[45] Refer to the 2010 Canadian Cardiovascular Society guidelines for a more complete discussion.[45]

Advise women with PPCM whose LVEF does not recover against any future pregnancy because of the high risk of cardiac mortality and morbidity.[45] Inform women who do recover about the high risk of recurrence of LV dysfunction in subsequent pregnancies.[45]

Sodium and fluid restrictions are recommended to minimize signs and symptoms of hypervolemia. Medications should be switched during pregnancy to those with better safety data.[45] **Beta-blockers** can be used during pregnancy.[45,46] $Beta_1$ selective agents are generally preferred to avoid increased uterine tone and decreased uterine perfusion.[45] Of the beta-blockers used in HF, **metoprolol** has been the most studied in pregnant women.[46] Monitor for fetal growth retardation.[46] Following delivery, monitor for hypoglycemia, bradycardia and hypotension in the newborn.[45,46] **Furosemide** can be used to maintain euvolemia in the mother, but take care to minimize the risk of dehydration which can lead to reduced placental perfusion.[45] **Digoxin** can also be used safely, but higher doses may be required in pregnant women because of the increased volume of distribution.[45] Reduce the dose of digoxin after delivery. **Hydralazine** in combination with **nitrates** can be also used to manage symptoms.[45] Hydralazine is also a treatment option in select patients with high blood pressure.[45,46] Avoid ACE inhibitors, ARBs and aldosterone antagonists during pregnancy because they are known teratogens.[45]

Heart Failure and Breastfeeding

In women with HF prior to pregnancy, maintain chronic treatment (or restart ACE inhibitors) following the pregnancy and continue indefinitely.

In women with PPCM, pharmacologic therapy should be continued and LV function and size periodically reassessed. In women in whom ventricular function does not normalize, continue treatment indefinitely. Although no formal guidelines exist, in women in whom the LV size and function normalize, diuretics can be stopped, and beta-blockers and ACE inhibitors slowly discontinued over months, or even years, with close monitoring to ensure that the ventricular function does not deteriorate.

Beta-blockers appear safe in breastfeeding.[46] Of the beta-blockers used in HF, **metoprolol** has been the most extensively studied in breastfeeding and may be preferred.[46] Limited data suggest that furosemide can be used in breastfeeding.[46] To minimize the transfer of drug into breast milk, the dose of furosemide should be taken right after breastfeeding.[46] The transfer of **spironolactone** into breast milk appears minimal; hence, it can be used during breastfeeding.[46] Current data for **captopril**, **enalapril**, **fosinopril**, **quinapril** and **ramipril** indicate that the quantity of these ACE inhibitor present in the milk is limited and they can be safely used while breastfeeding.[46] Data regarding ARBs are limited; hence, ACE inhibitors are preferred.[46]

A discussion of general principles on the use of medications in these special populations can be found in Appendix II and Appendix III. Other specialized reference sources are also provided in these appendices.

Therapeutic Tips

- The choice of whether to start an **ACE inhibitor** or a **beta-blocker** first in a HF patient is based on the vital signs, blood pressure and comorbidities. Most clinicians will start both agents simultaneously at low doses.
- If introduced sequentially, it is not necessary to reach the target doses of one agent before starting the other.
- The doses of ACE inhibitors and beta-blockers should generally not be increased simultaneously.
- Titrate ACE inhibitors, ARBs, beta-blockers and aldosterone antagonists to their target doses.
- Hypotension or worsening renal function when initiating or increasing the dose of an ACE inhibitor usually indicates the need to reduce the dose of a diuretic.
- The formulation of **metoprolol** available in Canada (metoprolol tartrate) has not been shown to reduce mortality in a randomized trial of patients with HF, is not available in a commercial dosage form that is suitable for initial treatment of HF and is not included in Canadian guidelines. Nevertheless, metoprolol tartrate is the preferred beta-blocker in pregnant and breastfeeding women.
- In patients with hypotension, consider administering antihypertensive drugs at different times during the day, rather than at the same time.
- Cough is a symptom of HF decompensation. Careful evaluation is necessary when evaluating a cough in a patient receiving an ACE inhibitor.
- Electrolyte abnormalities are common in patients with HF. Monitor patients closely, especially when taking combinations that have additive effects, for example, increased serum potassium due to the combination of an ACE inhibitor or ARB plus spironolactone. Measure serum creatinine and electrolytes 7–14 days after the initiation of ACE inhibitors, ARBs, aldosterone antagonists or diuretics, or following dosage changes.

Table 4: Outcomes Associated with Drugs Used for Systolic Heart Failure

Outcome	Intervention	Comparator	Relative Risk Reduction (%)	Absolute Risk Reduction (%)	Number Needed to Treat to Prevent One Outcome
Death prevented	ACE inhibitor[10]	Placebo	16	4.5	23
	Beta-blocker[15]	Placebo	32	5.5	29
	Aldosterone antagonist[26]	Placebo	30	11	10
	Hydralazine/isosorbide dinitrate (in addition to optimal therapy in black patients)[32]	Placebo	39	4	25
	ARB (ACE inhibitor-intolerant patients)[21]	Placebo	13[a]	N/A	N/A
Hospitalizations avoided	ACE inhibitor[10]	Placebo	30	10.8	9
	Beta-blocker[15]	Placebo	33	6	17
	Digoxin[28]	Placebo	28	7.9	13
	ARB (ACE inhibitor–intolerant patients; hospitalizations for HF only)[21]	Placebo	32	7.8	13

[a] Study size was not sufficient to produce a statistically significant value in an unadjusted analysis (p=0.11). This number was significant in an analysis adjusted for covariates (p=0.033).

Abbreviations: ACE = angiotensin converting enzyme; ARB = angiotensin II receptor blocker; N/A = not available

Table 5: **Drugs Used for Heart Failure**

Class	Drug	Dose	Adverse Effects	Drug Interactions	Comments	Cost[a]
ACE Inhibitors[b]	*captopril* generics	Initial: 6.25–12.5 mg TID po Target: 50 mg TID	Hypotension, hyperkalemia, dry cough, renal insufficiency, angioedema (rare), skin rashes, taste disturbance, proteinuria, neutropenia (rare), headache, dizziness.	Diuretics: hypotension (monitor BP). Potassium-sparing diuretics, potassium supplements, ARBs: hyperkalemia (monitor K^+). NSAIDs: reduced hypotensive effect (monitor BP), fluid retention, renal failure. Lithium: lithium toxicity (monitor lithium levels).	Monitor serum creatinine and potassium 7–14 days after initiation of therapy or dose changes. Some experienced clinicians use doses higher than usual target doses. Avoid in pregnancy.	$$$
	enalapril Vasotec, generics	Initial: 1.25–2.5 mg BID po Target: 10 mg BID	See captopril.	See captopril.	See captopril.	$
	lisinopril Prinivil, Zestril, generics	Initial: 2.5–5 mg once daily po Target: 20–35 mg once daily	See captopril.	See captopril.	See captopril.	$
	ramipril Altace, generics	Initial: 1.25–2.5 mg BID po Target: 5 mg BID	See captopril.	See captopril.	See captopril.	$
	trandolapril Mavik	Initial: 1 mg once daily po Target: 4 mg once daily	See captopril.	See captopril.	See captopril.	$$
Angiotensin Receptor Blockers	*candesartan* Atacand, generics	Initial: 4 mg once daily po Target: 32 mg once daily	Hypotension, hyperkalemia, renal insufficiency, angioedema (rare, less frequent than with ACE inhibitors), headache, dizziness.	Diuretics: hypotension (monitor BP). Potassium-sparing diuretics and ACE inhibitors: hyperkalemia (monitor K^+). Potassium: hyperkalemia (monitor K^+). NSAIDs: reduced hypotensive effect (monitor BP), fluid retention, renal failure. Lithium: lithium toxicity (monitor lithium levels).	Monitor serum creatinine and potassium 7–14 days after initiation of therapy or dose changes. Avoid in pregnancy.	$

Class	Drug	Dose	Adverse Effects	Drug Interactions	Comments	Cost[a]
	losartan Cozaar, generics	Initial: 12.5 mg once daily po Target: 150 mg once daily	See candesartan.	See candesartan.	See candesartan.	$
	valsartan Diovan, generics	Initial: 40 mg BID po Target: 160 mg BID	See candesartan.	See candesartan.	See candesartan.	$
Aldosterone Antagonists	*eplerenone* (renal-dose symbol) Inspra	Initial: 25 mg once daily po or every 2 days Target: 50 mg once daily	Hyperkalemia, dehydration, dizziness, diarrhea, nausea.	ACE inhibitors, ARBs, potassium supplements: hyperkalemia. NSAIDs: reduced diuretic effect, worsening renal function, hyperkalemia. Strong inhibitors/inducers of CYP3A4.	Monitor serum creatinine and potassium 3 and 7 days after initiating or titrating the dose. Repeat every 1–3 months once stable. Avoid in pregnancy.	$$$$
	spironolactone (renal-dose symbol) Aldactone, generics	Initial: 12.5 mg daily or every 2 days po Target (for mortality benefit): 25–50 mg/day	Hyperkalemia, dehydration, nausea, gynecomastia (usually reversible upon discontinuation).	ACE inhibitors, ARBs, potassium supplements: hyperkalemia. NSAIDs: reduced diuretic effect, worsening renal function, hyperkalemia.	See eplerenone.	$
$Beta_1$-adrenergic Antagonists	*bisoprolol* (renal-dose symbol) Sandoz Bisoprolol, other generics	Initial: 1.25 mg once daily po Target: 10 mg once daily	Orthostatic hypotension, worsening HF/fluid retention, bronchospasm (less with $beta_1$-selective), dyspnea, bradycardia, malaise, fatigue, asthenia, erectile dysfunction, may mask hypoglycemia.	Digoxin, amiodarone, diltiazem, verapamil: increased bradycardia. Nondihydropyridine calcium channel blockers: additive cardiodepressant effect.	Selective beta-blocker.	$
	carvedilol generics	Initial: 3.125 mg BID po Target: 25 mg BID	See bisoprolol. More likely to cause orthostatic hypotension than bisoprolol.	See bisoprolol. CYP2D6 inhibitors.	Nonselective beta-blocker with alpha-blocking activity. Has some vasodilating effects.	$
Calcium Channel Blockers	*amlodipine* Norvasc, generics	2.5–10 mg once daily po	Hypotension, constipation, peripheral edema, gingival hyperplasia, headache, dizziness.			$
	felodipine Plendil, generics	2.5–10 mg once daily po	See amlodipine.			$

(cont'd)

Table 5: **Drugs Used for Heart Failure** *(cont'd)*

Class	Drug	Dose	Adverse Effects	Drug Interactions	Comments	Cost[a]
Inotropic Agents	*digoxin* Toloxin	0.0625–0.25 mg once daily po (lower doses may be appropriate in select patients)	Anorexia, nausea, vomiting, visual disturbances, fatigue, dizziness, confusion, delirium. Cardiac arrhythmia. Noncardiovascular adverse effects do not always precede potentially fatal arrhythmias.	Amiodarone, clarithromycin, cyclosporine, erythromycin, itraconazole, propafenone, quinidine, ritonavir, tetracycline and verapamil increase digoxin serum levels. Antacids, cholestyramine, colestipol, neomycin, rifampin, St. John's wort and sulfasalazine reduce digoxin serum levels. Amiodarone, beta-blockers, diltiazem and verapamil increase risk of bradycardia.	Adjust dose based on patient's age, weight, renal function and concomitant drugs. Measure trough serum concentrations at least 8 hours after administration and adjust the dose to maintain the serum concentration between 0.6 and 1 nmol/L.	$
	milrinone generics	0.1–0.75 µg/kg/min iv	Tachyarrhythmias, hypotension, myocardial ischemia, thrombocytopenia.			$$$$$[c]
	dobutamine generics	2–20 µg/kg/min iv	Tachyarrhythmias, hypokalemia, myocardial ischemia.	Beta-blockers reduce positive inotropic effects of dobutamine.		$$$$$[c]
Loop Diuretics	*bumetanide* Burinex	1–4 mg/day po	Dehydration, hypokalemia, hypocalcemia, nausea, hypotension, azotemia, hypomagnesemia, anorexia, hyperglycemia (less than with thiazides), hyperuricemia, weakness, fatigue, rash, increased total cholesterol, ototoxicity with high doses.	Lithium: lithium toxicity (monitor lithium levels). Digoxin: digoxin toxicity if K^+ depleted (monitor K^+). Corticosteroids: hypokalemia (monitor K^+). NSAIDs: reduced diuretic effect; increased renal toxicity (monitor). Thiazide diuretics: hypokalemia, hypomagnesemia, dehydration, renal dysfunction (monitor).	1 mg is equivalent to 40 mg furosemide.	$$$
	furosemide Lasix, Lasix Special, generics	20–500 mg/day administered daily to BID po For decompensated HF: may be administered BID or TID	See bumetanide.	See bumetanide.		$

Class	Drug	Dose	Adverse Effects	Drug Interactions	Comments	Cost[a]
	ethacrynic acid Edecrin	50–200 mg daily po or divided BID	See bumetanide.	See bumetanide.	An alternative diuretic in patients with allergies to loop diuretics. Higher risk of ototoxicity than furosemide.	$$$$$
Thiazides and Related Diuretics	*chlorthalidone* generics	50–100 mg po once daily Maximum: 200 mg/day (use lower doses when used in combination with a loop diuretic)	Dehydration, hypokalemia, nausea, hypotension, azotemia, hypomagnesemia, hypercalcemia, hyponatremia, hyperglycemia (more with thiazides), hyperuricemia, rash, increased total cholesterol.	Lithium: lithium toxicity (monitor lithium levels). Digoxin: digoxin toxicity if K^+ depleted (monitor K^+). Corticosteroids: hypokalemia (monitor K^+). NSAIDs: reduced diuretic effect; increased renal toxicity (monitor). Loop diuretics: hypokalemia, hypomagnesemia, dehydration, renal dysfunction (monitor).	Use in patients with mild HF. May be combined with a loop diuretic by experienced clinicians.	$
	hydrochlorothiazide generics	25–100 mg/day po given in 1 or 2 divided doses Maximum: 200 mg/day (use lower doses in combination with a loop diuretic)	See chlorthalidone.	See chlorthalidone.	See chlorthalidone.	$
	metolazone Zaroxolyn	2.5–10 mg once daily po When combined with a loop diuretic, use lower doses (2.5–5 mg daily to weekly)	See chlorthalidone.	See chlorthalidone.	Experienced clinicians usually combine with a loop diuretic in those with refractory HF.	$
Vasodilators	*hydralazine* generics	Initial: 10–25 mg TID po Target: 75 mg TID–QID	Hypotension, GI complaints, SLE-like syndrome.		Used in combination with isosorbide dinitrate in black patients.	$$
	isosorbide dinitrate generics	Initial: 10–20 mg TID po Target: 40 mg TID–QID	Headache, hypotension.	Sildenafil, vardenafil and tadalafil: severe hypotension.	Use in combination with hydralazine in black patients.	$

(cont'd)

Table 5: **Drugs Used for Heart Failure** *(cont'd)*

Class	Drug	Dose	Adverse Effects	Drug Interactions	Comments	Cost[a]
	nitroglycerin generics	5–200 μg/min iv	Hypotension, headache, tachycardia, bradycardia.	See isosorbide dinitrate.		$$$[c]
	nitroprusside generics	0.1–5 μg/kg/min iv	Hypotension, cyanide toxicity, thiocyanate toxicity, methemoglobinemia, coronary artery steal, tachycardia, increased intracranial pressure.			$$$$$[c]

[a] Cost of 30-day supply for target doses; includes drug cost only.
[b] Only captopril, enalapril, ramipril and trandolapril have been shown to reduce morbidity and prolong survival in heart failure or in patients with LV dysfunction post-MI.
[c] Cost of 1-day supply for a 70 kg person.
Dosage adjustment may be required in renal impairment; see Appendix I
Abbreviations: HF = heart failure; SLE = systemic lupus erythematosus
Legend: $ < $25 $$ $25–50 $$$ $50–75 $$$$ $75–100 $$$$$ $100–125

Suggested Readings

Heart Failure Society of America, Lindenfeld J, Albert NM et al. HFSA 2010 comprehensive heart failure practice guideline. *J Card Fail* 2010;16(6):e1-194.

Howlett JG, McKelvie RS, Arnold JM et al. Canadian Cardiovascular Society Consensus Conference guidelines on heart failure, update 2009: diagnosis and management of right-sided heart failure, myocarditis, device therapy and recent important clinical trials. *Can J Cardiol* 2009;25(2):85-105.

McKelvie RS, Moe GW, Ezekowitz JA et al. The 2012 Canadian Cardiovascular Society heart failure management guidelines update: focus on acute and chronic heart failure. *Can J Cardiol* 2013;29(2):168-81.

McMurray JJ, Adamopoulos S, Anker SD et al. ESC guidelines for the diagnosis and treatment of acute and chronic heart failure 2012: the Task Force for the Diagnosis and Treatment of Acute and Chronic Heart Failure 2012 of the European Society of Cardiology. Developed in collaboration with the Heart Failure Association (HFA) of the ESC. *Eur Heart J* 2012;33(14):1787-847.

Yancy CW, Jessup M, Bozkurt B et al. 2013 ACCF/AHA guideline for the management of heart failure: a report of the American College of Cardiology Foundation/American Heart Association Task Force on practice guidelines. *Circulation* 2013;128(16):e240-319.

References

1. McKelvie RS, Moe GW, Ezekowitz JA et al. The 2012 Canadian Cardiovascular Society heart failure management guidelines update: focus on acute and chronic heart failure. *Can J Cardiol* 2013;29(2):168-81.
2. Jessup M, Brozena S. Heart failure. *N Engl J Med* 2003;348(20):2007-18.
3. McMurray JJ, Adamopoulos S, Anker SD et al. ESC Guidelines for the diagnosis and treatment of acute and chronic heart failure 2012: the Task Force for the Diagnosis and Treatment of Acute and Chronic Heart Failure 2012 of the European Society of Cardiology. Developed in collaboration with the Heart Failure Association (HFA) of the ESC. *Eur Heart J* 2012;33(14):1787-847.
4. Heart Failure Society of America, Lindenfeld J, Albert NM et al. HFSA 2010 comprehensive heart failure practice guideline. *J Card Fail* 2010;16(6):e1-194.
5. Yancy CW, Jessup M, Bozkurt B et al. 2013 ACCF/AHA guideline for the management of heart failure: a report of the American College of Cardiology Foundation/American Heart Association Task Force on practice guidelines. *Circulation* 2013;128(16):e240-319.
6. Mahé I, Chassany O, Grenard AS et al. Defining the role of calcium channel antagonists in heart failure due to systolic dysfunction. *Am J Cardiovasc Drugs* 2003;3(1):33-41.
7. Tang AS, Wells GA, Talajic M et al. Cardiac-resynchronization therapy for mild-to-moderate heart failure. *N Engl J Med* 2010;363(25):2385-95.
8. Ross H, Hendry P, Dipchand A et al. 2001 Canadian Cardiovascular Society Consensus Conference on cardiac transplantation. *Can J Cardiol* 2003;19(6):620-54.
9. Effects of enalapril on mortality in severe congestive heart failure. Results of the Cooperative North Scandinavian Enalapril Survival Study (CONSENSUS). The CONSENSUS Trial Study Group. *N Engl J Med* 1987;316(23):1429-35.
10. Effect of enalapril on survival in patients with reduced left ventricular ejection fractions and congestive heart failure. The SOLVD Investigators. *N Engl J Med* 1991;325(5):293-302.
11. Effect of enalapril on mortality and the development of heart failure in asymptomatic patients with reduced left ventricular ejection fractions. The SOLVD Investigators. *N Engl J Med* 1992;327(10):685-91.
12. Packer M, Poole-Wilson PA, Armstrong PW et al. Comparative effects of low and high doses of the angiotensin-converting enzyme inhibitor, lisinopril, on morbidity and mortality in chronic heart failure. ATLAS Study Group. *Circulation* 1999;100(23):2312-8.
13. de Denus S, Tardif JC, White M et al. Quantification of the risk and predictors of hyperkalemia in patients with left ventricular dysfunction: a retrospective analysis of the Studies of Left Ventricular Dysfunction (SOLVD) trials. *Am Heart J* 2006;152(4):705-12.
14. Effect of metoprolol CR/XL in chronic heart failure: Metoprolol CR/XL Randomised Intervention Trial in Congestive Heart Failure (MERIT-HF). *Lancet* 1999;353(9169):2001-7.
15. The Cardiac Insufficiency Bisoprolol Study II (CIBIS-II): a randomised trial. *Lancet* 1999;353(9146):9-13.
16. Packer M, Bristow MR, Cohn JN et al. The effect of carvedilol on morbidity and mortality in patients with chronic heart failure. U.S. Carvedilol Heart Failure Study Group. *N Engl J Med* 1996;334(21):1349-55.
17. Packer M, Coats AJ, Fowler MB et al. Effect of carvedilol on survival in severe chronic heart failure. *N Engl J Med* 2001;344(22):1651-8.
18. Poole-Wilson PA, Swedberg K, Cleland JG et al. Comparison of carvedilol and metoprolol on clinical outcomes in patients with chronic heart failure in the Carvedilol Or Metoprolol European Trial (COMET): randomised controlled trial. *Lancet* 2003;362(9377):7-13.
19. Gattis WA, O'Connor CM, Gallup DS et al. Predischarge initiation of carvedilol in patients hospitalized for decompensated heart failure: results of the Initiation Management Predischarge: Process for Assessment of Carvedilol Therapy in Heart Failure (IMPACT-HF) trial. *J Am Coll Cardiol* 2004;43(9):1534-41.
20. Brater DC. Diuretic therapy. *N Engl J Med* 1998;339(6):387-95.
21. Granger CB, McMurray JJ, Yusuf S et al. Effects of candesartan in patients with chronic heart failure and reduced left-ventricular systolic function intolerant to angiotensin-converting-enzyme inhibitors: the CHARM-Alternative trial. *Lancet* 2003;362(9386):772-6.
22. Pfeffer MA, McMurray JJ, Velazquez EJ et al. Valsartan, captopril, or both in myocardial infarction complicated by heart failure, left ventricular dysfunction, or both. *N Engl J Med* 2003;349(20):1893-906.
23. Konstam MA, Neaton JD, Dickstein K et al. Effects of high-dose versus low-dose losartan on clinical outcomes in patients with heart failure (HEAAL study): a randomised, double-blind trial. *Lancet* 2009;374(9704):1840-8.
24. McMurray JJ, Ostergren J, Swedberg K et al. Effects of candesartan in patients with chronic heart failure and reduced left-ventricular systolic function taking angiotensin-converting-enzyme inhibitors: the CHARM-Added trial. *Lancet* 2003;362(9386):767-71.

25. Cohn JN, Tognoni G. A randomized trial of the angiotensin-receptor blocker valsartan in chronic heart failure. *N Engl J Med* 2001;345(23):1667-75.
26. Pitt B, Zannad F, Remme WJ et al. The effect of spironolactone on morbidity and mortality in patients with severe heart failure. Randomized Aldactone Evaluation Study Investigators. *N Engl J Med* 1999;341(10):709-17.
27. Zannad F, McMurray JJ, Krum H et al. Eplerenone in patients with systolic heart failure and mild symptoms. *N Engl J Med* 2011;364(1):11-21.
28. The effect of digoxin on mortality and morbidity in patients with heart failure. The Digitalis Investigation Group. *N Engl J Med* 1997;336(8):525-33.
29. Gheorghiade M, van Veldhuisen DJ, Colucci WS. Contemporary use of digoxin in the management of cardiovascular disorders. *Circulation* 2006;113(21):2556-64.
30. Rathore SS, Curtis JP, Wang Y et al. Association of serum digoxin concentration and outcomes in patients with heart failure. *JAMA* 2003;289(7):871-8.
31. Adams KF, Gheorghiade M, Uretsky BF et al. Clinical benefits of low serum digoxin concentrations in heart failure. *J Am Coll Cardiol* 2002;39(6):946-53.
32. Taylor AL, Ziesche S, Yancy C et al. Combination of isosorbide dinitrate and hydralazine in blacks with heart failure. *N Engl J Med* 2004;351(20):2049-57.
33. Tavazzi L, Maggioni AP, Marchioli R et al. Effect of n-3 polyunsaturated fatty acids in patients with chronic heart failure (the GISSI-HF trial): a randomised, double-blind, placebo-controlled trial. *Lancet* 2008;372(9645):1223-30.
34. Howlett JG, McKelvie RS, Arnold JM et al. Canadian Cardiovascular Society Consensus Conference guidelines on heart failure, update 2009: diagnosis and management of right-sided heart failure, myocarditis, device therapy and recent important clinical trials. *Can J Cardiol* 2009;25(2):85-105.
35. Cohn JN, Ziesche S, Smith R et al. Effect of the calcium antagonist felodipine as supplementary vasodilator therapy in patients with chronic heart failure treated with enalapril: V-HeFT III. Vasodilator-Heart Failure Trial (V-HeFT) Study Group. *Circulation* 1997;96(3):856-63.
36. Packer M, O'Connor CM, Ghali JK et al. Effect of amlodipine on morbidity and mortality in severe chronic heart failure. Prospective Randomized Amlodipine Survival Evaluation Study Group. *N Engl J Med* 1996;335(15):1107-14.
37. Kober L, Torp-Pedersen C, McMurray J et al. Increased mortality after dronedarone therapy for severe heart failure. *N Engl J Med* 2008;358(25):2678-87.
38. Roy D, Talajic M, Nattel S et al. Rhythm control versus rate control for atrial fibrillation and heart failure. *N Engl J Med* 2008;358(25):2667-77.
39. Gissi-HF Investigators, Tavazzi L, Maggioni AP et al. Effect of rosuvastatin in patients with chronic heart failure (the GISSI-HF trial): a randomised, double-blind, placebo-controlled trial. *Lancet* 2008;372(9645):1231-9.
40. Kjekshus J, Apatrei E, Barrios V et al. Rosuvastatin in older patients with systolic heart failure. *N Engl J Med* 2007;357(22):2248-61.
41. Yusuf S, Pfeffer MA, Swedberg K et al. Effects of candesartan in patients with chronic heart failure and preserved left-ventricular ejection fraction: the CHARM-Preserved Trial. *Lancet* 2003;362(9386):777-81.
42. Massie BM, Carson PE, McMurray JJ et al. Irbesartan in patients with heart failure and preserved ejection fraction. *N Engl J Med* 2008;359(23):2456-67.
43. Cleland JG, Tendera M, Adamus J et al. The perindopril in elderly people with chronic heart failure (PEP-CHF) study. *Eur Heart J* 2006;27(19):2338-45.
44. Moioli M, Valenzano Menada M, Bentivoglio G et al. Peripartum cardiomyopathy. *Arch Gynecol Obstet* 2010;281(2):183-8.
45. Howlett JG, McKelvie RS, Costigan J et al. The 2010 Canadian Cardiovascular Society guidelines for the diagnosis and management of heart failure update: heart failure in ethnic minority populations, heart failure and pregnancy, disease management, and quality improvement/assurance programs. *Can J Cardiol* 2010;26(4):185-202.
46. Brochet MS, Louvigne C, Ferreira E. Hypertension artérielle. In: Ferreira E, ed. *Grossesse et allaitement: guide thérapeutique*. Montréal (QC): Éditions du CHU Sainte-Justine; 2007. p. 187-214.

Chapter 39
Hypertension

Norm R.C. Campbell, MD, FRCPC
Paul Gibson, MD, FRCPC and
Ross T. Tsuyuki, PharmD, MSc, FCSHP, FACC

Goals of Therapy

- Reduce the risk of premature cardiac, cerebrovascular, renal and other vascular morbidity and mortality
- Achieve blood pressure targets in treated patients. The targets presented in Table 1 are maximums; thus, the desired systolic blood pressure (SBP) and diastolic blood pressure (DBP) values are *below* these thresholds.

Investigations

- History:
  - duration of hypertension, usual level of blood pressure and any sudden change in severity of hypertension
  - history of antihypertensive drug use, reason for changing therapy, effectiveness, side effects and intolerance
  - drugs that may cause hypertension (Table 2)
  - drugs that may interact with antihypertensive drugs (those that induce or inhibit metabolism)
  - adherence with lifestyle recommendations and drug therapy
  - family history of hypertension, cardiovascular risk factors and premature cardiovascular disease
  - personal history of cigarette and alcohol use, usual physical activity, usual diet and sodium intake, current weight and recent weight change, waist circumference, diabetes and dyslipidemia
  - cerebrovascular, cardiac and peripheral vascular symptoms to assess for target organ damage
  - symptoms of secondary hypertension, which include, for example, pheochromocytoma (hyperadrenergic symptoms), hyper- and hypothyroidism, Cushing's syndrome, renal/urinary symptoms or a past history of renal disease

Table 1: **Blood Pressure Targets in Treated Patients**[1]

Setting	Target SBP/DBP (mm Hg)
Home[a]	<135/85
Office	
General patient population	<140/90
Isolated systolic hypertension	SBP <140 SBP <150 (if 80 y or older)
Diabetes mellitus	<130/80

[a] Measured by a validated home blood pressure monitor.
Abbreviations: DBP = diastolic blood pressure; SBP = systolic blood pressure

Table 2: **Drugs and Other Exogenous Factors That Can Induce or Aggravate Hypertension**[1]

Alcohol (excessive use)	NSAIDs including COX–2 inhibitors
Calcineurin inhibitors, e.g., cyclosporine, tacrolimus	Oral contraceptive and sex hormones
Corticosteroids and anabolic steroids	Salt (sodium—high intake)
Erythropoietin and analogues	Selective serotonin reuptake inhibitors (SSRIs)
Licorice root	Serotonin-norepinephrine reuptake inhibitors (SNRIs)
Midodrine	Stimulants, including cocaine
MAO inhibitors	Vasoconstricting, sympathomimetic decongestants

- Diagnosis:[1]
  - the diagnosis of hypertension is immediate in the case of hypertensive emergencies and urgencies. This includes patients with hypertension that is compromising vital organ function (encephalopathy, cardiac, or rapidly decreasing renal function), hypertension and a major artery dissection, or those with DBP ≥130 mm Hg
  - hypertension may be diagnosed in 2 office visits if blood pressure averages ≥180/110 mm Hg, or if it averages ≥140/90 mm Hg in the presence of diabetes, renal disease, atherosclerotic cardiovascular disease or cerebrovascular disease
  - the diagnosis may be arrived at after 2 visits if home or ambulatory blood pressure measurement is used
  - the diagnosis may require 3 visits if the blood pressure averages between 160/100 mm Hg and 180/110 mm Hg. However, 5 or more visits may be required to establish the diagnosis if the initial blood pressure average is between 140/90 mm Hg and 160/100 mm Hg and there is no target organ dysfunction. Attention to the details of measuring blood pressure is essential to making a valid diagnosis. Automated blood pressure measurements (using an approved monitor) in the office is recommended
  - home measurement of blood pressure can aid in the diagnosis of hypertension, identify white coat and masked hypertension, improve blood pressure control and improve medication adherence in poorly adherent patients
- Physical exam:
  - fundi for hypertensive retinopathy
  - bruits and peripheral pulses for vascular disease and renovascular hypertension
  - edema and lung fields for signs of heart failure
  - heart sounds (4th heart sound), sustained and displaced apex for left ventricular hypertrophy
  - abdominal mass for polycystic kidneys and aortic aneurysm
  - neurologic exam for cerebrovascular disease
- Initial laboratory testing:
  - serum potassium, sodium and creatinine
  - urinalysis
  - fasting glucose, total cholesterol, HDL-C, LDL-C, triglycerides
  - standard 12-lead ECG
  - select patients should have additional testing (Table 3)

Table 3: **Hypertensive Patients Requiring Additional Laboratory Testing**[1]

If these characteristics are present:	Check for:
• High serum creatinine (high normal in the elderly)	Renal disease
• Urinary albumin	Diabetes, renal disease
• Paroxysmal and/or severe sustained hypertension refractory to usual antihypertensive therapy • Hypertension and symptoms suggestive of catecholamine excess (2 or more of headaches, palpitations, sweating, etc.) • Hypertension triggered by beta-blockers, monoamine oxidase inhibitors, micturition or changes in abdominal pressure • Incidentally discovered adrenal adenoma • MEN 2A or 2B; von Recklinghausen's neurofibromatosis or von Hippel-Lindau disease	Pheochromocytoma
• Spontaneous hypokalemia • Profound diuretic-induced hypokalemia (K+ <3 mmol/L) • Hypertension refractory to treatment with ≥3 drugs • Incidental adrenal adenoma	Hyperaldosteronism
Two or more of: • Sudden onset or worsening of hypertension in patients aged >55 or <30 y • Abdominal bruit • Uncontrolled hypertension despite use of ≥3 drugs • Decreased renal function associated with use of an ACE inhibitor or ARB • Overt atherosclerotic vascular disease • Recurrent episodes of hypertension and flash pulmonary edema	Renovascular disease

Abbreviations: ARB = angiotensin receptor blocker; MEN = multiple endocrine neoplasia

Table 4: **Effect of Lifestyle Changes on Blood Pressure in Adults with Hypertension**

Intervention	Recommendation	Change in Blood Pressure (systolic/diastolic) mm Hg
Reduction in sodium intake	Reduce by 1800 mg (78 mmol) per day	−5.8/−2.5
Weight loss	Reduce weight by 4.5 kg	−7.2/−5.9
Reduction in alcohol intake	Reduce by 2.7 drinks/day	−4.6/−2.3
Exercise	3 times/week	−10.3/−7.5
Dietary modification	DASH eating plan[a]	−11.4/−5.5

[a] Available from: www.nhlbi.nih.gov/health/public/heart/hbp/dash/new_dash.pdf.
Adapted with permission from Campbell N. Canadian Hypertension Education Program. Brief overview of 2004 recommendations. *Can Fam Physician* 2004;50:1411-5.

Therapeutic Choices

Nonpharmacologic Choices

All individuals should be advised about a healthy lifestyle to prevent or control hypertension and cardiovascular disease (Table 4).

- Weight loss of 4 kg or more if overweight (target body mass index: 18.5–24.9 kg/m²; waist circumference <102 cm in men and <88 cm in women).
- Healthy diet—high in fresh fruits, vegetables, soluble fibre and low-fat dairy products, low in saturated fats and sodium, e.g., DASH eating plan available at www.nhlbi.nih.gov/health/public/heart/hbp/dash/new_dash.pdf.

- Sodium intake of 1500 mg (65 mmol) per day for those aged 19–50 years, 1300 mg (56 mmol) per day for those aged 51–70 years and 1200 mg (52 mmol) per day in those 71 years and older.
- Regular, moderate intensity cardiorespiratory physical activity for 30–60 minutes on most days.
- Low risk alcohol consumption (0 to 2 drinks/day, <9 drinks/week for women and <14 drinks/week for men).
- Smoke-free environment.

Pharmacologic Choices (Table 6)

If the average SBP/DBP is 140–159/90–99 mm Hg, treatment is recommended in the presence of either:

- hypertensive target organ damage or
- other independent risk factors for cardiovascular disease, e.g., cigarette smoking, dyslipidemia, strong family history of premature cardiovascular disease, truncal obesity, sedentary lifestyle, males older than 55 years, females older than 60 years.[1] More than 90% of patients with hypertension have other cardiovascular risks or overt cardiovascular disease so pharmacologic therapy is almost always recommended.[2]

If the average SBP/DBP is 140–159/90–99 mm Hg and the individual does not have additional risk factors, the short-term benefits of pharmacotherapy are small; discuss the risks and benefits of therapy with the patient. Monitor blood pressure and other risk factors regardless of whether such a patient chooses to begin drug therapy as generally the risks accumulate and blood pressure increases over time.

Consider low-dose **ASA** in patients over age 50 once blood pressure is controlled. Consider therapy for dyslipidemia if the patient meets the current Canadian criteria (see Chapter 37).

In general, the reduction in cardiovascular risk depends more on the extent of the reduction in blood pressure than on the specific blood pressure medication. Pharmacologic therapy should usually be started with a low dose of the initial drug. Consider concurrent risk factors and disease states when selecting initial therapy (Table 5). Dose titration to achieve goal blood pressure should be done every 4–8 weeks for all but those with severe hypertension or target organ damage or high cardiovascular risk, for whom closer follow-up and more frequent dosage titration is required. Lack of control over blood pressure is in most cases due to a failure to titrate therapy (adding drugs and/or increasing doses) in response to high office readings. Greater confidence in office readings can result from supplementing with home blood pressure measurements or ambulatory 24-hour monitors. Generally, high office readings should trigger a dosage increase, addition of another medication, investigations to identify the cause of the high readings or a follow-up appointment within 2–8 weeks to reassess blood pressure.

Diuretics

Extensive evidence supports low-dose thiazide or related diuretics (e.g., indapamide) as first-line therapy for uncomplicated hypertension. They should generally be selected unless there are specific indications for other drugs (see Table 5). Diuretics are inexpensive and well tolerated. They have proven antihypertensive effectiveness in patients with isolated systolic hypertension, the elderly and black patients.

Diuretics can cause hypokalemia that may be associated with adverse cardiovascular outcomes. Consider alternative first-line agents in those with or strongly predisposed to a serious arrhythmia, for example, prolonged QT syndrome. Consider using a combination product to minimize the risk of hypokalemia (hydrochlorothiazide plus a potassium-sparing diuretic—spironolactone, amiloride or triamterene). Reserve the use of high doses (e.g., >25 mg/day of hydrochlorothiazide) for patients with resistant hypertension unresponsive to treatment with multiple drugs or secondary to renal impairment. Consider using a loop diuretic in patients with renal impairment. Diuretics may worsen dysglycemia, although cardiovascular outcomes in patients with diabetes who are treated with diuretics are similar to those treated with ACE inhibitors.[3]

Beta-blockers

Beta-blockers are first-line therapy in patients who are younger than 60 years, or who have stable angina, heart failure or a history of MI. Beta-blockers are also useful in patients who have migraine headaches, tachycardia or essential tremor. However, beta-blockers are not as effective as angiotensin II receptor blockers (ARBs), calcium channel blockers (CCBs) or diuretics as initial therapy for primary prevention of cardiovascular events in patients over the age of 60 years. In addition, they may be ineffective in preventing cardiovascular events in people who smoke.[4]

Drugs that Act via the Renin Angiotensin Aldosterone System (RAAS)

The renin angiotensin aldosterone system (RAAS) plays a crucial role in modulating blood pressure, kidney function, electrolyte balance and vascular and cardiac structure. Drugs that act directly on this system include angiotensin-converting enzyme (ACE) inhibitors, angiotensin receptor antagonists, direct renin inhibitors and spironolactone. Antihypertensive drugs that stimulate the RAAS axis (e.g., diuretics) are as effective as those that block this system in preventing cardiovascular events in patients with hypertension. However, some inhibitors of the RAAS do provide additional benefits in certain patients, including those with heart failure, diabetes and/or chronic kidney disease. ACE inhibitors, ARBs and direct renin inhibitors are contraindicated in pregnant women.[5,6,7] Drugs from these classes should not be prescribed in women of child-bearing potential unless the risks are carefully weighed and adequate measures are taken to prevent pregnancy (see Choices during Pregnancy and Breastfeeding).

Angiotensin-converting Enzyme Inhibitors

Angiotensin-converting enzyme (ACE) inhibitors are first-line agents for non-black patients with uncomplicated hypertension and for patients with diabetes, ischemic heart disease, recent MI, heart failure or chronic kidney disease.

Angiotensin II Receptor Blockers

ARBs are first-line agents for patients with uncomplicated hypertension, for patients with diabetes or ischemic heart disease. They are good alternatives when ACE inhibitors are specifically indicated but not tolerated.

Direct Renin Inhibitors

Aliskiren, the first direct renin inhibitor, prevents renin from converting angiotensinogen to angiotensin I. The drug has a long duration of action and lowers blood pressure to the same extent as drugs from other antihypertensive classes. Until data become available on the effect of aliskiren on cardiovascular events the drug should be used only when first-line therapies cannot be used.

Long-acting Calcium Channel Blockers

Long-acting dihydropyridine CCBs can be used as first-line agents but in practice they are generally used in combination therapy. *Short-acting formulations* of these agents have caused an increase in cardiovascular events in randomized controlled trials and should *not* be used. Elderly patients with isolated systolic hypertension and black patients are particularly responsive to CCBs.

Other Antihypertensive Drugs

In general, other classes of antihypertensive drugs should not be prescribed unless there are specific indications (Table 5), contraindications or intolerance to first-line therapy, or a requirement for additional blood pressure lowering in combination with first-line antihypertensive drugs.

Combination Therapy

About 50% of patients will require more than one antihypertensive agent to achieve blood pressure targets. If the goal blood pressure is not achieved with moderate doses of a suitable first-line drug, add, rather than substitute, a second drug. Combining 2 drugs from different classes yields a 5 times greater incremental reduction in blood pressure than doubling the dose of 1 drug [Evidence: SORT C*].[8]

In high-risk patients (hypertension with diabetes or known cardiovascular disease) an ACE inhibitor (benazepril) with amlodipine was superior to an ACE inhibitor with a diuretic at preventing cardiovascular events. The Canadian Hypertension Education Program (CHEP) recommends consideration of an ACE inhibitor with amlodipine in high-risk patients whose blood pressure requires 2 or more medications for control.[9] CHEP recommends initiating therapy with a combination of 2 first-line agents if a patient's SBP is ≥20 or DBP is ≥10 mm Hg above the recommended target.[1] Use of a diuretic is desirable in combination with all other drug classes. In contrast, any combination of a beta-blocker, ACE inhibitor and/or an ARB has less than additive antihypertensive effects when combined in a 2-drug regimen. These combinations should be avoided unless there is a specific indication, for example, use of an ACE inhibitor and a beta-blocker in post-MI patients or in those with heart failure (Table 5).

All possible combinations of first-line agents are rational choices to lower blood pressure when 3 or 4 drugs are required, with the exception of the simultaneous prescription of ACE inhibitors and ARBs. A combination of ACE inhibitor plus ARB may further lower blood pressure but is associated with more adverse effects (e.g., hyperkalemia, renal impairment) and no clear benefit in terms of cardiovascular events.[10] This combination is generally not recommended for the treatment of hypertension, though it may be appropriate in some medical circumstances such as refractory heart failure.

Adherence

Medication adherence should be assessed at each visit. Poor adherence to therapy is a major cause of poor blood pressure control. Patients may admit to poor adherence when questioned in a nonthreatening manner, or it may be indicated by:

- Failure to keep scheduled appointments
- Poor blood pressure control
- Lack of secondary physiologic effects, e.g., decreased heart rate on beta-blocker
- Failure to renew prescriptions on time
- Lack of awareness of usual pill-taking routine and prescriptions

Poor adherence can be prevented. Routine care should include the following:

- Ensure patients are well informed about hypertension and its treatment, preferably verbally and with patient information pamphlets (available at www.hypertension.ca in the Public section)
- Include family or social support in lifestyle modification
- Use a simplified regimen of long-acting, once-daily drugs, and prescribe formulations that contain 2 drugs in combination when appropriate
- Ensure the patient can afford the prescribed drugs
- Advise the patient to establish a daily routine for pill-taking, e.g., putting their pills by their toothbrush and taking them every morning prior to brushing

Treat poor adherence:

- Determine the reason for poor adherence and tailor advice or interventions to the cause
- Increase the frequency of office visits
- Advise use of adherence-enhancing medication dispensers, e.g., dosette box
- Advise self-measurement of blood pressure

---

* SORT (Strength of Recommendation Taxonomy) is a rating system (A, B or C) that addresses the quality of available evidence. For more information consult **How to Use *Compendium of Therapeutic Choices*** on page xxv.

- Consider assessing adherence with an electronic pill dispenser
- Advise home-monitoring of adherence with pill counts and marking on a calendar when the prescription needs renewing
- Consider regular telephone contact with the patient if feasible

Resistant Hypertension

Many patients with hypertension require multiple drugs for blood pressure control. In those with resistant hypertension, investigate for a white coat effect, secondary hypertension, renal dysfunction, poor adherence, and in those with a poor response to an adequate combination of medications, consider the possibility of an "interfering lifestyle." Refer (to a hypertension specialist, nephrologist or internist) those who do not achieve blood pressure targets with medication regimens you feel comfortable prescribing.

Hypertensive Emergencies

It is uncommon for elevated blood pressure alone, without new or progressive target organ damage, to require emergency therapy. Refer true hypertensive emergencies to experienced centres with facilities to continuously monitor blood pressure. In stabilizing patients for transfer, the use of intermediate-acting drugs (e.g., felodipine) with close blood pressure monitoring is generally safer than using short-acting drugs that can rapidly produce hypotension with complications.

Choices during Pregnancy and Breastfeeding

Hypertension and Pregnancy

Inform women with pre-existing hypertension who are of child-bearing potential, particularly those who are considering pregnancy, that they are at an increased risk for adverse pregnancy outcomes including: intrauterine growth restriction; placental abruption; preterm delivery and the attendant neonatal risks of prematurity; and particularly a heightened risk of preeclampsia, with a crude risk of about 20–25% (varying with the severity and duration of the pre-existing hypertension). Enhanced surveillance is required during pregnancy to monitor for these complications. Prior to conception, or immediately upon recognition of an unplanned pregnancy, review the choice of antihypertensive medication for these women.

Management

While there remains a dearth of high quality data on the effects of many common antihypertensive medications on the developing fetus, international guidelines[11,12,13] have reached some consensus regarding a list of "preferred" medications for use in pregnancy, as well as a few "avoid" and "must avoid" drugs. Medications widely considered first-line for the management of hypertension in pregnancy include: **methyldopa** (250 mg BID to 1000 mg TID), **labetalol** (100 mg BID to 800 mg TID) and **nifedipine** XL (30 mg OD to 60 mg BID). These medications are preferred as they have evidence and/or a strong clinical record of safe and effective use in pregnancy,[14,15] as well as an absence of demonstrated adverse effects on subsequent neonatal and childhood development. Other antihypertensive medications considered appropriate for use in pregnancy include **clonidine**, **hydralazine** and other beta-blockers (**oxprenolol**, **pindolol**, **propranolol**, **metoprolol**). The data regarding the use of **nondihydropyridine calcium channel blockers**[16,17] and **alpha-blockers** in pregnancy is very limited, so these agents are typically deferred or exchanged for other preferred agents.

Avoid **atenolol**, as its use for the treatment of hypertension in pregnancy has been associated with fetal intrauterine growth restriction (IUGR).[18] The other beta-blockers, in contrast, are only weakly associated with IUGR and have been used widely in pregnancy for various indications. **Thiazides** and **loop diuretics** are other classes of medications which most experts caution to avoid during pregnancy. These medications may prevent the physiologic volume expansion seen in normal pregnancy, and thereby impair uteroplacental perfusion and fetal growth.[17] Available data do not support an adverse effect on perinatal outcome,[12] however, and these medications may therefore be considered or continued in women felt to have volume-dependent hypertension (renal impairment). They should be avoided in settings in which uteroplacental perfusion is already reduced (preeclampsia or IUGR). **Spironolactone** should not be used at all in pregnancy, due to its anti-androgenic effects.[19]

ACE inhibitors have been clearly shown to be fetotoxic when taken during the second and third trimesters,[20] leading to oligohydramnios, IUGR, fetal/neonatal renal failure and other growth effects. First trimester exposure has also been shown to lead to teratogenic effects, mainly to the fetal cardiovascular and central nervous system.[21] Discontinue these drugs prior to conception, or immediately upon discovery of an unplanned pregnancy. The data regarding the risk of fetal harm from **ARBs**[22] and **direct renin inhibitors**[23] are less robust (mainly animal data), but they appear to have similar harmful effects and should be avoided just as strictly as ACE inhibitors during pregnancy.

Most women with pre-existing hypertension, particularly those with long-standing, difficult-to-control hypertension or end-organ damage, should be followed throughout pregnancy by a specialist in obstetrics and gynecology. These clinicians are skilled at ongoing maternal management as well as appropriate monitoring of fetal growth and well being. Women with difficult-to-control hypertension or other medical issues benefit from assessment and follow-up with a hypertension specialist or obstetric medicine physician during their pregnancy.

Hypertension and Breastfeeding

Following the completion of a pregnancy, many women require ongoing antihypertensive therapy. The choice of antihypertensive agent may be influenced by whether or not the woman is breastfeeding her newborn child, as all oral medications appear in breast milk to some degree.[24] Breastfeeding women may safely continue treatment with any "pregnancy-preferred" drug. Most other antihypertensive medications may also be safely utilized, but a few choices to avoid in these women include diuretics (which may suppress lactation), atenolol and other beta-blockers with low serum protein-binding (which concentrate in breast milk), as well as long-acting ACE inhibitors and those for which there is little or no lactation data (ramipril, lisinopril, cilazapril and perindopril).

A discussion of general principles on the use of medications in these special populations can be found in Appendix II and Appendix III. Other specialized reference sources are also provided in these appendices.

Therapeutic Tips

- Prescribe a lower starting dose of antihypertensive drugs in elderly patients.
- Recent onset of hypertension or change in blood pressure control suggests an identifiable or secondary cause, such as drugs known to exacerbate hypertension or new onset of significant renal artery stenosis.
- Many drugs ineffective as monotherapy for hypertension are effective components in a rational combination regimen.
- Consider concurrent cardiovascular risk factors and disease states when prescribing therapy (Table 5).
- Cardiovascular risk can vary 10-fold in persons with the same blood pressure. Assess global cardiovascular risk in all hypertensive patients using a risk form, chart or computer program (see Chapter 37, Figure 2 as an example).
- Blood pressure measurements taken at home correlate better with cardiovascular outcomes than office-based measurements.[25,26] Recommend monitors endorsed by the Canadian Hypertension Society and train patients to use the proper technique. To allay anxiety, caution patients that some

variation throughout the day is normal. Patient instructions for selecting and using home blood pressure monitors can be found in the Public section of www.hypertension.ca.

- Pharmacists and nurses can play an important role in hypertension screening, medication selection, patient education, follow-up and adherence monitoring. Dietitians can assist patients in managing their sodium and caloric intake.
- A team approach to hypertension management is more effective than usual care. In patients with hypertension and diabetes, joint care by a family physician, community pharmacist and nurse resulted in an approximately 6 mm Hg greater reduction in SBP over 6 months, compared with usual physician-based care.[27]

Table 5: **Individualization of Antihypertensive Therapy**[1]

Category (BP Targets)	Risk Factor/Disease	Initial Therapy	Second-line Therapy	Notes/Cautions
Hypertension without other compelling indications (Target SBP/DBP <140/90 mm Hg. If isolated systolic hypertension and age ≥80 y, target SBP <150 mm Hg)	Diastolic ± systolic hypertension	Thiazide diuretic, beta-blocker, ACE inhibitor, ARB or long-acting CCB Consider ASA and statins in select patients Consider initiating therapy with a combination of first-line drugs if SBP is ≥20 mm Hg or DBP is ≥10 mm Hg above target	Combinations of first-line drugs	Beta-blockers are not recommended as initial therapy in patients over 60 years of age. Avoid hypokalemia in those who are prescribed diuretics as monotherapy by using K^+-sparing agents. ACE inhibitors are not recommended as initial therapy in black patients. ACE inhibitors, ARBs and direct renin inhibitors are teratogenic. Marked caution is required if prescribing to women of child-bearing potential. Combination of an ACE inhibitor with an ARB is not recommended.
	Isolated systolic hypertension without other compelling indications	Thiazide diuretic, ARB or long-acting dihydropyridine CCB	Combinations of first-line drugs	See diastolic ± systolic hypertension above.
Diabetes mellitus (Target SBP/DBP <130/80 mm Hg)	Diabetes mellitus with albuminuria, renal disease, CVD or additional cardiovascular risk factors	ACE inhibitor or ARB	Addition of a dihydropyridine CCB is preferred over thiazide diuretics	A loop diuretic could be considered in hypertensive CKD patients with extracellular fluid volume overload.
	Diabetes mellitus not included in the above category	ACE inhibitor, ARB, long-acting dihydropyridine CCB or thiazide diuretic	Combine first-line drugs If combination with ACE inhibitor is being considered, a dihydropyridine CCB is preferable to thiazide diuretics	Albuminuria is defined as an albumin to creatinine ratio (ACR) >2 mg/mmol in men and >2.8 mg/mmol in women.
Cardiovascular and cerebrovascular disease (Target SBP/DBP <140/90 mm Hg)	Coronary artery disease	ACE inhibitor or ARB (except in low-risk patients); beta-blocker for patients with stable angina	Long-acting CCB When combination therapy is being used for high-risk patients, an ACE inhibitor/dihydropyridine CCB is preferred	Avoid short-acting nifedipine. Combination of an ACE inhibitor with an ARB is specifically not recommended.
	Recent MI	Beta-blocker and ACE inhibitor (ARB if ACE inhibitor not tolerated)	Long-acting CCB	Non-dihydropyridine CCBs should not be used in the presence of concomitant heart failure.

Category (BP Targets)	Risk Factor/Disease	Initial Therapy	Second-line Therapy	Notes/Cautions
	Heart failure	ACE inhibitor and beta-blocker (ARB if ACE inhibitor not tolerated) Aldosterone antagonist in patients with a recent cardiovascular hospitalization, acute MI, elevated BNP, elevated NT-proBNP, or NYHA class II to IV symptoms	ARB added to ACE inhibitor Hydralazine/isosorbide dinitrate combined if black, or if ACE inhibitor and ARB contraindicated or not tolerated Thiazide or loop diuretic as additive therapy Dihydropyridine CCB (except nifedipine)	Titrate doses of ACE inhibitors and ARBs to those used in clinical trials. Monitor serum K^+ and SCr with the combination of ACE inhibitor, ARB or aldosterone antagonist.
	Left ventricular hypertrophy	ACE inhibitor, ARB, long-acting CCB or thiazide diuretic	Combination of additional agents	Hydralazine and minoxidil should not be used.
	Past stroke or TIA	ACE inhibitor/diuretic combination	Combination of additional agents	Hypertension should not be treated in acute stroke unless BP extremely elevated. Combination of an ACE inhibitor with an ARB is specifically not recommended.
Nondiabetic chronic kidney disease (Target SBP/DBP <140/90 mm Hg)	Nondiabetic chronic kidney disease with proteinuria	ACE inhibitor (ARB if ACE inhibitor not tolerated) diuretics as additive therapy	Combinations of additional agents	Carefully monitor serum K^+ and SCr in patients on an ACE inhibitor or an ARB. Combination of an ACE inhibitor with an ARB is specifically not recommended in patients with chronic kidney disease without proteinuria.
	Renovascular disease	Does not affect initial treatment recommendations	Combinations of additional agents	Avoid ACE inhibitors or ARBs in patients with bilateral renal artery stenosis or unilateral disease with a solitary kidney.
Other conditions (Target SBP/DBP <140/90 mm Hg)	Peripheral arterial disease	Does not affect initial treatment recommendations	Combinations of additional agents	Avoid beta-blockers in patients with severe disease.
	Dyslipidemia	Does not affect initial treatment recommendations	Combinations of additional agents	
	Overall vascular protection	Statin therapy for patients with hypertension and 3 or more cardiovascular risk factors or with atherosclerotic disease		
		Low-dose ASA in patients over 50 y with controlled blood pressure		Exercise caution if blood pressure is not controlled.

Adapted with permission from Canadian Hypertension Education Program.

Abbreviations: ACE = angiotensin-converting enzyme; ARB = angiotensin II receptor blocker; BNP = brain natriuretic peptide; CCB = calcium channel blocker; CKD = chronic kidney disease; CVD = cardiovascular disease; MI = myocardial infarction; NT-proBNP = N-terminal-proBNP; NYHA = New York Heart Association; SCr = serum creatinine; TIA = transient ischemic attack

Table 6: **Drugs Used for Hypertension**

Class	Drug	Dose	Adverse Effects	Drug Interactions	Comments	Cost[a]
ACE Inhibitors	*benazepril* ➔ Lotensin, generics	Initial: 10 mg/day Usual: 20 mg/day Maximum: 40 mg/day Once daily or divided BID po	Dry cough, hyperkalemia. Unusual: angioedema. Can precipitate renal failure in renovascular disease, volume depletion or those receiving NSAIDs.	Marked increase in serum K^+ in patients receiving K^+ supplements and/or K^+-sparing diuretics. Reduced hypotensive effect with NSAIDs and increased risk of renal dysfunction. Elevated Li^+ levels (potential toxicity).	**Contraindicated in pregnancy—caution when prescribing to women of child-bearing potential.**[5,6] Use lower (50%) initial doses if on diuretics (increased risk of hypotension with hypovolemia). Hyperkalemia usually occurs only in those on K^+ supplements or drugs that cause K^+ retention, those with renal impairment or diabetics with high serum K^+ levels. Assess SCr and K^+ after a few days, then regularly.	$$
	captopril ➔ generics	Initial: 25 mg/day Usual: 75 mg/day Maximum: 150 mg/day Divided BID or TID po	See benazepril.	See benazepril.	See benazepril.	$$
	cilazapril ➔ Inhibace, generics	Initial: 2.5 mg/day Usual: 2.5–5 mg/day Maximum: 10 mg/day Once daily or divided BID po	See benazepril.	See benazepril.	See benazepril.	$
	enalapril ➔ Vasotec, generics	Initial: 5 mg/day Usual: 10–40 mg/day Maximum: 40 mg/day Once daily or divided BID po	See benazepril.	See benazepril.	See benazepril.	$

Class	Drug	Dose	Adverse Effects	Drug Interactions	Comments	Cost[a]
	fosinopril generics	Initial: 10 mg/day Usual: 20 mg/day Maximum: 40 mg/day Once daily or divided BID po	See benazepril.	See benazepril.	See benazepril.	$
	lisinopril Prinivil, Zestril, generics	Initial: 10 mg/day Usual: 20 mg/day Maximum: 40 mg/day Once daily po	See benazepril.	See benazepril.	See benazepril.	$
	perindopril Coversyl, generics	Initial: 4 mg/day Maximum: 8 mg/day Once daily or divided BID po	See benazepril.	See benazepril.	See benazepril.	$$
	quinapril Accupril, generics	Initial: 10 mg/day Maximum: 40 mg/day Once daily or divided BID po	See benazepril.	See benazepril.	See benazepril.	$$
	ramipril Altace, generics	Initial: 2.5 mg/day Usual: 10 mg/day Maximum: 20 mg/day Once daily or divided BID po	See benazepril.	See benazepril.	See benazepril.	$
	trandolapril Mavik	Initial: 1 mg/day Maximum: 4 mg/day Once daily po	See benazepril.	See benazepril.	See benazepril.	$$
Alpha$_1$-adrenergic Antagonists	*doxazosin* Cardura, generics	Initial: 1 mg/day Usual: 1–8 mg/day Maximum: 16 mg/day Once daily po	Orthostatic hypotension, headache, drowsiness, palpitations, nasal congestion. Syncope usually occurs at the start of therapy, with rapid dose titration or on addition of other agents. Titrate slowly. If interrupted for several days, restart at initial dose.	Caution when adding other hypotensive drugs, may cause syncope.	Not for initial therapy.	$

(cont'd)

Table 6: **Drugs Used for Hypertension** *(cont'd)*

Class	Drug	Dose	Adverse Effects	Drug Interactions	Comments	Cost[a]
	prazosin generics	Initial: 0.5 mg with p.m. meal (day 1), then 0.5 mg BID–TID po × 3 days and gradually increase as required Maximum: 20 mg/day	See doxazosin.	See doxazosin.	Not for initial therapy.	$–$$
	terazosin Hytrin, generics	Initial: 1 mg QHS po Usual: 1–5 mg/day Maximum: 20 mg/day Once daily or divided BID po	See doxazosin.	See doxazosin. Verapamil increases serum concentrations of terazosin.	Not for initial therapy.	$
Angiotensin Receptor Blockers (ARB)	*azilsartan* Edarbi	Initial: 40 mg/day Maximum: 80 mg/day Once daily po	Hyperkalemia. Can precipitate renal failure in susceptible patients (bilateral renovascular disease, those with volume depletion or with concurrent NSAID use). Angioedema has been reported, but a causal association has not been established.	Marked increase in serum K^+ in patients receiving K^+ supplements and/or K^+-sparing diuretics. May elevate Li^+ levels (monitor Li^+ levels, adjust dose).	**Contraindicated in pregnancy—caution when prescribing to women of child-bearing potential.**[7] Use lower initial doses in patients who are volume depleted or on diuretics (increased risk of hypotension in hypovolemia). Hyperkalemia usually occurs only in those on K^+ supplements or drugs that cause K^+ retention, those with renal impairment or diabetics with high serum K^+ levels. Assess SCr and K^+ after a few days, then regularly.	$$
	candesartan Atacand, generics	Initial: 8 mg/day Usual: 8–16 mg/day Once daily po	See azilsartan.	See azilsartan.	See azilsartan.	$
	eprosartan Teveten	Initial: 600 mg/day Maximum: 800 mg/day Once daily or divided BID po	See azilsartan.	See azilsartan.	See azilsartan.	$$

Class	Drug	Dose	Adverse Effects	Drug Interactions	Comments	Cost[a]
	irbesartan Avapro, generics	Initial: 150 mg/day Usual: 150–300 mg/day Once daily po	See azilsartan.	See azilsartan.	See azilsartan.	$
	losartan Cozaar, generics	Initial: 50 mg/day Usual: 25–100 mg/day Maximum: 100 mg/day Once daily or divided BID po	See azilsartan.	See azilsartan.	See azilsartan.	$
	olmesartan Olmetec	Initial: 20 mg/day Maximum: 40 mg/day Once daily po	See azilsartan.	See azilsartan.	See azilsartan.	$$
	telmisartan Micardis, generics	Initial: 80 mg/day Usual: 80 mg/day Once daily po	See azilsartan.	See azilsartan.	See azilsartan.	$
	valsartan Diovan, generics	Initial: 80 mg/day Usual: 80–320 mg/day Once daily po	See azilsartan.	See azilsartan.	See azilsartan.	$
$Beta_1$-adrenergic Antagonists, nonselective	*nadolol* generics	Initial: 20 mg/day Usual: 160 mg/day Maximum: 320 mg/day Once daily po	Fatigue, bradycardia, decreased exercise capacity, headache, impotence, vivid dreams. Less common: hyperglycemia, depression, heart failure, heart block.	Bradycardia with digoxin or nondihydropyridine CCBs. Cardiodepressant effects with nondihydropyridine CCBs and amiodarone.	Beta-blockers should not be used as initial therapy in patients aged >60 y unless specifically indicated. Avoid in patients with asthma.[28] Avoid abrupt withdrawal (may precipitate rebound hypertension and ischemia). Taper the dose before discontinuation. Avoid in patients with severe PAD. Contraindicated in patients with 2nd or 3rd degree heart block in the absence of a pacemaker.	$$

(cont'd)

Table 6: **Drugs Used for Hypertension** *(cont'd)*

Class	Drug	Dose	Adverse Effects	Drug Interactions	Comments	Cost[a]
	propranolol, controlled release Inderal-LA	Initial: 80 mg/day Usual: 320 mg/day Maximum: 480 mg/day SR (once daily po) formulation recommended	See nadolol.	See nadolol. CYP2D6 inhibitors increase levels of propranolol. Propranolol increases serum levels of rizatriptan.	See nadolol. Propranolol is more likely to cause CNS side effects (insomnia, depression, vivid dreams) than other agents because of greater lipid solubility.	$$$$
	timolol generics	Initial: 5 mg BID Usual: 20 mg BID Maximum: 30 mg BID po	See nadolol.	See nadolol.	See nadolol.	$$
Beta$_1$-adrenergic Antagonists, β$_1$-selective	*atenolol* Tenormin, generics	Initial: 25 mg/day Usual: 50 mg/day Maximum: 100 mg/day Once daily or divided BID po	See nadolol. Fewer noncardiac effects due to cardioselectivity.	See nadolol.	See nadolol.	$
	bisoprolol Sandoz Bisoprolol, generics	Initial: 5 mg/day Usual: 10 mg/day Maximum: 20 mg/day Once daily po	See nadolol. Fewer noncardiac effects due to cardioselectivity.	See nadolol.	See nadolol.	$
	metoprolol, Lopresor, generics	Initial: 50 mg/day Usual: 100–200 mg/day Maximum: 400 mg/day Give regular formulations BID po; SR formulations once daily po	See nadolol. Fewer noncardiac effects due to cardioselectivity.	See nadolol. CYP2D6 inhibitors increase levels of metoprolol.	See nadolol.	$
	nebivolol Bystolic	Initial: 5 mg/day Usual: 10 mg/day Maximum: 20 mg/day Once daily po	See nadolol. Fewer noncardiac effects due to cardioselectivity.	See nadolol. CYP2D6 inhibitors increase levels of nebivolol.	See nadolol.	$$
Beta$_1$-adrenergic Antagonists, nonselective with intrinsic sympathomimetic activity (ISA)	*pindolol* Visken, generics	Initial: 5 mg BID po Usual: 15 mg BID po Maximum: 60 mg/day	See nadolol.	See nadolol.	See nadolol. Agents with ISA have less effect on resting heart rate than those without ISA.	$$

Class	Drug	Dose	Adverse Effects	Drug Interactions	Comments	Cost[a]
Beta$_1$-adrenergic Antagonists, β_1-selective with ISA	*acebutolol* Sectral, generics	Initial: 100 mg/day Usual: 400 mg/day Maximum: 800 mg/day Once daily or divided BID po	See nadolol. Fewer noncardiac effects due to cardioselectivity.	See nadolol.	See nadolol. Agents with ISA have less effect on resting heart rate than those without ISA.	$
Beta$_1$-adrenergic Antagonists with alpha$_1$-blocking activity	*labetalol* Trandate, generics	Initial: 50 mg BID po Usual: 200 mg BID po Maximum: 1200 mg/day	See nadolol. Edema, dizziness and nasal congestion and postural hypotension due to alpha$_1$ antagonism.	See nadolol.	See nadolol.	$$
Calcium Channel Blockers, dihydropyridine	*amlodipine* Norvasc, generics	Initial: 2.5 mg/day Maximum: 10 mg/day Once daily po	Ankle edema, flushing, headache and palpitations.	CYP3A4 substrate (many potential interactions). Strong inhibitors include azole antifungals, protease inhibitors, macrolides and quinidine. Grapefruit juice may increase serum concentrations.		$
	felodipine Plendil, generics	Initial: 2.5 mg/day Usual: 10 mg/day Maximum: 20 mg/day Once daily po	See amlodipine.	See amlodipine.	Grapefruit juice causes marked elevations in felodipine serum levels and adverse events.	$$
	nifedipine, extended release Adalat XL, generics	Initial: 30 mg/day Usual: 60 mg/day Maximum: 120 mg/day Once daily po	See amlodipine.	See amlodipine.	Do not use short-acting nifedipine formulations for treatment of essential hypertension.	$$
Calcium Channel Blockers, nondihydropyridine	*diltiazem* Cardizem CD, Tiazac, Tiazac XC, generics	Initial: 120 mg/day Usual: 240–360 mg/day Maximum: 360 mg/day Give CD or XC formulation once daily po, SR formulation divided BID po	Headache, dizziness, bradycardia, heart block, new onset or worsening of heart failure.	See amlodipine. Nondihydropyridines inhibit the metabolism of carbamazepine, cyclosporine, lovastatin, simvastatin. Rifampin induces metabolism of nondihydropyridines. Additive negative inotropic effects with amiodarone, beta-blockers and digoxin.	Caution in patients with heart failure, or 2nd or 3rd degree heart block without a functioning pacemaker.	$$

(cont'd)

Table 6: **Drugs Used for Hypertension** *(cont'd)*

Class	Drug	Dose	Adverse Effects	Drug Interactions	Comments	Cost[a]
	verapamil Isoptin SR, generics	Initial: 80 mg TID po Maximum:160 mg TID po SR (once daily or divided BID po): Initial: 180 mg/day; Usual: 180–480 mg/day; Maximum: 480 mg/day	See diltiazem. Constipation.	See amlodipine. See diltiazem. Verapamil increases digoxin levels by 50–75% within 1 wk (monitor levels).	See diltiazem.	$–$$
Centrally Acting Antihypertensive Agents	*methyldopa* generics	Initial: 500 mg/day Usual: 2000 mg/day Maximum: 3000 mg/day Divided BID or TID po	Drowsiness, dry mouth, nasal congestion, depression, orthostatic hypotension, palpitations, sexual dysfunction, sodium and water retention.	Iron salts reduce absorption (separate administration). Additive hypotension with levodopa. May exacerbate Li^+ adverse events without increasing Li^+ levels.	Positive Coombs' test is common, but usually unimportant; hemolytic anemia is rare. Drug fever with or without an influenza-like illness; hepatic disorders have occurred.	$$
Direct Renin Inhibitors	*aliskiren* Rasilez	Initial: 150 mg/day Maximum: 300 mg/day Once daily po	Diarrhea. The incidence of dry cough and hyperkalemia is low compared with ACE inhibitors.	Avoid combining with an ACE inhibitor or ARB in patients with significant renal impairment.	May take 4 wk to realize maximum antihypertensive effect. Effect on cardiovascular outcomes not yet established. Limited data in patients with greater than moderate renal dysfunction. Avoid use in pregnancy.	$$
Diuretics	*hydrochlorothiazide* generics	Initial: 12.5 mg/day Usual: 25 mg/day Once daily po	Hypotension, weakness, muscle cramps, impotence. Hypokalemia, hyponatremia, hyperuricemia, hyperglycemia, hyperlipidemia. Rare: azotemia, blood dyscrasias, allergic reactions (potential cross sensitivity with other sulfonamide derivatives), photosensitivity, fatigue.	Li^+ excretion reduced (monitor Li^+ levels, adjust dose). NSAIDs reduce hypotensive efficacy. Diuretic-induced hypokalemia increases the risk of digoxin toxicity. Reduced efficacy of antihyperglycemic agents.	Particularly effective in ISH, the elderly and black patients. Monitor SCr and K^+. Consider alternatives in patients with or predisposed to arrhythmias. Can exacerbate gout and diabetes (biochemical abnormalities are less frequent at low doses). Ineffective in patients with ClCr <30 to 40 mL/min.	$

Class	Drug	Dose	Adverse Effects	Drug Interactions	Comments	Cost[a]
	chlorthalidone ➔ generics	Initial: 12.5 mg/day Usual: 12.5–25 mg/day Once daily po	See hydrochlorothiazide.	See hydrochlorothiazide.	Lowest available tablet strength is 50 mg. Tablet (or "pill") splitters, widely available in pharmacies, can be used to derive a dose of 12.5 mg (one-quarter tablet) with reasonable accuracy. See hydrochlorothiazide.	$
	indapamide ➔ Lozide, generics	Initial: 1.25 mg/day Usual: 2.5 mg/day Once daily po	See hydrochlorothiazide.	See hydrochlorothiazide.	See hydrochlorothiazide.	$
	metolazone ➔ Zaroxolyn	Initial: 2.5 mg/day Usual: 5 mg/day Maximum: 10 mg/day Once daily po	See hydrochlorothiazide.	See hydrochlorothiazide.	See hydrochlorothiazide. Metolazone is effective in patients with moderate to severe renal dysfunction.	$
ACE Inhibitor/ Calcium Channel Blocker Combinations	*trandolapril/ verapamil*[b] ➔ Tarka	Trandolapril 1–4 mg/day plus verapamil 180–480 mg/day. Once daily or divided BID po[c]	See benazepril. See diltiazem. Constipation.	See benazepril. See amlodipine. Inhibits metabolism of carbamazepine, cyclosporine, lovastatin, simvastatin. Rifampin increases metabolism of verapamil. Additive negative inotropic effects with amiodarone, beta-blockers, digoxin. Verapamil increases digoxin levels by 50–75% within 1 wk (monitor levels).	See benazepril. See diltiazem.	$$$
ACE Inhibitor/ Diuretic Combinations	*cilazapril/hydro-chlorothiazide*[b] ➔ Inhibace Plus, generics	5/12.5 mg once daily po[c]	See benazepril. See hydrochlorothiazide.	See benazepril. See hydrochlorothiazide.	See benazepril. See hydrochlorothiazide.	$
	enalapril/hydro-chlorothiazide[b] ➔ Vaseretic, generics	5/12.5 mg or 10/25 mg once daily po[c]	See benazepril. See hydrochlorothiazide.	See benazepril. See hydrochlorothiazide.	See benazepril. See hydrochlorothiazide.	$$

(cont'd)

Table 6: **Drugs Used for Hypertension** *(cont'd)*

Class	Drug	Dose	Adverse Effects	Drug Interactions	Comments	Cost[a]
	lisinopril/hydro-chlorothiazide[b] Prinzide, Zestoretic, generics	10/12.5 mg, 20/12.5 mg or 20/25 once daily po[c]	See benazepril. See hydrochlorothiazide.	See benazepril. See hydrochlorothiazide.	See benazepril. See hydrochlorothiazide.	$–$$
	perindopril/ indapamide[b] Coversyl Plus, Coversyl Plus LD	4/1.25 mg once daily po[c]	See benazepril. See hydrochlorothiazide.	See benazepril. See hydrochlorothiazide.	See benazepril. See hydrochlorothiazide.	$$
	quinapril/hydro-chlorothiazide[b] Accuretic, generics	10/12.5 mg, 20/12.5 mg or 20/25 mg once daily po[c]	See benazepril. See hydrochlorothiazide.	See benazepril. See hydrochlorothiazide.	See benazepril. See hydrochlorothiazide.	$–$$
	ramipril/hydro-chlorothiazide[b] Altace HCT, generics	2.5/12.5 mg, 5/12.5 mg, 10/12.5 mg, 5/25 mg or 10/25 mg once daily po[c]	See benazepril. See hydrochlorothiazide.	See benazepril. See hydrochlorothiazide.	See benazepril. See hydrochlorothiazide.	$
ARB/ Diuretic Combinations	*azilsartan/chlorthali-done*[b] Edarbyclor	40/12.5 mg, 40/25 mg or 80/12.5 mg once daily po	See azilsartan. See hydrochlorothiazide.	See azilsartan. See hydrochlorothiazide.	See azilsartan. See hydrochlorothiazide.	$$
	candesartan/hydro-chlorothiazide[b] Atacand Plus, generics	16/12.5 mg once daily po[c]	See azilsartan. See hydrochlorothiazide.	See azilsartan. See hydrochlorothiazide.	See azilsartan. See hydrochlorothiazide.	$
	eprosartan/hydro-chlorothiazide[b] Teveten Plus	600/12.5 mg once daily po[c]	See azilsartan. See hydrochlorothiazide.	See azilsartan. See hydrochlorothiazide.	See azilsartan. See hydrochlorothiazide.	$$
	irbesartan/hydro-chlorothiazide[b] Avalide, generics	150/12.5 mg or 300/12.5 mg once daily po[c]	See azilsartan. See hydrochlorothiazide.	See azilsartan. See hydrochlorothiazide.	See azilsartan. See hydrochlorothiazide.	$
	losartan/hydro-chlorothiazide[b] Hyzaar, Hyzaar DS, generics	50/12.5 mg or 100/25 mg once daily po[c]	See azilsartan. See hydrochlorothiazide.	See azilsartan. See hydrochlorothiazide.	See azilsartan. See hydrochlorothiazide.	$
	olmesartan/hydro-chlorothiazide[b] Olmetec Plus	20/12.5 mg, 40/12.5 mg or 40/25 mg once daily po[c]	See azilsartan. See hydrochlorothiazide.	See azilsartan. See hydrochlorothiazide.	See azilsartan. See hydrochlorothiazide.	$$

Class	Drug	Dose	Adverse Effects	Drug Interactions	Comments	Cost[a]
	telmisartan/hydrochlorothiazide[b] Micardis Plus, generics	80/12.5 mg or 80/25 mg once daily po[c]	See azilsartan. See hydrochlorothiazide.	See azilsartan. See hydrochlorothiazide.	See azilsartan. See hydrochlorothiazide.	$
	valsartan/hydrochlorothiazide[b] Diovan-HCT, generics	80/12.5 mg, 160/12.5 mg or 160/25 mg once daily po[c]	See azilsartan. See hydrochlorothiazide.	See azilsartan. See hydrochlorothiazide.	See azilsartan. See hydrochlorothiazide.	$
Beta$_1$-adrenergic Antagonist/ Diuretic Combinations	*atenolol/chlorthalidone*[b] Tenoretic, generics	50/25 mg, or 100/25 mg once daily po[c]	See nadolol. See hydrochlorothiazide.	See nadolol. See hydrochlorothiazide.	See nadolol. See hydrochlorothiazide.	$
	pindolol/hydrochlorothiazide[b] Viskazide	10/25 mg or 10/50 mg once daily po[c]	See nadolol. See hydrochlorothiazide.	See nadolol. See hydrochlorothiazide.	See nadolol. See hydrochlorothiazide.	$$
Calcium Channel Blocker/ Anti-platelet Combinations	*nifedipine XL/ASA* Adalat XL Plus	nifedipine 20 mg, 30 mg or 60 mg with ASA 81 mg once daily po	See amlodipine. Bleeding, gastric intolerance.	See amlodipine. Increased bleeding risk with anticoagulants.	See nifedipine.	$–$$
Calcium Channel Blocker/ ARB Combinations	*amlodipine/ telmisartan*[b] Twynsta	5/40 mg, 5/80 mg, 10/40 mg or 10/80 mg once daily po[c]	See amlodipine. See azilsartan.	See amlodipine. See azilsartan.	See azilsartan.	$$
Calcium Channel Blocker/ HMG-CoA Reductase Inhibitor Combinations	*amlodipine/ atorvastatin* Caduet, generics	Amlodipine 5 or 10 mg plus atorvastatin 10, 20, 40 or 80 mg once daily po[c]	See amlodipine. Adverse effects of atorvastatin include constipation, flatulence, dyspepsia, abdominal pain and myalgia.	See amlodipine. Amlodipine and atorvastatin are both substrates of CYP3A4.	For patients with hypertension and an indication for an HMG-CoA inhibitor.	$–$$
Direct Renin Inhibitor/ Diuretic Combinations	*aliskiren/hydrochlorothiazide* Rasilez HCT	150/12.5 mg, 150/25 mg, 300/12.5 mg or 300/25 mg once daily po[c]	See aliskiren. See hydrochlorothiazide.	See aliskiren. See hydrochlorothiazide.	See aliskiren. See hydrochlorothiazide.	$$
Diuretic Combinations	*hydrochlorothiazide/ amiloride* (50/5) generics	One-half tablet once daily po	See hydrochlorothiazide.	See hydrochlorothiazide. May exacerbate ACE inhibitor-induced hyperkalemia.	See hydrochlorothiazide. Lower incidence of hypokalemia than with hydrochlorothiazide alone.	$

(cont'd)

Table 6: **Drugs Used for Hypertension** *(cont'd)*

Class	Drug	Dose	Adverse Effects	Drug Interactions	Comments	Cost[a]
	hydrochlorothiazide/ triamterene ◗ (25/50) generics	Initial: One-half tablet Usual: 1 tablet Once daily po	See hydrochlorothiazide.	See hydrochlorothiazide/amiloride.	See hydrochlorothiazide/amiloride.	$
	hydrochlorothiazide/ spironolactone ◗ (25/25) Aldactazide, generics	Initial: One-half tablet Usual: 1 tablet Once daily po	See hydrochlorothiazide. Gynecomastia in men and breast tenderness in women.	See hydrochlorothiazide/amiloride.	See hydrochlorothiazide/amiloride.	$

[a] Cost of 30-day supply of usual dose of drug; includes drug cost only.
[b] The Canadian Hypertension Education Program recommends initiating therapy with a combination of two first-line agents if a patient's SBP is ≥20 or DBP is ≥10 mm Hg above the recommended target.
[c] It is generally recommended that the dose of each component is titrated before starting a combination product.
◗ Dosage adjustment may be required in renal impairment; see Appendix I.
Abbreviations: CV = cardiovascular; IR = immediate-release; ISA = intrinsic sympathomimetic activity; ISH = isolated systolic hypertension; PAD = peripheral arterial disease; SCr = serum creatinine; SR = sustained-release; TCA = tricyclic antidepressant
Legend: $ <$20 $-$$ <$20–40 $$ $20–40 $$$ $40–60 $$$$ $60–80

Suggested Readings

Adrogue HJ, Madias NE. Sodium and potassium in the pathogenesis of hypertension. *N Engl J Med* 2007;356(19):1966-78.

Canadian recommendations on the management of hypertension are updated annually. A summary of the important and new recommendations can be found at www.hypertension.ca/ in the *Professional* section and is also broadly published in multidisciplinary journals annually.

References

1. Hypertension Canada. Canadian Hypertension Education Program (CHEP). *2014 CHEP recommendations*. Available from: hypertension.ca/en/chep. Accessed April 24, 2014.
2. Khan N, Chockalingam A, Campbell NR. Lack of control of high blood pressure and treatment recommendations in Canada. *Can J Cardiol* 2002;18(6):657-61.
3. ALLHAT Officers and Coordinators for the ALLHAT Collaborative Research Group. The Antihypertensive and Lipid-Lowering Treatment to Prevent Heart Attack Trial. Major outcomes in high-risk hypertensive patients randomized to angiotensin-converting enzyme inhibitor or calcium channel blocker vs diuretic: the Antihypertensive and Lipid-Lowering Treatment to Prevent Heart Attack Trial (ALLHAT). *JAMA* 2002;288(23):2981-97.
4. MRC trial of treatment of mild hypertension: principal results. Medical Research Council Working Party. *Br Med J (Clin Res Ed)* 1985;291(6488):97-104.
5. Cooper WO, Hernandez-Diaz S, Arbogast PG et al. Major congenital malformations after first-trimester exposure to ACE inhibitors. *N Engl J Med* 2006;354(23):2443-51.
6. Friedman JM. ACE inhibitors and congenital anomalies. *N Engl J Med* 2006;354(23):2498-500.
7. Alwan S, Polifka JE, Friedman JM. Angiotensin II receptor antagonist treatment during pregnancy. *Birth Defects Res A Clin Mol Teratol* 2005;73(2):123-30.
8. Wald DS, Law M, Morris JK et al. Combination therapy versus monotherapy in reducing blood pressure: meta-analysis on 11,000 participants from 42 trials. *Am J Med* 2009;122(3):290-300.
9. Weber MA, Bakris GL, Dahlof B et al. Baseline characteristics in the Avoiding Cardiovascular events through Combination therapy in Patients Living with Systolic Hypertension (ACCOMPLISH) trial: a hypertensive population at high cardiovascular risk. *Blood Press* 2007;16(1):13-9.
10. Mann JF, Schmieder RE, McQueen M et al. Renal outcomes with telmisartan, ramipril, or both, in people at high vascular risk (the ONTARGET study): a multicentre, randomised, double-blind, controlled trial. *Lancet* 2008;372(9638):547-53.
11. Magee LA, Helewa M, Moutquin JM et al. Diagnosis, evaluation, and management of hypertensive disorders of pregnancy. *J Obstet Gynaecol Can* 2008;30(3 Suppl):S1-48.
12. American College of Obstetricians and Gynecologists; Task Force on Hypertension in Pregnancy. Hypertension in pregnancy. Report of the American College of Obstetricians and Gynecologists' Task Force on Hypertension in Pregnancy. *Obstet Gynecol* 2013;122(5):1122-31.
13. U.K. National Institute for Health and Care Excellence (NICE). Clinical guidelines. *Hypertension in pregnancy (CG107)*. Available from: www.nice.org.uk/guidance/CG107.
14. Podymow T, August P. Update on the use of antihypertensive drugs in pregnancy. *Hypertension* 2008;51(4):960-9.
15. Magee LA. Drugs in pregnancy. Antihypertensives. *Best Pract Res Clin Obstet Gynaecol* 2001;15(6):827-45.
16. Magee LA, Schick B, Donnenfeld AE et al. The safety of calcium channel blockers in human pregnancy: a prospective, multicentre cohort study. *Am J Obstet Gynecol* 1996;174(3):823-8.
17. Papatsonis DN, Lok CA, Bos JM et al. Calcium channel blockers in the management of preterm labor and hypertension in pregnancy. *Eur J Obstet Gynecol Reprod Biol* 2001;97(2):122-40.
18. Butters L, Kennedy S, Rubin PC. Atenolol in essential hypertension during pregnancy. *BMJ* 1990;301(6752):587-9.
19. Groves TD, Corenblum B. Spironolactone therapy during human pregnancy. *Am J Obstet Gynecol* 1995;172(5):1655-6.
20. Shotan A, Widerhorn J, Hurst A et al. Risks of angiotensin-converting enzyme inhibition during pregnancy: experimental and clinical evidence, potential mechanisms, and recommendations for use. *Am J Med* 1994;96(5):451-6.
21. Cooper WO, Hernandez-Diaz S, Arbogast PG et al. Major congenital malformations after first trimester exposure to ACE inhibitors. *N Engl J Med* 2006;354(23):2443-51.
22. Lambot MA, Vermeylen D, Noel JC. Angiotensin-II-receptor inhibitors in pregnancy. *Lancet* 2001;357(9268):1619-20.
23. Cheng JW. Aliskiren: renin inhibitor for hypertension management. *Clin Ther* 2008;30(1):31-47.
24. Beardmore KS, Morris JM, Gallery ED. Excretion of antihypertensive medication into human breast milk: a systematic review. *Hypertens Pregnancy* 2002;21(1):85-95.
25. Ohkubo T, Imai Y, Tsuji I et al. Home blood pressure measurement has a stronger predictive power for mortality than does screening blood pressure measurement: a population-based observation in Ohasama, Japan. *J Hypertens* 1998;16(7):971-5.
26. Ohkubo T, Asayam K, Kikuya M et al. How many times should blood pressure be measured at home for better prediction of stroke risk? Ten-year follow-up results from the Ohasama study. *J Hypertens* 2004;22(6):1099-104.
27. McLean DL, McAlister FA, Johnson JA et al. A randomized trial of the effect of community pharmacist and nurse care on improving blood pressure management in patients with diabetes mellitus: Study of Cardiovascular Risk Intervention by Pharmacists-Hypertension (SCRIP-HTN). *Arch Intern Med* 2008;168(21):2355-61.
28. Salpeter S, Ormiston T, Salpeter E. Cardioselective beta-blockers for chronic obstructive pulmonary disease. *Cochrane Database Syst Rev* 2005;(4):CD003566.

Chapter 40
Intermittent Claudication

Richard I. Ogilvie, MD, FRCPC, FACP

Goals of Therapy

- Improve mobility and quality of life
- Increase walking distance and time to claudication
- Increase capacity for regular dynamic leg exercise
- Prevent associated cardiovascular events

Investigations

- History with special attention to cardiovascular disease risk factors and associated conditions:
  - hypertension
  - diabetes mellitus
  - smoking
  - dyslipidemia
  - angina pectoris/MI
  - TIA/stroke
- Define walking time to claudication (*severe* = <one-half city block; *moderate* = one-half to 1 block; *mild* = >1 block)
- Define duration of symptoms (a period of 6–12 months is required to develop collateral circulation)
- Physical examination:
  - signs of hypertension, dyslipidemia, diabetes mellitus, atherosclerosis (aortic aneurysm, bruits), heart failure
  - signs of peripheral artery obstruction as indicated by diminished pulses in the femoral, popliteal, posterior tibial and/or dorsalis pedis arteries. Conversely, the absence of a decreased pulse or bruit indicates lower likelihood of obstruction
  - evidence of acute peripheral artery occlusion (acute onset of continuous pain, pale and cool limb or mottled discolouration, thickened, swollen, stiff muscles plus pain over the muscle)
  - resting pain, dependent rubor, cyanosis, muscle atrophy and/or trophic ulcers suggest severe obstruction
- Laboratory tests:
  - fasting blood glucose, serum creatinine and lipid profile
  - hemoglobin (anemia may exacerbate symptoms), hematocrit, platelet count
  - increased levels of D-dimer and inflammatory markers (C-reactive protein, amyloid A) are associated with higher short-term (within 1–2 years) risk of cardiovascular and all-cause mortality[1]
  - resting Doppler-derived or sphygmomanometric ankle/arm systolic pressure index[2] (*ankle-brachial index*); see Figure 1

- consider invasive angiography for patients with signs of severe limb ischemia (resting pain, muscle atrophy, cyanosis, nonhealing ischemic ulcers or gangrene) in preparation for possible angioplastic or surgical revascularization

Therapeutic Choices

The treatment of intermittent claudication is summarized in Figure 1.

Figure 1: Treatment of Intermittent Claudication

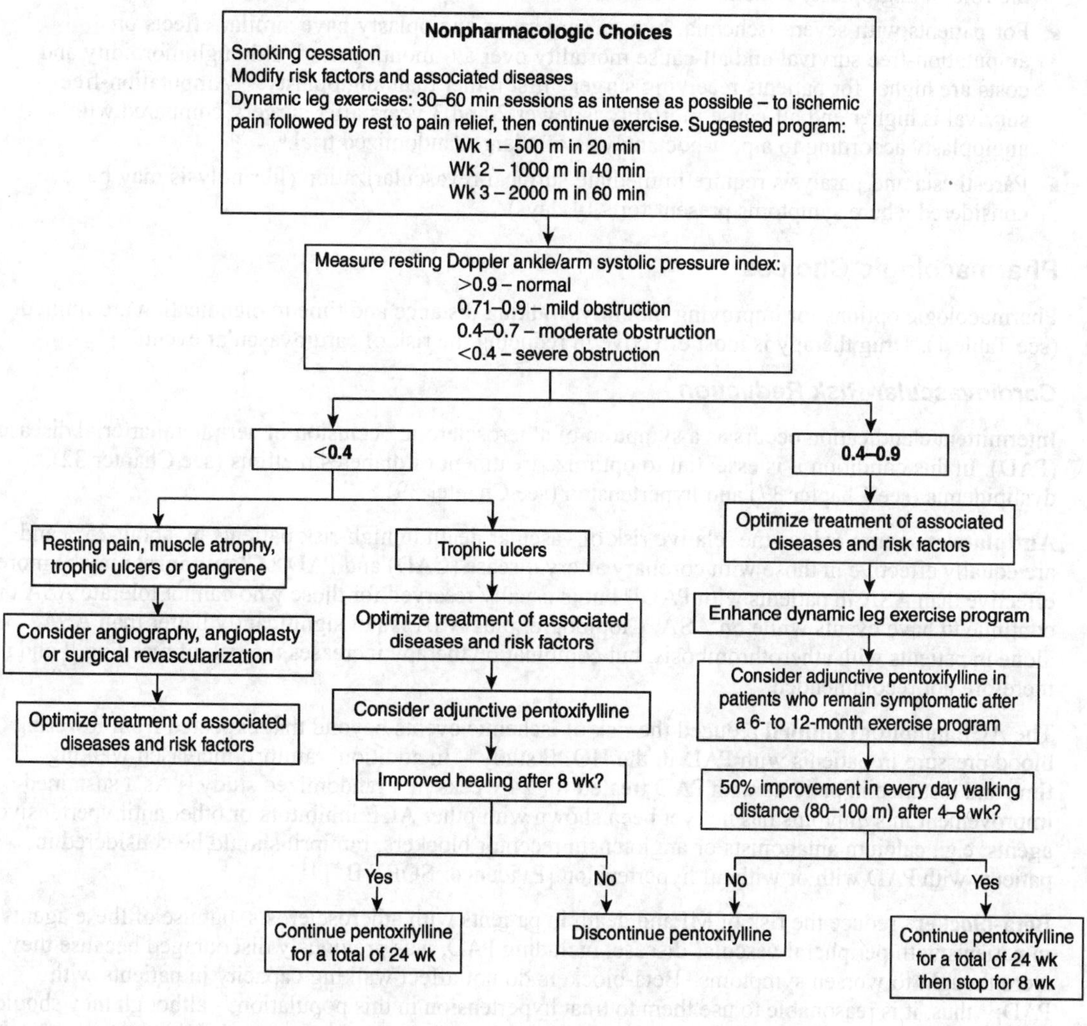
Nonpharmacologic Choices
Smoking cessation
Modify risk factors and associated diseases
Dynamic leg exercises: 30–60 min sessions as intense as possible – to ischemic pain followed by rest to pain relief, then continue exercise. Suggested program:
Wk 1 – 500 m in 20 min
Wk 2 – 1000 m in 40 min
Wk 3 – 2000 m in 60 min
Measure resting Doppler ankle/arm systolic pressure index:
>0.9 – normal
0.71–0.9 – mild obstruction
0.4–0.7 – moderate obstruction
<0.4 – severe obstruction
<0.4
0.4–0.9
Resting pain, muscle atrophy, trophic ulcers or gangrene
Trophic ulcers
Optimize treatment of associated diseases and risk factors
Consider angiography, angioplasty or surgical revascularization
Optimize treatment of associated diseases and risk factors
Enhance dynamic leg exercise program
Optimize treatment of associated diseases and risk factors
Consider adjunctive pentoxifylline
Consider adjunctive pentoxifylline in patients who remain symptomatic after a 6- to 12-month exercise program
Improved healing after 8 wk?
50% improvement in every day walking distance (80–100 m) after 4–8 wk?
Yes
No
No
Yes
Continue pentoxifylline for a total of 24 wk
Discontinue pentoxifylline
Continue pentoxifylline for a total of 24 wk then stop for 8 wk

Nonpharmacologic Choices

- Discontinuation of smoking (active and passive) (see Chapter 13).
- Time (collateral flow develops over 6–12 months).
- Nondrug treatment of obesity (see Chapter 33), lipid disorders (see Chapter 37), hypertension (see Chapter 39) and associated conditions.
- Regular dynamic leg exercise (5 times per week for 8 weeks initially).[3,4,5] Dynamic leg exercise for 6–12 months after the onset of claudication allows collateral circulation to develop; continued exercise 3 or more times a week over 24–36 months slows functional decline.[3]
- For patients with chronic intermittent claudication, and without signs of severe arterial obstruction, the role of angioplasty remains to be defined.
- For patients with severe ischemia, bypass surgery or angioplasty have similar effects on amputation-free survival and all-cause mortality over a 6-month period, although morbidity and costs are higher for patients receiving surgery first rather than angioplasty.[6,7] Amputation-free survival is higher and all-cause mortality is lower 2 and 3 years after surgery compared with angioplasty according to a post-hoc analysis of a large randomized trial.[6]
- Paresthesia and paralysis require immediate surgical revascularization (fibrinolysis may be considered where symptoms present for <14 days).

Pharmacologic Choices

Pharmacologic options for improving mobility, walking distance and time to claudication are limited (see Table 1). Drug therapy is most effective in reducing the risk of cardiovascular events.

Cardiovascular Risk Reduction

Intermittent claudication occurs as a symptom of atherosclerotic occlusion in peripheral arterial disease (PAD). In this condition it is essential to optimize treatment of diabetes mellitus (see Chapter 32), dyslipidemia (see Chapter 37) and hypertension (see Chapter 39).[8]

Antiplatelet agents reduce the relative risk of vascular death in high-risk patients by about 25% and are equally effective in those with coronary artery disease (CAD) and PAD.[9] **Clopidogrel** may be more effective than **ASA** in patients with PAD[10] but is usually reserved for those who cannot tolerate ASA or continue to have events while on ASA. Clopidogrel plus ASA is not significantly better than ASA alone in patients with atherothrombosis, but combination therapy increases the risk of bleeding,[11] and is therefore not recommended.

The ACE inhibitor **ramipril** reduced the risk of ischemic events beyond that expected from lowering blood pressure in patients with PAD in the HOPE study.[12] In addition, ramipril increased walking time and distance in patients with PAD treated for 24 weeks in a randomized study.[13] As a sustained improvement in symptoms has not yet been shown with other ACE inhibitors or other antihypertensive agents, e.g., calcium antagonists or angiotensin receptor blockers, ramipril should be considered in patients with PAD with or without hypertension [Evidence: SORT B*].[13]

Beta-blockers reduce the risk of MI and death in patients with atherosclerosis, but use of these agents in patients with peripheral vascular disease, including PAD, was previously discouraged because they were thought to worsen symptoms. Beta-blockers do not affect walking capacity in patients with PAD;[14] thus, it is reasonable to use them to treat hypertension in this population,[15] although they should be used cautiously in those with severe PAD.[15] Beta-blockers are not recommended for the treatment of

---

* SORT (Strength of Recommendation Taxonomy) is a rating system (A, B or C) that addresses the quality of available evidence. For more information consult **How to Use *Compendium of Therapeutic Choices*** on page xxv.

hypertension in patients over 60 years of age unless there are other compelling indications such as angina, recent MI or a supraventricular arrhythmia.

Lipid-lowering drugs reduce the risk of cardiovascular events in patients with atherosclerosis and may improve symptoms and increase walking distance in patients with intermittent claudication.[16,17]

Specific Therapy for Intermittent Claudication

Pentoxifylline, a methylxanthine derivative, alters erythrocyte deformability and reduces blood viscosity, platelet reactivity and plasma hypercoagulability.[18] Pentoxifylline produces marginal but statistically significant improvement in pain-free and maximal walking distance and thus is not indicated for *mild* claudication. Smoking cessation and regular dynamic leg exercise are probably more beneficial than pentoxifylline for *moderate* claudication. If pentoxifylline is used, a total of 24 weeks of therapy followed by an 8-week drug-free period (as exercise tolerance increases) can decrease or eliminate the need for pentoxifylline.

Pentoxifylline may be beneficial adjunctive therapy for *trophic ulcers* in diabetic and nondiabetic patients.[19] Assess therapy at 4-week intervals. Cost of therapy is unlikely to be justified beyond 24 weeks of treatment.

Cilostazol inhibits platelet aggregation by selectively inhibiting phosphodiesterase III and is a vasodilator that improves maximal treadmill walking distance.[20,21] It is not available in Canada.

Other Therapies

The role of vasoactive agents, buflomedil,[22] prostaglandin analogues,[23,24] L-carnitine or arterial gene therapy[25] has not been defined by adequate clinical trials. Low molecular weight heparin, oral anticoagulants, vitamin E and chelation therapy are not effective for PAD.

Table 1: **Drug Therapy for Intermittent Claudication**

Class	Drug	Dose	Adverse Effects	Comments	Drug Interactions	Cost[a]
Antiplatelet Agents	*ASA* Aspirin, Coated Aspirin, generics	80–325 mg daily po	GI intolerance, GI bleeding, nausea, heartburn.		Increased bleeding risk with anticoagulants and clopidogrel.	$
	clopidogrel Plavix, generics	75 mg daily po	Skin rash, diarrhea, bleeding.		Increased bleeding risk with ASA. PPI use may reduce clopidogrel efficacy.	$$
Rheologic Modifiers	*pentoxifylline* generics	400 mg SR TID po	Nausea, vomiting, dizziness, headache, flushing.	Clinical effectiveness is marginal. Not recommended in patients with marked hepatic or renal dysfunction. Contraindications: acute MI, hemorrhage, peptic ulcer disease, xanthine intolerance.	Reduced effect of adenosine; Increased effect of theophylline, warfarin, sympathomimetics, antihypertensives, hypoglycemics.	$$

[a] Cost of 30-day supply; includes drug cost only.
Abbreviations: SR = sustained-release
Legend: $ <$10 $$ $10–20

Suggested Readings

Ankle Brachial Index Collaboration, Fowkes FG, Murray GD et al. Ankle brachial index combined with Framingham Risk Score to predict cardiovascular events and mortality: a meta-analysis. *JAMA* 2008;300(2):197-208.

Gardner AW, Montgomery PS, Afaq A. Exercise performance in patients with peripheral arterial disease who have different types of exertional leg pain. *J Vasc Surg* 2007;46(1):79-86.

Rowlands TE, Donnelly R. Medical therapy for intermittent claudication. *Eur J Vasc Endovasc Surg* 2007;34(3):314-21.

Sumner AD, Khalil YK, Reed JF. The relationship of peripheral artery disease and metabolic syndrome prevalence in asymptomatic US adults 40 years and older: Results from the National Health and Nutrition Examination Survey (1999-2004). *J Clin Hypertension*2012;14(3):144-8.

Sutton-Tyrrell K, Venkitachalam L, Kanaya AM et al. Relationship of ankle blood pressures to cardiovascular events in older adults. *Stroke* 2008;39(3):863-9.

White C. Clinical practice. Intermittent claudication. *N Engl J Med* 2007;356(12):1241-50.

References

1. Vidula H, Tian L, Liu K et al. Biomarkers of inflammation and thrombosis as predictors of near-term mortality in patients with peripheral arterial disease: a cohort study. *Ann Intern Med* 2008;148(2):85-93.
2. Feringa HH, Bax JJ, Hoeks S et al. A prognostic risk index for long-term mortality in patients with peripheral arterial disease. *Arch Intern Med* 2007;167(22):2482-9.
3. McDermott MM, Liu K, Ferrucci L et al. Physical performance in peripheral arterial disease: a slower rate of decline in patients who walk more. *Ann Intern Med* 2006;144(1):10-20.
4. Kim DH. Exercise and peripheral arterial disease. *Ann Intern Med* 2006;144(9):699-700.
5. Wind J, Koelemay MJ. Exercise therapy and the additional effect of supervision on exercise therapy in patients with intermittent claudication. Systematic review of randomised controlled trials. *Eur J Vasc Endovasc Surg* 2007;34(1):1-9.
6. Adam DJ, Beard JD, Cleveland T et al. Bypass versus angioplasty in severe ischaemia of the leg (BASIL): multicentre, randomised controlled trial. *Lancet* 2005;366(9501):1925-34.
7. Goy JJ, Urban P. Life and limb: bypass versus angioplasty in the ischaemic limb. *Lancet* 2005;366(9501):1905-6.
8. Hirsch AT, Haskal ZJ, Hertzer NR et al. ACC/AHA 2005 practice guidelines for the management of patients with peripheral arterial disease (lower extremity, renal, mesenteric, and abdominal aortic). *Circulation* 2006;113(11):e463-654.
9. Collaborative overview of randomised trials of antiplatelet therapy--I: Prevention of death, myocardial infarction, and stroke by prolonged antiplatelet therapy in various categories of patients. Antiplatelet Trialists' Collaboration. *BMJ* 1994;308(6921):81-106.
10. A randomised, blinded, trial of clopidogrel versus aspirin in patients at risk of ischaemic events (CAPRIE). CAPRIE Steering Committee. *Lancet* 1996;348(9038):1329-39.
11. Bhatt DL, Fox KA, Hacke W et al. Clopidogrel and aspirin versus aspirin alone for the prevention of atherothrombotic events. *N Engl J Med* 2006;354(16):1706-17.
12. Yusuf S, Sleight P, Pogue J et al. Effects of an angiotensin-converting-enzyme inhibitor, ramipril, on cardiovascular events in high-risk patients. The Heart Outcomes Prevention Evaluation Study Investigators. *N Engl J Med* 2000;342(3):145-53.
13. Ahimastos AA, Walker PJ, Askew C et al. Effect of ramipril on walking times and quality of life among patients with peripheral artery disease and intermittent claudication: a randomized controlled trial. *JAMA* 2013;309(5):453-60.
14. Radack K, Deck C. Beta-adrenergic blocker therapy does not worsen intermittent claudication in subjects with peripheral arterial disease. A meta-analysis of randomized controlled trials. *Arch Intern Med* 1991;151(9):1769-76.
15. Heintzen MP, Strauer BE. Peripheral vascular effects of beta-blockers. *Eur Heart J* 1994;15(Suppl C):2-7.
16. Mohler ER, Hiatt WR, Creager MA. Cholesterol reduction with atorvastatin improves walking distance in patients with peripheral arterial disease. *Circulation* 2003;108(12):1481-6.
17. Mondillo S, Ballo P, Barbati R et al. Effects of simvastatin on walking performance and symptoms of intermittent claudication in hypercholesterolemic patients with peripheral vascular disease. *Am J Med* 2003;114(5):359-64.
18. Hood SC, Moher D, Barber GG. Management of intermittent claudication with pentoxifylline: meta-analysis of randomized controlled trials. *CMAJ* 1996;155(8):1053-9.
19. Jull A, Waters J, Arroll B. Pentoxifylline for treatment of venous leg ulcers: a systematic review. *Lancet* 2002;359(9317):1550-4.
20. Stevens JW, Simpson E, Harnan S et al. Systematic review of the efficacy of cilostazol, naftidrofuryl oxalate and pentoxifylline for the treatment of intermittent claudication. *Br J Surg* 2012;99(12):1630-8.
21. Rowlands TE, Donnelly R. Medical therapy for intermittent claudication. *Eur J Vasc Endovasc Surg* 2007;34(3):314-21.
22. de Backer TL, Bogaert M, Vander Stichele R. Buflomedil for intermittent claudication. *Cochrane Database Syst Rev* 2008;(1):CD000988.
23. Milio G, Mina C, Cospite V et al. Efficacy of the treatment with prostaglandin E-1 in venous ulcers of the lower limbs. *J Vasc Surg* 2005;42(2):304-8.
24. Robertson L, Andras A. Prostanoids for intermittent claudication. *Cochrane Database Syst Rev* 2012;4:CD000986.
25. Lederman RJ, Mendelsohn FO, Anderson RD et al. Therapeutic angiogenesis with recombinant fibroblast growth factor-2 for intermittent claudication (the TRAFFIC study): a randomised trial. *Lancet* 2002;359(9323):2053-8.

Chapter 41
Post-myocardial Infarction

Derek Y. F. So, MD, FRCPC, FACC

The term post-myocardial infarction applies to patients who experienced either ST-elevation myocardial infarction (STEMI) or non-ST-elevation myocardial infarction (NSTEMI). While the early management differs, the long-term therapeutic goals are similar. For details on early management see Chapter 35.

For patients with STEMI, initial acute reperfusion strategies, consisting of primary percutaneous coronary intervention (PCI) and thrombolytic therapy, enable restoration of patency to the occluded culprit artery and offer improved prognosis compared to patients treated conservatively.[1] For patients receiving primary PCI, early risk stratification is accomplished at angiography with evaluation of the nonculprit arteries and preliminary assessment of left ventricular function. For those receiving thrombolytic therapy, early assessment of reperfusion success is imperative, as transfer for urgent angiography is indicated for failed reperfusion.[2,3] Emerging evidence suggests the need for early cardiac catheterization even among those with successful reperfusion.[4] This is especially evident in individuals with large infarcts, where a pharmacoinvasive approach (transfer immediately after thrombolysis) prevents subsequent recurrent ischemia and infarction and allows early risk stratification.[5,6] While STEMI requires more urgent upfront treatment, NSTEMI actually has higher long-term morbidity and mortality.[7] Accordingly, the need for risk stratification early after NSTEMI is essential. An "invasive approach" of early angiography with subsequent revascularization with PCI or coronary bypass surgery, has been shown to reduce recurrent morbidity and mortality in high-risk NSTEMI patients.[8]

Management of patients following STEMI or NSTEMI is similar, with the overall aim of returning patients to an ideal quality of life and preventing progression of disease and repeat infarction.

Goals of Therapy

- Evaluate for the presence of complications associated with MI:
  - left ventricular (LV) dysfunction (cause of heart failure or arrhythmias)
  - LV clot (cause of stroke or other embolic events)
  - late or nonreperfused MI (cause of mechanical complications e.g., ventricular septal defects, mitral regurgitation)
- Target modifiable risk factors for secondary prevention
- Restore quality of life and facilitate return to work
- Monitor for potential arrhythmias (bradyarrythmias and ventricular arrythmias)

Investigations

- Determine risk for ongoing ischemia:
  - *coronary angiography*—evidence supports early angiography for most STEMI and NSTEMI patients. Angiography should be considered for patients not initially triaged to angiography, especially if they develop recurrent chest pain, heart failure or hemodynamic compromise.
  - *stress testing*—exercise or pharmacologic stress testing can be conducted for lower risk patients with NSTEMI or successfully reperfused STEMI patients without ready access to angiography. Coronary angiography should be performed if high-risk test result.

- Evaluation of infarct size (or left ventricular function):
  - patients with significantly diminished ejection fraction (EF) are at risk of LV thrombus formation, heart failure and arrhythmia.
    - left ventriculography can be conducted at coronary angiogram and provide an early evaluation of LV function.
    - echocardiogram, radionuclide imaging or magnetic resonance imaging can also measure infarct size. Echocardiogram is the modality of choice to assess for presence of LV clot.
  - repeat LV function evaluation should be conducted ≥1 month in nonrevascularized patients and ≥3 months in revascularized patients to determine LV recovery and the need for implantable defibrillator[9] (if LVEF <30%)
- Evaluate modifiable risk factors:
  - history, particularly of smoking
  - physical examination: blood pressure, BMI, waist circumference
  - blood work: fasting cholesterol and glucose measurements

Therapeutic Choices

The overall goals after MI are to address the consequences of the infarct, prevent reinfarction and deter progression of atherosclerosis. To address these goals, a combination of pharmacologic therapies and lifestyle management strategies are required.

Nonpharmacologic Choices

- In patients not initially triaged for coronary angiography, indications for subsequent angiography and revascularization include recurrent ischemic symptoms, heart failure or a high-risk stress test.
- Weight management. Target values are BMI 18.5–25, waist circumference <100 cm (male) and <90 cm (female).[9] Goal in general is to sustain 5–10% decrease in body weight. Nutritional counselling is an important tool for patients attempting to lose weight.
- Regular exercise (aerobic exercise and resistance training) with an individual prescription that accounts for age, obesity, level of fitness and biomechanical capability. Generally, the goal of burning off 1000 kcal/week can be attained by engaging in 30–45 minutes of moderate aerobic activity 3 or 4 times per week.[10]
- Individual or group counselling has a role in managing significant psychosocial issues (e.g. anxiety, social support).
- Implantable cardioverter/defibrillator (ICD) is indicated in selected patients (see Investigations) with significant residual LV dysfunction despite aggressive medical therapies for 3 or more months.[11]

Pharmacologic Choices

After MI, patients are at substantial risk for subsequent major adverse cardiovascular events (MACE), such as nonfatal MI, death or stroke. Secondary prevention with several classes of drugs independently reduces incidence of MACE by approximately 25%[12] (Table 1). An overview of individual agents is provided in Table 2.

Antiplatelet Agents

MI is a consequence of an acute plaque rupture, in which activated platelets play an integral role. Consequently, after reperfusion therapy early inhibition of platelets with ASA and an adenosine $P2Y_{12}$ receptor inhibitor is required to maintain vessel patency and prevent reinfarction.[13] Dual antiplatelet therapy is also required for prevention of acute occlusion of stents after PCI,[14,15] or in patients managed medically.[16] Long-term antiplatelet therapy is effective in preventing MACE.[9] Currently available $P2Y_{12}$ inhibitory drugs include the thienopyridines (clopidogrel, prasugrel) and ticagrelor.

In patients who have received thrombolytic therapy, clopidogrel is the $P2Y_{12}$ inhibitor of choice.[16] For most other infarct patients, the first-line $P2Y_{12}$ inhibitor is either prasugrel or ticagrelor. Irrespective of the choice of $P2Y_{12}$ inhibitor, the ideal duration of therapy should be at least 1 year after MI.[16] In certain patients, e.g., those at a high risk of bleeding, earlier discontinuation of the $P2Y_{12}$ inhibitor might be considered in consultation with their cardiologist.

ASA

ASA is the antiplatelet agent of choice for long-term secondary prevention due to its effectiveness and low cost. Indefinite therapy is indicated in all postinfarct patients; low-dose therapy (75–100 mg) is as effective as higher doses (300–325 mg).[17] Low-dose ASA is generally better tolerated, with lower bleeding risk.[18] ASA is used in combination with a $P2Y_{12}$ inhibitor when indicated (see Figure 1).

Figure 1: Management of Patients Post-myocardial Infarction

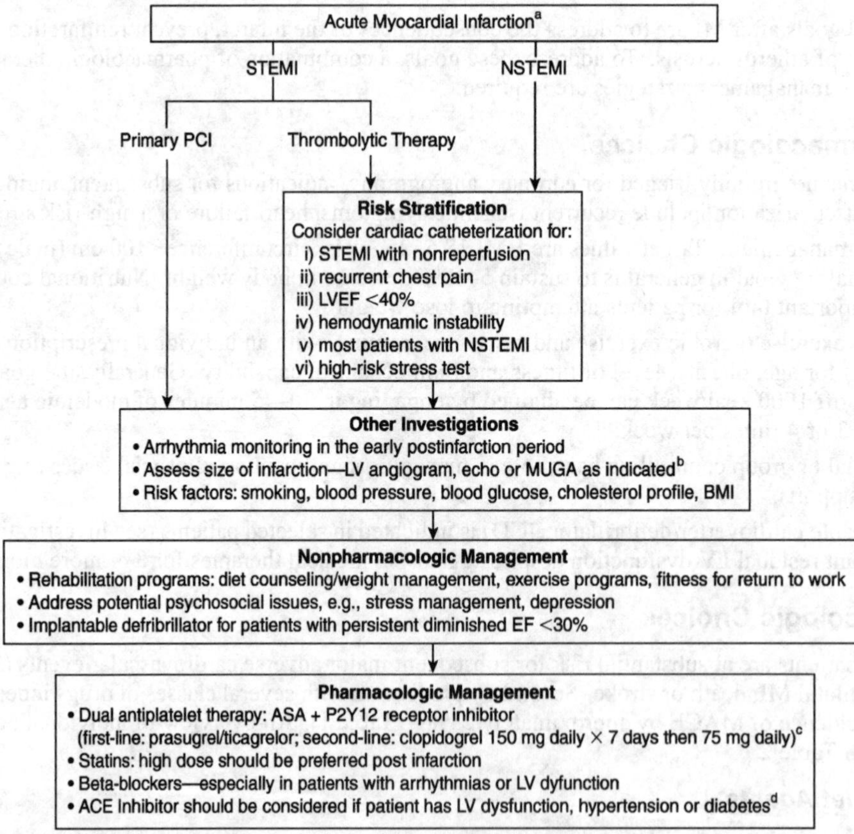

[a] For details of acute management see Chapter 35.
[b] Repeat testing in 3 months for reperfused patients with large anterior infarction to assess ejection fraction.
[c] Treatment duration: Bare metal stent—minimum of 4 weeks, ideally 1 year. Drug eluting stent—1 year. Consult with cardiologist if discontinuation before 1 year is considered.
[d] Substitute with an angiotensin receptor blocker if there is a history of ACE inhibitor induced cough.

Abbreviations ACE = angiotensin-converting enzyme; BMI = body mass index; EF = ejection fraction; LV = left ventricular; LVEF = left ventricular ejection fraction; MUGA = multiple-gated acquisition scan; NSTEMI = non-ST segment elevation myocardial infarction; PCI = percutaneous coronary intervention; STEMI = ST segment elevation myocardial infarction

Table 1: **Individual and Cumulative Impact of 4 Treatments for Secondary Prevention of Cardiovascular Events**

Drug Therapy	Relative Risk Reduction	2-year Event Rate (death, MI or stroke)
None		8%
ASA	25%	6%
Beta-blocker	25%	4.5%
Lipid lowering (reduce LDL-C by 1.5 mmol/L)	30%	3%
ACE inhibitor	25%	2.3%
Cumulative relative risk reduction if all 4 drugs are used	≈75%	

To calculate the cumulative risk reduction a multiplicative scale was used. For example, 2 interventions, each reducing the risk of an event by 30%, would be expected to have about a 50% relative risk reduction (1–[0.7 × 0.7]). No interactions in treatment effects are observed in trials, suggesting that the proportionate risk reduction of a specific drug in the presence or absence of other effective interventions would be expected to be similar. Smoking cessation lowers the risk of recurrent MI by about half after 2 years. In a smoker with vascular disease, quitting smoking and the use of the 4 preventive strategies could theoretically have a large potential benefit (approximately 80% relative risk reduction)

Reprinted from Yusuf S. Two decades of progress in preventing vascular disease. *Lancet* 2002;360(9326):2-3. Copyright 2002. With permission from Elsevier.

Clopidogrel

The thienopyridine **clopidogrel** continues to be commonly used after PCI. In MI patients receiving clopidogrel after PCI, a dose of 150 mg daily for the first 6 days has been shown to be superior and should be considered.[16,19] A daily dose of 75 mg should be used after the initial 6 days of high dose therapy or for those patients deemed not to require the initial high-dose therapy. For patients with ASA allergy, chronic clopidogrel therapy may be a substitute.

Prasugrel

Prasugrel is a thienopyridine with an active metabolite that binds irreversibly to the $P2Y_{12}$ receptor. Prasugrel has a faster onset of action with increased potency in platelet inhibition compared to clopidogrel. In patients with MI undergoing PCI, prasugrel reduced MACE compared to clopidogrel.[20] Current guidelines suggest prasugrel or ticagrelor as first-line agents after NSTEMI or STEMI.[16,21] Increased bleeding has been associated with prasugrel among patients who are elderly (>75 years), have a history of stroke or TIA or have low body weight (<60 kg). Accordingly, guidelines suggest a reduced dose of prasugrel in patients ≥75 years or weight ≤60 kg,[16] though this dose may be difficult to obtain with the formulation marketed in Canada. Prasugrel should be avoided in patients with previous stroke or TIA.

Ticagrelor

Ticagrelor, a cyclopentyltriazolopyrimidine, is a direct, reversible inhibitor of the $P2Y_{12}$ receptor. It is more effective in acute coronary syndrome when compared to clopidogrel.[22] Ticagrelor is endorsed as first-line therapy in current guidelines.[16,21] Bleeding is increased among patients treated medically or with PCI when compared to clopidogrel.[22] Dyspnea may occur in approximately 14% of patients treated with ticagrelor.[22]

Beta-Blockers

In the absence of contraindications, consider this class of medication in all patients after STEMI or NSTEMI, as they have been proven to reduce MACE post infarct.[9,21] In particular, beta-blockers play a role in the reduction of reinfarction and prevention of ventricular arrhythmia in the early phase after infarction.[23] Beta-blockers should be started within a few days of infarction and the dose titrated to maximally tolerated doses with heart rate not >70 bpm. However, intravenous beta-blockers should be used cautiously in the early acute phase as they may contribute to hemodynamic instability in patients suffering large infarcts.[23] Avoid beta-blockers in patients with hypotension, bradycardia and active heart failure. Patients with reduced LV function derive significant benefit from beta-blockers, but should be monitored closely especially in the postinfarction period. This benefit extends to those already treated with ACE inhibitors. If tolerated, beta-blockers should be continued indefinitely, especially in patients with reduced LV function. However, they can be stopped at follow up in patients with normal LV function if fatigue or other side effects are encountered.

Inhibition of the Renin–Angiotensin–Aldosterone Pathway

ACE Inhibitors

ACE inhibitors should be considered in all post-MI patients, especially in those with LV dysfunction (LVEF <40%), hypertension or diabetes mellitus.[9,21] The relative benefits of ACE inhibitors are greater among those with LV dysfunction, as they play a role in LV remodeling post-MI. Long-term treatment with ACE inhibitors reduces cardiovascular death and MI among those with atherosclerosis and multiple risk factors.[24] In patients with significant renal dysfunction or those with hyperkalemia, avoid ACE inhibitors.[9] Titration to evidence-based dosages is important and should be evaluated at follow-up visits.[24,25]

Angiotensin Receptor Blockers (ARB)

ARBs may be used instead of ACE inhibitors in those intolerant of the latter because of cough. In a randomized control study, valsartan demonstrated equivalent benefit to captopril among post-MI patients with heart failure and LV dysfunction.[26] However, combination therapy with ACE inhibitor and ARB increases adverse events and has no evidence of benefit.[27]

Aldosterone Antagonists

Consider using a selective aldosterone antagonist in patients post-MI with significant LV dysfunction. **Eplerenone**, when added to other post-MI evidenced-based therapies, has demonstrated a reduction in mortality and hospitalization for cardiovascular events (heart failure, re-infarction, stroke and ventricular arrhythmia).[28] Similarly, **spironolactone** had previously been proven beneficial in patients with severe LV dysfunction when used in conjunction with an ACE inhibitor and diuretic.[29] Comparative data are limited, so choice is based on tolerability and availability. Closely monitor electrolytes as eplerenone and spironolactone are associated with a risk of hyperkalemia.

HMG-CoA Reductase Inhibitors (Statins)

Starting a statin early after MI decreases both early and late adverse events. Guidelines suggest documenting the cholesterol profile within 24 hours as LDL cholesterol may be falsely low for up to 4 weeks postinfarction.[21,30] Evidence suggests that intensive treatment with higher dose statins (e.g., atorvastatin 80 mg/day or rosuvastatin 40 mg/day) early after MI confer additional benefits compared with moderate dosages.[31] The benefit extends beyond lowering of LDL cholesterol levels alone and contributes to plaque stabilization by preventing future acute coronary syndromes.[32]

Indefinite continuation of statin therapy is integral to the prevention of ischemic events. Following MI, all patients are considered to be in the high-risk group for subsequent events.[33] Current Canadian Cardiovascular Society guidelines advocate a minimum target LDL-C of <2 mmol/L[33] (see Chapter 37). Muscle discomfort may occur in up to 5% of patients.[34] In patients intolerant of statins, alternative cholesterol-lowering agents such as **niacin** or **ezetimibe** may be considered. For patients not achieving target levels despite maximal statin therapy or for those intolerant of higher statin doses, attempt combination therapy with a statin and extended-release niacin.[35]

Oral Anticoagulants

Oral anticoagulants are recommended in post-MI patients with paroxysmal or persistent atrial fibrillation, demonstrable LV thrombus or large infarcts with extensive dyskinetic or aneurysmal segments.[9] **Warfarin** is the oral anticoagulant of choice for patients with LV thrombus.

There is a significant increase in bleeding risk when warfarin is used concurrently with dual antiplatelet therapy.[21] This is of particular concern when combining prasugrel or ticagrelor with warfarin as there may be an even higher risk of bleeding compared to clopidogrel.[36] Accordingly, most patients receiving warfarin should use clopidogrel as the $P2Y_{12}$ inhibitory drug. Close monitoring of INR in these patients is imperative, with consideration of shorter duration of antiplatelet therapy if indefinite warfarin therapy is indicated. In those treated with warfarin for LV thrombus post-MI, repeat echocardiography should be performed after 3 months of treatment.[9] If the thrombus has resolved, consider discontinuation of warfarin therapy. Avoid using new oral anticoagulants, e.g. **dabigatran**, **rivaroxaban**, for treatment of atrial fibrillation in combination with prasugrel or ticagrelor as there is little evidence to support the safety of combining these drugs.

Therapeutic Tips

- Close adherence to evidenced-based therapies is correlated with improved long-term outcomes.[37,38] Institution of these therapies early post-MI during initial hospitalization may confer higher adherence rates. Ongoing titration to evidence-based dosages of beta-blockers and ACE inhibitors is important.
- *Smoking cessation* programs and *cardiac rehabilitation* referral should be offered early post-MI to all motivated patients. Use of nicotine replacement strategies, bupropion or varenicline can be safely offered in the early post-MI period.[9,21]
- Treat blood pressure using drug therapy to a target of <140/90 and for diabetics to <130/80.[39]
- Initiate hypoglycemic therapy to attain a HbA_{1C} of <7%.[9] Avoid thiazolidinediones in post-MI patients.
- Give sublingual **nitrates** to all post-MI patients with clear instructions for proper use and response in the setting of recurrent chest discomfort.
- Encourage post-MI patients to receive annual influenza vaccination.
- Depression is common in post-MI patients. Maintain a high level of awareness for the psychosocial status of patients with inquiries about depression, anxiety, sleep disorder and social support. Treatment with cognitive behavioural therapy or pharmacotherapy may be indicated especially in the first year after MI.[9] Use of an SSRI reduces symptoms of depression and may improve cardiovascular outcomes.[40]
- **Hormone therapy** is not indicated and may be harmful for secondary prevention of cardiovascular events in postmenopausal women.[9]
- Routine use of **antioxidant vitamins** for prevention of cardiovascular events is not recommended.[9]
- **Celecoxib** and some nonselective **NSAIDs** such as **ibuprofen** may increase atherothrombotic complications. In addition, ibuprofen may reduce the antiplatelet effect of low-dose ASA. Avoid NSAIDs if possible, especially in those with significant LV dysfunction [Evidence: SORT B*].[41] Two meta-analyses suggest that **naproxen** is the NSAID with the least adverse cardiovascular effects [Evidence: SORT B*].[42,43]

---

* SORT (Strength of Recommendation Taxonomy) is a rating system (A, B or C) that addresses the quality of available evidence. For more information consult **How to Use *Compendium of Therapeutic Choices*** on page xxv.

Table 2: Drugs Used Post-myocardial Infarction

Drug Class	Drug	Dose	Adverse Effects	Drug Interactions	Comments	Cost[a]
ACE Inhibitors[b]	*captopril* generics	Initial: 6.25 mg TID po Target dose: 50 mg TID	Dry cough, hyperkalemia, angioedema (unusual). Can precipitate renal failure in patients with renovascular disease, volume depletion or in those receiving NSAIDs.	Marked increase in serum K^+ in patients receiving K^+ supplements and/or K^+-sparing diuretics. Reduced hypotensive effect and increased risk of renal dysfunction with NSAIDs. Elevated Li^+ levels (potential toxicity).	Use lower (i.e., 50%) initial doses in patients taking diuretics (increased risk of hypotension with hypovolemia). Hyperkalemia usually occurs only in patients taking K^+ supplements or drugs that cause K^+ retention, patients with renal impairment or those with diabetes and high serum K^+ levels. Assess SCr and K^+ after a few days, then regularly.	$$
	cilazapril Inhibace, generics	Initial: 0.5 mg daily po Target dose in HF: 2.5–5 mg daily	See captopril.	See captopril.	See captopril.	$
	enalapril Vasotec, generics	Initial: 2.5 mg BID po Target dose in HF: 10 mg BID	See captopril.	See captopril.	See captopril.	$
	fosinopril generics	Initial: 10 mg daily po Target dose: 20–40 mg once daily	See captopril.	See captopril.	See captopril.	$
	lisinopril Zestril, Prinivil, generics	Initial: 2.5 mg daily po Target dose: 35–40 mg once daily	See captopril.	See captopril.	See captopril.	$
	perindopril Coversyl	Initial: 2 mg daily po Target dose for CAD: 8 mg daily	See captopril.	See captopril.	See captopril.	$$
	quinapril Accupril, generics	Initial: 5 mg daily po Target dose: 20–40 mg BID	See captopril.	See captopril.	See captopril.	$$
	ramipril Altace, generics	Initial: 2.5 mg daily po Target dose: 5 mg BID or 10 mg daily	See captopril.	See captopril.	See captopril.	$
	trandolapril Mavik	Initial: 1 mg daily po Target dose: 4 mg daily	See captopril.	See captopril.	See captopril.	$$

Drug Class	Drug	Dose	Adverse Effects	Drug Interactions	Comments	Cost[a]
Aldosterone Antagonists	*eplerenone* Inspra	Initial: 25 mg daily or every 2 days po Target: 50 mg daily	Hyperkalemia, dehydration, dizziness, diarrhea, nausea.	ACE inhibitors, ARBs, potassium supplements: hyperkalemia. NSAIDs: Reduced diuretic effect, worsening renal function, hyperkalemia. Strong inhibitors/inducers of CYP3A4.	Monitor serum creatinine and potassium 3 and 7 days after initiating or titrating the dose. Repeat every 1–3 months once stable.	$$$
	spironolactone Aldactone, generics	Initial: 12.5 mg daily or every 2 days po Target (for mortality benefit): 25–50 mg/day	Hyperkalemia, dehydration, nausea, gynecomastia (usually reversible upon discontinuation).	ACE inhibitors, ARBs, potassium supplements: hyperkalemia. NSAIDs: reduce diuretic effect, worsening renal function, hyperkalemia.	See eplerenone.	$
Angiotensin Receptor Blockers	*candesartan* Atacand, generics	Initial: 4 or 8 mg daily po Target dose in HF: 32 mg once daily	Hyperkalemia. Can precipitate renal failure in susceptible patients (bilateral renovascular disease, those with volume depletion or with concurrent NSAID use). Angioedema has been reported, but a causal association has not been established.	Marked increase in serum K^+ in patients receiving K^+ supplements and/or K^+-sparing diuretics. May elevate Li^+ levels (potential toxicity).	Use lower (i.e., 50%) initial doses in patients on diuretics (increased risk of hypotension with hypovolemia). Hyperkalemia usually occurs only in patients taking K^+ supplements or drugs that cause K^+ retention, those with renal impairment or patients with diabetes and high serum K^+ levels. Assess SCr and K^+ after a few days, then regularly.	$
	losartan Cozaar, generics	Initial: 50 mg daily po Target dose in HF: 150 mg daily	See candesartan.	See candesartan.	See candesartan.	$
	valsartan Diovan, generics	Initial dose: 20 mg BID po Target dose:[23] 160 mg BID	See candesartan.	See candesartan.	See candesartan.	$
Antiplatelet Agents	*ASA* Aspirin, Coated Aspirin, generics	80–325 mg daily po	Nausea, vomiting, GI hemorrhage, tinnitus, vertigo, hypersensitivity.	Increased risk of bleeding when antiplatelets are given with anticoagulants (e.g., warfarin). Caution with NSAIDs.		$
	clopidogrel Plavix, generics	75 mg daily po	Rash, purpura, diarrhea, bleeding.	Caution with NSAIDs. PPI use may reduce clopidogrel efficacy.	Consider an initial dose of 150 mg daily po x 6 days in STEMI and NSTEMI patients after PCI	$

(cont'd)

Table 2: **Drugs Used Post-myocardial Infarction** *(cont'd)*

Drug Class	Drug	Dose	Adverse Effects	Drug Interactions	Comments	Cost[a]
	prasugrel Effient	Loading dose: 60 mg, then 10 mg daily po	Increased risk of bleeding, rash.	Caution with NSAIDs.	Caution in patients >75 y, body weight <60 kg. Consider 5 mg daily if available. Contraindicated if history of ischemic stroke.	$$$
	ticagrelor Brilinta	Loading dose: 180 mg, then 90 mg BID po	Increased risk of bleeding, bradycardia, headache, nausea, transient dyspnea (>13%).	Caution with NSAIDs. Avoid strong CYP3A4 inhibitors (e.g., clarithromycin). Digoxin level increased.	Reversible increase in serum creatine or uric acid in some patients.	$$$$
	ticlopidine generics	250 mg BID po	Diarrhea, rash, bleeding, neutropenia (usually reversible), purpura.	Caution with NSAIDs.	Rarely used. Must monitor neutrophil counts Q2 wk for the first 3 months.	$$
Beta$_1$-adrenergic Antagonists, selective	*atenolol* Tenormin, generics	Initial: 50 mg daily po Usual: 100 mg daily	Fatigue, bradycardia, Reduced exercise capacity, headache, impotence, vivid dreams. Less common: hyperglycemia, depression, heart failure, heart block.	Bradycardia with digoxin or nondihydropyridine CCBs. Cardiodepressant effects with nondihydropyridine CCBs, antiarrhythmics, anesthetics.	Start with low dose and increase at weekly intervals to maintain heart rate <70 bpm. Contraindications: heart rate <50–60 bpm, systolic BP <90–100 mmHg, severe heart failure, cardiogenic shock, severe reactive airway disease, 2nd or 3rd degree AV block.	$
	bisoprolol Sandoz Bisoprolol, other generics	Initial: 2.5 mg daily po Usual: 10 mg daily	See atenolol.	See atenolol.	See atenolol.	$
	metoprolol Lopresor, generics	Initial: 50 mg daily po Usual: 200 mg daily IR: give in 2 divided doses SR: give once daily	See atenolol.	See atenolol. CYP2D6 inhibitors increase levels of propranolol and metoprolol.	See atenolol.	$
Beta$_1$-adrenergic Antagonists, selective with ISA	*acebutolol* Sectral, generics	Initial: 100–200 mg BID po Usual: 400 mg BID	See atenolol.	See atenolol.	See atenolol. Agents with ISA have less effect on resting heart rate than those without ISA.	$$
Beta$_1$-adrenergic Antagonists with alpha$_1$-blocking activity	*carvedilol* generics	Initial: 3.125 mg BID po Usual: 25 mg BID	See atenolol. Edema, dizziness, nasal congestion and postural hypotension due to alpha$_1$ antagonism.	See atenolol.	See atenolol.	$$

Drug Class	Drug	Dose	Adverse Effects	Drug Interactions	Comments	Cost[a]
HMG-CoA Reductase Inhibitors (Statins)	*atorvastatin* Lipitor, generics	Initial: 10 or 20 mg daily po Maximum: 80 mg/day Once daily with or without meals	GI disturbances, sleep disturbances, headache, rash, myalgia (with and without increased CK levels), increased CK and transaminase levels (reversible). Rare: myopathy, rhabdomyolysis.	CYP3A4 inhibitors (e.g., amiodarone, cyclosporine, macrolides, protease inhibitors, gemfibrozil, grapefruit juice, azole antifungals, verapamil): Increased serum levels of atorvastatin, lovastatin and simvastatin.	Start with 40 mg/day if the desired reduction in LDL-C is >45%. Maximum response is usually evident within 4 wk.	$
	fluvastatin Lescol, generics	Initial: 20 or 40 mg daily po Maximum: 80 mg/day Once daily with or without meals	See atorvastatin.	Fluconazole inhibits the metabolism and increases serum levels of fluvastatin.	Start with 40 mg/day if the desired reduction in LDL-C is >25%.	$
	lovastatin Mevacor, generics	Initial: 20 mg daily po Maximum: 80 mg/day Take with the evening meal	See atorvastatin.	See atorvastatin.		$$
	pravastatin Pravachol, generics	Initial: 20 mg daily po Maximum: 80 mg/day Take at bedtime	See atorvastatin.	Low potential for drug interactions (not metabolized by CYP450 isozymes).		$
	rosuvastatin Crestor, generics	10–40 mg daily po	See atorvastatin.	May increase INR in patients taking warfarin.		$
	simvastatin Zocor, generics	10–80 mg daily po with the evening meal	See atorvastatin.	See atorvastatin.		$

[a] Cost of 30-day supply of usual or target doses; includes drug cost only.
[b] Only captopril, enalapril, ramipril and trandolapril have been shown to reduce morbidity and prolong survival in heart failure or in patients with LV dysfunction post-MI.
Dosage adjustment may be required in renal impairment; see Appendix I.
Abbreviations: ARBs = angiotensin receptor blockers; CAD = coronary artery disease; CCB = calcium channel blocker; CK = creatine kinase; HF = heart failure; IR = immediate release; ISA = intrinsic sympathomimetic activity; NSTEMI = non-ST segment elevation myocardial infarction; PCI = percutaneous coronary intervention; PPI = proton pump inhibitor; SCr = serum creatinine; SR = sustained release; STEMI = ST segment elevation myocardial infarction
Legend: $ < $25 $$ $25–50 $$$ $50–75 $$$$ $75–100

Suggested Readings

2012 Writing Committee Members, Jneid H, Anderson JL et al. 2012 ACCF/AHA focused update of the guideline for the management of patients with unstable angina/Non-ST-elevation myocardial infarction (updating the 2007 guideline and replacing the 2011 focused update): a report of the American College of Cardiology Foundation/American Heart Association Task Force on practice guidelines.*Circulation* 2012;126(7):875-910.

O'Gara PT, Kushner FG, Ascheim DD et al. 2013 ACCF/AHA guideline for the management of ST-elevation myocardial infarction: executive summary: a report of the American College of Cardiology Foundation/American Heart Association Task Force on Practice Guidelines.*Circulation* 2013;127(4):529-55.

Tanguay JF, Bell AD, Ackman ML et al. Focused 2012 update of the Canadian Cardiovascular Society guidelines for the use of antiplatelet therapy. *Can J Cardiol* 2013;29(11):1334-45.

References

1. Barron HV, Bowlby LJ, Breen T et al. Use of reperfusion therapy for acute myocardial infarction in the United States: data from the National Registry of Myocardial Infarction. *Circulation* 1998;97(12):1150-6.
2. Gershlick AH, Stephens-Lloyd A, Hughes S et al. Rescue angioplasty after failed thrombolytic therapy for acute myocardial infarction. *N Engl J Med* 2005;353(26):2758-68.
3. Wijeysundera HC, Vijayaraghavan R, Nallamothu BK et al. Rescue angioplasty or repeat fibrinolysis after failed fibrinolytic therapy for ST-segment myocardial infarction: a meta-analysis of randomized trials. *J Am Coll Cardiol* 2007;49(4):422-30.
4. Armstrong PW; WEST Steering Committee. A comparison of pharmacologic therapy with/without timely coronary intervention vs. primary percutaneous intervention early after ST-elevation myocardial infarction: the WEST (Which Early ST-elevation myocardial infarction Therapy) study. *Eur Heart J* 2006;27(13):1530-8.
5. Le May MR, Wells GA, Labinaz M et al. Combined angioplasty and pharmacological intervention versus thrombolysis alone in acute myocardial infarction (CAPITAL AMI study). *J Am Coll Cardiol* 2005;46(3):417-24.
6. Cantor WJ, Fitchett D, Borgundvaag B et al. Routine early angioplasty after fibrinolysis for acute myocardial infarction. *N Engl J Med* 2009;360(26):2705-18.
7. Chan MY, Sun JL, Newby LK et al. Long-term mortality of patients undergoing cardiac catheterization for ST-elevation and non-ST-elevation myocardial infarction. *Circulation* 2009;119(24):3110-7.
8. Cannon CP, Weintraub WS, Demopoulos LA et al. Comparison of early invasive and conservative strategies in patients with unstable coronary syndromes treated with the glycoprotein IIb/IIIa inhibitor tirofiban. *N Engl J Med* 2001;344(25):1879-87.
9. O'Gara PT, Kushner FG, Ascheim DD et al. 2013 ACCF/AHA guideline for the management of ST-elevation myocardial infarction: executive summary: a report of the American College of Cardiology Foundation/American Heart Association Task Force on Practice Guidelines.*Circulation* 2013;127(4):529-55.
10. Ades PA. Cardiac rehabilitation and secondary prevention of coronary heart disease. *N Engl J Med* 2001;345(12):892-902.
11. Moss AJ, Zareba W, Hall WJ et al. Prophylactic implantation of a defibrillator in patients with myocardial infarction and reduced ejection fraction. *N Engl J Med* 2002;346(12):877-83.
12. Yusuf S. Two decades of progress in preventing vascular disease. *Lancet* 2002;360(9326):2-3.
13. Sabatine MS, Cannon CP, Gibson CM et al. Effect of clopidogrel pretreatment before percutaneous coronary intervention in patients with ST-elevation myocardial infarction treated with fibrinolytics: the PCI-CLARITY study. *JAMA* 2005;294(10):1224-32.
14. Schomig A, Neumann FJ, Kastrati A et al. A randomized comparison of antiplatelet and anticoagulant therapy after the placement of coronary-artery stents. *N Engl J Med* 1996;334(17):1084-9.
15. Hall P, Nakamura S, Maiello L et al. A randomized comparison of combined ticlopidine and aspirin therapy versus aspirin therapy alone after successful intravascular ultrasound-guided stent implantation. *Circulation* 1996;93(2):215-22.
16. Tanguay JF, Bell AD, Ackman ML et al. Focused 2012 update of the Canadian Cardiovascular Society guidelines for the use of antiplatelet therapy. *Can J Cardiol* 2013;29(11):1334-45.
17. CURRENT-OASIS 7 Investigators, Mehta SR, Bassand JP et al. Dose comparisons of clopidogrel and aspirin in acute coronary syndromes. *N Engl J Med* 2010;363(10):930-42.
18. Peters RJ, Mehta SR, Fox KA et al. Effects of aspirin dose when used alone or in combination with clopidogrel in patients with acute coronary syndromes: observations from the Clopidogrel in Unstable angina to prevent Recurrent Events (CURE) study. *Circulation* 2003;108(14):1682-7.
19. Mehta SR, TanguayJF, Eikelboom JW et al. Double-dose versus standard-dose clopidogrel and high-dose versus low-dose aspirin in individuals undergoing percutaneous coronary intervention for acute coronary syndromes (CURRENT-OASIS 7): a randomised factorial trial. *Lancet* 2010;376(9748):1233-43.
20. Wiviott SD, Braunwald E, McCabe CH et al. Prasugrel versus clopidogrel in patients with acute coronary syndromes. *N Engl J Med* 2007;357(20):2001-15.
21. 2012 Writing Committee Members, Jneid H, Anderson JL et al. 2012 ACCF/AHA focused update of the guideline for the management of patients with unstable angina/Non-ST-elevation myocardial infarction (updating the 2007 guideline and replacing the 2011 focused update): a report of the American College of Cardiology Foundation/American Heart Association Task Force on practice guidelines.*Circulation* 2012;126(7):875-910.
22. Wallentin L, Becker RC, Budaj A et al. Ticagrelor versus clopidogrel in patients with acute coronary syndromes. *N Engl J Med* 2009;361(11):1045-57.
23. Chen ZM, Pan HC, Chen YP et al. Early intravenous then oral metoprolol in 45,852 patients with acute myocardial infarction: randomised placebo-controlled trial. *Lancet* 2005;366(9497):1622-32.

24. Yusuf S, Sleight P, Pogue J et al. Effects of an angiotensin-converting-enzyme inhibitor, ramipril, on cardiovascular events in high-risk patients. The Heart Outcomes Prevention Evaluation Study Investigators. *N Engl J Med* 2000;342(3):145-53.
25. Fox KM; EURopean trial On reduction of cardiac events with Perindopril in stable coronary Artery disease Investigators. Efficacy of perindopril in reduction of cardiovascular events among patients with stable coronary artery disease: randomised, double-blind, placebo-controlled, multicentre trial (the EUROPA study). *Lancet* 2003;362(9386):782-8.
26. Pfeffer MA, McMurray JJ, Velazquez EJ et al. Valsartan, captopril, or both in myocardial infarction complicated by heart failure, left ventricular dysfunction, or both. *N Engl J Med* 2003;349(20):1893-906.
27. ONTARGET Investigators, Yusuf S, Teo KK et al. Telmisartan, ramipril, or both in patients at high risk for vascular events. *N Engl J Med* 2008;358(15):1547-59.
28. Pitt B, Remme W, Zannad F et al. Eplerenone, a selective aldosterone blocker, in patients with left ventricular dysfunction after myocardial infarction. *N Engl J Med* 2003;348(14):1309-21.
29. Pitt B, Zannad F, Remme WJ et al. The effect of spironolactone on morbidity and mortality in patients with severe heart failure. Randomized Aldactone Evaluation Study Investigators. *N Engl J Med* 1999;341(10):709-17.
30. Mehta RH, Eagle KA. Secondary prevention in acute myocardial infarction. *BMJ* 1998;316(7134):838-42.
31. Cannon CP, Braunwald E, McCabe CH et al. Intensive versus moderate lipid lowering with statins after acute coronary syndromes. *N Engl J Med* 2004;350(15):1495-504.
32. Libby P. Current concepts of the pathogenesis of the acute coronary syndromes. *Circulation* 2001;104(3):365-72.
33. Anderson TJ, Grégoire J, Hegele RA et al. 2012 update of the Canadian Cardiovascular Society guidelines for the diagnosis and treatment of dyslipidemia for the prevention of cardiovascular disease in the adult. *Can J Cardiol* 2013;29(2):151-67.
34. Genest J, McPherson R, Frohlich J et al. 2009 Canadian Cardiovascular Society/Canadian guidelines for the diagnosis and treatment of dyslipidemia and prevention of cardiovascular disease in the adult—2009 recommendations. *Can J Cardiol* 2009;25(10):567-79.
35. Taylor AJ, Villines TC, Stanek EJ et al. Extended-release niacin or ezetimibe and carotid intima-media thickness. *N Engl J Med* 2009;361(22):2113-22.
36. Sarafoff N, Martischnig A, Wealer J et al. Triple therapy with aspirin, prasugrel, and vitamin K antagonists in patients with drug-eluting stent implantation and an indication for oral anticoagulation. *J Am Coll Cardiol* 2013;61(20):2060-6.
37. Mukherjee D, Fang J, Chetcuti S et al. Impact of combination evidence-based medical therapy on mortality in patients with acute coronary syndromes. *Circulation* 2004;109(6):745-9.
38. Allen LA, O'Donnell CJ, Giugliano RP et al. Care concordant with guidelines predicts decreased long-term mortality in patients with unstable angina pectoris and non-ST-elevation myocardial infarction. *Am J Cardiol* 2004;93(10):1218-22.
39. Hackam DG, Quinn RR, Ravani P et al. The 2013 Canadian Hypertension Education Program recommendations for blood pressure measurement, diagnosis, assessment of risk, prevention, and treatment of hypertension. *Can J Cardiol* 2013;29(5):528-42.
40. Pizzi C, Rutjes AW, Costa GM et al. Meta-analysis of selective serotonin reuptake inhibitors in patients with depression and coronary heart disease. *Am J Cardiol* 2011;107(7):972-9.
41. Antman EM, Bennett JS, Daugherty A et al. Use of nonsteroidal antiinflammatory drugs: an update for clinicians: a scientific statement from the American Heart Association. *Circulation* 2007;115(12):1634-42.
42. Fosbol EL, Folke F, Jacobsen S et al. Cause-specific cardiovascular risk associated with nonsteroidal antiinflammatory drugs among healthy individuals. *Circ Cardiovasc Qual Outcomes* 2010;3(4):395-405.
43. Trelle S, Reichenbach S, Wandel S et al. Cardiovascular safety of non-steroidal anti-inflammatory drugs: network meta-analysis. *BMJ* 2011;342:c7086.

Chapter 42
Prevention of Ischemic Stroke

Robert Côté, MD, FRCPC, FAHA

The occurrence of a first transient ischemic attack (TIA) or ischemic stroke increases the risk of experiencing a second ischemic event. Patients experiencing a TIA or mild stroke (without disabling deficits) may derive the most long-term benefit from full investigation and treatment. Secondary prevention of ischemic stroke is the main subject of this chapter. Primary prevention of stroke is covered in detail elsewhere (see Chapter 43).

The short-term prognosis after a first TIA is worse for patients with certain characteristics and symptoms; 8% of these individuals will present with a stroke within 2 days.[1] Adverse prognostic indicators include age >60 years, blood pressure ≥140/90 mm Hg, diabetes mellitus, speech and/or motor symptoms and duration of symptoms >10 minutes. Accordingly, these higher-risk patients should be promptly investigated and treated, optimally within 48–72 hours of the initial ischemic event.

Goals of Therapy

- Prevent disabling neurologic deficits (stroke) and recurrent TIA
- Prevent cerebrovascular and cardiovascular mortality

Investigations

- Complete history with attention to:
  - nature, frequency, duration and distribution of symptoms (cerebral localization)
  - identification of vascular risk factors
- Physical examination:
  - complete neurologic assessment
  - visual assessment including eye movements, visual fields, acuity and funduscopy
  - complete vascular examination including auscultation (cranium, neck, cardiac), palpation (temporal artery, peripheral pulses) and blood pressure in both arms
- Laboratory tests—indicated in most patients with TIAs or mild strokes:
  - CT scan of brain (to exclude a hemorrhagic process and/or TIA mimics) and neck ultrasonography
  - CBC, coagulation parameters, blood glucose, renal, lipid and hepatic enzyme profile
  - in select patients (young patients or older patients with possible arteritis), more specialized blood tests may be indicated (e.g., ESR, immunologic work-up, hypercoagulable screen, antiphospholipid antibodies, homocysteine)
  - baseline ECG (exclude atrial fibrillation or other contributing arrhythmia)
  - other cardiac tests (e.g., transthoracic or transesophageal echocardiography, 24-hour Holter monitoring) may be indicated (usually have a higher yield in patients with established cardiac disease or in young stroke patients)
  - MRI, MR angiography (MRA) or CT angiography is often required to confirm the degree of arterial occlusion and/or exclude other neurologic conditions mimicking cerebral ischemia. Cerebral angiography may be required in select patients to confirm occlusive vascular disease or vasculitis and appropriateness of endarterectomy.

Figure 1: **Secondary Prevention of Cerebral Ischemia**

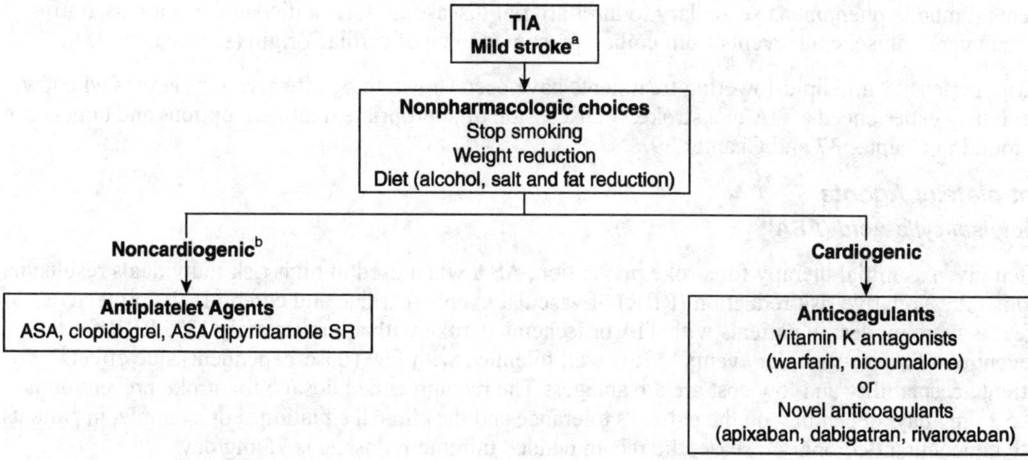

[a] Mild stroke = No substantial impact on activities of daily living.
[b] If symptomatic carotid stenosis, consider surgery.

Therapeutic Choices

Therapeutic options for preventing the recurrance of ischemic stroke are summarized in Figure 1.

Nonpharmacologic Choices

- Stop smoking (see Chapter 13).
- Control vascular risk factors through weight reduction, diet modification (reducing alcohol, fat and salt consumption) and diabetes management if required (see Chapter 32, Chapter 33).
- Start rehabilitative therapy (physiotherapy, occupational and speech therapy) within 24–48 hours if there are residual neurologic deficits.

Carotid Endarterectomy

- The prevalence of asymptomatic carotid disease in patients aged >65 years can be as high as 10% for the presence of a stenosis (≥50%). The risk of ischemic stroke increases with the degree of stenosis, progression of the stenosis and with the presence of coronary disease, hypertension and/or peripheral vascular disease.[2] The annual rate of unheralded stroke ipsilateral to a substantial (≥50%) asymptomatic stenosis is about 1.5%.[2] The presence of carotid disease is a marker of concomitant coronary disease which accounts for about half of all ischemic events in these individuals.[2] Presently, no evidence supports the use of **ASA** for ischemic stroke prevention in this clinical context although it may be required for its cardioprotective effects in patients with evidence of coronary disease. The role of prophylactic carotid endarterectomy for asymptomatic carotid disease may be considered in select individuals with a high degree (≥60%) of stenosis and when performed by surgeons with low complication rates (≤3%).[3] In many cases, however, it is also acceptable to inform the patient about potential neurologic symptoms and provide follow-up to eliminate or control vascular risk factors.
- Consider carotid endarterectomy in addition to long-term antithrombotic therapy for patients with carotid symptoms that are ipsilateral to a significant (≥70%) carotid stenosis documented by angiography, cervical duplex, MRA or CT angiography.

Pharmacologic Choices

Antiplatelet agents (Table 1) are the drugs of choice for long-term prevention of atherothrombotic events (embolic phenomena secondary to intra-arterial disease).[4,5] Oral anticoagulants are used to prevent cerebral ischemic events from emboli presumed to be of cardiac origin (see Chapter 45).

Antihypertensive and lipid-lowering treatments have been shown to be effective for patients who have previously experienced a TIA or a stroke.[6,7] Discussion of appropriate treatment options and targets can be found in Chapter 37 and Chapter 39.

Antiplatelet Agents

Acetylsalicylic Acid (ASA)

Often given as initial therapy for stroke prevention, **ASA** when used in high-risk individuals results in about a 25% relative risk reduction (RRR) of vascular events (cardiac and cerebral). Its protective effect is more modest in patients with TIA or ischemic stroke with approximately 13% RRR for the prevention of major vascular events.[4,8] It is well tolerated with few (dose-dependent) side effects. Patient acceptability and low cost are advantages. The recommended dosage for stroke prevention is 50–325 mg/day, depending on the patient's tolerance and the clinical situation. For example, in patients with concomitant coronary disease, the recommended minimum dosage is 75 mg/day.

When combined with an oral anticoagulant, ASA 100 mg/day provides better protection against cardioembolic events than an anticoagulant alone in patients with prosthetic heart valves.[9,10] However, this combination does increase the risk of systemic bleeding and should be used with caution.

Thienopyridines

Clopidogrel 75 mg daily is somewhat more effective than ASA for the prevention of ischemic events, including stroke, in patients at high risk of ischemic events.[11] The absolute difference in annual rate of ischemic stroke, MI or vascular death between clopidogrel and ASA is 0.5%, corresponding to an 8.7% RRR in favour of clopidogrel. Thus clopidogrel is an alternative antiplatelet agent in patients who are allergic to or cannot tolerate ASA.[11] It can be prescribed in patients who have new cerebral ischemic events while on ASA, although there are no clinical trials to support this.

In patients with a history of stroke or TIA, combined use of **low-dose ASA and clopidogrel** is associated with a significantly increased risk of bleeding, including intracranial hemorrhage, and long-term use does not significantly reduce the rate of ischemic events including stroke.[12,13,14] The role of short-term combined treatment is under investigation; long-term use of ASA plus clopidogrel is not routinely recommended for secondary prevention of ischemic events in patients with a history of stroke or TIA, but may be warranted in patients with other compelling indications such as recent MI [Evidence: SORT B*].[12,15]

Ticlopidine 250 mg twice daily is comparable to ASA for prevention of all vascular events in patients at risk and may be slightly superior for stroke prevention.[16] Diarrhea and skin rash are common adverse events of ticlopidine. Neutropenia occurs infrequently but is potentially serious and requires frequent monitoring (every 2 weeks for the first 3 months). For these reasons, ticlopidine is not recommended for routine use in stroke prevention. Clopidogrel is as effective as ticlopidine and is better tolerated.

Dipyridamole/ASA

Dipyridamole/ASA (200/25 mg) given twice daily reduces the relative risk of stroke by 23% (mostly for ischemic strokes) when compared with ASA in patients with cerebral ischemic symptoms.[17] This finding was confirmed in a randomized controlled trial in which the incidence of death, stroke, MI or

* SORT (Strength of Recommendation Taxonomy) is a rating system (A, B or C) that addresses the quality of available evidence. For more information consult **How to Use *Compendium of Therapeutic Choices*** on page xxv.

major bleeding complications occurred significantly less often in patients with cerebral ischemia treated with dipyridamole/ASA than ASA alone (absolute risk reduction 3%, RRR 19% and NNT 34 over a mean of 3.5 years).[18] No increased risk of cardiac events was reported in the dipyridamole/ASA groups in either study; however, a higher daily dose of ASA may be desirable in patients with concomitant coronary artery disease. The addition of ASA 81 mg to the dipyridamole/ASA combination appears reasonable in these patients, though the efficacy and safety of this measure are unknown.

Anticoagulants

Vitamin K Antagonists

Oral anticoagulants prevent cerebral and systemic emboli in patients with acute MI, valvular and nonvalvular atrial fibrillation and prosthetic cardiac valves. The risk of bleeding is influenced by many factors (e.g., the intensity of anticoagulation, concomitant use of high doses of ASA or other drugs with antiplatelet effects).[19] Vitamin K antagonist (**nicoumalone, warfarin**) therapy is superior to clopidogrel plus ASA for prevention of vascular events in patients with atrial fibrillation at high risk for stroke.[20] Patients with nonvalvular atrial fibrillation and prior TIA/stroke may require a higher target INR of 3 instead of 2.5.[21]

Novel Anticoagulants

Dabigatran, a direct thrombin inhibitor, is approved for the prevention of systemic embolism in patients with nonvalvular atrial fibrillation based on the results of the RE-LY study.[22] **Rivaroxaban** and **apixaban**, oral factor Xa inhibitors, are also approved for this indication.[23,24] Most clinical practice guidelines[5,25,26] consider these novel anticoagulants useful alternatives to warfarin for stroke prevention. In many cases, these agents are suggested as a first choice, especially for patients in whom anticoagulant therapy needs to be initiated. Overall, they have similar or superior efficacy for the prevention of ischemic events and a comparable if not better safety profile, in particular for hemorrhagic strokes. Cautious patient selection is important, especially in elderly patients with renal insufficiency in whom renal function monitoring is advised. The absence of a specific agent to reverse the antithrombotic effect of these agents could be problematic in certain circumstances (e.g., urgent surgery).

Therapeutic Tips

- In most cases, antithrombotic treatment should be continued long term, especially in older individuals with atherosclerosis and vascular risk factors.
- **Dipyridamole/ASA** appears to be more protective than ASA alone in patients with a *recent* cerebral ischemic event. For the prevention of *recurrent* stroke, **dipyridamole/ASA** and **clopidogrel** appear to provide comparable protection.[27]
- It is common practice to switch treatment to **dipyridamole/ASA** or **clopidogrel** in patients who experience *recurrent* attacks of cerebral ischemia while on low-dose ASA (325 mg/day or less), although this has not been validated in clinical trials.
- It is common practice to prescribe the combination of **low-dose ASA** (81 mg/day) **plus an oral anticoagulant** in patients who have *new events* on an anticoagulant alone and who are at risk for a cardioembolic stroke, although this has not been validated in clinical trials. Follow such patients very closely, as the risk for hemorrhagic complications is increased.
- Combination therapy (**oral anticoagulant plus low-dose ASA**) is superior to anticoagulant alone in patients with prosthetic heart valves but carries an increased risk of bleeding episodes. For patients *intolerant* of ASA, **dipyridamole** (400 mg/day) plus an oral anticoagulant may be used. This approach has not been validated in clinical trials.
- In healthy postmenopausal women, the risks associated with combination **estrogen/progestin** therapy (increased risk of coronary heart disease and breast cancer and a 40% increase in stroke risk) exceed the beneficial effects on colorectal cancer and hip fracture.[28]

- In postmenopausal women who have suffered a recent stroke or TIA, hormonal therapy with **estrogen** does not have a protective effect.[29]
- The risk of ischemic stroke is increased in users of **low-dose oral contraceptives** compared with nonusers. This translates into a relatively small increase in the absolute risk of stroke,[30] except possibly in the presence of other risk factors such as hypertension, smoking and prior thromboembolic events. In these settings, oral contraceptives should probably be avoided. See Chapter 70 for a full discussion of contraceptive options.

Suggested Readings

Antithrombotic Trialists' Collaboration. Collaborative meta-analysis of randomised trials of antiplatelet therapy for prevention of death, myocardial infarction, and stroke in high risk patients. *BMJ* 2002;324(7329):71-86.

Furie KL, Kasner SE, Adams RJ et al. Guidelines for the prevention of stroke in patients with stroke or transient ischemic attack: a guideline for healthcare professionals from the American Heart Association/American Stroke Association. *Stroke* 2011;42(1):227-76.

Goldstein LB, Bushnell CD, Adams RJ et al. Guidelines for the primary prevention of stroke: a guideline for healthcare professionals from the American Heart Association/American Stroke Association. *Stroke* 2011;42(2):517-84.

Hart RG, Pearce LA, Aguilar MI. Meta-analysis: antithrombotic therapy to prevent stroke in patients who have nonvalvular atrial fibrillation. *Ann Intern Med* 2007;146(12):857-67.

Katsnelson M, Sacco RL, Moscucci M. Progress for stroke prevention with atrial fibrillation: emergence of alternative oral anticoagulants. *Circulation* 2012;125(12):1577-83.

Lansberg MG, O'Donnell MJ, Khatri P et al. Antithrombotic and thrombolytic therapy for ischemic stroke: Antithrombotic Therapy and Prevention of Thrombosis, 9th ed: American College of Chest Physicians Evidence-Based Clinical Practice Guidelines. *Chest* 2012;141(2 Suppl):e601S-36S.

Table 1: **Drugs Used in Secondary Prevention of Stroke**

Class	Drug	Dose	Adverse Effects	Drug Interactions	Comments	Cost[a]
Anticoagulants	*apixaban* Eliquis	Usual: 5 mg BID po If serum creatinine >133 mmol/L and patient either >80 years of age or ≤60 kg: 2.5 mg BID po	Bleeding.	Contraindicated in combination with strong inhibitors of both CYP3A4 and P-gp, e.g., itraconazole, ritonavir.	Not recommended when ClCr <15 mL/min or in patients undergoing dialysis.	$$$$$
	dabigatran Pradaxa	Usual: 150 mg BID po Patients with increased bleeding risk or >80 years of age: 110 mg BID po	Bleeding, gastric intolerance.	Combination with strong inhibitors of P-gp (e.g., ketoconazole) contraindicated. Caution with other drugs acting on P-gp.	Contraindicated when ClCr <30 mL/min.	$$$$$
	nicoumalone Sintrom	Oral: Dose to maintain INR between 2 and 3 for most cerebrovascular indications; for stroke prevention in certain **high-risk patients with mechanical heart valves**, maintain INR between 2.5 and 3.5	Bleeding. Skin necrosis.	Many potential interactions. Substrate for CYP2C9 and other isoenzymes.[b]	Coumarin anticoagulants are contraindicated in pregnancy.	$$$
	rivaroxaban Xarelto	20 mg daily po Use 15 mg daily po if ClCr 30–49 mL/min	Bleeding.	Contraindicated in combination with strong inhibitors of both CYP3A4 and P-gp, e.g., itraconazole, ritonavir.	Not recommended when ClCr <30 mL/min.	$$$$
	warfarin Coumadin, generics	Oral: Dose to maintain INR between 2 and 3 for most cerebrovascular indications; for stroke prevention in certain **high-risk patients with mechanical heart valves**, maintain INR between 2.5 and 3.5	See nicoumalone.	See nicoumalone.	See nicoumalone.	$
Antiplatelet Agents	*ASA* Aspirin, Coated Aspirin, generics	50–325 mg/day po	Bleeding, usually minor (epistaxis, etc.). Gastric intolerance, GI bleeding (gastric ulcers, erosions), nausea, heartburn, constipation, tinnitus usually dose-related.	Hemorrhagic risk increased with concomitant use of anticoagulants.		$

(cont'd)

Table 1: Drugs Used in Secondary Prevention of Stroke *(cont'd)*

Class	Drug	Dose	Adverse Effects	Drug Interactions	Comments	Cost[a]
	clopidogrel Plavix, generics	75 mg daily po	Bleeding, usually minor. Skin rash (4%), diarrhea (5%).	See ASA.		$$
	dipyridamole/ASA 200/25 mg Aggrenox	1 capsule BID po	Bleeding, usually minor. Headache, diarrhea.	See ASA.		$$$
	ticlopidine generics	250 mg BID po	Bleeding, usually minor. Diarrhea (up to 20%), skin rash, neutropenia.	See ASA. Reduced digoxin levels. Absorption reduced by antacids.	Contraindicated in severe hepatic impairment.	$$

[a] Cost of 30-day supply of usual dose; includes drug cost only.
[b] Clinically significant warfarin interactions listed in Chapter 48, Table 3.
Dosage adjustment may be required in renal impairment; see Appendix I.
Abbreviations: ASA = acetylsalicylic acid; ClCr = creatine clearance; CYP = cytochrome P450; GI = gastrointestinal; INR = International Normalized Ratio; P-gp = P-glycoprotein
Legend: $ <$10 $$ $10–40 $$$ $40–70 $$$$ $70–100 $$$$$ $100–130

References

1. Johnston SC, Rothwell PM, Nguyen-Huynh MN et al. Validation and refinement of scores to predict very early stroke risk after transient ischaemic attack. *Lancet* 2007;369(9558):283-92.
2. Mackey AE, Abrahamowicz M, Langlois Y et al. Outcome of asymptomatic patients with carotid disease. Asymptomatic Cervical Bruit Study Group. *Neurology* 1997;48(4):896-903.
3. Goldstein LB, Bushnell CD, Adams RJ et al. Guidelines for the primary prevention of stroke: a guideline for healthcare professionals from the American Heart Association/American Stroke Association. *Stroke* 2011;42(2):517-84.
4. Antithrombotic Trialists' Collaboration. Collaborative meta-analysis of randomised trials of antiplatelet therapy for prevention of death, myocardial infarction, and stroke in high risk patients. *BMJ* 2002;324(7329):71-86.
5. Lansberg MG, O'Donnell MJ, Khatri P et al. Antithrombotic and thrombolytic therapy for ischemic stroke: Antithrombotic Therapy and Prevention of Thrombosis, 9th ed: American College of Chest Physicians Evidence-Based Clinical Practice Guidelines. *Chest* 2012;141(2 Suppl):e601S-36S.
6. Amarenco P, Bogousslavsky J, Callahan A et al. High-dose atorvastatin after stroke or transient ischemic attack. *N Engl J Med* 2006;355(6):549-59.
7. Chapman N, Huxley R, Anderson C et al. Effects of a perindopril-based blood pressure-lowering regimen on the risk of recurrent stroke according to stroke subtype and medical history: the PROGRESS Trial. *Stroke* 2004;35(1):116-21.
8. Algra A, van Gijn J. Cumulative meta-analysis of aspirin efficacy after cerebral ischemia of arterial origin. *J Neurol Neurosurg Psychiatry* 1999;66(2):255.
9. Dentali F, Douketis JD, Lim W et al. Combined aspirin-oral anticoagulant therapy compared with oral anticoagulant therapy alone among patients at risk for cardiovascular disease: a meta-analysis of randomized trials. *Arch Intern Med* 2007;167(2):117-24.
10. Whitlock RP, Sun JC, Fremes SE et al. Antithrombotic and thrombolytic therapy for valvular disease: Antithrombotic Therapy and Prevention of Thrombosis, 9th ed: American College of Chest Physicians Evidence-Based Clinical Practice Guidelines. *Chest* 2012;141(2 Suppl):e576S-e600S.
11. CAPRIE Steering Committee. A randomised, blinded, trial of clopidogrel versus aspirin in patients at risk of ischaemic events (CAPRIE). *Lancet* 1996;348(9038):1329-39.
12. Diener HC, Bogousslavsky J, Brass LM et al. Aspirin and clopidogrel compared with clopidogrel alone after recent ischaemic stroke or transient ischaemic attack in high-risk patients (MATCH): randomised, double-blind, placebo-controlled trial. *Lancet* 2004;364(9431):331-7.
13. Bhatt DL, Fox KA, Hacke W et al. Clopidogrel and aspirin versus aspirin alone for the prevention of atherothrombotic events. *N Engl J Med* 2006;354(16):1706-17.
14. SPS3 Investigators, Benavente OR, Hart RG et al. Effects of clopidogrel added to aspirin in patients with recent lacunar stroke. *N Engl J Med* 2012;367(9):817-25.
15. Canadian Stroke Network. *Canadian best practice recommendations for stroke care.* 4th ed. Available from: www.strokebestpractices.ca/wp-content/uploads/2012/10/20120BPR_Ch2_Prevention_Final-Version_20Sept-2012F-12.pdf. Accessed November 8, 2013.
16. Hass WK, Easton JD, Adams HP et al. A randomized trial comparing ticlopidine hydrochloride with aspirin for the prevention of stroke in high-risk patients. Ticlopidine Aspirin Stroke Study Group. *N Engl J Med* 1989;321(8):501-7.
17. Diener HC, Cunha L, Forbes C et al. European Stroke Prevention Study. 2. Dipyridamole and acetylsalicylic acid in the secondary prevention of stroke. *J Neurol Sci* 1996;143(1-2):1-13.
18. ESPRIT Study Group; Halkes PH, van Gijn J et al. Aspirin plus dipyridamole versus aspirin alone after cerebral ischaemia of arterial origin (ESPRIT): randomised controlled trial. *Lancet* 2006;367(9523):1665-73.
19. You JJ, Singer DE, Howard PA et al. Antithrombotic therapy for atrial fibrillation: Antithrombotic Therapy and Prevention of Thrombosis, 9th ed: American College of Chest Physicians Evidence-Based Clinical Practice Guidelines. *Chest* 2012;141(2 Suppl):e531S-75S.
20. ACTIVE Writing Group of the ACTIVE Investigators, Connolly S, Pogue J et al. Clopidogrel plus aspirin versus oral anticoagulation for atrial fibrillation in the Atrial fibrillation Clopidogrel Trial with Irbesartan for prevention of Vascular Events (ACTIVE W): a randomised controlled trial. *Lancet* 2006;367(9526):1903-12.
21. The European Atrial Fibrillation Trial Study Group. Optimal oral anticoagulant therapy in patients with nonrheumatic atrial fibrillation and recent cerebral ischemia. *N Engl J Med* 1995;333(1):5-10.
22. Connolly SJ, Ezekowitz MD, Yusuf S et al. Dabigatran versus warfarin in patients with atrial fibrillation. *N Engl J Med* 2009;361(12):1139-51.
23. Patel MR, Mahaffey KW, Garg J et al. Rivaroxaban versus warfarin in nonvalvular atrial fibrillation. *N Engl J Med* 2011;365(10):883-91.
24. Granger CB, Alexander JH, McMurray JJ et al. Apixaban versus warfarin in patients with atrial fibrillation. *N Engl J Med* 2011;365(11):981-92.
25. Skanes AC, Healey JS, Cairns JA et al. Focused 2012 update of the Canadian Cardiovascular Society atrial fibrillation guidelines: recommendations for stroke prevention and rate/rhythm control. *Can J Cardiol* 2012;28(2):125-36.
26. De Caterina R, Husted S, Wallentin L et al. New oral anticoagulants in atrial fibrillation and acute coronary syndromes. *J Am Coll Cardiol* 2012;59(16):1413-25.
27. Sacco RL, Diener HC, Yusuf S et al. Aspirin and extended-release dipyridamole versus clopidogrel for recurrent stroke. *N Engl J Med* 2008;359(12):1238-51.
28. Rossouw JE, Anderson GL, Prentice RL et al. Risks and benefits of estrogen plus progestin in healthy postmenopausal women: principal results from the Women's Health Initiative randomized controlled trial. *JAMA* 2002;288(3):321-33.
29. Viscoli CM, Brass LM, Kernan WN et al. A clinical trial of estrogen-replacement therapy after ischemic stroke. *N Engl J Med* 2001;345(17):1243-9.
30. Gillum LA, Mamidipudi SK, Johnston SC. Ischemic stroke risk with oral contraceptives: a meta-analysis. *JAMA* 2000;284(1):72-8.

Chapter 43
Primary Prevention of Vascular Disease

Tania Mysak, BSP, PharmD

Vascular disease remains a top contributor to morbidity and mortality in Canada. Although improvements have been made, it is well recognized that many modifiable risk factors are undertreated, leaving a care gap with costly consequences for our health care system.[1,2]

Prevention of morbidity and mortality from vascular disease requires early recognition and management of modifiable risk factors such as poor diet, sedentary lifestyle, obesity, elevated blood pressure, elevated cholesterol, diabetes mellitus and smoking.

Primary prevention of vascular disease involves management of risk factors before the patient suffers a vascular event such as MI or stroke.[3] While the data supporting pharmacologic therapies in secondary prevention of vascular disease (management of risk factors after the patient has suffered a vascular event) are fairly robust, evidence supporting primary prevention strategies is relatively sparse in comparison.

Goals of Therapy

- Prevent vascular events, including MI, stroke or amputation
- Prevent vascular mortality
- Minimize adverse effects from drug therapy
- Preserve quality of life

Investigations

- For all adults >18 years, determine the following at all appropriate visits:[4]
  - blood pressure using standardized techniques[5]
  - smoking status[3]
  - patient weight, waist circumference and body mass index (BMI)[3,4]
- All men ≥40 years, all women who are postmenopausal or ≥50 years, and any adult with vascular risk factors such as diabetes mellitus, cigarette smoking, hypertension, obesity and/or a family history of premature coronary artery disease should:
  - have a lipid profile done every 1–3 years. More frequent screening is recommended for patients with abnormal values or those requiring treatment[6]
  - be screened for peripheral arterial disease (PAD) on the basis of symptoms and measurement of the ankle-brachial index (ABI).[6,7,8] This recommendation is controversial. The ABI is the ratio of systolic blood pressure in the dorsalis pedis or posterior tibial artery to the systolic blood pressure in the brachial artery and is performed using a blood pressure cuff assisted by an ultrasound Doppler device instead of a stethoscope. An ABI <0.9 is indicative of PAD
- Screen all individuals ≥40 years for type 2 diabetes by measuring fasting plasma glucose every 3 years. Consider more frequent and/or earlier testing in people with first-degree relatives with diabetes, members of high-risk populations (e.g., Aboriginal, Hispanic, Asian, South Asian or African) and those with hypertension, dyslipidemia, obesity or schizophrenia[9]

- Calculate the patient's cardiovascular risk (see Chapter 37, Figure 2). Management of the patient depends on their risk score. Individuals over age 40 with diabetes mellitus type 1 or type 2 or those >30 years with a >15-year history of diabetes are considered "high-risk".[6,9]
- Rule out secondary causes of elevated blood glucose (see Chapter 32), dyslipidemia (see Chapter 37) and hypertension (see Chapter 39)

Therapeutic Choices

Nonpharmacologic Choices

- Lifestyle modification including weight loss, increased physical activity, reduced sodium intake and adherence to the DASH (Dietary Approaches to Stop Hypertension) diet can improve control of risk factors and potentially reduce vascular risk.[10,11,12,13,14,15]
- Based primarily on observational studies and supported by a recent randomized trial,[16] current guidelines recommend a diet that emphasizes fruits, vegetables, fish, whole grains and low-fat dairy products, and limits intake of saturated and trans fatty acids, simple sugars and refined carbohydrates.[5,6,7,11,17]
- Encourage regular physical activity to maintain physical fitness, vascular health and optimal body weight and to sustain weight loss. Most guidelines suggest 30–60 minutes of moderate intensity exercise (walking, jogging, cycling or swimming) 4–7 days of the week.[18]
- Encourage patients to achieve and maintain a healthy body weight (BMI of 18.5–24.9 kg/m^2).[3,5,6] Bariatric surgery may be required for the morbidly obese.[19]
- Counsel patients to stop using tobacco and minimize exposure to second-hand smoke.[20] Nonpharmacologic therapies may include psychological counselling.
- Limit alcohol intake to a maximum of 2 standard drinks per day for men and 1 standard drink per day for women.[3]

Pharmacologic Choices

Absolute risk reductions (ARR) for primary preventive strategies are small compared with secondary preventive strategies. Refer to Table 1 for the ARR and number needed to treat (NNT) to prevent vascular events with the pharmacologic therapies discussed below.

Hypertension

Lowering blood pressure (BP) with antihypertensive therapy reduces the relative risk of a first major vascular event by ~20–40% when compared with placebo.[21,22] Larger reductions in BP produce larger reductions in risk.[23] ARR are small (Table 1); however, the higher the baseline BP, the greater the potential benefits of reduction.[24] In the absence of other vascular risk factors (e.g., age >55, male gender, positive family history, abdominal obesity) or macrovascular target organ damage, antihypertensive treatment should be initiated if the average BP is ≥160/100 mm Hg. In the presence of target organ damage or other vascular risk factors, treatment should be initiated if the average BP is ≥140/90 mm Hg. The target BP is <140/90 mm Hg, except in patients with diabetes mellitus where the target BP is <130/80 mm Hg.[5] The choice of antihypertensive agent is less important than achieving target BP. See Chapter 39 for current recommendations on the choice of antihypertensive agents.

Dyslipidemia

Cholesterol-lowering therapy with **HMG-CoA reductase inhibitors (statins)** reduces the relative risk of a first major vascular event by ~15–30% (Table 1) when compared with placebo.[25,26,27,28] Statins provide similar relative risk reductions in primary and secondary prevention trials, but with smaller absolute reductions in primary prevention, resulting in larger NNTs.[25,26,27,28] The primary goal of therapy is reduction of LDL-C, with the specific target number based on individual patient risk (see Chapter 37, Figure 1). While controversial, current guidelines recommend patients at low risk should target an LDL-C reduction of >50%, and for those at intermediate or high risk the target LDL-C is <2 mmol/L or, if that cannot be achieved, a reduction of >50% from baseline.[6] The lower LDL target for high-risk individuals is based on secondary prevention trials, and the routine use of statins in low and intermediate-risk individuals is controversial.[6,25,26,27,28] Data for aggressive LDL reduction in primary prevention are limited.

Most patients are able to achieve target levels of LDL-C on statin monotherapy, however, some patients may require combination therapy to achieve targets. Evidence is lacking for the use of agents other than statins in primary prevention. See Chapter 37 for current recommendations on the choice of antihyperlipidemic agents.

Diabetes Mellitus

The target HbA_{1c} for most patients with type 1 or type 2 diabetes is ≤7%.[9] Such tight control of blood glucose reduces the risk of microvascular complications (e.g., retinopathy or nephropathy), but evidence linking tight glycemic control to prevention of macrovascular complications is less robust, particularly in type 2 diabetes.[29,30,31,32] The Canadian Diabetes Association guidelines provide an algorithm to assist in evidence-based choices for drug therapy.[9] See Chapter 32 for current recommendations on the choice of antihyperglycemic agents.

Antithrombotics

The role of antiplatelet therapy in primary prevention of vascular disease is controversial. A meta-analysis of data from 6 major primary prevention trials suggests that **ASA** reduces the annual risk of a "serious vascular event" from 0.57% to 0.51%, primarily due to a reduction in the annual risk of MI from 0.23% to 0.18%. This benefit is offset by an increase in the annual risk of major GI and extracranial bleeding from 0.07% to 0.1%. The risk of stroke or vascular mortality was not significantly reduced by ASA.[33] Various guidelines make weak to moderate recommendations for using ASA 75–162 mg/day in some patients at "moderate risk" (defined as 10-year CV risk >10% according to Framingham Risk Score) if or when the potential benefit outweighs the risk of bleeding.[3,34,35] Risk factors for bleeding include age, sex, upper GI pain, history of ulcers, NSAID use, uncontrolled hypertension and concomitant use of anticoagulants.[35]

The lack of agreement and clarity in the guidelines reflect the current controversies. The impact of age, gender and diabetes on potential benefits and risks of ASA in primary prevention are still unclear.[33,36,37] At this time a standard recommendation for use of ASA that applies to all persons cannot be made.

Patients with atrial fibrillation are at high risk for cardioembolic stroke and may be candidates for anticoagulation (**apixaban**, **dabigatran**, **rivaroxaban** or **warfarin**) therapy to prevent a first stroke or transient ischemic attack (TIA). $CHADS_2$ is a risk assessment tool that can be used to stratify patients by their risk of stroke on the basis of risk factors including congestive heart failure ("C"), hypertension ("H"), age >75 years ("A"), diabetes mellitus ("D") and history of stroke or TIA ("S").[38] ASA 75–325 mg daily is an alternative to warfarin for low-risk patients.[38,39] A complete description of $CHADS_2$ is provided in Chapter 45.

Smoking Cessation

Observational studies suggest that the elevated vascular risk induced by cigarette smoking can be decreased by quitting and reversed after 5 years of abstinence.[40] Successful smoking cessation can be enhanced by **nicotine replacement therapy** (NRT) (gum, patch, inhalers, lozenges), **bupropion** and **varenicline**. Bupropion and NRT are roughly equivalent in terms of efficacy, and either varenicline or the combination of bupropion and NRT may provide higher success rates.[41,42,43]

Nonpharmacologic interventions, in combination with pharmacologic therapies, are effective in optimizing success rates and may be superior to pharmacologic therapies alone.[42] See Chapter 13 for current recommendations on the choice of nonpharmacologic and pharmacologic therapies.

Obesity

Orlistat is approved for obesity management. It produces a 5–10% weight loss that is maintained over 2 years in ~60% of patients; however, the impact of drug-induced weight loss of this magnitude on vascular morbidity and mortality is unknown.[44] Discontinuation of orlistat generally leads to weight regain; therefore, effective management must focus on lifestyle changes. Drug therapy should be regarded as a therapeutic trial and stopped if significant weight loss is not achieved after several months.[45] See Chapter 33 for current recommendations on the choice of nonpharmacologic and pharmacologic therapies.

Nutritional Supplements

There is no conclusive evidence that omega-3 fatty acid supplementation reduces vascular risk, although dietary recommendations suggest including foods rich in omega-3 fatty acids in a balanced diet.[46,47] Interpretation of data regarding **omega-3 fatty acids** (found in oily fish and plants) is hindered by poor study design. Reduction of risk by vitamin therapy (e.g., folic acid, vitamin E) in patients with established vascular disease has largely been shown to be ineffective, and current data do not support supplementation in primary prevention.[48,49,50,51,52,53,54,55]

Hormone Therapy (HT)

Women should not be encouraged to continue HT if the sole reason is vascular protection. While observational data suggested a vascular risk reduction benefit of hormone therapy in postmenopausal women, experimental data have refuted that claim.[56] Further discussion of hormone therapy can be found in Chapter 75.

Therapeutic Tips

- View every patient encounter as an opportunity to identify risk factors, discuss risk factor modification and encourage patient progress. Recent guidelines emphasize an approach that is multifaceted and includes cognitive and behavioural therapies, individual and group-based strategies, and consideration of cultural and social context variables that may influence behavioural change.[57]
- Consider nonpharmacologic management to be the most essential component of risk reduction strategies. Drugs can have adverse effects. Patients suitable for primary prevention have not yet experienced symptoms of disease and may not wish to be "medicalized."
- Individualize patient goals based on the risk of having an event. The comparatively small absolute benefits of many drug therapies for primary prevention warrant discussion with patients regarding their personal health goals. Long-term adherence to drug therapy will be required to obtain any significant benefit.
- Patients must make the link between risk factors and potential consequences (major vascular events). Stress the importance of risk factor reduction to prevent MI and stroke, not simply to reduce surrogate markers (e.g., cholesterol, blood pressure).
- Pharmacologic choices should include consideration of significant cost differences among therapies that are equally effective.

Table 1: **Primary Prevention of Coronary Events and Stroke**

Outcome Prevented	Intervention	Comparator	ARR (%)	NNT	Potential Risks
Coronary event[58]	Antihypertensive therapy	Placebo	0.7[a]	143 over 4–5 years	Symptoms of hypotension Side effects of drug therapy
Coronary event[26]	Statin	Placebo	1.3	77 over 4–5 years	Rhabdomyolysis 0.2% per year[59]
Coronary event[33]	ASA	Placebo	0.06	1666 over 1 year	GI bleed 1% per year[60]
Stroke[58]	Antihypertensive therapy	Placebo	1.3	77 over 4–5 years	Symptoms of hypotension Side effects of drug therapy
Stroke[26]	Statin	Placebo	0.4	250 over 4 years	Rhabdomyolysis 0.2% per year[59]
Stroke[33]	ASA	Placebo	NS	NS	GI bleed 1% per year[60]

[a] Absolute benefits are correlated with baseline risk.[24]
Abbreviations: ARR = absolute risk reduction; NNT = number needed to treat to prevent one outcome; NS = not significant

Suggested Readings

Abramson BL, Huckell V, Anand S et al. Canadian Cardiovascular Society Consensus Conference: peripheral arterial disease—executive summary. *Can J Cardiol* 2005;21(12):997-1006.

Anderson TJ, Gregoire J, Hegele RA et al. 2012 update of the Canadian Cardiovascular Society guidelines for the diagnosis and treatment of dyslipidemia for the prevention of cardiovascular disease in the adult. *Can J Cardiol* 2013;29(2):151-67.

Canadian Diabetes Association Clinical Practice Guidelines Expert Committee. Canadian Diabetes Association 2013 clinical practice guidelines for the prevention and management of diabetes in Canada. *Can J Diabetes* 2013;37(Suppl 1):S1-212.

Hypertension Canada. *Canadian Hypertension Education Program (CHEP) 2013 recommendations*. Available from: www.hypertension.ca.

Lau DC, Douketis JD, Morrison KM et al. 2006 Canadian clinical practice guidelines on the management and prevention of obesity in adults and children [summary]. *CMAJ* 2007;176(8):S1-13.

References

1. Wilkins K, Campell N, Joffres M et al. Blood pressure in Canadian adults. Ottawa (ON): Statistics Canada. *Health Reports* 2010;21(1):1-11. Available from: www.statcan.gc.ca/pub/82-003-x/2010001/article/11118-eng.pdf. Accessed March 30, 2011.
2. McLean DL, Simpson SH, McAlister FA et al. Treatment and blood pressure control in 47,964 people with diabetes and hypertension: a systematic review of observational studies. *Can J Cardiol* 2006;22(10):855-60.
3. Pearson TA, Blair SN, Daniels SR et al. AHA Guidelines for Primary Prevention of Cardiovascular Disease and Stroke: 2002 Update: Consensus Panel Guide to Comprehensive Risk Reduction for Adult Patients Without Coronary or Other Atherosclerotic Vascular Diseases. American Heart Association Science Advisory and Coordinating Committee. *Circulation* 2002;106(3):388-91.
4. Redberg RF, Benjamin EJ, Bittner V et al. AHA/ACCF 2009 Performance measures for primary prevention of cardiovascular disease in adults: a report of the American College of Cardiology Foundation/American Heart Association Task Force on performance measures (writing committee to develop performance measures for primary prevention of cardiovascular disease). *Circulation* 2009;120(13):1296-336.
5. Hypertension Canada. *Canadian Hypertension Education Program (CHEP) 2013 recommendations*. Available from: www.hypertension.ca. Accessed April 23, 2013.
6. Anderson TJ, Gregoire J, Hegele RA et al. 2012 update of the Canadian Cardiovascular Society guidelines for the diagnosis and treatment of dyslipidemia for the prevention of cardiovascular disease in the adult. *Can J Cardiol* 2013;29(2):151-67.
7. Abramson BL, Huckell V, Anand S et al. Canadian Cardiovascular Society Consensus Conference: peripheral arterial disease-executive summary. *Can J Cardiol* 2005;21(12):997-1006.
8. Beckman JA, Jaff MR, Creager MA. The United States preventive services task force recommendation statement on screening for peripheral arterial disease: more harm than benefit? *Circulation* 2006;114(8):861-6.
9. Canadian Diabetes Association Clinical Practice Guidelines Expert Committee. Canadian Diabetes Association 2013 clinical practice guidelines for the prevention and management of diabetes in Canada. *Can J Diabetes* 2013;37(Suppl 1):S1-212.
10. Elmer PJ, Obarzanek E, Vollmer WM et al. Effects of comprehensive lifestyle modification on diet, weight, physical fitness and blood pressure control: 18-month results of a randomized trial. *Ann Intern Med* 2006;144(7):485-95.
11. Appel LJ, Moore TJ, Obarzanek E et al. A clinical trial of the effects of dietary patterns on blood pressure. DASH Collaborative Research Group. *N Engl J Med* 1997;336(16):1117-24.
12. Diabetes Prevention Program Research Group, Knowler WC, Fowler SE et al. 10-year follow-up of diabetes incidence and weight loss in the Diabetes Prevention Program Outcomes Study. *Lancet* 2009;374(9702):1677-86.
13. Forman JP, Stampfer MJ, Curhan GC. Diet and lifestyle risk factors associated with incident hypertension in women. *JAMA* 2009;302(4):401-11.
14. Blumenthal J, Babyak M, Hinderliter A et al. Effects of the DASH diet alone and in combination with exercise and weight loss on blood pressure and cardiovascular biomarkers in men and women with high blood pressure: the ENCORE study. *Arch Intern Med* 2010;170(2):126-35.
15. Maruthur N, Wang NY, Appel JL. Lifestyle interventions reduce coronary heart disease risk: results from the PREMIER trial. *Circulation* 2009;119(15):2026-31.
16. Estruch R, Ros E, Salas-Salvadó J et al. Primary prevention of cardiovascular disease with a Mediterranean diet. *N Engl J Med* 2013;368(14):1279-90.
17. Health Canada. *Eating well with Canada's food guide*. Ottawa (ON): Health Canada; 2007. Available from: www.hc-sc.gc.ca/fn-an/food-guide-aliment/index-eng.php. Accessed March 30, 2011.
18. American Heart Association Nutrition Committee; Lichtenstein AH, Appel LJ, Brands M et al. Diet and lifestyle recommendations revision 2006: a scientific statement from the American Heart Association Nutrition Committee. *Circulation* 2006;114(1):82-96.
19. Kral JG. ABC of obesity. Management part III–surgery. *BMJ* 2006;333(7574):900-3.
20. A clinical practice guideline for treating tobacco use and dependence: A US Public Health Service report. The Tobacco Use and Dependence Clinical Practice Guideline Panel, Staff, and Consortium Representatives. *JAMA* 2000;283(24):3244-54.
21. Neal B, MacMahon S, Chapman N et al. Effects of ACE inhibitors, calcium antagonists, and other blood-pressure-lowering drugs: results of prospectively designed overviews of randomised trials. Blood Pressure Lowering Treatment Trialists' Collaboration. *Lancet* 2000;355(9246):1955-64.
22. Turnbull F; Blood Pressure Lowering Treatment Trialists' Collaboration. Effects of different blood-pressure-lowering regimens on major cardiovascular events: results of prospectively designed overviews of randomized trials. *Lancet* 2003;632(9395):1527-35.
23. Law MR, Morris JK, Wald NJ. Use of blood pressure lowering drugs in the prevention of cardiovascular disease: meta-analysis of 147 randomised trials in the context of expectations from prospective epidemiological studies. *BMJ* 2009;338:b1665.
24. Ogden L, He J, Lydick E et al. Long-term absolute benefit of lowering blood pressure in hypertensive patients according to JNC VI risk stratification. *Hypertension* 2000;35(2):539-43.

25. Cholesterol Treatment Trialists' (CTT) Collaborators, Mihaylova B, Emberson J et al. The effects of lowering LDL cholesterol with statin therapy in people at low risk of vascular disease: meta-analysis of individual data from 27 randomised trials. *Lancet* 2012;380(9841):581-90.
26. Brugts JJ, Yetgin T, Hoeks SE et al. The benefits of statins in people without established cardiovascular disease but with cardiovascular risk factors : meta-analysis of randomised controlled trials. *BMJ* 2009;330:b2376.
27. Mills EJ, Rachlis B, Wu P et al. Primary prevention of cardiovascular mortality and events with statin treatments: a network meta-analysis involving more than 65,000 patients. *J Am Coll Cardiol* 2008;52(22):1769-81.
28. Ray KK, Seshasai SR, Erqou S et al. Statins and all-cause mortality in high-risk primary prevention. *Arch Intern Med* 2010;170(12):1024-31.
29. Intensive blood-glucose control with sulphonylureas or insulin compared with conventional treatment and risk of complications in patients with type 2 diabetes (UKPDS 33). UK Prospective Diabetes Study (UKPDS) Group. *Lancet* 1998;352(9131):837-53.
30. Nathan DM, Cleary PA, Blacklund JY et al. Intensive diabetes treatment and cardiovascular disease in patients with type 1 diabetes. *N Eng J Med* 2005;353(25):2643-53.
31. ADVANCE Collaborative Group, Patel A, MacMahon et al. Intensive blood glucose control and vascular outcomes in patients with type 2 diabetes. The ADVANCE Collaborative Group. *N Engl J Med* 2008;358(24):2560-72.
32. Action to Control Cardiovascular Risk in Diabetes Study Group, Gerstein HC, Miller ME et al. Effects of intensive glucose lowering in type 2 diabetes. *N Engl J Med* 2008;358(24):2545-59.
33. Antithrombotic Trialists' (ATT) Collaboration, Baigent C, Blackwell L et al. Aspirin in the primary and secondary prevention of vascular disease: collaborative meta-analysis of individual participant data from randomised trials. *Lancet* 2009;373(9678):1849-60.
34. Vandvik PO, Lincoff AM, Gore JM et al. Primary and secondary prevention of cardiovascular disease: Antithrombotic Therapy and Prevention of Thrombosis, 9th ed: American College of Chest Physicians Evidence-Based Clinical Practice Guidelines. *Chest* 2012;141(2 Suppl):e637S-68S.
35. U.S. Preventive Services Task Force. Aspirin for the prevention of cardiovascular disease: U.S. Preventive Services Task Force recommendation statement. *Ann Intern Med* 2009;150(6):396-404.
36. Berger JS, Roncaglioni MC, Avanzini F et al. Aspirin for the primary prevention of cardiovascular events in women and men; a sex specific meta-analysis of randomized controlled trials. *JAMA* 2006;295(3):306-13.
37. Pignone M, Alberts MJ, Colwell JA et al. Aspirin for primary prevention of cardiovascular events in people with diabetes: a position statement of the American Diabetes Association, a scientific statement of the American Heart Association, and an expert consensus document of the American College of Cardiology Foundation. *Circulation* 2010;121(24):2694-701.
38. Goldstein LB, Bushnell CD, Adams RJ et al. Guidelines for the primary prevention of stroke: a guideline for healthcare professionals from the American Heart Association/American Stroke Association. *Stroke* 2011;42(2):517-84.
39. Lansberg MG, O'Donnell MJ, Khatri P et al. Antithrombotic and thrombolytic therapy for ischemic stroke: Antithrombotic Therapy and Prevention of Thrombosis, 9th ed: American College of Chest Physicians Evidence-Based Clinical Practice Guidelines. *Chest* 2012;141(2 Suppl):e601S-36S.
40. Wolf PA, D'Agostino RB, Kannel WB et al. Cigarette smoking as a risk factor for stroke. The Framingham Study. *JAMA* 1988;259(7):1025-9.
41. Okuyemi KS, Nollen NL, Ahluwalia JS. Interventions to facilitate smoking cessation. *Am Fam Physician* 2006;74(2):262-71.
42. Ranney L, Melvin C, Lux L et al. Systematic review: smoking cessation intervention strategies for adults and adults in special populations. *Ann Intern Med* 2006;145(11):845-56.
43. Wu P, Wilson K, Dimoulas P et al. Effectiveness of smoking cessation therapies: a systematic review and meta-analysis. *BMC Public Health* 2006;6:300.
44. Padwal RS, Majumdar SR. Drug treatments for obesity: orlistat, sibutramine, and rimonabant. *Lancet* 2007;369(9555):71-7.
45. Lean M, Finer N. ABC of obesity. Management: part II—drugs. *BMJ* 2006;333(7572):794-7.
46. Hooper L, Thompson RL, Harrison RA et al. Omega 3 fatty acids for prevention and treatment of cardiovascular disease. *Cochrane Database Syst Rev* 2004;(4):CD003177.
47. Rizos E, Ntzani EE, Bika E et al. Association between omega-3 fatty acid supplementation and risk of major cardiovascular disease events: a systematic review and meta-analysis. *JAMA* 2012;308(10):1024-33.
48. Toole JF, Malinow MR, Chambless LE et al. Lowering homocysteine in patients with ischemic stroke to prevent recurrent stroke, myocardial infarction, and death: the Vitamin Intervention for Stroke Prevention (VISP) randomized controlled trial. *JAMA* 2004;291(5):565-75.
49. Bonaa KH, Njolstad I, Ueland PM et al. Homocysteine lowering and cardiovascular events after acute myocardial infarction. *N Engl J Med* 2006;354(15):1578-88.
50. Lonn E, Yusuf S, Arnold MJ et al. Homocysteine lowering with folic acid and B vitamins in vascular disease. *N Engl J Med* 2006;354(15):1567-77.
51. Lonn E, Bosch J, Yusuf S et al. Effects of long-term vitamin E supplementation on cardiovascular events and cancer: a randomized controlled trial. *JAMA* 2005;293(11):1338-47.
52. Sesso HD, Buring JE, Christen WG et al. Vitamins E and C in the prevention of cardiovascular disease in men: the Physicians' Health Study II randomized controlled trial. *JAMA* 2008;300(18):2123-33.
53. Neuhouser ML, Wassertheil-Smoller S, Thomson C et al. Multivitamin use and risk of cancer and cardiovascular disease in the Women's Health Initiative cohorts. *Arch Intern Med* 2009;169(3):294-304.
54. Pittas AG, Chung M, Trikalinos T et al. Systematic review: vitamin D and cardiometabolic outcomes. *Ann Intern Med* 2010;152(5):307-14.
55. Myung SK, Ju W, Cho B et al. Efficacy of vitamin and antioxidant supplements in prevention of cardiovascular disease: systematic review and meta-analysis of randomised controlled trials. *BMJ* 2013;346:f10.
56. Gabriel SR, Carmona L, Roque M et al. Hormone replacement therapy for preventing cardiovascular disease in post-menopausal women. *Cochrane Database Syst Rev* 2005;(2):CD002229.
57. Artinian NT, Fletcher GF, Mozaffarian D et al. Interventions to promote physical activity and dietary lifestyle changes for cardiovascular risk factor reduction in adults: A scientific statement from the American Heart Association. *Circulation* 2010;122(4):406-41.
58. Herbert PR, Moser M, Mayer J et al. Recent evidence on drug therapy of mild to moderate hypertension and decreased risk of coronary heart disease. *Arch Intern Med* 1993;153(5):578-81.
59. Kashani A, Phillips CO, Foody JM et al. Risks associated with statin therapy: a systematic overview of randomized clinical trials. *Circulation* 2006;114(25):2788-97.
60. Derry S, Loke YK. Risk of gastrointestinal hemorrhage with long term use of aspirin: meta-analysis. *BMJ* 2000;321(7270):1183-7.

Chapter 44
Raynaud's Phenomenon

André Roussin, MD, FRCPC

Goals of Therapy

- Reduce the frequency and severity of attacks
- Decrease symptoms (cold-induced blanching of the fingers) in patients with primary or secondary Raynaud's phenomenon
- Prevent local and systemic deterioration in secondary Raynaud's phenomenon
- Heal lesions in patients with secondary Raynaud's phenomenon

Investigations

The investigation of Raynaud's phenomenon is summarized in Figure 1.

- Thorough history to differentiate between:
  - *primary* Raynaud's phenomenon (no associated illness or trauma)
  - *secondary* Raynaud's phenomenon (secondary to occupational hazards, vascular diseases, connective tissue diseases [CTD], e.g., systemic sclerosis, carpal tunnel syndrome, hypothyroidism or other disorders)
  - secondary Raynaud's phenomenon that may be *drug-induced* (see Table 1)
- Physical examination for:
  - altered pulsations
  - abnormal Allen's test, which is done by compressing both the radial and ulnar arteries while clenching the hand, then releasing compression alternately to demonstrate the patency of the arteries
  - local signs of CTD (e.g., sclerodactyly) and carpal tunnel syndrome
  - systemic signs of CTD (e.g., telangiectasis, pulmonary fibrosis), vascular diseases and hypothyroidism
  - evidence of digital ischemic lesions
- Laboratory tests:
  - nailfold capillary microscopy where available to detect megacapillaries and other abnormalities suggestive of systemic sclerosis. Capillaroscopy will help to diagnose early systemic sclerosis in patients with recent onset of Raynaud's phenomenon, especially when the presentation is atypical or if symptoms suggestive of collagen vascular disease are suspected
  - antinuclear antibodies (ANA), extractable nuclear antibodies (ENA) and rheumatoid factor to detect CTD. ACA (anticentromere antibodies) are specific for systemic sclerosis and, together with capillaroscopy, are the best markers to predict evolution towards systemic sclerosis[1]
  - other tests (ESR, serum electrophoresis, cryoglobulins and all other immunologic tests) are less useful as early markers of secondary Raynaud's phenomenon
  - normal test results suggest primary Raynaud's phenomenon

Figure 1: Investigation and Management of Raynaud's Phenomenon

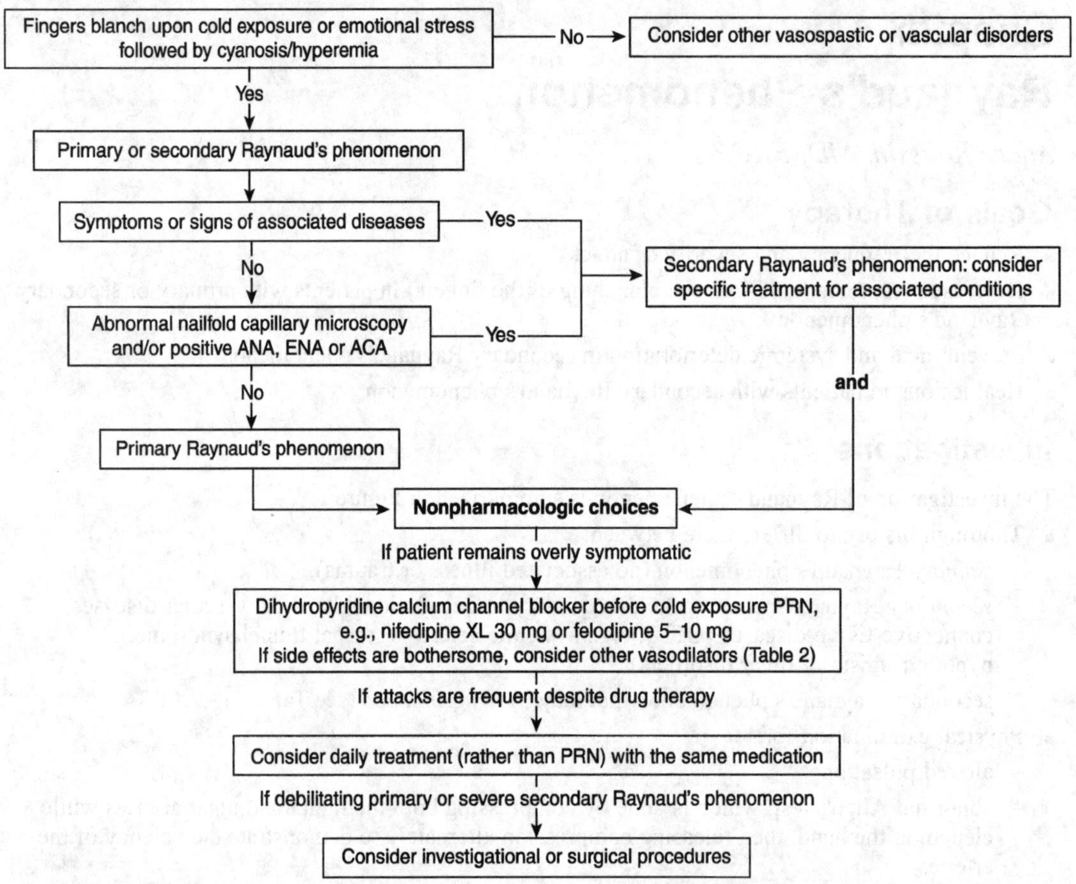

Abbreviations: ACA = anticentromere antibodies; ANA = antinuclear antibodies; ENA = extractable nuclear antibodies

Table 1: Drugs Implicated in Secondary Raynaud's Phenomenon

Drug	Comment
Antineoplastic agents	Bleomycin-, vinblastine- and cisplatin-containing regimens have been associated with Raynaud's phenomenon
Beta-blockers	Unlikely but controversial. Evidence implicating beta-blockers in Raynaud's phenomenon is equivocal[2]
Cyclosporine	Not dose related
Ergot derivatives	Bromocriptine, ergonovine maleate, methysergide
Interferon alfa, beta	When used for treatment of cancer, viral hepatitis and multiple sclerosis. May persist for several months after withdrawal

Therapeutic Choices

The management of Raynaud's phenomenon is summarized in Figure 1.

Nonpharmacologic Choices

- Minimize cold exposure.
- Avoid prescribing medications with vasoconstrictive potential (e.g., ergot derivatives, beta-blockers) unless there is a compelling reason, such as use of a beta-blocker in a patient with coronary artery disease.
- Reassure patients that no complications arise from primary Raynaud's phenomenon.
- Teach warming exercises such as swinging the arms vigorously (windmill effect).
- Instruct patients to dress warmly (including the head and neck) to avoid a sympathetically mediated vasoconstrictive reflex and use warming devices in mittens or boots if appropriate and affordable.
- Encourage patients to stop smoking and to avoid using vibrating tools (grinders, pneumatic hammers, drills, chain saws).
- Acupuncture was ineffective in patients with secondary Raynaud's phenomenon in a randomized, double-blind, placebo-controlled trial.[3]

Pharmacologic Choices

Many negative studies of pharmacologic therapy for Raynaud's phenomenon have never been published. This complicates the interpretation of the numerous small studies and case reports that report positive outcomes for a variety of drugs.

There are no evidence-based or consensus-based guidelines for the pharmacologic treatment of Raynaud's phenomenon. Figure 1 and the drugs chosen for Table 2 are based on available evidence and the clinical experience of the author.

Dihydropyridine **calcium channel blockers** (CCB) reduce the frequency and severity of attacks and are first-line agents in patients with primary and secondary Raynaud's phenomenon.[4,5] **Nifedipine** is the best studied in this class.[6]

Patients with primary or secondary Raynaud's phenomenon may be advised to use a CCB of the dihydropyridine class (e.g., **nifedipine XL** 30 mg or **felodipine** 5–10 mg) 30–60 minutes before cold exposure, or regularly during the winter months. If a dihydropyridine (including **amlodipine**) is not well tolerated, nondihydropyridine CCBs may be considered, although they are less effective for Raynaud's phenomenon.[4,6] Higher doses may be used in patients with severe primary or secondary Raynaud's phenomenon, or if ulcers are present, e.g., systemic sclerosis.

Peripheral **alpha-blockers** (e.g., **prazosin**) are less effective than calcium channel blockers, although there are no head-to-head data to substantiate this opinion. Prazosin was more effective than placebo in patients with systemic sclerosis secondary to Raynaud's phenomenon in 2 randomized trials.[7] However, the dosage is limited by side effects in nonhypertensive patients.[7]

Angiotensin converting enzyme inhibitors, angiotensin II receptor blockers, antiplatelet agents and pentoxifylline are generally not effective for Raynaud's phenomenon. Topical nitrate formulations with minimal systemic effects are currently being investigated, but are not commercially available.

Intravenous **iloprost**, a PGI_2 analogue, may be useful for short-term treatment of severe secondary Raynaud's phenomenon, to reduce the frequency and severity of attacks and in some cases increase the rate of digital ulcer healing; oral iloprost is less effective.[8,9] Oral **ketanserin** (a serotonin receptor antagonist) reduces the duration of symptoms somewhat.[10] Neither drug is commercially available in Canada.

Bosentan, an endothelin-1 inhibitor, heals digital ulcers and reduces the Raynaud's phenomenon in select patients with systemic sclerosis.[11]

Phosphodiesterase type 5 inhibitors reduce the severity of Raynaud's phenomenon and may be effective in healing digital ulcers [Evidence: SORT B*].[12] **Sildenafil** 50 mg twice daily reduced the frequency and duration of Raynaud's attacks in patients with severe secondary Raynaud's phenomenon resistant to vasodilator therapy.[13] **Vardenafil** 10 mg twice daily has been effective[14] as well as **tadalafil** 20 mg on alternate days.[15] Reducing the tadalafil dose to 5 mg daily improves tolerability and may still provide benefit.

Phosphodiesterase type 5 inhibitors and bosentan should be considered only for patients with severe secondary Raynaud's phenomenon. These drugs are not currently approved for this indication, are costly and have a number of contraindications and significant side effects. Specialist consultation is recommended before prescribing them.

Surgical Choices

- Extremity sympathectomy, particularly by thoracoscopy, is not effective in the long term in patients with difficult secondary Raynaud's phenomenon with digital ulcers.
- Digital sympathectomy may be more effective, although the evidence is very limited.

Choices during Pregnancy and Breastfeeding

Both primary and secondary Raynaud's phenomenon usually decrease substantially in frequency and intensity during pregnancy and for at least a few months after delivery. Most patients return to their pre-pregnancy state afterwards.

Management during Pregnancy and Postpartum Period

For the majority of women whose Raynaud's phenomenon improves during pregnancy, nonpharmacologic measures suffice (see Nonpharmacologic Choices). For women with persistent severe Raynaud's, usually related to systemic sclerosis, **nifedipine** can be considered if previous clear benefit has been experienced with 30 mg of the long-acting formulation. Nifedipine, although causing fetal malformations in rodents at high dosage, has not resulted in such problems in humans. Nevertheless, the fact that nifedipine reduces only symptoms and does not reduce complications such as digital ulcers should be discussed with the pregnant patient, especially since nifedipine is not approved in Canada for use during pregnancy.

Raynaud's and Breastfeeding

Nonpharmacologic measures are the mainstay of management of Raynaud's phenomenon during breastfeeding. Calcium channel blockers are passed on to the newborn via breast milk so their use during this period should be avoided. Other classes of drugs have no proven benefit.

A discussion of general principles on the use of medications in these special populations can be found in Appendix II and Appendix III. Other specialized reference sources are also provided in these appendices.

Therapeutic Tips

- Since pharmacologic prophylaxis of Raynaud's phenomenon is effective in only 60% of patients at most (usually 40%), it is important to stress nonpharmacologic approaches and reassure patients.

---

* SORT (Strength of Recommendation Taxonomy) is a rating system (A, B or C) that addresses the quality of available evidence. For more information consult **How to Use *Compendium of Therapeutic Choices*** on page xxv.

Only about 5% of patients with primary Raynaud's phenomenon will go on to develop secondary Raynaud's phenomenon. It is the underlying disease itself rather than the phenomenon that causes complications.

- Taking medication daily rather than as needed during the winter will increase tolerance to side effects, e.g., headaches.
- If dihydropyridines are ineffective, other vasodilators are not likely to be effective.
- Patients with primary and secondary Raynaud's phenomenon generally respond equally well to medications; it is the frequency of attacks, rather than intensity and duration, that is most likely to be reduced with effective drug therapy.

Table 2: Drugs Used for the Treatment of Raynaud's Phenomenon

Class	Drug	Dose	Adverse Effects	Cost[a]
Alpha$_1$-Adrenergic Antagonists	*prazosin* Minipress generics	1–2 mg BID po (regular dosage, to avoid risk of syncope with irregular use)	Most common: dizziness, drowsiness, lightheadedness, lack of energy, weakness, palpitations, nausea. Less frequent adverse effects include syncope, edema and angina.	$
Calcium Channel Blockers, dihydropyridines	*nifedipine, extended-release* Adalat XL, generics	Extended-release: 30 mg po 30–60 min before cold exposure	Tachycardia, flushing, headache, dizziness, orthostatic hypotension and edema.	$$
	felodipine, extended-release Plendil, generics	Extended-release: 5–10 mg po 60 min before cold exposure	See nifedipine.	$$
	amlodipine Norvasc, generics	5 mg po 60 min before cold exposure	See nifedipine.	$
Calcium Channel Blockers, nondihydropyridines	*diltiazem, extended-release* Cardizem CD, Tiazac, Tiazac XC, generics	Extended-release: 180–240 mg po 60–90 min before cold exposure	Usually well tolerated. Occasional hypotension or orthostatic hypotension, flushing, arrhythmia and bradycardia. Use with caution in patients with heart disease.	$$

[a] Cost per dose; includes drug cost only.
Legend: $ <$0.50 $$ $0.50–1.00 $$$ $1.00–1.50

Suggested Readings

Goundry B, Bell L, Langtree M et al. Diagnosis and management of Raynaud's phenomenon. *BMJ* 2012;344:e289.

Herrick AL. Management of Raynaud's phenomenon and digital ischemia. *Curr Rheumatol Rep* 2013;15(1):303.

Herrick AL. The pathogenesis, diagnosis and treatment of Raynaud phenomenon. *Nat Rev Rheumatol* 2012;8(8):469-79.

Stewart M, Morling JR. Oral vasodilators for primary Raynaud's phenomenon. *Cochrane Database Syst Rev* 2012;7:CD006687.

References

1. Koenig M, Joyal F, Fritzler MJ et al. Autoantibodies and microvascular damage are independent predictive factors for the progression of Raynaud's phenomenon to systemic sclerosis: a twenty-year prospective study of 586 patients, with validation of proposed criteria for early systemic sclerosis. *Arthritis Rheum* 2008;58(12):3902-12.
2. Franssen C, Wollersheim H, de Haan A et al. The influence of different beta-blocking drugs on the peripheral circulation in Raynaud's phenomenon and in hypertension. *J Clin Pharmacol* 1992;32(7):652-9.
3. Hahn M, Steins A, Mohrle M et al. Is there a vasospasmolytic effect of acupuncture in patients with secondary Raynaud phenomenon? *J Dtsch Dermatol Ges* 2004;2(9):758-62.
4. Thompson AE, Pope JE. Calcium channel blockers for primary Raynaud's phenomenon: a meta-analysis. *Rheumatology (Oxford)* 2005;44(2):145-50.
5. Ennis H, Anderson ME, Wilkinson J et al. Calcium channel blockers for primary Raynaud's phenomenon. *Cochrane Database Syst Rev* 2014;1:CD002069.
6. Thompson AE, Shea B, Welch V et al. Calcium-channel blockers for Raynaud's phenomenon in systemic sclerosis. *Arthritis Rheum* 2001;44(8):1841-7.
7. Harding SE, Tingey PC, Pope J et al. Prazosin for Raynaud's phenomenon in progressive systemic sclerosis. *Cochrane Database Syst Rev* 1998;(2):CD000956.
8. Pope J, Fenlon D, Thompson A et al. Iloprost and cisaprost for Raynaud's phenomenon in progressive systemic sclerosis. *Cochrane Database Syst Rev* 2000;(2):CD000953.
9. Wigley FM, Wise RA, Seibold JR et al. Intravenous iloprost infusion in patients with Raynaud phenomenon secondary to systemic sclerosis. A multicenter, placebo-controlled, double-blind study. *Ann Intern Med* 1994;120(3):199-206.
10. Pope J, Fenlon D, Thompson A et al. Ketanserin for Raynaud's phenomenon in progressive systemic sclerosis. *Cochrane Database Syst Rev* 2000;(2):CD000954.
11. Launay D, Diot E, Pasquier E et al. [Bosentan for treatment of active digital ulcers in patients with systemic sclerosis]. *Presse Med* 2006;35(4 Pt 1):587-92. [French].
12. Roustit M, Blaise S, Allanore Y et al. Phosphodiesterase-5 inhibitors for the treatment of secondary Raynaud's phenomenon: systematic review and meta-analysis of randomised trials. *Ann Rheum Dis* 2013;72(10):1696-9.
13. Fries R, Shariat K, von Wilmowsky H et al. Sildenafil in the treatment of Raynaud's phenomenon resistant to vasodilatory therapy. *Circulation* 2005;112(19):2980-5.
14. Caglayan E, Huntgeburth M, Karasch T et al. Phosphodiesterase type 5 inhibition is a novel therapeutic option in Raynaud disease. *Arch Intern Med* 2006;166(2):231-3.
15. Shenoy PD, Kumar S, Jha LK et al. Efficacy of tadalafil in secondary Raynaud's phenomenon resistant to vasodilator therapy: a double-blind randomized cross-over trial. *Rheumatology (Oxford)* 2010;49(12):2420-8.

Chapter 45
Supraventricular Tachycardia

David Birnie, MD and
Pablo Nery, MD

Supraventricular tachycardia (SVT) includes all tachyarrhythmias arising from above the ventricles. SVT usually has a narrow QRS width (≤120 ms). Occasionally the QRS complex during tachycardia is broad because there is coexistent bundle branch block. In this situation, the initial step is to exclude ventricular tachycardia, after which a differential diagnosis of SVT is performed (see Figure 1).

The classification of common forms of SVT is shown in Table 1.

The terms "paroxysmal," "persistent" and "permanent" are now used to classify atrial fibrillation and flutter; the older term "chronic atrial fibrillation" is obsolete (Table 2).

Figure 1: Differential Diagnosis of Supraventricular Tachycardia

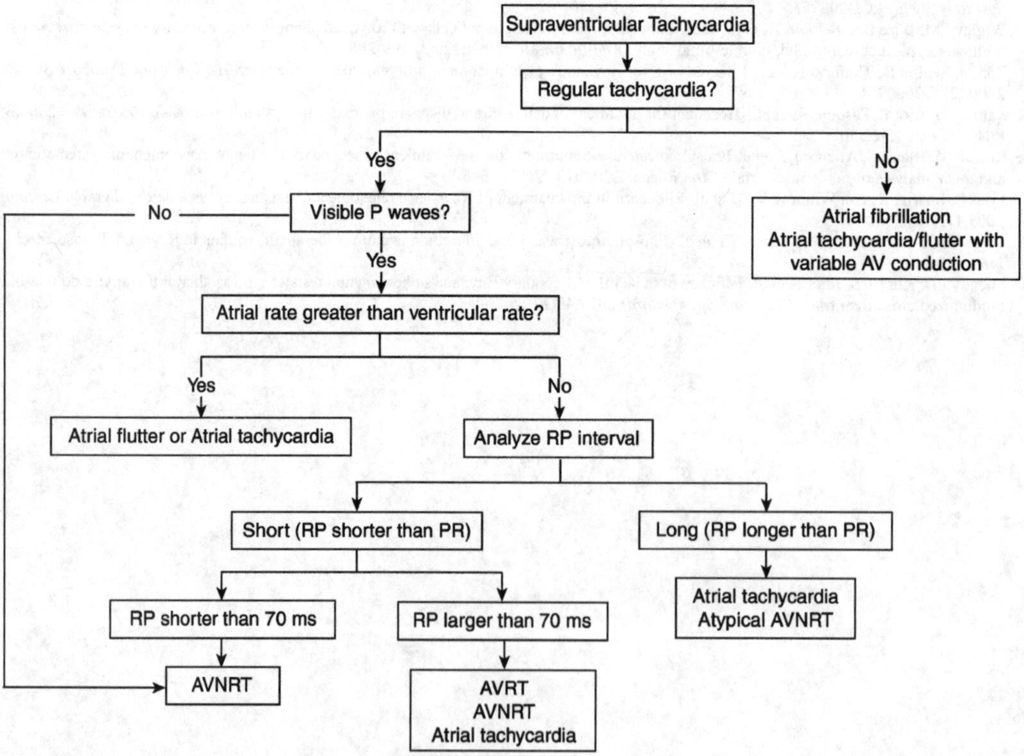

Abbreviations: AV = atrioventricular; AVNRT = atrioventricular nodal re-entry tachycardia; AVRT = atrioventricular re-entry tachycardia; ms = millisecond
Modified from *Circulation* 2003;108(15):1871-909 with permission of the American Heart Association.

Management of atrial fibrillation and atrial flutter is similar. The risk of thromboembolic complications should be assessed in both situations. Many patients have a combination of both arrhythmias, but there are some important differences in the management of the two. Firstly, it is often more difficult to achieve heart rate control in patients with atrial flutter than atrial fibrillation. Secondly, the threshold for using catheter ablation is lower for atrial flutter than for atrial fibrillation.

An algorithm for the management of newly discovered atrial fibrillation or flutter is provided in Figure 2.

The heart is usually structurally normal in patients with atrioventricular re-entry tachycardia (AVRT), atrioventricular nodal re-entry tachycardia (AVNRT) and focal atrial tachycardia (AT). AVRT is due to a congenital accessory bypass tract between the atria and ventricles. The circuit usually follows an antegrade limb through the atrioventricular (AV) node and a retrograde limb through the accessory pathway, although the opposite occasionally occurs. If the accessory pathway is capable of antegrade conduction during sinus rhythm, it usually manifests on the resting ECG as a delta wave and is known as Wolff-Parkinson-White (WPW) syndrome. AVNRT involves a localized short circuit within the AV node. Focal AT arises from a localized area of atrial myocardium that is capable of accelerated automatic firing.

Goals of Therapy

- In the acute stage, the goal is to restore sinus rhythm. Rhythm control should always be possible in re-entrant arrhythmias (AVRT or AVNRT)
- Rhythm control may not be possible or desirable in some patients with atrial fibrillation, atrial flutter or atrial tachycardia. In these situations, the goal is to control the rate of the SVT
- In the longer term, the goal is to prevent arrhythmia recurrence, or substantially reduce the overall arrhythmia burden
- Reduce the risk of thromboembolic events (stroke) in patients with atrial fibrillation/atrial flutter

Table 1: **Classification of Supraventricular Tachycardia**

Arrhythmia	Clinical Significance of Arrhythmia
Atrial fibrillation	Significant because of thromboembolic risk
Atrial flutter	Probably similar thromboembolic risk to atrial fibrillation
Atrioventricular nodal re-entry tachycardia (AVNRT)	Usually benign
Atrioventricular re-entry tachycardia (AVRT)	Usually benign. There is a risk of sudden death if AVRT degenerates into pre-excited SVT (rare)
Atrial tachycardia (AT)	Usually benign unless it persists for prolonged period (rare)

Table 2: **Classification of Atrial Fibrillation or Flutter**[1]

Paroxysmal	Recurrent self-limiting episodes (lasting less than 7 days)
Persistent	Episodes lasting more than 7 days and sinus rhythm achievable (spontaneously or by cardioversion)
Permanent	Cardioversion failed or not attempted/planned

Investigations

- Detailed history including a description of the onset, frequency and duration of episodes and identification of possible triggers, e.g., alcohol, caffeine, exercise, hyperthyroidism. In most patients, there are no consistent triggers.
- Document the arrhythmia, ideally on 12-lead ECG, but a Holter or loop monitor is also acceptable.
- Echocardiography to assess left ventricular function, left atrial size and valvular status.

Therapeutic Choices

Nonpharmacologic Choices

Cardioversion

In general, any tachycardia that produces hemodynamic compromise, heart failure or angina, and is resistant to prompt medical management, should be terminated electrically. Most supraventricular arrhythmias, with the exception of atrial flutter and fibrillation, are usually responsive to medical therapy and hence cardioversion is seldom necessary. Furthermore, cardioversion can be a useful adjunctive measure in patients with persistent atrial fibrillation or flutter. A synchronized shock on the R wave is used, and there is no evidence that any paddle position is more effective than another. It is normal to start with the anterior-apex position, and if this is unsuccessful, then another position, usually antero-posterior, is tried. The initial success rate of cardioversion for atrial fibrillation is 70–90% but only about 20% of patients will remain in sinus rhythm at 12-month follow up. Using additional antiarrhythmic therapy can improve maintenance of sinus rhythm. For example, 50–70% of patients treated with amiodarone are still in sinus rhythm at 12 months. Direct current cardioversion has a low incidence of side effects. Arrhythmias induced by the cardioversion are generally caused by inadequate synchronization.

Figure 2: **Therapy of Newly Discovered Atrial Fibrillation or Flutter**

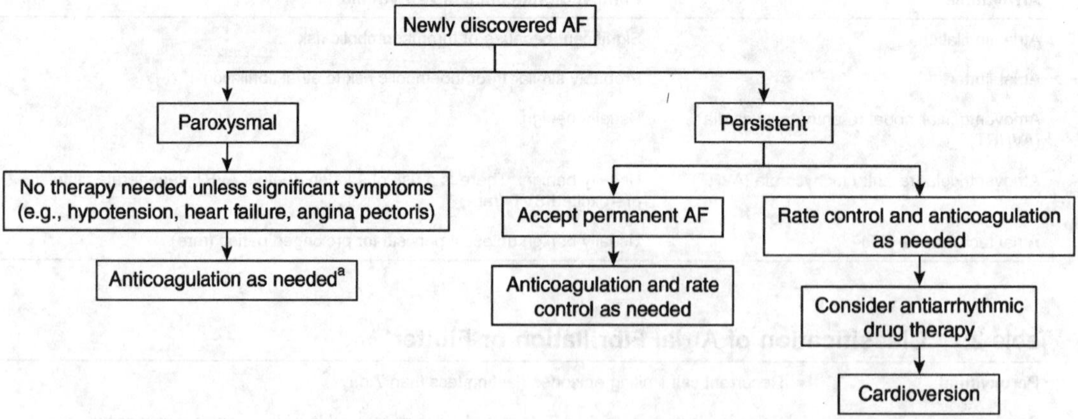

[a] See Table 3 for details of the $CHADS_2$ criteria used to estimate stroke risk.
Abbreviations: AF = atrial fibrillation or flutter
Modified from *Circulation* 2006;114(7):e257-354 with permission of the American Heart Association.

Catheter Ablation

The success rate for catheter ablation of typical atrial flutter is usually about 95% with a low rate of complications; hence, ablation should be considered as first-line treatment for most patients with typical atrial flutter. Suitable patients can usually be rate controlled while awaiting elective ablation. If patients cannot be rate controlled, expedited ablation or electrical cardioversion are reasonable options.

Catheter ablation for atrial fibrillation is an option for patients who have failed at least one antiarrhythmic drug. Ablation is often not a complete cure for atrial fibrillation, but can significantly reduce the arrhythmia burden. Success rates vary from 30–90% depending on technique, atrial fibrillation subtype and the extent of structural heart disease. Patients with paroxysmal atrial fibrillation have the highest success rates. In contrast, patients with persistent, long-lasting (>3–5 years) atrial fibrillation have much lower success rates. The technique involves extensive ablation of the left atrium, primarily focusing on the areas around the pulmonary veins. The success of ablation seems to relate to disconnection of atrial fibrillation triggers arising from the pulmonary veins and/or modification of the arrhythmogenic left atrial substrate. Procedural complications specifically related to atrial fibrillation ablation include a 2% risk of vascular access complications, 1–2% risk of tamponade, 0.25% risk of stroke and a 0.15% risk of death, usually due to atrial esophageal fistula.

In patients with re-entrant tachycardias or focal atrial tachycardia, the reported cure rates after catheter ablation range from 90–98%. The associated risk is much less than the risk with catheter ablation for atrial fibrillation. Hence, the threshold for nonpharmacologic management of these arrhythmias is low. Catheter ablation is strongly recommended for patients with WPW and rapidly conducted pre-excited SVT. Catheter ablation should be considered as a first-line treatment option in patients with recurrent symptomatic AVRT, AVNRT or focal atrial tachycardia. Catheter ablation is also an option for patients with occasional episodes of AVNRT who desire complete rhythm control and for patients with asymptomatic pre-excitation.

Pharmacologic Choices

Long-term Management of Atrial Fibrillation or Flutter

This first decision is whether to choose rate control (leaving atrial arrhythmia as the permanent rhythm) or to actively pursue sinus rhythm (rhythm control). The AFFIRM Study compared these 2 treatment strategies in 4060 patients and found no difference in stroke or death rates between the 2 groups.[2] However, patients in the AFFIRM study were elderly (mean age 69.7) and were either asymptomatic or had minimal symptoms. Therefore, rhythm control should be actively pursued in patients with more than minimal symptoms, in asymptomatic young patients and in those with possible tachycardia-related cardiomyopathy. Data suggest that this latter diagnosis is a more frequent problem than previously thought.[3]

An overview of the rhythm control management of patients with atrial fibrillation is provided in Figure 3. Selection of antiarrhythmic drug therapy is determined by coexisting structural heart disease. **Amiodarone** is more effective than sotalol or propafenone for the prevention of recurrences of atrial fibrillation as shown by the Canadian Trial of Atrial Fibrillation (CTAF).[6] However, amiodarone may require discontinuation due to side effects in up to 18% of patients. Breakthrough episodes can be terminated by either electrical or chemical cardioversion. Options for chemical cardioversion include oral **flecainide** or **propafenone**, **intravenous amiodarone**, **ibutilide** or **procainamide** (Table 6). The Canadian Cardiovascular Society (CCS) recommends catheter ablation when a rhythm-control strategy is desired but the patient remains symptomatic following adequate trials of antiarrhythmic drug therapy.[7]

Figure 3: **Methods to Maintain Sinus Rhythm (Rhythm Control) in Patients with Atrial Fibrillation**[4,5]

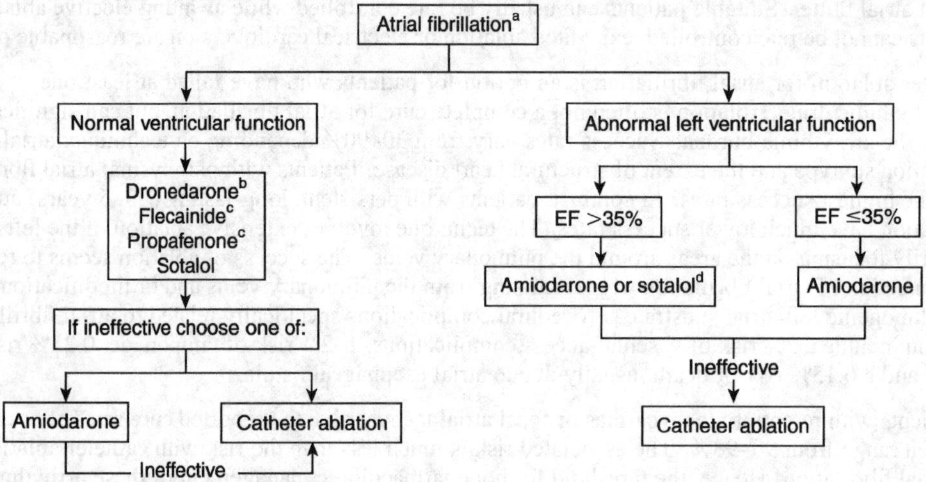

[a] A similar algorithm can be followed for atrial flutter. However, catheter ablation for atrial flutter should be considered first-line.
[b] Use caution when combining dronedarone with digoxin.
[c] An AV nodal blocking agent should always be coprescribed with propafenone or flecainide. Avoid using in coronary artery disease.
[d] Use sotalol with caution when EF 35–40%. Do not use in women >65 years who are taking diuretics.
Abbreviations: EF = ejection fraction

Dronedarone is a class III antiarrhythmic drug, a benzofuran derivative structurally related to amiodarone but without iodine-related organ toxicity. The ATHENA trial evaluated the effect of dronedarone in 4628 patients with atrial fibrillation or flutter and additional risk factors for death.[8] Dronedarone was associated with a 24% relative risk reduction in the combined endpoint of cardiovascular (CV) hospitalization or death. This was mainly driven by reduced hospitalization for atrial fibrillation or flutter and reduced arrhythmic death. Of note, dronedarone may not be as efficacious as amiodarone in preventing atrial fibrillation recurrences. The DYONISOS trial[9] compared amiodarone 200 mg daily (after appropriate loading dose) with dronedarone 400 mg twice daily in maintaining sinus rhythm in 504 patients with atrial fibrillation. More patients given dronedarone had a recurrence of atrial fibrillation or discontinued the drug at 12 months (75.1% vs. 58.8%). Based on the results of the ANDROMEDA[10] and PALLAS[11] trials, Health Canada recommends that dronedarone not be prescribed for patients with heart failure, left ventricular dysfunction or permanent atrial fibrillation.

Heart Rate Control in Patients with Persistent or Permanent Atrial Fibrillation or Flutter

Most patients will need drugs to achieve rate control, with the exception of some patients with intrinsic AV nodal disease (usually elderly individuals). Pharmacologic control of heart rate should initially be attempted with a **beta-blocker** or a **calcium channel blocker** (**diltiazem** or **verapamil**) (Table 7). **Digoxin** is usually inadequate alone for rate control. Because of its potential toxicity, **amiodarone** should be used only as a last resort.

The medication dose should be titrated to achieve a resting heart rate of <80 bpm and a mean heart rate of <100 bpm on 24-hour Holter monitoring. A randomized study suggests that these criteria may be too strict.[12] However, these findings need to be confirmed by further research. Finally, if rate control cannot be achieved with medication, consider AV nodal ablation and permanent pacemaker implantation.

Anticoagulation for Paroxysmal, Persistent and Permanent Atrial Fibrillation or Flutter

Use of an oral anticoagulant is recommended for the prevention of thromboembolic stroke in patients who have atrial flutter or fibrillation and are at high risk for stroke [Evidence: SORT A].[13] Estimate stroke risk using the $CHADS_2$ tool outlined in Table 3 [Evidence: SORT A].[14] The estimated annual risk of stroke in a patient with a $CHADS_2$ score of 0 who is not receiving an antithrombotic is 1.9%.[14] In the absence of antithrombotic therapy, the risk of stroke increases by a factor of about 1.5 for each 1-unit increase in $CHADS_2$ score in patients with atrial fibrillation. In patients with a $CHADS_2$ score of 0, additional risk factors (female gender, age >65 and diagnosis of vascular disease), which are part of the CHADS-VASc score,[15] can further define risk. The recommendations of the CCS for choosing an antithrombotic agent for stroke prevention are summarized in Figure 4.[13] Estimate the risk of bleeding when choosing a treatment by using the HAS-BLED score [Evidence: SORT A].[16] See Table 4.

Warfarin and **ASA** have been used for many years, although ASA is less effective than warfarin. **Apixaban, dabigatran** and **rivaroxaban** are approved for prevention of systemic embolism in patients with atrial fibrillation (see Table 8). Approval of dabigatran was based largely on the RE-LY study, which randomized patients to warfarin or dabigatran.[17] Dabigatran 150 mg twice a day was superior to warfarin in preventing stroke and systemic embolism. Rivaroxaban was compared to warfarin in the ROCKET-AF trial and was found noninferior to warfarin.[18] Apixaban was shown to be superior to ASA in the AVERROES study[19] and to warfarin in the ARISTOTLE study.[20] CCS guidelines suggest that when an oral anticoagulant is indicated, most patients should receive apixaban, dabigatran or rivaroxaban.[5] The preference for 1 of the new oral anticoagulants over warfarin is less marked among patients already receiving warfarin with stable INRs and no bleeding complications. Other factors (e.g., cost, renal function) may also influence drug choice.

The combination of **clopidogrel** and **ASA** is recommended by the CCS for stroke prevention in low-risk patients with stable coronary artery disease, acute coronary syndrome or percutaneous coronary intervention.[13] The summary of recommendations for antithrombotic therapy in patients with atrial fibrillation or atrial flutter and coronary artery disease is shown in Figure 5.

Figure 4: **Using the $CHADS_2$ Score to Select an Antithrombotic Agent**

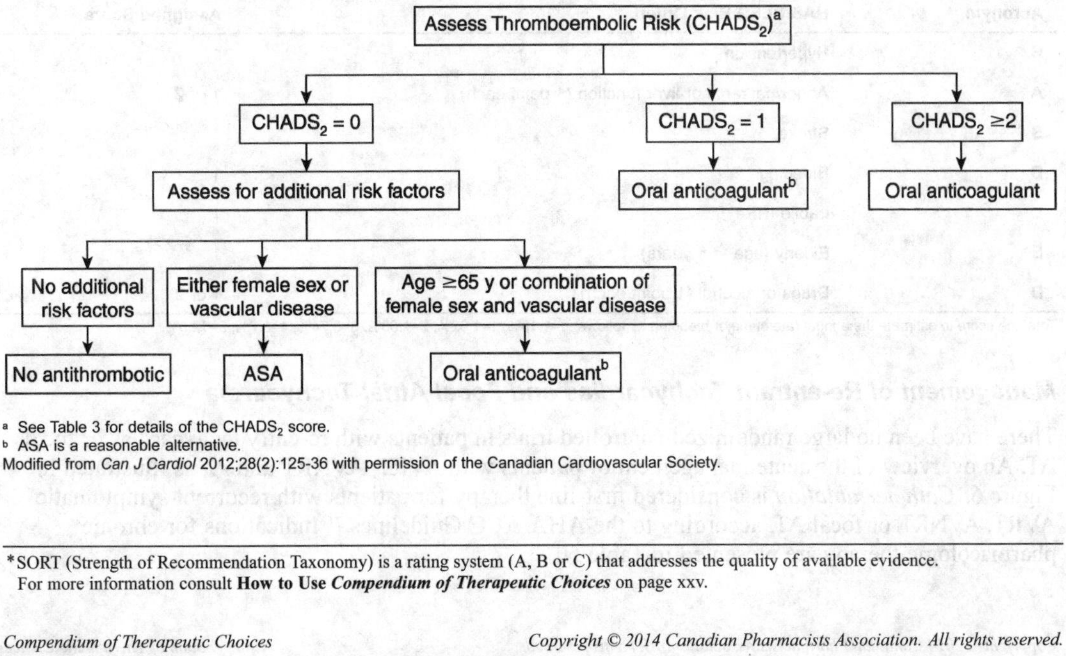

a See Table 3 for details of the $CHADS_2$ score.
b ASA is a reasonable alternative.
Modified from *Can J Cardiol* 2012;28(2):125-36 with permission of the Canadian Cardiovascular Society.

*SORT (Strength of Recommendation Taxonomy) is a rating system (A, B or C) that addresses the quality of available evidence. For more information consult **How to Use *Compendium of Therapeutic Choices*** on page xxv.

Figure 5: **Summary of Recommendations for Antithrombotic Management in Patients with Coronary Artery Disease**

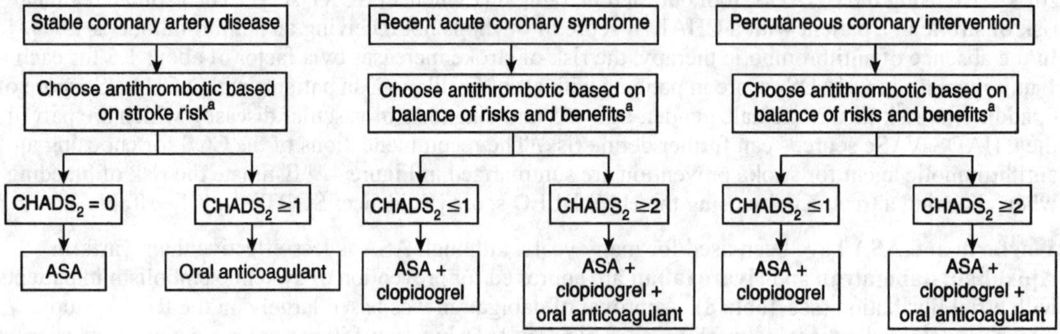

[a] See Table 3 for details of the $CHADS_2$ criteria used to estimate stroke risk.
Reproduced from *Can J Cardiol* 2012;28(2):125-36 with permission of the Canadian Cardiovascular Society.

Table 3: **Stroke Risk in Patients with Nonvalvular Atrial Fibrillation or Flutter[14]**

Acronym	$CHADS_2$ Risk Criteria	Assigned Score
C	Congestive heart failure	1
H	Hypertension	1
A	Age >75 years	1
D	Diabetes mellitus	1
S	Prior stroke or transient ischemic attack	2

Table 4: **Estimating Bleeding Risk in Patients with Atrial Fibrillation[16]**

Acronym	HAS-BLED Risk Criteria	Assigned Score
H	Hypertension	1
A	Abnormal renal or liver function (1 point each)	1 or 2
S	Stroke	1
B	Bleeding	1
L	Labile INRs	1
E	Elderly (age >65 years)	1
D	Drugs or alcohol (1 point each)	1 or 2

Total the score to estimate the annual rate of major bleeding as follows: 0=1.13%, 1=1.02%, 2=1.88%, 3=3.74%, 4=8.7%, 5=12.5%.

Management of Re-entrant Tachycardias and Focal Atrial Tachycardia

There have been no large randomized controlled trials in patients with re-entry tachycardias or focal AT. An overview of the acute management of patients with AVRT, AVNRT and AT is illustrated in Figure 6. *Catheter ablation* is considered first-line therapy for patients with recurrent symptomatic AVRT, AVNRT or focal AT, according to the AHA/ACC Guidelines.[21] Indications for chronic pharmacologic therapy are presented in Table 5.

Figure 6: **Acute Management of Atrioventricular Re-entry Tachycardia, Atrioventricular Nodal Re-entry Tachycardia and Atrial Tachycardia**

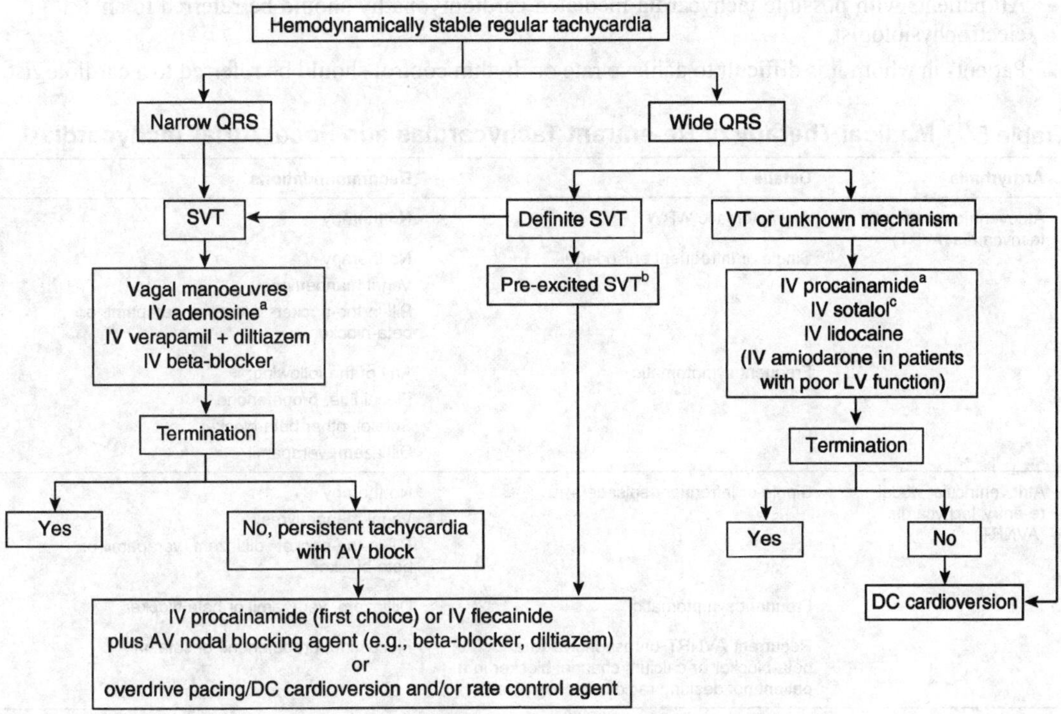

[a] Drugs are listed in order of preference starting with the first choice agent.
[b] Pre-excited SVT is an extremely rare and occasionally lethal arrhythmia due to rapid conduction down an accessory pathway.
[c] IV sotalol is not available in Canada.
Abbreviations: AV = atrioventricular; DC = direct current; LV = left ventricular; SVT = supraventricular tachycardia; VT = ventricular tachycardia
Modified from *Circulation* 2003;108(15):1871-909 with permission of the American Heart Association.

Therapeutic Tips

- Either rate or rhythm control is reasonable for elderly asymptomatic or mildly symptomatic patients with atrial fibrillation or atrial flutter.
- Rhythm control should be pursued in younger patients or symptomatic older patients with atrial fibrillation or atrial flutter.
- Rhythm control for atrial fibrillation should initially be with antiarrhythmic drugs.
- Rhythm control with catheter ablation should be considered second- or third-line in atrial fibrillation and first-line in atrial flutter.
- Rhythm control with catheter ablation for paroxysmal atrial fibrillation has a high success rate; results in patients with persistent or permanent atrial fibrillation are more modest.
- Rhythm control should *always* be the objective in patients with re-entry tachycardia (AVRT or AVNRT). Rhythm control should be attempted with either antiarrhythmic drugs or catheter ablation.
- Rhythm control should usually be the objective in patients with AT. Rate control is acceptable if rhythm control cannot be achieved.
- Avoid use of flecainide and propafenone in patients with structural heart disease.

- Use only immediate-release dosage forms when prescribing single-dose pill-in-the-pocket oral therapy.
- All patients with a possible indication for ablation should be referred to an electrophysiologist.
- All patients with possible tachycardia-mediated cardiomyopathy should be referred to an electrophysiologist.
- Patients in whom it is difficult to achieve rate or rhythm control should be referred to a cardiologist.

Table 5: **Medical Therapy of Re-entrant Tachycardias and Focal Atrial Tachycardia**[21]

Arrhythmia	Details	Recommendations
Atrioventricular re-entry tachycardia (AVRT)	Asymptomatic WPW	No therapy
	Single or infrequent episode(s)	No therapy Vagal manoeuvres Pill-in-the-pocket[a] diltiazem, verapamil or beta-blocker
	Frequent symptomatic	Any of the following: Flecainide, propafenone Sotalol, other beta-blocker Diltiazem, verapamil
Atrioventricular nodal re-entry tachycardia (AVNRT)	Single or infrequent episode(s)	No therapy Vagal manoeuvres Pill-in-the-pocket[a] diltiazem, verapamil or beta-blocker
	Frequent symptomatic	Diltiazem, verapamil or beta-blocker
	Recurrent AVNRT unresponsive to a beta-blocker or calcium channel blocker in a patient not desiring radiofrequency ablation	Flecainide, propafenone or sotalol
Focal atrial tachycardia (AT)	Single or infrequent episode(s)	No therapy Pill-in-the-pocket[a] diltiazem, verapamil or beta-blocker
	Recurrent symptomatic	Any of the following: Diltiazem, verapamil or beta-blocker Flecainide, propafenone[b] Sotalol, amiodarone[c]

[a] The single dose oral pill-in-the-pocket approach is an option in carefully selected patients. Suitable candidates should not have significant LV dysfunction or sinus bradycardia. Intermittent single-dose therapy minimizes exposure to unnecessary therapy between events.
[b] Flecainide and propafenone should not be used in patients with coronary artery disease or structural heart disease.
[c] Ablation should be considered before amiodarone.
Abbreviations: WPW = Wolff-Parkinson-White

Table 6: **Drug Therapy for Control of Heart Rhythm in Patients with Supraventricular Tachycardia**

Class	Drug	Dose	Adverse Effects	Drug Interactions	Comments	Cost[a]
Antiarrhythmics, Class IA	*procainamide* Procainamide Hydrochloride Injection USP	15–17 mg/kg over 30 min iv	Hypotension, torsades de pointes.	Risk of arrhythmias with drugs that also prolong the QT_c interval, e.g., erythromycin, phenothiazines.	For chemical cardioversion.	$15/dose
Antiarrhythmics, Class IC	*flecainide* generics	50 mg Q12H po Titration: Increase by 50 mg increments based on QRS intervals. Reduce dose if QRS increases >20% from baseline Maximum: 200 mg Q12H po Renal dysfunction: Reduce initial dose by 50% Pill-in-the-pocket: 300 mg × 1 po (if weight >70 kg) 200 mg × 1 po (if weight <70 kg)	VT proarrhythmia, tremor, blurred vision, HF.	Metabolized by CYP2D6 (many potential interactions, e.g., celecoxib, desipramine, risperidone).	In patients with atrial fibrillation and/or atrial flutter, a beta-blocker or nondihydropyridine calcium channel blocker *should always be* coprescribed with a Class IC agent. Not to be used in patients with coronary artery disease or structural heart disease.	$
	propafenone Rythmol, generics	150 mg Q8H po Reduce dose if QRS prolonged >20% from baseline Maximum: 300 mg Q8H po Renal/hepatic dysfunction: Reduce initial dose by 50% and increase dosing interval to Q12H Pill-in-the-pocket: 600 mg × 1 po (if weight >70 kg) 450 mg × 1 po (if weight <70 kg)	Constipation, headache, metallic taste, VT proarrhythmia.	Reduce digoxin dose by 25–50%. Metabolized by CYP2D6 (many potential interactions, e.g., celecoxib, desipramine, risperidone).	Active metabolites accumulate in rapid metabolizers. Monitor QRS duration carefully. See flecainide.	$
Antiarrhythmics, Class III	*amiodarone* Cordarone, generics	Usually 200 mg TID po × 2 wk then 200 mg daily po when treating atrial arrhythmias Intravenous loading: 150 mg iv over 10 min followed by iv infusion of 1.2–1.8 g/day to a total of 10 g Loading doses may vary	Various gastrointestinal, dermatologic, neurologic, ophthalmologic and thyroid abnormalities. Pulmonary fibrosis, hepatic dysfunction and aggravation of arrhythmias are rare but potentially life-threatening.	Reduce doses of beta-blockers, digoxin, procainamide, quinidine and warfarin by 50%.	Monitor transaminases and thyroid function Q6 months, CXR annually.	po: $ iv: $330/1g dose

(cont'd)

Table 6: Drug Therapy for Control of Heart Rhythm in Patients with Supraventricular Tachycardia *(cont'd)*

Class	Drug	Dose	Adverse Effects	Drug Interactions	Comments	Cost[a]
	dofetilide ➔ Tikosyn	125–500 µg BID po Reduce dose if QT_c interval prolonged by >15% after first dose	Headache, nausea, torsades de pointes.	Increased plasma levels with cimetidine, ketoconazole, trimethoprim (alone or combined with sulfamethoxazole), verapamil.	Requires prescription by an electrophysiologist; must be initiated in hospital.[b]	[b]
	dronedarone Multaq	400 mg BID po	Diarrhea, dyspepsia, nausea, hepatic dysfunction (rare). Slight increase in plasma creatinine related to inhibition of secretion, no change in GFR.	Drugs metabolized by CYP3A4 (e.g., diltiazem, simvastatin).	Contraindicated with: – severe heart failure (NYHA class IV) – strong CYP3A4 inhibitors, e.g., azole antifungals, macrolide antibiotics. Not recommended in patients with permanent atrial fibrillation.	$$$$$
	ibutilide ➔ Corvert	Patients ≥60 kg: 1 mg × 1 iv over 10 min Patients <60 kg: 0.01 mg/kg × 1 iv over 10 min May repeat dose once after 10 min	Hypotension, torsades de pointes.	Risk of arrhythmias with drugs that also prolong the QT interval, e.g., erythromycin, phenothiazines.	For chemical cardioversion. Correct any hypokalemia or hypomagnesemia prior to administering ibutilide.	$300/dose
	sotalol ➔ generics	80 mg Q12H po Titration: Increase by 80 mg increments if QT_c <460 ms Reduce dose if QT_c ≥500 ms Maximum: 240 mg Q12H po Elderly: Reduce initial dose to 40 mg Q12H po Renal dysfunction: Reduce initial dose in renal failure	Hypotension, bradycardia, wheezing, VT proarrhythmia. Torsades de pointes, especially at higher doses or with renal dysfunction.	Digoxin, diltiazem, verapamil, other beta-blockers: May cause AV block, bradycardia.	Since sotalol is a beta-blocker, use with great caution in view of the risk of QT_c prolongation and torsades de pointes.	$

[a] Cost of 30-day supply based on 70 kg body weight; includes drug cost only.
[b] Available through Special Access Programme, Health Canada.
➔ Dosage modification may be required in renal dysfunction; see Appendix I.
Abbreviations: AV = atrioventricular; CXR = chest x-ray; GFR = glomerular filtration rate; HF = heart failure; ms = millisecond; NYHA = New York Heart Association; VT = ventricular tachycardia
Legend: $ < $30 $$ $30–60 $$$ $60–90 $$$$ $90–120 $$$$$ $120–150

Table 7: **Drug Therapy for Control of Heart Rate in Patients with Supraventricular Tachycardia**

Class	Drug	Dose	Adverse Effects	Drug Interactions	Comments	Cost[a]
Beta$_1$-adrenergic Antagonists[c]	*propranolol* Inderal-LA, generics	1–3 mg Q2 min × 2 iv. May repeat in 4 h 80–240 mg/day po	Bradycardia, hypotension, dyspnea, fatigue, depression.	With digoxin, calcium channel blockers, amiodarone: Reduce dose 25–50%. Hypoglycemic agents.	Monitor carefully in diabetic patients; use with caution in patients with HF or bronchospastic lung disease.	iv: $$ po: $
	atenolol (renal) Tenormin, generics	50–150 mg/day po	See propranolol. Less likely to cause CNS effects, e.g., depression.	See propranolol.	See propranolol. Beta$_1$ selective.	$
	metoprolol Lopresor, generics	5–10 mg Q5 min × 3 iv 100–400 mg/day po	See propranolol.	See propranolol.	See propranolol. Beta$_1$ selective.	$
	nadolol (renal) generics	20–160 mg/day po	See propranolol. Less likely to cause CNS effects, e.g., depression.	See propranolol.	See propranolol.	$
Calcium Channel Blockers, non-dihydropyridine	*verapamil* Isoptin SR, generics	5–10 mg iv. May give extra 10 mg iv in 30 min Usual starting dose: 120 mg/day po; maximum: 480 mg/day po. IR given in divided doses TID–QID; SR given daily or divided doses BID	Bradycardia, hypotension, constipation, flushing.	Beta-blockers, digoxin, amiodarone.	Use with caution in patients with HF.	iv: $$$ po: $$
	diltiazem Cardizem CD, Tiazac, Tiazac XC, generics	0.25 mg/kg iv. May give another 0.35 mg/kg iv after 15 min if necessary 180–540 mg/day po. IR given in divided doses TID–QID; SR in divided doses BID; CD and Tiazac given daily	Bradycardia, hypotension.	See verapamil.	See verapamil.	iv[b]: $ po: $
Cardiac Glycosides	*digoxin* (renal) Toloxin	Loading: 1–1.5 mg in divided doses po/iv Maintenance: 0.125–0.375 mg/day po/iv	Bradycardia, nausea, vomiting, visual disturbances, proarrhythmia.	With beta-blockers, calcium channel blockers, amiodarone, propafenone, quinidine: Reduce digoxin dose by 25–50%.	Rarely indicated. Check serum potassium, correct hypokalemia if present.	$

[a] Cost of 30-day supply of oral doses and 1-day supply for iv doses; includes drug cost only.
[b] Cost based on 70 kg body weight.
[c] The beta-blockers suggested are examples only. Acebutolol, labetalol and timolol would also be effective. Some agents are available as sustained-release preparations.
(renal) Dosage adjustment may be required in renal impairment; see Appendix I.
Abbreviations: CD = controlled delivery; HF = heart failure; IR = immediate release; SR = sustained release
Legend: $ < $25 $$ $25–50 $$$ $50–75

Table 8: **Drug Therapy for Prevention of Systemic Embolism in Patients with Supraventricular Tachycardia**

Class	Drug	Dose	Adverse Effects	Drug Interactions	Cost[a]
Antiplatelet Agents	*ASA* Aspirin, generics	81–325 mg/day po	Bleeding, usually minor (e.g., epistaxis), gastric intolerance, GI bleeding (gastric ulcers, erosions), tinnitus usually dose related.	Hemorrhagic risk increased with concomitant use of anticoagulants.	$
	clopidogrel Plavix, generics	75 mg daily po	Bleeding, usually minor. Skin rash (4%); diarrhea (5%).	Hemorrhagic risk increased with concomitant use of anticoagulants.	$$
Direct Factor Xa Inhibitors	*apixaban* Eliquis	Usual: 5 mg BID po If serum creatinine >133 mmoL/L and patient either >80 y or ≤60 kg: 2.5 mg BID po	Bleeding.	Contraindicated in combination with strong inhibitors of both CYP3A4 and P-gp (e.g., itraconazole, ritonavir).	$$$$
	rivaroxaban ❥ Xarelto	20 mg daily po Moderate renal impairment (ClCr 30–49 mL/min): 15 mg daily po	Bleeding.	See apixaban.	$$$
Direct Thrombin Inhibitors	*dabigatran* ❥ Pradaxa	Usual: 150 mg BID po Patients with increased bleeding risk or >80 y: 110 mg BID po	Bleeding, gastric intolerance.	Contraindicated in combination with strong inhibitors of P-gp (e.g., ketoconazole). Caution with other drugs acting on P-gp.	$$$$
Vitamin K Antagonists	*warfarin* Coumadin, generics	Dose to maintain INR between 2 and 3	Bleeding, skin necrosis. Contraindicated in pregnancy.	Many potential interactions. Substrate for CYP2C9 and other isoenzymes.	$
	nicoumalone Sintrom	Dose to maintain INR between 2 and 3	See warfarin.	See warfarin.	$$$

[a] Cost of 30-day supply; includes drug cost only.

❥ Dosage adjustment may be required in renal impairment; see Appendix I.

Abbreviations: CYP = cytochrome P450; P-gp = P-glycoprotein

Legend: $ <$10 $$ $10–50 $$$ $50–90 $$$$ $90–130

Suggested Readings

Delacretaz E. Clinical practice. Supraventricular tachycardia. *N Engl J Med* 2006;354(10):1039-51.

Dewire J, Calkins H. State-of-the-art and emerging technologies for atrial fibrillation ablation. *Nat Rev Cardiol* 2010;7(3):129-38.

Fox DJ, Tischenko A, Krahn AD et al. Supraventricular tachycardia: diagnosis and management. *Mayo Clin Proc* 2008;83(12):1400-11.

Fuster V, Ryden LE, Cannom DS et al. ACC/AHA/ESC 2006 Guidelines for the Management of Patients with Atrial Fibrillation: a report of the American College of Cardiology/American Heart Association Task Force on Practice Guidelines and the European Society of Cardiology Committee for Practice Guidelines (Writing Committee to Revise the 2001 Guidelines for the Management of Patients With Atrial Fibrillation). *Circulation* 2006;114(7):e257-354.

Prystowsky EN, Camm J, Lip GY et al. The impact of new and emerging clinical data on treatment strategies for atrial fibrillation. *J Cardiovasc Electrophysiol* 2010;21(8):946-58.

References

1. Fuster V, Ryden LE, Cannom DS et al. ACC/AHA/ESC 2006 guidelines for the management of patients with atrial fibrillation: full text. *Europace* 2006;8(9):651-745.
2. Wyse DG, Waldo AL, DiMarco JP et al. A comparison of rate control and rhythm control in patients with atrial fibrillation. *N Engl J Med* 2002;347(23):1825-33.
3. Umana E, Solares CA, Alpert MA. Tachycardia-induced cardiomyopathy. *Am J Med* 2003;114(1):51-5.
4. Gillis AM, Verma A, Talajic M et al. Canadian Cardiovascular Society atrial fibrillation guidelines 2010: rate and rhythm management. *Can J Cardiol* 2011;27(1):47-59.
5. Skanes AC, Healey JS, Cairns JA et al. Focused 2012 update of the Canadian Cardiovascular Society atrial fibrillation guidelines: recommendations for stroke prevention and rate/rhythm control. *Can J Cardiol* 2012;28(2):125-36.
6. Roy D, Talajic M, Dorian P et al. Amiodarone to prevent recurrence of atrial fibrillation. Canadian Trial of Atrial Fibrillation Investigators. *N Engl J Med* 2000;342(13):913-20.
7. Verma A, Macle L, Cox J et al. Canadian Cardiovascular Society atrial fibrillation guidelines 2010: catheter ablation for atrial fibrillation/atrial flutter. *Can J Cardiol* 2011;27(1):60-6.
8. Hohnloser SH, Crijns HJ, van Eickels M et al. Effect of dronedarone on cardiovascular events in atrial fibrillation. *N Engl J Med* 2009;360(7):668-78.
9. Le Heuzey JY, De Ferrari GM, Radzik D et al. A short-term, randomized, double-blind, parallel-group study to evaluate the efficacy and safety of dronedarone versus amiodarone in patients with persistent atrial fibrillation: the DIONYSOS Study. *J Cardiovasc Electrophysiol* 2010;21(6):597-605.
10. Kober L, Torp-Pedersen C, McMurray JJ et al. Increased mortality after dronedarone therapy for severe heart failure. *N Engl J Med* 2008;358(25):2678-87.
11. Connolly SJ, Camm AJ, Halperin JL et al. Dronedarone in high-risk permanent atrial fibrillation. *N Engl J Med* 2011;365(24):2268-76.
12. Van Gelder IC, Groenveld HF, Crijns HJ et al. Lenient versus strict rate control in patients with atrial fibrillation. *N Engl J Med* 2010;362(15):1363-73.
13. Cairns JA, Connolly S, McMurty S et al. Canadian Cardiovascular Society atrial fibrillation guidelines 2010: prevention of stroke and systemic thromboembolism in atrial fibrillation and flutter. *Can J Cardiol* 2011;27(1):74-90.
14. Gage BF, Waterman AD, Shannon W et al. Validation of clinical classification schemes for predicting stroke: results from the National Registry of Atrial Fibrillation. *JAMA* 2001;285(22):2864-70.
15. Lip GY, Nieuwlaat R, Pisters R et al. Refining clinical risk stratification for predicting stroke and thromboembolism in atrial fibrillation using a novel risk factor-based approach: the Euro Heart Survey on atrial fibrillation. *Chest* 2010;137(2):263-72.
16. Pisters R, Lane DA, Nieuwlaat R et al. A novel user-friendly score (HAS-BLED) to assess 1-year risk of major bleeding in patients with atrial fibrillation: the Euro Heart Survey. *Chest* 2010;138(5):1093-100.
17. Connolly SJ, Ezekowitz MD, Yusuf S et al. Dabigatran versus warfarin in patients with atrial fibrillation. *N Engl J Med* 2009;361(12):1139-51.
18. Patel MR, Mahaffey KW, Garg J et al. Rivaroxaban versus warfarin in nonvalvular atrial fibrillation. *New Engl J Med* 2011;365(10):883-91.
19. Connolly SJ, Eikelboom J, Joyner C et al. Apixaban in patients with atrial fibrillation. *N Engl J Med* 2011;364(9):806-17.
20. Granger CB, Alexander JH, McMurray JJ et al. Apixaban versus warfarin in patients with atrial fibrillation. *N Engl J Med* 2011;365(11):981-92.
21. Blomstrom-Lundqvist C, Scheinman MM, Aliot EM et al. ACC/AHA/ESC guidelines for the management of patients with supraventricular arrhythmias—executive summary. *Circulation* 2003;108(15):1871-909.

Chapter 46
Stable Angina

Michael Froeschl, MD, MSc, FRCPC, FACC

Angina pectoris is a discomfort, classically described as a "squeezing", felt in the chest and/or an adjacent area caused by myocardial ischemia, i.e., an inadequate supply of blood and oxygen to the heart muscle. Coronary artery disease (CAD)—the build-up of cholesterol plaque in the walls of the vessels that feed the heart—is the most common underlying cause of myocardial ischemia. The therapeutic discussions in this chapter assume that CAD is the etiology, unless indicated otherwise. However, other conditions that can produce or exacerbate myocardial ischemia must be considered when evaluating a patient with angina pectoris, e.g., tachyarrhythmia, severe aortic stenosis, hypertrophic cardiomyopathy and anemia. Identifying these alternative causes of angina is important not only to allow appropriate treatments to be administered, but also to ensure that inappropriate treatments are not (e.g., a patient with angina due to hypertrophic cardiomyopathy may be harmed by long-acting nitrate therapy).

Goals of Therapy

- Improve quality of life by decreasing or preventing angina and improving exercise tolerance
- Minimize the risk of cardiovascular death and nonfatal MI
- Treat the modifiable risk factors that promote the development and progression of CAD

Investigations

- History:
  - a thorough history focusing on the patient's age and sex as well as the details of the chest discomfort (its character, location, precipitating and alleviating factors) is the most important tool for estimating the likelihood that obstructive CAD is the cause of the patient's discomfort (Table 1)
  - identify modifiable risk factors for CAD (e.g., diabetes mellitus, dyslipidemia, hypertension, obesity, smoking, diet, lack of exercise, unhealthy alcohol use, psychosocial stress)
- Physical examination to assess for:
  - tachycardia
  - hypertension
  - evidence of atherosclerotic disease, e.g., arterial bruits
- Laboratory tests:
  - complete blood count
  - serum creatinine and electrolytes
  - fasting glucose and cholesterol panel
- Noninvasive cardiovascular testing:
  - resting electrocardiogram (ECG)
  - echocardiogram if important valvular heart disease, left ventricular systolic dysfunction or a cardiomyopathy is suspected

- stress-testing is usually indicated to confirm the diagnosis of myocardial ischemia and to risk stratify the patient; the "stress" can take the form of either exercise or a pharmacologic agent (e.g., adenosine, dipyridamole or dobutamine) and the "test" consists of either an ECG, nuclear myocardial perfusion imaging or echocardiography

Therapeutic Choices

Nonpharmacologic Choices

- *Aggressive lifestyle intervention.* Counsel patients to undertake regular aerobic exercise (e.g., walking, jogging, cycling, swimming); consume a heart-healthy diet low in processed foods and sodium; quit smoking; consume alcohol in moderation only; take advantage of stress management techniques. High-risk patients (e.g., those with concomitant heart failure) should ideally be referred to a medically supervised program (cardiac rehabilitation).
- *Revascularization*, in the form of either percutaneous coronary intervention (PCI, also known as coronary angioplasty) or coronary artery bypass graft surgery (CABG). Revascularization is indicated to improve quality of life in medically refractory patients and to prolong life in patients with high-risk coronary anatomy (e.g., >50% stenosis of the left main artery; >70% stenosis of all 3 coronary arteries, particularly with a left ventricular ejection fraction <50%).
- For patients who fail to respond to medical therapy and for whom coronary revascularization is not possible, additional nonpharmacologic treatments are being investigated. These include enhanced external counterpulsation (EECP), spinal cord stimulation and angiogenesis.

Pharmacologic Choices

Drugs that Decrease or Prevent Angina

A paucity of randomized controlled trials compare anti-ischemic drugs (nitrates, beta-blockers and calcium channel blockers) in patients with angina.[1,2] As such, it is reasonable to use any of these drugs, and the choice of which drug to start with should include consideration of patient-specific factors (Figure 1, Table 2). That said, it is also reasonable to provide all patients with sublingual nitroglycerin as acute treatment for an angina attack.

Table 1: Likelihood of Significant Coronary Artery Disease According to Age, Sex and Character of Symptoms

	Nonanginal[a] (%)		Atypical Angina[a] (%)		Typical Angina[a] (%)	
Age (y)	**Men**	**Women**	**Men**	**Women**	**Men**	**Women**
30–39	5	1	22	4	70	26
40–49	14	3	46	13	87	55
50–59	22	8	59	32	92	79
60–69	28	19	67	54	94	91

[a] The following 3 questions establish whether the discomfort is considered nonanginal chest pain, atypical angina or typical angina.

1. Is the discomfort substernal?
2. Are the symptoms precipitated by exertion?
3. Are the symptoms relieved within ten minutes of rest?

Patients who respond "yes" to all 3 questions have typical angina. Patients who respond "yes" to 2 questions have atypical angina. Patients who respond "yes" to 1 question or no questions have nonanginal chest pain.

Adapted with permission from Diamond GA, Forrester JS. Analysis of probability as an aid in the clinical diagnosis of coronary-artery disease. *N Engl J Med* 1979;300(24):1350-8. Copyright © 1979 Massachusetts Medical Society. All rights reserved.

Figure 1: Medical Management of Stable Angina Pectoris

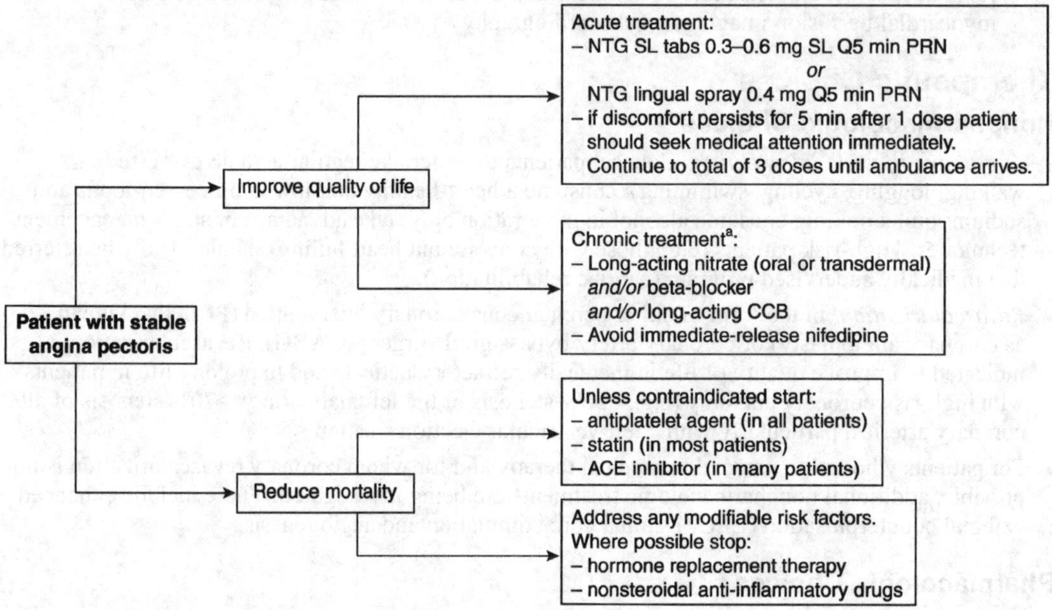
Acute treatment:
– NTG SL tabs 0.3–0.6 mg SL Q5 min PRN
or
NTG lingual spray 0.4 mg Q5 min PRN
– if discomfort persists for 5 min after 1 dose patient should seek medical attention immediately. Continue to total of 3 doses until ambulance arrives.
Improve quality of life
Chronic treatment[a]:
– Long-acting nitrate (oral or transdermal) and/or beta-blocker and/or long-acting CCB
– Avoid immediate-release nifedipine
Patient with stable angina pectoris
Unless contraindicated start:
– antiplatelet agent (in all patients)
– statin (in most patients)
– ACE inhibitor (in many patients)
Reduce mortality
Address any modifiable risk factors.
Where possible stop:
– hormone replacement therapy
– nonsteroidal anti-inflammatory drugs

[a] Agents are not listed in order of preference.
Abbreviations: ACE = angiotensin-converting enzyme; CCB = calcium channel blocker; NTG = nitroglycerin

Nitrates

Nitrates are primarily venodilators. As a consequence, they reduce cardiac preload and, with it, myocardial oxygen demand. Nitrates are effective both for acute and chronic angina. Sublingual nitroglycerin tablets or spray alleviate anginal pain and, if taken in advance, can prevent symptoms that occur with activity.

Advise patients to sit when taking sublingual nitrates to reduce the risk of syncope. Long-acting nitrate preparations prevent angina but frequently cause headaches. Tolerance to the antianginal effects of nitrates develops unless a nitrate-free period of 10–12 hours is prescribed each day.

Beta-blockers

Beta-blockers decrease heart rate, contractility and blood pressure (the major determinant of left ventricular afterload). Therefore, they prevent or decrease angina by decreasing myocardial oxygen demand. Both nonselective and beta$_1$-selective beta-blockers are effective. In patients with recent prior MI and/or depressed left ventricular systolic function, beta-blockers also reduce mortality.

Calcium Channel Blockers

Practically speaking, there are 2 classes of calcium channel blockers. The nondihydropyridines **verapamil** and **diltiazem** act more centrally and thus behave similarly to beta-blockers: they decrease myocardial oxygen demand by lowering heart rate, contractility and blood pressure. The dihydropyridines exert their effects primarily by arterial dilation. **Amlodipine**, **felodipine**, and **nifedipine** have been effective in stable angina, though felodipine does not have Health Canada approval for this indication. They reduce blood pressure and, consequently, myocardial oxygen demand. Furthermore, by dilating coronary arteries, dihydropyridines may also increase myocardial oxygen supply.

Drugs that Decrease the Risk of Cardiovascular Death and Nonfatal MI

Stable coronary artery disease has a relatively benign prognosis. It is the destabilization of coronary plaques that commonly results in MI and/or death. Therefore, it stands to reason that agents that promote stabilization of coronary plaques, along with those that limit the thrombotic consequences when plaque rupture occurs, would be protective. Indeed, there is evidence from large, randomized controlled trials that patients with stable CAD, including those with angina pectoris, can benefit from antiplatelet therapy, HMG-CoA reductase inhibition (statin therapy) and angiotensin-converting enzyme (ACE) inhibition.

Antiplatelet Agents

A systematic review of randomized controlled trials has demonstrated that antiplatelet agents decrease the relative risk of cardiovascular death, nonfatal MI or nonfatal stroke by 30% compared with placebo.[3] It also showed that **ASA** 80–160 mg daily is as effective as higher doses. **Clopidogrel**, a $P2Y_{12}$ adenosine receptor antagonist, has been compared to ASA in the management of patients with vasculopathy (CAPRIE trial).[4] Although there was a reduction of ischemic endpoints in favour of clopidogrel, it was limited to the subgroup of patients with peripheral arterial disease; patients with CAD did not benefit from clopidogrel over ASA. The addition of clopidogrel to ASA alone has also been compared to ASA in a heterogeneous population of individuals with, or at risk for, vascular disease. Although there was no benefit to combination therapy in the overall trial,[5] there was benefit in the large subgroup of patients with established vasculopathy, including CAD.[5,6] Today, in the absence of a recent acute coronary syndrome or PCI with stent implantation, clopidogrel is reserved for stable angina patients who cannot take ASA. Because of its GI and hematologic side effects (including rare but potentially fatal thrombotic thrombocytic purpura), **ticlopidine** is rarely used. Newer $P2Y_{12}$ adenosine receptor antagonists, such as **prasugrel** and **ticagrelor**, do not have evidence to support their use in patients with stable angina, although studies are being conducted.

HMG-CoA Reductase Inhibitors (Statins)

The mechanism of action of statins is not limited to reducing cholesterol levels but includes improving endothelial function.

The randomized Heart Protection Study enrolled patients at high risk for vascular disease complications and demonstrated that **simvastatin** 40 mg daily decreased the relative risk of death by 13% and nonfatal MI by 37% compared with placebo.[7] Furthermore, the TNT trial compared atorvastatin 80 mg to atorvastatin 10 mg in a population with stable CAD. The 80 mg dose resulted in a relative risk reduction of 22% for major cardiovascular events (absolute rates of 8.7% for 80 mg vs. 10.9% for 10 mg).[8] All patients with established vascular disease, including those with stable CAD and angina, are at high risk for vascular complications. Current Canadian guidelines recommend that these patients should be treated to ensure that their LDL is below 2 mmol/L or that it has fallen at least 50% on statin therapy.[9] For more information on statins, see Chapter 37.

ACE Inhibitors

ACE inhibitors have a number of potential anti-ischemic mechanisms including decreasing sympathetic adrenergic transmission, reducing afterload and blood pressure and improving coronary flow reserve. ACE inhibitors have been shown to prevent major cardiovascular events in patients with stable angina who do not have heart failure or left ventricular systolic dysfunction.[10]

In the HOPE trial, which enrolled patients at high risk of cardiovascular events, **ramipril** 10 mg/day decreased the relative risk of cardiovascular death, nonfatal MI or nonfatal stroke by 20% compared with placebo in the subgroup of patients with angina.[11] Other large, placebo-controlled clinical trials of ACE-inhibitors in lower risk populations have yielded variable results.[12,13] Therefore, the decision to deploy these agents should be made in the context of the patient's risk.[14]

Other Agents

In addition to standard pharmacologic interventions, other agents have demonstrated efficacy in the treatment of angina. **Nicorandil**[15] dilates both arterioles and, via its nitrate moiety, veins. **Ranolazine**[16,17] reduces calcium overload in the ischemic myocyte by inhibiting the late sodium current (I_{Na}). **Ivabradine**[18] inhibits the I_f current in the sinus node to reduce heart rate. None of the above agents are approved for use in Canada.

Drugs that Increase the Risk of Cardiovascular Death and Nonfatal MI

Based on the results of the Heart and Estrogen/progestin Replacement Study (HERS trial) and the Women's Health Initiative trial, the need for hormone therapy in postmenopausal women should be carefully considered.[19,20] If hormone replacement is deemed necessary to treat menopausal symptoms, keep the duration of therapy to a minimum (see Chapter 75). Similarly, COX-2 inhibitors and most nonselective NSAIDs increase the risk of vascular events to varying degrees.[21] If the use of NSAIDs is required to maintain an adequate quality of life, administer the lowest dose for the shortest possible duration.

Treat Modifiable Risk Factors

Observational studies have demonstrated that smoking cessation is associated with decreased mortality and morbid cardiac events. Pharmacologic interventions that improve smoking cessation rates include **nicotine replacement therapy**, **bupropion**, **nortriptyline**, **clonidine** and **varenicline** (see Chapter 13).

The aggressive treatment of comorbid hypertension and diabetes mellitus is warranted. The reader is referred to the respective chapters on these subjects (see Chapter 32 and Chapter 39) along with the current Canadian guidelines.[22,23]

Although observational studies have suggested that lower homocysteine levels and vitamin E therapy are beneficial for patients with angina, large randomized controlled trials have not shown any benefit to folic acid, B vitamins and vitamin E in patients with angina.[24,25]

Therapeutic Tips

- When prescribing organic **nitrates**, ensure a 10- to 12-hour nitrate-free period each day to avoid the development of tolerance. Schedule the nitrate-free period for a time when minimal symptoms are expected, usually at night.
- Although heart rate lowering anti-anginal drugs, **beta-blockers**, **diltiazem** or **verapamil**, are best titrated to heart rate during exertion, in clinical practice they are usually titrated to resting heart rate with a target between 50 and 60 bpm. Titrate the dose of dihydropyridines (e.g., **amlodipine**, **nifedipine**) to achieve maximum symptom relief with minimal adverse effects.
- Do not withdraw **beta-blocker** therapy abruptly in patients who have been on chronic high dose therapy, as this may precipitate rebound tachycardia and a worsening of anginal symptoms; taper the dose over a 10- to 14-day period.
- If the use of a beta-blocker is desired in a patient with resting bradycardia, an agent with intrinsic sympathomimetic activity (e.g., **acebutolol**, **pindolol**) may be considered.
- Avoid beta-blocker therapy in patients with suspected or documented coronary arterial spasm (Prinzmetal's angina); **calcium channel blockers** and **nitrates** are the agents of choice in such cases.
- Avoid verapamil and diltiazem in patients with left ventricular systolic dysfunction and use with caution in patients with AV nodal disease.[26]
- When using a calcium channel blocker to treat angina in a patient who is already on a beta-blocker, a peripherally acting dihydropyridine is preferred; close monitoring of heart rate and AV nodal function is required if verapamil or diltiazem is combined with a beta-blocker.

- If a patient who is prescribed an ACE inhibitor for vascular protection does not tolerate this medication due to cough, substitution with an **angiotensin receptor blocker** (ARB) is reasonable.[27]

Suggested Readings

Fox K, Garcia MA, Ardissino D et al. Guidelines on the management of stable angina pectoris: executive summary: The Task Force on the Management of Stable Angina Pectoris of the European Society of Cardiology. *Eur Heart J* 2006;27(11):1341-81.

Fraker TD, Fihn SD; 2002 Chronic Stable Angina Writing Committee et al. 2007 chronic angina focused update of the ACC/AHA 2002 guidelines for the management of patients with chronic stable angina: a report of the American College of Cardiology/American Heart Association Task Force on Practice Guidelines Writing Group to develop the focused update of the 2002 guidelines for the management of patients with chronic stable angina. *J Am Coll Cardiol* 2007;50(23):2264-74.

Gibbons RJ, Abrams J, Chatterjee K et al. ACC/AHA 2002 guideline update for the management of patients with chronic stable angina--summary article: a report of the American College of Cardiology/American Heart Association Task Force on practice guidelines (Committee on the Management of Patients With Chronic Stable Angina). *J Am Coll Cardiol* 2003;41(1):159-68.

Table 2: Drugs to Treat Stable Angina

Class	Drug	Dose	Adverse Effects	Drug Interactions	Comments	Cost[a]
Antiplatelet Agents	*ASA* Aspirin, Coated Aspirin, generics	80–325 mg once daily po	Nausea, vomiting, gastritis, bleeding (epistaxis to major GI bleeds), rash.	Increased risk of bleeding when combined with other antiplatelets or anticoagulants.	Serious GI bleeding is less common with lower doses (80–160 mg/day).	$
	clopidogrel Plavix, generics	75 mg once daily po	Bleeding, diarrhea, rash.	See ASA. PPI use may reduce clopidogrel efficacy.		$
	ticlopidine generics	250 mg BID po	Bleeding, diarrhea, rash, purpura, neutropenia.	See ASA.	Monitor neutrophils every 2 wk for the first 3 months of therapy.	$
Beta$_1$-adrenergic Antagonists, nonselective	*nadolol* generics	Initial: 20 mg/day po Maximum: 320 mg/day Once daily	Fatigue, hypotension, bradycardia, impotence, sleep disorders. Less common: hyperglycemia, depression, heart failure, heart block.	Bradycardia with digoxin or nondihydropyridine CCBs. Cardiodepressant effects with nondihydropyridine CCBs and amiodarone.	Avoid abrupt withdrawal (may precipitate ischemia). Taper the dose before discontinuation. Contraindicated in asthma and in 2nd or 3rd degree heart block in the absence of a pacemaker.	$
	propranolol, immediate release generics	Initial: 40–60 mg QID po Usual: 80–320 mg/day (divided BID–QID)	See nadolol.	See nadolol. CYP2D6 inhibitors increase levels of propranolol and metoprolol. Propranolol increases serum levels of rizatriptan.	See nadolol. More likely to cause CNS side effects (insomnia, depression, vivid dreams) than other agents because of greater lipid solubility.	$
	propranolol, controlled release Inderal-LA	60–320 mg/day po	See nadolol.	See propranolol.		$$$
	timolol generics	Initial: 10 mg BID po Maximum: 30 mg BID	See nadolol.	See nadolol.	See nadolol.	$
Beta$_1$-adrenergic Antagonists, selective	*atenolol* Tenormin, generics	Initial: 25 mg/day po Maximum: 200 mg/day Once daily or divided BID	See nadolol.	See nadolol.	See nadolol.	$

Class	Drug	Dose	Adverse Effects	Drug Interactions	Comments	Cost[a]
	bisoprolol ❸ Sandoz Bisoprolol, other generics	Initial: 2.5 mg daily po Maximum: 20 mg daily	See nadolol.	See nadolol.	See nadolol.	$
	metoprolol Lopresor, generics	Initial: 50 mg/day po Maximum: 400 mg/day Give regular formulations in divided doses BID; SR once daily	See nadolol.	See nadolol. CYP2D6 inhibitors increase levels of propranolol and metoprolol.	See nadolol.	$
Beta$_1$-adrenergic Antagonists, non-selective with ISA	*pindolol* Visken, generics	Initial: 5 mg TID po Maximum: 15 mg TID or QID	See nadolol.	See nadolol.	See nadolol. Agents with ISA have less effect on resting heart rate than those without ISA.	$$
Beta$_1$-adrenergic Antagonists, selective with ISA	*acebutolol* ❸ Sectral, generics	Initial: 200 mg BID po Maximum: 400 mg BID	See nadolol.	See nadolol.	See nadolol. Agents with ISA have less effect on resting heart rate than those without ISA.	$
Calcium Channel Blockers, dihydropyridine	*amlodipine* Norvasc, generics	Initial: 2.5 mg/day po Maximum: 10 mg/day Once daily	Ankle edema, flushing, headache, hypotension and tachycardia.	CYP3A4 substrate (many potential interactions). Strong inhibitors include azole antifungals, protease inhibitors, macrolides. Grapefruit may increase serum concentrations.		$
	nifedipine, extended-release XL Adalat XL, generics	Initial: 30 mg/day po Maximum: 120 mg/day Once daily	See amlodipine.	See amlodipine.		$$
Calcium Channel Blockers, nondihydro-pyridine	*diltiazem* Cardizem CD, Tiazac, Tiazac XC, generics	Initial: 120 mg/day po Maximum: 360 mg/day Give CD and XC formulations once daily	Headache, dizziness, bradycardia, heart block, new onset or worsening of heart failure.	See amlodipine. Inhibits metabolism of carbamazepine, cyclosporine, lovastatin, simvastatin. Additive negative inotropic effects with amiodarone, beta-blockers and digoxin.	Caution in patients with heart failure or 2nd or 3rd degree heart block without a functioning pacemaker.	$

(cont'd)

Table 2: **Drugs to Treat Stable Angina** *(cont'd)*

Class	Drug	Dose	Adverse Effects	Drug Interactions	Comments	Cost[a]
	verapamil Isoptin SR, generics	Initial: 80 mg Maximum: 160 mg TID po SR (once daily or divided BID): Initial: 180 mg/day Maximum: 480 mg/day	See diltiazem. Constipation.	See amlodipine. See diltiazem. Verapamil increases digoxin levels by 50–75% within 1 wk (monitor levels).	See diltiazem.	$$
Nitrates	*nitroglycerin, sublingual* Nitrolingual Pumpspray, Nitrostat, generics	SL tablet: 0.3–0.6 mg SL PRN Q5 min Spray: 0.4 mg PRN Q5 min	Headache (usually resolves if the patient persists with therapy), tachycardia, hypotension, syncope (rare), dizziness, flushing.	Potentiates the hypotensive effects of vasodilators. Potentially fatal hypotension with sildenafil, tadalafil and vardenafil.	If discomfort persists for 5 min after 1 dose, patient should seek medical attention immediately. Continue to total of 3 doses until ambulance arrives.	$
	nitroglycerin, topical Nitrol	Ointment: 1.25–5 cm applied BID–TID Remove at end of the dosing interval	See nitroglycerin, sublingual.	See nitroglycerin, sublingual.	Ensure a 10–12 h nitrate-free period daily to prevent tolerance.	$$$
	nitroglycerin, transdermal Minitran, Nitro-Dur, Transderm-Nitro, Trinipatch, generics	Initial: 0.2 mg/h patch applied and removed daily Maximum: 0.8 mg/h patch	See nitroglycerin, sublingual. Contact dermatitis.	See nitroglycerin, sublingual.	See nitroglycerin, topical.	$
	isosorbide dinitrate generics	SL: 5 mg PRN Q5 min IR: 10–30 mg TID po (allow for a 10–12 h nitrate-free period)	See nitroglycerin, sublingual.	See nitroglycerin, sublingual.	See nitroglycerin, topical.	$
	isosorbide-5-mononitrate Imdur, generics	Initial: 30 or 60 mg/day po daily Maximum: 240 mg daily	See nitroglycerin, sublingual.	See nitroglycerin, sublingual.	To minimize headache, start with 30 mg once daily.	$

[a] Cost of a 30-day supply of usual dose of drug; includes drug cost only.
Dosage adjustment may be required in renal impairment; see Appendix I.
Abbreviations: CCB = calcium channel blocker; IR = immediate release; ISA = intrinsic sympathomimetic activity; PPI = proton pump inhibitor
Legend: $ < $20 $$ $20–40 $$$ $40–60

References

1. Dargie HJ, Ford I, Fox KM. Total Ischaemic Burden European Trial (TIBET). Effects of ischaemia and treatment with atenolol, nifedipine SR and their combination on outcome in patients with chronic stable angina. The TIBET Study Group. *Eur Heart J* 1996;17(1):104-12.
2. Rehnqvist N, Hjemdahl P, Billing E et al. Effects of metoprolol vs verapamil in patients with stable angina pectoris. The Angina Prognosis Study in Stockholm (APSIS). *Eur Heart J* 1996;17(1):76-81.
3. Antithrombotic Trialists' Collaboration. Collaborative meta-analysis of randomised trials of antiplatelet therapy for prevention of death, myocardial infarction, and stroke in high risk patients. *BMJ* 2002;324(7329):71-86.
4. A randomised, blinded, trial of clopidogrel versus aspirin in patients at risk of ischaemic events (CAPRIE). CAPRIE Steering Committee. *Lancet* 1996;348(9038):1329-39.
5. Bhatt DL, Fox KA, Hacke W et al. Clopidogrel and aspirin versus aspirin alone for the prevention of atherothrombotic events. *N Engl J Med* 2006;354(16):1706-17.
6. Bhatt DL, Flather MD, Hacke W et al. Patients with prior myocardial infarction, stroke, or symptomatic peripheral arterial disease in the CHARISMA trial. *J Am Coll Cardiol* 2007;49(19):1982-8.
7. Heart Protection Study Collaborative Group. MRC/BHF Heart Protection Study of cholesterol lowering with simvastatin in 20,536 high-risk individuals: a randomised placebo-controlled trial. *Lancet* 2002;360(9326):7-22.
8. LaRosa JC, Grundy SM, Waters DD et al. Intensive lipid lowering with atorvastatin in patients with stable coronary disease. *N Engl J Med* 2005;352(14):1425-35.
9. Anderson TJ, Gregoire J, Hegele RA et al. 2012 update of the Canadian Cardiovascular Society guidelines for the diagnosis and treatment of dyslipidemia for the prevention of cardiovascular disease in the adult. *Can J Cardiol* 2013;29(2):151-67.
10. Danchin N, Cucherat M, Thuillez C et al. Angiotensin-converting enzyme inhibitors in patients with coronary artery disease and absence of heart failure or left ventricular systolic dysfunction: an overview of long-term randomized controlled trials. *Arch Intern Med* 2006;166(7):787-96.
11. Yusuf S, Sleight P, Pogue J et al. Effects of an angiotensin-converting-enzyme inhibitor, ramipril, on cardiovascular events in high-risk patients. The Heart Outcomes Prevention Evaluation Study Investigators. *N Engl J Med* 2000;342(3):145-53.
12. Fox KM; EURopean trial On reduction of cardiac events with Perindopril in stable coronary Artery disease Investigators. Efficacy of perindopril in reduction of cardiovascular events among patients with stable coronary artery disease: randomised, double-blind, placebo-controlled, multicentre trial (the EUROPA study). *Lancet* 2003;362(9386):782-8.
13. Braunwald E, Domanski MJ, Fowler SE et al. Angiotensin-converting-enzyme inhibition in stable coronary artery disease. *N Engl J Med* 2004;351(20):2058-68.
14. Remuzzi G, Ruggenenti P. Overview of randomized trials of ACE inhibitors. *Lancet* 2006;368(9535):555-6.
15. IONA Study Group. Effect of nicorandil on coronary events in patients with stable angina: the Impact Of Nicorandil in Angina (IONA) randomized trial. *Lancet* 2002;359(9314):1269-75.
16. Chaitman BR, Skettino SL, Parker JO et al. Anti-ischemic effects and long-term survival during ranolazine monotherapy in patients with chronic severe angina. *J Am Coll Cardiol* 2004;43(8):1375-82.
17. Chaitman BR, Pepine CJ, Parker JO et al. Effects of ranolazine with atenolol, amlodipine, or diltiazem on exercise tolerance and angina frequency in patients with severe chronic angina: a randomized controlled trial. *JAMA* 2004;291(3):309-16.
18. Borer JS, Fox K, Jaillon P et al. Antianginal and antiischemic effects of ivabradine, an I(f) inhibitor, in stable angina: a randomized, double-blind, multicentered, placebo-controlled trial. *Circulation* 2003;107(6):817-23.
19. Hulley S, Grady D, Bush T et al. Randomized trial of estrogen plus progestin for secondary prevention of coronary heart disease in postmenopausal women. Heart and Estrogen/progestin Replacement Study (HERS) Research Group. *JAMA* 1998;280(7):605-13.
20. Rossouw JE, Anderson GL, Prentice RL et al. Risks and benefits of estrogen plus progestin in healthy postmenopausal women: principal results from the Women's Health Initiative randomized controlled trial. *JAMA* 2002;288(3):321-33.
21. Kearney PM, Baigent C, Godwin J et al. Do selective cyclo-oxygenase-2 inhibitors and traditional non-steroidal anti-inflammatory drugs increase the risk of atherothrombosis? Meta-analysis of randomised trials. *BMJ* 2006;332(7553):1302-8.
22. Hackam DG, Quinn RR, Rayani P et al. The 2013 Canadian Hypertension Education Program recommendations for blood pressure measurement, diagnosis, assessment of risk, prevention and treatment of hypertension. *Can J Cardiol* 2013;29(5):528-42.
23. Canadian Diabetes Association Clinical Practice Guidelines Expert Committee. Canadian Diabetes Association 2013 clinical practice guidelines for the prevention and management of diabetes in Canada. *Can J Diabetes* 2013;37(Suppl 1):S1-S212. Available from: guidelines.diabetes.ca/App_Themes/CDACPG/resources/cpg_2013_full_en.pdf.
24. Lonn E, Yusuf S, Arnold MJ et al. Homocysteine lowering with folic acid and B vitamins in vascular disease. *N Engl J Med* 2006;354(15):1567-77.
25. Yusuf S, Dagenais G, Pogue J et al. Vitamin E supplementation and cardiovascular events in high-risk patients. The Heart Outcomes Prevention Evaluation Study Investigators. *N Engl J Med* 2000;342(3):154-60.
26. Opie LH, Yusuf S, Kubler W. Current status of safety and efficacy of calcium channel blockers in cardiovascular diseases: a critical analysis based on 100 studies. *Prog Cardiovasc Dis* 2000;43(2):171-96.
27. ONTARGET Investigators, Yusuf S, Teo KK et al. Telmisartan, ramipril, or both in patients at high risk for vascular events. *N Engl J Med* 2008;358(15):1547-59.

Chapter 47
Syncope

Monica Solbiati, MD and
Robert Sheldon, MD, PhD

Syncope is defined as a reversible loss of consciousness not requiring specific resuscitative measures, and not associated with generalized seizures. Probably over 50% of people faint at least once in their life, and many faint recurrently.[1,2] Most people who faint have a benign cause but a few are at risk of death. Common causes of syncope are listed in Table 1.

Table 1: **Common Causes of Syncope**

Category	Causes
Volume depletion and drugs	**Volume depletion** Diarrhea Diminished oral intake Polyuria **Drugs** ACE inhibitors Alcohol Alpha- and beta-adrenergic blockers Antiparkinsonian drugs Diuretics Nitrates Phosphodiesterase type 5 inhibitors (sildenafil, tadalafil, vardenafil) Vasodilators
Orthostatic intolerance disorders	**Reflex syncope syndromes** Carotid sinus hypersensitivity Situational syncope syndromes, e.g., cough and gelastic syncope Vasovagal syncope syndromes **Autonomic neuropathies** Primary autonomic failure syndromes Degenerative neurologic diseases, e.g., pure autonomic failure, multiple system atrophy, Parkinson's disease, Lewy body dementia Secondary autonomic failure (amyloidosis, diabetes, uremia)
Arrhythmias	**Bradycardias** Complete (third degree) and bifasicular heart block Sinus node disease **Tachycardias** Supraventricular arrhythmias (uncommon) Torsades de pointes polymorphic ventricular tachycardia Ventricular tachycardia
Obstruction	Aortic stenosis Pulmonary emboli Many other rare causes

Goals of Therapy

- Identify potentially fatal causes of syncope
- Aggressively investigate and treat high-risk patients
- Remove reversible causes of syncope
- Treat patients with therapies appropriate to the degree of their symptoms

Investigations

- In patients with transient loss of consciousness perform a complete cardiovascular and neurologic history and physical examination.[3,4,5] Exclude nonsyncopal causes of loss of consciousness. In the case of suspected seizures refer to a neurologist. Remember that cerebrovascular disorders rarely cause loss of consciousness without other neurologic symptoms. Screen for life-threatening causes such as ventricular outflow tract obstruction, aortic dissection, major bleeding, ventricular tachycardia and asystole or heart block (Figure 1)
- Tailor laboratory investigations to the individual patient:
  - ECG (most patients)
  - older patients (>50 years) should have ambulatory ECG monitoring unless the history is strongly persuasive for vasovagal syncope. Implanted patient-activated loop recorders may be useful in patients with infrequent syncope that eludes conventional attempts at diagnosis[6]
  - ambulatory ECGs and stress tests are of limited use in younger patients
  - echocardiogram or other noninvasive measure of left ventricular function if structural heart disease is suspected
  - coronary angiography as indicated
  - refer patients with structural heart disease for electrophysiologic assessment
  - unless contraindicated, carotid sinus massage should be performed in patients >50 years to screen for carotid sinus hypersensitivity (do not perform in patients with carotid bruits)
  - tilt table testing might be useful in diagnosing vasovagal syncope in patients with atypical symptoms[7,8]
- After potentially fatal causes are eliminated and reversible causes are removed, most patients will have one of several syndromes of orthostatic intolerance:[3]
  - reflex syncope syndromes
    - vasovagal syncope
    - carotid sinus hypersensitivity in the elderly
  - primary or secondary autonomic failure syndromes. Consider a neurologic consult only in the case of primary autonomic failure
- The orthostatic intolerance syndromes can be distinguished based on history and a simple *stand test* in the office. To perform the stand test, first measure blood pressure and heart rate after the patient has been supine for 5 minutes, then after 2 and 4 minutes of standing. The following responses may be seen:
  - *normal and vasovagal syncope:* modest rises in heart rate (about 10 BPM) and blood pressure (about 10 mm Hg).
  - *autonomic failure:* progressive fall in blood pressure of ≥20 mm Hg systolic or ≥10 mm Hg diastolic with development of presyncope; often no increase in heart rate.

Figure 1: **Diagnostic Approach to the Patient with Syncope**

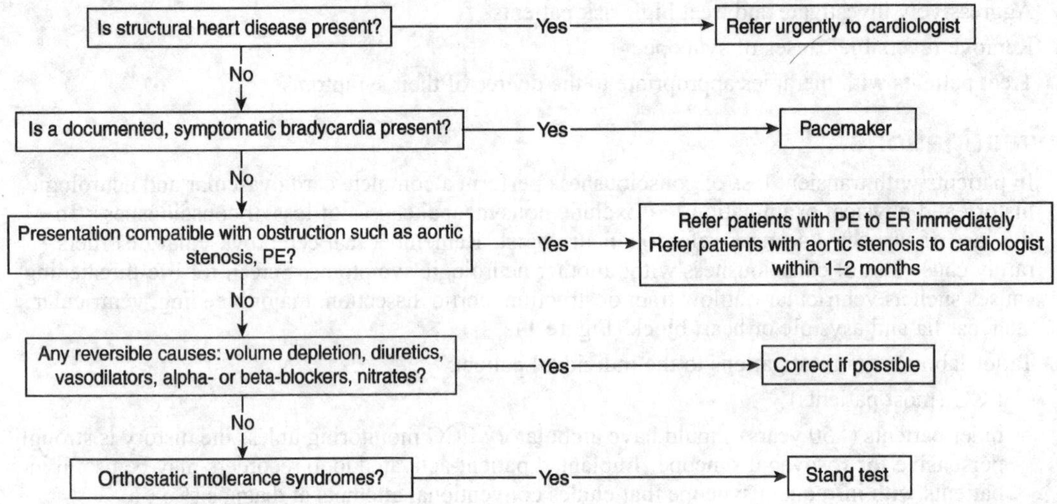

Abbreviations: ER = emergency room; PE = pulmonary emboli

Treatment

Treatment is directed at the cause of syncope. Treat any reversible causes. Refer patients with syncope secondary to bradycardia (asystole or complete heart block) for a permanent pacemaker. Refer patients with suspected or diagnosed ventricular tachycardia, an abnormal ECG (including signs of old infarction, conduction system disease and genetic arrhythmias) and all patients with structural heart disease to a cardiologist, preferably an electrophysiologist. The following addresses treatment of syndromes of orthostatic intolerance.

Vasovagal Syncope

Therapeutic Choices

Nonpharmacologic Choices

- Reassure the patient that vasovagal syncope is not life threatening and that it is a physical problem, not a psychiatric disorder. Encourage increased dietary salt (3–5 g daily) and fluid (up to 2.5 litres daily) in the absence of contraindications such as hypertension or heart failure.[5,8]
- Teach the patient to use physical counterpressure manoeuvres at the onset of presyncope.[9,10] These include squatting, crossing the legs with isometric contraction if standing, and vigorous hand clenching with upper girdle isometric contraction. All should be tried. The evidence is based on a good physiologic study[10] and an open label randomized clinical trial.[9]
- Pacemaker therapy remains controversial in patients with vasovagal syncope. The first adequately powered randomized placebo-controlled trial of patients with vasovagal syncope and a positive tilt table test failed to show any benefit with pacing.[11] However, a more recent study has shown that a pacemaker might be effective in older patients with spontaneous asystolic vasovagal syncope.[12] These patients should be assessed at a tertiary referral clinic.

Pharmacologic Choices

Drug therapy may be effective in some, although the evidence is mixed. Few drugs have been evaluated in large randomized trials. Drugs that might be considered are shown in Table 2. Therapy may be unnecessary in patients with infrequent vasovagal syncope who have recognizable premonitory symptoms.

Fludrocortisone can be tried if simple salt supplements are ineffective. The goal is fluid retention, which may precipitate heart failure. A single randomized trial in children was negative.[13] Data from a recent unpublished trial shows that fludrocortisone reduced the likelihood of syncope by 35% in adults.

Alpha-agonists increase venous return, thereby preventing the onset of vasovagal syncope. The evidence supporting **midodrine** is inconclusive. Symptoms improved in patients enrolled in small randomized trials,[14,15] including one that showed midodrine to be more effective after 6 months than salt and fluid supplementation.[14] A randomized cross-over trial showed that midodrine seems to have no additional benefit over placebo in patients unresponsive to nonpharmacologic treatment.[16] Supine hypertension may complicate treatment.

SSRIs are of uncertain benefit in preventing vasovagal syncope. **Paroxetine** significantly reduced the frequency of spontaneous syncope over 2 years compared with placebo in one randomized trial,[17] although it was not helpful in a second trial.[18]

Beta-blockers are no longer indicated as first-line treatment for vasovagal syncope. This is based on one adequately powered, randomized placebo-controlled trial[19] and 4 smaller studies.[5] There may be an age-dependent benefit of **metoprolol**. Combined data from an observational cohort study and a randomized controlled trial suggest it may be effective in patients aged ≥42 years.[20]

Orthostatic Hypotension

The goal of therapy is to relieve symptoms of cerebral hypoperfusion while avoiding treatment side effects. Orthostatic hypotension is often associated with supine hypertension, which complicates its therapy.

Therapeutic Choices

Nonpharmacologic Choices

Remove as many hypotensive and volume-depleting drugs as possible. Increase dietary salt and fluid intake if not contraindicated. Elevate the head of the bed on blocks or bricks by 15–30 cm (this is often not well tolerated). Instruct patients to avoid hemodynamic stress such as getting up quickly, eating large meals, warm environments or hot baths, and heavy exertion.

Pharmacologic Choices

Sodium and water retention may be beneficial in patients with orthostatic hypotension. **Fludrocortisone** increases blood volume and sensitizes peripheral alpha receptors (see Table 2). **NSAIDs** promote fluid retention and also indirectly cause vasoconstriction. Try **indomethacin** 25–50 mg 3 times daily or equivalent doses of related drugs.

Midodrine (see Table 2) is a pressor amine that causes both venoconstriction (thereby increasing venous return) and arteriolar constriction (which directly increases blood pressure). Midodrine significantly increased standing blood pressure and decreased the severity of symptoms in placebo-controlled trials.[21,22] As noted above, supine hypertension may complicate treatment.

The acetylcholinesterase inhibitor **pyridostigmine**, given alone or in combination with midodrine, significantly improved standing blood pressure without increasing supine blood pressure in a short-term randomized placebo-controlled trial.[23] Further study is needed before this agent can be recommended.

Nonselective beta-blockers (e.g., **propranolol**, **timolol**, **nadolol**) block vasodilatory β_2-receptors and reduce or abolish the fall in blood pressure upon standing in patients with orthostatic hypotension. They may be helpful if indicated for another reason and if tolerated.[24]

Therapeutic Tips

- All physicians treating patients with syncope should be familiar with relevant provincial driving regulations. The regulations vary with the cause of syncope and with the therapy. The Canadian Cardiovascular Society has guidelines on the fitness of patients with syncope to drive.[25]

Table 2: **Drugs for Treatment of Syndromes of Orthostatic Intolerance**

Class	Drug	Dose	Adverse Effects	Drug Interactions	Comments	Cost[a]
Alpha$_1$-adrenergic Agonists	*midodrine* generics	Initial: 2.5–5 mg TID po ac; none after 5 pm Increase by 2.5 mg TID Q1–2 wk (Maximum: 15 mg TID)	Supine hypertension, shivering, paresthesias, piloerection, pruritus, dysuria.	Digoxin (bradycardia, arrhythmia); sympathomimetics (increased pressor effect); sympatholytics (reduced effect).	Careful adjustment of dosage or dosing intervals required. Check supine BP 2 h after any dosage increase. Increase dose until effective or limited by adverse effects.	$$$
Electrolytes	*sodium chloride*	3–5 g elemental Na^+ daily	Gastric upset, fluid retention.	Diuretics interfere with effect.	Fluid retention may precipitate HF in susceptible patients.	$
Mineralocorticoids	*fludrocortisone* Florinef	Initial: 0.1 mg daily po Increase by 0.1 mg Q1–2 wk to 0.4 mg daily	Mild edema, supine hypertension, hypokalemia, eczema, thin skin.	Diuretics interfere with effect.	Check serum K^+ and supine BP 1 wk after each dosage increase; K^+ supplements are often necessary. Fluid retention may precipitate HF in susceptible patients.	$$

[a] Cost of 30-day supply; includes drug cost only.

Dosage adjustment may be required in renal impairment; see Appendix I.

Abbreviations: HF = heart failure

Legend: $ < $10 $$ $10–50 $$$ $50–90

Suggested Readings

Grubb BP, Karas B. Clinical disorders of the autonomic nervous system associated with orthostatic intolerance: an overview of classification, clinical evaluation, and management. *Pacing Clin Electrophysiol* 1999;22(5):798-810.

Guzman JC, Armaganijan LV, Morillo CA. Treatment of neurally mediated reflex syncope.*Cardiol Clin* 2013;31(1):123-9.

Kuriachan V, Sheldon RS, Platonov M. Evidence-based treatment for vasovagal syncope. *Heart Rhythm* 2008;5(11):1609-14.

Sheldon R, Morillo CA, Krahn A. Management of vasovagal syncope: 2004. *Expert Rev Cardiovasc Ther* 2004;2(6):915-23.

Task Force for the Diagnosis and Management of Syncope; European Society of Cardiology (ESC); European Heart Rhythm Association (EHRA) et al. Guidelines for the diagnosis and management of syncope (version 2009). *Eur Heart J* 2009;30(21):2631-71.

References

1. Serletis A, Rose S, Sheldon AG et al. Vasovagal syncope in medical students and their first-degree relatives. *Eur Heart J* 2006;27(16):1965-70.
2. Colman N, Nahm K, Ganzeboom KS et al. Epidemiology of reflex syncope. *Clin Auton Res* 2004;14(Suppl 1):9-17.
3. Task Force for the Diagnosis and Management of Syncope; European Society of Cardiology (ESC); European Heart Rhythm Association (EHRA) et al. Guidelines for the diagnosis and management of syncope (version 2009). *Eur Heart J* 2009;30(21):2631-71.
4. Sheldon R, Rose S, Connolly S et al. Diagnostic criteria for vasovagal syncope based on a quantitative history. *Eur Heart J* 2006;27(3):344-50.
5. Sheldon R, Morillo CA, Krahn A. Management of vasovagal syncope: 2004. *Expert Rev Cardiovascular Ther* 2004;2(6):915-23.
6. Moya A, Brignole M, Menozzi C et al. Mechanism of syncope in patients with isolated syncope and in patients with tilt-positive syncope. *Circulation* 2001;104(11):1261-7.
7. Sheldon R. Tilt testing for syncope: a reappraisal. *Curr Opin Cardiol* 2005;20(1):38-41.
8. Kuriachan V, Sheldon RS, Platonov M. Evidence-based treatment for vasovagal syncope. *Heart Rhythm* 2008;5(11):1609-14.
9. van Dijk N, Quartieri F, Blanc JJ et al. Effectiveness of physical counterpressure maneuvers in preventing vasovagal syncope: the Physical Counterpressure Maneuvers Trial (PC-Trial). *J Am Coll Cardiol* 2006;48(8):1652-7.
10. Krediet CT, van Dijk N, Linzer M et al. Management of vasovagal syncope: controlling or aborting faints by leg crossing and muscle tensing. *Circulation* 2002;106(13):1684-9.
11. Connolly SJ, Sheldon R, Thorpe KE et al. Pacemaker therapy for prevention of syncope in patients with recurrent severe vasovagal syncope: Second Vasovagal Pacemaker Study (VPS II): a randomized trial. *JAMA* 2003;289(17):2224-9.
12. Brignole M, Menozzi C, Moya A et al. Pacemaker therapy in patients with neurally mediated syncope and documented asystole: Third International Study on Syncope of Uncertain Etiology (ISSUE-3): a randomized trial. *Circulation* 2012;125(21):2566-71.
13. Salim MA, Di Sessa TG. Effectiveness of fludrocortisone and salt in preventing syncope recurrence in children: a double-blind, placebo-controlled, randomized trial. *J Am Coll Cardiol* 2005;45(4):484-8.
14. Perez-Lugones A, Schweikert R, Pavia S et al. Usefulness of midodrine in patients with severely symptomatic neurocardiogenic syncope: a randomized control study. *J Cardiovasc Electrophysiol* 2001;12(8):935-8.
15. Ward CR, Gray JC, Gilroy JJ et al. Midodrine: a role in the management of neurocardiogenic syncope. *Heart* 1998;79(1):45-9.
16. Romme JJ, van Dijk N, Go-Schön IK et al. Effectiveness of midodrine treatment in patients with recurrent vasovagal syncope not responding to non-pharmacological treatment (STAND-trial). *Europace* 2011;13(11):1639-47.
17. Di Girolamo E, Di Iorio C, Sabatini P et al. Effects of paroxetine hydrochloride, a selective serotonin reuptake inhibitor, on refractory vasovagal syncope: a randomized, double-blind, placebo-controlled study. *J Am Coll Cardiol* 1999;33(5):1227-30.
18. Theodorakis GN, Leftheriotis D, Livanis EG et al. Fluoxetine vs. propranolol in the treatment of vasovagal syncope: a prospective, randomized, placebo-controlled study. *Europace* 2006;8(3):193-8.
19. Sheldon R, Connolly S, Rose S et al. Prevention of Syncope Trial (POST): a randomized, placebo-controlled study of metoprolol in the prevention of vasovagal syncope. *Circulation* 2006;113(9):1164-70.
20. Sheldon RS, Morillo CA, Klingenheben T et al. Age-dependent effect of β-blockers in preventing vasovagal syncope. *Circ Arrhythm Electrophysiol* 2012;5(5):920-6.
21. Low PA, Gilden JL, Freeman R et al. Efficacy of midodrine vs placebo in neurogenic orthostatic hypotension. A randomized, double-blind multicenter study. Midodrine Study Group. *JAMA* 1997;277(13):1046-51.
22. Wright RA, Kaufmann HC, Perera R et al. A double-blind, dose-response study of midodrine in neurogenic orthostatic hypotension. *Neurology* 1998;51(1):120-4.
23. Singer W, Sandroni P, Opfer-Gehrking TL et al. Pyridostigmine treatment trial in neurogenic orthostatic hypotension. *Arch Neurol* 2006;63(4):513-8.
24. Cleophas TJ, Kauw FH, Bijl C et al. Effects of beta adrenergic receptor agonists and antagonists in diabetics with symptoms of postural hypotension: a double-blind, placebo-controlled study. *Angiology* 1986;37(11):855-62.
25. Simpson C, Dorian P, Gupta A et al. Assessment of the cardiac patient for fitness to drive: drive subgroup executive summary. *Can J Cardiol* 2004;20(13):1314-20.

Cardiovascular Disorders

Chapter 48
Venous Thromboembolism

Philip S. Wells, MD, FRCP(C), MSc

This chapter addresses both the treatment and prophylaxis of venous thromboembolism.

Treatment of Venous Thromboembolism

Goals of Therapy

Deep Vein Thrombosis (DVT)

- Prevent major pulmonary embolism
- Prevent thrombus extension
- Prevent post-thrombotic syndrome
- Reduce morbidity of the acute event

Pulmonary Embolism (PE)

- Prevent death
- Prevent recurrent thromboembolism
- Prevent chronic thromboembolic pulmonary hypertension

Investigations

The signs and symptoms of DVT and PE are insensitive and nonspecific. To help stratify patient risk when PE or DVT are considered possibilities, it is widely recommended that a validated clinical rule (e.g., Wells[1] or Modified Geneva[2] rule) be applied after the history, physical exam and routine tests such as chest x-ray and ECG. To select patients who require additional imaging procedures, the next test should be a D-dimer. VTE can reliably be excluded without imaging tests for patients with pretest probabilities of low, moderate or "unlikely," in combination with a negative D-dimer test.[3,4] In all others imaging is important for optimal management. The following tests should be selected based on availability and ease of use:

- DVT: B-mode compression ultrasound, colour duplex ultrasound, ascending contrast venography, CT contrast venography
- PE: Contrast pulmonary angiography, ventilation-perfusion lung scan, CT, pulmonary angiography, magnetic resonance pulmonary angiography, tests for DVT as described above

If distal DVT is diagnosed and symptoms are not severe, treatment may not be necessary. Repeat imaging at 1 week to identify any clot extension requiring treatment.[5]

Screen for thrombophilia in patients under the age of 40 with recurrent venous thromboembolism (VTE) or a family history.

Therapeutic Choices

General Measures

The majority of patients with DVT can be treated as outpatients. Likewise, many patients with PE—best estimates are about 50% of all cases of PE—who do not have compromised cardiopulmonary function may also be treated as outpatients.[6,7] Ideally an organized outpatient treatment program should be utilized to ensure safe and effective patient management. Other general measures are specific to DVT or PE.

Deep Vein Thrombosis

- Rest if symptoms warrant (reduces pain and swelling), but evidence suggests early ambulation is safe and may actually be preferred as resolution of pain and swelling may be faster.[8,9]
- Elevating the swollen limb while resting may hasten resolution of edema.
- **Analgesics** may be prescribed for pain. NSAIDs are effective but may increase the risk of bleeding, especially when used with anticoagulants. Start with acetaminophen, but opioids may be required for a few days.

Pulmonary Embolism

- Oxygen as indicated for hypoxia.
- Intravenous fluids if hypotensive or volume contracted.
- Vasopressor agents if hypotensive and organ hypoperfusion is detected (shock).
- **Analgesics** may be prescribed for pain. NSAIDs are effective but may increase the risk of bleeding, especially when used with anticoagulants. Start with acetaminophen, but opioids may be required for a few days.

Nonpharmacologic Choices

Elastic Stockings and Compression Bandages

The post-thrombotic syndrome (PTS) is a clinically important and frequent complication of DVT developing in as many as 60% of patients after proximal DVT. The most prominent symptoms are chronic swelling and pain, discomfort when walking and skin discolouration.[5] Precise prediction of which patients will develop PTS is not possible although some data support a higher probability for those with iliofemoral DVT and recurrent DVT. It was thought that graduated compression stockings that apply an ankle pressure of 30–40 mm Hg and a lower pressure higher up the leg reduced the risk of PTS following DVT. This was shown to not be the case in a large, placebo controlled trial.[10] The SOX study enrolled over 800 patients with DVT. The cumulative incidence of PTS was 14.2% in the active stocking group (30–40 mmHg compression stockings) and 12.7% in the placebo stocking group, which was not a statistically significant difference.

Graduated compression stockings can improve edema and pain in the acute stage of DVT. They can also relieve symptoms in patients who develop PTS but do not prevent the development of PTS. Use of compression stockings is not appropriate when there is pre-existing peripheral vascular disease.

Pharmacologic Choices

Subcutaneous **low molecular weight heparin (LMWH), fondaparinux**, or **unfractionated heparin (UFH)** is recommended for the initial treatment of established DVT or PE (Figure 1, Table 5). UFH can be administered iv or in a monitored or fixed-dose sc regimen. Oral vitamin K antagonists such as **warfarin** are started at the same time and administered concurrently for several days. LMWH, fondaparinux or UFH is continued for a minimum of 5 days or until the INR is ≥2 for 24–48 hours. The duration of oral anticoagulation is dependent on the risk of recurrence of VTE (Table 1). Treatment of a first episode in a patient with a transient risk factor should continue for just 3 months.[11] In those with unprovoked VTE or irreversible risk factors, treatment with oral anticoagulants for an indefinite period may be considered because of lifelong increased risk of recurrence. The risk is highest in males. This risk should be balanced against the treatment-related risk of bleeding.[5] LMWH is generally the treatment of choice in cancer-associated thrombosis and may be used as an alternative to warfarin in circumstances in which warfarin therapy is contraindicated, inconvenient or impractical to manage, such as poor venous access for INR testing.[12] ASA was the least effective agent in a network meta-analysis, though it might be considered where bleeding is a concern.[13]

Low Molecular Weight Heparins

The pharmacokinetics of LMWHs are more predictable than those of UFH, and their elimination half-life is longer. These properties make weight-adjusted fixed dosing of sc LMWHs an excellent alternative to adjusted-dose iv UFH in the initial treatment of VTE. Meta-analyses suggest similar or superior efficacy with LMWH.[14] One systematic review suggests that 6 months of therapeutic doses of tinzaparin was more effective than vitamin K antagonist therapy in reducing the risk of PTS.[15] LMWHs, as a single daily dose, have become the management of choice for initial treatment of DVT for many outpatients.[16] They are also effective in the treatment of PE.

Unfractionated Heparin

If UFH is used for the treatment of VTE, it is most commonly given by iv infusion in a dose adjusted to prolong the activated partial thromboplastin time (aPTT) to a time that corresponds to a heparin anti-Xa level of 0.3–0.7. In general this is an aPTT of 1.5–2.5 times control (target therapeutic range should be determined by an institution's coagulation laboratory). A practical weight-based nomogram has been developed for adjusting iv UFH[17] (Table 2).

Figure 1: Management of Venous Thromboembolism

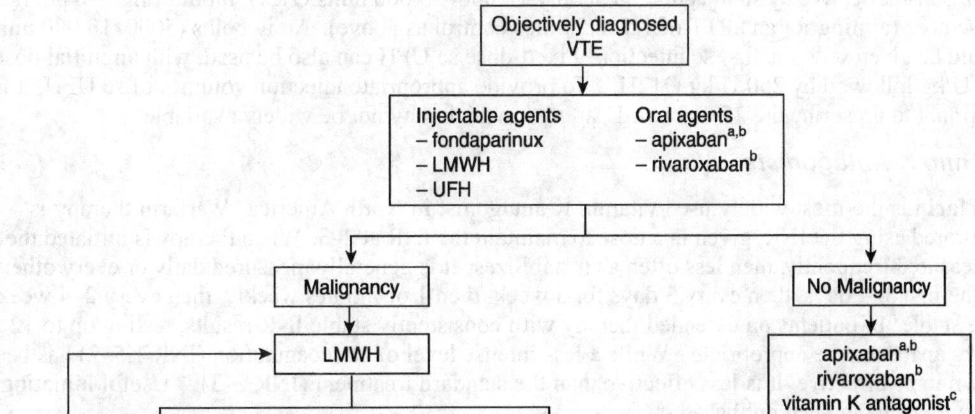

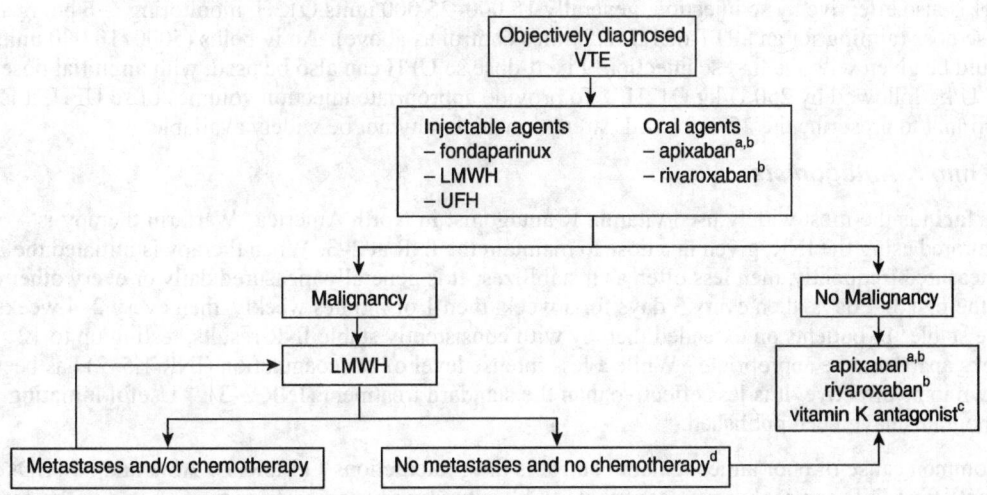

[a] Not Health Canada-approved for this indication.
[b] If malignancy not suspected and patient hemodynamically stable.
[c] Start vitamin K antagonist concomitantly with the injectable anticoagulant. Stop the injectable agent when INR ≥2 for 24–48 hours.
[d] Although studies are lacking in cancer patients, anticoagulation is generally continued until cancer resolves or cancer treatment is completed. After 6 months of LMWH the use of VKA is an option, especially in lower risk patients (e.g., those with early stage cancer).

Abbreviations: INR = international normalized ratio; LMWH = low molecular weight heparin; UFH = unfractionated heparin; VTE = venous thromboembolism

Table 1: **Duration of Treatment for Symptomatic Venous Thromboembolism**[5]

Duration of Treatment	Clinical Setting
3 months	First event with reversible or time-limited risk factor such as surgery First episode of unprovoked distal DVT
Minimum of 3 months (consider extended treatment)	First unprovoked event
Extended treatment	Cancer (until resolved) Second episode of unprovoked VTE

Table 2: **Body Weight-based Dosing of Intravenous Heparin in Adults**[a]

aPTT (seconds)	Dose Change (units/kg/h)	Additional Action	Next aPTT (h)
<35 (<1.2 × mean normal)	+4	Rebolus with 80 units/kg	6
35–45 (1.2–1.5 × mean normal)	+2	Rebolus with 40 units/kg	6
46–70[b] (1.5–2.3 × mean normal)	0	None	6[c]
71–90 (2.3–3 × mean normal)	−2	None	6
>90 (>3 × mean normal)	−3	Stop infusion for 1 h	6

[a] Initial dosing: 80 units/kg iv bolus; maintenance infusion of heparin, at a rate dictated by body weight through an infusion apparatus calibrated for low flow rates: 18 units/kg/h (aPTT in 6 hours).
[b] The therapeutic range in seconds should correspond to a plasma heparin level of 0.2–0.4 units/mL by protamine sulfate titration. When aPTT is checked at 6 hours or longer, steady-state kinetics can be assumed.
[c] During the first 24 hours, repeat aPTT every 6 hours. Thereafter, monitor aPTT once every morning unless it is outside the therapeutic range.
Adapted with permission from Hyers TM et al. Antithrombotic therapy for venous thromboembolic disease. *Chest* 1998;114(5 Suppl):561S-578S.

UFH is also effective by sc injection, generally 15 000–25 000 units Q12H, monitoring 4–6 hours after the sc dose (aiming for an aPTT of 1.5–2.5 times control as above). An iv bolus (5000–10 000 units) should be given with the first sc injection. Fixed-dose sc UFH can also be used, with an initial dose of 333 U/kg followed by 250 U/kg Q12H.[18] To provide appropriate injection volumes of sc UFH, it is important to prescribe the 25 000 U/mL strength, which may not be widely available.

Vitamin K Antagonists

Warfarin is the most widely used vitamin K antagonist in North America. Warfarin therapy is monitored using the INR, given in a dose to maintain the INR at 2–3. When therapy is initiated the INR is measured frequently, then less often as it stabilizes. It is generally measured daily or every other day for the first 3–4 days, then every 3 days for a week, then 1 or 2 times weekly, then every 2–4 weeks once stable. In patients on extended therapy with consistently stable INR results, testing up to 12 weeks apart may be appropriate.[5] While a less intense level of anticoagulation (INR 1.5–2) has been shown to be effective, it is less effective than the standard treatment (INR 2–3).[19] Useful initiating nomograms have been published.[20]

A common cause of poor anticoagulant control is drug interactions[21] (Table 3). ASA and NSAIDs do not affect INR control but may contribute to bleeding by causing gastric irritation and in the case of ASA by inhibiting platelet function. Several herbal or alternative products interact with warfarin, for example ginkgo, ginseng and St. John's wort. Advise patients to avoid using such products. The Thrombosis Interest Group of Canada provides information that can be used for patient education (available at www.tigc.org/clinical-guides/For-Patients-Taking-Oral-Anticoagulants.aspx).

If an alternative vitamin K antagonist is required, **nicoumalone (acenocoumarol)** is available (see Table 5). It is used in a similar way to warfarin, with a similar drug interaction profile, but a much shorter half-life.

Table 3: Clinically Significant Warfarin Drug Interactions[a]

Category of Interaction	Class		Drug
Drugs that increase INR and potentiate the effects of warfarin	Anti-inflammatory Analgesics and Immunologics		Acetaminophen,[b] ASA, celecoxib, interferon, phenylbutazone, piroxicam, sulfinpyrazone, tramadol
	Antimicrobials		
		Azole antifungals	Fluconazole, itraconazole, miconazole (including vaginal preparations), voriconazole
		Fluoroquinolones	Ciprofloxacin, levofloxacin
		Macrolides	Azithromycin, clarithromycin, erythromycin
		Others	Amoxicillin/clavulanate, isoniazid, metronidazole, ritonavir, sulfamethoxazole/trimethoprim, tetracycline
	Cardiovascular Drugs		
		Fibrates	Fenofibrate
		Statins	Fluvastatin, simvastatin
		Others	Amiodarone, diltiazem, propafenone, propranolol, quinidine
	CNS Drugs		
		Antiparkinsonian drugs	Entacapone, ropinirole
		SSRIs	Citalopram, fluvoxamine, sertraline
		Others	Alcohol (large amounts; patients with liver disease), chloral hydrate, disulfiram, phenytoin (acute administration)
	Gastrointestinal Drugs		Cimetidine, omeprazole
	Foods, Chinese Medicines, Herbs		Boldo-fenugreek,[c] Danshen,[d] Dong quai,[e] fish oil, grapefruit juice, *Lycium barbarum*, mango fruit, PC-SPES, Quilinggao[f]
	Others		Anabolic steroids, fluorouracil, gemcitabine, levamisole/fluorouracil, paclitaxel, tamoxifen, tolterodine, zileuton
Drugs that decrease INR and diminish the effects of warfarin	Antimicrobials		Ribavirin, rifampin, ritonavir
	Cardiovascular Drugs		Bosentan, cholestyramine
	CNS Drugs		Barbiturates, carbamazepine, chlordiazepoxide
	Gastrointestinal Drugs		Azathioprine, mesalamine (5-aminosalicylic acid), sucralfate
	Foods and Herbs		Avocado (large amounts); ginseng; foods, enteral feeds or multivitamins that contain large amounts of vitamin K
	Others		Chelation therapy, mercaptopurine, raloxifene

[a] Rated as "highly-probably" or "probably" clinically significant according to a systematic review.[21]
[b] Doses >2 g/day.[22]
[c] A herbal combination of boldo (*Peumus boldus*) and fenugreek (*Trigonella foenum-graecum*).
[d] A Chinese medicine derived from *Salvia miltiorrhiza*.
[e] A Chinese medicine derived from Chinese Angelica (*Angelica sinensis*).
[f] A Chinese medicine that contains several herbs. Composition varies among manufacturers.

New Oral Anticoagulants

Newer oral anticoagulants are characterized broadly as small molecules that directly inhibit the active site of thrombin or factor Xa. They have rapid onset of action, with peak drug levels in 3–4 hours, and relatively short half-lives of 6–12 hours. Importantly, they are given in a fixed dose and no monitoring of anticoagulant effect is required. These drugs have few drug interactions and no significant food interactions.[23] **Apixaban**, **dabigatran** and **rivaroxaban** (see Table 5) have been compared to standard VTE treatment and found to be at least noninferior.[24,25,26] Apixaban and rivaroxaban were started and used as a single agent throughout avoiding the need for injectable heparin. Only rivaroxaban is approved for treatment of DVT or PE. Currently the management of major hemorrhage in patients taking these agents is complicated by the lack of a specific antidote.

Thrombolytic Agents

The use of thrombolytic therapy for the treatment of acute DVT or PE is uncommon as benefits are uncertain and there is a significant risk of intracranial hemorrhage.

Less than 10% of patients with VTE are eligible for thrombolytic therapy (young patients with massive ileofemoral vein thrombosis or patients with hemodynamically unstable PE). Though not approved by Health Canada, **alteplase** is recommended by the American College of Chest Physicians when indicated.[5] The best results are obtained with recent thrombi (symptoms for <14 days) Thrombolysis should probably not be considered in those with short life expectancy and poor functional status. Some data suggest catheter-directed lysis may be superior to systemically administered thrombolysis but local technical expertise is required.

Thrombolytic-associated reductions in PTS were seen in a randomized trial comparing catheter-directed thrombolysis to standard therapy for iliofemoral DVT.[27] Thrombolytic therapy increased vein patency at 6 months (66% vs. 47%) and there was significantly less PTS at 24 months (41% vs. 56%). Thrombolysis was associated with more bleeding complications, did not prevent recurrent events and mortality was no different in the 2 groups, and as a consequence it is unclear if the advantages outweigh the cost and risk of therapy.

Thrombolytics are rarely required for DVT and use should generally be reserved for those patients with life- or limb-threatening VTE and no bleeding contraindications. Though there is some consensus in the treatment of PE,[5] there is no agreement on the appropriate dose of alteplase for DVT.

Prophylaxis of Venous Thromboembolism

Venous thromboembolism (VTE) is a common cause of morbidity and mortality in hospitalized patients; the frequency varies according to patients' risk. The risk of VTE is probably increased in the presence of factors related to venous stasis and coagulopathy, but few of these factors have been demonstrated to increase postoperative risk of thrombosis. Therefore recommendations for thrombosis prophylaxis are currently based on the type of surgery (Table 4).[28,29] Certain acutely ill hospitalized medical patients (e.g., those with acute infection, heart failure or respiratory failure) may also be candidates for thrombosis prophylaxis.[30]

Duration of prophylaxis depends upon the surgery and medical condition. Prophylaxis should generally be continued for at least 10–14 days. In high-risk situations such as hip/knee arthroplasty and some gynecologic procedures, prophylaxis has been suggested beyond discharge from hospital, especially in cases of early discharge or continued immobility. Further research is needed to develop criteria for selection of patients who require an extended duration of prophylaxis.

Table 4: **Surgeries with Level 1B Evidence[a] for Postoperative Prophylaxis with Pharmacologic Agents[b,28,29]**

Elective total hip replacement	Hip fracture surgery
Elective total knee replacement	High risk general and abdominal surgery

[a] Level 1B is a strong recommendation with moderate quality evidence.
[b] In patients at very high bleeding risk, mechanical prophylaxis may be preferable.

Goals of Therapy

- Prevent deep vein thrombosis (DVT) and pulmonary embolism (PE)
- Reduce mortality
- Prevent the postphlebitic syndrome
- Prevent chronic thromboembolic pulmonary hypertension

Therapeutic Choices

Nonpharmacologic Choices

Graduated compression stockings and intermittent pneumatic compression devices (sleeves placed on the legs and inflated with a programmable pump) reduce the risk of VTE, but to a lesser degree than pharmacologic methods. Their use should be limited to clinical settings where the risk of bleeding is high (e.g., after neurosurgery). Some guidelines suggest the combination of pharmacologic and nonpharmacologic methods in patients at high risk for VTE, but the quality of evidence is poor. Ensure proper use and adherence.

Interruption of the inferior vena cava through the use of a filter that prevents embolization is rarely indicated for primary prophylaxis but should be considered in patients in whom anticoagulants have failed or are absolutely contraindicated. A variety of retrievable filters are now available and are often preferred over the permanent ones.

Pharmacologic Choices

Dalteparin, **enoxaparin**, **nadroparin** and **tinzaparin** are low molecular weight heparins approved for both the treatment and prophylaxis of VTE (see Table 6).[31] **Unfractionated heparin** is effective as prophylaxis only for procedures with moderate risk. **Fondaparinux** is a specific factor Xa inhibitor approved for the prophylaxis of VTE in high-risk orthopedic patients.[32] All these agents prevent VTE with minimal risk of bleeding in older acute medical patients. **Vitamin K antagonists** are used with the dose adjusted to target an INR of 2–3. Some evidence suggests that **ASA** may be effective for VTE prophylaxis following orthopedic surgery, but its use for this indication is controversial.[28] **Apixaban**, **dabigatran** and **rivaroxaban** are new oral anticoagulants that can be used for VTE prophylaxis following elective total hip or total knee replacement surgery. Apixaban and rivaroxaban have demonstrated superiority over enoxaparin.[33,34]

Choices during Pregnancy and Breastfeeding

VTE during pregnancy and the postpartum period is an important cause of maternal morbidity and mortality. Anticoagulants may be required for the treatment of new episodes of VTE, or for prophylaxis in mothers with a history of prior VTE.[35]

- LMWH is the anticoagulant of choice during pregnancy. UFH is used when LMWH is not available. LMWH induces less bone loss than UFH and can be used daily. UFH and LMWHs do not cross the placental barrier. Warfarin is usually avoided during pregnancy because of the potential for teratogenic effects.[35]

- It has been recommended that use of LMWH to treat VTE during pregnancy should include monitoring of anti-Xa levels to achieve a target of 0.5–1 U/mL 3–6 hours postdose, but no study has compared monitoring to no monitoring.[36]
- Subcutaneous injections of UFH twice daily can be monitored and adjusted to achieve therapeutic levels (mid-interval anti-Xa 0.35–0.7 U/mL).
- Warfarin, sc UFH or LMWH may be used for about 6 weeks after delivery for secondary prevention. This applies to treatment doses used in women with new VTE during pregnancy, or lower prophylactic doses used for other indications.
- Women can breastfeed while being treated with warfarin, UFH or LMWH.
- The management of pregnant women with a previous DVT or PE is controversial with no large studies to date; UFH 5000 units sc Q12H or LMWH throughout pregnancy is recommended in some women, e.g., those with a prior history of VTE or with a high-risk thrombophilia.
- Fondaparinux should be used in pregnant or breastfeeding women only if other agents cannot be used.
- Apixaban, dabigatran and rivaroxaban should not be used in pregnant and breastfeeding women.

A discussion of general principles on the use of medications in these special populations can be found in Appendix II and Appendix III. Other specialized reference sources are also provided in these appendices.

Therapeutic Tips

- **Argatroban** and **danaparoid** are approved for treatment of heparin-induced thrombocytopenia (HIT) in Canada. Limited data indicate that **bivalirudin** and **fondaparinux** may also be effective.

Suggested Readings

Bates SM, Jaeschke R, Stevens SM et al. Diagnosis of DVT: Antithrombotic Therapy and Prevention of Thrombosis, 9th ed: American College of Chest Physicians Evidence-Based Clinical Practice Guidelines. *Chest* 2012;141(2 Suppl):e351S-418S.

Gandara E, Wells PS. Diagnosis: use of clinical probability algorithms. *Clin Chest Med* 2010;31(4):629-39.

Qaseem A, Snow V, Barry P et al. Current diagnosis of venous thromboembolism in primary care: a clinical practice guideline from the American Academy of Family Physicians and the American College of Physicians. *Ann Fam Med* 2007;5(1):57-62.

Table 5: Drugs for Treatment of Venous Thromboembolism

Class	Drug	Dose	Adverse Effects	Comments	Cost[a]
Direct Factor Xa Inhibitors	*rivaroxaban* Xarelto	15 mg BID po × 3 weeks, then 20 mg po daily First DVT with reversible or time-limited risk factor: × 3 months First idiopathic DVT: × 6 months	Bleeding.	Contraindicated in combination with strong inhibitors of both CYP3A4 and P-gp, e.g., itraconazole, ritonavir. Not recommended when ClCr <30 mL/min.	$$
Indirect Factor Xa Inhibitors	*fondaparinux* Arixtra, generics	<50 kg: 5 mg daily sc 50–100 kg: 7.5 mg daily sc >100 kg: 10 mg daily sc	Bleeding; thrombocytopenia; allergic reactions (rare).	Use caution in patients with renal dysfunction. Use with caution in patients with a history of HIT.	$$$
Low-Molecular-Weight Heparins	*dalteparin* Fragmin	100 IU/kg BID sc or 200 IU/kg Q24H sc Maximum: 18 000 IU/day	Bleeding; HIT and osteoporosis are both less common than with UFH.	Contraindicated in those with a history of HIT; caution in those with renal dysfunction.	$$$
	enoxaparin Lovenox	1 mg/kg BID sc or 1.5 mg/kg Q24H sc Maximum: 180 mg/day	See dalteparin.	See dalteparin. 1 mg = 100 IU.	$$$$
	nadroparin Fraxiparine, Fraxiparine Forte	86 IU/kg BID sc or 171 IU/kg Q24H sc Maximum: 17 100 IU/day	See dalteparin.	See dalteparin.	$$
	tinzaparin Innohep	175 IU/kg Q24H sc Maximum: 18 000 IU/day	See dalteparin.	See dalteparin.	$$$
Thrombolytics	*alteplase* Activase rt-PA	PE: 100 mg iv over 2 hours	Bleeding (can be fatal). Significant bleeding associated with: aortic dissection, previous intracranial hemorrhage or other intracerebral pathology. Other bleeding risks: uncontrolled HTN (BP >180/110 mm Hg); traumatic or prolonged (>10 min) CPR or major surgery (<3 wk); noncompressible venous punctures; recent (2–4 wk) internal bleeding; pregnancy; active peptic ulcer.	Not a Health Canada-approved indication. Dose for PE recommended by American College of Chest Physicians guidelines.[5]	$2746/ 100 mg vial

(cont'd)

Table 5: **Drugs for Treatment of Venous Thromboembolism** *(cont'd)*

Class	Drug	Dose	Adverse Effects	Comments	Cost[a]
Unfractionated Heparin (UFH)	*heparin, unfractionated* Heparin Leo, generics	Treatment: iv infusion most common (see Table 2 for dosing nomogram). Also can use sc 5000–10 000 units iv followed by 15 000–20 000 units Q12H sc adjusted to maintain therapeutic aPTT	Bleeding, HIT, osteoporosis.	Monitor platelets. Contraindicated in patients with a history of HIT.	$$
Vitamin K Antagonists	*warfarin* Coumadin, generics	Usual dose: 0.5–6 mg daily po Adjust dose to maintain INR 2–3; higher doses may be necessary in some patients	Bleeding; hair loss, blue fingers and toes (uncommon); skin necrosis (rare).	See Table 3 for drug interactions.	$
	nicoumalone Sintrom	Usual dose: 0.5–4 mg daily po Adjust dose to maintain INR 2–3; higher doses may be necessary in some patients	See warfarin.	See Table 3 for drug interactions.	$

[a] Costs provided are for the first week of therapy based on 50 kg unless otherwise specified; includes drug cost only.

Dosage adjustment may be required in renal impairment; see Appendix I.

Abbreviations: aPTT = activated partial thromboplastin time; HIT = heparin-induced thrombocytopenia; HTN = hypertension; INR = international normalized ratio; PE = pulmonary emboli; UFH = unfractionated heparin

Legend: $ < $25 $$ $25–75 $$$ $75–125 $$$$ $125–175

Table 6: Drugs for Prophylaxis of Venous Thromboembolism[a]

Class	Drug	Dose	Adverse Effects	Comments	Cost[b]
Direct Factor Xa Inhibitors	*apixaban* Eliquis	2.5 mg BID po starting 12–24 h after surgery THR surgery: × 32–38 days TKR surgery: × 14 days	Bleeding.	Contraindicated in combination with strong inhibitors of both CYP3A4 and P-gp, e.g., itraconazole, ritonavir.	$
	rivaroxaban (renal) Xarelto	10 mg daily po starting 6–10 h after surgery THR surgery: × 35 days TKR surgery: × 14 days	Bleeding.	See apixaban. Not recommended in severe renal impairment.	$
Direct Thrombin Inhibitors	*dabigatran* (renal) Pradaxa	110 mg 1–4 h after surgery, then 220 mg daily po THR surgery: × 28–35 days TKR surgery: × 10 days	Bleeding, dyspepsia.	Contraindicated in combination with strong inhibitors of P-gp, e.g., quinidine. Caution with other drugs acting on P-gp. Reduce dose if >75 years of age and moderate renal impairment.	$
Indirect Factor Xa Inhibitors	*fondaparinux* (renal) Arixtra, generics	Patients ≥50 kg: 2.5 mg daily sc after high-risk orthopedic surgery Patients <50 kg: not recommended	Bleeding, allergic reactions (rare).	Not recommended in patients with renal dysfunction.	$$$
Low Molecular Weight Heparins	*dalteparin* (renal) Fragmin	General surgery: 2500 IU daily sc Orthopedics: 5000 IU daily sc	Bleeding, HIT (rare) and osteoporosis (less common than UFH).	Contraindicated in those with a history of HIT.	$$-$$$
	enoxaparin (renal) Lovenox	General surgery: 40 mg Q24H sc Orthopedics: 30 mg Q12H sc	See dalteparin.	See dalteparin. 1 mg = 100 IU.	$$$
	nadroparin (renal) Fraxiparine, Fraxiparine Forte	General surgery: 2850 IU daily sc Orthopedics: 38 IU/kg Q12H sc × 2; then 38 IU/kg Q24H sc through postoperative day 3, then 57 IU/kg Q24H sc	See dalteparin.	See dalteparin.	$$$
	tinzaparin (renal) Innohep	General surgery: 3500 IU Q24H sc Orthopedics: 50–75 IU/kg Q24H sc	See dalteparin.	See dalteparin.	$$
Unfractionated Heparin (UFH)	*heparin, unfractionated* Heparin Leo, generics	General surgery: 5000 units Q12H or Q8H sc	Bleeding, HIT, osteoporosis.	Monitor platelets closely during first week of therapy. Contraindicated in those with a history of HIT.	$$

[a] For vitamin K antagonist information see Table 5.
[b] Costs provided are for 10 days of therapy, based on 50 kg; includes drug cost only.
(renal) Dosage adjustment may be required in renal impairment; see Appendix I.
Abbreviations: HIT = heparin-induced thrombocytopenia; THR = total hip replacement; TKR = total knee replacement
Legend: $ < $40 $$ $40–80 $$-$$$ $40–120 $$$ $80–120

References

1. Wells PS, Anderson DR, Rodger M et al. Evaluation of D-dimer in the diagnosis of suspected deep-vein thrombosis. *N Engl J Med* 2003;349(13):1227-35.
2. Klok FA, Mos IC, Nijkeuter M et al. Simplification of the revised Geneva score for assessing clinical probability of pulmonary embolism. *Arch Intern Med* 2008;168(19):2131-6.
3. Gandara E, Wells PS. Diagnosis: use of clinical probability algorithms. *Clin Chest Med* 2010;31(4):629-39.
4. Wells PS. Integrated strategies for the diagnosis of venous thromboembolism. *J Thromb Haemos* 2007;5(Suppl 1):41-50.
5. Kearon C, Akl EA, Comerota AJ et al. Antithrombotic therapy for VTE disease: Antithrombotic Therapy and Prevention of Thrombosis, 9th ed: American College of Chest Physicians Evidence-Based Clinical Practice Guidelines. *Chest* 2012;141(2 Suppl):e419S-94S.
6. Scarvelis D, Wells PS. Diagnosis and treatment of deep-vein thrombosis. *CMAJ* 2006;175(9):1087-92.
7. Baglin T. Fifty percent of patients with pulmonary embolism can be treated as outpatients. *J Thromb Haemost* 2010;8(11):2404-5.
8. Aissaoui N, Martins E, Mouly S et al. A meta-analysis of bed rest versus early ambulation in the management of pulmonary embolism, deep vein thrombosis, or both. *Int J Cardiol* 2009;137(1):37-41.
9. Kahn SR, Shrier I, Kearon C. Physical activity in patients with deep venous thrombosis: a systematic review. *Thromb Res* 2008;122(6):763-73.
10. Kahn SR, Shapiro S, Wells PS et al. Compression stockings to prevent post-thrombotic syndrome: a randomised placebo-controlled trial. *Lancet* 2014;383(9920):880-8.
11. Iorio A, Kearon C, Filippucci E et al. Risk of recurrence after a first episode of symptomatic venous thromboembolism provoked by a transient risk factor: a systematic review. *Arch Intern Med* 2010;170(19):1710-6.
12. Andras A, Sala Tenna A, Crawford F. Vitamin K antagonists or low-molecular-weight heparin for the long term treatment of symptomatic venous thromboembolism. *Cochrane Database Syst Rev* 2012;10:CD002001.
13. Castellucci LA, Cameron C, Le Gal G et al. Efficacy and safety outcomes of oral anticoagulants and antiplatelet drugs in the secondary prevention of venous thromboembolism: systematic review and network meta-analysis. *BMJ* 2013;347:f5133.
14. Erkens PM, Prins MH. Fixed dose subcutaneous low-molecular-weight heparins versus adjusted dose unfractionated heparin for venous thromboembolism. *Cochrane Database Syst Rev* 2010;(9):CD001100.
15. Hull RD, Liang J, Townshend G. Long-term low-molecular-weight heparin and the post-thrombotic syndrome: a systematic review. *Am J Med* 2011;124(8):756-65.
16. Bhutia S, Wong PF. Once versus twice daily low-molecular-weight heparin for the initial treatment of venous thromboembolism. *Cochrane Database Syst Rev* 2013;7:CD003074.
17. Raschke RA, Reilly BM, Guidry JR et al. The weight-based heparin dosing nomogram compared with a "Standard care" nomogram. A randomized controlled trial. *Ann Intern Med* 1993;119(9):874-81.
18. Kearon C, Ginsberg JS, Julian JA et al. Comparison of fixed-dose weight-adjusted unfractionated heparin and low-molecular-weight heparin for acute treatment of venous thromboembolism. *JAMA* 2006;296(8):935-42.
19. Kearon C, Ginsberg JS, Kovacs MJ et al. Comparison of low-intensity warfarin therapy with conventional-intensity warfarin therapy for long-term prevention of recurrent venous thromboembolism. *N Engl J Med* 2003;349(7):631-9.
20. Le Gal G, Carrier M, Tierney S et al. Prediction of the warfarin maintenance dose after completion of the 10 mg initiation nomogram: do we really need genotyping? *J Thromb Haemost* 2010;8(1):90-4.
21. Holbrook AM, Pereira JA, Labiris R et al. Systematic overview of warfarin and its drug and food interactions. *Arch Intern Med* 2005;165(10):1095-106.
22. Gebauer MG, Nyfort-Hansen K, Henschke PJ et al. Warfarin and acetaminophen interaction. *Pharmacotherapy* 2003;23(1):109-12.
23. Garcia DA, Libby E, Crowther MA. The new oral anticoagulants. *Blood* 2010;115(1):15-20.
24. Agnelli G, Buller HR, Cohen A et al. Oral apixaban for the treatment of acute venous thromboembolism. *N Engl J Med* 2013;369(9):799-808.
25. EINSTEIN Investigators, Bauersachs R, Berkowitz SD et al. Oral rivaroxaban for symptomatic venous thromboembolism. *N Engl J Med* 2010;363(26):2499-510.
26. Schulman S, Kearon C, Kakkar AK et al. Dabigatran versus warfarin in the treatment of acute venous thromboembolism. *N Engl J Med* 2009;361(24):2342-52.
27. Enden T, Haig Y, Klow NE et al. Long-term outcome after additional catheter-directed thrombolysis versus standard treatment for acute iliofemoral deep vein thrombosis (the CaVenT study): a randomised controlled trial. *Lancet* 2012;379(9810):31-8.
28. Falck-Ytter Y, Francis CW, Johanson NA et al. Prevention of VTE in orthopedic surgery patients: Antithrombotic Therapy and Prevention of Thrombosis, 9th ed: American College of Chest Physicians Evidence-Based Clinical Practice Guidelines. *Chest* 2012;141(2 Suppl):e278S-325S.
29. Gould MK, Garcia DA, Wren SM et al. Prevention of VTE in nonorthopedic surgical patients: Antithrombotic Therapy and Prevention of Thrombosis, 9th ed: American College of Chest Physicians Evidence-Based Clinical Practice Guidelines. *Chest* 2012;141(2 Suppl):e227S-77S.
30. Kahn SR, Lim W, Dunn AS et al. Prevention of VTE in nonsurgical patients: Antithrombotic Therapy and Prevention of Thrombosis, 9th ed: American College of Chest Physicians Evidence-Based Clinical Practice Guidelines. *Chest* 2012;141(2 Suppl):e195S-226S.
31. Weitz JI. Low-molecular-weight heparins. *N Engl J Med* 1997;337(10):688-98.
32. Turpie AG, Bauer KA, Eriksson BI et al. Fondaparinux vs enoxaparin for the prevention of venous thromboembolism in major orthopedic surgery: a meta-analysis of 4 randomized double-blind studies. *Arch Intern Med* 2002;162(16):1833-40.
33. Lassen MR, Gallus A, Raskob GE et al. Apixaban versus enoxaparin for thromboprophylaxis after hip replacement. *N Engl J Med* 2010;363(26):2487-98.
34. Eriksson BI, Kakkar AK, Turpie AG et al. Oral rivaroxaban for the prevention of symptomatic venous thromboembolism after elective hip and knee replacement. *J Bone Joint Surg Br* 2009;91(5):636-44.
35. Bates SM, Greer IA, Pabinger I et al. Venous thromboembolism, thrombophilia, antithrombotic therapy, and pregnancy: American College of Chest Physicians Evidence-Based Clinical Practice Guidelines (8th edition). *Chest* 2008;133(6 Suppl):844S-886S.
36. Bourjeily G, Paidas M, Khalil H et al. Pulmonary embolism in pregnancy. *Lancet* 2010;375(9713):500-12.

Chapter 49
Ventricular Tachyarrhythmias

Paul Dorian, MD, MSc, FRCPC

Ventricular tachycardia (VT) is defined as ≥3 consecutive ventricular complexes at a rate >100 bpm on an ECG recording. *Ventricular fibrillation* (VF) is defined as a rapid, disorganized rhythm without recognizable QRS complexes on the ECG. VF is invariably associated with cardiovascular collapse and is almost always fatal unless the patient is electrically defibrillated.

This chapter describes a diagnostic and therapeutic approach for patients with documented VF, VT or cardiac arrest.

Goals of Therapy

- Relieve symptoms, including restoring a perfusing rhythm as quickly as possible in cases of sustained VT, VF or cardiac arrest[1,2]
- Prevent the potentially fatal occurrence or recurrence of sustained VT or VF[1,2]

Investigations[3,4]

- Careful history with special reference to:
  - syncope or severe presyncope
  - angina, heart failure symptoms
  - history suggesting structural heart disease, especially prior MI, or heart failure
  - symptom correlation with exercise or stress
  - recent ingestion of medications that might cause or contribute to arrhythmias, e.g., antiarrhythmics, drugs that prolong the QT_c interval (see Suggested Readings)
  - family history of sudden death (or VT/VF) at age <65
- Physical examination for signs of structural heart disease
- 12-lead ECG:
  - signs of prior MI
  - repolarization abnormalities (short or prolonged QT_c interval, ECG signs of Brugada syndrome, early repolarization syndrome)
  - *Note:* A 12-lead ECG documenting VT is very helpful. If available, an ECG at tachycardia onset (or offset) is also very useful
- Echocardiogram with special reference to:
  - left ventricular size and function
  - right ventricular size
- Consider Holter or loop event recorder monitoring with special reference to:
  - presence and morphology of ventricular ectopy and symptom-rhythm correlation
- Treadmill exercise test with special reference to:
  - exercise-induced VT

- ECG signs and symptoms of myocardial ischemia (or scintigraphic evidence of ischemia if necessary)
- consider signal-averaged ECG, MRI, provocative drug testing (isoproterenol for long QT, procainamide for Brugada syndrome) if structural heart disease is absent

All wide-complex tachycardias (QRS duration ≥0.12 seconds) in patients over the age of 50 years should be considered to be VT until proven otherwise. Wide-complex tachycardia in an older patient with a history of heart disease is almost always VT, regardless of the morphology of ECG complexes. Most wide-complex tachycardias in any patient of any age group are due to VT.

Significance of VT/VF

The clinical and prognostic importance and management of VT depends on whether it is sustained or nonsustained and whether there is associated structural heart disease, particularly left ventricular systolic dysfunction.

Asymptomatic: Asymptomatic VT usually consists of nonsustained short episodes (3–10 beats). It is often discovered during routine screening ECG or other electrocardiographic monitoring. In the presence of structural heart disease, especially left ventricular dysfunction, asymptomatic VT (usually nonsustained) may indicate a risk of future serious, symptomatic, sustained VT or VF.[3]

Symptomatic: Symptoms may include palpitations, dyspnea, chest discomfort, presyncope, loss of consciousness or cardiac arrest. The severity of symptoms does not determine the prognostic importance of VT and its management (e.g., even severe symptoms in a patient with nonsustained VT and no structural heart disease are prognostically benign; such patients require reassurance, but not necessarily specific antiarrhythmic therapy).[5]

Cardiac arrest: Most episodes of out-of-hospital cardiac arrest are likely the result of VF, although the initial cardiac rhythm documented by first responders is often asystole. VF almost always leads to cardiac arrest, whereas sustained VT may lead to cardiac arrest after a variable duration, usually one to several minutes.

Sustained VT: Lasts ≥30 seconds or requires immediate medical intervention. For management decisions, >15 beats is a reasonable working definition. It is most often associated with structural heart disease, typically coronary disease with previous MI. Sustained VT requires investigation and therapy with antiarrhythmic drugs, an implanted cardioverter defibrillator or antitachycardia surgery.

Nonsustained VT: Lasts <30 seconds, usually only a few seconds. Most commonly there are <10 consecutive ventricular complexes. Unless symptomatic, it requires treatment only if the likelihood of subsequent sustained VT or cardiac arrest is high (ejection fraction <35%, or associated with marked QT prolongation).

VT associated with structural heart disease (e.g., coronary, valvular or hypertensive heart disease): Is usually symptomatic and associated with a high risk of sudden death or recurrence (if sustained), or is asymptomatic and associated with at least a moderate risk of sudden death (if nonsustained). The magnitude of left ventricular dysfunction is the most important prognostic factor.

VT associated with a structurally normal heart: May be symptomatic but rarely is life-threatening even if sustained; it requires no therapy if asymptomatic and nonsustained.[5]

Monomorphic VT: Usually implies an abnormal automatic focus in the ventricle or a fixed re-entrant pathway associated with a scar. It does not by itself suggest prognosis or therapy.

Polymorphic VT: Usually presents as long runs of nonsustained VT. Consider myocardial ischemia and abnormalities of repolarization (torsades de pointes VT associated with QT_c prolongation and a characteristic long-short initiating sequence).[4]

VF may complicate acute MI. However, the prognosis for resuscitated patients with VF occurring during the first 48 hours post-MI is similar to that in patients with an infarction of equivalent severity uncomplicated by VF.

The most common underlying cause is coronary artery disease (CAD), often with prior MI, with or without acute ischemia or infarction.

Most patients with VF are at high risk of recurrence. These individuals should be investigated in a similar fashion to patients with sustained VT and should be treated to prevent recurrences.[1,2,3]

Therapeutic Choices

Immediate Therapy for Sustained VT or VF

If a patient with sustained monomorphic VT is unstable (e.g., has hypotension, angina, heart failure or marked symptoms), cardioversion is effective and safe.[1,6] A synchronized biphasic shock of 120 J or more is usually effective for VT. If immediate conversion to sinus rhythm is not considered necessary, antiarrhythmic drug therapy can be given.[6]

For polymorphic VT or VF, an immediate nonsynchronized shock of 120–200 J (biphasic) is required, repeated as necessary (with minimum interruptions in CPR) until defibrillation is achieved.

Amiodarone: IV amiodarone is effective in terminating VT and is especially effective in preventing early recurrence. It is likely the most effective therapy for electrical storm (characterized by frequent recurrences of VT/VF) and is useful in shock-resistant VF.[6,7,8,9] The usual dose is 3–5 mg/kg iv over 5–10 minutes followed by a 0.5–1 mg/min infusion. There are few randomized studies to guide dosing, but the product monograph recommends 150 mg iv over 10 minutes followed by 1 mg/min for 6 hours then 0.5 mg/min for 18 hours.[10] If necessary, an ongoing infusion of 0.5–1 mg/min can be continued for 24–48 hours. Hypotension may occur, especially if the drug is administered very rapidly.

Procainamide: 10–15 mg/kg iv over 30–45 minutes will often slow VT and terminate tachycardia. Hypotension may occur, especially at more rapid infusion rates, and blood pressure should be carefully monitored.[6,9]

Magnesium: 2–5 g iv over 3–5 minutes is the treatment of choice for torsades de pointes VT, and may be useful in the presence of myocardial ischemia. It is probably of no benefit in monomorphic VT.[4,11] Magnesium is generally safe, but may rarely cause hypotension.

Beta-blockers (e.g., **metoprolol**, **propranolol**, **esmolol**): IV beta-blockers can prevent VT or VF in the setting of acute myocardial ischemia, recent MI or electrical storm.[1,4,9] Bradycardia or hypotension may occur.

Lidocaine: 1–1.5 mg/kg iv followed by a 1–3 mg/minute infusion is occasionally effective (in <20% of cases of sustained monomorphic VT).[2] If conversion does not occur within 10–15 minutes, lidocaine will probably not be effective. There is no good evidence that lidocaine is useful in shock-resistant VF.[2,6,9] Lidocaine rarely causes hypotension and at high doses can cause CNS adverse events.

Chronic Therapy—Prevention of VT/VF Recurrence

Therapeutic choices for long-term management of sustained VT/VF (Figure 1, Figure 2) include both drug therapy (Table 1)[1,2,4,9] and nondrug therapy (implanted cardioverter defibrillator, ICD, map-guided endocardial resection, catheter ablation).[5,12,13,14,15,16]

Figure 1: **Management of Nonsustained Ventricular Tachycardia (<15 beats)**

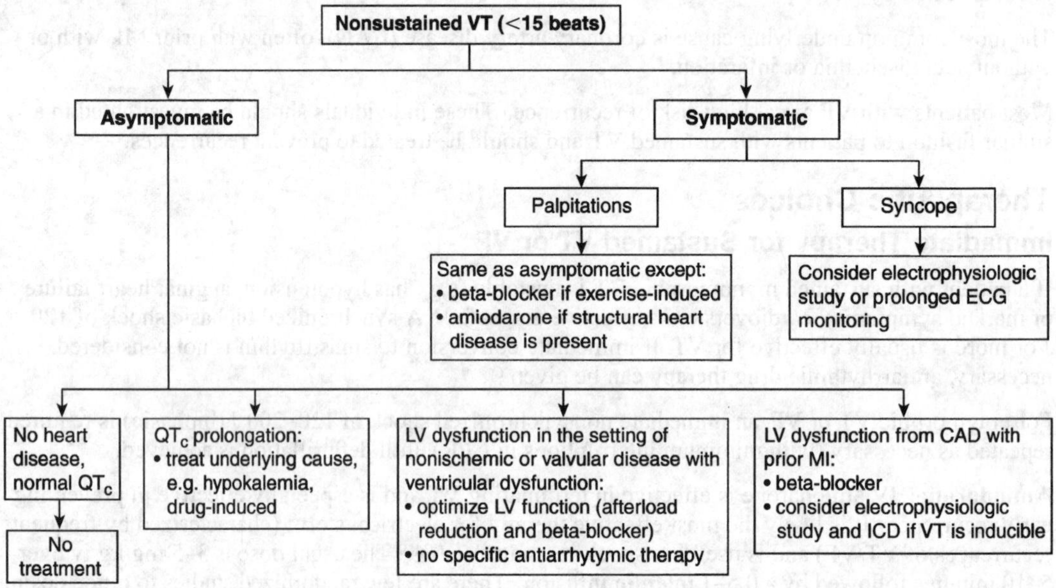

Abbreviations: CAD = coronary artery disease; ICD = implanted cardioverter defibrillator; LV = left ventricular; VT = ventricular tachycardia

Sustained monomorphic VT/VF is likely to recur in the absence of treatment. Objective documentation of efficacy (e.g., electrophysiologic testing or reduction of VT episodes on Holter monitoring) can be considered. In patients with LV dysfunction, drug therapy should rarely be used as the only therapy for the prevention of recurrent sustained VT or prevention of first occurrence of VT in at-risk patients (primary prophylaxis).

Indicators that have been used to assess efficacy of drugs in individual patients include the ability to prevent induction of VT during an electrophysiologic study or with exercise, and elimination or marked reduction in the frequency of nonsustained VT episodes or premature ventricular contractions (PVCs). The latter indicator is unproven and is not recommended.

Patients with a history of VF or cardiac arrest are at risk of recurrence of VF or VT, since their original arrhythmia may have been VT degenerating to VF. Their treatment is similar to that of patients with sustained VT, although markers to judge drug efficacy (inducible VT or VF; PVCs or nonsustained VT on Holter monitoring) are present less often.[18]

Beta-blockers, if tolerated, should be administered to all patients in whom drug therapy is used (and will be indicated in any event in almost all patients with CAD or severe LV dysfunction). They are particularly useful in patients with exercise-, stress- or ischemia-induced VT.

Amiodarone and **sotalol** are effective in preventing VT or VF but almost all studies show they are less effective than implanted defibrillators in preventing sudden death and decreasing all-cause mortality in patients at high risk for sustained VT or VF.[2,5,12,13,14,15,16,17,18] No randomized study has shown that antiarrhythmic drugs reduce mortality. However, amiodarone or sotalol can be used as an adjunct to ICD implantation to prevent ICD shocks, which are painful.[19]

In patients with multiple, frequent recurrences of VT or VF (electrical storm) resistant to the combination of a beta-blocker and amiodarone, or if amiodarone is ineffective or not tolerated, Class I agents such as **mexiletine**, **quinidine** or **procainamide** can be cautiously added. Such combinations are entirely empiric and should be used only as a last resort.[4] In highly selected cases, empiric combinations of sotalol and quinidine or procainamide,[20] or quinidine and mexiletine,[21] or other combinations of drugs with class Ia, Ib, and III activity can be considered. Quinidine is available only through the Health Canada Special Access Programme and is rarely used.

Figure 2: Long-term Management of Sustained Ventricular Tachycardia (>15 beats), Ventricular Fibrillation or Resuscitated Cardiac Arrest[a]

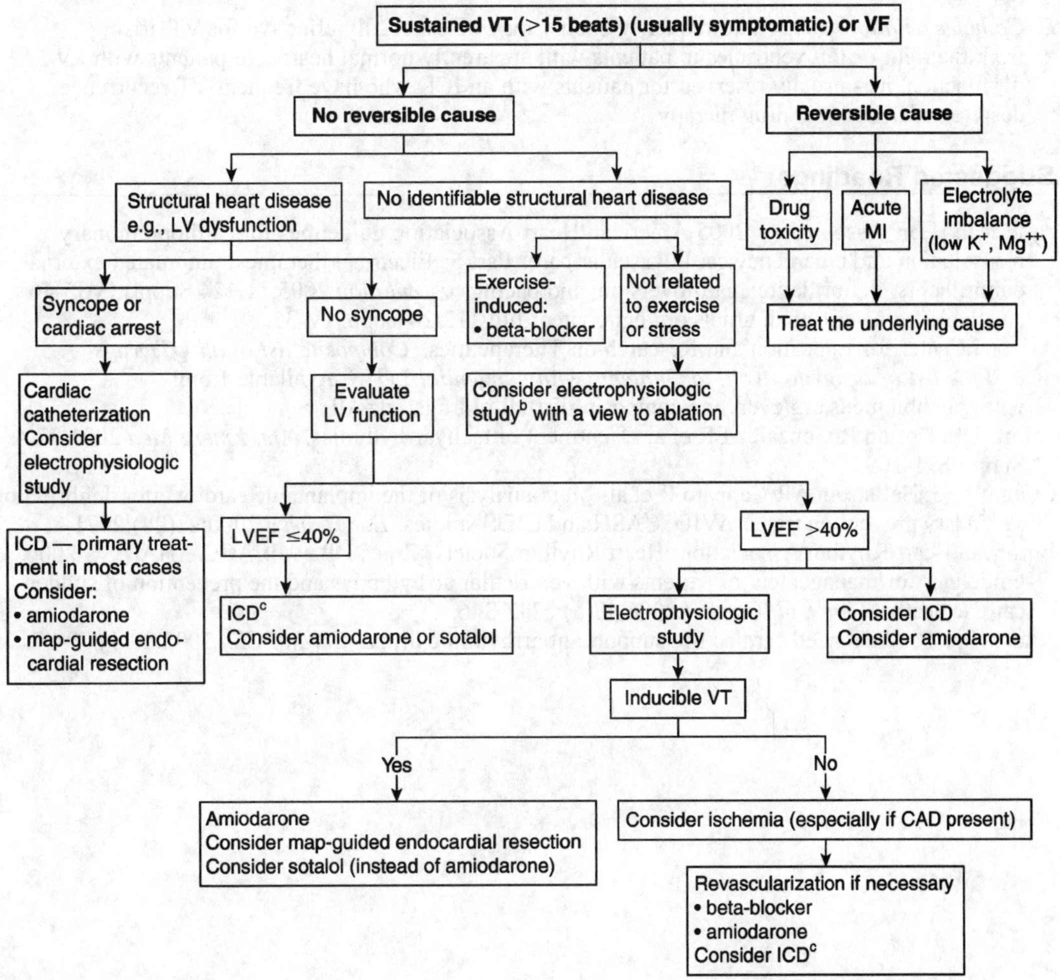

[a] Current guidelines[24] indicate that in most cases an ICD is the preferred therapy for any patient with sustained VT and symptoms in the presence of structural heart disease (with no reversible cause). Electrophysiologic studies are not necessarily indicated in such patients. Cardiac catheterization may be reasonable but is also not necessarily indicated in such patients.

[b] Patients with monomorphic VT.

[c] An ICD may be considered for any patient with sustained VT, and most patients with VF or cardiac arrest. In addition to the therapies listed, all patients should receive beta-blockers unless contraindicated.

Abbreviations: CAD = coronary artery disease; ICD = implanted cardioverter defibrillator; LV = left ventricular; LVEF = LV ejection fraction; VF = ventricular fibrillation; VT = ventricular tachycardia

Nonpharmacologic Choices for VT

- *An implanted cardioverter defibrillator* (ICD) is very effective in treating VT or VF but requires complex evaluation and follow-up.[12,13,14,15,16,17] The AVID trial reported a 39% reduction in total mortality after one year in ICD-treated patients relative to antiarrhythmic therapy (primarily amiodarone).[15] Current guidelines recommend an ICD as preferred treatment in patients with a history of cardiac arrest, VF or sustained VT with no reversible cause.[22,23]
- *Map-guided endocardial ablation (catheter ablation) or surgical ablation* requires careful patient selection, specialized facilities and complex mapping equipment. It may be very effective in certain patient subsets.
- *Catheter ablation* using radiofrequency energy may be especially effective for VT arising from the right or left ventricles in patients with apparently normal hearts. In patients with LV dysfunction, it is usually reserved for patients with an ICD who have frequent VT recurrences despite antiarrhythmic drug therapy.

Suggested Readings

American Heart Association. 2005 American Heart Association guidelines for cardiopulmonary resuscitation and emergency cardiovascular care. Part 5: Electrical therapies: automated external defibrillators, defibrillation, cardioversion, and pacing. *Circulation* 2005;112(24 Suppl):IV35-46. Available from: circ.ahajournals.org/cgi/content/full/112/24_suppl/IV-35.

Arizona Center for Education and Research on Therapeutics. *Composite list of all QTDrugs and the list of drugs to avoid for patients with congenital LQTS*. Available from: www.crediblemeds.org/everyone/composite-list-all-qtdrugs/?rf=All.

Atkins DL, Dorian P, Gonzalez ER et al. Treatment of tachyarrhythmias. *Ann Emerg Med* 2001;37(4 Suppl):S91-109.

Connolly SJ, Hallstrom AP, Cappato R et al. Meta-analysis of the implantable cardioverter defibrillator secondary prevention trials. AVID, CASH and CIDS studies. *Eur Heart J* 2000;21(24):2071-8.

European Heart Rhythm Association; Heart Rhythm Society; Zipes DP et al. ACC/AHA/ESC 2006 guidelines for management of patients with ventricular arrhythmias and the prevention of sudden cardiac death. *J Am Coll Cardiol* 2006;48(5):e247-346.

Kudenchuk PJ. Advanced cardiac life support antiarrhythmic drugs. *Cardiol Clin* 2002;20(1):79-87.

Table 1: Drug Therapy for Ventricular Tachycardia and Ventricular Fibrillation

Class	Drug	Dose	Drug Interactions	Adverse Effects	Comments	Cost[a]
Beta$_1$-adrenergic Antagonists[d]	*metoprolol* Lopresor, generics	100–400 mg/day po	With digoxin, Ca^{++} channel blockers, amiodarone, reduce dose 25–50%.	Fatigue, bradycardia, AV block, decreased exercise capacity, headache, erectile dysfunction, vivid dreams. Less common: hyperglycemia, depression, heart failure.	Monitor carefully in patients with diabetes who are prone to hypoglycemia. Caution in patients with HF. Especially useful in exercise-induced VT, with ischemia, or VT in the absence of structural heart disease. Of probable but unclear benefit in patients with sustained VT and prior MI. May enhance efficacy of other antiarrhythmic drugs in this setting. Very low proarrhythmic risk. Contraindicated in asthma.	$
Class IA Antiarrhythmics[b]	*quinidine* generics	Usual: 800–1600 mg/day (sulfate equivalent) po	Reduce digoxin dose by 50%. Inhibits CYP2D6 (many potential interactions).	Frequent GI intolerance. Rare fever, thrombocytopenia. Torsades de pointes; (proarrhythmic) VT.	Active metabolites accumulate in renal failure, but therapeutic blood monitoring is not readily available. Monitor ECG intervals to guide dosing decisions.	[c]
	procainamide Procan SR	Usual: 2–4 g/day po. Administer Q6H if using an SR preparation	Amiodarone may increase procainamide plasma level.	Frequent arthralgias after long-term use. May cause SLE syndrome. Rare granulocytopenia. Occasional torsades de pointes.	Metabolism depends on rate of acetylation. The active metabolite NAPA accumulates in fast acetylators and in renal failure. Monitor procainamide and NAPA levels; monitor ECG intervals.	$$$$
Class IB Antiarrhythmics[b]	*mexiletine* generics	Usual: 600–900 mg/day po	Phenytoin and rifampin may reduce effect (may need to increase mexiletine dose).	Frequent CNS side effects.	Rarely used as monotherapy.	$$$
Class IC Antiarrhythmics[b]	*flecainide* generics	Usual: 100–200 mg/day po	Metabolized by CYP2D6 (many potential interactions).	Dizziness and visual disturbances common.	Titrate dose based on QRS intervals. Do not use in patients with LV dysfunction, especially prior MI (increases mortality in patients who have frequent PVCs after MI).	$$

(cont'd)

Table 1: Drug Therapy for Ventricular Tachycardia and Ventricular Fibrillation *(cont'd)*

Class	Drug	Dose	Drug Interactions	Adverse Effects	Comments	Cost[a]
	propafenone Rythmol, generics	Usual: 600–900 mg/day po Hepatic failure: Reduce initial dose by 50% and increase dosing interval to Q12H	Reduce digoxin dose by 25–50%. Metabolized by CYP2D6.	Depresses LV function.	Weak beta-blocking effect. Use with care, if at all, in patients with LV dysfunction, especially prior MI. Active metabolites accumulate in rapid metabolizers. Monitor QRS duration.	$$
Class III Antiarrhythmics	*sotalol* ❥ generics	Usual: 160–480 mg/day po Elderly: Reduce initial dose to 40 mg Q12H po	Digoxin, verapamil, other beta-blockers may cause AV block, bradycardia. See metoprolol.	Torsades de pointes, especially at higher doses or with renal dysfunction. See metoprolol.	Sotalol is a beta-blocker. May be especially effective in exercise-related arrhythmias. Likely more effective than other drugs in suppressing inducibility of VT. Contraindicated in asthma.	$
	amiodarone Cordarone, generics	Loading dose: 800–1600 mg/day po for 7–10 days Maintenance dose: 200–400 mg/day po Avoid high loading dose in setting of sinus bradycardia (HR <50 BPM)	Reduce digoxin dose by 50%. Reduce beta-blocker dose by 50%. Reduce quinidine or procainamide dose by 50%. Reduce warfarin dose by 50%.	Various gastrointestinal, dermatologic, neurologic, ophthalmologic and thyroid abnormalities. Pulmonary fibrosis, hepatic dysfunction and aggravation of arrhythmias are rare but potentially life-threatening.	Slows conduction, blocks adrenergic activity, blocks Ca^{++} channels. Very long half-life. Likely the most effective antiarrhythmic drug. Usually used empirically.	$

[a] Cost of 30-day supply of mean dose; includes drug cost only.
[b] There is no evidence that any drug with primarily class I activity is of long-term benefit in reducing mortality from VT or VF; in particular, Class I drugs are not recommended in patients with VT or VF and structural heart disease (in the absence of an ICD).
[c] Available through the Special Access Programme, Therapeutic Products Directorate, Health Canada.
[d] The $beta_1$-adrenergic antagonist suggested is an example only. Other $beta_1$-adrenergic antagonists may be used.
❥ Dosage adjustment may be required in renal impairment; see Appendix I.
Abbreviations: HF = heart failure; LV = left ventricular; NAPA = N-acetylprocainamide; PVC = premature ventricular contraction; SLE = systemic lupus erythematosus; VF = ventricular fibrillation; VT = ventricular tachycardia
Legend: $ < $25 $$ $25–100 $$$ $100–175 $$$$ $175–250

References

1. Atkins DL, Dorian P, Gonzalez ER et al. Treatment of tachyarrhythmias. *Ann Emerg Med* 2001;37(4 Suppl):S91-109.
2. Dorian P, Philippon F. The management of acute ventricular tachycardia or fibrillation. *Can J Cardiol* 2000;16(Suppl C):16C-9C.
3. Green MS, Ricci J, Wolfe K. The appropriate evaluation of the patient at risk for sudden death from ventricular arrhythmias. *Can J Cardiol* 2000;16(Suppl C):13C-5C.
4. Gillis AM. Intractable ventricular tachyarrhythmias: immediate evaluation and management, role of pharmacological therapy. *Card Electrophysiol Rev* 2001;5:354-8.
5. Gillis AM, Hamilton RM, LeFeuvre CA. Unusual causes of sudden cardiac death due to ventricular tachyarrhythmias. *Can J Cardiol* 2000;16(Suppl C):34C-40C.
6. Guidelines 2000 for Cardiopulmonary Resuscitation and Emergency Cardiovascular Care. Part 6: advanced cardiovascular life support: section 1: Introduction to ACLS 2000: overview of recommended changes in ACLS from the guidelines 2000 conference. The American Heart Association in collaboration with the International Liaison Committee on Resuscitation. *Circulation* 2000;102(8 Suppl):I86-9.
7. Dorian P, Cass D, Schwartz B et al. Amiodarone as compared with lidocaine for shock-resistant ventricular fibrillation. *N Engl J Med* 2002;346(12):884-90.
8. Kowey PR, Levine JH, Herre JM et al. Randomized, double-blind comparison of intravenous amiodarone and bretylium in the treatment of patients with recurrent, hemodynamically destabilizing ventricular tachycardia or fibrillation. The Intravenous Amiodarone Multicenter Investigators Group. *Circulation* 1995;92(11):3255-63.
9. Kudenchuk PJ. Advanced cardiac life support antiarrhythmic drugs. *Cardiol Clin* 2002;20(1):79-87.
10. Amiodarone Hydrochloride for Injection Sandoz Standard [product monograph]. In: Jovaisas B, ed. *Compendium of pharmaceuticals and specialties: Canada's trusted drug reference.* Ottawa (ON): CPhA; 2014. p. 183-8.
11. Tzivoni D, Banai S, Schuger C et al. Treatment of torsade de pointes with magnesium sulfate. *Circulation* 1988;77(2):392-7.
12. Buxton AE, Lee KL, Fisher JD et al. A randomized study of the prevention of sudden death in patients with coronary artery disease. Multicenter Unsustained Tachycardia Trial Investigators. *N Engl J Med* 1999;341(25):1882-90.
13. Moss AJ, Zareba W, Hall WJ et al. Prophylactic implantation of a defibrillator in patients with myocardial infarction and reduced ejection fraction. *N Engl J Med* 2002;346(12):877-83.
14. Connolly SJ, Gent M, Roberts RS et al. Canadian implantable defibrillator study (CIDS): a randomized trial of the implantable cardioverter defibrillator against amiodarone. *Circulation* 2000;101(11):1297-302.
15. A comparison of antiarrhythmic-drug therapy with implantable defibrillators in patients resuscitated from near-fatal ventricular arrhythmias. The Antiarrhythmics versus Implantable Defibrillators (AVID) Investigators. *N Engl J Med* 1997;337(22):1576-83.
16. Moss AJ, Hall WJ, Cannom DS et al. Improved survival with an implanted defibrillator in patients with coronary disease at high risk for ventricular arrhythmia. Multicenter Automatic Defibrillator Implantation Trial Investigators. *N Engl J Med* 1996;335(26):1933-40.
17. Connolly SJ, Krahn A, Klein G. Long term management of the survivor of ventricular fibrillation or sustained ventricular tachycardia. *Can J Cardiol* 2000;16(Suppl C):20C-2C.
18. Connolly SJ, Hallstrom AP, Cappato R et al. Meta-analysis of the implantable cardioverter defibrillator secondary prevention trials. AVID, CASH and CIDS studies. Antiarrhythmics vs Implantable Defibrillator study. Cardiac Arrest Study Hamburg. Canadian Implantable Defibrillator Study. *Eur Heart J* 2000;21(24):2071-8.
19. Connolly SJ, Dorian P, Roberts RS et al. Comparison of beta-blockers, amiodarone plus beta-blockers, or sotalol for prevention of shocks from implantable cardioverter defibrillators: the OPTIC Study: a randomized trial. *JAMA* 2006;295(2):165-71.
20. Lee SD, Newman D, Ham M et al. Electrophysiologic mechanisms of antiarrhythmic efficacy of a sotalol and class Ia drug combination: elimination of reverse use dependence. *J Am Coll Cardiol* 1997;29(1):100-5.
21. Duff HJ, Mitchell LB, Wyse DG et al. Mexiletine/quinidine combination therapy: electrophysiologic correlates of anti-arrhythmic efficacy. *Clin Invest Med* 1991;14(5):476-83.
22. Kusumoto F. A comprehensive approach to management of ventricular arrhythmias. *Cardiol Clin* 2008;26(3):481-96.
23. Goldberger JJ, Cain ME, Hohnloser SH et al. American Heart Association/American College of Cardiology Foundation/Heart Rhythm Society scientific statement on noninvasive risk stratification techniques for identifying patients at risk for sudden cardiac death: a scientific statement from the American Heart Association Council on Clinical Cardiology Committee on Electrocardiography and Arrhythmias and Council on Epidemiology and Prevention. *J Am Coll Cardiol* 2008;52(14):1179-99.
24. European Heart Rhythm Association; Heart Rhythm Society; Zipes DP et al. ACC/AHA/ESC 2006 guidelines for management of patients with ventricular arrhythmias and the prevention of sudden cardiac death: a report of the American College of Cardiology/American Heart Association Task Force and the European Society of Cardiology Committee for Practice Guidelines (Writing Committee to Develop Guidelines for Management of Patients With Ventricular Arrhythmias and the Prevention of Sudden Cardiac Death). *J Am Coll Cardiol* 2006;48(5):e247-346.

Chapter 50

Allergic Rhinitis

Paul Keith, MD, MSc, FRCPC

CPhA acknowledges the contribution of Dr. D. William Moote as the previous author of this chapter.

Goals of Therapy

- Prevent allergic symptoms from occurring by avoiding exposure to allergens
- Suppress and control symptoms produced by the allergic response
- Avoid/minimize medication side effects including negative impact on activities of daily living, e.g., minimal interference with school or work performance or attendance, leisure activities, sleep

Investigations

- Clinical history (Table 1) with particular attention to:
  - symptoms, frequency and severity
  - duration and pattern of symptoms (intermittent, persistent)
  - precipitating factors, e.g., environmental allergens such as animal and pollen triggers
  - personal or family history of allergy
- Physical examination (Table 1):
  - View nasal mucosa (e.g., colour, anatomy) using ordinary otoscope
- Objective measurements:
  - Skin testing confirms allergic sensitivity, if present. There is little benefit in measuring total serum IgE or eosinophils, which do not correlate well with presence of allergic disease. In vitro measurements of specific allergen sensitivity such as enzyme-linked immunosorbent assay are acceptable, but more expensive. Skin testing is generally preferred unless conditions exist that make it unsatisfactory, e.g., widespread skin disease or inability to stop antihistamine therapy. Discontinue antihistamines temporarily for at least 3 days prior to skin testing. Tricyclic antidepressants and phenothiazines as well as other drugs with antihistaminic effect (e.g., dimenhydrinate) will also interfere with skin testing, but should only be discontinued after discussion with the patient.

Therapeutic Choices

Figure 1 provides an algorithm for the treatment of allergic rhinitis.

Nonpharmacologic Choices

- Avoid exposure to allergens to which a patient is sensitized. This reduces medication use.[1,2]
  - Air conditioning reduces pollen exposure.
  - Removing pets from the home will reduce perennial symptoms caused by animal dander.
  - Dust avoidance measures can reduce dust mite exposure; however, evidence has not shown benefit in reducing symptoms.[2,3]

Table 1: **Differential Diagnosis of Rhinitis**

Condition	Characteristics
Seasonal or perennial allergic rhinitis	Nasal obstruction and rhinorrhea are common. Often conjunctival symptoms, paroxysmal sneezing, itching of the nasal mucosa and the oropharynx. Seasonal patterns may be recognized, or perennial symptoms may flare up after exposure to allergens like dust mites or animal danders. Nasal mucosa is swollen, often pale or bluish, and moist.
Upper respiratory infections	More episodic, often associated with sore throat or fever and not associated with itch. Nasal mucosa is often red.
Vasomotor rhinitis	Obstruction and rhinorrhea are prominent and other symptoms infrequent. May be triggered by irritant exposures such as smoke, temperature changes, strong odours, cold air and other factors such as exercise, eating hot or spicy foods.
Nasal polyps	Obstruction is the main complaint. Anosmia and reduced taste perception are almost always present. Nasal exam will usually detect a polyp.

Pharmacologic Choices

Information on drugs used in the management of allergic rhinitis can be found in Table 2.

Saline nose sprays or irrigation systems can help relieve symptoms by washing out mucus and the inhaled allergen. Similarly, **lubricant eyedrops** or cold compresses can reduce conjunctival symptoms.

Antihistamines

Antihistamines help relieve most symptoms of acute allergic rhinitis such as sneezing, rhinorrhea, nasal itch and conjunctivitis, but are not usually recommended for the treatment of nasal congestion. **Desloratadine** has demonstrated modest improvement in the symptom of nasal congestion, and is indicated for relief of this symptom.[4] There is some evidence to suggest similar results for **fexofenadine**;[5] however, fexofenadine is not indicated for the relief of congestion. Antihistamines are most effective if used prophylactically; however, onset of action is fast enough such that they are also effective when used on an as-needed basis. Once-daily dosing of the newer antihistamines is usually sufficient.

Although sedation and anticholinergic side effects are common with the older antihistamines (also known as first-generation or sedating antihistamines), these side effects are usually not seen with newer agents (second-generation or nonsedating antihistamines). Patients who are unaware of sedation may be impaired with respect to attention, memory, vigilance and speed. These effects persist into the next day. Caution is advised in the elderly as they may be more susceptible to the anticholinergic effects of the first-generation antihistamines. Patients whose occupations require vigilance or concentration should receive only nonsedating antihistamines, as they do not affect performance and have no anticholinergic effects.[2,6,7,8,9] Of the newer antihistamines, **cetirizine** is more likely to cause some sedation, especially at higher doses. Patients with hepatic impairment may be at increased risk of adverse effects, and dosage modification may be required (see Table 2). The currently available second-generation antihistamines have not caused QT_c interval prolongation.[2]

Although older studies of long-term dosing with first-generation antihistamines have demonstrated loss of effectiveness, they are flawed by lack of evidence of adherence to therapy. No loss of effectiveness has been shown up to 1 year.[10]

Figure 1: **Management of Allergic Rhinitis**

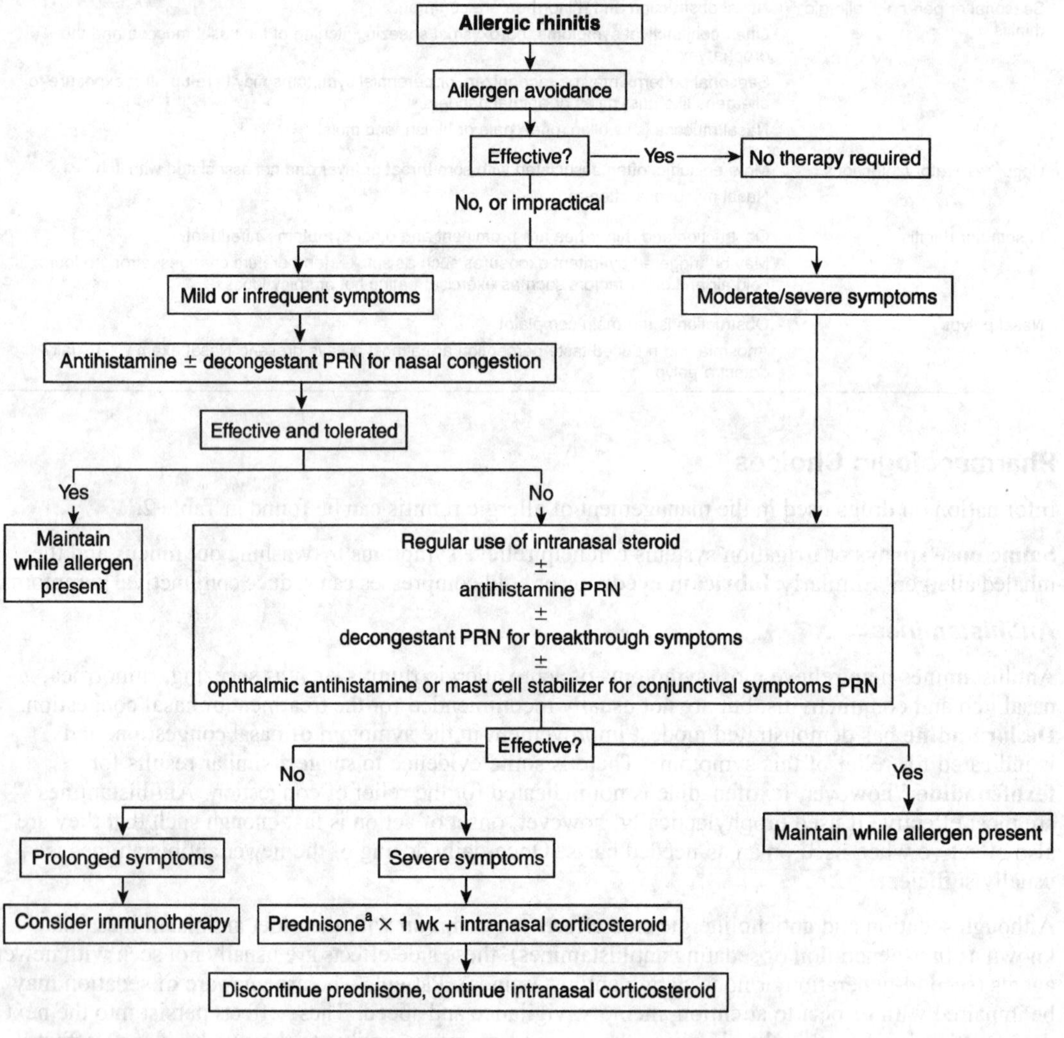

[a] Adults: prednisone 50 mg/day (or 0.5 mg/kg/day) po for 1 week; children: 1 mg/kg/day (maximum 50 mg) po for 5 days.

Decongestants (Alpha-adrenergic Agonists)

Oral decongestants (pseudoephedrine, phenylephrine) relieve nasal obstruction; however, the effectiveness of phenylephrine in improving nasal congestion has not been well established, and unlike pseudoephedrine is not available as a single-entity product or in combination with a second-generation antihistamine.[11] Some individuals are intolerant of the stimulant side effects of decongestants. Avoid oral decongestants in those receiving monamine oxidase inhibitors. Use decongestants with caution in patients with controlled hypertension, hyperthyroidism or ischemic heart disease, though evidence of an associated risk is weak when they are used at recommended doses.[12] Use of **topical nasal decongestants** for more than 3–7 days may result in rhinitis medicamentosa (rebound congestion); thus, they should be avoided in allergic rhinitis because long-term therapy is often required.

Antihistamine-Decongestant Combinations

Antihistamines and decongestants have complementary effects and patients taking both drugs may find combination tablets convenient. Combinations which include the nonsedating second-generation antihistamines are preferred. Avoid antihistamine-decongestant combinations with additional ingredients, such as analgesics and expectorants, e.g., cold preparations, which have not been found to be helpful in allergic rhinitis.

Intranasal Therapy

Intranasal corticosteroids are the mainstay of therapy for moderate to severe rhinitis symptoms. Indeed, intranasal corticosteroids as monotherapy have been shown to be more effective than combined use of an antihistamine and leukotriene antagonist.[11] They can be given on an as-needed basis in seasonal allergic rhinitis; however, continuous use more effectively provides symptom relief. In addition, they are effective in managing ocular symptoms associated with allergic rhinitis. Newer preparations have a lower spray volume, which may be preferred by some. **Budesonide** is available as a dry powder nasal inhaler and offers an alternative for those who dislike aqueous sprays. A 2- to 4-week trial may be needed to see maximal effect although benefit is seen in the first day of therapy compared to placebo in controlled trials.

Intranasal corticosteroids act locally and are quickly metabolized once absorbed. Adrenal suppression has not been seen at therapeutic dosages.[9,13,14] However, high-dose **beclomethasone** nasal spray (168 µg BID) has been shown to cause mild growth suppression in children, averaging 0.9 cm after 1 year of continuous use.[15] **Mometasone** aqueous nasal spray 100 µg daily and **fluticasone propionate** 100 µg daily had no effect on growth over 1 year of therapy.[16,17] Although there have been case reports of nasal septal perforation in patients using intranasal corticosteroids, this potential adverse effect has not been confirmed in controlled studies.[18] Nevertheless, instruct patients to aim the spray at the turbinates, i.e., inside the nose, pointing upwards and angled laterally towards the tip of the ear, not at the septum.

Sodium cromoglycate (cromolyn sodium) nasal sprays have an excellent safety profile but are less effective than corticosteroids and usually need QID dosing, at least initially. Onset of action is 4–7 days but full benefit may not be evident for weeks.[11]

Levocabastine, an antihistamine nasal spray, has a rapid onset and is effective PRN and for daily use. Systemic effects are minimal compared to oral antihistamines but it is less potent than intranasal corticosteroids and is not effective for treatment of congestion.[11,19]

Intranasal **ipratropium** 0.03% solution reduces the volume of watery nasal discharge.[20] It may be used when rhinorrhea is the only symptom or when rhinorrhea is refractory to topical intranasal corticosteroids and/or antihistamines. This may be especially helpful in some types of vasomotor rhinitis, e.g., "skier's nose."

Intranasal medications for the treatment of allergic rhinitis are described in Table 3.

Leukotriene Receptor Antagonists

Montelukast has a modest effect on allergic rhinitis showing similar benefit to antihistamines but less benefit than intranasal corticosteroids in improving symptoms and quality of life in patients with seasonal allergic rhinitis.[21,22,23] It may be especially helpful in patients with concomitant asthma or nasal polyps. Montelukast is approved for the treatment of seasonal allergic rhinitis when other medications are ineffective or poorly tolerated.

Ophthalmic Preparations

Oral antihistamines, intranasal corticosteroids and leukotriene receptor antagonists may also improve conjunctival symptoms. When these are insufficient, topical ophthalmic antihistamines such as

olopatadine or **ketotifen** provide relief in minutes with duration of effect of about 12 hours. Olopatadine is also available in a once-daily formulation. Topical mast cell stabilizers such as **cromoglycate**, **nedocromil** or **lodoxamide**, require several days for onset and are administered QID initially. Regular use of topical vasoconstrictors is discouraged because of development of rebound vasodilation. Once opened, cromoglycate should be discarded within a month. Olopatadine or ketotifen eyedrops are more stable once opened. See Table 4 for available ophthalmic preparations.

Immunotherapy

Desensitization (immunotherapy; "allergy shots") is useful, especially for symptoms caused by pollen or dust mites.[24,25] Immunotherapy is indicated only when there is evidence of IgE-dependent sensitivity to a specific antigen the patient cannot effectively avoid and when frequency and severity of symptoms are difficult to control with conventional drug therapy and allergen avoidance.[25,26] A long-term follow up of children who received immunotherapy for 3 years showed long-term clinical benefits and reduced risk of asthma development up to 7 years after cessation of immunotherapy.[27] Sublingual immunotherapy is now available in Canada for grass pollen allergy and will soon be available for other inhalant allergens. This therapy may be administered at home after an initial dose under medical supervision. Like sc immunotherapy, it has a persistent benefit after being administered for 3 years.[28]

Allergic Rhinitis in Children

Poorly controlled rhinitis impacts significantly on learning performance in children.[29] Treatment of rhinitis symptoms in children is hampered by the difficulty of administering nose sprays of any kind; most children simply don't like the idea of spraying something into their noses. If antihistamines are sufficient, they are the ideal choice. **Second-generation antihistamines** are preferred, as **first-generation antihistamines** are associated with sedation and learning impairment.[2] In addition, oral cough and cold preparations containing **decongestants** with or without first-generation antihistamines are not to be used in children younger than 6 years.[30] Health Canada came to this decision based on limited evidence of efficacy in viral rhinitis and reported adverse effects. Among the nasal preparations, **cromoglycate** is safe and may be tried. **Intranasal corticosteroids** are more effective.[2] **Mometasone**, **fluticasone propionate** and **fluticasone furoate** have usually been recommended because of low oral bioavailability and absence of growth suppression with long-term use. However, fluticasone propionate is scented and many children prefer unscented preparations. Mometasone and fluticasone furoate are available unscented. If liquid sprays are not tolerated, dry powder formulations of **budesonide** may be tried (turbuhaler). Once-daily dosing of intranasal corticosteroids in the morning seems to reduce risk of growth suppression.[9] Any risk is increased when total corticosteroid use is increased, e.g., intranasal use plus inhaled corticosteroids for asthma; therefore, care must be taken to use medication at the lowest effective dose.

Choices during Pregnancy and Breastfeeding

Rhinitis is common in pregnancy. Pregnant women are also more likely to complain of congestion, even in the absence of allergic rhinitis, i.e., rhinitis of pregnancy.[31,32,33] As with all medications in pregnancy, it is ideal to discuss the relative risks and benefits with the patient. All antihistamines cross the placenta. Unfortunately, there are very few clinical trials in pregnant patients with rhinitis. From historical data and extrapolation from asthma studies, there is satisfactory evidence for safe use of **beclomethasone**,[34] **budesonide**,[35] **cromoglycate**[36] and **chlorpheniramine**.[37] Second-generation antihistamines are considered probably safe for use during pregnancy.[11] **Montelukast** is considered safe for the treatment of allergic rhinitis during pregnancy. **Intranasal corticosteroids** are associated with minimal systemic effects in adults and are more effective than antihistamines or leukotriene receptor antagonists for allergic rhinitis. Risk-benefit considerations thus favour their first-line use during pregnancy.[38]

Avoid use of **oral decongestants** during the first trimester of pregnancy.[11]

Pseudoephedrine concentrates in breast milk although there are no reports of adverse effects on the breastfed infant. Recommendations for use of this drug during breastfeeding are similar to those for the general population.

A discussion of general principles on the use of medications in these special populations can be found in Appendix II and Appendix III. Other specialized reference sources are also provided in these appendices.

Therapeutic Tips

- Evidence is insufficient to support a significant difference in quality of life measures or symptom scores between **intranasal corticosteroid** monotherapy and **intranasal corticosteroid/oral antihistamine** combination therapy.[39,40,41] Results are mixed; some studies found superiority for the combination in some patient-rated nasal symptoms but not quality of life scores.[39,40] A more recent study found that adding an antihistamine over the first 2 weeks of therapy did not result in a difference that was clinically meaningful in any measure.[41] If allergic rhinitis is not adequately controlled with intranasal corticosteroid monotherapy the addition of an antihistamine may be considered but should be discontinued if no benefit is observed within 2–4 weeks [Evidence: SORT C*].[11]
- Intranasal corticosteroids will shrink nasal polyps, but long-term treatment is required. Anosmia is not usually improved. If surgery is considered, the use of topical corticosteroids after surgery may decrease the recurrence rate.
- A short course (5–7 days) of **oral corticosteroids** may be used for very severe nasal symptoms.[11]
- Many antihistamine preparations are available as syrups for children but are not convenient for portable PRN dosing. **Loratadine** tablets are tasteless and can be chewed.
- Start medications at the maximum tolerated dose and then taper to the minimum required for maintenance.
- Patients with predictable seasonal allergic rhinitis can start medications such as intranasal corticosteroids before the allergen exposure period and take them regularly until the end of the season for maximum effectiveness.
- If desired results are not achieved with once-daily dosing of newer intranasal corticosteroids, a twice-daily regimen may be more effective, even at the same total daily dose.
- Antihistamines are not contraindicated in asthmatic patients; many have a slightly beneficial effect on asthma symptoms.
- Refer patient to an allergist or immunologist in the following clinical situations:[11]
  - inadequate control of symptoms despite adherence and correct use of therapies
  - adverse reactions to medications
  - reduced quality of life and/or the ability to function secondary to the condition
  - desire to identify the sensitizing allergens and to receive advice on environmental control
  - comorbid conditions such as asthma and recurrent sinusitis
  - allergen immunotherapy

* SORT (Strength of Recommendation Taxonomy) is a rating system (A, B or C) that addresses the quality of available evidence. For more information consult **How to Use *Compendium of Therapeutic Choices*** on page xxv.

Table 2: Oral Drugs Used in Allergic Rhinitis

Class	Drug	Dose	Adverse Effects	Drug Interactions	Comments	Cost[a]
Antihistamines, Alkylamines, first-generation	*chlorpheniramine* Chlor-Tripolon, generics[b]	Adults and children ≥12 y: 4 mg Q4–6H; maximum 24 mg/day Children 6–11 y: 2 mg Q4–6H; maximum 12 mg/day	CNS: sedation, fatigue, dizziness, impairment of cognition and performance (the patient may be unaware of impairment).[2] Anticholinergic: dryness of the mouth and eyes, constipation, inhibition of micturition, potential precipitation of narrow-angle glaucoma, thickening of bronchial secretions.	Increased CNS depression: alcohol, sedatives, tranquilizers, barbiturates. Increased anticholinergic side effects: TCAs, scopolamine. Moderate CYP2D6 inhibitors, e.g., amiodarone, celecoxib: may increase chlorpheniramine levels. Strong CYP2D6 inhibitors, e.g., bupropion, paroxetine; avoid combination.	Use with caution in the elderly as they may be more susceptible to side effects such as sedation and syncope. Avoid in patients with narrow-angle glaucoma (increased IOP), urinary obstruction (prostatic hypertrophy), bladder neck obstruction (can cause urinary retention), GI obstruction. Observe infants and young children for paradoxical excitation. Discontinue 3 days before skin testing procedure for allergy. Administer with food to decrease GI distress.	$
Antihistamines, Ethanolamines, first-generation	*diphenhydramine* Benadryl Preparations, generics[b]	Adults and children ≥12 y: 25–50 mg TID–QID; maximum 4 doses/day or 300 mg/day Children 6–<12 y: 12.5–25 mg Q4–6H; maximum 150 mg/day Children 2–5 y: 6.25 mg Q4–6H; maximum 37.5 mg/day	See chlorpheniramine.	Increased CNS depression: alcohol, sedatives, tranquilizers, barbiturates. Increased anticholinergic side effects: TCAs, scopolamine. May increase levels of CYP2D6 substrates, e.g., metoprolol, venlafaxine.	See chlorpheniramine. Thickening of bronchial secretions. Available in chewable tablets, elixir and liquid.	$

Class	Drug	Dose	Adverse Effects	Drug Interactions	Comments	Cost[a]
Antihistamines, Piperidines, second-generation	*cetirizine* Reactine, generics[b]	Adults and children >12 y: 5–10 mg/day; maximum 20 mg/day Children 6–12 y: 5–10 mg/day 2–6 y: 2.5–5 mg/day 12–23 months: 2.5 mg once daily; maximum 2.5 mg BID Infants 6–11 months: 0.25 mg/kg Q12H[42] **Moderate renal/hepatic impairment**: ≥12 y: 5 mg/day 6–11 y: <2.5 mg/day	Somnolence (with high dose), fatigue, dry mouth, dizziness, headache, diarrhea, nausea, vomiting, pharyngitis.	Increased CNS depression: alcohol, sedatives, tranquilizers, barbiturates. Increased anticholinergic side effects: TCAs, scopolamine.	Safe and well tolerated in children. Discontinue 3 days before skin testing procedure for allergy. Metabolite of hydroxyzine. Avoid in patients with a hypersensitivity to hydroxyzine.	$
	fexofenadine Allegra[b]	Adults and children ≥12 y: 60 mg Q12H; maximum 180 mg daily *or* 120 mg once daily Children 6–11 y: 30 mg BID **Renal impairment**: ≥12 y: Initial dose 60 mg once daily 6–11 y: Initial dose 30 mg once daily	Headache, nausea.	Decreased fexofenadine level: aluminum- and magnesium-containing antacids; ingestion of fruit juices such as apple, grapefruit or orange may decrease bioavailability.	Safe and well tolerated in children. Discontinue 3 days before skin testing procedure for allergy.	$
	loratadine Claritin, generics[b]	Adults and children ≥10 y (>30 kg): 10 mg once daily Children 2–9 y (≤30 kg): 5 mg once daily **ClCr <30 mL/min or severe liver impairment**: ≥6 y: Initial dose 10 mg every other day 2–5 y: 5 mg every other day	≥12 y: headache, fatigue, xerostomia. 6–12 y: nervousness, wheezing, fatigue.	QT_c prolongation reported with concomitant use of loratadine and amiodarone. Caution is advised. P-gp inhibitors (e.g., erythromycin, ketoconazole) may increase loratadine levels while P-gp inducers (e.g., carbamazepine, dexamethasone) may decrease loratadine levels; clinical effect probably minimal.	Safe and well tolerated in children. Discontinue 3 days before skin testing procedure for allergy. Clearance decreased in patients with severe liver impairment—use lower initial doses. Patients with renal impairment—drug accumulation and increased risk of CNS side effects. Rapid dissolve tablets recommended to be taken on an empty stomach.	$

(cont'd)

Table 2: **Oral Drugs Used in Allergic Rhinitis** *(cont'd)*

Class	Drug	Dose	Adverse Effects	Drug Interactions	Comments	Cost[a]
Antihistamines, Piperidines, third-generation	*desloratadine* Aerius, generics[b]	Adults and children ≥12 y: 5 mg daily Children 6–11 y: 2.5 mg daily Children 1–5 y: 1.25 mg daily Children 6–11 months: 1 mg daily **Renal or hepatic impairment (adults)**: initial dose 5 mg every other day	Headache, pharyngitis, dyspepsia. Incidence of diarrhea in children reported as 15–20%.	P-gp inhibitors (e.g., erythromycin, ketoconazole) may increase loratadine levels while P-gp inducers (e.g., carbamazepine, dexamethasone) may decrease loratadine levels; clinical effect probably minimal.	Avoid in patients with hypersensitivity to loratadine. Safe and well tolerated in children. Discontinue 3 days before skin testing procedure for allergy.	$
Antihistamine/ Decongestant Combinations, second-generation	*cetirizine/ pseudoephedrine* Reactine Allergy & Sinus[b]	Adults and children ≥12 y: 1 tab (5 mg/120 mg) Q12H	See cetirizine. See pseudoephedrine.	See cetirizine. See pseudoephedrine.	See cetirizine. See pseudoephedrine.	$$
	desloratadine/ pseudoephedrine Aerius Dual Action 12 Hour[b]	Adults and children ≥12 y: 1 tab (2.5 mg/120 mg) Q12H	See desloratadine. See pseudoephedrine.	See desloratadine. See pseudoephedrine.	See desloratadine. See pseudoephedrine.	$$
	fexofenadine/ pseudoephedrine Allegra-D[b]	Adults and children ≥12 y: 1 tab (60 mg/120 mg) BID	See fexofenadine. See pseudoephedrine.	See fexofenadine. See pseudoephedrine.	To be taken on an empty stomach. See fexofenadine. See pseudoephedrine.	$
	loratadine/ pseudoephedrine Claritin Allergy & Sinus, Claritin Allergy & Sinus Extra Strength[b]	Adults and children ≥12 y: 5 mg/120 mg: 1 tab BID 10 mg/240 mg: 1 tab daily, preferably upon waking	See loratadine. See pseudoephedrine.	See loratadine. See pseudoephedrine.	See loratadine. See pseudoephedrine.	$$

Class	Drug	Dose	Adverse Effects	Drug Interactions	Comments	Cost[a]
Decongestants, single-entity	*pseudoephedrine* ◗ Eltor 120, Sudafed, generics[b]	Adults and children ≥12 y: 60 mg Q4–6H or 120 mg SR Q12H; maximum 240 mg/day Children 6–11 y: 30 mg Q4–6H PRN; maximum 120 mg/day SR formulations are not recommended in children <12 y	Insomnia, tremor, irritability, headache, palpitations, tachycardia, urinary retention.	Beta-blockers: antihypertensive effects may be reduced. Contraindicated with MAOIs and ergot derivatives. Avoid use with phenothiazines and selective serotonin reuptake inhibitors.	No published evidence supports use of oral cough and cold products in children <6 y for viral rhinitis. Therefore, these products are not recommended in this age group. Contraindicated in patients with severe hypertension and coronary artery disease. Use with caution in CVD, diabetes, hyperthyroidism, prostatic hypertrophy and angle-closure glaucoma.	$
Leukotriene Receptor Antagonists	*montelukast* Singulair, generics	Adults and children ≥15 y: 10 mg QHS 6–14 y: 5 mg QHS 2–5 y: 4 mg QHS	Headache, abdominal pain, flu-like symptoms.	Strong CYP2C9 and 3A4 inducers (e.g., carbamazepine, phenobarbital, phenytoin, rifampin) may decrease montelukast levels whereas, strong CYP2C9 inhibitors (e.g., sulfadiazine) may increase montelukast levels; clinical significance is uncertain; however, monitor for reduced efficacy or adverse effects.		$$

[a] Cost of 10-day supply; includes drug cost only.
[b] Available without a prescription.
◗ Dosage adjustment may be required in renal impairment; see Appendix I.
Abbreviations: CNS = central nervous system; CVD = cardiovascular disease; IOP = intraocular pressure; GI = gastrointestinal; MAOI = monoamine oxidase inhibitor; P-gp = P-glycoprotein; SR = sustained-release; TCA = tricyclic antidepressant
Legend: $ < $10 $$ $10–20

Table 3: Intranasal Drugs Used in Allergic Rhinitis

Class	Drug	Dose	Adverse Effects	Comments	Cost[a]
Antihistamines	*levocabastine* Livostin Nasal Spray	12–65 y: 2 sprays (50 µg/spray) per nostril BID, may increase to 2 sprays TID–QID	Nasal irritation.	Shake well before use. Priming necessary for first time. Discontinue if no improvement seen within 3 days.	$$$
Anticholinergics	*ipratropium* Atrovent Nasal Spray, generics	0.03%: 2 sprays per nostril BID–TID	Nosebleeds, nasal dryness, dry mouth or throat, headache.	Avoid accidental release of nasal spray into eyes. Optimal dose based on specific patient's symptoms and response.	$$
Corticosteroids	*beclomethasone* Mylan-Beclo AQ, other generics	Adults and children ≥6 y: 2 sprays (50 µg/spray) in each nostril BID Adults: maximum 12 sprays/day Children: maximum 8 sprays/day Use lowest effective dose for maintenance therapy	Burning or stinging, nosebleeds. May cause mild growth suppression with prolonged use.[15]	Use at regular intervals. Slow onset (7–14 days for maximal effect). Drug may fail to reach the site of action if excessive nasal mucus secretion or edema of the nasal mucosa is present. May use a vasoconstrictor (intranasal decongestant) 2–3 days prior to the suspension. Aim spray up towards turbinates and away from septum. Liquid forms may be more effective than metered-dose inhalers.	$$
	budesonide Rhinocort Aqua, Rhinocort Turbuhaler, generics	Nasal suspension: Adults and children ≥6 y (64 µg/metered dose): initial dose 2 sprays in each nostril daily or 1 spray in each nostril BID; may decrease maintenance dose to 1 spray in each nostril daily Nasal powder: Adults and children ≥6 y (100 µg/dose): initial dose: 2 applications in each nostril in the morning or 1 application in each nostril BID; maximum 400 µg/day	Burning or stinging, nosebleeds.	See beclomethasone. For the nasal suspension, initial priming needed. Re-prime if not used ≥4 days.	$$-$$$
	ciclesonide Omnaris	Adults and children ≥12 y: 2 sprays (50 µg/spray) in each nostril daily; maximum 200 µg/day	See budesonide.	See beclomethasone. Initial priming needed.	$$$

Class	Drug	Dose	Adverse Effects	Comments	Cost[a]
	flunisolide generics	Adults: 2 sprays (25 µg/metered spray) in each nostril BID, may increase to TID if needed; maximum 300 µg/day Children 6–14 y: 1 spray in each nostril TID; maximum 150 µg/day	See budesonide.	See beclomethasone.	$$
	fluticasone propionate Flonase, generics	Adults and children ≥12 y: 2 sprays (50 µg/spray) in each nostril daily, may increase to BID in severe situations; maximum 400 µg/day Children 4–11 y: 1–2 sprays in each nostril daily; maximum 200 µg/day	See budesonide.	See beclomethasone.	$$$
	fluticasone furoate Avamys	Adults and children ≥12 y: 2 sprays (27.5 µg/spray) in each nostril once daily; maximum 110 µg/day Children ≥2 y to <12 y: 1 spray in each nostril once daily, may increase to 2 sprays in each nostril once daily if needed. Decrease to 1 spray in each nostril daily for maintenance; maximum 110 µg/day	See budesonide.	See beclomethasone. Initial priming needed. Re-prime if not used ≥30 days or if cap let off for ≥5 days.	$$$
	mometasone Nasonex	Adults and children ≥12 y: 2 sprays (50 µg/spray) in each nostril daily, may decrease to 1 spray in each nostril daily for maintenance, may increase to BID in severe situations Children 3–11 y: 1 spray in each nostril daily	See budesonide.	See beclomethasone. Initial priming needed. Re-prime if not used ≥14 days.	$$$
	triamcinolone Nasacort AQ	Adults and children ≥12 y: 2 sprays (55 µg/spray) in each nostril once daily, may decrease to 1 spray in each nostril once daily Children 4–11 y: 1 spray in each nostril daily	See budesonide.	See beclomethasone.	$$$
Mast Cell Stabilizers	*sodium cromoglycate* Rhinaris CS Anti-allergic,[b]	Adults and children ≥2 y: 1 spray in each nostril QID, may increase to 6 times daily Use lowest effective dose for maintenance therapy	Nasal stinging, burning, irritation, sneezing.	Dosing must be repeated at 6 h intervals to maintain the effect.	$$

[a] Cost of 1 unit (spray pump); includes drug cost only.
[b] Available without a prescription.
Legend: $ < $10 $$ $10–20 $$-$$$ $10–30 $$$ $20–30

Table 4: Ophthalmic Preparations Used in Allergic Conjunctivitis

Class	Drug	Dose	Adverse Effects	Comments	Cost[a]
Antihistamines and Mast Cell Stabilizers	*ketotifen* Zaditor, generics[b]	≥3 y: 1 drop into affected eye Q8–12H	Conjunctival injection, headache.	May be used for acute or chronic symptoms.	$$$
	olopatadine Patanol, Pataday, generics[b]	≥3 y: 1–2 drops into affected eye BID *or* ≥12 y: 1 drop into affected eye once daily (Pataday formulation)	Mild transient burning or stinging, pruritus, hyperemia, photophobia, headache.	See ketotifen.	$$$
Mast Cell Stabilizers	*lodoxamide* Alomide[b]	>2 y: 1–2 drops into affected eye QID at regular intervals	Mild and transient discomfort upon instillation—burning, stinging, itching, tearing.	Improvement in signs and symptoms in response to therapy evident in a few days; longer treatment for up to 4 wk may be required.	$$
	nedocromil Alocril[b]	≥3 y: 1–2 drops into each eye BID	Headache, eye burning, eye stinging, taste perversion.	Use regularly to ensure optimal control of symptoms. Initiate treatment at the start of the symptoms.	$$$
	sodium cromoglycate Opticrom, generics[b,c]	≥5 y: 2 drops in each eye QID at regular intervals	Transient ocular stinging, eye burning.	Use regularly to ensure optimal control of symptoms. Initiate treatment at the start of the symptoms. Onset of symptomatic improvement occurs in 2–3 days.	$

[a] Cost of smallest available pack size; includes drug cost only.
[b] Contains benzalkonium chloride. Remove soft contact lenses prior to instillation of drops and wait at least 10 minutes after instilling the solution before inserting the contact lenses.
[c] Available without a prescription.
Legend: $ < $10 $$ $10–20 $$$ $20–30

Suggested Readings

Brozek JL, Bousquet J, Baena-Cagnani CE et al. Allergic rhinitis and its impact on asthma (ARIA) guidelines: 2010 revision. *J Allergy Clin Immunol* 2010;126(3):466-76.

Juniper EF, Stahl E, Doty RL et al. Clinical outcomes and adverse effect monitoring in allergic rhinitis. *J Allergy Clin Immunol* 2005;115(3 Suppl 1):S390-413.

Keith PK, Desrosiers M, Laister T et al. The burden of allergic rhinitis (AR) in Canada: perspectives of physicians and patients. *Allergy Asthma Clin Immunol* 2012;8(1):7.

Milgrom H, Bender B. Adverse effects of medications for rhinitis. *Ann Allergy Asthma Immunol* 1997;78(5):439-44.

Plaut M, Valentine MD. Clinical practice. Allergic rhinitis. *N Engl J Med* 2005;353(18):1934-44.

Wallace DV, Dykewicz MS, Bernstein DI et al. The diagnosis and management of rhinitis: an updated practice parameter. *J Allergy Clin Immunol* 2008;122(2 Suppl):S1-84.

References

1. Asher I, Baena-Cagnani C, Boner A et al. World Allergy Organization guidelines for prevention of allergy and allergic asthma. *Int Arch Allergy Immunol* 2004;135(1):83-92.
2. Brozek JL, Bousquet J, Baena-Cagnani CE et al. Allergic rhinitis and its impact on asthma (ARIA) guidelines: 2010 revision. *J Allergy Clin Immunol* 2010;126(3):466-76.
3. Arroyave WD, Rabito FA, Carlson JC et al. Impermeable dust mite covers in the primary and tertiary prevention of allergic disease: a meta-analysis. *Ann Allergy Asthma Immunol* 2014;112(3):237-48.
4. Horak F, Stubner UP, Zieglmayer R et al. Effect of desloratadine versus placebo on nasal airflow and subjective measures of nasal obstruction in subjects with grass pollen-induced allergic rhinitis in an allergen-exposure unit. *J Allergy Clin Immunol* 2002;109(6):956-61.
5. Wilson AM, Haggart K, Sims EJ et al. Effects of fexofenadine and desloratadine on subjective and objective measures of nasal congestion in seasonal allergic rhinitis. *Clin Exp Allergy* 2002;32(10):1504-9.
6. Kay GG. The effects of antihistamines on cognition and performance. *J Allergy Clin Immunol* 2000;105(6 Pt 2):S622-7.
7. O'Hanlon JF, Ramaekers JG. Antihistamine effects on actual driving performance in a standard test: a summary of Dutch experience, 1989-94. *Allergy* 1995;50(3):234-42.
8. Howarth PH. Assessment of antihistamine efficacy and potency. *Clin Exp Allergy* 1999;29(Suppl 3):87-97.
9. Juniper EF, Stahl E, Doty RL et al. Clinical outcomes and adverse effect monitoring in allergic rhinitis. *J Allergy Clin Immunol* 2005;115(3 Pt 2):S390-413.
10. Simons KJ, Simons FE. The effect of chronic administration of hydroxyzine on hydroxyzine pharmacokinetics in dogs. *J Allergy Clin Immunol* 1987;79(6):928-32.
11. Wallace DV, Dykewicz MS, Bernstein DI et al. The diagnosis and management of rhinitis: an updated practice parameter. *J Allergy Clin Immunol* 2008;122(2 Suppl):S1-84.
12. Radack K, Deck CC. Are oral decongestants safe in hypertension? An evaluation of the evidence and a framework for assessing clinical trials. *Ann Allergy* 1986;56(5):396-401.
13. Boner AL. Effects of intranasal corticosteroids on the hypothalamic-pituitary-adrenal axis in children. *J Allergy Clin Immunol* 2001;108(1 Suppl):S32-9.
14. Wilson AM, Sims EJ, McFarlane LC et al. Effects of intranasal corticosteroids on adrenal, bone, and blood markers of systemic activity in allergic rhinitis. *J Allergy Clin Immunol* 1998;102(4 Pt 1):598-604.
15. Skoner DP, Rachelefsky GS, Meltzer EO et al. Detection of growth suppression in children during treatment with intranasal beclomethasone dipropionate. *Pediatrics* 2000;105(2):E23.
16. Schenkel EJ, Skoner DP, Bronsky EA et al. Absence of growth retardation in children with perennial allergic rhinitis after one year of treatment with mometasone furoate aqueous nasal spray. *Pediatrics* 2000;105(2):E22.
17. Allen DB, Meltzer EO, Lemanske RF et al. No growth suppression in children treated with the maximum recommended dose of fluticasone propionate aqueous nasal spray for one year. *Allergy Asthma Proc* 2002;23(6):407-13.
18. LaForce C. Use of nasal steroids in managing allergic rhinitis. *J Allergy Clin Immunol* 1999;103(3 Pt 2):S388-94.
19. Lange B, Lukat KF, Rettig K et al. Efficacy, cost-effectiveness, and tolerability of mometasone furoate, levocabastine, and disodium cromoglycate nasal sprays in the treatment of seasonal allergic rhinitis. *Ann Allergy Asthma Immunol* 2005;95(3):272-82.
20. Grossman J, Banov C, Boggs P et al. Use of ipratropium bromide nasal spray in chronic treatment of nonallergic perennial rhinitis, alone and in combination with other perennial rhinitis medications. *J Allergy Clin Immunol* 1995;95(5 Pt 2):1123-7.
21. Rodrigo GJ, Yanez A. The role of antileukotriene therapy in seasonal allergic rhinitis: a systematic review of randomized trials. *Ann Allergy Asthma Immunol* 2006;96(6):779-86.
22. Wilson AM, O'Byrne PM, Parameswaran K. Leukotriene receptor antagonists for allergic rhinitis: a systematic review and meta-analysis. *Am J Med* 2004;116(5):338-44.
23. Saengpanich S, deTineo M, Naclerio RM et al. Fluticasone nasal spray and the combination of loratadine and montelukast in seasonal allergic rhinitis. *Arch Otolaryngol Head Neck Surg* 2003;129(5):557-62.
24. Durham SR, Walker SM, Varga EM et al. Long-term clinical efficacy of grass-pollen immunotherapy. *N Engl J Med* 1999;341(7):468-75.
25. Joint Task Force on Practice Parameters. Allergen immunotherapy: a practice parameter. American Academy of Allergy, Asthma and Immunology. American College of Allergy, Asthma and Immunology. *Ann Allergy Asthma Immunol* 2003;90(1 Suppl 1):1-40.
26. Guidelines for the use of allergen immunotherapy. Canadian Society of Allergy and Clinical Immunology. *CMAJ* 1995;152(9):1413-9.
27. Jacobsen L, Niggemann B, Dreborg S et al. Specific immunotherapy has long-term preventive effect of seasonal and perennial asthma: 10-year follow-up on the PAT study. *Allergy* 2007;62(8):943-8.
28. Ott H, Sieber J, Brehler R et al. Efficacy of grass pollen sublingual immunotherapy for three consecutive seasons and after cessation of treatment: the ECRIT study. *Allergy* 2009;64(9):1394-401.

29. Meltzer EO. Quality of life in adults and children with allergic rhinitis. *J Allergy Clin Immunol* 2001;108(1 Suppl):S45-53.
30. Health Canada. *Health Canada releases decision on the labelling of cough and cold products for children.* December 18, 2008. Available from: www.healthycanadians.gc.ca/recall-alert-rappel-avis/hc-sc/2008/13267a-eng.php. Accessed May 9, 2014.
31. Incaudo GA, Takach P. The diagnosis and treatment of allergic rhinitis during pregnancy and lactation. *Immunol Allergy Clin North Am* 2006;26(1):137-54.
32. Ellegard EK. Pregnancy rhinitis. *Immunol Allergy Clin North Am* 2006;26(1):119-35, vii.
33. Ellegard EK. Clinical and pathogenetic characteristics of pregnancy rhinitis. *Clin Rev Allergy Immunol* 2004;26(3):149-59.
34. Piette V, Daures JP, Demoly P. Treating allergic rhinitis in pregnancy. *Curr Allergy Asthma Rep* 2006;6(3):232-8.
35. Norjavaara E, de Verdier MG. Normal pregnancy outcomes in a population-based study including 2,968 pregnant women exposed to budesonide. *J Allergy Clin Immunol* 2003;111(4):736-42.
36. Schatz M, Zeiger RS, Harden K et al. The safety of asthma and allergy medications during pregnancy. *J Allergy Clin Immunol* 1997;100(3):301-6.
37. Diav-Citrin O, Shechtman S, Aharonovich A et al. Pregnancy outcome after gestational exposure to loratadine or antihistamines: a prospective controlled cohort study. *J Allergy Clin Immunol* 2003;111(6):1239-43.
38. Gilbert C, Mazzotta P, Loebstein R et al. Fetal safety of drugs used in the treatment of allergic rhinitis: a critical review. *Drug Saf* 2005;28(8):707-19.
39. Di Lorenzo G, Pacor ML, Pellitteri ME et al. Randomized placebo-controlled trial comparing fluticasone aqueous nasal spray in mono-therapy, fluticasone plus cetirizine, fluticasone plus montelukast and cetirizine plus montelukast for seasonal allergic rhinitis. *Clin Exp Allergy* 2004;34(2):259-67.
40. Ratner PH, van Bavel JH, Martin BG et al. A comparison of the efficacy of fluticasone propionate aqueous nasal spray and loratadine, alone and in combination, for the treatment of seasonal allergic rhinitis. *J Fam Pract* 1998;47(2):118-25.
41. Barnes ML, Ward JH, Fardon TC et al. Effects of levocetirizine as add-on therapy to fluticasone in seasonal allergic rhinitis. *Clin Exp Allergy* 2006;36(5):676-84.
42. Simons FE, Silas P, Portnoy JM et al. Safety of cetirizine in infants 6 to 11 months of age: a randomized, double-blind, placebo-controlled study. *J Allergy Clin Immunol* 2003;111(6):1244-8.

Chapter 51
Asthma in Adults

David G. McCormack, MD, FRCPC, FCCP

Asthma is a respiratory disorder characterized by:

- Paroxysmal or persistent symptoms (dyspnea, chest tightness, wheezing, sputum production and cough)
- Variable airflow limitation
- Airway inflammation
- Airway hyper-responsiveness

Goals of Therapy

- Prevent asthma-related mortality
- Maintain normal activity levels, e.g., avoid absenteeism from work or school, ability to exercise without limitations
- Prevent daytime and nocturnal symptoms (cough, wheezing, dyspnea)
- Maintain normal (or near normal) spirometry
- Prevent exacerbations
- Provide optimal pharmacotherapy and avoid side effects

According to Canadian guidelines, the definition of controlled asthma includes occurrence of daytime symptoms <4 days/week or nighttime symptoms <1 night/week and the need for <4 doses/week of a fast-acting $beta_2$-agonist.[1]

Investigations

- Thorough history with particular attention to:
  - symptoms, frequency and severity
  - pattern of symptoms (seasonal, perennial, diurnal variation, etc.)
  - precipitating factors (environmental allergens, occupational exposures, irritants such as smoke, exercise, drugs such as ASA or beta-blockers, preservatives such as sulfites, viral respiratory infections, rhinitis, sinusitis, gastroesophageal reflux)
  - previous hospitalizations, emergency room visits and intensive care admissions
- Physical examination:
  - wheezing, nasal polyps
- Objective measurements needed to confirm diagnosis and assess severity include:
  - spirometry (preferred method of diagnosis): reduced expiratory flow rates
  - home peak flow monitoring can be used to diagnose asthma or to monitor patients with severe asthma or poor perception of airway obstruction
  - bronchoprovocation challenge test, using methacholine or histamine, if diagnosis in doubt

- Sputum eosinophil counts may be used in specialized centres to monitor effectiveness of anti-inflammatory therapy and guide dosage adjustments in individuals with moderate to severe asthma[1]

Therapeutic Choices

Nonpharmacologic Choices

- Identify and avoid precipitating factors such as environmental allergens and occupational irritants.
- Smoking cessation is essential[2] (see Chapter 13). Also important is the avoidance of exposure to second-hand smoke whenever possible.
- Hyposensitization therapy to allergens generally is not useful in the management of asthma.[3]
- Use of home air cleaners/purifiers is not supported by evidence.[4]

Pharmacologic Choices

Choose the initial level of treatment with medication after an assessment of asthma severity and previous treatment (Figure 1).[1] Review treatment every 3–6 months and if control is achieved, try a stepwise reduction in treatment.

Figure 1: Pharmacologic Management of Asthma in Adults

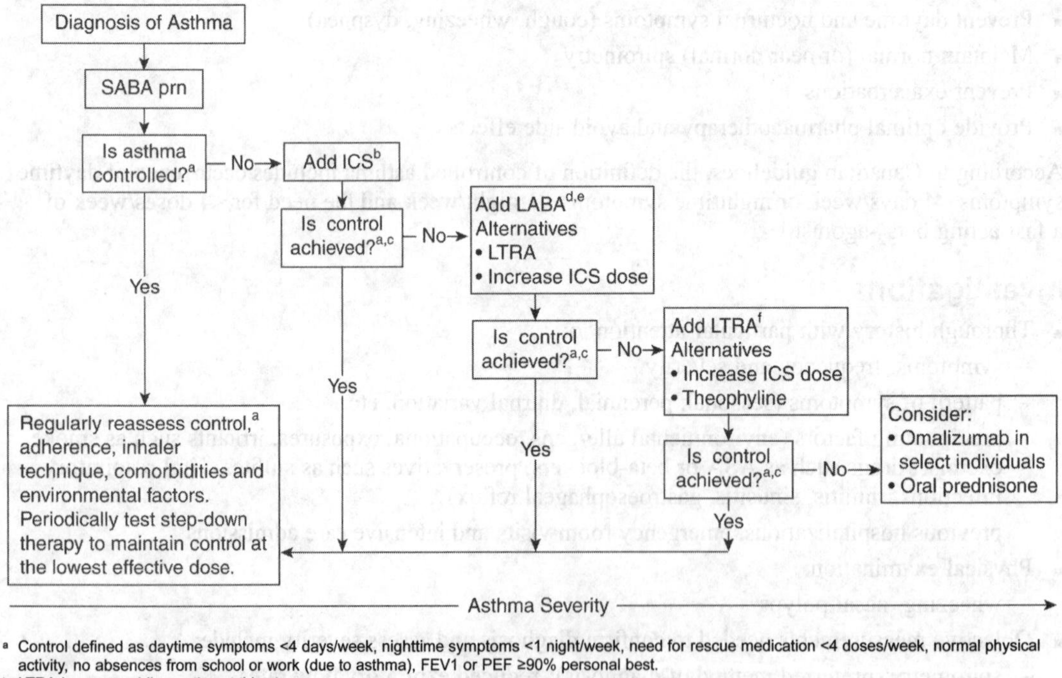

a Control defined as daytime symptoms <4 days/week, nighttime symptoms <1 night/week, need for rescue medication <4 doses/week, normal physical activity, no absences from school or work (due to asthma), FEV1 or PEF ≥90% personal best.
b LTRA is a second-line option at this stage.
c Ensure adherence and inhaler technique before stepping up therapy. If control is not achieved despite adherence to low dose ICS, confirm diagnosis.
d LABAs must always be used in combination with an ICS. If budesonide/formoterol is used as the controller it may also be used as a reliever in place of a SABA.
e Although LABA is the preferred adjunct therapy, other options include LTRA or increasing to medium dose of ICS.
f Alternatives include increasing ICS dose or adding theophylline (fourth-line option). If a LABA was not chosen previously it would be a preferred option over increasing the ICS dose or adding theophylline at this stage.

Abbreviations: ICS = inhaled corticosteroid; LABA = long-acting $beta_2$-agonist; LTRA = leukotriene receptor antagonist; SABA = short-acting $beta_2$-agonist

Inhaled therapy that maximizes delivery of drugs to the respiratory tract and minimizes systemic side effects is the cornerstone of asthma management. Pressurized metered dose inhalers (pMDI) with spacers or dry powder inhalers (DPI) deliver drugs as effectively as nebulized therapy. Medications include bronchodilators and anti-inflammatory agents (Table 2).

Bronchodilators

Short-acting Inhaled Beta$_2$-agonists (SABAs)

Salbutamol and **terbutaline** are selective beta$_2$-agonists and are agents of first choice for treatment of acute exacerbations and for prevention of exercise-induced asthma. They are best used as required rather than on a fixed schedule. Although potent bronchodilators, they have little effect on the late (inflammatory) phase of an exacerbation. If patients use a short-acting beta$_2$-agonist 4 or more times per week (including any doses used to prevent or treat exercise-induced symptoms), initiate therapy with an anti-inflammatory agent.[5] Isoproterenol and epinephrine are not recommended for the treatment of asthma because of lack of beta$_2$-selectivity and potential for excessive cardiac stimulation, especially at high doses.

Long-acting Inhaled Beta$_2$-agonists (LABAs)

Salmeterol and **formoterol** are long-acting beta$_2$-agonists for regular twice daily treatment of asthma. These drugs should be used only in patients already taking inhaled corticosteroids and may be particularly useful for the prevention of nocturnal symptoms. Adding LABAs to inhaled corticosteroids may permit decreasing the dose of the latter.[6] In adults, consider adding a LABA when low-dose inhaled corticosteroids fail to provide adequate control of asthma.[1] LABAs also help to prevent *exercise-induced bronchospasm*.[7]

Salmeterol has a slow onset of action and should not be used for immediate relief of bronchospasm. Formoterol has a rapid onset and although it is effective for rescue therapy it should only be used for rescue treatment when combined with budesonide.[1] See Combination Inhaled Corticosteroids and Long-acting Bronchodilators.

Indacaterol, a LABA approved for use in chronic obstructive pulmonary disease, is not indicated for asthma as data on safety and efficacy are lacking.

Oral Beta$_2$-agonists

Oral **orciprenaline** and **salbutamol** offer less bronchodilation, more systemic side effects and a slower onset of action than the inhaled preparations and are therefore not recommended.

Anticholinergic Agents

Anticholinergics are not routinely indicated in asthma but may have a role in certain circumstances. **Ipratropium** is a useful alternative for patients who are unusually susceptible to tremor or tachycardia from beta$_2$-agonists. Although the onset of action is delayed compared to beta$_2$-agonists, the bronchodilator effect lasts longer. It may also be useful in beta-blocker-induced bronchospasm.[8] **Tiotropium** is an alternative to ipratropium bromide although its indications are not identical. Unlike ipratropium bromide, tiotropium should not be used for relief of acute bronchospasm but as maintenance therapy. The advantage over ipratropium bromide is that tiotropium is administered once a day instead of 3 or 4 times a day.

Theophylline Products

Oral **theophylline** and **oxtriphylline** are uncommonly used due to systemic toxicity and only mild bronchodilator activity. Aminophylline is no longer available in an oral formulation. Administer carefully according to standard regimens and monitor blood levels. In theophylline-naïve patients, titrate the dose slowly to minimize side effects.

Anti-inflammatory Agents

Inhaled Corticosteroids (ICS)

Inhaled **beclomethasone**, **budesonide**, **ciclesonide**, **fluticasone** and **mometasone** are safe, effective, and cost-effective drugs that treat the inflammatory component of asthma.[1,6] They are the preferred agents for maintenance treatment and should be used regularly at the lowest effective dose rather than "as needed" to maintain good asthma control. ICS have a higher ratio of topical to systemic activity than do oral corticosteroids. The incidence of pharyngeal candidiasis from deposition of the inhaled corticosteroid in the pharynx can be reduced by rinsing the mouth after use and/or using a spacer device. Dose equivalencies for inhaled corticosteroids are listed in Table 1.

In the past it has been suggested to "double" the dose of inhaled corticosteroids in response to a worsening of asthma symptoms. However, available evidence does not demonstrate a benefit from this strategy and it is no longer recommended.[1,9] There is evidence from a post hoc, modified intention-to-treat, subgroup analysis that quadrupling versus doubling the dose of ICS (up to 1000 μg/day beclomethasone-HFA equivalent) reduces the risk of an exacerbation requiring oral corticosteroids (odds ratio = 0.27; NNT = 4).[9] The authors call for confirmatory data. Nevertheless, the Canadian Thoracic Society suggests adults with a history of severe exacerbations in the past year requiring systemic corticosteroids may initiate a trial with a four or fivefold increase in ICS dose for 7–14 days as part of an action plan for acute loss of asthma control.[1]

Combination Inhaled Corticosteroids and Long-acting Bronchodilators

As long-acting beta$_2$-agonists (LABAs) should only be given to patients already on inhaled corticosteroids, combination products of inhaled corticosteroids and LABAs have been developed. **Fluticasone/salmeterol** and **mometasone/formoterol** are given on a regular BID schedule. **Budesonide/formoterol** can be used as both maintenance and reliever medication.[10,11]

Table 1: Comparative Dose Equivalencies for Inhaled Corticosteroids for Adults[1,4,6]

Class	Drug	Dose
Inhaled Corticosteroids	*beclomethasone pMDI (HFA)* Qvar	Low: ≤250 μg/day Moderate: 251–500 μg/day High: >500 μg/day
	budesonide DPI Pulmicort Turbuhaler	Low: ≤400 μg/day Moderate: 401–800 μg/day High: >800 μg/day
	budesonide nebulizer Pulmicort Nebuamp	Low: ≤1000 μg/day Moderate: 1001–2000 μg/day High: >2000 μg/day
	ciclesonide pMDI Alvesco	Low: ≤200 μg/day Moderate: 201–400 μg/day High: >400 μg/day
	fluticasone DPI or pMDI plus spacer Flovent Diskus, Flovent HFA	Low: ≤250 μg/day Moderate: 251–500 μg/day High: >500 μg/day
	mometasone furoate DPI Asmanex	Low: ≤200 μg/day Moderate: 400–800 μg/day High: >800 μg/day

Abbreviations: DPI = dry powder inhaler; HFA = hydrofluoroalkane; pMDI = pressurized metered dose inhaler

Systemic Corticosteroids

These are useful in both preventing and treating acute exacerbations. Optimal dosage has not been established. Side effects are significant: fluid retention, glucose intolerance, hypertension, increased appetite, mood alterations and weight gain in the short term and adrenal axis suppression, avascular necrosis of the hip, cataracts, dermal thinning, diabetes, glaucoma, hypertension, myopathy, and osteoporosis in the long term. Reduce side effects by limiting treatment to short periods (1–2 weeks) following an acute exacerbation. Side effects with long-term use may be minimized by using alternate-day dosing regimens.

Leukotriene Receptor Antagonists (LTRAs)

Zafirlukast and **montelukast** have anti-inflammatory properties; however, evidence suggests that leukotriene receptor antagonists (LTRAs) are not as effective as low dose inhaled corticosteroids (ICS) for improving symptoms or preventing exacerbations.[12] Consequently, they are second-line monotherapy after ICS for asthma control [Evidence: SORT B*].[5,12] Although ICS with a long-acting $beta_2$-agonist is more effective than ICS with an LTRA for preventing exacerbations in adults,[13] LTRAs may be considered as add-on therapy with an ICS [Evidence: SORT C*].[1] See Figure 1.

IgE-Neutralizing Antibody

Omalizumab, a monoclonal antibody that binds IgE, may be considered for patients with moderate to severe persistent asthma in those who have had a positive skin test or in vitro reactivity to a perennial aeroallergen and whose symptoms are inadequately controlled with high-dose inhaled corticosteroids and add-on therapy. In these patients, it significantly decreases the incidence of asthma exacerbations and improves overall asthma control.[14,15] Therapy should be initiated by a specialist.

Choices during Pregnancy and Breastfeeding

Asthma and Pregnancy

Pregnancy does not affect asthma in any predictable manner, with some patients noticing disease worsening and others noting improvement in symptoms.[6] Much more important is the effect of asthma on the outcome of the pregnancy. Inadequate control of asthma during pregnancy is associated with worse outcomes, such as pre-term birth, low birth weight, congenital anomalies, pre-eclampsia and placenta previa. Conversely, good control of asthma during pregnancy is associated with a normal outcome.

Management of Asthma during Pregnancy

The best outcome for pregnancy complicated by asthma occurs with optimal management of asthma using the same stepwise approach as in nonpregnant patients.[4] Short-acting inhaled **$beta_2$-agonists**, **theophylline** and **inhaled corticosteroids** (particularly **budesonide**) have been used extensively and are considered safe for use in pregnancy.[16] However, theophylline may worsen gastroesophageal reflux and can cause nausea, so avoid if possible. Accumulating evidence indicates **montelukast** may be used safely during pregnancy.[17] There is limited experience with the use of **LABAs** during pregnancy. The risk of using medications to control asthma during pregnancy appears to be much less than the risk of adverse outcomes related to severe uncontrolled asthma.[18]

Asthma and Breastfeeding

Breastfeeding has no known effect on the severity of asthma. When asthma medication is required for a breastfeeding mother, **bronchodilators** (SABAs, LABAs and anticholinergics) are considered

* SORT (Strength of Recommendation Taxonomy) is a rating system (A, B or C) that addresses the quality of available evidence. For more information consult **How to Use *Compendium of Therapeutic Choices*** on page xxv.

safe.[19] Further, both **inhaled** and **oral corticosteroids** are considered safe for breastfeeding mothers. Although **theophylline** is also considered safe, maintain blood theophylline levels in the low end of the therapeutic range in the mother. There is no information concerning the use of **leukotriene receptor antagonist** therapy during breastfeeding, so alternate drugs for the control of asthma may be appropriate.

A discussion of general principles on the use of medications in these special populations can be found in Appendix II and Appendix III. Other specialized reference sources are also provided in these appendices.

Emergency Treatment of Asthma

See Figure 2 for the emergency management of acute asthma.

- Priorities include oxygenation, rehydration, bronchodilation and use of anti-inflammatory medications.
- Bronchodilation using a metered dose inhaler with a spacer is equivalent to nebulized therapy.[20,21]
- Additive bronchodilator effect of **ipratropium bromide** and the **beta$_2$-agonists** supports administering these 2 medications concomitantly.[22]
- Use oral or parenteral **corticosteroids** early in most patients.[23]
- Avoid iv **aminophylline** in acute asthma.[24,25]

Therapeutic Tips

- Avoid ASA and NSAIDs in patients with ASA-induced asthma and in high-risk patients (severe asthma symptoms, nasal polyps, urticaria or chronic rhinitis).[26] Exercise caution in all patients.
- Exercise caution with beta-blockers.
- Treat conditions that may affect asthma control such as rhinitis, sinusitis and GERD.
- Patient education about asthma symptoms and therapy is essential for optimal management.
  - Provide a written action plan for self-management based on peak expiratory flow rates and/or signs and symptoms for each patient. An example of an asthma action plan developed by the Canadian Lung Association is available from: www.lung.ca/_resources/asthma_action_plan.pdf.
  - Review inhaler technique regularly.

Figure 2: Emergency Treatment of Asthma in Adults

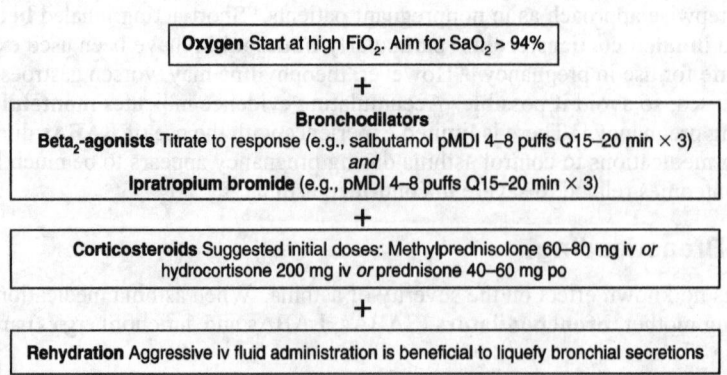

Oxygen Start at high FiO_2. Aim for SaO_2 > 94%

+

Bronchodilators
Beta$_2$-agonists Titrate to response (e.g., salbutamol pMDI 4–8 puffs Q15–20 min × 3)
and
Ipratropium bromide (e.g., pMDI 4–8 puffs Q15–20 min × 3)

+

Corticosteroids Suggested initial doses: Methylprednisolone 60–80 mg iv *or* hydrocortisone 200 mg iv *or* prednisone 40–60 mg po

+

Rehydration Aggressive iv fluid administration is beneficial to liquefy bronchial secretions

Abbreviations: FiO_2 = fraction of inspired oxygen; pMDI = pressurized metered dose inhaler; SaO_2 = arterial oxygen percent saturation

Table 2: Drugs for the Treatment of Chronic Asthma in Adults

Class	Drug	Dose	Adverse Effects	Comments	Cost[a]
Anticholinergic Agents, long-acting	*tiotropium* Spiriva	DPI: 18 µg (1 capsule) inhaled once daily	See ipratropium.		$$$
Anticholinergic Agents, short-acting	*ipratropium* Atrovent HFA, generics	pMDI 20 µg/puff: 2 puffs Q6–8H PRN; maximum 240 µg/day Nebules: 250–500 µg Q4–6H PRN	Dry mouth, metallic taste; mydriasis and glaucoma if released into eye.		$
Anticholinergic/SABA Combinations	*ipratropium/salbutamol* Combivent UDV, generics	Individualize dose. Nebules: 2.5 mL (0.5 mg/2.5 mg) Q6H PRN	See ipratropium. See salbutamol.		$
	ipratropium/fenoterol Duovent UDV	Nebules: 4 mL (0.5/1.25 mg) Q6H PRN	See ipratropium. See salbutamol.		$
Beta$_2$-adrenergic Agonists, long-acting (LABAs)	*formoterol fumarate* Foradil	DPI 12 µg/capsule: 1 capsule BID; maximum 48 µg/day	See salbutamol.	Recommended only if confident patient will use prescribed inhaled corticosteroid as well. Combination LABA/corticosteroid product preferred. Not for reliever therapy.	$$$
	formoterol fumarate dihydrate Oxeze Turbuhaler	DPI: 6–12 µg Q12H; maximum 48 µg/day	See salbutamol.	See formoterol fumarate.	$$
	salmeterol Serevent	Diskhaler 50 µg/blister: 1 blister BID Diskus 50 µg/inhalation: 1 inhalation BID	See salbutamol.	See formoterol fumarate.	$$$
Beta$_2$-adrenergic Agonists, short-acting (SABAs)	*salbutamol* Airomir pMDI, Ventolin Diskus, Ventolin HFA, Ventolin Nebules P.F., generics	pMDI 100 µg/puff: 1–2 puffs TID–QID PRN; maximum 8 puffs/day Diskus: 200 µg TID–QID PRN; maximum 800 µg/day Nebules: 2.5–5 mg QID PRN	Nervousness, tremor, tachycardia, palpitations.		$
	terbutaline Bricanyl Turbuhaler	DPI 0.5 mg/inhalation: 1 inhalation Q4–6H PRN; maximum 6 inhalations/day	See salbutamol.		$

(cont'd)

Table 2: **Drugs for the Treatment of Chronic Asthma in Adults** *(cont'd)*

Class	Drug	Dose	Adverse Effects	Comments	Cost[a]
Corticosteroids, inhaled	*beclomethasone* Qvar	pMDI: 100–800 µg/day divided BID; usual starting dose ≤200 µg/day[b]	Sore mouth, sore throat, dysphonia, oral thrush (can be reduced by rinsing mouth or using spacer).	Bone densitometry is suggested in patients who require high doses or have risk factors for osteoporosis. Patients with personal or family history of glaucoma (and need high-dose inhaled corticosteroids) should have IOP checked soon after starting therapy and periodically thereafter.	$$$
	budesonide Pulmicort Turbuhaler, Pulmicort Nebuamp	DPI: 400–2400 µg/day divided BID; usual starting dose 400 µg/day[b] Nebules: 0.125–2 mg/dose; dose is individualized	See beclomethasone.	See beclomethasone.	DPI: $$$$$ Nebule: $
	ciclesonide Alvesco	pMDI: 100–800 µg daily; usual starting dose 200 µg/day[b] At 800 µg/day, divide dose BID	See beclomethasone.	See beclomethasone.	$$
	fluticasone Flovent HFA, Flovent Diskus	pMDI/DPI: 200–1000 µg/day divided BID; may increase to 1000 µg BID if very severe; usual starting dose 200 or 250 µg/day[b]	See beclomethasone.	See beclomethasone.	$$
	mometasone furoate Asmanex	DPI: 200–400 µg daily; usual starting dose 200 µg/day[b]; maximum 400 µg BID	See beclomethasone.	See beclomethasone.	$$
Corticosteroid/LABA Combinations	*budesonide/formoterol fumarate dihydrate* Symbicort	Maintenance therapy: DPI 100/6 µg or 200/6 µg: 1–2 inhalations daily–BID; maximum 4 inhalations/day. May temporarily increase to 4 inhalations BID for worsening asthma Maintenance and reliever therapy: 1–2 inhalations BID or 2 inhalations once daily. Inhale 1 additional inhalation PRN in response to symptoms; if symptoms persist after a few min, an additional dose should be taken; maximum 6 inhalations on any single occasion; maximum 8 inhalations/day	See beclomethasone. See salbutamol.	See beclomethasone. Fixed-dose combination inhalers are more convenient, enhance adherence, ensure the patient receives their inhaled corticosteroid with their LABA, and are less expensive than the individual agents combined. A disadvantage is a loss in dosing flexibility.	$$$

Class	Drug	Dose	Adverse Effects	Comments	Cost[a]
	fluticasone/salmeterol Advair pMDI, Advair Diskus	pMDI 125/25 µg or 250/25 µg: 2 puffs BID Diskus 100/50 µg, 250/50 µg or 500/50 µg: 1 inhalation BID	See beclomethasone. See salbutamol.	See budesonide/formoterol. Not for reliever therapy.	$$$$
	mometasone/formoterol fumarate dihydrate Zenhale	pMDI 50/5 µg, 100/5 µg or 200/5 µg: 2 puffs BID	See beclomethasone. See salbutamol.	See budesonide/formoterol. Not for reliever therapy.	$$$
IgE-Neutralizing Antibody	*omalizumab* Xolair	150–375 mg sc every 2–4 wk (based on patient's weight and pretreatment serum IgE level)	Injection site reactions (45%), viral infections (24%), upper respiratory tract infections (19%), headache (15%), sinusitis (16%), pharyngitis (10%).	Store at 2–8°C. Reconstituted product may be stored for up to 8 h at 2–8°C. Do not inject more than 150 mg at one site. After start of treatment, do not use serum IgE for dose adjustment. Omalizumab raises IgE levels which may persist for up to a year after ending the treatment.	$630/150 mg vial
Leukotriene Receptor Antagonists	*montelukast* Singulair, generics	10 mg QHS po	Headache (common), abdominal pain, flu-like symptoms.	Reduced montelukast levels: carbamazepine, rifampin, phenobarbital, phenytoin.	$$$
	zafirlukast Accolate	20 mg BID po, at least 1 h before or 2 h after meals	Headache (common), nausea, diarrhea.	ASA may increase zafirlukast levels. Zafirlukast may potentiate effect of warfarin; may increase theophylline levels. Reduced zafirlukast levels: carbamazepine, erythromycin, phenobarbital, phenytoin, rifampin, theophylline.	$$

(cont'd)

Table 2: **Drugs for the Treatment of Chronic Asthma in Adults** *(cont'd)*

Class	Drug	Dose	Adverse Effects	Comments	Cost[a]
Methylxanthines	*oxtriphylline* Choledyl elixir, generics	Initial: 200 mg QID po Maintenance dose: 800–1200 mg/day po given in 3–4 divided doses	Nausea, vomiting, abdominal cramps, headache, palpitations, CNS stimulation.	Monitor serum levels. Multiple drug interactions: e.g., phenytoin, carbamazepine and rifampin reduce theophylline levels, whereas macrolides, oral contraceptives and quinolones increase theophylline levels. Theophylline levels may increase if patient stops smoking. Oxtriphylline available as elixir only.	$$
	theophylline Uniphyl, Apo-Theo LA, other generics	Initial: 400–600 mg/day po, given in 1–3 divided doses depending on preparation used	See oxtriphylline.	See oxtriphylline. Extended-release tablets should not be chewed, crushed or dissolved.	$

[a] Cost of inhaled agents is per unit (1 inhaler, nebule or vial); cost of oral medications is per 30-day supply; includes drug cost only.
[b] Usual starting dose based on published guidelines[5,6] and may differ from product monographs.
Abbreviations: DPI = dry powder inhaler; IOP = intraocular pressure; LABA = long-acting inhaled $beta_2$-agonist; pMDI = pressurized metered dose inhaler; SABA = short-acting inhaled $beta_2$-agonist
Legend: $ < $25 $$ $25–50 $$$ $50–75 $$$$ $75–100 $$$$$ $100–125

Suggested Readings

Balter MS, Bell AD, Kaplan AG et al. Management of asthma in adults. *CMAJ* 2009;181(12):915-22.

Global Initiative for Asthma. *GINA report, global strategy for asthma management and prevention*. Updated May 2014. Available from: www.ginasthma.org/guidelines-gina-report-global-strategy-for-asthma.html.

Global Initiative for Asthma. *Pocket guide for asthma management and prevention (for adults and children older than 5 years): a pocket guide for physicians and nurses*. Updated May 2014. Available from: www.ginasthma.org/guidelines-pocket-guide-for-asthma-management.html.

Lougheed MD, Lemiere C, Dell SD et al. Canadian Thoracic Society Asthma Management Continuum—2010 Consensus Summary for children six years of age and over, and adults. *Can Respir J* 2010;17(1):15-24.

Lougheed MD, Lemiere C, Ducharme FM et al. Canadian Thoracic Society 2012 guideline update: diagnosis and management of asthma in preschoolers, children and adults. *Can Respir J* 2012;19(2):127-64.

References

1. Lougheed MD, Lemiere C, Ducharme FM et al. Canadian Thoracic Society 2012 guideline update: diagnosis and management of asthma in preschoolers, children and adults. *Can Respir J* 2012;19(2):127-64.
2. Chaudhuri R, Livingston E, McMahon AD et al. Effects of smoking cessation on lung function and airway inflammation in smokers with asthma. *Am J Respir Crit Care Med* 2006;174(2):127-33.
3. Adkinson NF, Eggleston PA, Eney D et al. A controlled trial of immunotherapy for asthma in allergic children. *N Engl J Med* 1997;336(5):324-31.
4. Boulet LP, Becker A, Berube D et al. Summary of recommendations from the Canadian Asthma Consensus Report, 1999. Canadian Asthma Consensus Group. *CMAJ* 1999;161(11 Suppl):1-12. Available from: www.cmaj.ca/cgi/content/full/161/11_suppl_2/S1. Accessed April 4, 2011.
5. Lougheed MD, Lemiere C, Dell SD et al. Canadian Thoracic Society Asthma Management Continuum—2010 Consensus Summary for children six years of age and over, and adults. *Can Respir J* 2010;17(1):15-24.
6. Global Initiative for Asthma. *GINA report, global strategy for asthma management and prevention*. Updated May 2014. Available from: www.ginasthma.org/guidelines-gina-report-global-strategy-for-asthma.html.
7. Nelson JA, Strauss L, Skowronski M et al. Effect of long-term salmeterol treatment on exercise-induced asthma. *N Engl J Med* 1998;339(3):141-6.
8. Ind PW, Dixon CM, Fuller RW et al. Anticholinergic blockade of beta-blocker-induced bronchoconstriction. *Am Rev Respir Dis* 1989;139(6):1390-4.
9. Quon BS, Fitzgerald JM, Lemiere C et al. Increased versus stable doses of inhaled corticosteroids for exacerbations of chronic asthma in adults and children. *Cochrane Database Syst Rev* 2010;(12):CD007524.
10. O'Byrne PM, Bisgaard H, Godard PP et al. Budesonide/formoterol combination therapy as both maintenance and reliever medication in asthma. *Am J Resp Crit Care Med* 2005;171(2):129-36.
11. Scicchitano R, Aablers R, Ukena D et al. Efficacy and safety of budesonide/formoterol single inhaler therapy versus a higher dose budesonide in moderate to severe asthma. *Curr Med Res Opin* 2004;20(9):1403-8.
12. Chauhan BF, Ducharme FM. Anti-leukotriene agents compared to inhaled corticosteroids in the management of recurrent and/or chronic asthma in adults and children. *Cochrane Database Syst Rev* 2012;5:CD002314.
13. Chauhan BF, Ducharme FM. Addition to inhaled corticosteroids of long-acting beta2-agonists versus anti-leukotrienes for chronic asthma. *Cochrane Database Syst Rev* 2014;1:CD003137.
14. Chapman KR, Cartier A, Hebert J et al. The role of omalizumab in the treatment of severe allergic asthma. *Can Respir J* 2006;13(Suppl B):1B-9B.
15. Karpel J, Massanari M, Geba GP et al. Effectiveness of omalizumab in reducing corticosteroid burden in patients with moderate to severe persistent allergic asthma. *Ann Allergy Asthma Immunol* 2010;105(6):465-70.
16. Briggs GG, Freeman RK, Yaffe SJ. *Drugs in pregnancy and lactation: a reference guide to fetal and neonatal risk*. 9th ed. Philadelphia (PA): Lippincott Williams & Wilkins; 2011.
17. Koren G, Sarkar M, Einarson A. Safety of using montelukast during pregnancy. *Can Fam Physician* 2010;56(9):881-2.
18. Schatz M. Interrelationships between asthma and pregnancy: a literature review. *J Allergy Clin Immunol* 1999;103(2 Pt 2):S330-6.
19. Drugs and Lactation Database (LactMed). Bethesda (MD): U.S. National Library of Medicine. Available from toxnet.nlm.nih.gov/cgi-bin/sis/htmlgen?LACT. Accessed August 26, 2013.
20. Turner MO, Patel A, Ginsburg S et al. Bronchodilator delivery in acute airflow obstruction. A meta-analysis. *Arch Intern Med* 1997;157(15):1736-44.
21. Cates CJ, Welsh EJ, Rowe BH. Holding chambers (spacers) versus nebulizers for beta-agonist treatment of acute asthma. *Cochrane Database Syst Rev* 2013;9:CD000052.
22. Rodrigo GJ, Castro-Rodriguez JA. Anticholinergics in the treatment of children and adults with acute asthma: a systematic review with meta-analysis. *Thorax* 2005;60(9):740-6.
23. Rowe BH, Spooner CH, Ducharme FM et al. Early emergency department treatment of acute asthma with systemic corticosteroids. *Cochrane Database Syst Rev* 2001;(1):CD002178.
24. Littenberg B. Aminophylline treatment in severe, acute asthma. A meta-analysis. *JAMA* 1988;259(11):1678-84.

25. Nair P, Milan SJ, Rowe BH. Addition of intravenous aminophylline to beta(2)-agonists in adults with acute asthma. *Cochrane Database Syst Rev* 2012;12:CD002742.
26. Jenkins C, Costello J, Hodge L. Systematic review of prevalence of aspirin induced asthma and its implications for clinical practice. *BMJ* 2004;328(7437):434-41.

Chapter 52
Asthma in Infants and Children

Mary Noseworthy, MD, FRCPC and
Mark Montgomery, MD, FRCPC

Goals of Therapy

- Prevent cough, wheeze or shortness of breath that interferes with daytime activities, exercise, school attendance or sleep
- Reduce use of $beta_2$-agonists for symptom relief to <4 doses/week
- Prevent exacerbations requiring emergency room visits, hospitalizations or systemic corticosteroids
- Achieve normal measures of expiratory airflow such as peak flows or pulmonary function studies, e.g., forced expiratory volume in 1 second (FEV_1)
- Avoid/minimize medication side effects, especially interference with normal growth and development

Investigations

- Diagnosis of asthma in children <6 years depends on history and physical examination since pulmonary function tests are not easily obtained[1]
- History:
  - evidence suggesting airway hyperreactivity, e.g., wheeze or chest tightness that limits activities, cough that is worse at night, cough with duration longer than or of greater severity than usual for an upper respiratory tract infection (URTI)
  - evidence of inherited hyperreactivity, e.g., eczema, multiple food or inhalant allergies, positive family history of asthma, atopy
  - past history of admission to hospital due to respiratory syncytial virus bronchiolitis (risk of future asthma 39% vs. 9% for controls)[2]
  - consider features that suggest the cough or respiratory concern is related to conditions other than asthma:
    - associated evidence of malabsorption or failure to thrive, e.g., cystic fibrosis
    - associated swallowing difficulties or choking, e.g., vascular compression of the airway or congenital malformation
    - shortness of breath that is associated with weak voice and/or is absent at night or with sleep, e.g., vocal cord dysfunction[3]
    - recurrent otitis media and sinusitis, e.g., primary ciliary dyskinesia
- Physical examination:
  - presence of eczema and allergic rhinitis suggest that the child has inherited the atopic tendency and that the cause of cough or wheeze is related to asthma
  - hyperexpansion of thorax, increased nasal secretion, pale mucosal swelling, or sounds of wheezing during normal breathing or a forced exhalation
  - nasal polyps in a prepubertal child or finger clubbing in an individual of any age suggest that the primary cause of the cough is more likely related to cystic fibrosis, not asthma

- localized findings on exam, particularly if the wheeze or cough had a sudden onset, suggest aspiration of a foreign body

- Objective measurements needed to confirm diagnosis and assess severity include:
  - perform spirometry at least annually on all children >6 years of age who are using asthma medication regularly to maintain asthma control. Peak flow rates in children are an insensitive indicator of airflow limitation. There may be significant airflow limitation in the presence of normal peak flows
  - explore specific allergies to inhalants by history and/or skin testing[4]

Therapeutic Choices

Nonpharmacologic Choices

- Avoid exposure to cigarette smoke.[5,6,7,8,9]
- Avoid known allergens.[5,6,10] Evaluate and individualize environmental control measures.
- Recommend annual influenza vaccine for children with asthma.[11]
- Educate patients and children regarding chronicity of asthma and proper use of inhaler devices.

Pharmacologic Choices

See Figure 1 for an asthma management algorithm and Table 2 for detailed drug information.

Principles of Management

Asthma symptoms are due to airway hyperreactivity and narrowing. Airway obstruction is due to a combination of bronchospasm and airway inflammation. **Beta$_2$-agonists** provide short-term relief from bronchospasm and have no effect on airway inflammation. Regular use of an **inhaled corticosteroid** to treat airway inflammation is required if a beta$_2$-agonist is needed regularly for relief or provides inadequate relief of wheeze or shortness of breath. Inhaled corticosteroids control airway obstruction within weeks of initiation of therapy. Regular use for months or years is required to control airway inflammation.[12,13] The episodic use of inhaled corticosteroids for a few weeks at a time may reduce cough, but is unlikely to reduce airway hyperreactivity.

Drug Delivery Devices

Inhalation is the preferred route of administration because therapeutic effect is maximized and systemic side effects minimized. The hydrofluoroalkane propellants (HFA) used in pressurized metered dose inhalers (pMDIs) demonstrate excellent lung deposition of active ingredients.[14]

Review inhalation technique regularly. For infants and young children (<5 years), a pMDI and spacer device (also called a holding chamber) with mask attachment improves ability to correctly use the device. Assess very young infants for their ability to produce sufficient respiratory effort to open and close the valves of a spacer device. Drug deposition with a pMDI and spacer in infants and young children is generally 10–20% of the deposition in adults.[15] Therefore, adult doses may be required in children.[16] In older children (≥5 years), either a dry powder system (e.g., Diskus, Turbuhaler) or a pMDI with spacer device may be used. Adherence may be enhanced if the child participates in the selection of the device that works best for them.

Wet nebulization is a less attractive alternative due to difficulties with portability, time required for therapy and cost.[17] Furthermore, lung deposition of drug is compromised if technique is not meticulous, for example when the mask is not on the child's face, if tubing is used rather than the mask or if a soother is in the infant's mouth.

Incentive spirometers provide visual feedback to children about their inspiratory flows and can be invaluable teaching devices.

Figure 1: **Maintenance Therapy of Asthma in Children**

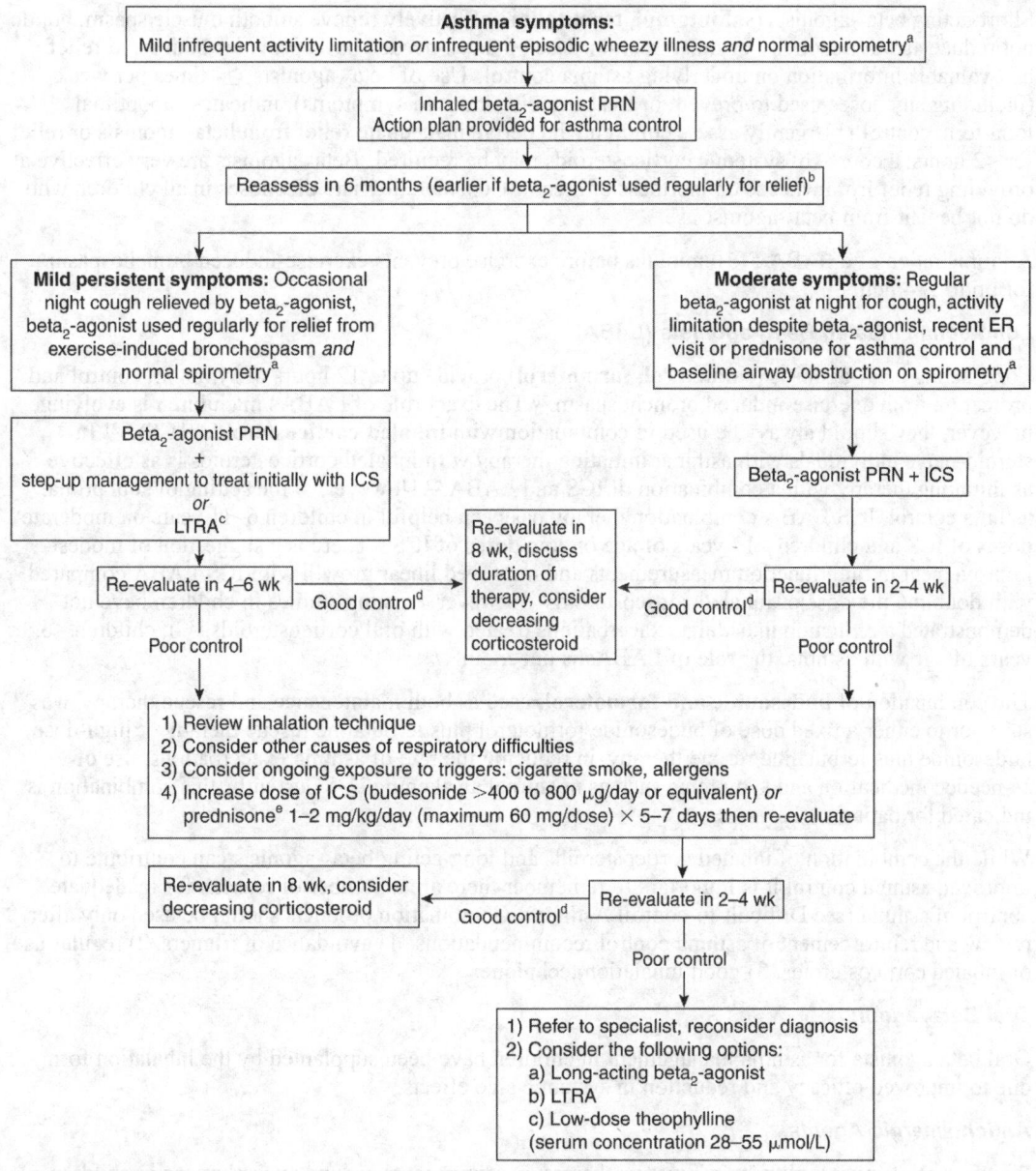

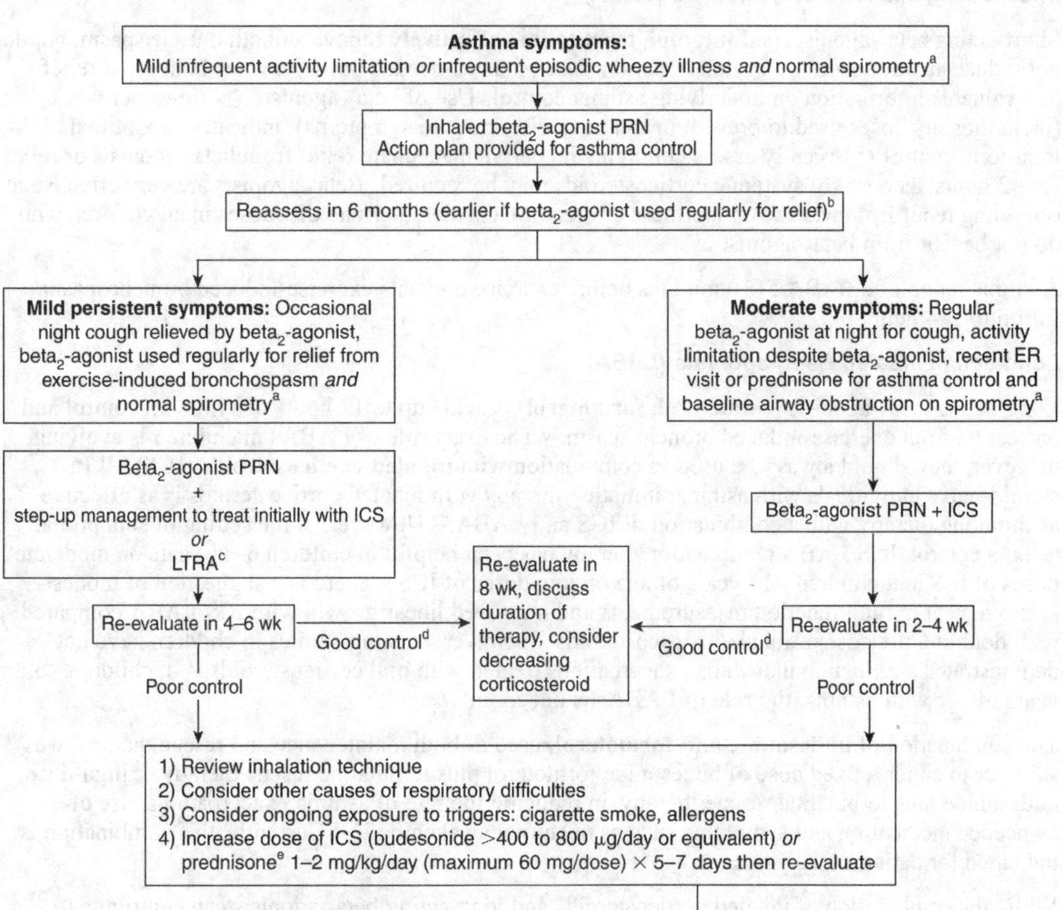

[a] Spirometry is used in children >6 years.
[b] Regular use of beta$_2$-agonist: use >4 times/week for relief.
[c] Reserve LTRA for patients who cannot or are not willing to use inhaled corticosteroids.
[d] Good asthma control: see Goals of Therapy.
[e] Or prednisolone which is available in a liquid formulation for young children.

Abbreviations: ER = emergency room; ICS = inhaled corticosteroid; LTRA = leukotriene receptor antagonist

Bronchodilator Agents

Short-acting Inhaled Beta$_2$-agonists (SABA)

Short-acting beta$_2$-agonists (**salbutamol**, **terbutaline**) effectively relieve smooth muscle spasm, but do not reduce airway reactivity or inflammation. Use on an as-needed basis provides both rapid relief and valuable information on underlying asthma control. Use of beta$_2$-agonists, ≥4 times per week (including any doses used to prevent or treat exercise-induced symptoms), indicates suboptimal long-term control.[18] Urgently assess children who derive inadequate relief from beta$_2$-agonists or relief for <2 hours; a course of systemic corticosteroids may be required. Beta$_2$-agonists are very effective at providing relief from wheeze or shortness of breath. Consider alternate diagnoses in all children who do not benefit from beta$_2$-agonist use.

Administration of a SABA 5–10 minutes before exercise prevents exercise-induced bronchospasm for up to 2–4 hours.[19]

Long-acting Inhaled Beta$_2$-agonists (LABA)

Long-acting beta$_2$-agonists (**salmeterol**, **formoterol**) provide up to 12 hours of symptom control and protection from exercise-induced bronchospasm.[20] The exact role of LABAs in children is evolving, however, they should always be used in combination with **inhaled corticosteroids (ICS)**.[6,21] In steroid-naïve individuals with asthma, initiating therapy with inhaled corticosteroids is as effective as initiating therapy with a combination of ICS and LABA.[22] However, in the setting of suboptimal asthma control, ICS/LABA combination therapy has been helpful in children 6–11 years on moderate doses of ICS and children >12 years of age on low doses of ICS.[6] There is a suggestion of modest improvement in lung function measurements and improved linear growth with ICS/LABA compared with doubling the dose of inhaled corticosteroids. However, existing studies in children have not demonstrated a reduction in asthma exacerbations treated with oral corticosteroids.[23] In children <6 years of age with asthma, the role of LABAs is uncertain.

The combination of **budesonide and formoterol**, used as both maintenance and rescue therapy, was superior to either a fixed dose of budesonide/formoterol plus terbutaline rescue therapy or high-dose budesonide plus terbutaline rescue therapy, in reducing the rate of asthma exacerbations, use of as-needed medication and symptoms such as nocturnal awakening.[24,25] Currently, this combination is indicated for patients ≥12 years.

While the combination of inhaled corticosteroids and long-acting beta$_2$-agonists can contribute to improved asthma control it is important to remember there are a number of reasons for inadequate control of asthma (see Difficult-to-control Asthma). Combination products should be used only after review and reinforcement of asthma control recommendations: 1) avoidance of triggers, 2) regular use of inhaled corticosteroids, 3) good inhalation technique.

Oral Beta$_2$-agonists

Oral beta-agonists for asthma management in children have been supplanted by the inhalation form, due to improved efficacy and reduction in systemic side effects.

Anticholinergic Agents

Restrict use of **ipratropium** to adjunctive therapy in severe acute asthma exacerbations in children.

Methylxanthines

Theophylline preparations, used as add-on therapy, may have an additional anti-inflammatory role in adult patients already using inhaled corticosteroid therapy.[26,27] The anti-inflammatory effect of theophylline occurs at serum levels lower than those employed in an attempt to relieve bronchospasm.[28] Theophylline is rarely used for routine maintenance of asthma in children because of the potential for toxicity, numerous drug interactions and the need for monitoring of serum levels.

Anti-inflammatory Agents

Inhaled Corticosteroids (ICS)

Inhaled corticosteroids (**beclomethasone, budesonide, ciclesonide, fluticasone, mometasone**) are the cornerstone of asthma management in infants and children, both to reduce and control symptoms and to prevent airway remodeling.[4] Regular use of ICS reduces mortality and asthma exacerbations, improves pulmonary function and controls symptoms, reduces the need for rescue bronchodilator treatment, reduces the need for oral corticosteroids to treat exacerbations and may decrease airway remodeling. ICS do not cure asthma and do not prevent development of asthma in preschool children at high risk.[29] Cessation following months of regular use may result in return of airway hyperreactivity to the previous status.

Symptom control generally occurs within days with low doses (e.g., budesonide 400 µg/day, see Table 1);[30] however, reduction in airway hyperreactivity may require months of regular use.[12,13] The majority of children with asthma experience good control with low doses of ICS.[31,32,33,34,35] Reconsider the diagnosis in children whose asthma is poorly controlled at moderate doses.

Doubling the dose of ICS in response to a viral respiratory tract infection or to control an exacerbation of asthma is a common practice. However, the early signs of an exacerbation are poorly defined and often underappreciated.[36] Moreover, the dose response relationship of inhaled corticosteroids has not been consistent.[37] Consequently, the benefits of this approach are inconsistent. The episodic doubling of ICS with exacerbations is not supported by evidence or by Canadian guidelines.[6,38,39] Emphasize regular use of ICS in a dose sufficient to control airway hyperreactivity rather than episodic short-term doubling of ICS in response to asthma symptoms. Temporary increases in ICS to high doses, e.g., fluticasone 750 µg BID, may reduce the need for oral corticosteroids used for viral-associated wheeze in preschool children. However, the long-term safety of this approach is uncertain and therefore it is not recommended.[6,40]

Doses of budesonide ≤400 µg/day or equivalent (see Table 1) have minimal systemic side effects. Most studies indicate there is an initial decrease in growth rate during the first year of inhaled corticosteroid use, but it is not sustained with long-term therapy and has minimal effect on final adult height.[41,42,43,44] In one study, regular use of budesonide 400 µg/day for 4–6 years was found to reduce adult height by approximately 1 cm.[45] There is a lack of data regarding higher doses of ICS or the impact of ICS "holidays" (e.g., discontinuation during the summer months). Always titrate to the lowest effective dose that maintains asthma control.

Table 1: Dosage Equivalencies for Inhaled Corticosteroids in Children (6–11 years)[a,b,6]

Drug	Low Dose	Moderate Dose	High Dose
Beclomethasone dipropionate pMDI	≤200 µg/day	201–400 µg/day	>400 µg/day
Budesonide DPI	≤400 µg/day	401–800 µg/day	>800 µg/day
Ciclesonide	≤200 µg/day	201–400 µg/day	>400 µg/day
Fluticasone propionate DPI or pMDI plus spacer	≤200 µg/day	201–400 µg/day	>400 µg/day

[a] Dosage equivalencies in children <6 years are similar due to smaller tidal volumes and, consequently, reduced lung deposition in this younger age group. Young children should use a pMDI with a spacer.
[b] For dosage equivalencies in children ≥12 years see Chapter 51.
Abbreviations: pMDI = pressurized metered dose inhaler; DPI = dry powder inhaler

Leukotriene Receptor Antagonists (LTRAs)

Leukotriene receptor antagonists (**montelukast, zafirlukast**) may provide bronchoprotection with exercise and in patients with ASA-sensitive asthma;[4,12] however, these patients should still avoid the use of NSAIDs when on LTRAs. These agents may have corticosteroid-sparing properties, allowing improved control of asthma at a reduced dose of inhaled corticosteroid.[46,47,48] As monotherapy, they provide control of airway inflammation that is approximately equivalent to fluticasone 100 µg/day.[49] Monotherapy with montelukast has resulted in improved asthma control and reduced exacerbations in preschool children.[50,51] Montelukast effectively reduced asthma exacerbations in September in school-aged children and adolescents.[52] However, LTRAs are not recommended as first-choice monotherapy in place of ICS due to inferior efficacy in preventing acute exacerbations that require oral corticosteroids and in improving other parameters of lung function.[53]

LTRAs can be used as adjunctive therapy with moderate to high doses of inhaled corticosteroids to achieve control of persistent asthma or in patients who cannot or will not use inhaled corticosteroids.

Reports of development of Churg-Strauss syndrome, an eosinophilic vasculitis, with use of LTRAs likely represents an unmasking of the vasculitis as doses of systemic corticosteroids are reduced.[54,55,56]

Anti-IgE Therapy

Omalizumab, a recombinant humanized monoclonal antibody that binds IgE receptors, thus impeding the IgE-mediated allergic response, has reduced asthma exacerbations and allowed reduction in the dose of inhaled corticosteroid, with improved asthma symptom control.[57,58] Its use is restricted to children >12 years with moderate to severe asthma inadequately controlled with ICS and evidence of allergic IgE-mediated asthma. Therapy should be initiated by a specialist.

Difficult-to-control Asthma

The majority of children with asthma can be well controlled with regular use of inhaled corticosteroids and beta$_2$-agonists for occasional relief.[18,59] If there is ongoing difficulty with asthma control, as evidenced by persistent symptoms, need for systemic corticosteroids or exacerbations of asthma necessitating an emergency department visit, consider several factors before concluding the child has difficult-to-control asthma; reconsider/confirm the diagnosis of asthma, ensure correct inhaler technique, ensure adherence to medical therapy,[60,61] ensure adequate irritant and allergen avoidance strategies and rule out comorbidities. Rhinitis and postnasal drip, particularly common comorbidities, will produce persistent cough, primarily during the day without associated symptoms of wheeze or shortness of breath. Consider the role of intercurrent infection, as with pertussis, or contribution of gastroesophageal reflux. Evaluation of the multifactorial nature of difficult-to-control asthma often requires a team approach, including a physician, nurse, asthma educator and psychologist.

An association between vitamin D deficiency and increased asthma symptoms or exacerbations in children has been observed.[62,63] However, RCTs demonstrating improvement in asthma control with vitamin D supplementation are lacking. It would be reasonable to consider the possibility of vitamin D deficiency in poorly controlled asthma and ensure adequate vitamin D supplementation in the patient (see Appendix IV). The use of systemic corticosteroids may have long-term consequences on adrenal function and on bone health. The use of 4 short courses of systemic corticosteroids over 2.5 years has been associated with an increased risk of fractures.[64]

Acute Asthma Management

An exacerbation of asthma requiring an emergency room visit, unscheduled doctor visit or hospitalization is a failure of long-term management. Immediate care for respiratory distress, evaluation of the cause of the exacerbation and intensification of long-term management are indicated. See Figure 2 for an approach to acute asthma management.

Manage acute severe asthma as a pediatric emergency. Initial therapy should be aggressive and then reduced as the exacerbation settles. Ideally, a child with asthma should not deteriorate once in hospital. Perform pulse oximetry or measure arterial blood gases and initiate supplemental oxygen in all children with respiratory distress.

Figure 2: **Treatment of Acute Asthma in Children**

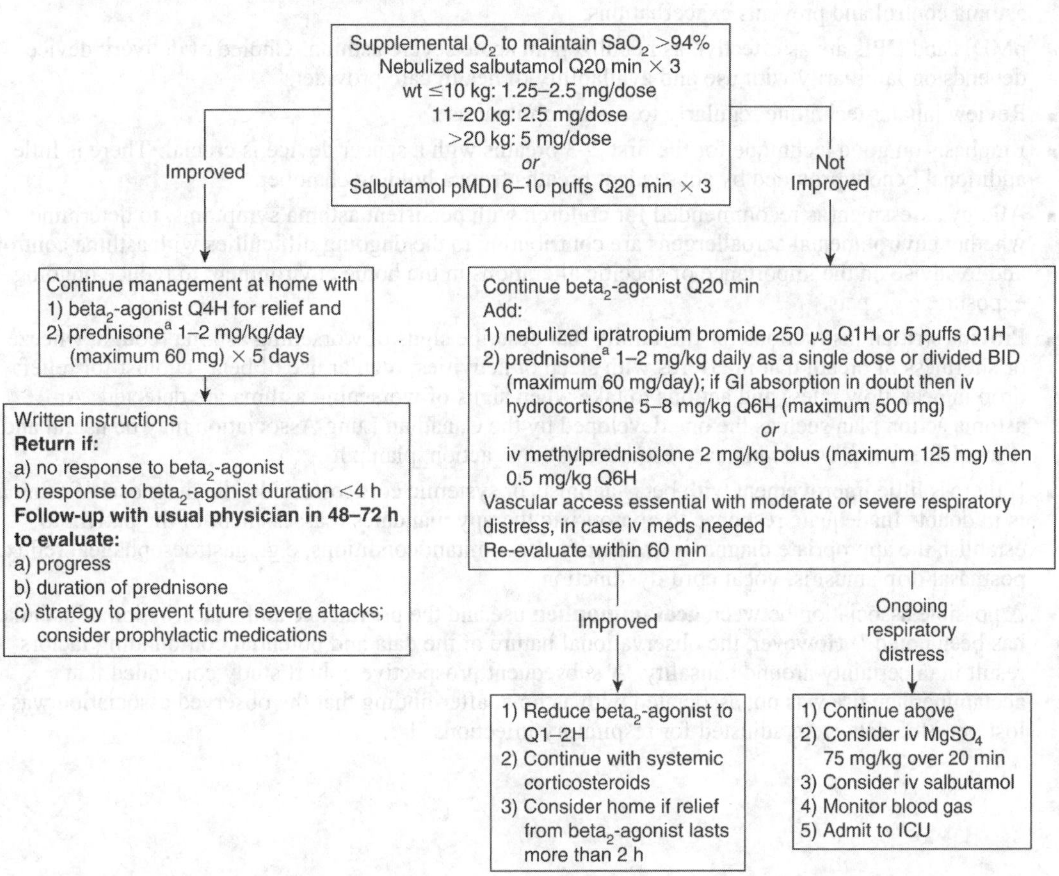
Supplemental O_2 to maintain SaO_2 >94%
Nebulized salbutamol Q20 min × 3
wt ≤10 kg: 1.25–2.5 mg/dose
11–20 kg: 2.5 mg/dose
>20 kg: 5 mg/dose
or
Salbutamol pMDI 6–10 puffs Q20 min × 3
Improved
Not Improved
Continue management at home with
1) $beta_2$-agonist Q4H for relief and
2) prednisone[a] 1–2 mg/kg/day (maximum 60 mg) × 5 days
Written instructions
Return if:
a) no response to $beta_2$-agonist
b) response to $beta_2$-agonist duration <4 h
Follow-up with usual physician in 48–72 h to evaluate:
a) progress
b) duration of prednisone
c) strategy to prevent future severe attacks; consider prophylactic medications
Continue $beta_2$-agonist Q20 min
Add:
1) nebulized ipratropium bromide 250 µg Q1H or 5 puffs Q1H
2) prednisone[a] 1–2 mg/kg daily as a single dose or divided BID (maximum 60 mg/day); if GI absorption in doubt then iv hydrocortisone 5–8 mg/kg Q6H (maximum 500 mg)
or
iv methylprednisolone 2 mg/kg bolus (maximum 125 mg) then 0.5 mg/kg Q6H
Vascular access essential with moderate or severe respiratory distress, in case iv meds needed
Re-evaluate within 60 min
Improved
Ongoing respiratory distress
1) Reduce $beta_2$-agonist to Q1–2H
2) Continue with systemic corticosteroids
3) Consider home if relief from $beta_2$-agonist lasts more than 2 h
1) Continue above
2) Consider iv $MgSO_4$ 75 mg/kg over 20 min
3) Consider iv salbutamol
4) Monitor blood gas
5) Admit to ICU

[a] Or prednisolone which is available in a liquid formulation for young children.
Abbreviations: GI = gastrointestinal; ICU = intensive care unit; pMDI = pressurized metered dose inhaler; SaO_2 = arterial oxygen percent saturation

The cornerstones of therapy are supplemental oxygen, frequent high-dose **inhaled $beta_2$-agonist** and **systemic corticosteroids** (e.g., prednisolone). **Ipratropium bromide** may provide additional bronchodilation.[65,66,67] IV **magnesium** or **salbutamol** are adjunctive therapies for more severe attacks.[68,69] There is little evidence that the routine use of **aminophylline** is required in the management of acute severe asthma.[70,71] The use of aminophylline may be considered in the setting of ongoing deterioration and impending respiratory failure despite intensive therapy with inhaled $beta_2$-agonists, anticholinergics and systemic corticosteroids. Avoid sedation. Correct mild to moderate dehydration if present. If there is acute severe asthma, always anticipate the possible need for airway control and subsequent difficult ventilatory management. Controlled rather than emergent airway procedures are preferred.

Close observation and frequent reassessment of all children with acute severe asthma is mandatory. Arrange for follow-up care for all children discharged home from the emergency department.

Therapeutic Tips

- Prolonged use of **inhaled corticosteroids** for a minimum of months or seasons is required to control airway hyperreactivity in children.

- Frequent re-evaluation of asthma control is essential. These visits provide a good opportunity to determine if the ICS dose can be reduced to achieve the lowest daily dose that provides excellent asthma control and prevents exacerbations.
- pMDIs and DPIs are as effective as nebulizers in acute severe asthma. Choice of delivery device depends on familiarity with use and availability of health care providers.
- Review inhaler technique regularly to ensure optimal use.
- Emphasis on good technique for the first 2–3 breaths with a spacer device is crucial. There is little additional benefit provided by subsequent breaths from a holding chamber.[72]
- Allergy assessment is recommended for children with persistent asthma symptoms, to determine whether environmental aeroallergens are contributing to the ongoing difficulties with asthma control and to advise on the importance of specific alterations in the home environment to reduce ongoing exposure, e.g., pets.
- Provide written instructions for the family that describe signs of worsening asthma (cough, wheeze or shortness of breath that interferes with sleep or activities; regular use of beta$_2$-agonist for relief; drop in peak flow rates) and actions to take when signs of worsening asthma are detected. An asthma action plan such as the one developed by the Canadian Lung Association may be useful and is available from: www.lung.ca/_resources/asthma_action_plan.pdf.
- If there is little improvement with beta$_2$-agonists or systemic corticosteroids, the diagnosis of asthma is in doubt. Inadequate response to appropriate therapy mandates reassessment of the patient to establish the appropriate diagnosis or identify concomitant conditions, e.g., gastroesophageal reflux, postnasal drip/sinusitis, vocal cord dysfunction.
- A possible association between **acetaminophen** use and the prevalence and exacerbation of asthma has been noted.[73] However, the observational nature of the data and potential confounding factors result in uncertainty around causality. A subsequent prospective cohort study concluded that acetaminophen use was not associated with asthma, after finding that the observed association was lost once the data were adjusted for respiratory infections.[74]

Table 2: Drugs Used for Maintenance Therapy for Asthma in Children

Class	Drug	Dose	Adverse Effects	Comments	Cost[a]
$Beta_2$-Agonists, long-acting (LABA)	*formoterol fumarate* Foradil	DPI 12 µg/capsule: 6–16 y: 1 capsule inhaled BID; maximum 24 µg/day	Tachycardia, palpitations, nervousness, tremor, hypokalemia. Possibility of tolerance with regular use.	**LABAs are not to be used as monotherapy.** Provides protection from exercise-induced bronchospasm for 10 h. Combination LABA/corticosteroid product preferred to ensure LABA is not used as monotherapy.	$$
	formoterol fumarate dihydrate Oxeze Turbuhaler	DPI 6 or 12 µg/inhalation: 6–16 y: 1 inhalation BID; maximum 24 µg/day	See formoterol fumarate.	See formoterol fumarate.	$$
	salmeterol Serevent	Diskhaler 50 µg/blister: ≥4 y: 1 blister BID Diskus 50 µg/inhalation: ≥4 y: 1 inhalation BID	See formoterol fumarate.	See formoterol fumarate.	$$
$Beta_2$-Agonists, short-acting (SABA)	*salbutamol* Airomir pMDI, Ventolin Diskus, Ventolin HFA, Ventolin Nebules P.F., generics	pMDI 100 µg/puff: adult doses may be required due to poor deposition[16,17] 4–11 y: 1 puff TID–QID PRN; maximum 400 µg/day ≥12 y: 1–2 puffs TID–QID PRN; maximum 800 µg/day Diskus 200 µg/blister: ≥4 y: 1 inhalation TID–QID PRN; maximum 800 µg/day Nebules: 5–12 y: 1.25–2.5 mg as a single dose; maximum 5 mg. May repeat QID PRN	Tachycardia, palpitations, nervousness, tremor, hypokalemia.	Prevents exercise-induced bronchospasm for up to 2–4 h. Provides relief and information on asthma control in that regular use indicates poor control, use of ≥1 canister per month associated with increased risk of asthma mortality. pMDI plus spacer may be used in children <4 y, though no trials have been done to assess optimal dose.	$
	terbutaline Bricanyl Turbuhaler	DPI 0.5 mg/inhalation: ≥6 y: 1 inhalation PRN; maximum 6 inhalations/day	See salbutamol.	See salbutamol.	$

(cont'd)

Table 2: **Drugs Used for Maintenance Therapy for Asthma in Children** *(cont'd)*

Class	Drug	Dose	Adverse Effects	Comments	Cost[a]
Corticosteroids, inhaled	*beclomethasone* Qvar	Individualize dose. Adult doses may be required due to poor deposition.[16,17] pMDI: ≥12 y: 50–400 µg BID 5–11 y: 50 µg BID; maximum 100 µg BID	Oral thrush, dysphonia.	Follow linear growth every 3–6 months with regular asthma reassessments. Short-term growth rate may be slowed during first year of inhaled corticosteroid use but is not sustained. Inhaled corticosteroids have minimal impact on final adult height. Dysphonia and candidiasis can be decreased by use of spacer with pMDI and rinsing after use. Most of the corticosteroid effect on asthma control is achieved with doses <400 µg/day of budesonide or equivalent;[33] children requiring more than this on a regular basis should be assessed by a specialist. Regular re-evaluation required to ensure that lowest effective dose of inhaled corticosteroid is being used to maintain control.	$$
	budesonide Pulmicort Turbuhaler, Pulmicort Nebuamp	Individualize dose. DPI: ≥12 y: 200–400 µg BID 6–12 y: 100–200 µg BID Nebules: Individualize dose. 3 months–12 y: 0.25–0.5 mg BID; may increase to 1 mg BID	See beclomethasone.	See beclomethasone.	$$-$$$
	ciclesonide Alvesco	Individualize dose. pMDI: ≥12 y: 100–800 µg daily 6–11 y: 100–200 µg daily	See beclomethasone.	See beclomethasone.	$$-$$$
	fluticasone Flovent HFA, Flovent Diskus	Individualize dose. Adult doses may be required due to poor deposition.[16,17] pMDI, DPI: >16 y: 100–500 µg BID; maximum 1000 µg BID 4–16 y: 50–100 µg BID; may increase to 200 µg BID pMDI: 1–4 y: 100 µg BID via pediatric spacer device with face mask	See beclomethasone.	See beclomethasone.	$$-$$$
	mometasone furoate Asmanex	DPI: ≥12 y: 200–400 µg daily; maximum 400 µg BID	See beclomethasone.	See beclomethasone.	$$-$$$

Class	Drug	Dose	Adverse Effects	Comments	Cost[a]
Corticosteroid/ LABA Combinations	*budesonide/formoterol fumarate dihydrate* Symbicort	DPI 100/6 µg or 200/6 µg: **Maintenance therapy:** ≥12 y: 1–2 inhalations daily–BID; maximum 4 inhalations/day. May temporarily increase to 4 inhalations BID for worsening asthma **Maintenance and reliever therapy:** ≥12 y: 1–2 inhalations BID or 2 inhalations once daily. May use 1 additional inhalation in response to symptoms; if symptoms persist after a few minutes, an additional dose may be taken; maximum 6 inhalations on any single occasion; maximum 8 inhalations/day	See beclomethasone. See formoterol fumarate dihydrate.	Fixed-dose combination inhalers are more convenient, enhance adherence, ensure the patient receives their inhaled corticosteroid with their LABA and are less expensive than the individual agents combined. See beclomethasone.	$$$
	fluticasone/salmeterol Advair pMDI, Advair Diskus	pMDI 125/25 µg or 250/25 µg: ≥12 y: 2 puffs BID Diskus 100/50 µg: 4–11 y: 1 inhalation BID Diskus 100/50, 250/50 or 500/50 µg: ≥12 y: 1 inhalation BID	See beclomethasone. See salmeterol.	See budesonide/formoterol fumarate dihydrate. Not for rescue therapy.	$$$$-$$$$$
	mometasone/formoterol fumarate dihydrate Zenhale	pMDI 50/5 µg, 100/5 µg or 200/5 µg: ≥12 y: 2 puffs BID	See beclomethasone. See formoterol fumarate dihydrate.	See budesonide/formoterol fumarate dihydrate. Not for rescue therapy.	$$$$
IgE-Neutralizing Antibody	*omalizumab* Xolair	≥12 y: Dose is titrated based on body weight and serum IgE level. Administer sc injection Q2–4 wk	Common: injection site reactions, viral infections, upper respiratory tract infections, headache, sinusitis, pharyngitis. Rare: urticaria.	Store at 2–8°C. Reconstituted product may be stored for up to 8 h at 2–8°C. Do not inject more than 150 mg at one site. After start of treatment, do not use serum IgE for dose adjustment. Omalizumab raises IgE levels which may persist for up to a year after end of treatment.	$630/150 mg vial

(cont'd)

Table 2: **Drugs Used for Maintenance Therapy for Asthma in Children** *(cont'd)*

Class	Drug	Dose	Adverse Effects	Comments	Cost[a]
Leukotriene Receptor Antagonists	*montelukast* Singulair, generics	≥15 y: 10 mg QHS po 6–14 y: 5 mg (chewable tablet) QHS po 2–5 y: 4 mg (chewable tablet or granules) QHS po	Headache, abdominal pain, flu-like symptoms, hepatotoxicity (rare). Reports of neuropsychiatric effects, e.g., depression, agitation.	Decreased montelukast levels: carbamazepine, rifampin, phenobarbital, phenytoin.	$$
	zafirlukast Accolate	≥12 y: 20 mg BID 1 h before or 2 h after meals po	Common: headache, nausea, diarrhea. Rare: hepatotoxicity, including some fatalities; neuropsychiatric effects.	May potentiate effect of warfarin, monitor INR and adjust dose as necessary; may increase theophylline levels. Decreased zafirlukast levels: erythromycin, carbamazepine, rifampin, phenobarbital, phenytoin.	$$

[a] Includes drug cost only. Cost of inhaled agents is per unit (1 inhaler, nebule or vial); oral medications is per 30-day supply.
Abbreviations: DPI = dry powder inhaler; LABA = long-acting beta$_2$-agonist; pMDI = pressurized metered dose inhaler
Legend: $ < $30 $$ $30–60 $$-$$$ $30–90 $$$ $60–90 $$$$ $90–120 $$$$-$$$$$ $90–150 $$$$$ $120–150

Suggested Readings

Global Initiative for Asthma. *Pocket guide for asthma management and prevention in children 5 years and younger: a pocket guide for physicians and nurses* [updated 2009]. Available from: www.ginasthma.org/guidelines-pocket-guide-for-asthma-management-and-prevention-in.html.

Hedlin G, Konradsen J, Bush A. An update on paediatric asthma. *Eur Respir Rev* 2012;21(125):175-85.

Kovesi T, Schuh S, Spier S et al. Achieving control of asthma in preschoolers. *CMAJ* 2010;182(4):E172-83.

Lougheed MD, Lemiere C, Dell SD et al. Canadian Thoracic Society Asthma Management Continuum—2010 Consensus Summary for children six years of age and over, and adults. *Can Respir J* 2010;17(1):15-24.

Lougheed MD, Lemiere C, Ducharme FM et al. Canadian Thoracic Society 2012 update: diagnosis and management of asthma in preschoolers, children and adults. *Can Respir J* 2012;19(2):127-64.

National Asthma Education and Prevention Program. *Expert panel report 3: guidelines for the diagnosis and management of asthma.* Bethesda (MD): National Heart, Lung, and Blood Institute; 2007. (NIH publication no. 08-4051). Available from: www.nhlbi.nih.gov/guidelines/asthma/asthgdln.pdf.

Ortiz-Alvarez O, Mikrogianakis A; Canadian Paediatric Society, Acute Care Committee. Managing the paediatric patient with an acute asthma exacerbation. *Paediatr Child Health* 2012;17(5):251-62.

References

1. Respiratory Review Panel. *Respiratory (asthma and COPD) guidelines for family practice.* Toronto (ON): MUMS Guidelines Clearinghouse; 2007.
2. Sigurs N, Aljassim F, Kjellman B et al. Asthma and allergy patterns over 18 years after severe RSV bronchiolitis in the first year of life. *Thorax* 2010;65(12):1045-52.
3. Tilles SA. Vocal cord dysfunction in children and adolescents. *Curr Allergy Asthma Rep* 2003;3(6):467-72.
4. Djukanovic R. Airway inflammation in asthma and its consequences: implications for treatment in children and adults. *J Allergy Clin Immunol* 2002;109(6 Suppl):S539-48.
5. Global Initiative for Asthma. *GINA Report, Global strategy for asthma management and prevention.* Updated 2014. Available from: www.ginasthma.org/guidelines-gina-report-global-strategy-for-asthma.html.
6. Lougheed MD, Lemiere C, Ducharme FM et al. Canadian Thoracic Society 2012 update: diagnosis and management of asthma in preschoolers, children and adults. *Can Respir J* 2012;19(2):127-64.
7. Strachan DP, Cook DG. Health effects of passive smoking. 5. Parental smoking and allergic sensitisation in children. *Thorax* 1998;53(2):117-23.
8. Cook DG, Strachan DP. Health effects of passive smoking. 3. Parental smoking and prevalence of respiratory symptoms and asthma in school age children. *Thorax* 1997;52(12):1081-94.
9. Strachan DP, Cook DG. Health effects of passive smoking. 1. Parental smoking and lower respiratory illness in infancy and early childhood. *Thorax* 1997;52(10):905-14.
10. Morgan WJ, Crain EF, Gruchalla RS et al. Results of a home-based environmental intervention among urban children with asthma. *N Engl J Med* 2004;351(11):1068-80.
11. National Advisory Committee on Immunization (NACI). Statement on seasonal Trivalent Inactivated Influenza vaccine (TIV) for 2010-2011. An Advisory Committee Statement (ACS). *Can Commun Dis Rep* 2010;36(ACS-6):1-49. Available from: www.phac-aspc.gc.ca/publicat/ccdr-rmtc/10pdf/36-acs-6.pdf. Accessed April 4, 2011.
12. Haahtela T, Jarvinen M, Kava T et al. Comparison of a beta 2-agonist, terbutaline, with an inhaled corticosteroid, budesonide, in newly detected asthma. *N Engl J Med* 1991;325(6):388-92.
13. Nielsen KG, Bisgaard H. The effect of inhaled budesonide on symptoms, lung function, and cold air and methacholine responsiveness in 2- to 5-year-old asthmatic children. *Am J Respir Crit Care Med* 2000;162(4 Pt 1):1500-6.
14. Pedersen S, Warner J, Wahn U et al. Growth, systemic safety, and efficacy during 1 year of asthma treatment with different beclomethasone dipropionate formulations: an open-label, randomized comparison of extrafine and conventional aerosols in children. *Pediatrics* 2002;109(6):e92.
15. Salmon B, Wilson NM, Silverman M. How much aerosol reaches the lungs of wheezy infants and toddlers? *Arch Dis Child* 1990;65(4):401-3.
16. Tal A, Golan H, Grauer N et al. Deposition pattern of radiolabeled salbutamol inhaled from a metered-dose inhaler by means of a spacer with mask in young children with airway obstruction. *J Pediatr* 1996;128(4):479-84.
17. Castro-Rodriguez JA, Rodrigo GJ. beta-agonists through metered-dose inhaler with valved holding chamber versus nebulizer for acute exacerbation of wheezing or asthma in children under 5 years of age: a systematic review with meta-analysis. *J Pediatr* 2004;145(2):172-7.
18. Lougheed MD, Lemiere C, Dell SD et al. Canadian Thoracic Society Asthma Management Continuum—2010 Consensus Summary for children six years of age and over, and adults. *Can Respir J* 2010;17(1):15-24.
19. Anderson SD, Seale JP, Rozea P et al. Inhaled and oral salbutamol in exercise-induced asthma. *Am Rev Respir Dis* 1976;114(3):493-500.
20. Green CP, Price JF. Prevention of exercise induced asthma by inhaled salmeterol xinafoate. *Arch Dis Child* 1992;67(8):1014-7.
21. Lemanske RF, Mauger DT, Sorkness CA et al. Step-up therapy for children with uncontrolled asthma receiving inhaled corticosteroids. *N Engl J Med* 2010;362(11):975-85.
22. Lemiere C, Becker A, Boulet LP et al. Should combination therapy with inhaled corticosteroids and long-acting beta2-agonists be prescribed as initial maintenance treatment for asthma? *CMAJ* 2002;167(9):1008-9.
23. Ni Chroinin M, Lasserson TJ, Greenstone I et al. Addition of long-acting beta-agonists to inhaled corticosteroids for chronic asthma in children. *Cochrane Database Syst Rev* 2009;(3):CD007949.
24. O'Byrne PM, Bisgaard H, Godard PP et al. Budesonide/formoterol combination therapy as both maintenance and reliever medication in asthma. *Am J Respir Crit Care Med* 2005;171(2):129-36.

25. Bisgaard H, Le Roux P, Bjamer D et al. Budesonide/formoterol maintenance plus reliever therapy: a new strategy in pediatric asthma. *Chest* 2006;130(6):1733-43.
26. Evans DJ, Taylor DA, Zetterstrom O et al. A comparison of low-dose inhaled budesonide plus theophylline and high-dose inhaled budesonide for moderate asthma. *N Engl J Med* 1997;337(20):1412-8.
27. Ukena D, Harnest U, Sakalauskas R et al. Comparison of addition of theophylline to inhaled steroid with doubling of the dose of inhaled steroid in asthma. *Eur Respir J* 1997;10(12):2754-60.
28. Weinberger M, Hendeles L. Theophylline in asthma. *N Engl J Med* 1996;334(21):1380-8.
29. Guilbert TW, Morgan WJ, Zeiger RS et al. Long-term inhaled corticosteroids in preschool children at high risk for asthma. *N Engl J Med* 2006;354(19):1985-97.
30. Shapiro G, Bronsky EA, LaForce CF et al. Dose-related efficacy of budesonide administered via a dry powder inhaler in the treatment of children with moderate to severe persistent asthma. *J Pediatr* 1998;132(6):976-82.
31. Bisgaard H. Delivery of inhaled medication to children. *J Asthma* 1997;34(6):443-67.
32. Bisgaard H, Gillies J, Groenewald M et al. The effect of inhaled fluticasone propionate in the treatment of young asthmatic children: a dose comparison study. *Am J Respir Crit Care Med* 1999;160(1):126-31.
33. Pedersen S, Hansen OR. Budesonide treatment of moderate and severe asthma in children: a dose-response study. *J Allergy Clin Immunol* 1995;95(1 Pt 1):29-33.
34. Visser MJ, Postma DS, Arends LR et al. One-year treatment with different dosing schedules of fluticasone propionate in childhood asthma. Effects on hyperresponsiveness, lung function, and height. *Am J Respir Crit Care Med* 2001;164(11):2073-7.
35. Chauhan BF, Chartrand C, Ducharme FM. Intermittent versus daily inhaled corticosteroids for persistent asthma in children and adults. *Cochrane Database Syst Rev* 2013;2:CD009611.
36. Rivera-Spoljaric K, Chinchilli VM, Camera LJ et al. Signs and symptoms that precede wheezing in children with a pattern of moderate-to-severe intermittent wheezing. *J Pediatr* 2009;154(6):877-81.
37. Zhang L, Axelsson I, Chung M et al. Dose response of inhaled corticosteroids in children with persistent asthma: a systematic review. *Pediatrics* 2011;127(1):129-38.
38. Garrett J, Williams S, Wong C et al. Treatment of acute asthmatic exacerbations with an increased dose of inhaled steroid. *Arch Dis Child* 1998;79(1):12-7.
39. Hendeles L, Sherman J. Are inhaled corticosteroids effective for acute exacerbations of asthma in children? *J Pediatr* 2003;142(2 Suppl):S26-32.
40. Ducharme FM, Lemire C, Noya FJ et al. Preemptive use of high-dose fluticasone for virus-induced wheezing in young children. *N Engl J Med* 2009;360(4):339-53.
41. Agertoft L, Pedersen S. Effect of long-term treatment with inhaled budesonide on adult height in children with asthma. *N Engl J Med* 2000;343(15):1064-9.
42. Pedersen S. Do inhaled corticosteroids inhibit growth in children? *Am J Respir Crit Care Med* 2001;164(4):521-35.
43. Silverstein MD, Yunginger JW, Reed CE et al. Attained adult height after childhood asthma: effect of glucocorticoid therapy. *J Allergy Clin Immunol* 1997;99(4):466-74.
44. Leone FT, Fish JE, Szefler SJ et al. Systematic review of the evidence regarding potential complications of inhaled corticosteroid use in asthma: collaboration of American College of Chest Physicians, American Academy of Allergy, Asthma, and Immunology, and American College of Allergy, Asthma, and Immunology. *Chest* 2003;124(6):2329-40.
45. Kelly HW, Sternberg AL, Lescher R et al. Effect of inhaled glucocorticoids in childhood on adult height. *N Engl J Med* 2012;367(10):904-12.
46. Ducharme FM. Anti-leukotrienes as add-on therapy to inhaled glucocorticoids in patients with asthma: systematic review of current evidence. *BMJ* 2002;324(7353):1545.
47. Lofdahl CG, Reiss TF, Leff JA et al. Randomised, placebo controlled trial of effect of a leukotriene receptor antagonist, montelukast, on tapering inhaled corticosteroids in asthmatic patients. *BMJ* 1999;319(7202):87-90.
48. Tamaoki J, Kondo M, Sakai N et al. Leukotriene antagonist prevents exacerbation of asthma during reduction of high-dose inhaled corticosteroid. The Tokyo Joshi-Idai Asthma Research Group. *Am J Respir Crit Care Med* 1997;155(4):1235-40.
49. Busse W, Raphael GD, Galant S et al. Low-dose fluticasone propionate compared with montelukast for first-line treatment of persistent asthma: a randomized clinical trial. *J Allergy Clin Immunol* 2001;107(3):461-8.
50. Bisgaard H, Zielen S, Garcia-Garcia ML et al. Montelukast reduces asthma exacerbations in 2- to 5-year-old children with intermittent asthma. *Am J Respir Crit Care Med* 2005;171(4):315-22.
51. Straub DA, Moeller A, Minocchieri S et al. The effect of montelukast on lung function and exhaled nitric oxide in infants with early childhood asthma. *Eur Respir J* 2005;25(2):289-94.
52. Johnston NW, Mandhane PJ, Dai J et al. Attenuation of the September epidemic of asthma exacerbations in children: a randomized, controlled trial of montelukast added to usual therapy. *Pediatrics* 2007;120(3):e702-12.
53. Chauhan BF, Ducharme FM. Anti-leukotriene agents compared to inhaled corticosteroids in the management of recurrent and/or chronic asthma in adults and children. *Cochrane Database Syst Rev* 2012;5:CD002314.
54. Boccagni C, Tesser F, Mittino D et al. Churg-Strauss syndrome associated with the leukotriene antagonist montelukast. *Neurol Sci* 2004;25(1):21-2.
55. Tang MB, Yosipovitch G. Acute Churg-Strauss syndrome in an asthmatic patient receiving montelukast therapy. *Arch Dermatol* 2003;139(6):715-8.
56. Turvey SE, Vargas SO, Phipatanakul W. Churg-Strauss syndrome in a 7-year-old receiving montelukast and inhaled corticosteroids. *Ann Allergy Asthma Immunol* 2003;90(2):274.
57. Ruffin CG, Busch BE. Omalizumab: a recombinant humanized anti-IgE antibody for allergic asthma. *Am J Health Syst Pharm* 2004;61(14):1449-59.
58. Normansell R, Walker S, Milan SJ et al. Omalizumab for asthma in adults and children. *Cochrane Database Syst Rev* 2014;1:CD003559.
59. Kovesi T, Schuh S, Spier S et al. Achieving control of asthma in preschoolers. *CMAJ* 2010;182(4):E172-83.
60. Bracken M, Fleming L, Hall P et al. The importance of nurse-led home visits in the assessment of children with problematic asthma. *Arch Dis Child* 2009;94(10):780-4.
61. Pando S, Lemiere C, Beauchesne MF et al. Suboptimal use of inhaled cortiocosteroids in children with persistent asthma: inadequate prescription, poor drug adherence or both? *Pharmacotherapy* 2010;30(11):1109-16.
62. Brehm JM, Schuemann B, Fuhlbrigge AL et al. Serum vitamin D levels and severe asthma exacerbations in the Childhood Asthma Management Program study. *J Allergy Clin Immunol* 2010;126(1):52-8.

63. Litonjua AA. Vitamin D deficiency as a risk factor for childhood allergic disease and asthma. *Curr Opin Allergy Clin Immunol* 2012;12(2):179-85.
64. van Staa TP, Cooper C, Leufkens HG et al. Children and the risk of fractures caused by oral corticosteroids. *J Bone Miner Res* 2003;18(5):913-8.
65. Rodrigo GJ, Castro-Rodriguez JA. Anticholinergics in the treatment of children and adults with acute asthma: a systematic review with meta-analysis. *Thorax* 2005;60(9):740-6.
66. Plotnick LH, Ducharme FM. Should inhaled anticholinergics be added to beta2 agonists for treating acute childhood and adolescent asthma? A systematic review. *BMJ* 1998;317(7164):971-7.
67. Griffiths B, Ducharme FM. Combined inhaled anticholinergics and short-acting beta-agonists for initial treatment of acute asthma in children. *Cochrane Database Syst Rev* 2013;8:CD000060.
68. Browne GJ, Penna AS, Phung X et al. Randomised trial of intravenous salbutamol in early management of acute severe asthma in children. *Lancet* 1997;349(9048):301-5.
69. Mohammed S, Goodacre S. Intravenous and nebulised magnesium sulphate for acute asthma: systematic review and meta-analysis. *Emerg Med J* 2007;24(12):823-30.
70. DiGiulio GA, Kercsmar CM, Krug SE et al. Hospital treatment of asthma: lack of benefit from theophylline given in addition to nebulized albuterol and intravenously administered corticosteroid. *J Pediatr* 1993;122(3):464-9.
71. Strauss RE, Wertheim DL, Bonagura VR et al. Aminophylline therapy does not improve outcome and increases adverse effects in children hospitalized with acute asthmatic exacerbations. *Pediatrics* 1994;93(2):205-10.
72. Schultz A, Le Souef TJ, Venter A et al. Aerosol inhalation from spacers and valved holding chambers requires few tidal breaths for children. *Pediatrics* 2010;126(6):e1493-8.
73. McBride JT. The association of acetaminophen and asthma prevalence and severity. *Pediatrics* 2011;128(6):1181-5.
74. Lowe AJ, Carlin JB, Bennett CM et al. Paracetamol use in early life and asthma: prospective birth cohort study. *BMJ* 2010;341:c4616.

Chapter 53
Chronic Cough in Adults

Pearce Wilcox, MD, FRCP, FACP

Chronic cough (cough lasting >8 weeks) adversely affects quality of life and has an estimated prevalence of up to 20% in adults.[1] There is a very broad differential diagnosis given the ubiquitous distribution of cough receptors in the upper and lower respiratory tracts and other anatomic compartments. However, in nonsmokers with a negative chest radiograph who are not taking an ACE inhibitor, chronic cough can be attributed to upper airway cough syndrome (UACS; formerly known as postnasal drip syndrome), asthma, gastroesophageal reflux disease (GERD) or nonasthmatic eosinophilic bronchitis in the majority of cases (see Table 1).[1,2,3,4] Nonetheless, cough is refractory to therapy in up to 40% of cases referred to specialty clinics.[9] Chronic cough results from an interplay between airway inflammation, airway hyperresponsiveness and cough reflex hypersensitivity.

Acute cough is most often infectious, contributes to clearing secretions, and does not generally require antitussive therapy.[1,2,4] Postinfectious cough is a persistent cough that lasts >3 weeks after acute symptoms of an upper respiratory tract infection (e.g., *Mycoplasma pneumoniae*, *Bordetella pertussis*, *B. parapertussis*). Postinfectious cough does not usually last for >8 weeks.[10] The cough is generally self-limited and resolves on its own.[10] Pertussis is a well-recognized exception where cough is often prolonged.

Goals of Therapy

- Choose appropriate and effective therapy based on cough etiology
- Resist nonspecific cough suppression therapy, which may delay diagnosis of a curative cause
- Prevent complications attributable to cough, e.g., rib fractures, syncope, loss of sleep, aggravation of stress incontinence, exercise intolerance, emesis, epistaxis
- Ensure uncommon but more serious causes such as lung cancer are not missed

Investigations

A standardized approach will lead to identifiable cause(s) of cough in most patients[11,12] (Figure 1). More detailed testing (e.g., CT scan, bronchoscopy) should be reserved for those with no overt cause detected on initial evaluation and cough refractory to empiric therapeutic trials for the most common etiologies.

- History and physical exam, with special attention to:
  - duration of cough (variation in cough over the day), history of smoking (tobacco, cannabis) and medication use (ACE inhibitor), signs and symptoms of asthma, upper airway symptoms, GERD. Examine nasal cavities, oropharynx and otic canals, respiratory and cardiac systems
  - consider occupational and environmental causes, e.g., nonspecific irritants or allergens
  - personal or family history of atopy/asthma
- Objective measurements needed to confirm diagnosis:
  - chest x-ray (CXR)
  - spirometry to evaluate for asthma (pre-/post-bronchodilator) and COPD
  - challenge testing (e.g., methacholine) to detect airway hyper-responsiveness. However, this can be false-positive in up to 20% of cases in the investigation of cough

- nonasthmatic eosinophilic bronchitis: consider in patients with normal spirometry, normal CXR, negative methacholine challenge and sputum eosinophilia, elevated exhaled nitric oxide or a response to inhaled corticosteroids (Table 1)
- investigations for GERD—ambulatory pH monitoring most sensitive but still has limited predictability for detecting acid related cough.[13] Nonacid reflux can be detected by impedance monitoring but not widely available and not well validated. Upper GI and endoscopy often normal, laryngoscopy can be suggestive[14]
- investigation of less common causes of cough, e.g., carcinoma of respiratory tract, chronic lung infection, interstitial lung disease, occult left heart failure, irritable larynx syndrome, bronchiectasis; include CT and bronchoscopy
- although frequently benign, the presence of hemoptysis requires investigation; consider bronchiectasis, chronic bronchitis, chronic infection, malignancy or causes of pulmonary hemorrhage. Investigations include sputum for acid fast staining and culture, sputum cytology, CXR and CT scan of the chest. Refer to a respirologist for fibre optic bronchoscopy

Pertussis, a highly contagious infection, leads to severe paroxysms of cough with frequent complications. Early administration of antibiotics is crucial. Clinical features include a 2-week virus-like illness with symptoms such as conjunctivitis, rhinorrhea, fever and malaise. Later, cough is followed by the paroxysmal phase characterized by worsening cough associated with post-tussive emesis and/or inspiratory whooping sound.[10] Nasopharyngeal swab for culture is used to confirm pertussis and if available, polymerase chain reaction. Do not delay antimicrobial treatment; initiate at the time of diagnostic testing.

Table 1: Chronic Cough: Common Causes, Clinical Features and Investigations

Common Causes	Clinical Features	Investigations
Upper airway cough syndrome	Postnasal drainage; cobblestoning and mucus in oropharynx Nasal discharge Throat clearing	Sinus x-rays often unhelpful CT scan of paranasal sinuses Nasal endoscopy
Cough variant asthma	Typical features of asthma, such as wheezing, often absent	Spirometry pre-/post-bronchodilator Methacholine challenge (sensitivity 60–80%, specificity >90%), induced sputum eosinophilia, exhaled nitric oxide
Gastroesophageal reflux disease	Consider after exclusion of other etiologies Up to 50% of cases not associated with typical reflux symptoms[5,6]	Therapeutic trial of H_2-receptor antagonist or a proton pump inhibitor (PPI) × 3 months Gold standard for diagnosis lacking Upper GI series (limited sensitivity) pH monitoring/impedance (good sensitivity, moderate to poor specificity) Endoscopy an option if pH monitoring not available (less sensitive)
ACE inhibitor[7]	Dry, nonproductive cough Onset hours-months post-initiation No predisposing factors Class effect of ACE inhibitors	Drug withdrawal; resolution or marked improvement of symptoms within 4 weeks
Nonasthmatic eosinophilic bronchitis[8]	Often prolonged in postinfectious setting	Normal spirometry and chest x-ray, negative challenge testing, induced sputum eosinophilia, exhaled nitric oxide (if available) Therapeutic trial of inhaled corticosteroid

Abbreviations: ACE = angiotensin-converting enzyme; GI = gastrointestinal

Therapeutic Choices

Nonpharmacologic Choices

- Advise on smoking cessation (see Chapter 13). A temporary worsening of cough may occur due to transient bronchorrhea.
- Avoid exposure to allergens and irritants.
- Lifestyle modifications for GERD, e.g., weight loss, specific food/beverage avoidance, nocturnal elevation of head of bed.
- Saline nasal irrigation for chronic rhinosinusitis.[15] Emphasize the importance of using distilled or boiled water in preparing saline for irrigation.[16]
- Speech and behavioural therapy can be beneficial in laryngeal dysfunction.[17]

Pharmacologic Choices

Therapy of chronic cough is directed at the cause, once identified (Figure 1, Table 2).

- *Chronic upper airway cough syndrome* (UACS), previously referred to as *postnasal drip syndrome*, secondary to rhinosinus diseases: Choose treatment according to the specific cause of UACS-induced cough if known.[18] If the cause is not apparent, the combination of a **first-generation antihistamine** and a **decongestant** is recommended empirically for cough related to *postnasal drip*; first-generation antihistamines are usually more effective than the newer antihistamines in this setting.
  - *Nonallergic rhinitis:* Appropriate therapy may include **intranasal corticosteroids** or **intranasal ipratropium.**[19]
  - *Allergic rhinitis:* Appropriate therapy may include **antihistamines, intranasal corticosteroids** or **leukotriene receptor antagonists** (see Chapter 50).
  - *Chronic sinusitis:* Appropriate therapy may include **antibiotics, short-course oral prednisone, intranasal corticosteroids** or **decongestants**[18] (see Chapter 121).
- *Asthma:* Appropriate therapy includes **short-acting beta$_2$-agonist** PRN and inhaled **corticosteroids.**[20] If asthma is not well controlled, consider adding **long-acting beta$_2$-agonists, leukotriene receptor antagonists** or a 1- to 2-week pulse of **oral corticosteroids** (see Chapter 51). In patients with asthma who are not responsive to conventional therapy, the potential role of neutrophilic airway inflammation has been considered. Long-term low-dose macrolide therapy (erythromycin) reduced neutrophil counts, but showed no benefit in cough symptoms in a group with otherwise unexplained cough.[21] Elevated exhaled nitric oxide has been shown to predict likelihood of response of cough to inhaled corticosteroids independent of other symptoms.[22]
- *Nonasthmatic eosinophilic bronchitis:* Responds to **inhaled corticosteroids.**[8]
- *GERD:* If nonpharmacologic (dietary and lifestyle) approaches fail to control symptoms in patients with GERD-associated chronic cough, guidelines suggest a trial of an **H$_2$-receptor antagonist** or **proton pump inhibitor (PPI)** for a minimum of 2–3 months (see Chapter 61) [Evidence: SORT C*].[1] Though a Cochrane review found insufficient evidence of benefit in patients with nonspecific chronic cough,[23] a more recent systematic review identified a benefit with PPI therapy in a subset of patients with pathologic acid exposure confirmed through pH monitoring, although statistical analysis was not possible.[24] Despite a lack of conclusive evidence, a trial of acid suppression is reasonable in patients with chronic cough in whom GERD is suspected as a contributing cause, since a proportion of patients may respond.
- *ACE inhibitor-induced cough:* Consider cough due to **ACE inhibitor**, whatever the temporal onset. Stop ACE inhibitor.[25] The median time to resolution is usually within 1 week but may it take up

---

* SORT (Strength of Recommendation Taxonomy) is a rating system (A, B or C) that addresses the quality of available evidence. For more information consult **How to Use *Compendium of Therapeutic Choices*** on page xxv.

to 4 weeks. Cough usually recurs with rechallenge. An angiotensin receptor blocker may be an appropriate substitution and is generally not associated with cough.

- *Pertussis:* If probable or confirmed pertussis, isolate patients for 5 days and treat with **macrolide** antibiotics.[10,26] Administer a booster **pertussis vaccine** once in all adults.[27]

Figure 1: Management of Chronic Cough

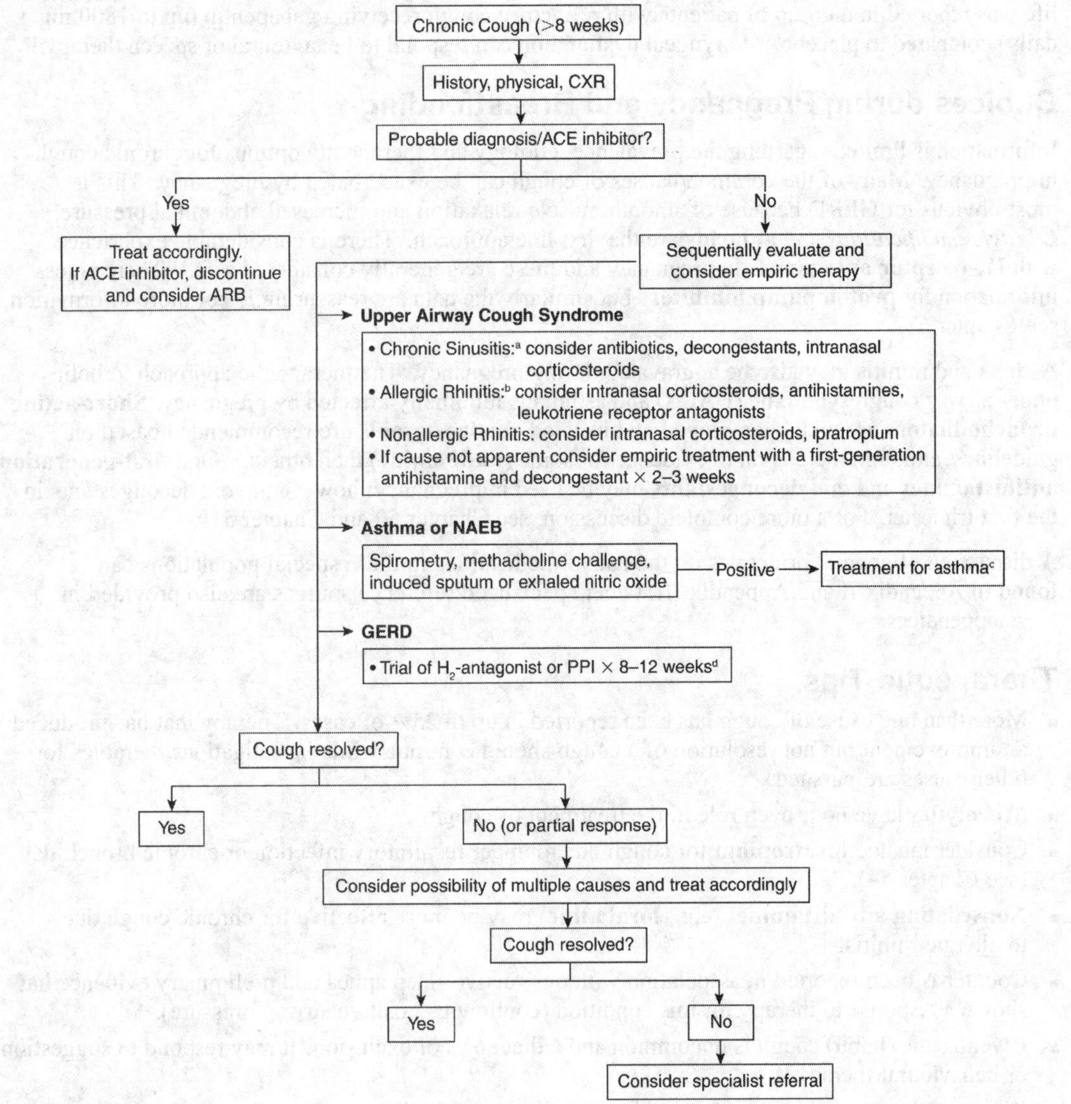

[a] See Chapter 121.
[b] See Chapter 50.
[c] See Chapter 51.
[d] See Chapter 61.

Abbreviations: ACE = angiotensin-converting enzyme; ARB = angiotensin receptor blocker; CXR = chest x-ray; GERD = gastroesophageal reflux disease; NAEB = nonasthmatic eosinophilic bronchitis; PPI = proton pump inhibitor

Antitussives have a limited role in the management of chronic cough. However, they may sometimes be used to enable sleep or in certain social settings (e.g., live theatre) if the cough cannot be controlled by measures targeted at a specific diagnosis. Use with caution when cough is productive.

Refractory cough is common and is observed in up to 40% of cases referred to specialty clinics.[28] The term *cough hypersensitivity syndrome* is being advocated to account for persistent cough induced by triggers that in most individuals would produce at most a more short-lived manifestation.[29] Hypersensitivity of afferent receptors may combine with central mechanisms to augment and perpetuate the cough. This has lead to new approaches to therapy. Improved cough-specific quality of life was reported in a group of patients with refractory cough receiving gabapentin (up to 1800 mg daily) compared to placebo.[30] Laryngeal dysfunction can respond to behavioural or speech therapy.[17]

Choices during Pregnancy and Breastfeeding

Information is limited regarding the prevalence, etiology and therapeutic options for chronic cough in pregnancy. Many of the common causes of cough can be exacerbated by pregnancy. This is most obvious for GERD because of smooth muscle relaxation and increased abdominal pressure. *Lifestyle modifications* and **antacids** are the first line approach. There is considerable experience with **H_2-receptor antagonists** in pregnancy and these are generally considered safe.[31] There is less information for **proton pump inhibitors** but similarly the data are reassuring.[32] For more information, see Chapter 61.

Asthma and rhinitis may also be aggravated during pregnancy. The therapeutic approach to both upper airway cough syndrome (UACS) and asthma is minimally affected by pregnancy. **Short-acting bronchodilators** are widely employed and **inhaled corticosteroids** are recommended based on guidelines, although there is more evidence for some (**budesonide**) than others.[33] Oral **first-generation antihistamines** and oral **decongestants** may be used in pregnancy; however, avoid decongestants in the first trimester. For a more complete discussion, see Chapter 50 and Chapter 51.

A discussion of general principles on the use of medications in these special populations can be found in Appendix II and Appendix III. Other specialized reference sources are also provided in these appendices.

Therapeutic Tips

- More than one cause of cough has been reported in up to 25% of cases. Therapy that has produced an improvement but not resolution of a cough should continue while investigations/therapies for other causes are pursued.
- **Mucolytics** have no proven role in the treatment of cough.[1]
- Consider inhaled **ipratropium** for cough due to upper respiratory infection or chronic bronchitis[1] (see Chapter 54).
- **Nonsedating antihistamines** (e.g., **loratadine**) may be more effective for chronic cough due to allergic rhinitis.[18]
- Cough has been reported in association with obstructive sleep apnea and preliminary evidence has shown a response to therapy for this condition (continuous positive airway pressure).[34,35]
- Psychogenic (habit) cough is uncommon and a diagnosis of exclusion. It may respond to suggestion or behavioural therapy.[36]
- When employing a cough diagnostic/therapeutic algorithm (in pre-screened patients), nonphysician respiratory educators have achieved comparable outcomes to subspecialists, with reduced referral wait times.[37]

Table 2: **Drugs for Cough Suppression**

Class	Drug	Adult Dose	Adverse Effects	Comments	Cost[a]
Anticholinergic Agents	*ipratropium bromide* Atrovent Nasal Spray, Atrovent HFA, generics	Nasal spray (0.03%): 2 sprays BID–TID in each nostril. Dose is individualized. pMDI: 2–4 puffs QID	Nosebleeds, nasal dryness, dry mouth or throat, metallic taste.	Avoid accidental release of nasal spray into eyes. pMDI: For cough due to upper respiratory infection or chronic bronchitis.	$$$/nasal spray $$$$/inhaler
Antihistamines, first-generation	*chlorpheniramine* Chlor-Tripolon, generics	4–8 mg HS po	Sedation, anticholinergic effects.	For cough associated with nonallergic rhinitis, used in combination with a decongestant. Available without prescription.	$
Antihistamines, second-generation	*loratadine* Claritin, generics	10 mg daily po	Little to no sedation or anticholinergic effects.	For cough associated with allergic rhinitis. Available without prescription.	$
Antitussives	*codeine* generics	5–20 mg Q4–8H po Maximum: 120 mg/day	Constipation, drowsiness, nausea.	May be used if analgesia and sedation desired. Short-term symptomatic relief of coughing. For patients with upper respiratory infections or chronic bronchitis. Not recommended for ACE inhibitor-induced cough.	$
	dextromethorphan Benylin DM, Delsym DM (sustained-release), Robitussin DM, Koffex DM, Balminil DM, others	*Immediate-release*: 15–30 mg Q6–8H po *Sustained-release:* 60 mg Q12H po Maximum: 120 mg/day	Drowsiness, GI upset, blurred vision and urinary hesitancy in patients who metabolize DM slowly.	For patients with upper respiratory infections or chronic bronchitis. Not recommended for ACE inhibitor-induced cough. Available without prescription.	$

(cont'd)

Table 2: Drugs for Cough Suppression *(cont'd)*

Class	Drug	Adult Dose	Adverse Effects	Comments	Cost[a]
	hydrocodone (kidney symbol) Hycodan	5 mg Q4–6H po Maximum: 30 mg/24 h	See codeine.	May be used if analgesia and sedation desired. Short-term symptomatic relief of coughing. For patients with upper respiratory infections or chronic bronchitis. Not recommended for ACE inhibitor-induced cough.	$$$$
Decongestants	*pseudoephedrine* (kidney symbol) Sudafed, generics	60 mg Q4–6H po *or* 120 mg SR Q12H po Maximum 240 mg/24 h	Insomnia, tremor, irritability, headache, palpitations, tachycardia, urinary retention.	For cough associated with nonallergic rhinitis, used in combination with a first-generation antihistamine. Available without prescription. Contraindicated in patients with severe hypertension and coronary artery disease. Use with caution in CVD, diabetes, hyperthyroidism, prostatic hypertrophy and angle-closure glaucoma.	$

[a] Cost of 100 mL or 15 tablets unless otherwise specified; includes drug cost only.

(kidney symbol) Dosage adjustment may be required in renal impairment; see Appendix I.

Abbreviations: CVD = cardiovascular disease; DM = dextromethorphan; HFA = hydrofluoroalkane; pMDI = pressurized metered dose inhaler; SR = sustained release

Legend: $ < $5 $$ $5–10 $$$ $10–15 $$$$ $15–20

Suggested Readings

Birring SS. Controversies in the evaluation and management of chronic cough. *Am J Respir Crit Care Med* 2011;183(6):708-15.

Boulet, LP, Côté G. Canadian Thoracic Society. *Cough: etiology, evaluation and treatments. Update 2012*. Available from: www.respiratoryguidelines.ca/cough-etiology-evaluation-and-treatments.

Irwin RS, Baumann MH, Bolser DC et al. Diagnosis and management of cough: ACCP evidence-based clinical practice guidelines. *Chest* 2006;129(1 Suppl):1S-287S.

Irwin RS, Madison JM. The persistently troublesome cough. *Am J Respir Crit Care Med* 2002;165(11):1469-74.

Morice AH, Fontana GA, Sovijarvi AR et al. The diagnosis and management of chronic cough. *Eur Respir J* 2004;24(3):481-92.

Simpson CB, Amin MR. Chronic cough: state-of-the-art review. *Otolaryngol Head Neck Surg* 2006;134(4):693-700.

References

1. Irwin RS, Baumann MH, Bolser DC et al. Diagnosis and management of cough executive summary: ACCP evidence-based clinical practice guidelines. *Chest* 2006;129(1 Suppl):1S-23S.
2. Carney IK, Gibson PG, Murree-Allen K et al. A systematic evaluation of mechanisms in chronic cough. *Am J Respir Crit Care Med* 1997;156(1):211-6.
3. Morice AH, Kastelik JA. Cough. 1: Chronic cough in adults. *Thorax* 2003;58(10):901-7.
4. Irwin RS, Madison JM. The persistently troublesome cough. *Am J Respir Crit Care Med* 2002;165(11):1469-74.
5. Poe RH, Kallay MC. Chronic cough and gastroesophageal reflux disease: experience with specific therapy for diagnosis and treatment. *Chest* 2003;123(3):679-84.
6. Ing AJ, Ngu MC, Breslin AB. Chronic persistent cough and clearance of esophageal acid. *Chest* 1992;102(6):1668-71.
7. Dykewicz MS. Cough and angioedema from angiotensin-converting enzyme inhibitors: new insights into mechanisms and management. *Curr Opin Allergy Clin Immunol* 2004;4(4):267-70.
8. Gibson PG, Fujimura M, Niimi A. Eosinophilic bronchitis: clinical manifestations and implications for treatment. *Thorax* 2002;57(2):178-82.
9. McGarvey LP. Does idiopathic cough exist? *Lung* 2008;186(Suppl 1):S78-81.
10. Braman SS. Postinfectious cough: ACCP evidence-based clinical practice guidelines. *Chest* 2006;129(1 Suppl):138S-146S.
11. Irwin RS, Zawacki JK. Accurately diagnosing and successfully treating chronic cough due to gastroesophageal reflux disease can be difficult. *Am J Gastroenterol* 1999;94(11):3095-8.
12. Pratter MR, Brightling CE, Boulet LP et al. An empiric integrative approach to the management of cough: ACCP evidence-based clinical practice guidelines. *Chest* 2006;129(1 Suppl):222S-31S.
13. Ours TM, Kavuru MS, Schilz RJ et al. A prospective evaluation of esophageal testing and a double-blind, randomized study of omeprazole in a diagnostic and therapeutic algorithm for chronic cough. *Am J Gastroenterol* 1999;94(11):3131-8.
14. Morice AH, McGarvey L, Pavord I; British Thoracic Society Cough Guideline Group. Recommendations for the management of cough in adults. *Thorax* 2006;61(Suppl 1):i1-24.
15. Harvey R, Hannan SA, Badia L et al. Nasal saline irrigations for the symptoms of chronic rhinosinusitis. *Cochrane Database Syst Rev* 2007;(3):CD006394.
16. Yoder JS, Straif-Bourgeois S, Roy SL. Primary amebic meningoencephalitis deaths associated with sinus irrigation using contaminated tap water. *Clin Infect Dis* 2012;55(9):e79-85.
17. Vertigan AE, Theodoros DG, Gibson PG et al. Efficacy of speech pathology management for chronic cough: a randomised placebo controlled trial of treatment efficacy. *Thorax* 2006;61(12):1065-9.
18. Pratter MR. Chronic upper airway cough syndrome secondary to rhinosinus diseases (previously referred to as postnasal drip syndrome): ACCP evidence-based clinical practice guidelines. *Chest* 2006;129(1 Suppl):63S-71S.
19. Wallace DV, Dykewicz MS, Bernstein DI et al. The diagnosis and management of rhinitis: an updated practice parameter. *J Allergy Clin Immunol* 2008;122(2 Suppl):S1-84.
20. Lougheed MD, Lemiere C, Ducharme FM et al. Canadian Thoracic Society 2012 guideline update: diagnosis and management of asthma in preschoolers, children and adults. *Can Respir J* 2012;19(2):127-64.
21. Yousaf N, Monteiro W, Parker D et al. Long-term low-dose erythromycin in patients with unexplained cough: a double-blind placebo controlled trial. *Thorax* 2010:65(12):1107-10.
22. Hahn PY, Morgenthaler TY, Kim KG. Use of exhaled nitric oxide in predicting response to inhaled corticosteroids for chronic cough. *Mayo Clin Proc* 2007;82(11):1350-5.
23. Chang AB, Lasserson TJ, Gaffney J et al. Gastro-oesophageal reflux treatment for prolonged non-specific cough in children and adults. *Cochrane Database Syst Rev* 2011;(1):CD004823.
24. Kahrilas PJ, Howden CW, Hughes N et al. Response of chronic cough to acid-suppressive therapy in patients with gastroesophageal reflux disease. *Chest* 2013;143(3):605-12.
25. Irwin RS, Boulet LP, Cloutier MM et al. Managing cough as a defense mechanism and as a symptom. A consensus panel report of the American College of Chest Physicians. *Chest* 1998;114(2 Suppl Managing):133S-181S.
26. Hewlett EL, Edwards KM. Clinical practice. Pertussis—not just for kids. *N Engl J Med* 2005;352(12):1215-22.
27. National Advisory Committee on Immunization (NACI). Public Health Agency of Canada. *Canadian immunization guide*. Evergreen ed. Available from: www.phac-aspc.gc.ca/publicat/cig-gci/index-eng.php. Accessed September 30, 2013.
28. Haque RA, Usmani OS, Barnes PJ. Chronic idiopathic cough: a discrete clinical entity? *Chest* 2005;127(5):1710-3.
29. Chung KF. Chronic 'cough hypersensitivity syndrome': a more precise label for chronic cough. *Pulm Pharmacol Ther* 2011;24(3):267-71.

30. Ryan NM, Birring SS, Gibson PG. Gabapentin for refractory chronic cough: a randomised, double-blind, placebo-controlled trial. *Lancet* 2012;380(9853):1583-9.
31. Larson JD, Patatanian E, Miner PB et al. Double-blind, placebo-controlled study of ranitidine for gastroesophageal reflux symptoms during pregnancy. *Obstet Gynecol* 1997;90(1):83-7.
32. Gill SK, O'Brien L, Einarson TR et al. The safety of proton pump inhibitors (PPIs) in pregnancy: a meta-analysis. *Am J Gastroenterol* 2009;104(6):1541-5.
33. National Heart, Lung, and Blood Institute; National Asthma Education and Prevention Program Asthma and Pregnancy Working Group. NAEPP expert panel report. Managing asthma during pregnancy: recommendations for pharmacologic treatment—2004 update. *J Allergy Clin Immunol* 2005;115(1):34-46.
34. Chan KK, Ing AJ, Laks L et al. Chronic cough in patients with sleep-disordered breathing. *Eur Respir J* 2010;35(2):368-72.
35. Birring SS, Ing AJ, Chan K et al. Obstructive sleep apnoea: a cause of chronic cough. *Cough* 2007;3:7.
36. Weinberger M. The habit cough syndrome and its variations. *Lung* 2012;190(1):45-53.
37. Field SK, Conley DP, Thawer AM et al. Assessment and management of patients with chronic cough by Certified Respiratory Educators: a randomized controlled trial. *Can Respir J* 2009;16(2):49-54.

Chapter 54
Chronic Obstructive Pulmonary Disease

R. Andrew McIvor, MD, MSc, FRCPC

Chronic obstructive pulmonary disease (COPD) is a chronic, systemic disease largely caused by smoking and characterized by progressive, partially reversible airway limitation, systemic manifestations (e.g., altered nutrition) and increasing frequency and severity of exacerbations. COPD is preventable and treatable. The cardinal symptoms are shortness of breath and activity limitation.[1,2]

Goals of Therapy[1,2]

- Prevent disease progression
- Decrease or abolish breathlessness and other respiratory symptoms
- Improve exercise tolerance
- Reduce the frequency and severity of exacerbations
- Improve health-related quality of life
- Reduce impairment and disability
- Reduce mortality

Investigations

- History with particular attention to:[1,2]
  - symptoms and their pattern: dyspnea (insidious at onset and progressive), chronic cough (seldom entirely nocturnal), sputum production, limitations to physical activity
  - assess degree of shortness of breath and disability: use the Medical Research Council's Dyspnea Scale (Table 1)[1,3] or the CAT test
    - the COPD Assessment Test (CAT) is a new questionnaire for people with COPD. It is designed to measure the impact of COPD on a person's life, and how this changes over time. The CAT is very simple to administer and aims to help clinicians optimally manage a patient's COPD. It is available from www.catestonline.org
  - precipitating factors and triggers: cigarette smoking, heavy exposure to occupational dusts and chemicals, air pollution, alpha$_1$-antitrypsin deficiency
  - signs/symptoms that suggest other comorbidities or systemic manifestations such as cardiovascular disease, osteoporosis, skeletal muscle dysfunction, pulmonary embolism, secondary polycythemia, depression, altered nutrition, pneumonia, malignancy, metabolic syndrome
  - previous history of acute exacerbations of COPD: hospitalizations, emergency room visits, use of oral corticosteroids and antibiotics
  - impact on daily life and social supports available
- Physical examination is relatively insensitive for diagnosis
  - late clinical findings: signs of hyperinflation, hypoxemia and pulmonary hypertension

- Objective measurements needed to confirm diagnosis and assess severity include:
  - spirometry, the gold standard for diagnosis and risk stratification of COPD.[2] Baseline postbronchodilator FEV_1 <80% of the predicted value and an FEV_1/FVC <0.7 are both necessary to establish the diagnosis.[1,2,4,5] Approximately 30% of patients thought to have COPD will have an increase of 12% and >200 mL in FEV_1 after salbutamol
  - assessment of lung volumes and carbon monoxide diffusion
  - CBC to assess for polycythemia indicating chronic hypoxia or anemia that can worsen dyspnea
  - chest x-ray to rule out lung cancer, bronchiectasis, tuberculosis
  - pulse oximetry ± arterial blood gases if FEV_1 <1 L or <40% predicted or SaO_2 <92% or clinical signs of respiratory failure or right heart failure[1,2]
  - $alpha_1$-antitrypsin level if patient <45 years old presents with COPD or has a strong family history of COPD[2]

Therapeutic Choices

Nonpharmacologic Choices

- Recommend smoking cessation to stop COPD progression, reduce the risk of developing COPD[1,2,6,7,8,9,10] and decrease mortality[11] (see Chapter 13).
- Minimize/eliminate exposure to air pollution and occupational dusts and chemicals.[12,13]
- Educate patients and their families to enhance patient outcomes and reduce costs by improving skills, ability to cope with the illness and health status.[2,14]
- Encourage physical activity to prevent decrease in mobility and increase in dyspnea. Patients with a lower activity level at 1 month after hospital discharge were more likely to be readmitted in the following year.[15]
- Consider early referral of symptomatic patients to **pulmonary rehabilitation** programs providing respiratory, physical and occupational therapy, exercise conditioning, nutritional assistance and psychosocial and vocational rehabilitation. Although a limited resource, patients benefit from pulmonary rehabilitation in all stages of COPD.[16,17,18,19]

Pharmacologic Choices

A small improvement in airflow may be of significant clinical benefit in COPD patients with severe obstruction. Initial therapy commences with a **short-acting $beta_2$-agonist** as needed and may be supplemented by regular **long-acting bronchodilators**.[1,2,20] Maximum bronchodilation may be obtained with a combination of long-acting $beta_2$-agonists and anticholinergics.[1,2]

Table 1: **Modified Medical Research Council Questionnaire for Assessing the Severity of Breathlessness**[a,b,3]

Grade 1	I only get breathless with strenuous exercise.	□
Grade 2	I get short of breath when hurrying on the level or walking up a slight hill.	□
Grade 3	I walk slower than people of the same age on the level because of breathlessness, or I have to stop for breath when walking on my own pace on the level.	□
Grade 4	I stop for breath after walking about 100 meters or after a few minutes on the level.	□
Grade 5	I am too breathless to leave the house or I am breathless when dressing or undressing.	□

[a] Patient can only tick 1 response at one time.

[b] The mMRC scale can be used on follow-up visits to monitor progress or response to therapy. Spirometry is the gold standard for diagnosis of COPD.

COPD is characterized by persistent inflammation even in early disease.[1] However, **inhaled corticosteroids** (ICS) do not affect the neutrophilic response in COPD as significantly as in asthma. In addition, the TORCH study showed increased mortality with ICS monotherapy.[21] Their main role in COPD is in combination with long-acting $beta_2$-agonists in moderate to severe disease.[1]

COPD exacerbations become more frequent and more severe as a patient's disease worsens and the strongest predictor of exacerbations is a prior history of exacerbation, irrespective of disease severity. This suggests that the "frequent exacerbator" is a distinct subgroup (or phenotype) of patients who could be identified and targeted with specific exacerbation prevention strategies.[22]

See Table 3 and Table 4 for the available agents for COPD treatment and Figure 1 for a step-wise approach to COPD management.

Delivery Systems

Inhaled bronchodilators are delivered via pressurized metered-dose inhaler (pMDI) with or without a spacer device, dry powder inhaler (DPI) or nebulizer.[25] If pMDI technique is inadequate or ineffective, consider a spacer device to improve deposition of the medication to the lower respiratory tract and to avoid problems in coordinating the time of inhaler actuation with inhalation. DPIs do not present the problems with hand-breath coordination seen with pMDIs. Appropriate use of pMDIs (with or without spacer devices) or DPIs provides optimal drug delivery and should be encouraged over nebulizers. Nebulizers may be used in patients who remain symptomatic despite maximal treatment with handheld inhalers.

The choice of delivery device (pMDI or DPI) for patients with COPD depends on the patient's age, preference and ability to correctly use the device, and on convenience, ease of use and affordability.[25,26]

The proper use of inhalers is not intuitive. Careful instruction and demonstration of correct inhaler technique is essential before therapy is initiated and should be reinforced at each visit. Various manufacturers of DPIs have been developing their own "trademarked" devices to deliver their proprietary medications. Patients will therefore have to become familiar with the individual requirements of multiple devices to optimize the clinical benefits.

COPD Strategies and Guidelines

COPD is a global problem and various national and international bodies are reviewing the evidence and suggesting various management strategies. Guideline development has advanced significantly; precise criteria have been developed for reviewing evidence-based data for guidelines to avoid observer bias. The Canadian Thoracic Society produces guidelines[1] which are currently awaiting update, but Canadian experts also acknowledge the GOLD COPD Strategy (Global Obstructive Lung Disease).[1,2] The GOLD Strategy is no longer considered a guideline as its development and recommendations do not meet the modern guideline definition.[27]

In its latest update GOLD has evolved its recommendations beyond simply classifying COPD as mild, moderate, severe or very severe based on the progressive impairment of FEV_1.[2] GOLD now categorizes patients by combining the spirometric classification and/or the number of exacerbations or hospitalizations in the preceding year, with a symptomatic assessment (CAT score or mMRC score), to stratify patients as Group A, B, C or D, where D is the most severe. GOLD has also launched an App to facilitate integration of this approach into clinical practice (available from itunes.apple.com/us/app/gold-copd-strategy/id576193649?mt=8).

Stable COPD

Bronchodilators, the mainstay of pharmacotherapy, decrease air trapping, improve FEV_1, reduce symptoms (e.g., dyspnea) and improve exercise capacity and quality of life in stable COPD and in acute exacerbations of COPD. Inhaled bronchodilators can be used as needed for occasional symptoms or regularly for symptom prevention and/or reduction.

Short-acting Bronchodilators

Recommend PRN use of a short-acting beta$_2$-agonist (SABA) such as **salbutamol** or **terbutaline** in all stages of disease severity for immediate symptom relief.[1] SABAs have approximately equal efficacy, side effects, onset and duration of action (4–6 hours).[2] Recommended doses of beta$_2$-agonists result in less than maximal bronchodilation; the dose may be doubled or tripled, although tachycardia, tremor and potential hypokalemia must be recognized and monitored in patients at risk.

The short-acting anticholinergic **ipratropium bromide** has a slower onset of action than inhaled beta$_2$-agonists but a longer duration of action (up to 8 hours).[2] The recommended dose of 40 µg, 3–4 times per day, produces less than maximal bronchodilation and may be doubled or tripled without notable side effects. The role of ipratropium monotherapy is limited because it is less effective than tiotropium bromide and salbutamol has a more rapid onset of action.

Salbutamol and **ipratropium** *in combination* produce greater and more sustained improvement in FEV$_1$ and a greater degree of bronchodilation with a lower or similar incidence of side effects compared with either drug alone.[2] The combination also confers greater improvement in lung function than doubling the dose of a single bronchodilator.[28,29,30]

Oral beta$_2$-agonists offer few advantages and are associated with an increased incidence of side effects. They have no role in the routine management of COPD.

Long-acting Bronchodilators

Use a long-acting bronchodilator in patients with persistent symptoms and moderate to severe airflow obstruction. There are 2 types of long-acting bronchodilators available, **long-acting muscarinic antagonists/anticholinergics (LAMA)** and **long-acting beta$_2$-agonists (LABA)**.

The **LAMA tiotropium bromide** is a first-line agent for managing persistent symptoms and moderate to severe airflow obstruction as it decreases exacerbations and hospitalizations.[1,31] Compared with ipratropium, it deposits more successfully in the airways of patients with very low inspiratory flow rates. A single daily 18 µg dose gives maximal anticholinergic activity for a full 24 hours.[32] More sustained effects on pulmonary function, activity-related dyspnea and quality of life are noted when compared to ipratropium. When given in combination with pulmonary rehabilitation, tiotropium improved treadmill walking endurance time.[33] It is available as a breath-activated dry powder inhaler.

Retrospective studies have shown an increased risk of cardiovascular death, MI or stroke associated with both the long- and short-acting inhaled muscarinic antagonists/anticholinergics (**ipratropium, tiotropium**).[34,35,36] This was not confirmed in a 4-year randomized controlled trial which evaluated efficacy of tiotropium but also included safety parameters as secondary endpoints.[37] The FDA and others have extensively reviewed available data and have concluded there is no increased risk of stroke, MI or death associated with tiotropium HandiHaler.[38,39] However, ipratropium appears to be associated with an increase in cardiovascular events.[40,41] There are no data for LAMAs other than tiotropium.

Glycopyrronium bromide is the first rapid-onset LAMA DPI having a faster onset of action than tiotropium. The currently licensed dose is 50 µg once daily. Phase III studies have established improvement in dyspnea, quality of life and reduced risk of exacerbation compared with placebo and results similar to that seen with tiotropium with a similar safety profile.[42,43,44] The bronchodilation effect is seen on day 1 of administration; however, improvements in exercise endurance and quality of life are seen over time.

The LAMA **aclidinium bromide** is dosed twice daily and has effects similar to those of tiotropium and glycopyrronium on lung function.[45,46,47]

The inhaled **LABAs salmeterol** and **formoterol** offer sustained improvements in pulmonary function, dyspnea and quality of life compared with SABAs.[1,48,49] Unlike salmeterol, formoterol has the advantage of rapid onset of bronchodilation in addition to the 12-hour duration of action.[48,50,51]

Indacaterol is a once-daily rapid-acting ultra-long-acting beta$_2$-adrenergic agonist, which has shown bronchodilation similar to tiotropium.[52,53] This is the first once-daily LABA available and represents a new option for patients who either cannot tolerate an anticholinergic agent due to adverse effects or demonstrate poor adherence with twice daily LABA regimens.

Combination Long-acting Bronchodilators

Offer the combination of a LAMA and LABA if disability persists despite monotherapy. The combination maximizes bronchodilation and lung deflation and is recommended in moderate to severe disease with persistent symptoms and infrequent exacerbations (<1 per year for at least 2 consecutive years).[1]

The combination of a LAMA and a LABA in a single inhaler is now available (**glycopyrronium/indacaterol, umeclidinium/vilanterol**). Studies show an acceptable safety profile and superior bronchodilation when compared with both placebo and individual components.[54,55,56] Cardiovascular safety was acceptable in studies up to 24 or 52 weeks.[55,57,58]

Combination Inhaled Corticosteroids and Long-acting Bronchodilators

Inhaled corticosteroids (ICS) are not recommended as monotherapy in the management of COPD symptoms.[1] ICS and long-acting beta$_2$-agonists (LABAs) in combination are more effective than either drug alone in terms of exercise endurance, symptom control, lung function and exacerbation rates in patients with moderate to very severe COPD.[59,60,61,62] An increased rate of pneumonia diagnosis without expected increases in morbidity and mortality has been noted in patients on combination therapy compared with LABA monotherapy.[21,62,63]

Recommend the addition of a combined ICS/LABA to tiotropium (triple therapy) for patients with moderate to severe COPD and repeated exacerbations (≥1 per year for at least 2 consecutive years). This combination improves bronchodilation and lung deflation, reduces frequency and severity of exacerbations, improves health and reduces hospitalization.[1,21,64]

The availability of new bronchodilators and combination LAMA/LABA therapy may reduce the use of triple therapy. Although the practice of triple therapy is common, there is currently insufficient evidence to determine if triple therapy is clinically superior to dual bronchodilator therapy or combination ICS/LABA therapy.[65]

Phosphodiesterase 4 (PDE4) Inhibitors

Roflumilast (Table 4) is an oral medication that suppresses the release of inflammatory mediators through inhibition of cyclic AMP breakdown. It is indicated as add-on therapy with bronchodilators for maintenance treatment of severe COPD associated with chronic bronchitis (history of chronic cough and sputum) in adult patients with a history of frequent exacerbations.[66] Roflumilast has demonstrated a significant improvement in prebronchodilator FEV_1 (48–80 mL increase) along with a small reduction in exacerbations requiring systemic corticosteroids (8%), even for patients who were also taking long-acting beta$_2$-agonists.[67,68,69] A Cochrane review found that patients were 23% less likely to experience an exacerbation over the study period (≤1 year) with an NNT of 20; however, quality of life and symptoms scores were not greatly improved.[70] Data support addition of roflumilast to foundation bronchodilatory therapy to reduce exacerbations, either before or in addition to introduction of ICS/LABA. Nausea, diarrhea and weight loss were the most common adverse effects reported, but were generally mild to moderate in intensity and usually occurred in the first weeks of treatment. Neuropsychiatric effects (e.g., anxiety, depression, insomnia, headache) are reported. Patients with a history of depression with suicidal ideation should not receive roflumilast.

Theophylline

Long-acting preparations of theophylline (Table 4) may be used in patients with severe symptoms of COPD despite use of a LAMA plus LABA/ICS combination[1] (Figure 1). Consult a specialist when a patient reaches this stage of disease. Clinically, little bronchodilator effect is observed beyond that of optimal dosing of inhaled bronchodilators. Because of theophylline's narrow therapeutic index and complex pharmacokinetics, serum levels should be measured and adjusted to the low therapeutic range (55–85 μmol/L) to minimize adverse effects. Theophylline has significant drug interactions, e.g., levels may be doubled if the patient stops smoking or with the addition of medications commonly used during acute exacerbations of COPD, e.g., antibiotics such as clarithromycin.

Oxygen Therapy

Oxygen therapy reduces the risk of death in select patients. In COPD patients with severe hypoxemia (PaO_2 ≤55 mm Hg or SaO_2 <88%), long-term oxygen therapy may prolong life by 6–7 years.[2] Improved survival has been seen only when oxygen is administered for ≥15 hours per day.[71] Continuously administered oxygen provides the greatest survival benefit. A patient whose PaO_2 is between 55 and 59 mm Hg may benefit from oxygen therapy if there is evidence of bilateral ankle edema, cor pulmonale or a hematocrit greater than 56%.[1] Oxygen therapy is usually administered via Venturi facemask or nasal prongs at a flow rate sufficient to produce a resting PaO_2 between 65 and 80 mm Hg. Flow rates are often increased by 1 or 2 L/min during exercise and sleep. If hypoventilation ($PaCO_2$ >45 mm Hg) is present, the titration of oxygen may worsen hypercarbic hypoxia, thus monitoring is advised.

Vaccines

Vaccinate annually against influenza early in the fall. **Influenza vaccine** reduces exacerbations and death in patients with COPD.[1,2,72,73] Recommend pneumococcal vaccination to all patients with COPD who have no contraindications.[74] Efficacy studies of **pneumococcal vaccine** in patients with COPD yield conflicting results.[75,76] However, because patients with COPD are at increased risk of hospitalization and mortality from pneumonia, pneumococcal vaccination is recommended; consider repeating pneumococcal vaccine in high-risk patients in 5–10 years.[1,2]

Acute Exacerbations of COPD

Acute exacerbations are the most frequent cause of medical visits, hospital admissions and death among COPD patients. Characterized by sustained worsening of dyspnea, cough or sputum production,[1,2] acute exacerbations of COPD contribute to the accelerated rate of decline in lung function. In addition, acute exacerbations lead to an increase in the use of maintenance medications and/or initiation of systemic corticosteroids and/or inhaled oxygen.[1,2] In acute exacerbations of COPD, bronchodilation is optimized by increasing the dose and/or frequency of existing bronchodilator treatment.[2] Treat dyspnea with a **short-acting beta$_2$-agonist** and **ipratropium**. Apart from optimizing the bronchodilator, patients with purulent acute exacerbations benefit from antibiotics.[1,2] Severe COPD patients gain additional benefit from a short course of systemic corticosteroids.[1,2]

Systemic Corticosteroids

Oral corticosteroids (Table 4) improve lung function and shorten length of hospital stay in all patients and reduce risk of early relapse.[1,2] There is no advantage to using intravenous steroids. A 10- to 14-day course of oral **prednisone** 30–40 mg/day or equivalent is sufficient, although a 5-day course of corticosteroids was shown to be noninferior to 14 days of treatment and may be used.[2,77] Tapering is unnecessary for oral corticosteroid courses that last <2 weeks. There is no role for oral corticosteroid maintenance therapy for patients with COPD.

Antibiotics

The most common infectious agents in exacerbations are viruses. Consider rapid virology and antivirals for influenza during the influenza season (see Chapter 116). Routine use of antibiotics in acute exacerbations of COPD is not recommended because of inconsistent study results in nonsevere exacerbations and concerns about increasing prevalence of antimicrobial resistance.[78] Antibiotics are indicated in all patients with severe exacerbations requiring invasive mechanical ventilation, or if the exacerbation is accompanied by 2–3 of the following cardinal signs: increased dyspnea, increased sputum or increased sputum purulence (Table 2).[2,80]

The common bacterial pathogens causing acute exacerbations of COPD are *Streptococcus pneumoniae, Haemophilus influenzae* and *Moraxella catarrhalis*.[1,2,81] In complicated patients, *Klebsiella* species and other gram-negative organisms including *Pseudomonas aeruginosa* can also be involved.[81]

Empiric choice of an antibiotic (Table 2) should take into account individual risk stratification, previous antibiotic use and the prevalence of antimicrobial resistance in the area. Consider a change in antibiotic class if the same class has been used within the previous 3 months. Re-evaluate patients who do not respond within 24–36 hours. See Table 5 for antibiotic dosing information.

Table 2: **Empiric Antibiotic Therapy for Acute Exacerbation of COPD**[1,79]

Group	Symptoms and Risk Factors	Probable Pathogens	Antibiotic of First Choice[a]
Simple exacerbations (COPD without risk factors[b])	↑ sputum purulence ***plus*** at least 1 of: ↑ sputum volume ↑ dyspnea	*Haemophilus* spp., *M. catarrhalis,* *S. pneumoniae*	Amoxicillin, doxycycline, trimethoprim/sulfamethoxazole or extended-spectrum macrolide
Complicated exacerbations (COPD with risk factors[b])	As in simple exacerbation above ***plus*** at least 1 of: • FEV_1 <50% predicted • ≥4 exacerbations per year • ischemic heart disease • use of home O_2 • chronic oral corticosteroid use • antibiotic use in previous 3 months	As for simple exacerbations ***plus*** *Klebsiella* spp. ***plus*** other gram-negative pathogens *Pseudomonas* spp. Higher probability of β-lactam resistance	Beta-lactam/beta-lactamase inhibitor (e.g., amoxicillin/clavulanate), 2nd generation cephalosporin or fluoroquinolone

[a] Use an antibiotic from a different class, if used within the last 3 months.
[b] Risk factors for treatment failure and/or resistant organisms.

Oxygen Therapy

Arterial blood gas determination is the gold standard to assess oxygenation and ventilation during an exacerbation.

Therapeutic Tips

- Promote smoking cessation at each visit. See Chapter 13.
- Perform spirometry with bronchodilator assessment in the following patients:[4]
  - all smokers ≥35 years
  - past smokers with a ≥20 pack-year history of smoking, whether or not the patient complains of symptoms
  - patients with recurrent or chronic respiratory symptoms including cough and breathlessness on exertion
  - patients with a family history of COPD
  - patients who have significant occupational exposure to respiratory irritants
- Encourage physical activity to prevent a vicious cycle of decreasing mobility and increasing dyspnea.
- Ensure patient and family are aware of warning signs of a COPD exacerbation and have a written action plan for initial management. A COPD action plan has been developed and is available from www.respiratoryguidelines.ca/updated-cts-copd-action-plan.
- Review inhaler technique at each visit.

- Encourage adherence to therapy by using a stepwise approach to treatment with positive reinforcement at all stages.
- Consider combining tiotropium and a LABA for maximal bronchodilation in patients with moderate to severe persistent symptoms and exercise intolerance.[1,2] Add a SABA PRN for acute symptom relief and to improve exercise tolerance.[1,2]
- Recognize and treat COPD comorbidities (e.g., cardiovascular disease, depression, osteoporosis, smoking-related malignancies).
- Involve helpline groups including the Lung Association (New Patient Information number 1-866-717-COPD [2673]).
- Although studies indicate continuous use of a macrolide may reduce exacerbations in patients with severe COPD and/or a history of frequent exacerbations, concerns regarding antibiotic resistance and adverse effects such as hearing loss preclude recommending continuous use at this time.[83]

Figure 1: **Pharmacologic Management of COPD**[1]

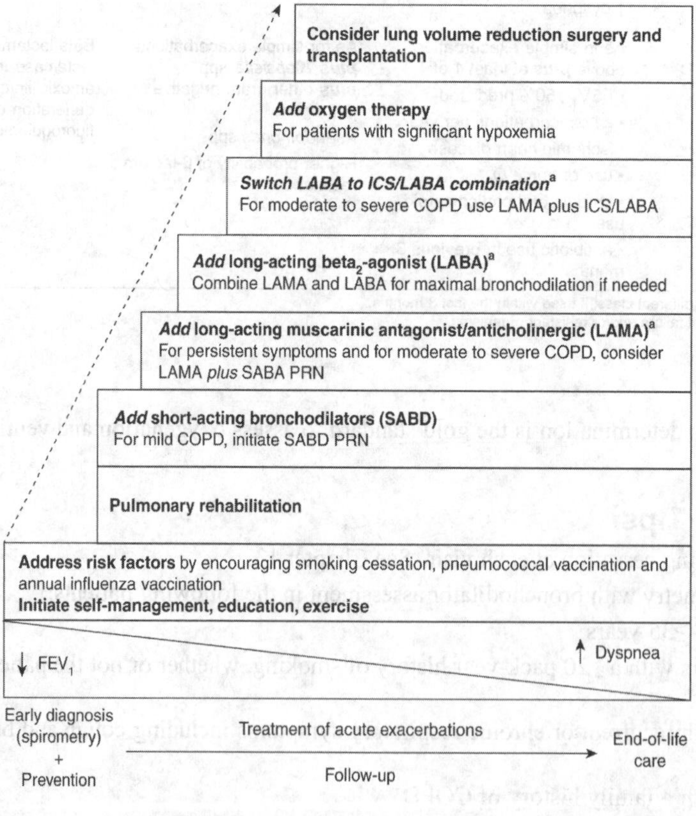
Consider lung volume reduction surgery and transplantation
Add oxygen therapy
For patients with significant hypoxemia
Switch LABA to ICS/LABA combination[a]
For moderate to severe COPD use LAMA plus ICS/LABA
Add long-acting beta$_2$-agonist (LABA)[a]
Combine LAMA and LABA for maximal bronchodilation if needed
Add long-acting muscarinic antagonist/anticholinergic (LAMA)[a]
For persistent symptoms and for moderate to severe COPD, consider LAMA *plus* SABA PRN
Add short-acting bronchodilators (SABD)
For mild COPD, initiate SABD PRN
Pulmonary rehabilitation
Address risk factors by encouraging smoking cessation, pneumococcal vaccination and annual influenza vaccination
Initiate self-management, education, exercise
↓ FEV$_1$
↑ Dyspnea
Early diagnosis (spirometry) + Prevention
Treatment of acute exacerbations
Follow-up
End-of-life care

[a] Consider adding roflumilast to long-acting bronchodilators (± inhaled corticosteroids) to reduce exacerbation frequency in those with severe COPD, frequent exacerbations and chronic bronchitis.

Abbreviations: COPD = chronic obstructive pulmonary disease; FEV$_1$ = forced expiratory volume in 1 second; ICS = inhaled corticosteroid; LABA = long-acting beta$_2$-agonist; LAMA = long-acting muscarinic antagonist/anticholinergic; SABA = short-acting beta$_2$-agonist; SABD = short-acting bronchodilator

Table 3: **Inhaled Drugs Used for the Treatment of COPD**

Class	Drug	Dose	Adverse Effects	Cost[a]
Anticholinergics,[b] long-acting (LAMA)	*aclidinium* Tudorza Genuair	DPI 400 µg/actuation: 1 inhalation BID	Dry mouth, metallic taste, mydriasis and glaucoma if released into eye, urinary retention.	$$$
	glycopyrronium Seebri Breezhaler	DPI 50 µg/capsule: 1 capsule inhaled once daily	See aclidinium.	$$
	tiotropium Spiriva	DPI 18 µg/capsule: 1 capsule inhaled once daily	See aclidinium.	$$$
Anticholinergics,[b] short-acting	*ipratropium* Atrovent HFA, generics	Individualize dose. May use PRN or regularly scheduled. pMDI 20 µg/puff: 2–4 puffs Q6–8H up to 6–8 puffs Q6–8H, if tolerated; maximum 12 puffs/day Nebules: 250–500 µg TID–QID	Dry mouth, metallic taste, mydriasis and glaucoma if released into eye, urinary retention. Possible increased risk of cardiovascular events.	$
Anticholinergic[b]/ Beta$_2$-adrenergic Agonist Combinations, long-acting (LAMA/LABA)	*glycopyrronium/indacaterol* Ultibro Breezhaler	DPI 50/110 µg/capsule: 1 inhalation once daily	See aclidinium. See formoterol fumarate.	$$$
	umeclidinium/vilanterol Anoro Ellipta	DPI 62.5/25 µg: 1 inhalation once daily	See aclidinium. See formoterol fumarate.	$$$
Anticholinergic[b]/ Beta$_2$-adrenergic Agonist Combinations, short-acting	*ipratropium/fenoterol* Duovent UDV	Individualize dose. Nebules 0.5 mg/1.25 mg per 4 mL: 4 mL Q6H PRN	See ipratropium. See salbutamol.	$$$
	ipratropium/salbutamol Combivent UDV, generics	Individualize dose. Nebules 0.5 mg/2.5 mg per 2.5 mL: 2.5 mL Q6H PRN	See ipratropium. See salbutamol.	$
Beta$_2$-adrenergic Agonists, long-acting (LABA)	*formoterol fumarate* Foradil	DPI 12 µg/capsule: 1 capsule inhaled BID; maximum 48 µg/day. May increase to 2 inhalations BID, if required	Tremor, nervousness, hypokalemia, tachycardia, palpitations.	$$
	formoterol fumarate dihydrate Oxeze Turbuhaler	DPI 6 or 12 µg/inhalation: 1 inhalation Q12H; maximum 48 µg/day	See formoterol fumarate.	$$

(cont'd)

Table 3: **Inhaled Drugs Used for the Treatment of COPD** *(cont'd)*

Class	Drug	Dose	Adverse Effects	Cost[a]
	indacaterol Onbrez Breezhaler	DPI 75 µg/capsule: 1 capsule inhaled once daily	See formoterol fumarate.	$$
	salmeterol Serevent	Diskhaler 50 µg/blister: 1 blister BID Diskus 50 µg/inhalation: 1 inhalation BID	See formoterol fumarate.	$$
Beta$_2$-adrenergic Agonists, short-acting (SABA)	*salbutamol* Airomir, Ventolin Diskus, Ventolin HFA, Ventolin Nebules P.F., generics	pMDI 100 µg/puff: 1–2 puffs TID–QID PRN; maximum 8 puffs/day Diskus: 200 µg TID–QID PRN; maximum 800 µg/day Nebules: 2.5–5 mg QID PRN	Tremor, nervousness, hypokalemia, tachycardia, palpitations.	$
	terbutaline Bricanyl Turbuhaler	Individualize dose. DPI 0.5 mg/inhalation: 1 inhalation Q4–6H PRN; maximum 6 inhalations/day	See salbutamol.	$
Corticosteroid/ LABA Combinations	*budesonide/formoterol fumarate dihydrate*[c] Symbicort Turbuhaler	DPI 100/6 µg or 200/6 µg: 2 inhalations BID; maximum 4 inhalations/day	Corticosteroid: Oropharyngeal candidiasis and hoarseness can be prevented by using a spacer with pMDI or by using DPI, and by rinsing mouth after use. Skin bruising,[23] posterior subcapsular and nuclear cataracts,[24] possible worsening of glaucoma. May decrease bone mineral density and increase fracture risk. Consider monitoring bone mineral density in individuals at high risk, e.g., osteoporosis. LABA: See formoterol fumarate.	$$$
	fluticasone/salmeterol Advair, Advair Diskus	pMDI 125/25 or 250/25 µg: 2 puffs BID Diskus DPI 100/50 µg or 250/50 µg or 500/50 µg: 1 inhalation BID	See budesonide/formoterol fumarate dihydrate.	$$$$$
	fluticasone/vilanterol Breo Ellipta	DPI 100/25 µg: 1 inhalation daily	See budesonide/formoterol fumarate dihydrate.	$$$

[a] Cost of inhaled agents is per unit; cost of inhaled solutions is per 20 vials; includes drug cost only.
[b] Also referred to as a muscarinic antagonist.
[c] Not approved for the relief of acute bronchospasm in COPD.
Abbreviations: DPI = dry powder inhaler; pMDI = pressurized metered dose inhaler
Legend: $ < $30 $$ $30–60 $$$ $60–90 $$$$ $90–120 $$$$$ 120–150

Table 4: Oral Drugs Used in the Treatment of COPD

Class	Drug	Dose	Adverse Effects	Drug Interactions	Cost[a]
Corticosteroids, systemic	*prednisone* generics	For acute exacerbation of COPD: 30–40 mg once daily po × 5–14 days	GI upset, fluid/electrolyte imbalance, pituitary-adrenal suppression, hypertension, cutaneous effects (dermal thinning, easy bruising, acne), hyperglycemia, glycosuria, peptic ulcer, behavioural disturbances (insomnia, euphoria), posterior subcapsular cataracts, glaucoma, myopathy, decreased bone mineral density, cushingoid syndrome, avascular necrosis of bone including hip (rare).	Increased GI ulceration with NSAIDs. Decreased efficacy of prednisone with barbiturates, phenytoin, rifampin. Increased levels with CYP3A4 inhibitors, e.g., clarithromycin, erythromycin, ketoconazole. Hypokalemia with concomitant diuretics, e.g., thiazides. Prednisone decreases response to vaccines.	$
Methylxanthines	*theophylline* Uniphyl, Apo-Theo LA, other generics	Initial: 400–600 mg once daily po with food, usually with the evening meal. Monitor and adjust based on serum levels	Nausea, vomiting, abdominal cramps, headaches, nervousness, tremor, insomnia, tachycardia.	Many drugs can affect theophylline serum levels. Decreased theophylline serum levels: e.g., alcohol, carbamazepine, phenobarbital, phenytoin, rifampin, tobacco smoking. Increased theophylline serum levels: e.g., amiodarone, cimetidine, ciprofloxacin, clarithromycin, erythromycin, fluvoxamine, isoniazid, mexiletine, verapamil.	$
Phosphodiesterase (PDE4) Inhibitors	*roflumilast* Daxas	500 µg once daily po	Nausea, vomiting, diarrhea, decreased appetite, weight decrease, abdominal pain, headache, insomnia, anxiety, depression.	Strong CYP450 inducers (e.g., carbamazepine, phenobarbital, phenytoin, rifampin) may reduce the therapeutic effect of roflumilast and are not recommended in combination with roflumilast.	$$$

[a] Cost of 14-day supply; includes drug cost only.
Abbreviations: NSAID = nonsteroidal anti-inflammatory drug
Legend: $ < $10 $$ $10–20 $$$ $20–30

Table 5: **Oral Antibiotics for Treatment of Acute Exacerbations of COPD**

Class	Drug	Dose[79,82]	Adverse Effects	Drug Interactions	Cost[a]
Cephalosporins	*cefprozil* Cefzil, generics	500 mg BID po × 5–10 days	GI intolerance, anaphylaxis (rare), rash.	No major drug interactions but enhanced anticoagulant effect of warfarin possible.	$$
	cefuroxime axetil Ceftin, generics	500 mg BID po × 5–10 days	See cefprozil.	See cefprozil.	$$$
Fluoroquinolones	*ciprofloxacin* Cipro, generics	Patients at risk of *P. aeruginosa:* 500–750 mg BID po × 7–14 days	Usually well tolerated. Headache, dizziness may occur. Peripheral neuropathy, tendon rupture (rare). May worsen symptoms of myasthenia gravis and should not be used in this population.	Antacids, sucralfate, metal cations decrease fluoroquinolone absorption. May increase theophylline levels; may decrease warfarin effect.	$$-$$$
	levofloxacin Levaquin, generics	750 mg once daily po × 5 days *or* 500 mg once daily po × 7 days	See ciprofloxacin. QT_c prolongation. Cases of severe liver injury including liver failure have been reported.	Antacids, sucralfate, metal cations decrease fluoroquinolone absorption. Avoid using with drugs that prolong the QT_c interval such as Class IA or Class III antiarrhythmics. May increase warfarin effect.	$$
	moxifloxacin Avelox	400 mg once daily po × 5 days	See ciprofloxacin. QT_c prolongation. Cases of severe liver injury including liver failure have been reported.	Antacids, sucralfate, metal cations decrease fluoroquinolone absorption. Avoid using with drugs that prolong the QT_c interval such as Class IA or Class III antiarrhythmics.	$$$
Macrolides, extended spectrum	*azithromycin* Zithromax, Zmax SR, generics	500 mg po × 1 day, then 250 mg once daily × 4 days or 500 mg once daily po × 3 days Zmax SR: 2 g po single dose	GI intolerance, QT_c prolongation.	Coadministration with pimozide is contraindicated. Use cautiously with other drugs that cause QT_c prolongation such as Class IA or Class III antiarrhythmics. May increase effects of digoxin and warfarin.	$$-$$$
	clarithromycin Biaxin BID, Biaxin XL, generics	Biaxin BID: 500 mg BID po × 5–10 days Biaxin XL: 1000 mg once daily po × 5–10 days	Bitter taste, gastrointestinal intolerance, QT_c prolongation.	See azithromycin. Inhibitor of CYP3A4 enzymes therefore many potential interactions (e.g., atorvastatin, some benzodiazepines, buspirone, carbamazepine, colchicine, cyclosporine, ergots, glyburide, lovastatin, simvastatin, sirolimus, tacrolimus, theophylline). Inhibitor of P-gp and may therefore increase levels of P-gp substrates, e.g., colchicine, dabigatran.	$$$-$$$$

Class	Drug	Dose[79,82]	Adverse Effects	Drug Interactions	Cost[a]
Penicillins	*amoxicillin* ❥ generics	500 mg TID po × 5–7 days	Rash, anaphylaxis (rare).	May increase serum levels of methotrexate. May enhance anticoagulant effect of warfarin.	$
	amoxicillin/ clavulanate ❥ Clavulin, generics	500 mg TID po or 875 mg BID po × 5–10 days	Anaphylaxis, GI upset, diarrhea.	See amoxicillin.	$$
Sulfonamide Combinations	*sulfamethoxazole/ trimethoprim* ❥ generics	800/160 mg (2 regular-strength tablets or 1 DS tablet) BID po × 5–7 days	Nausea, skin rash, Stevens-Johnson syndrome (rare).	May increase warfarin effect, increased phenytoin levels. May increase methotrexate toxicity.	$
Tetracyclines	*doxycycline* Vibramycin, generics	100 mg BID po × 1 day, then 100 mg once daily × 4–6 days	GI upset, photosensitivity.	Iron or antacids decrease doxycycline absorption. Carbamazepine, phenytoin, rifampin, may decrease doxycycline levels.	$

[a] Cost is for one course of therapy; includes drug cost only.
❥ Dosage adjustment may be required in renal impairment; see Appendix I.
Abbreviations: DS = double strength; P-gp = P-glycoprotein
Legend: $ < $10 $$ $10–25 $$-$$$ $10–50 $$$ $25–50 $$$-$$$$ $25–75 $$$$ $50–75

Suggested Readings

Bourbeau J, Julien M, Maltais F et al. Reduction of hospital utilization in patients with chronic obstructive pulmonary disease: a disease-specific self-management intervention. *Arch Intern Med* 2003;163(5):585-91.

Global Initiative for Chronic Obstructive Lung Disease (GOLD). *Global strategy for the diagnosis, management and prevention of COPD*. Updated January 2014. Available from: www.goldcopd.org.

Hurst JR, Vestbo J, Anzueto A et al. Susceptibility to exacerbation in chronic obstructive pulmonary disease. *N Engl J Med* 2010; 363:1128-38.

Jones PW, Harding G, Berry P et al. Development and first validation of the COPD Assessment Test. *Eur Respir J* 2009;34(3):648-54.

McIvor A, Little P. Chronic obstructive pulmonary disease. *BMJ* 2007;334(7597):798.

Niewoehner DE. Clinical practice. Outpatient management of severe COPD. *N Engl J Med* 2010;362(15):1407-16.

O'Donnell DE, Hernandez P, Kaplan A et al. Canadian Thoracic Society recommendations for management of chronic obstructive pulmonary disease–2008 update–highlights for primary care. *Can Respir J* 2008;15(Suppl A):1A-8A.

References

1. O'Donnell DE, Aaron S, Bourbeau J et al. Canadian Thoracic Society recommendations for the management of chronic obstructive pulmonary disease–2007 update. *Can Respir J* 2007;14(Suppl B):5B-32B. Available from: www.respiratoryguidelines.ca/sites/all/files/CTS_COPD_Guidelines_2007_Update.pdf. Accessed September 24, 2013.
2. Global Initiative for Chronic Obstructive Lung Disease (GOLD). *Global strategy for the diagnosis, management and prevention of COPD*. Updated January 2014. Available from: www.goldcopd.org. Accessed February 7, 2014.
3. Bestall JC, Paul EA, Garrod R et al. Usefulness of the Medical Research Council (MRC) dyspnoea scale as a measure of disability in patients with chronic obstructive pulmonary disease. *Thorax* 1999;54(7):581-6.
4. McIvor RA, Tashkin DP. Underdiagnosis of chronic obstructive pulmonary disease: a rationale for spirometry as a screening tool. *Can Respir J* 2001;8(3):153-8.
5. Johannessen A, Lehmann S, Omenaas ER et al. Post-bronchodilator spirometry reference values in adults and implications for disease management. *Am J Respir Crit Care Med* 2006;173(12):1316-25.
6. Kanner RE, Connett JE, Williams DE et al. Effects of randomized assignment to a smoking cessation intervention and changes in smoking habits on respiratory symptoms in smokers with early chronic obstructive pulmonary disease: the Lung Health Study. *Am J Med* 1999;106(4):410-6.
7. Stang P, Lydick E, Silberman C et al. The prevalence of COPD: using smoking rates to estimate disease frequency in the general population. *Chest* 2000;117(5 Suppl 2):354S-9S.
8. Wagena EJ, van der Meer RM, Ostelo RJ et al. The efficacy of smoking cessation strategies in people with chronic obstructive pulmonary disease: results from a systematic review. *Respir Med* 2004;98(9):805-15.
9. Scanlon PD, Connett JE, Waller LA et al. Smoking cessation and lung function in mild-to-moderate chronic obstructive pulmonary disease. The Lung Health Study. *Am J Respir Crit Care Med* 2000;161(2 Pt 1):381-90.
10. Anthonisen NR, Connett JE, Kiley JP et al. Effects of smoking intervention and the use of an inhaled anticholinergic bronchodilator on the rate of decline of FEV1. The Lung Health Study. *JAMA* 1994;272(19):1497-505.
11. Anthonisen NR, Skeans MA, Wise RA et al. The effects of a smoking cessation intervention on 14.5-year mortality: a randomized clinical trial. *Ann Intern Med* 2005;142(4):233-9.
12. Becklake MR. Occupational exposures: evidence for a causal association with chronic obstructive pulmonary disease. *Am Rev Respir Dis* 1989;140(3 Pt 2):S85-91.
13. Matheson MC, Benke G, Raven J et al. Biological dust exposure in the workplace is a risk factor for chronic obstructive pulmonary disease. *Thorax* 2005;60(8):645-51.
14. Bourbeau J, Julien M, Maltais F et al. Reduction of hospital utilization in patients with chronic obstructive pulmonary disease: a disease-specific self-management intervention. *Arch Intern Med* 2003;163(5):585-91.
15. Pitta F, Troosters T, Probst VS et al. Physical activity and hospitalization for exacerbation of COPD. *Chest* 2006;129(3):536-44.
16. Lacasse Y, Wong E, Guyatt GH et al. Meta-analysis of respiratory rehabilitation in chronic obstructive pulmonary disease. *Lancet* 1996;348(9035):1115-9.
17. Lacasse Y, Goldstein R, Lasserson TJ et al. Pulmonary rehabilitation for chronic obstructive pulmonary disease. *Cochrane Database Syst Rev* 2006;(4):CD003793.
18. Nici L, Donner C, Wouters E et al. American Thoracic Society/European Respiratory Society statement on pulmonary rehabilitation. *Am J Respir Crit Care Med* 2006;173(12):1390-413.
19. Man WD, Polkey MI, Donaldson N et al. Community pulmonary rehabilitation after hospitalisation for acute exacerbations of chronic obstructive pulmonary disease: randomised controlled study. *BMJ* 2004;329(7476):1209.
20. Tashkin DP, Cooper CB. The role of long-acting bronchodilators in the management of stable COPD. *Chest* 2004;125(1):249-59.
21. Calverley PM, Anderson JA, Celli B et al. Salmeterol and fluticasone propionate and survival in chronic obstructive disease. *N Engl J Med* 2007;356(8):775-89.
22. Hurst JR, Vestbo J, Anzueto A et al. Susceptibility to exacerbation in chronic obstructive pulmonary disease. *N Engl J Med* 2010;363(12):1128-38.
23. Tashkin DP, Murray HE, Skeans M et al. Skin manifestations of inhaled corticosteroids in COPD patients: results from Lung Health Study II. *Chest* 2004;126(4):1123-33.
24. Cumming RG, Mitchell P, Leeder SR. Use of inhaled corticosteroids and the risk of cataracts. *N Engl J Med* 1997;337(1):8-14.

25. Dolovich MB, Ahrens RC, Hess DR et al. Device selection and outcomes of aerosol therapy: evidence-based guidelines: American College of Chest Physicians/American College of Asthma, Allergy, and Immunology. *Chest* 2005;127(1):335-71.
26. Rau JL. Practical problems with aerosol therapy in COPD. *Respir Care* 2006;51(2):158-72.
27. Institute of Medicine. Clinical Practice Guidelines We Can Trust. Washington, DC: The National Academies Press, 2011. Available from: www.iom.edu/Reports/2011/Clinical-Practice-Guidelines-We-Can-Trust/Standards.aspx. Accessed: June 6, 2014
28. Ikeda A, Nishimura K, Koyama H et al. Bronchodilating effects of combined therapy with clinical dosages of ipratropium bromide and salbutamol for stable COPD: comparison with ipratropium bromide alone. *Chest* 1995;107(2):401-5.
29. Campbell S. For COPD a combination of ipratropium bromide and albuterol sulfate is more effective than albuterol base. *Arch Intern Med* 1999;159(2):156-60.
30. Tashkin DP, Celli B, Decramer M et al. Bronchodilator responsiveness in patients with COPD. *Eur Respir J* 2008;31(4):742-50.
31. Niewoehner DE, Rice K, Cote C et al. Prevention of exacerbations of chronic obstructive pulmonary disease with tiotropium, a once-daily inhaled anticholinergic bronchodilator: a randomized trial. *Ann Intern Med* 2005;143(5):317-26.
32. Littner MR, Ilowite JS, Tashkin DP et al. Long-acting bronchodilation with once-daily dosing of tiotropium (Spiriva) in stable chronic obstructive pulmonary disease. *Am J Respir Crit Care Med* 2000;161(4 Pt 1):1136-42.
33. Casaburi R, Kukafka D, Cooper CB et al. Improvement in exercise tolerance with the combination of tiotropium and pulmonary rehabilitation in patients with COPD. *Chest* 2005;127(3):809-17.
34. U.S. Food and Drug Administration. *Early communication about an ongoing safety review of tiotropium (marketed as Spiriva HandiHaler)*; created March 18, 2008, updated October 7, 2008. Available from: www.fda.gov/Drugs/DrugSafety/PostmarketDrugSafetyInformationforPatientsandProviders/DrugSafetyInformationforHeathcareProfessionals/ucm070651.htm. Accessed March 21, 2011.
35. Lee TA, Pickard AS, Au DH et al. Risk for death associated with medications for recently diagnosed chronic obstructive pulmonary disease. *Ann Intern Med* 2008;149(6):380-90.
36. Singh S, Loke YK, Furberg CD. Inhaled anticholinergics and risk of major adverse cardiovascular events in patients with chronic obstructive pulmonary disease: a systematic review and meta-analysis. *JAMA* 2008;300(12):1439-50.
37. Tashkin DP, Celli B, Senn S et al. A 4-year trial of tiotropium in chronic obstructive pulmonary disease. *N Engl J Med* 2008;359(15):1543-54.
38. Michele TM, Pinheiro S, Iyasu S. The safety of tiotropium—the FDA's conclusions. *N Engl J Med* 2010;363(12):1097-9.
39. Celli B, Decramer M, Leimer I et al. Cardiovascular safety of tiotropium in patients with COPD. *Chest* 2010;137(1):20-30.
40. Lee TA, Pickard AS, Au DH et al. Risk for death associated with medications for recently diagnosed chronic obstructive pulmonary disease. *Ann Intern Med* 2008;149(6):380-90.
41. Ogale SS, Lee TA, Au DH et al. Cardiovascular events associated with ipratropium bromide in COPD. *Chest* 2010;137(1):13-9.
42. D'Urzo A, Ferguson GT, van Noord JA et al. Efficacy and safety of once-daily NVA237 in patients with moderate-to-severe COPD: the GLOW1 trial. *Respir Res* 2011;12:156.
43. Kerwin E, Hébert J, Gallagher N et al. Efficacy and safety of NVA237 versus placebo and tiotropium in patients with moderate-to-severe COPD: The GLOW2 study. *Eur Respir J* 2012;40(5):1106-14.
44. Beeh KM, Singh D, Di Scala L et al. Once-daily NVA237 improves exercise tolerance from the first dose in patients with COPD: the GLOW3 trial. *Int J Chron Obstruct Pulmon Dis* 2012;7:503-13.
45. Jones PW, Singh D, Bateman ED et al. Efficacy and safety of twice-daily aclidinium bromide in COPD patients: the ATTAIN study. *Eur Respir J* 2012;40(4):830-6.
46. Fuhr R, Magnussen H, Sarem K et al. Efficacy of aclidinium bromide 400 μg twice daily compared with placebo and tiotropium in patients with moderate to severe COPD. *Chest* 2012;141(3):745-52.
47. Karabis A, Lindner L, Mocarski M et al. Comparative efficacy of aclidinium versus glycopyrronium and tiotropium, as maintenance treatment of moderate to severe COPD patients: a systematic review and network meta-analysis. *Int J Chron Obstruct Pulmon Dis* 2013;8:405-23.
48. Mahler DA, Donohue JF, Barbee RA et al. Efficacy of salmeterol xinafoate in the treatment of COPD. *Chest* 1999;115(4):957-65.
49. Rennard SI, Anderson W, Zuwallack R et al. Use of a long-acting inhaled beta2-adrenergic agonist, salmeterol xinafoate, in patients with chronic obstructive pulmonary disease. *Am J Respir Crit Care Med* 2001;163(5):1087-92.
50. Maesen BL, Westermann CJ, Duurkens VA et al. Effects of formoterol in apparently poorly reversible chronic obstructive pulmonary disease. *Eur Respir J* 1999;13(5):1103-8.
51. Partridge MR, Schuermann W, Beckman O et al. Effect on lung function and morning activities of budesonide/formoterol versus salmeterol/fluticasone in patients with COPD. *Ther Adv Respir Dis* 2009;3(4):1-11.
52. Kerwin EM, Williams J. Indacaterol 75 μg once daily for the treatment of patients with chronic obstructive pulmonary disease: a North American perspective. *Ther Adv Respir Dis* 2013;7(1):25-37.
53. Donohue JF, Fogarty C, Lotvall J et al. Once-daily bronchodilators for chronic obstructive pulmonary disease: indacaterol versus tiotropium. *Am J Respir Crit Care Med* 2010;182(2):155-62.
54. van Noord JA, Buhl R, Laforce C et al. QVA149 demonstrates superior bronchodilation compared with indacaterol or placebo in patients with chronic obstructive pulmonary disease. *Thorax* 2010;65(12):1086-91.
55. Donohue JF, Maleki-Yazdi MR, Kilbride S et al. Efficacy and safety of once-daily umeclidinium/vilanterol 62.5/25 mcg in COPD. *Respir Med* 2013;107(10):1538-46.
56. Celli B, Crater G, Kilbride S et al. Once-daily umeclidinium/vilanterol 125/25 mcg in COPD: a randomized, controlled study. *Chest* 2014 Jan 2. [Epub ahead of print].
57. van de Maele B, Fabbri LM, Martin C et al. Cardiovascular safety of QVA149, a combination of indacaterol and NVA237, in COPD patients. *COPD* 2010;7(6):418-27.
58. Dahl R, Chapman KR, Rudolf M et al. Safety and efficacy of dual bronchodilation with QVA149 in COPD patients: The ENLIGHTEN study. *Respir Med* 2013;107(10):1558-67.
59. Calverley P, Pauwels R, Vestbo J et al. Combined salmeterol and fluticasone in the treatment of chronic obstructive disease: a randomised controlled trial. *Lancet* 2003;361(9356):449-56.
60. O'Donnell DE, Sciurba F, Celli B et al. Effect of fluticasone propionate/salmeterol on lung hyperinflation and exercise endurance in COPD. *Chest* 2006;130(3):647-56.
61. Nannini LJ, Poole P, Milan SJ et al. Combined corticosteroid and long-acting beta2-agonist in one inhaler versus inhaled corticosteroids alone for chronic obstructive pulmonary disease. *Cochrane Database Syst Rev* 2013;8:CD006826.
62. Nannini LJ, Lasserson TJ, Poole P et al. Combined corticosteroid and long-acting beta(2)-agonist in one inhaler versus long-acting beta(2)-agonists for chronic obstructive pulmonary disease. *Cochrane Database Syst Rev* 2012;9:CD006829.

63. Kew KM, Seniukovich A. Inhaled steroids and risk of pneumonia for chronic obstructive pulmonary disease. *Cochrane Database Syst Rev* 2014;3:CD010115.
64. Aaron SD, Vandemheen KL, Fergusson D et al. Tiotropium in combination with placebo, salmeterol, or fluticasone-salmeterol for treatment of chronic obstructive pulmonary disease: a randomized trial. *Ann Intern Med* 2007;146(8):545-55.
65. Gaebel K, McIvor RA, Xie F et al. Triple therapy for the management of COPD: a review. *COPD* 2011;8(3):206-43.
66. McIvor RA. Future options for disease intervention: important advances in phosphodiesterase 4 inhibitors. *Eur Respir Rev* 2007;16(105):105-12. Available from: err.ersjournals.com/content/16/105/105.full.pdf. Accessed September 24, 2013.
67. Calverley PM, Sanchez-Toril F, McIvor A et al. Effect of 1-year treatment with roflumilast in severe chronic obstructive pulmonary disease. *Am J Respir Crit Care Med* 2007;176(2):154-61.
68. Calverley PM, Rabe KF, Goehring UM et al. Roflumilast in symptomatic chronic obstructive pulmonary disease: two randomised clinical trials. *Lancet* 2009;374(9691):685-94.
69. Fabbri LM, Calverley PM, Izquierdo-Alonso JL et al. Roflumilast in moderate-to-severe chronic obstructive pulmonary disease treated with long acting bronchodilators: two randomised clinical trials. *Lancet* 2009;374(9691):695-703.
70. Chong J, Poole P, Leung B et al. Phosphodiesterase 4 inhibitors for chronic obstructive pulmonary disease. *Cochrane Database Syst Rev* 2011;(5):CD002309.
71. Ringbaek TJ. Continuous oxygen therapy for hypoxic pulmonary disease: guidelines, compliance and effects. *Treat Respir Med* 2005;4(6):397-408.
72. Poole PJ, Chacko E, Wood-Baker RW et al. Influenza vaccine for patients with chronic obstructive pulmonary disease. *Cochrane Database Syst Rev* 2006;(1):CD002733.
73. Wongsurakiat P, Maranetra KN, Wasi C et al. Acute respiratory illness in patients with COPD and the effectiveness of influenza vaccination: a randomized controlled study. *Chest* 2004;125(6):2011-20.
74. Respiratory Review Panel. *Respiratory (asthma and COPD) guidelines for family practice*. Toronto (ON): MUMS Guidelines Clearinghouse; 2007.
75. Jackson LA, Neuzil KM, Yu O et al. Effectiveness of pneumococcal polysaccharide vaccine in older adults. *N Engl J Med* 2003;348(18):1747-55.
76. Alfageme I, Vazquez R, Reyes N et al. Clinical efficacy of anti-pneumococcal vaccination in patients with COPD. *Thorax* 2006;61(3):189-95.
77. Leuppi JD, Schuetz P, Bingisser R et al. Short-term vs conventional glucocorticoid therapy in acute exacerbations of chronic obstructive pulmonary disease: the REDUCE randomized clinical trial. *JAMA* 2013;309(21):2223-31.
78. Vollenweider DJ, Jarrett H, Steurer-Stey CA et al. Antibiotics for exacerbations of chronic obstructive pulmonary disease. *Cochrane Database Syst Rev* 2012;12:CD010257.
79. Blondel-Hill E, Fryters S. *Bugs & drugs 2012*. Edmonton (AB): Alberta Health Services; 2012.
80. Anthonisen NR, Manfreda J, Warren CP et al. Antibiotic therapy in exacerbations of chronic obstructive pulmonary disease. *Ann Intern Med* 1987;106(2):196-204.
81. Saint S, Bent S, Vittinghoff E et al. Antibiotics in chronic obstructive pulmonary disease exacerbations. A meta-analysis. *JAMA* 1995;273(12):957-60.
82. Anti-infective Review Panel. *Anti-infective guidelines for community-acquired infections*. Toronto (ON): MUMS Guideline Clearinghouse; 2012.
83. Herath SC, Poole P. Prophylactic antibiotic therapy for chronic obstructive pulmonary disease (COPD). *Cochrane Database Syst Rev* 2013;11:CD009764.

Respiratory Disorders

Chapter 55
Croup

Candice Bjornson, MD, MSc, FRCPC and
David W. Johnson, MD

Croup (laryngotracheobronchitis) is a common cause of upper airway obstruction in children. It is most prevalent in the late fall to early winter months. The annual incidence of croup is 1.5–6 per 100 in children <6 years.[1] Though common in children between 6 months and 3 years of age, it can also occur in children as young as 3 months and as old as 15 years.[1] It is rarely reported in adults.[2] Boys are affected more often than girls. Viruses are the most common cause, particularly parainfluenza virus types 1 and 3. Influenza A and B, adenovirus, respiratory syncytial virus (RSV), metapneumovirus, coronavirus and mycoplasma have also been isolated.[3,4]

Croup hospitalizations demonstrate a seasonal pattern, proposed to be related to the temporal prevalence of parainfluenza virus in circulation in the community.[5] In Canada, peak hospitalizations occur in October of odd-numbered years, with smaller peaks in February of alternate years. Although croup incidence is greatest between 2 and 3 years of age, infants under one year are at highest risk of hospitalization compared with older children. In Ontario, croup hospitalization rates reached over 250 per 100 000 children in the fall of 1993, and thereafter showed sharp decreases coinciding with the widespread introduction of corticosteroid treatment for croup in subsequent years.

The majority of affected children can be safely managed at home. Very few require artificial support of their airway.[6] More than 60% of children diagnosed with croup have mild symptoms, about 4% are hospitalized and approximately 1 in 5000 children are intubated (approximately 1 in 200 hospitalized children).[6]

Goals of Therapy

- Decrease the duration and severity of symptoms
- Minimize anxiety of the child and parent(s)
- Decrease intubations, hospitalizations and return visits to physicians

Investigations

- Diagnosis of croup, which is most commonly due to a viral infection, requires no specific laboratory or radiologic investigation (see Table 1 for Differential Diagnosis)
- History with particular attention to symptoms:
  - *seal-like barky cough* may be preceded by nonspecific cough, rhinorrhea and fever (up to 40°C)
  - symptoms are substantially worse at night and improve during the day, and are aggravated by agitation and crying
  - obstructive symptoms generally resolve within 48 hours; a small percentage of children remain symptomatic for up to 5–6 days[7]
- Physical examination for *stridor*, *chest wall retractions*, *respiratory distress*:
  - stridor: typically occurs during inspiration but may occur during expiration if severe
  - chest wall retractions and respiratory distress: occur to varying degrees and are indicative of severity

- respiratory failure occurs over several hours. Signs include reduced respiratory effort, lethargy, pallor, cyanosis, dusky appearance, decreased breath sounds
- Objective measurements:
  - lateral and anteroposterior (AP) soft tissue neck films may clarify diagnosis in patients with atypical croup-like disease or in cases where a child is not responding to treatment as expected
  - pulse oximetry is indicated in patients with more severe croup
  - Westley croup score[9] stratifies croup severity into mild (1–2), moderate (3–8) or severe (>8); however, objective scoring systems have little utility in clinical practice. Assessment of symptoms (barky cough, stridor, chest wall indrawing and agitation/fatigue) are useful for determination of severity (see Figure 1).

Table 1: Differential Diagnosis for Children Who Present with Acute Onset of Stridor

Differential Diagnosis	Characteristics
Croup	Symptoms (seal-like barky cough, hoarseness, inspiratory stridor, chest wall retractions) usually worse at night. May have fever
Bacterial tracheitis most common diagnosis after croup	High fever, toxic appearance, poor response to nebulized epinephrine. Often presents following a viral-like illness after which a child becomes suddenly worse. Respiratory distress is due to thick, membranous tracheal secretions which may result in acute airway obstruction
Epiglottitis relatively rare since introduction of *Haemophilus influenzae* type b vaccine	Absence of barky cough, sudden onset of high fever, dysphagia, drooling, toxic appearance, anxious appearance and sitting slightly forward in the "sniffing" position. There is risk of progression to complete upper airway obstruction. This is an airway emergency
Allergic reactions, angioedema rare	May present at any age; rapid onset of dysphagia, stridor, and possible cutaneous manifestations (urticarial rash); may be personal or family history of allergy
Diphtheria[8] rare	Extremely rare airway emergency. May present at any age in individual with a history of inadequate immunization. Prodromic symptoms of pharyngitis, low-grade fever, hoarse voice, dysphagia, potentially barky cough and/or inspiratory stridor. Membranous pharyngitis on examination is characteristic
Upper-airway abscess (peritonsillar, retropharyngeal)[8] rare	Dysphagia, drooling, occasionally stridor, dyspnea, tachypnea, neck stiffness, unilateral cervical adenopathy; onset is typically more gradual, often accompanied by fever
Occult foreign object very rare	Acute onset of stridor, presence of occult foreign body, most commonly lodged in the upper esophagus and causing secondary airway compression

Therapeutic Choices

Patients with mild croup can be managed in the office setting, while those with moderate or severe croup should be referred to an emergency department for treatment and observation (Figure 1).

Nonpharmacologic Choices

- Keep children calm by ensuring a calm and reassuring atmosphere. This will minimize oxygen demand and respiratory muscle fatigue.
- Evidence establishes that mist (bedside humidified air, mist tents) is not effective at reducing respiratory distress and should not be used.[10,11,12,13] Placing children in mist tents—a wet, cold, confined environment separated from their parents—may provoke anxiety and agitation.[14]
- Oxygen therapy in conjunction with corticosteroids and epinephrine is reserved for children with hypoxia and significant respiratory distress. It should never be forced on a child, especially if it results in significant agitation. Administration of oxygen through a plastic hose with the end

opening held near the child's nose and mouth (called "blow-by" oxygen), is often the most beneficial way of administering oxygen.

- It is thought that the lower density of a helium-oxygen mixture (relative to nitrogen in room air) allows laminar flow and decreases turbulence in narrowed airways, thus potentially improving ventilation and reducing respiratory distress. Helium-oxygen mixtures (heliox) may benefit children with severe respiratory distress; however, study results have been mixed. There is insufficient evidence to advocate its general use.[15,16,17,18,19]

Figure 1: Management of Croup in the Outpatient Setting

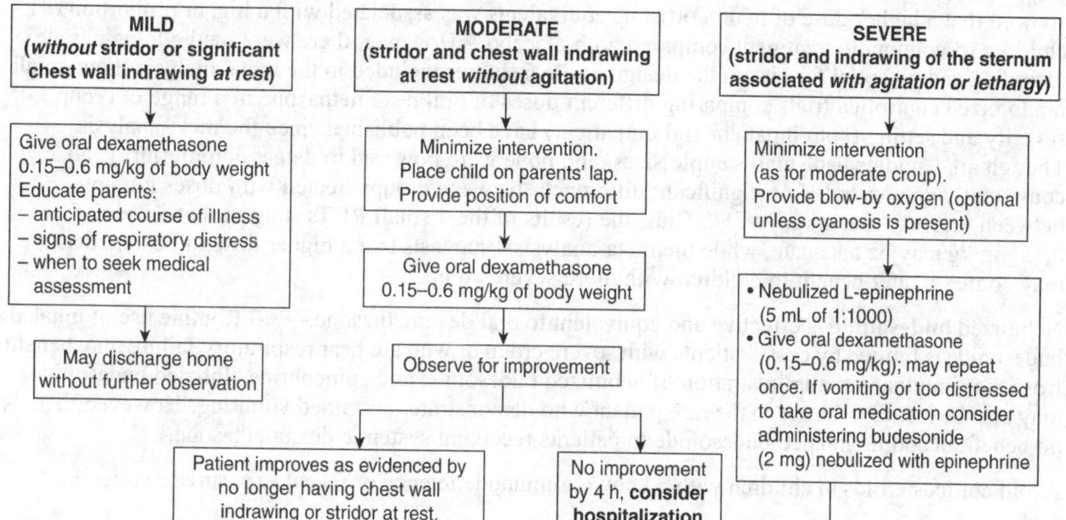

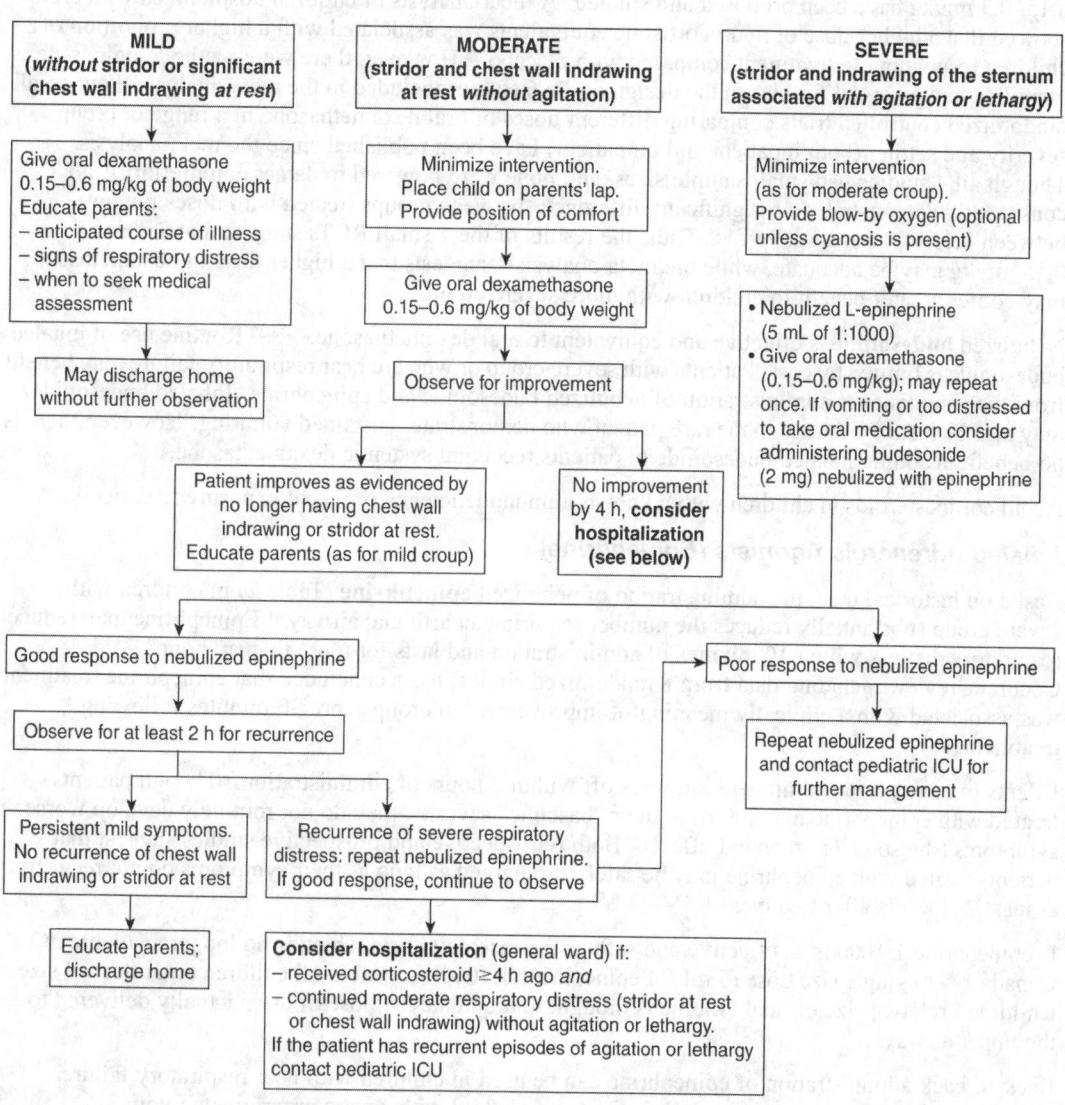

Modified with permission. Toward Optimized Practice (TOP) Working Group for Croup. *Guideline for the diagnosis and management of croup*. July 2003 [Revised 2008]. Edmonton (AB): TOP; c2008. Algorithm, Croup in the out-patient setting; p. 11. Available from: www.topalbertadoctors.org/download/252/croup_guideline.pdf.

Pharmacologic Choices

Corticosteroids

Corticosteroids (Table 2) are the mainstay of therapy for croup, irrespective of clinical severity.[20] Corticosteroids have been shown to reduce intubations, duration of intubation, need for re-intubation, rate of hospitalization, duration of hospitalization, need for additional inhaled epinephrine and rate of return to a health care practitioner for persistent croup symptoms.[20,21,22,23,24,25,26,27,28,29] Dexamethasone and budesonide relieve symptoms of croup 2–3 hours after treatment.[23]

Dexamethasone, 0.6 mg/kg, is effective when given orally or parenterally.[30,31] The optimal dose is unknown. The traditional dose of dexamethasone has been 0.6 mg/kg; however, doses of 0.15–0.3 mg/kg have been proposed and studied. A meta-analysis of children hospitalized with croup showed that a higher dose of hydrocortisone equivalents was associated with a higher proportion of children responding to treatment compared with placebo.[22] However, there were methodologic issues identified and potential for bias in the design of the 6 studies included in the meta-analysis. Four small randomized controlled trials comparing different doses of oral dexamethasone in a range of croup severity and setting (both inpatient and outpatient) have been published since the meta-analysis. Though all 4 studies had small sample sizes, and none were powered to detect noninferiority, all consistently demonstrated no significant differences between groups treated with doses ranging between 0.15 to 0.6 mg/kg.[32,33,34,35] Thus, the results of the 4 small RCTs suggest that a dose of 0.15 mg/kg may be adequate, while the meta-analysis[22] suggests that a higher dose of dexamethasone may confer greater benefit to children with more severe croup.

Nebulized **budesonide** is effective and equivalent to oral dexamethasone.[23,36,37] Routine use of inhaled budesonide is limited by cost. Patients with severe croup or who are near respiratory failure may benefit from the simultaneous administration of nebulized budesonide and epinephrine. Inhaled budesonide may also be justified for use in the rare patient who demonstrates sustained vomiting. However, there is no benefit in adding inhaled budesonide to patients receiving systemic dexamethasone.[38]

Avoid corticosteroids in children with a known immunodeficiency or recent exposure to varicella.[39,40]

Inhaled Adrenergic Agonists (Epinephrine)

Based on historical data, the administration of nebulized **epinephrine** (Table 2) in children with severe croup substantially reduces the number requiring an artificial airway.[41] Epinephrine may reduce respiratory distress within 10 minutes of administration and lasts for more than an hour.[9,42,43,44,45] A Cochrane review including data from 8 randomized clinical trials concluded that epinephrine treatment was associated with a clinically meaningful improvement in croup score 30 minutes following treatment.[46]

Effects of epinephrine administration wear off within 2 hours of administration.[9] Though patients treated with epinephrine may return to their "baseline" severity, they do not routinely develop worse symptoms (the so-called rebound effect).[9] Both retrospective and prospective studies suggest that patients treated with epinephrine may be safely discharged as long as their symptoms do not recur for at least 2–3 hours after treatment.[46,47,48,49,50,51]

L-epinephrine 1:1000 is as effective and safe as the racemate form which is no longer available in Canada.[46,52] A single size dose (5 mL of epinephrine 1:1000) is used in all children regardless of size. Children's relative size of tidal volume is thought to modulate the dose of drug actually delivered to the upper airway.

Back-to-back administration of epinephrine can be used in children with near respiratory failure. However, there is one report of an otherwise normal child with severe croup treated with 3 nebulizations of epinephrine within 1 hour who developed ventricular tachycardia and a myocardial infarction.[53] Therefore, administer repeated doses of epinephrine only if a child is near respiratory failure and close cardiac monitoring is possible. If back-to-back epinephrine is considered necessary, the treating physician should contact a pediatric intensivist as soon as possible regarding further treatment and transport.

Inhaled Beta$_2$-agonists

There are no randomized controlled trials assessing the use of beta$_2$-agonists (e.g., salbutamol) in the treatment of croup. However, as these agents have no inherent effect on upper airways which contain no smooth muscle, benefit is unlikely and therefore these agents are not recommended in the treatment of croup.

Analgesics

Analgesics may provide some degree of increased comfort by reducing fever and pain.

Antitussives and Decongestants

No studies have been published regarding the potential benefit of antitussives or decongestants in children with croup. There is no rational basis for their use.

Antibiotics

As croup is a viral disease antibiotics are not effective in the treatment of croup. However, in rare instances, a bacterial superinfection such as bacterial tracheitis or an alternate diagnosis of epiglottitis or upper airway abscess may be suspected. These infections pose serious potential for rapid deterioration and airway obstruction, and as such, treatment includes monitoring of the airway by skilled personnel in an ICU setting and broad-spectrum iv antibiotic treatment.

Therapeutic Tips

- Children with mild to moderate croup may derive adequate relief from breathing in cool air. This can be achieved by dressing them warmly and opening a bedroom window or freezer door for a few minutes while allowing them to breath in the cool air. The child should not be left alone.
- Oral **dexamethasone** is the preferred corticosteroid treatment. If the child is severely ill, vomiting or too distressed to be given oral dexamethasone, consider parenteral dexamethasone or nebulized **budesonide**. While nebulized budesonide is expensive, im or iv administration of dexamethasone may be upsetting to an already distressed child.

Table 2: Drugs Used for Croup

Drug Class	Drug	Dose and Duration	Comments	Cost[a]
Adrenergic Agonists	*L-epinephrine* Adrenalin, Epinephrine, generics	5 mL of 1:1000 (1 mg/mL) solution via nebulizer	Use for rapid response in children with severe respiratory distress. Positive effects of epinephrine last up to 2 h; patients should be observed for at least 2 h before discharge.	$$
Corticosteroids	*dexamethasone* generics	0.15–0.6 mg/kg po/im/iv once[22,32] May supplement initial dose in 6–24 h as necessary to a maximum daily dose of 0.6 mg/kg or 10 mg whichever is less	Benefit demonstrated for all patients diagnosed with croup regardless of severity (mild-severe); reduces symptoms, sleep loss and parental anxiety, rate and duration of intubation, rate and duration of hospitalization and rate of return to medical care. While both oral and parenteral dexamethasone are effective, oral is preferred as it is less distressing for the child. Onset of action: 2–3 h after treatment. No evidence to suggest multiple doses provide additional benefit over a single dose.	$
	budesonide Pulmicort Nebuamp	2 mg (4 mL of 0.5 mg/mL) solution via nebulizer May repeat dose in 6–24 h if necessary	Inhaled budesonide has been shown in several studies to be equivalent to oral dexamethasone but is more expensive. A good option for patients with vomiting or severe respiratory distress (may be nebulized together with epinephrine).	$$

[a] Cost of one dose; includes drug cost only.
Legend: $ < $1 $$ $1–5

Suggested Readings

Alberta Medical Association. *Guideline for the diagnosis and management of croup*. Edmonton (AB): Toward Optimized Practice; 2008. Available from: www.topalbertadoctors.org/download/252/croup_guideline.pdf.

Bjornson CL, Johnson DW. Croup. *Lancet* 2008;371(9609):329-39.

Bjornson CL, Johnson DW. Croup in children. *CMAJ* 2013;185(15):1317-23.

Bjornson CL, Johnson DW. Croup-treatment update. *Pediatr Emerg Care* 2005;21(12):863-73.

Johnson D. Croup. *Clin Evid (Online)* 2009;pii:0321.

References

1. Denny FW, Murphy TF, Clyde WA et al. Croup: an 11-year study in a pediatric practice. *Pediatrics* 1983;71(6):871-6.
2. Tong MC, Chu MC, Leighton SE et al. Adult croup. *Chest* 1996;109(6):1659-62.
3. Ho HK. Human metapneumovirus and lower respiratory tract disease in children. *N Engl J Med* 2004;350(17):1788-90.
4. Sung JY, Lee HJ, Eun BW et al. Role of human coronavirus NL63 in hospitalized children with croup. *Pediatr Infect Dis J* 2010;29(9):822-6.
5. Segal AO, Crighton EJ, Moineddin R et al. Croup hospitalizations in Ontario: a 14-year time-series analysis. *Pediatrics* 2005;116(1):51-5.
6. Brown JC. The management of croup. *Br Med Bull* 2002;61:189-202.
7. Johnson D, Williamson J. Croup: duration of symptoms and impact on family functioning. *Pediatr Res* 2001;49:83A.
8. Tunnessen W. Respiratory system: stridor. In: *Signs and symptoms in pediatrics*. Philadelphia (PA): Lippincott; 1983.
9. Westley CR, Cotton EK, Brooks JG. Nebulized racemic epinephrine by IPPB for the treatment of croup: a double-blind study. *Am J Dis Child* 1978;132(5):484-7.
10. Chin R, Browne GJ, Lam LT et al. Effectiveness of a croup clinical pathway in the management of children with croup presenting to an emergency department. *J Paediatr Child Health* 2002;38(4):382-7.
11. Lavine E, Scolnik D. Lack of efficacy of humidification in the treatment of croup: why do physicians persist in using an unproven modality? *CJEM* 2001;3(3):209-12.
12. Scolnik D, Coates AL, Stephens D et al. Controlled delivery of high vs low humidity vs mist therapy for croup in emergency departments: a randomized controlled trial. *JAMA* 2006;295(11):1274-80.
13. Moore M, Little P. Humidified air inhalation for treating croup. *Cochrane Database Syst Rev* 2006;(3):CD002870.
14. Henry R. Moist air in the treatment of laryngotracheitis. *Arch Dis Child* 1983;58(8):577.
15. Duncan PG. Efficacy of helium-oxygen mixtures in the management of severe viral and post-intubation croup. *Can Anaesth Soc J* 1979;26(3):206-12.
16. McGee DL, Wald DA, Hinchliffe S. Helium-oxygen therapy in the emergency department. *J Emerg Med* 1997;15(3):291-6.
17. Terregino CA, Nairn SJ, Chansky ME et al. The effect of heliox on croup: a pilot study. *Acad Emerg Med* 1998;5(11):1130-3.
18. Weber JE, Chudnofsky CR, Younger JG et al. A randomized comparison of helium-oxygen mixture (Heliox) and racemic epinephrine for the treatment of moderate to severe croup. *Pediatrics* 2001;107(6):E96.
19. Moraa I, Sturman N, McGuire T et al. Heliox for croup in children. *Cochrane Database Syst Rev* 2013;12:CD006822.
20. Russell KF, Liang Y, O'Gorman K et al. Glucocorticoids for croup. *Cochrane Database Syst Rev* 2011;(1):CD001955.
21. Ausejo M, Saenz A, Pham B et al. The effectiveness of glucocorticoids in treating croup: meta-analysis. *BMJ* 1999;319(7210):595-600.
22. Kairys SW, Olmstead EM, O'Connor GT. Steroid treatment of laryngotracheitis: a meta-analysis of the evidence from randomized trials. *Pediatrics* 1989;83(5):683-93.
23. Johnson DW, Jacobson S, Edney PC et al. A comparison of nebulized budesonide, intramuscular dexamethasone, and placebo for moderately severe croup. *N Engl J Med* 1998;339(8):498-503.
24. Bjornson C, Klassen T, Williamson J et al. A randomized trial of a single dose of oral dexamethasone for mild croup. *N Engl J Med* 2004;351(13):1306-13.
25. Tibballs J, Shann FA, Landau LI et al. Placebo-controlled trial of prednisolone in children intubated for croup. *Lancet* 1992;340(8822):745-8.
26. Geelhoed GC. Sixteen years of croup in a Western Australian teaching hospital: effects of routine steroid treatment. *Ann Emerg Med* 1996;28(6):621-6.
27. Geelhoed GC, Turner J, Macdonald WB. Efficacy of a small single dose of oral dexamethasone for outpatient croup: a double blind placebo controlled clinical trial. *BMJ* 1996;313(7050):140-2.
28. Luria JW, Gonzalez-del-Rey JA, DiGiulio GA et al. Effectiveness of oral or nebulized dexamethasone for children with mild croup. *Arch Pediatr Adolesc Med* 2001;155(12):1340-5.
29. Klassen TP, Feldman ME, Watters LK et al. Nebulized budesonide for children with mild-to-moderate croup. *N Engl J Med* 1994;331(5):285-9.
30. Donaldson D, Poleski D, Knipple E et al. Intramuscular versus oral dexamethasone for the treatment of moderate-to-severe croup: a randomized, double-blind trial. *Acad Emerg Med* 2003;10(1):16-21.
31. Rittichier KK, Ledwith CA. Outpatient treatment of moderate croup with dexamethasone: intramuscular versus oral dosing. *Pediatrics* 2000;106(6):1344-8.
32. Geelhoed GC, Macdonald WB. Oral dexamethasone in the treatment of croup: 0.15 mg/kg versus 0.3 mg/kg versus 0.6 mg/kg. *Pediatr Pulmonol* 1995;20(6):362-8.
33. Chub-Uppakarn S, Sangsupawanich P. A randomized comparison of dexamethasone 0.15 mg/kg for the treatment of moderate to severe croup. *Int J Pediatr Otorhinolaryngol* 2007;71(3):473-7.
34. Fifoot AA, Ting JY. Comparison between single-dose oral prednisolone and oral dexamethasone in the treatment of croup: a randomized, double-blinded clinical trial. *Emerg Med Australas* 2007;19(1):51-8.
35. Alsheri M, Almegamsi T, Hammdi A. Efficacy of a small dose of oral dexamethasone in croup. *Biomed Res (Aligarh)* 2005;16:65-72.
36. Klassen TP, Craig WR, Moher D et al. Nebulized budesonide and oral dexamethasone for treatment of croup: a randomized controlled trial. *JAMA* 1998;279(20):1629-32.
37. Geelhoed GC, Macdonald WB. Oral and inhaled steroids in croup: a randomized, placebo-controlled trial. *Pediatr Pulmonol* 1995;20(6):355-61.
38. Geelhoed GC. Budesonide offers no advantage when added to oral dexamethasone in the treatment of croup. *Pediatr Emerg Care* 2005;21(6):359-62.

39. Johnson DW, Schuh S, Koren G et al. Outpatient treatment of croup with nebulized dexamethasone. *Arch Pediatr Adolesc Med* 1996;150(4):349-55.
40. Patel H, Macarthur C, Johnson D et al. Recent corticosteroid use and the risk of complicated varicella in otherwise immunocompetent children. *Arch Pediatr Adolesc Med* 1996;150(4):409-14.
41. Adair JC, Ring WH, Jordan WS et al. Ten-year experience with IPPB in the treatment of acute laryngotracheobronchitis. *Anesth Analg* 1971;50(4):649-55.
42. Gardner HG, Powell KR, Roden VJ et al. The evaluation of racemic epinephrine in the treatment of infectious croup. *Pediatrics* 1973;52(1):52-5.
43. Fogel JM, Berg IJ, Gerber MA et al. Racemic epinephrine in the treatment of croup: nebulization alone versus nebulization with intermittent positive pressure breathing. *J Pediatr* 1982;101(6):1028-31.
44. Corkey CW, Barker GA, Edmonds JF et al. Radiographic tracheal diameter measurements in acute infectious croup: an objective scoring system. *Crit Care Med* 1981;9(8):587-90.
45. Taussig LM, Castro O, Beaudry PH et al. Treatment of laryngotracheobronchitis (croup). Use of intermittent positive-pressure breathing and racemic epinephrine. *Am J Dis Child* 1975;129(7):790-3.
46. Bjornson C, Russell KF, Vandermeer T et al. Nebulized epinephrine for croup in children. *Cochrane Database Syst Rev* 2013;10:CD006619.
47. Rizos JD, DiGravio BE, Sehl MJ et al. The disposition of children with croup treated with racemic epinephrine and dexamethasone in the emergency department. *J Emerg Med* 1998;16(4):535-9.
48. Corneli HM, Bolte RG. Outpatient use of racemic epinephrine in croup. *Am Fam Physician* 1992;46(3):683-4.
49. Kelley PB, Simon JE. Racemic epinephrine use in croup and disposition. *Am J Emerg Med* 1992;10(3):181-3.
50. Ledwith CA, Shea LM, Mauro RD. Safety and efficacy of nebulized racemic epinephrine in conjunction with oral dexamethasone and mist in the outpatient treatment of croup. *Ann Emerg Med* 1995;25(3):331-7.
51. Kunkel NC, Baker MD. Use of racemic epinephrine, dexamethasone, and mist in the outpatient management of croup. *Pediatr Emerg Care* 1996;12(3):156-9.
52. Waisman Y, Klein BL, Boenning DA et al. Prospective randomized double-blind study comparing L-epinephrine and racemic epinephrine aerosols in the treatment of laryngotracheitis (croup). *Pediatrics* 1992;89(2):302-6.
53. Butte MJ, Nguyen BX, Hutchison TJ et al. Pediatric myocardial infarction after racemic epinephrine administration. *Pediatrics* 1999;104(1):e9.

Respiratory Disorders

Chapter 56
Viral Rhinitis

Timothy P. Lynch, MD, FRCPC

Goals of Therapy

- Lessen interference with activities of daily living
- Reduce the discomfort and emotional distress of rhinorrhea
- Relieve the discomfort of nasal congestion
- Minimize the potential adverse effects of pharmacologic agents
- Prevent infection
- Prevent person-to-person transmission

Investigations

- Diagnosis of the common cold, which is most commonly due to a rhinovirus infection, requires no specific laboratory investigation
- The incubation period for rhinovirus illness is short, generally 1–2 days. Virus shedding coincides with the onset of illness or may begin shortly before symptoms develop
- History with particular attention to intensity, frequency and severity of symptoms
  - early symptoms of a cold include headache, chills, sneezing and sore throat. Later symptoms include nasal discharge, nasal obstruction, cough and malaise. Symptoms may last from a few days to 2 weeks[1]
  - symptoms of the flu are more severe than those of colds and typically include abrupt onset of fever, severe myalgias, anorexia, sore throat, headache and cough.[2] See Chapter 116
  - symptoms of sinus headache, difficulty breathing or chest pain suggest bacterial infection

Therapeutic Choices

Viral rhinitis is usually a benign, self-limited condition. Typical symptoms of rhinorrhea and nasal congestion resolve untreated in 7–10 days. There is no evidence that treatment of the rhinitis lessens the risk of developing a complication such as middle ear effusion, otitis media, sinusitis, a febrile seizure or an asthma exacerbation.[3] To improve these symptoms and the patient's quality of life, nonpharmacologic and pharmacologic approaches are available. Each pharmacologic agent employed should be directed against a specific symptom.

Nonpharmacologic Choices

- Avoiding close contact with someone who has a cold is key to prevention.[3]
- Limit the risk of inoculation and transmission by adhering to strict hand-washing techniques,[4] abstaining from touching eyes or nose, and sneezing or coughing into the elbow or into a facial tissue which is then discarded immediately.
- Maintain usual fluid intake.[5]
- Encourage rest.

Pharmacologic Choices

Figure 1 provides an approach to the symptomatic treatment of viral rhintis. Dosing information for the medications discussed can be found in Table 1.

Decongestants (Alpha-adrenergic Agents)

Decongestants are used to relieve nasal congestion and improve rhinorrhea. They help most adults by improving nasal air flow. A single dose is effective for the short-term relief (3–10 hours) of congestion in adults.[6] There is insufficient evidence to support their use in children under the age of 12 years.[7] Decongestants are available in oral or intranasal dosage forms. **Pseudoephedrine** is an effective oral treatment for nasal congestion in adults.[8,9] Multiple doses of pseudoephedrine over a 3-day period are safe.[9] Evaluations of the effectiveness of oral **phenylephrine** have yielded conflicting results.[10,11]

Anticholinergic Agents

Intranasal **ipratropium** blocks cholinergic-mediated vasodilatation. It is effective for rhinorrhea and relief of sneezing but does not improve nasal congestion.[12] Adverse effects include nasal dryness, blood-tinged mucous and epistaxis.

Antihistamines

The anticholinergic effects of some first-generation antihistamines may reduce nasal secretions, but there is no evidence in children or adults that they improve recovery time from colds when used as monotherapy. In addition, the incidence of sedation is higher than with placebo for these medications.[13] **Antihistamine/decongestant** combinations have been shown to improve short-term nasal symptoms in adolescents and adults with viral rhinitis.[14]

Figure 1: **Management of Viral Rhinitis**

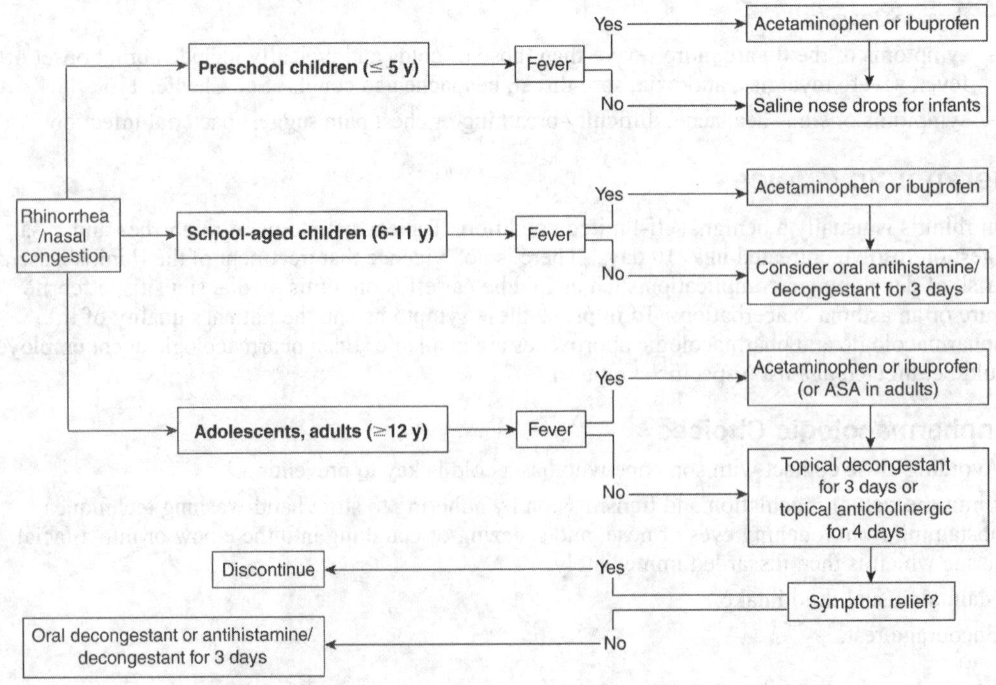

Second-generation or nonsedating antihistamines have no anticholinergic activity.[3] There is no evidence to support their use alone in controlling rhinorrhea or nasal congestion secondary to viral rhinitis.[15]

Vitamin C

Daily vitamin C (ascorbic acid) supplementation is not effective in the prevention of colds in the general population but may be useful in those exposed to brief periods of extreme physical stress (e.g., marathons, arctic expeditions).[16] However, daily supplementation (1 g) is associated with a reduction in duration and possibly severity of symptoms. Ingestion of high "treatment" doses (4–8 g) at the onset of cold symptoms has not been shown to reduce the duration of cold symptoms or their severity.[16]

Vitamin D

Randomized controlled trials have not shown a benefit of regular vitamin D supplementation on the incidence, severity or duration of upper respiratory tract infections.[17,18]

Zinc Lozenges

Zinc lozenges appear to reduce the duration of the common cold by 1–1.5 days when initiated within 24 hours of symptom onset, although this is based on low quality evidence and significant heterogeneity.[19,20] It is difficult to make recommendations with respect to its dose and duration. Zinc has an unpleasant taste and may cause nausea.

Antibiotics

Antibiotic use is not effective in the treatment of the common cold in children or adults. GI adverse effects are significantly increased in adults who take antibiotics for their colds.[21] In addition, their use may contribute to antibiotic resistance in the community.

Natural Health Products

Chinese Herbal Medicines

There are no studies to support the use of Chinese herbal medicines in the treatment of the common cold.[22]

Echinacea

Echinacea products are extracted from different species and parts of the plant, making it difficult to compare studies. A Cochrane review found that although none of 12 individual prevention studies using various *Echinacea* products demonstrated a significant difference in participants experiencing a cold, a significant 10–20% relative risk reduction was observed when the studies were pooled.[23] While statistically significant it is unclear if this small decrease is of clinical relevance. In the same review treatment trials were mixed with no clear conclusions. In addition, conclusions regarding its use in children could not be drawn from this review; however, one study reported a 5% increase in rash in the *Echinacea* treatment group.

Garlic

There is no evidence to support the use of garlic in the treatment of the common cold.[24]

North American Ginseng Extract

A systematic review of 5 heterogeneous trials found insufficient evidence that North American ginseng extract (*Panax quinquefolius*), or COLD-FX (Table 2), reduces the incidence or severity of the common cold.[25] However, ginseng may reduce the total number of days with upper respiratory tract symptoms by about 6 days if used daily for up to 4 months. The main side effect was GI upset. There are no efficacy studies for use of ginseng in children or for treatment of the common cold. In conclusion, evidence is insufficient to recommend ginseng for the prevention [Evidence: SORT B*] or treatment [Evidence: SORT C*] of the common cold.

Nonprescription Cough and Cold Medications

There is no evidence to support the use of these agents for the symptomatic treatment of *cough* in children and adults.[26] Furthermore, Health Canada now requires manufacturers to label nonprescription cough and cold medications to indicate they should not be used by children under 6 years of age.[27,28]

Appropriate Treatment for Specific Age Groups

Acetaminophen or **ibuprofen** may be helpful for fever or headache in *preschool children*. ASA should not be used in children due to the increased incidence of Reye's syndrome associated with its use during influenza virus infections. Breast- or bottle-fed infants who are obligate nose breathers may benefit from regular administration of **normal saline drops,** which aid in cleaning the nose and may improve mucociliary clearance in young infants.[29]

Studies examining the use of antihistamines, decongestants or antihistamine/decongestant combinations in children less than 6 years of age have failed to show benefit.[6,30] In addition, accidental ingestion and dosing errors with these products can do much harm.

There have been few trials in *school-aged children*. An antihistamine/decongestant/antitussive combination is superior to an antihistamine/expectorant combination in reducing nasal symptoms.[14] There are no published trials that evaluate topical nasal decongestants in children. Antihistamine/decongestant combinations may be of benefit but risks of treatment should be carefully considered.[13]

In *adolescents* and *adults*, decongestants (topical or oral) and antihistamine/decongestant combinations have been shown to improve short-term nasal symptoms.[14] Oral decongestants are associated with an increased number of adverse effects.[14] Prolonged use (usually over 5 days) of topical nasal decongestants is associated with rebound congestion (rhinitis medicamentosa).[31] Anticholinergic agents have also been shown to improve rhinorrhea.[15] A short course of topical decongestants or topical anticholinergic agents is first-line therapy.

Choices during Pregnancy and Breastfeeding

Women may experience symptoms of the common cold with increased frequency during their pregnancy.[32] The common cold in the first trimester may be a modest risk factor for birth defects.[33]

There are few trials that have studied the effects of viral rhinitis treatment during pregnancy. The first-generation antihistamines, **diphenhydramine** and **chlorpheniramine**, have not been shown to increase the risk of malformations.[34,35] Conflicting reports suggest a possible increased risk of malformations with first-trimester use of oral decongestants (**pseudoephedrine** and **phenylephrine**) and therefore they are best avoided in the first trimester.[36,37] Although data are limited, **oxymetazoline** and **xylometazoline** are considered relatively safe during pregnancy for short-term use and may be preferred over oral agents in the first trimester.[32,36] There are no published data regarding the use of **anticholinergics** during pregnancy for patients with asthma or rhinitis.[38]

The recommended dietary allowance of vitamin C increases in pregnancy (80–85 mg/day) and adequate intake is an important consideration in pregnancy.[39] However, a higher incidence of intrauterine growth restriction was observed in women taking **vitamin C** (1 g) in combination with **Vitamin E** (400 IU) in a study designed to evaluate their role in prevention of pre-eclampsia.[40,41] This brings into question the safety of high-dose vitamin C in pregnancy and therefore its use is not

* SORT (Strength of Recommendation Taxonomy) is a rating system (A, B or C) that addresses the quality of available evidence. For more information consult **How to Use *Compendium of Therapeutic Choices*** on page xxv.

recommended for this self-limiting condition. The safety of ***Echinacea*** use during pregnancy remains to be established.[42,43] The active component of **ginseng**, ginsenoside Rb1, was teratogenic in animal studies, therefore caution is advised in pregnancy.[44] There are no published studies of **zinc** therapy for viral rhinitis during pregnancy.

Though little evidence is available, most of the above agents are considered probably safe while breastfeeding with the exception of ***Echinacea*** and **ginseng** where insufficient data are available to assess. Caution is advised.

A discussion of general principles on the use of medications in these special populations can be found in Appendix II and Appendix III. Other specialized reference sources are also provided in these appendices.

Therapeutic Tips

- There is insufficient evidence to support the practice of inhaling steam.[45]
- There is evidence that single-dose **oral** or **nasal decongestants** are effective for the relief of congestion in adults.[6]
- There is no evidence to support the use of intranasal corticosteroids for the treatment of the common cold.[46]
- Inhaled **menthol** does not seem to affect nasal air flow.[47] However, it is associated with increased patient perception of nasal patency. No significant reduction in cough is observed.[48] A study in 138 children found that parents reported superior relief of their children's nocturnal cough, congestion and sleep difficulty caused by upper respiratory tract infection with vapor rub ointment (containing menthol, camphor and eucalyptus) compared to petrolatum and no treatment. The vapor rub was applied to the child's chest and neck before bedtime.[49] Due to concerns of increased production and decreased clearance of mucus potentially leading to respiratory distress in children, menthol and camphor rubs should never be placed directly under or in the nostrils.[50] In addition, menthol and camphor rubs should not be used in children under 2 years of age. Camphor-containing products can pose a risk of toxicity in children when used inappropriately.[51]

Table 1: Drugs Used in the Management of Symptoms of Viral Rhinitis

Class	Drug	Dose	Adverse Effects	Drug Interactions	Comments	Cost[a]
Anticholinergic Agents	*ipratropium bromide* Atrovent Nasal Spray, generics	Adults and children ≥12 y: 0.06%: 2 sprays in each nostril TID–QID PRN	Nosebleeds, nasal dryness, dry mouth or throat.		Avoid accidental release of nasal spray into eyes.	$$
Decongestants, oral	*pseudoephedrine* Eltor 120, Sudafed 12 Hour, generics	Adults and children ≥12 y: 60 mg Q4–6H PRN or 120 mg SR Q12H; maximum 240 mg/24h po Children 6–11 y: 30 mg Q4–6H PRN; maximum 120 mg/24h po	Insomnia, tremor, irritability, headache, palpitations, tachycardia, urinary retention.	Beta-blockers: antihypertensive effects may be reduced. MAOIs and ergot derivatives may enhance the hypertensive effect of pseudoephedrine. Concurrent use and use within 14 days of discontinuation of MAOIs is contraindicated. SNRIs (e.g., venlafaxine) may enhance the tachycardic and vasopressor effects of pseudoephedrine.	No published evidence to support use of antihistamines, decongestants or antihistamine-decongestant combinations in children <6 y of age. In addition, accidental ingestion and dosing errors can do much harm. Contraindicated in patients with severe hypertension and coronary artery disease. Use with caution in cardiovascular disease, diabetes, hyperthyroidism, prostatic hyperplasia and angle-closure glaucoma. Slow-release formulations are not recommended in children <12 y.	$
Decongestants, nasal	*oxymetazoline* Claritin Allergic Congestion Relief, Dristan Long Lasting Nasal Spray, Drixoral, generics	Adults and children ≥12 y: 0.05%: 2 or 3 sprays in each nostril Q10–12H PRN; maximum 2 doses/24h	Transient burning, stinging and dryness of nasal mucosa. Rebound congestion may occur with >3–5 days of continuous use. Topical products are associated with fewer systemic adverse effects than oral decongestants.	MAOIs: avoid combination. Risk persists for 2 weeks following discontinuation of nonselective MAOIs (e.g., phenelzine).	Use with caution in patients with hypertension, diabetes, cardiovascular disease, prostatic hyperplasia or hyperthyroidism. Caution is advised around young children as small amounts (1–2 mL) can lead to serious adverse events in children.[52]	$
	phenylephrine (ingredient in combination products) Dristan Nasal Mist, Soframycin Nasal Spray	Adults and children ≥12 y: 0.25% or 0.5%: 2–3 sprays in each nostril no more than Q4H; maximum 6 doses/24h	See oxymetazoline.	See oxymetazoline.	See oxymetazoline.	$

Class	Drug	Dose	Adverse Effects	Drug Interactions	Comments	Cost[a]
	xylometazoline Balminil Nasal Decongestant, Otrivin, generics	Adults and children ≥12 y: 0.05 % or 0.1%: 1–2 sprays or 2–3 drops each nostril Q8–10H PRN; maximum 3 doses/24h	See oxymetazoline.	See oxymetazoline.	See oxymetazoline.	$
Decongestant/ Antihistamine, first-generation Combinations	*phenylephrine/ brompheniramine* Dimetapp Preparations, generics	Consult individual product labels; dose based on phenylephrine content: Adults: 10 mg Q4H; maximum 60 mg/24h po Children 6–11 y: 5 mg Q4H; maximum 30 mg/24h po	Decongestant: See pseudoephedrine. Antihistamine: drowsiness, fatigue, anticholinergic effects such as dry eyes, dry mouth and urinary retention. Paradoxical stimulatory effects may occur in children and the elderly.	Decongestant: See pseudoephedrine. Antihistamine: additive CNS depressive effects with alcohol and other CNS depressants.	See pseudoephedrine.	$
	pseudoephedrine ● *(ingredient in combination products)* Drixoral Preparations, generics	Consult individual product labels; dose based on pseudoephedrine content: Adults and children ≥12 y: 60 mg Q4–6H PRN or 120 mg SR Q12H; maximum 240 mg/24h po Children 6–11 y: 30 mg Q4–6H PRN; maximum 120 mg/24h po	Decongestant: See pseudoephedrine. Antihistamine: drowsiness, fatigue, anticholinergic effects such as dry eyes, dry mouth and urinary retention. Paradoxical stimulatory effects may occur in children and the elderly.	Decongestant: See pseudoephedrine. Antihistamine: additive CNS depressive effects with alcohol and other CNS depressants.	See pseudoephedrine.	$

[a] Cost of one unit (spray pump, drops) or 100 mL of liquid or 12 tablets; includes drug cost only.

● Dosage adjustment may be required in renal impairment; see Appendix I.

Abbreviations: CNS = central nervous system; MAOI = monoamine oxidase inhibitor; SNRI = serotonin-norepinephrine reuptake inhibitor; SR = sustained release

Legend: $ < $10 $$ $10–20

Table 2: Natural Health Products Used in the Prevention of Viral Rhinitis

Class	Drug	Dose	Drug Interactions	Comments	Cost[a]
Natural Health Products	*North American ginseng—Panax quinquefolium* COLD-FX, generics	Prevention: 200 mg BID po for 4 months on an empty stomach at the onset of cold season[53]	Decreased INR with concomitant warfarin use.	May cause hypoglycemia; use with caution in diabetes.	$$

[a] Cost of 18 tablets; includes drug cost only.
Legend: $ < $5 $$ $5–10

Suggested Readings

Allan GM, Arroll B. Prevention and treatment of the common cold: making sense of the evidence. *CMAJ* 2014;186(3):190-9.

Arroll B. Non-antibiotic treatments for upper-respiratory tract infections (common cold). *Respir Med* 2005;99(12):1477-84.

Gentile DA, Skoner DP. Viral rhinitis. *Curr Allergy Asthma Rep* 2001;1(3):227-34.

Smith MB, Feldman W. Over-the-counter cold medications. A critical review of clinical trials between 1950 and 1991. *JAMA* 1993;269(17):2258-63.

References

1. Eccles R. Understanding the symptoms of the common cold and influenza. *Lancet Infect Dis* 2005;5(11):718-25.
2. Monto AS, Gravenstein S, Elliott M et al. Clinical signs and symptoms predicting influenza infection. *Arch Intern Med* 2000;160(21):3243-7.
3. Fireman P. Pathophysiology and pharmacotherapy of common upper respiratory diseases. *Pharmacotherapy* 1993;13(6 Pt 2):101S-9S.
4. Ryan MA, Christian RS, Wohlrabe J. Handwashing and respiratory illness among young adults in military training. *Am J Prev Med* 2001;21(2):79-83.
5. Guppy MP, Mickan SM, Del Mar CB et al. Advising patients to increase fluid intake for treating acute respiratory infections. *Cochrane Database Syst Rev* 2013;2:CD004419.
6. Arroll B. Non-antibiotic treatments for upper-respiratory tract infections (common cold). *Respir Med* 2005;99(12):1477-84.
7. Taverner D, Latte J. Nasal decongestants for the common cold. *Cochrane Database Syst Rev* 2007;(1):CD001953.
8. Latte J, Taverner D, Slobodian P et al. A randomized, double-blind, placebo-controlled trial of pseudoephedrine in coryza. *Clin Exp Pharmacol Physiol* 2004;31(7):429-32.
9. Eccles R, Jawad MS, Jawad SS et al. Efficacy and safety of single and multiple doses of pseudoephedrine in the treatment of nasal congestion associated with common cold. *Am J Rhinol* 2005;19(1):25-31.
10. Hatton RC, Winterstein AG, McKelvey RP et al. Efficacy and safety of oral phenylephrine: systematic review and meta-analysis. *Ann Pharmacother* 2007;41(3):381-90.
11. Kollar C, Schneider H, Waksman J et al. Meta-analysis of the efficacy of a single dose of phenylephrine 10 mg compared with placebo in adults with acute nasal congestion due to the common cold. *Clin Ther* 2007;29(6):1057-70.
12. Albalawi ZH, Othman SS, Alfaleh K. Intranasal ipratropium bromide for the common cold. *Cochrane Database Syst Rev* 2013;6:CD008231.
13. Sutter AI, Lemiengre M, Campbell H et al. Antihistamines for the common cold. *Cochrane Database Syst Rev* 2003;(3):CD001267.
14. De Sutter AI, van Driel ML, Kumar AA et al. Oral antihistamine-decongestant-analgesic combinations for the common cold. *Cochrane Database Syst Rev* 2012;2:CD004976.
15. Luks D, Anderson MR. Antihistamines and the common cold. A review and critique of the literature. *J Gen Intern Med* 1996;11(4):240-4.
16. Hemila H, Chalker E. Vitamin C for preventing and treating the common cold. *Cochrane Database Syst Rev* 2013;1:CD000980.
17. Murdoch DR, Slow S, Chambers ST et al. Effect of vitamin D3 supplementation on upper respiratory tract infections in healthy adults: the VIDARIS randomized controlled trial. *JAMA* 2012;308(13):1333-9.
18. Rees JR, Hendricks K, Barry EL et al. Vitamin D3 supplementation and upper respiratory tract infections in a randomized, controlled trial. *Clin Infect Dis* 2013;57(10):1384-92.
19. Singh M, Das RR. Zinc for the common cold. *Cochrane Database Syst Rev* 2013;6:CD001364.
20. Science M, Johnstone J, Roth DE et al. Zinc for the treatment of the common cold: a systematic review and meta-analysis of randomized controlled trials. *CMAJ* 2012;184(10):E551-61.
21. Kenealy T, Arroll B. Antibiotics for the common cold and acute purulent rhinitis. *Cochrane Database Syst Rev* 2013;6:CD000247.
22. Wu T, Zhang J, Qiu Y et al. Chinese medicinal herbs for the common cold. *Cochrane Database Syst Rev* 2007;(1):CD004782.
23. Karsch-Völk M, Barrett B, Kiefer D et al. Echinacea for preventing and treating the common cold. *Cochrane Database Syst Rev* 2014;2:CD000530.
24. Lissiman E, Bhasale AL, Cohen M. Garlic for the common cold. *Cochrane Database Syst Rev* 2012;3:CD006206.
25. Seida JK, Durec T, Kuhle S. North American (Panax quinquefolius) and Asian Ginseng (Panax ginseng) preparations for prevention of the common cold in healthy adults: a systematic review. *Evid Based Complement Alternat Med* 2011;2011:282151.
26. Smith SM, Schroeder K, Fahey T. Over-the-counter (OTC) medications for acute cough in children and adults in ambulatory settings. *Cochrane Database Syst Rev* 2012;8:CD001831.
27. Health Canada. *Health Canada releases decision on the labelling of cough and cold products for children*. Ottawa (ON): Health Canada; 2008. Available from: www.healthycanadians.gc.ca/recall-alert-rappel-avis/hc-sc/2008/13267a-eng.php. Accessed April 4, 2011.
28. Shefrin AE, Goldman RD. Use of over-the-counter cough and cold medications in children. *Can Fam Physician* 2009;55(11):1081-3.
29. Jones NS. Current concepts in the management of paediatric rhinosinusitis. *J Laryngol Otol* 1999;113(1):1-9.
30. Clemens CJ, Taylor JA, Almquist JR et al. Is an antihistamine-decongestant combination effective in temporarily relieving symptoms of the common cold in preschool children? *J Pediatr* 1997;130(3):463-6.
31. Graf P. Rhinitis medicamentosa: aspects of pathophysiology and treatment. *Allergy* 1997;52(40 Suppl):28-34.
32. Erebara A, Bozzo P, Einarson A et al. Treating the common cold during pregnancy. *Can Fam Physician* 2008;54(5):687-9.
33. Zhang J, Cai WW. Association of the common cold in the first trimester of pregnancy with birth defects. *Pediatrics* 1993;92(4):559-63.
34. Seto A, Einarson T, Koren G. Pregnancy outcome following first trimester exposure to antihistamines: meta-analysis. *Am J Perinatol* 1997;14(3):119-24.
35. Schatz M, Petitti D. Antihistamines and pregnancy. *Ann Allergy Asthma Immunol* 1997;78(2):157-9.
36. Wallace DV, Dykewicz MS, Bernstein DI et al. The diagnosis and management of rhinitis: an updated practice parameter. *J Allergy Clin Immunol* 2008;122(2 Suppl):S1-84.
37. Briggs GG, Freeman RK, Yaffe SJ. *Drugs in pregnancy and lactation: a reference guide to fetal and neonatal risk*. 9th ed. Philadelphia (PA): Wolters Kluwer Health; Lippincott Williams & Wilkins; 2011.

38. National Heart, Lung, and Blood Institute; National Asthma Education and Prevention Program Asthma and Pregnancy Working Group. NAEPP expert panel report. Managing asthma during pregnancy: recommendations for pharmacologic treatment-2004 update. *J Allergy Clin Immunol* 2005;115(1):34-46.
39. Health Canada. *Dietary reference intakes tables*. Available from: www.hc-sc.gc.ca/fn-an/nutrition/reference/table/index-eng.php. Accessed May 28, 2014.
40. Goh YI, Ungar W, Rovet J et al. Mega-dose vitamin C and E in preventing FASD: the decision to terminate the study prematurely. *J FAS Int* 2007;5:e3. Available from: www.motherisk.org/JFAS_documents/JFAS7002_5_e3.pdf. Accessed April 4, 2011.
41. Poston L, Briley AL, Seed PT et al. Vitamin C and vitamin E in pregnant women at risk for pre-eclampsia (VIP trial): randomised placebo-controlled trial. *Lancet* 2006:367(9517):1145-54.
42. Gallo M, Sarkar M, Au W et al. Pregnancy outcome following gestational exposure to echinacea: a prospective controlled study. *Arch Intern Med* 2000;160(20):3141-3.
43. Perri D, Dugoua JJ, Mills E et al. Safety and efficacy of echinacea (Echinacea angustifolia, e. purpurea and e. Pallida) during pregnancy and lactation. *Can J Clin Pharmacol* 2006;13(3):e262-7.
44. Liu P, Xu Y, Yin H et al. Developmental toxicity research of ginsenoside Rb1 using a whole mouse embryo culture model. *Birth Defects Res B Dev Reprod Toxicol* 2005;74(2):207-9.
45. Singh M, Singh M. Heated, humidified air for the common cold. *Cochrane Database Syst Rev* 2013;6:CD001728.
46. Hayward G, Thompson MJ, Perera R et al. Corticosteroids for the common cold. *Cochrane Database Syst Rev* 2012;8:CD008116.
47. Pereira EJ, Sim L, Driver H et al. The effect of inhaled menthol on upper airway resistance in humans: a randomized controlled crossover study. *Can Respir J* 2013;20(1):e1-4.
48. Kenia P, Houghton T, Beardsmore C. Does inhaling menthol affect nasal patency or cough? *Pediatr Pulmonol* 2008;43(6):532-7.
49. Paul IM, Beiler JS, King TS et al. Vapor rub, petrolatum, and no treatment for children with nocturnal cough and cold symptoms. *Pediatrics* 2010;126(6):1092-9.
50. Abanses JC, Arima S, Rubin BK. Vicks VapoRub induces mucin secretion, decreases ciliary beat frequency, and increases tracheal mucus transport in the ferret trachea. *Chest* 2009;135(1):143-8.
51. Camphor revisited: focus on toxicity. Committee on Drugs. American Academy of Pediatrics. *Pediatrics* 1994;94(1):127-8.
52. U.S. Food and Drug Administration. *FDA Drug Safety Communication: Serious adverse events from accidental ingestion of OTC eye drops and nasal sprays by children*. Available from: www.fda.gov/drugs/drugsafety/ucm325257.htm. Accessed May 14, 2014.
53. Predy GN, Goel V, Lovlin R et al. Efficacy of an extract of North American ginseng containing poly-furanosyl-pyranosyl-saccharides for preventing upper respiratory tract infections: a randomized controlled trial. *CMAJ* 2005;173(9):1043-8.

Chapter 57
Chronic Liver Diseases

Mark G. Swain, MSc, MD, FRCPC

This chapter discusses ascites, spontaneous bacterial peritonitis, hepatic encephalopathy, cholestatic disease (including symptom management), autoimmune chronic hepatitis, alcoholic liver disease (including alcoholic hepatitis), hemochromatosis and Wilson's disease. Management of esophageal varices is discussed in Chapter 65. Management of viral hepatitis is discussed in Chapter 66.

Goals of Therapy

- Manage symptoms associated with chronic liver conditions
- Treat complications of chronic disease, e.g., infection
- Prevent recurrence
- Delay or prevent disease progression
- Decrease liver-related mortality

Ascites (Portal Hypertension)

Investigations

- Thorough history with special attention to documented liver disease; rule out other causes of ascites
- Physical examination for features of chronic liver disease (e.g., cutaneous stigmata), hepatosplenomegaly, degree of ascites accumulation (shifting dullness, abdominal protuberance, eversion of umbilicus), signs of portal hypertension (caput medusae, venous hum) or other features of liver failure and related complications (GI bleeding, asterixis)
- Laboratory tests:
  - CBC, serum electrolytes, albumin, INR, bilirubin
  - ascitic tap (all patients with significant or worsening ascites) for neutrophil count, culture, protein/albumin
  - calculate serum-ascites albumin gradient (SAAG).[1] SAAG >11 g/L is most consistent with ascites secondary to portal hypertension and is typically responsive to diuretics, whereas a SAAG <11 g/L (infectious, malignant) is not typically responsive to diuretics.

Therapeutic Choices

Table 1 lists the drugs used to treat ascites and Figure 1 outlines the management of ascites secondary to portal hypertension.

High plasma aldosterone levels in patients with ascites result in sodium and fluid retention; thus, **spironolactone** (an aldosterone antagonist) is the diuretic of choice. The clearance of spironolactone and its active metabolites are impaired in advanced cirrhosis. Full therapeutic diuretic effects can take up to 2 weeks to be observed; adjust dose slowly in this setting. Add **furosemide** to enhance diuresis and/or control serum potassium levels. **Metolazone** can be added if ascites is refractory to spironolactone and furosemide. The combination of furosemide and metolazone can produce profound diuresis, causing volume depletion and electrolyte abnormalities (e.g., hypochloremic metabolic alkalosis, hypokalemia). Start with low doses and titrate up. **Amiloride** can be substituted for spironolactone if intolerable side effects develop.

Spontaneous Bacterial Peritonitis (SBP)

Investigations

- History of fever, abdominal pain or clinical deterioration (may present with minimal, nonspecific symptoms)
- Physical examination, other than to confirm the presence of ascites, is often unhelpful
- Laboratory tests: culture and polymorphonuclear (PMN) cell count of ascitic fluid; repeat after treatment to ensure resolution of the infection

Figure 1: Management of Ascites Secondary to Portal Hypertension

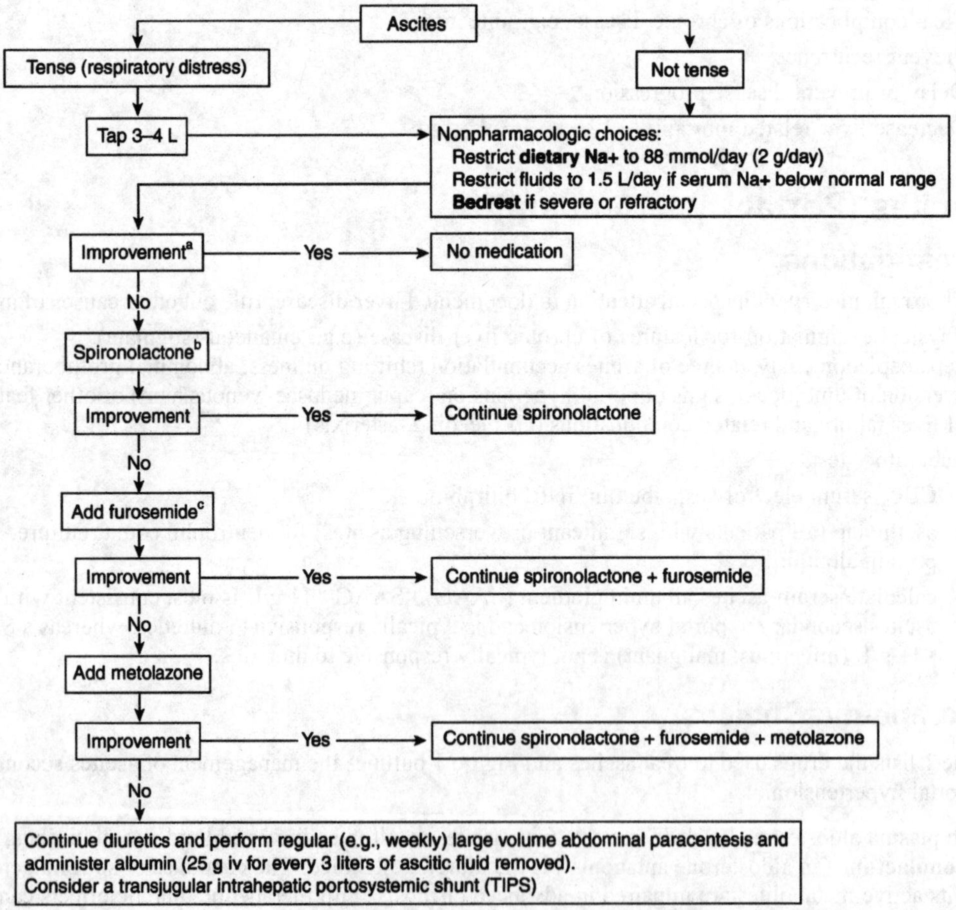

[a] Aim for weight loss of 1–1.5 kg/day in patients with peripheral edema, and 0.5–1 kg/day in patients without edema.
[b] If side effects occur (e.g., painful gynecomastia) switch to another potassium-sparing diuretic (e.g., amiloride).
[c] Spironolactone and furosemide can be started simultaneously, which often provides more predictable diuresis with better electrolyte balance. Give diuretics as single morning doses. Use the lowest effective dose to achieve adequate diuresis and monitor serum electrolytes, urea and creatinine before therapy, weekly until stabilized, then monthly. Doses can be reduced after diuresis is initiated.

Therapeutic Choices

If the PMN cell count in the ascitic fluid is $>0.25 \times 10^9$/L (250 cells/μL), treat with a third-generation cephalosporin (e.g., **cefotaxime** or **ceftriaxone**) for 5 days (Table 2) and commence intravenous infusion of **albumin** (1.5 g/kg of body weight at the time of diagnosis and 1 g/kg on day 3 of treatment).

Use prophylactic antibiotics after a patient has experienced 1 episode of SBP or in patients with renal impairment or severe liver disease (Child-Pugh score >9) whose ascites protein level is <15 g/L.[2] A patient with 1 episode of SBP has a 69% chance of recurrence within 1 year. Treatment with **sulfamethoxazole/trimethoprim**,[3] **norfloxacin**[4] or **ciprofloxacin**[5] (Table 2) decreases the rate of SBP recurrence, and, although it does not improve survival, is very cost effective.[6] Based on the best available evidence norfloxacin is considered the drug of choice.[7] Start prophylactic antibiotics after the completion of intravenous antibiotic therapy for the acute episode and continue until resolution of ascites, liver transplantation or death. Patients with an episode of SBP should be referred and considered for possible liver transplantation if eligible.

Hepatic Encephalopathy

Therapeutic Choices

Figure 2 outlines the management of hepatic encephalopathy and Table 3 lists the drugs used to treat hepatic encephalopathy. The antibiotic **rifaximin** is expensive and is indicated for the reduction in risk of overt hepatic encephalopathy recurrence in adults. It is reasonable to consider using rifaximin in individuals who are refractory to, or who cannot tolerate, **lactulose**.

Figure 2: Management of Hepatic Encephalopathy

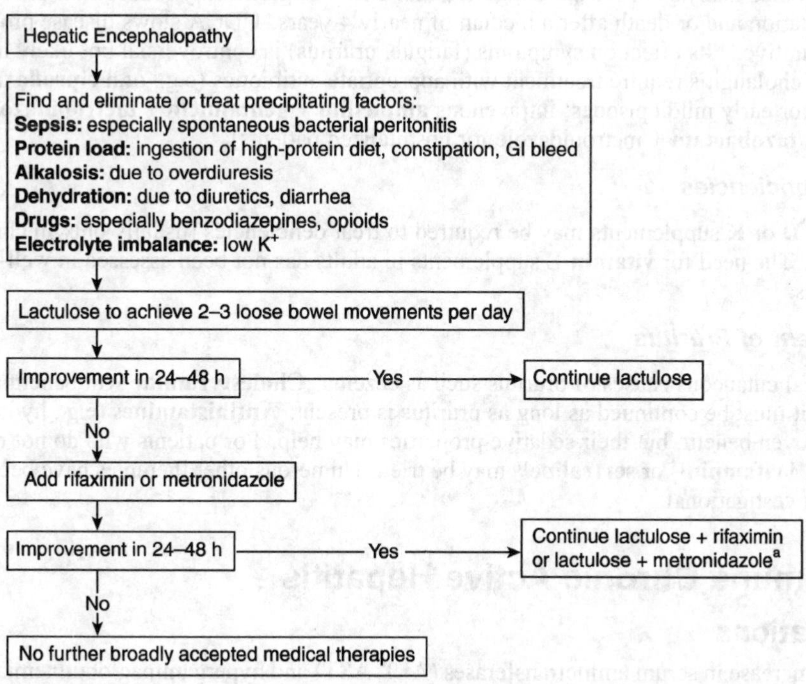

[a] Dose and duration of metronidazole should be minimized as much as possible to avoid peripheral neuropathy (usually <3 weeks).

Cholestatic Disease

Investigations

- Clinical/biochemical evidence of cholestasis (elevated alkaline phosphatase, gamma glutamyl transferase [GGT] and later bilirubin) with:
  - for *primary biliary cirrhosis (PBC):* positive antimitochondrial antibody (>95% of cases); can be confirmed by liver biopsy, although this is not absolutely required if a patient has a positive antimitochondrial antibody test and a cholestatic biochemical profile
  - for *primary sclerosing cholangitis (PSC):* ductular abnormalities (strictures, beading) on endoscopic retrograde cholangiopancreatography (ERCP) or magnetic resonance imaging (MRCP)
- Identify vitamin deficiencies by:
  - prothrombin time (elevated if vitamin K is deficient)
  - serum calcium and 25(OH)-vitamin D levels
  - serum vitamin A and/or beta-carotene levels

Therapeutic Choices

Figure 3 outlines the approach to the management of cholestatic symptoms and Table 4 lists drugs used to treat cholestatic liver disease.

Primary Biliary Cirrhosis (PBC) and Primary Sclerosing Cholangitis (PSC)

Ursodeoxycholic acid (UDCA) 13–15 mg/kg/day improves serum liver biochemical tests in patients with PBC[8,9,10] and PSC. It appears to have limited efficacy in preventing disease progression in PSC.[11] There is no benefit to using high dose UDCA (28–30 mg/kg/day) in the management of PSC.[12] In PBC, a combined analysis of 3 trials suggested that UDCA significantly reduced the probability of transplantation and/or death after a median of nearly 4 years. UDCA slows disease progression but is not curative.[13] Its effect on symptoms (fatigue, pruritus) is controversial but likely minimal. Episodes of cholangitis require treatment with appropriate antibiotics (e.g., oral **ciprofloxacin** in outpatients for early mild episodes; intravenous **ampicillin** + **gentamicin** + **metronidazole** or **piperacillin/tazobactam** + metronidazole for hospitalized patients).

Vitamin Deficiencies

Vitamin A, **D** or **K** supplements may be required to treat deficiencies (usually only in chronic cholestasis). The need for **vitamin E** supplements in adults has not been assessed in well-designed clinical trials.

Management of Pruritus

Rule out local cutaneous causes of pruritus such as eczema. **Cholestyramine** will benefit about 90% of patients; it must be continued as long as pruritus is present. **Antihistamines** (e.g., hydroxyzine) are of no proven benefit, but their sedative properties may help. For patients who do not respond, **naltrexone**,[14] **rifampin**[15] or **sertraline**[16] may be tried. Numerous other therapies have been evaluated, but all are investigational.

Autoimmune Chronic Active Hepatitis

Investigations

- Marked increase in serum aminotransferases (ALT, AST) and hypergammaglobulinemia; antinuclear antibody (ANA) is present in about 70% of patients (Type I autoimmune hepatitis)

- Diagnosis confirmed by liver biopsy

The classic patient is a young woman who presents with an acute or chronic illness characterized by lethargy, arthralgia, oligomenorrhea and fluctuating jaundice; however, symptoms and signs are often nonspecific and the disease is suspected by the findings of abnormal liver tests.

Therapeutic Choices

Immunosuppression with **corticosteroids** (Table 5), with or without **azathioprine**, prolongs life, decreases symptoms, improves serum biochemical abnormalities and diminishes hepatic inflammation on liver biopsy. The goal is to induce remission, defined as a decrease in serum aminotransferase levels to within the normal range, but at least to ≤2 times the upper limit of normal, and a follow-up liver biopsy that is normal or shows only chronic persistent hepatitis. Most patients will require therapy for up to 2 years before attempts at discontinuing **prednisone** should be considered; the majority will require lifelong therapy. If the dose of prednisone cannot be decreased below 10 mg/day, azathioprine may be added to the regimen. The combination of **mycophenolate mofetil** (up to 1 g BID po) and **prednisone** (Table 5) may be used in patients resistant to or intolerant of azathioprine.[17]

Figure 3: Management of Cholestatic Symptoms

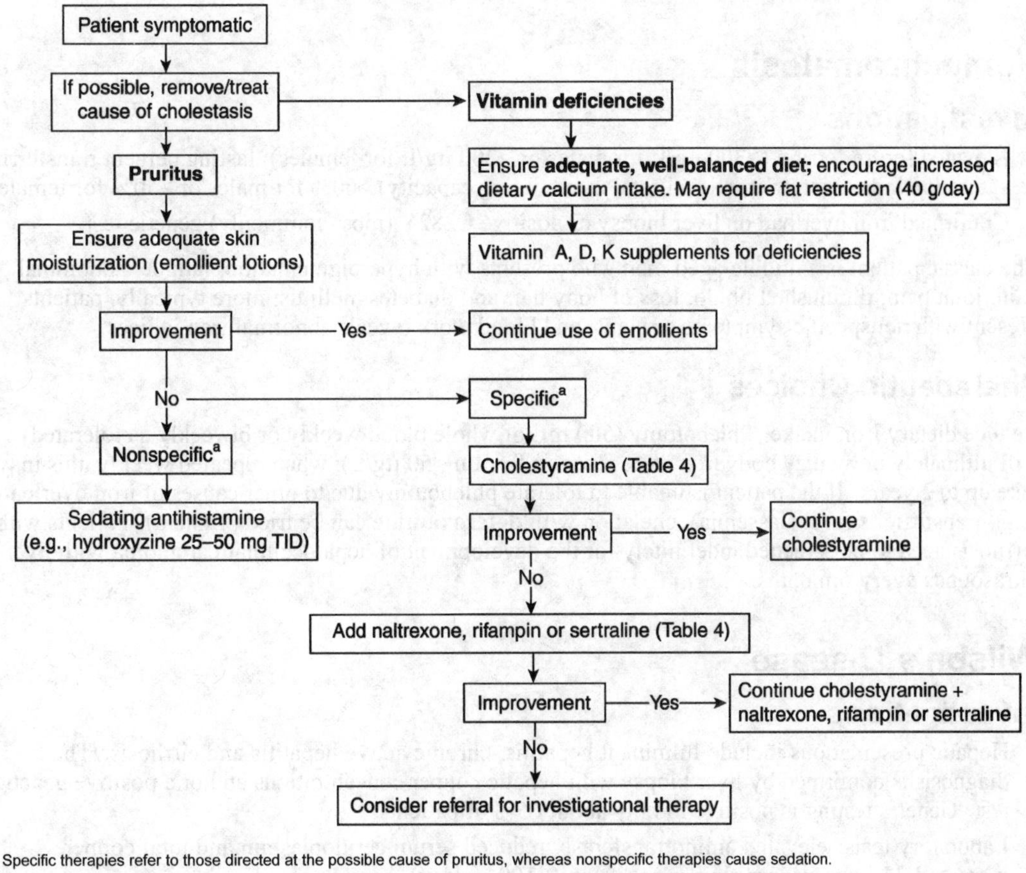

[a] Specific therapies refer to those directed at the possible cause of pruritus, whereas nonspecific therapies cause sedation.

Alcoholic Liver Disease

Investigations

- An AST to ALT ratio ≥2:1 and GGT ≥2 times the upper limit of normal strongly suggests alcohol abuse

Therapeutic Choices

Chronic Alcohol-related Liver Disease

There is no universally accepted medical therapy except *abstention from alcohol*. Long-term treatment with **propylthiouracil** or **colchicine** has been studied but results have not been encouraging.[18,19]

Alcoholic Hepatitis

Corticosteroids[20] and **pentoxifylline**[21] (Table 5) improve short-term survival in patients with severe biopsy-proven alcoholic hepatitis. Severe alcoholic hepatitis can be documented by calculating the Maddrey discriminant function: values >32 denote severe alcoholic hepatitis with a mortality rate approaching 50%.[22] Corticosteroid therapy for severe alcoholic hepatitis has been examined in numerous studies with variable results, whereas the beneficial effects of pentoxifylline have been documented in 2 studies.[21,23] A randomized controlled trial found pentoxifylline to be superior to **prednisolone** in patients with severe alcoholic hepatitis.[24]

Hemochromatosis

Investigations

- Elevated serum ferritin (>300 μg/L for males or >200 μg/L for females); fasting percent transferrin saturation index (serum iron level/total iron binding capacity) >60% for males or >50% for females.
- Confirmed iron overload on liver biopsy or positive C282Y (most commonly) genetic test.

The classic patient is a middle-aged man who presents with hyperpigmentation, fatigue, abdominal pain, joint pain, diminished libido, loss of body hair and diabetes mellitus; more typically, patients present with nonspecific symptoms or signs, and blood work reveals abnormal iron indices.

Therapeutic Choices

Reduce dietary iron intake. Phlebotomy (500 mL of whole blood weekly or biweekly as tolerated) will ultimately normalize body iron stores (serum ferritin <50 μg/L): when repeated weekly, this may take up to 2 years. If the patient is unable to tolerate phlebotomy due to other causes of iron overload (e.g., transfusions for thalassemia), chelation with **deferoxamine** can be tried (Table 6). Patients with cirrhosis need to be screened indefinitely for the development of hepatocellular carcinoma with liver ultrasounds every 6 months.

Wilson's Disease

Investigations

- Hepatic presentations include fulminant hepatitis, chronic active hepatitis and cirrhosis. The diagnosis is confirmed by liver biopsy with hepatic copper concentrations and/or a positive genetic test. Genetic testing is positive in only about 65% of patients
- Laboratory tests: elevated aminotransferase, reduced serum ceruloplasmin and total copper, increased 24-hour urinary copper excretion (>100 μg/day)

- Family history; most patients are diagnosed before age 30

Therapeutic Choices

Copper chelating agents (**penicillamine** or **trientine**) are the treatment of choice for Wilson's disease (Table 7), and treatment is lifelong. Trientine may be better tolerated, but is available only through the Special Access Programme; thus, penicillamine is the first-line agent in Canada. Give **pyridoxine** 25 mg daily with penicillamine to counteract its antipyridoxine effect. Twenty-four–hour urinary copper excretion and serum free copper levels can be monitored to ensure adequate removal of copper. Trientine may be used in patients intolerant of penicillamine. Elemental **zinc** is an option in patients intolerant of penicillamine and trientine. Recommend avoiding foods high in copper (e.g., peanuts, chocolate, liver, shellfish, mushrooms).

Choices during Pregnancy and Breastfeeding

Pregnancy in patients with chronic liver disease, especially if there is clinical evidence of liver failure (ascites, variceal bleeding, encephalopathy), is not a frequently encountered clinical issue, as in this setting conception can be very difficult if not impossible.

However, pregnancy is more commonly observed in patients with well controlled chronic liver diseases such as those caused by chronic cholestatic disorders, autoimmune hepatitis, Wilson's disease and hemochromatosis (especially in the absence of cirrhosis). There is limited available information on the effects of these diseases on pregnancy or breastfeeding.

Ursodeoxycholic acid (UDCA) has been used to treat pruritus in the setting of benign cholestasis of pregnancy. Previously, it was recommended that UDCA be avoided in the first trimester of pregnancy. Emerging evidence suggests that this medication can be used throughout pregnancy without untoward effects.[25] Avoid breastfeeding if a patient is taking UDCA.

Although **prednisone** may not cause major teratogenic defects, it may increase the risk of developing oral cleft palate and therefore is best avoided in the first trimester.[26] Prednisone is compatible with breastfeeding, and exposure of the nursing infant to this drug may be minimized if nursing is performed 3–4 h after the dose is taken by the mother.[27,28] **Azathioprine** is considered low risk in pregnancy[29] and is probably compatible with breastfeeding.[30]

The risks of using **penicillamine** in pregnancy remain unclear but the repercussions of discontinuing penicillamine in a pregnant patient with Wilson's disease may be serious. Therefore, these patients should remain on penicillamine during pregnancy but at a dose of <1 g/day. Avoid breastfeeding if the patient is receiving penicillamine; the consequences of therapy cessation are unclear.

A discussion of general principles on the use of medications in these special populations can be found in Appendix II and Appendix III. Other specialized reference sources are also provided in these appendices.

Table 1: Drugs Used to Treat Ascites

Class	Drug	Dose	Adverse Effects	Drug Interactions	Cost[a]
Diuretics	*amiloride* Midamor	Initial: 5 mg daily po May increase to 20 mg daily po	Hyperkalemia, gynecomastia, muscle cramps, hyperchloremic metabolic acidosis.	Increases serum K^+ when combined with ACE inhibitors, angiotensin receptor blockers or K^+ supplements.	$$$
	furosemide generics	Initial: 40 mg/day po Increase by 20–40 mg/day to achieve diuresis (up to 160 mg/day)	Nausea, anorexia, fatigue, weakness, decreased serum Na^+, Cl^-, K^+, Mg^{++}, hyperuricemia, hyperglycemia, volume depletion, metabolic alkalosis, rash.	Increases ototoxicity of aminoglycosides; increases digoxin toxicity (hypokalemia).	$
	metolazone Zaroxolyn	Initial: 2.5 mg/day po May increase up to 10 mg/day po	See furosemide.	Increases digoxin toxicity (hypokalemia).	$$
	spironolactone Aldactone, generics	Initial: 100–200 mg/day po Increase Q5–7 days to 400 mg/day po	Hyperkalemia, hyperchloremic metabolic acidosis, gynecomastia and mastalgia in men.	See amiloride.	$$$

[a] Cost of 30-day supply; includes drug cost only.

Dosage adjustment may be required in renal impairment; see Appendix I.

Legend: $ <$10 $$ $10–20 $$$ $20–30

Table 2: Drugs Used to Treat Spontaneous Bacterial Peritonitis

Class	Drug	Dose	Adverse Effects	Drug Interactions	Cost[a]
Cephalosporins, third-generation	*cefotaxime* ➊ Claforan	Treatment: 2 g Q8H iv × 5 days Reduce dose in severe renal impairment (ClCr <20 mL/min)	GI disturbances, hypersensitivity.		$$$$
	ceftriaxone generics	Treatment: 2 g Q24H iv × 5 days	GI disturbances, hypersensitivity, biliary pseudolithiasis (sludging).	Do not reconstitute or mix with calcium-containing solutions. Do not administer simultaneously with calcium-containing iv solutions via a Y-site. Administration may be done sequentially provided the infusion lines are thoroughly flushed between infusions.	$$$
Fluoroquinolones	*ciprofloxacin* ➊ Cipro, generics	Prophylaxis: 750 mg weekly po	GI disturbances, CNS effects, skin rash.	Absorption decreased by antacids, calcium and iron (separate administration). Increases theophylline and pentoxifylline levels.	$
	norfloxacin ➊ generics	Prophylaxis: 400 mg/day po	See ciprofloxacin.	Absorption decreased by antacids, calcium and iron (separate administration).	$
Sulfonamide Combinations	*sulfamethoxazole/trimethoprim* ➊ generics	Prophylaxis: 1 DS tablet 5 times weekly po	Nausea, vomiting, fever, hypersensitivity reactions (may be severe), blood dyscrasias.	Enhanced effect of sulfonylureas and warfarin. Increases phenytoin levels. Increases nephrotoxicity of cyclosporine.	$

[a] Cost of 30-day supply unless specified otherwise; includes drug cost.

➊ Dosage adjustment may be required in renal impairment; see Appendix I.

Legend: $ <$20 $$ $20–100 $$$ $100–200 $$$$ $200–300

Table 3: Drugs Used to Treat Hepatic Encephalopathy

Class	Drug	Dose	Adverse Effects	Drug Interactions	Cost[a]
Antibiotics	*metronidazole* Flagyl, generics	250–500 mg two or three times daily po	GI disturbances, headache, metallic taste.	Disulfiram-like reaction may be experienced with alcohol. Increases INR with warfarin. Barbiturates, phenytoin may increase metabolism of metronidazole.	$
	rifaximin Zaxine	550 mg BID po without food	Rifaximin is not significantly absorbed from the GI tract. However, absorption is increased in subjects with impaired hepatic function. Anemia, arthralgia, dizziness, dyspnea, muscle spasms, peripheral edema, pruritus, pyrexia, rash	May diminish the anticoagulant effect of warfarin.	Approx. $985
Hyperosmotic Agents	*lactulose* generics	45 mL every hour po until bowel movement and clinical improvement then maintain with 15–45 mL 1–4 times daily po (titrate to produce 2–3 loose bowel movements per day)	Bloating, flatulence, cramps, diarrhea.		$$-$$$

[a] Cost of 30-day supply; includes drug cost only.
Legend: $ <$15 $$ $15–30 $$-$$$ $15–45 $$$ $30–45

Table 4: **Drugs Used to Treat Cholestatic Liver Disease**

Class	Drug	Dose	Adverse Effects	Drug Interactions	Cost[a]
Bile Acids	*ursodiol* (ursodeoxy-cholic acid) Urso, generics	Primary biliary cirrhosis: 13–15 mg/kg/day po in 2–4 divided doses	Occasional diarrhea, leukopenia, rash.	Do not give with antacids.	$$$$
Bile Acid Sequestrants	*cholestyramine* Olestyr	Cholestatic pruritus: Initial: 4 g before and after breakfast po; may add additional 4 g doses at dinner and lunch if pruritus is not resolved	Constipation, heartburn, nausea, vomiting.	May bind other drugs given concurrently; separate doses (1 h before or 4–6 h after resin).	$$
Opiate Receptor Antagonists	*naltrexone* ReVia	Cholestatic pruritus: 50 mg daily po × 4 wk	Nausea, vomiting, headache, insomnia, dysphoria.	Precipitates opioid withdrawal in dependent patients.	$$$$$
Rifamycins	*rifampin* Rifadin, Rofact	Cholestatic pruritus: 150 mg daily po; can be increased up to 10 mg/kg/day in 2 divided doses	Rash (petechial rash may suggest thrombocytopenia), orange discolouration of body fluids (contact lens staining), GI upset, hematologic effects (e.g., thrombocytopenia).	Potent inducer of CYP450—evaluate when coadministered with other drugs (e.g., may reduce levels of cyclosporine, oral contraceptives, phenytoin, sirolimus, tacrolimus, warfarin).	$$
SSRIs	*sertraline* Zoloft, generics	Cholestatic pruritus: 50–100 mg daily po	Nausea, tremors, diarrhea, dry mouth, sexual dysfunction, increased risk of GI bleeding.	Contraindicated with MAO inhibitors (serotonin syndrome), increases risk of GI bleeding with NSAIDs. Increased levels of sertraline by CYP450 inhibitors (e.g., cimetidine, clarithromycin, erythromycin, fluconazole, itraconazole, ketoconazole, quinidine, ritonavir). Sertraline may reduce clearance of clozapine, methadone, mexiletine, phenytoin, pimozide, propafenone and reduce the activation of codeine and tamoxifen. Carbamazepine, phenobarbital and phenytoin can increase clearance of sertraline.	$
Vitamins, fat-soluble	*vitamin A*	Deficiency in patients with chronic cholestasis: 5000–10 000 IU/day po (aqueous). Use the minimum effective dose		Mineral oil decreases absorption.	$

(cont'd)

Table 4: Drugs Used to Treat Cholestatic Liver Disease *(cont'd)*

Class	Drug	Dose	Adverse Effects	Drug Interactions	Cost[a]
	vitamin D	Deficiency in patients with chronic cholestasis: 1000 IU Q2 days po (with 2–3 g elemental calcium/day)		Mineral oil decreases absorption.	$
	vitamin K	Deficiency in patients with chronic cholestasis: 10 mg monthly im		Antagonizes warfarin (decreases INR); decreased absorption with mineral oil.	$

[a] Cost of 30-day supply based on 70 kg body weight unless specified otherwise; includes drug cost only.
Legend: $ <$25 $$ $25–50 $$$ $50–100 $$$$ $100–150 $$$$$ $150–200

Table 5: Drugs Used to Treat Autoimmune Chronic Active Hepatitis and Alcoholic Hepatitis

Class	Drug	Dose	Adverse Effects	Drug Interactions	Cost[a]
Corticosteroids	*prednisone* generics	Autoimmune chronic active hepatitis: 60 mg/day po × 1 wk, then 40 mg/day × 1 wk, then 30 mg/day × 2 wk, then 20 mg/day Gradually taper from 20 mg/day over weeks to months using serum aminotransferase levels and clinical status as a guide Alcoholic hepatitis: 40 mg/day po × 28 days. Taper over 2 wk	Fluid/electrolyte imbalance, suppression of pituitary-adrenal function, hyperglycemia, peptic ulcer, behavioural disturbances, ocular cataracts, glaucoma, cushingoid syndrome, aseptic necrosis of hip. Increases risk of infections.	Increases GI ulceration with NSAID; decreased efficacy with barbiturates, phenytoin, rifampin; decreases effect of vaccines.	$
Immunosuppressants	*azathioprine* (kidney symbol) Imuran, generics	Autoimmune hepatitis: 50–150 mg/day po	Decreased appetite, leukopenia, thrombocytopenia (monitor CBC monthly), infection, biliary stasis, hypersensitivity reactions, rash, rare veno-occlusive disease, nausea, vomiting, pancreatitis.	Increased toxicity with allopurinol.	$$
	mycophenolate mofetil Cellcept, Apo-Mycophenolate, other generics	Autoimmune hepatitis: 500–1000 mg BID po	Anemia, leucopenia, thrombocytopenia.	Antacids, iron and cholestyramine decrease absorption of mycophenolate.	$60–120
Xanthines	*pentoxifylline* generics	Alcoholic hepatitis: 400 mg TID po × 4 wk	Dizziness, headache, nausea, vomiting, heartburn, chest pain, rash, tremor, flushing.	Cimetidine and ciprofloxacin increase pentoxifylline levels; increases theophylline levels.	$$$$

[a] Cost of 30-day supply unless specified otherwise; includes drug cost only.
(kidney symbol) Dosage adjustment may be required in renal impairment; see Appendix I.
Legend: $ <$15 $$ $15-30 $$$ $30-45 $$$$ $45-60

Table 6: Drugs Used to Treat Iron Overload in Hemochromatosis

Class	Drug	Dose	Adverse Effects	Drug Interactions	Cost[a]
Chelating Agents	*deferoxamine*[b] Desferal, generics	1–4 g sc by minipump over 12 h, adjusted on an individual basis	Allergic reactions, auditory/ocular toxicity, tachycardia, flushing, abdominal discomfort, pain at injection site, hypotension, skin rash, convulsions.	Loss of consciousness with prochlorperazine; cardiac impairment with vitamin C (>500 mg/day).	$500–2000

[a] Cost of 30-day supply; includes drug cost only.
[b] Phlebotomy is the preferred treatment for iron overload in hemochromatosis. Chelation with deferoxamine can be tried in patients unable to tolerate phlebotomy.

Table 7: Drugs Used to Treat Wilson's Disease

Class	Drug	Dose	Adverse Effects	Drug Interactions	Cost[a]
Chelating Agents	*penicillamine* Cuprimine	1–2 g/day po in 4 divided doses on an empty stomach	Proteinuria (nephrotoxic), hematologic effects, positive ANA, mouth ulcers, diarrhea, reduced sense of taste, decreased appetite, nausea, vomiting, hypersensitivity.	Decreased effect with antacids, iron, zinc; decreases levels of digoxin.	$425–850
	trientine Syprine	1–2 g/day po in 4 divided doses	Anemia.	Reduced effect with iron.	[b]
	zinc generics	50 mg (elemental zinc) TID po between meals	GI disturbances.	Decreases levels of quinolones, tetracycline, penicillamine.	$

[a] Cost of 30-day supply; includes drug cost only.
[b] Available through the Special Access Programme, Therapeutic Products Directorate, Health Canada.
Abbreviations: ANA = antinuclear antibody
Legend: $ <$10

Suggested Readings

Eaton JE, Talwalker JA, Lazaridis KN et al. Pathogenesis of primary sclerosing cholangitis and advances in diagnosis and management. *Gastroenterology* 2013;145(3):521-36.

European Association for the Study of the Liver. EASL clinical practice guidelines on the management of ascites, spontaneous bacterial peritonitis, and hepatorenal syndrome in cirrhosis. *J Hepatol* 2010;53(3):397-417.

European Association for Study of Liver. EASL clinical practice guidelines: Wilson's disease. *J Hepatol* 2012;56(3):671-85.

Gan EK, Powell LW, Olynyk JK. Natural history and management of HFE-hemochromatosis. *Semin Liver Dis* 2011;31(3):293-301.

Gao B, Bataller R. Alcoholic liver disease: pathogenesis and new therapeutic targets. *Gastroenterology* 2011;141(5):1572-85.

Lindor KD, Gershwin ME, Poupon R et al. Primary biliary cirrhosis. *Hepatology* 2009;50(1):291-308.

Manns MP, Czaja AJ, Gorham JD et al. Diagnosis and management of autoimmune hepatitis. *Hepatology* 2010;51(6):2193-213.

References

1. Runyon BA, Montano AA, Akriviadis EA et al. The serum-ascites albumin gradient is superior to the exudate-transudate concept in the differential diagnosis of ascites. *Ann Intern Med* 1992;117(3):215-20.
2. Leung W, Wong F. Medical management of ascites. *Exp Opin Pharmacother* 2011;12(8):1269-83.
3. Singh N, Gayowski T, Yu VL et al. Trimethoprim-sulfamethoxazole for the prevention of spontaneous bacterial peritonitis in cirrhosis: a randomized trial. *Ann Intern Med* 1995;122(8):595-8.
4. Gines P, Rimola A, Planas R et al. Norfloxacin prevents spontaneous bacterial peritonitis recurrence in cirrhosis: results of a double-blind, placebo-controlled trial. *Hepatology* 1990;12(4 Pt 1):716-24.
5. Rolachon A, Cordier L, Bacq Y et al. Ciprofloxacin and long-term prevention of spontaneous bacterial peritonitis: results of a prospective controlled trial. *Hepatology* 1995;22(4 Pt 1):1171-4.
6. Inadomi J, Sonnenberg A. Cost-analysis of prophylactic antibiotics in spontaneous bacterial peritonitis. *Gastroenterology* 1997;113(4):1289-94.
7. Segarra-Newnham M, Henneman A. Antibiotic prophylaxis for prevention of spontaneous bacterial peritonitis in patients without gastrointestinal bleeding. *Ann Pharmacother* 2010;44(12):1946-54.
8. Heathcote EJ, Cauch-Dudek K, Walker V et al. The Canadian Multicenter Double-blind Randomized Controlled Trial of ursodeoxycholic acid in primary biliary cirrhosis. *Hepatology* 1994;19(5):1149-56.
9. Lindor KD, Dickson ER, Baldus WP et al. Ursodeoxycholic acid in the treatment of primary biliary cirrhosis. *Gastroenterology* 1994;106(5):1284-90.
10. Poupon RE, Balkau B, Eschwege E et al. A multicenter, controlled trial of ursodiol for the treatment of primary biliary cirrhosis. UDCA-PBC Study Group. *N Engl J Med* 1991;324(22):1548-54.
11. Triantos CK, Koukias NM, Nikolopoulou VN et al. Meta-analysis: ursodeoxycholic acid for primary sclerosing cholangitis. *Aliment Pharmacol Ther* 2011;34(8):901-10.
12. Lindor KD, Kowdley KV, Luketic VA et al. High-dose ursodeoxycholic acid for the treatment of primary sclerosing cholangitis. *Hepatology* 2009;50(3):808-14.
13. Poupon RE, Lindor KD, Pares A et al. Combined analysis of the effect of treatment with ursodeoxycholic acid on histologic progression in primary biliary cirrhosis. *J Hepatol* 2003;39(1):12-6.
14. Wolfhagen FH, Sternieri E, Hop WC et al. Oral naltrexone treatment for cholestatic pruritus: a double-blind, placebo-controlled study. *Gastroenterology* 1997;113(4):1264-9.
15. Bachs L, Pares A, Elena M et al. Effects of long-term rifampicin administration in primary biliary cirrhosis. *Gastroenterology* 1992;102(6):2077-80.
16. Browning J, Combes B, Mayo MJ. Long-term efficacy of sertraline as a treatment for cholestatic pruritus in patients with primary biliary cirrhosis. *Am J Gastroenterol* 2003;98(12):2736-41.
17. Richardson PD, James PD, Ryder SD. Mycophenolate mofetil for maintenance of remission in autoimmune hepatitis in patients resistant to or intolerant of azathioprine. *J Hepatol* 2000;33(3):371-5.
18. Rambaldi A, Gluud C. Colchicine for alcoholic and non-alcoholic liver fibrosis and cirrhosis. *Cochrane Database Syst Rev* 2005;(2):CD002148.
19. Rambaldi A, Gluud C. Propothiouracil for alcoholic liver disease. *Cochrane Database Syst Rev* 2005;(4):CD002800.
20. Ramond MJ, Poynard T, Rueff B et al. A randomized trial of prednisolone in patients with severe alcoholic hepatitis. *N Engl J Med* 1992;326(8):507-12.
21. Akriviadis E, Botla R, Briggs W et al. Pentoxifylline improves short-term survival in severe acute alcoholic hepatitis: a double-blind, placebo-controlled trial. *Gastroenterology* 2000;119(6):1637-48.
22. Haber PS, Warner R, Seth D et al. Pathogenesis and management of alcoholic hepatitis. *J Gastroenterol Hepatol* 2003;18(12):1332-44.
23. Sidhu S, Singla M, Bhatia K et al. Pentoxifylline reduces disease severity and prevents renal impairment in severe acute alcoholic hepatitis: a double-blind, placebo-controlled trial. *Hepatology* 2006;44(Suppl 1A):373A-374A.
24. De BK, Gangopadhyay S, Dutta D et al. Pentoxifylline versus prednisolone for severe alcoholic hepatitis: a randomized controlled trial. *World J Gastroenterol* 2009;15(13):1613-9.
25. Wellge BE, Sterneck M, Teufel A et al. Pregnancy in primary sclerosing cholangitis. *Gut* 2011;60(8):1117-21.
26. Park-Wyllie L, Mazzotta P, Pastuszak A et al. Birth defects after maternal exposure to corticosteroids: prospective cohort study and meta-analysis of epidemiological studies. *Teratology* 2000;62(6):385-92.

27. Greenberger PA, Odeh YK, Frederiksen MC et al. Pharmacokinetics of prednisolone transfer to breast milk. *Clin Pharmacol Ther* 1993;53(3):324-8.
28. Ost L, Wettrell G, Bjorkhem I et al. Prednisolone excretion in human milk. *J Pediatr* 1985;106(6):1008-11.
29. Coelho J, Beaugerie L, Colombel JF et al. Pregnancy outcome in patients with inflammatory bowel disease treated with thiopurines: cohort from the CESAME Study. *Gut* 2011;60(2):198-203.
30. Mahadevan U, Kane S. American gastroenterological association institute medical position statement on the use of gastrointestinal medications in pregnancy. *Gastroenterology* 2006;131(1):278-82.

Chapter 58
Constipation in Adults

Hugh Chaun, MA, BM, FRCP, FRCP(Ed), FACG, AGAF

Constipation is a symptom, not a disease. Establishing the potential cause and correcting it are the primary objectives of treatment.

Chronic constipation may be defined as outlined in Table 1.

Table 1: Diagnostic Criteria for Constipation[1]

The presence of 2 or more of the following symptoms for the last 3 months and symptom onset at least 6 months before diagnosis:
• Lumpy or hard stools in >25% of defecations
• <3 evacuations per week
• Straining in >25% of defecations
• A sensation of incomplete evacuation in >25% of defecations
• A sensation of anorectal obstruction or blockade in >25% of defecations
• Manual manoeuvres to facilitate >25% of defecations, e.g., digital evacuation, support of the pelvic floor
Loose stools (including laxative-induced) are not present and the criteria for irritable bowel syndrome are not met.

Adapted with permission from Longstreth GF, Thompson WG, Chey WD et al. Functional bowel disorders. *Gastroenterology* 2006;130(5):1480-91.

Goals of Therapy

- Establish regular bowel function
- Abolish the need to strain and prevent the adverse effects of straining, e.g., hernia, coronary and cerebrovascular dysfunction in the elderly, gastroesophageal reflux, rectal prolapse, aggravation of bladder or uterine prolapse in females
- Prevent complications, e.g., hemorrhoids, anal fissure, rectal prolapse, stercoral ulcer (ulcer of the colon/rectum caused by fecal pressure and irritation), fecal impaction, fecal incontinence
- Treat complications, e.g., fecal impaction, intestinal obstruction
- Prevent adverse effects of laxative dependence, e.g., cathartic colon
- Determine "normal" bowel routine for each patient, e.g., some patients may feel a bowel movement every day is a sign of normal health, but this may not be "normal" for everyone

Investigations

- Thorough history with special attention to:
  - duration of constipation
  - the most distressing features of constipation: infrequency, straining, hard stool, unusual toilet postures to facilitate stool expulsion, digital manipulation, feeling of incomplete bowel evacuation, bloating, pain
  - previous laxative use
  - structural abnormalities (previous surgery)

- dietary fibre and fluid
- physical inactivity or immobilization (more common with increased age)
- drugs with constipating effects (see Table 2)
- symptoms of obstructive disease (colonic neoplasm or stricture, anal stricture), painful hemorrhoid or fissure, pregnancy, neuromuscular disease, endocrine disorder (hypothyroidism, diabetes mellitus), collagen vascular disease (progressive systemic sclerosis)

Table 2: **Drugs with Constipating Effects**

Antacids containing aluminum or calcium	Antispasmodics	Resins (e.g., cholestyramine)
Anticholinergic agents	Bismuth preparations	Serotonin receptor antagonists (e.g., ondansetron)
Anticonvulsant agents	Diuretics that cause hypokalemia	Sucralfate
Antiparkinsonian agents	Iron-containing products	Verapamil
Antipsychotic agents	Opioids (e.g., codeine, morphine)	

- Physical examination:
  - abdominal/perineal/rectal examination looking for abdominal and rectal masses, anorectal fissures and hemorrhoids
- Laboratory tests:
  - CBC
  - serum electrolytes and creatinine
  - thyroid-stimulating hormone
  - fecal occult blood
- *Routine* use of lower endoscopy (colonoscopy or sigmoidoscopy) is *not* recommended. Consider colonoscopy, double contrast barium enema (now less readily available) or, rarely, CT colonography if:
  - recent onset of symptoms in patients over 50 years old[2]
  - severe symptoms
  - symptoms do not resolve with simple measures
  - the cause of rectal bleeding is not demonstrated on sigmoidoscopy
  - alarm features are present (e.g., weight loss, anemia, unexplained positive fecal occult blood test)
  - family history of colorectal cancer
- Psychological assessment when appropriate
- Transit studies (radiopaque markers,[3] defecography,[4] anorectal manometry[5]) and anorectal and pelvic floor tests in selected (usually <5%) patients

Therapeutic Choices

Figure 1 outlines the management of constipation in adults.

Figure 1: Management of Constipation in Adults

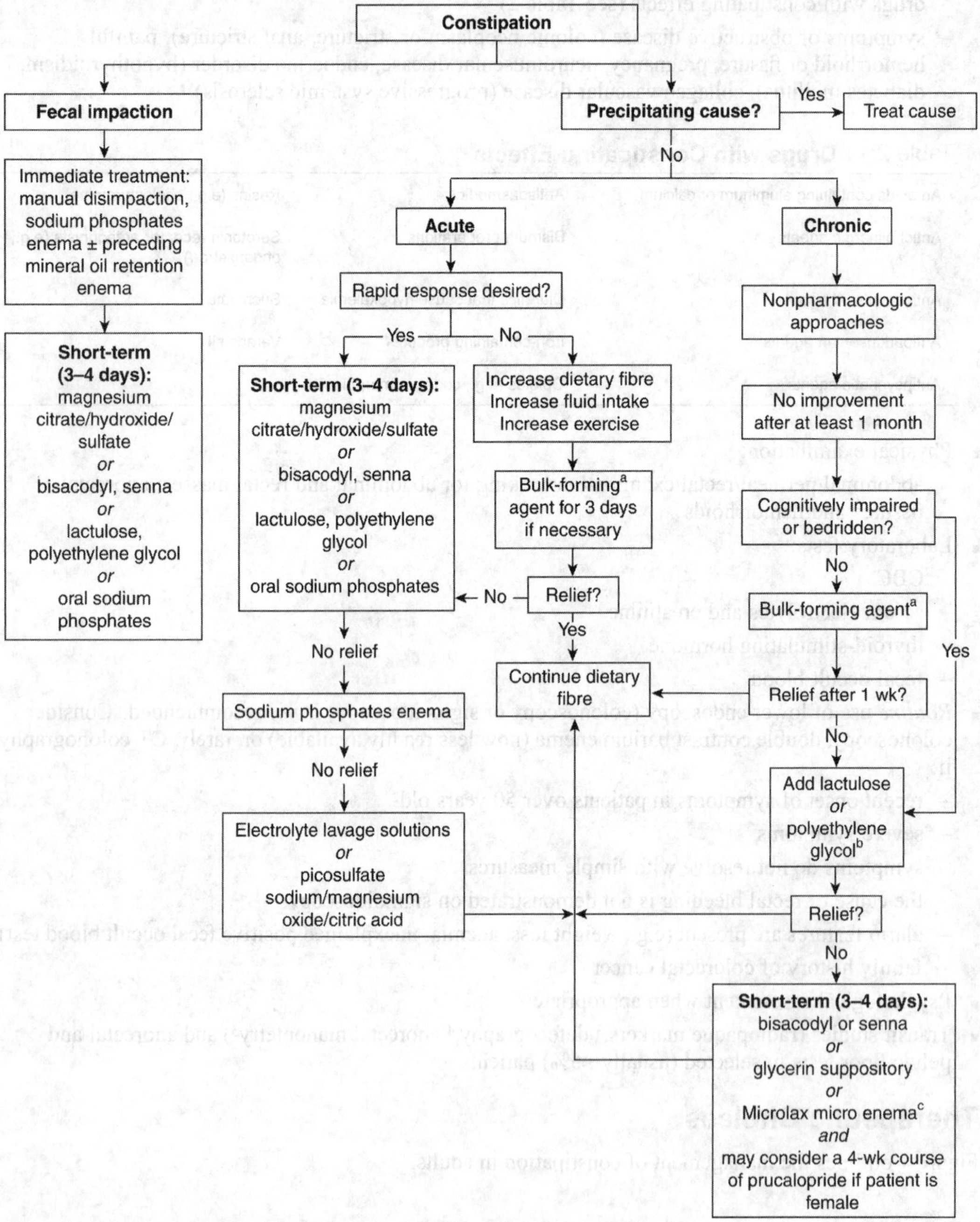

a Do not use bulk-forming agents in patients with inadequate fluid intake or those unable to express thirst, e.g., cognitively impaired, bedbound.

b Polyethylene glycol is preferred over lactulose if cost is not a limiting factor.

c Microlax micro-enema is composed of sodium citrate, sodium lauryl sulfoacetate, sorbitol, glycerin and sorbic acid.

Nonpharmacologic Choices

- Discontinue drugs with constipating effects when possible (see Investigations).
- Encourage dietary fibre (14 g/1000 kcal),[6] flax seeds, psyllium,[7] unprocessed bran,[8] whole grains, fruits and vegetables. Increase the daily amount gradually to minimize side effects such as flatulence, bloating and unpleasant taste. Raising the daily intake of fibre to >30 g daily increases side effects without added benefit.[9]
- Increase fluid intake to supplement the high-fibre diet.
- Recommend prune juice, stewed prunes or figs.
- Encourage regular scheduled time for toilet use, e.g., after breakfast, to develop a conditioned gastrocolic reflex.
- Advise patients not to ignore the urge to defecate.
- Advise avoidance of prolonged straining.
- Encourage physical exercise.[11]
- For constipation due to defecatory disorders, recommend relaxation exercises for the pelvic floor and external anal sphincter muscles in conjunction with biofeedback.[12,13]
- Digital manipulation of the anal sphincter may help in patients with motility problems, e.g., those with spina bifida.

Pharmacologic Choices

Table 3 details the drugs used in the management of constipation.

- In general, use drug therapy only when nonpharmacologic approaches have failed. Moreover, continue and reinforce nonpharmacologic therapy when drug therapy is initiated.
- Bulk-forming agents (e.g., **psyllium**) may be effective[7,14] and can be safely used for long-term therapy, but must be taken with adequate fluids. Fibre is not useful in the treatment of constipation caused by pelvic floor dysfunction.[15]
- Osmotic laxatives (e.g., **lactulose**, **polyethylene glycol 3350**) are safe and effective for long-term use.[7,16] Polyethylene glycol (PEG) is also safe and effective for use in pediatric and geriatric patients.[17,18] Whenever possible, use PEG instead of lactulose for the treatment of chronic constipation since it results in greater improvements in stool frequency, stool form and relief of abdominal pain and reduces the need for additional laxatives [Evidence: SORT A*].[19]
- Some stimulant laxatives (e.g., **bisacodyl**, **picosulfate sodium**, **senna**) have been shown to be effective for the treatment of acute or chronic constipation.[20,21,22,23,24]
- Some geriatric patients may benefit from using a combination of laxatives with different mechanisms of action (e.g., bulk-forming plus stimulant laxatives).[25]
- The stool softeners **docusate sodium** and **docusate calcium** have not been shown to be effective in the management of constipation and most probably exert a placebo effect.[9,10]
- Seek the patient's understanding and cooperation regarding general principles of therapy, and monitor laxative tolerance.
- A new 5-HT_4 receptor agonist, **prucalopride**, is approved for the treatment of idiopathic chronic constipation in females who have failed to respond to other laxatives (prucalopride has not been adequately studied in male patients).[26,27,28] Prucalopride should be prescribed by a clinician with experience in treating chronic constipation.[29]

---

* SORT (Strength of Recommendation Taxonomy) is a rating system (A, B or C) that addresses the quality of available evidence. For more information consult **How to Use *Compendium of Therapeutic Choices*** on page xxv.

- To discontinue chronic laxative use, gradually reduce the frequency of use over 3–4 weeks, while optimizing nonpharmacologic approaches; use an osmotic laxative (e.g., lactulose, polyethylene glycol) intermittently until bowel regularity is achieved.
- Start patients on a stimulant (e.g., bisacodyl, senna) or osmotic (e.g., lactulose, polyethylene glycol) laxative at the time of prescribing an opioid, if they have a history of opioid-induced constipation or are experiencing constipation.
- **Methylnaltrexone**, a μ-opioid receptor antagonist, is indicated for the treatment of opioid-induced constipation in patients receiving palliative care. It is used as an adjunctive treatment when response to laxatives has been insufficient; however, more data are needed to determine its place in therapy.[31]

Choices during Pregnancy and Breastfeeding

Constipation is a common condition during pregnancy; a greater prevalence is observed during the first 2 trimesters relative to the third trimester and the postpartum period.[32,33] In late pregnancy, constipation is attributed to increased circulating progesterone which reduces gastrointestinal motility.[34] Constipation in pregnancy is commonly associated with symptoms of straining, hard stools and incomplete evacuation but not infrequent defecation.[32] Iron supplementation during pregnancy may cause constipation.

Management of Constipation during Pregnancy

Encourage nonpharmacologic approaches for the treatment of constipation in pregnant women (see Nonpharmacologic Choices). Because they are not systemically absorbed, bulk-forming agents containing **psyllium** are considered first-line in pregnancy.[35] With adequate hydration, they increase defecation frequency and soften the stools.[36] If constipation persists, especially as heartburn is frequent during the third trimester, the laxative effect of a **magnesium-containing** liquid **antacid** may be helpful. Stimulant laxatives such as **senna** or **bisacodyl** may be recommended short-term.[35]

Consider **lactulose** and **polyethylene glycol** if constipation is refractory to dietary fibre and stimulant laxatives.[35]

Avoid **castor oil** because it can induce premature uterine contractions.[35] Chronic use of emollient laxatives such as **mineral oil** can interfere with absorption of fat-soluble vitamins[35] and in rare cases can cause lipoid pneumonia due to aspiration.

Docusate, a commonly prescribed stool softener, is probably ineffective.[35,37]

Management of Constipation during Breastfeeding

As in pregnancy, offer nonpharmacologic choices in breastfeeding women.

Bulk-forming agents are preferred as they are not systemically absorbed, cost less and have a favourable side effect profile. **Magnesium hydroxide** is considered second-line. **Senna** and **bisacodyl** are acceptable to use during breastfeeding;[38] however, stimulant laxatives are recommended only for short-term use. The stool softener **docusate** is probably ineffective.[37]

There is a paucity of data regarding transfer of other laxatives into breast milk.

A discussion of general principles on the use of medications in these special populations can be found in Appendix II and Appendix III. Other specialized reference sources are also provided in these appendices.

Therapeutic Tips

- Perform careful history to determine any potential cause and whether colonic investigation is indicated.
- Encourage optimum dietary and supplementary fibre along with increased daily fluid intake and regular physical exercise.
- Encourage patient to seek medical advice if constipation worsens or if new symptoms (e.g., rectal bleeding) develop.
- Use laxatives wisely to minimize side effects.

Table 3: Drugs Used to Treat Constipation

Class	Drug	Adult Dose	Onset of Action	Adverse Effects	Comments	Cost[a]
5-HT$_4$ Receptor Agonists	*prucalopride* Resotran	Adult women <65 years: 2 mg once daily po Women >65 years: 1 mg once daily po; increase to 2 mg once daily po if needed	Within 4 wk	Abdominal pain, diarrhea, headache, nausea.	Indicated for chronic idiopathic constipation in adult females in whom laxatives failed to provide adequate relief. Lack of data in pregnancy, breastfeeding and male patients. Should be prescribed by a clinician with experience in treating chronic constipation.[29] If there is no bowel movement in 3–4 days after starting prucalopride consider an add-on laxative for rescue treatment of acute constipation.[30] Discontinue prucalopride if ineffective after 4 wk of treatment.[30]	$$
Bulk-forming Agents	*polycarbophil calcium* Prodiem Caplets	1250 mg (2 caplets) once daily to QID po, not to exceed 8 caplets/24 h	12–72 h	Bloating, flatulence, abdominal discomfort, allergic reactions (rare), esophageal and colonic obstruction (rare).	Increases stool weight and consistency, decreases GI transit time and increases the frequency of defecation. Take with plenty of fluids (at least 250 mL) to prevent esophageal obstruction and/or fecal impaction. Can be used long term. Advise patients to not take psyllium within 2 h of taking any other medications.	$
	psyllium hydrophilic mucilloid Metamucil, generics	3.4 g once daily to TID po	12–72 h	See polycarbophil calcium.	See polycarbophil calcium.	$
	sterculia gum Normacol	One 7 g sachet once daily to BID po	12–72 h	See polycarbophil calcium.	See polycarbophil calcium.	$
Hyperosmotic Agents	*glycerin* Glycerin Suppositories, generics	2.6 g (1 adult suppository) once daily to BID or PRN pr	15 min–1 h	Rectal discomfort or burning.	Stimulates peristalsis. Insert high into rectum and retain for 15 min if possible.	$

Class	Drug	Adult Dose	Onset of Action	Adverse Effects	Comments	Cost[a]
	lactulose generics	15–30 mL once daily to BID po	24–48 h	Bloating, flatulence, cramps, diarrhea.	Induces bowel water retention, improves stool consistency and increases the frequency of defecation.	$
Lavage Solutions	*electrolyte solutions* PegLyte, Colyte, Klean-Prep, generics	1000–4000 mL po prior to gastrointestinal examinations or procedures	30 min–1 h	Retching, nausea, abdominal fullness and bloating.	Contain mainly sodium sulfate and polyethylene glycol. Excellent cleansing for colonoscopy.	$$$$$
	picosulfate sodium/magnesium oxide/citric acid Pico-Salax, generics	2 sachets po: taken on day **before** procedure at 8:00 am and then between 2:00 pm and 4:00 pm	<3–6 h	See electrolyte solutions.	Excellent cleansing for colonoscopy (better tolerated than polyethylene glycol).[39]	$$$
Lubricants	*glycerin-mineral oil oral emulsion* Agarol, generics	10–20 mL QHS po; may repeat next morning 2 h after breakfast	6–8 h	Lipoid pneumonia if aspirated. Seepage from rectum causing pruritus and irritation.	Use the oral dosage form with extreme caution because of the risk of aspiration pneumonia. There is insufficient evidence for the use of mineral or paraffin oil to treat chronic constipation in adults.[40] Stool softeners increase absorption of mineral oil (do not use together). Use only for short periods. Decreases absorption of fat-soluble vitamins.	$
	mineral oil Fleet Enema Mineral Oil, Lansoyl, generics	15–45 mL daily po Enema: 120 mL as a single dose pr	po: 6–8 h Enema: 2–15 min	See Glycerin-mineral oil oral emulsion.	See Glycerin-mineral oil oral emulsion.	Oral: $ Enema: $$$

(cont'd)

Table 3: **Drugs Used to Treat Constipation** *(cont'd)*

Class	Drug	Adult Dose	Onset of Action	Adverse Effects	Comments	Cost[a]
μ-opioid Receptor Antagonists	*methylnaltrexone* Relistor	33–<38 kg: 6 mg every 2nd day sc 38–<62 kg: 8 mg every 2nd day sc 62–114 kg: 12 mg every 2nd day sc 115–126 kg: 18 mg every 2nd day sc 0.15 mg/kg for all other weights. Consider discontinuing treatment in patients who fail to show an adequate response after 4 doses (1 week)	4 h	Abdominal pain, flatulence, nausea, increased body temperature, dizziness. Bowel perforation (use with extreme caution in patients at increased risk of perforation such as those with tumour infiltration, acute inflammation of the intestine, or those receiving corticosteroids, NSAIDs or biologics).[41]	For the treatment of opioid-induced constipation in patients with advanced illness receiving palliative care.	$40/dose
Osmotic Agents	*magnesium citrate* Citro-Mag, generics	3.75–7.5 g (75–150 mL) daily po. Follow doses with 250 mL water	30 min–6 h	Hypermagnesemia in renal dysfunction.	Osmotic agents stimulate peristalsis and are useful when rapid response is required (e.g., colonoscopy, preoperatively). Avoid in renal failure (risk of hypermagnesemia); decreases absorption of quinolones and tetracyclines (administer at separate times).	$$
	magnesium hydroxide Milk of Magnesia, generics	2.4–4.8 g (30–60 mL) once daily or in divided doses po	30 min–6 h	See magnesium citrate.	See magnesium citrate.	$
	magnesium sulfate Epsom Salts, generics	10–30 g (dissolved in 240 mL water or juice) once daily or in divided doses po	30 min–6 h	See magnesium citrate.	See magnesium citrate.	$

Class	Drug	Adult Dose	Onset of Action	Adverse Effects	Comments	Cost[a]
	polyethylene glycol 3350 Lax-A-Day, Pegalax, Restoralax	17 g once daily po	2–4 days[42]	Common: nausea, cramping, diarrhea Rare: hives, skin rash.	May require treatment for 2–4 days to produce a bowel movement. Add powder to 250 mL of water, juice, soda, coffee or tea and stir until completely dissolved. Polyethylene glycol is not absorbed. May consider in patients with renal or cardiac dysfunction as it does not contain electrolytes. Effective in the management of opioid-induced constipation.	$
	sodium citrate/sodium lauryl sulfoacetate/sorbitol/glycerin/sorbic acid, enema Microlax micro-enema	5 mL (1 tube) once pr	5–20 min	Slight cramps or tenesmus.	Useful for rectal constipation. May also be used to facilitate rectoscopic or sigmoidoscopic examination.	$$
	sodium phosphates, enema Fleet Enema, generics	120 mL (26.4 g) as a single dose pr	2–15 min	Hyperphosphatemia in patients with renal dysfunction.	Avoid in renal failure (risk of hyperphosphatemia).	$$
	sodium phosphates, oral generics	20 mL once daily po Dilute in 120 mL cool water or clear liquid. Follow with 240 mL cool water or clear liquid.	30 min–6 h	Hyperphosphatemia in patients with renal dysfunction. Risk of arrhythmias if exceed recommended daily dose.	Associated with decline in glomerular filtration rate in the elderly.[43] Use as bowel cleanser not recommended.[44] Avoid in renal failure (risk of hyperphosphatemia).	$$
Stimulant Agents	*bisacodyl* Dulcolax, Carters Little Pills, generics	5–10 mg once daily or PRN po Suppository: 10 mg daily or PRN pr	po: 6–12 h pr: 15 min–1 h	Abdominal pain, cramps, cathartic colon. Rectal microscopic mucosal changes with suppository and enema.	Stimulates colonic peristalsis. Usually short-term use only but long-term use may be necessary in patients on long-term opioid therapy, e.g., cancer patients.	$
	senna Senokot Preparations, others	16.2–32.4 mg (2–4 tablets) at bedtime po (maximum 8 tablets/day)	6–12 h	Abdominal pain, cramps, cathartic colon. Melanosis coli (anthraquinone derivatives).	See bisacodyl. Some senna preparations have high sugar content.	$

(cont'd)

Table 3: Drugs Used to Treat Constipation *(cont'd)*

Class	Drug	Adult Dose	Onset of Action	Adverse Effects	Comments	Cost[a]
Stool Softeners	*docusate calcium* generics	240 mg once daily to BID po	12–72 h		Acts as a surfactant. Often used as a stool softener after rectal surgery and in long-term opioid users, but there are no documented beneficial effects. May exert a placebo effect.	$
	docusate sodium Colace, generics	100 mg once daily to BID po	12–72 h		See docusate calcium.	$

[a] Cost per day; includes drug cost only.

Dosage adjustment may be required in renal impairment; see Appendix I

Legend: $ <$1 $$ $1–5 $$$ $5–10 $$$$ $10–15 $$$$$ $15–20

Suggested Readings

American College of Gastroenterology Chronic Constipation Task Force. An evidence-based approach to the management of chronic constipation in North America. *Am J Gastroenterol* 2005;100(Suppl 1):S1-4.

Ford AC, Suares NC. Effect of laxatives and pharmacological therapies in chronic idiopathic constipation: systematic review and meta-analysis. *Gut* 2011;60(2):209-18.

Gallegos-Orozco JF, Foxx-Orenstein AE, Sterler SM et al. Chronic constipation in the elderly. *Am J Gastroenterol* 2012;107(1):18-25.

Gandell D, Straus SE, Bundookwala M et al. Treatment of constipation in older people. *CMAJ* 2013;185(8):663-70.

Pare P. The approach to diagnosis and treatment of chronic constipation: suggestions for a general practitioner. *Can J Gastroenterol* 2011;25(Suppl B):36B-40B.

Tack J. Current and future therapies for chronic constipation. *Best Pract Res Clin Gastroenterol* 2011;25(1):151-8.

References

1. Longstreth GF, Thompson WG, Chey WD et al. Functional bowel disorders. *Gastroenterology* 2006;130(5):1480-91.
2. Locke GR, Pemberton JH, Phillips SF. American Gastroenterological Association medical position statement: guidelines on constipation. *Gastroenterology* 2000;119(6):1761-6.
3. Szarka LA, Camilleri M. Methods for the assessment of small-bowel and colonic transit. *Semin Nucl Med* 2012;42(2):113-23.
4. Kim AY. How to interpret a functional or motility test - defecography. *J Neurogastroenterol Motil* 2011;17(4):416-20.
5. Pucciani F, Ringressi MN. Obstructed defecation: the role of anorectal manometry. *Tech Coloproctol* 2012;16(1):67-72.
6. Anderson JW, Baird P, Davis RH et al. Health benefits of dietary fiber. *Nutr Rev* 2009;67(4):188-205.
7. Ramkumar D, Rao SS. Efficacy and safety of traditional medical therapies for chronic constipation: systematic review. *Am J Gastroenterol* 2005;100(4):936-71.
8. Badiali D, Corazziari E, Habib FI et al. Effect of wheat bran in treatment of chronic nonorganic constipation. A double-blind controlled trial. *Dig Dis Sci* 1995;40(2):349-56.
9. Pare P. The approach to diagnosis and treatment of chronic constipation: suggestions for a general practitioner. *Can J Gastroenterol* 2011;25(Suppl B):36B-40B.
10. Tarumi Y, Wilson MP, Szafran O et al. Randomized, double-blind, placebo-controlled trial of oral docusate in the management of constipation in hospice patients. *J Pain Symptom Manage* 2013;45(1):2-13.
11. De Schryver AM, Keulemans YC, Peters HP et al. Effects of regular physical activity on defecation pattern in middle-aged patients complaining of chronic constipation. *Scand J Gastroenterol* 2005;40(4):422-9.
12. Chiarioni G, Salandini L, Whitehead WE. Biofeedback benefits only patients with outlet dysfunction, not patients with isolated slow transit constipation. *Gastroenterology* 2005;129(1):86-97.
13. Chiarioni G, Whitehead WE, Pezza V et al. Biofeedback is superior to laxatives for normal transit constipation due to pelvic floor dyssynergia. *Gastroenterology* 2006;130(3):657-64.
14. Suares NC, Ford AC. Systematic review: the effects of fibre in the management of chronic idiopathic constipation. *Aliment Pharmacol Ther* 2011;33(8):895-901.
15. Gallegos-Orozco JF, Foxx-Orenstein AE, Sterler SM et al. Chronic constipation in the elderly. *Am J Gastroenterol* 2012;107(1):18-25.
16. Dipalma JA, Cleveland MV, McGowan J et al. A randomized, multicenter, placebo-controlled trial of polyethylene glycol laxative for chronic treatment of chronic constipation. *Am J Gastroenterol* 2007;102(7):1436-41.
17. Gordon M, Naidoo K, Akobeng AK et al. Osmotic and stimulant laxatives for the management of childhood constipation. *Cochrane Database Syst Rev* 2012;7:CD009118.
18. Zurad EG, Johanson JF. Over-the-counter laxative polyethylene glycol 3350: an evidence-based appraisal. *Curr Med Res Opin* 2011;27(7):1439-52.
19. Lee-Robichaud H, Thomas K, Morgan J et al. Lactulose versus polyethylene glycol for chronic constipation. *Cochrane Database Syst Rev* 2010;(7):CD007570.
20. Kamm MA, Mueller-Lissner S, Wald A et al. Oral bisacodyl is effective and well-tolerated in patients with chronic constipation. *Clin Gastroenterol Hepatol* 2011;9(7):577-83.
21. Mueller-Lissner S, Kamm MA, Wald A et al. Multicenter, 4-week, double-blind, randomized, placebo-controlled trial of sodium picosulfate in patients with chronic constipation. *Am J Gastroenterol* 2010;105(4):897-903.
22. Kienzle-Horn S, Vix JM, Schuijt C et al. Efficacy and safety of bisacodyl in the acute treatment of constipation: a double-blind, randomized, placebo-controlled study. *Aliment Pharmacol Ther* 2006;23(10):1479-88.
23. Wulkow R, Vix JM, Schuijt C et al. Randomised, placebo-controlled, double-blind study to investigate the efficacy and safety of the acute use of sodium picosulphate in patients with chronic constipation. *Int J Clin Pract* 2007;61(6):944-50.
24. Kienzle-Horn S, Vix JM, Schuijt C et al. Comparison of bisacodyl and sodium picosulphate in the treatment of chronic constipation. *Curr Med Res Opin* 2007;23(4):691-9.
25. Fleming V, Wade WE. A review of laxative therapies for treatment of chronic constipation in older adults. *Am J Geriatr Pharmacother* 2010;8(6):514-50.
26. Quigley EM, Vandeplassche L, Kerstens R et al. Clinical trial: the efficacy, impact on quality of life, and safety and tolerability of prucalopride in severe chronic constipation--a 12-week, randomized, double-blind, placebo-controlled study. *Aliment Pharmacol Ther* 2009;29(3):315-28.
27. Camilleri M, Kerstens R, Rykx A et al. A placebo-controlled trial of prucalopride for severe chronic constipation. *N Engl J Med* 2008;358(22):2344-54.

28. Camilleri M, Van Outryve MJ, Beyens G et al. Clinical trial: the efficacy of open-label prucalopride treatment in patients with chronic constipation - follow-up of patients from the pivotal studies. *Aliment Pharmacol Ther* 2010;32(9):1113-23.
29. U.K. National Health Service. National Institute for Health and Clinical Excellence. *Prucalopride for the treatment of chronic constipation in women*. London (GB): NICE; 2010. Available from: www.nice.org.uk/nicemedia/live/13284/52078/52078.pdf. Accessed July 3, 2012.
30. e-CPS. Ottawa (ON): Canadian Pharmacists Association. *Resotran* [product monograph]. Available from: e-therapeutics.ca. Subscription required.
31. McNicol ED, Boyce D, Schumann R et al. Mu-opioid antagonists for opioid-induced bowel dysfunction. *Cochrane Database Syst Rev* 2008;(2):CD006332.
32. Bradley CS, Kennedy CM, Turcea AM et al. Constipation in pregnancy: prevalence, symptoms, and risk factors. *Obstet Gynecol* 2007;110(6):1351-7.
33. Derbyshire E, Davies J, Costarelli V et al. Diet, physical inactivity and the prevalence of constipation throughout and after pregnancy. *Matern Child Nutr* 2006;2(3):127-34.
34. Chiloiro M, Darconza G, Piccioli E et al. Gastric emptying and orocecal transit time in pregnancy. *J Gastroenterol* 2001;36(8):538-43.
35. American College of Gastroenterology. *Pregnancy in gastrointestinal disorders*. Bethesda (MD): ACG; 2007. Available from: s3.gi.org/physicians/PregnancyMonograph.pdf. Accessed February 21, 2012.
36. Prather CM. Pregnancy-related constipation. *Curr Gastroenterol Rep* 2004;6(5):402-4.
37. Singh S, Rao SS. Pharmacologic management of chronic constipation. *Gastroenterol Clin North Am* 2010;39(3):509-27.
38. American Academy of Pediatrics Committee on Drugs. The transfer of drugs and other chemicals into human milk. *Pediatrics* 2001;108(3):776-89.
39. Turner D, Benchimol EI, Dunn H et al. Pico-Salax versus polyethylene glycol for bowel cleanout before colonoscopy in children: a randomized controlled trial. *Endoscopy* 2009;41(12):1038-45.
40. Pare P, Bridges R, Champion MC et al. Recommendations on chronic constipation (including constipation associated with irritable bowel syndrome) treatment. *Can J Gastroenterol* 2007;21(Suppl B):3B-22B.
41. Bader S, Jaroslawski K, Blum HE et al. Opioid-induced constipation in advanced illness: safety and efficacy of methylnaltrexone bromide. *Clin Med Insights Oncol* 2011;5:201-11.
42. e-CPS. Ottawa (ON): Canadian Pharmacists Association. *Lax-A-Day* [product monograph]. Available from: e-therapeutics.ca. Subscription required.
43. Khurana A, McLean L, Atkinson S et al. The effect of oral sodium phosphate drug products on renal function in adults undergoing bowel endoscopy. *Arch Intern Med* 2008;168(6):593-7.
44. Health Canada. *Health Canada warns that use of oral sodium phosphate products for bowel cleansing may lead to kidney injury*. Ottawa (ON): Health Canada. Available from: healthycanadians.gc.ca/recall-alert-rappel-avis/hc-sc/2009/13368a-eng.php. Accessed March 31, 2011.

Gastrointestinal Disorders

Chapter 59
Diarrhea

Dina Kao, MD, FRCPC

Clinically, diarrhea is present when an alteration in a normal bowel habit occurs; it is characterized by a decrease in consistency to soft or liquid and an increase in frequency to ≥3 stools/day. Increased loss of fecal water and electrolytes occurs with the increased excretion of fecal matter. Patients who have other gastrointestinal symptoms, such as fecal incontinence or fecal urgency or who notice a change in stool consistency, may refer to it as "diarrhea". These symptoms will need to be ruled out before a diagnosis of "true diarrhea" is given.

Diarrhea may be *acute* (<14 days in duration) or *chronic* (>30 days in duration). Acute diarrhea may be caused by infections, medications, food intolerance and intestinal disease (Table 1). Causes of chronic diarrhea include postinfectious irritable bowel syndrome and persistent and/or repeated infections.

Goals of Therapy

- Reduce symptoms and re-establish normal fecal weight (volume)
- Prevent and treat complications, i.e., dehydration, electrolyte depletion, nutrient malabsorption, hemorrhoids, rectal prolapse
- Remove or eradicate the cause of diarrhea where applicable

Investigations

Key questions prior to treatment:[1,2,3]

- *What is the patient's history?* Obtain a thorough history that includes the following clinical and epidemiologic features:
  - when and how the illness began (duration of symptoms; abrupt or gradual onset)
  - are the stools pale or difficult to flush? Do they float or have a particularly foul smell (suggestive of steatorrhea)?
  - sexual history (diarrhea is common in patients with HIV/AIDS)
  - family history of inflammatory bowel disease, colorectal cancer or celiac disease
  - stool characteristics (watery, bloody, mucousy, greasy)
  - frequency of bowel movements and quantity of stool produced
  - symptoms of volume depletion (thirst, tachycardia, orthostatic hypotension, decreased urination, lethargy, decreased skin turgor)
  - associated systemic symptoms and their frequency and intensity (nausea, vomiting, abdominal pain, cramps, headache, fever, myalgias, altered sensorium)
  - changes in diet
  - medication history including use of prescription and nonprescription drugs, herbal or "natural" products and dietary supplements
  - recent travel history (see Chapter 123), locale of employment and residence and other family members or co-workers that have a similar illness

- *Is this true diarrhea?* Many people who complain of diarrhea actually have a motility disturbance, e.g., irritable bowel syndrome. They experience an increased frequency of very small bowel movements, but the 24-hour stool weight does not exceed normal amounts. When clinically indicated, measuring fecal fat, osmolarity and bile acid levels can also help determine specific etiologies.
- *Is the diarrhea acute or chronic?* In the absence of fever, dehydration or bloody stools, the management of acute diarrhea should alleviate symptoms rather than provide a specific diagnosis or therapy. Acute diarrhea (Figure 1, Figure 2, Table 1) is frequently caused by viral agents, drugs or food toxins for which there is no specific therapy, and usually remits spontaneously within 1 week. Acute infectious diarrhea of a bacterial or parasitic etiology should be identified early to permit early successful intervention. Evaluate chronic diarrhea as in Figure 3.

Acute Diarrhea

Etiology

Critical to therapy is identifying the etiology of acute diarrhea as presented in Table 1.

Table 1: **Etiology of Acute Diarrhea**

Etiology	Examples
Infectious	
Bacterial	*Shigella*, *Salmonella* (*typhi*, *enteritidis*), *Campylobacter*, *Yersinia*, *Escherichia coli* (EHEC 0157:H7, ETEC, EPEC), *Clostridium* (*difficile*, *perfringens*) *Vibrio* (*cholerae*, *parahaemolyticus*), *Staphylococcus aureus*, *Bacillus cereus*
Viral	Norovirus (Norwalk virus), rotavirus, adenovirus, cytomegalovirus, herpes simplex virus
Parasitic	*Cryptosporidium*, Microsporidia, *Entamoeba histolytica*, *Giardia lamblia*, *Cyclospora*
Medications	Antibiotics, colchicine, laxatives, magnesium-containing antacids
Food Intolerance	Lactose, fructose in soft drinks, sorbitol in diet candy, coffee
Intestinal Disease	Celiac disease, inflammatory bowel disease (ulcerative colitis, Crohn's disease)

Infectious Diarrhea

- Proctitis can be diagnosed with sigmoidoscopy. Involvement of only the distal 15 cm suggests herpesvirus, gonococcal, chlamydial or syphilitic infection. Colitis extending more proximally suggests *Campylobacter*, *Shigella*, *Clostridium difficile* or chlamydial (LGV serotype) infection.
- An inflammatory etiology (e.g., invasive colitis due to *Salmonella*, *Shigella* or *Campylobacter*, *C. difficile* colitis, inflammatory bowel disease) can be suspected on the basis of fever, tenesmus or bloody stools. Microscopy for fecal leukocytes or fecal lactoferrin testing may confirm inflammation. A meta-analysis and a recent review of the diagnostic accuracy for fecal leukocyte testing demonstrated a sensitivity of only 70% and a specificity ranging from 50–84%.[1,3] Fecal lactoferrin has a higher sensitivity and specificity of 90% and 79%, respectively, but is not widely available.[4]
- Consider tests for parasitic causes of diarrhea including fluorescence and enzyme immunoassay for *Giardia* and *Cryptosporidium* and acid-fast stains for *Cryptosporidium*, *Cyclospora*, *Isospora* or *Mycobacterium* species.
- Any diarrheal illness accompanied by fever, bloody stools, systemic illness, recent use of antibiotics, daycare centre attendance, hospitalization or dehydration should prompt evaluation of a fecal specimen, including stool cultures plus other investigations as noted below and in Figure 1. In patients who do not appear unwell or do not have the above symptoms, the necessity of documenting

a pathogen is often not needed, since acute diarrheal episodes are generally self-limiting and resolve within several days.

- Selective fecal testing can improve the yield and usefulness of stool testing and should be adopted whenever possible using the following guidelines:
  - consider *E. coli* 0157 in persons with a history of undercooked red meat ingestion and acute bloody diarrhea or hemolytic uremic syndrome, as well as those with marked abdominal pain and bloody diarrhea but without high fever
  - consider *Vibrio parahaemolyticus* in persons who have ingested shellfish within the 3 days before the illness began
  - consider *Yersinia enterocolitica* in fall or winter and in certain at-risk populations (e.g., Asians and African-American infants), as well as those with persistent abdominal pain and fever
  - consider *C. difficile* toxin assay in all patients with diarrhea
  - immunocompromised patients or those with significant comorbidities that increase the risk for complications
  - patients with inflammatory bowel disease in whom distinction between a flare and superimposed infection is critical
  - fecal specimens from patients with diarrhea that develops after 3 days of hospitalization have a very low yield when cultured for standard bacterial pathogens (*Campylobacter*, *Salmonella*, *Shigella*, etc.) or examined for ova and parasites
  - consider *Norwalk* virus (a norovirus) in patients with nausea, vomiting, intense cramping and watery diarrhea. The disease is self-limited and usually lasts 48–72 hours. The virus is spread by ingestion of feces-contaminated water (including that in swimming pools) or food, contact with contaminated environments or individuals with the illness. The virus is shed in vomitus and the stool for at least 24–48 hours after the onset of illness. Given the classic clinical presentation and rapid recovery, the specific viral diagnosis is not necessary in adult gastroenteritis.
- Ask patients about potential epidemiologic risk factors for particular diarrheal diseases or for their spread:
  - travel to a developing country (see Chapter 123)
  - daycare centre attendance or employment
  - visitation or employment in acute-care or long-term care facilities
  - ingestion of unsafe foods (e.g., raw meats, eggs or shellfish; unpasteurized milk or juices)
  - swimming in or drinking untreated water
  - visiting a farm or petting zoo or having contact with pets with diarrhea
  - knowledge of other ill family members or co-workers
  - recent antibiotic use
  - underlying medical conditions predisposing to infectious diarrhea (e.g., AIDS, immunosuppressive therapies, previous gastrectomy, extremes of age)
  - occupation as a food-handler or caregiver
  - where appropriate, inquire about receptive anal intercourse or oral-anal sexual contact

For persons with AIDS, a modified algorithm for the investigation and management of diarrhea is available.[3]

Figure 1: **Evaluation and Management of Acute Diarrhea**

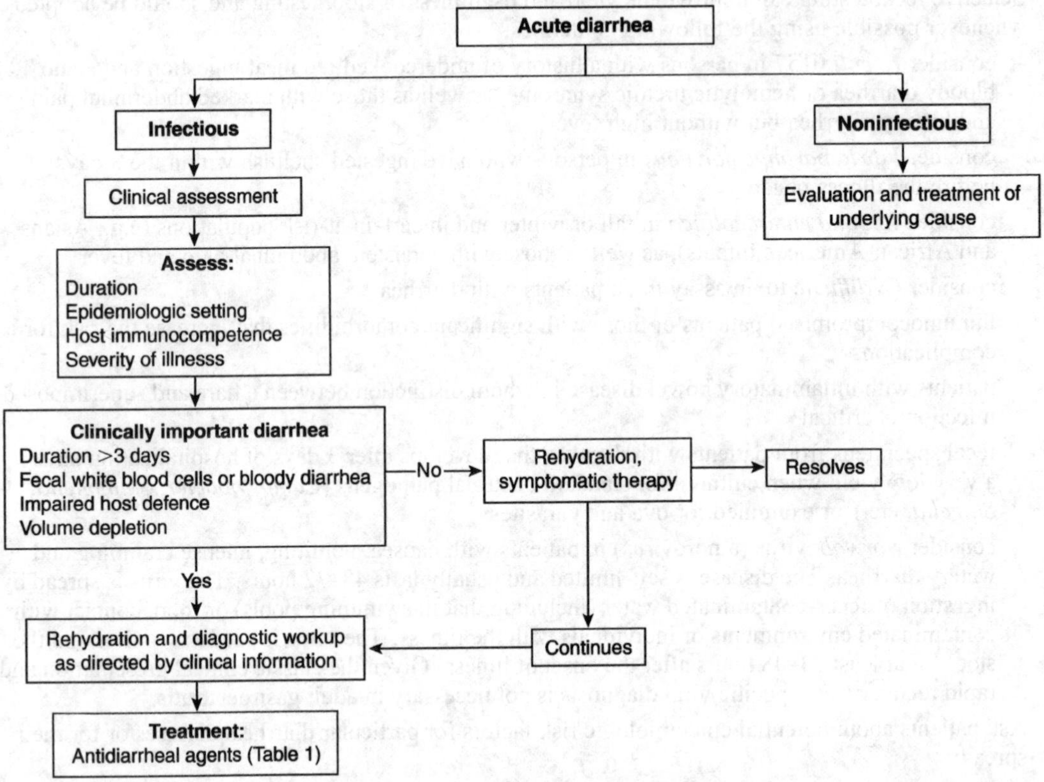

Antibiotic-associated Diarrhea

- Antibiotic-associated diarrhea occurs during or shortly after administration of an antibiotic. The use of any antibiotic can alter the commensal gastrointestinal microflora and lead to diarrhea in approximately 5–35% of patients.[5] Most cases of antibiotic-associated diarrhea are mild and resolve spontaneously. The pathogenesis of antibiotic-associated diarrhea can vary and includes accelerated gastrointestinal motility (e.g., erythromycin), osmotic diarrhea due to decreased carbohydrate metabolism by colonic anaerobes or opportunistic infections, alterations in intestinal absorption and/or secretion, bacterial overgrowth syndromes and *C. difficile* infection (CDI).
- *C. difficile* is the most common bacterium responsible for antibiotic-associated infectious diarrhea. Other rare infections described include *S. aureus*, *Salmonella*, *C. perfringens* and *Candida* species.
- The spectrum of symptoms associated with CDI range from no symptoms (carrier state) through watery diarrhea to toxic megacolon.
- Diagnosis consists of detection of *C. difficile* toxin in the stool or presence of characteristic pseudomembranous colitis on endoscopy. Since pseudomembranes can be limited to the right side of the colon a full colonoscopy is recommended. Stool culture is the most sensitive test, though it has a slow turnaround time. Enzyme immunoassay testing for *C. difficile* toxins A and B is rapid, but less sensitive. There is limited value in repeat testing during the same episode of diarrhea.[6]

Figure 2: **Management of Antibiotic-associated Diarrhea[6]**

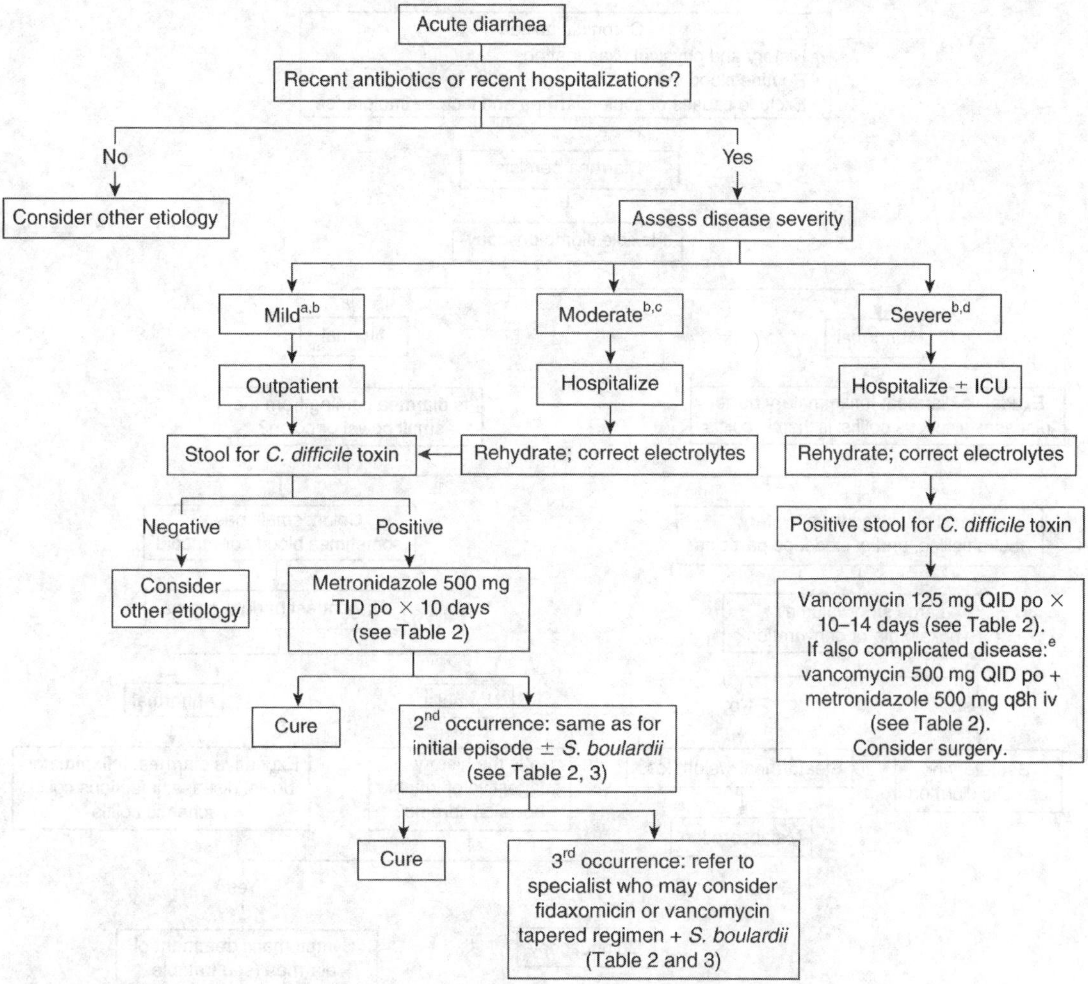

a Mild = <5 stools/day, + abdominal pain, leukocytosis with a white blood cell count <15 000 cells/µL and serum creatinine level <1.5 times the premorbid level.

b In patients >65 y and/or with comorbidities, consider more aggressive management (e.g., earlier hospitalization).

c Moderate = febrile, ++ abdominal pain, signs of dehydration (dry mucous membranes, tachycardia, and decreased urine output), leukocytosis with a white blood cell count <15 000 cells/µL and serum creatinine level <1.5 times the premorbid level.

d Severe = febrile, +++ abdominal pain (or peritonitis), signs of sepsis (e.g., confusion), leukocytosis with a white blood cell count ≥15 000 cells/µL or serum creatinine level ≥1.5 times the premorbid level.

e Complicated disease = severe signs and symptoms with ileus, shock, hypotension or megacolon. Antibiotics should be started even in the absence of confirmed *C. difficile* infection.

Chronic Diarrhea

Figure 3 illustrates the evaluation of chronic diarrhea. For information on diarrhea related to inflammatory bowel disease and irritable bowel syndrome, see Chapter 62 and Chapter 63.

Figure 3: **Evaluation of Chronic Diarrhea**

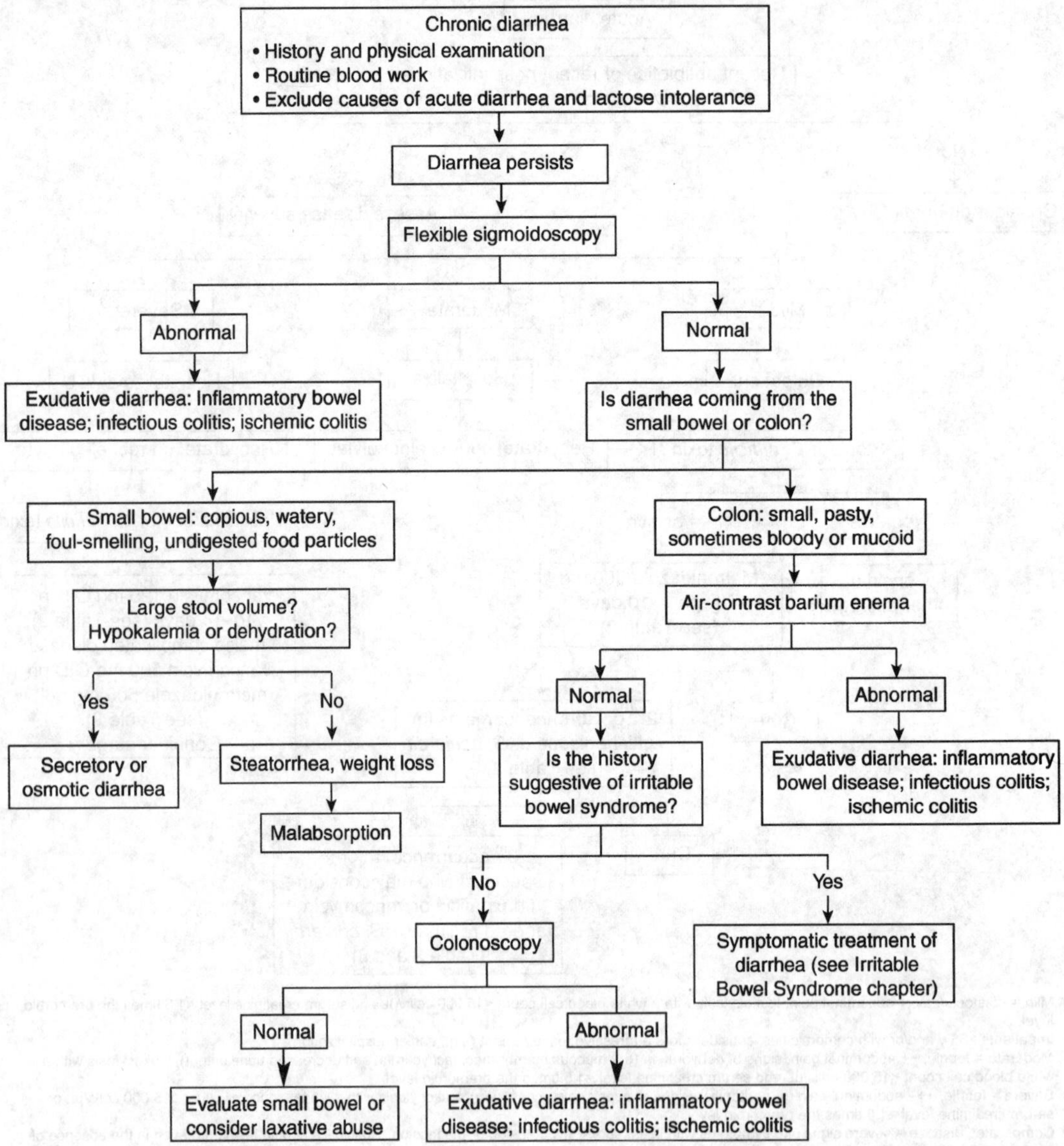

Therapeutic Choices

Nonpharmacologic Choices

- Discontinue medications that cause diarrhea (e.g., acarbose, antacids containing magnesium, antibiotics, cholinergic drugs, diuretics, fluorouracil, irinotecan, laxatives, orlistat, promotility agents, prostaglandins, theophylline).[2]
- Stop ingestion of poorly absorbed carbohydrates (e.g., dietetic candies and jams containing sorbitol, mannitol or xylitol, beverages and foods containing fructose, or lactose-containing dairy products).

If the history is compatible with lactose intolerance, a 2-week trial of a lactose-restricted diet can avoid costly diagnostic work-ups.[2]

- Reduce food intake for 12–24 hours. This will improve the symptoms of acute diarrhea. Maintenance of adequate fluid and electrolyte intake is important and a bland diet (low fat, low carbohydrate including, for example, bananas, rice, unsweetened applesauce, clear soup) can be reintroduced once bowel motions have subsided.[2]
- Prevent *C. difficile* spread via direct contact. Prevention of spread consists of educating patients and health care providers, good hand hygiene (frequent handwashing) and patient isolation in hospital setting (until symptom free for 48 hours post initiation of treatment), protective clothing (gowns and gloves) and environmental control (cleaning of medical equipment).[7]
- In the case of *Norwalk* virus, identifying the causative agent allows for institution of appropriate control measures:
  - frequent handwashing with soap
  - wearing of protective barriers such as gloves
  - careful washing of all fruits and vegetables
  - appropriate disposal of vomitus (in toilet) and disinfection of potentially contaminated surfaces
  - infected persons should not prepare foods while they are symptomatic and for 3 days after they have recovered

Pharmacologic Choices

Table 2 lists the agents used in the management of diarrhea.

Acute Diarrhea

Infectious Diarrhea

Use **oral rehydration therapy** (ORT) to prevent dehydration and electrolyte loss in both acute and chronic diarrhea (see Chapter 101). Oral rehydration solutions should have a balanced sodium-to-glucose ratio. Excess glucose, for example in Jell-O and soft drinks, or excess sodium, for example in Gatorade or other "sports drinks," may aggravate diarrhea as a consequence of their osmotic effect. Early use of ORT is essential for young children and the elderly.

Balanced electrolyte oral rehydration solutions are available commercially without prescription (e.g., Gastrolyte, Pedialyte). If necessary, a similar solution can be made by adding 1 level teaspoon (5 mL) of salt and 6 teaspoons (30 mL) of sugar to 1 litre of water.[8]

Aside from travellers' diarrhea (see Chapter 123), *empiric* **antibiotic** treatment is not generally recommended for acute diarrhea because of the self-limiting nature of most illnesses, the cost of treatment, the potential for promoting antimicrobial resistance and the possibility of adverse drug reactions.[8,9]

Bismuth subsalicylate has been shown to be effective in small cohort studies in the treatment of idiopathic diarrhea and diarrhea caused by microscopic colitis (Table 2). Although frequently used in acute diarrheas, there is no firm evidence for its efficacy. The salicylate component can cause gastric and duodenal mucosal damage, particularly in patients who are also using ASA or NSAIDs. At high doses, the calcium carbonate in the tablet formation can cause hypercalcemia, hypercalciuria and associated metabolic symptoms. Bismuth-related encephalopathy can result from the use of doses 10 times those recommended, or after years of use. Black stools due to bismuth may be confused with melena.

Available opioids (**codeine**, **diphenoxylate** and **loperamide**) are very effective for symptomatic use in both acute and chronic diarrhea (Table 2); however, side effects limit their acute use and tolerance usually occurs with chronic use. Antimotility effects are not desired if the diarrhea is caused by microorganisms because gastrointestinal stasis may enhance their invasion.[8,10] Diphenoxylate and loperamide have fewer CNS side effects than other opioids. Diphenoxylate is combined with atropine to limit its potential for abuse. Loperamide has the lowest incidence of side effects and abuse potential, is available without prescription and is effective in patients with radiotherapy- and chemotherapy-induced diarrhea and in patients with ileorectal pouch incontinence. Combining loperamide with simethicone provides faster and more complete relief of acute diarrhea associated with gas-related abdominal discomfort.[11] Consider codeine if sedation or analgesia is also desired.

Probiotics are nonpathogenic microorganisms that, when present in the gut, improve intestinal microbial balance. Multiple clinical trials have looked at the use of probiotics in the prevention and treatment of gastrointestinal infections in adults and children. Use probiotic mixtures described in clinical trials (Table 3) since not all probiotics have the same therapeutic effect.

- In children and adults <65 years of age, probiotics *prevent* antibiotic- and *C. difficile*-associated diarrhea.[12,15,16,17,18,19,20]
- In children and adults, probiotics shorten the duration and reduce stool frequency in acute infectious diarrhea.[21] In children, probiotics may be effective in treating persistent diarrhea lasting >14 days[22] and may reduce the severity and duration of acute rotavirus-induced diarrhea.[12,23,24,25] There is no conclusive evidence for the effectiveness of probiotics in the management of travellers' diarrhea.[26]

Antibiotic-associated Diarrhea

Management of *C. difficile*-associated diarrhea consists of the following key steps: prompt diagnosis, prevention of spread, cessation of causative antibiotic, supportive measures in severe cases (hospitalization, rehydration, correction of electrolyte imbalances) and eradication of CDI (Figure 2).

Eradication therapy is required in patients with symptoms (usually diarrhea) *and* confirmed diagnosis of CDI (positive stool test for toxigenic *C. difficile* or its toxins) or visual confirmation of pseudomembranous colitis. Therapy may be initiated in the absence of a firm diagnosis and in the presence of high suspicion and severe symptoms. Asymptomatic *C. difficile* carriers do not benefit from eradication therapy and should not be treated.[6]

Use **metronidazole** for mild-moderate initial episodes of *C. difficile*-associated diarrhea (Figure 2, Table 2).[6] Use **oral vancomycin** for severe initial episodes or if patient is unable to take metronidazole.[6] Use high-dose oral vancomycin plus iv metronidazole for severe *and* complicated disease (e.g., hypotension, shock, ileus, megacolon).[6] First CDI relapse occurs in 10–25% of patients and should be managed based on its severity by repeating the first line of therapy used.[6] Second relapse should be investigated for other causes of diarrhea and, if *C. difficile* is confirmed, treat with tapered or pulsed vancomycin oral regimen.[6] Use metronidazole with caution after the first recurrence due to potential for cumulative neurotoxicity.[6,13] For the third or subsequent recurrences consider longer treatment periods with vancomycin or refer to an infectious disease specialist.

Fidaxomicin, a poorly absorbed antibiotic, has similar efficacy to vancomycin for the treatment of a first occurrence of *C. difficile* infection (CDI) and lower recurrence rates than vancomycin for non-hypervirulent strains [Evidence: SORT B*].[29,30] Fidaxomicin's high cost may offset its advantages over vancomycin[31] making its precise role in the treatment of CDI uncertain. It is reasonable to consider fidaxomicin in those patients who have more than 2 occurrences of CDI or in those who require ongoing therapy with other antibiotics [Evidence: SORT C*].[32] Fidaxomicin is usually administered in a hospital setting on the advice of an infectious disease specialist or gastroenterologist.

Rifampin can be utilized for the treatment of recurrent CDI, but there is a rising concern about rifampin-resistance.[33]

* SORT (Strength of Recommendation Taxonomy) is a rating system (A, B or C) that addresses the quality of available evidence. For more information consult **How to Use *Compendium of Therapeutic Choices*** on page xxv.

Investigational treatment options include fecal transplantation,[34] intravenous immunoglobulins[35,36,37] and nitazoxanide.[38]

Patients requiring treatment with antimicrobials during or shortly after the completion of their *C. difficile* therapy should receive concomitant oral vancomycin until the antimicrobials are stopped; however, it is unknown if this regimen results in reduced recurrence of CDI.[6]

There is no role for **probiotic** monotherapy in the acute treatment or prevention of CDI in adults and children,[14] however, the probiotic *Saccharomyces boulardii* may be marginally effective when used in conjunction with antibiotic treatment to prevent *C. difficile* recurrence (Table 3).[27,28] There is also no evidence that adding **cholestyramine** or **colestipol** to the antibiotic treatment regimen decreases the risk of further recurrence. In fact, resins are contraindicated with antibiotics since they can bind to and sequester antibiotics in the gut.[6]

Antimotility agents such as **loperamide** are not used in symptomatic CDI because their use increases the risk of toxin retention and precipitation of toxic megacolon.[39]

Chronic Diarrhea

See Oral Rehydration Therapy and Opioids discussion in the Acute Diarrhea section.

Hydrophilic Bulking Agents

Although **psyllium** may reduce nonspecific diarrheal symptoms, its role in the management of diarrhea is limited. Many psyllium-containing products are combined with laxatives; avoid these products in patients with diarrhea.

Cholestyramine resin is useful in treating bile acid–induced diarrhea due to malabsorption of bile acids in diseased ileum (e.g., Crohn's disease) or in some cases of irritable bowel syndrome where rapid transit results in loss of bile acids into the colon.

Alpha$_2$-adrenergic Agonists

Clonidine may be effective for opioid-withdrawal diarrhea and diarrhea associated with diabetic autonomic neuropathy.[40] Unfortunately, the dose required to achieve an antidiarrheal effect is often associated with sedation, dry mouth and symptomatic orthostatic hypotension.

Somatostatin Analogues

Somatostatin analogues can be administered sc daily (**octreotide**) or im monthly (**octreotide acetate**, **lanreotide acetate**). These agents have been used to control diarrhea caused by neuroendocrine tumors (VIPoma, carcinoid, medullary carcinoma of the thyroid). Octreotide also limits idiopathic and infant secretory diarrhea, as well as diarrhea associated with ileostomy, short bowel syndrome, diabetic neuropathy, chemotherapy, bone marrow transplant, cryptosporidia, graft versus host disease and HIV disease.

Somatostatin has a short half-life and requires continuous iv infusion, which limits its role in the management of diarrhea.

Probiotics

VSL#3 may decrease the occurrence and severity of postradiation diarrhea.[41]

Public Health Considerations

- Food-handlers in the food service industry and health care workers with direct patient contact and diarrhea should be tested for parasitic and bacterial pathogens due to their potential to transmit the infections to large numbers of persons.

- Similarly, daycare attendees and employees, or residents of an institutional facility (nursing home, psychiatric hospital, prison) with diarrhea should be tested for bacterial, parasitic or viral pathogens since the diarrhea may be an indicator of an endemic outbreak.
- Physicians who suspect an endemic diarrheal disease outbreak should report their concern to public health authorities and work with them to initiate appropriate diagnostic testing to identify the pathogen and define the extent of the outbreak.
- Follow-up testing is not generally recommended. However, since food handlers and healthcare workers can transmit bacterial and parasitic diseases even if they are asymptomatic, they should, before returning to their jobs, have 2 consecutive negative stool samples taken 24 hours apart and be symptom free for at least 48 hours.

Choices during Pregnancy and Breastfeeding

Loperamide can be used safely in pregnancy and is compatible with breastfeeding.[42] **Diphenoxylate with atropine** should not be used during pregnancy or breastfeeding since it has been found to be teratogenic in animals[43] and its active metabolite is probably excreted in breast milk.[43] **Cholestyramine** is used to treat cholestasis of pregnancy and can be used to manage diarrhea resulting from ileal resection or cholecystectomy.[44] Use it with caution during pregnancy or breastfeeding since fat-soluble vitamin deficiency and coagulopathy can occur. Avoid **bismuth subsalicylate** in pregnancy because salicylates can be absorbed and may lead to increased perinatal mortality, premature closure of the ductus arteriosus, neonatal hemorrhage, decreased birth weight, prolonged gestation and labour and possible teratogenicity.[45] Salicylates should be used cautiously while breastfeeding since they are excreted in breast milk.

Metronidazole is not associated with congenital malformations.[46,47,48] It is excreted in breast milk and breastfeeding should be suspended until treatment with this drug is completed.[49] **Vancomycin** has not been shown to have adverse effects in pregnant women. There is limited human data on its use while breastfeeding but it is probably safe.

Therapeutic Tips

- Infectious diarrhea can be prevented by following simple rules of personal hygiene and safe food preparation. Handwashing with soap is an effective step in preventing spread of the illness and should be emphasized for both patients and their caregivers.
- It is critical that patients understand the importance of a balanced electrolyte **oral rehydration solution** in preventing dehydration, and are aware of the inability of non-balanced electrolyte solutions to achieve rehydration.
- Repeated diarrheal illnesses in young children can lead to malnutrition and physical and cognitive growth impairment.
- Specific **vaccines** are available for prevention of diarrhea due to cholera (*V. cholerae*) and enterotoxigenic *E. coli* in adults and children (see Chapter 123), typhoid fever (*S. typhi*) in adults and children, and rotavirus in infants.

Table 2: Drugs Used to Treat Diarrhea

Class	Drug	Dose	Adverse Effects	Drug Interactions	Comments	Cost[a]
Alpha$_2$-adrenergic Agonists	*clonidine* Catapres, generics	0.1–0.6 mg Q12H po	Centrally mediated sedation and hypotension.	Additive effects with drugs that cause hypotension.		$
Antibacterial Agents	*fidaxomicin* Dificid	200 mg BID po × 10 days	Constipation (1.2%), nausea (2.7%), rash (2.8%), vomiting (1.2%).	No significant drug interactions.	Expensive. May be considered in patients experiencing more than 2 occurrences of *C. difficile*-associated diarrhea (see Figure 2).	$240/day
	metronidazole Flagyl, generics	First or second occurrence of mild-moderate *C. difficile* diarrhea: 500 mg TID po × 10–14 days ± *S. boulardii* (Table 3) Severe and complicated *C. difficile* diarrhea: 500 mg Q8H iv in combination with vancomycin	Nausea, headache, anorexia, dry mouth, metallic taste in mouth.	Metronidazole may potentiate warfarin; monitor INR when metronidazole is added or discontinued and adjust warfarin dose accordingly. Disulfiram-like reaction with alcohol: avoid alcohol intake during treatment and for 48 h after treatment.	Refrain from using metronidazole for third or subsequent occurrences to avoid drug accumulation and neurotoxicity.	$
	vancomycin Vancocin, generics	First or second occurrence of severe *C. difficile* diarrhea: 125 mg QID po × 10–14 days First episode of severe and complicated *C. difficile* diarrhea: 500 mg QID po in combination with metronidazole; consider adding vancomycin retention enema if complete ileus Third or later occurrence of *C. difficile* diarrhea: 125 mg QID po × 10–14 days then 125 mg BID po × 7 days, then 125 mg daily po × 7 days, then	Bitter taste, nausea, vomiting, stomatitis, chills, drug fever, eosinophilia.	Minimal with oral administration.	Vancomycin is poorly absorbed after oral administration.	$$$$

(cont'd)

Table 2: **Drugs Used to Treat Diarrhea** *(cont'd)*

Class	Drug	Dose	Adverse Effects	Drug Interactions	Comments	Cost[a]
		125 mg po every 2–3 days × 2–8 wk in combination with *S. boulardii* (Table 3)				
Hydrophilic Bulking Agents	*psyllium hydrophilic mucilloid* Metamucil Preparations, generics	1 teaspoon (5–6 g) Q12H po	Inhalation of psyllium powder may cause allergic reactions.		Take with fluids. Avoid combinations with laxatives.	$
Intestinal Adsorbants	*bismuth subsalicylate* Pepto-Bismol generics	30 mL (17.6 mg BSS/mL) Q30 min po to a maximum of 8 doses/day	Salicylate toxicity, black tongue, black stool, bismuth-induced encephalopathy.	Decreases absorption of fluoroquinolones, doxycycline and tetracycline.		$
	bismuth subsalicylate with calcium carbonate Pepto-Bismol Chewable Tablets	2 tablets (262 mg BSS/tablet) Q30 min po to a maximum of 8 doses/day	See bismuth subsalicylate. Hypercalcemia, hypercalciuria.	See bismuth subsalicylate.		$
Opioids	*codeine* ● generics	30–60 mg Q4H PRN po	Sedation, nausea, tolerance, potentially addictive.	Additive CNS depression with CNS depressants.	Elderly may be particularly susceptible to the adverse effects.	$
	diphenoxylate with atropine sulfate ● Lomotil	5 mg po initially then 2.5 mg po after each loose bowel movement (maximum of 20 mg/day)	Sedation, nausea, abdominal cramps, dry skin and mucous membranes (from atropine), some addiction potential.	Additive anticholinergic effects with other anticholinergic agents.	The elderly are more susceptible to the antimuscarinic effects of atropine, e.g., agitation, drowsiness, increased intraocular pressure.	$
	loperamide Imodium, Riva-Loperamide, other generics	2 mg po after each loose bowel movement (maximum of 16 mg/day)	Sedation, nausea, abdominal cramps. Lowest addiction potential of all opioids.			$
Resins	*cholestyramine resin* Olestyr	4 g Q12H po	Nausea, fat soluble vitamin deficiency with long-term use, constipation.	May bind drugs, e.g., digoxin, in GI tract; do not take within 1 h before or 4–6 h after other medications.	Take with fluids.	$
Somatostatin Analogues	*lanreotide acetate* Somatuline autogel	60 mg monthly im	Pain at injection site, nausea, mild diarrhea.			$1100/month

Class	Drug	Dose	Adverse Effects	Drug Interactions	Comments	Cost[a]
	octreotide acetate Sandostatin, generics	50–500 µg Q12H sc	See lanreotide acetate.	May decrease insulin resistance; increases risk of hypoglycemia with concurrent use of antihyperglycemic agents.		$$$
	octreotide acetate long-acting Sandostatin LAR	10–30 mg monthly im	See lanreotide acetate.			$1325–$2195/ month

[a] Cost of 1-day supply unless otherwise specified; includes drug cost only.
Abbreviations: BSS = bismuth subsalicylate; INR = international normalized ratio; LAR = long-acting release
Legend: $ <$5 $$ $5–15 $$$ $15–30 $$$$ $30–45

Table 3: Probiotic Products Used to Treat Diarrhea

Class	Drug	Dose	Adverse Effects	Drug Interactions	Comments	Cost[a]
Probiotics	*lactic acid bacterial mixture* VSL#3	Packets contain 450×10^9 freeze-dried lactic acid bacteria (*Bifidobacterium breve, B. longum, B. infantis, L. acidophilus, L. plantarum, L. casei, L. bulgaricus, Streptococcus thermophilus*) in a defined ratio. The dose is based on the frequency of BM Adults: 1–2 packets/day po if <5 BM; 2–4 packets/day po if 5–8 BM; 4 packets/day po if >8 BM	No evidence of adverse health effects.	A mixture of bacteria; therefore, do not administer with antibiotics.	Has been studied in patients with radiation-induced diarrhea, Crohn's disease, ulcerative colitis, ileal pouch anastomosis and IBS.	$$
	Lactobacillus GG Culturelle	1 capsule contains at least 10 billion bacteria Adults: 1–2 capsules daily po	~2% of patients report bloating and gas for a few days.	A bacterium; therefore, do not administer with antibiotics.	May contain traces of casein or whey. Does not ferment lactose; unhelpful for lactose intolerance.	$$
	Saccharomyces boulardii Florastor	1 capsule (250 mg) contains 5 billion organisms 1 capsule BID po × 3–5 days, maximum 3 capsules per day In combination with metronidazole, for recurrence of *C. difficile*-associated diarrhea: 2 capsules BID po × 14–21 days In combination with vancomycin for second recurrence of *C. difficile* diarrhea: 2 capsules BID po × 12 months	Constipation, bloating.	A yeast; therefore, do not administer with antifungal agents.	There have been rare reports of fungemia in patients with a central venous catheter.	$

[a] Cost of 1-day supply.
Abbreviations: BM = bowel movement; IBS = irritable bowel syndrome
Legend: $ <$5 $$ $5–15

Suggested Readings

Aranda-Michel J, Giannella RA. Acute diarrhea: a practical review. *Am J Med* 1999;106(6):670-6.

Fedorak RN. Anti-diarrheal therapy. In: Friedman G, Jacobson ED, McCallum RW, eds. *Gastrointestinal pharmacology and therapeutics*. Philadelphia (PA): Lippincott-Raven; 1997. p. 175-93.

Fine KD, Schiller LR. AGA technical review on the evaluation and management of chronic diarrhea. *Gastroenterology* 1999;116(6):1464-86.

Theilman NM, Guerrant RL. An algorithmic approach to the workup and management of HIV-related diarrhea. *J Clin Outcomes Manag* 1997;4:36-47.

Thielman NM, Guerrant RL. Clinical practice. Acute infectious diarrhea. *N Engl J Med* 2004;350(1):38-47.

References

1. DuPont HL. Guidelines on acute infectious diarrhea in adults. The Practice Parameters Committee of the American College of Gastroenterology. *Am J Gastroenterol* 1997;92(11):1962-75.
2. Schiller LR. Chronic diarrhea. *Gastroenterology* 2004;127(1):287-93.
3. Thielman NM, Guerrant RL. Clinical practice. Acute infectious diarrhea. *N Engl J Med* 2004;350(1):38-47.
4. Kane SV, Sandborn WJ, Rufo PA et al. Fecal lactoferrin is a sensitive and specific marker in identifying intestinal inflammation. *Am J Gastroenterol* 2003;98(6):1309-14.
5. McFarland LV. Antibiotic-associated diarrhea: epidemiology, trends and treatment. *Future Microbiol* 2008;3(5):563-78.
6. Cohen SH, Gerding DN, Johnson S et al. Clinical practice guidelines for Clostridium difficile infection in adults: 2010 update by the Society for Healthcare Epidemiology of America (SHEA) and the Infectious Diseases Society of America (IDSA). *Infect Control Hosp Epidemiol* 2010;31(5):431-55.
7. Vonberg RP, Kuijper EJ, Wilcox MH et al. Infection control measured to limit the spread of Clostridium difficile. *Clin Microbiol Infect* 2008;14(Suppl 5):2-20.
8. Committee to Advise on Tropical Medicine and Travel (CATMAT). An Advisory Committee Statement (ACS). Statement on travellers' diarrhea. *Can Commun Dis Rep* 2001;27(ACS-3):1-12.
9. Sirinavin S, Garner P. Antibiotics for treating salmonella gut infections. *Cochrane Database Syst Rev* 2000;(2):CD001167.
10. Molbak K, Mead PS, Griffin PM. Antimicrobial therapy in patients with Escherichia coli O157:H7 infection. *JAMA* 2002;288(8):1014-6.
11. Hanauer SB, DuPont HL, Cooper KM et al. Randomized, double-blind, placebo-controlled clinical trial of loperamide plus simethicone versus loperamide alone and simethicone alone in the treatment of acute diarrhea with gas-related abdominal discomfort. *Curr Med Res Opin* 2007;23(5):1033-43.
12. NASPGHAN Nutrition Report Committee; Michail S, Sylvester F et al. Clinical efficacy of probiotics: review of the evidence with focus on children. *J Pediatr Gastroenterol Nutr* 2006;43(4):550-7.
13. Kapoor K, Chandra M, Nag D et al. Evaluation of metronidazole toxicity: a prospective study. *Int J Clin Pharmacol Res* 1999;19(3):83-8.
14. Pillai A, Nelson R. Probiotics for treatment of Clostridium difficile-associated colitis in adults. *Cochrane Database Syst Rev* 2008;(1):CD004611.
15. Allen SJ, Wareham K, Wang D et al. Lactobacilli and bifidobacteria in the prevention of antibiotic-associated diarrhoea and Clostridium difficile diarrhoea in older inpatients (PLACIDE): a randomised, double-blind, placebo-controlled, multicentre trial. *Lancet* 2013;382(9900):1249-57.
16. Johnston BC, Goldenberg JZ, Vandvik PO et al. Probiotics for the prevention of pediatric antibiotic-associated diarrhea. *Cochrane Database Syst Rev* 2011;(11):CD004827.
17. Goldenberg JZ, Ma SS, Saxton JD et al. Probiotics for the prevention of Clostridium difficile-associated diarrhea in adults and children. *Cochrane Database Syst Rev* 2013;5:CD006095.
18. Hempel S, Newberry SJ, Maher AR et al. Probiotics for the prevention and treatment of antibiotic-associated diarrhea: a systematic review and meta-analysis. *JAMA* 2012;307(18):1959-69.
19. Johnston BC, Ma SS, Goldenberg JZ et al. Probiotics for the prevention of Clostridium difficile-associated diarrhea: a systematic review and meta-analysis. *Ann Intern Med* 2012;157(12):878-88.
20. Videlock EJ, Cremonini F. Meta-analysis: probiotics in antibiotic-associated diarrhoea. *Aliment Pharmacol Ther* 2012;35(12):1355-69.
21. Allen SJ, Martinez EG, Gregorio GV et al. Probiotics for treating acute infectious diarrhoea. *Cochrane Database Syst Rev* 2010;(11):CD003048.
22. Bernaola Aponte G, Bada Mancilla CA, Carreazo NY et al. Probiotics for treating persistent diarrhoea in children. *Cochrane Database Syst Rev* 2013;8:CD007401.
23. Dalgic N, Sancar M, Bayraktar B et al. Probiotic, zinc and lactose-free formula in children with rotavirus diarrhea: are they effective? *Pediatr Int* 2011;53(5):677-82.
24. Erdoğan O, Tanyeri B, Torun E et al. The comparition of the efficacy of two different probiotics in rotavirus gastroenteritis in children. *J Trop Med* 2012;2012:787240.
25. Grandy G, Medina M, Soria R et al. Probiotics in the treatment of acute rotavirus diarrhoea. A randomized, double-blind, controlled trial using two different probiotic preparations in Bolivian children. *BMC Infect Dis* 2010;10:253.
26. Ritchie ML, Romanuk TN. A meta-analysis of probiotic efficacy for gastrointestinal diseases. *PLoS One* 2012;7(4):e34938.
27. Surawicz CM, McFarland LV, Greenberg RN et al. The search for a better treatment for recurrent Clostridium difficile disease: use of high-dose vancomycin combined with Saccharomyces boulardii. *Clin Infect Dis* 2000;31(4):1012-7.
28. McFarland LV, Surawicz CM, Greenberg RN et al. A randomized placebo-controlled trial of Saccharomyces boulardii in combination with standard antibiotics for Clostridium difficile disease. *JAMA* 1994;271(24):1913-8.
29. Louie TJ, Miller MA, Mullane KM et al. Fidaxomicin versus vancomycin for Clostridium difficile infection. *N Engl J Med* 2011;364(5):422-31.
30. Cornely OA, Crook DW, Esposito R et al. Fidaxomicin versus vancomycin for infection with Clostridium difficile in Europe, Canada, and the USA: a double-blind, non-inferiority, randomised controlled trial. *Lancet Infect Dis* 2012;12(4):281-9.
31. Bartsch SM, Umscheid CA, Fishman N et al. Is fidaxomicin worth the cost? An economic analysis. *Clin Infect Dis* 2013;57(4):555-61.

32. Mullane KM, Miller MA, Weiss K et al. Efficacy of fidaxomicin versus vancomycin as therapy for Clostridium difficile infection in individuals taking concomitant antibiotics for other concurrent infections. *Clin Infect Dis* 2011;53(5):440-7.
33. Curry SR, Marsh JW, Shutt KA et al. High frequency of rifampin resistance identified in an epidemic Clostridium difficile clone from a large teaching hospital. *Clin Infect Dis* 2009;48(4):425-9.
34. Brandt LJ, Aroniadis OC, Mellow M et al. Long-term follow-up of colonoscopic fecal microbiota transplant for recurrent Clostridium difficile infection. *Am J Gastroenterol* 2012;107(7):1079-87.
35. Giannasca PJ, Warny M. Active and passive immunization against Clostridium difficile diarrhea and colitis. *Vaccine* 2004;22(7):848-56.
36. Wilcox MH. Descriptive study of intravenous immunoglobulin for the treatment of recurrent Clostridium difficile diarrhoea. *J Antimicrob Chemother* 2004;53(5):882-4.
37. Salcedo J, Keates S, Pothoulakis C et al. Intravenous immunoglobulin therapy for severe Clostridium difficile colitis. *Gut* 1997;41(3):366-70.
38. Musher DM, Logan N, Hamill RJ et al. Nitazoxanide for the treatment of Clostridium difficile colitis. *Clin Infect Dis* 2006;43(4):421-7.
39. Fekety R. Guidelines for the diagnosis and management of Clostridium difficile-associated diarrhea and colitis. American College of Gastroenterology, Practice Parameters Committee. *Am J Gastroenterol* 1997;92(5):739-50.
40. Fedorak RN, Field M. Antidiarrheal therapy. Prospects for new agents. *Dig Dis Sci* 1987;32(2):195-205.
41. Delia P, Sansotta G, Donato V et al. Prevention of radiation-induced diarrhea with the use of VSL#3, a new high-potency probiotic preparation. *Am J Gastroenterol* 2002;97(8):2150-2.
42. Einarson A, Mastroiacovo P, Arnon J et al. Prospective, controlled, multicentre study of loperamide in pregnancy. *Can J Gastroenterol* 2000;14(3):185-7.
43. Product information. *Lomotil*. G.D. Searle and Company; 2000.
44. Jenkins JK, Boothby LA. Treatment of itching associated with intrahepatic cholestasis of pregnancy. *Ann Pharmacother* 2002;36(9):1462-5.
45. Collins E. Maternal and fetal effects of acetaminophen and salicylates in pregnancy. *Obstet Gynecol* 1981;58(5 Suppl):57S-62S.
46. Burtin P, Taddio A, Ariburnu O et al. Safety of metronidazole in pregnancy: a meta-analysis. *Am J Obstet Gynecol* 1995;172(2 Pt 1):525-9.
47. Caro-Paton T, Carvajal A, Martin de Diego I et al. Is metronidazole teratogenic? A meta-analysis. *Br J Clin Pharmacol* 1997;44(2):179-82.
48. Diav-Citrin O, Shechtman S, Gotteiner T et al. Pregnancy outcome after gestational exposure to metronidazole: a prospective controlled cohort study. *Teratology* 2001;63(5):186-92.
49. Stewart JJ. Gastrointestinal drugs. In: Wilson JT, ed. *Drugs in breast milk*. New York (NY): ADIS Press Australasia; 1981. p. 71.

Gastrointestinal Disorders

Chapter 60
Dyspepsia and Peptic Ulcer Disease

Laura Targownik, MD, MSHS, FRCPC

CPhA acknowledges the contribution of Dr. A.B.R. Thomson as a previous author of this chapter.

Dyspepsia, defined as pain or discomfort located in the upper abdomen, is one of the most common complaints bringing patients to consult their family physician.[1] Other upper GI symptoms associated with dyspepsia may include nausea, vomiting, fullness, early satiety and bloating. Dyspepsia is the cardinal symptom of peptic ulcer disease (PUD) which refers to the development of breaks in the mucosa of the stomach (gastric ulcers; GU) and/or proximal duodenum (duodenal ulcers; DU).

Dyspepsia occurs in about 25% of people over the course of any year.[2,3] Organic findings accounting for dyspeptic symptoms will be present in approximately 25% of persons with dyspepsia where erosive esophagitis and PUD are the most common causes.[4] Other less common findings include upper GI tract Crohn's disease, celiac disease, eosinophilic esophagitis, esophageal candidiasis and cytomegalovirus related ulceration. In the absence of alarm symptoms (see Investigations), the likelihood of detecting malignancy as a cause of the dyspepsia is very low.[5,6]

Approximately 75% of patients with chronic dyspepsia will have a normal upper GI tract upon endoscopic examination. This group of subjects with chronic dyspepsia and normal endoscopic findings are often referred to as having nonulcer dyspepsia (NUD) or functional dyspepsia. As the nature and severity of the symptoms do not significantly differ between persons with PUD and NUD, it is not possible to reliably differentiate between these syndromes without performing endoscopy or other imaging. However, differentiation of NUD from PUD is not crucial to the initial management of persons with dyspepsia and may not be necessary if symptoms resolve as a result of the initial management.[7]

Lifetime prevalence of PUD is about 10% in North Americans and the incidence is decreasing.[8,9] The most common risk factors for the development of chronic PUD are *Helicobacter pylori* infections and use of medications such as NSAIDs or antiplatelets (e.g., ASA, clopidogrel, ticagrelor). However, 5–20% of patients with GU/DU have no evidence of either *H. pylori* or ASA/NSAID use.[10]

This chapter considers the management of:

1. Uninvestigated dyspepsia
2. Dyspepsia with normal endoscopy (functional dyspepsia or nonulcer dyspepsia)
3. Treatment of PUD due to *H. pylori* infection
4. Prevention and treatment of PUD during ASA or NSAID therapy

GERD is addressed in Chapter 61.

Goals of Therapy

- Relieve and prevent symptoms of dyspepsia
- Treat underlying PUD if present
- Prevent recurrence of PUD
- Prevent PUD-related complications in users of NSAIDs and ASA

Investigations

- History and physical examination:
  - exclude non-GI sources of pain or discomfort in the upper abdomen, e.g., ischemic heart disease, pulmonary disease.
  - "red flags" such as age >50 years and alarm signs such as abdominal mass, vomiting, bleeding, dysphagia, anemia or unexplained weight loss occurring with symptoms may be associated with rare but serious causes such as esophageal or gastric cancer.
  - identify those with predominant reflux-like symptoms (e.g., heartburn, regurgitation) because they are more likely to respond to empiric proton pump inhibitor (PPI) therapy.
  - take a drug history focusing on NSAID or ASA use (including low-dose ASA), antiplatelet agents (e.g., clopidogrel, ticagrelor) as well as other medications that may cause or aggravate dyspepsia such as bisphosphonates, tetracyclines, calcium channel blockers, iron salts and opioids, particularly codeine.
  - physical examination will usually be normal. Epigastric tenderness is a common but nonspecific finding.
- Investigations for dyspepsia:
  - endoscopy is the most sensitive and specific means to diagnose the cause of dyspepsia. However, not every person with dyspeptic symptoms requires prompt endoscopy.[7,11] Endoscopy is most appropriate in dyspeptic patients with 1 or more of the following red flags: age >50 years, alarm signs such as vomiting, bleeding, anemia, weight loss and dysphagia, and failure to respond to initial management strategies (see below). The disadvantages of endoscopy include scarcity of gastroenterologists to perform the procedure, cost, time lost from work and risk of complications such as aspiration or perforation (about 1 in 5000 procedures).
  - upper GI barium study has an approximately 20% false-positive and false-negative rate for detection of ulcer disease and is generally not recommended, especially in those with red flags.[12,13] However, barium studies are often more readily available than upper endoscopy and are still used to reassure the physician that nothing serious has been missed as a cause of the dyspepsia.
  - consider a CT scan of the abdomen if patient experiences weight loss, jaundice or pain radiating to the back, to rule out the presence of chronic pancreatitis or pancreatic cancer.
- Investigations for *H. pylori* infection:
  - *H. pylori* infection may cause or worsen dyspepsia and its complications. About 25% of Canadians with uninvestigated dyspepsia will have evidence of active *H. pylori* infection in the stomach.
  - a "test-and-treat" strategy for *H. pylori* is advocated as first-line management since approximately 50% of persons with dyspepsia who are *H. pylori*-positive will respond to eradicative therapy.[14]
  - noninvasive tests for *H. pylori* include:
    - serology: assessment of *H. Pylori* serology in drawn serum is appropriate if there has been no prior attempt at *H. pylori* eradication, since serology may remain persistently positive for several years after successful eradication and therefore may represent a false-positive result.[15]
    - urea breath testing (UBT): the UBT is a highly sensitive and specific test for *H. pylori*. A patient is given a solution of radiolabelled urea (^{13}C or ^{14}C) to drink, and if *H. pylori* is present the urea is metabolized to radiolabelled carbon dioxide which can be detected in the breath.[16] The main disadvantages of UBT are that patients must be off antibiotics or bismuth for 1 month and PPIs or histamine H_2-receptor antagonists for at least 1 week prior to the urea breath test, to avoid a false-negative test result [Evidence: SORT C*].[17,18,19,20,21,22,23] UBT is available

* SORT (Strength of Recommendation Taxonomy) is a rating system (A, B or C) that addresses the quality of available evidence. For more information consult **How to Use *Compendium of Therapeutic Choices*** on page xxv.

only at centres that have nuclear medicine facilities. However, the Helikit, a ^{13}C UBT can be used at home by the patient to collect a breath sample which is then sent to a lab for analysis.
  - stool antigen testing: *H. pylori* antigens can be detected in the stool in the presence of active infection. Stool antigen testing is very specific but is slightly less sensitive than UBT. The main disadvantage of this test is that it requires collection of a stool specimen.[24] Its accuracy is also affected by concomitant acid-inhibiting therapy.
- endoscopy: biopsy samples can either be examined histologically or by indirect methods for the presence of *H. pylori*. Endoscopy is considered the gold standard for detection of *H. pylori*, but noninvasive testing is preferred unless the endoscopy is being performed for other reasons.

Uninvestigated Dyspepsia

Therapeutic Choices

Figure 1 presents an approach to the management of uninvestigated dyspepsia.

Figure 1: **Management of Dyspepsia**

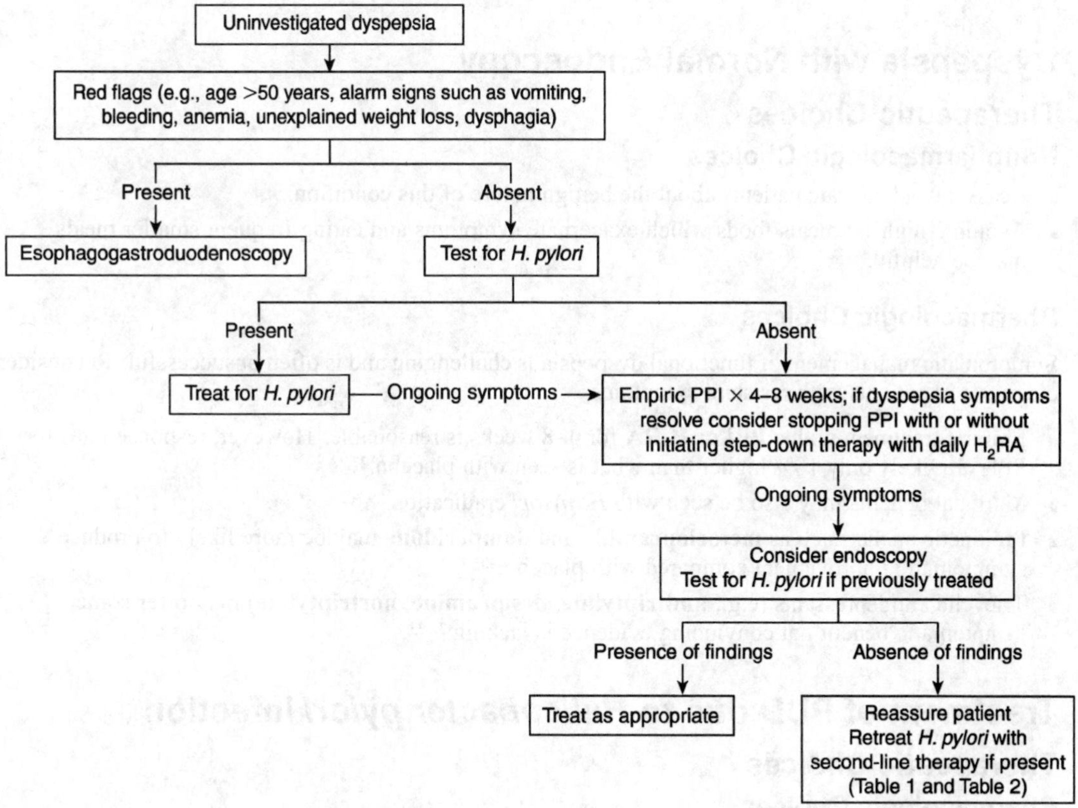

Abbreviations: H_2RA = histamine H_2–receptor antagonist; PPI = proton pump inhibitor

Nonpharmacologic Choices

General lifestyle modification is the first approach for the management of uninvestigated dyspepsia.

- Recommend moderation if a food or beverage (e.g., coffee, orange juice, spicy foods, fatty foods or large meals) or eating on the run worsens dyspepsia.
- Recommend avoiding use of nonprescription medications containing NSAIDs or ASA, which may cause dyspepsia or PUD.

Pharmacologic Choices

- Initial pharmacologic management of dyspepsia in the absence of alarm symptoms focuses on testing for *H. pylori* and eradicating it if present, or empirically treating symptoms with a standard-dose PPI for 4–8 weeks. The "test-and-treat" strategy is cost effective if the pretest probability of active *H. pylori* infection exceeds 20%.[15]
- If dyspepsia resolves after eradication of *H. pylori*, no further therapy is required.
- If dyspepsia resolves following empiric PPI therapy, consider discontinuing the PPI with or without initiating step-down therapy with a daily H_2-receptor antagonist (H_2RA).[25] If dyspepsia symptoms persist or if there are frequent recurrences, investigate for *H. pylori* infection with a UBT or with prompt endoscopy. UBT for *H. pylori* is safe, effective, more comfortable and less distressing for the patient than endoscopy.[26]

Dyspepsia with Normal Endoscopy

Therapeutic Choices

Nonpharmacologic Choices

- Reassure and educate patients about the benign nature of this condition.
- Avoiding high-fat meals/foods which exacerbate symptoms and eating frequent smaller meals may be helpful.

Pharmacologic Choices

Symptomatic management of functional dyspepsia is challenging and is often unsuccessful. Reconsider diagnosis in patients with resistant symptoms.

- Empiric treatment with a **PPI** or **H_2RA** for 4–8 weeks is reasonable. However, response rates for PPIs are likely only 10% higher than what is seen with placebo.[27,28]
- Marginal benefits may also be seen with *H. pylori* eradication.[29,30]
- Prokinetic agents such as **metoclopramide** and **domperidone** may be more likely to produce symptomatic improvement compared with placebo.[30,31]
- Tricyclic antidepressants (e.g., **amitriptyline**, **desipramine**, **nortriptyline**) may offer some symptomatic benefit but convincing evidence is lacking.[32,33]

Treatment of PUD due to *Helicobacter pylori* Infection

Therapeutic Choices

Pharmacologic Choices

Successful treatment of *H. pylori* (see Table 1) will result in ulcer healing and will prevent the development of recurrent PUD (in the absence of concomitant ASA or NSAID use).

Table 1: ***Helicobacter pylori* Eradication Regimens**

Regimen	Dose	Treatment Period	Cost[a]
Triple Therapy			
PPI	BID	10–14 days	$$$
clarithromycin	500 mg BID		
amoxicillin	1 g BID		
Hp-PAC, Losec 1-2-3 A, Nexium 1-2-3 A			
PPI	BID	10–14 days	$$$
clarithromycin	250 mg BID		
metronidazole	500 mg BID		
Losec 1-2-3 M			
Quadruple Therapy			
PPI	BID	10–14 days	$$$
bismuth subsalicylate	2 tabs QID		
metronidazole	250 mg QID		
tetracycline	500 mg QID		
Sequential Therapy			
PPI	BID	5–7 days	$$$
amoxicillin	1 g BID		
followed by			
PPI	BID	5–7 days	
clarithromycin	500 mg BID		
metronidazole	500 mg BID		

[a] Cost per treatment period; includes drug cost only.
[b] Dose may be increased to 500 mg clarithromycin twice daily.
Dosage adjustment may be required in renal impairment; see Appendix I.
Abbreviations: PPI = proton pump inhibitor
Legend: $ <$15 $$ $15–30 $$$ $30–45

Eradication of Helicobacter pylori

- First-line *triple* therapy consists of any **PPI** plus **clarithromycin** and **amoxicillin** administered BID for 10–14 days (Table 1).[15] Therapy for 10–14 days leads to 10% higher eradication rates than 7-day therapy.[34]
- Amoxicillin can be replaced with **metronidazole** if a beta-lactam allergy is present.
- *Quadruple* therapy consisting of any **PPI** taken BID combined with **bismuth subsalicylate**, **metronidazole** and **tetracycline** taken QID for 10–14 days is also considered to be a first-line treatment option (Table 1). Quadruple therapy may be used for triple therapy failures, if patient is intolerant of macrolide antibiotics or if resistance to clarithromycin in the geographic treatment area is known to be high (>15% of *H. pylori* isolates).[35]
- The above regimens are approved by the Canadian Helicobacter Study Group and achieve a minimum eradication rate (on an intention-to-treat basis) of at least 80%.[36]
- After successful *H. pylori* eradication, the risk of reinfection is about 1% per year.
- Following completion of *H. pylori* eradicative therapy, perform follow-up testing with either UBT, stool antigen testing or histology to confirm eradication (see Investigations).
- In patients with complicated ulcers (e.g., bleeding, perforation, severe symptoms), continue therapy with PPIs until eradication of *H. pylori* is confirmed.
- If *H. pylori* is not successfully eradicated, second-line options include:
  - Quadruple therapy with a PPI + bismuth + metronidazole + tetracycline × 10–14 days
  - Quadruple therapy with a PPI + amoxicillin + metronidazole + clarithromycin × 10–14 days

- Sequential therapy with a PPI + amoxicillin × 5–7 days followed by a PPI + metronidazole + clarithromycin × 5–7 days
- In the absence of other indications (e.g., ongoing ASA or NSAID use, GERD, severe symptoms, bleeding ulcers), continued therapy with a PPI is not required once eradication of *H. pylori* is confirmed.

Prevention of PUD during ASA or NSAID Therapy

Therapeutic Choices

- Consider using a gastroprotective agent for all patients on chronic ASA or NSAID therapy who have risk factors for PUD:[37]
  - age >65 years
  - use of high-dose or multiple NSAIDs
  - concomitant use of corticosteroids, antiplatelet agents (e.g., clopidogrel), anticoagulants (e.g., warfarin, heparin) or SSRIs
  - severe medical comorbidity (e.g., heart failure, COPD, chronic renal or hepatic disease, advanced malignancy)
  - history of gastric or duodenal ulcer or GI bleeding
- Accepted gastroprotective strategies include once-daily **PPIs**, **misoprostol** 800 µg daily (in 4 divided doses) and substitution of a traditional NSAID with a COX-2 inhibitor.[38]
- Standard-dose PPIs are more efficacious than standard-dose **H_2RAs** or misoprostol 400 µg daily (in 2 divided doses) but not misoprostol 800 µg daily (in 4 divided doses) for the prevention of NSAID-associated gastric and duodenal ulcers.[39,40]
- Eradication of *H. pylori* prior to the initiation of ASA or NSAID therapy may reduce the risk of symptomatic ulcers.[41]
- Compared with regular NSAIDs, COX-2 inhibitors may have a 50–70% lower risk of causing complicated peptic ulcer bleeding.[42,43] However, reports of cardiovascular complications with the use of COX-2 inhibitors have limited their use and challenged their safety.[44] Celecoxib (the only available COX-2 inhibitor in Canada) should not be used in persons with established cardiovascular disease. However, all NSAIDs have been linked to an increased risk of cardiovascular complications.

Treatment of PUD during ASA or NSAID Therapy

Therapeutic Choices

- When appropriate, stop ASA or the NSAID.
- Treat PUD in those using ASA or NSAIDs with standard-dose **PPIs**. **H_2RAs** and **misoprostol** are less effective alternatives.[39,40]
- Treatment may be stopped 8 weeks after discontinuation of ASA or NSAIDs.
- If low-dose ASA is indicated for cardiovascular prophylaxis it should not be discontinued. However, concomitant PPI therapy should continue as long as the patient remains on ASA.[45,46]
- Continue PPI therapy if NSAIDs cannot be discontinued.
- If PUD was associated with bleeding, continuation of an NSAID is associated with a 5% risk of recurrent bleeding ulcer at 1 year despite PPI use.[47] Use of a COX-2 inhibitor with a PPI affords the greatest protection against recurrent PUD.[47]
- All patients with PUD (including those using ASA or an NSAID) should be tested for *H. pylori* infection and treated if present.

Choices during Pregnancy and Breastfeeding

Dyspepsia may appear for the first time during pregnancy but usually resolves afterwards. Some patients with dyspepsia, including women of reproductive potential, may try to manage their symptoms with nonprescription **antacids**, **barrier agents** (e.g., alginates), **H_2RAs** and **PPIs**. These medications are considered to be generally safe to use during pregnancy.[48,49,50,51,52,53,54]

Limited data suggest that maternal ingestion of **esomeprazole**, **omeprazole** and **pantoprazole** produces low levels of these drugs in breast milk and would not be expected to cause adverse effects in breastfed infants. No information is available on the use of **rabeprazole**, **lansoprazole** or **dexlansoprazole** during breastfeeding. Similarly, the available information indicates that maternal ingestion of **cimetidine**, **famotidine**, **nizatidine** and **ranitidine** while breastfeeding results in infant dosages much less than those given directly to neonates; these agents would not be expected to cause adverse effects in breastfed infants. However, because of cimetidine's potential to cause hepatic enzyme inhibition, other drugs in this class might be preferred.

Treat a pregnant woman with uninvestigated dyspepsia as outlined in the section "Uninvestigated Dyspepsia" above. If a diagnostic test for *H. pylori* (serology, endoscopy, urea breath test with the ^{13}C isotope) was done during pregnancy or breastfeeding, postpone treatment for the *H. pylori* infection until after pregnancy and breastfeeding. There is no need to test the infant for *H. pylori* if the mother is infected. It has been proposed that the ^{14}C (radioactive) and the ^{13}C (nonradioactive) urea breath tests are acceptable to use during pregnancy, since the radioactivity delivered to the fetus from the ^{14}C is very low and is estimated to be less than the total amount of natural radioactivity the fetus is exposed to in 1 day.[55]

The synthetic prostaglandin E_1 analogue **misoprostol** must not be used during pregnancy. If ASA, NSAIDs or COX-2 inhibitors are absolutely indicated during pregnancy, the guidance given in "Uninvestigated Dyspepsia" may be followed. Exposure to NSAIDs after 30 weeks' gestation is associated with an increased risk of premature closure of the fetal ductus arteriosus and oligohydramnios (amniotic fluid volume that is less than expected for gestational age).[56,57]

A discussion of general principles on the use of medications in these special populations can be found in Appendix II and Appendix III. Other specialized reference sources are also provided in these appendices.

Table 2: Drugs Used for Dyspepsia and Peptic Ulcer Disease

Class	Drug	Dose	Adverse Effects	Drug Interactions	Cost[a]
Histamine H_2-Receptor Antagonists	*cimetidine* generics	Treatment:[b] 800 mg QHS po, *or* 300 mg QID po, *or* 600 mg BID po Maintenance: 400 mg QHS po, *or* 300 mg BID po	Diarrhea, constipation, headache, fatigue, confusion (most likely in elderly or in poor renal function), cardiac effects, rash, gynecomastia, impotence (rare).	Cimetidine decreases cytochrome P450 metabolism of other drugs (e.g., phenytoin, theophylline, warfarin). Other H_2RAs (ranitidine or famotidine) have minimal effects.	$
	famotidine Pepcid, generics	Treatment:[b] 20 mg BID po, *or* 40 mg QHS po Maintenance: 20 mg QHS po	Diarrhea, constipation, headache, fatigue, confusion (most likely in elderly and those with poor renal function), cardiac effects, rash.		$
	nizatidine Axid, generics	Treatment:[b] 150 mg BID po, *or* 300 mg QHS po Maintenance: 150 mg QHS po	See famotidine.		$
	ranitidine Zantac, generics	Treatment:[b] 150 mg BID po, *or* 300 mg QHS po Maintenance: 150 mg QHS po	See famotidine.		$
Mucosal Protective Agents	*misoprostol* generics	Treatment: 200 µg QID po	Diarrhea (dose-related), abdominal cramps, flatulence. **Contraindicated in pregnancy** (abortifacient).	Increased risk of diarrhea if used with magnesium-based antacids.	$$$$
Proton Pump Inhibitors	*esomeprazole* Nexium, generics	20 mg daily AC breakfast po[b] 20 mg BID po if part of *H. pylori* eradication regimen	Abdominal pain, diarrhea, flatulence, hypomagnesemia, decreased serum vitamin B_{12} level.	Monitor for decreased efficacy of drugs requiring an acidic medium for dissolution or absorption (e.g., itraconazole). Esomeprazole may interfere with cytochrome P450-metabolism of other drugs (e.g., diazepam, phenytoin, warfarin). Adjust dosages as needed when esomeprazole is added or discontinued.	$$$$

Class	Drug	Dose	Adverse Effects	Drug Interactions	Cost[a]
	lansoprazole Prevacid, generics	Treatment: 15–30 mg daily AC breakfast po[b] Maintenance: 15 mg daily AC breakfast po 30 mg BID po if part of *H. pylori* eradication regimen	See esomeprazole.	Monitor for decreased efficacy of drugs requiring an acidic medium for dissolution or absorption (e.g., itraconazole).	$
	omeprazole Losec Capsules, Losec Tablets, generics	20–40 mg daily AC breakfast po[b] 20 mg BID po if part of *H. pylori* eradication regimen	See esomeprazole.	See esomeprazole.	$
	pantoprazole magnesium Tecta	40 mg daily AC breakfast po[b] 40 mg BID po if part of *H. pylori* eradication regimen	See esomeprazole.	See lansoprazole.	$$
	pantoprazole sodium Pantoloc, generics	40 mg daily AC breakfast po[b] 40 mg BID po if part of *H. pylori* eradication regimen	See esomeprazole.	See lansoprazole.	$
	rabeprazole Pariet, generics	20 mg daily AC breakfast po[b] 20 mg BID po if part of *H. pylori* eradication regimen	See esomeprazole.	See lansoprazole.	$

[a] Cost of 30-day (treatment dosages) supply; includes drug cost only.
[b] Duration of treatment for duodenal ulcer is 4–8 wk. Duration of treatment for gastric ulcer is 8–12 wk.
Dosage adjustment may be required in renal impairment; see Appendix I.
Abbreviations: H_2RA = H_2-receptor antagonist
Legend: $ <$15 $$ $15–30 $$$ $30–45 $$$$ $45–60

Suggested Readings

Ford AC, Moayyedi P. Managing dyspepsia. *Curr Gastroenterol Rep* 2009;11(4):288-94.

Graham DY, Rugge M. Clinical practice: diagnosis and evaluation of dyspepsia. *J Clin Gastroenterol* 2010;44(3):167-72.

Lacy BE, Talley NJ, Locke GR et al. Review article: current treatment options and management of functional dyspepsia. *Aliment Pharmacol Ther* 2012;36(1):3-15.

Malfertheiner P, Chan FK, McColl KE. Peptic ulcer disease. *Lancet* 2009;374(9699):1449-61.

McColl KE. Clinical practice. Helicobacter pylori infection. *N Engl J Med* 2010;362(17):1597-604.

Selgrad M, Kandulski A, Malfertheiner P. Dyspepsia and Helicobacter pylori. *Dig Dis* 2008;26(3):210-4.

Suzuki H, Nishizawa T, Hibi T. Helicobacter pylori eradication therapy. *Future Microbiol* 2010;5(4):639-48.

References

1. Chiba N, Bernard L, O'Brien BJ et al. A Canadian physician survey of dyspepsia management. *Can J Gastroenterol* 1998;12(1):83-90.
2. Talley NJ, Zinsmeister AR, Schleck CD et al. Dyspepsia and dyspepsia subgroups: a population-based study. *Gastroenterology* 1992;102(4 Pt 1):1259-68.
3. Tack J, Talley NJ, Camilleri M et al. Functional gastroduodenal disorders. *Gastroenterology* 2006;130(5):1466-79.
4. Ford AC, Bercik P, Morgan DG et al. The Rome III criteria for the diagnosis of functional dyspepsia in secondary care are not superior to previous definitions. *Gastroenterology* 2014;146(4):932-40.e1.
5. Williams B, Luckas M, Ellingham JH et al. Do young patients with dyspepsia need investigation? *Lancet* 1988;2(8624):1349-51.
6. Vakil N, Talley N, van Zanten SV et al. Cost of detecting malignant lesions by endoscopy in 2741 primary care dyspeptic patients without alarm symptoms. *Clin Gastroenterol Hepatol* 2009;7(7):756-61.
7. Talley NJ, Vakil N. Guidelines for the management of dyspepsia. *Am J Gastroenterol* 2005;100(10):2324-37.
8. el-Serag HB, Sonnenberg A. Opposing time trends of peptic ulcer and reflux disease. *Gut* 1998;43(3):327-33.
9. Sung JJ, Kuipers EJ, El-Serag HB. Systematic review: the global incidence and prevalence of peptic ulcer disease. *Aliment Pharmacol Ther* 2009;29(9):938-46.
10. Musumba C, Jorgensen A, Sutton L et al. The relative contribution of NSAIDs and Helicobacter pylori to the aetiology of endoscopically-diagnosed peptic ulcer disease: observations from a tertiary referral hospital in the UK between 2005 and 2010. *Aliment Pharmacol Ther* 2012;36(1):48-56.
11. Veldhuyzen van Zanten SJ, Flook N, Chiba N et al. An evidence-based approach to the management of uninvestigated dyspepsia in the era of Helicobacter pylori. Canadian Dyspepsia Working Group. *CMAJ* 2000;162(12 Suppl):S3-23.
12. Dooley CP, Larson AW, Stace NH et al. Double-contrast barium meal and upper gastrointestinal endoscopy. A comparative study. *Ann Intern Med* 1984;101(4):538-45.
13. Rich M, Scheiman JM, Tierney W et al. Is upper gastrointestinal radiography a cost-effective alternative to a Helicobacter pylori "test and treat" strategy for patients with suspected peptic ulcer disease? *Am J Gastroenterol* 2000;95(3):651-8.
14. Chiba N, Van Zanten SJ, Sinclair P et al. Treating Helicobacter pylori infection in primary care patients with uninvestigated dyspepsia: the Canadian adult dyspepsia empiric treatment-Helicobacter pylori positive (CADET-Hp) randomised controlled trial. *BMJ* 2002;324(7344):1012-6.
15. Malfertheiner P, Megraud F, O'Morain CA et al. Management of Helicobacter pylori infection--the Maastricht IV/ Florence Consensus Report. *Gut* 2012;61(5):646-64.
16. Gisbert JP, Pajares JM. Review article: 13C-urea breath test in the diagnosis of Helicobacter pylori infection--a critical review. *Aliment Pharmacol Ther* 2004;20(10):1001-17.
17. Laine L, Estrada R, Trujillo M et al. Effect of proton-pump inhibitor therapy on diagnostic testing for Helicobacter pylori. *Ann Intern Med* 1998;129(7):547-50.
18. Chey WD, Spybrook M, Carpenter S et al. Prolonged effect of omeprazole on the 14C-urea breath test. *Am J Gastroenterol* 1996;91(1):89-92.
19. Connor SJ, Seow F, Ngu MC et al. The effect of dosing with omeprazole on the accuracy of the 13C-urea breath test in Helicobacter pylori-infected subjects. *Aliment Pharmacol Ther* 1999;13(10):1287-93.
20. Savarino V, Tracci D, Dulbecco P et al. Negative effect of ranitidine on the results of urea breath test for the diagnosis of Helicobacter pylori. *Am J Gastroenterol* 2001;96(2):348-52.
21. Chey WD, Woods M, Scheiman JM et al. Lansoprazole and ranitidine affect the accuracy of the 14C-urea breath test by a pH-dependent mechanism. *Am J Gastroenterol* 1997;92(3):446-50.
22. Savarino V, Bisso G, Pivari M et al. Effect of gastric acid suppression on 13C-urea breath test: comparison of ranitidine with omeprazole. *Aliment Pharmacol Ther* 2000;14(3):291-7.
23. Bravo LE, Realpe JL, Campo C et al. Effects of acid suppression and bismuth medications on the performance of diagnostic tests for Helicobacter pylori infection. *Am J Gastroenterol* 1999;94(9):2380-3.
24. Gisbert JP, de la Morena F, Abraira V. Accuracy of monoclonal stool antigen test for the diagnosis of H. pylori infection: a systematic review and meta-analysis. *Am J Gastroenterol* 2006;101(8):1921-30.
25. Inadomi JM, Jamal R, Murata GH et al. Step-down management of gastroesophageal reflux disease. *Gastroenterology* 2001;121(5):1095-100.
26. McColl KE, Murray LS, Gillen D et al. Randomised trial of endoscopy with testing for Helicobacter pylori compared with non-invasive H pylori testing alone in the management of dyspepsia. *BMJ* 2002;324(7344):999-1002.
27. Wang WH, Huang JQ, Zheng GF et al. Effects of proton-pump inhibitors on functional dyspepsia: a meta-analysis of randomized placebo-controlled trials. *Clin Gastroenterol Hepatol* 2007;5(2):178-85.
28. Abraham NS, Moayyedi P, Daniels B et al. Systematic review: the methodological quality of trials affects estimates of treatment efficacy in functional (non-ulcer) dyspepsia. *Aliment Pharmacol Ther* 2004;19(6):631-41.

29. McColl K, Murray L, El-Omar E et al. Symptomatic benefit from eradicating Helicobacter pylori infection in patients with nonulcer dyspepsia. *N Engl J Med* 1998;339(26):1869-74.

30. Moayyedi P, Soo S, Deeks J et al. Eradication of Helicobacter pylori for non-ulcer dyspepsia. *Cochrane Database Syst Rev* 2006;(2):CD002096.

31. Veldhuyzen van Zanten SJ, Jones MJ, Verlinden M et al. Efficacy of cisapride and domperidone in functional (nonulcer) dyspepsia: a meta-analysis. *Am J Gastroenterol* 2001;96(3):689-96.

32. Jackson JL, O'Malley PG, Tomkins G et al. Treatment of functional gastrointestinal disorders with antidepressant medications: a meta-analysis. *Am J Med* 2000;108(1):65-72.

33. Lacy BE, Talley NJ, Locke GR et al. Review article: current treatment options and management of functional dyspepsia. *Aliment Pharmacol Ther* 2012;36(1):3-15.

34. Fuccio L, Minardi ME, Zagari RM et al. Meta-analysis: duration of first-line proton-pump inhibitor based triple therapy for Helicobacter pylori eradication. *Ann Intern Med* 2007;147(8):553-62.

35. Sun Q, Liang X, Zheng Q et al. High efficacy of 14-day triple therapy-based, bismuth-containing quadruple therapy for initial Helicobacter pylori eradication. *Helicobacter* 2010;15(3):233-8.

36. Hunt R, Fallone C, Veldhuyzan van Zanten S et al. Canadian Helicobacter Study Group Consensus Conference: Update on the management of Helicobacter pylori--an evidence-based evaluation of six topics relevant to clinical outcomes in patients evaluated for H pylori infection. *Can J Gastroenterol* 2004;18(9):547-54.

37. Bhatt DL, Scheiman J, Abraham NS et al. ACCF/ACG/AHA 2008 expert consensus document on reducing the gastrointestinal risks of antiplatelet therapy and NSAID use: a report of the American College of Cardiology Foundation Task Force on Clinical Expert Consensus Documents. *Circulation* 2008;118(18):1894-909.

38. Lanza FL, Chan FK, Quigley EM. Guidelines for prevention of NSAID-related ulcer complications. *Am J Gastroenterol* 2009;104(3):728-38.

39. Yeomans ND, Tulassay Z, Juhasz L et al. A comparison of omeprazole with ranitidine for ulcers associated with nonsteroidal antiinflammatory drugs. Acid Suppression Trial: Ranitidine versus Omeprazole for NSAID-associated Ulcer Treatment (ASTRONAUT) Study Group. *N Engl J Med* 1998;338(11):719-26.

40. Hawkey CJ, Karrasch JA, Szczepanski L et al. Omeprazole compared with misoprostol for ulcers associated with nonsteroidal antiinflammatory drugs. Omeprazole versus Misoprostol for NSAID-induced Ulcer Management (OMNIUM) Study Group. *N Engl J Med* 1998;338(11):727-34.

41. Huang JQ, Sridhar S, Hunt RH. Role of Helicobacter pylori infection and non-steroidal anti-inflammatory drugs in peptic-ulcer disease: a meta-analysis. *Lancet* 2002;359(9300):14-22.

42. Bombardier C, Laine L, Reicin A et al. Comparison of upper gastrointestinal toxicity of rofecoxib and naproxen in patients with rheumatoid arthritis. VIGOR Study Group. *N Engl J Med* 2000;343(21):1520-8.

43. Silverstein FE, Faich G, Goldstein JL et al. Gastrointestinal toxicity with celecoxib vs nonsteroidal anti-inflammatory drugs for osteoarthritis and rheumatoid arthritis: the CLASS study: A randomized controlled trial. Celecoxib Long-term Arthritis Safety Study. *JAMA* 2000;284(10):1247-55.

44. Bresalier RS, Sandler RS, Quan H et al. Cardiovascular events associated with rofecoxib in a colorectal adenoma chemoprevention trial. *N Engl J Med* 2005;352(11):1092-102.

45. Sung JJ, Lau JY, Ching JY et al. Continuation of low-dose aspirin therapy in peptic ulcer bleeding: a randomized trial. *Ann Intern Med* 2010;152(1):1-9.

46. Lai KC, Lam SK, Chu KM et al. Lansoprazole for the prevention of recurrences of ulcer complications from long-term low-dose aspirin use. *N Engl J Med* 2002;346(26):2033-8.

47. Chan FK, Wong VW, Suen BY et al. Combination of a cyclo-oxygenase-2 inhibitor and a proton-pump inhibitor for prevention of recurrent ulcer bleeding in patients at very high risk: a double-blind, randomised trial. *Lancet* 2007;369(9573):1621-6.

48. Pasternak B, Hviid A. Use of proton-pump inhibitors in early pregnancy and the risk of birth defects. *N Engl J Med* 2010;363(22):2114-23.

49. Law R, Maltepe C, Bozzo P et al. Treatment of heartburn and acid reflux associated with nausea and vomiting during pregnancy. *Can Fam Physician* 2010;56(2):143-4.

50. Gill SK, O'Brien L, Koren G. The safety of histamine 2 (H2) blockers in pregnancy: a meta-analysis. *Dig Dis Sci* 2009;54(9):1835-8.

51. Matok I, Levy A, Wiznitzer A et al. The safety of fetal exposure to proton-pump inhibitors during pregnancy. *Dig Dis Sci* 2012;57(3):699-705.

52. Gill SK, O'Brien L, Einarson TR et al. The safety of proton pump inhibitors (PPIs) in pregnancy: a meta-analysis. *Am J Gastroenterol* 2009;104(6):1541-5.

53. Nikfar S, Abdollahi M, Moretti ME et al. Use of proton pump inhibitors during pregnancy and rates of major malformations: a meta-analysis. *Dig Dis Sci* 2002;47(7):1526-9.

54. Majithia R, Johnson DA. Are proton pump inhibitors safe during pregnancy and lactation? Evidence to date. *Drugs* 2012;72(2):171-9.

55. Bentur Y, Matsui D, Koren G. Safety of 14C-UBT for diagnosis of Helicobacter pylori infection in pregnancy. *Can Fam Physician* 2009;55(5):479-80.

56. Antonucci R, Zaffanello M, Puxeddu E et al. Use of non-steroidal anti-inflammatory drugs in pregnancy: impact on the fetus and newborn. *Curr Drug Metab* 2012;13(4):474-90.

57. Koren G, Florescu A, Costei AM et al. Nonsteroidal antiinflammatory drugs during third trimester and the risk of premature closure of the ductus arteriosus: a meta-analysis. *Ann Pharmacother* 2006;40(5):824-9.

Chapter 61
Gastroesophageal Reflux Disease

Eldon A. Shaffer, MD, DipABIM, FACP, FRCPC

Gastroesophageal reflux disease (GERD) refers to the troublesome symptoms (primarily heartburn, regurgitation) and/or complications that result from an excessive reflux of gastric contents into the esophagus, oropharynx or lungs.[1] Reflux may cause inflammation (*erosive esophagitis*) and complications such as the development of an ulcer, bleeding or stricture. Chronic esophagitis can further evolve through attempted repair into metaplastic columnar epithelium (*Barrett's esophagus*) and the development of esophageal adenocarcinoma. However, the majority of GERD patients (55–80%) have no erosive disease on endoscopy. GERD with no demonstrable esophageal disease (a normal esophagus at endoscopy while not on any treatment) is termed *nonerosive reflux disease* (NERD) and is sometimes referred to as functional heartburn. GERD may be associated with several extraesophageal syndromes such as chronic cough, asthma, laryngitis, oropharyngeal ulceration and dental erosions.

GERD symptoms range from mild (trivial) to severe. The severity of symptoms and esophageal mucosal injury correlate with the total time the esophageal mucosa is in direct contact with acid (at pH <4) per 24-hour period.[1,2] Mild symptoms do not interfere with daily activity and are usually of low intensity, short in duration, *not* nocturnal, infrequent (<3 times weekly) and without major complications. Severe symptoms regularly interfere with daily activities and are usually of high intensity, persistent (>6 months), nocturnal, frequent and often associated with complications. Dysphagia, defined as difficulty in swallowing solids or liquids (experienced anywhere from the mouth to the stomach), is an ominous symptom that often necessitates endoscopic evaluation. In contrast, the more common GERD symptom of globus (a continuous feeling of a lump in the throat that does not interfere with swallowing) is a benign occurrence in acid reflux, does not require investigation and usually responds to effective acid reduction.

Goals of Therapy

- Relieve symptoms, particularly heartburn, and improve quality of life
- Promote healing of esophagitis
- Prevent complications (stricture formation, bleeding, progression to Barrett's epithelium or extraesophageal problems)
- Prevent recurrences

Investigations

- History:
  - common symptoms of GERD: heartburn, regurgitation of acid or bile, hypersalivation (water brash) or noncardiac chest pain. The history is usually sufficient for diagnosis. Heartburn or acid regurgitation has a high specificity (89% and 95%, respectively), but a low sensitivity (38% and 6%) for GERD[4]
  - extraesophageal manifestations: airway symptoms (e.g., cough, asthma), laryngitis, oropharyngeal symptoms (globus sensation) or ulceration, dental caries, or the burning mouth syndrome
  - complications: dysphagia from a peptic stricture, ulceration causing GI bleeding, or pain on swallowing (odynophagia)

- predisposing/associated conditions: pregnancy, obesity, scleroderma

- Upper endoscopy is not required in typical GERD. Consider endoscopy in patients with heartburn refractory to optimal therapy with a proton pump inhibitor (Figure 1) or if concerned about:
  - "Alarm features" suggesting an upper GI malignancy: dysphagia (especially for solids), weight loss (>5%), epigastric mass, GI bleeding, anemia
  - Other causes of esophagitis (eosinophilic, "pill" or infectious esophagitis)
  - Barrett's esophagus. Risk factors for development of cancer in Barrett's esophagus include chronic GERD (>5–10 years), hiatal hernia, advanced age (>50 years), male gender, white ethnicity, cigarette smoking and elevated BMI (as abdominal obesity). The utility of endoscopic screening for Barrett's esophagus is controversial because there is no demonstrated decrease in mortality as a result of screening[3]
- Ambulatory 24-hour pH and impedance (detecting reflux by changes in intraluminal resistance) monitoring are indicated in patients with atypical reflux symptoms suggesting questionable GERD diagnosis, for those who fail standard medical therapy (but have a normal endoscopy), and as a preoperative evaluation (especially with NERD) before antireflux surgery
- Testing for *H. pylori* infection in GERD patients is not necessary due to the low prevalence of this infection in Canada.[5] Further, *H. pylori* infection does not cause and has little impact on GERD.[6] *H. pylori* eradication has only modest effects on GERD symptoms, resulting in a slight worsening in patients with corpus-predominant gastritis (acid hyposecretors) and improvement in those with antral-predominant gastritis (hypersecretors)

Therapeutic Choices

Nonpharmacologic Choices

There is little evidence to support the effectiveness of lifestyle changes, except as initial therapy in mild cases. However, recommending them provides broad health care benefits and carries no risk.

- Modify diet (avoid chocolate, caffeine, acidic citrus juices, large fatty meals)
- Reduce body weight if BMI >30 kg/m^2 or recently gained weight[7,8,9,10]
- Avoid eating for up to 3 hours before bedtime[11]
- Avoid lying down after meals
- Elevate the head of the bed by 10–20 cm particularly if nocturnal reflux symptoms are present.[12,13] This is best achieved by elevating the bed frame itself rather than with pillows or a wedge
- Stop smoking[14] (see Chapter 13)
- Avoid tight clothing

Pharmacologic Choices

When possible and appropriate, eliminate drugs that impair esophageal motility and lower esophageal sphincter tone (e.g., anticholinergic agents, beta-blockers, calcium channel blockers, theophylline, tricyclic antidepressants).

Trivial to Mild Gastroesophageal Reflux Disease

Most people with mild symptoms do not seek medical attention and will obtain symptomatic relief with **antacids**, **alginates** or **histamine H_2-receptor antagonists** (H_2RAs). Additional therapy becomes necessary if GERD severity increases (Figure 1).

Figure 1: **Management of Gastroesophageal Reflux Disease**

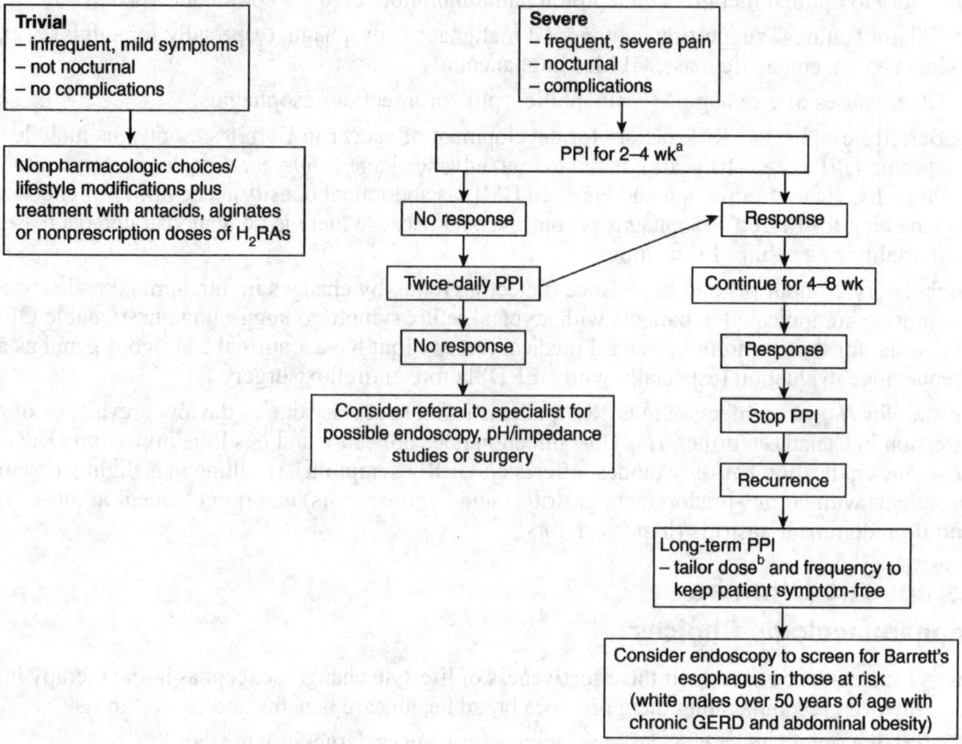

a For suspected GERD and those with noncardiac chest pain, an empiric trial of a proton pump inhibitor twice daily for 2–4 weeks (up to 8 weeks) also can be diagnostic.
b It may be possible to step down to H_2RAs in some with nonerosive GERD.
Abbreviations: H_2RA = histamine H_2-receptor antagonist; PPI = proton pump inhibitor

Moderate to Severe Gastroesophageal Reflux Disease

Antacids or H_2RAs alone are generally *not* effective. The most effective and common approach is an 8-week course of a **proton pump inhibitor** (PPI) to effectively raise the gastric pH above 4. The goal is to eliminate symptoms, heal erosive esophagitis and prevent complications (Figure 1).[2]

Histamine H_2-receptor Antagonists

Cimetidine, **famotidine**, **nizatidine** and **ranitidine** are equally effective. Their rapid onset of action makes them attractive for "on-demand" use by some patients with *mild* GERD (mild symptoms <3 times per week). This class of drugs is not always effective for severe esophagitis (Table 1). Twice-daily doses relieve symptoms in 60% with moderate to severe disease and heal histologically mild esophagitis in over 40% of patients. Bedtime dosing of H_2RAs may improve nocturnal reflux as an adjunct to daytime PPI therapy.[15] Their safety profile is excellent. Efficacy of H_2RAs is limited by the swift development of tachyphylaxis and their inability to adequately suppress meal-related acid secretion.

When initial therapy is beneficial, maintenance will be necessary if symptoms recur and cannot be controlled by nonpharmacologic means. Use the lowest effective dose to control symptoms and prevent complications (Table 2).

Proton Pump Inhibitors

The PPIs (**dexlansoprazole**, **esomeprazole**, **lansoprazole**, **omeprazole**, **pantoprazole magnesium**, **pantoprazole sodium** and **rabeprazole**) effectively block acid secretion by irreversibly binding to and inhibiting the hydrogen-potassium ATPase (the proton pump) on the apical surface of the parietal cell membrane. PPIs are more effective than H_2RAs (Table 1), providing more rapid relief of symptoms and twice the healing rates for esophagitis at standard once-daily doses (up to 90% by 12 weeks).[2,16] PPIs are prodrugs requiring proton pump activation for optimal efficacy, hence they are best administered 30–60 minutes before a meal. Initial therapy should be once a day before breakfast. For those with a partial response, consider twice-daily dosing (30–60 minutes before meals) or switching to a different PPI. PPIs are the drugs of choice in most GERD patients with or without mucosal injury and for extraesophageal manifestations.[17,18] Though PPIs can heal ulceration, they do not reverse epithelial changes in patients with Barrett's esophagus. Tachyphylaxis does not develop with continued PPI use. Acid rebound occurs with their discontinuation and may be a factor in GI symptoms recurring after PPIs are withdrawn.[19] At equivalent doses, available PPIs offer similar symptom relief, mucosal healing, tolerability and safety (Table 2).[20] Apparent differences in bioavailability and antisecretory potency upon initial dosing have no clinical importance in most settings; cost is the major factor to consider when selecting a PPI. Compared with other PPIs, esomeprazole is only slightly more effective in healing erosive esophagitis and relieving GERD symptom.[21] Dexlansoprazole (an enantiomer of lansoprazole) uses a delayed-release formulation to prolong the plasma half-life and reduce the duration of acid secretion. Marketed at a higher dose than lansoprazole, it may offer an advantage over lansoprazole in healing erosive esophagitis.[22] Less clear is the effectiveness of substituting one PPI for another in patients who have initially responded but then developed further GERD symptoms despite continued treatment.[23] The occasional use of a PPI taken "as needed" does not reliably provide adequate acid inhibition and does not produce a consistent or satisfactory clinical response; therefore, a trial at adequate doses is necessary to gauge efficacy. GERD symptoms that persist despite adequate PPI therapy are likely due to functional heartburn rather than acid reflux, or may represent an overlap with functional dyspepsia.

Prokinetic Agents

Although the basis for acid reflux is incompetence of the antireflux barrier, impaired esophageal clearance of acid and delayed gastric emptying, no effective motility agent is available at this time.

Table 1: **Efficacy of Drugs Used to Treat Gastroesophageal Reflux Disease**

	Acute Treatment		
	Symptoms	**Esophagitis**	**Prevention of Recurrences**
Antacids	+	–	–
Alginates/antacids	+	–	–
Histamine H_2-receptor antagonists	++	+	±
Proton pump inhibitors	+++	+++	+++

Legend:
+ Drug of proven value (controlled trials).
– Not established (negative trial or not tested).
± Conflicting data.

Maintenance Therapy for Severe Gastroesophageal Reflux Disease

The recurrence rate following discontinuation of successful therapy is extremely high: almost 100% of patients with erosive esophagitis and 65% with NERD will relapse.[18] PPIs maintain remission far more effectively than H_2RAs and are cost-effective.[24] Maintenance therapy for such severe disease appears to be long term and is especially important in severe erosive esophagitis and Barrett's esophagus.

Step-down therapy: Once symptomatic relief has been achieved with full strength PPIs, gradually decrease the intensity of acid suppression in NERD patients until breakthrough symptoms occur, i.e., lowest dose that provides symptom relief. Half of the healing PPI dose may suffice. Some can transition to H_2RAs once symptomatic relief has been achieved with PPIs, without adversely affecting quality of life.[25]

Intermittent (on-demand): PPI therapy is an alternative to a continuous maintenance regimen particularly in those with NERD in whom symptom control is paramount.[26] On-demand therapy constitutes daily PPI use for a period of time sufficient to achieve resolution of the reflux symptoms at which time the patient discontinues the drug with a subsequent drug-free remission which may last months. On-demand therapy is ineffective for healing erosive esophagitis.

As-needed therapy: Sporadic use for very short treatment periods is not suitable for PPIs. The response to PPIs does not have a rapid enough onset as only 30% experience heartburn relief with their first PPI dose.[27] However, H_2RAs may have a role in as-needed therapy for mild and chronic GERD although nonpharmacologic measures usually suffice.

The safety record of PPIs overall is excellent, even with long-term use over many years. Potential concerns include the development of osteoporosis, magnesium deficiency (rare), nosocomial pneumonia and enteric infections such as *C. difficile*.[28,29]

Management of the Refractory Patient

Despite their potent antisecretory properties, PPIs may not provide symptomatic relief or heal esophagitis; 10–40% of patients with GERD will have continuing symptoms despite standard-dose PPI therapy.[30] PPI failure (best defined after twice daily use) may relate to:

- functional heartburn, e.g., NERD or esophageal hypersensitivity
- incorrect diagnosis, e.g., functional dyspepsia or achalasia
- other causes of esophagitis: alkali (bile) reflux, eosinophilic esophagitis or pill esophagitis
- inadequate acid suppression:
  - improper use
    - nonadherence—sporadic use
    - taking PPIs with or after meals or in combination with H_2RAs (PPIs are most effective when proton pumps are most active)
  - genetic differences leading to rapid metabolism via CYP2C19 (less common)

Additional investigations such as endoscopy with biopsies, 24-hour pH monitoring and/or esophageal impedance testing may be warranted to identify the cause of refractory esophagitis.

In addition to the above, management of GERD that is refractory to PPIs must ensure patient adherence and ingestion of the drug 30 minutes before a meal. Double-dose PPI (before breakfast and again before supper) is common practice;[31,32] further escalation has no value. Another option for those patients with symptoms refractory to a PPI, though not completely substantiated, is to switch to another PPI as some individuals may be more responsive to one PPI than another.

Nocturnal acid breakthrough with gastric pH <4 can occur in up to 70% of patients on twice-daily PPI therapy, but may not necessarily be associated with nighttime heartburn or refractory GERD.

Supplementary bedtime H_2RA therapy may temporarily improve nocturnal GERD, but tachyphylaxis limits its use.[33,34,35]

Antireflux Surgery

Though it may feel intuitive that failure of optimal medical therapy suggests refractory GERD that would benefit from surgery to restore the physiological equivalent of the lower esophageal sphincter, complete response to medical therapy is actually the best predictor of surgical success. Laparoscopic antireflux surgery is effective for reflux control in well-selected cases; following fundoplication, complaints like dysphagia and the gas-bloat syndrome remain a problem. Indications for surgery include intractable reflux esophagitis (particularly in a young person) despite optimal medical therapy, or complications such as severe erosive esophagitis, stricture formation or recurrent lung disease (e.g., aspiration pneumonia). Long-term outcome studies show little difference between surgically and medically treated patients.[36] In fact, drug therapy may be less expensive than surgery.[37,38] Novel endoluminal approaches such as natural orifice transluminal endoscopic surgery (NOTES) employ endoscopic sewing of the upper stomach or implant full-thickness biopolymer devices, aiming to tighten the gastroesophageal junction. Such endoscopic therapies show variable outcomes for reduced need of antisecretory medications and harbor trial design flaws.[39]

Choices during Pregnancy and Breastfeeding

During pregnancy, increased intra-abdominal pressure (caused mechanically by the growing fetus) and reduced tone in the lower esophageal sphincter (progesterone-mediated) increase the risk of gastroesophageal reflux. GERD symptoms (heartburn, regurgitation and dyspepsia) occur in 30–80% of pregnancies, increasing during the pregnancy and leading to a decreased quality of life.[40] The risk of heartburn increases when heartburn exists before pregnancy and with increasing gestational age and parity. Although the heartburn of pregnancy can be relentless, esophagitis and its complications are infrequent in the absence of pre-existing GERD.[41] However, aspiration is a major risk during labour and immediately after delivery, presumably from the mechanical and physiological consequences of the pregnant state, compounded by delivery that entails assumption of a recumbent position or any sedation/anesthesia/intubation. GERD tends to resolve postpartum, but often recurs in subsequent pregnancies.[40]

Lifestyle modification is the cornerstone for treating mild symptoms.[42] This involves elevating the head of the bed,[12,13] consuming small frequent meals and refraining from eating at least 3 hours before bedtime. If this fails, begin nonsystemic drug therapy with **antacids**, which generally provide immediate relief and are quite safe except for sodium bicarbonate, which can cause fluid retention and metabolic alkalosis.[43] Do not use magnesium trisilicate (found in alginic acid) long-term and in high doses as it can lead to fetal nephrolithiasis, hypotonia and respiratory distress. None of the antacids concentrate in breast milk and are acceptable when breastfeeding. **Sucralfate**, a mucosal protectant with minimal absorption, is also acceptable during pregnancy and when breastfeeding.[43] Sucralfate has no role in nonpregnant patients with GERD.

Use of systemic acid-inhibiting drugs represents the next step in more resistant cases, beginning with histamine H_2-receptor antagonists. **Ranitidine** is effective and safe during pregnancy and when breastfeeding even with some passage into breast milk.[43] In more refractory cases, **proton pump inhibitors** may become necessary, and appear to be safe in pregnancy.[44,45] PPIs are *not* recommended for breastfeeding mothers because of a paucity of information.

A discussion of general principles on the use of medications in these special populations can be found in Appendix II and Appendix III. Other specialized reference sources are also provided in these appendices.

Therapeutic Tips

- PPIs are superior to H_2RAs for reduction of heartburn and healing of esophagitis in patients with moderate to severe GERD. H_2RAs may be instituted after achieving symptomatic relief with PPIs.
- The recurrence rate of GERD is extremely high and long-term maintenance therapy is often necessary. PPIs maintain remission far more effectively than H_2RAs. On-demand (intermittent) therapy with PPIs may be effective in select patients such as those with NERD.

Table 2: Drugs Used in the Management of Gastroesophageal Reflux Disease

Class	Drug	Dose	Adverse Effects	Drug Interactions	Comments	Cost[a]
Alginates	*alginate/aluminum hydroxide* Gaviscon Liquid, generics	10–20 mL PRN after meals	Nausea, vomiting, eructation, flatulence.	Decreased bioavailability of digoxin, tetracycline, quinolone antibiotics; separate dosing by 2 h.	Alginates and some antacids contain significant amounts of sodium. A significant source of aluminum.	$
	alginate/magnesium carbonate Gaviscon Tablets, generics	2–4 tablets chewed PRN after meals followed by a drink of water	See alginate/aluminum hydroxide.	See alginate/aluminum hydroxide.	See alginate/aluminum hydroxide. Aluminum free. A significant source of magnesium.	$
Antacids	*aluminum hydroxide/magnesium hydroxide combinations* Diovol	30 mL (regular strength) PRN after meals	Constipation, diarrhea.	See alginate/aluminum hydroxide.	Avoid antacids containing magnesium or aluminum in renal dysfunction.	$
Histamine H_2-receptor Antagonists	*cimetidine* generics	800 mg once daily po *or* 600 mg BID po *or* 300 mg QID po	Diarrhea, constipation, headache, fatigue, confusion (most likely in elderly and those with poor renal function), cardiac effects, rash. Also gynecomastia, impotence (rare).	Cimetidine increases serum concentration of several drugs (e.g., alprazolam, amiodarone, carbamazepine, carvedilol, citalopram, clonazepam, diazepam, diltiazem, flurazepam, labetalol, metformin, metoprolol, midazolam, mirtazapine, nifedipine, paroxetine, phenytoin, propranolol, theophylline, triazolam, tricyclic antidepressants, warfarin)—use another H_2RA. Decreased bioavailability of ketoconazole and itraconazole. Decreased cimetidine levels with simultaneous administration of antacids.		$
	famotidine Pepcid AC, Maximum Strength, generics	20–40 mg BID po	See ranitidine.	Decreased bioavailability of ketoconazole and itraconazole.	Also available without a prescription. Typical nonprescription dose is 20-40 mg per day. Antacids may be given concomitantly if needed.	$$

(cont'd)

Table 2: **Drugs Used in the Management of Gastroesophageal Reflux Disease** *(cont'd)*

Class	Drug	Dose	Adverse Effects	Drug Interactions	Comments	Cost[a]
	nizatidine Axid, generics	150 mg BID po	See ranitidine.	Reduces bioavailability of cefuroxime axetil, itraconazole and ketoconazole. Increases serum cyclosporine and salicylate concentration.		$
	ranitidine Zantac, Zantac Maximum Strength Non-Prescription, generics	150 mg BID–QID po *or* 300 mg QHS po	Diarrhea, constipation, headache, fatigue, confusion (most likely in elderly and those with poor renal function), cardiac effects, rash.	May alter prothrombin time when warfarin is used—monitor. Decreased bioavailability of itraconazole and ketoconazole. Increases absorption of midazolam and triazolam. Sucralfate coadministration decreases absorption of ranitidine.	Also available without a prescription. Typical nonprescription dose is 75–150 mg per day.	$
Proton Pump Inhibitors	*dexlansoprazole* Dexilant	30–60 mg once daily po	Headache, nausea, diarrhea, rash.	May decrease absorption of ampicillin esters, atazanavir, digoxin, iron salts, ketoconazole. Decreases theophylline levels. Decreased bioavailability by sucralfate. Increases blood levels of tacrolimus. Data is conflicting regarding interaction with clopidogrel.[46]	Can be taken without regard to food or the timing of food. Antacids may be used concomitantly if required.	$$$$$
	esomeprazole Nexium, generics	20–40 mg once daily po ½ hour before food	See dexlansoprazole.	Inhibits CYP2C19: increases level of carbamazepine, diazepam, digoxin, triazolam, warfarin. When esomeprazole is added or removed, these drugs may require dosage adjustment. Increased esomeprazole levels with clarithromycin. May decrease absorption of ampicillin esters, atazanavir, digoxin, iron salts, ketoconazole. Data is conflicting regarding interaction with clopidogrel.[46]	Commonly used at 40 mg daily.	$$$$
	lansoprazole Prevacid, generics	15–30 mg once daily po ½ h before food	See dexlansoprazole.	See dexlansoprazole.	If partial or no response, give usual dose BID AC. Giving half the usual dose may be useful for maintenance in some patients with less severe symptoms or who have gone into remission on standard dosages.	$
	omeprazole Losec Capsules, Losec Tablets, generics	20–40 mg once daily po ½ h before food[b]	See dexlansoprazole.	See esomeprazole.	See lansoprazole.	$

Class	Drug	Dose	Adverse Effects	Drug Interactions	Comments	Cost[a]
	pantoprazole magnesium Tecta	40 mg once daily po ½ h before food	See dexlansoprazole.	See dexlansoprazole.	See lansoprazole.	$$
	pantoprazole sodium Pantoloc, generics	20–40 mg once daily po ½ h before food	See dexlansoprazole.	See dexlansoprazole.	See lansoprazole.	$
	rabeprazole Pariet, generics	10–20 mg once daily po ½ h before food	See dexlansoprazole.	See dexlansoprazole. Digoxin levels may increase moderately in some patients.	See lansoprazole.	$

[a] Cost of 30-day supply, includes drug cost only.
[b] Not to exceed 20 mg/day in hepatic impairment.
Dosage adjustment may be required in renal impairment; see Appendix I.
Legend: $ <$15 $$ $15–30 $$$ $30–45 $$$$ $45–60 $$$$$ $60–75

Suggested Readings

Armstrong D, Marshall JK, Chiba N et al. Canadian Consensus Conference on the management of gastroesophageal reflux disease in adults—update 2004. *Can J Gastroenterol* 2005;19(1):15-35.

Flook N, Jones R, Vakil N. Approach to gastroesophageal reflux disease in primary care: putting the Montreal definition into practice. *Can Fam Physician* 2008;54(5):701-5.

Hershcovici T, Fass R. Management of gastroesophageal reflux disease that does not respond well to proton pump inhibitors. *Curr Opin Gastroenterol* 2010;26(4):367-78.

Katz PO, Gerson LB, Vela MF. Guidelines for the diagnosis and management of gastroesophageal reflux disease. *Am J Gastroenterol* 2013;108(3):308-28.

Moayyedi P, Talley NJ. Gastro-oesophageal reflux disease. *Lancet* 2006;367(9528):2086-100.

Tytgat GN, McColl K, Tack J et al. New algorithm for the treatment of gastro-oesophageal reflux disease. *Aliment Pharmacol Ther* 2008;27(3):249-56.

References

1. Vakil N , van Zanten SV, Kahrilas P et al. The Montreal definition and classification of gastroesophageal reflux disease: a global evidence-based consensus. *Am J Gastroenterol* 2006;101(8):1900-20.
2. Hunt RH. Importance of pH control in the management of GERD. *Arch Intern Med* 1999;159(7):649-57.
3. Sikkema M, de Jonge PJ, Steyerberg EW et al. Risk of esophageal adenocarcinoma and mortality in patients with Barrett's esophagus: a systematic review and meta-analysis. *Clin Gastroenterol Hepatol* 2010;8(3):235-44.
4. Klauser AG, Schindlbeck NE, Muller-Lissner SA. Symptoms in gastro-oesophageal reflux disease. *Lancet* 1990;335(8683):205-8.
5. Thomson AB, Barkun AN, Armstrong D et al. The prevalence of clinically significant endoscopic findings in primary care patients with uninvestigated dyspepsia: the Canadian Adult Dyspepsia Empiric Treatment-Prompt Endoscopy (CADET-PE) study. *Aliment Pharmacol Ther* 2003;17(12):1481-91.
6. Raghunath AS, Hungin AP, Wooff D et al. Systematic review: the effect of Helicobacter pylori and its eradication on gastro-oesophageal reflux disease in patients with duodenal ulcers or reflux esophagitis. *Aliment Pharmacol Ther* 2004;20(7):733-44.
7. Ness-Jensen E, Lindam A, Lagergren J et al. Weight loss and reduction in gastroesophageal reflux. A prospective population-based cohort study: the HUNT study. *Am J Gastroenterol* 2013;108(3):376-82.
8. Hampel H, Abraham NS, El-Serag HB. Meta-analysis: obesity and the risk for gastroesophageal reflux disease and its complications. *Ann Intern Med* 2005;143(3):199-211.
9. Nocon M, Labenz J, Jaspersen D et al. Association of body mass index with heartburn, regurgitation and esophagitis: results of the Progression of Gastroesophageal Reflux Disease study. *J Gastroenterol Hepatol* 2007;22(11):1728-31.
10. El-Serag HB, Graham DY, Satia JA et al. Obesity is an independent risk factor for GERD symptoms and erosive esophagitis. *Am J Gastroenterol* 2005;100(6):1243-50.
11. Yamamichi N, Mochizuki S, Asada-Hirayama I et al. Lifestyle factors affecting gastroesophageal reflux disease symptoms: a cross-sectional study of healthy 19864 adults using FSSG scores. *BMC Med* 2012;10:45.
12. Gerson LB, Fass R. A systematic review of the definitions, prevalence, and response to treatment of nocturnal gastroesophageal reflux disease. *Clin Gastroenterol Hepatol* 2009;7(4):372-8.
13. Khan BA, Sodhi JS, Zargar SA et al. Effect of bed head elevation during sleep in symptomatic patients of nocturnal gastroesophageal reflux. *J Gastroenterol Hepatol* 2012;27(6):1078-82.
14. Pandolfino JE, Kahrilas PJ. Smoking and gastro-oesophageal reflux disease. *Eur J Gastroenterol Hepatol* 2000;12(8):837-42.
15. Mainie I, Tutuian R, Castell DO. Addition of a H2 receptor antagonist to PPI improves acid control and decreases nocturnal acid breakthrough. *J Clin Gastroenterol* 2008;42(6):676-9.
16. Khan M, Santana J, Donnellan C et al. Medical treatments in the short term management of reflux oesophagitis. *Cochrane Database Syst Rev* 2007;(2):CD003244.
17. Richter JE, Campbell DR, Kahrilas PJ et al. Lansoprazole compared with ranitidine for the treatment of nonerosive gastroesophageal reflux disease. *Arch Intern Med* 2000;160(12):1803-9.
18. Donnellan C, Sharma N, Preston C et al. Medical treatments for the maintenance therapy of reflux oesophagitis and endoscopic negative reflux disease. *Cochrane Database Syst Rev* 2005;(2):CD003245.
19. Howden CW, Kahrilas PJ. Editorial: just how "difficult" is it to withdraw PPI treatment? *Am J Gastroenterol* 2010;105(7):1538-40.
20. Vakil N, Fennerty MB. Direct comparative trials of the efficacy of proton pump inhibitors in the management of gastro-oesophageal reflux disease and peptic ulcer disease. *Aliment Pharmacol Ther* 2003;18(6):559-68.
21. Gralnek IM, Dulai GS, Fennerty MB et al. Esomeprazole versus other proton pump inhibitors in erosive esophagitis: a meta-analysis of randomized clinical trials. *Clin Gastroenterol Hepatol* 2006;4(12):1452-8.
22. Sharma P, Shaheen NJ, Perez MC et al. Clinical trials: healing of erosive oesophagitis with dexlansoprazole MR, a proton pump inhibitor with a novel dual delayed-release formulation—results from two randomized controlled studies. *Aliment Pharmacol Ther* 2009;29(7):731-41.
23. Nelson WW, Vermeulen LC, Geurkink EA et al. Clinical and humanistic outcomes in patients with gastroesophageal reflux disease converted from omeprazole to lansoprazole. *Arch Intern Med* 2000;160(16):2491-6.
24. Vigneri S, Termini R, Leandro G et al. A comparison of five maintenance therapies for reflux esophagitis. *N Engl J Med* 1995;333(17):1106-10.
25. Inadomi JM, Jamal R, Murata GH et al. Step-down management of gastroesophageal reflux disease. *Gastroenterology* 2001;121(5):1095-100.
26. Pace F, Tonini M, Pallotta S et al. Systematic review: maintenance treatment of gastro-oesophageal reflux disease with proton pump inhibitors taken 'on-demand'. *Aliment Pharmacol Ther* 2007;26(2):195-204.
27. McQuaid KR, Laine L. Early heartburn relief with proton pump inhibitors: a systematic review and meta-analysis of clinical trials. *Clin Gastroenterol Hepatol* 2005;3(6):553-63.

28. U.S. Food and Drug Administration. *Proton Pump Inhibitor drugs (PPIs): drug safety communication—low magnesium levels can be associated with long-term use*. Available from: www.fda.gov/Safety/MedWatch/SafetyInformation/SafetyAlertsforHumanMedicalProducts/ucm245275.htm. Accessed November 23, 2011.
29. Johnson DA, Oldfield EC. Reported side effects and complications of long-term proton pump inhibitor use: dissecting the evidence. *Clin Gastroenterol Hepatol* 2013;11(5):458-64.
30. Fass R, Sifrim D. Management of heartburn not responding to proton pump inhibitors. *Gut* 2009;58(2):295-309.
31. Johnson DA, Katz PO. Nocturnal gastroesophageal reflux disease: issues, implications, and management strategies. *Rev Gastroenterol Disord* 2008;8(2):98-108.
32. Hammer J, Schmidt B. Effect of splitting the dose of esomeprazole on gastric acidity and nocturnal acid breakthrough. *Aliment Pharmacol Ther* 2004;19(10):1105-10.
33. Fackler WK, Ours TM, Vaezi MF et al. Long-term effect of H2RA therapy on nocturnal gastric acid breakthrough. *Gastroenterology* 2002;122(3):625-32.
34. Rackoff A, Agrawal A, Hila I et al. Histamine-2 receptor antagonists at night improve gastroesophageal reflux disease symptoms for patients on proton pump inhibitor therapy. *Dis Esophagus* 2005;18(6):370-3.
35. Wang Y, Pan T, Wang Q et al. Additional bedtime H2-receptor antagonist for the control of nocturnal gastric acid breakthrough. *Cochrane Database Syst Rev* 2009;(4):CD004275.
36. Spechler SJ, Lee E, Ahnen D et al. Long-term outcome of medical and surgical therapies for gastroesophageal reflux disease: follow-up of a randomized controlled trial. *JAMA* 2001;285(18):2331-8.
37. Myrvold HE, Lundell L, Miettinen P et al. The cost of long term therapy for gastro-oesophageal reflux disease: a randomised trial comparing omeprazole and open antireflux surgery. *Gut* 2001;49(4):488-94.
38. Romagnuolo J, Meier MA, Sadowski DC. Medical or surgical therapy for erosive reflux esophagitis: cost-utility analysis using a Markov model. *Ann Surg* 2002;236(2):191-202.
39. Rothstein RI. Endoscopic therapy of gastroesophageal reflux disease: outcomes of the randomized-controlled trials done to date. *J Clin Gastroenterol* 2008;42(5):594-602.
40. Rey E, Rodriguez-Artalejo F, Herraiz MA et al. Gastroesophageal reflux symptoms during and after pregnancy: a longitudinal study. *Am J Gastroenterol* 2007;102(11):2395-400.
41. Castro Lde P. Reflux esophagitis as the cause of heartburn in pregnancy. *Am J Obstet Gynecol* 1967;98(1):1-10.
42. Richter JE. Review article: the management of heartburn in pregnancy. *Aliment Pharmacol Ther* 2005;22(9):749-57.
43. Mahadevan U. Gastrointestinal medications in pregnancy. *Best Pract Res Clin Gastroenterol* 2007;21(5):849-77.
44. Diav-Citrin O, Arnon J, Shechtman S et al. The safety of proton pump inhibitors in pregnancy: a multicenter prospective controlled study. *Aliment Pharmacol Ther* 2005;21(3):269-75.
45. Gill SK, O'Brien L, Einarson TR et al. The safety of proton pump inhibitors (PPIs) in pregnancy: a meta-analysis. *Am J Gastroenterol* 2009;104(6):1541-5.
46. Chua D, Shalansky SJ, Legal MG et al. Conflicting evidence surrounding the clopidogrel and proton pump inhibitor drug interaction. *Arch Intern Med* 2010;170(16):1507-8.

Chapter 62
Inflammatory Bowel Disease

George Chami, MD, FRCPC

The idiopathic inflammatory bowel diseases (IBD) consist of Crohn's disease (CD) and ulcerative colitis (UC). CD may involve any part of the GI tract while UC is restricted to the colon, with a variable extent of involvement. UC of the distal colon is termed ulcerative proctosigmoiditis.

Investigations

Refer all patients to specialist care for confirmation of diagnosis, initial treatment and management of exacerbations.

- History:
  - diarrhea, abdominal pain, rectal bleeding and weight loss are the most frequent symptoms
  - presence of nocturnal diarrhea usually indicates "organic" pathology as opposed to functional disorders such as irritable bowel syndrome
  - extraintestinal manifestations, e.g., aphthous ulcers, arthritis, erythema nodosum, iritis, perianal disease, fever
  - family history of IBD
  - previous endoscopic/radiologic test results
  - previous medical (drugs, dose, duration) or surgical treatment (type and number of surgeries)
- Physical examination:
  - weight, nutritional assessment, abdominal tenderness, presence of abdominal mass, perianal disease (fistulae, abscess)
  - growth failure in children (chart height and weight, growth curve Tanner stage)
  - extraintestinal manifestations (e.g., peripheral arthritis, sacroiliitis, ankylosing spondylitis, osteoporosis, erythema nodosum, pyoderma gangrenosum, oral aphthous ulcers, stomatitis, uveitis, scleritis, episcleritis, primary sclerosing cholangitis, nephrolithiasis and thromboembolic events)
- Laboratory tests:
  - hemoglobin, electrolytes, renal function, liver function tests and liver enzymes
  - measures of inflammation (white blood cell and platelet count, erythrocyte sedimentation rate, C-reactive protein, albumin)
  - stool testing to exclude other diagnoses or concomitant infections (*Clostridium difficile*, culture, ova and parasites)
- Further investigations to establish a precise diagnosis:
  - endoscopy (gastroscopy, ileocolonoscopy, capsule endoscopy, balloon assisted enteroscopy)
  - imaging studies (CT/MR enterography, small bowel follow through)
  - biopsy/histopathology (presence of small bowel involvement; granulomata are characteristic of CD)
  - 10% of cases with colonic disease cannot be classified and are termed *colitis not yet determined*

- A definitive diagnosis is important since:
  - IBD is treated differently from other similar diseases (e.g., IBS)
  - colectomy cures UC; CD recurs after surgery
  - the conditions respond differently to drug therapy (especially to aminosalicylates)
  - precise anatomic localization is necessary for selecting drug therapy and planning surgery

Goals of Therapy

- Induce and maintain clinical and endoscopic remission
- Improve nutritional status and growth (children/adolescents)
- Prevent development of colon cancer, which is associated with UC and colonic CD
- Identify and treat extraintestinal manifestations (e.g., arthritis, arthralgia, iritis, uveitis)

Therapeutic Choices

Therapy is determined by the site and extent of disease, and by the severity of symptoms. Patients with mild to moderate disease activity are managed as outpatients, whereas those with severe symptoms may require hospitalization. Therapy is sequential in first inducing and then maintaining remission.

Pharmacologic Choices

Pharmacologic management of IBD includes the use of aminosalicylates, corticosteroids, immunosuppressives, antidiarrheals, antibiotics and, to a limited degree, opioid analgesics (Table 1). In selecting therapy, consider efficacy, the route of administration (oral, iv, rectal) and potential adverse events.

Inflammatory bowel disease has been associated with a higher rate of infections, many of which may be preventable with appropriate vaccination.[1] Determining the immunization status of patients prior to receiving immunomodulators or anti-TNF-α agents is an important part of initial management. While on immunosuppressive treatment, patients have an increased risk of opportunistic infections, a blunted response to immunization, and live-attenuated vaccines are contraindicated. During initial assessment obtain a history of past chicken pox infection as well as serologies for varicella zoster virus (VZV), hepatitis B virus (HBV) and hepatitis C virus. In those patients who are VZV negative, vaccination is recommended followed by a minimum of 3 weeks' wait prior to starting an immunomodulator or anti-TNF-α agent. Yearly vaccination against influenza virus is recommended, as is vaccination against pneumococcus every 3–5 years. In young females vaccination against human papilloma virus is recommended if not already done. Immunization against HBV is recommended in patients who are HBV-negative. In patients who are HBV-positive, antiviral therapy should start at least 2 weeks prior to initiation of immunomodulators or anti-TNF-α agents. Contraindicated live vaccines in immunosuppressed IBD patients include anthrax, intranasal influenza, measles-mumps-rubella, polio live oral, smallpox, tuberculosis BCG, typhoid live oral, yellow fever and varicella.[2]

Aminosalicylates

5-aminosalicylic acid is also known as 5-ASA, mesalamine or mesalazine. It is available for oral or rectal administration (see Ulcerative Proctosigmoiditis section). Oral preparations are formulated to release 5-ASA at specific sites in the gastrointestinal tract since efficacy is dependent on luminal concentration. **Salofalk**, **Mesasal** and **Pentasa** release 5-ASA in the small bowel, allowing 5-ASA to be available in the small bowel and the colon. **Sulfasalazine**, **olsalazine**, **Asacol** and **Mezavant** release 5-ASA primarily in the colon.

All 5-ASA compounds, irrespective of their formulation, are equally effective and safe for induction of remission and prevention of relapse of mild to moderate UC.[3] 5-ASA is ineffective for induction or maintenance of pharmacologically or surgically induced remission of CD while sulfasalazine may have a modest benefit for induction of remission in mild CD.[4,5] Sulfasalazine has the least favourable adverse effect profile, which includes nausea, headache, rash, hemolytic anemia and hepatotoxicity. However, many of these effects are minor and dose-related. The majority of these events (>90%) are related to the sulfapyridine moiety which is not present in 5-ASA preparations. Reversible oligospermia has been reported with sulfasalazine, but has not been associated with 5-ASA.

Corticosteroids

Corticosteroids are effective for induction of remission in npatients with CD and UC.[6,7] Patients with moderately severe exacerbations of CD or UC are treated initially with oral **prednisone** 40–60 mg/day.[8] In those with more severe disease, hospitalization and treatment with iv corticosteroids (e.g., **hydrocortisone**, **methylprednisolone**) may be necessary. Patients who respond to iv therapy are switched to oral prednisone once stabilized. Taper the prednisone dose as improvement occurs (see Table 1).[8,9] Oral **budesonide** is not useful in the treatment of active UC[10] but is effective for induction of remission of mild to moderate ileocecal CD,[11] but to a lesser extent than conventional corticosteroids.[7,12] However, budesonide *enemas* are as effective as other corticosteroid enemas for the treatment of left-sided UC and have a lower incidence of side effects, but are more costly.[13] Budesonide is rapidly inactivated in the liver, resulting in lower systemic bioavailability and lower adrenal suppression compared with conventional corticosteroids.[11,12]

Avoid long-term use of corticosteroids and reserve for patients unresponsive to other drugs. Oral corticosteroids are not recommended for maintenance of remission of IBD.[12,14] Inform patients of the possible side effects and obtain informed consent. Osteoporosis is a concern with long-term therapy. To maintain bone health, supplemental calcium and vitamin D, smoking cessation and exercise are useful interventions; bisphosphonates are helpful in select individuals.[15] Use of corticosteroids is also associated with avascular necrosis of the femoral head.

Immunosuppressive Agents

Azathioprine and **6-mercaptopurine (6-MP)** are used in patients with refractory IBD to reduce the dose of prednisone and maintain remission of quiescent disease[16,17,18,19,20] but they are ineffective in inducing remission of active IBD.[20] Limited evidence and expert consensus suggest that weekly im injections of **methotrexate** can induce remission in patients with CD,[21,22,23] but the usual recommendation is to start it at the same time as corticosteroids to maintain remission of CD, particularly when azathioprine or 6-MP are contraindicated or not tolerated.[21,23,24] Data are lacking regarding usefulness of methotrexate in UC.

All immunosuppressive drugs have significant side effects (e.g., bone marrow suppression, cytopenias and infections). Hypersensitivity pneumonitis and hepatotoxicity are the most important adverse effects of methotrexate. Coadministration of folic acid (1 mg daily) is recommended with methotrexate. Pancreatitis occurs in approximately 3% of patients treated with azathioprine or 6-MP.[25] IBD therapy with thiopurines is also associated with a four- to sixfold increased risk of lymphoproliferative disorders (typically as a result of B-cell clonal proliferation) and this risk is dependent on the patient's age, disease duration and duration of thiopurine treatment.[26,27] Despite this, the benefits of thiopurines in the management of IBD outweigh the risks, particularly in young patients.[26] Although the development of nonmelanoma skin cancer is an uncommon complication of treatment with thiopurines, ongoing and past exposure to these medications significantly increases the risk in all patients with IBD.[28,29] Recommend yearly skin checks and UV protection in patients treated with azathioprine or 6-MP.[28] No strong evidence exists to support a similar relationship with methotrexate.

Biologic Response Modifiers

Anti-tumor necrosis factor alpha (TNF-α) antibodies useful in the management of IBD (particularly fistulizing CD) are **adalimumab**, **certolizumab pegol**, **golimumab** and **infliximab**. Infliximab, an iv chimeric (murine/human) antibody, can provoke minor (headache, flushing, lightheadedness) or major (manifestations of anaphylaxis) infusion reactions. Adalimumab, certolizumab pegol and golimumab are administered sc and are effective in patients with CD who are refractory to or intolerant of infliximab. Any of these drugs is a potential first-line choice depending on cost, safety, route of administration and patient's preference.[30,31,32]

Usually, induction doses of all anti-TNF-α agents are given on weeks 0 and 2 with additional doses at week 4 for certolizumab or week 6 for infliximab. Maintenance doses are usually given every 4 weeks thereafter except for adalimumab (every 2 weeks) and infliximab (every 8 weeks). Up to half of patients with UC or CD do not initially respond to the anti-TNF-α medications and a significant proportion of responders relapse during therapy. To address therapy failure or persistent inflammation, standard doses may be increased, dosing frequencies may be shortened or the anti-TNF-α agent may be replaced with another agent from the same or different class.

Formation of anti-nuclear antibodies, a rare lupus-like syndrome, lymphoma, nonmelanoma skin cancer, cervical dysplasia and worsening of heart failure are important concerns associated with anti-TNF-α therapies. Bacterial pneumonia and sepsis in the pelvis are the most common serious infections associated with anti-TNF-α use. Opportunistic infections and tuberculosis have occurred during anti-TNF-α treatment.[33] Screen for tuberculosis prior to treatment by obtaining a history of exposure, chest x-ray and by performing tuberculin skin testing. Manage patients who are infected with tuberculosis in collaboration with an infectious disease specialist.

Antibiotics

Short courses (2–4 weeks) of **metronidazole** and/or **ciprofloxacin** are useful for the treatment of patients with CD and perianal fistulae or isolated colonic CD.[34] Metronidazole may cause a disulfiram-like reaction in some patients if alcohol is ingested and neuropathy may occur with long-term use.

Antidiarrheals

Use antidiarrheals with caution and avoid in severe disease because of the risk of toxic megacolon. **Diphenoxylate with atropine** is a combination of an opiate and an anticholinergic drug which can cause CNS side effects. **Loperamide** acts on both cholinergic and opiate receptors, but has a lower incidence of adverse effects than diphenoxylate.

Opiate Analgesics

Opiates decrease gastrointestinal motility. Chronic use may lead to narcotic bowel syndrome (chronic or frequently recurring abdominal pain that worsens with continued or escalating dosages of narcotics), increased risk for habituation and, in some individuals, worsened IBD symptoms.

Codeine is useful for pain control and decreasing the number of bowel movements (although approximately 10% of patients may not respond to the drug because of a genetic polymorphism; see the section on analgesics in Chapter 85). Avoid use of morphine or meperidine; if necessary to use, restrict to short-term treatment in select patients.

Crohn's Disease

Therapeutic Choices

Nonpharmacologic Choices

- Encourage smoking cessation since smoking may worsen CD.[35]

- Advise patients not to arbitrarily limit food groups. The goal is to ensure an adequate caloric intake. Nutritional supplements or parenteral nutrition may be necessary in select patients who are malnourished.
- Surgery may be necessary to treat strictures, abscesses, fistulae or for patients refractory to medical management. Recurrence after surgery is almost universal, so conservative surgical management with resection of a minimum amount of bowel is favoured. Since the introduction of the anti-TNF-α agents, surgery as a management option for CD has declined.[36] However, preoperative use of anti-TNF-α drugs may increase the occurrence of postoperative complications (particularly infectious) in CD patients.[37,38]
- Limited evidence indicates that psychological therapy may be beneficial in adolescent IBD patients and shows most promise in reducing pain, fatigue, relapse rate and hospitalisation as well as improving adherence to medication.[39,40] However, there is no evidence to support psychological therapy in adult IBD patients.[40]

Pharmacologic Choices

See the previous general discussion of pharmacologic choices in inflammatory bowel diseases. Figure 1 outlines the pharmacologic management of CD and Table 1 lists the drugs used in the treatment of IBD.

- **Corticosteroids** are most effective for the *induction of remission* (70% response rate). **Prednisone** (40–60 mg/day for 12–16 weeks) is the most commonly used drug.[8]
- Chronic low-dose corticosteroid therapy is ineffective for the *maintenance of remission*.[41]
- The antimetabolites **azathioprine** and **6-mercaptopurine** are ineffective for induction of remission in active Crohn's disease but are effective in maintaining remission [Evidence: SORT A*].[42,43] In patients intolerant to azathioprine, a trial of 6-mercaptopurine may be safely attempted before abandoning this class of medications.[44]
- **5-ASA** is ineffective for maintenance of pharmacologically or surgically induced remission of CD while **sulfasalazine** may have a modest benefit for induction of remission in mild CD.[4,8,45]
- Limited and weak evidence suggests that im **methotrexate** at 25 mg/week may be useful in maintaining remission in severe CD.[22,23]
- **Infliximab**,[46] **adalimumab**[47,48,49] and **certolizumab pegol**[50,51,52,53] are effective in inducing and maintaining remission in patients with moderate to severe CD (infliximab has the best evidence for inducing fistula closure).[54,55,56] Certolizumab pegol is not approved for use in CD patients in Canada. Combining infliximab with azathioprine is more effective than infliximab monotherapy[57] suggesting that initial dual therapy may be preferable for high-risk patients. Whether these findings can be extrapolated to the other biologic agents is unclear.

Therapeutic Tips

- A rare hypersensitivity reaction to **5-ASA** preparations can worsen symptoms.
- 5-ASA does not have a corticosteroid-sparing effect.
- Bile salt–induced diarrhea may occur in patients who have had resection of their terminal ileum. This usually responds to **cholestyramine** or **antidiarrheals**. Vitamin B_{12} deficiency may occur in this setting.
- Infusion reactions from **infliximab** may require treatment with epinephrine, antihistamines and corticosteroids.
- Not all patients with IBD experience worsening symptoms with NSAIDs. Advise patients to stop using NSAIDs if these agents cause disease flares.

* SORT (Strength of Recommendation Taxonomy) is a rating system (A, B or C) that addresses the quality of available evidence. For more information consult **How to Use *Compendium of Therapeutic Choices*** on page xxv.

Figure 1: **Management of Crohn's Disease**

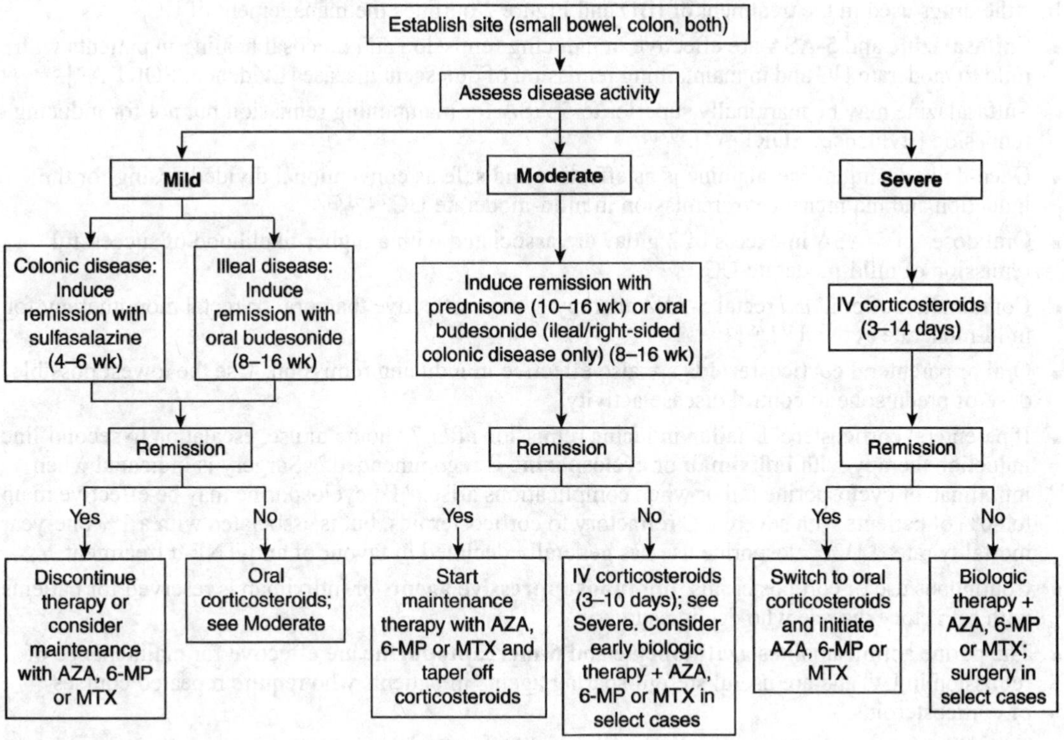

Abbreviations: 5-ASA = 5-aminosalicylic acid; 6-MP = 6-mercaptopurine; AZA = azathioprine; MTX = methotrexate

Ulcerative Colitis

Therapeutic Choices

Nonpharmacologic Choices

- Advise patients not to arbitrarily limit food groups. Watch for dehydration and electrolyte abnormalities especially during disease flares.
- Surgery (colectomy) may be used to treat patients who are refractory to medical therapy or who have pre-cancerous or cancerous changes in the colon. Since the introduction of the anti-TNF-α agents, however, surgery as a management option for ulcerative colitis (UC) has declined.[36]
- Start colon cancer surveillance with colonoscopy within 8 years of diagnosis of pancolitis and within 15 years of diagnosis of left-sided colitis. Consider an early start in those with history of severe inflammation or primary sclerosing cholangitis, and if date of disease onset is uncertain.[58]
- Although colectomy "cures" UC, pouchitis, a chronic inflammatory condition which occurs after ileal-anal reservoir construction, can be troublesome.[34] Symptoms of pouchitis include tenesmus (feeling of constantly needing to pass stools despite an empty colon), diarrhea and bleeding.

Pharmacologic Choices

See the previous general discussion of pharmacologic choices in inflammatory bowel diseases. Table 1 lists the drugs used in the treatment of IBD and Figure 2 outlines the management of UC.

- **Sulfasalazine** and **5-ASA** are effective in inducing remission and mucosal healing in patients with mild to moderate UC and in maintaining remission of quiescent disease [Evidence: SORT A*].[59,60,61]
- Sulfasalazine may be marginally superior to 5-ASA for maintaining remission but not for inducing remission [Evidence: SORT A*].[59,60]
- Once-daily dosing of mesalamine is as effective and safe as conventional divided dosing for the induction and maintenance of remission in mild-moderate UC.[62,63,64,65]
- Oral doses of 5-ASA in excess of 2 g/day are associated with a higher likelihood of successful remission of mild-moderate UC.[66,67]
- Combination of oral *and* rectal 5-ASA therapy is more effective than oral or rectal monotherapy for mild-moderate active UC.[68,69]
- Oral or parenteral **corticosteroids** are also effective in inducing remission. Use the lowest possible dose of prednisone to control disease activity.
- If parenteral corticosteroids fail in inducing remission after 72 hours of use, escalation to second-line induction therapy with **infliximab** or **cyclosporine** is recommended.[70] Surgery is indicated when infliximab or cyclosporine fail or when complications arise.[70] IV cyclosporine may be effective in up to 80% of patients with severe UC refractory to corticosteroids, but is associated with a 1% one-year mortality rate.[71] IV cyclosporine use has generally declined in favour of anti-TNF-α treatment.
- Continuous use of corticosteroids, **immunosuppressive agents** or infliximab is reserved for patients with refractory disease who decline surgery.
- The purine antimetabolites **azathioprine** and **6-mercaptopurine** are effective for maintenance of remission in UC and are useful steroid-sparing agents in patients who require repeated courses of corticosteroids.[72]
- The efficacy of **methotrexate** in the treatment of UC is not known.[73,74]
- The anti-TNF-α agents infliximab, **adalimumab** and **golimumab** are equally effective in inducing and maintaining remission in patients with UC including those refractory to conventional medical therapy.[75,76,77] Adalimumab may be less effective in those patients who had prior exposure to infliximab.[78,79,80]

Therapeutic Tips

- Use extreme caution when prescribing opioids and anticholinergic drugs for patients with active UC due to the risk of toxic megacolon. Use these drugs only when all other alternatives have failed.
- Weak evidence suggests that folate supplementation and high adherence to aminosalicylate maintenance therapy may reduce the risk of colon cancer.[81,82]
- Patients with severe colitis often will not tolerate tube feeds due to diarrhea.
- Avoid NSAIDs because they may exacerbate symptoms or precipitate relapse.
- Be aware that *C. difficile* may cause severe exacerbations of IBD, including megacolon. Independent risk factors include antibiotic exposure, colonic involvement and immunosuppressive drug therapy.

* SORT (Strength of Recommendation Taxonomy) is a rating system (A, B or C) that addresses the quality of available evidence. For more information consult **How to Use *Compendium of Therapeutic Choices*** on page xxv.

Figure 2: **Management of Ulcerative Pancolitis**

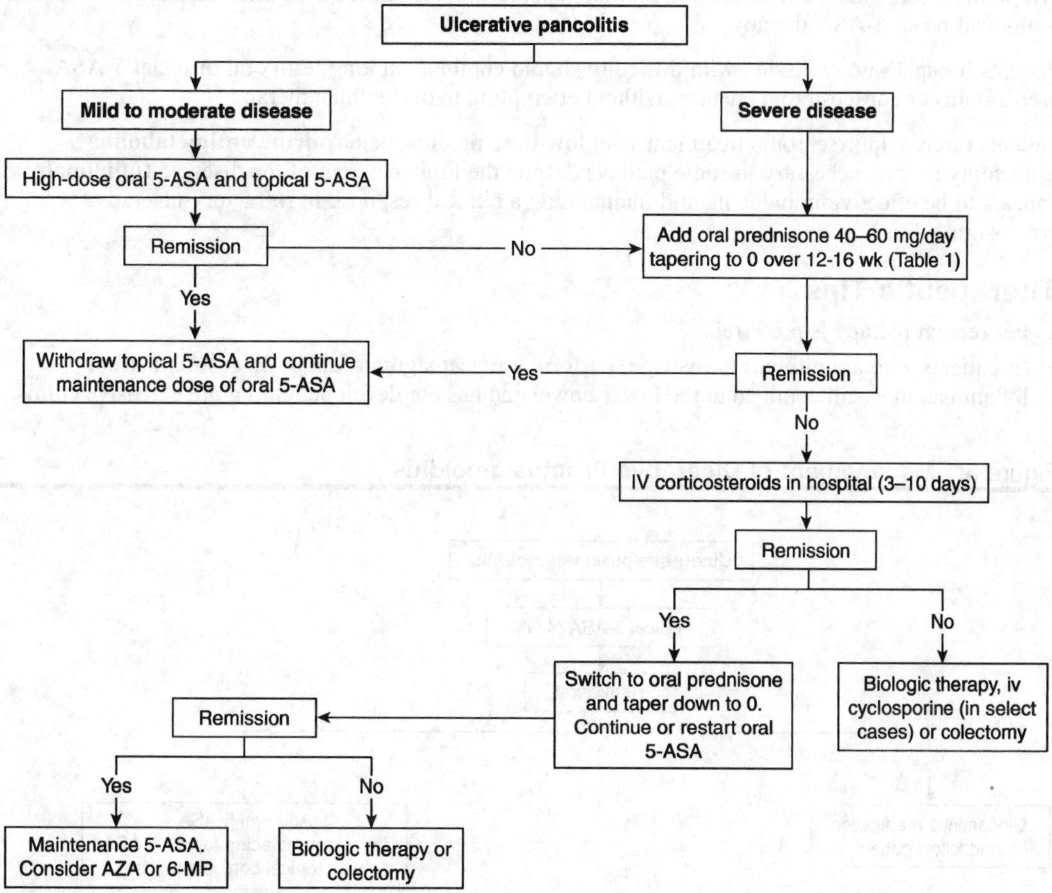

Abbreviations: 5-ASA = 5-aminosalicylic acid; 6-MP = 6-mercaptopurine; AZA = azathioprine

Ulcerative Proctosigmoiditis

Therapeutic Choices

Pharmacologic Choices

Given the limited extent of the inflammation (rectum/sigmoid colon), the focus is on rectally administered therapy (Table 1, Figure 3).[68] **5-ASA** preparations (suppositories, enemas) administered at bedtime are the initial treatment of choice. Alternatively, **rectal corticosteroids** can be used. If a response is not achieved with one of these strategies, switching to the other is advised. Suppositories are effective only for proctitis, whereas enemas can be used to treat disease in the descending colon and rectum from the splenic flexure distally.

If remission is not induced within 2–4 weeks, oral 5-ASA can be added. Limited data suggest that there is an additive benefit of combined oral and rectal 5-ASA induction therapy.[83] Rectal 5-ASA monotherapy may be effective for maintenance of remission of mild to moderate distal disease.[83,84] Switch patients unresponsive to these measures to **prednisone** or (rarely) iv corticosteroids.

Discontinue all medications if patients are brought into remission easily after a first episode (within 4–8 weeks). Follow-up is essential; place patients on chronic maintenance therapy with 5-ASA if symptoms recur. Most patients prefer oral maintenance therapy, although in practice many will require prolonged rectal 5-ASA therapy.

Patients brought into remission with difficulty should continue on long-term oral or rectal 5-ASA preparations or corticosteroid enemas, without attempting to discontinue therapy.

Patients rarely require chronic treatment with low-dose prednisone or **purine antimetabolites**. Colectomy may be necessary in some patients despite the limited extent of the disease. **Infliximab** appears to be effective in inducing and maintaining a clinical response in refractory ulcerative proctosigmoiditis.[85]

Therapeutic Tips

- Per rectum therapy is preferred.
- In patients who are difficult to manage, perform a repeat sigmoidoscopy to ensure that the inflammation is still confined to the lower bowel and has not developed into more extensive colitis.

Figure 3: Management of Ulcerative Proctosigmoiditis

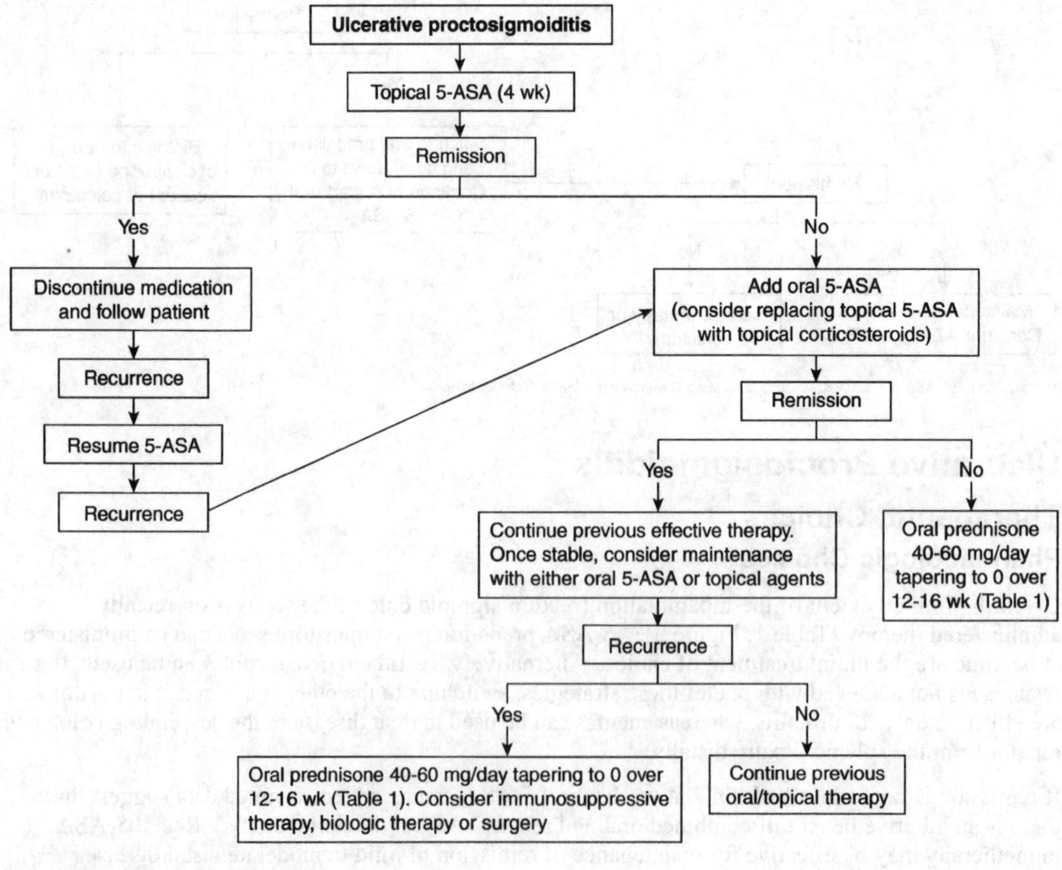

Abbreviations: 5-ASA = 5-aminosalicylic acid

Choices during Pregnancy and Breastfeeding

Inflammatory bowel disease (IBD) in pregnant women increases the risk of preterm birth, low birth weight and miscarriages.[86] However, the evidence is not as strong for an increased risk of congenital abnormalities.[86] Pregnant IBD patients in remission at the time of conception are likely to remain in remission during pregnancy but up to one-third may relapse during the pregnancy.[87,88] Advise women with IBD who are planning a pregnancy to try conceiving at a time when the disease is in remission.[89] Advise female and male IBD patients that their disease does not reduce fertility; the observed childlessness in IBD patients is due to voluntary choices based on incorrect patient beliefs rather than physiologic or organic causes.[90] Most IBD medications (except methotrexate) should not be discontinued at conception or while breastfeeding since their cessation might lead to disease flare; the risk of the untreated disease (preterm birth, miscarriage) is often greater than the risk of most available medications.[86]

- **Methotrexate** is contraindicated in pregnancy and breastfeeding owing to its teratogenic and cytotoxic effects.[91] Recommend effective contraception if patient is receiving methotrexate. Discontinue the drug 3–6 months prior to attempted conception.
- **Azathioprine** and **6-mercaptopurine** use during pregnancy is considered low risk despite the conflicting safety data.[86] Azathioprine and 6-mercaptopurine are generally considered compatible with breastfeeding but it is considered safest to separate breastfeeding by a few hours from dosing.[92]
- **Cyclosporine** is not usually used for treatment of IBD but is considered to have an overall low risk during pregnancy. Do not use cyclosporine during breastfeeding; anti-TNF-α agents are safer in this situation.[93]
- **Corticosteroids** are considered safe and may be continued in pregnancy if indicated. However, use them with caution in the first trimester since they have been associated with an increased (though still low) risk of oral clefts in the newborn.[94] Corticosteroids may be used at any stage of pregnancy (including first trimester) if benefits outweigh potential risks (e.g., during disease flares). **Prednisone** and **prednisolone** are considered compatible with breastfeeding.[86]
- **Aminosalicylates** are considered low risk for use in pregnancy or while breastfeeding.[95] Due to potential anti-folate effects, women taking **sulfasalazine** may be safely switched to 5-ASA or are generally advised to supplement with 2 mg daily of folic acid starting before conception and continuing throughout their pregnancy.[86]
- **Metronidazole** has a low teratogenic risk when used during pregnancy but do not use while patient is breastfeeding because it transfers to breast milk.[86] Avoid prolonged metronidazole use in pregnant patients.
- The **fluoroquinolones** can be regarded as safe during pregnancy when used for short periods.[86] Fluoroquinolones are probably safe to use while breastfeeding if necessary.
- **Infliximab**, **adalimumab**, **certolizumab pegol** and **golimumab** are considered low risk in pregnancy[96] during at least the first 2 trimesters.[97] Carefully time infusions of infliximab, adalimumab and golimumab in the third trimester since they are actively transported across the placenta. Certolizumab pegol is not transferred across the placenta and hence may be a better choice than the other anti-TNF-α agents for use in pregnancy, particularly in the third trimester.[98] For those anti-TNF-α agents that are known to cross the placenta, fetal serum levels have been detected for up to 6 months. Therefore, delay administration of any live or live-attenuated vaccinations to the newborn until after 6 months of age, unless serum anti-TNF-α levels are proven negative.[99] Infliximab and certolizumab pegol are compatible with breastfeeding, whereas adequate safety data for adalimumab and golimumab are not available.

A discussion of general principles on the use of medications in these special populations can be found in Appendix II and Appendix III. Other specialized reference sources are also provided in these appendices.

Table 1: **Drugs Used for the Treatment of Inflammatory Bowel Disease**

Class	Drug	Dose	Adverse Effects	Drug Interactions	Comments	Cost[a]
Aminosalicylates	*5-aminosalicylic acid (5-ASA), oral* 5-ASA, Asacol, Asacol 800, Mesasal, Pentasa, Salofalk Tablets, generics	**5-ASA:** Active disease: up to 4.8 g/day in divided doses Maintenance: 0.8–3.2 g/day in divided doses **Asacol:** Active disease: up to 4.8 g/day in divided doses Maintenance: 1.6 g/day in divided doses **Mesasal:** Active disease: 1.5–3 g/day in divided doses Maintenance: 1.5 g/day in divided doses **Mezavant:** Active disease: 2.4–4.8 g once daily Maintenance: 2.4 g once daily **Pentasa:** Active disease: 2–4 g/day in divided doses Maintenance: 1.5–3 g/day in divided doses **Salofalk:** Active disease: 3–4 g/day in divided doses Maintenance: 1.5–3 g/day in divided doses	Abdominal pain, cramps, diarrhea, headache, nausea, rash including urticaria, vomiting. Rare hypersensitivity reactions, including pneumonitis, hepatitis and worsening of colitis.	Increases risk of myelosuppression when coadministered with azathioprine or 6-mercaptopurine. Increased risk of renal failure when coadministered with other nephrotoxic agents such as NSAIDs and azathioprine.	All aminosalicylates are equally effective in UC. The value of 5-ASA as maintenance therapy in CD is controversial. Abrupt discontinuation of 5-ASA is not recommended, and may result in relapse. Best evidence for Asacol 2.4 g/day and Pentasa 3 g/day.	$
	5-aminosalicylic acid, rectal Pentasa, Salofalk Enema,Salofalk Suppositories	Active disease: Enema: 4 g QHS Suppositories: 1 g QHS Maintenance: Enema: 2 g QHS or 4 g every 2nd or 3rd night Suppositories: 1 g every 2nd or 3rd night based on patient's response	Local reactions (e.g., pruritus, rectal discomfort and urgency), fever, flu-like symptoms, worsening of hemorrhoids, abdominal pain, cramps or discomfort.		Enemas and suppositories effective in ulcerative proctitis.	$
	olsalazine Dipentum	Active disease: 500 mg QID po Maintenance: 500 mg BID po	Secretory diarrhea; may be minimized by increasing dose gradually.			$

Class	Drug	Dose	Adverse Effects	Drug Interactions	Comments	Cost[a]
	sulfasalazine Salazopyrin, generics	Active disease: 1000–2000 mg 3–4 times daily po Maintenance: 1000 mg 2–3 times daily po	Dose-related adverse effects: nausea, vomiting, diarrhea, anorexia, headache. Hypersensitivity reaction (rash, fever), hemolytic anemia (particularly in patients with G6PD deficiency), oligospermia (reversible). Maintain adequate fluid intake to prevent crystalluria and stone formation.	Reduced absorption of folic acid and digoxin.	All aminosalicylates are equally effective in UC.	$
Biologic Response Modifiers	*adalimumab* Humira	CD: Active disease: 160 mg sc at wk 0 (given as 4 injections in a single day or as 2 injections/day × 2 days), then 80 mg sc at wk 2 (given as 2 injections) Maintenance: 40 mg sc every other wk beginning at wk 4	Nausea, injection site reactions (e.g., erythema, itching, pain, swelling), tuberculosis, opportunistic infections, upper respiratory tract infections, abdominal pain, reactivation of hepatitis B infection, formation of antinuclear antibodies, reversible lupus-like syndrome, worsening heart failure, lymphoma, CNS demyelinating disorders.	Patients should not receive live vaccines during treatment.	Evaluate patients for risk of tuberculosis, hepatitis B, hepatitis C and varicella (if no history of disease) before starting therapy.	$775/ dose
	certolizumab pegol Cimzia	CD: Active disease: 400 mg sc at wk 0, 2 and 4 Maintenance: 400 mg sc every 4 wk	See adalimumab.	See adalimumab.	See adalimumab. Not a Health Canada–approved indication.	$700/ dose
	golimumab Simponi	Active disease: 200 mg sc at wk 0, 100 mg at wk 2 Maintenance: 50 mg sc every 4 wk	Upper respiratory tract infections, viral infections, bronchitis, sinusitis, superficial fungal infections, abscess, liver test abnormalities, anemia, leukopenia, autoantibody positive, constipation, rash, pyrexia, injections site reaction.	See adalimumab.	See adalimumab.	~$1600/ 50 mg dose

(cont'd)

Table 1: **Drugs Used for the Treatment of Inflammatory Bowel Disease** *(cont'd)*

Class	Drug	Dose	Adverse Effects	Drug Interactions	Comments	Cost[a]
	infliximab Remicade	CD (luminal or fistulizing) or UC: Active disease: 5 mg/kg iv at 0, 2 and 6 wk; consider increasing dose up to 10 mg/kg if no response Maintenance: 5 mg/kg iv every 8 wk	See adalimumab.	See adalimumab.	See adalimumab.	~$1000/ 100 mg dose
Corticosteroids, systemic	*budesonide, oral* Entocort Capsules	Acute exacerbation: 9 mg QAM po before food Maintenance (maximum of 3 months): 6 mg QAM po before food	Dyspepsia, muscle cramps, palpitations, blurred vision, rash, urticaria, suppression of the hypothalamic pituitary adrenal axis, hypokalemia, osteoporosis.	CYP3A4 inhibitors: budesonide is metabolized via CYP3A4. Inhibitors of CYP3A4 (e.g., clarithromycin, erythromycin, grapefruit juice, itraconazole, ketoconazole) increase plasma levels of budesonide. Antidiabetic agents: corticosteroids may increase blood glucose. NSAIDs: may increase the risk of GI ulceration. Thiazide and loop diuretics also deplete potassium.	Controlled-release capsule for treating CD in the ileum and/or ascending colon. Benefits are mostly due to its topical action since it is rapidly and almost completely degraded by hepatic 1st pass metabolism. Exhibits somewhat fewer adverse effects than conventional corticosteroids. Can be used up to 3 months for maintenance therapy.	$
	hydrocortisone sodium succinate Solu-Cortef, generics	Acute exacerbation: 300–400 mg/day iv until patient is stable then switch to prednisone po	Acne, glucose intolerance, weight gain, hypertension, hypokalemia, osteoporosis, aseptic necrosis of femoral head, suppression of the hypothalamic pituitary adrenal axis, impaired wound healing. Caution in hyperthyroidism, osteoporosis, peptic ulcer, cirrhosis.	Clearance may decrease with estrogens; may increase digitalis toxicity secondary to hypokalemia.	Avoid immunization during corticosteroid use. No role in maintenance therapy.	$$

Class	Drug	Dose	Adverse Effects	Drug Interactions	Comments	Cost[a]
	methylprednisolone sodium succinate Solu-Medrol, generics	Acute exacerbation: 40–60 mg/day iv until patient is stable then switch to prednisone po	See hydrocortisone sodium succinate.	See hydrocortisone sodium succinate.	No advantage over hydrocortisone. No role in maintenance therapy.	$
	prednisone generics	Acute exacerbation: 40–60 mg QAM po for 2–4 wk, then taper the daily dose by 5 mg each week until a daily dose of 20 mg is reached, then taper by 2.5 mg each week until prednisone is discontinued	See hydrocortisone sodium succinate.	See hydrocortisone sodium succinate. Phenobarbital, phenytoin, and rifampin may increase metabolism which may necessitate increased maintenance dose. Increased risk of hypokalemia with coadministration of diuretics.	Useful in moderately severe and severe UC and CD. No role in maintenance therapy.	$
Corticosteroids, topical	*betamethasone, enema* Betnesol	Acute exacerbation: 5 mg (100 mL) QHS pr	Topical therapy, in general, has less severe adverse effects than systemic therapy.		Enemas effective in ulcerative proctitis. Useful in UC; role in CD not well established. As much as 75% of administered topical dose may be absorbed if the lower colon is severely inflamed.	$$
	budesonide, enema Entocort Enema	Acute exacerbation: 2 mg (100 mL) QHS pr	See betamethasone enema.		See betamethasone enema.	$$
	hydrocortisone, enema Cortenema, Cortifoam, Hycort	Acute exacerbation: 80–100 mg QHS as enema	See betamethasone enema.		See betamethasone enema.	$$

(cont'd)

Table 1: **Drugs Used for the Treatment of Inflammatory Bowel Disease** *(cont'd)*

Class	Drug	Dose	Adverse Effects	Drug Interactions	Comments	Cost[a]
Immunomodulators	*6-mercaptopurine* ❥ Purinethol	100 mg daily po	Nausea, stomatitis, GI discomfort, arthralgias, diarrhea, anorexia, increased risk of opportunistic infection, blood dyscrasias, and rarely pancreatitis, hepatotoxicity.	Oral anticoagulants: mercaptopurine may inhibit hypoprothrombinemic response to warfarin and possibly other anticoagulants. Allopurinol may increase azathioprine toxicity; dosage adjustment may be necessary (1/4 of regular dose); similar interaction with mercaptopurine. ACE inhibitors may increase the likelihood of neutropenia when combined with azathioprine or mercaptopurine.	Low risk in pregnancy and breastfeeding. Metabolism of azathioprine and mercaptopurine is influenced by a genetic polymorphism.	$$
	azathioprine ❥ Imuran, generics	1–2.5 mg/kg daily po	See 6-mercaptopurine.	See 6-mercaptopurine. Concurrent use with ACE inhibitors may induce severe leukopenia; may increase levels of methotrexate metabolites.	See 6-mercaptopurine. Reduce dose in oliguric patients.	$

Class	Drug	Dose	Adverse Effects	Drug Interactions	Comments	Cost[a]
	cyclosporine Sandimmune	2–5 mg/kg daily iv	Renal toxicity (monitor renal function), hypertension, hypertrichosis, cytopenia, gum hyperplasia, electrolyte imbalances, nausea, diarrhea, seizures, opportunistic infection.	Metabolized by CYP450: many possible drug interactions (e.g., erythromycin, ketoconazole, rifampin, St. John's wort).	May help avoid colectomy in select patients with severe disease not responding to other therapies. Do not use in pregnancy.	$$$$
	methotrexate (kidney symbol) Methotrexate Injection USP, Metoject, other generics	25 mg im weekly	Nausea, flu-like aches, headache, oral ulcers, bone marrow and liver toxicity, pneumonitis, immunosuppression, lymphoma.	Alcohol restriction may minimize hepatotoxicity. NSAIDs may increase methotrexate serum concentrations (probably not significant with low once-weekly methotrexate doses). Some penicillins may decrease methotrexate clearance.	Potentially hepatotoxic. Oral methotrexate has not been evaluated in controlled trials. Do not use in pregnancy.	$$

[a] Cost of 1-day supply for 70 kg person unless otherwise specified; includes drug cost only.

(kidney symbol) Dosage adjustment may be required in renal impairment; see Appendix I.

Abbreviations: CD = Crohn's disease; G6PD = glucose-6-phosphate dehydrogenase; UC = ulcerative colitis

Legend: $ <$5 $$ $5–10 $$$ $10–20 $$$$ $20–30

Suggested Readings

Baumgart DC, Carding SR. Inflammatory bowel disease: cause and immunobiology. *Lancet* 2007;369(9573):1627-40.

Baumgart DC, Sandborn WJ. Inflammatory bowel disease: clinical aspects and established and evolving therapies. *Lancet* 2007;369(9573):1641-57.

Colombel JF, Sandborn WJ, Reinisch W et al. Infliximab, azathioprine, or combination therapy for Crohn's disease. *N Engl J Med* 2010;362(15):1383-95.

Hanauer SB. Inflammatory bowel disease: epidemiology, pathogenesis, and therapeutic opportunities. *Inflamm Bowel Dis* 2006;12(Suppl 1):S3-9.

Kornbluth A, Sachar DB, Practice Parameters Committee of the American College of Gastroenterology. Ulcerative colitis practice guidelines in adults: American College Of Gastroenterology, Practice Parameters Committee. *Am J Gastroenterol* 2010;105(3):501-23.

Mahadevan U, Cucchiara S, Hyams JS et al. The London Position Statement of the World Congress of Gastroenterology on Biological Therapy for IBD With the European Crohn's and Colitis Organisation: pregnancy and pediatrics. *Am J Gastroenterol* 2011;106(2):214-23.

Nguyen GC, Bernstein CN, Bitton A et al. Consensus statements on the risk, prevention, and treatment of venous thromboembolism in inflammatory bowel disease: Canadian Association of Gastroenterology. *Gastroenterology* 2014;146(3):835-848.e6.

Panaccione R, Rutgeerts P, Sandborn WJ et al. Review article: treatment algorithms to maximize remission and minimize corticosteroid dependence in patients with inflammatory bowel disease. *Aliment Pharmacol Ther* 2008;28(6):674-88.

References

1. Lodhia N. The appropriate use of vaccines in patients with inflammatory bowel disease. *J Clin Gastroenterol* 2014;48(5):395-401.
2. Sánchez-Tembleque MD, Corella C, Pérez-Calle JL. Vaccines and recommendations for their use in inflammatory bowel disease. *World J Gastroenterol* 2013;19(9):1354-8.
3. Feagan BG, Chande N, MacDonald JK. Are there any differences in the efficacy and safety of different formulations of Oral 5-ASA used for induction and maintenance of remission in ulcerative colitis? evidence from Cochrane Reviews. *Inflamm Bowel Dis* 2013;19(9):2031-40.
4. Akobeng AK, Gardener E. Oral 5-aminosalicylic acid for maintenance of medically-induced remission in Crohn's Disease. *Cochrane Database Syst Rev* 2005;(1):CD003715.
5. Lim WC, Hanauer S. Aminosalicylates for induction of remission or response in Crohn's disease. *Cochrane Database Syst Rev* 2010;(12):CD008870.
6. Benchimol EI, Seow CH, Steinhart AH et al. Traditional corticosteroids for induction of remission in Crohn's disease. *Cochrane Database Syst Rev* 2008;(2):CD006792.
7. Ford AC, Bernstein CN, Khan KJ et al. Glucocorticosteroid therapy in inflammatory bowel disease: systematic review and meta-analysis. *Am J Gastroenterol* 2011;106(4):590-9.
8. Summers RW, Switz DM, Sessions JT et al. National Cooperative Crohn's Disease Study: results of drug treatment. *Gastroenterology* 1979;77(4 Pt 2):847-69.
9. Jani N, Regueiro MD. Medical therapy for ulcerative colitis. *Gastroenterol Clin North Am* 2002;31(1):147-66.
10. Sherlock ME, Seow CH, Steinhart AH et al. Oral budesonide for induction of remission in ulcerative colitis. *Cochrane Database Syst Rev* 2010;(10):CD007698.
11. Seow CH, Benchimol EI, Griffiths AM et al. Budesonide for induction of remission in Crohn's disease. *Cochrane Database Syst Rev* 2008;(3):CD000296.
12. Kane SV, Schoenfeld P, Sandborn WJ et al. The effectiveness of budesonide therapy for Crohn's disease. *Aliment Pharmacol Ther* 2002;16(8):1509-17.
13. Hanauer SB, Robinson M, Pruitt R et al. Budesonide enema for the treatment of active, distal ulcerative colitis and proctitis: a dose-ranging study. U.S. Budesonide enema study group. *Gastroenterology* 1998;115(3):525-32.
14. Benchimol EI, Seow CH, Otley AR et al. Budesonide for maintenance of remission in Crohn's disease. *Cochrane Database Syst Rev* 2009;(1):CD002913.
15. Melek J, Sakuraba A. Efficacy and safety of medical therapy for low bone mineral density in patients with inflammatory bowel disease: a meta-analysis and systematic review. *Clin Gastroenterol Hepatol* 2014;12(1):32-44.e5.
16. Candy S, Wright J, Gerber M et al. A controlled double blind study of azathioprine in the management of Crohn's disease. *Gut* 1995;37(5):674-8.
17. Feagan BG, Rochon J, Fedorak RN et al. Methotrexate for the treatment of Crohn's disease. The North American Crohn's Study Group Investigators. *N Engl J Med* 1995;332(5):292-7.
18. Pearson DC, May GR, Fick GH et al. Azathioprine and 6-mercaptopurine in Crohn disease. A meta-analysis. *Ann Intern Med* 1995;123(2):132-42.
19. Prefontaine E, Macdonald JK, Sutherland LR. Azathioprine or 6-mercaptopurine for induction of remission in Crohn's disease. *Cochrane Database Syst Rev* 2010;(6):CD000545.
20. Khan KJ, Dubinsky MC, Ford AC et al. Efficacy of immunosuppressive therapy for inflammatory bowel disease: a systematic review and meta-analysis. *Am J Gastroenterol* 2011;106(4):630-42.

21. Dassopoulos T, Sultan S, Falck-Ytter YT et al. American Gastroenterological Association Institute technical review on the use of thiopurines, methotrexate, and anti-TNF-α biologic drugs for the induction and maintenance of remission in inflammatory Crohn's disease. *Gastroenterology* 2013;145(6):1464-78.e1-5.
22. McDonald JW, Tsoulis DJ, Macdonald JK et al. Methotrexate for induction of remission in refractory Crohn's disease. *Cochrane Database Syst Rev* 2012;12:CD003459.
23. Terdiman JP, Gruss CB, Heidelbaugh JJ et al. American Gastroenterological Association Institute guideline on the use of thiopurines, methotrexate, and anti-TNF-α biologic drugs for the induction and maintenance of remission in inflammatory Crohn's disease. *Gastroenterology* 2013;145(6):1459-63.
24. U.K. National Institute for Health and Care Excellence. *Crohn's disease: management in adults, children and young people.* October 2012. Available from: www.nice.org.uk/nicemedia/live/13936/61001/61001.pdf.
25. Present DH, Meltzer SJ, Krumholz MP et al. 6-Mercaptopurine in the management of inflammatory bowel disease: short- and long-term toxicity. *Ann Intern Med* 1989;111(8):641-9.
26. Subramaniam K, D'Rozario J, Pavli P. Lymphoma and other lymphoproliferative disorders in inflammatory bowel disease: a review. *J Gastroenterol Hepatol* 2013;28(1):24-30.
27. Health Canada. Healthy Canadians. Imuran (azathioprine) or Purinethol (mercaptopurine)—association with a type of blood cancer—hepatosplenic t-cell lymphoma—for health professionals. March 26, 2014. Available from: healthycanadians.gc.ca/recall-alert-rappel-avis/hc-sc/2014/38691a-eng.php.
28. Peyrin-Biroulet L, Khosrotehrani K, Carrat F et al. Increased risk for nonmelanoma skin cancers in patients who receive thiopurines for inflammatory bowel disease. *Gastroenterology* 2011;141(5):1621-28.e5
29. Singh H, Nugent Z, Demers AA et al. Increased risk of nonmelanoma skin cancers among individuals with inflammatory bowel disease. *Gastroenterology* 2011;141(5):1612-20.
30. Sandborn WJ, Rutgeerts P, Enns R et al. Adalimumab induction therapy for Crohn disease previously treated with infliximab: a randomized trial. *Ann Intern Med* 2007;146(12):829-38.
31. Da W, Zhu J, Wang L et al. Adalimumab for Crohn's disease after infliximab treatment failure: a systematic review. *Eur J Gastroenterol Hepatol* 2013;25(8):885-91.
32. Sandborn WJ, Abreu MT, D'Haens G et al. Certolizumab pegol in patients with moderate to severe Crohn's disease and secondary failure to infliximab. *Clin Gastroenterol Hepatol* 2010;8(8):688-95.e2.
33. Ford AC, Peyrin-Biroulet L. Opportunistic infections with anti-tumor necrosis factor-α therapy in inflammatory bowel disease: meta-analysis of randomized controlled trials. *Am J Gastroenterol* 2013;108(8):1268-76.
34. Shen B, Achkar JP, Lashner BA et al. A randomized clinical trial of ciprofloxacin and metronidazole to treat acute pouchitis. *Inflamm Bowel Dis* 2001;7(4):301-5.
35. Sutherland LR, Ramcharan S, Bryant H et al. Effect of cigarette smoking on recurrence of Crohn's disease. *Gastroenterology* 1990;98(5 Pt 1):1123-8.
36. Costa J, Magro F, Caldeira D, Alarcão J et al. Infliximab reduces hospitalizations and surgery interventions in patients with inflammatory bowel disease: a systematic review and meta-analysis. *Inflamm Bowel Dis* 2013;19(10):2098-110.
37. Billioud V, Ford AC, Tedesco ED et al. Preoperative use of anti-TNF therapy and postoperative complications in inflammatory bowel diseases: a meta-analysis. *J Crohns Colitis* 2013;7(11):853-67.
38. Narula N, Charleton D, Marshall JK. Meta-analysis: peri-operative anti-TNFα treatment and post-operative complications in patients with inflammatory bowel disease. *Aliment Pharmacol Ther* 2013;37(11):1057-64.
39. McCombie AM, Mulder RT, Gearry RB. Psychotherapy for inflammatory bowel disease: a review and update. *J Crohns Colitis* 2013;7(12):935-49.
40. Timmer A, Preiss JC, Motschall E et al. Psychological interventions for treatment of inflammatory bowel disease. *Cochrane Database Syst Rev* 2011;(2):CD006913.
41. Steinhart AH, Ewe K, Griffiths AM et al. Corticosteroids for maintenance of remission in Crohn's disease. *Cochrane Database Syst Rev* 2003;(4):CD000301.
42. Chande N, Tsoulis DJ, MacDonald JK. Azathioprine or 6-mercaptopurine for induction of remission in Crohn's disease. *Cochrane Database Syst Rev* 2013;4:CD000545.
43. Prefontaine E, Sutherland LR, Macdonald JK et al. Azathioprine or 6-mercaptopurine for maintenance of remission in Crohn's disease. *Cochrane Database Syst Rev* 2009;(1):CD000067.
44. Kennedy NA, Rhatigan E, Arnott ID et al. A trial of mercaptopurine is a safe strategy in patients with inflammatory bowel disease intolerant to azathioprine: an observational study, systematic review and meta-analysis. *Aliment Pharmacol Ther* 2013;38(10):1255-66.
45. Hanauer SB, Stromberg U. Oral Pentasa in the treatment of active Crohn's disease: a meta-analysis of double-blind, placebo-controlled trials. *Clin Gastroenterol Hepatol* 2004;2(5):379-88.
46. Hanauer SB, Feagan BG, Lichtenstein GR et al. Maintenance infliximab for Crohn's disease: the ACCENT I randomised trial. *Lancet* 2002;359(9317):1541-9.
47. Hanauer SB, Sandborn WJ, Rutgeerts P et al. Human anti-tumor necrosis factor monoclonal antibody (adalimumab) in Crohn's disease: the CLASSIC-I trial. *Gastroenterology* 2006;130(2):323-33.
48. Sandborn WJ, Hanauer SB, Rutgeerts P et al. Adalimumab for maintenance treatment of Crohn's disease: results of the CLASSIC II trial. *Gut* 2007;56(9):1232-9.
49. Colombel JF, Sandborn WJ, Rutgeerts P et al. Adalimumab for maintenance of clinical response and remission in patients with Crohn's disease: the CHARM trial. *Gastroenterology* 2007;132(1):52-65.
50. Schreiber S, Khaliq-Kareemi M, Lawrance IC et al. Maintenance therapy with certolizumab pegol for Crohn's disease. *N Engl J Med* 2007;357(3):239-50.
51. Shao LM, Chen MY, Cai JT. Meta-analysis: the efficacy and safety of certolizumab pegol in Crohn's disease. *Aliment Pharmacol Ther* 2009;29(6):605-14.
52. Kawalec P, Mikrut A, Wiśniewska N et al. Tumor necrosis factor-α antibodies (infliximab, adalimumab and certolizumab) in Crohn's disease: systematic review and meta-analysis. *Arch Med Sci* 2013;9(5):765-79.
53. Lichtenstein GR, Thomsen OØ, Schreiber S et al. Continuous therapy with certolizumab pegol maintains remission of patients with Crohn's disease for up to 18 months. *Clin Gastroenterol Hepatol* 2010;8(7):600-9.
54. Present DH, Rutgeerts P, Targan S et al. Infliximab for the treatment of fistulas in patients with Crohn's disease. *N Engl J Med* 1999;340(18):1398-405.

55. Colombel JF, Schwartz DA, Sandborn WJ et al. Adalimumab for the treatment of fistulas in patients with Crohn's disease. *Gut* 2009;58(7):940-8.
56. Peyrin-Biroulet L, Deltenre P, de Suray N et al. Efficacy and safety of tumor necrosis factor antagonists in Crohn's disease: meta-analysis of placebo-controlled trials. *Clin Gastroenterol Hepatol* 2008;6(6):644-53.
57. Colombel JF, Sandborn WJ, Reinisch W et al. Infliximab, azathioprine, or combination therapy for Crohn's disease. *N Engl J Med* 2010;362(15):1383-95.
58. Winawer S, Fletcher R, Rex D et al. Colorectal cancer screening and surveillance: clinical guidelines and rationale. Update based on new evidence. *Gastroenterology* 2003;124(2):544-60.
59. Feagan BG, Macdonald JK. Oral 5-aminosalicylic acid for maintenance of remission in ulcerative colitis. *Cochrane Database Syst Rev* 2012;(10):CD000544.
60. Feagan BG, Macdonald JK. Oral 5-aminosalicylic acid for induction of remission in ulcerative colitis. *Cochrane Database Syst Rev* 2012;(10):CD000543.
61. Römkens TE, Kampschreur MT, Drenth JP et al. High mucosal healing rates in 5-ASA-treated ulcerative colitis patients: results of a meta-analysis of clinical trials. *Inflamm Bowel Dis* 2012;18(11):2190-8.
62. Feagan BG, MacDonald JK. Once daily oral mesalamine compared to conventional dosing for induction and maintenance of remission in ulcerative colitis: a systematic review and meta-analysis. *Inflamm Bowel Dis* 2012;18(9):1785-94.
63. Sandborn WJ, Korzenik J, Lashner B et al. Once-daily dosing of delayed-release oral mesalamine (400-mg tablet) is as effective as twice-daily dosing for maintenance of remission of ulcerative colitis. *Gastroenterology* 2010;138(4):1286-96, 1296.e1-3.
64. Zhu Y, Tang RK, Zhao P et al. Can oral 5-aminosalicylic acid be administered once daily in the treatment of mild-to-moderate ulcerative colitis? A meta-analysis of randomized-controlled trials. *Eur J Gastroenterol Hepatol* 2012;24(5):487-94.
65. Tong JL, Huang ML, Xu XT et al. Once-daily versus multiple-daily mesalamine for patients with ulcerative colitis: a meta-analysis. *J Dig Dis* 2012;13(4):200-7.
66. Gracie DJ, Ford AC. Evidence-based management of ulcerative colitis. *Minerva Gastroenterol Dietol* 2012;58(2):87-99.
67. Ford AC, Achkar JP, Khan KJ et al. Efficacy of 5-aminosalicylates in ulcerative colitis: systematic review and meta-analysis. *Am J Gastroenterol* 2011;106(4):601-16.
68. Ford AC, Khan KJ, Achkar JP et al. Efficacy of oral vs. topical, or combined oral and topical 5-aminosalicylates, in ulcerative colitis: systematic review and meta-analysis. *Am J Gastroenterol* 2012;107(2):167-76.
69. Marshall JK, Thabane M, Steinhart AH et al. Rectal 5-aminosalicylic acid for maintenance of remission in ulcerative colitis. *Cochrane Database Syst Rev* 2012;11:CD004118.
70. Bitton A, Buie D, Enns R et al. Treatment of hospitalized adult patients with severe ulcerative colitis: Toronto consensus statements. *Am J Gastroenterol* 2012;107(2):179-94
71. Lichtiger S, Present DH, Kornbluth A et al. Cyclosporine in severe ulcerative colitis refractory to steroid therapy. *N Engl J Med* 1994;330(26):1841-5.
72. Timmer A, McDonald JW, Tsoulis DJ et al. Azathioprine and 6-mercaptopurine for maintenance of remission in ulcerative colitis. *Cochrane Database Syst Rev* 2012;9:CD000478.
73. Oren R, Arber N, Odes S et al. Methotrexate in chronic active ulcerative colitis: a double-blind, randomized, Israeli multicenter trial. *Gastroenterology* 1996;110(5):1416-21.
74. Herfarth HH, Osterman MT, Isaacs KL et al. Efficacy of methotrexate in ulcerative colitis: failure or promise. *Inflamm Bowel Dis* 2010;16(8):1421-30.
75. Thorlund K, Druyts E, Mills EJ et al. Adalimumab versus infliximab for the treatment of moderate to severe ulcerative colitis in adult patients naïve to anti-TNF therapy: An indirect treatment comparison meta-analysis. *J Crohns Colitis* 2014. pii: S1873-9946(14)00014-2.
76. Lv R, Qiao W, Wu Z et al. Tumor necrosis factor alpha blocking agents as treatment for ulcerative colitis intolerant or refractory to conventional medical therapy: a meta-analysis. *PLoS One* 2014;9(1):e86692.
77. Stidham RW, Lee TC, Higgins PD et al. Systematic review with network meta-analysis: the efficacy of anti-tumour necrosis factor-alpha agents for the treatment of ulcerative colitis. *Aliment Pharmacol Ther* 2014;39(7):660-71.
78. Adalimumab in the treatment of moderate-to-severe ulcerative colitis: ULTRA 2 trial results. *Gastroenterol Hepatol (N Y)* 2013;9(5):317-20.
79. Reinisch W, Sandborn WJ, Hommes DW et al. Adalimumab for induction of clinical remission in moderately to severely active ulcerative colitis: results of a randomised controlled trial. *Gut* 2011;60(6):780-7.
80. Sandborn WJ, van Assche G, Reinisch W et al. Adalimumab induces and maintains clinical remission in patients with moderate-to-severe ulcerative colitis. *Gastroenterology* 2012;142(2):257-65.e1-3.
81. Bernstein CN, Eaden J, Steinhart AH et al. Cancer prevention in inflammatory bowel disease and the chemoprophylactic potential of 5-aminosalicylic acid. *Inflamm Bowel Dis* 2002;8(5):356-61.
82. Lashner BA, Heidenreich PA, Su GL et al. Effect of folate supplementation on the incidence of dysplasia and cancer in chronic ulcerative colitis. A case-control study. *Gastroenterology* 1989;97(2):255-9.
83. Marshall JK, Thabane M, Steinhart AH et al. Rectal 5-aminosalicylic acid for maintenance of remission in ulcerative colitis. *Cochrane Database Syst Rev* 2012;(11):CD004118.
84. Ford AC, Khan KJ, Sandborn WJ et al. Efficacy of topical 5-aminosalicylates in preventing relapse of quiescent ulcerative colitis: a meta-analysis. *Clin Gastroenterol Hepatol* 2012;10(5):513-9.
85. Bouguen G, Roblin X, Bourreille A et al. Infliximab for refractory ulcerative proctitis. *Aliment Pharmacol Ther* 2010;31(11):1178-85.
86. Kwan LY, Mahadevan U. Inflammatory bowel disease and pregnancy: an update. *Expert Rev Clin Immunol* 2010;6(4):643-57.
87. Hanan IM, Kirsner JB. Inflammatory bowel disease in the pregnant woman. *Clin Perinatol* 1985;12(3):669-82.
88. Pedersen N, Bortoli A, Duricova D et al. The course of inflammatory bowel disease during pregnancy and postpartum: a prospective European ECCO-EpiCom Study of 209 pregnant women. *Aliment Pharmacol Ther* 2013;38(5):501-12.
89. Abhyankar A, Ham M, Moss AC. Meta-analysis: the impact of disease activity at conception on disease activity during pregnancy in patients with inflammatory bowel disease. *Aliment Pharmacol Ther* 2013;38(5):460-6.
90. Tavernier N, Fumery M, Peyrin-Biroulet L et al. Systematic review: fertility in non-surgically treated inflammatory bowel disease. *Aliment Pharmacol Ther* 2013;38(8):847-53.
91. Briggs GG, Freeman RK, Yaffe SJ. *Drugs in pregnancy and lactation: a reference guide to fetal and neonatal risk.* 9th ed. Baltimore (MD): Lippincott Williams & Wilkins; 2011.
92. Christensen LA, Dahlerup JF, Nielsen MJ et al. Azathioprine treatment during lactation. *Aliment Pharmacol Ther* 2008;28(10):1209-13.
93. Nielsen OH, Maxwell C, Hendel J. IBD medications during pregnancy and lactation. *Nat Rev Gastroenterol Hepatol* 2014;11(2):116-27.
94. Carmichael SL, Shaw GM. Maternal corticosteroid use and risk of selected congenital anomalies. *Am J Med Genet* 1999;86(3):242-4.

95. Diav-Citrin O, Park YH, Veerasuntharam G et al. The safety of mesalamine in human pregnancy: a prospective controlled cohort study. *Gastroenterology* 1998;114(1):23-8.
96. Schnitzler F, Fidder H, Ferrante M et al. Outcome of pregnancy in women with inflammatory bowel disease treated with antitumor necrosis factor therapy. *Inflamm Bowel Dis* 2011;17(9):1846-54.
97. Mahadevan U, Kane S. American Gastroenterological Association Institute technical review on the use of gastrointestinal medications in pregnancy. *Gastroenterology* 2006;131(1):283-311.
98. El Mourabet M, El-Hachem S, Harrison JR et al. Anti-TNF antibody therapy for inflammatory bowel disease during pregnancy: a clinical review. *Curr Drug Targets* 2010;11(2):234-41.
99. Mahadevan U, Wolf DC, Dubinsky M et al. Placental transfer of anti-tumor necrosis factor agents in pregnant patients with inflammatory bowel disease. *Clin Gastroenterol Hepatol* 2013;11(3):286-92.

Chapter 63
Irritable Bowel Syndrome

W. Grant Thompson, MD, FRCPC, FACG

The irritable bowel syndrome (IBS) is a collection of symptoms attributed to the intestine, related to defecation and unpredictable bowel habit (Table 1). Since there is no known pathology or pathophysiology, IBS can only be recognized by its characteristic pattern of abdominal pain and discomfort, which is relieved by defecation or associated with a change in bowel habit.[1,2] A substantial number of IBS patients date the onset of their symptoms to an attack of bacterial enteritis.[3] While subgroups have been proposed according to whether constipation, diarrhea or both are present, these are intermittent and it is very common for the predominant bowel habit to change from time to time.

In Canadian adults, the one-year prevalence is about 12%,[4] and females with IBS outnumber males 4:1. Because the symptoms come and go, the lifetime prevalence is much higher. Most people who have these symptoms do not consult physicians. Nevertheless, IBS accounts for 30% of gut complaints in primary care (approximately 2% of all adult patient visits), and the few that are referred to specialists are about 20% of a gastroenterologist's practice. While the syndrome occurs at all ages, more young IBS sufferers see physicians.[2,5] IBS is the fourth most expensive digestive disease in Canada with an economic and health care burden in excess of $6.5 billion per year.[6]

Goals of Therapy

- Establish caring relationship with patient
- Conduct a thorough interview and examination to establish the diagnosis and rule out serious pathology
- Reassure the patient through a confident diagnosis. Address fears of serious disease
- Alleviate symptoms while establishing realistic expectations. Patients have a greater expectation of deriving benefit from lifestyle modification than from drug therapy[7]
- Promote coping and normal social and occupational functioning
- Treat psychosocial comorbidity if present

Investigations

Thorough history with particular attention to abdominal pain and its relationship with diet, defecation and altered stool frequency and form (Table 1, Figure 1, Figure 2).[8] Pelvic pain (actually lower abdominal pain) may be due to IBS rather than a gynecologic cause.[9] However, potential gynecologic causes of pain must be ruled out. Physical findings or alarm symptoms such as rectal bleeding, anemia, fever or profound weight loss are not explained by IBS (Table 2). The history should also explore the patient's psychosocial circumstances and the reasons that the patient has chosen to consult a physician. A recent history of bacterial gastroenteritis may explain self-limiting IBS-like symptoms. Difficult, chronic constipation or persistent diarrhea are not likely due to IBS and raise different diagnostic and treatment issues that are discussed elsewhere (see Chapter 58 and Chapter 59).

Table 1: Diagnostic Criteria for Irritable Bowel Syndrome[1] (Rome III)[a,b,c]

Recurrent abdominal pain or discomfort[d] at least 3 days per month in the last 3 months associated with 2 or more of the following:

1. Improvement with defecation
2. Onset associated with a change in frequency of stool
3. Onset associated with a change in form (appearance) of stool

[a] Criteria fulfilled for the last 3 months with symptom onset at least 6 months prior to diagnosis.
[b] Supportive symptoms that are not part of the diagnostic criteria include abnormal stool frequency (a) <3 bowel movements per week or (b) >3 bowel movements per day; abnormal stool form (c) lumpy/hard stool or (d) loose/watery stool; (e) defecation straining; (f) urgency or also feeling of incomplete bowel movement, passing mucus and bloating.
[c] In the absence of structural or metabolic abnormalities to explain the symptoms.
[d] "Discomfort" means an uncomfortable sensation not described as pain.

Figure 1: Bristol Stool Form Scale

Stool form	Appearance	Type
Separate hard lumps like nuts, (hard to pass). Result of slow transit.	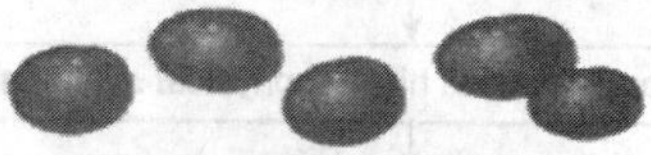	1
Sausage-shaped but lumpy.	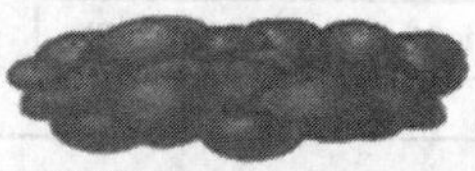	2
Like a sausage but cracks on its surface.		3
Like a sausage or snake — smooth and soft.	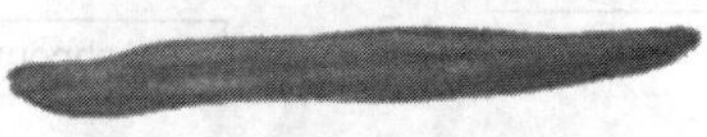	4
Soft blobs with clear cut edges (easy to pass).	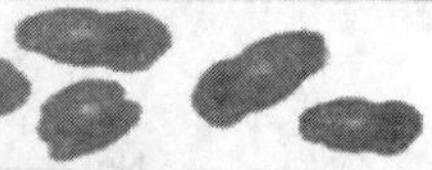	5
Fluffy pieces with ragged edges, a mushy stool.	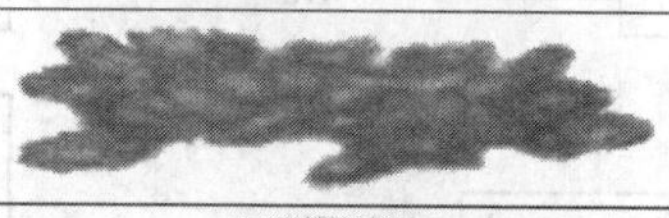	6
Watery, no solid pieces. Result of very fast transit.	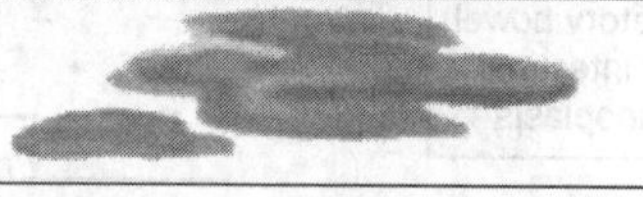	7

Reproduced with permission from Thompson WG, Heaton KW. *Fast facts: irritable bowel syndrome*. 2nd ed. Oxford (GB): Health Press Limited; 2003.

Tests may be unnecessary in a young person with chronic and typical symptoms of IBS (Table 1), no alarm symptoms and no family history of colon cancer or inflammatory bowel disease (Table 2).[9,10] However, prevalence of celiac disease may be increased in patients with IBS.[11,12] Since celiac disease is treatable, celiac serology testing is advisable in those patients with diarrhea predominant IBS[12] and are at high risk of developing celiac disease (northern European descendants). Patients over the age of 50 are candidates for colon cancer screening, which could be performed through fecal occult blood testing, sigmoidoscopy or colonoscopy.[13,14,15,16]

Table 2: Alarm Symptoms That Cannot be Explained by Irritable Bowel Syndrome

Fever
Anemia
Bleeding from the gut
Significant weight loss
Family history of cancer, inflammatory bowel disease or celiac disease
Recent consistent change in bowel habit
Persistent, daily diarrhea or constipation
Abnormal physical findings, e.g., abdominal mass or malnutrition

Figure 2: Investigating a Patient with Recurrent Abdominal Pain or Discomfort and Disordered Bowel Habit

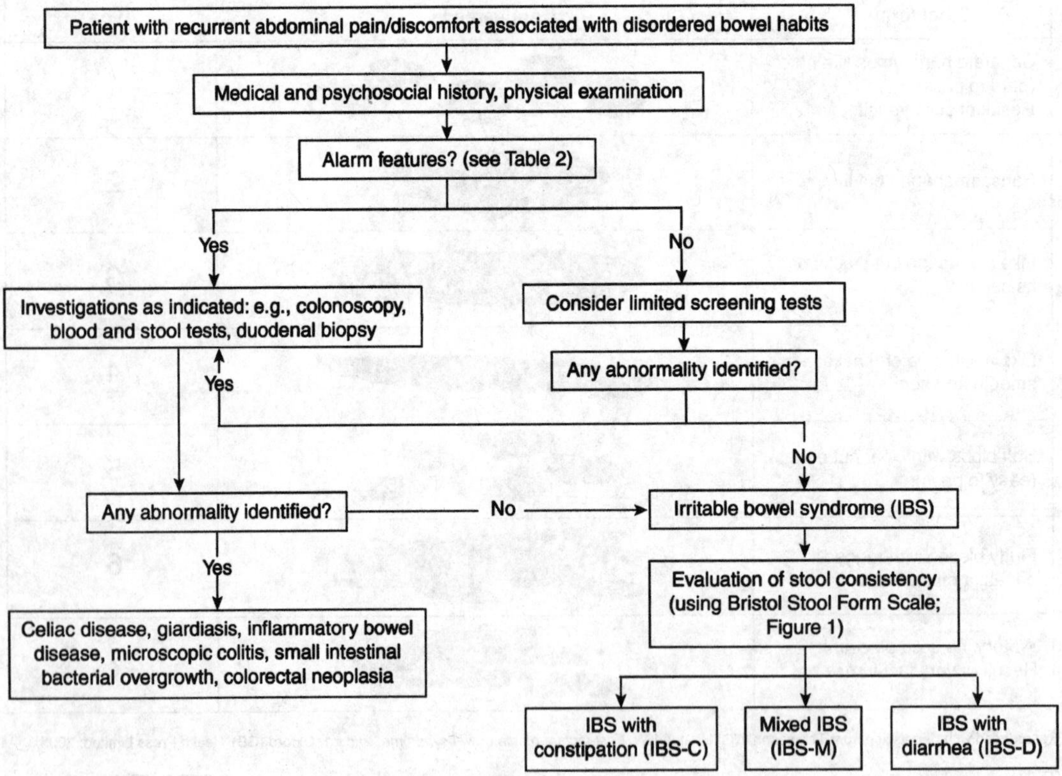

Therapeutic Choices

Table 3 discusses the management of IBS and Table 4 lists the drugs used when addressing IBS symptoms.

Table 3: **Management of Irritable Bowel Syndrome**

Diagnosis: It is essential to make a positive diagnosis, rather than a diagnosis of exclusion, and to convincingly convey this to the patient

Education/reassurance: Explain the pathophysiology and natural history of IBS

- Physiological abnormalities include altered intestinal motility and visceral hypersensitivity
- IBS can be precipitated by a previous enteric infection
- Diet has no causal role, but may exacerbate IBS
- Emotional stress does not cause IBS, but psychosocial factors may exacerbate the symptoms and/or contribute to the distress they cause
- Validate symptoms. The symptoms are real, not imagined. Gut and brain interact to alter motility (muscle contractions) and/or increase bowel sensation
- **IBS is a chronic, relapsing, but benign disorder**

Healthy lifestyle: Provide advice regarding the importance of a balanced diet, exercise and time for toilet each morning

Diet: Advise patients about potentially aggravating foods

- Follow Eating Well with Canada's Food Guide (www.hc-sc.gc.ca/fn-an/food-guide-aliment/index-eng.php)
- Limit intake of alcohol, caffeine, fat and sorbitol. They do not cause IBS, but may exacerbate the symptoms
- Restrict lactose consumption in patients who seem to improve with a trial of lactose restriction
- Refer problem eaters to a dietitian

Psychosocial issues: Explore in select patients

"Indicators" of difficulty coping with IBS:

- Poor insight
- Inability to express emotions
- Comorbid conditions
- History of physical or sexual abuse or other major life stresses
- Multiple somatic complaints or abnormal illness behaviour
- "Catastrophizing" symptoms, e.g., "First sign of pain means my day is ruined"
- Poor coping mechanisms
- Inadequate social supports

A 2-week symptom diary may assist select patients in connecting diet and stress with aggravation of symptoms

Consider cognitive behavioural therapy or hypnosis and relaxation therapy for patients with severe IBS

Drug Therapy: Explain the role of drug therapy in IBS

- Most patients will not require drug therapy
- No single drug has been shown to be beneficial for the IBS symptom complex
- *Specific* IBS symptoms may be amenable to drug therapy (Table 4)—first identify the predominant symptom (Figure 1, Figure 2)

Abbreviations: IBS = irritable bowel syndrome
Adapted with permission from Paterson WG et al. *CMAJ* 1999;161(2):154-60.

Nonpharmacologic Choices

- Discuss the diagnosis and prognosis with the patient.
- Address the patient's fears and provide reassurance.
- A good doctor-patient relationship maximizes placebo effects[17] and improves long-term outcomes.[18]
- Patients generally expect to derive more benefit from lifestyle modification than from drug therapy.[7]
- Encourage consumption of a healthy diet (*Eating Well with Canada's Food Guide*)[10,19] and sufficient fluid intake.
- Encourage patients to avoid food fads and to keep a diary of life stressors as well as foods that trigger or relieve symptoms.
- Advise patients to avoid excessive caffeine, alcohol, sorbitol (in gums and candies) and fructose (or sucrose, from which fructose may be released).

- Many treatments proposed by alternative practitioners or the media have no proven efficacy and some proposed diets may be nutritionally unsound or unnecessary (e.g., benefits of gluten-free diets in relieving IBS symptoms are controversial; before trying a gluten-free diet, determine if celiac disease is present).
- Be alert to gut symptoms that may be caused by adverse effects of drugs or alternative health products such as herbal medicines.
- If constipated, ensure sufficient dietary fibre.
- Lifestyle adjustment: stress management, relaxation advice, quiet time for eating and defecation.
- Treat comorbid conditions: depression,[20] anxiety,[20] panic, life stress.[21,22]
- Psychological treatments may require the involvement of a mental health professional, and the benefits in patients with IBS are difficult to prove.[23] The following may help in refractory cases, or when psychopathology is evident: psychopharmacotherapy,[24] individual or group psychotherapy,[25] cognitive behavioural therapy,[26] hypnosis[27] (if available) and stress management or relaxation techniques including audio and video tapes.
- Avoid inappropriate referral and unnecessary surgery. IBS symptoms are sometimes mistaken for gynecologic or gallbladder diseases.

Pharmacologic Choices

- No one drug is effective for the entire IBS symptom complex.
- For the purposes of treatment, patients are grouped by their predominant bowel habit: IBS with constipation, IBS with diarrhea or IBS alternating between constipation and diarrhea (mixed IBS). Since this may change from time to time, use laxatives and antidiarrheal agents cautiously and monitor their effects.
- When nonpharmacologic measures fail, target the most troublesome symptom (Table 4).
- The *Bristol Stool Form Scale* (Figure 1)[28] can be used to identify patients who suffer from constipation or diarrhea.[7,29] Selection of pharmacotherapy depends largely upon the predominant symptom.
- For patients who have IBS with *predominant diarrhea* (Bristol Stool Form Scale type 6 or 7): **loperamide** PRN[30] may be recommended, especially if the patient is concerned about incontinence.[31] **Diphenoxylate with atropine** may also be used; rarely, a patient may improve on **cholestyramine**. For patients who have IBS with *predominant constipation* (pellety stools, Bristol Stool Form Scale type 1): recommend 2–4 tablespoons of raw bran or **psyllium** daily with plenty of fluids. **Calcium polycarbophil** may also be used.[32] If this fails, laxatives such as **bisacodyl**, **lactulose**, **magnesium hydroxide** or **polyethylene glycol** may be tried. If the constipation does not respond to these measures, consider alternative diagnoses such as functional constipation (see Chapter 58).
- **Linaclotide** is a first-in-class orally administered peptide agonist of guanylate cyclase C. It acts topically on the intestinal enterocytes leading to release of chloride and bicarbonate into the intestinal lumen. As a consequence, intestinal fluid secretion is increased and intestinal transit is accelerated. Linaclotide (290 μg/day) is approved for the treatment of IBS with predominant constipation but the available evidence for its efficacy in this patient population is relatively weak. Linaclotide is minimally absorbed, has no drug interactions and does not interact with the cytochrome P450 enzyme system. Its most common side effects include diarrhea, abdominal pain, flatulence and bloating. Given the lack of comparative data with other treatments for IBS, absence of long-term safety and teratogenic data, the drug's relatively high cost (several dollars per day) and the frequent side effect of diarrhea leading to therapy discontinuation, linaclotide is considered to have a low place in IBS therapy and is best reserved for occasional specialist initiation when conventional treatments are ineffective. This author does not endorse the use of linaclotide in the treatment of IBS with constipation.

- "Colonic spasm" does not explain IBS symptoms and therefore drugs that "relieve spasm" are unlikely to be helpful. Antispasmodic drugs approved by Health Canada for IBS include **dicyclomine**, **pinaverium** and **trimebutine**. Weak evidence suggests that pinaverium and trimebutine may, at best, exert modest improvement in abdominal pain.[33] If at all, prescribe these drugs for only a few weeks at a time to be taken before meals for patients with postprandial pain or as needed for acute attacks. This author endorses none of them.
- For patients with chronic abdominal pain that impairs normal functioning: **amitriptyline**[35] or **desipramine**[26,35] may be useful, and may be effective in doses lower than those used for depression.[36,37]
- Data evaluating the use of SSRIs in the treatment of IBS-related symptoms are conflicting.[38]

There is much interest in the use of **probiotics** for IBS, but the quality and viability of most individual products is unknown and the supporting evidence is meagre.[39] Promising results were demonstrated using *Bifidobacterium infantis* in a small study of patients with IBS where symptomatic improvement after 8 weeks correlated with normalization of the IL-10/IL-12 ratio (an indicator of a pro-inflammatory state that was elevated at baseline).[40,41]

Bacterial overgrowth is a supposed cause of IBS, but is likely not an important factor for many patients. A consensus questions the evidence for this hypothesis and recommends against the use of antibiotics with their attendant potential for harm.[7]

Prognosis

- Usually recurrent and lifelong; no effect upon life expectancy.[34]
- The bowel habit may change from time to time.
- If the diagnosis of IBS is carefully made, there is a low risk of missing underlying structural disease.
- There is no predisposition to structural disease such as diverticular disease, cancer or inflammatory bowel disease.[34]

The Difficult-to-Treat Patient

Complicated patients who tend to be referred to specialists often have comorbid conditions such as depression or a history of serious emotional trauma (e.g., sexual abuse). Such patients are best managed with regularly scheduled visits for a sympathetic discussion.[42] If necessary, a gastroenterology consultation may support the primary care physician's diagnosis and management plan, and reduce future IBS-related costs.[43] A mental health professional may assist with a severe comorbid psychological disorder. Long-term cure is unlikely, particularly in severely affected patients, so the emphasis should be on coping and normal occupational and social functioning.

Choices during Pregnancy and Breastfeeding

IBS and pregnancy are independent, i.e., there is no evidence that one affects the other. A prominent feature of IBS is its unpredictable, chronic and relapsing nature. Therefore, in a woman with IBS, pregnancy may be accompanied with worsened, improved or unchanged IBS symptoms.

IBS does not contraindicate pregnancy, nor are there any precautions beyond those recommended above prior to pregnancy. Management of IBS during pregnancy or breastfeeding entails addressing the symptoms when necessary as described above. In principle, no drug should be used unless absolutely necessary and only then after all nondrug therapies have been tried. Although **loperamide** has not been associated with teratogenic effects, its safe use during pregnancy has not been established. Small amounts of loperamide appear in breast milk making its use inadvisable during breastfeeding. While **calcium polycarbophil** and **psyllium** are unabsorbed and safe, withhold **antidepressants** unless there is a psychiatric indication.

A discussion of general principles on the use of medications in these special populations can be found in Appendix II and Appendix III. Other specialized reference sources are also provided in these appendices.

Therapeutic Tips

- The efficacy of many drugs proposed for IBS is unproven or varies greatly.[33,44,45]
- No medication has been proven beneficial for bloating.

Table 4: Drugs Used for the Management of Irritable Bowel Syndrome

Drug Class	Drug	Dose	Adverse Effects	Drug Interactions	Comments	Cost[b]
Antidiarrheals	*cholestyramine* Olestyr	**For diarrhea:** 4 g Q12H po	Nausea, fat soluble vitamin deficiency with long-term use, constipation.	May bind drugs, e.g., digoxin, in GI tract; do not take within 1 h before or 4–6 h after other medications.	Take with fluids.	$$$
	diphenoxylate with atropine sulfate Lomotil	**For diarrhea:** 5 mg (diphenoxylate) po initially then 2.5 mg po after each loose bowel movement (maximum 20 mg/day)	Sedation, nausea, abdominal cramps, dry skin and mucous membranes (from atropine), some addiction potential.	Additive anticholinergic effects with other anticholinergic agents.	The elderly are more susceptible to the antimuscarinic effects of atropine, e.g., agitation, drowsiness, increased intraocular pressure.	$$$
	loperamide Imodium, Riva-Loperamide, other generics	**For diarrhea:** 2–4 mg PRN po (maximum 12 mg/day)	Abdominal cramps, dizziness, dry mouth.		Nonprescription. Generally regarded as first-line pharmacologic option for the management of diarrhea due to its high efficacy, low side effect profile, low cost, ease of use, common availability and low abuse potential.	$-$$
Bulk-forming Agents[a]	*polycarbophil calcium* Prodiem Fibre Therapy	**For constipation:** 625 mg caplets: 2 caplets daily to QID po; not to exceed 8 caplets/24 h	Cramps, bloating, flatulence.	Advise patients not to take within 3 h of other drugs, to minimize interference with absorption.	Take with fluids. Nonprescription.	$
	psyllium hydrophilic mucilloid Metamucil Preparations, generics	**For constipation:** 15 g BID with meals po, then adjust (varies with product)	See polycarbophil calcium.	See polycarbophil calcium.	See polycarbophil calcium.	$

(cont'd)

Table 4: Drugs Used for the Management of Irritable Bowel Syndrome *(cont'd)*

Drug Class	Drug	Dose	Adverse Effects	Drug Interactions	Comments	Cost[b]
Tricyclic Antidepressants	*amitriptyline* generics	**For abdominal pain:** 25–100 mg QHS po	Drowsiness, dry mouth, headache.	Possible CNS excitation with serotonergic agents. Avoid combined use with other agents that prolong QT_c.	Use low doses for select patients with intractable pain. Numerous other agents are available.	$
	desipramine generics	**For abdominal pain:** 25–100 mg QHS po	See amitriptyline.	See amitriptyline.	See amitriptyline.	$

[a] Information on laxatives can be found in Chapter 58.
[b] Cost per day includes drug cost only.
Legend: $ <$1 $-$$ <$1–2 $$ $1–2 $$$ $2–4

Suggested Readings

American College of Gastroenterology Task Force on Irritable Bowel Syndrome, Brandt LJ, Chey WD et al. An evidence-based position statement on the management of irritable bowel syndrome. *Am J Gastroenterol* 2009;104(Suppl 1):S1-35.

Longstreth GF, Thompson WG, Chey WD et al. Functional bowel disorders. *Gastroenterology* 2006;130(5):1480-91.

Thompson WG. *The placebo effect in health: combining science & compassionate care*. Amherst (NY): Prometheus Books; 2005.

Thompson WG. *Understanding the irritable gut: the functional gastrointestinal disorders*. McLean (VA): Degnon Associates; 2008.

References

1. Longstreth GF, Thompson WG, Chey WD et al. Functional bowel disorders. *Gastroenterology* 2006;130(5):1480-91.
2. Thompson WG. *Understanding the irritable gut: the functional gastrointestinal disorders*. McLean (VA): Degnon Associates; 2008.
3. Spiller R, Garsed K. Postinfectious irritable bowel syndrome. *Gastroenterology* 2009;136(6):1979-88.
4. Thompson WG, Irvine EJ, Pare P et al. Functional gastrointestinal disorders in Canada: first population-based survey using Rome II criteria with suggestions for improving the questionnaire. *Dig Dis Sci* 2002;47(1):225-35.
5. Drossman DA. The functional gastrointestinal disorders and the Rome III process. *Gastroenterology* 2006;103(5):1377-90.
6. Canadian Digestive Health Foundation. *Irritable bowel syndrome*. Available from: www.cdhf.ca/en/statistics#Irritable Bowel Syndrome. Accessed May 5, 2014.
7. Whitehead WE, Levy RL, Von Korff M et al. The usual medical care for irritable bowel syndrome. *Aliment Pharmacol Ther* 2004;20(11-12):1305-15.
8. Spiller RC, Thompson WG. Bowel disorders. *Am J Gastroenterol* 2010;105(4):775-85.
9. Thompson WG, Heaton KW, Smyth GT et al. Irritable bowel syndrome in general practice: prevalence, characteristics, and referral. *Gut* 2000;46(1):78-82.
10. Paterson WG, Thompson WG, Vanner SJ et al. Recommendations for the management of irritable bowel syndrome in family practice. IBS Consensus Conference Participants. *CMAJ* 1999;161(2):154-60.
11. Ford AC, Chey WD, Talley NJ et al. Yield of diagnostic tests for celiac disease in individuals with symptoms suggestive of irritable bowel syndrome: systematic review and meta-analysis. *Arch Intern Med* 2009;169(7):651-8.
12. Spiegel BM, DeRosa VP, Gralnek IM et al. Testing for celiac sprue in irritable bowel syndrome with predominant diarrhea: a cost-effectiveness analysis. *Gastroenterology* 2004;126(7):1721-32.
13. Winawer S, Fletcher R, Rex D et al. Colorectal cancer screening and surveillance: clinical guidelines and rationale-Update based on new evidence. *Gastroenterology* 2003;124(2):544-60.
14. Winawer SJ, Fletcher RH, Miller L et al. Colorectal cancer screening: clinical guidelines and rationale. *Gastroenterology* 1997;112(2):594-642.
15. U.S. Preventive Services Task Force. Screening for colorectal cancer: U.S. Preventive Services Task Force recommendation statement. *Ann Intern Med* 2008;149(9):627-37.
16. Leddin D, Hunt R, Champion M et al. Canadian Association of Gastroenterology and the Canadian Digestive Health Foundation: guidelines on colon cancer screening. *Can J Gastroenterol* 2004;18(2):93-9.
17. Thompson WG. Placebos: a review of the placebo response. *Am J Gastroenterol* 2000;95(7):1637-43.
18. Owens DM, Nelson DK, Talley NJ. The irritable bowel syndrome: long-term prognosis and the physician-patient interaction. *Ann Intern Med* 1995;122(2):107-12.
19. *Eating well with Canada's food guide*. Ottawa (CA): Health Canada; 2011. Available from: www.hc-sc.gc.ca/fn-an/food-guide-aliment/index-eng.php.
20. Tollefson GD, Tollefson SL, Pederson M et al. Comorbid irritable bowel syndrome in patients with generalized anxiety and major depression. *Ann Clin Psychiatry* 1991;3:215-22.
21. Craig TK, Brown GW. Goal frustration and life events in the aetiology of painful gastrointestinal disorder. *J Psychosom Res* 1984;28(5):411-21.
22. Creed F. Life events and appendicectomy. *Lancet* 1981;1(8235):1381-5.
23. Talley NJ, Owen BK, Boyce P et al. Psychological treatments for irritable bowel syndrome: a critique of controlled treatment trials. *Am J Gastroenterol* 1996;91(2):277-83.
24. Potter WZ, Rudorfer MV, Manji H. The pharmacologic treatment of depression. *N Engl J Med* 1991;325(9):633-42.
25. Guthrie E, Creed F, Dawson D et al. A randomised controlled trial of psychotherapy in patients with refractory irritable bowel syndrome. *Br J Psychiatry* 1993;163:315-21.
26. Drossman DA, Toner BB, Whitehead WE et al. Cognitive-behavioral therapy versus education and desipramine versus placebo for moderate to severe functional bowel disorders. *Gastroenterology* 2003;125(1):19-31.
27. Gonsalkorale WM, Houghton LA, Whorwell PJ. Hypnotherapy in irritable bowel syndrome: a large-scale audit of a clinical service with examination of factors influencing responsiveness. *Am J Gastroenterol* 2002;97(4):954-61.
28. Heaton KW, O'Donnell LJ. An office guide to whole-gut transit time. Patients' recollection of their stool form. *J Clin Gastroenterol* 1994;19(1):28-30.
29. Thompson WG, Heaton KW. *Fast facts: irritable bowel syndrome*. 2nd ed. Oxford (GB): Health Press; 2003.
30. Thompson WG. Nonulcer dyspepsia. *Can Med Assoc J* 1984;130(5):565-9.
31. Read M, Read NW, Barber DC et al. Effects of loperamide on anal sphincter function in patients complaining of chronic diarrhea with fecal incontinence and urgency. *Dig Dis Sci* 1982;27(9):807-14.
32. Toskes PP, Connery KL, Ritchey TW. Calcium polycarbophil compared with placebo in irritable bowel syndrome. *Aliment Pharmacol Ther* 1993;7(1):87-92.
33. Ruepert L, Quartero AO, de Wit NJ et al. Bulking agents, antispasmodics and antidepressants for the treatment of irritable bowel syndrome. *Cochrane Database Syst Rev* 2011;(8):CD003460.

34. Thompson WG. The treatment of irritable bowel syndrome. *Aliment Pharmacol Ther* 2002;16(8):1395-406.
35. Jackson JL, O'Malley PG, Tomkins G et al. Treatment of functional gastrointestinal disorders with antidepressant medications: a meta-analysis. *Am J Med* 2000;108(1):65-72.
36. Halpert A, Dalton CB, Diamant NE et al. Clinical response to tricyclic antidepressants in functional bowel disorders is not related to dosage. *Am J Gastroenterol* 2005;100(3):664-71.
37. Chao GQ, Zhang S. A meta-analysis of the therapeutic effects of amitriptyline for treating irritable bowel syndrome. *Intern Med* 2013;52(4):419-24.
38. Bundeff AW, Woodis CB. Selective serotonin reuptake inhibitors for the treatment of irritable bowel syndrome. *Ann Pharmacother* 2014;48(6):777-784.
39. Moayyedi P, Ford AC, Talley NJ et al. The efficacy of probiotics in the treatment of irritable bowel syndrome: a systematic review. *Gut* 2010;59(3):325-32.
40. O'Mahony L, McCarthy J, Kelly P et al. Lactobacillus and bifidobacterium in irritable bowel syndrome: symptom responses and relationship to cytokine profiles. *Gastroenterology* 2005;128(3):541-51.
41. Breener DM, Moeller MJ, Chey WD et al. The utility of probiotics in the treatment of irritable bowel syndrome: a systematic review. *Am J Gastroenterol* 2009;104(4):1033-49.
42. Drossman DA. Struggling with the "controlling" patient. *Am J Gastroenterol* 1994;89(9):1441-6.
43. Ilnyckyj A, Graff LA, Blanchard JF et al. Therapeutic value of a gastroenterology consultation in irritable bowel syndrome. *Aliment Pharmacol Ther* 2003;17(7):871-80.
44. Akehurst R, Kaltenthaler E. Treatment of irritable bowel syndrome: a review of randomised controlled trials. *Gut* 2001;48(2):272-82.
45. Klein KB. Controlled treatment trials in the irritable bowel syndrome: a critique. *Gastroenterology* 1988;95(1):232-41.

Chapter 64
Nausea in Adults

Cathy MacLean, MD, FCFP

Nausea is a symptom (not a diagnosis) that refers to the unpleasant sensation experienced prior to vomiting. It may be a transient symptom secondary to a self-limited condition such as viral gastroenteritis or a part of more complex medical issues. Attempt to determine the underlying cause when possible. Nausea may be of short duration or may be defined as chronic if it lasts >1 month. Many causes of nausea are iatrogenic but approaches to its treatment are dependent on the associated diagnosis such as postoperative nausea and vomiting (PONV), chemotherapy-induced nausea and vomiting (CINV), metabolic, GI, vestibular or neurologic causes such as motion sickness.[1] This chapter does not address treatment of nausea in children. For the management of cancer chemotherapy- or radiation-induced nausea and vomiting, see Chapter 126 and Chapter 127.

Causes of nausea include:

- Neurologic/vestibular: stroke, increased intracranial pressure, migraine, neoplasm, pain, head injury, labyrinthitis, Ménière's disease, motion sickness
- Drugs/toxins: alcohol, antibiotics, bacterial food poisoning, chemotherapy, hormones, opioids, NSAIDs, antiarrhythmics, anticonvulsants, digoxin, benzodiazepines, SSRIs, noxious odours, anesthesia, radiation therapy, or medication initiation, withdrawal or toxicity
- GI: viral gastroenteritis, constipation, diseases of the liver (including hepatitis), cholecystitis, pancreatitis, chronic idiopathic nausea, chronic intestinal pseudo-obstruction, gastroparesis, irritable bowel syndrome, nonulcer dyspepsia, gastroesophageal reflux, GI motility disorders
- Psychiatric: anxiety, depression, fear, grief, eating disorders, functional nausea, anticipatory nausea (situations in which patients are conditioned by previous experience of nausea and vomiting)
- Medical conditions: Addison's disease, diabetic ketoacidosis, hormonal effects of pregnancy, severe heart failure, hypercalcemia, hyponatremia, hypothyroidism, malignancy (including metastasis), MI, uremia, acute infections

Goals of Therapy

- Rule out acute emergencies or causes that require hospitalization and/or surgery
- Diagnose and remove or treat the underlying cause of nausea
- Correct any consequences of persistent nausea (with or without vomiting) such as electrolyte abnormalities or nutritional compromise. Control nausea and provide patient comfort (nausea can be more distressing to some patients than actual vomiting and interferes significantly with quality of life)
- Prevent the development of anticipatory nausea
- Balance the benefit of symptomatic treatment with cost and potential adverse effects of medications
- Control nausea so patients can resume treatment of other conditions

Investigations

- History:[1]
  - determine whether patient is at increased risk of experiencing nausea or vomiting, to help decide whether antiemetics should be prescribed. Risk factors for PONV are female gender, history of PONV or motion sickness, nonsmoker status, younger age in adults, duration of anesthesia with volatile anesthetics and postoperative opioid use[2]
  - determine whether the nausea is acute or chronic
  - ascertain the frequency and severity of nausea as well as the timing in relation to meals, time of day, emotions or stresses
  - explore possible underlying causes, and whether they are simple versus complex or chronic
  - establish the onset, progression and temporal sequence of associated events, e.g., surgery
  - identify other symptoms, e.g., headache, pain, vertigo
  - clarify the relationship between nausea and vomiting; if vomiting is occurring, determine the amount and nature of the vomitus
  - complete an appropriate GI functional inquiry including frequency and nature of bowel movements, early satiety, postprandial symptoms, abdominal pain or weight loss
  - inquire about diet history including any new foods, food allergies or intolerances and if potentially infected food has been consumed
  - establish any exposure to, or other symptoms of, infection such as gastroenteritis or exposure to others who are ill
  - in all women of reproductive age, inquire about last menstrual period to rule out pregnancy
  - obtain a thorough medication history including use of prescription, nonprescription, herbal or recreational drugs as well as alcohol, nutritional supplements and vitamins
  - inquire about recent changes to drug regimens (dosage increases or withdrawal) and correlation with nausea
  - inquire about past history of migraine headaches, endocrine disorders, malignancy
  - explore possible psychosocial stressors, conflicts, sources of emotional pain or loss
  - inquire about the patient's feelings, concerns, ideas, functional impairment and expectations of treatment
- Physical examination:
  - vital signs including blood pressure, pulse, respiratory rate and temperature
  - determine severity and consequences of symptoms—assess hydration including JVP, mucous membranes, skin turgor and postural changes in blood pressure and heart rate
  - assess systems related to the probable underlying cause when apparent, e.g., perform neurologic exam for a migraine patient, examine for bowel obstruction if the patient has a malignancy or is postsurgical, check for nystagmus in vertigo-associated nausea, inspect fundi for papilledema
  - if no specific cause is identified in the history, use the physical exam to rule out other potential causes, e.g., abdominal mass
- Other investigations:
  - laboratory investigations are determined by the history and physical exam
  - test females of childbearing age for pregnancy
  - electrolytes may be indicated if metabolic disturbances are suspected, e.g., test for hypercalcemia in a patient with a malignancy, glucose in a diabetic patient, hypokalemia or hyponatremia in a patient on diuretics, serum lipase/amylase levels if pancreatitis is suspected
  - CBC and differential if an infective cause is suspected

- serum creatinine and urea to determine whether there is a renal cause and assess degree of dehydration
- drug levels in select cases, e.g., digoxin, anticonvulsants
- lipase and amylase levels
- liver function tests
- thyroid function or fasting cortisol levels may be helpful for ruling out endocrine disorders
- x-rays may also be indicated; an abdominal x-ray if a bowel obstruction is suspected or an upper GI series with motility studies if gastroesophageal reflux or gastroparesis is suspected
- ultrasound of the liver, gallbladder or pancreas may be useful in some patients
- upper GI endoscopy or CT of the abdomen may be required in select patients as determined by the history and physical
- CT of the head should be considered if an intracranial cause is suspected

Therapeutic Choices

Nonpharmacologic Choices

- When appropriate, minimize baseline risk factors to reduce patient's chances of experiencing PONV:[3]
  - use regional anesthesia instead of general anesthesia
  - avoid use of nitrous oxide
  - avoid use of volatile anesthetics
  - minimize use of perioperative opioids
  - provide adequate hydration
- In adult or pediatric patients, P6 acupoint stimulation may be as effective as antiemetic drugs in preventing and treating PONV and may reduce the need for rescue antiemetics.[4,5]
- Inhalation of isopropyl alcohol vapour may be effective in reducing PONV but is less effective than standard antiemetics.[6] Effectiveness of inhaled essential oils vapour (e.g., peppermint or ginger) in the prevention or treatment of PONV is not consistently demonstrated in the literature.[6,7,8]
- Ensure adequate oral hydration in surgical and nonsurgical patients.
- Dietary interventions may be important for nausea associated with certain food intolerances.
- Recommend consumption of frequent small meals and snacks rather than large meals at infrequent intervals.
- Consult a dietitian when necessary.
- Advise patients to avoid smells and foods that cause nausea.
- Recommend controlled breathing for motion sickness.
- Relaxation therapy and cognitive behavioural therapies may be useful in the treatment of nausea associated with irritable bowel syndrome and anticipatory nausea.[1]
- Engage the patient in the decisions around treatment. Not every patient will want treatment; watchful waiting is an alternative to medication for these individuals.
- Reassure patient when the underlying cause is self-limited.

Pharmacologic Choices

Although antiemetics are widely prescribed (Table 1), there is a paucity of randomized controlled trials examining their effectiveness, with the exception of serotonin (5-HT_3) antagonists for CINV (see Chapter 126) and PONV. When selecting a drug, consider whether the nausea is acute or chronic, review concurrent medications and attempt to identify the underlying cause of nausea (Figure 1). Many patients cannot tolerate oral medications when nauseated, and alternative routes of administration (im, iv, sc, rectal or transdermal) may be more suitable.

In an emergency room setting, iv **droperidol** may be more effective than iv **metoclopramide** or iv **prochlorperazine** for relief of moderate to severe nausea and/or vomiting of any etiology.[9] However, due to concerns regarding QT_c interval prolongation and severe cardiac arrhythmias, use iv droperidol only for the prevention or treatment of PONV when other treatments are ineffective or inappropriate, and use the lowest effective dose.[10] **Promethazine** has similar efficacy but is more sedating when compared to **ondansetron** for undifferentiated nausea managed in emergency settings.[11]

Standardized **ginger** (*Zingiber officinale*) could be considered an alternative to established antiemetics in the management of pregnancy-induced[12,13,14,15,16] and postoperative[17] nausea and vomiting [Evidence: SORT B*].

Figure 1: Management of Nausea

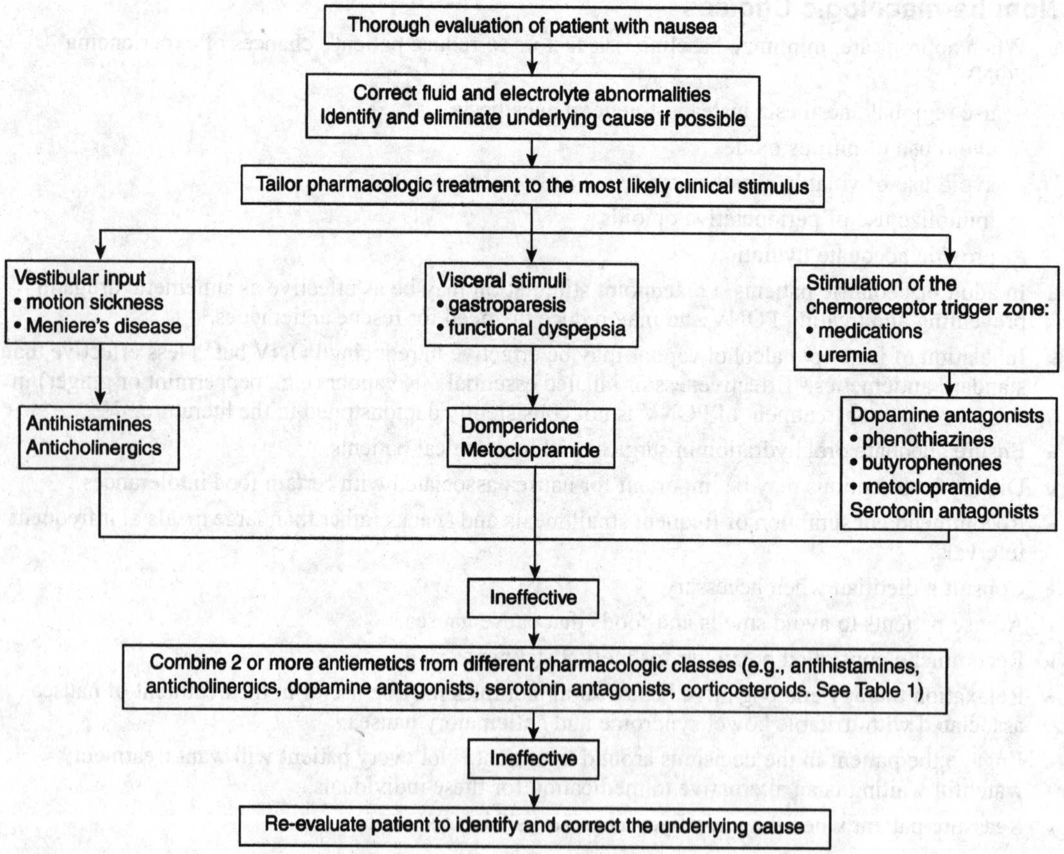

Abbreviations: CTZ = chemoreceptor trigger zone

* SORT (Strength of Recommendation Taxonomy) is a rating system (A, B or C) that addresses the quality of available evidence. For more information consult **How to Use *Compendium of Therapeutic Choices*** on page xxv.

A preventive approach may be appropriate in certain situations, for example, in the management of motion sickness.

If nausea is associated with peptic ulcer disease (see Chapter 60) or gastroesophageal reflux (see Chapter 61), treat the underlying cause.

Choices during Pregnancy and Breastfeeding

Nausea and vomiting of pregnancy (NVP) is common and can often be controlled effectively. Approximately 70% of all pregnant women experience varying degrees of nausea and vomiting, usually in the first 16 weeks of pregnancy, and 1% of pregnant women may experience hyperemesis gravidarum which may require hospitalization and iv therapy.[18] NVP can occur throughout the day despite the common expression "morning sickness." Assess and treat NVP in all pregnancies to avoid significant psychosocial morbidity resulting in disruption of work, home life, relationships, nutritional status and well-being. Consider other causes of nausea and vomiting not due to pregnancy as in the nonpregnant patient. A full assessment is especially appropriate for those pregnant women who first experience nausea and vomiting after the first trimester or have additional symptoms such as pain or fever which do not normally accompany NVP.

There is insufficient strong evidence to recommend one pharmacologic or nonpharmacologic intervention over another for the management of nausea and vomiting in early pregnancy (NVP).[19] However, the best available evidence suggests that **acupressure**, **ginger** and **pyridoxine** (10–20 mg QID po) are likely beneficial for mild nausea [Evidence: SORT B*].[16] In Canada, **Diclectin** (doxylamine + pyridoxine) is the only medication specifically approved for the treatment of NVP. Although limited scientific evidence suggests that Diclectin is only marginally superior to placebo,[22] clinical experience indicates that it is effective and safe in the management of NVP. Expert opinion suggests that first-line options for NVP include Diclectin, **dimenhydrinate** and **promethazine**; second-line agents such as **chlorpromazine**, **methylprednisolone**, **metoclopramide**, **ondansetron** and **prochlorperazine** may also be effective and safe [Evidence: SORT C*].[20,21] Reserve corticosteroids for treatment of resistant cases after the first trimester and limit use of metoclopramide to 5 days since it may cause oculogyric crisis.[21] Though concerns were previously raised, ondansetron does not appear to be associated with a significantly increased risk of adverse fetal outcomes.[23] These drugs can also be used safely while breastfeeding. An algorithm for management of nausea and vomiting during pregnancy is presented in Figure 2.

A discussion of general principles on the use of medications in these special populations can be found in Appendix II and Appendix III. Other specialized reference sources are also provided in these appendices.

Therapeutic Tips

- Preemptive treatment may reduce nausea with certain procedures (e.g., insertion of a nasogastric tube).
- When a more complex cause is suspected, antiemetics may provide some symptomatic relief. However, when possible, determine and treat the underlying cause.[24]
- Start with a low dose and increase the dose slowly when prescribing for the elderly.
- Combination antiemetic therapy may be required for treatment of moderate-severe nausea and vomiting. Use combination therapy to prevent PONV if the patient has multiple risk factors (see Investigations).

* SORT (Strength of Recommendation Taxonomy) is a rating system (A, B or C) that addresses the quality of available evidence. For more information consult **How to Use *Compendium of Therapeutic Choices*** on page xxv.

- If management of a nauseated patient fails to provide some symptomatic relief, reassess the patient and look for other causes.
- Know a few medications well. If one medication fails, try a different class of antiemetics or try an alternative route of administration.
- Start with less expensive choices unless there is a preferred antiemetic for a specific disorder.

Figure 2: Treatment of Nausea and Vomiting during Pregnancy[a]

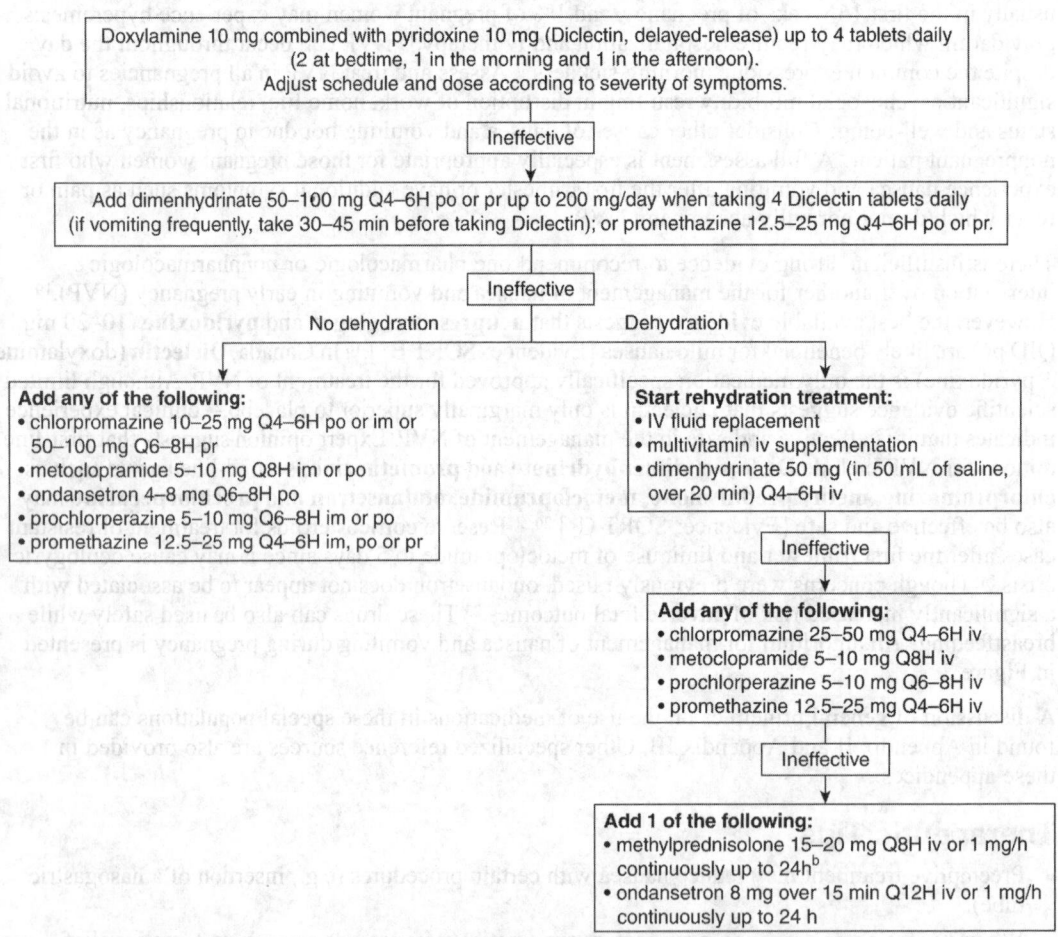

Doxylamine 10 mg combined with pyridoxine 10 mg (Diclectin, delayed-release) up to 4 tablets daily (2 at bedtime, 1 in the morning and 1 in the afternoon).
Adjust schedule and dose according to severity of symptoms.

↓ Ineffective

Add dimenhydrinate 50–100 mg Q4–6H po or pr up to 200 mg/day when taking 4 Diclectin tablets daily (if vomiting frequently, take 30–45 min before taking Diclectin); or promethazine 12.5–25 mg Q4–6H po or pr.

↓ Ineffective

No dehydration

Add any of the following:
- chlorpromazine 10–25 mg Q4–6H po or im or 50–100 mg Q6–8H pr
- metoclopramide 5–10 mg Q8H im or po
- ondansetron 4–8 mg Q6–8H po
- prochlorperazine 5–10 mg Q6–8H im or po
- promethazine 12.5–25 mg Q4–6H im, po or pr

Dehydration

Start rehydration treatment:
- IV fluid replacement
- multivitamin iv supplementation
- dimenhydrinate 50 mg (in 50 mL of saline, over 20 min) Q4–6H iv

↓ Ineffective

Add any of the following:
- chlorpromazine 25–50 mg Q4–6H iv
- metoclopramide 5–10 mg Q8H iv
- prochlorperazine 5–10 mg Q6–8H iv
- promethazine 12.5–25 mg Q4–6H iv

↓ Ineffective

Add 1 of the following:
- methylprednisolone 15–20 mg Q8H iv or 1 mg/h continuously up to 24h[b]
- ondansetron 8 mg over 15 min Q12H iv or 1 mg/h continuously up to 24 h

[a] Use of this algorithm assumes that other causes of nausea and vomiting during pregnancy have been ruled out. At any step, when indicated consider total parenteral nutrition.

[b] Corticosteroids are not recommended during the first 10 wk of pregnancy because of possible increased risk for oral clefts.

Reproduced with permission from: Einarson A, Maltepe C, Boskovic R, et al. Treatment of nausea and vomiting in pregnancy. An updated algorithm. *Can Fam Physician*. 2007;53:2109–11.

Table 1: **Drugs Used to Treat Nausea**

Class	Drug	Adult Dose	Adverse Effects	Drug Interactions	Cost[a]
Antacids	*aluminum hydroxide/ magnesium hydroxide combinations* Diovol, various others	GI-related nausea: 15–30 mL Q2–4H PRN po	Diarrhea (magnesium-containing), constipation (aluminum-containing).	May decrease bioavailability of some drugs (e.g., digoxin); separate dosing by 2 h.	$
Anticholinergics	*scopolamine* Transderm V	Motion sickness or PONV: 1.5 mg (1 transdermal patch) Q72H PRN Patch could be applied the night before or on the day of surgery[25]	Constipation, dry mouth. Confusion (especially in the elderly).	Additive sedation with alcohol or other sedating medications.	$
Antihistamines	*dimenhydrinate* Gravol Preparations, generics	Motion sickness or gastroenteritis: Immediate-release formulations: 50–100 mg Q4–6H PRN po/pr/im/iv (maximum 400 mg/day) Long-acting formulation: 100 mg Q8–12H PRN po (maximum 300 mg/day)	Sedation, anticholinergic effects, confusion. The elderly may be particularly susceptible.	Additive sedation with alcohol or other sedating medications. May increase absorption of digoxin.	po: $ rectal: $ iv: $$
	diphenhydramine Benadryl Preparations, generics	Motion sickness or gastroenteritis: 25–50 mg TID–QID PRN po 10–50 mg TID–QID PRN im/iv	See dimenhydrinate.	See dimenhydrinate. Inhibits CYP2D6 and can increase serum levels of many drugs including antidepressants and cardiovascular drugs.	po: $ iv: $$$
	doxylamine succinate/ pyridoxine Diclectin	Nausea and vomiting of pregnancy: 2 tablets QHS po, plus 1 tablet QAM po, plus 1 tablet mid afternoon po The 4 tablets may be scheduled differently according to timing, duration, severity and frequency of the symptoms experienced by the patient. Since Diclectin is a delayed-release formulation it should not be prescribed on an as needed basis and should be taken daily on a regular basis for optimal effect.	Diarrhea, disorientation, drowsiness, epigastric pain, headache, insomnia, irritability, nervousness, palpitation, urinary retention, vertigo.	MAO inhibitors may prolong and intensify the effects of doxylamine. There is an increased risk of antimuscarinic side effects when doxylamine is given with other antimuscarinic drugs. Doxylamine may increase the CNS depressant effects of other drugs (e.g., alcohol, barbiturates, opioid analgesics).	$$
	hydroxyzine Atarax, generics	Motion sickness or gastroenteritis: 25–100 mg TID–QID PRN po/im	See dimenhydrinate.	See dimenhydrinate.	po: $ iv: $$$

(cont'd)

Table 1: **Drugs Used to Treat Nausea** *(cont'd)*

Class	Drug	Adult Dose	Adverse Effects	Drug Interactions	Cost[a]
Benzamides	*domperidone*[b] generics	Gastroparesis, functional dyspepsia: 10 mg QID po	Diarrhea, abdominal cramps and distention, headache, hyperprolactinemia.	See chlorpromazine.	$
	metoclopramide Metonia, other generics	Drug-induced nausea, migraine-related nausea, gastroparesis: 10–20 mg TID–QID PRN po/sc/iv	Diarrhea, abdominal cramps and distention, headache, hyperprolactinemia, drowsiness, fatigue, EPS.	See chlorpromazine.	po: $ iv: $$$
Butyrophenones	*droperidol* generics	PONV only: Adults: 0.625–1.25 mg Q4–6H iv Elderly: 0.625 mg Q4–6H iv Children over 2 years: 20–50 μg/kg (maximum 1.25 mg) Q4–6H iv Doses of 1 mg or less may be as effective as higher doses.[10] Administer at end of surgery	Sedation, extrapyramidal effects. QT_c interval prolongation and severe arrhythmia.	Additive sedation with alcohol or other CNS depressants. Caution if used with other drugs that prolong the QT_c interval.	iv: $$
	haloperidol generics	Drug-induced nausea, PONV: 0.5–2 mg Q12H PRN po/im/iv	QT_c prolongation.	See droperidol.	$
Corticosteroids	*dexamethasone* generics	PONV: 4–8 mg iv at start of surgery	May increase risk of postoperative infection, may raise blood glucose.		$
	methylprednisolone Solu-Medrol, generics	PONV: 40 mg iv	See dexamethasone.		$
Natural Health Products	*ginger (zingiber officinale)* Gravol Natural Source, others	Nausea and vomiting of pregnancy (mild): 250 mg QID[26,27,28,29] or 500 mg BID[30] po PONV: 1000–1500 mg 1 hour before induction of anesthesia po[31,32,33,34,35]	Abdominal discomfort, diarrhea, heartburn, pepper-like irritant effect in the mouth and throat.	May inhibit in vitro CYP2C19; clinical significance unknown.	$
Phenothiazines	*chlorpromazine* generics	Labyrinthitis: 10–25 mg Q4–6H PRN po 25–50 mg Q3–4H PRN im/iv	Sedation, anticholinergic effects, EPS. Hypotension with im/iv administration.	Additive sedation with alcohol or other CNS depressants.	po: $ iv: $$$
	perphenazine generics	PONV: 2–4 mg Q8H PRN po	See chlorpromazine.	See chlorpromazine.	$

Class	Drug	Adult Dose	Adverse Effects	Drug Interactions	Cost[a]
	prochlorperazine generics	Drug-induced nausea, migraine-related nausea, PONV, vertigo-related nausea: 5–10 mg TID–QID PRN po/pr 5–10 mg BID–TID PRN im/iv	See chlorpromazine.	See chlorpromazine.	po: $ rectal/iv: $$
	promethazine Histantil, generics	Motion sickness, PONV or gastroenteritis: 12.5–25 mg Q4–6H PRN po	See dimenhydrinate.	See dimenhydrinate.	$$
Serotonin Antagonists[b]	*granisetron* generics	PONV: 1–2 mg once or twice daily po 0.35–3 mg iv Administer at end of surgery	Headache, constipation, diarrhea, weakness, QT_c prolongation.	Potential serotonin syndrome or neuroleptic malignant syndrome-like events when taken in combination with other serotonergic or neuroleptic drugs.	$$$$$
	ondansetron Ondissolve ODF, Zofran, Zofran ODT, generics	po: 16–24 mg per day iv: up to 16 mg initially infused over no less than 15 min (do not exceed 8 mg if ≥75 years). Subsequent iv doses must not exceed 8 mg/dose and may be given 4 and 8 hours after the initial dose.	Headache, constipation, diarrhea, sedation, bradycardia, dizziness. Transient ECG changes, QT_c prolongation.	See granisetron. May decrease analgesic effect of tramadol. CYP3A4 inducers (e.g., carbamazepine, phenytoin, rifampin) decrease ondansetron's blood concentrations.	$$$
	palonosetron Aloxi	PONV: 0.075 mg iv administered at start of surgery	Constipation, headache.	See granisetron.	$90/vial

[a] Cost of 1-day supply unless otherwise specified; includes drug cost only.
[b] Non-sedating.
Dosage adjustment may be required in renal impairment; see Appendix I.
Abbreviations: CINV = chemotherapy-induced nausea and vomiting; ECG = electrocardiogram; EPS = extrapyramidal symptoms; PONV = postoperative nausea and vomiting
Legend: $ <$5 $$ $5–10 $$$ $10–20 $$$$ $20–30 $$$$$ $30–40

Suggested Readings

Anderson WD, Strayer SM. Evaluation of nausea and vomiting: a case-based approach. *Am Fam Physician* 2013;88(6):371-9.

Gan TJ, Diemunsch P, Habib AS et al. Consensus guidelines for the management of postoperative nausea and vomiting. *Anesth Analg* 2014;118(1):85-113.

Metz A, Hebbard G. Nausea and vomiting in adults: a diagnostic approach. *Aust Fam Physician* 2007;36(9):688-92.

Scorza K, Williams A, Phillips JD et al. Evaluation of nausea and vomiting. *Am Fam Physician* 2007;76(1):76-84.

Tack J, Talley NJ, Camilleri M et al. Functional gastroduodenal disorders. *Gastroenterology* 2006;30(5):1466-79.

References

1. Quigley EM, Hasler WL, Parkman HP. AGA technical review on nausea and vomiting. *Gastroenterology* 2001;120(1):263-86.
2. Apfel CC, Heidrich FM, Jukar-Rao S et al. Evidence-based analysis of risk factors for postoperative nausea and vomiting. *Br J Anaesth* 2012;109(5):742-53.
3. Gan TJ, Diemunsch P, Habib AS et al. Consensus guidelines for the management of postoperative nausea and vomiting. *Anesth Analg* 2014;118(1):85-113.
4. Cheong KB, Zhang JP, Huang Y et al. The effectiveness of acupuncture in prevention and treatment of postoperative nausea and vomiting—a systematic review and meta-analysis. *PLoS One* 2013;8(12):e82474.
5. Lee A, Fan LT. Stimulation of the wrist acupuncture point P6 for preventing postoperative nausea and vomiting. *Cochrane Database Syst Rev* 2009;(2):CD003281.
6. Hines S, Steels E, Chang A et al. Aromatherapy for treatment of postoperative nausea and vomiting. *Cochrane Database Syst Rev* 2012;4:CD007598.
7. Lua PL, Zakaria NS. A brief review of current scientific evidence involving aromatherapy use for nausea and vomiting. *J Altern Complement Med* 2012;18(6):534-40.
8. Hunt R, Dienemann J, Norton HJ et al. Aromatherapy as treatment for postoperative nausea: a randomized trial. *Anesth Analg* 2013;117(3):597-604.
9. Braude D, Soliz T, Crandall C et al. Antiemetics in the ED: a randomized controlled trial comparing 3 common agents. *Am J Emerg Med* 2006;24(2):177-82.
10. Schaub I, Lysakowski C, Elia N et al. Low-dose droperidol (≤1 mg or ≤15 μg kg-1) for the prevention of postoperative nausea and vomiting in adults: quantitative systematic review of randomised controlled trials. *Eur J Anaesthesiol* 2012;29(6):286-94.
11. Braude D, Crandall C. Ondansetron versus promethazine to treat acute undifferentiated nausea in the emergency department: a randomized, double-blind, noninferiority trial. *Acad Emerg Med* 2008;15(3):209-15.
12. Borrelli F, Capasso R, Aviello G et al. Effectiveness and safety of ginger in the treatment of pregnancy-induced nausea and vomiting. *Obstet Gynecol* 2005;105(4):849-56.
13. Viljoen E, Visser J, Koen N et al. A systematic review and meta-analysis of the effect and safety of ginger in the treatment of pregnancy-associated nausea and vomiting. *Nutr J* 2014;13(1):20.
14. Thomson M, Corbin R, Leung L. Effects of ginger for nausea and vomiting in early pregnancy: a meta-analysis. *J Am Board Fam Med* 2014;27(1):115-22.
15. Ding M, Leach M, Bradley H. The effectiveness and safety of ginger for pregnancy-induced nausea and vomiting: a systematic review. *Women Birth* 2013;26(1):e26-30.
16. Festin M. Nausea and vomiting in early pregnancy. *Clin Evid (Online)* 2014;2014. pii: 1405.
17. Chaiyakunapruk N, Kitikannakorn N, Nathisuwan S et al. The efficacy of ginger for the prevention of postoperative nausea and vomiting: a meta-analysis. *Am J Obstet Gynecol* 2006;194(1):95-9.
18. Einarson TR, Piwko C, Koren G. Prevalence of nausea and vomiting of pregnancy in the USA: a meta analysis. *J Popul Ther Clin Pharmacol* 2013;20(2):e163-70.
19. Matthews A, Haas DM, O'Mathúna DP et al. Interventions for nausea and vomiting in early pregnancy. *Cochrane Database Syst Rev* 2014;(3):CD007575.
20. Einarson A, Maltepe C, Boskovic R et al. Treatment of nausea and vomiting in pregnancy: an updated algorithm. *Can Fam Physician* 2007;53(12):2109-11.
21. Jarvis S, Nelson-Piercy C. Management of nausea and vomiting in pregnancy. *BMJ* 2011;342:d3606.
22. Koren G, Clark S, Hankins GD, et al. Effectiveness of delayed-release doxylamine and pyridoxine for nausea and vomiting of pregnancy: a randomized placebo controlled trial. *Am J Obstet Gynecol* 2010;203(6):571.e1-577.e1.
23. Pasternak B1, Svanström H, Hviid A. Ondansetron in pregnancy and risk of adverse fetal outcomes. *N Engl J Med* 2013;368(9):814-23.
24. Ozucelik DN, Karaca MA, Sivri B. Effectiveness of pre-emptive metoclopramide infusion in alleviating pain, discomfort and nausea associated with nasogastric tube insertion: a randomised, double-blind, placebo-controlled trial. *Int J Clin Pract* 2005;59(12):1422-7.
25. Apfel CC, Zhang K, George E et al. Transdermal scopolamine for the prevention of postoperative nausea and vomiting: a systematic review and meta-analysis. *Clin Ther* 2010;32(12):1987-2002.
26. Fischer-Rasmussen W, Kjaer SK, Dahl C et al. Ginger treatment of hyperemesis gravidarum. *Eur J Obstet Gynecol Reprod Biol* 1991;38(1):19-24.
27. Vutyavanich T, Kraisarin T, Ruangsri R. Ginger for nausea and vomiting in pregnancy: randomized, double-masked, placebo-controlled trial. *Obstet Gynecol* 2001;97(4):577-82.
28. Smith C, Crowther C, Wilson K et al. A randomized controlled trial of ginger to treat nausea and vomiting in pregnancy. *Obstet Gynecol* 2004;103(4):639-45.

29. Pongrojpaw D, Somprasit C, Chanthasenanont A. A randomized comparison of ginger and dimenhydrinate in the treatment of nausea and vomiting in pregnancy. *J Med Assoc Thai* 2007;90(9):1703-9.
30. Chittumma P, Kaewkiattikun K, Wiriyasiriwach B. Comparison of the effectiveness of ginger and vitamin B6 for treatment of nausea and vomiting in early pregnancy: a randomized double-blind controlled trial. *J Med Assoc Thai* 2007;90(1):15-20.
31. Phillips S, Ruggier R, Hutchinson SE. Zingiber officinale (ginger)—an antiemetic for day case surgery. *Anaesthesia* 1993;48(8):715-7.
32. Bone ME, Wilkinson DJ, Young JR et al. Ginger root—a new antiemetic. The effect of ginger root on postoperative nausea and vomiting after major gynaecological surgery. *Anaesthesia* 1990;45(8):669-71.
33. Ernst E, Pittler MH. Efficacy of ginger for nausea and vomiting: a systematic review of randomized clinical trials. *Br J Anaesth* 2000;84(3):367-71.
34. Visalyaputra S, Petchpaisit N, Somcharoen K et al. The efficacy of ginger root in the prevention of postoperative nausea and vomiting after outpatient gynaecological laparoscopy. *Anaesthesia* 1998;53(5):506-10.
35. Chaiyakunapruk N, Kitikannakorn N, Nathisuwan S et al. The efficacy of ginger for the prevention of postoperative nausea and vomiting: a meta-analysis. *Am J Obstet Gynecol* 2006;194(1):95-9.

Gastrointestinal Disorders

Chapter 65
Upper Gastrointestinal Bleeding

Alan Barkun, MD, CM, FRCPC, FACP, FACG, AGAF, MSc (Clinical Epidemiology)

CPhA acknowledges the contribution of Dr. A.B.R. Thomson as a previous author of this chapter.

Upper GI bleeding (UGIB) is a common medical emergency, with a mortality rate of about 3%,[1] especially in older persons with comorbid conditions. Common nonvariceal causes include duodenal ulcer (DU), gastric ulcer (GU) and gastric or esophageal erosions. Esophageal and gastric varices represent about 10% of all causes of UGIB in Canada. Less frequent sources include a malignancy affecting the GI tract, an eroded gastric blood vessel (Dieulafoy's lesion) or a tear of the gastroesophageal junction (Mallory-Weiss tear).[2]

Goals of Therapy

- Resuscitate (ABCs)
- Prevent hypoxia-related damage to other organs
- Heal the underlying lesion
- Prevent recurrences of UGIB by managing, when appropriate, the cause of the bleed (e.g., *H. pylori*, NSAIDs)

Investigations

- History and physical examination:
  - resuscitate immediately to ensure the patient is breathing and to restore circulating blood volume, while quickly taking a focused history and performing a physical examination, especially to exclude signs of chronic liver disease
  - recent data suggest improved outcomes by adopting a more restrictive transfusional policy (e.g., transfusing patients when the Hb level falls below 70 g/L)[3]
  - the cause of bleeding may be suggested by the history: Patients with *ulcer disease* may present with a history of pain, a past history of ulcer and/or use of ASA/NSAIDs or clopidogrel.[4,5] Patients with *varices* present with signs of liver disease (jaundice, ascites, hepatosplenomegaly, coagulopathy, hepatic encephalopathy, skin changes suggestive of liver disease) and/or have risk factors (e.g., alcohol abuse, infectious hepatitis B or C). Retching or vomiting followed by bleeding is suggestive of a Mallory-Weiss tear
  - the prognosis is usually worse if the patient has multiple comorbidities, especially a malignancy or renal/liver disease. Higher risk is also associated with vomiting fresh red blood, passing red blood per rectum, advanced age, tachycardia or hypotension. Formal risk stratification scales such as the Glasgow Blatchford scale and the Rockall score facilitate prediction of interventions and outcomes[6]
- Draw venous blood for STAT type and crossmatch (usually 4 units of packed red blood cells or more depending on the severity of bleeding), Hb concentration or hematocrit, electrolytes, renal function (serum creatinine or urea) and coagulation studies (platelet count, INR and PTT)
- A rapid estimate of blood loss can be made at the bedside: 50% loss of blood volume is suggested by systolic pressure <100 mm Hg, a pulse rate >100 bpm and a Hb <100 g/L

- The role of the nasogastric tube:
  - there is no need to insert a nasogastric (NG) tube if the patient is currently or was previously witnessed vomiting blood
  - in patients with melena or hematochezia, the discovery of fresh red blood in the NG tube aspirate indicates more severe bleeding and points to the cause being in the upper GI tract.[7] In about 10% of patients with clinically unsuspected UGIB, a positive NG aspirate points to bleeding from the upper rather than the lower GI tract. Melena, age <50 years and urea (mmol/L):creatinine (µmol/L) ratio ≥0.12 predict a UGIB source[8]
  - the absence of fresh blood in the NG tube aspirate may be a false negative finding if the tip of the NG tube has not been placed in the pool of blood in the stomach or duodenum, or if the source of bleeding is beyond a closed pylorus
  - NG lavage is no longer performed and has been supplanted by the use of prokinetics, which do not compromise the airway. In those patients with red blood in the hematemesis or the NG tube aspirate, **erythromycin** 250 mg iv as a single dose can be administered 20–90 minutes prior to the esophagogastroduodenoscopy, as it decreases the need for a repeat endoscopy to find the source of bleeding and improves visibility by clearing blood from the stomach[9]
- An ECG is useful in older patients with suspected or possible ischemic heart disease and prior to the administration of erythromycin, to rule out a prolonged QTc interval
- An upper GI series (e.g., barium swallow) must not be performed in the patient with UGIB. The diagnostic accuracy is poor in this setting; it may obscure a clear field for subsequent esophagogastroduodenoscopy, and endoscopic hemostatic therapy (EHT) cannot be performed if the field of vision is obscured by barium
- Esophagogastroduodenoscopy (EGD):
  - refer all patients with UGIB for EGD after they are stabilized. The timing will depend on the suspected severity of bleeding, the likely cause and the patient's general condition, but ideally should be done within 12–24 hours of the patient presenting.[10] An earlier timing of endoscopy is recommended for patients suspected to be bleeding from varices. Some experts suggest an earlier EGD in more severely ill patients
  - prompt EGD will identify the lesion in about 90% of patients. The most common EGD finding is a peptic ulcer or erosions.[11] Inability to make a diagnosis is usually due to profuse bleeding and may require a repeat EGD or, rarely, angiography
  - prognosis may be established at the time of EGD. A patient with a clean-based ulcer (an ulcer exhibiting no stigma of recent bleeding) who is stable, reliable and otherwise healthy and who has family support and transportation available may be discharged home from the emergency room after endoscopy. In contrast, an older person with multiple comorbidities and an actively bleeding ulcer or a patient presenting with a visible vessel or adherent clot at the time of endoscopy is at significant risk of rebleeding and therefore should be admitted to hospital
  - a diagnostic test for *H. pylori* should be considered (high false negative rate when performed in the context of acute bleeding)

Therapeutic Choices

Figure 1 illustrates the approach to the management of acute nonvariceal UGIB and Figure 2 outlines the management of acute variceal UGIB. Table 1 details the parenteral drugs used in the management of UGIB.

Figure 1: Management of Acute Nonvariceal Upper Gastrointestinal Bleeding[6]

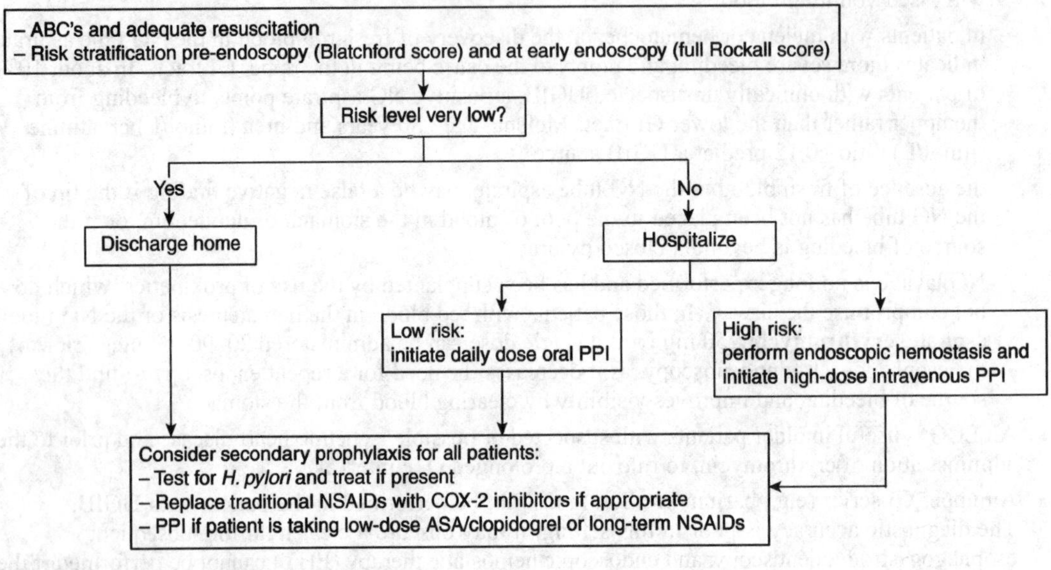

Abbreviations: COX-2 = cyclooxygenase type 2; PPI = proton pump inhibitor

Figure 2: Management of Acute Variceal Upper Gastrointestinal Bleeding[36,49]

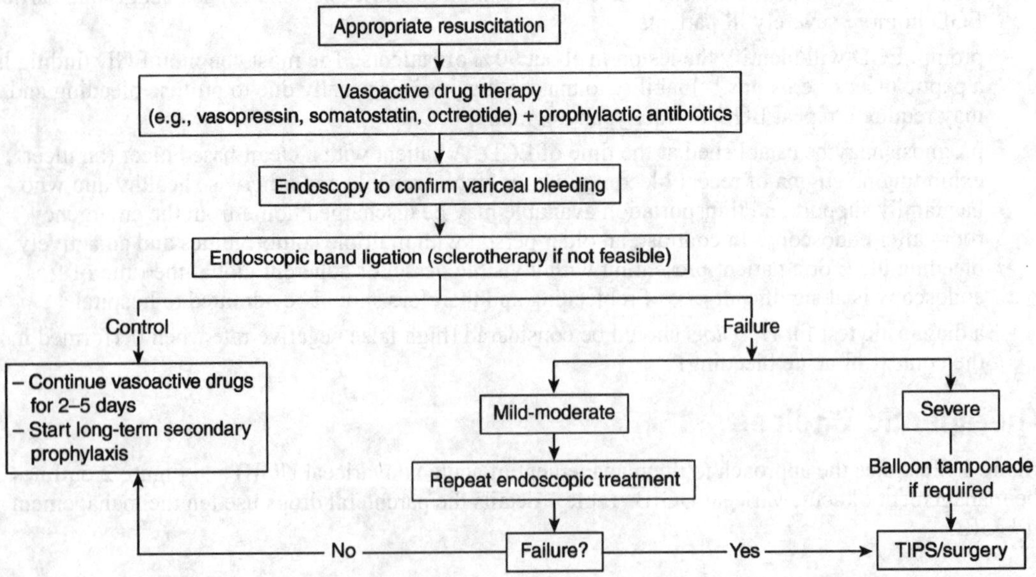

Abbreviations: TIPS = transjugular intrahepatic portosystemic shunt

Nonpharmacologic Choices

Protect the airway, provide supplementary nasal oxygen and insert at least 2 large-bore (18 gauge or larger) iv lines. Fluid resuscitation and hemodynamic stability are essential before attempting endoscopy. In the patient with severe and continued active bleeding, intubation may be needed prior to patient sedation, in order to prevent aspiration.

Endoscopic Hemostatic Treatment (EHT)

Endoscopic triage provides for assessment of the risk of the UGIB.[12] In the more serious lesions seen in EGD, such as an ulcer with an adherent clot, visible vessel or active bleeding (oozing or spurting), EHT must be used.[13] EHT involves coaptive thermal coagulation, injection of a large volume (30 mL) of 1:10 000 or 1:20 000 epinephrine in saline[14] and/or mechanical techniques (banding, hemoclip, staples, sutures).[2] Hemostatic powders have become available, although their optimal role remains unclear.[15] Angiographic embolization is usually reserved for patients failing a second attempt of EHT, and surgery is reserved for refractory or special cases.[16] A routine second-look endoscopy is suggested only in select patients at very high risk for rebleeding.

In *nonvariceal* bleeding, single or multiple therapeutic modalities may be indicated, although injection of epinephrine alone is inferior and should no longer be practised.[17] Gastric and duodenal ulcers are the most common lesions in Canadian patients with nonvariceal UGIB. After EHT, the early rates of rebleeding, surgery and mortality are respectively reported to be 14.1%, 6.5% and 5.4%.[18]

In nonvariceal UGIB, endoscopy can be considered in patients who are anticoagulated (as long as the INR is not supratherapeutic) and in patients exhibiting a platelet count of at least 50–100 × 10^9/L. In patients with supratherapeutic INR, consider administering fresh frozen plasma or clotting factor concentrate. Consider platelet transfusion if the platelet count is <50 × 10^9/L, though the necessity of this has not been specifically studied. The optimal timing of EGD in patients receiving the newer target-specific anticoagulants remains unstudied.

In bleeding *esophageal varices*, endoscopic variceal band ligation or sclerotherapy is highly effective in stopping bleeding and preventing rebleeding.[19,20] Band ligation is preferred because there are fewer complications. For bleeding *gastric varices*, the tissue adhesive **cyanoacrylate** may be carefully applied.

Pharmacologic Choices

When primary endoscopic treatment is indicated in patients with variceal or nonvariceal bleeding, pharmacologic therapy can be considered as adjuvant treatment to yield further improvement in outcomes.

Nonvariceal Upper GI Bleeding

Optimal therapy for nonvariceal UGIB (Figure 1) includes early EGD (within 24 hours of the initial bleeding episode) and appropriate EHT (depending on the nature of the bleeding site). Acid inhibition with oral **proton pump inhibitors** (PPIs) is usually sufficient but iv PPIs (preferably high-dose) are required if EHT is performed for active bleeding or a visible nonbleeding vessel. This pharmacologic therapy further reduces the relative risk of rebleeding by >50%.[21] Use of oral or iv **H_2-receptor antagonists** is not recommended.

In patients with nonvariceal UGIB, PPIs significantly reduce rebleeding, the need for surgery or repeat endoscopic treatment, and mortality among patients at highest risk (having first undergone successful endoscopic hemostasis for active bleeding, a nonbleeding visible vessel or an adherent clot).[22,23,24,25,26] Oral PPIs, including **lansoprazole**, given by NG tube may be as effective as iv PPIs in nonvariceal UGIB, though this is controversial.[26,27] Since most episodes of recurrent bleeding occur during the first 3 days after successful treatment, evidence supports the use of iv PPIs after EHT for 72 hours (e.g., high-dose iv pantoprazole 80 mg bolus followed by a 72-hour continuous infusion of 8 mg/h).[28] The benefit of using PPIs before endoscopy is to begin the ulcer-healing process, resulting in a lower proportion of more severe lesions seen on subsequent prompt EGD. In circumstances where urgent endoscopy is not available, cost analysis supports the use of iv PPIs before EGD.[29] In patients presenting with a bleeding ulcer while on cardioprotective doses of ASA, reintroduction of ASA within 3–5 days post-endoscopy (once iv pantoprazole infusion has stopped) is favoured.[30,31]

Pantoprazole and **omeprazole** are the most extensively studied parenteral PPIs for UGIB, but iv omeprazole is not approved in Canada. IV pantoprazole is administered by continuous infusion (see Table 1). After 3 days of iv therapy, switch to an oral PPI to heal the associated ulcer or esophagitis. Where iv PPIs are not available, oral **omeprazole** 40 mg (or the equivalent dose of another oral PPI) may be administered BID although the data supporting this option are weak. Following discharge, the PPI is continued at a dose and duration determined by the cause of bleeding and the presence of ongoing risk factors for recurrent bleeding (e.g., ongoing ASA or NSAID use).

Somatostatin and its analogue **octreotide** reduce acid and pepsin secretion as well as mucosal blood flow. Their exact role in the management of peptic ulcer bleeding remains largely undefined. More evidence for their efficacy and safety is required before widespread use can be recommended.[32]

In the case of bleeding ulcers, treat *H. pylori*-positive patients with triple therapy (PPI plus 2 appropriate antibiotics taken BID for 10–14 days).[33] It is not always necessary to continue the PPI for longer. Confirmation of eradication with a urea breath test or gastric biopsy is required because of high rebleeding rate in patients with a history of bleeding ulcer.[34] Following successful eradication, no further PPI treatment is needed if the patient had no other cause for the bleeding ulcer. If the *H. pylori* has not cleared, use a different triple therapy or quadruple therapy and repeat the urea breath test to confirm eradication of *H. pylori*. If the ulcer is not associated with *H. pylori* or if the use of ASA/NSAIDs cannot be stopped, continue PPI maintenance therapy for life to reduce the risk of rebleeding (see Chapter 60). The long-term management of patients with UGIB while on anticoagulants remains poorly studied. These patients are often managed on a case-by-case basis, weighing the risk of thromboembolism with that of rebleeding.

Bleeding Esophageal Varices

Antibiotic prophylaxis to decrease the incidence of bacterial infections is an integral part of therapy for patients with cirrhosis presenting with UGIB and should be started at time of admission. Antibiotics reduce bacterial infections, all-cause mortality, rebleeding events and length of hospitalisation.[35] The most common infections are urinary tract infections, spontaneous bacterial peritonitis, respiratory infections and primary bacteremia. Oral fluoroquinolones are recommended for most patients (**norfloxacin** 400 mg twice daily for seven days), but iv **ceftriaxone** (1 g daily for seven days) is considered in patients with advanced cirrhosis, in hospital settings with high prevalence of quinolone-resistant bacterial infections and in patients on previous quinolone prophylaxis.[36,37]

For bleeding esophageal varices, EHT (banding/sclerotherapy) should be supplemented with pharmacologic agents aimed at reducing portal pressure (Figure 2). The long-acting somatostatin analogue **octreotide** reduces portal pressure and bleeding and is given iv for 5 days following esophageal banding.[36] **Vasopressin** reduces splanchnic blood flow and portal pressure, but causes vasoconstriction in other vascular beds. Thus, caution is advised in patients with myocardial ischemia or peripheral vascular disease. Where octreotide or banding/sclerotherapy is not available, vasopressin may be used. IV **nitroglycerin** mitigates the adverse vasoconstrictive effects of vasopressin.

Placement of a transjugular intrahepatic portosystemic shunt (TIPS) within 72 h (ideally within 24 h) should be considered in patients at high risk of treatment failure (e.g., Child-Pugh class C <14 points or class B with active bleeding) after initial pharmacologic and endoscopic therapy.

Prevention of Variceal Bleeding

Nonselective beta-blockers (e.g., **propranolol, nadolol**) may be used to prevent an initial bleed (primary prophylaxis) or to reduce the risk of recurrent bleeding in patients with *portal hypertension* and *esophageal varices* (secondary prophylaxis; see Figure 2). However, beta-blockers do not prevent the development of varices in patients with cirrhosis.[38] Prophylaxis must be continued indefinitely as the risk of hemorrhage returns to that of an untreated patient if beta-blocker therapy is stopped.[39] In patients with high-risk (large) esophageal varices, endoscopic ligation of the varices is more effective than propranolol for the primary prevention of variceal bleeding.[40] A potential harmful effect of propranolol in patients with cirrhosis with refractory ascites deserves further confirmation.[41] PPIs do not play a role in the care of the patient with bleeding esophageal varices. PPIs may be used after sclerotherapy to prevent or to treat injection-associated esophageal ulceration.

Several clinical trials reported that **carvedilol** is more effective than propranolol in lowering the hepatic vein pressure gradient, while one suggested it was as effective as nadolol plus isosorbide mononitrate in preventing variceal rebleeding with fewer severe adverse events and a similar rate of survival. Carvedilol also appears to lower variceal bleeding rates more than endoscopic band ligation but without any differences in mortality. Further studies are required to confirm these results and to analyze the role of carvedilol in secondary prophylaxis.[41,42]

Choices during Pregnancy and Breastfeeding

Perform endoscopic hemostatic therapy in the pregnant patient with an upper GI bleed even though EGD has a higher risk during pregnancy. Suitable monitoring of the fetus is necessary and obstetrical assistance must be immediately available. **PPIs** are considered safe for use in pregnancy[43,44,45,46] and may be utilized based on the endoscopic nature of the lesion. There is little available evidence on the safety of PPIs during breastfeeding. However, based on low concentration of PPIs in breast milk and the destruction of ingested PPIs in the infant's acidic stomach, it is unlikely that PPIs in breast milk affect the infant's development. Based on limited data, **omeprazole** or **pantoprazole** may be used while breastfeeding if a PPI is necessary.[47,48]

A discussion of general principles on the use of medications in these special populations can be found in Appendix II and Appendix III. Other specialized reference sources are also provided in these appendices.

Therapeutic Tips

- Early appropriate resuscitation and risk assessment of patients with UGIB is critical.
- Early EGD is recommended within 12–24 hours with appropriate treatment of variceal or high-risk nonvariceal lesions.
- Attention to long-term prophylaxis, when indicated, is critical in decreasing rebleeding.

Table 1: Parenteral Drugs Used in the Management of Upper Gastrointestinal Bleeding

Class	Drug	Indication	Dose	Adverse Effects	Comments	Cost[a]
Proton Pump Inhibitors	*pantoprazole* Panto IV, generics	Nonvariceal bleeding	80 mg bolus over 2 h then 8 mg/h continuous infusion × 3 days[b]	Abdominal pain, chest pain, rash, pruritus, anaphylaxis.	Metabolized via cytochrome P450. No significant drug interactions with diazepam, phenytoin or warfarin.	$100
Somatostatin Analogues	*octreotide* Sandostatin, generics	Bleeding esophageal varices	50–100 µg bolus in 0.9% NaCl, then 25–50 µg/h infusion for up to 2 days after bleeding stops	Abdominal pain, nausea, diarrhea, hyperglycemia, headache, flushing.	May inhibit morphine analgesia.	$100
Vasopressin Receptor Agonists	*vasopressin* Pressyn AR, generics	Bleeding esophageal varices	20 units in 20 mL D5W bolus over 20 minutes then 0.2–0.4 units/min infusion for up to 2 days	Tremor, sweating, vertigo, nausea, anaphylaxis, water intoxication (early signs are drowsiness, listlessness, headache). Patients with vascular disease may experience angina or even MI.	Consider use of iv nitroglycerin to minimize ischemia. Ganglionic blocking agents may increase sensitivity to pressor effects.	$600

[a] Cost for bolus and 48 h infusion.
[b] May be infused over 15 minutes.
Abbreviations: PPI = proton pump inhibitor

Suggested Readings

Barkun A, Fallone CA, Chiba N et al. A Canadian clinical practice algorithm for the management of patients with nonvariceal upper gastrointestinal bleeding. *Can J Gastroenterol* 2004;18(10):605-9.

Barkun AN, Bardou M, Kuipers EJ et al. International consensus recommendations on the management of patients with nonvariceal upper gastrointestinal bleeding. *Ann Intern Med* 2010;152(2):101-13.

Sreedharan A, Martin J, Leontiadis GI et al. Proton pump inhibitor treatment initiated prior to endoscopic diagnosis in upper gastrointestinal bleeding. *Cochrane Database Syst Rev* 2010;(7):CD005415.

Toubia N, Sanyal AJ. Portal hypertension and variceal hemorrhage. *Med Clin North Am* 2008;92(3):551-74.

References

1. Taefi A, Cho WK, Nouraie M. Decreasing trend of upper gastrointestinal bleeding mortality risk over three decades. *Dig Dis Sci* 2013;58(10):2940-8.
2. Dallal HJ, Palmer KR. ABC of the upper gastrointestinal tract: Upper gastrointestinal haemorrhage. *BMJ* 2001;323(7321):1115-7.
3. Villanueva C, Colomo A, Bosch A et al. Transfusion strategies for acute upper gastrointestinal bleeding. *N Engl J Med* 2013368(1):11-21.
4. Rahme E, Barkun A, Nedjar H et al. Hospitalizations for upper and lower GI events associated with traditional NSAIDs and acetaminophen among the elderly in Quebec, Canada. *Am J Gastroenterol* 2008;103(4):872-82.
5. Ibanez L, Vidal X, Vendrell L et al. Upper gastrointestinal bleeding associated with antiplatelet drugs. *Aliment Pharmacol Ther* 2006;23(2):235-42.
6. Barkun AN, Bardou M, Kuipers EJ et al. International consensus recommendations on the management of patients with nonvariceal upper gastrointestinal bleeding. *Ann Intern Med* 2010;152(2):101-13.
7. Byers SE, Chudnofsky CR, Sorondo B et al. Incidence of occult upper gastrointestinal bleeding in patients presenting to the ED with hematochezia. *Am J Emerg Med* 2007;25(3):340-4.
8. Witting MD, Magder L, Heins AE et al. ED predictors of upper gastrointestinal tract bleeding in patients without hematemesis. *Am J Emerg Med* 2006;24(3):280-5.
9. Barkun AN, Bardou M, Martel M et al. Prokinetics in acute upper GI bleeding: a meta-analysis. *Gastrointest Endosc* 2010;72(6):1138-45.
10. da Silveira EB, Lam E, Martel M et al. The importance of process issues as predictors of time to endoscopy in patients with acute upper-GI bleeding using the RUGBE data. *Gastrointest Endosc* 2006;64(3):299-309.
11. Enestvedt BK, Gralnek IM, Mattek N et al. An evaluation of endoscopic indications and findings related to nonvariceal upper-GI hemorrhage in a large multicenter consortium. *Gastrointest Endosc* 2008;67(3):422-9.
12. Gisbert JP, Legido J, Castel I et al. Risk assessment and outpatient management in bleeding peptic ulcer. *J Clin Gastroenterol* 2006;40(2):129-34.
13. Lau JY, Sung JJ, Lam YH et al. Endoscopic retreatment compared with surgery in patients with recurrent bleeding after initial endoscopic control of bleeding ulcers. *N Engl J Med* 1999;340(10):751-6.
14. Liou TC, Chang WH, Wang HY et al. Large-volume endoscopic injection of epinephrine plus normal saline for peptic ulcer bleeding. *J Gastroenterol Hepatol* 2007;22(7):996-1002.
15. Barkun AN, Moosavi S, Martel M. Topical hemostatic agents: a systematic review with particular emphasis on endoscopic application in GI bleeding. *Gastrointest Endosc* 2013;77(5):692-700.
16. Lu Y, Loffroy R, Lau JY et al. Multidisciplinary management strategies for acute non-variceal upper gastrointestinal bleeding. *Br J Surg* 2014;101(1):e34-50.
17. Marmo R, Rotondano G, Piscopo R et al. Dual therapy versus monotherapy in the endoscopic treatment of high-risk bleeding ulcers: a meta-analysis of controlled trials. *Am J Gastroenterol* 2007;102(2):279-89.
18. Barkun AN, Thomson A, Marshall J et al. Response to "Potentially flawed interpretation of data by Andriulli et al." *Am J Gastroenterol* 2005;100(9):2133; author reply 2133-4.
19. Sharara AI, Rockey DC. Gastroesophageal variceal hemorrhage. *N Engl J Med* 2001;345(9):669-81.
20. Ferguson JW, Tripathi D, Hayes PC. Review article: the management of acute variceal bleeding. *Aliment Pharmacol Ther* 2003;18(3):253-62.
21. Zargar SA, Javid G, Khan BA et al. Pantoprazole infusion as adjuvant therapy to endoscopic treatment in patients with peptic ulcer bleeding: prospective randomized controlled trial. *J Gastroenterol Hepatol* 2006;21(4):716-21.
22. Leontiadis GI, Sharma VK, Howden CW. Proton pump inhibitor therapy for peptic ulcer bleeding: Cochrane collaboration meta-analysis of randomized controlled trials. *Mayo Clin Proc* 2007;82(3):286-96.
23. Andriulli A, Annese V, Caruso N et al. Proton-pump inhibitors and outcome of endoscopic hemostasis in bleeding peptic ulcers: a series of meta-analyses. *Am J Gastroenterol* 2005;100(1):207-19.
24. Bardou M, Toubouti Y, Benhaberou-Brun D et al. Meta-analysis: proton-pump inhibition in high-risk patients with acute peptic ulcer bleeding. *Aliment Pharmacol Ther* 2005;21(6):677-86.
25. Khuroo MS, Yattoo GN, Javid G et al. A comparison of omeprazole and placebo for bleeding peptic ulcer. *N Engl J Med* 1997;336(15):1054-8.
26. Lau JY, Sung JJ, Lee KK et al. Effect of intravenous omeprazole on recurrent bleeding after endoscopic treatment of bleeding peptic ulcers. *N Engl J Med* 2000;343(5):310-6.
27. Laine L, Shah A, Bemanian S. Intragastric pH with oral vs intravenous bolus plus infusion proton-pump inhibitor therapy in patients with bleeding ulcers. *Gastroenterology* 2008;134(7):1836-41.
28. van Rensburg CJ, Cheer S. Pantoprazole for the Treatment of Peptic Ulcer Bleeding and Prevention of Rebleeding. *Clin Med Insights Gastroenterol* 2012;5:51-60.
29. Tsoi KK, Lau JY, Sung JJ. Cost-effectiveness analysis of high-dose omeprazole infusion before endoscopy for patients with upper-GI bleeding. *Gastrointest Endosc* 2008;67(7):1056-63.
30. Masterton GS, Plevris JN. Recommencing aspirin following a peptic ulcer bleed: when is the time right? *Ann Gastroenterol* 2011;24(4):331-332.

31. Sung JJ, Lau JY, Ching JY et al. Continuation of low-dose aspirin therapy in peptic ulcer bleeding: a randomized trial. *Ann Intern Med* 2010;152(1):1-9.
32. Sgouros SN, Bergele C, Viazis N et al. Somatostatin and its analogues in peptic ulcer bleeding: facts and pathophysiological aspects. *Dig Liver Dis* 2006;38(2):143-8.
33. Yuan Y, Ford AC, Khan KJ et al. Optimum duration of regimens for Helicobacter pylori eradication. *Cochrane Database Syst Rev* 2013;12:CD008337.
34. Gisbert JP, Abraira V. Accuracy of Helicobacter pylori diagnostic tests in patients with bleeding peptic ulcer: a systematic review and meta-analysis. *Am J Gastroenterol* 2006;101(4):848-63.
35. Chavez-Tapia NC, Barrientos-Gutierrez T, Tellez-Avila F et al. Meta-analysis: antibiotic prophylaxis for cirrhotic patients with upper gastrointestinal bleeding—an updated Cochrane review. *Aliment Pharmacol Ther* 2011;34(5):509-18.
36. de Franchis R; Baveno V Faculty. Revising consensus in portal hypertension: report of the Baveno V consensus workshop on methodology of diagnosis and therapy in portal hypertension. *J Hepatol* 2010;53(4):762-8.
37. Garcia-Tsao G, Sanyal AJ, Grace ND et al. Prevention and management of gastroesophageal varices and variceal hemorrhage in cirrhosis. *Hepatology* 2007;46(3):922-38.
38. Groszmann RJ, Garcia-Tsao G, Bosch J et al. Beta-blockers to prevent gastroesophageal varices in patients with cirrhosis. *N Engl J Med* 2005;353(21):2254-61.
39. Abraczinskas DR, Ookubo R, Grace ND et al. Propranolol for the prevention of first esophageal variceal hemorrhage: a lifetime commitment? *Hepatology* 2001;34(6):1096-102.
40. Garcia-Tsao G. Portal hypertension. *Curr Opin Gastroenterol* 2002;18(3):351-9.
41. Giannelli V, Lattanzi B, Thalheimer U et al. Beta-blockers in liver cirrhosis. *Ann Gastroenterol* 2014;27(1):20-26.
42. Sinagra E1, Perricone G, D'Amico M et al. Systematic review with meta-analysis: the haemodynamic effects of carvedilol compared with propranolol for portal hypertension in cirrhosis. *Aliment Pharmacol Ther* 2014;39(6):557-68.
43. Gill SK, O'Brien L, Einarson TR et al. The safety of proton pump inhibitors (PPIs) in pregnancy: a meta-analysis. *Am J Gastroenterol* 2009;104(6):1541-5.
44. Pasternak B, Hviid A. Use of proton-pump inhibitors in early pregnancy and the risk of birth defects. *N Engl J Med* 2010;363(22):2114-23.
45. Nava-Ocampo AA, Velazquez-Armenta EY, Han JY et al. Use of proton pump inhibitors during pregnancy and breastfeeding. *Can Fam Physician* 2006;52:853-4.
46. Pasternak B, Hviid A. Use of proton-pump inhibitors in early pregnancy and the risk of birth defects. *N Engl J Med* 2010;363(22):2114-23.
47. Broussard CN, Richter JE. Treating gastro-oesophageal reflux disease during pregnancy and lactation: what are the safest therapy options? *Drug Saf* 1998;19(4):325-37.
48. Marshall JK, Thompson AB, Armstrong D. Omeprazole for refractory gastroesophageal reflux disease during pregnancy and lactation. *Can J Gastroenterol* 1998;12(3):225-7.
49. de Franchis R. Evolving consensus in portal hypertension. Report of the Baveno IV consensus workshop on methodology of diagnosis and therapy in portal hypertension. *J Hepatol* 2005;43(1):167-76.

Chapter 66
Viral Hepatitis

Kevork M. Peltekian, MD and
Geralynn Hirsch, RN-NP, MSN

Hepatitis A virus (HAV), hepatitis B virus (HBV), hepatitis C virus (HCV), hepatitis D virus (HDV) and hepatitis E virus (HEV) cause 95% of acute viral hepatitis cases observed in North America (Table 1).[1] Other causes of viral hepatitis include adenovirus, Coxsackie virus, cytomegalovirus, Epstein-Barr virus and, rarely, herpes simplex virus or parvovirus B19 infection. Over 500 million people around the world and >500 000 Canadians are infected chronically with HBV or HCV making chronic viral hepatitis a major public health concern.[2,3]

Table 1: **Characteristics of Hepatitis Viruses[4,5]**

Characteristics	HAV	HBV	HCV	HDV[a]	HEV
Virus type	RNA	DNA	RNA	RNA	RNA
Incubation (days)	15–45	30–180	15–60	21–140	15–65
Transmission	Fecal-oral	Percutaneous, sexual, perinatal	Percutaneous, perinatal (uncommon)	Percutaneous, sexual, perinatal	Fecal-oral
Acute hepatitis progressing to chronic disease	No	Adults 2–7%, preschoolers 25%, neonates 90%	70–80%	In superinfection; rare in coinfection	No
Prevention	Pre/postexposure immunization	Pre/postexposure immunization	Blood donor screening, risk behaviour modification	HBV immunization prevents HDV infection	Ensure safe drinking water

[a] Requires coexisting HBV infection; HDV may infect a chronic HBV carrier (superinfection) or may infect a subject at the same time as HBV (co-infection).
Abbreviations: HAV = hepatitis A virus; HBV = hepatitis B virus; HCV = hepatitis C virus; HDV = hepatitis D virus; HEV = hepatitis E virus

Patients diagnosed with hepatitis B or C generally require referral to specialists with expertise in the treatment of viral hepatitis and the management of liver disease. If untreated, chronic viral hepatitis may lead to the development of cirrhosis, hepatocellular carcinoma and decompensation with end-stage liver disease requiring transplantation.

Viral hepatitis is considered chronic when present for ≥6 months. It can progress to cirrhosis, decompensation (liver failure) and hepatoma (primary liver cancer). HBV and HCV are the most common causes. HAV and HEV do not cause chronic infections.

This chapter focuses on:

- prevention of viral hepatitis
- treatment of viral hepatitis
- recognition of acute and chronic viral hepatitis
- short- and long-term monitoring of chronic hepatitis B and C

Goals of Therapy

General

- Prevent spread of infection
- Improve quality of life
- Minimize liver damage, reduce liver inflammation, prevent cirrhosis, hepatic failure and hepatocellular carcinoma

Specific

- Sustained suppression of hepatitis B viral replication, ensuring undetectable serum HBV DNA (<10–15 IU/mL) with normalization of alanine aminotransferase (ALT) leading to improvement in liver histology. While hepatitis B surface antigen (HBsAg) seroconversion (loss of HBsAg and appearance of hepatitis B surface antibodies [anti-HBs]) is the most desirable goal of therapy, it is a rare event and not the specific goal of most treatments.[3]
- Eradicate the virus in the case of acute or chronic hepatitis C infection.[6] The desired outcome in chronic hepatitis C is sustained virologic response (SVR), defined as undetectable serum HCV RNA (<10–15 IU/mL) 12–24 weeks after the end of treatment.

Prevention of Viral Hepatitis

Specific vaccines are available for *hepatitis A and B viruses* but not for *hepatitis C, D or E viruses* (Table 4). HDV is a defective RNA virus that requires HBsAg for entry into and exit from hepatocytes; thus, vaccination against HBV confers immunity against coinfection with HBV and HDV.

Vaccinate individuals at high risk of contracting hepatitis A or B (Table 2). Immunoglobulins obtained from pooled human plasma exhibiting anti-HAV activity and **hepatitis B immunoglobulin** (HBIg) provide immediate short-term passive immunity against HAV and HBV, respectively (Table 4).

Hepatitis A vaccine (inactivated) is the preferred agent for pre-exposure prophylaxis and has largely replaced pooled immunoglobulins for postexposure prophylaxis.[7] It is very effective (up to 10 years) and is recommended for high-risk groups. Detectable antibody is present at 1 month in 96–100% of recipients after the first dose and in 100% after the booster dose, given 6–12 months later. Hepatitis A vaccines are well tolerated and safe.

Hepatitis B (HB) vaccines induce anti-HBs production. Antibody response in general decreases with age. Children 2–19 years of age have the highest response rate (99%). The response rate for those older than 60 years is 50–70%.[9] In most preparations, the antigen is adsorbed onto aluminum hydroxide with thimerosal as a preservative. A preparation of HB vaccine without thimerosal is recommended for immunization of infants at birth. Revaccinating with a single booster dose, a complete 3-dose vaccination series or using a vaccine formulation with higher concentration of HBsAg may be needed in hyporesponders or nonresponders (e.g., elderly or those with diminished immune function including patients on hemodialysis). HBV vaccines are well tolerated and safe. Although sustainable anti-HBs levels may diminish 10–15 years following vaccination, long-lasting protection remains due to "immunologic memory."[10] There is no need for routine booster doses of HBV vaccine in immunocompetent persons after successful vaccination.

Hepatitis B immune globulin (HBIg) is prepared from pooled human plasma from select donors who have a high level of anti-HBs and are seronegative for bloodborne infections. It provides immediate short-term passive immunity. HBIg administered concurrently with the vaccine, but at a different site, does not interfere with the antibody response to the vaccine.

Table 2: Recommendations for Hepatitis A and B Vaccinations[8]

Patient Characteristics	Hepatitis A Vaccine	Hepatitis B Vaccine
Infants and pre-adolescent children[a]		x
Persons with end-stage renal disease or recipients of dialysis		x
Persons with clotting factor disorders	x	x
Persons with HIV infection		x
Persons with chronic liver disease including HCV	x	x
Health care and emergency service workers who have exposure to blood in the workplace		x
Persons handling HAV-infected primates or involved in research on HAV	x	
Persons in training in schools of dentistry, laboratory technology, medicine, nursing and other allied health professions		x
Injection drug users and persons snorting cocaine and other illicit drugs		x
Persons with multiple sex partners and all clients in STI clinics		x
Men who have sex with men	x	x
Household and sexual contacts of persons identified as HBsAg positive		x
Staff and inmates of long-term correctional facilities	?	x
Clients and staff of institutions for the developmentally challenged	?	x
International travellers to HAV- or HBV-endemic areas	x	x

[a] Public health guidelines vary among Canadian provinces and territories.
Abbreviations: HAV = hepatitis A virus; HBV = hepatitis B virus; HCV = hepatitis C virus; HIV = human immunodeficiency virus; STI = sexually transmitted infection
Legend: x = Highly recommended; ? = Recommended when there is evidence for sustained HAV transmission

Acute Viral Hepatitis

Introduction

Acute viral hepatitis is a systemic viral infection that by definition has been present for <6 months (often <6 weeks) and causes inflammatory necrosis of the liver. Although most cases of acute viral hepatitis are asymptomatic, the infection could rarely cause acute liver failure particularly in pregnant women.[5,11] Immediately refer patients with a prolonged INR, jaundice and encephalopathy to a liver transplantation centre since massive necrosis may occur, potentially resulting in liver failure and death.

Investigations

Figure 1 depicts the approach to a patient presenting with hepatitis symptoms (acute rise in serum aminotransferases, viral-like illness including fever, muscle and joint pain, headaches, general sense of feeling unwell, constant fatigue, jaundice).

- Monitor liver aminotransferases (ALT, AST) and liver function tests (total bilirubin, serum albumin and INR). Urgently refer to a specialist patients with severe liver dysfunction and elevations in both INR and total bilirubin.
- Ask about risk factors such as injection drug use, high-risk sexual behaviour, travel history or daycare exposure.

- Rule out drug-induced hepatitis, including that caused by acetaminophen or herbal products such as buckthorn, chaparral, comfrey, germander, nutmeg or valerian. The initial presentation of autoimmune hepatitis and Wilson's disease (especially in children and young adults) may mimic acute viral hepatitis.
- Identify hepatitis viruses by the presence of serologic markers:
  - anti-HAV (antibody to hepatitis A virus) represents total IgG and IgM antibodies. Presence of anti-HAV indicates either acute or resolved HAV infection. Presence of IgM anti-HAV indicates acute HAV infection.
  - HBsAg indicates either acute or chronic HBV infection. Persistence of HBsAg beyond 6 months signifies chronic HBV infection. While the absence of IgM antibodies to hepatitis B core antigen (HBcAg) excludes acute hepatitis B, its presence cannot distinguish between an acute HBV infection and a flare-up of chronic HBV infection. Anti-HBs is a marker of hepatitis B immunity. Hepatitis B e antigen (HBeAg) is a marker of a high degree of HBV infectivity and correlates with a high level of HBV replication. Presence of anti-HBe in a person with chronic HBV infection suggests a low degree of infectivity. HBV-DNA is a marker of viral replication/infectivity and is used to assess and monitor the treatment of chronic HBV infection.
  - Acute hepatitis C can be identified by a positive HCV RNA test as early as 2–3 weeks after infection. Anti-HCV antibodies may not be detected for up to 20 weeks after exposure to the virus, but are usually present by 8 weeks.
- Most cases of acute HCV infection are asymptomatic and are usually diagnosed under 3 circumstances—documented seroconversion, known exposure (e.g., needle-stick exposure) and acute clinical hepatitis with jaundice.

Therapeutic Choices

In most cases specific antiviral therapy is not indicated for acute viral hepatitis (Figure 1). With appropriate supportive care, the majority of patients with acute hepatitis A or B recover completely and do not experience chronic complications. Acute hepatitis C is rarely diagnosed and most patients with acute HCV become chronically infected. But when acute HCV infection is diagnosed, pharmacologic treatment leads to favourable outcomes.

Nonpharmacologic Choices

- Avoid alcohol for at least 3 months or until complete normalization of liver enzymes and hepatic function.
- No dietary restrictions are necessary.
- No restriction of physical activities is needed.

Pharmacologic Choices

Stop all hepatotoxic drugs. For patients with a prolonged INR (>1.4), administer **vitamin K** 10 mg orally or subcutaneously (avoid plasma unless there is active bleeding). If the patient develops encephalopathy heralding fulminant liver failure, start **lactulose** to achieve 2–3 loose bowel movements per day.

Nucleos(t)ide analogues or **peginterferons** are ineffective in managing acute hepatitis B infections except in *severe* acute hepatitis B where the nucleos(t)ide analogues may prevent the progression to fulminant liver failure and death.[12] However, some patients may still require liver transplantation despite antiviral therapy.[12] Effective and specific antiviral therapy is available only for acute hepatitis C.

Women, younger patients and icteric patients are more likely to clear the virus than other patients with acute hepatitis C. A single negative HCV RNA test result is insufficient to confirm viral clearance in a patient with acute hepatitis C; repeat the test at least once. If HCV RNA persists beyond 12 weeks of symptom onset, consider interferon-based antiviral treatment (see discussion of peginterferon alfa in the section on chronic hepatitis C and in Table 5). Treatment is most effective if started by 24 weeks. SVR rates of >90% have been obtained with peginterferon monotherapy. Treat patients infected with HCV genotypes 2 or 3 for 12 weeks; treat those infected with other genotypes for 24 weeks.[13]

Chronic Hepatitis B

Introduction

HBV infection becomes chronic in 5–10% of infected teenagers or adults, 90% of infected infants and 25–50% of infected children <5 years of age.[14] Among those with chronic hepatitis B, about 1% will seroconvert spontaneously each year from an HBsAg-positive to an anti-HBs-positive state (become immune).

Figure 1: Approach to a Patient Presenting with Acute Viral Hepatitis

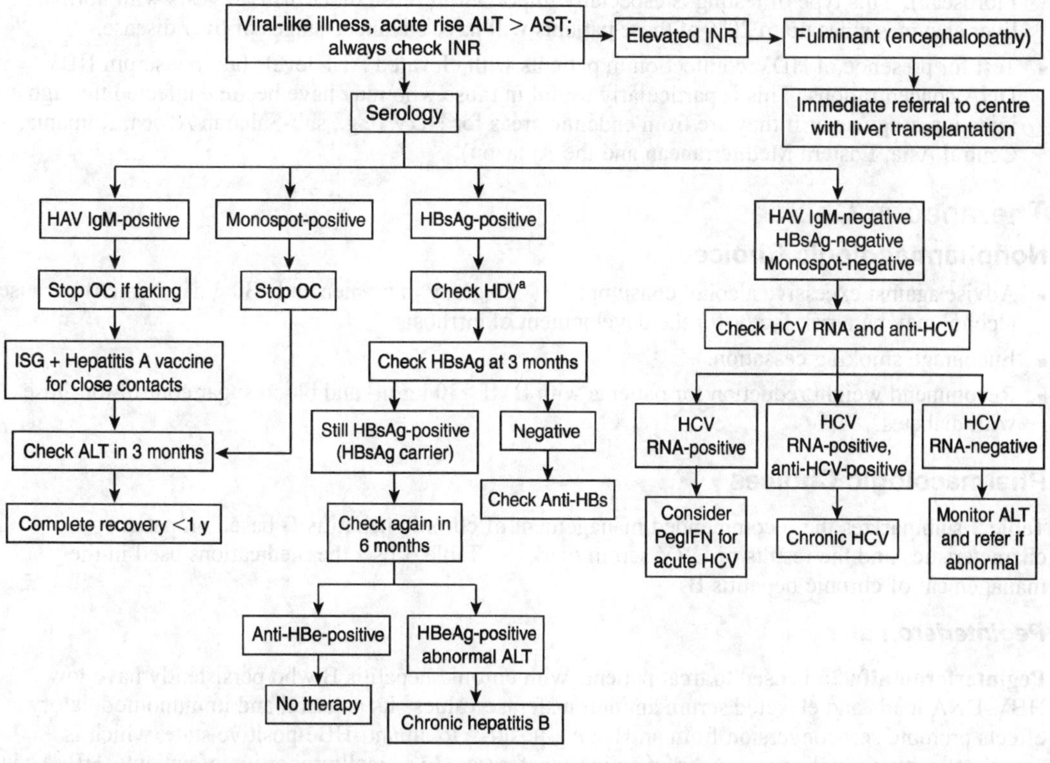

[a] Note: Coinfection with HDV does not change treatment course, but is generally more severe.

Abbreviations: ALT = alanine aminotransferase; Anti-HBe = antibody to HBeAg; Anti-HBs = antibody to hepatitis B surface antigen; Anti-HCV = antibody to HCV; AST = aspartate aminotransferase; HAV IgM = hepatitis A IgM; HBeAg = hepatitis B e antigen; HBsAg = hepatitis B surface antigen; HCV = hepatitis C virus; HCV RNA = hepatitis C virus RNA; HDV = hepatitis D (delta) virus; INR = International Normalized Ratio; ISG = immune serum globulin; OC = oral contraceptive; PegIFN = peginterferon alfa

Investigations

- Persistence of HBsAg for >6 months defines chronic hepatitis B infection.
- If not already done, test all household members of patients with chronic HBV infection for HBsAg and anti-HBs status. If household members are negative for both HBsAg and anti-HBs, offer all hepatitis B vaccine and test for anti-HBs 1 month after the last dose to ensure response to the vaccine.
- Since HBV and HIV may be acquired by the same transmission routes, test patients with HBV for HIV coinfection, especially when considering nucleos(t)ide analogues for HBV.
- Monitor liver aminotransferases (ALT, AST) and liver function tests (total bilirubin, serum albumin, INR and platelets).

When patients with chronic HBV infection are referred to the specialist, the decision to start treatment is based on many investigative considerations:

- Measurement of HBV DNA in serum, which is a predictor of progression to cirrhosis and development of hepatocellular carcinoma. Monitor HBV DNA levels every 3–6 months.[3]
- HBeAg and antibody to HBeAg (anti-HBe) help determine the replicative state of HBV and the presence of a mutant HBV lacking production of HBeAg.
- Liver biopsy is not generally recommended and has been largely replaced by noninvasive tests (e.g., Fibroscan). This type of testing is especially important in those older than 40 years with normal liver enzymes since up to 20% of these patients will have advanced stages of liver disease.
- Test for presence of HDV coinfection in patients with elevated ALT levels but low serum HBV DNA concentrations. This is particularly useful in those who may have become infected through injection drug use or if they are from endemic areas for HDV (e.g., sub-Saharan Africa, Romania, Central Asia, Eastern Mediterranean and the Amazon).

Therapeutic Choices

Nonpharmacologic Choices

- Advise against excessive alcohol consumption (>20 g/day in women and >30 g/day in men) because alcohol may be a risk factor for the development of cirrhosis.[15]
- Encourage smoking cessation.
- Recommend weight reduction for patients with BMI >30 kg/m² and blood sugar control for those with diabetes.

Pharmacologic Choices

Table 3 summarizes the recommended management of chronic hepatitis B based on patient characteristics and the results of HBV serum markers. Table 5 lists the medications used in the management of chronic hepatitis B.

Peginterferon alfa

Peginterferon alfa 2a is used to treat patients with chronic hepatitis B who persistently have low HBV-DNA loads and elevated serum aminotransferase values. Its antiviral and immunomodulatory effects promote seroconversion from an HBeAg-positive to an anti-HBe-positive state, which is associated with normalization of serum aminotransferases. In a small proportion of patients, HBsAg is also lost. Do not use peginterferon alfa in decompensated cirrhosis because of the increased risk of life-threatening infections and possible worsening of hepatic decompensation.[16] HIV-positive and other immunosuppressed patients with chronic hepatitis B respond poorly to peginterferon alfa.

Table 3: **Management of Chronic Hepatitis B**[3]

Patient Characteristics	HBV Serum Markers					Recommended Management[a]
	Anti-HBs	**HBsAg**	**Anti-HBe**	**ALT Status**	**HBV DNA, IU/mL**	
Immune	+	−	+	↔	−	Antiviral therapy is not indicated
Low-replicating	−	+	+/−	↔	<1000	No antiviral therapy. Monitor ALT Q6 months
Immune- tolerant						
HBeAg(+)	−	+	−	↔	>10 000	No antiviral therapy. Monitor ALT Q3 months × 1 year, then Q6–12 months thereafter
High-replicating						
Wild type	−	+	−	↑	>10 000	Consider therapy with peginterferon or nucleos(t)ide analogues (adefovir, entecavir, lamivudine, telbivudine or tenofovir). The goal is to suppress HBV DNA replication below the limit of detection until HBe seroconversion occurs
Precore mutant (HBeAg negative)	−	+	+	↑	>1000	Consider long-term therapy with nucleos(t)ide analogues (adefovir, entecavir, lamivudine, telbivudine or tenofovir)
Lamivudine resistant[b]	−	+	+/−	↑	>10 000	Add adefovir or switch to tenofovir or entecavir at 1 mg/day
Decompensated cirrhosis	−	+	+/−	↑	>100	Nucleos(t)ide analogues therapy (entecavir or tenofovir)
Post-liver transplant	−	+	+/−	↔/↑	+	Lamivudine plus HBIg[c]

[a] Where >1 nucleoside analogue is presented, the presentation is alphabetical and does not imply the order of choice. Drug doses are presented in Table 5.

[b] HBV species with mutations in the tyrosine-methionine-aspartate-aspartate (YMDD) locus of the HBV-RNA-dependent DNA polymerase resulting in resistance to lamivudine.

[c] HBIg is generally given during the anhepatic phase (10 000 IU iv bolus), then daily during the first week to ensure an anti-HBs titre >100 IU/mL, and then either at a dose of 5 mL im monthly or adjusted to maintain an anti-HBs titre >100 IU/mL.

Abbreviations: + = positive (marker is present); – = negative (marker is absent); ↔ = not elevated above the upper limit of normal; ↑ = elevated above the upper limit of normal; HBIg = hepatitis B immune globulin

Nucleos(t)ide Analogues

Nucleoside analogues include **lamivudine**, **telbivudine** and **entecavir** and the nucleotide analogues include **adefovir** and **tenofovir**. Of these agents, tenofovir and entecavir are first-line therapies based on efficacy, safety, development of viral resistance and tolerability. Nucleos(t)ide analogues effectively inhibit replication of HBV in patients who are HBeAg-positive or HBeAg-negative and should be given only to patients who have ongoing hepatitis (persistent ALT and HBV DNA elevations). Inhibition of HBV replication with nucleos(t)ide analogues is associated with significant reductions in hepatic necroinflammation, increased rates of HBe seroconversion and a reduced risk of developing hepatocellular carcinoma.[17]

Resistance to nucleos(t)ide analogues is an important issue. Among these agents, lamivudine is associated with the highest rates of resistance (up to 70% after 5 years of therapy)[18] while entecavir and tenofovir are associated with almost no resistance even after years of therapy.[19,20]

Lamivudine improves outcomes in patients with decompensated cirrhosis and is primarily used to prevent disease reactivation in patients on immunosuppressive therapy.

Adefovir dipivoxil has activity against wild-type, precore mutant (HBV not capable of producing HBeAg) and lamivudine-resistant HBV. Adefovir dipivoxil in high doses is associated with nephrotoxicity. Monitoring liver function tests may be necessary immediately after discontinuation since severe acute exacerbations of hepatitis have been reported in patients stopping treatment.

Entecavir[21,22] and **telbivudine**[23] produce significantly greater reductions in HBV DNA levels than lamivudine in both HBeAg-positive and HBeAg-negative patients.

Tenofovir disoproxil is active against HIV and HBV including lamivudine-resistant HBV. It has been approved as monotherapy for chronic hepatitis B, based on studies in both HBeAg-positive and HBeAg-negative adults.[24] It has also been studied in patients with HIV-HBV coinfection receiving combination antiretroviral regimens.

Chronic Hepatitis C

Introduction

About 75–85% of acute HCV infections in adults become chronic (the rate is somewhat lower in children).[25,26] HCV is acquired most frequently through illicit drug use (e.g., snorting cocaine, injection drug use), blood transfusion (prior to 1992), tattooing and needle-stick injuries. Risk factors for progressive fibrosis and cirrhosis in patients with chronic hepatitis C include male gender, age >40 years at acquisition, duration of infection, alcohol consumption >50 g daily, coinfection with HIV, immune suppression, diabetes and higher BMI.[27]

In line with the Centers for Disease Control and Prevention and the US Preventive Services Task Force recommendations in the United States,[28,29] the Canadian Liver Foundation recommends one-time HCV testing for all persons born between 1945 and 1975 irrespective of their risk factors.[30] The Public Health Agency of Canada recommends testing only those patients with identified risk factors.[31]

Investigations

- Unlike HAV and HBV, anti-HCV is a marker for exposure to HCV, not immunity; tests are false-positive in <4% of patients, but may be false-negative in immunocompromised individuals (in this group the presence of HCV may be detected only by HCV RNA assay).
- HCV RNA detection by PCR to confirm the diagnosis.

Prior to starting treatment, specialists reviewing the case will test for HCV RNA viral load, HCV genotype and hepatic inflammatory grade and fibrosis stage (via liver biopsy or non-invasive tests; not required if cirrhosis is obvious). Cirrhosis affects response to treatment and duration of therapy. HCV-infected patients require treatment if they exhibit advanced fibrosis involving numerous septa or cirrhosis (F3 and F4 on the Metavir scale). In patients with HCV genotype 1, the IL28B genotype is the strongest pretreatment predictor of response to peginterferon and ribavirin dual therapy (the favourable CC genotype is highly prevalent in Asians but relatively uncommon in Africans). Although not available in routine practice in Canada, testing for the IL28B genotype is most useful in treatment-naïve patients and those with HCV genotypes 1 and 4.

All patients who complete treatment must return 12–24 weeks after completion of therapy for a qualitative HCV RNA test to determine SVR status.

Therapeutic Choices

Nonpharmacologic Choices

- Moderate (1–19 g/day) and excessive (≥30 g/day) alcohol consumption may raise the risk of mortality in chronic HCV patients.[32] Advise minimal alcohol use.

- Advise weight loss in obese patients to reduce progression to liver fibrosis and cirrhosis.

Pharmacologic Choices

Up to 72% of HCV infections in North America are caused by the difficult-to-treat genotype 1 HCV. Patients most likely to have an SVR are those infected with genotype 2 or 3, individuals with a low baseline HCV RNA level and those without advanced hepatic fibrosis.

An overview of the properties of antiviral agents used for chronic hepatitis C is provided in Table 5. SVR is associated with clinically significant outcomes including improvements in liver histology and health-related quality of life, reductions in liver-related morbidity and mortality and is durable.[33]

The pharmacologic treatment options for HCV infections are rapidly evolving and future drug combinations are expected to eventually replace what is currently approved and discussed in this chapter (up-to-date recommendations for testing, managing and treating HCV infections can be found at hcvguidelines.org/). Dual therapy with peginterferon and ribavirin is no longer the standard of care for patients with chronic HCV infection.[6] Future drug combination regimens are expected to be all oral and free of ribavirin and peginterferon. Such achievements would allow this disease to be effectively managed in the primary care setting thus allowing the large number of undiagnosed and untreated patients to receive appropriate, safe and relatively quick care.

Polymerase Inhibitors

In Canada, **sofosbuvir** is currently the only available nucleoside inhibitor of the HCV polymerase (the enzyme mediating HCV RNA replication; also commonly known as NS5B). It is indicated in combination with peginterferon and ribavirin for the treatment of genotypes 1 and 4 chronic HCV infections and with ribavirin alone for the treatment of genotypes 2 and 3 infections. Compared with peginterferon + ribavirin dual therapy, triple therapy with sofosbuvir raises the average cure rate of chronic HCV genotype 1 infections from 40–50% to >90%.[34] Sofosbuvir must not be administered as monotherapy and is dosed once daily for a duration of 12 weeks when treating HCV genotype 1, 2 and 4 infections and 16–24 weeks when treating HCV genotype 3 infection. No dose adjustment is needed for mild-to-moderate renal impairment or with hepatic impairment. The combination of sofosbuvir with other anti-HCV agents is currently being explored in clinical trials and new drug cocktails are expected to eventually replace what is currently approved.

Sofosbuvir is generally well tolerated and the most common adverse effects are fatigue and headache when combined with ribavirin and fatigue, anemia, neutropenia, insomnia, headache and nausea when combined with peginterferon and ribavirin. Sofosbuvir is a substrate of drug transporter P-gp. Potent P-gp inducers in the intestine (e.g., rifampin, St. John's wort) may decrease sofosbuvir plasma concentration leading to reduced therapeutic effect. However, P-gp inhibitors may be coadministered with sofosbuvir (see Table 5).

In summary, sofosbuvir has a number of ideal properties including pangenotypic activity, once-daily dosing, low pill burden, no meal restrictions, few drug-specific adverse effects (seen mostly in combination therapy), minimal drug-drug interactions, high genetic barrier to viral resistance, good safety and efficacy in patients with advanced liver disease and excellent SVR rates in patients with unfavourable baseline characteristics. It is highly anticipated that sofosbuvir may play a key role in future all-oral regimens for the treatment of genotype 1 HCV infections. The major negative aspect of this drug is its high cost (see Table 5).

Protease Inhibitors

The protease inhibitors (PIs) **boceprevir**, **simeprevir** and **telaprevir** inhibit HCV replication and are only licensed for the treatment of chronic HCV genotype 1 infections in combination with peginterferon alfa and ribavirin.[6]

Treatment success rates have improved drastically since the introduction of the PIs. Compared with peginterferon + ribavirin dual therapy, triple therapy that includes a PI raises the average cure rate of chronic HCV genotype 1 infections from 40–50% to 70–80% and shortens the duration of therapy from 1 year to 6 months for about 50% of HCV-infected patients.[6,34] Boceprevir is taken every 8 hours, telaprevir twice daily (10–14 hours apart) and simeprevir once daily (Table 5). All 3 agents should be taken with food. Boceprevir is initiated after a 4-week lead-in period of peginterferon alfa and ribavirin while telaprevir and simeprevir are started simultaneously with peginterferon alfa and ribavirin and given for the initial 12 weeks of therapy only.[6] Response-guided therapy (RGT) tailors treatment duration based on early viral kinetics, and in appropriate patients it reduces treatment duration from 48 weeks to 24–28 weeks. The RGT and stopping rules differ for each PI (refer to boceprevir, simeprevir and telaprevir drug monographs for details). Strict adherence to these rules will limit exposure to potential side effects of these costly therapies in patients who would not achieve SVR, and will likely reduce the emergence of antiviral resistance.

The most important adverse effects of boceprevir are anemia and abnormal taste sensation which occur in about half of the patients. For telaprevir, anemia, skin rash, and anorectal burning and pruritus occur in about one-third of patients. The most common adverse effects attributable to simeprevir are rash (including a potentially serious photosensitivity reaction), pruritus and nausea. Patients taking simeprevir should limit sun exposure, use protective sun exposure measures and avoid use of any tanning device. Triple therapy with PIs may cause higher rates of treatment discontinuation compared to dual therapy with peginterferon and ribavirin. Boceprevir and telaprevir increase the frequency of anemia and therefore close monitoring of hemoglobin levels is recommended (weekly for at least the first 2 months of therapy).The first-line approach in managing the anemia is to reduce ribavirin dose. Alternative strategies include transfusion of packed red blood cells and/or erythropoietin administration.

The PIs are substrates and inhibitors of CYP3A4. Therefore, substantial potential for drug-drug interactions exists. Moderate or strong inducers or inhibitors of CYP3A4 should not be coadministered with the PIs. PIs could reduce the efficacy of oral contraceptives and therefore a second method of contraception should be used during treatment with these agents. Use boceprevir and telaprevir with caution in patients with long QT syndromes and in patients receiving drugs that are known to prolong the QT interval.

In summary, treatment regimen with PIs is complex and efficacy is monitored with regular measurements of viral load.[6] Simeprevir has the advantage of once daily dosing, lower pill burden and less adverse effects compared to the other PIs. Until treatment with PIs is simplified, long-term safety data become available, and newer antivirals with comparatively lesser adverse effects are developed, it may be best if patients receiving triple therapy are followed by clinicians experienced in the treatment of hepatitis C infection.

Combination Peginterferon plus Ribavirin

The combination of peginterferon alfa plus ribavirin is still the cornerstone of dual or triple pharmacologic therapy for chronic hepatitis C. Pegylation of interferon reduces its clearance and allows for once-weekly administration. Peginterferon alfa monotherapy is significantly less effective than combination therapy and is appropriate only for patients who have a contraindication to or cannot tolerate ribavirin. Do not administer ribavirin without peginterferon alfa because ribavirin monotherapy is ineffective. Infection with genotypes other than 1–3 are much less common and outcomes are less well defined. SVR rates in these individuals are more similar to genotype 1 than to genotype 2 or 3; therefore, manage them in a manner similar to genotype 1. The duration of dual therapy is usually 48 weeks (range 24–72 weeks) for genotypes 1, 4, 5 and 6, and 24 weeks (range 16–24 weeks) for genotypes 2 and 3. Ribavirin is contraindicated in patients with renal failure in which case peginterferon monotherapy should be given for at least 48 weeks (see Table 5 for drug dosing details).

Choices during Pregnancy and Breastfeeding

Hepatitis A Infection

Management of hepatitis A during pregnancy or breastfeeding is mainly supportive. Advise pregnant women of the increased risk of miscarriage or premature labour. Breastfeeding can be continued.

Hepatitis B Infection

Hepatitis B infection during pregnancy does not exert teratogenic effects on the fetus and treatment of pregnant women with acute hepatitis B is mainly supportive. Hospitalization may be required if liver damage leads to coagulopathy, encephalopathy or severe debilitation. In general, pregnant women with chronic hepatitis B do well during pregnancy and require no specific treatment but they may experience an increased rate of miscarriage or premature labour similar to that seen in hepatitis A infections.[35]

In the absence of intervention, the rate of vertical transmission (mother to infant) of infection may be as high as 90% if the mother is HBeAg-positive.[36] Mode of delivery (vaginal, caesarean section) does not influence the likelihood of HBV transmission[36] and most infants (>90%) become chronic carriers if infected.[37] The risk of transmission is greatly reduced if the newborn is immunized at birth with **hepatitis B specific immunoglobulin** (HBIg) and **hepatitis B surface antigen vaccine** (the standard of care).[38,39] The failure rate of such strategy is about 1–14% and appears to be associated with situations when the fetus is already infected or when the mother exhibits a high viral load and infectiousness.[40] When used to further reduce the risk of in utero and vertical transmission in pregnant women with high viral loads, **lamivudine**, **telbivudine** and **tenofovir** are usually started at 28 weeks' gestation and continued for 1 month postpartum.[40,41,42] These agents are not specifically licensed for use during pregnancy and there is currently no universally accepted HBV viral load threshold for starting antiviral therapy. Tenofovir has the advantage of better efficacy and higher barrier to viral resistance compared to lamivudine and telbivudine but its safety is less well characterized.[40,43,44,45,46]

Peginterferon alfa may have abortifacient effects and its efficacy and safety have not been studied adequately in pregnant women. Until more data become available, do not use peginterferon alfa during pregnancy unless the potential benefits to the mother clearly outweigh the potential risks to the fetus.[37]

HBV infection is not a contraindication to breastfeeding of infants who receive HBIg and HBV vaccines within 12 hours of birth.[47] Therefore, infected mothers should continue to breastfeed as there is no additional risk of transmitting the virus, but breastfeeding should be stopped if the mother experiences cracking and bleeding of the nipples.[47] Breastfeeding can be resumed once bleeding stops and the cracked nipples heal.

Lamivudine and tenofovir are both excreted into human breast milk but there are no data about telbivudine. Although lamivudine and tenofovir use may be considered appropriate in breastfeeding mothers with HIV, little is known about the long-term effects of these drugs on the nursing infant of HBV infected mothers. Experts are divided over whether they recommend breastfeeding while mothers take these antivirals.[48] Until more long-term data become available, it would not be wise to routinely recommend using these drugs to breastfeeding mothers and the risks/benefits would have to be carefully evaluated on a case by case basis.[43,49,50]

Hepatitis C Infection

Treatment of pregnant women infected with hepatitis C is mainly supportive and antiviral therapy is usually delayed until the postpartum period. Sperm abnormalities are seen in men with HCV while on antiviral therapy; in addition **ribavirin** concentrations are twofold higher in seminal fluid compared with serum levels. This reinforces the need for contraception during antiviral combination therapy and for at least 6 months after cessation of ribavirin therapy.[51] If absolutely necessary and only when treatment outweighs side effects, interferon monotherapy may be attempted during pregnancy with close monitoring of mother and baby.

Vertical transmission of hepatitis C virus occurs in about 5% of cases but higher rates are seen if the woman is coinfected with HIV.[52] There is at present no effective way of reducing the risk of vertical transmission of HCV and mode of delivery (vaginal, caesarean section) does not modify the risk of transmission.[36] Routine testing of pregnant women for HCV is not recommended nor cost effective.[53]

The available evidence suggests that breastfeeding does not transmit HCV; however, to be cautious, an infected mother should avoid breastfeeding if her nipples are cracked and bleeding.[36] It is not known if ribavirin or interferon is excreted in human breast milk but ribavirin has been shown to be toxic in nursing animals.[36] At present, ribavirin and peginterferon are not recommended during breastfeeding because the benefits to the mother do not outweigh the potential harms to the infant.

A discussion of general principles on the use of medications in these special populations can be found in Appendix II and Appendix III. Other specialized reference sources are also provided in these appendices.

Therapeutic Tips

- Hepatitis B viral load rises when patients are started on immunosuppressive drugs, including **prednisone**. Many hepatitis B carriers experience a flare-up later in the course of treatment and after withdrawal of the immunosuppressive drugs with rise in serum aminotransferases and conversion from an anti-HBe-positive to an HBeAg-positive state.[21]
- The sexual transmission rate of HCV appears to be extremely low among monogamous heterosexual couples in which one partner has chronic HCV infection.[54] Presence of HIV coinfection appears to increase the probability of sexual transmission of HCV.[55]
- Do not use nucleos(t)ide analogues as monotherapy for HBV in HIV-positive patients because of the potential for development of resistant HIV strains.
- Treatment of HBV and HCV in patients who have decompensated cirrhosis or have undergone liver transplantation should be handled by or in consultation with transplant hepatologists.
- In patients with addiction problems, delay treatment of HCV until appropriate interventions have been initiated for the addiction.
- Coinfection with HCV and/or HBV in HIV-positive patients should be handled by infectious disease specialists.[56]
- Adherence to medication and follow-up visits are very important.[57,58]
- Depression is a major complication of interferon-based therapy in patients with chronic hepatitis C infections even in those without a history of a psychiatric disorder. SSRIs are effective for treating[59,60] or preventing[61,62,63] interferon-induced depression without affecting the sustained virologic response or adherence to antiviral medications [Evidence: SORT B*].
- Hemolytic anemia is a common and dose-limiting side effect of **ribavirin** that is managed by dosage reductions. As dosage reductions reduce the likelihood of achieving an SVR, **erythropoietin** may be an effective means of maintaining the dose of ribavirin (see Chapter 99).[64]

---

* SORT (Strength of Recommendation Taxonomy) is a rating system (A, B or C) that addresses the quality of available evidence. For more information consult **How to Use *Compendium of Therapeutic Choices*** on page xxv.

Table 4: Hepatitis A and Hepatitis B Immunizing Agents

Class	Vaccine	Dose	Cost[a]
Passive Immunizing Agents	*hepatitis B immune globulin* Hyperhep B S/D	**Postexposure prophylaxis for hepatitis B:** 0.06 mL/kg im Combined with active hepatitis B vaccine to achieve short- and long-term protection. Indicated for: • acute exposure to blood containing HBsAg (e.g., accidental inoculations with HBV contaminated medical instruments) • patients unwilling to take the hepatitis B vaccine regimen or those who were not protected against HBV prior to HBV exposure • perinatal exposure of infants born to HBsAg-positive mothers • sexual exposure to an HBsAg-positive person • household exposure to persons with acute HBV infection (e.g., infant <1 year, if the primary caregiver has acute HBV infection)	$$$$[b]
	pooled immunoglobulins with activity against hepatitis A GamaSTAN S/D	**Postexposure prophylaxis for hepatitis A within 2 weeks of exposure (if exposure is continuous, repeat in 5 months):** **Adults:** 0.08–0.12 mL/kg im **Children:** 0.02–0.04 mL/kg im Consider for postexposure prophylaxis when: • hepatitis A vaccine for active immunization is not available or contraindicated • hepatitis A vaccine had not been used prior to exposure to HAV • age is <1 year • patient is immunocompromised • patient has chronic liver disease	$$[b]
Viral Vaccines, combinations	*combined hepatitis A and B* Twinrix	**Adults ≥19 y:** 1 mL (720 ELISA units plus 20 µg HBsAg) im × 3 at 0, 1 and 6 months *or* × 4 at 0, 7, 21 and 365 days **Children 1–18 y:** 0.5 mL (360 ELISA units plus 10 µg HBsAg) im × 3 at 0, 1 and 6 months **Children 1–15 y (alternative 2-dose schedule):** 1 mL (720 ELISA units plus 20 µg HBsAg) im × 2 at 0 and 6–12 months	$$
	combined hepatitis A and Salmonella Typhi Vivaxim	**≥16 y:** 1 mL (160 AU plus 25 µg *S. typhi* Vi capsular polysaccharide) im × 2 at 0 and 6–12 months	$$$

(cont'd)

Table 4: Hepatitis A and Hepatitis B Immunizing Agents *(cont'd)*

Class	Vaccine	Dose	Cost[a]
Viral Vaccines, single component	*hepatitis A vaccine* Avaxim, Avaxim-Pediatric, Havrix 1440, Havrix 720 Junior, Vaqta, Vaqta pediatric	**Avaxim: Adults and children ≥12 y:** 0.5 mL (160 AU) im × 2 at 0 and 6–12 months **Avaxim-Pediatric: Children 1–15 y:** 0.5 mL (80 AU) im × 2 at 0 and 6–12 months Avaxim or Avaxim-Pediatric may be used in children 12–15 y. **Havrix 1440: Adults ≥19 y:** 1 mL (1440 ELISA units) im × 2 at 0 and 6–12 months **Havrix 720 Junior: Children 1–18 y:** 0.5 mL (720 ELISA units) im × 2 at 0 and 6–12 months **Vaqta: Adults ≥18 y:** 1 mL (50 units) im × 2 at 0 and 6 months	$–$$
	hepatitis B vaccine Engerix-B, Recombivax HB	**Engerix-B:** **Adults ≥20 y:** 1 mL (20 μg HBsAg) im × 3 at 0, 1 and 6 months *or* × 4 at 0, 1, 2 and 12 months, or 0, 7, 21 and 365 days **Adults (dialysis ≥16 y):** 2 mL (40 μg HBsAg) im × 4 at 0, 1, 2 and 6 months **Children 0–19:** 0.5 mL (10 μg HBsAg) im × 3 at 0, 1 and 6 months *or* × 4 at 0, 1, 2 and 12 months **Children 11–15 y (alternative 2-dose schedule):** 1 mL (20 μg HBsAg) im × 2 at 0 and 6 months **Immunocompromised patients:** 2 mL (40 μg HBsAg) im. Monitor anti-HBsAg titre annually and give boosters as needed **Recombivax HB:** **Adults ≥20 y:** 1 mL (10 μg HBsAg) im × 3 at 0, 1 and ≥2 months **Adults (predialysis or dialysis):** 1 mL (40 μg HBsAg) of dialysis presentation vial im × 3 at 0, 1 and 6 months **Children 11–19 y:** 0.5 mL (5 μg HBsAg) im × 3 at 0, 1 and ≥2 months **Infants and children 0 to <11 y:** 0.25 mL (2.5 μg HBsAg) im × 3 at 0, 1 and ≥2 months **Children 11–15 y (alternative 2-dose schedule):** 1 mL (10 μg HBsAg) im × 2 at 0 and 4–6 months	$

[a] Vaccine cost only.
[b] Available through Canadian Blood Services.
Abbreviations: Anti-HBsAg = antibody to HBsAg; AU = antigen units; ELISA = enzyme-linked immunosorbent assay; HBsAg = hepatitis B surface antigen
Legend: $ <$25 $–$$ <$25–50 $$ $25–50 $$$ $50–75 $$$$ $75–100

Table 5: **Drugs Used in Viral Hepatitis**

Class	Drug	Indication and Dose	Adverse Effects	Comments	Cost[a]
Immunomodulators	*peginterferon alfa-2a* Pegasys	**Chronic hepatitis B:** 180 µg once weekly sc × 48 wk	Flu-like syndrome, bacterial infections, fatigue, fever, muscle aches, asthenia, weight loss, diarrhea, nausea, headaches, irritability, depression, anxiety, difficulty concentrating and sleeping, memory loss, hair loss, retinopathy (particularly in those with pre-existing hypertension),[65,66] soreness and redness at injection site, neutropenia and thrombocytopenia.	Neutropenia (<0.75 × 10^9/L) and thrombocytopenia (<50 × 10^9/L) are managed by dose reductions. Neutropenia associated with peginterferon does not appear to increase susceptibility to infection.[67] Contraindications include pregnancy, decompensated liver disease, severe cardiac disease, solid organ transplant (except liver), ongoing/untreated alcohol abuse or injection drug use, severe/untreated major depression or psychosis, renal failure.[6]	$$$$
Nucleoside Analogues	*entecavir* Baraclude	**Chronic hepatitis B:** Nucleoside-naïve patients: 0.5 mg once daily po Lamivudine-experienced patients: 1 mg once daily po Administered on an empty stomach	Increased aminotransferase levels.	Do not use nucleoside analogues as monotherapy for HBV in patients with HIV coinfection: can select resistant HIV variants. Acute exacerbations of HBV disease evidenced by marked ALT elevation have occurred after discontinuing nucleoside analogues.	$$$
	lamivudine Heptovir	**Chronic hepatitis B:** 100 mg once daily po	See entecavir.	See entecavir.	$
	telbivudine Sebivo	**Chronic hepatitis B:** 600 mg once daily po	Increased aminotransferase levels. Elevated creatine kinase levels and myopathy. Peripheral neuropathy if given with peginterferon.	See entecavir.	$$
Nucleotide Analogues	*adefovir dipivoxil* Hepsera	**Chronic hepatitis B:** 10 mg once daily po 10 mg every 48 h po if ClCr 30–50 mL/min 10 mg every 72 h po if ClCr 10–30 mL/min	Increased aminotransferase levels, nephrotoxicity (increased serum creatinine). Lactic acidosis and severe hepatomegaly with steatosis.	See entecavir.	$$$
	tenofovir disoproxil fumarate Viread	**Chronic hepatitis B:** 300 mg once daily po	Renal toxicity. Monitor renal function and serum phosphorus. Lactic acidosis and severe hepatomegaly with steatosis have been reported.	See entecavir.	$$

(cont'd)

Table 5: **Drugs Used in Viral Hepatitis** *(cont'd)*

Class	Drug	Indication and Dose	Adverse Effects	Comments	Cost[a]
Nucleoside Analogue and Immunomodulator Combinations	*ribavirin/peginterferon alfa-2a* Pegasys RBV	**Chronic hepatitis C:** peginterferon alfa-2a 180 µg once weekly sc with ribavirin; dose depends on genotype Genotype 1, 4, 5, 6: ribavirin 1000 mg/day if <75 kg; 1200 mg/day if ≥75 kg Genotype 2 or 3: ribavirin 800 mg/day Divide total daily dose BID, take with food	Ribavirin: Hemolytic anemia (reduce dose), rash. See peginterferon alfa-2a.	Monotherapy with peginterferon should only be used in patients with contraindications or intolerance to ribavirin. Contraindicated in pregnancy (teratogenic); effective contraception during treatment is mandatory. Anemia (Hb <100 g/L) is managed by dose reductions. See peginterferon alfa-2a.	$$$$[b]
	ribavirin/peginterferon alfa-2b Pegetron	**Chronic hepatitis C:** peginterferon alfa-2b 1.5 µg/kg once weekly sc with ribavirin 13.5 mg/kg (800–1400 mg/day) divided BID po with food	See ribavirin/peginterferon alfa-2a.	See ribavirin/peginterferon alfa-2a.	$$$$[b]
Polymerase Inhibitors	*sofosbuvir* Sovaldi	**Chronic hepatitis C genotypes 1 and 4 (with ribavirin and peginterferon alfa-2a or 2b) and genotypes 2 and 3 (with ribavirin):** 400 mg once daily po	Most common include anemia, fatigue, headache, insomnia, nausea, neutropenia. Most of the observed adverse effects are due to combination with ribavirin or peginterferon.	Minimal interaction with other drugs. Do not administer with carbamazepine, modafinil, oxcarbazepine, phenobarbital, phenytoin, rifampin or St. John's wort.	$21 000
Protease Inhibitors	*boceprevir* Victrelis, Victrelis Triple	**Chronic hepatitis C genotype 1 (with ribavirin and peginterferon alfa-2b):** 800 mg TID po with a meal or light snack. Doses are spaced 7–9 h apart	Anemia, diarrhea, dysgeusia, nausea, neutropenia, pruritus, rash.	Response-Guided Therapy is recommended for most individuals, but longer dosing is recommended in target groups (e.g., patients with cirrhosis). Refer to product monograph for details on treatment duration. Always administered with peginterferon alfa and ribavirin.	$5000

Class	Drug	Indication and Dose	Adverse Effects	Comments	Cost[a]
	simeprevir Galexos	**Chronic hepatitis C genotype 1 (with ribavirin and peginterferon alfa-2a or 2b):** 150 mg once daily po with food	Most common adverse effects include nausea, photosensitivity, pruritus, rash, transient increase in serum bilirubin levels.	Dose of simeprevir does not need adjusting in patients with mild hepatic impairment (Child-Pugh Class A). Refer to product monograph for details on length of treatment. Always administered with peginterferon alfa and ribavirin.	$13 000
	telaprevir Incivek	**Chronic hepatitis C genotype 1 (with ribavirin and peginterferon alfa-2a or 2b):** 1125 mg (3 tablets) BID po with a meal (not low fat). Doses are spaced 10–14 h apart	See boceprevir. Anorectal adverse drug reactions including anal pruritus, anorectal discomfort, hemorrhoids and rectal burning.	Not recommended for use in patients with moderate or severe hepatic impairment (Child-Pugh B or C, score ≥7) or decompensated liver disease. Refer to product monograph for details on length of treatment. Always administered with peginterferon alfa and ribavirin.	$13 000

[a] Cost of 30-day supply; includes drug cost only.
[b] Ribavirin is available only in combination with peginterferon alfa-2a or peginterferon alfa-2b.
Dosage adjustment may be required in renal impairment; see Appendix I.
Abbreviations: ALT = alanine aminotransferase; HBV = hepatitis B virus; HIV = human immunodeficiency virus
Legend: $ <$250 $$ $250–750 $$$ $750–1250 $$$$ $1250–1750

Suggested Readings

Coffin CS, Fung SK, Ma MM et al. Management of chronic hepatitis B: Canadian Association for the Study of the Liver consensus guidelines. *Can J Gastroenterol* 2012;26(12):917-38.

Jayakumar S, Chowdhury R, Ye C et al. Fulminant viral hepatitis. *Crit Care Clin* 2013;29(3):677-97.

Myers RP, Ramji A, Bilodeau M et al. An update on the management of hepatitis C: consensus guidelines from the Canadian Association for the Study of the Liver. *Can J Gastroenterol* 2012;26(6):359-75.

National Advisory Committee on Immunization. *Canadian immunization guide.* Evergreen ed. Ottawa (ON): Public Health Agency of Canada; 2013. Available from: www.phac-aspc.gc.ca/publicat/cig-gci/index-eng.php.

Pawlotsky JM. New hepatitis C therapies: the toolbox, strategies, and challenges. *Gastroenterology* 2014;146(5):1176-92.

References

1. Alter MJ, Mast EE. The epidemiology of viral hepatitis in the United States. *Gastroenterol Clin North Am* 1994;23(3):437-55.
2. Parry J. At last a global response to viral hepatitis. *Bull World Health Organ* 2010;88(11):801-2.
3. Sherman M, Shafran S, Burak K et al. Management of chronic hepatitis B: consensus guidelines. *Can J Gastroenterol* 2007;21(Suppl C):5C-24C.
4. Centers for Disease Control and Prevention. *Viral hepatitis*. Atlanta (GA): CDC; 2014. Available from: www.cdc.gov/Hepatitis/. Accessed April 22, 2014.
5. Ryder SD, Beckingham IJ. ABC of diseases of liver, pancreas, and biliary system: acute hepatitis. *BMJ* 2001;322(7279):151-3.
6. Myers RP, Ramji A, Bilodeau M et al. An update on the management of hepatitis C: consensus guidelines from the Canadian Association for the Study of the Liver. *Can J Gastroenterol* 2012;26(6):359-75.
7. Victor JC, Monto AS, Surdina TY et al. Hepatitis A vaccine versus immune globulin for postexposure prophylaxis. *N Engl J Med* 2007;357(17):1685-94.
8. National Advisory Committee on Immunization. *Canadian immunization guide*. Evergreen ed. Ottawa (ON): Public Health Agency of Canada; 2013. Available from: www.phac-aspc.gc.ca/publicat/cig-gci/index-eng.php. Accessed December 12, 2013.
9. National Advisory Committee on Immunization. Part 4. Active vaccines. In: *Canadian immunization guide*. Evergreen ed. Ottawa (ON): Public Health Agency of Canada; 2012. Available from: www.phac-aspc.gc.ca/publicat/cig-gci/p04-hepb-eng.php. Accessed December 12, 2013.
10. Su FH, Chu FY, Bai CH et al. Efficacy of hepatitis B vaccine boosters among neonatally vaccinated university freshmen in Taiwan. *J Hepatol* 2013;58(4):684-9.
11. Sookoian S. Liver disease during pregnancy: acute viral hepatitis. *Ann Hepatol* 2006;5(3):231-6.
12. Tillmann HL, Zachou K, Dalekos GN. Management of severe acute to fulminant hepatitis B: to treat or not to treat or when to treat? *Liver Int* 2012;32(4):544-53.
13. Liang TJ, Ghany MG. Current and future therapies for hepatitis C virus infection. *N Engl J Med* 2013;368(20):1907-17.
14. Jonas MM, Block JM, Haber BA et al. Treatment of children with chronic hepatitis B virus infection in the United States: patient selection and therapeutic options. *Hepatology* 2010;52(6):2192-205.
15. Lok AS, McMahon BJ. Chronic hepatitis B. *Hepatology* 2007;45(2):507-39.
16. Crippin JS, McCashland T, Terrault N et al. A pilot study of the tolerability and efficacy of antiviral therapy in hepatitis C virus-infected patients awaiting liver transplantation. *Liver Transpl* 2002;8(4):350-5.
17. Gordon SC, Lamerato LE, Rupp LB et al. Antiviral therapy for chronic hepatitis B virus infection and development of hepatocellular carcinoma in a US population. *Clin Gastroenterol Hepatol* 2014;12(5):885-93.
18. Lai CL, Chien RN, Leung NW et al. A one-year trial of lamivudine for chronic hepatitis B. Asia Hepatitis Lamivudine Study Group. *N Engl J Med* 1998;339(2):61-8.
19. Colonno RJ, Rose R, Baldick CJ et al. Entecavir resistance is rare in nucleoside naive patients with hepatitis B. *Hepatology* 2006;44(6):1656-65.
20. Kitrinos KM, Corsa A, Liu Y et al. No detectable resistance to tenofovir disoproxil fumarate after 6 years of therapy in patients with chronic hepatitis B. *Hepatology* 2014;59(2):434-42.
21. Chang TT, Gish RG, de Man R et al. A comparison of entecavir and lamivudine for HBeAg-positive chronic hepatitis B. *N Engl J Med* 2006;354(10):1001-10.
22. Lai CL, Shouval D, Lok AS et al. Entecavir versus lamivudine for patients with HBeAg-negative chronic hepatitis B. *N Engl J Med* 2006;354(10):1011-20.
23. Dienstag J, Easley C, Kirkpatrick P. Telbivudine. *Nat Rev Drug Discov* 2007;6(4):267-8.
24. *Viread product monograph (tenofovir)*. Mississauga (ON): Gilead Sciences Canada, Inc.; August 14, 2008.
25. Guido M, Rugge M, Jara P et al. Chronic hepatitis C in children: the pathological and clinical spectrum. *Gastroenterology* 1998;115(6):1525-9.
26. Chen SL, Morgan TR. The natural history of hepatitis C virus (HCV) infection. *Int J Med Sci* 2006;3(2):47-52.
27. Poynard T, Afdhal NH. Perspectives on fibrosis progression in hepatitis C: an à la carte approach to risk factors and staging of fibrosis. *Antivir Ther* 2010;15(3):281-91.
28. Centers for Disease Control and Prevention (CDC). Testing for HCV infection: an update of guidance for clinicians and laboratorians. *MMWR Morb Mortal Wkly Rep* 2013;62(18):362-5.
29. Moyer VA, U.S. Preventive Services Task Force. Screening for hepatitis C virus infection in adults: U.S. Preventive Services Task Force recommendation statement. *Ann Intern Med* 2013;159(5):349-57.
30. Canadian Liver Foundation. *Hepatitis C testing*. Markham (ON): CLF; 2012. Available from: www.liver.ca/support-liver-foundation/advocate/clf-position-statements/hepatitis_C_testing.aspx. Accessed January 13, 2014.

31. Public Health Agency of Canada. *Frequently asked questions about hepatitis C.* Ottawa (ON): Public Health Agency of Canada; 2012. Available from: www.phac-aspc.gc.ca/hepc/faq-eng.php. Accessed January 13, 2014.
32. Younossi ZM, Zheng L, Stepanova M et al. Moderate, excessive or heavy alcohol consumption: each is significantly associated with increased mortality in patients with chronic hepatitis C. *Aliment Pharmacol Ther* 2013;37(7):703-9.
33. Dienstag JL, McHutchison JG. American Gastroenterological Association technical review on the management of hepatitis C. *Gastroenterology* 2006;130(1):231-64.
34. Dugum M, O'Shea R. Hepatitis C virus: here comes all-oral treatment. *Cleve Clin J Med* 2014;81(3):159-72.
35. Elina E, Ben-Dov IZ, Shapira Y et al. Acute hepatitis A infection in pregnancy is associated with high rates of gestational complications and preterm labor. *Gastroenterology* 2006;130(4):1129-34.
36. Fiore S, Savasi V. Treatment of viral hepatitis in pregnancy. *Expert Opin Pharmacother* 2009;10(17):2801-9.
37. Tran TT. Management of hepatitis B in pregnancy: weighing the options. *Cleve Clin J Med* 2009;76(Suppl 3):S25-9.
38. Lee C, Gong Y, Brok J et al. Hepatitis B immunisation for newborn infants of hepatitis B surface antigen-positive mothers. *Cochrane Database Syst Rev* 2006;(2):CD004790.
39. European Association For The Study Of The Liver. EASL clinical practice guidelines: management of chronic hepatitis B virus infection. *J Hepatol* 2012;57(1):167-85.
40. Wong F, Pai R, Van Schalkwyk J et al. Hepatitis B in pregnancy: a concise review of neonatal vertical transmission and antiviral prophylaxis. *Ann Hepatol* 2014;13(2):187-95.
41. Shi Z, Yang Y, Ma L et al. Lamivudine in late pregnancy to interrupt in utero transmission of hepatitis B virus: a systematic review and meta-analysis. *Obstet Gynecol* 2010;116(1):147-59.
42. Han L, Zhang HW, Xie JX et al. A meta-analysis of lamivudine for interruption of mother-to-child transmission of hepatitis B virus. *World J Gastroenterol* 2011;17(38):4321-33.
43. Bzowej NH. Hepatitis B therapy in pregnancy. *Curr Hepat Rep* 2010;9(4):197-204.
44. Antiretroviral Pregnancy Registry. Available from: www.apregistry.com. Accessed September 27, 2011.
45. Munderi P, Wilkes H, Tumukunde D et al. *Pregnancy rates and outcomes among women on triple-drug antiretroviral therapy (HAART) in the DART trial.* 5th International AIDS Society Conference; 2009 Jul 19-22; Cape Town (ZA). Poster abstract WEPEB261.
46. Celen MK, Mert D, Ay M et al. Efficacy and safety of tenofovir disoproxil fumarate in pregnancy for the prevention of vertical transmission of HBV infection. *World J Gastroenterol* 2013;19(48):9377-82.
47. American College of Obstetricians and Gynecologists. *Viral hepatitis in pregnancy.* Washington (DC): ACOG; updated 2012. Available from: www.guideline.gov/content.aspx?id=12627.
48. Ahn J, Salem SB, Cohen SM. Evaluation and management of hepatitis B in pregnancy: a survey of current practices. *Gastroenterol Hepatol (N Y)* 2010;6(9):570-8.
49. Borgia G, Carleo MA, Gaeta GB et al. Hepatitis B in pregnancy. *World J Gastroenterol* 2012;18(34):4677-83.
50. Tran TT. Management of hepatitis B in pregnancy: weighing the options. *Cleve Clin J Med* 2009;76(Suppl 3):S25-9.
51. Hofer H, Donnerer J, Sator K et al. Seminal fluid ribavirin level and functional semen parameters in patients with chronic hepatitis C on antiviral combination therapy. *J Hepatol* 2010;52(6):812-6.
52. Mast EE, Hwang LY, Seto DS et al. Risk factors for perinatal transmission of hepatitis C virus (HCV) and the natural history of HCV infection acquired in infancy. *J Infect Dis* 2005;192(11):1880-9.
53. Plunkett BA, Grobman WA. Routine hepatitis C virus screening in pregnancy: a cost-effectiveness analysis. *Am J Obstet Gynecol* 2005;192(4):1153-61.
54. Terrault NA, Dodge JL, Murphy EL et al. Sexual transmission of hepatitis C virus among monogamous heterosexual couples: the HCV partners study. *Hepatology* 2013;57(3):881-9.
55. Filippini P, Coppola N, Scolastico C et al. Does HIV infection favor the sexual transmission of hepatitis C? *Sex Transm Dis* 2001;28(12):725-9.
56. Adeyemi OM. Hepatitis C in HIV-positive patients–treatment and liver disease outcomes. *J Clin Gastroenterol* 2007;41(1):75-87.
57. Lo Re V, Amorosa VK, Localio AR et al. Adherence to hepatitis C virus therapy and early virologic outcomes. *Clin Infect Dis* 2009;48(2):186-93.
58. Lo Re V, Teal V, Localio AR et al. Relationship between adherence to hepatitis C virus therapy and virologic outcomes: a cohort study. *Ann Intern Med* 2011;155(6):353-60.
59. Gupta RK, Kumar R, Bassett M. Interferon-induced depressive illness in hep C patients responds to SSRI antidepressant treatments. *Neuropsychiatr Dis Treat* 2006;2(3):355-8.
60. Kraus MR, Schafer A, Schottker K et al. Therapy of interferon-induced depression in chronic hepatitis C with citalopram: a randomised, double-blind, placebo-controlled study. *Gut* 2008;57(4):531-6.
61. Ehret M, Sobieraj DM. Prevention of interferon-alpha-associated depression with antidepressant medications in patients with hepatitis C virus: a systematic review and meta-analysis. *Int J Clin Pract* 2014;68(2):255-61.
62. Jiang HY, Deng M, Zhang YH et al. Specific serotonin reuptake inhibitors prevent interferon-α-induced depression in patients with hepatitis C: a meta-analysis. *Clin Gastroenterol Hepatol* 2013 May 4. pii:S1542-3565(13)00605-8. [Epub ahead of print].
63. Hou XJ, Xu JH, Wang J et al. Can antidepressants prevent pegylated interferon-α/ribavirin-associated depression in patients with chronic hepatitis C: meta-analysis of randomized, double-blind, placebo-controlled trials? *PLoS One* 2013;8(10):e76799.
64. Sherman M, Cohen L, Cooper MA et al. Clinical recommendations for the use of recombinant human erythropoietin in patients with hepatitis C virus being treated with ribavirin. *Can J Gastroenterol* 2006;20(7):479-85.
65. Fouad YM, Khalaf H, Ibraheem H et al. Incidence and risk factors of retinopathy in Egyptian patients with chronic hepatitis C virus treated with pegylated interferon plus ribavirin. *Int J Infect Dis* 2012;16(1):e67-71.
66. Vujosevic S, Tempesta D, Noventa F et al. Pegylated interferon-associated retinopathy is frequent in hepatitis C virus patients with hypertension and justifies ophthalmologic screening. *Hepatology* 2012;56(2):455-63.
67. Cooper CL, Al-Bedwawi S, Lee C et al. Rate of infectious complications during interferon-based therapy for hepatitis C is not related to neutropenia. *Clin Infect Dis* 2006;42(12):1674-8.

Chapter 67
Lower Urinary Tract Symptoms and Benign Prostatic Hyperplasia

Richard W. Norman, MD, FRCSC

Goals of Therapy

- Improve or abolish lower urinary tract symptoms (LUTS)
- Prevent or delay clinical progression of benign prostatic hyperplasia (BPH)
- Reduce the risk of surgical intervention
- Prevent the sequelae of long-term bladder outlet obstruction (urinary tract infections, bladder stones, hydronephrosis)

Investigations

- Thorough history with attention to:
  - voiding (weak/interrupted stream, dribbling, hesitancy, straining) and storage (nocturia, frequency, urgency) symptoms
  - onset and progression of LUTS and degree of inconvenience or bother to the patient (International Prostate Symptom Score) is recommended—available at www.urospec.com/uro/Forms/ipss.pdf
  - details of urethral infection, instrumentation or injury (e.g., surgery, radiation)
  - episodes of urinary tract infection, hematuria or urinary retention
- Physical examination:
  - abdomen (bladder distention, flank tenderness)
  - external genitalia (phimosis, meatal stenosis, urethral mass/induration)
  - digital rectal examination (DRE). Document prostate size, consistency, symmetry and tenderness
- Laboratory tests:
  - urinalysis (and urine culture if pyuria)
  - prostate specific antigen (PSA); recommended in patients who have a life expectancy >10 years and for whom knowledge of the presence of prostate cancer would change management.[1] PSA can be used as a surrogate marker of prostate size in benign disease and may predict the risk of BPH progression.[1] The Canadian Cancer Society recommends that patients discuss the potential benefits and harms of PSA testing with their family physician[2]
- Other diagnostic tests are occasionally required when the history is not clear, physical examination or laboratory tests reveal abnormalities, or the response to treatment is unsatisfactory:
  - serum creatinine
  - cystourethroscopy
  - urodynamic studies
  - renal/bladder/transrectal ultrasonography
  - iv urography
  - CT abdomen and pelvis

Therapeutic Choices

Nonpharmacologic Choices

- Manage minimal symptoms with reassurance and active surveillance (regular reassessment).
- Advise patients with problematic nocturia to avoid caffeine-containing beverages and alcohol in the evening.
- Advise patients with pedal edema to elevate legs prior to retiring.

Pharmacologic Choices

The $alpha_1$-adrenergic antagonists, **alfuzosin**, **doxazosin**, **silodosin**, **tamsulosin** and **terazosin**, and the 5-alpha-reductase inhibitors, **dutasteride** and **finasteride**, are all useful in improving symptoms (Figure 1, Table 2).

Figure 1: Management of Benign Prostatic Hyperplasia

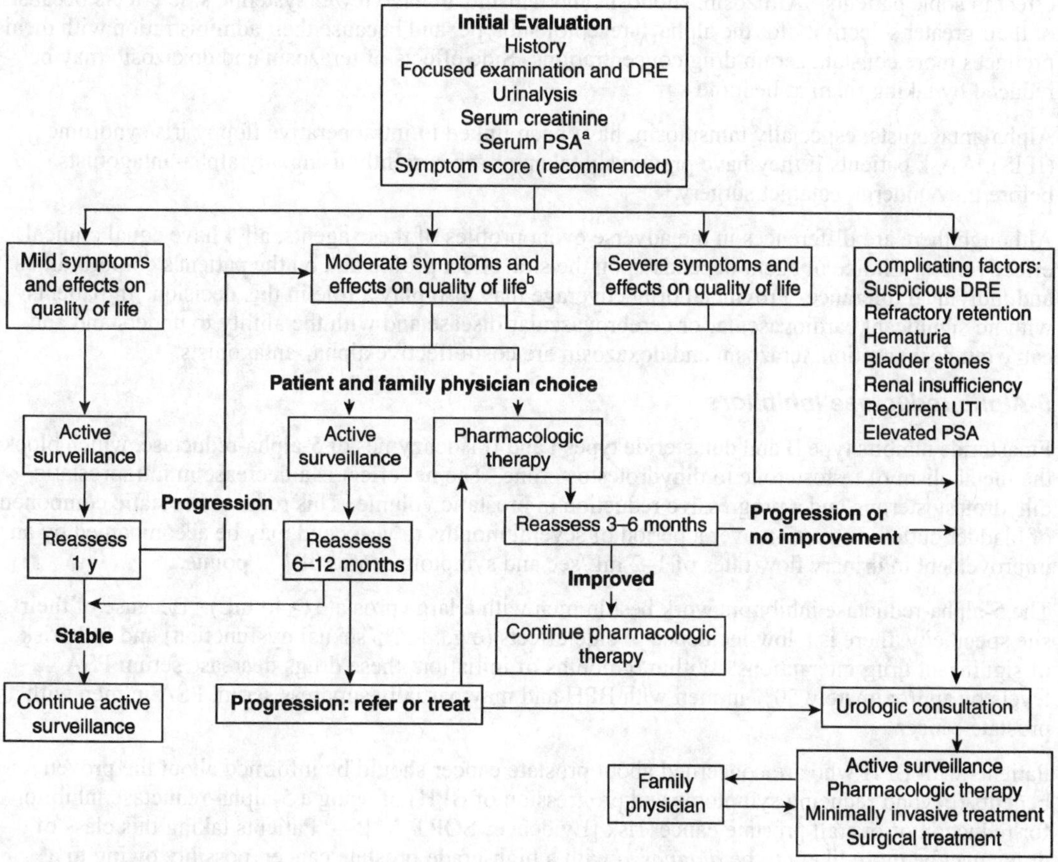

Abbreviations: DRE = digital rectal examination; PSA = prostate specific antigen; UTI = urinary tract infection

[a] Routine PSA testing in men without symptoms (screening) is not recommended (see Investigations)

[b] Consultation with a urologist at this juncture is an option depending on the comfort level of the treating physician

Alpha$_1$-adrenergic Antagonists

Alfuzosin, doxazosin, silodosin, tamsulosin and terazosin are the agents most commonly used to block alpha$_1$-adrenergic receptors that mediate muscular activity in the bladder neck, prostate and prostatic capsule, reducing the dynamic component of bladder outlet obstruction. Over a period of days to weeks, this may improve urinary flow rates by 1–3 mL/sec and symptom scores by 1–3 points. The effectiveness of the alpha$_1$-adrenergic antagonists is not influenced by prostate size.

To avoid first-dose syncope, start doxazosin and terazosin at a low dosage and gradually increase until symptomatic improvement or intolerance occurs. Dose titration is not necessary with alfuzosin, silodosin and tamsulosin because of their greater selectivity for the alpha$_{1A}$-receptor subtype which predominates in the prostate, bladder neck and urethra.

Side effects of alpha-antagonists include dizziness (10–20%), headaches (15%), asthenia (5–15%) and nasal congestion (5–10%). Retrograde ejaculation develops in 28% of men taking silodosin and 5–10% taking tamsulosin. Alpha-antagonists may potentiate other antihypertensive medications, and caution should be used when they are added to an ongoing regimen, particularly in the elderly. Doxazosin and sildenafil, taken within hours of each other, may result in an undesirable hypotensive effect in some patients.[3] Alfuzosin, silodosin and tamsulosin have fewer systemic side effects because of their greater selectivity for the alpha$_{1A}$-receptor subtype, and because their administration with meals produces more constant serum drug concentrations. Side effects of terazosin and doxazosin may be reduced by taking them at bedtime.

Alpha-antagonists, especially tamsulosin, have been linked to intraoperative floppy iris syndrome (IFIS).[4,5] Ask patients if they have previously taken or are currently using any alpha-antagonists before they undergo cataract surgery.[4]

Although there are differences in the adverse event profiles of these agents, all 4 have equal clinical effectiveness. Choice of agent depends upon the side effect profile and on the patient's comorbidities and individual tolerance. Provincial drug coverage may also play a role in this decision. In patients with no significant cardiovascular or cerebrovascular disease and with the ability to understand and carry out dose titration, terazosin and doxazosin are cost-effective alpha$_1$-antagonists.

5-Alpha-reductase Inhibitors

Finasteride inhibits type II and dutasteride types I and II isoenzymes of 5-alpha-reductase, which blocks the metabolism of testosterone to dihydrotestosterone. The net effect is a decrease in intraprostatic dihydrotestosterone and a progressive reduction in prostatic volume. This reduces the static component of bladder outlet obstruction over a period of several months to years and may be accompanied by an improvement in urinary flow rates of 1–2 mL/sec and symptom scores of 1–2 points.

The 5-alpha-reductase inhibitors work best in men with a large prostate (≥40 mL).[6] Because of their site specificity, there is a low incidence of side effects (e.g., 3–4% sexual dysfunction) and little risk of significant drug interactions. Within 6 months of initiation, these drugs decrease serum PSA levels by approximately 50% in men with BPH and may partially suppress serum PSA in men with prostate cancer.

Patients with BPH who are concerned about prostate cancer should be informed about the proven benefits (beyond reducing symptoms and progression of BPH) of using a 5-alpha-reductase inhibitor for reduction of overall prostate cancer risk [Evidence: SORT A*].[7,8,9] Patients taking this class of drugs may be more likely to be *diagnosed* with a high-grade prostate cancer, possibly owing to a

* SORT (Strength of Recommendation Taxonomy) is a rating system (A, B or C) that addresses the quality of available evidence. For more information consult **How to Use *Compendium of Therapeutic Choices*** on page xxv.

detection bias caused by the reduction in prostate volume and the improved performance of the PSA test.[10,11] Neither finasteride nor dutasteride is approved for prevention of prostate cancer in Canada.[12]

Combination Alpha$_1$-adrenergic Antagonist and 5-Alpha-reductase Inhibitor Therapy

The combination of an alpha$_1$-adrenergic antagonist and a 5-alpha-reductase inhibitor is an appropriate and effective treatment for patients with LUTS associated with demonstrable prostatic enlargement.[13]

Give patients who are successfully treated with combination therapy the option of discontinuing the alpha-antagonist after 6–12 months.[14] If symptoms recur, restart the alpha-antagonist.

Antimuscarinics

Antimuscarinic agents (alone or in combination with an alpha$_1$-adrenergic antagonist) are safe and effective in men with predominant or persistently bothersome storage symptoms.[15] These agents are associated with a minimal risk of urinary retention which tends to occur during the first month of treatment.[15,16] Use these drugs with caution in patients with residual urine volume >200 mL and a history of spontaneous episodes of urinary retention. There are numerous drug choices and some effort may be required to find the one that works best in an individual patient with the least side effects and at the best cost (see Chapter 68).

Phosphodiesterase Type 5 Inhibitors

Tadalafil is the only phosphodiesterase type 5 inhibitor (PDE5I) indicated for the daily management of erectile dysfunction, LUTS associated with BPH or both. Its precise mechanism in improving LUTS is unknown but several trials have shown the benefit of 5 mg daily based upon a reduction in total International Prostate Symptom Scores.[17,18,19,20] Men taking nitrate-based drugs, such as nitroglycerin, should not take tadalafil as it can lead to a dangerous decrease in blood pressure. Use of a PDE5I and an alpha$_1$-adrenergic antagonist in combination leads to improved LUTS compared to alpha$_1$-adrenergic antagonist monotherapy.[21]

Phytotherapeutic Agents

Saw palmetto is the most popular and studied plant extract used to reduce symptoms related to BPH. Some patients report a favourable response but published trials fail to show any benefit greater than placebo.[22,23] Identification and pharmacokinetics of active ingredients are often unclear in phytotherapeutic mixtures. Until more information regarding their mode of action and long-term efficacy and safety becomes available in quality studies, their use cannot be recommended.[24]

Procedures

While transurethral resection of the prostate (TURP) and retropubic prostatectomy are traditional means of dealing with an enlarged and obstructing prostate gland, transurethral incision of the prostate (TUIP) and various forms of laser prostatectomy are useful in some patients (Table 1). Long-term catheter drainage or clean intermittent catheterization are appropriate options for patients who are not candidates for any other intervention.

Therapeutic Tips

- Patients with minimal symptoms that do not interfere with their normal activities should be managed by active surveillance and regular follow-up.
- Patients starting to develop progressive symptoms or who are moderately inconvenienced or bothered by them are candidates for pharmacologic intervention.
- Continue drug therapy indefinitely since symptoms recur when medication is stopped.
- Complicating factors or unexpected (or lack of) response to any intervention are indications for urologic consultation.

- Avoid decongestants and other drugs with alpha-adrenergic activity because they can stimulate smooth muscle in the bladder neck and prostate, and increase obstruction.
- Drugs with anticholinergic activity may reduce detrusor contractility. Although they may be less problematic than previously thought in patients with symptoms of bladder outlet obstruction, these agents should be used with caution.[25]

Table 1: **Procedures for Benign Prostatic Hyperplasia**

Procedure	Description/Efficacy	Adverse Effects	Comments
Laser prostatectomy (various types)	1-day hospital stay; 80% reduction in symptoms.	Little or no bleeding.	Preferred technique for patients requiring anticoagulants or with uncorrected coagulopathies; long-term data awaited.
Retropubic prostatectomy	Open surgery; 3–5 days in hospital; similar efficacy to TURP.	Retrograde ejaculation (80–90%); bladder neck contracture (2–3%).	For very enlarged prostates or when required to correct other bladder pathology.
Transurethral incision of prostate (TUIP)	Outpatient; 80% reduction in symptoms.	Retrograde ejaculation (6–55%).	Useful for smaller prostates.
Transurethral resection of prostate (TURP)	1–2 days in hospital; gold standard for efficacy (85–90% reduction in symptoms).	Retrograde ejaculation (50–95%), urethral strictures (3%), bladder neck contracture (3–10%), re-resection (3–8%).	For moderately enlarged prostates.

Table 2: **Drugs Used in The Management of Benign Prostatic Hyperplasia**

Class	Drug	Dose	Adverse Effects	Drug Interactions	Comments	Cost[a]
5-Alpha-reductase Inhibitors	*dutasteride* Avodart	0.5 mg once daily po	Sexual dysfunction (3–4%).	Combination with strong CYP3A4 inhibitors (e.g., ketoconazole, ritonavir) may increase serum concentration of dutasteride. Monitor for increased adverse reactions, e.g., erectile dysfunction, decreased libido.	Blocks types I and II isoenzymes. Decreases prostate-specific antigen. Early response seen in 6 months.	$$$
	finasteride Proscar, generics	5 mg once daily po	See dutasteride.	No known clinically significant drug interactions.	Blocks type II isoenzyme. Decreases prostate-specific antigen. Early response seen in 6 months.	$$
$Alpha_1$-adrenergic Antagonists, nonselective	*doxazosin* Cardura, generics	1–12 mg QHS po Dose titrated weekly to desired response	Dizziness, headaches, asthenia and nasal congestion (5–20%); syncope (<1%).	Possible additive hypotension when combined with beta-blockers. Monitor blood pressure. May precipitate hypotension in conjunction with phosphodiesterase type 5 inhibitors (e.g., sildenafil).	Maximal response seen in weeks. May rarely cause intraoperative floppy iris syndrome. Patients undergoing cataract surgery should inform their ophthalmologist if they are or were using an α_1-adrenergic antagonist.[5]	$-$$
	terazosin Hytrin, generics	1–10 mg QHS po Dose titrated weekly to desired response	See doxazosin.	See doxazosin.	See doxazosin.	$-$$
$Alpha_{1A}$-adrenergic Antagonists, selective	*alfuzosin* Xatral, generics	10 mg once daily po after the same meal each day	Constipation (1.1%), dizziness (5.7%), fatigue (2.7%), headache (3%), nausea (1.1%), upper respiratory tract infection (6.1%).	Possible additive hypotension when combined with beta blockers. Monitor blood pressure. Avoid combination with potent CYP3A4 inhibitors (e.g., ketoconazole, ritonavir). Excessive hypotension may occur.	See doxazosin. Shown to have a role in management of acute urinary retention.	$

(cont'd)

Table 2: **Drugs Used in The Management of Benign Prostatic Hyperplasia** *(cont'd)*

Class	Drug	Dose	Adverse Effects	Drug Interactions	Comments	Cost[a]
	silodosin Rapaflo	8 mg once daily po after the same meal each day. 4 mg once daily in patients with moderate renal impairment (ClCr 30–50 mL/min)	Diarrhea (2.6%), dizziness (3.2%), headache (2.4%), nasal congestion (2.1%), orthostatic hypotension (2.6%), retrograde ejaculation (28%).	Increased silodosin blood levels when combined with P-glycoprotein inhibitors (e.g., cyclosporine) or potent CYP3A4 inhibitors (e.g., clarithromycin, itraconazole, ketoconazole, ritonavir). No dose adjustment is required if combined with moderate CYP3A4 inhibitors (e.g., diltiazem).	See doxazosin. Contraindicated in patients with severe renal impairment (ClCr <30 mL/min). Not recommended in severe hepatic insufficiency or if also using potent CYP3A4 inhibitors.	$$$
	tamsulosin controlled-release Flomax CR, generics	0.4 mg once daily po at the same time each day, with or without food	Dizziness (1–10%), retrograde ejaculation (5–10%).	No known clinically significant drug interactions.	See doxazosin. Swallow pills whole; do not crush or chew.	$
5-Alpha-reductase Inhibitors and Alpha$_{1A}$-adrenergic Antagonists Combinations	*dutasteride/tamsulosin modified release* Jalyn	0.5 mg dutasteride/ 0.4 mg tamsulosin (1 capsule) po 30 minutes after the same meal each day	Breast disorders (1%), decreased libido (5%), dizziness (1%), ejaculation disorders (8%), impotence (5%). All are most pronounced within first 6 months of treatment.	See dutasteride.	See dutasteride. See tamsulosin controlled-release. Contact with the contents of the dutasteride soft gelatin capsule contained within the hard-shell capsule may irritate the oropharyngeal mucosa. Indicated for the treatment of moderate to severe symptomatic benign prostatic hyperplasia in men with enlarged prostates.	$$$
Phosphodi-esterase Type 5 Inhibitors	*tadalafil* Cialis	5 mg once daily po	Back pain (2%), dyspepsia (3%), flushing (2%), headache (3%), myalgia (2%), nasal congestion (2%). Rare: visual disturbances, permanent vision loss.	Contraindicated with nitrates (seek emergency care if chest pain presents within 24–48 hours of taking tadalafil; not to be given for 5 days after stopping long-acting nitrates). May cause hypotension if used with nonselective alpha-adrenergic antagonists (e.g., doxazosin).	Not recommended for those with severe renal or hepatic impairment.	$$$$$

[a] Cost of 30-day supply; includes drug cost only.
Legend: $ <$25 $-$$ <$25–50 $$ $25–50 $$$ $50–75 $$$$ $75–100 $$$$$ $100–125

Suggested Readings

Abrams P, Chapple C, Khoury S et al. Evaluation and treatment of lower urinary tract symptoms in older men. *J Urol* 2013;189(1 Suppl):S93-S101.

Burnett AL,Wein AJ. Benign prostatic hyperplasia in primary care: what you need to know. *J Urol* 2006;175(3 Pt 2):S19-24.

Carson CC. Combination of phosphodiesterase-5 inhibitors and alpha-blockers in patients with benign prostatic hyperplasia: treatments of lower urinary tract symptoms, erectile dysfunction, or both? *BJU Int* 2006;97(Suppl 2):39-43.

Hao N, Tian Y, Liu W et al. Antimuscarinics and α-blockers or α-blockers monotherapy on lower urinary tract symptoms—a meta-analysis. *Urology* 2014;83(3):556-62.

Lee SW, Choi JB, Lee KS et al. Transurethral procedures for lower urinary tract symptoms resulting from benign prostatic enlargement: a quality and meta-analysis. *Int Neurourol J* 2013;17(2):59-66.

Oelke M, Bachmann A, Descazeaud A et al. EAU guidelines on the treatment and follow-up of non-neurogenic male lower urinary tract symptoms including benign prostatic obstruction. *Eur Urol* 2013;64(1):118-40.

References

1. Nickel JC, Mendez-Probst CE, Whelan TF et al. 2010 Update: guidelines for the management of benign prostatic hyperplasia. *Can Urol Assoc J* 2010;4(5):310-6.
2. Canadian Cancer Society. *About PSA testing*. Available from: /www.cancer.ca/en/prevention-and-screening/early-detection-and-screening/finding-cancer-early/finding-prostate-cancer/about-psa-testing/?region=nl. Accessed March 7, 2014.
3. Pfizer. *Viagra (sildenafil citrate) tablets*. New York (NY): Pfizer Labs; 2011. Available from: www.pfizer.com/files/products/uspi_viagra.pdf. Accessed March 7, 2014.
4. Chaga DF, Braga-Mele R, Mamalis N et al. ASCRS White Paper: clinical review of intraoperative floppy-iris syndrome. *J Cataract Refract Surg* 2008;34(12):2153-62.
5. Chatziralli IP, Sergentanis TN. Risk factors for intraoperative floppy iris syndrome: a meta-analysis. *Ophthalmology* 2011;118(4):730-5.
6. McConnell JD, Roehrborn CG, Bautista OM et al. The long-term effect of doxazosin, finasteride, and combination therapy on the clinical progression of benign prostatic hyperplasia. *N Engl J Med* 2003;349(25):2387-98.
7. Thompson IM, Goodman PJ, Tangen CM et al. The influence of finasteride on the development of prostate cancer. *N Engl J Med* 2003;349(3):215-24.
8. Andriole GL, Bostwick DG, Brawley OW et al. Effect of dutasteride on the risk of prostate cancer. *N Engl J Med* 2010;362(13):1192-202.
9. Wilt TJ, Macdonald R, Hagerty K et al. 5-α-Reductase inhibitors for prostate cancer chemoprevention: an updated Cochrane systematic review. *BJU Int* 2010;106(10):1444-51.
10. Klotz L, Saad F; PCPT-MTOPS Consensus Panel. PCPT, MTOPS and the use of 5-ARIs: a Canadian consensus regarding implications for clinical practice. *Can Urol Assoc J* 2007;1(1):17-21.
11. Klotz L, Chetner M, Chin J et al. Canadian Consensus Conference: The FDA decision on the use of 5ARIs. *Can Urol Assoc J* 2012;6(2):83-8.
12. Health Canada. *Finasteride (Proscar, Propecia) and dutasteride (Avodart, Jalyn): may increase the risk of high-grade prostate cancer*. Available from: www.healthycanadians.gc.ca/recall-alert-rappel-avis/hc-sc/2012/13665a-eng.php. Accessed March 7, 2014.
13. Füllhase C, Chapple C, Cornu JN et al. Systematic review of combination drug therapy for non-neurogenic male lower urinary tract symptoms. *Eur Urol* 2013;64(2):228-43.
14. Baldwin KC, Ginsberg PC, Roehrborn CG et al. Discontinuation of alpha-blockade after initial treatment with finasteride and doxazosin in men with lower urinary tract symptoms and clinical evidence of benign prostatic hyperplasia. *Urology* 2001;58(2):203-9.
15. Kaplan SA, Roehrborn CG, Abrams P et al. Antimuscarinics for treatment of storage lower urinary tract symptoms in men: a systematic review. *Int J Clin Pract* 2011;65(4):487-507.
16. Filson CP, Hollingsworth JM, Clemens JQ et al. The efficacy and safety of combined therapy with α-blockers and anticholinergics for men with benign prostatic hyperplasia: a meta-analysis. *J Urol* 2013;190(6):2153-60.
17. Andersson KE, de Groat WC, McVary KT et al. Tadalafil for the treatment of lower urinary tract symptoms secondary to benign prostatic hyperplasia: pathophysiology and mechanism(s) of action. *Neurourol Urodyn* 2011;30(3):292-301.
18. Egerdie RB, Auerbach S, Roehrborn CG et al. Tadalafil 2.5 or 5 mg administered once daily for 12 weeks in men with both erectile dysfunction and signs and symptoms of benign prostatic hyperplasia: results of a randomized, placebo-controlled, double-blind study. *J Sex Med* 2012;9(1):271-81.
19. Porst H, Kim ED, Casabé AR et al. Efficacy and safety of tadalafil once daily in the treatment of men with lower urinary tract symptoms suggestive of benign prostatic hyperplasia: results of an international randomized, double-blind, placebo-controlled trial. *Eur Urol* 2011;60(5):1105-13.
20. Oelke M, Giuliano F, Mirone V et al. Monotherapy with tadalafil or tamsulosin similarly improved lower urinary tract symptoms suggestive of benign prostatic hyperplasia in an international, randomised, parallel, placebo-controlled clinical trial. *Eur Urol* 2012;61(5):917-25.
21. Gacci M, Corona G, Salvi M et al. A systematic review and meta-analysis on the use of phosphodiesterase 5 inhibitors alone or in combination with α-blockers for lower urinary tract symptoms due to benign prostatic hyperplasia. *Eur Urol* 2012;61(5):994-1003.
22. Tacklind J, MacDonald R, Rutks I et al. Serenao repens for benign prostatic hyperplasia. *Cochrane Database Syst Rev* 2012;12:CD001423.
23. Bent S, Kane C, Shinohara K et al. Saw palmetto for benign prostatic hyperplasia. *N Engl J Med* 2006;354(6):557-66.
24. Dedhia RC, McVary KT. Phytotherapy for lower urinary tract symptoms secondary to benign prostatic hyperplasia. *J Urol* 2008;179(6):2119-25.
25. Blake-James BT, Rashidian A, Ikeda Y et al. The role of anticholinergics in men with lower urinary tract symptoms suggestive of benign prostatic hyperplasia: a systematic review and meta-analysis. *BJU Int* 2007;99(1):85-96.

Chapter 68
Urinary Incontinence in Adults

Cheryl A. Sadowski, B.Sc.(Pharm), PharmD, FCSHP

Urinary incontinence (UI) is the complaint of involuntary leakage of urine.[1] The lower urinary tract symptoms can be broadly described as relating to storage dysfunction or voiding dysfunction.[2,3] There are a number of types of urinary incontinence: stress, urge and overflow.[4] *Stress incontinence* is the most common form of UI in women. It is due to the loss of small amounts of urine secondary to an increase in intra-abdominal pressure (e.g., cough, exercise). In urethral hypermobility the urethra drops below the pelvic floor muscles when the support provided by those muscles is relaxed or lost thus exerting pressure on the bladder neck exceeding that on the urethra which in turn may cause urine leakage. Intrinsic sphincter deficiency is a less common form of stress incontinence and may occur after pelvic surgery or irradiation, anti-incontinence procedure, vaginal birth or in conjunction with a neurologic problem. *Urge incontinence* usually involves leakage of moderate to large amounts of urine due to inability to delay voiding when an urge is perceived. Overactive bladder is a syndrome that includes urgency and can lead to urge incontinence. Causes include bladder wall hyperactivity or instability and CNS disorders (e.g., parkinsonism, stroke, spinal cord injury, multiple sclerosis). *Mixed incontinence* is a common type of UI in women and includes features of both stress and urge incontinence. Chronic retention of urine often involves leakage of urine due to a distended bladder, commonly due to detrusor underactivity, neurogenic bladder (e.g., diabetic neuropathy) or outlet obstruction (e.g., prostatic hyperplasia), which leads to *overflow incontinence* when the amount of urine retained produces pressure beyond the sphincter or obstruction pressure. *Functional incontinence* is the loss of urine caused by the inability to get to or use the toilet, and does not involve changes in the lower urinary tract. Causes include physical constraints (e.g., restricted mobility, difficulty removing clothing), cognitive factors (e.g., depression, dementia) and environmental barriers (access to toilet, positioning).

Goals of Therapy

- Relieve urinary symptoms
- Prevent complications (e.g., skin breakdown, urinary tract infections)
- Improve quality of life
- Avoid treatment side effects
- Increase functional capacity of the bladder

Investigations

Screening questions:[5,6,7,8,9,10,11]

- In the past 3 months, did you leak urine?
- Do you ever lose urine when you don't want to?
- How often do you leak urine?
- Do you ever leak urine when you cough, laugh or exercise?
- Do you ever leak urine on the way to the bathroom?
- Do you have difficulty getting to the toilet?

- Do you ever use pads, tissue or cloth in your underwear to catch urine?
- Do you ever feel that you are unable to completely empty your bladder?

If positive:[2,12,13,14]

- Thorough history with attention to:
  - previous treatments (medical and surgical) for urinary symptoms
  - medical and surgical history (including obstetric history)
  - characteristics of symptoms (e.g., onset, frequency and severity of symptoms, degree of bother)
  - possible causes such as diabetes, depression, mobility or cognitive limitations, previous bladder surgeries or neurologic conditions such as multiple sclerosis, stroke or spinal cord injury
  - modifiable risk factors (Table 1)
  - bladder diary for 3 days to determine fluid intake, frequency, timing and amount of voiding and urine leakage
  - bowel habits
  - medications
- Physical examination:
  - review of systems
  - mental status, cognition
  - pelvic examination (to rule out pelvic masses, organ prolapse, latent stress incontinence)
  - neurologic examination (if patient has symptoms of a neurologic disease)
  - rectal examination
  - physical impairment (dexterity, mobility, vision)
- Investigations:
  - cough test (to detect stress incontinence)
  - urinalysis (to rule out infection, glucosuria, hematuria)
  - renal function tests (urea, serum creatinine, glucose and calcium) if renal dysfunction suspected or polyuria present
  - urodynamic testing may be used to measure detrusor compliance and contractility, postvoid residual volume and bladder capacity

Table 1: **Modifiable Risk Factors for Urinary Incontinence in Adults**[7,8,10,15,16,17,18]

Caffeine intake
Benign prostatic hyperplasia in men
Bowel problems (constipation, fecal impaction)
Fluid intake (1.5–2 L/day is considered appropriate)
Lower urinary tract conditions (urinary tract infection, urogenital atrophy)
Obesity (notably abdominal)
Smoking[7]
Medications (alcohol, alpha-agonists, alpha-antagonists, anticholinergics, cholinergic agonists, diuretics, psychotropics, sedative hypnotics, sympatholytics)
Restricted mobility/environmental issues (includes dexterity in clothing removal, accessibility to toilets)

Stress Incontinence

Therapeutic Choices

Due to safety concerns and, in some cases, limited clinical benefit of pharmacologic efficacy, nonpharmacologic interventions are first line. If behavioural therapies are ineffective, surgery may be considered in some cases (Figure 1).

Figure 1: Management of Urinary Incontinence in Adults[12]

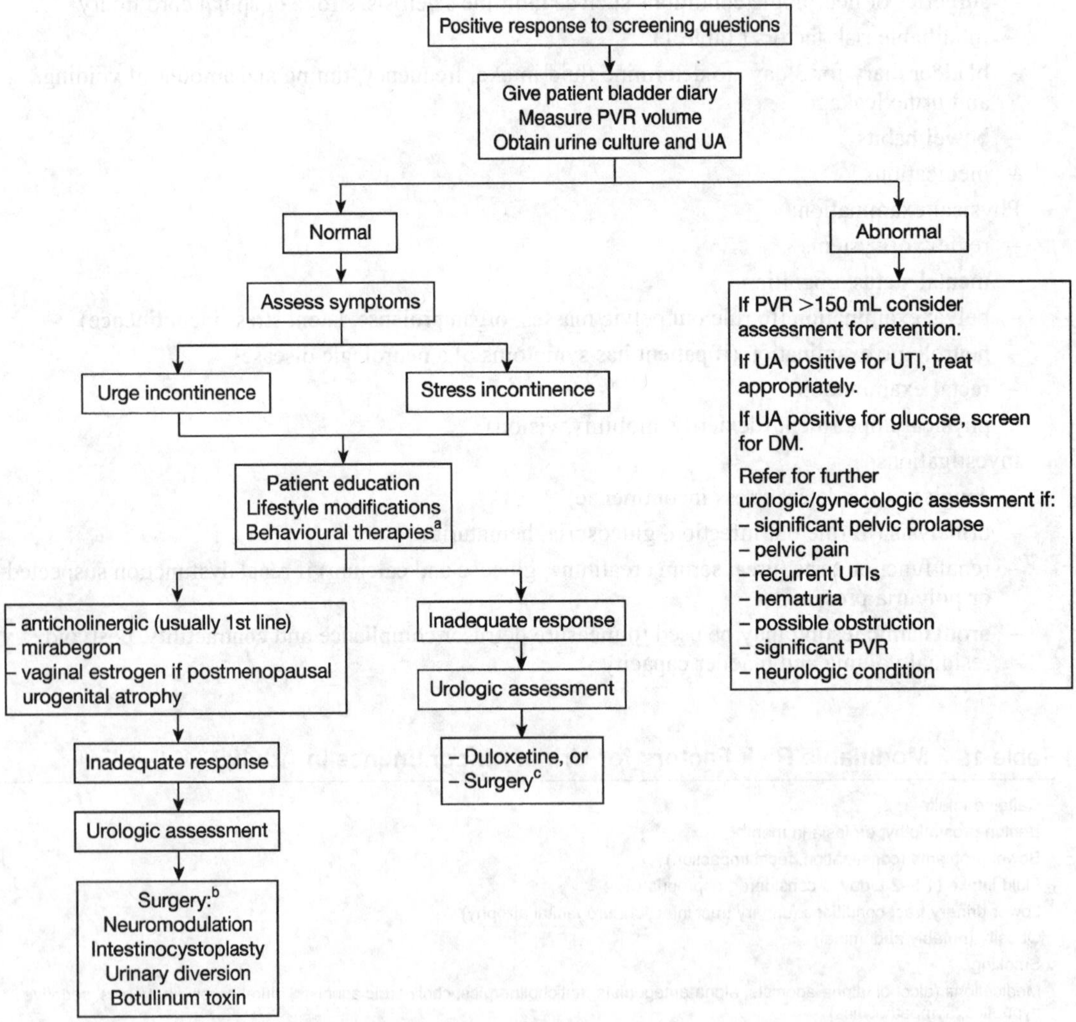

[a] In most circumstances it is appropriate to initiate treatment without referral for urologic testing.
[b] In the management of urge incontinence, consider surgical options only after failure of noninvasive treatments, including pharmacotherapy.
[c] In the management of stress incontinence, surgery may be recommended first-line due to limited efficacy of pharmacotherapy.
Abbreviations: DM = diabetes mellitus; PVR = postvoid residual; TVT = tension-free vaginal tape; UA = urinalysis
Adapted with permission from Culligan PJ. Urinary incontinence in women: evaluation and management. *Am Fam Physician* 2000;62(11):2433-44,2447,2452.

Nonpharmacologic Choices

When secondary causes have been ruled out or treated, initiate behavioural therapy:[12,14,19,20,21,22,23,24,25,26]

- *Pelvic floor muscle training (Kegel exercises):* 12–20 muscle contractions 3–5 times per day (goal of 10 seconds for each contraction); may take 6–8 weeks to see results[27,28]
- *Bladder training (timed voiding):* maintain a voiding schedule (e.g., 1-hour voiding interval) which is gradually (e.g., weekly) increased to a reasonable interval (e.g., voiding every 2–3 hours) with minimal incontinence episodes[22]
- *Biofeedback* and/or *electrical stimulation therapy:* stimulation that teaches the patient to isolate and control pelvic floor muscles

In some women with vaginal prolapse, a pessary may be appropriate.[29] Weighted vaginal cones are also an option, which result in pelvic floor muscle training similar to Kegel exercises.

Surgical options depend on the etiology. In females, bladder neck slings are most often used for intrinsic sphincter deficiency while mid-urethral slings are most common for urethral hypermobility.[30,31,32,33,34,35] However, the American Urologic Association Guidelines do not recommend one therapy over the other.[36] Alternatives include bulking agents, although this procedure is less effective and does not last as long as a surgical intervention.[36] As a last line, retropubic suspension may be considered for some patients.[37] For males who have undergone prostatectomy, sling procedures are first-line interventions. Alternatives include artificial sphincters and, as a last line, bulking agents.

Pharmacologic Choices

Table 3 details the drugs used in the management of stress incontinence.

While *vaginal* **estrogen** therapy has been shown in some trials to improve symptoms of stress incontinence, the overall supporting evidence is weak and the benefit is not significant.[38] However, vaginal estrogen therapy may be considered in select cases if the postmenopausal patient is diagnosed with mixed urinary incontinence and vaginal atrophy. *Systemic* estrogen therapy (transdermal or oral administration) does not offer benefits and may worsen symptoms of UI.[39,40,41,42,43] The decision to use estrogen therapy must be discussed with the patient in the context of her individual health needs and risk factors (e.g., breast cancer, venous thromboembolism, MI).

Adrenergic agonists are ineffective in the treatment of stress UI and are associated with toxicities (e.g., cardiac), which is of concern in older adults.[19,44]

Duloxetine, a serotonin-norepinephrine reuptake inhibitor approved for use in depression, anxiety, fibromyalgia and neuropathic pain, has also been studied for the treatment of stress incontinence. This medication influences the micturition reflex centrally.[45,46] Duloxetine decreases the rate of UI and improves quality of life scores (Table 3).[19,47] Duloxetine is generally well tolerated with minor adverse effects. However, all antidepressants in Canada have a warning regarding self-harm. In addition, duloxetine has the potential for numerous drug interactions, may cause hepatotoxicity and is not indicated in Canada for the treatment of UI.

Urge Incontinence

Therapeutic Choices

Figure 1 outlines the management of urinary incontinence in adults and Table 4 details the medications available for the treatment of urge incontinence.

Nonpharmacologic Choices

When secondary causes have been ruled out or treated, initiate behavioural therapy:

- *Pelvic floor muscle training:* although primarily prescribed for stress UI, Kegel exercises (as described under stress incontinence) may also benefit urge UI
- *Bladder training (timed voiding):* as described under stress incontinence
- *Biofeedback training:* as described under stress incontinence

Pharmacologic Choices

Antimuscarinics (**darifenacin, fesoterodine, oxybutynin, solifenacin, tolterodine, trospium**) are first-line treatment for urge incontinence (Table 4). These medications have been shown to increase bladder capacity, improve urge symptoms, enhance quality of life and reduce incontinence episodes up to 50%.[19,48,49] However, the clinical significance in some patients may be small.[49,50,51] They can be combined with nonpharmacologic therapies for added benefit.[49,52,53,54]

Anticholinergic effects from these antimuscarinic products include dry mouth, delirium, increased intraocular pressure and worsening glaucoma, slowing of gastric motility (including constipation), decreased secretions (including dry eyes) and the potential for changes in heart rate and rhythm, all of which are of greater concern in older adults and often lead to early discontinuation of therapy.[24,50,55,56] To minimize side effects start at a low dose and titrate slowly. Vigilant monitoring is required when using antimuscarinic medications in older adults, since these patients are more susceptible to their adverse effects. The newer agents (darifenacin, solifenacin, trospium) and new formulations (oxybutynin *patch* and *gel*) demonstrate reduced side effects compared with traditional anticholinergic therapy and may improve adherence.[57,58,59,60]

Currently, systemic **estrogen** does not have a place in therapy in the treatment of postmenopausal urge incontinence.[2,12,19,61] A secondary analysis of the Women's Health Initiative trial[62] found an increased risk of urge incontinence with oral estrogen. *Vaginal* estrogen for women with postmenopausal urogenital atrophy may be an option as an adjunct to behavioural or pharmacologic treatment (Table 3).[38,41,42,61] The decision to use estrogen therapy must be discussed with the patient in the context of her individual health needs and risk factors (e.g., breast cancer, venous thromboembolism, MI).

Mirabegron is a beta$_3$-adrenergic agonist indicated for the treatment of urge incontinence. Compared to placebo, mirabegron is effective in reducing the number of incontinence and micturition episodes (about 1 less episode of each every 2 days).[63,64,65] The most common adverse effects of mirabegron include hypertension, tachycardia, nasopharyngitis and urinary tract infections. Uncommon but significant adverse effects include QTc prolongation. Due to its potentially significant cardiac adverse effects, high cost and lack of long-term data especially in frail older adults, consider mirabegron in patients who have failed first-line therapies [Evidence: SORT C*].[63,64,65]

Tricyclic antidepressants (e.g., **desipramine, doxepin, imipramine, nortriptyline**) are not recommended for the management of urinary incontinence.[66,67]

Intravesicular **botulinum toxin** decreases urge incontinence and has become increasingly common as a therapy for individuals who cannot tolerate or do not respond to first-line antimuscarinic therapies.[68,69] Although this is a relatively noninvasive procedure compared to surgery its long term safety requires further study.

Mixed Incontinence

Treat patients with mixed UI for the predominant symptom (e.g., stress or urge symptoms). See Stress Incontinence and Urge Incontinence.

* SORT (Strength of Recommendation Taxonomy) is a rating system (A, B or C) that addresses the quality of available evidence. For more information consult **How to Use *Compendium of Therapeutic Choices*** on page xxv.

Chronic Retention of Urine

Therapeutic Choices

Nonpharmacologic Choices

- Chronic retention of urine due to a contractile bladder is poorly responsive to behavioural or surgical therapy.[70]
- Surgery is the treatment of choice in many men with chronic urinary retention due to benign prostatic hyperplasia (see Chapter 67).[71]
- Use catheterization only for well-documented indications because it is associated with urinary tract infections (UTIs) and sepsis. For individuals who are either waiting for surgery or are not surgical candidates, catheterization may be a temporary or permanent option:
  - intermittent catheterization[72]
  - indwelling catheter: when intermittent catheterization is not possible for those in urinary retention[73]
- Discontinue drugs reported to induce or aggravate urinary retention (Table 2) if possible.

Pharmacologic Choices

Chronic retention of urine due to acontractile bladder is poorly responsive to pharmacologic therapy. A review found no support for the cholinergic agonist, **bethanechol**, for urinary retention in older adults.[75] Bethanechol has primarily been studied for postsurgical urinary retention.[76] For management of benign prostatic hyperplasia, see Chapter 67.

Choices during Pregnancy and Breastfeeding

Urinary Incontinence during Pregnancy

Urinary incontinence before pregnancy is extremely rare, affecting <1% of women.[77] However, during pregnancy stress incontinence is quite common.[78,79] The reports of urgency and frequency increase from the 1st to 3rd trimester, with rates of >80% by week 36.[80,81,82,83] The mechanism is thought to be increased maternal weight gain, mechanical pressure on the bladder and increased urine production.[84,85,86] Risk factors associated with urinary incontinence during pregnancy include advanced maternal age and higher BMI.[87]

Table 2: **Drugs that May Cause or Aggravate Urinary Retention[70,74]**

Antiarrhythmics	**Antihistamines**	**Sedatives/Hypnotics**
disopyramide	chlorpheniramine	diazepam
procainamide	diphenhydramine	flurazepam
quinidine	hydroxyzine	**Sympathomimetics (alpha-agonists)**
Anticholinergics	**Antiparkinsonian Agents**	ephedrine
benztropine	amantadine	phenylephrine
oxybutynin	bromocriptine	pseudoephedrine
scopolamine	levodopa	**Sympathomimetics (beta-agonists)**
tolterodine	**Antipsychotics**	isoproterenol
trihexyphenidyl	chlorpromazine	orciprenaline
Antidepressants	prochlorperazine	terbutaline
amitriptyline	**Muscle Relaxants**	**Miscellaneous**
doxepin	baclofen	carbamazepine
imipramine	cyclobenzaprine	nifedipine
	NSAIDs	

Many women report a resolution of urinary symptoms after delivery. However, pregnancy increases the prevalence of long-term stress incontinence and nocturia in women, especially those who have had >1 child.[88,89] The hypothesized mechanism is damage from childbirth to the urinary tract, pelvic floor musculature or the nervous system.[84,90] In addition, exposure to oxytocin in labour increases the risk of urinary incontinence in later life.[89] Episiotomy and operative vaginal delivery also increase the risk of subsequent pelvic floor dysfunction.[84] The nocturia may be due primarily to the endocrinologic changes.[90]

Management

The emphasis in pregnancy is on preventative measures. Use of oxytocin or a procedure such as an episiotomy may increase the risk of subsequent incontinence and should be discussed prior to the delivery.[84]

Treatment of urinary incontinence during pregnancy involves pelvic floor rehabilitation.[7,85] Multiple studies have demonstrated that incontinence could be prevented by starting pelvic floor muscle strengthening during pregnancy and in the early postpartum period.[91,92] Women may be referred to a physiotherapist or participate in a home-based exercise program.[85]

Urinary Incontinence during Breastfeeding

Many women will have resolution of urinary symptoms post-delivery. However, if pelvic floor injury occurs, symptoms may persist. While disruptive for the mother, this condition does not significantly impact the nursing child. While fluid intake has been considered by some to be the cause of urinary frequency, this is not supported by the medical literature.[85] However, this common misconception may affect the fluid intake of women who are nursing, thereby affecting milk production.

Management

The recommendations for management of postpartum urinary incontinence primarily focus on pelvic floor rehabilitation.[7,85]

A discussion of general principles on the use of medications in these special populations can be found in Appendix II and Appendix III. Other specialized reference sources are also provided in these appendices.

Therapeutic Tips

- Provide patient education regarding management alternatives (risks, benefits, realistic outcomes), determine patient expectations and involve the patient in the decision-making process.
- None of the pharmacologic interventions provides complete relief from incontinence episodes. Effectiveness is limited to reduction in incontinence episodes and severity of symptoms.
- Treat all secondary causes (e.g., UTI, lifestyle factors, medications or poor mobility) either before or concurrently with other management strategies.
- Several weeks of therapy may be required to achieve maximum effect.
- As initial therapy, recommend the strategy that is the least invasive, is reversible and has the fewest side effects.
- Scheduled toileting (at fixed times every 2–4 hours, based on individual toilet habits), habit training (toileting based on individual voiding patterns) and prompted voiding (checking for dryness, regular reminders and praising) are toileting assistance strategies that will help to keep chronically incontinent patients, particularly those in institutional settings, drier.
- Stress the importance of using absorbent products designed specifically for bladder problems, as they reduce odour and prevent skin breakdown. These products are not considered first-line

management but rather as adjuncts to other treatment measures. A thorough assessment is key in providing optimal continence care.

- Be attentive to medication persistence and adherence. The anticholinergic side effect of dry mouth is a common cause of patient-initiated dosage reduction or drug discontinuation.

Table 3: **Drug Therapy for Stress Incontinence in Women**

Class	Drug	Dose	Adverse Effects	Drug Interactions	Comments	Cost[a]
Estrogens, vaginal	*conjugated estrogens, vaginal cream* 0.625 mg/g Premarin Vaginal Cream	1.25–2.5 mg (2–4 g cream) daily pv (3 wk on, 1 wk off)	Abdominal pain (7.7%), breast pain (5.6%), migraine headaches (1.4%), peripheral edema (1.4%), vaginitis (5.6%), weight gain (2.1%); although systemic estrogen absorption occurs, the incidence of adverse effects varies with dose, drug and duration of therapy.	Systemic absorption variable; no serious interactions reported.	Although progestin administration is not required for occasional estrogen cream use, routine endometrial surveillance is recommended.[93] Adjust dosage and frequency of application as needed.	$$
	estradiol-17β, vaginal ring 2 mg Estring	1 ring Q3 months pv (delivers 7.5 µg daily)	See conjugated estrogens, vaginal cream.	See conjugated estrogens, vaginal cream.	Progestin administration is not necessary with estrogen vaginal rings. Routine endometrial surveillance is recommended.	$$$
	estradiol-17β, vaginal tablet Vagifem 10	1 tablet daily pv × 2 wk then 1 tablet twice weekly thereafter	See conjugated estrogens, vaginal cream.	See conjugated estrogens, vaginal cream.	Progestin administration is not necessary with estrogen vaginal tablets. Routine endometrial surveillance is recommended. Adjust dosage and frequency of application as needed.	$$$
	estrone, vaginal cream Estragyn Vaginal Cream	2–4 g daily pv (3 wk on, 1 wk off)	See conjugated estrogens, vaginal cream.	See conjugated estrogens, vaginal cream.	Adjust dosage and frequency of application as needed.	$$
Serotonin-Norepinephrine Reuptake Inhibitors	*duloxetine* Cymbalta	60 mg daily po A starting dose of 30 mg daily po × 1–2 wk may be considered for tolerability reasons in some patients, with a target dose of 60 mg/day	Tachycardia, blood pressure, palpitations; nausea, dry mouth, constipation, erectile dysfunction, flushing.	Substrate and inhibitor of CYP2D6. Contraindicated with MAO inhibitors (increased risk of serotonin syndrome). CYP1A2 or CYP2D6 inhibitors (e.g., bupropion, ciprofloxacin, fluoxetine, fluvoxamine, ketoconazole, norfloxacin, ofloxacin, paroxetine, quinidine and terbinafine) may decrease metabolism of duloxetine. CYP1A2 and CYP2D6 inducers (carbamazepine, phenobarbital, primidone, rifampin and smoking tobacco) may increase the metabolism of duloxetine.	Duloxetine is not approved for treatment of stress urinary incontinence in Canada. The doses available, 30 mg and 60 mg, are not consistent with the studied doses of 80 mg once daily or 40 mg twice daily. Duloxetine is not recommended for patients with end-stage renal disease (requiring dialysis) or in severe renal impairment (estimated ClCr <30 mL/min).	$$$$

[a] Cost of 30-day supply; includes drug cost only.
Legend: $ <$25 $$ $25–50 $$$ $50–75 $$$$ $75–100

Table 4: Drug Therapy for Urge Incontinence

Class	Drug	Dose	Adverse Effects	Drug Interactions	Comments	Cost[a]
Anticholinergics	*darifenacin, extended-release* Enablex	7.5 mg daily po After 2 weeks, may increase to 15 mg daily po if necessary	Primarily anticholinergic effects (dry mouth, constipation, tachycardia).	Potential additive anticholinergic effects with other drugs. Do not exceed 7.5 mg daily with potent inhibitors of CYP3A4 such as erythromycin, itraconazole, ketoconazole, nelfinavir, ritonavir. Caution with other substrates of CYP2D6 that have narrow therapeutic indices (e.g., TCAs as their clearance may be decreased).	Avoid in patients with severe hepatic insufficiency. There are no special dosing requirements for patients with renal impairment.	$$
	fesoterodine fumarate extended-release Toviaz	4 mg daily po May increase to 8 mg daily po if needed Limit dose to 4 mg daily if ClCr <30 mL/min or if strong CYP3A4 inhibitors are used concomitantly See Drug Interactions	Back pain (2%), constipation (4–6%), cough (2%), dry eyes (1–4%), dry mouth (19–34%).	Potential additive effects with other anticholinergic drugs. Potent CYP3A4 inhibitors (e.g., clarithromycin, itraconazole, ketoconazole) increase the concentration of the active metabolite of fesoterodine. CYP3A4 inducers (e.g., carbamazepine, rifampin) reduce the concentration of the active metabolite of fesoterodine and concomitant use is not recommended.	Should not be crushed or chewed. Avoid in severe hepatic Impairment. No dosing adjustment of fesoterodine is necessary if CYP450 inducers are used concomitantly.	$$$
	oxybutynin, immediate-release generics	2.5–5 mg daily–QID po	See darifenacin, extended-release.	Potential additive effects with other anticholinergic drugs.	Use with caution in patients with renal impairment. In older adults, prescribe the lowest recommended starting dose; when switching from immediate-release to extended-release formulation, use closest equivalent dose.	$
	oxybutynin, extended-release Ditropan XL	5–30 mg daily po	See darifenacin, extended-release.	See oxybutynin, immediate-release.	See oxybutynin, immediate-release. Extended-release formulation must not be divided, chewed or crushed.	$$$$

(cont'd)

Table 4: **Drug Therapy for Urge Incontinence** *(cont'd)*

Class	Drug	Dose	Adverse Effects	Drug Interactions	Comments	Cost[a]
	oxybutynin, 10% transdermal gel Gelnique	1 g (contents of 1 sachet or 1 metered-dose pump) applied once daily to dry, intact skin on the abdomen, thighs or upper arms/shoulders	Application site pruritus (2.1%), dizziness (1.5%), dry mouth (6.9%).	See oxybutynin, immediate-release.	Rotate application sites. Do not apply to a recently shaved skin surface or skin areas with eczema, seborrhea or psoriasis. Steady-state concentrations are achieved within 7 days of continuous dosing.	$$$
	oxybutynin, transdermal patch Oxytrol	1 patch applied to skin twice weekly (alternating sites); delivers 3.9 mg per day	See darifenacin, extended-release. Application site reactions.	See oxybutynin, immediate-release.	In older adults, prescribe the lowest recommended starting dose. Associated with a decreased incidence of anticholinergic side effects compared to oral oxybutynin and tolterodine. Use with caution in patients with hepatic or renal impairment.	$$
	solifenacin Vesicare	5 mg daily po May increase to 10 mg daily po if tolerated	See darifenacin, extended-release.	See oxybutynin, immediate-release. Do not exceed 5 mg daily with potent CYP3A4 inhibitors, e.g., erythromycin, itraconazole, nelfinavir, ritonavir.	Avoid in patients with severe hepatic insufficiency. Do not exceed 5 mg daily in severe renal impairment. Doses >5 mg are not recommended in patients with severe renal impairment (ClCr <30 mL/min).	$$
	tolterodine, immediate-release Detrol	1–2 mg BID po	See darifenacin, extended-release.	Potential additive effects with other anticholinergic drugs. CYP3A4 metabolism becomes significant in CYP2D6 poor metabolizers—maximum dose of 2 mg per day in patients taking potent inhibitors of CYP3A4 (e.g., erythromycin, itraconazole, ketoconazole, nelfinavir, ritonavir).	In older adults and those with severe renal impairment, prescribe the lowest recommended starting dose.	$$
	tolterodine, extended-release Detrol LA	2–4 mg once daily po	See darifenacin, extended-release.	See tolterodine, immediate-release. Coadministration of Detrol LA with antacid results in increased C_{max} of tolterodine and the potential for "dose-dumping." Tolterodine extended-release products may also be affected by PPI treatment.[94,95]	See tolterodine, immediate-release.	$$

Class	Drug	Dose	Adverse Effects	Drug Interactions	Comments	Cost[a]
	trospium Trosec	20 mg BID on an empty stomach In older patients or those with severe renal impairment do not exceed 20 mg QHS	See darifenacin, extended-release.	See oxybutynin, immediate-release.	Although it has been suggested that trospium may produce less central nervous system side effects than other anticholinergics, this advantage has not been demonstrated in clinical trials.	$$
Beta$_3$-adrenergic agonists	*mirabegron, extended release* Myrbetriq	25–50 mg once daily po In patients with severe renal impairment, moderate hepatic impairment or taking drugs metabolized by CYP2D6 and with a narrow therapeutic index, do not exceed 25 mg once daily po	Hypertension (11.3%), nasopharyngitis (3.5%), urinary tract infection (4.2%), tachycardia (1.6%).	Moderate inhibitor of CYP2D6 and weak inhibitor of P-gp. May increase level of substrates of CYP2D6 (desipramine, metoprolol) and Pg-p (digoxin, dabigatran). Coadministration with antimuscarinic agents may increase risk of urinary retention.	Should not be crushed or chewed. Should not be used in severe uncontrolled hypertension.	$$

[a] Cost of 30-day supply; includes drug cost only.
Legend: $ <$30 $$ $30–60 $$$ $60–90 $$$$ $90–120

Suggested Readings

Bettez M, Tu le M, Carlson K et al. 2012 update: guidelines for adult urinary incontinence collaborative consensus document for the Canadian Urological Assocation. *Can Urol Assoc J* 2012;6(5):354-63.

Cameron AP, Heidelbaugh JJ, Jimbo M. Diagnosis and office-based treatment of urinary incontinence in adults. Part one: diagnosis and testing. *Ther Adv Urol* 2013;5(4):181-7.

Cameron AP, Jimbo M, Heidelbaugh JJ. Diagnosis and office-based treatment of urinary incontinence in adults. Part two: treatment. *Ther Adv Urol* 2013;5(4):189-200.

Hersh L, Salzman B. Clinical management of urinary incontinence in women. *Am Fam Physician* 2013;87(9):634-40.

Marinkovic SP, Rovner ES, Moldwin RM et al. The management of overactive bladder syndrome. *BMJ* 2012;344:e2365.

Thirugnanasothy S. Managing urinary incontinence in older people. *BMJ* 2010;341:c3835.

References

1. Abrams P, Cardozo L, Fall M et al. The standardisation of terminology of lower urinary tract function: report from the Standardisation Sub-committee of the International Continence Society. *Neurourol Urodyn* 2002;21(2):167-78.
2. Abrams P, Andersson KE, Birder L et al. Fourth International Consultation on Incontinence Recommendations of the International Scientific Committee: Evaluation and treatment of urinary incontinence, pelvic organ prolapse, and fecal incontinence. *Neurourol Urodyn* 2010;29(1):213-40.
3. Vella M, Robinson D, Staskin D. A reappraisal of storage and voiding dysfunction. *Curr Urol Rep* 2012;13(6):482-7.
4. Haylen BT, de Ridder D, Freeman RM et al. An International Urogynecological Association (IUGA)/International Continence Society (ICS) joint report on the terminology for female pelvic floor dysfunction. *Int Urogynecol J* 2010;21(1):5-26.
5. Canadian Continence Foundation. *Initial management of UI in women, men and frail elderly*. Available from: www.canadiancontinence.ca/images/chart-initial-management-of-ui.gif. Accessed March 31, 2011.
6. Farrell SA, Epp A, Flood C et al. The evaluation of stress incontinence prior to primary surgery. *J Obstet Gynaecol Can* 2003;25(4):313-24.
7. Landefeld CS, Bowers BJ, Feld AD et al. National Institutes of Health state-of-the-science conference statement: prevention of fecal and urinary incontinence in adults. *Ann Intern Med* 2008;148(6):449-58.
8. Gibbs CF, Johnson TM, Ouslander JG. Office management of geriatric urinary incontinence. *Am J Med* 2007;120(3):211-20.
9. Holroyd-Leduc JM, Tannenbaum C, Thorpe KE et al. What type of urinary incontinence does this woman have? *JAMA* 2008;299(12):1446-56.
10. Cameron AP, Heidelbaugh JJ, Jimbo M. Diagnosis and office-based treatment of urinary incontinence in adults. Part one: diagnosis and testing. *Ther Adv Urol* 2013;5(4):181-7.
11. Brown JS, Bradley CS, Subak LL et al. The sensitivity and specificity of a simple test to distinguish between urge and stress urinary incontinence. *Ann Intern Med* 2006;144(10):715-23.
12. Bettez M, Tu le M, Carlson K et al. 2012 update: guidelines for adult urinary incontinence collaborative consensus document for the Canadian Urological Association. *Can Urol Assoc J* 2012;6(5):354-63.
13. Guzzo TJ, Drach GW. Major urologic problems in geriatrics: assessment and management. *Med Clin North Am* 2011;95(1):253-64.
14. Thirugnanasothy S. Managing urinary incontinence in older people. *BMJ* 2010;341:c3835.
15. Finkelstein MM. Medical conditions, medications, and urinary incontinence. Analysis of a population-based survey. *Can Fam Physician* 2002;48:96-101.
16. Landi F, Cesari M, Russo A et al. Potentially reversible risk factors and urinary incontinence in frail older people living in community. *Age Ageing* 2003;32(2):194-9.
17. Offermans MP, Du Moulin MF, Hamers JP et al. Prevalence of urinary incontinence and associated risk factors in nursing home residents: a systematic review. *Neurourol Urodyn* 2009;28(4):288-94.
18. Hall SA, Yang M, Gates MA et al. Associations of commonly used medications with urinary incontinence in a community based sample. *J Urol* 2012;188(1):183-9.
19. Shamliyan TA, Kane RL, Wyman J et al. Systematic review: randomized, controlled trials of nonsurgical treatments for urinary incontinence in women. *Ann Intern Med* 2008;148(6):459-73.
20. Griebling TL. Urinary incontinence in the elderly. *Clin Geriatr Med* 2009;25(3):445-57.
21. Neumann PB, Grimmer KA, Deenadayalan Y. Pelvic floor muscle training and adjunctive therapies for the treatment of stress urinary incontinence in women: a systematic review. *BMC Womens Health* 2006;6:11.
22. Wallace SA, Roe B, Williams K et al. Bladder training for urinary incontinence in adults. *Cochrane Database Syst Rev* 2004;(1):CD001308.
23. Dumoulin C, Hay-Smith EJ, Mac Habée-Séguin G. Pelvic floor muscle training versus no treatment, or inactive control treatments, for urinary incontinence in women. *Cochrane Database Syst Rev* 2014;(5):CD005654.
24. Wagg AS. Antimuscarinic treatment in overactive bladder: special considerations in elderly patients. *Drugs Aging* 2012;29(7):539-48.
25. Cameron AP, Jimbo M, Heidelbaugh JJ. Diagnosis and office-based treatment of urinary incontinence in adults. Part two: treatment. *Ther Adv Urol* 2013;5(4):189-200.
26. Seehusen DA. Treatments for urinary incontinence in women. *Am Fam Physician* 2013;87(10):726-8.
27. Canadian Continence Foundation. *Pelvic muscle exercises, Kegel exercises for urinary incontinence*. Available from: www.canadiancontinence.ca/pdf/pelvicmuscleexercises.pdf. Accessed March 31, 2011.
28. Greer JA, Smith AL, Arya LA. Pelvic floor muscle training for urgency urinary incontinence in women: a systematic review. *Int Urogynecol J* 2012;23(6):687-97.
29. Bugge C, Adams EJ, Gopinath D et al. Pessaries (mechanical devices) for pelvic organ prolapse in women. *Cochrane Database Syst Rev* 2013;2:CD004010.
30. Jain P, Jirschele K, Botros SM et al. Effectiveness of midurethral slings in mixed urinary incontinence: a systematic review and meta-analysis. *Int Urogynecol J* 2011;22(8):923-32.

31. Pradhan A, Jain P, Latthe PM. Effectiveness of midurethral slings in recurrent stress urinary incontinence: a systematic review and meta-analysis. *Int Urogynecol J* 2012;23(7):831-41.
32. Mischinger J, Amend B, Reisenauer C et al. Different surgical approaches for stress urinary incontinence in women. *Minerva Ginecol* 2013;65(1):21-8.
33. Novara G, Artibani W, Barber MD et al. Updated systematic review and meta-analysis of the comparative data on colposuspensions, pubovaginal slings, and midurethral tapes in the surgical treatment of female stress urinary incontinence. *Eur Urol* 2010;58(2):218-38.
34. Rehman H, Bezerra CC, Bruschini H et al. Traditional suburethral sling operations for urinary incontinence in women. *Cochrane Database Syst Rev* 2011;(1):CD001754.
35. Richter HE, Albo ME, Zyczynski HM et al. Retropubic versus transobturator midurethral slings for stress incontinence. *N Engl J Med* 2010;362(22):2066-76.
36. Dmochowski RR, Blaivas JM, Gormley EA et al. Update of AUA guideline on the surgical management of female stress urinary incontinence. *J Urol* 2010;183(5):1906-14.
37. Kirchin V, Page T, Keegan PE et al. Urethral injection therapy for urinary incontinence in women. *Cochrane Database Syst Rev* 2012;2:CD003881.
38. National Institute for Health and Care Excellence. National Collaborating Centre for Women's and Children's Health. *Urinary incontinence in women: the management of urinary incontinence in women.* London (GB): Royal College of Obtetricians and Gynaecologists; 2013. Available from: www.nice.org.uk/nicemedia/live/14271/65144/65144.pdf.
39. Cody JD, Jacobs ML, Richardson K et al. Oestrogen therapy for urinary incontinence in post-menopausal women. *Cochrane Database Syst Rev* 2012;10:CD001405.
40. Nappi RE, Davis SR. The use of hormone therapy for the maintenance of urogynecological and sexual health post WHI. *Climacteric* 2012;15(3):267-74.
41. Hillard T. The postmenopausal bladder. *Menopause Int* 2010;16(2):74-80.
42. Ewies AA, Alfhaily F. Topical vaginal estrogen therapy in managing postmenopausal urinary symptoms: a reality or a gimmick? *Climacteric* 2010;13(5):405-18.
43. Nelson HD, Walker M, Zakher B et al. Menopausal hormone therapy for the primary prevention of chronic conditions: a systematic review to update the U.S. Preventive Services Task Force recommendations. *Ann Intern Med* 2012;157(2):104-13.
44. Alhasso A, Glazener CM, Pickard R et al. Adrenergic drugs for urinary incontinence in adults. *Cochrane Database Syst Rev* 2005;(3):CD001842.
45. Thor KB, Kirby M, Viktrup L. Serotonin and noradrenaline involvement in urinary incontinence, depression and pain: scientific basis for overlapping clinical efficacy from a single drug, duloxetine. *Int J Clin Pract* 2007;61(8):1349-55.
46. McCormack PL, Keating GM. Duloxetine: in stress urinary incontinence. *Drugs* 2004;64(22):2567-73.
47. Mariappan P, Ballantyne Z, N'Dow JM et al. Serotonin and noradrenaline reuptake inhibitors (SNRI) for stress urinary incontinence in adults. *Cochrane Database Syst Rev* 2005;(3):CD004742.
48. Andersson KE. Antimuscarinics for treatment of overactive bladder. *Lancet Neurol* 2004;3(1):46-53.
49. Rai BP, Cody JD, Alhasso A et al. Anticholinergic drugs versus non-drug active therapies for non-neurogenic overactive bladder syndrome in adults. *Cochrane Database Syst Rev* 2012;12:CD003193.
50. Shamliyan T, Wyman JF, Ramakrishnan R et al. Benefits and harms of pharmacologic treatment for urinary incontinence in women: a systematic review. *Ann Intern Med* 2012;156(12):861-74.
51. Nabi G, Cody JD, Ellis G et al. Anticholinergic drugs versus placebo for overactive bladder syndrome in adults. *Cochrane Database Syst Rev* 2006;(4):CD003781.
52. Chapple CR, Khullar V, Gabriel Z et al. The effects of antimuscarinic treatments in overactive bladder: an update of a systematic review and meta-analysis. *Eur Urol* 2008;54(3):543-62.
53. Madhuvrata P, Cody JD, Ellis G et al. Which anticholinergic drug for overactive bladder symptoms in adults. *Cochrane Database Syst Rev* 2012;1:CD005429.
54. Andersson KE, Chapple CR, Cardozo L et al. Pharmacological treatment of overactive bladder: report from the International Consultation on Incontinence. *Curr Opin Urol* 200;19(4):380-94.
55. Chancellor M, Boone T. Anticholinergics for overactive bladder therapy: central nervous system effects. *CNS Neurosci Ther* 2012;18(2):167-74.
56. Gopal M, Haynes K, Bellamy SL et al. Discontinuation rates of anticholinergic medications used for the treatment of lower urinary tract symptoms. *Obstet Gynecol* 2008;112(6):1311-8.
57. Leone Roberti Maggiore U, Salvatore S, Alessandri F et al. Pharmacokinetics and toxicity of antimuscarinic drugs for overactive bladder treatment in females. *Expert Opin Drug Metab Toxicol* 2012;8(11):1387-408.
58. Weiss BD. Selecting medications for the treatment of urinary incontinence. *Am Fam Physician* 2005;71(2):315-22.
59. Dull P. Transdermal oxybutynin (oxytrol) for urinary incontinence. *Am Fam Physician* 2004;70(12):2351-2.
60. Gomelsky A, Dmochowski RR. Update on the management of overactive bladder: patient considerations and adherence. *Open Access J Urol* 2011;3:7-17.
61. DuBeau CE. Estrogen treatment for urinary incontinence: never, now, or in the future? *JAMA* 2005;293(8):998-1001.
62. Hendrix SL, Cochrane BB, Nygaard IE et al. Effects of estrogen with and without progestin on urinary incontinence. *JAMA* 2005;293(8):935-48.
63. Caremel R, Loutochin O, Corcos J. What do we know and not know about mirabegron, a novel β3 agonist, in the treatment of overactive bladder? *Int Urogynecol J* 2013 Aug 7. [Epub ahead of print].
64. Cui Y, Zong H, Yang C et al. The efficacy and safety of mirabegron in treating OAB: a systematic review and meta-analysis of phase III trials. *Int Urol Nephrol* 2013 Jul 30. [Epub ahead of print].
65. Bridgeman MB, Friia NJ, Taft C et al. Mirabegron: β3-adrenergic receptor agonist for the treatment of overactive bladder. *Ann Pharmacother* 2013;47(7-8):1029-38.
66. Haeusler G, Leitich H, van Trotsenburg M et al. Drug therapy of urinary urge incontinence: a systematic review. *Obstet Gynecol* 2002;100(5 Pt 1):1003-16.
67. American Geriatrics Society 2012 Beers Criteria Update Expert Panel. American Geriatrics Society updated Beers Criteria for potentially inappropriate medication use in older adults. *J Am Geriatr Soc* 2012;60(4):616-31.
68. Duthie JB, Vincent M, Herbison GP et al. Botulinum toxin injections for adults with overactive bladder syndrome. *Cochrane Database Syst Rev* 2011;(12):CD005493.
69. Karsenty G, Denys P, Amarenco G et al. Botulinum toxin A (Botox) intradetrusor injections in adults with neurogenic detrusor overactivity/neurogenic overactive bladder: a systematic literature review. *Eur Urol* 2008;53(2):275-87.

70. Selius BA, Subedi R. Urinary retention in adults: diagnosis and initial management. *Am Fam Physician* 2008;77(5):643-50.
71. Wilt TJ, N'Dow J. Benign prostatic hyperplasia. Part 2—management. *BMJ* 2008;336(7637):206-10.
72. Niël-Weise BS, van den Broek PJ. Urinary catheter policies for short-term bladder drainage in adults. *Cochrane Database Syst Rev* 2005;(3):CD004203.
73. Jahn P, Beutner K, Langer G. Types of indwelling urinary catheters for long-term bladder drainage in adults. *Cochrane Database Syst Rev* 2012;10:CD004997.
74. Curtis LA, Dolan TS, Cespedes RD. Acute urinary retention and urinary incontinence. *Emerg Med Clin North Am* 2001;19(3):591-619.
75. Taylor JA, Kuchel GA. Detrusor underactivity: clinical features and pathogenesis of an underdiagnosed geriatric condition. *J Am Geriatr Soc* 2006;54(12):1920-32.
76. Buckley BS, Lapitan MC. Drugs for treatment of urinary retention after surgery in adults. *Cochrane Database Syst Rev* 2010;(10):CD008023.
77. Casey BM, Schaffer JI, Bloom SL et al. Obstetric antecedents for postpartum pelvic floor dysfunction. *Am J Obstet Gynecol* 2005;192(5):1655-62.
78. Viktrup L, Lose G, Rolff M et al. The symptom of stress incontinence caused by pregnancy or delivery in primiparas. *Obstet Gynecol* 1992;79(6):945-9.
79. Thorp JM, Norton PA, Wall LL et al. Urinary incontinence in pregnancy and the puerperium: a prospective study. *Am J Obstet Gynecol* 1999;181(2):266-73.
80. Cutner A, Cardozo LD, Benness CJ. Assessment of urinary symptoms in early pregnancy. *Br J Obstet Gynaecol* 1991;98(12):1283-6.
81. Cutner A, Cardozo LD, Benness CJ. Assessment of urinary symptoms in the second half of pregnancy. *Int Urogynecol* 1992;3:30-2.
82. van Brummen HJ, Bruinse HW, van der Bom JG et al. How do the prevalences of urogenital symptoms change during pregnancy? *Neurourol Urodyn* 2006;25(2):135-9.
83. Thom DH, Rortveit G. Prevalence of postpartum urinary incontinence: a systematic review. *Acta Obstet Gynecol Scand* 2010;89(12):1511-22.
84. Rogers RG, Leeman LL. Postpartum genitourinary changes. *Urol Clin North Am* 2007;34(1):13-21.
85. FitzGerald MP, Graziano S. Anatomic and functional changes of the lower urinary tract during pregnancy. *Urol Clin North Am* 2007;34(1):7-12.
86. Jeyabalan A, Lain KY. Anatomic and functional changes of the upper urinary tract during pregnancy. *Urol Clin North Am* 2007;34(1):1-6.
87. Cerruto MA, D'Elia C, Aloisi A et al. Prevalence, incidence and obstetric factors' impact on female urinary incontinence in Europe: a systematic review. *Urol Int* 2013;90(1):1-9.
88. Groutz A, Gordon D, Keidar R et al. Stress urinary incontinence: prevalence among nulliparous compared with primiparous and grand multiparous premenopausal women. *Neurourol Urodyn* 1999;18(5):419-25.
89. Thom DH, van den Eeden SK, Brown JS. Evaluation of parturition and other reproductive variables as risk factors for urinary incontinence in later life. *Obstet Gynecol* 1997;90(6):983-9.
90. Lose G, Alling-Moller L, Jennum P. Nocturia in women. *Am J Obstet Gynecol* 2001;185(2):514-21.
91. Allahdin S, Kambhampati L. Stress urinary incontinence in continent primigravidas. *J Obstet Gynaecol* 2012;32(1):2-5.
92. Boyle R, Hay-Smith EJ, Cody JD et al. Pelvic floor muscle training for prevention and treatment of urinary and fecal incontinence in antenatal and postnatal women: a short version Cochrane review. *Neurourol Urodyn* 2013 Apr 24. [Epub ahead of print].
93. Willhite LA, O'Connell MB. Urogenital atrophy: prevention and treatment. *Pharmacotherapy* 2001;21(4):464-80.
94. Sathyan G, Dmochowski RR, Appell RA et al. Effect of antacid on the pharmacokinetics of extended-release formulations of tolterodine and oxybutynin. *Clin Pharmacokinet* 2004;43(14):1059-68.
95. Dmochowski R, Chen A, Sathyan G et al. Effect of the proton pump inhibitor omeprazole on the pharmacokinetics of extended-release formulations of oxybutynin and tolterodine. *J Clin Pharmacol* 2005;45(8):961-8.

Chapter 69
Urinary Incontinence in Children

Fabian P. Gorodzinsky, MD, AAPD, FRCP

Urinary incontinence in children is defined as the repeated daytime or nighttime voiding of urine into the bed or clothes at least twice per week for at least 3 consecutive months, in a child who is at least 5 years of age.[1] Most children are successfully toilet trained by around the age of 3 years, with a wide range of 0.75–5.25 years. Girls are usually trained earlier than boys.[2]

Enuresis is bedwetting, or wetting during sleep (e.g., nap time), more than twice weekly beyond the age of 5 years for girls and 6 years for boys. In primary enuresis bladder control has never been achieved, and in secondary enuresis loss of bladder control occurs after at least 6 months without bedwetting.[3] Primary enuresis, which is more common in boys, occurs in 15–20% of 5-year-olds and 5% of 10-year-olds, and declines to <2% in those 15 years or older.[4] There are 2 subtypes of primary enuresis: volume-dependent enuresis (associated with nocturnal polyuria; a normal nocturnal rise in antidiuretic hormone [ADH] secretion may not occur in these children) and detrusor-dependent enuresis (associated with daytime frequency, urgency or incontinence).[5] Possible causes of enuresis include developmental delay (immaturity of CNS control over bladder contractions and/or responsiveness to bladder filling), genetics (molecular linkage to chromosome 8q, 12q, 13q) and obstructive sleep apnea[6,7] (very rare). Lack of sufficient ADH release, bladder overactivity and failure to wake up can also cause enuresis.[3]

Daytime incontinence occurs in about 10% of children 4–6 years old, declining to 4% in adolescents. Girls are affected twice as often as boys. It is considered a problem in a child 4 years or older who wets daily (primary) or who relapses after 6 consecutive months without daytime wetting (secondary). Possible functional or organic causes of daytime incontinence are listed in Table 1.

There is no evidence that urinary incontinence is associated with any specific behavioural or psychological problems, yet most affected children are clearly distressed by their condition. The parents' supportive role in treatment is crucial; an intolerant attitude on the part of the parents predicts early drop-out from treatment.[8]

Table 1: Possible Causes of Daytime Incontinence

Functional	Constipation (as defined by the Rome III diagnostic criteria for functional gastrointestinal disorders—See www.romecriteria.org/assets/pdf/19_RomeIII_apA_885-898.pdf)[9]
	Deferral of voiding ("holding it in until the last minute")
	Fusion of labia minora
	Urinary tract infection
	Urge syndrome (unstable bladder; sudden attacks of uncontrollable urge to void; characteristic squatting to avoid detrusor contractions)
	Stress incontinence
	Giggle incontinence
	Emotional stress
	Daytime frequency syndrome
Organic	Neurogenic bladder
	Partial urethral obstruction, e.g., posterior urethral valve, congenital strictures
	Ectopic ureter

Goals of Therapy

- Identify and/or manage serious causes
- Minimize symptoms
- Provide reassurance and guidance

Investigations

- History with attention to:
  - family history (often present in enuresis)
  - bowel function; constipation is frequently associated with urinary incontinence that is due to decreased bladder capacity
  - pattern of wetting
  - history of urinary tract infections (UTI) or urologic surgery
  - psychological status of child and family dynamics
- Physical examination with attention to:
  - perineal sensation, perineal reflexes, sphincter tone (to rule out neurogenic bladder)
  - genitalia, particularly the urethral meatus (to rule out anatomical causes such as meatal stenosis in boys or labial fusion in girls)
  - possible neurologic disorders that relate to malformations of the spinal cord such as tethered spinal cord syndrome, a congenital spinal cord abnormality that can cause progressive neurologic damage. Signs include the presence of a hair tuft, dimple, pigmented lesion or subcutaneous lipoma over the lower spine, or asymmetry of the gluteal cleft (refer to pediatric neurosurgeon)
  - direct observation of voiding, if possible, to rule out abnormalities of urinary stream
- Other investigations as indicated:
  - diary to record voiding pattern and/or bowel movements
  - urinalysis and urine culture; no other investigations are necessary for primary enuresis
  - voiding cystourethrogram (to detect vesicoureteral reflux, partial urethral obstruction or neurogenic bladder) as well as ultrasound of kidneys and bladder are recommended if history of UTI
  - if voiding cystourethrogram is abnormal, a referral to a urologist is indicated[3]

Therapeutic Choices

Figure 1 depicts the management of urinary incontinence in children. Without treatment, 15% of affected children are expected to become dry each year. Tailor therapy to etiologic factors. Combinations of different interventions may be useful.

Nonpharmacologic Choices

- In cases of daytime incontinence, advise parents to refrain from humiliating or punishing the child, and to support the child's efforts with positive reinforcement, e.g., reassurance, diary of dry days, facilitated access to bathroom at home and school.
- Have the child avoid excessive intake of fluids within 2 hours of bedtime and empty the bladder before going to bed.
- Encourage the child to avoid deferral of micturition.
- *Enuresis alarms* are effective for enuresis when used properly for 3–4 months.[10] Enuresis alarms, which are highly sensitive to moisture, attach to underpants or an absorbent pad and either vibrate or produce sound at the first sign of voiding. Because children with enuresis are usually very deep

sleepers, the parent must often be the one to wake the child when the alarm sounds. The child then completes voiding in the toilet and returns to sleep after changing the underwear or bedding. Alarm therapy may be effective in children with a normal urine output and a small or normal bladder capacity.[11,12] Enuresis alarms (e.g., Malem, Dri Sleeper, Nytone) are inexpensive (e.g., $80–120) relative to medications and are available at medical supply stores. Alarms may be tried in motivated and committed patients as young as 5 years old with consistent parental involvement and support. However, in the author's experience, best results are achieved in children 7 years or older. Relapse rates were lower when dry bed training (following a strict schedule for waking the child up at night until he or she learns to wake up alone when needed), reward systems (e.g., star chart) or overlearning (child drinks 4–6 oz of water in the hour before going to bed while continuing to use the alarm) were added to alarm treatment.[4,10,13]

- Encourage bladder training exercises for daytime incontinence, e.g., scheduled voiding routine, abdominal or pelvic floor muscle exercises.
- There is no evidence of effectiveness for complementary therapies such as hypnosis, acupuncture, chiropractic, faradization (electric shock to the genital area), homeopathy, diet or restricted foods.[14]

Figure 1: Management of Urinary Incontinence in Children

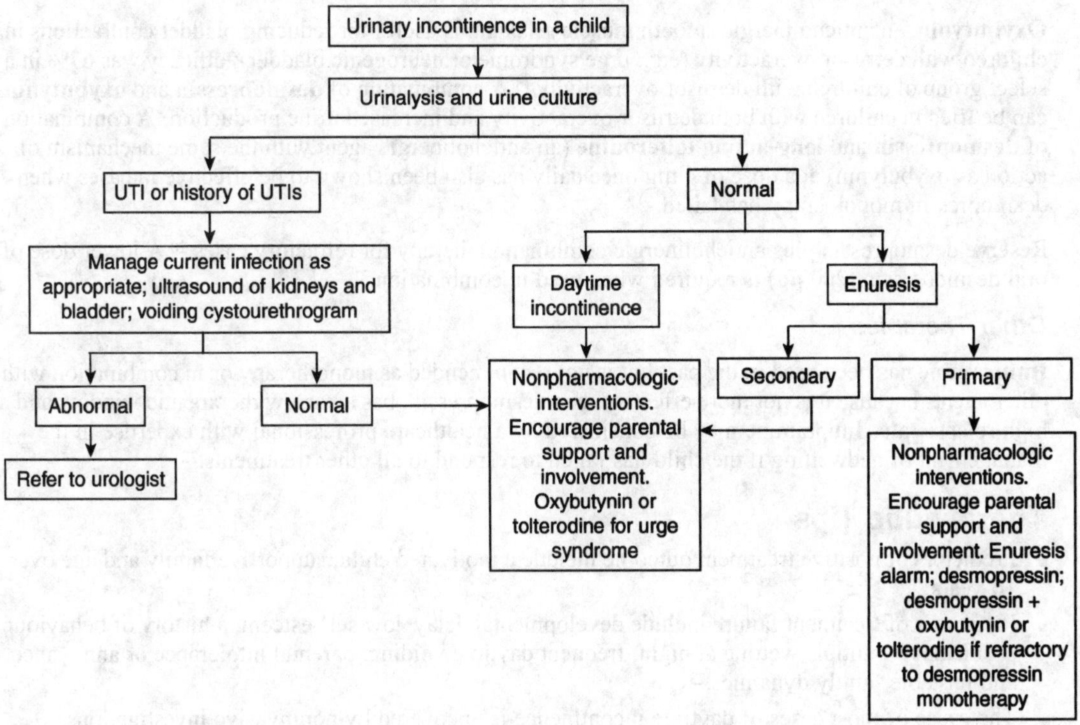

Abbreviations: UTI = urinary tract infection

Pharmacologic Choices

Table 2 lists medications used in the management of urinary incontinence in children ≥5 years of age.

Antidiuretic Hormone Analogues

Desmopressin, an analogue of human ADH, decreases urine production when given at bedtime and reduces the number of wet nights in 75% of children, with complete cessation in about 50% of those who respond.[15] Desmopressin is used when a rapid response is required. There is limited evidence of long-term success with desmopressin use.[10] If successful, consider a 1-week interruption every 3 months to see if treatment is no longer needed.[16] Desmopressin may be most effective in children with a normal bladder capacity but with a large urine output.[12,16,17] Patients with high urine output and *reduced* bladder capacity may require combination treatment with desmopressin and enuresis alarms.[14] If cost is a concern, reserve desmopressin for special occasions such as overnight visits or camp. The risk of overhydration and hyponatremia associated with desmopressin necessitates limiting fluid intake to <500 mL for children >12 years and <250 mL for children <12 years, within 1 hour of going to bed.[18]

Desmopressin nasal spray is no longer indicated for the management of primary enuresis. Compared to oral formulations, it is associated with a higher incidence of hyponatremia, which may result in seizures and death.[18]

Smooth Muscle Relaxants

Oxybutynin, an anticholinergic smooth muscle relaxant, is useful for reducing bladder contractions in children with detrusor overactivity (e.g., urge syndrome or neurogenic bladder); efficacy was 67% in a select group of children with detrusor overactivity.[15] A combination of **desmopressin** and **oxybutynin** can be tried in children with both detrusor overactivity and increased urine production. A combination of **desmopressin** and **long-acting tolterodine** (an anticholinergic agent with the same mechanism of action as oxybutynin) at a dose of 4 mg once daily has also been shown to be effective in cases when desmopressin monotherapy has failed.[19]

Reserve desmopressin plus anticholinergic combination therapy for refractory cases.[20] A lower dose of oral desmopressin (200 µg) is required when used in combination.[21]

Other Therapies

Imipramine has been used in the past but is not recommended as monotherapy or in combination with other agents because it is not more effective than desmopressin, has a narrow therapeutic window and a high relapse rate. Imipramine may be considered by a healthcare professional with expertise in the management of bedwetting if the child has failed to respond to all other treatments.[22]

Therapeutic Tips

- Predictors of positive treatment outcome include a motivated child, supportive family and age over 10 years.
- Predictors of treatment failure include developmental delay, low self-esteem, a history of behaviour problems or multiple wetting at night, frequent daytime voiding, parental intolerance or annoyance and unstable family dynamics.[23]
- The cause of most cases of daytime incontinence is uncovered by noninvasive investigations (history, physical exam, urinalysis, urine culture and ultrasound of kidney and bladder).
- Relative to desmopressin, enuresis alarms are superior in that once the child achieves dryness, there is less chance of relapse.[10] The effects of desmopressin are immediate, whereas enuresis alarms take longer to reduce frequency of bedwetting.

Table 2: Drug Therapy for Urinary Incontinence in Children ≥5 Years of Age

Class	Drug	Dose	Adverse Effects	Comments	Cost[a]
Antidiuretic Hormone Analogues	*desmopressin* DDAVP Melt, DDAVP Tablets, Minirin generics	Dose is individualized. Tablets: 200–600 µg QHS po (start with 200 µg 1 hour before HS. If no response, increase by 200 µg increments every 3 days). Fast-melting formulation: 120–240 µg QHS sl (start with 120 µg 1 hour before HS. If no response, increase by 120 µg increments every 3 days). May continue treatment for 6 months.	Headache (transient), abdominal pain, water intoxication, hyponatremia-related seizures (rare).	For enuresis. Used in conjunction with nonpharmacologic treatment. Desmopressin should not be used in children with kidney disease, heart failure, diabetes, ileitis or cystic fibrosis. The fast-melting formulation of desmopressin is effective for 7–11 h.[24] Withhold desmopressin in the case of an acute illness leading to decreased fluid intake. Combination therapy of low-dose desmopressin (e.g., 200 µg of tablet formulation) and smooth muscle relaxants can be used in cases refractory to desmopressin monotherapy.	$$-$$$$
Smooth Muscle Relaxants	*oxybutynin* generics	Dose is individualized. >5 y: 5 mg TID po	Dry mouth, constipation, flushing and occasional mood changes.[15]	Available as syrup. Combination therapy with desmopressin and oxybutynin can be used in cases refractory to desmopressin monotherapy.	$
	tolterodine extended-release Detrol LA	Children 6–17 y: 2–4 mg QHS po	See oxybutynin.	Combination of desmopressin plus extended-release tolterodine is used in cases refractory to desmopressin monotherapy.	$$$$$

[a] Cost of 30-day supply; includes drug cost only.
Legend: $ <$15 $$ $15–30 $$-$$$$ $15–60 $$$ $30–45 $$$$ $45–60 $$$$$ $60–75

Suggested Readings

Caldwell PH, Nankivell G, Sureshkumar P. Simple behavioural interventions for nocturnal enuresis in children. *Cochrane Database Syst Rev* 2013;7:CD003637.

Management of primary nocturnal enuresis. *Paediatr Child Health* 2005;10(10):611-4.

Robson WL. Clinical practice. Evaluation and management of enuresis. *N Engl J Med* 2009;360(14):1429-36.

Russell K, Kiddoo D. The Cochrane Library and nocturnal enuresis; an umbrella review. *Evid Based Child Health* 2006;1(1):5-8.

von Gontard A. Urinary incontinence in children with special needs. *Nat Rev Urol* 2013;10(11):667-74.

References

1. Fritz G, Rockney R, Bernet W et al. Practice parameter for the assessment and treatment of children and adolescents with enuresis. *J Am Acad Child Adolesc Psychiatry* 2004;43(12):1540-50.
2. Schulpen TW. The burden of nocturnal enuresis. *Acta Paediatr* 1997;86(9):981-4.
3. Bloom DA, Butler RJ, Djurhuus JC et al. *Conservative management in children*. In: Incontinence. First International Consultation on Incontinence; 1998 June 28-July 1. Monaco: World Health Organization, International Union Against Cancer (UICC); 1999.
4. Kiddoo D. Nocturnal enuresis. *Clin Evid (Online)* 2011;2011:0305.
5. Management of primary nocturnal enuresis. *Paediatr Child Health* 2005;10(10):611-4.
6. Alexopoulos EI, Kaditis AG, Kostadima E et al. Resolution of nocturnal enuresis in snoring children after treatment with nasal budesonide. *Urology* 2005;66(1):194.
7. Basha S, Bialowas C, Ende K et al. Effectiveness of adenotonsillectomy in the resolution of nocturnal enuresis secondary to obstructive sleep apnea. *Laryngoscope* 2005;115(6):1101-3.
8. Butler RJ, Redfern EJ, Forsythe I. The Maternal Tolerance Scale and nocturnal enuresis. *Behav Res Ther* 1993;31(4):433-6.
9. Rome Foundation. *Appendix A: Rome III diagnostic criteria for functional gastrointestinal disorders*. Available from: www.romecriteria.org/assets/pdf/19_RomeIII_apA_885-898.pdf.
10. Glazener CM, Evans JH, Peto RE. Alarm interventions for nocturnal enuresis in children. *Cochrane Database Syst Rev* 2005;(2):CD002911.
11. Hjalmas K, Arnold T, Bower W et al. Nocturnal enuresis: an international evidence based management strategy. *J Urol* 2004;171(6 Pt 2):2545-61.
12. Vande Walle J, Rittig S, Bauer S et al. Practical consensus guidelines for the management of enuresis. *Eur J Pediatr* 2012;171(6):971-83.
13. Robertson B, Yap K, Schuster S. Effectiveness of an alarm intervention with overlearning for primary nocturnal enuresis. *J Pediatr Urol* 2013 Sep 10. [Epub ahead of print].
14. Huang T, Shu X, Huang YS et al. Complementary and miscellaneous interventions for nocturnal enuresis in children. *Cochrane Database Syst Rev* 2011;(12):CD005230.
15. Butler R, Stenberg A. Treatment of childhood nocturnal enuresis: an examination of clinically relevant principles. *BJU Int* 2001;88(6):563-71.
16. Hjalmas K, Hanson E, Hellstrom AL et al. Long-term treatment with desmopressin in children with primary monosymptomatic nocturnal enuresis: an open multicentre study. Swedish Enuresis Trial (SWEET) Group. *Br J Urol* 1998;82(5):704-9.
17. Neveus T. Osmoregulation and desmopressin pharmacokinetics in enuretic children. *Scand J Urol Nephrol Suppl* 1999;202:52.
18. Lucchini B, Simonetti GD, Ceschi A et al. Severe signs of hyponatremia secondary to desmopressin treatment for enuresis: a systematic review. *J Pediatr Urol* 2013;9(6 Pt B):1049-53.
19. Austin PF, Ferguson G, Yan Y et al. Combination therapy with desmopressin and an anticholinergic medication for nonresponders to desmopressin for monosymptomatic nocturnal enuresis: a randomized, double-blind, placebo-controlled trial. *Pediatrics* 2008;122(5):1027-32.
20. Vermandel A, de Wachter S, Wyndaele JJ. Refractory monosymptomatic nocturnal enuresis: a combined stepwise approach in childhood and follow-up into adolescence, with attention to the clinical value of normalizing bladder capacity. *BJU Int* 2005;96(4):629-33.
21. Lee T, Suh HJ, Lee HJ et al. Comparison of effects of treatment of primary nocturnal enuresis with oxybutynin plus desmopressin, desmopressin alone or imipramine alone: a randomized controlled clinical trial. *J Urol* 2005;174(3):1084-7.
22. National Clinical Guideline Centre at the Royal College of Physicians. *Nocturnal enuresis: the management of bedwetting in children and young people*. Available from: www.nice.org.uk/nicemedia/live/13246/51365/51365.pdf.
23. Moffatt ME, Cheang M. Predicting treatment outcome with conditioning alarms. *Scand J Urol Nephrol Suppl* 1995;173:119-22.
24. Vande Walle JG, Bogaert GA, Mattsson S et al. A new fast-melting oral formulation of desmopressin: a pharmacodynamic study in children with primary nocturnal enuresis. *BJU Int* 2006;97(3):603-9.

Sexual Health

Chapter 70
Contraception

Gillian Graves, MD, FRCSC

Goals of Therapy

- Prevent pregnancy
- Individualize contraceptive method based on specific needs, lifestyle, age, parity and desire for future fertility

Investigations

Prior to initiating contraceptive methods, certain baseline measures are required.

- Pregnancy test
- Weight
- Blood pressure in women considering combined estrogen-and progestin-containing contraceptives (COCs)
- Bimanual examination and cervical inspection for women considering intrauterine devices (copper-IUD or LNG-IUS), cervical cap or diaphragm
- STI screening for women considering intrauterine devices

Therapeutic Choices

Assess the woman's contraceptive needs. Effective contraception and education reduce rates of maternal and child mortality, as well as population growth. Individual contraceptive needs change over time. Preferred contraceptive methods for young women are reversible, affordable and have good safety profiles and low failure rates. The method chosen should not interfere with other physiologic processes, e.g., vaginal lubrication, spontaneity or pleasure of either partner. Present contraceptive choices along with appropriate counselling to each individual. Many newer options are available such as route of delivery, dosage, regimens and generic products.

Nonpharmacologic Choices

Nonhormonal contraceptive options such as natural timing, barrier methods, spermicides, IUDs and surgical sterilization are included in Table 3.

Pharmacologic Choices

Hormonal contraceptive options are presented in Table 4.

Combined Estrogen- and Progestin-containing Contraceptives

Combined Oral Contraceptives (COCs)

COCs combined with male condoms (for STI protection) are the method of choice for most young couples, including teens. COCs containing synthetic estrogen and progestogen (progestin) have been modified as a result of synthesis of more potent steroids. This has led to dose reduction, increased safety and reliability and decreased adverse effects. Absolute contraindications of COCs are listed in Table 1.

Table 1: **Absolute Contraindications to Combined Oral Hormonal Contraception**[12,13]

- Breast cancer or hormone-dependent cancer
- Cerebrovascular disease, history of cerebrovascular accident
- Complicated valvular heart disease
- Current or past history of venous thromboembolism or pulmonary embolism, known thrombogenic mutations (e.g., factor V Leiden), prothrombin mutation, protein S, protein C and antithrombin deficiencies or other known coagulation-factor deficiency
- Diabetes with microvascular complications
- History of or current MI or ischemic heart disease, vascular disease
- <6 weeks postpartum if breastfeeding
- Migraines with aura at any age
- Hypertension (SBP ≥160 mm Hg or DBP ≥100 mm Hg)
- Severe cirrhosis or liver tumour
- Smoker >35 years of age (≥15 cigarettes/day)

SBP = systolic blood pressure; DBP = diastolic blood pressure

Significant differences have not been shown between monophasic and triphasic COCs in regard to bleeding pattern or efficacy.[14] Fixed-dose (monophasic) COCs are easier to manipulate than triphasic COCs. Low-dose COCs with 20–25 µg EE are effective contraceptive agents with pregnancy rates between 0.07 and 2.1 pregnancies per 100 woman-years of treatment.[15] They demonstrate reduced symptoms of bloating and breast tenderness[16] and may be used in individuals who experience adverse effects with higher EE doses. However, low dose COCs may be associated with more bleeding pattern abnormalities.[17]

Most COCs are available in 28-day cycles (21 days of active medication with a 7-day hormone-free interval); for other regimens, see Extended or Continuous Use of Combined Hormonal Contraceptives (CHC).

The progestin component of COCs may vary among different products; see Table 2 for a list of COCs divided by progestin type. Products containing *third-generation progestins* (e.g., desogestrel, norgestimate) are less androgenic and may be useful in acne. While not approved by Health Canada for contraception, **cyproterone acetate** is a progestin with antiandrogenic activity that is used in combination with ethinyl estradiol (EE) for the treatment of moderate to severe acne. However, most oral contraceptives improve mild to moderate acne (see Chapter 88).

Drospirenone is related to the aldosterone antagonist spironolactone and has both progestational and antiandrogenic activity.[18] A Cochrane review of 5 trials shows drospirenone-containing COCs may benefit women with premenstrual dysphoric disorder (PMDD), but there is limited evidence of benefit for milder disease or for greater than 3 cycles of use.[19] Several observational studies concluded that drospirenone-containing COCs may confer a higher risk of venous thromboembolism than COCs containing other progestins (see Risks Associated with Hormonal Contraception).[20,21,22]

Table 2 lists the relative hormonal activity of various oral contraceptive products.

Contraceptive Vaginal Ring

An estrogen/progestin-releasing vaginal ring (NuvaRing) provides a more uniform contraceptive hormone concentration throughout the day,[23] thus avoiding daily hormonal fluctuations. Since both hepatic first-pass and gastrointestinal metabolism are avoided, lower doses of hormones can be used. Cycle control is good, with irregular bleeding in 5.5% of cycles and withdrawal bleeding in 98.5% of cycles.[24,25] One case of mesenteric vein thrombosis has been reported.[26] The ring can be used without interfering with intercourse. Failure rate is 0.65 per 100 woman-years.[15] A randomized controlled trial of 3 vaginal ring regimens (49, 91 or 364 days) compared with the usual 28-day cycle of ring use showed the frequency of breast tenderness, weight changes, headache and mood change were similar in all groups. Breast soreness was more frequent with continuous use than cyclic use. Compared with

28-day regimens of ring use, a 49-day extended use showed a mean decrease of 2% in bleeding/spotting days. Using it for 91 or 364 days increased the mean days of bleeding by 3.5 and 7.1 % respectively; more women discontinued therapy with the longer extended regimens.[27]

Table 2: Hormonal Activity of Combined Oral Contraceptives

Oral Contraceptive Products	Components	Relative Hormonal Activity: Estrogen	Progestin	Androgen
Products with first-generation progestins				
Minestrin 1/20	ethinyl estradiol 20 µg/norethindrone 1 mg	+	+++	+++
Loestrin 1.5/30	ethinyl estradiol 30 µg/norethindrone 1.5 mg	+	+++	++++
Demulen 30	ethinyl estradiol 30 µg/ethynodiol diacetate 2 mg	+	++++	+++
Brevicon 0.5/35, Ortho 0.5/35	ethinyl estradiol 35 µg/norethindrone 0.5 mg	+++	+	+
Synphasic (biphasic)	ethinyl estradiol 35 µg/norethindrone 0.5/1 mg	+++	++	++
Brevicon 1/35, Ortho 1/35, Select 1/35	ethinyl estradiol 35 µg/norethindrone 1 mg	+++	++	+++
Ortho 7/7/7 (triphasic)	ethinyl estradiol 35 µg/norethindrone 0.5/0.75/1 mg	++++	++	++
Products with second-generation progestins				
Alesse, Alysenna	ethinyl estradiol 20 µg/levonorgestrel 0.1 mg	+	+	++
Triquilar (triphasic)	ethinyl estradiol 30/40/30 µg/levonorgestrel 0.05/0.075/0.125 mg	++	+	++
Min-Ovral, Portia, Seasonale, Seasonique	ethinyl estradiol 30 µg/levonorgestrel 0.15 mg	++	++	+++
Products with third-generation progestins				
Apri, Marvelon, Ortho-Cept	ethinyl estradiol 30 µg/desogestrel 0.15 mg	++	+++	+
Cyclen	ethinyl estradiol 35 µg/norgestimate 0.25 mg	+++	+	+
Linessa	ethinyl estradiol 25 µg/desogestrel 0.1/0.125/0.15 mg	++	+++	+
Tri-Cyclen Lo (triphasic)	ethinyl estradiol 25 µg/norgestimate 0.18/0.215/0.25 mg	+++	+	+
Tri-Cyclen (triphasic)	ethinyl estradiol 35 µg/norgestimate 0.18/0.215/0.25 mg	+++	+	+
Products containing drospirenone (antiandrogenic)				
Yasmin, Zarah	ethinyl estradiol 30 µg/drospirenone 3 mg	++	++[a]	—
Yaz, Yaz Plus	ethinyl estradiol 20 µg/drospirenone 3 mg	+	++[a]	—

[a] Best estimate; data lacking.

Adapted with permission from Regier L, Downey S. Contraceptive, combination hormonal products—Prescription. In: *RxFiles. Drug comparison charts.*. 8th ed., 3rd printing, Jan. 2014. Available from: www.rxfiles.ca. Subscription required.

Transdermal Contraceptives

A transdermal estrogen/progestin patch (Evra) has similar contraceptive efficacy, cycle control and ovulation suppression to COCs,[28,29] and better adherence (88% vs. 78% for COCs).[30,31] The pregnancy rate is between 0.70 and 0.88 pregnancies per 100 woman-years of treatment.[15,32] For women weighing 90 kg or more, this method may not be effective. Obesity may also affect follicular development through various mechanisms in patients taking oral contraceptives.[33,34]

Extended or Continuous Use of Combined Hormonal Contraceptives (CHC)

Use of extended cycles (with planned hormone-free intervals) or continuous use of pills, rings or patches without a hormone-free interval may provide patients with relief from severe dysmenorrhea, heavy flow or socially undesirable flow.[35] This can be achieved with products marketed for extended use (84 active tablets and 7 placebo tablets) or by the use of any pill, patch or ring in a continuous regimen (users take no break in between packages). Hormone-free intervals between cycles of any length should not exceed 7 days.

Compared with a 28-day cycle, extended cycles or continuous use of CHCs results in fewer bleeding days, decreased likelihood of side effects (e.g., pelvic pain, headache, bloating, swelling and tenderness) and helps improve symptoms of endometriosis and polycystic ovary syndrome.[35] One of the side effects or disadvantages of extended/continuous use is irregular unscheduled bleeding. If an inadvertent pregnancy occurs (due to several missed pills or forgotten change of patch or ring) a woman may not realize she is pregnant without the amenorrhea that might otherwise alert a cyclic contraception user that she could be pregnant.

Progestin-only Contraceptives

Oral Progestin

Norethindrone (Micronor) inhibits cervical sperm penetration by thickening the cervical mucus. Regular and consistent use is necessary to maintain contraceptive efficacy since effect on cervical mucus decreases rapidly 22 hours after dosing. A backup method for the first month of use is recommended by the manufacturer, although some experts agree that 2 days of backup may be sufficient.[36] If a dose is missed by more than 3 hours, a backup method is required. Norethindrone can be used in women >35 years of age who smoke, who cannot tolerate estrogen, have unwanted side effects with COCs, experience migraine headaches with neurologic symptoms or in women who are breastfeeding.

Depot Medroxyprogesterone Acetate (DMPA)

Medroxyprogesterone acetate given by depot injection (DMPA) produces amenorrhea in the majority of women, but some women experience irregular bleeding and side effects such as bloating, weight gain or loss and mood swings. DMPA can be used after abortion (5 days postpartum) or during breastfeeding (6 weeks postpartum). It may be a viable option for women over 35 who smoke and in women who cannot tolerate estrogen. When DMPA is discontinued, ovulation and regular menstrual periods may not resume for up to a year after the last injection. Failure rate is <0.3% per year.[32]

A large cross-sectional study of women (18–54 years of age) noted a 7.2% lower spinal bone mineral density (BMD) in users of DMPA than in nonusers. The rate of loss was higher for women who started using DMPA before age 21 and in those using it for longer duration (≥15 years). Because the loss may not be completely reversible, the clinical significance of low BMD, especially in adolescents who have not yet reached peak bone mass, needs to be elucidated.[37] Continuous losses at both hip and spine were seen in a small study of adolescent women (14–18 years of age) over 36 months of DMPA use, but significant gains after discontinuation indicate this is likely reversible.[38] Small double-blind trials suggest that estrogen supplementation is protective of bone in adolescents who are on DMPA.[39]

Levonorgestrel Intrauterine System (LNG-IUS)

After insertion of the IUS into the uterus, a low dose of **levonorgestrel** is released continuously over a period of at least 5 years. LNG-IUS is associated with low systemic levels of levonorgestrel and is highly efficacious (≤0.2 pregnancy rate per year[15]). It can reduce menstrual blood loss, fibroid growth, dysmenorrhea and endometriosis pain; it may also reduce the risk of developing precancerous cells in the uterus. This method requires a clinician visit for initiation and discontinuation. Twenty to 30% of women will stop having periods while using LNG-IUS. In fibroid-related menorrhagia, menstrual bleeding was reduced by 90% with LNG-IUS compared with a 13% reduction with COCs.[40] Normal menstruation restarts within 1–3 months of IUS removal.

The most common adverse effect is occasional bleeding or spotting for the first 3 months after insertion. Treatment for LNG-IUS-related spotting with NSAIDs, tranexamic acid or estrogen supplementation has demonstrated mixed results.[41,42] For information on other intrauterine devices, see Table 3.

Risks Associated with Hormonal Contraception

Cardiovascular Risks

Long-term studies are required to quantify cardiovascular risk for users of third-generation combined oral contraceptives (COCs) compared with COCs containing older progestins. It is important to note that pregnancy confers appreciably higher cardiovascular risks than low-dose COCs.

Smoking and hypertension increase the risk of ischemic stroke in COC users.[43,44,45,46,47] Women who have migraine with aura are at a higher risk of ischemic stroke than women who have migraine without aura.[46,48,49,50,51,52] COC users with migraine and aura who also smoked had a further increase in the risk of stroke.[52] The risk of stroke does not differ among generations of progestins contained in COCs.[53] Consider alternative contraceptive methods in women who suffer from migraines with focal neurologic signs, smoke cigarettes or are hypertensive.[11,12,54]

The risk of MI is compounded in COC users ≥35 years who have other CV disease risk factors such as smoking, hypertension and diabetes[37,43,55,56] and in those whose blood pressure has not been effectively screened.[37,43,44,49,47] Increased risk of MI is associated with increasing number of cigarettes smoked per day.[11] No increase in risk of MI is found in women under 35 years of age who have no additional CV risk factors.[44] A large prospective study of Swedish women aged 30–49 years who used COCs containing <50 µg EE with 11 years of follow-up showed no increased risk of MI compared to nonusers.[57] Consider alternative contraceptive methods in women >35 years who have additional cardiovascular risk factors.

The risk of venous thromboembolism (VTE) increases with age and with COC use, but to a lesser extent than the increased risk associated with pregnancy.[58,59,60] The incidence of VTE in women not on oral contraceptives is 0.19–0.37 per 1000 woman years, but this increases to 6–10-fold in pregnancy.[60] Two large systematic reviews found a 1.5 to 3-fold increased risk of VTE among current COC users compared to nonusers.[61,62,63]

The risk of VTE increases with higher estrogen doses[64,65] but the VTE risk associated with COCs containing 20 µg EE is equivalent to that of COCs containing 30–35 µg EE.[50] COCs containing drospirenone[20,21,22] or desogestrel may confer a 50–80% higher VTE risk compared to those containing levonorgestrel.[61,62] Non oral hormonal contraception, including the vaginal ring and transdermal patch, may also confer a slightly higher risk of VTE compared to COCs; this risk was not observed with the LNG-IUS.[66]

Inherited hypercoagulable states such as Factor V Leiden mutation, protein C or S deficiency[11] or acquired conditions such as immobility, trauma or surgery are associated with an increased risk of VTE. Obese COC users are at an increased risk of VTE compared to obese nonusers.[67,68] Women with Factor V Leiden who use COCs experience a VTE risk 30 times higher than that of COC users without the mutation.[64,69,70] Broad-based screening for this or other thrombophilias (protein C or S deficiency) is not appropriate because of the rarity of these conditions and the high screening costs. If there is a strong family or personal history of VTE, screening is recommended.[71,72] COCs are contraindicated in women with a history of VTE and hypercoagulable states.

In summary, the risk of CV disease in nonsmoking normotensive women under the age of 35 is so small that there is no health impact related to the choice of a second- versus third-generation progestin. Individualize COC selection based on history, also considering noncontraceptive benefits, and control the individual's risk factors for CV disease such as obesity, smoking and hypertension.

Breast Cancer Risk

The effect of COCs on the risk of breast cancer is controversial. Studies of COC use and breast cancer find no overall risk or a slight increase in risk.[12] In women under the age of 35, the baseline risk is 2 in 1000. COC use increases the risk 1.5 to 3-fold in 1000. As women age the risk increases. One of the risk factors for breast cancer is not having a baby by the age of 25. It is uncertain whether the risk is associated with use of a COC or the delay in pregnancy. In women with a positive family history of breast cancer, COC use has been associated with increase in baseline risk;[73] thus early screening is advised.

A prospective study that followed 116 608 female nurses from 1989-2001 found that past use of OCs was not associated with an increased risk of breast cancer. Current use conferred a small increase in relative risk (RR 1.33 95% CI 1.03-1.73).[74]

Management of Breakthrough Bleeding

Breakthrough bleeding is a common and self-resolving adverse effect of hormonal contraceptive therapy, occurring within the first 3–6 months of treatment.[75] Causes of breakthrough bleeding include pregnancy, STIs, nonadherence to contraceptives, drug interactions, smoking, abnormal cervical cytology and pre-existing gynecological problems. Progestin-only contraceptives and COCs with 20–25 μg EE are associated with more breakthrough bleeding than other oral contraceptive methods.[17]

Management of breakthrough bleeding should not be attempted until after at least 3 months of therapy. COC-related breakthrough bleeding may be managed by increasing the dose to a maximum of 35 μg EE or the changing type of progestin in the COC.[75,76] Preliminary studies indicate that progestin-only-related breakthrough bleeding may be managed with supplemental estrogen or COCs, NSAIDs, tranexamic acid, mifepristone/estrogen and doxycycline.[76,77]

HIV and Contraception

Correct and consistent use of latex male condoms is the most effective way to reduce risk of acquisition and transmission of HIV. Regardless of formulation or dosage, spermicides containing nonoxynol-9 do not provide any protection against HIV.[78,79]

Copper-IUDs do not confer a greater risk of acquiring HIV than if no contraceptive method is used.[78] Although there is concern about the theoretical risk of pelvic infection in women with HIV/AIDS who use IUDs and about transmission to uninfected partners, evidence is lacking. People who engage in sexual intercourse with partners who may be HIV-infected should consistently and correctly use latex condoms regardless of other contraceptive methods used.

No studies of hormone use have directly addressed whether COC use enhances disease progression in women with HIV/AIDS. For women at high risk of contracting HIV, evidence showing any increase in that risk for COC users compared to nonusers is inconsistent. For women infected with HIV, evidence is limited but there appears to be no correlation between COC use and changes in CD4 counts or RNA levels.[80] Some antiretroviral drugs may interact with OCs (see Table 4). There is no strong evidence of association between use of OCs or DMPA and HIV infection.[37,81]

Emergency Postcoital Contraception

A single dose of **levonorgestrel** 1.5 mg used within 24 hours of unprotected intercourse prevents 95% of expected pregnancies.[82] Efficacy is highest if treatment is provided within 24 hours; it can be taken up to 5 days after unprotected intercourse though the effectiveness declines with increasing delay between unprotected intercourse and treatment initiation.[83] Unprotected intercourse is defined as no contraceptive method used, condom breakage, more than 2 OC-pills missed any time during the cycle, 1 pill missed in the first week, more than 7-day pill-free interval, more than 13-week interval between DMPA injections, ejaculation on external genitalia or sexual assault.

The efficacy of levonorgestrel may be reduced with increased BMI.[84] Health Canada issued an advisory in March 2014 to inform women and healthcare providers that levonorgestrel emergency contraceptives are less effective in women weighing 75–80 kg and ineffective in women weighing more than 80 kg.[85] However, women who do not have access to or do not wish to use alternative emergency contraceptive methods such as copper IUD insertion should not be discouraged from using levonorgestrel.[86]

Levonorgestrel emergency contraception (EC) has a good safety record. There was no diagnosis of DVT or PE within 45 days of the prescription in a large UK study of EC users.[87] Side effects include nausea, vomiting, dizziness and fatigue. EC has no effect on an established postimplantation pregnancy.

Postcoital insertion of a **copper IUD** can be considered up to 7 days after unprotected intercourse. Prior to insertion, it is important to exclude pre-existing pregnancy. A meta-analysis demonstrated a failure rate of 0.1% from more than 8400 insertions of postcoital IUDs.[88,89] Though the exact mechanism of action is unknown, copper is postulated to impair implantation.[90] In addition to a high efficacy rate, the copper IUD is the only method to provide ongoing contraception to prevent future need for emergency contraception.[91]

See Table 5 for more information on emergency contraceptive choices.

Contraceptive Choices during Breastfeeding and the Postpartum Period

After delivery, it is highly unpredictable when fertility will be restored in breastfeeding mothers. Within 6 weeks of delivery there can be ovulation and pregnancy and these issues can be addressed at the postpartum visit. If coitus has resumed before the 6 week visit, exclude pregnancy before initiating a hormonal method of contraception.

Breastfeeding does not provide reliable contraceptive efficacy without a back up barrier method or alternative, as lactational amenorrhea is difficult to maintain (depends on the mother ensuring consistent, exclusive breastfeeding, with no supplemental food or fluids given; additionally, menses must not have returned and the baby must be <6 months old).

Barrier methods and **spermicide** can provide lubrication to the hypoestrogenic vagina but are not as effective for contraception as other methods.

The current Canadian Contraception Consensus guidelines recommend **progestin-only** methods of contraception in postpartum mothers regardless of breastfeeding status.[32] These methods can be introduced immediately after delivery. Since expulsion rates are higher for **LNG-IUS** when inserted immediately postpartum compared to 6 weeks after delivery, guidelines recommend waiting before insertion.[32] However, immediate insertion appears to be safe and effective, and provides convenience and assurance of contraception postpartum [Evidence: SORT B*].[93,94]

* SORT (Strength of Recommendation Taxonomy) is a rating system (A, B or C) that addresses the quality of available evidence. For more information consult **How to Use *Compendium of Therapeutic Choices*** on page xxv.

Progestin-based methods are recommended during breastfeeding due to the reduced risk of thromboembolism in the puerperium and their neutral effect on milk supply and establishment of breastfeeding. There is limited evidence of safety with regards to growth, health and development of infants exposed to progestin-only oral contraceptives. Oral formulations must be taken every day at the same time, without missing a pill, to minimize spotting and maintain contraceptive efficacy.

Avoid use of **COCs** in the first 6 weeks postpartum due to an increase in thrombotic risk in this period related to coagulation changes of the puerperium. There is also a concern about establishing an adequate milk supply. There are insufficient data to establish an effect of hormonal contraception on milk quality or quantity.[95]

An IUD[96] or COCs may be started immediately after first-trimester abortion or loss.

An IUD can be inserted immediately[97] or up to 6 weeks postpartum once involution has occurred and the uterus is firm enough to minimize the risk of insertional perforation. Ensure good fundal placement; this can be difficult in the immediate postpartum state with the larger uterine cavity.

Therapeutic Tips

- Hormonal contraceptives help regulate cycles and decrease menstrual flow. This may help to control anemia in women with heavy or irregular periods. In nonsmoking women with no cardiovascular risk factors, COCs may be considered for contraception or control of dysfunctional uterine bleeding until menopause. For more information, see Chapter 71.
- Noncontraceptive health benefits attributed to hormonal contraceptives use include a decrease in the frequency of fibroids, endometriosis pain, benign breast disease, functional ovarian cysts, ectopic pregnancy, dysmenorrhea, pelvic inflammatory disease and perimenopausal symptoms. COC use is also associated with a reduced incidence of endometrial and ovarian cancers compared to nonusers.[15] For more information, see Chapter 72.
- Hormonal contraception does not protect against acquisition of sexually transmitted infections. Educate patients on use of male latex condoms.
- Long-acting reversible contraception (LNG-IUS or copper-IUD) is the preferred form of contraception in adolescents at high risk of contraception failure due to incorrect use.[98,99] These devices are safe for use in nulliparous adolescents.[100]

Table 3: Nonhormonal Contraceptive Methods

Class	Contraceptive Method	Contraindications	Adverse Effects	Comments	Cost[a]
Barrier Methods	*cervical cap* FemCap	Absolute: cervical deformity (inability to obtain suitable fit), current PID, current vaginal or cervical infection, cervical or uterine cancer, cervical intraepithelial neoplasia, recurrent vaginal, urinary tract or cervical infections. Relative: abnormal cervical cytology, chronic cervicitis, recurrent salpingitis. Postpartum use unsuitable prior to uterine involution.	Common: vaginal discharge, vaginal odour, cervical or fornices ulceration, hypersensitivity (cap or spermicide). Infection if not used/cleaned properly, vaginitis. Rare: toxic shock syndrome.	**Failure rate:**[b,1] Typical use: 20% (nulliparous), 40% (parous). Perfect use: 9% (nulliparous), 26% (parous). Can be left in place for up to 48 h for multiple acts of intercourse. Use with spermicide, placed inside cap prior to insertion. Can be used in breastfeeding women (not within 6 weeks of delivery). Manufacturer recommends refitting after miscarriage, term delivery, abortion, or if lose/gain ≥3 kg.	$90/cap
	condoms, male (latex, polyurethane, lambskin) Trojan, Lifestyles, various	Relative: hypersensitivity to latex, polyurethane, or lanolin (in case of lambskin condoms).	Common: hypersensitivity to latex in either partner (may use polyurethane type).	**Failure rate:**[b,2] Typical use: 18%. Perfect use: 2%. Protects against STI including HIV (except lambskin condoms which do *not* protect against STI); best suited to infrequent intercourse; may use with a separately provided vaginal spermicide; check expiry date; latex condom integrity is degraded by miconazole and oil-based lubricants (use water-based lubricants).	$0.35–1.00/ male condom
	condoms, female (polyurethane) FC 2	Relative: hypersensitivity to polyurethane, vaginal anatomical abnormalities that make fitting difficult.	Discomfort.	**Failure rate:**[b,2] Typical use: 21%. Perfect use: 5%. Inserted up to 8 h prior to intercourse and removed immediately after. Not to be used with male condoms, potential for displacement; best suited for women who find spermicide irritating or who dislike messiness of other vaginal barrier methods; shelf-life of up to 5 years. This product is not available in pharmacies; may need to be purchased from sexual health clinics (e.g., Planned Parenthood).	$2.00/female condom

(cont'd)

Table 3: **Nonhormonal Contraceptive Methods** *(cont'd)*

Class	Contraceptive Method	Contraindications	Adverse Effects	Comments	Cost[a]
	diaphragm, silicone Wide Seal, Caya	Absolute: inability to achieve proper fit, marked uterine prolapse, large cystocele/rectocele, vaginal deformity, recurrent UTI. Relative: hypersensitivity, inability to insert. Postpartum use unsuitable prior to uterine involution.	Common: hypersensitivity to diaphragm and/or spermicide. Infection if diaphragm not used/cleaned properly. Less common: increased incidence of UTI Rare: toxic shock syndrome.	**Failure rate:**[b,2] Typical use: 12%. Perfect use: 6%. Best suited to infrequent intercourse. Use with spermicide. Can be inserted 6 h before intercourse. Refit after childbirth, surgery, or if lose/gain ≥4 kg. Can be used in breastfeeding women.	$55/diaphragm
	sponge Today Sponge	Absolute: inability to achieve proper fit, recurrent UTI. Relative: hypersensitivity, inability to insert.	Common: hypersensitivity. Rare: toxic shock syndrome.	**Failure rate:**[b,2] Typical use: 12% (nulliparous), 24% (parous). Perfect use: 9% (nulliparous), 20% (parous). Spermicide is released in a sustained fashion for up to 12 h. May increase HIV transmission by damaging vaginal mucosa; in women at high risk of HIV infection, this risk must be balanced against risk of pregnancy. Do not use during menstruation.[3]	$6/unit
Intrauterine Devices (IUD)	*copper-T IUD* Nova-T, Flexi-T	Absolute: pregnancy, undiagnosed vaginal bleeding, stenosed cervix, copper allergy, current PID or STI, cervical or endometrial cancer, copper allergy, inability to place or retain device.[7] Relative: 2–28 days postpartum (to decrease risk of expulsion).[8]	Major: salpingitis, uterine perforation, cervical perforation, endometrial embedding, menorrhagia, pain, infection, ectopic pregnancy.	**Failure rate:**[b,2] 0.6–0.8%. Excellent for spacing children in a stable relationship; risk of PID and tubal infections; immediate risks are insertional infection or perforation; late risks are infection and ectopic pregnancy. May be used post abortion. Although AHA guidelines suggest it is no longer mandatory to use endocarditis prophylaxis for IUD insertion in women with complicated valvular heart disease, clinical judgment should be used based on the complexity of the heart lesion.	$70–180 (lasts 3–10y)[5]
Natural Methods	*coital timing*	Relative: irregular cycle.	None.	**Failure rate:**[b,2] Typical use: 24%. Perfect use: 0.4–5%. Fertility awareness methods require high motivation; depends on identification of mucus and temperature patterns to identify fertile time; very difficult if there is an irregular cycle or ovulation defects; high pregnancy rates.	None

Class	Contraceptive Method	Contraindications	Adverse Effects	Comments	Cost[a]
Spermicides	*nonoxynol-9* Vaginal Contraceptive Film (VCF), others	Relative: hypersensitivity.	Common: hypersensitivity.	**Failure rate:**[b,2] (when used alone) Typical use: 28%. Perfect use: 18%. Not effective against HIV or STI. Increased risk of HIV transmission due to increased risk of genital lesions with regular use;[4] in women at high risk of HIV infection, this risk must be balanced against risk of pregnancy.	$1/unit
Sterilization, Surgical	*tubal ligation*	Pregnancy, systemic conditions (e.g., cardiopulmonary) that can be aggravated by general anesthesia, pelvic infection.	Cumulative 10-year probability of ectopic pregnancy post tubal ligation: 7.3 per 1000.[9]	**Failure rate:**[b,2] 0.5%. Method of choice for couples with completed family. Reversible only if salpingectomy not performed and sufficient length of undamaged tubal remnants remain. Cost of reversal surgery: $3000–5000.	Cost-insured service in Canada.
	vasectomy	Systemic conditions (e.g., acute infectious diseases), local infection, sexual dysfunction, local genital abnormalities (e.g., hernia).	Local pain, scrotal ecchymosis, swelling.	**Failure rate:**[b,2] 0.1–0.15%. Method of choice for couples with completed family; reversible with more surgery if <10 years since procedure. Cost of reversal surgery: $3000–5000.	Cost-insured service in Canada.

[a] Approximate cost per unit (condom, tube, canister, package); includes drug or contraceptive cost only. Mark-up is not included.
[b] Percentage of women with unintended pregnancy within 1st year of use.
Abbreviations: HIV = human immunodeficiency virus; PID = pelvic inflammatory disease ; STI = sexually transmitted infection; UTI = urinary tract infection

Table 4: **Hormonal Contraceptive Methods**

Class	Drug	Contraindications	Adverse Effects	Drug Interactions	Comments	Cost[a]
Contraceptives, oral – combined estrogen (35 µg EE) and progestin, Monophasic	*EE 35 µg/ norethindrone 1 mg* Brevicon 1/35, Ortho 1/35, Select 1/35	Absolute: history of MI or ischemic heart disease, cerebrovascular disease, complicated valvular heart disease, current or past history of VTE, known thrombogenic mutation, severe cirrhosis, liver tumour, breast cancer, diabetes with microvascular complications, migraines with aura, <6 weeks postpartum if breastfeeding, smoker >35 years (≥15 cigarettes/day), hypertension (systolic BP ≥160 mm Hg or diastolic BP ≥100 mm Hg), known coagulation-factor deficiency.[11] Relative: estrogen hypersensitivity, migraine, gallbladder disease, high BMI/weight. Low-dose COCs are relatively contraindicated if BP ≥140/90.	Major: thromboembolism (rare), stroke, retinal artery thrombosis, MI, benign liver tumour, cholelithiasis, hypertension. Watch for danger signals: ACHES—**a**bdominal pain, **c**hest pain, **h**eadaches, **e**ye problems, **s**evere leg pain. Advise patient to consult physician. Common: breakthrough bleeding/spotting, amenorrhea, nausea/vomiting, bloating, chloasma, breast tenderness, mood changes such as depression, headaches.	May increase cyclosporine levels or hepatotoxicity; may decrease lamotrigine levels. Significant pharmacokinetic interaction with rifampin, griseofulvin (advise backup barrier method during therapy). Monitor INR with concurrent oral anticoagulant use. Carbamazepine, modafinil, phenytoin, protease inhibitors, phenobarbital, St. John's wort, topiramate may decrease EE/progestin serum concentrations. Reports of COC failure with concomitant ampicillin, amoxicillin, tetracycline, erythromycin, sulfamethoxazole/ trimethoprim or nitrofurantoin.	**Failure rate:**[b,2] Typical use: 9%. Perfect use: 0.3%. Lower-dose COCs are method of choice for most young couples, especially for teens, if combined with condoms; products with lower dose of EE have increased safety, decreased side effects; condoms needed for STI protection. Patients with diarrhea or breakthrough bleeding may be at higher risk of contraceptive failure.	$
	EE 35 µg/ norethindrone 0.5 mg Brevicon 0.5/35, Ortho 0.5/35	See EE 35 µg/ norethindrone 1 mg.	See EE 35 µg/ norethindrone 1 mg.	See EE 35 µg/ norethindrone 1 mg.	See EE 35 µg/ norethindrone 1 mg.	$$
	EE 35 µg/ norgestimate 0.25 mg Cyclen	See EE 35 µg/ norethindrone 1 mg.	See EE 35 µg/ norethindrone 1 mg.	See EE 35 µg/ norethindrone 1 mg.	See EE 35 µg/ norethindrone 1 mg.	$$$

Class	Drug	Contraindications	Adverse Effects	Drug Interactions	Comments	Cost[a]
Contraceptives, oral – combined estrogen (30 µg EE) and progestin, Monophasic	*EE 30 µg/ desogestrel 0.15 mg* Marvelon, Ortho-Cept, Apri, Freya, Mirvala	See EE 35 µg/ norethindrone 1 mg.	See EE 35 µg/ norethindrone 1 mg.	See EE 35 µg/ norethindrone 1 mg.	See EE 35 µg/ norethindrone 1 mg.	$
	EE 30 µg/ drospirenone 3 mg Yasmin, Zamine, Zarah	See EE 35 µg/ norethindrone 1 mg.	See EE 35 µg/ norethindrone 1 mg. Risk of hyperkalemia in patients prone to increased K^+ (e.g., renal disease, concomitant ACEI, ARB, potassium-sparing diuretics, NSAID). Check K^+ after 1st cycle. May increase risk of VTE compared to LNG-containing OCs.	See EE 35 µg/ norethindrone 1 mg.	See EE 35 µg/ norethindrone 1 mg. Also indicated for acne treatment.	$$
	EE 30 µg/ ethynodiol diacetate 2 mg Demulen 30	See EE 35 µg/ norethindrone 1 mg.	See EE 35 µg/ norethindrone 1 mg.	See EE 35 µg/ norethindrone 1 mg.	See EE 35 µg/ norethindrone 1 mg.	$$
	EE 30 µg/ levonorgestrel 0.15 mg, 1-month Min-Ovral, Portia	See EE 35 µg/ norethindrone 1 mg.	See EE 35 µg/ norethindrone 1 mg.	See EE 35 µg/ norethindrone 1 mg.	See EE 35 µg/ norethindrone 1 mg.	$$
	EE 30 µg/ levonorgestrel 0.15 mg, 3-month Seasonale, Seasonique	See EE 35 µg/ norethindrone 1 mg.	See EE 35 µg/ norethindrone 1 mg.	See EE 35 µg/ norethindrone 1 mg.	See EE 35 µg/ norethindrone 1 mg. Seasonale and Seasonique are packaged for 3 months of continuous use, with 84 active tablets and 7 inert (Seasonale) or ultra-low dose (0.01 mg) EE tablets (Seasonique).	$59/ 3 months
	EE 30 µg/ norethindrone acetate 1.5 mg Loestrin 1.5/30	See EE 35 µg/ norethindrone 1 mg.	See EE 35 µg/ norethindrone 1 mg.	See EE 35 µg/ norethindrone 1 mg.	See EE 35 µg/ norethindrone 1 mg.	$$

(cont'd)

Table 4: **Hormonal Contraceptive Methods** *(cont'd)*

Class	Drug	Contraindications	Adverse Effects	Drug Interactions	Comments	Cost[a]
Contraceptives, oral – combined estrogen (20 µg EE) and progestin, Monophasic	*EE 20 µg/ drospirenone 3 mg* Yaz, MYA	See EE 35 µg/ norethindrone 1 mg.	See EE 35 µg/ norethindrone 1 mg. Risk of hyperkalemia in patients prone to increased K^+ (e.g., renal disease, concomitant ACEI, ARB, potassium-sparing diuretics, NSAID). Check K^+ after 1st cycle. May increase risk of VTE compared to LNG-containing OCs.	See EE 35 µg/ norethindrone 1 mg.	See EE 35 µg/ norethindrone 1 mg. Also indicated for acne treatment. Packaged with active tablets × 24 days, inert tablets × 4 days.	$$
	EE 20 µg/ drospirenone 3 mg/levomefolate calcium 0.451 mg Yaz Plus	See EE 20 µg/ drospirenone 3 mg.	See EE 20 µg/ drospirenone 3 mg.	See EE 20 µg/ drospirenone 3 mg.	See EE 20 µg/ drospirenone 3 mg. First 24 tablets contain all 3 ingredients; last 4 tablets contain levomefolate calcium only.	$$
	EE 20 µg/ levonorgestrel 0.1 mg Alesse, Alysena, Aviane, ESME, Lutera	See EE 35 µg/ norethindrone 1 mg.	See EE 35 µg/ norethindrone 1 mg.	See EE 35 µg/ norethindrone 1 mg.	See EE 35 µg/ norethindrone 1 mg. Also indicated for acne treatment.	$
	EE 20 µg/ norethindrone1 mg Minestrin 1/20	See EE 35 µg/ norethindrone 1 mg.	See EE 35 µg/ norethindrone 1 mg.	See EE 35 µg/ norethindrone 1 mg.	See EE 35 µg/ norethindrone 1 mg.	$$
Contraceptives, oral – combined estrogen and progestin, Triphasic	*EE 25 µg/ desogestrel 0.1 mg/ 0.125 mg/0.15 mg* Linessa	See EE 35 µg/ norethindrone 1 mg.	See EE 35 µg/ norethindrone 1 mg.	See EE 35 µg/ norethindrone 1 mg.	See EE 35 µg/ norethindrone 1 mg. EE dose stays constant, desogestrel dose increases Q7 days.	$$
	EE 35 µg/ norethindrone 0.5 mg/0.75 mg/1 mg Ortho 7/7/7	See EE 35 µg/ norethindrone 1 mg.	See EE 35 µg/ norethindrone 1 mg.	See EE 35 µg/ norethindrone 1 mg.	See EE 35 µg/ norethindrone 1 mg. EE dose stays constant, norethindrone dose increases Q7 days.	$$

Class	Drug	Contraindications	Adverse Effects	Drug Interactions	Comments	Cost[a]
	EE 35 μg/ norethindrone 0.5 mg/1 mg/0.5 mg Synphasic	See EE 35 μg/ norethindrone 1 mg.	See EE 35 μg/ norethindrone 1 mg.	See EE 35 μg/ norethindrone 1 mg.	See EE 35 μg/ norethindrone 1 mg. EE dose stays constant, norethindrone dose increases between days 8–16 of 21-day cycle.	$$
	EE 35 μg/ norgestimate 0.18 mg/0.215 mg/ 0.25 mg Tri-Cyclen	See EE 35 μg/ norethindrone 1 mg.	See EE 35 μg/ norethindrone 1 mg.	See EE 35 μg/ norethindrone 1 mg.	See EE 35 μg/ norethindrone 1 mg. EE dose stays constant, norgestimate dose increases Q7 days. Also indicated for acne treatment.	$$$
	EE 25 μg/ norgestimate 0.18 mg/0.215 mg/ 0.25 mg Tri-Cyclen Lo, Tricira Lo	See EE 35 μg/ norethindrone 1 mg.	See EE 35 μg/ norethindrone 1 mg.	See EE 35 μg/ norethindrone 1 mg.	See EE 35 μg/ norethindrone 1 mg. EE dose stays constant, norgestimate dose increases Q7 days.	$$
	EE 30 μg/40 μg/ 30 μg, levonorgestrel 0.05 mg/0.075 mg/ 0.125 mg Triquilar	See EE 35 μg/ norethindrone 1 mg.	See EE 35 μg/ norethindrone 1 mg.	See EE 35 μg/ norethindrone 1 mg.	See EE 35 μg/ norethindrone 1 mg. Both EE and levonorgestrel doses vary at days 7 and 12 of 21-day cycle.	$$
Contraceptives, transdermal	*EE 600 μg/ norelgestromin 6 mg per weekly patch* *(releases approximately EE 35 μg/day, norelgestromin 200 μg/day)* Evra	See EE 35 μg/ norethindrone 1 mg. Relative: body weight ≥90 kg (decreased efficacy).	See EE 35 μg/ norethindrone 1 mg. Breast discomfort (19%) is more common than with COC in 1st 2 months of use; headache (22%), skin reaction under patch (20%), nausea (20%), dysmenorrhea. 2–3% detachment rate from skin. Studies assessing the risk of VTE in transdermal vs. COC users are conflicting.	See EE 35 μg/ norethindrone 1 mg.	**Failure rate:**[b,2] Typical use: 9%. Perfect use: 0.3%. Condoms needed for STI protection. Apply once weekly × 3 weeks (on same day each week), followed by 1 patch-free week. Apply to dry intact skin of buttock, abdomen, upper outer arm or upper torso. If off for >24 h, apply new patch and use backup method × 7 days. To switch from COC, apply initial patch on 1st day of withdrawal	$$

(cont'd)

Table 4: **Hormonal Contraceptive Methods** *(cont'd)*

Class	Drug	Contraindications	Adverse Effects	Drug Interactions	Comments	Cost[a]
					bleeding. If applied later than 1st day, use backup method × 7 days. To switch from DMPA, apply 1st patch on day of scheduled injection.	
Contraceptives, vaginal ring	*EE 15 μg/day, etonorgestrel 120 μg/day* NuvaRing	See EE 35 μg/ norethindrone 1 mg. Relative: uterovaginal prolapse, vaginal stenosis (prevent retention of ring).	See EE 35 μg/ norethindrone 1 mg. Common: vaginal discomfort, vaginitis (5%), headache (6.6%), leukorrhea (5.3%), decreased libido, nausea, breast tenderness.	See EE 35 μg/ norethindrone 1 mg. May interfere with the correct placement and position of diaphragm or cervical cap—do not use these methods as backup. Concurrent use of vaginal tampons not recommended (ring can be expelled when removing tampon); can use tampons after vaginal ring is removed.	**Failure rate:**[b,2] Typical use: 9%. Perfect use: 0.3%. Can be self-inserted and removed; is worn vaginally continuously × 3 weeks then removed × 1 week. Systemic absorption occurs. If ring is left out of the vagina for >3 h use backup method × 7 days. May not provide adequate contraception if left in place longer than 4 weeks. Some reports suggest efficacy lasts up to 6 weeks.[6] Condoms needed for STI protection. May leave at room temperature for up to 4 months prior to insertion. Can be expelled from vagina while emptying bladder or bowel, especially during severe straining.	$$

Class	Drug	Contraindications	Adverse Effects	Drug Interactions	Comments	Cost[a]
Contraceptives, progestin-only, oral	*norethindrone* Micronor	Absolute: pregnancy, current breast cancer. Relative: active viral hepatitis, liver tumours.	Higher incidence of ectopic pregnancy compared to COC. Irregular bleeding (~12% of users in the first months, <3% in 18 months).	Significant pharmacokinetic interaction with griseofulvin (advise backup barrier method during therapy). Carbamazepine, modafinil, phenytoin, protease inhibitors, phenobarbital, St. John's wort, topiramate may decrease progestin serum concentrations.	**Failure rate:**[b,2] Typical use: 9%. Perfect use: 0.3%. Preferred in lactating women or if contraindication to estrogen; condoms needed for STI protection; packaged as active tablets × 28 days.	$$$
Contraceptives, progestin-only, injectable	*medroxyprogesterone acetate* Depo-Provera, generics	Absolute: pregnancy, unexplained vaginal or urinary tract bleeding, current diagnosis of breast cancer, known sensitivity to MPA or to the vehicle. Relative: severe cirrhosis, active viral hepatitis, benign hepatic adenoma.	Breast tenderness, insomnia or somnolence, fatigue, mood changes, e.g., depression or irritability, weight gain, menstrual irregularities, decreased libido, skin sensitivity reactions, hyperpyrexia, acne. Long-term: decrease in BMD, delayed return of fertility.	See norethindrone.	**Failure rate:**[b,2] Typical use: 6%. Perfect use: 0.2%. Inject 150 mg within first 5 days of onset of menses (to be effective immediately). Interval between injections must not exceed 13 weeks. Excellent for women who should avoid high estrogen doses, e.g., migraine sufferers. Consider other options in women with risk factors for osteoporosis. Condoms needed for STI protection.	$$$/3 months

(cont'd)

Table 4: **Hormonal Contraceptive Methods** *(cont'd)*

Class	Drug	Contraindications	Adverse Effects	Drug Interactions	Comments	Cost[a]
Contraceptives, progestin-only, intrauterine system (IUS)	*levonorgestrel 20 μg/day* Mirena	Pregnancy, current or recurrent PID, genital infection, postpartum endometritis, undiagnosed abnormal uterine bleeding, uterine or cervical malignancy, cervicitis, acute liver disease, hypersensitivity to components of system, hematologic malignancies, uterine anomaly, <4 weeks postpartum.	Spotting for first 3 months after insertion; eventual amenorrhea in 20–30% of women. Expelled in 6% of women.	See norethindrone	**Failure rate:**[b,2] 0.2%. Condoms needed for STI protection. Remains in place for 5 years. Insert within 7 days of onset of menses (to be effective immediately). Although AHA guidelines suggest it is no longer mandatory to use endocarditis prophylaxis for IUDinsertion in women with complicated valvular heart disease, use clinical judgment based on the complexity of the heart lesion. May be used postabortion (no difference in safety or expulsion rate compared to copper IUD).[8]	$350 (lasts 5 years)
	levonorgestrel 14 μg/day Jaydess	See levonorgestrel 20 μg/day.	Prolonged and frequent bleeding and/or spotting for the first 3–6 months of therapy. Over time, infrequent bleeding and amenorrhea may occur. Expelled in 3% of women.	See norethindrone	**Failure rate:**[b,10] 0.4–0.9%. Condoms needed for STI protection. Remains in place for 3 years. Insert within 7 days of onset of menses (to be effective immediately). May be used postabortion.	$285 (lasts 3 years)

[a] Approximate cost per 1 package for 1 month unless otherwise indicated; includes drug or contraceptive cost only. Mark-up is not included.
[b] Percentage of women with unintended pregnancy within 1st year of use.
Abbreviations: ACEI = angiotensin-converting enzyme inhibitor; AHA = American Heart Association; ARB = angiotensin receptor blocker; BMD = bone mineral density; BMI = body mass index; BP = blood pressure; COC = combined oral contraceptive; DMPA = depot medroxyprogesterone acetate; EE = ethinyl estradiol; IUD = intrauterine device; IUS = intrauterine system; LNG = levonorgestrel; MI = myocardial infarction; MPA = medroxyprogesterone acetate; NSAID = nonsteroidal anti-inflammatory drug; PID = pelvic inflammatory disease; STI = sexually transmitted infection; VTE = venous thromboembolism
Legend: $ < $10 $$ $10–20 $$$ $20–30

Table 5: Emergency Contraceptive Methods

Class	Drug	Contraindications	Adverse Effects	Drug Interactions	Comments	Cost[a]
Contraceptives, intrauterine device (IUD): emergency postcoital	*copper-T IUD* Nova-T, Flexi-T	See Table 3, Intrauterine Devices.	See Table 3, Intrauterine Devices.	None.	Use within 7 days of unprotected intercourse as an emergency contraceptive. Interferes with implantation after fertilization. Can be used as ongoing method of contraception.	$70–$180
Contraceptives, oral progestin: emergency postcoital	*levonorgestrel 0.75 mg* Plan B, NorLevo, generics	Pregnancy.	Nausea (23.1%), vomiting (5.6%), dizziness, fatigue.	Griseofulvin, carbamazepine, modafinil, phenytoin, protease inhibitors, phenobarbital, St. John's wort, topiramate may decrease levonorgestrel serum concentrations.	Dose: 1.5 mg (2 × 0.75 mg tablets taken together) as soon as possible after unprotected intercourse (most effective if taken within 72 h). 0.75 mg Q12H × 2 doses is equally effective. (Second dose can be taken up to 24 h after 1st dose without significant change in pharmacokinetics.[92]) Heath Canada advisory regarding reduced effectiveness in women weighing 75–80 kg and lack of effectiveness in women weighing ≥80 kg.[85]	$19

[a] Cost of 1 dose; includes drug cost only.
Abbreviations: ECP = emergency contraceptive pill; EE = ethinyl estradiol

Suggested Readings

Black A, Francoeur D, Rowe T et al. SOGC clinical practice guidelines: Canadian contraception consensus. *J Obstet Gynaecol Can* 2004;26(3):219-96.

Division of Reproductive Health, National Center for Chronic Disease Prevention and Health Promotion, Centers for Disease Control and Prevention (CDC). U.S. Selected Practice Recommendations for Contraceptive Use, 2013: adapted from the World Health Organization selected practice recommendations for contraceptive use, 2nd edition. *MMWR Recomm Rep* 2013;62(RR-05):1-60.

Dunn S, Guilbert E. Emergency contraception. *J Obstet Gynaecol Can* 2012;34(9):870-8.

Faculty of Family Planning & Reproductive Health Care. FFPRHC Guidance (July 2004). Contraceptive choices for breastfeeding women. *J Fam Plann Reprod Health Care* 2004;30(3):181-9.

Stegeman BH, de Bastos M, Rosendaal FR et al. Different combined oral contraceptives and the risk of venous thrombosis: systematic review and network meta-analysis. *BMJ* 2013;347:f5298.

References

1. Society of Obstetricians and Gynecologists of Canada. SexualityandU.ca. *Non-hormonal methods: Cervical cap*. Available from: www.sexualityandu.ca/birth-control/non-hormonal-methods. Accessed February 6, 2014.
2. Trussell J. Contraceptive efficacy. In: Hatcher RA, Trussel J, Nelson AL et al. *Contraceptive technology: twentieth revised edition*. New York (NY): Ardent Media; 2011. Available from: www.contraceptivetechnology.org/wp-content/uploads/2013/09/CTFailureTable.pdf. Accessed February 6, 2014.
3. Faich G, Pearson K, Fleming D et al. Toxic shock syndrome and the vaginal contraceptive sponge. *JAMA* 1986;255(2):216-8.
4. Workowski KA, Berman S; Centers for Disease Control and Prevention (CDC). Sexually transmitted diseases treatment guidelines, 2010. *MMWR Recomm Rep* 2010;59(RR-12):1-110.
5. Medisafe Distribution. *Liberté TT 380: Information leaflet for the doctor*. Available from: medisafecanada.com/ns/wp-content/uploads/2012/08/TT380-DoctorLeafletWEB.pdf. Accessed on December 12, 2013.
6. Dragoman M, Petrie K, Torgal A et al. Contraceptive vaginal ring effectiveness is maintained during 6 weeks of use: a prospective study of normal BMI and obese women. *Contraception* 2013;87(4):432-6.
7. Nelson AL. Contraindications to IUD and IUS use. *Contraception* 2007;75(6 Suppl):S76-81.
8. World Health Organization. Intrauterine devices (IUDs). In: *Medical eligibility criteria for contraceptive use*. Geneva (CH): Department of Reproductive Health, WHO; 2010. p. 65-78. Available from: whqlibdoc.who.int/publications/2010/9789241563888_eng.pdf. Accessed July 5, 2013.
9. Peterson HB, Xia Z, Hughes JM et al. The risk of pregnancy after tubal sterilization: findings from the U.S. Collaborative Review of Sterilization. *Am J Obstet Gynecol* 1996;174(4):1161-8.
10. Health Canada. Drug Product Database Online Query. Bayer Inc. *Jaydess* [product monograph]. Available from: webprod5.hc-sc.gc.ca/dpd-bdpp/newSearch-nouvelleRecherche.do?lang=eng.
11. World Health Organization. *Medical eligibility criteria for contraceptive use*. Geneva (CH): Department of Reproductive Health, WHO; 2010. Available from: whqlibdoc.who.int/publications/2010/9789241563888_eng.pdf. Accessed July 5, 2013.
12. Seibert C, Barbouche E, Fagan J et al. Prescribing oral contraceptives for women older than 35 years of age. *Ann Intern Med* 2003;138(1):54-64.
13. Boukes FS, Beijderwellen L, van der Does FE et al. [Summary of the practice guideline 'Hormonal contraception' (second revision) from the Dutch College of General Practitioners]. *Ned Tijdschr Geneeskd* 2004;148(26):1285-9. [Dutch].
14. Van Vliet HA, Grimes DA, Helmerhorst FM et al. Biphasic versus monophasic oral contraceptives for contraception. *Cochrane Database Syst Rev* 2006;(3):CD002032.
15. Practice Committee of the American Society for Reproductive Medicine. Hormonal contraception: recent advances and controversies. *Fert Steril* 2004;82(Suppl 1):S26-32.
16. Rosenberg MJ, Meyers A, Roy V. Efficacy, cycle control and side effects of low- and lower-dose oral contraceptives: a randomized trial of 20 micrograms and 35 micrograms estrogen preparations. *Contraception* 1999;60(6):321-9.
17. Gallo MF, Nanda K, Grimes DA et al. 20 µg versus >20 µg estrogen combined oral contraceptives for contraception. *Cochrane Database Syst Rev* 2013;8:CD003989.
18. Keam SJ, Wagstaff AJ. Ethinylestradiol/drospirenone: a review of its use as an oral contraceptive. *Treat Endocrinol* 2003;2(1):49-70.
19. Lopez LM, Kaptein AA, Helmerhorst FM. Oral contraceptives containing drospirenone for premenstrual syndrome. *Cochrane Database Syst Rev* 2012;(2):CD006586.
20. Jick SS, Hernandez RK. Risk of non-fatal venous thromboembolism in women using oral contraceptives containing drospirenone compared with women using oral contraceptives containing levonorgestrel: case-control study using United States claims data. *BMJ* 2011;342:d2151.
21. Parkin L, Sharples K, Hernandez RK et al. Risk of venous thromboembolism in users of oral contraceptives containing drospirenone or levonorgestrel: nested case-control study based on UK General Practice Research Database. *BMJ* 2011;342:d2139.
22. Wu CQ, Grandi SM, Fillion KB et al. Drospirenone-containing oral contraceptive pills and the risk of venous and arterial thrombosis: a systematic review. *BJOG* 2013;120(7):801-10.
23. Oddsson K, Leifels-Fischer B, de Melo NR et al. Efficacy and safety of a contraceptive vaginal ring (NuvaRing) compared with a combined oral contraceptive: a 1-year randomized trial. *Contraception* 2005;71(3):176-82.
24. Roumen FJ, Apter D, Mulders TM et al. Efficacy, tolerability and acceptability of a novel contraceptive vaginal ring releasing etonogestrel and ethinyl oestradiol. *Hum Reprod* 2001;16(3):469-75.
25. Dieben TO, Roumen FJ, Apter D. Efficacy, cycle control, and user acceptability of a novel combined contraceptive vaginal ring. *Obstet Gynecol* 2002;100(3):585-93.

26. Voora D, Vijayan A. Mesenteric vein thrombosis associated with intravaginal contraceptives: a case report and review of the literature. *J Thromb Thrombolysis* 2003;15(2):105-8.
27. Miller L, Verhoeven CH, Hout J. Extended regimens of the contraceptive vaginal ring: a randomized trial. *Obstet Gynecol* 2005;106(3):473-82.
28. Sicat BL. Ortho Evra, a new contraceptive patch. *Pharmacotherapy* 2003;23(4):472-80.
29. Lopez LM, Grimes DA, Gallo MF et al. Skin patch and vaginal ring versus combined oral contraceptives for contraception. *Cochrane Database Syst Rev* 2013;4:CD003552.
30. Audet MC, Moreau M, Koltun WD et al. Evaluation of contraceptive efficacy and cycle control of a transdermal contraceptive patch vs an oral contraceptive: a randomized controlled trial. *JAMA* 2001;285(18):2347-54.
31. Gomes MP, Deitcher SR. Risk of venous thromboembolic disease associated with hormonal contraceptives and hormone replacement therapy: a clinical review. *Arch Intern Med* 2004;164(18):1965-76.
32. Black A, Francoeur D, Rowe T et al. SOGC clinical practice guidelines: Canadian contraception consensus. *J Obstet Gynaecol Can* 2004;26(3):219-96.
33. Westhoff CL, Torgal AH, Mayeda ER et al. Ovarian suppression in normal-weight and obese women during oral contraceptive use: a randomized controlled trial. *Obstet Gynecol* 2010;116(2 Pt 1):275-83.
34. Lopez LM, Grimes DA, Chen-Mok M et al. Hormonal contraceptives for contraception in overweight or obese women. *Cochrane Database Syst Rev* 2013;4:CD008452.
35. Guilbert E, Boroditsky R, Black A et al. Canadian consensus guideline on continuous and extended hormonal contraception, 2007. *J Obstet Gynaecol Can* 2007;29(7 Suppl 2):S1-32.
36. Division of Reproductive Health, National Center for Chronic Disease Prevention and Health Promotion, Centers for Disease Control and Prevention (CDC). U.S. Selected Practice Recommendations for Contraceptive Use, 2013: adapted from the World Health Organization selected practice recommendations for contraceptive use, 2nd edition. *MMWR Recomm Rep* 2013;62(RR-05):1-60.
37. Curtis KM, Chrisman CE, Peterson HB et al. Contraception for women in selected circumstances. *Obstet Gynecol* 2002;99(6):1100-12.
38. Scholes D, LaCroix AZ, Ichikawa LE et al. Change in bone mineral density among adolescent women using and discontinuing depot medroxyprogesterone acetate contraception. *Arch Pediatr Adolesc Med* 2005;159(2):139-44.
39. Cromer BA, Lazebnik R, Rome E et al. Double-blinded randomized controlled trial of estrogen supplementation in adolescent girls who receive depot medroxyprogesterone acetate for contraception. *Am J Obstet Gynecol* 2005;192(1):42-7.
40. Sayed GH, Zakherah MS, El-Nashar SA et al. A randomized clinical trial of a levonorgestrel-releasing intrauterine system and a low-dose combined oral contraceptive for fibroid-related menorrhagia. *Int J Gynaecol Obstet* 2011;112(2):126-30.
41. Sordal T, Inki P, Draeby J et al. Management of initial bleeding or spotting after levonorgestrel-releasing intrauterine system placement: a randomized controlled trial. *Obstet Gynecol* 2013;121(5):934-41.
42. Madden T, Proehl S, Allsworth JE et al. Naproxen or estradiol for bleeding and spotting with the levonorgestrel intrauterine system: a randomized controlled trial. *Am J Obstet Gynecol* 2012;206(2):129.e1-8.
43. Farley TM, Collins J, Schlesselman JJ. Hormonal contraception and risk of cardiovascular disease. An international perspective. *Contraception* 1998;57(3):211-30.
44. Acute myocardial infarction and combined oral contraceptives: results of an international multicentre case-control study. WHO Collaborative Study of Cardiovascular Disease and Steroid Hormone Contraception. *Lancet* 1997;349(9060):1202-9.
45. Chan WS, Ray J, Wai EK et al. Risk of stroke in women exposed to low-dose oral contraceptives: a critical evaluation of the evidence. *Arch Intern Med* 2004;164(7):741-7.
46. Schwartz SM, Petitti DB, Siscovick DS et al. Stroke and use of low-dose oral contraceptives in young women: a pooled analysis of two US studies. *Stroke* 1998;29(11):2277-84.
47. Schwartz SM, Siscovick DS, Longstreth WT et al. Use of low-dose oral contraceptives and stroke in young women. *Ann Intern Med* 1997;127(8 Pt 1):596-603.
48. Chang CL, Donaghy M, Poulter N. Migraine and stroke in young women: case-control study. The World Health Organisation Collaborative Study of Cardiovascular Disease and Steroid Hormone Contraception. *BMJ* 1999;318(7175):13-8.
49. Curtis KM, Mohllajee AP, Peterson HB. Use of combined oral contraceptives among women with migraine and nonmigrainous headaches: a systematic review. *Contraception* 2006;73(2):189-94.
50. Spitzer WO, Faith JM, MacRae KD. Myocardial infarction and third generation oral contraceptives: aggregation of recent studies. *Hum Reprod* 2002;17(9):2307-14.
51. Etminan M, Takkouche B, Isorna FC et al. Risk of ischaemic stroke in people with migraine: systematic review and meta-analysis of observational studies. *BMJ* 2005;330(7482):63.
52. MacClellan LR, Giles W, Cole J et al. Probable migraine with visual aura and risk of ischemic stroke: the stroke prevention in young women study. *Stroke* 2007;38(9):2438-45.
53. Kemmeren JM, Tanis BC, van den Bosch MA et al. Risk of Arterial Thrombosis in Relation to Oral Contraceptives (RATIO) study: oral contraceptives and the risk of ischemic stroke. *Stroke* 2002;33(5):1202-8.
54. Schiff I, Bell WR, Davis V et al. Oral contraceptives and smoking, current considerations: recommendations of a consensus panel. *Am J Obstet Gynecol* 1999;180(6 Pt 2):S383-4.
55. Petitti DB. Clinical practice. Combination estrogen-progestin oral contraceptives. *N Engl J Med* 2003;349(15):1443-50.
56. Ahmed SB, Hovind P, Parving HH et al. Oral contraceptives, angiotensin-dependent renal vasoconstriction, and risk of diabetic nephropathy. *Diabetes Care* 2005;28(8):1988-94.
57. Margolis KL, Adami HO, Luo J et al. A prospective study of oral contraceptive use and risk of acute myocardial infarction among Swedish women. *Fertil Steril* 2007;88(2):310-6.
58. Farmer RD, Lawrenson RA, Thompson CR et al. Population-based study of risk of venous thromboembolism associated with various oral contraceptives. *Lancet* 1997;349(9045):83-8.
59. Farmer RD, Lawrenson RA, Todd JC et al. A comparison of the risks of venous thromboembolic disease in association with different combined oral contraceptives. *Br J Clin Pharmacol* 2000;49(6):580-90.
60. Kujovich JL. Hormones and pregnancy: thromboembolic risks for women. *Br J Haematol* 2004;126(4):443-54.
61. de Bastos M, Stegeman BH, Rosendaal FR et al. Combined oral contraceptives: venous thrombosis. *Cochrane Database Syst Rev* 2014;3:CD010813.
62. Stegeman BH, de Bastos M, Rosendaal FR et al. Different combined oral contraceptives and the risk of venous thrombosis: systematic review and network meta-analysis. *BMJ* 2013;347:f5298.

63. Peragallo Urrutia R, Coeytaux RR, McBroom AJ et al. Risk of acute thromboembolic events with oral contraceptive use: a systematic review and meta-analysis. *Obstet Gyn* 2013;122(2 Pt 1):380-9.
64. Bloemenkamp KW, Rosendaal FR, Buller HR et al. Risk of venous thrombosis with use of current low-dose oral contraceptives is not explained by diagnostic suspicion and referral bias. *Arch Intern Med* 1999;159(1):65-70.
65. Lidegaard O, Edstrom B, Kreiner S. Oral contraceptives and venous thromboembolism: a five-year national case-control study. *Contraception* 2002;65(3):187-96.
66. Lidegaard O, Nielsen LH, Skovlund CW et al. Venous thrombosis in users of non-oral hormonal contraception: follow-up study, Denmark 2001-10. *BMJ* 2012;344:e2990.
67. Middeldorp S. Oral contraceptives and the risk of venous thromboembolism. *Gend Med* 2005;2(Suppl A):S3-S9.
68. Nightingale AL, Lawrenson RA, Simpson EL et al. The effects of age, body mass index, smoking and general health on the risk of venous thromboembolism in users of combined oral contraceptives. *Eur J Contracept Reprod Health Care* 2000;5(4):265-74.
69. Vandenbroucke JP, Koster T, Briet E et al. Increased risk of venous thrombosis in oral-contraceptive users who are carriers of factor V Leiden mutation. *Lancet* 1994;344(8935):1453-7.
70. Bloemenkamp KW, Rosendaal FR, Helmerhorst FM et al. Enhancement by factor V Leiden mutation of risk of deep-vein thrombosis associated with oral contraceptives containing a third-generation progestagen. *Lancet* 1995;346(8990):1593-6.
71. Wu O, Robertson L, Twaddle S et al. Screening for thrombophilia in high-risk situations: systematic review and cost-effectiveness analysis. The Thrombosis: Risk and Economic Assessment of Thrombophilia Screening (TREATS) study. *Health Technol Assess* 2006;10(11):1-110.
72. Wu O, Robertson L, Twaddle S et al. Screening for thrombophilia in high-risk situations: a meta-analysis and cost-effectiveness analysis. *Br J Haematol* 2005;131(1):80-90.
73. Borgelt-Hansen L. Oral contraceptives: an update on health benefits and risks. *J Am Pharm Assoc (Wash)* 2001;41(6):875-86.
74. Hunter DJ, Colditz GA, Hankinson SE et al. Oral contraceptive use and breast cancer: a prospective study of young women. *Cancer Epidemiol Biomarkers Prev* 2010;19(10):2496-502.
75. Lumsden MA, Gebbie A, Holland C. Managing unscheduled bleeding in non-pregnant premenopausal women. *BMJ* 2013;346:f3251.
76. U.K. Royal College of Obstetricians and Gynaecologists. Faculty of Sexual and Reproductive Healthcare clinical guidance. *Management of unscheduled bleeding in women using hormonal contraception.* 2009. Available from: www.fsrh.org/pdfs/UnscheduledBleedingMay09.pdf. Accessed on December 13, 2013.
77. Abdel-Aleem H, d'Arcangues C, Vogelsong KM et al. Treatment of vaginal bleeding irregularities induced by progestin only contraceptives. *Cochrane Database Syst Rev* 2013;10:CD003449.
78. Cates W. Review of non-hormonal contraception (condoms, intrauterine devices, nonoxynol-9 and combos) on HIV acquisition. *J Acquir Immune Defic Syndr* 2005;38(Suppl 1):S8-10.
79. Roddy RE, Zekeng L, Ryan KA et al. A controlled trial of nonoxynol-9 film to reduce male-to-female transmission of sexually transmitted diseases. *N Engl J Med* 1998;339(8):504-10.
80. World Health Organization. *Medical eligibility criteria for contraceptive use* 4th ed. Geneva (CH): Department of Reproductive Health, WHO; 2009. Available from: www.who.int/reproductivehealth/publications/family_planning/9789241563888/en/index.html.
81. Polis CB, Curtis KM. Use of hormonal contraceptives and HIV acquisition in women: a systematic review of the epidemiological evidence. *Lancet Infect Dis* 2013;13(9):797-808.
82. von Hertzen H, Piaggio G, Ding J et al. Low dose mifepristone and two regimens of levonorgestrel for emergency contraception: a WHO multicenter randomised trial. *Lancet* 2002;360(9348):1803-10.
83. Rodrigues I, Grou F, Joly J. Effectiveness of emergency contraceptive pills between 72 and 120 hours after unprotected sexual intercourse. *Am J Obstet Gynecol* 2001;184(4):531-7.
84. Glasier A, Cameron ST, Blithe D et al. Can we identify women at risk of pregnancy despite using emergency contraception? Data from randomized trials of ulipristal acetate and levonorgestrel. *Contraception* 2011;84(4):363-7.
85. Health Canada. *Emergency contraceptive pills to carry warnings for reduced effectiveness in women over a certain body weight.* Available from: healthycanadians.gc.ca/recall-alert-rappel-avis/hc-sc/2014/38701a-eng.php.
86. Society of Obstetricians and Gynaecologists of Canada. Position statement [in response to Health Canada's Emergency contraceptive pills to carry warnings for reduced effectiveness in women over a certain body weight]. May 2014. Available from: sogc.org/wp-content/uploads/2014/05/medStatementEC_BMI_1400502E.pdf.
87. Vasilakis C, Jick SS, Jick H. The risk of venous thromboembolism in users of postcoital contraceptive pills. *Contraception* 1999;59(2):79-83.
88. Trussell J, Ellerston C. Efficacy of emergency contraception. *Fertil Control Rev* 1995;4:8-11.
89. Cleland K, Zhu H, Goldstuck N et al. The efficacy of intrauterine devices for emergency contraception: a systematic review of 35 years of experience. *Hum Reprod* 2012;27(7):1994-2000.
90. Thomas MA. Postcoital contraception. *Clin Obstet Gynecol* 2001;44(1):101-5.
91. Cheng L, Che Y, Gulmezoglu AM. Interventions for emergency contraception. *Cochrane Database Syst Rev* 2012;8:CD001324.
92. Tremblay D, Gainer E, Ulmann A. The pharmacokinetics of 750 microg levonorgestrel following administration of one single dose or two doses at 12- or 24-h interval. *Contraception* 2001;64(6):327-31.
93. Grimes DA, Lopez LM, Schulz KF et al. Immediate post-partum insertion of intrauterine devices. *Cochrane Database Syst Rev* 2010;(5):CD003036.
94. Chen BA, Reeves MF, Hayes JL et al. Postplacental or delayed insertion of the elevonorgestrel intrauterine device after vaginal delivery: a randomized controlled trial. *Obstet Gynecol* 2010;116(5):1079-87.
95. Truitt ST, Fraser AB, Grimes DA et al. Combined hormonal versus nonhormonal versus progestin-only contraception in lactation. *Cochrane Database Syst Rev* 2003;(2):CD003988.
96. Bednarek PH, Creinin MD, Reeves MF et al. Immediate versus delayed IUD insertion after uterine aspiration. *N Engl J Med* 2011;364(23):2208-17.
97. Centers for Disease Control and Prevention (CDC). Update to CDC's U.S. medical eligibility criteria for contraceptive use, 2010: revised recommendations for the use of contraceptive methods during the postpartum period. *MMWR Morb Mortal Wkly Rep* 2011;60(26):878-83.
98. Winner B, Peipert JF, Zhao Q et al. Effectiveness of long-acting reversible contraception. *N Engl J Med* 2012;366(21):1998-2007.
99. Committee opinion no. 539: adolescents and long-acting reversible contraception: implants and intrauterine devices. *Obstet Gynecol* 2012;120(4):983-8.
100. Berenson AB, Tan A, Hirth JM et al. Complications and continuation of intrauterine device use among commercially insured teenagers. *Obstet Gynecol* 2013;121(5):951-8.

Chapter 71
Dysmenorrhea

Margaret Burnett, MD, FRCSC, FACOG

Dysmenorrhea is abdominal and pelvic pain associated with menses. More than half of menstruating women are affected to some degree and 15% are incapacitated for 1–3 days per month.[1,2] Primary dysmenorrhea occurs in the absence of organic pathology, while secondary dysmenorrhea results from an underlying cause such as endometriosis, adenomyosis or obstructed uterine outflow (Table 1).

Table 1: **Characteristics of Dysmenorrhea**[1,2,3]

Primary	Secondary
No identifiable pelvic pathology Occurs in ovulatory cycles Most severe in young, nulliparous women Onset within 2 y after menarche; tendency to improve with age More common in smokers Pain due to myometrial contractions induced by prostaglandin production in the secretory endometrium Pain is ameliorated by empiric therapy with anti-prostaglandins and/or ovulation suppression	Associated with pelvic pathology, e.g., endometriosis, adenomyosis, submucous uterine myoma, endometrial polyp, intrauterine device, pelvic inflammatory disease, vaginal septum, imperforate hymen, congenital Mullerian malformations, post-ablation syndrome Diagnostic clues include pain onset premenstrually, pain lasting throughout the menses, infertility, dyspareunia, abnormal uterine bleeding Onset immediately at menarche or after age 25 A component of pain may be due to endometrial prostaglandins; therefore, partial response may be seen to NSAID therapy

Goals of Therapy

- Decrease or abolish distressing menstrual pain
- Target and treat the specific underlying causes of secondary dysmenorrhea

Investigations

- A thorough history to determine the severity, timing, chronicity and manifestations of the pain as well as aggravating and relieving factors. As a general rule, the pain of primary dysmenorrhea starts within several hours before the onset of bleeding up to a few hours after the start of menses,[1] and:
  - lasts a maximum of a few days
  - is described as crampy, located in the lower mid-abdomen and/or pelvis
  - other symptoms of prostaglandin excess may be present, e.g., nausea, vomiting, diarrhea, backache, thigh pain, headache, dizziness
- Physical examination of the abdomen and pelvis to identify potential causes of secondary dysmenorrhea. In virginal women an abdominal examination and inspection of the external genitalia are sufficient. In sexually active women, a single digit vaginal examination can be a useful addition to the exam. Each pelvic structure should be carefully palpated in order to isolate potential areas of tenderness, masses or nodules (best performed when the woman is not experiencing pain).

  In the absence of abnormal findings, diagnostic imaging is unlikely to be helpful and may be misleading if noncontributory abnormalities are discovered. Pelvic ultrasound or MRI is indicated if the physical examination is suggestive of a pelvic mass or uterine outflow obstruction. If an adequate physical examination is not possible, e.g., in obese patients or if the patient refuses, a pelvic ultrasound or MRI can be useful.

- Laparoscopy is reserved for those women whose dysmenorrhea does not respond to medical therapy
- No laboratory tests are required

Therapeutic Choices

An algorithm for the management of dysmenorrhea is shown in Figure 1.

Figure 1: Management of Dysmenorrhea

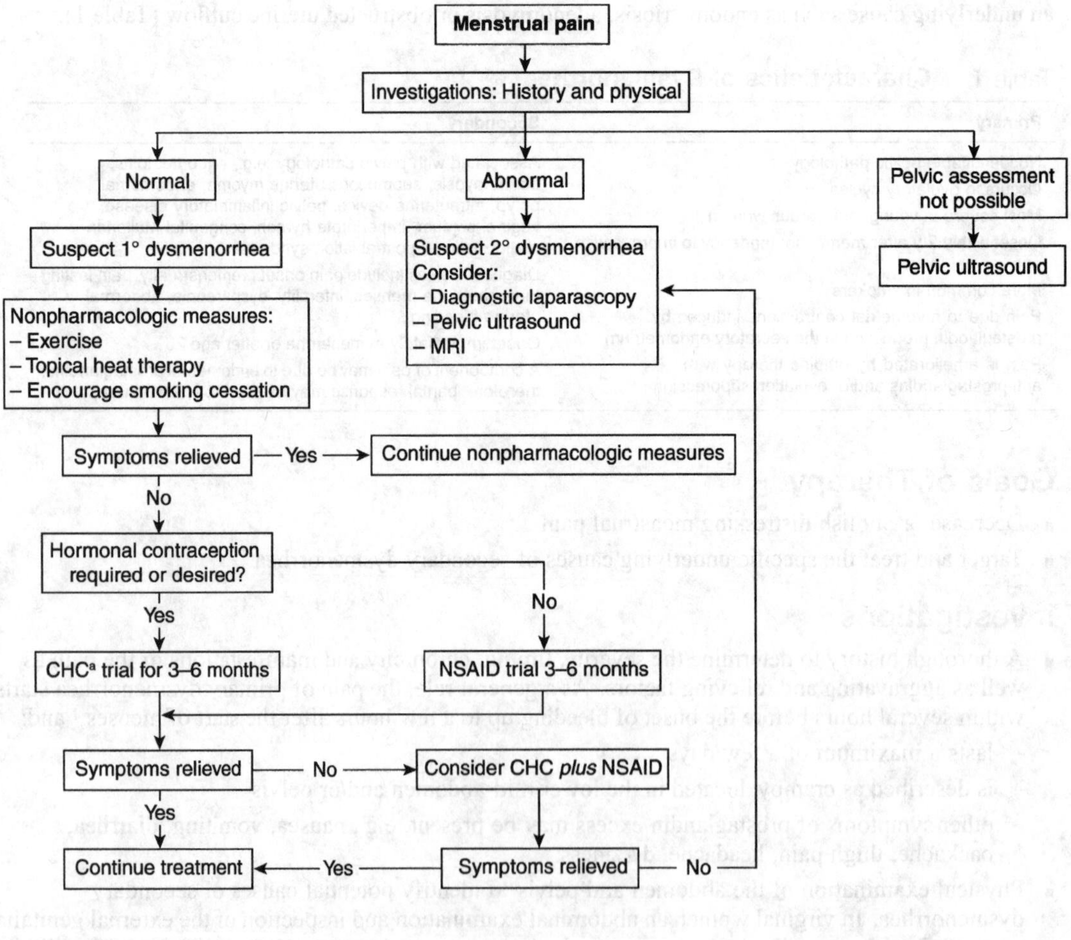

[a] Consider levonorgestrel IUS or depot medroxyprogesterone in certain situations (see text).

Abbreviations: CHC = combined hormonal contraceptive; IUS = intrauterine system; NSAID = nonsteroidal anti-inflammatory drug

Nonpharmacologic Choices

- Explain that primary dysmenorrhea is a common, frequently distressing phenomenon; reassure patient that pain does not indicate an organic process or abnormality in most cases. If an organic cause is suspected, institute appropriate investigation and targeted therapy.
- Topical heat therapy, e.g., heating pads, may be useful.[3]
- Regular exercise may provide some relief.[4]
- Yoga[5]
- Acupressure[6,7] and acupuncture are potential options for women with dysmenorrhea.[8,9,10]
- High-frequency transcutaneous electrical nerve stimulation (TENS) has shown promise in the management of dysmenorrhea.[11]
- Facilitate smoking cessation.[2]

Pharmacologic Choices

Drug therapies for the management of dysmenorrhea are presented in Table 2.

Nonsteroidal Anti-inflammatory Drugs (NSAIDs)

Primary dysmenorrhea is caused by abnormal uterine contractions as a result of increased prostaglandin production by the endometrium in ovulatory cycles. NSAIDs, which are prostaglandin synthetase inhibitors, are the treatment of choice. All NSAIDs except ASA have been shown to be effective in about 80% of cases of dysmenorrhea [Evidence: SORT A*].[12,13] In practice, there appears to be minimal difference among NSAIDs.[12] With short-term use, side effects of all NSAIDs are generally minor. **Ibuprofen** and **naproxen sodium** are available without a prescription. The choice depends more on tolerability, duration of action, cost and availability [Evidence: SORT B*].[3,12] NSAIDs should be taken with food, starting immediately at the onset of symptoms or menses and continued on a *regular schedule* for 2–3 days. An initial loading dose may help obtain faster relief of symptoms [Evidence: SORT C*].[3] Although all NSAIDs demonstrate an increased risk of cardiovascular events (e.g., MI or stroke), studies indicate that **diclofenac** and high-dose **ibuprofen** are associated with the highest risk of cardiovascular events.[14,15] However, it should be noted that cardiovascular events are likely to be extremely rare in young women using NSAIDs on an intermittent basis.

Acetaminophen demonstrates minimal analgesic effect in dysmenorrhea[13] and inferior pain relief compared to NSAIDs.[12] Consider acetaminophen only for patients with contraindications to NSAIDs.

Montelukast

A preliminary double-blind trial conducted in Japan suggests that the leukotriene receptor antagonist, **montelukast** may benefit some women with dysmenorrhea.[16] However, overall pain reduction and NSAID use were not significantly different between treatment and placebo groups.

Combined Hormonal Contraceptives

Combined hormonal contraceptives (CHCs) are available as oral, vaginal or transdermal formulations. CHCs inhibit ovulation, which limits endometrial growth and decreases menstrual blood flow, thereby suppressing prostaglandin production at menses. CHCs effectively treat dysmenorrhea; however, no large, well-designed studies have been undertaken to prove the effectiveness of low-dose CHCs.[17] Combined oral contraceptives (COCs), the contraceptive patch or the vaginal ring are ideal first-line choices for women wishing contraception. *Continuous* or *extended-cycle regimens* may decrease the frequency of menstrual periods and the prevalence of pain. These regimens may also ameliorate

* SORT (Strength of Recommendation Taxonomy) is a rating system (A, B or C) that addresses the quality of available evidence. For more information consult **How to Use *Compendium of Therapeutic Choices*** on page xxv.

dysmenorrhea due to endometriosis and adenomyosis. Continuous use of COCs is often successful if cyclic use fails. Extended or continuous use of the contraceptive ring or patch may be another alternative.

For prescribing information on contraceptives, see Chapter 70.

Progestin-only Contraceptives

The **levonorgestrel intrauterine system (LNG IUS)** reduces menstrual bleeding and is highly effective for dysmenorrhea associated with heavy menstrual flow.[18,19,20,21] A low dose of levonorgestrel is released continuously over a period of at least 3 years, causing the endometrium to become atrophic and inactive.

Depot medroxyprogesterone (DMPA) intramuscular injections suppress ovulation, induce endometrial atrophy and produce amenorrhea. Consider DMPA as a treatment option in the management of primary dysmenorrhea[3] in women who cannot tolerate estrogen and in women over 35 years who smoke. DMPA can also be useful in treating secondary dysmenorrhea caused by endometriosis, adenomyosis or structural abnormalities of the uterus. Although bone mineral density may return to baseline on discontinuation of therapy, use DMPA with caution in adolescents 12–18 years as they have not yet attained their peak bone mass. To promote overall bone health, encourage adequate **calcium** (total of 1200 mg daily from all sources, preferably through dietary intake) and **vitamin D** (1000 IU supplement daily) in women on DMPA therapy.[22]

For prescribing information on contraceptives, see Chapter 70.

Nutritional Supplements

Magnesium, vitamin B_1, omega-3 fatty acids, ginger, Chinese herbs[23] and **valerian**[24] have shown promise in the management of dysmenorrhea, but further randomized controlled trials are necessary.[26,27]

Therapeutic Tips

- A therapeutic trial of 3–6 months with either an NSAID (on a regular schedule) or a CHC is usually sufficient to demonstrate effectiveness. Although there are no clinical trials to support the combination, if either fails it is reasonable to consider a trial of NSAID + CHC before commencing further investigation.
- Pharmacotherapy fails in 20% of patients. These patients often have secondary dysmenorrhea and require further investigation. Ultrasound and diagnostic laparoscopy are useful to differentiate primary from secondary dysmenorrhea. Therapy can then be directed to the underlying cause and may involve surgery, e.g., laser ablation or electrofulguration of endometriosis. Dysmenorrhea resulting from menorrhagia will improve if the heavy bleeding is controlled.[25]
- In a small percentage of patients, pharmacotherapy and/or conservative surgery fail to relieve menstrual pain. These patients may require surgical intervention such as hysterectomy with or without oophorectomy to obtain relief.

Table 2: **Nonsteroidal Anti-inflammatory Drugs (NSAIDs)[a] for the Management of Dysmenorrhea**

Class	Drug	Dose	Adverse Effects	Comments	Cost[b]
COX-2 Inhibitors	*celecoxib* Celebrex	200 mg/day in 1 or 2 doses with food	Very common (>10%): dyspepsia, nausea/vomiting. Common (5–10%): nonspecific rash, pruritus, dizziness, headache. NSAIDs may be nephrotoxic and should not be used in severe renal impairment. May be useful in women at high risk for GI adverse effects.	First line in the management of dysmenorrhea. Begin at onset of symptoms or menses and continue for 2–3 days. Prescribe hormonal contraceptives if contraception is required or desired. Can be given in combination if treatment with NSAIDs is inadequate. SSRIs may increase risk of gastrointestinal bleeding when used with NSAIDs. Contraindications: hypersensitivity to ASA, active pelvic inflammatory bowel disease, existing renal disease, clotting disorders. Contraindicated if sulfonamide allergy.	$$
NSAIDs, acetic acid derivatives	*diclofenac potassium* Voltaren Rapide, generics	Loading dose of 100 mg po then 50 mg Q6–8H with food. Maximum daily dose: 150 mg	Very common (>10%): dyspepsia, nausea/vomiting. Common (5–10%): nonspecific rash, pruritus, dizziness, headache. NSAIDs may be nephrotoxic and should not be used in severe renal impairment.	First line in the management of dysmenorrhea. Begin at onset of symptoms or menses and continue for 2–3 days. Prescribe hormonal contraceptives if contraception is required or desired. Can be given in combination if treatment with NSAIDs is inadequate. SSRIs may increase risk of gastrointestinal bleeding when used with NSAIDs. Contraindications: hypersensitivity to ASA, active pelvic inflammatory bowel disease, existing renal disease, clotting disorders.	$$$

(cont'd)

Table 2: **Nonsteroidal Anti-inflammatory Drugs (NSAIDs)[a] for the Management of Dysmenorrhea** *(cont'd)*

Class	Drug	Dose	Adverse Effects	Comments	Cost[b]
	diclofenac sodium Voltaren, Voltaren SR, generics	Immediate-release: 50 mg BID–TID po with food Sustained-release: 75 mg BID po with food Maximum daily dose: 150 mg	See diclofenac potassium.	See diclofenac potassium.	$
NSAIDs, fenamates	*mefenamic acid* Ponstan, generics	Loading dose of 500 mg then 250 mg Q6H with food	See diclofenac potassium.	See diclofenac potassium. Theoretically, the fenamates should be the most effective pain relievers; they also bind to prostaglandin receptors and have an antagonistic effect.	$$$
NSAIDs, propionic acid derivatives	*ibuprofen* Advil, Motrin, Motrin Liquid Gels, generics	200–600 mg Q6H po with food Maximum daily dose: 2400 mg	See diclofenac potassium.	See diclofenac potassium. Available without prescription.	$
	ketoprofen generics	50 mg TID po with food	See diclofenac potassium.	See diclofenac potassium.	$$
	naproxen Naprosyn, generics	Loading dose of 500 mg po then 250 mg Q6–8H or 500 mg BID with food Maximum daily dose: 1250 mg	See diclofenac potassium.	See diclofenac potassium.	$
	naproxen sodium Anaprox, Aleve, generics	220–550 mg BID po with food	See diclofenac potassium.	See diclofenac potassium. 220 mg tablets are available without prescription.	$$

[a] NSAIDs listed are examples. For a comprehensive listing of NSAIDs, see Chapter 82.
[b] Cost of 7-day supply; includes drug cost only.
Legend: $ < $5 $$ $5–10 $$$ $10–15

Suggested Readings

Dawood MY. Primary dysmenorrhea: advances in pathogenesis and management. *Obstet Gynecol* 2006;108(2):428-41.

Lefebvre G, Pinsonneault O, Antao V et al. Primary dysmenorrhea consensus guideline. *J Obstet Gynaecol Can* 2005;27(12):1117-46.

References

1. Dawood MY. Primary dysmenorrhea: advances in pathogenesis and management. *Obstet Gynecol* 2006;108(2):428-41.
2. Burnett MA, Antao V, Black A et al. Prevalence of primary dysmenorrhea in Canada. *J Obstet Gynaecol Can* 2005;27(8):765-70.
3. Lefebvre G, Pinsonneault O, Antao V et al. Primary dysmenorrhea consensus guideline. *J Obstet Gynaecol Can* 2005;27(12):1117-46.
4. Brown J, Brown S. Exercise for dysmenorrhea. *Cochrane Database Syst Rev* 2010;(2):CD004142.
5. Rakhshaee Z. Effect of three yoga poses (cobra, cat and fish poses) in women with primary dysmenorrhea: a randomized clinical trial. *J Pediatr Adolesc Gynecol* 2011;24(4):192-6.
6. Smith CA, Zhu X, He L et al. Acupuncture for primary dysmenorrhoea. *Cochrane Database Syst Rev* 2011;(1):CD007854.
7. Chung YC, Chen HH, Yeh ML. Acupoint stimulation intervention for people with primary dysmenorrhea: systematic review and meta-analysis of randomized trials. *Complement Ther Med* 2012;20(5):353-63.
8. Yang H, Liu CZ, Chen X et al. Systematic review of clinical trial of acupuncture-related therapies for primary dysmenorrhea. *Acta Obstet Gynecol Scand* 2008;87(11):1114-22.
9. Witt CM, Reinhold T, Brinkhaus B et al. Acupuncture in patients with dysmenorrhea: a randomized study on clinical effectiveness and cost-effectiveness in usual care. *Am J Obstet Gynecol* 2008;198(2):166.e1-8.
10. Cho SH, Hwang EW. Acupuncture for primary dysmenorrhoea: a systematic review. *BJOG* 2010;117(5):509-21.
11. Proctor ML, Smith CA, Farquhar CM et al. Transcutaneous electrical nerve stimulation and acupuncture for primary dysmenorrhoea. *Cochrane Database Syst Rev* 2002;(1):CD002123.
12. Marjoribanks J, Proctor ML, Farquhar C. Nonsteroidal anti-inflammatory drugs for dysmenorrhoea. *Cochrane Database Syst Rev* 2010;(1):CD001751.
13. Zhang WY, Li Wan Po A. Efficacy of minor analgesics in primary dysmenorrhoea: a systematic review. *Br J Obstet Gynaecol* 1998;105(7):780-9.
14. Trelle S, Reichenbach S, Wandel S et al. Cardiovascular safety of non-steroidal anti-inflammatory drugs: network meta-analysis. *BMJ* 2011;342:c7086.
15. McGettigan P, Henry D. Cardiovascular risk with non-steroidal anti-inflammatory drugs: systematic review of population-based controlled observational studies. *PLoS Med* 2011;8(9):e1001098.
16. Fujiwara H, Konno R, Netsu S et al. Efficacy of montelukast, a leukotriene receptor antagonist, for the treatment of dysmenorrhea: a prospective, double-blind, randomized placebo-controlled study. *Eur J Obstet Gynecol Reprod Biol* 2010;148(2):195-8.
17. Wong CL, Farquhar C, Roberts H et al. Oral contraceptive pill for primary dysmenorrhoea. *Cochrane Database Syst Rev* 2009;(4):CD002120.
18. Barrington JW, Bowen-Simpkins P. The levonorgestrel intrauterine system in the management of menorrhagia. *Br J Obstet Gynaecol* 1997;104(5):614-6.
19. Andersson JK, Rybo G. Levonorgestrel-releasing intrauterine device in the treatment of menorrhagia. *Br J Obstet Gynaecol* 1990;97(8):690-4.
20. Aslam N, Blunt S, Latthe P. Effectiveness and tolerability of levonorgestrel intrauterine system in adolescents. *J Obstet Gynaecol* 2010;30(5):489-91.
21. Lindh I, Milsom I. The influence of intrauterine contraception on the prevalence and severity of dysmenorrhea: a longitudinal population study. *Hum Reprod* 2013;28(7):1953-60.
22. Black A; Ad Hoc DMPA Committee of the Society of Obstetricians and Gynaecologists of Canada. Canadian contraception consensus—update on Depot Medroxyprogesterone Acetate (DMPA). *J Obstet Gynaecol Can* 2006;28(4):305-8.
23. Zhu X, Proctor M, Bensoussan A et al. Chinese herbal medicine for primary dysmenorrhea. *Cochrane Database Syst Rev* 2008;(2):CD005288.
24. Mirabi P, Dolatian M, Mojab F et al. Effects of valerian on the severity and systemic manifestations of dysmenorrhea. *Int J Gynaecol Obstet* 2011;115(3):285-8.
25. Chapa HO, Venegas G, Antonetti AG et al. In-office endometrial ablation and clinical correlation of reduced menstrual blood loss and effects on dysmenorrheal and premenstrual symptomatology. *J Reprod Med* 2009;54(4):232-8.
26. Proctor ML, Murphy PA. Herbal and dietary therapies for primary and secondary dysmenorrhoea. *Cochrane Database Syst Rev* 2001;(3):CD002124.
27. Zhu X, Proctor M, Bensoussan A et al. Chinese herbal medicine for primary dysmenorrhea. *Cochrane Database Syst Rev* 2008;(2):CD005288.

Chapter 72
Endometriosis

G. Barry Gilliland, MD, FRCSC, FACOG

Endometriosis, diagnosed by finding tissue that histologically resembles endometrium at sites outside the uterine cavity, can cause pelvic pain, dysmenorrhea and infertility. Histological confirmation requires at least 2 of the following: endometrial epithelium, endometrial glands, endometrial stroma and hemosiderin-laden macrophages. Although endometriosis is most often classified according to the revised American Fertility Sterility Classification (r-AFS),[1] there is no direct correlation between the volume of endometriotic tissue, i.e., stage of disease, and either pregnancy rates or severity of symptoms.

There is a higher incidence of endometriosis in Caucasian women, particularly those who are 25–29 years old and those with high alcohol intake.[2] Cigarette smoking is associated with increased risk of endometriosis in women who never reported infertility. However, in women who are concurrently infertile, cigarette smoking is associated with reduced risk of endometriosis. Similarly, there is an inverse relationship between diagnosis of endometriosis and BMI in women who are concurrently infertile.[2]

Endometriosis-associated pain is frequently recurrent. After treatment with gonadotropin-releasing hormone (GnRH) analogues, the rate of recurrent pelvic pain over 5 years ranges from 37% in patients with mild endometriosis to 74% in those with severe disease.[3] Following surgical ablation/resection of endometriosis, the risk of recurrence of pain is estimated to be as high as 40% at 10 years of follow-up.[4] Many patients have persistent pain due to other pelvic pathology, notably interstitial cystitis and irritable bowel syndrome or regional sympathetic syndrome.

Endometriosis may be treated with drugs, surgery or both. Individualize treatment according to age, duration of infertility, severity of pelvic pain, response to previous therapies, anticipated side effects and cost.

This chapter discusses endometriosis-associated pain and endometriosis-associated infertility.

Goals of Therapy

- Relieve pain
- Treat infertility
- Prevent recurrence

Investigations

Diagnosis of endometriosis is difficult due to its variable presentation. Significant overlap with other conditions, e.g., irritable bowel syndrome, has been observed.[5]

- History of pelvic pain (cyclical at first, becomes continuous as endometriosis worsens), dysmenorrhea (does not diminish after menstrual day 2), deep dyspareunia or infertility suggests endometriosis
- Physical examination: a pelvic examination with tenderness, particularly in the uterosacral ligament area and especially around the time of menses, suggests endometriosis

- Objective measurements:
  - the gold standard for diagnosis of endometriosis is laparoscopy ± biopsy. Appearance of endometriotic tissue may be typical or atypical. Focal deposits may have the classic blue or black appearance. They may also appear yellow, brown, white or red—81% of such areas show histological evidence of endometriosis[6]
  - serum CA 125 (a tumor-associated protein) levels are often significantly elevated (>35 IU/mL) but not always found with endometriosis. Other causes of elevated serum CA 125 levels include pelvic inflammatory disease, epithelial ovarian cancer and pregnancy. Serum CA 125 levels should not be performed as part of routine diagnostic work-up but are useful for treatment follow up and may aid in identifying infertile women with severe endometriosis who could benefit from surgery[7]
  - ultrasound reliably identifies masses with features of endometriomas;[8] however, these features are nonspecific. The use of color velocity imaging and pulsed Doppler does not improve the diagnostic accuracy of transvaginal ultrasonography alone in the diagnosis of ovarian endometrioma.[9] Sensitivity of ultrasound is poor for the detection of focal implants[10]
  - MRI may be useful for identifying deep subperitoneal lesions and for monitoring residual or recurrent disease after surgery

Endometriosis-associated Pain

Therapeutic Choices

An algorithm for the management of endometriosis is shown in Figure 1.

Figure 1: Endometriosis Management

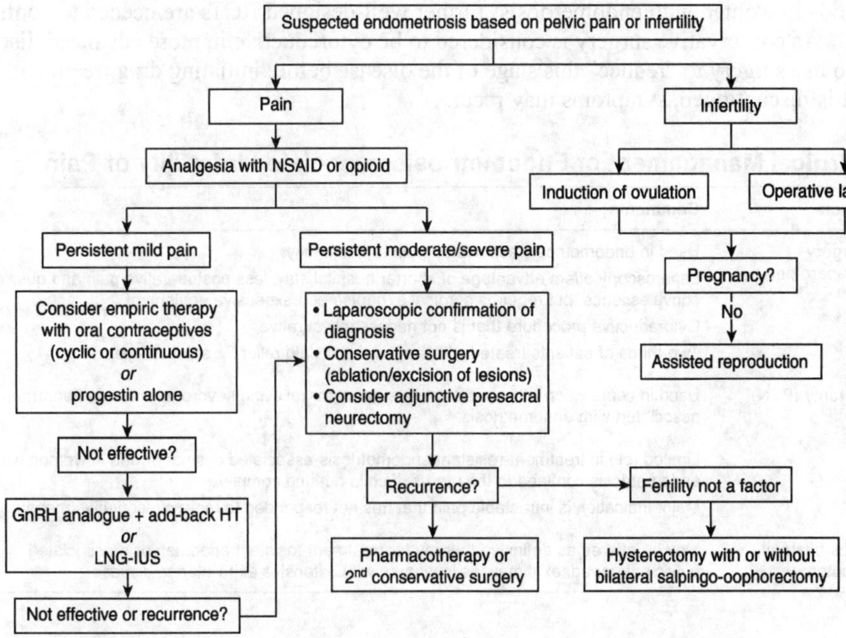

Abbreviations: GnRH = gonadotropin-releasing hormone; HT = hormone therapy; LNG-IUS = levonorgestrel intrauterine system; MPA = medroxyprogesterone acetate; NSAID = nonsteroidal anti-inflammatory drug; OC = oral contraceptive

Nonpharmacologic Choices

The primary goals in the surgical treatment of endometriosis-associated pain (Table 1) include the removal of typical and atypical endometriotic implants and the restoration of pelvic anatomy. After any form of surgery residual disease may be left behind.

Conservative surgery or ablative surgery for endometriosis is a cytoreductive procedure that is not necessarily curative. It may be considered for recurrent disease, if pain relief is required,[11] or if a patient declines definitive surgery. Sixty to 100% of patients experience decreased severity of pain after ablative surgery.[12] Recurrence rates range from 13.5–40.3% at 5 years.[11,13] Pregnancy does not influence the average time to recurrence of symptoms.[14]

Conservative surgery can be performed by laparoscopy or laparotomy; both procedures are equally effective.[15] Potential advantages of laparoscopy include the ability to treat the disease at the time of diagnosis, enhanced removal and ablation of endometriosis, reduced morbidity, shorter hospital stay, rapid recovery and potential decrease in the rate of postoperative adhesion formation.[16]

One randomized controlled trial with follow up showed that laser ablation with laparascopic uterosacral nerve ablation (LUNA) effectively relieved pain in 62.5% of treated patients, compared to 22.6% in the control group (no treatment).[17,18] However, a later Cochrane review concluded that the addition of LUNA to surgical treatment for secondary causes of dysmenorrhea (including endometriosis) did not aid pain relief.[19] Current guidelines suggest that LUNA alone does not provide significant pain relief in patients with endometriosis.[20]

Presacral neurectomy, in conjunction with conservative surgery for endometriosis, may be effective in relieving severe midline dysmenorrhea associated with endometriosis if the surgeon completely resects the presacral nerve plexus.[21] Results of adding this procedure to conservative surgery are mixed.

Following conservative surgery for endometriosis, pain relief may be maximized and relapse/symptom recurrence may be reduced by long-term oral contraceptive therapy (see Hormonal Therapies).[22,23] There is limited but consistent evidence showing that postoperative LNG-IUD reduces the recurrence of painful periods in women with endometriosis; further well-designed RCTs are needed to confirm these findings.[24] As conservative surgery is considered to be cytoreductive in more advanced disease, it is reasonable to use surgery to "reduce" this stage of the disease before initiating drug treatment. Once drug treatment is discontinued, symptoms may recur.

Table 1: **Surgical Management of Endometriosis-associated Infertility or Pain**

Surgical Approach	Comments
Conservative surgery (laparoscopy or laparotomy)	Used in endometriosis-associated pain and infertility Laparoscopy offers advantage of shorter hospital stay, less postoperative pain and quicker convalescence, but requires surgical expertise and expensive equipment Cytoreductive procedure that is not necessarily curative Two-thirds of patients treated with surgery have pain relief for at least 1 year
Presacral neurectomy (PSN)	Used in conjunction with conservative surgery for relieving severe midline dysmenorrhea associated with endometriosis
Hysterectomy	Limited role in treatment-resistant endometriosis-associated dysmenorrhea in women with endometriosis confined to the uterus, if child bearing complete Major indication is intractable pain that has not responded to more conservative measures
Hysterectomy plus bilateral salpingo-oophorectomy	May be offered as definitive therapy for treatment-resistant endometriosis-associated pelvic pain or adnexal masses in women with extensive extra-uterine disease

Definitive surgical therapy of endometriosis-associated pain requires total abdominal hysterectomy with or without bilateral salpingo-oophorectomy, with complete excision or ablation of endometriosis. The major indication for definitive therapy is intractable pain in patients who have not responded to more conservative measures or who have completed their families. It is considered 90–95% effective for pain relief.[25]

A retrospective study of recurrence of symptoms after definitive surgery, with a mean follow up of 4 years and 10 months, showed that 62% of patients with ovarian conservation had recurrent symptoms and 31% required further surgery. In women with bilateral oophorectomy, 10% had recurrent symptoms and 3.7% required further surgery.[26] Postoperative **estrogen** replacement therapy is associated with minimal (1–3%) risk of disease recurrence.[27,28] There is no advantage in delaying the introduction of estrogen replacement therapy after surgery.[26]

Pharmacologic Choices (Table 2)

Analgesics

NSAIDs inhibit endometrial prostaglandins (which cause abnormal uterine contractions) and are recommended as first-line treatment of mild endometriosis-associated pelvic pain and dysmenorrhea (see Chapter 71). NSAIDs can be used as an adjunct to combined oral contraceptives, progestin-only contraceptives, GnRH analogues or danazol, if needed.[29] They are most effective if started at the onset of menstrual symptoms and given throughout the menstrual period. NSAIDs are well tolerated, safe and inexpensive. However, the efficacy of NSAIDs for managing pain caused by endometriosis, rather than dysmenorrhea, has not been sufficiently studied.[30] There is no evidence one NSAID is more effective than another.

Opioid analgesics may be used but their effect on bowel motility may contribute to pelvic pain. Although long-term use may lead to addiction, opioids may be appropriate in select patients with intractable chronic pain and no history of drug abuse (for a listing of opioids, see Chapter 80). Avoid opioids with short half-lives as they are associated with rebound pain. **Fentanyl** transdermal patches may be a good choice as more consistent serum levels are maintained.[31]

Consider prescribing analgesics if necessary for pain relief while awaiting resolution of symptoms from other treatments (both medical and surgical).[20]

Hormonal Therapies

Combined Hormonal Contraceptives

Combined oral contraceptives (COC) relieve symptoms in 75–100% of cases of endometriosis-associated pain, reduce menstrual blood flow and suppress ovulation. When used continuously, monophasic COCs produce amenorrhea,[29,32] and pain (associated with estrogen and progestin withdrawal) may be suppressed.[29,32,33] Low-dose COCs can be used for an unlimited time.

The **contraceptive vaginal ring** and **transdermal contraceptives** may also help in symptomatic endometriosis.[34] However, both systems were associated with irregular bleeding when used continuously.

Progestin-only Contraceptives

When used continuously, **progestins** inhibit ovulation and suppress gonadotropin secretion thereby inducing a hypoestrogenic, acyclic hormonal environment.

Injectable depot **medroxyprogesterone acetate (MPA)**, 150 mg every 6–12 weeks intramuscularly, significantly reduces pain and induces amenorrhea.[35,36] Do not use depot MPA in younger women who wish to become pregnant immediately after stopping treatment because resumption of ovulation is delayed following cessation of therapy. Depot MPA may decrease bone mineral density;[37,38,39] reserve use for patients >18 years who do not want to conceive and wish to avoid surgery.

Continuous oral **MPA** 20–40 mg daily, **norethindrone** 5–15 mg daily or **dienogest** 2 mg daily[40,41] relieve endometriosis-associated pain. Ovulation resumes promptly after discontinuation of oral therapy. High-dose progestin therapy may cause spotting/irregular bleeding, weight gain and mood changes (e.g., depression).

The **levonorgestrel intrauterine system (LNG-IUS)** delivers the drug directly into the uterine cavity at a steady rate of 20 µg/day over a 5-year period.[42] An effective hormonal option for the treatment of symptomatic endometriosis (mild to moderate disease), LNG-IUS alters the staging of disease[43] and has been effective in symptom control for up to 3 years.[44,45] Advantages include lower cost, no repeated treatments and fewer side effects. Breakthrough bleeding is common especially in the first 3 months. Amenorrhea occurs in up to 35% of patients at 1 year.

Androgen Agonists

Danazol inhibits ovarian estrogen production and causes atrophy of endometrial deposits. It is highly effective in the treatment of endometriosis-associated dysmenorrhea but less effective in the management of chronic pelvic pain.[46] Endometriomas >1 cm in diameter respond poorly to danazol. Doses of 600–800 mg/day for 6 months effectively alleviate symptoms of endometriosis, particularly in the earlier stages of the disease.[47] Although effective, its use is limited by its adverse effect profile: androgenic side effects, e.g., hirsutism and acne, and a negative impact on lipids are common with danazol therapy.[48]

Gonadotropin-releasing Hormone (GnRH) Analogues

GnRH analogues inhibit the hypothalamic-pituitary-gonadal axis, reducing the secretion of LH and FSH required for follicular development and resulting in a markedly hypoestrogenic state, which induces atrophy and regression of endometriotic implants.[49] GnRH analogues are not more effective than COCs[50] or progestins[36,51] in managing endometriosis-associated pain. Endometriomas respond poorly to GnRH analogues.

Use **nafarelin** 200 µg intranasally twice daily, **goserelin** 3.6 mg subcutaneously monthly or **leuprolide** 3.75 mg intramuscularly monthly. There is no advantage of one GnRH analogue over another. No significant differences in pain relief or clinical symptoms were observed using GnRH analogue therapy for 3 months vs. 6 months.[52] Hypoestrogenic adverse effects are common and include hot flashes, insomnia, mood changes and vaginal atrophy. Decrease in bone mineral density of 1–3% is seen when a GnRH analogue is taken for 3–6 months.[53] Recurrence of endometriosis symptoms commonly occurs within 9–12 months after completion of therapy.

Add-back **hormone therapy** (HT) is used to mitigate the hypoestrogenic symptoms and bone density loss that occur with GnRH analogues. Add-back therapy consists of continuous administration of **estrogen** (Canadian guidelines suggest any standard HT regimen containing estradiol-17β 1 mg or equivalent would be adequate[20]) plus **medroxyprogesterone acetate** (MPA) 2.5 mg once daily.[54] **Norethindrone acetate** 5 mg once daily is an alternative to estrogen plus MPA[55] and is approved by Health Canada for add-back therapy. Micronized progesterone has not been studied for this use.

A GnRH analogue plus add-back hormone therapy is as effective as GnRH analogue therapy alone for relieving pelvic symptoms in endometriosis.[56] Add-back hormone therapy does not increase the recurrence rate of endometriosis. Efficacy of GnRH analogue treatment is not reduced, and adverse hypoestrogenic effects are decreased although not abolished.[57] GnRH analogues plus add-back hormone therapy may be used for 6–12 months.[55] The risks of breast cancer and cardiovascular disease associated with hormone therapy are low given this relatively short-term use in young women. However, add-back hormones should not be used in women with risk factors for thromboembolic disease.

Others

Patients with endometriosis have a high level of aromatase P450 expression in eutopic and ectopic endometrium. Aromatase P450 inhibitors (**anastrozole**, **letrozole**) reduce estrogen produced from sources other than the ovary such as the adrenal gland. Aromatase inhibitors are used with oral contraceptives, GnRH analogues or a progestin to reduce the risk of developing ovarian cysts.[58] Aromatase inhibitors represent a promising new approach to the therapy for endometriosis,[58,59,60,61] but remain investigational.[62]

Mifepristone (RU-486) shows promise in the management of pain in endometriosis but larger controlled clinical trials are needed to establish the role of antiprogestins in the management of endometriosis.[63] Mifepristone is not available in Canada.

Selective progesterone receptor modulators (SPRMs) such as **ulipristal**, have been used successfully in pilot studies for treatment of endometriosis.[64] However, more clinical trials are needed before they can be recommended for this indication.

Recurrent Disease

Combined oral contraceptives reduce symptoms of mild disease (suggested by pelvic tenderness, no nodularity) and may be used for an unlimited time. Use MPA, danazol or a GnRH analogue if low-dose COC therapy is ineffective.

MPA, danazol or a GnRH analogue may also be used to relieve the pain of advanced disease (suggested by an adnexal mass, a fixed uterus or obliteration of the cul-de-sac) but may not affect the disease process. Although these drugs may reduce the size of endometriomas, their use does not necessarily reduce the length of surgery or affect its eventual outcome.

Use danazol or a progestin as alternative treatment when there has been marked unrecovered bone loss with GnRH analogue therapy, when bone density is not being evaluated or if the patient has other risk factors for osteoporosis.

Choices during Pregnancy and Breastfeeding

Women with endometriosis may have difficulty conceiving (see Endometriosis-associated Infertility). In women who become pregnant, symptoms of endometriosis are suppressed and thus treatment is not required; however, the disease may recur after childbirth.

During breastfeeding, symptoms may remain in remission, at least initially; treatment is not required as long as breastfeeding is frequent and intense enough to inhibit estrogen release from the ovaries. Symptoms may recur during long-term breastfeeding.

Prolonged breastfeeding and multiple pregnancies protect against the development of endometriosis.[65]

Endometriosis-associated Infertility

Therapeutic Choices

An algorithm for the management of endometriosis is shown in Figure 1.

Nonpharmacologic Choices

Surgery (Table 1)

Drug treatment of endometriosis does not improve fecundity.[66] Laparoscopy and laparotomy are equally successful in the surgical treatment of endometriosis-associated infertility.[15,67] Laparoscopy offers the advantage of a shorter hospital stay, less pain and quicker convalescence but requires surgical expertise and expensive equipment.

Laparoscopic resection or ablation of minimal or mild endometriosis enhances fecundity in infertile women.[25] There is no relative advantage to any of the various cytoreductive techniques (coagulation, laser vaporization or excision of endometriosis).

The addition of postsurgical GnRH analogue therapy offers no advantage over surgery alone in terms of pain relief or increased fertility.[27]

Assisted Reproductive Technologies

The efficacy of in vitro fertilization-embryo transfer (IVF-ET) in treating endometriosis-associated infertility has not been evaluated based on severity of disease or other important prognostic variables such as age and duration of infertility. With improvements in IVF programs, this therapy may be considered in milder forms of endometriosis-associated infertility.

Pharmacologic Choices (Table 2, Table 3)

Ovulation Induction

Clomiphene 50 mg daily for 5 days, administered on days 3–7 of the menstrual cycle, is simple and inexpensive. Clomiphene use for ovulation induction with or without intrauterine insemination does not significantly increase pregnancy rates but helps with timing intercourse or intrauterine insemination. **Human chorionic gonadotropin (hCG)** is sometimes added in a dose of 5000–10 000 units im at midcycle, with or without intrauterine insemination.

A Cochrane review concluded that administering GnRH analogues for 3–6 months prior to IVF or intracytoplasmic sperm injection (ICSI) in women with endometriosis results in a fourfold increase in the odds of clinical pregnancy.[68] Use gonadotropin therapy, referred to as superovulation or controlled ovarian hyperstimulation, together with intrauterine insemination to treat minimal or mild endometriosis-associated infertility.[69] Live birth rates diminish with successive treatments. Because of its cost, limit gonadotropin therapy to 3 cycles.

As fecundity significantly decreases and spontaneous abortion rate increases in women >35 years, these patients may benefit from an aggressive therapeutic plan with superovulation/intrauterine insemination or IVF-ET.[66]

Ovarian Suppression

Ovarian suppression is inappropriate to use for endometriosis-associated infertility as it prevents pregnancy. It may be an option if there is severe coexisting endometriosis-associated pain.[70,71]

Therapeutic Tips

- Chronic pelvic pain is a diagnosis in itself, and should be treated as such.
- Hormonal treatment may be used prior to surgery to reduce the size of endometrial implants; however, this strategy does not prolong pain-free interval, decrease recurrence rates or increase pregnancy rates.
- After surgery (laparotomy, laparoscopic conservative or definitive surgical treatment), residual disease treated with progestin, danazol or GnRH analogue results in prolonged pain-free interval and delayed recurrence.[72]
- To promote bone health, encourage adequate **calcium** intake (1200 mg/day total intake, preferably through dietary intake) and **vitamin D** supplementation (400–1000 units daily) for women taking **GnRH analogues** with add-back **hormone therapy**.

Table 2: Drugs Used for Endometriosis-associated Pain

Class	Drug	Dose	Adverse Effects	Comments	Cost[a]
Contraceptives, oral—combined estrogen (≤35 µg EE) and progestin, monophasic	*EE 35 µg/ norethindrone 1 mg* Brevicon 1/35, Ortho 1/35, Select 1/35	1 tablet daily po	Common: breakthrough bleeding/spotting, amenorrhea, nausea/vomiting, bloating, chloasma, breast tenderness, mood changes such as depression, headaches. Major: thromboembolism (rare), stroke, retinal artery thrombosis, myocardial infarction, benign liver tumour, cholelithiasis, hypertension.	Continuous use (no break for menstrual period) of COCs produces anovulation and amenorrhea. Cyclic or continuous use of COCs may delay onset or recurrence of disease. If used continuously, may consider short breaks Q3 months. Watch for danger signals: ACHES—**a**bdominal pain, **c**hest pain, **h**eadaches, **e**ye problems, **s**evere leg pain. Advise physician consult. *Absolute contraindications:* History of MI or ischemic heart disease, cerebrovascular disease, complicated valvular heart disease, current or past history of VTE, known thrombogenic mutation, severe cirrhosis, liver tumour, breast cancer, diabetes with microvascular complications, migraines with aura, <6 weeks postpartum if breastfeeding, smoker >35 y (≥15 cigarettes/day), hypertension (SBP ≥160 mm Hg or DBP ≥100 mm Hg), known coagulation-factor deficiency.	$
	EE 35 µg/ norethindrone 0.5 mg Brevicon 0.5/35, Ortho 0.5/35	1 tablet daily po	See EE 35 µg /norethindrone 1 mg.	See EE 35 µg /norethindrone 1 mg.	$
	EE 35 µg/ norgestimate 0.25 mg Cyclen	1 tablet daily po	See EE 35 µg /norethindrone 1 mg.	See EE 35 µg /norethindrone 1 mg.	$$

(cont'd)

Table 2: Drugs Used for Endometriosis-associated Pain *(cont'd)*

Class	Drug	Dose	Adverse Effects	Comments	Cost[a]
	EE 30 µg/ desogestrel 0.15 mg Marvelon, Ortho-Cept, Apri, Freya 21, Mirvala	1 tablet daily po	See EE 35 µg/ norethindrone 1 mg.	See EE 35 µg/ norethindrone 1 mg.	$
	EE 30 µg/ drospirenone 3 mg Yasmin, Zamine, Zarah	1 tablet daily po	See EE 35 µg/ norethindrone 1 mg. Risk of hyperkalemia in patients prone to increased K^+ (e.g., renal disease, concurrent use of ACEIs, ARBs, potassium-sparing diuretics, NSAIDs). Check K^+ after 1st cycle. May increase risk of VTE compared to levonorgestrel-containing COCs.	See EE 35 µg/ norethindrone 1 mg.	$
	EE 30 µg/ ethynodiol diacetate 2 mg Demulen 30	1 tablet daily po	See EE 35 µg/ norethindrone 1 mg.	See EE 35 µg/ norethindrone 1 mg.	$
	EE 30 µg/ levonorgestrel 0.15 mg, 1-month Min-Ovral, Portia	1 tablet daily po	See EE 35 µg/ norethindrone 1 mg.	See EE 35 µg/ norethindrone 1 mg.	$
	EE 30 µg/ levonorgestrel 0.15 mg, 3-month Seasonale, Seasonique	1 tablet daily po	See EE 35 µg/ norethindrone 1 mg.	See EE 35 µg/ norethindrone 1 mg. Seasonale and Seasonique are packaged for 3 months of continuous use, with 84 active tablets and 7 inert (Seasonale) or ultra-low dose (0.01 mg) EE tablets (Seasonique).	$$$/3 months
	EE 30 µg/ norethindrone acetate 1.5 mg Loestrin 1.5/30	1 tablet daily po	See EE 35 µg/ norethindrone 1 mg.	See EE 35 µg/ norethindrone 1 mg.	$

Class	Drug	Dose	Adverse Effects	Comments	Cost[a]
	EE 20 μg/ drospirenone 3 mg Yaz, MYA	1 tablet daily po	See EE 35 μg/ norethindrone 1 mg. Risk of hyperkalemia in patients prone to increased K^+ (e.g., renal disease, concurrent use of ACEIs, ARBs, potassium-sparing diuretics, NSAIDs). Check K^+ after 1st cycle. May increase risk of VTE compared to levonorgestrel-containing COCs.	See EE 35 μg/ norethindrone 1 mg.	$
	EE 20 μg/ norethindrone acetate 1 mg Minestrin 1/20	1 tablet daily po	See EE 35 μg/ norethindrone 1 mg.	See EE 35 μg/ norethindrone 1 mg.	$
	EE 20 μg/ levonorgestrel 0.1 mg Alesse, Alysena, Aviane, ESME, Lutera	1 tablet daily po	See EE 35 μg/ norethindrone 1 mg.	See EE 35 μg/ norethindrone 1 mg.	$
Contraceptives, progestin-only, injectable	*medroxyprogesterone acetate* Depo-Provera, generics	150 mg Q6–12 weeks im	Breast tenderness, insomnia or somnolence, fatigue, mood changes (e.g., depression, irritability), dizziness, headache, skin sensitivity reactions, hyperpyrexia, weight changes, acne. Long-term: decrease in BMD, delayed return of fertility.	Not recommended for women who wish to become pregnant immediately after stopping treatment as resumption of ovulation is significantly delayed after stopping treatment. Consider other options in women <18 y and those with risk factors for osteoporosis.	$$/3 months
Contraceptives, progestin-only, intrauterine system (IUS)	*levonorgestrel IUS* Mirena	Insert every 5 years. Releases levonorgestrel 20 μg/day into uterine cavity	Spotting for first 3 monthsafter insertion; menstrual changes such as amenorrhea.	Inserted within 7 days of onset of menses. Intrauterine levonorgestrel has been shown to be effective in symptom control for at least 3 y.[45]	$350/unit

(cont'd)

Table 2: **Drugs Used for Endometriosis-associated Pain** *(cont'd)*

Class	Drug	Dose	Adverse Effects	Comments	Cost[a]
Gonadotropin Inhibitors, pituitary	*danazol* Cyclomen	600–800 mg daily po divided BID–QID without interruption for 3–6 months	Androgenic side effects: voice deepening (irreversible), decrease breast size, increase weight, hirsutism, increase LDL, decrease HDL. Menopausal symptoms: hot flashes, vaginal dryness.	Avoid in patients with dyslipidemia or liver disease. Use limited by poor tolerability. Effective contraception necessary for duration of treatment.	$250
Gonadotropin-releasing Hormone Analogues (GnRH analogues)	*buserelin acetate* Suprefact	200 µg (2 sprays) TID into each nostril × 6 months	Bone loss (if used for 6 months, reversible upon cessation of treatment). Vasomotor symptoms: hot flashes, vaginal dryness, insomnia, loss of libido, emotional lability.	A temporary increase in pain upon initiation of therapy may occur. Usually given for 6 months as long-term use is associated with significant decrease in BMD. Symptoms may recur within 9–12 months after stopping therapy; *add-back* hormonal therapy improves hypoestrogenic symptoms and controls bone loss.	$85/unit
	goserelin acetate Zoladex	3.6 mg monthly sc × 6 months	See buserelin acetate.	See buserelin acetate.	$420/unit
	goserelin acetate long-acting Zoladex LA	10.8 mg Q12 weeks sc × 6 months	See buserelin acetate.	See buserelin acetate.	$1195/unit
	leuprolide acetate Lupron Depot	3.75 mg monthly im × 6 months or 11.25 mg Q3 months im × 6 months	See buserelin acetate.	See buserelin acetate.	3.75 mg: $365/unit 11.25 mg: $1090/unit
	nafarelin acetate Synarel	200 µg (1 spray) into one nostril QAM and 200 µg into the other nostril QPM × 6 months Total daily dose: 400 µg	See buserelin acetate.	See buserelin acetate.	$230/unit
	triptorelin pamoate ◗ Trelstar	3.75 mg Q28 days im × 6 months	See buserelin acetate.	See buserelin acetate.	$345/unit

Class	Drug	Dose	Adverse Effects	Comments	Cost[a]
NSAIDs, propionic acid derivatives	*ibuprofen* Advil, Motrin, Motrin Liquid Gels, generics	400 mg Q4–6H po Maximum daily dose: 2400 mg	Very common (>10%): dyspepsia, nausea/vomiting. Common (5–10%): nonspecific rash, pruritus, dizziness, headache.	First line in the management of mild endometriosis-associated pelvic pain and dysmenorrhea. May start treatment at the onset of symptoms. Do not take on an as-needed basis during this time. Contraindications: hypersensitivity to ASA, active pelvic inflammatory bowel disease, existing renal disease, clotting disorders. SSRIs may increase risk of gastrointestinal bleeding when used with NSAIDs.	$
	naproxen Naprosyn, generics	250 mg Q6–8H po Maximum daily dose: 1250 mg	See ibuprofen.	See ibuprofen.	$
Progestins, oral	*dienogest* Visanne	2 mg daily po	Headache, breast discomfort (engorgement, pain), weight gain, mood changes, breakthrough bleeding.	Ovulation resumes promptly after discontinuation. Metabolized by CYP3A4; effect may be increased if given concomitantly with CYP3A4 inhibitors (azole antifungals, grapefruit juice, macrolide antibiotics, protease inhibitors) or decreased if given with CYP3A4 inducers (antiepileptic drugs, dexamethasone, rifampin).	$$$
	medroxyprogesterone acetate Provera, generics	20–40 mg daily po	Well tolerated. Breakthrough bleeding, weight gain, fluid retention, mood swings.	Ovulation resumes promptly after discontinuation of oral (but not depot) MPA.	$
	norethindrone acetate Norlutate	Treatment: 5 mg once daily; increase by 2.5 mg daily every 2 weeks up to 15 mg daily. Add-back: 5 mg once daily	Breakthrough bleeding, spotting, weight gain, mood changes (e.g., depression, irritability).	See dienogest.	$$$

[a] Cost of 28-day supply unless otherwise specified; includes drug cost only.
Abbreviations: ACEI = ACE inhibitor; ARB = angiotensin II receptor blocker; ASA = acetylsalicylic acid; BMD = bone mineral density; COC = combined oral contraceptive; DBP = diastolic blood pressure; EE = ethinyl estradiol; HDL = high-density lipoprotein; LDL = low-density lipoprotein; MI = myocardial infarction; MPA = medroxyprogesterone acetate; NSAID = nonsteroidal anti-inflammatory drug; SSRI = selective serotonin receptor inhibitor; SBP = systolic blood pressure; VTE = venous thromboembolism
Legend: $ <$20 $$ $20–40 $$$ $40–60

Table 3: Drugs Used for Endometriosis-associated Infertility

Class	Drug	Dose	Comments	Cost[a]
Ovulation Stimulators	*clomiphene* Serophene, Clomid	50 mg daily po × 5 days. Start on 5th day of menstrual cycle if bleeding occurs. May start at any time if no recent uterine bleeding. Can increase dose to 100 mg daily po × 5 days, if ovulation does not occur after initial course within 30 days of previous course.	Repeat regimen for 3 or 4 cycles if conception does not occur with ovulation.	$30

[a] Cost of 5-day supply; includes drug cost only.

Suggested Readings

Ferrero S, Remorgida V, Venturini PL. Current pharmacotherapy for endometriosis. *Expert Opin Pharmacother* 2010;11(7):1123-34.

Johnson NP, Hummelshoj L. Consensus on current management of endometriosis. *Human Reproduction* 2013;28(6):1552-68.

Schrager S, Falleroni J, Edgoose J. Evaluation and treatment of endometriosis. *Am Fam Physician* 2013;87(2):107-13.

Brown J, Farquhar C. Endometriosis: an overview of Cochrane Reviews. *Cochrane Database Syst Rev* 2014 Mar 10;3:CD009590

References

1. Revised American Fertility Society classification of endometriosis: 1985. *Fertil Steril* 1985;43(3):351-2.
2. Missmer SA, Hankinson SE, Spiegelman D et al. Incidence of laparoscopically confirmed endometriosis by demographic, anthropometric, and lifestyle factors. *Am J Epidemiol* 2004;160(8):784-96.
3. Waller KG, Shaw RW. Gonadotropin-releasing hormone analogues for the treatment of endometriosis: long-term follow-up. *Fertil Steril* 1993;59(3):511-5.
4. Wheeler JM, Malinak LR. Recurrent endometriosis: incidence, management, and prognosis. *Am J Obstet Gynecol* 1983;146(3):247-53.
5. Zondervan KT, Yudkin PL, Vessey MP et al. Patterns of diagnosis and referral in women consulting for chronic pelvic pain in UK primary care. *Br J Obstet Gynaecol* 1999;106(11):1156-61.
6. Nisolle M, Paindaveine B, Bourdon A et al. Histologic study of peritoneal endometriosis in infertile women. *Fertil Steril* 1990;53(6):984-8.
7. Mol BW, Bayram N, Lijmer JG et al. The performance of CA-125 measurement in the detection of endometriosis: a meta-analysis. *Fertil Steril* 1998;70(6):1101-8.
8. Guerriero S, Mais V, Ajossa S et al. The role of endovaginal ultrasound in differentiating endometriomas from other ovarian cysts. *Clin Exp Obstet Gynecol* 1995;22(1):20-2.
9. Alcazar JL, Laparte C, Jurado M et al. The role of transvaginal ultrasonography combined with color velocity and pulsed Doppler in the diagnosis of endometrioma. *Fertil Steril* 1997;67(3):487-91.
10. Friedman H, Vogelzang RL, Mendelson EB et al. Endometriosis detection by US with laparoscopic correlation. *Radiology* 1985;157(1):217-20.
11. Redwine DB. Conservative laparoscopic excision of endometriosis by sharp dissection: life table analysis of reoperation and persistent or recurrent disease. *Fertil Steril* 1991;56(4):628-34.
12. Lu PY, Ory SJ. Endometriosis: current management. *Mayo Clin Proc* 1995;70(5):453-63.
13. Revelli A, Modotti M, Ansaldi C et al. Recurrent endometriosis: a review of biological and clinical aspects. *Obstet Gynecol Surv* 1995;50(10):747-54.
14. Wheeler JM, Malinak LR. Recurrent endometriosis: incidence, management, and prognosis. *Am J Obstet Gynecol* 1983;146(3):247-53.
15. Crosignani PG, Vercellini P, Biffignandi F et al. Laparoscopy versus laparotomy in conservative surgical treatment for severe endometriosis. *Fertil Steril* 1996;66(5):706-11.
16. Cook AS, Rock JA. The role of laparoscopy in the treatment of endometriosis. *Fertil Steril* 1991;55(4):663-80.
17. Sutton CJ, Ewen SP, Whitelaw N et al. Prospective, randomized, double-blind, controlled trial of laser laparoscopy in the treatment of pelvic pain associated with minimal, mild, and moderate endometriosis. *Fertil Steril* 1994;62(4):696-700.
18. Sutton CJ, Pooley AS, Ewen SP et al. Follow-up report on a randomized controlled trial of laser laparoscopy in the treatment of pelvic pain associated with minimal to moderate endometriosis. *Fertil Steril* 1997;68(6):1070-4.
19. Proctor ML, Latthe PM, Farquhar CM et al. Surgical interruption of pelvic nerve pathways for primary and secondary dysmenorrhoea. *Cochrane Database Syst Rev* 2005;(4):CD001896.
20. Leyland N, Casper R, Laberge P et al. SOGC Clinical Practice Guideline No. 244. Endometriosis: diagnosis and management. *J Obstet Gynaecol Can* 2010;32(7 Suppl 2):S1-28.
21. Candiani GB, Fedele L, Vercellini P et al. Presacral neurectomy for the treatment of pelvic pain associated with endometriosis: a controlled study. *Am J Obstet Gynecol* 1992;167(1):100-3.
22. Giudice LC. Clinical practice. Endometriosis. *N Engl J Med* 2010;362(25):2389-98.
23. Seracchioli R, Mabrouk M, Manuzzi L et al. Post-operative use of oral contraceptive pills for prevention of anatomical relapse or symptom-recurrence after conservative surgery for endometriosis. *Hum Reprod* 2009;24(11):2729-35.
24. Abou-Setta AM, Houston B, Al-Inany HG et al. Levonorgestrel-releasing intrauterine device (LNG-IUD) for symptomatic endometriosis following surgery. *Cochrane Database Syst Rev* 2013;1:CD005072.
25. Olive DL, Schwartz LB. Endometriosis. *N Engl J Med* 1993;328(24):1759-69.
26. Namnoum AB, Hickman TN, Goodman SB et al. Incidence of symptom recurrence after hysterectomy for endometriosis. *Fertil Steril* 1995;64(5):898-902.
27. Malinak LR. Surgical treatment and adjunct therapy of endometriosis. *Int J Gynaecol Obstet* 1993;40(Suppl):S43-7.
28. Al Kadri H, Hassan S, Al-Fozan HM et al. Hormone therapy for endometriosis and surgical menopause. *Cochrane Database Syst Rev* 2009;(1):CD005997.
29. Jarrell JF, Vilos GA, Allaire C et al. Consensus guidelines for the management of chronic pelvic pain. *J Obstet Gynaecol Can* 2005;27(8):781-826.
30. Allen C, Hopewell S, Prentice A et al. Nonsteroidal anti-inflammatory drugs for pain in women with endometriosis. *Cochrane Database Syst Rev* 2009;(2):CD004753.
31. Caplin RA et al. Transdermal fentanyl: an overview of clinical progress. In: Estafanous FG, ed. *Opioids in anesthesia II*. Boston (MA): Butterworth-Heinemann; 1991.
32. Vercellini P, De Giorgi O, Mosconi P et al. Cyproterone acetate versus a continuous monophasic oral contraceptive in the treatment of recurrent pelvic pain after conservative surgery for symptomatic endometriosis. *Fertil Steril* 2002;77(1):52-61.
33. Harada T, Momoeda M, Taketani Y et al. Low-dose oral contraceptive pill for dysmenorrhea associated with endometriosis: a placebo-controlled, double-blind, randomized trial. *Fertil Steril* 2008;90(5):1583-8.

34. Vercellini P, Barbara G, Somigliana S et al. Comparison of contraceptive ring and patch for the treatment of symptomatic endometriosis. *Fertil Steril* 2010;93(7):2150-61.
35. Vercellini P, De Giorgi O, Oldani S et al. Depot medroxyprogesterone acetate versus an oral contraceptive combined with very-low-dose danazol for long-term treatment of pelvic pain associated with endometriosis. *Am J Obstet Gynecol* 1996;175(2):396-401.
36. Vercellini P, Cortesi I, Crosignani PG. Progestins for symptomatic endometriosis: a critical analysis of the evidence. *Fertil Steril* 1997;68(3):393-401.
37. Curtis KM, Chrisman CE, Peterson HB et al. Contraception for women in selected circumstances. *Obstet Gynecol* 2002;99(6):1100-12.
38. Scholes D, LaCroix AZ, Ichikawa LE et al. Change in bone mineral density among adolescent women using and discontinuing depot medroxyprogesterone acetate contraception. *Arch Pediatr Adolesc Med* 2005;159(2):139-44.
39. Cromer BA, Lazebnik R, Rome E et al. Double-blinded randomized controlled trial of estrogen supplementation in adolescent girls who receive depot medroxyprogesterone acetate for contraception. *Am J Obstet Gynecol* 2005;192(1):42-7.
40. Strowitzki T, Marr J, Gerlinger C et al. Dienogest is as effective as leuprolide acetate in treating the painful symptoms of endometriosis: a 24-week, randomized, multicentre, open-label trial. *Hum Reprod* 2010;25(3):633-41.
41. Schindler AE. Dienogest in long-term treatment of endometriosis. *Int J Womens Health* 2011(3);175-84.
42. Andersson K, Odlind V, Rybo G. Levonorgestrel-releasing and copper-releasing (Nova T) IUDs during five years of use: a randomized comparative trial. *Contraception* 1994;49(1):56-72.
43. Lockhat FB, Emembolu JO, Konje JC. The evaluation of the effectiveness of an intrauterine-administered progestogen (levonorgestrel) in the symptomatic treatment of endometriosis and in the staging of the disease. *Hum Reprod* 2004;19(1):179-84.
44. Lockhat FB, Emembolu JE, Konje JC. Serum and peritoneal fluid levels of levonorgestrel in women with endometriosis who were treated with an intrauterine contraceptive device containing levonorgestrel. *Fertil Steril* 2005;83(2):398-404.
45. Lockhat FB, Emembolu JO, Konje JC. The efficacy, side-effects and continuation rates in women with symptomatic endometriosis undergoing treatment with an intra-uterine administered progestogen (levonorgestrel): a 3-year follow-up. *Hum Reprod* 2005;20(3):789-93.
46. Barbieri RL, Evans S, Kistner RW. Danazol in the treatment of endometriosis: analysis of 100 cases with a 4-year follow-up. *Fertil Steril* 1982;37(6):737-46.
47. Dmowski WP. Danazol. A synthetic steroid with diverse biologic effects. *J Reprod Med* 1990;35(1 Suppl):69-74.
48. Selak V, Farquhar C, Prentice A et al. Danazol for pelvic pain associated with endometriosis. *Cochrane Database Syst Rev* 2007;(4):CD000068.
49. Bergqvist IA. Hormonal regulation of endometriosis and the rationales and effects of gonadotrophin-releasing hormone agonist treatment: a review. *Hum Reprod* 1995;10(2):446-52.
50. Davis L, Kennedy SS, Moore J et al. Modern combined oral contraceptives for pain associated with endometriosis. *Cochrane Database Syst Rev* 2007;(3):CD001019.
51. Brown J, Pan A, Hart RJ. Gonadotrophin releasing hormone analogues for pain associated with endometriosis. *Cochrane Database Syst Rev* 2010;(12):CD008475.
52. Heinrichs WL, Henzl MR. Human issues and medical economics of endometriosis. Three- vs. six-month GnRH-agonist therapy. *J Reprod Med* 1998;43(3 Suppl):299-308.
53. Dawood MY, Ramos J, Khan-Dawood FS. Depot leuprolide acetate versus danazol for treatment of pelvic endometriosis: changes in vertebral bone mass and serum estradiol and calcitonin. *Fertil Steril* 1995;63(6):1177-83.
54. Friedman AJ, Hornstein MD. Gonadotropin-releasing hormone agonist plus estrogen-progestin "add-back" therapy for endometriosis-related pelvic pain. *Fertil Steril* 1993;60(2):236-41.
55. Hornstein MD, Surrey ES, Weisberg GW et al. Leuprolide acetate depot and hormonal add-back in endometriosis: a 12-month study. Lupron Add-Back Study Group. *Obstet Gynecol* 1998;91(1):16-24.
56. Surrey ES, Hornstein MD. Prolonged GnRH agonist and add-back therapy for symptomatic endometriosis: long-term follow-up. *Obstet Gynecol* 2002;99(5 Pt 1):709-19.
57. Howell R, Edmonds DK, Dowsett M et al. Gonadotropin-releasing analogue (goserelin) plus hormone replacement therapy for the treatment of endometriosis: a randomized controlled trial. *Fertil Steril* 1995;64(3):474-81.
58. Amsterdam LL, Gentry W, Jobanputra S et al. Anastrazole and oral contraceptives: a novel treatment for endometriosis. *Fertil Steril* 2005;84(2):300-4.
59. Soysal S, Soysal ME, Ozer S et al. The effects of post-surgical administration of goserelin plus anastrozole compared to goserelin alone in patients with severe endometriosis: a prospective randomized trial. *Hum Reprod* 2004;19(1):160-7.
60. Ailawadi RK, Jobanputra S, Kataria M et al. Treatment of endometriosis and chronic pelvic pain with letrozole and norethindrone acetate: a pilot study. *Fertil Steril* 2004;81(2):290-6.
61. Nawathe A, Patwardhan S, Yates D et al. Systematic review of the effects of aromatase inhibitors on pain associated with endometriosis. *BJOG* 2008;115(7):818-22.
62. Attar E, Bulun SE. Aromatase inhibitors: the next generation of therapeutics for endometriosis? *Fertil Steril* 2006;85(5):1307-18.
63. Kettel LM, Murphy AA, Morales AJ et al. Preliminary report on the treatment of endometriosis with low-dose mifepristone (RU 486). *Am J Obstet Gynecol* 1998;178(6):1151-6.
64. Chwalisz K, Perez MC, Demanno D et al. Selective progesterone receptor modulator development and use in the treatment of leiomyomata and endometriosis. *Endocr Rev* 2005;26(3):423-38.
65. Missmer SA, Hankinson SE, Spiegelman D et al. Incidence of laparoscopically confirmed endometriosis by demographic, anthropometric, and lifestyle factors. *Am J Epidemiol* 2004;160(8):784-96.
66. Practice Committee of the American Society for Reproductive Medicine. Endometriosis and infertility. *Fertil Steril* 2006;86(5 Suppl):S156-60.
67. Adamson GD, Pasta DJ. Surgical treatment of endometriosis-associated infertility: meta-analysis compared with survival analysis. *Am J Obstet Gynecol* 1994;171(6):1488-504.
68. Sallam HN, Garcia-Velasco JA, Dias S et al. Long-term pituitary down-regulation before in vitro fertilization (IVF) for women with endometriosis. *Cochrane Database Syst Rev* 2006;(1):CD004635.
69. Tummon IS, Asher LJ, Martin JS et al. Randomized controlled trial of superovulation and insemination for infertility associated with minimal or mild endometriosis. *Fertil Steril* 1997;68(1):8-12.
70. Hughes EG, Fedorkow DM, Collins JA. A quantitative overview of controlled trials in endometriosis-associated infertility. *Fertil Steril* 1993;59(5):963-70.
71. Hughes E, Brown J, Collins JJ et al. Ovulation suppression for endometriosis. *Cochrane Database Syst Rev* 2007;(3):CD000155.
72. Kennedy S, Bergqvist A, Chapron C et al. ESHRE guideline for the diagnosis and treatment of endometriosis. *Hum Reprod* 2005;20(10):2698-704.

Sexual Health

Chapter 73
Female Sexual Dysfunction

Rosemary Basson, MD, FRCP (UK)

Ongoing sexual difficulties causing distress affect 10–15% of sexually active women.[1,2,3] Women (and men) have sex for many reasons.[4,5] Sexual response results from the brain's appraisal of sexual stimuli, to trigger feelings of sexual excitement, arousal and desire as well as physical responses including genital congestion (Figure 1). Multiple factors influence a woman's motivation to begin a sexual encounter[6,7,8] and to attend to the stimulation, and also determine whether or not she becomes aroused. Frequently the degree of subjective arousal and genital congestion are poorly correlated.[9] A lack of subjective arousal commonly occurs despite a normal genital vasocongestive response.[9] A woman's awareness of the engorgement of the genitalia is often minimal. Her subjective experience is influenced more consistently by concurrent thoughts and emotions than by feedback from the vasocongesting genitalia.[10] Although the major factors influencing women's sexual response are mood, stress,[11] feelings for the partner and past sexual experiences,[6,7,12] medical conditions, obesity,[13] medications, surgery, radiation or aging may contribute to impairment.[14,15,16,17] In assessing a woman's sexual problems, it is recommended to interview both partners (preferably together and separately).[18]

This chapter addresses 3 disorders of female sexual function: female sexual interest/arousal disorder, female orgasmic disorder and genito-pelvic pain/penetration disorder.

Figure 1: Model of Female Sexual Response Cycle

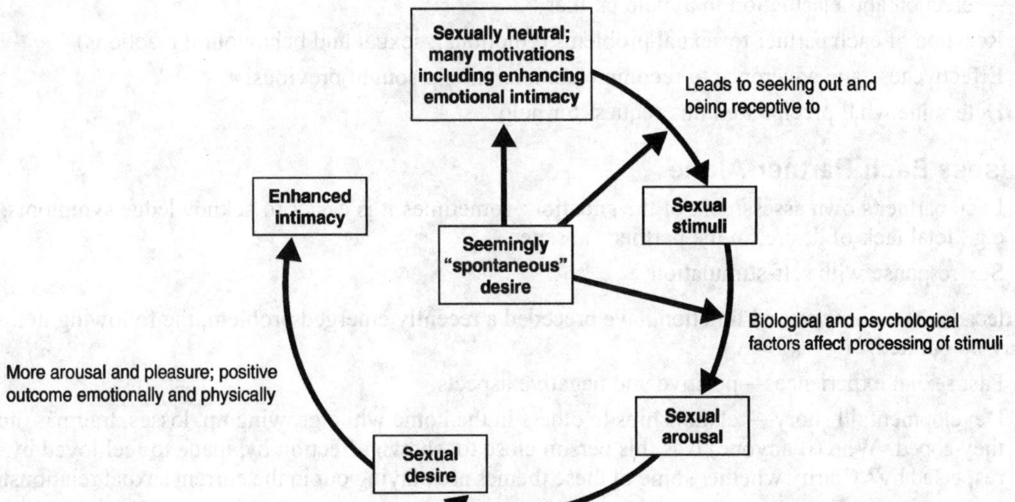

Adapted with permission from Lippincott Williams & Wilkins. Basson R. Female sexual response: the role of drugs in the management of sexual dysfunction. *Obstet Gynecol* 2001;98(2):350-3.

Interviewing for Female Sexual Dysfunction

Assess Partners Together

- Description of sexual problems in the patient's own words. Clarify with direct questions; give options rather than asking leading questions
- Description of duration, consistency of problem(s) and priority if more than 1 problem
- Context of sexual problems:
  - emotional intimacy with partner
  - activity/behaviour just prior to sexual activity
  - privacy
  - safety
  - birth control
  - risk of sexually transmitted infections (STIs)
  - usefulness of sexual stimulation
  - sexual skills of partner
  - sexual communication
  - time of day
  - cultural context
- Other aspects of each partner's sexual response (currently and prior to the onset of the sexual problems)—check:
  - sexual motivation
  - subjective arousal
  - enjoyment
  - orgasm
  - pain
  - erection and ejaculation in a male partner
- Reaction of each partner to sexual problems (emotional, sexual and behavioural reactions)
- Effectiveness and adherence to recommendations if help sought previously
- Determine what precipitated this request for help

Assess Each Partner Alone

- Each partner's own assessment of the situation: sometimes it is easier to acknowledge symptoms, e.g., total lack of desire, in the partner's absence
- Sex response with self-stimulation

If decades of healthy sexual function have preceded a recently emerged problem, the following items may be omitted:

- Past sexual experiences—positive and negative aspects
- Developmental history—relationships to others in the home while growing up, losses, traumas, how they coped. Who (if anyone) was this person close to, shown affection by, made to feel loved by, respected by? Clarify whether some of these themes are playing out in the current sexual relationship
- Enquire regarding sexual, emotional and physical abuse; explain that questions about abuse are routine and do not necessarily imply causation of the problems

Female Sexual Interest/Arousal Disorder

To make this diagnosis, a lack of sexual interest/arousal for a minimum duration of approximately 6 months as manifested by at least 3 of the following indicators must be present:[19]

- Absent/reduced interest in sexual activity
- Absent/reduced sexual/erotic thoughts or fantasies
- No/reduced initiation of sexual activity and typically unreceptive to a partner's attempts to initiate
- Absent/reduced sexual excitement/pleasure during sexual activity in all or almost all (approximately 75%) sexual encounters
- Absent/reduced sexual interest/arousal in response to any internal or external sexual/erotic cues (e.g., written, verbal, visual)
- Absent/reduced genital and/or nongenital sensations during sexual activity in all or almost all (approximately 75%) sexual encounters

Goals of Therapy

- Provide patient and partner with knowledge and understanding of sexual response cycle (Figure 1).[20] Address problematic areas
- Identify need for psychological or psychiatric consultation for deep-seated issues that prevent the woman from responding to sexual stimuli or that result in her experiencing negative emotions such as shame, guilt or disgust with arousal

Investigations

- Sexual history including current and past sexual function of both partners (see Interviewing for Female Sexual Dysfunction). Past sexual function strongly modulates current sexual function[7]
- Medical history including mood—the factor most consistently correlated with sexual function of both well and chronically ill women[6,7,21]
- Address factors impairing subjective arousal: psychological (e.g., distractions, sexual anxiety, stressors, relationship issues, previous abuse) and biological (e.g., fatigue, depression)
- Relationship details, both past and present, focusing on nonsexual intimacy, trust and respect, safety, birth control, fertility and stressors
- Address medications that may impair subjective arousal or interfere with genital vasocongestion (Table 1)
- Address any lack of required auditory, visual or physical sexual stimuli
- Genital examination: although physical examination in premenopausal women is usually normal, a reported lack of genital response may be the result of conditions such as lichen sclerosus. Post menopause, vulvovaginal atrophy is common but physical signs correlate poorly with sexual symptoms[22,23]
- Address conditions that may be impairing genital vasocongestion, e.g., estrogen deficiency, vaginitis
- Lab investigations only as indicated by medical history. No correlation has been found between androgen levels and sexual function, even when using mass spectrometry methods which avoid the difficulties with previous assays of testosterone in women.[24] In the past, lack of correlation was thought to be in part because about 50% of testosterone is made within cells and not reflected in serum levels. However, in a study of women with and without low sexual desire, no correlation was found between sexual desire and total testosterone as measured by serum androgen metabolites[24]

Table 1: **Drugs Associated with Female Sexual Dysfunction**[a,20,21,24,25,26]

Alcohol at higher doses	Antiandrogens	Beta-blockers
Alkylating agents	Cimetidine	Clonidine
Amphetamines	Spironolactone	Digoxin
Anticholinergics	Antiepileptic drugs	GnRH agonists
Antidepressants[b]	Antihistamines	Ketoconazole
MAOIs	Antipsychotics[c]	Lithium
SNRIs	Aromatase inhibitors	Methadone
SSRIs	Barbiturates	Metoclopramide
TCAs	Benzodiazepines	Trazodone

[a] This list is not exhaustive. A trial off the drug may help determine whether or not the drug is contributing to the problem.
[b] Achieving remission of depression improves sexual desire and function beyond treatment-emergent sexual dysfunction due to the medications.[25]
[c] Olanzapine may impair sexual response less than risperidone.[26]
Abbreviations: GnRH = gonadotropin-releasing hormone; MAOI = monoamine oxidase inhibitor; SNRI = serotonin and norepinephrine reuptake inhibitor; SSRI = selective serotonin reuptake inhibitor; TCA = tricyclic antidepressant

Therapeutic Choices

Nonpharmacologic Choices

- Screen for and treat mood disorders, especially depression. Achieving remission of depression improves sexual desire and function beyond treatment-emergent sexual dysfunction due to medications (Table 1).[25]
- Counsel or refer the couple when their emotional intimacy is insufficient to motivate her sexually and/or impairs her subjective arousal/pleasure.
- Address lack of stimuli, e.g., insufficient nongenital stimuli or insufficient nonpenetrative genital stimuli or lack of appropriate sexual context.
- Address psychological factors that are inhibiting the effectiveness of sexual stimulation:
  - distractions/nonsexual stressors
  - dysphoric arousal (may indicate previous abuse)
  - constant sexual self-monitoring
  - low self-esteem/poor body image/feeling sexually substandard
  - past experience of pain—a past history of dyspareunia can interfere with the processing of sexual stimuli, even if pain is currently absent
  - negative outcome, e.g., partner's sexual dysfunction, dyspareunia from provoked vestibulodynia (see Genito-pelvic Pain/Penetration Disorder) and subsequent sexual avoidance. In this situation, address the primary problem.
  - negative emotions with arousal
  - suppressed anger and therefore suppressed sexual emotions
  - learned pattern of feeling emotions minimally
- Address biological factors limiting the effectiveness of stimulation (other than depression):
  - dyspareunia from vulvovaginal atrophy, endometriosis, provoked vestibulodynia (see Genito-pelvic Pain/Penetration Disorder)
  - medications (Table 1)
  - fatigue, e.g., chronic ill health, sleep disorder, shift work, disturbed nights
  - irregular or absent menstrual cycles indicative of hyperprolactinemia
  - hypothyroidism
  - urinary incontinence and fear of incontinence during sexual activity

- Standard therapy includes cognitive behavioural therapy (CBT), sexual therapy and, more recently, mindfulness.[27,28]

Pharmacologic Choices

There are no approved pharmacologic treatments for female sexual interest/arousal disorder.

Use **local estrogen** when lack of genital congestion, loss of pleasure from genital stimulation, loss of lubrication or dyspareunia are associated with estrogen-deficient states (see Chapter 75). **Vaginal lubricants** used with intercourse (e.g., Gyne-Moistrin, Astroglide) or **moisturizers** (e.g., Replens) used regularly improve lubrication but may not remove pain from lost elasticity.

There are no approved androgen formulations for women in North America. Transdermal testosterone for postmenopausal women receiving systemic estrogen has been withdrawn from Europe due to low sales and recent RCTs showing no benefit.[29] While in the past testosterone therapy has been prescribed off-label with careful follow up for postmenopausal women, there is now evidence that low desire in women is not related to testosterone levels.[24,30] Although several RCTs show positive results with testosterone, the trials were underpowered[31] and lacked appropriate inclusion criteria[32] and long-term safety data.[33] Until further safety and efficacy data become available, there is insufficient evidence to recommend testosterone in women for female sexual dysfunction [Evidence: SORT C*].[34]

For more information see also Female Orgasmic Disorder, Pharmacologic Choices; and Genito-Pelvic Pain/Penetration Disorder, Pharmacologic Choices.

Female Orgasmic Disorder

To make this diagnosis, at least one of the 2 following symptoms must have been present for a minimum duration of approximately 6 months and be experienced on all or almost all (approximately 75%) occasions of sexual activity:[19]

- Marked delay in, infrequency or absence of orgasm
- Markedly reduced intensity of orgasmic sensation.

While the most common complaint is low desire and low arousal with rare or absent orgasms, some women have healthy arousal but do not experience orgasm.

Goals of Therapy

- Identify need for psychological or psychiatric consultation for deep-seated issues regarding control and vulnerability.
- See also Goals of Therapy in female sexual/interest arousal disorder.

Investigations

- Address lack of trust of others, including the partner
- Address fear of closeness because of fear of loss of partner
- See also Investigations in female sexual/interest arousal disorder.

* SORT (Strength of Recommendation Taxonomy) is a rating system (A, B or C) that addresses the quality of available evidence. For more information consult **How to Use *Compendium of Therapeutic Choices*** on page xxv.

Therapeutic Choices

While etiology and therapy are similar to that of female sexual interest/arousal disorder, there are additional therapeutic choices.

Nonpharmacologic Choices

- Guided self-stimulation involves education and information followed by body awareness exercises designed to enhance women's awareness of their genitals and to challenge any negative or distorted thoughts that might emerge. Explain that vulnerability is needed to let go control so that orgasm occurs. This is very difficult for many women such that learning to orgasm alone may be the first step. See Suggested Readings below.
- Coital Alignment Technique is a behavioral technique which allows more pubis-to-pubis contact between partners during intercourse. It may only be possible to obtain after a male partner's ejaculation and partial detumescence.
- Vibrostimulation involves the patient using a vibrator during partner sex or self-stimulation. It may be especially useful in patients with nerve damage (e.g., from multiple sclerosis or diabetes).
- Clarify range of stimuli that are often needed including nonphysical (e.g., erotic conversation or music), nongenital (e.g., caressing/kissing neck, breasts, thighs, toes) and genital but nonpenetrative (e.g., manual, oral or vibrator stimulation of mons pubis and all parts of the vulva).
- Referral to mental health professional if the following issues are identified: lack of trust, fear of closeness or fear of losing control.

Pharmacologic Choices

- One small randomized controlled trial investigated use of **sildenafil** (50–100 mg as needed prior to sexual activity) to benefit antidepressant-induced female sexual dysfunction.[35] Among other aspects of female sexual dysfunction, sildenafil demonstrated the greatest improvement in ability and time to reach orgasm.
- Investigational intravaginal **dehydroepiandrosterone** (DHEA) 6.5–13 mg at night increased genital sexual sensitivity, improving orgasmic function in RCTs in postmenopausal women who were prescribed DHEA for vaginal atrophy.[36]

For more information see also Sexual Interest/Arousal Disorder, Pharmacologic Choices; and Genito-Pelvic Pain/Penetration Disorder, Pharmacologic Choices

Genito-pelvic Pain/Penetration Disorder

To make this diagnosis, persistent or recurrent difficulties for a minimum duration of approximately 6 months with one or more of the following must be present:[19]

- Marked difficulty with vaginal penetration during intercourse
- Marked vulvovaginal or pelvic pain during vaginal intercourse/penetration attempts
- Marked fear or anxiety about vulvovaginal or pelvic pain in anticipation of, during, or as a result of vaginal penetration
- Marked tensing or tightening of the pelvic floor muscles during attempted vaginal penetration.

Dyspareunia is persistent or recurrent pain with attempted or complete vaginal entry and/or penile vaginal intercourse.[20]

Vaginismus is the persistent or recurrent difficulty of the woman to allow vaginal entry of a penis, a finger and/or any object, despite the woman's expressed wish to do so. There is often phobic avoidance and anticipation/fear/experience of pain, along with variable and involuntary pelvic muscle contraction.

Vaginismus and dyspareunia are now merged under genito-pelvic pain/penetration disorder due to clinical overlap.

Provoked vestibulodynia is pain with touch to the vaginal opening (including attempted vaginal penetration), associated with allodynia (pain sensation from a touch stimulus) around the outer edge of the hymen and no abnormal physical signs other than variable redness. Provoked vestibulodynia is the most common type of dyspareunia, affecting about 16% of women.[37,38,39] Some women with phobic avoidance of penetration such that penile introital contact has never been possible, have no abnormal findings on examination. With other women, examination confirms allodynia of the vestibule thus diagnosing vaginismus by history, but current provoked vestibulodynia.

Goals of Therapy

- Explain current understanding of chronic pain—a composite experience of physical sensations, emotions and thoughts as confirmed by brain imaging
  - outline how parts of the pain experience can be altered, i.e., explain CBT
- Address biological factors:
  - estrogen deficiency
  - infection, e.g., chronic vaginitis, chronic pelvic inflammatory disease
  - pelvic pathology, e.g., endometriosis, interstitial cystitis, inflammatory bowel disease
  - rare congenital abnormalities, e.g., vaginal septum
- Address personal psychological factors:
  - fear of pain or being damaged by something entering the vagina, difficulty with relinquishing control causing reflexive pelvic muscle tightening on introital contact (vaginismus)
  - ambivalence about being sexual with intercourse (the pain may be solely from *appropriate* tightening of perivaginal muscles)
  - psychological distress associated with intense fear of negative evaluation, anxiety, somatization and catastrophization as shown by a majority of women with provoked vestibulodynia
- Address psychosexual factors:
  - lowered sexual self-confidence
  - avoiding sexual stimuli or finding stimuli ineffective because of the focus on negative outcome
  - feelings of being extremely sexually abnormal, shame, guilt and fears of permanent infertility especially when intercourse has never been possible
  - lack of sexual arousal and therefore lack of increased elasticity, lubrication and expansion of proximal vagina
  - partner may be confused, feel unattractive and withdraw emotionally, compounding the woman's low sexual self-image

Investigations

- Determine timing of pain. Pain may occur with:
  - external contact, minimal entry of penis, dildo, finger (compatible with vaginismus)
  - partial entry of penis, compatible with vaginismus, provoked vestibulodynia, vulvovaginal atrophy, tears of posterior fourchette
  - full entry and thrusting (compatible with lack of arousal, provoked vestibulodynia, vulvovaginal atrophy, pelvic pathology including endometriosis)
  - penile movement (typical of provoked vestibulodynia, vulvovaginal atrophy, infection)

- postcoital urination, partner's ejaculation (typical of provoked vestibulodynia but also compatible with vulvovaginal atrophy and with tears of posterior fourchette)
- any of the above and lasts for hours after intercourse (typical of provoked vestibulodynia, endometriosis)

- Gynecologic and medical history
- Physical exam looking for:
  - abdominal tenderness, masses
  - vulvar atrophy (associated with estrogen deficiency)
  - interlabial fissures (associated with estrogen deficiency or candidiasis)
  - signs of past tears of posterior fourchette
  - adhesions between labia minora which preclude penile entry and require surgical division
  - tight posterior fourchette requiring simple perineoplasty
  - abnormal discharge (vaginal infection or possibly more serious pelvic pathology)
  - erythema of introital margin (consistent with but not diagnostic of provoked vestibulodynia)
  - allodynia of introital margin (diagnostic of provoked vestibulodynia)
  - lichen sclerosus involving the introitus
  - bimanual exam: pain on palpation of uterus, cervix or adnexae, nodularity along uterosacral ligaments or in the pouch of Douglas, all evidence of possible pelvic pathology; pelvic muscle hypertonicity with "trigger points" in deep levator ani muscles; abnormalities in urethra, bladder or rectum
  - woman unable to be examined: encourage "practising" at home in private for 10 minutes daily. She should recline on couch or bed, or in the bathtub, partially abducting her thighs and learning to tolerate self-touch to the vulva, ultimately to the introitus, spreading the labia so the introitus can be examined. When she is ready for the exam, allow her to be in control, separating her labia, and any touch (e.g., with a Q-tip for provoked vestibulodynia) can be done by her. Full examination is preferably delayed to a subsequent visit
- Laboratory investigations as indicated by history and physical examination
  - KOH whiff test (fishy odour intensified by addition of a few drops of potassium hydroxide 10% to vaginal secretions on speculum or smear) to detect bacterial vaginosis
  - microscopy and pH for bacterial vaginosis, candidiasis, trichomoniasis
  - fasting glucose and HIV status if chronic candidiasis present
  - biopsy of any vulval area with abnormal appearance
  - DNA and/or culture for gonococcus and chlamydia

Therapeutic Choices

Nonpharmacologic Choices

- Advise couples to focus on nonpenetrative sex and avoid actual intercourse to break cycle of pain.
- Address concomitant lack of arousal and desire.
- Identify nonpharmacologic means of addressing pain, e.g., mindfulness,[40] CBT.[41]
- Assess pelvic muscle hypertonicity[42] and identify physical methods (including pelvic muscle physiotherapy and biofeedback) to address the associated hypertonicity of pelvic muscles.
  - refer to pelvic muscle physiotherapist or teach "reverse Kegel exercises" with use of conical vaginal inserts of gradually increasing diameter
- Refer for definitive treatment if pelvic pathology suspected.
- Refer if conservative therapy for recurrent tearing of posterior fourchette fails.

- Explain role of stress in chronic pain, and counsel on management.

Pharmacologic Choices

There is minimal good evidence for treatment of genito-pelvic pain/penetration disorder (dyspareunia/vaginismus). The following recommendations are based on the author's experience and an international consensus.[43]

Local **estrogen** is beneficial for vulvovaginal atrophy (see Chapter 75).

Treat any STIs that are identified (see Chapter 120).

Topical **estrogen cream** can be used for recurrent posterior fourchette tearing. Topical **testosterone** 2% (compounded in a vehicle such as Glaxal Base) is also helpful. Apply sparingly daily to the posterior fourchette and review in 3 months.

Vaginal lubricants and **vaginal moisturizers** can be helpful (see Chapter 75).

In association with psychological approaches to chronic pain, consider prescribing medical adjuncts for provoked vestibulodynia. There is no good evidence of their efficacy when prescribed alone, but the following agents have been studied: **tricyclic antidepressants**, **antiepileptic drugs**, topical anti-inflammatory **cromolyn** (to limit the activity of the mast cells present in biopsies of areas of allodynia) and topical **local anesthetics**.[42,44] There is consensus to recommend against the use of topical steroids[44] and botulinum toxins.[45]

For more information see also Sexual Interest/Arousal Disorder, Pharmacologic Choices; and Female Orgasmic Disorder, Pharmacologic Choices.

Therapeutic Tips

- Information is often therapeutic, especially for changes in sexual function and needs in both men and women with life cycle changes and aging. Women's desire "normally" lessens with duration of relationships. The need for orgasm with each sexual interaction "normally" lessens with age in men and women. Gradual loss of spontaneous/initial desire, but the ability to become aroused and trigger desire "once into it" is "normal" for all men and women but especially common for middle-aged and older women.
- Loss of sexual desire is a common symptom of depression. Successful treatment of the depression is the most important aspect of improving sexual desire and function[25] despite the fact that many antidepressants can cause not only orgasmic dysfunction but loss of desire. **Bupropion, mirtazapine** and **moclobemide** appear to be less likely to cause sexual dysfunction.[46,47] There is some evidence that adding on bupriopion 150 mg twice daily may benefit patients with SSRI-induced sexual dysfunction.[48,49]
- For the woman complaining of low sexual desire or arousal or orgasmic dysfunction, construct her sex response cycle (Figure 1) to identify the breaks. This logic is therapeutic as she may feel less dysfunctional and become aware of the contextual and interpersonal changes needed to restore her motivation and ability to become sexually aroused and satisfied.
- Most women complaining of lack of arousal have normal vulval and vaginal congestion. Focus assessment and therapy on the adequacy of stimuli and context and the biological and psychological factors interfering with arousability of her mind.
- When the etiology of desire and arousal disorders appears to stem from deep-seated themes in childhood and adolescence and/or there is a history of abuse (mental, emotional, physical), refer to a psychiatrist or psychologist. When the relevant factors are lack of useful sexual contexts, stimuli, sexual information, needed eroticism and attractive behaviours of partners, consider referral to a sex therapist.

Suggested Readings

Basson R. The recurrent pain and sexual sequelae of provoked vestibulodynia: a perpetuating cycle. *J Sex Med* 2012;9(8):2077-92.

Basson R. Sexual function of women with chronic illness and cancer. *Womens Health (Lond Engl)* 2010;6(3):407-29.

Basson R. Testosterone therapy for reduced libido in women. *Ther Adv Endocrinol Metab* 2010;1(4):155-64.

Bhasin S, Enzlin P, Coviello A et al. Sexual dysfunction in men and women with endocrine disorders. *Lancet* 2007;369(9561):597-611.

Heiman J, LoPiccolo J. *Becoming orgasmic: a sexual and personal growth program for women.* New York (NY): Prentice Hall; 1987.

Meston CM, Buss DM. Why humans have sex. *Arch Sex Behav* 2007;36(4):477-507.

References

1. Lutfey KE, Link CL, Rosen RC et al. Prevalence and correlates of sexual activity and function in women: results from the Boston Area Community Health (BACH) Survey. *Arch Sex Behav* 2009;38(4):514-27.
2. Mitchell KR, Mercer CH, Wellings K et al. Prevalence of low sexual desire among women in Britain: associated factors. *J Sex Med* 2009;6(9):2434-44.
3. Basson R. Pharmacotherapy for women's sexual dysfunction. *Expert Opin Pharmacother* 2009;10(10):1631-48.
4. Meston CM, Buss DM. Why humans have sex. *Arch Sex Behav* 2007;36(4):477-507.
5. Toates F. An integrative theoretical framework for understanding sexual motivation, arousal, and behaviour. *J Sex Res* 2009;46(2-3):168-93.
6. Bancroft J, Loftus J, Long JS. Distress about sex: a national survey of women in heterosexual relationships. *Arch Sex Behav* 2003;32(3):193-208.
7. Dennerstein L, Guthrie JR, Hayes RD et al. Sexual function, dysfunction, and sexual distress in a prospective, population-based sample of mid-aged, Australian-born women. *J Sex Med* 2008;5(10):2291-9.
8. Sanders SA, Graham CA, Milhausen RR. Predicting sexual problems in women: the relevance of sexual excitation and sexual inhibition. *Arch Sex Behav* 2008;37(2):241-51.
9. Chivers ML, Seto MC, Lalumiere ML et al. Agreement of self-reported and genital measures of sexual arousal in men and women: a meta-analysis. *Arch Sex Behav* 2010;39(1):5-56.
10. van Lunsen RH, Laan E. Genital vascular responsiveness and sexual feelings in midlife women: psychophysiologic, brain, and genital imaging studies. *Menopause* 2004;11(6 Pt 2):741-8.
11. Maserejian NN, Shifren JL, Parish J et al. The presentation of hypoactive sexual desire disorder in premenopausal women. *J Sex Med* 2010;7(10):3439-48.
12. Laumann EO, Waite LJ. Sexual dysfunction among older adults: prevalence and risk factors from a nationally representative U.S. probability sample of men and women 57-85 years of age. *J Sex Med* 2008;5(10):2300-11.
13. Kolotkin RL, Zunker C, Ostbye T. Sexual functioning and obesity: a review. *Obesity (Silver Spring)* 2012;20(12):2325-33.
14. Mitchell KR, Mercer CH, Ploubidis GB et al. Sexual function in Britain: findings from the third National Survey of Sexual Attitudes and Lifestyles (Natsal-3). *Lancet* 2013;382(9907):1817-29.
15. Basson R, Schultz WW. Sexual sequelae of general medical disorders. *Lancet* 2007;369(9559):409-24.
16. Rees PM, Fowler CJ, Maas CP. Sexual function in men and women with neurological disorders. *Lancet* 2007;369(9560):512-25.
17. Bhasin S, Enzlin P, Coviello A et al. Sexual dysfunction in men and women with endocrine disorders. *Lancet* 2007;369(9561):597-611.
18. Chevret-Measson M, Lavallee E, Troy S et al. Improvement in quality of sexual life in female partners of men with erectile dysfunction treated with sildenafil citrate: findings of the Index of Sexual Life (ISL) in a couple study. *J Sex Med* 2009;6(3):761-9.
19. American Psychiatric Association. Task Force on DSM-5. *Diagnostic and statistical manual of mental disorders: DSM-5.* Washington (DC): American Psychiatric Association; 2013.
20. Basson R, Leiblum S, Brotto L et al. Definitions of women's sexual dysfunction reconsidered: advocating expansion and revision. *J Psychosom Obstet Gynaecol* 2003;24(4):221-9.
21. Basson R. Sexual function of women with chronic illness and cancer. *Womens Health (Lond Engl)* 2010;6(3):407-29.
22. Huang AJ, Moore EE, Boyko EJ et al. Vaginal symptoms in postmenopausal women: self-reported severity, natural history, and risk factors. *Menopause* 2010;17(1):121-6.
23. Davila GW, Singh A, Karapanagiotou I et al. Are women with urogenital atrophy symptomatic? *Am J Obstet Gynecol* 2003;188(2):382-8.
24. Basson R, Brotto LA, Petkau J et al. Role of androgens in women's sexual dysfunction. *Menopause* 2010;17(5):962-71.
25. Clayton A, Kornstein S, Prakash A et al. Changes in sexual functioning associated with duloxetine, escitalopram, and placebo in the treatment of patients with major depressive disorder. *J Sex Med* 2007;4(4 Pt 1):917-29.
26. Schmidt HM, Hagen M, Kriston L et al. Management of sexual dysfunction due to antipsychotic therapy. *Cochrane Database Syst Rev* 2012;11:CD003546.
27. Brotto LA, Basson R, Luria M. A mindfulness-based group psychoeducational intervention targeting sexual arousal disorder in women. *J Sex Med* 2008;5(7):1646-59.
28. Gunzler C, Berner MM. Efficacy of psychosocial interventions in men and women with sexual dysfunctions--a systematic review of controlled clinical trials: part 2--the efficacy of psychosocial interventions for female sexual dysfunction. *J Sex Med* 2012;9(12):3108-25.
29. Snabes MC, Zborowski J, Simes S. Libigel (testosterone gel) does not differentiate from placebo therapy in the treatment of hypoactive sexual desire disorder in postmenopausal women. 11th Annual Meeting of the International Society for the Study of Women's Sexual Health; Jerusalem, IL. *J Sex Med* 2012;9:171.
30. Basson R. Testosterone therapy for reduced libido in women. *Ther Adv Endocrinol Metab* 2010;1(4):155-64.
31. Kingsberg S, Shifren J, Wekselman K et al. Evaluation of the clinical relevance of benefits associated with transdermal testosterone treatment in postmenopausal women with hypoactive sexual desire disorder. *J Sex Med* 2007;4(4 Pt 1):1001-8.

32. Davis SR, van der Mooren MJ, van Lunsen RH et al. Efficacy and safety of a testosterone patch for the treatment of hypoactive sexual desire disorder in surgically menopausal women: a randomized placebo-controlled trial. *Menopause* 2006;13(3):387-96.
33. Davis SR, Moreau M, Kroll R et al. Testosterone for low libido in postmenopausal women not taking estrogen. *N Engl J Med* 2008;359(19):2005-17.
34. Wierman ME, Basson R, Davis SR et al. Androgen therapy in women: an Endocrine Society Clinical Practice guideline. *J Clin Endocrinol Metab* 2006;91(10):3697-710.
35. Nurnberg HG, Hensley PL, Heiman JR et al. Sildenafil treatment of women with antidepressant-associated sexual dysfunction: a randomized controlled trial. *JAMA* 2008;300(4):395-404.
36. Labrie F, Archer D, Bouchard C et al. Effect on intravaginal dehydroepiandrosterone (Prasterone) on libido and sexual dysfunction in postmenopausal women. *Menopause* 2009;16(5):923-31.
37. Harlow BL, Wise LA, Stewart EG. Prevalence and predictors of chronic lower genital tract discomfort. *Am J Obstet Gynecol* 2001;185(3):545-50.
38. Landry T, Bergeron S. How does vulval vaginal pain begin? Prevalence and characteristics of dyspareunia in adolescence. *J Sex Med* 2009;6(4):927-35.
39. Arnold LD, Bachmann GA, Rosen R et al. Assessment of vulvodynia symptoms in a sample of US women: a prevalence survey with a nested case control study. *Am J Obstet Gynecol* 2007;196(2):128.e1-6.
40. Fortney L, Taylor M. Meditation in medical practice: a review of the evidence and practice. *Prim Care* 2010;37(1):81-90.
41. Bergeron S, Khalifé S, Glazer HI et al. Surgical and behavioral treatments for vestibulodynia: two-and-one-half year follow-up and predictors of outcome. *Obstet Gynecol* 2008;111(1):159-66.
42. Gunter J. Vulvodynia: new thoughts on a devastating condition. *Obstet Gynecol Surv* 2007;62(12):812-9.
43. van Lankveld JJ, Granot M, Weijmar Schultz WC et al. Women's sexual pain disorders. *J Sex Med* 2010;7(1 Pt 2):615-31.
44. Landry T, Bergeron S, Dupuis MJ et al. The treatment of provoked vestibulodynia: a critical review. *Clin J Pain* 2008;24(2):155-71.
45. Petersen CD, Giraldi A, Lundvall L et al. Botulinum toxin type A—a novel treatment for provoked vestibulodynia? Results from a randomized, placebo controlled, double blinded study. *J Sex Med* 2009;6(9):2523-37.
46. Gregorian RS, Golden KA, Bahce A et al. Antidepressant-induced sexual dysfunction. *Ann Pharmacother* 2002;36(10):1577-89.
47. Baldwin DS. Sexual dysfunction associated with antidepressant drugs. *Expert Opin Drug Saf* 2004;3(5):457-70.
48. Safarinejad MR. Reversal of SSRI-induced female sexual dysfunction by adjunctive bupropion in menstruating women: a double-blind, placebo-controlled and randomized study. *J Psychopharmacol* 2011;25(3):370-8.
49. Taylor MJ, Rudkin L, Bullemor-Day P et al. Strategies for managing sexual dysfunction induced by antidepressant medication. *Cochrane Database Syst Rev* 2013;(5):CD003382.

Chapter 74
Male Sexual Dysfunction

Rosemary Basson, MD, FRCP(UK)

This chapter addresses erectile dysfunction, premature ejaculation and low sexual desire. A careful sexual history is required to distinguish these 3 conditions since more than one may be present in one patient.

Erectile dysfunction (ED) is the inability to obtain or maintain an erection sufficiently firm for satisfactory sexual activity on all or almost all occasions. Addressing sexual function is an integral part of general medical assessment, not only in men with chronic illness[1] but in apparently well men as impairment can signal serious disease. Of note is the frequency with which vascular ED heralds asymptomatic coronary artery disease[2] and is a potent predictor of "all cause" mortality, cardiovascular death, MI, stroke and heart failure in men with cardiovascular disease.[3] Recent evidence suggests that this is also true for self-stimulated erections and that nonpartnered men should be asked about erections with masturbation.[4] There is a strong multidimensional relationship between ED, coronary artery disease and depression such that the presence of one of the triad necessitates inquiry about the other two.[5]

Premature ejaculation (PE) is defined as ejaculation that occurs within a minute of vaginal penetration and before the person wishes it. This definition needs to be expanded to apply to gay men. Although orgasm and ejaculation are separate physiological events, they occur simultaneously even when delayed by medication. PE may be acquired or lifelong.

Low sexual desire, now called male *hypoactive sexual desire disorder* (HSDD), is a persistent or recurrent lack of sexual thoughts, fantasies and desire. However, as is well recognized in women, men's desire and subjective arousal are experienced together.[6] Typically, sex with the partner becomes extremely infrequent or stops when the man in a heterosexual relationship loses desire. Depression, anxiety, insomnia, age, insufficient physical activity and lower alcohol intake are associated with lower male sexual desire.[7]

Goals of Therapy

- Treat underlying conditions and reversible causes of ED, PE or HSDD
- Address contributing psychological and interpersonal factors
- Assess the safety of resuming intercourse and orgasm after serious illness
- Choose safe and appropriate therapy for the man's or couple's circumstances
- Provide knowledge, understanding and reassurance; encourage realistic expectations focused on pleasure and mutual enjoyment
- Restore sexual intimacy

Investigations

Assessment and management of erectile dysfunction is presented in Figure 1.

Obtain details of chief complaint and psychosexual history (Table 1), preferably from each partner individually, with attention to:

- description of the problem and previously tried interventions

- potentially reversible causes (Table 2)
- childhood experiences that may have affected ability to be intimate or to feel emotions, especially for long-term dysfunction
- past sexual experiences both positive and negative
- sexual context, i.e., partner's arousal and enthusiasm, erotic stimuli
- negative thoughts during sexual engagement
  - for ED, e.g., fear of loss of erection, anger, resentment, distractions
  - for PE, e.g., fear of intimacy or of causing pain to the partner, lack of sexual skill, feelings of guilt or shame associated with sex
- other personal, psychological and interpersonal issues that may contribute, or may hinder the efficacy of pharmacotherapy

Figure 1: **Assessment and Management of Acquired Erectile Dysfunction**

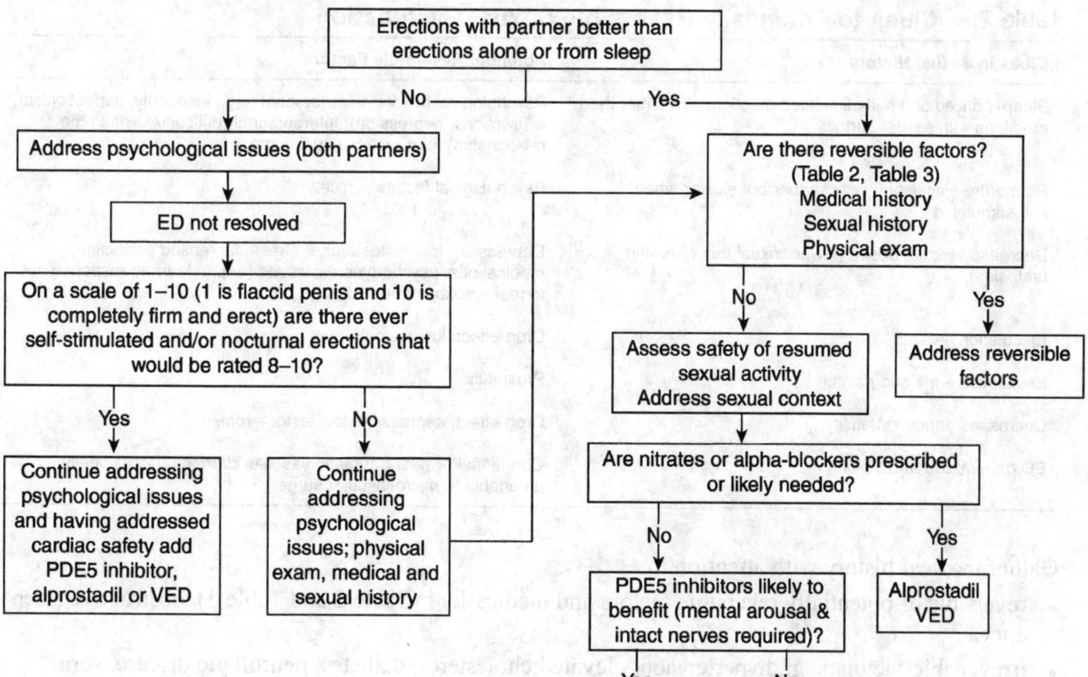

Abbreviations: ED = erectile dysfunction; PDE5 inhibitor = phosphodiesterase type 5 inhibitor; VED = vacuum erection device

Table 1: Questions to Clarify Sexual History and Current Sexual Status

For patients with erectile dysfunction and hypoactive sexual desire disorder:

- For how long have you had difficulty with sexual desire and/or getting and keeping erections?
- Do you still have sexual thoughts or fantasies? Have they reduced markedly? Do you still have the desire to self-stimulate/masturbate? Do you become aroused mentally if you see or hear something erotic? How sexually excited (in your mind) are you when sexually active with your partner?
- On a scale of 1–10/10 where 1/10 is a flaccid penis, 10/10 is completely firm and erect and 6/10 allows (but only just allows) intercourse, how firm are erections when you have sexual play with your partner, when you attempt intercourse, as intercourse proceeds, when you waken from sleep (typically deep sleep) and when you self-stimulate?
- Your experience of orgasm—has that changed?
- Are you reaching ejaculation—and has that changed?
- How rewarding is partnered sex on the occasions it is still occurring or when it was occurring?
- *For ED:* despite these changes, are you both still stimulating each other in sexual ways and being a sexual couple with nonpenetrative sex?
- Does your partner have sexual difficulties? Will I be able to interview your partner? Is your partner in agreement with reinstituting sexual activity including intercourse?
- What effects have these difficulties had on you, on your relationship and on your partner?

Table 2: Clues to Potentially Reversible Sexual Dysfunction

Clues in Sexual History	Potential Reversible Factors
Sleep-induced and self-stimulated erections are firmer than erections with sexual partner	Psychological factors: intrapersonal (e.g., insecurity, perfectionism, distractions, depression); interpersonal (difficulties within the relationship); non-erotic sexual context
Premature ejaculation with partner but slower when self-stimulated	Psychological factors: anxiety
Decreased sexual desire (fewer sexual thoughts and fantasies)	Depression, low testosterone, stress, increased prolactin, medications, psychodynamic issues (e.g., a learned response not to feel emotions generally)
Ejaculation delayed	Drug effect, low testosterone
Ejaculation early and painful	Prostatitis
Decreased orgasm intensity	Drug effect, depression, low testosterone
ED generalized and lifelong	Congenital or past traumatic vascular damage, occasionally amenable to microvascular surgery

Gather medical history with attention to:

- reversible or potentially reversible factors and medications (Table 2 and Table 3), obstructive sleep apnea
- irreversible factors, e.g., hypertension, elevated cholesterol, diabetes, neurologic disease, some penile structural problems, pelvic surgery or trauma damaging pelvic autonomic nerves
- factors of questionable reversibility such as: Peyronie's disease; first 3–4 years after nerve-sparing radical prostatectomy; smoking; chronic illness affecting energy, self-image, ability to pleasure the partner; lifestyle issues including lack of exercise, obesity, fatigue
- cardiovascular risk assessment (Table 4) and discussion of risks associated with resumption of sexual activity, e.g., cardiac events or, less commonly, respiratory or other physical compromise or recurrent cerebral bleed

Table 3: Drugs Associated with Hypoactive Sexual Desire Disorder and Erectile Dysfunction[8,9,10]

Sexual Disorder	Potential Drug Causes		
Hypoactive sexual desire	5-alpha reductase inhibitors	Carbamazepine	Phenytoin
	Alcohol (chronic)	GnRH analogues	Spironolactone
	Anti-androgens	Ketoconazole	SSRIs
	Barbiturates	MAOIs	Tricyclic antidepressants
	Beta blockers	Opioids	
Erectile dysfunction (in addition to the above drugs)	Acetazolamide	Clofibrate	Metoclopramide
	Alcohol (acute)	Clonidine	Phenothiazines
	Alpha blockers	Digoxin	Thiazide diuretics
	Cimetidine	Lithium	

Abbreviations: GnRH = gonadotropin-releasing hormone; MAOI = monoamine oxidase inhibitor

Table 4: Management Recommendations Based on Graded Cardiovascular Risk Assessment[11]

Grade of Risk	Categories of Cardiovascular Disease	Management Recommendations
Low-risk	• Asymptomatic, <3 major risk factors for CAD excluding age and gender • Controlled hypertension • Mild, stable angina • Post successful coronary revascularization • Uncomplicated past MI (>6–8 wk) • Mild valvular disease • LVD/HF (NYHA Class I) • Pericarditis • Mitral valve prolapse • Atrial fibrillation with controlled ventricular response	• Primary-care management • Consider all first-line therapies • Reassess at regular intervals (6–12 months)
Intermediate-risk	• Asymptomatic, ≥3 major risk factors for CAD, excluding gender • Moderate, stable angina • Recent MI (2–6 wk) • LVD/HF (NYHA Class II) • Noncardiac sequelae of atherosclerotic disease (e.g., stroke, peripheral vascular disease)	• Evaluation by a cardiologist prior to initiation of any therapy for erectile dysfunction, due to risk of myocardial ischemia during sexual activity and orgasm • Specialized CV testing, e.g., ETT, echocardiogram • Restratification into high risk or low risk based on the results of CV assessment
High-risk	• Unstable or refractory angina • Uncontrolled hypertension • LVD/HF (NYHA Class III/IV) • Recent MI (<2 wk), stroke • High-risk arrhythmias • Obstructive hypertrophic cardiomyopathies • Moderate/severe valvular disease	• Priority referral for specialized CV management • Treatment for sexual dysfunction to be deferred until cardiac condition stabilized and dependent on specialist recommendations

Abbreviations: CAD = coronary artery disease; HF = heart failure; ETT = exercise tolerance test; LVD = left ventricular dysfunction; NYHA = New York Heart Association

Perform physical examination with attention to:

- cardiovascular (CV) signs that may indicate irreversible vascular cause, e.g., bruits, hypertension, fundal changes, poor peripheral pulses, heart failure. Normal CV exam does not exclude vascular etiology (e.g., endothelial cells lining corpora cavernosal sinusoids cannot be examined)
- CNS signs that may indicate irreversible neurologic damage, e.g., multiple sclerosis, dementia, Parkinson's disease, peripheral neuropathy, spinal cord injury or diabetic neuropathy. Note: A normal CNS exam in the context of autonomic nerve impairment (e.g., diabetic neuropathy or past Guillain-Barré syndrome) does not exclude neurologic etiology (autonomic nerves cannot be tested clinically)
- late signs of hypotestosteronism including fine body hair, smooth skin, testicular atrophy, lessening of beard, gynecomastia, hepatomegaly
- rectal exam to detect signs of prostate pathology (having discussed advantages and disadvantages of routine prostate examination)
- when indicated, stress testing to 4 metabolic equivalents (METs) to identify silent or symptomatic cardiac ischemia that could occur with sexual intercourse and orgasm

Laboratory investigations with attention to:

- total testosterone, calculated free testosterone or bioavailable testosterone and prolactin levels, if the patient is identified as having a primary decrease in sexual desire
  - if testosterone is low, LH and FSH
  - if LH/FSH low, investigate hypothalamic-pituitary function; consider hemochromatosis (imaging, transferrin saturation)
- fasting blood glucose, lipid profile, CBC and liver function tests as needed (abnormalities in these parameters may clarify etiology of ED, but correcting them is unlikely to improve it)
- serum creatinine and calculated GFR
- *for PE:* urinalysis and pelvic ultrasound if infection or bladder calculus suspected. Cystoscopy may be indicated if other underlying pathology is suspected or ultrasound findings require clarification.
- *for HSDD:* TSH (free T4 if LH/FSH low and hypopituitary state is in question)

Erectile Dysfunction

Therapeutic Choices

Nonpharmacologic Choices

Address sexual avoidance by reminding couples that reinstating sexual intimacy requires effort:

- the first priority is to make time to be together, away from responsibilities, to create a context appropriate for reinstituting sex
- reintroduce sexual/sensual/intimate remarks and behaviours throughout the day to allow each individual to once again view the other as a potential sexual partner
- address perceived negative consequences of attempting to be sexual together, e.g., performance failure, pregnancy, moral issues, dyspareunia in the woman
- normalize nonpenetrative sex

Address lack of subjective sexual arousal:

- address intra- and interpersonal psychological issues identified in history that are contributing to the ED and/or would likely preclude benefit from pharmacologic intervention
- address partner sexual dysfunction/lack of enjoyment
- address lack of useful stimulation/contexts

Address lifestyle factors:

- exercise programs, active lifestyle and healthy diet have been shown to benefit men with ED[12]

Vacuum erection devices (VEDs), also known as vacuum constrictive devices, create a vacuum and draw venous blood back into the penis. The blood is then trapped by the use of a retaining band around the base of the penis, to attain adequate firmness for intercourse. There is a learning curve with the use of VEDs. Warn patients that the tightness of the retention band is critical and the band must be removed within 30 minutes after being applied. Some men cannot tolerate the degree of tightness required. Any condition that predisposes to priapism (e.g., leukemia, polycythemia, myelofibrosis and sickle cell disease) is a contraindication to the use of a VED, as is warfarin therapy or other causes of increased INR.

Pharmacologic Choices

Table 6 details the drugs used in the management of ED.

Phosphodiesterase Type 5 Inhibitors

Given their safety, efficacy and oral administration, **sildenafil**, **tadalafil** and **vardenafil** are the drugs of first choice for ED, including antidepressant-induced ED.[13,14,15,16] PDE5 inhibitors can only enhance an erection that is partially developing as a result of effective sexual stimulation and mental sexual arousal (or reflex erection in men with spinal cord injury). Benefit is less in men with diabetes; some evidence supports the addition of folic acid 5 mg daily to increase endothelial nitric oxide production.[17]

Duration of action is longest with tadalafil (up to 36 h); however, the effect of sildenafil[18] and vardenafil[19] may last longer (8–12 hours) than previously thought. Vardenafil and sildenafil have some affinity for PDE_6 in the retina, accounting for occasional visual side effects. Tadalafil has some affinity for PDE_{11A} which may underlie myalgia associated with this drug. Absorption of sildenafil is delayed by high-fat meals. All 3 PDE5 inhibitors have comparable efficacy and side effect profiles in the treatment of ED.[20,21,22,23,24,25]

Contraindications to the use of PDE5 inhibitors include concurrent use of nitrates, symptomatic hypotension (PDE5 inhibitors are mildly hypotensive drugs), any condition in which even a slight lowering of systemic pressure is poorly tolerated (e.g., conditions restricting aortic outflow and volume depletion states), previous priapism and conditions predisposing to priapism (e.g., leukemia, polycythemia, myelofibrosis and sickle cell disease).

Careful concomitant use of PDE5 inhibitors with selective alpha-blockers (alfuzosin, tamsulosin) may benefit ED and lower urinary tract symptoms more than either drug alone.[26,27,28] Caution is needed when using nonselective alpha-blockers due to increased risk of hypotension when combined with PDE5 inhibitors.

Daily or on-demand dosing of PDE5 inhibitors may improve erectile recovery after bilateral nerve-sparing radical prostatectomy[29] but proof is lacking.[30]

Prostaglandin E_1 Analogues

Alprostadil Intracavernosal Injection

If sufficient corporal erectile tissue is still present, injected alprostadil will cause erections even in the absence of mental sexual arousal.[31]

Because alprostadil directly stimulates nociceptors, the technique, dose and dilution are critical for efficacy, safety and comfort of erection. Proper dilution and measurement of the dose are particularly important in neurogenic ED, which often requires doses of only 1–3 µg. Doses up to 40–60 µg may be needed for vascular ED.[31] Priapism (a persistent and painful erection lasting >4 hours in the absence of sexual stimulation or desire) is most commonly caused by intracavernosal injections. Priapism is considered a urologic emergency and should be treated quickly (within hours of presentation) to avoid permanent penile damage. Risk of developing priapism is minimized by slow and careful dose titration of injected drugs.

Contraindications to the use of intracavernosal alprostadil include anticoagulation, previous priapism, symptomatic thrombocytopenia, conditions predisposing to priapism (e.g., leukemia, polycythemia, myelofibrosis, sickle cell disease and valve lesions with significant risk of subacute bacterial endocarditis).

Alprostadil by Urethral Instillation

Instilling alprostadil in the form of a pellet into the urethra allows the drug to enter the corpus spongiosum. Retrograde venous passage from spongiosum to cavernosa is unpredictable and depends on the individual's venous anatomy.[32] Therefore, a trial of intraurethral alprostadil pellets is necessary to determine efficacy in a particular patient.

By entering the communicating veins between the corpora, the drug is introduced into the systemic circulation, and hypotensive systemic side effects are possible.[32]

Contraindications to the use of intraurethral alprostadil include symptomatic hypotension, previous priapism, conditions predisposing to priapism (e.g., leukemia, polycythemia, myelofibrosis and sickle cell disease) and distal urethral pathology.

Other

Treating cardiovascular risk factors with statins may benefit ED.[12]

Premature Ejaculation

Therapeutic Choices

Nonpharmacologic Choices

The following sex therapy techniques must include suggestions for pleasuring the partner, to avoid feelings of being used. They are not appropriate for couples with poor relationships for whom referral for relationship counselling is the appropriate therapy.

- Adaptation
  - ejaculation resulting from partner's manual or oral stimulation can be the beginning of a more leisurely sexual experience for the younger man with PE. If the couple then proceeds towards mutual sexual touching and then intercourse, his erection will return but his orgasmic response will be slower with the "second" erection.
- The following 3 techniques emphasize the appreciation of low intensity sexual arousal without a "goal", e.g., of intercourse.
  - Stop/start technique: the couple has a series of experiences (6–12) where low-key stimulation, e.g., his partner's hand is used. When he reaches moderate mental sexual arousal, the stimulation is deliberately stopped for 1 minute. It is then continued, to be stopped and restarted 4 times before he moves on to ejaculation. These exercises can be used to slow down his self-stimulated response but typically the difficulty occurs mostly with the partner. The objective is for him to learn to focus and enjoy lower degrees of sexual arousal.
  - Squeeze technique: the stop/start method is modified to include a brief, firm squeeze to the glans with the "stop." This will decrease his excitement more than just discontinuing the stimulus. Most clinicians do not recommend this addition because of the negative/painful aspects of the intervention.

- Quiet vagina: to decrease the immediate excitement (and ejaculation) resulting from vaginal stimulation with movement, the woman sits astride her partner, her vagina containing his penis, but with minimal movement for the first 4–5 minutes.

Address possible sequelae of PE in both the patient and his partner (Table 5).

Table 5: Sequelae of Premature Ejaculation for Both Patient and Partner

- Low sexual self-confidence (which creates more anxiety, compounding premature ejaculation and possibly provoking erectile dysfunction)
- Arousal, desire or orgasmic disorder in female or male partner resulting from rushing on to (brief) intercourse, or simply discontinuing sexual engagement as soon as the early ejaculation occurs
- Intercourse itself never resulting in partner's orgasm
- Dyspareunia from premature entry into vagina without woman's arousal

Pharmacologic Choices

Medications to slow down the ejaculatory reflex by increasing serotonergic transmission are commonly used. Ejaculation may be delayed eightfold by **paroxetine** (10–40 mg daily) and fourfold to fivefold by **clomipramine** (12.5–50 mg daily), **sertraline** (50–200 mg daily) and **fluoxetine** (20–40 mg daily).[33,34,35] On-demand therapy 1–2 hours before sexual activity is generally less effective and may result in bothersome side effects. Most common side effects with these agents include fatigue, nausea, diarrhea, decreased sexual desire and erectile dysfunction. Relapse is likely when medication is discontinued. Combining pharmacologic and behavioural techniques is recommended to prolong benefit and ultimately allow withdrawal of medication.

Evidence supporting the effectiveness of PDE5 inhibitors in the treatment of PE is weak.[36,37,38] If tried, it is best to combine PDE5 inhibitors with a medication used in the management of PE (e.g., paroxetine) or target those patients with coincident ED.[36,37]

Although not generally recommended, intracavernosal therapy in those with severe PE may improve partner satisfaction due to erectile persistence after ejaculation.

Numbing the penile skin with local anesthetic reinforces the man's inability to recognize lower states of sexual arousal and is generally not advised.

Hypoactive Sexual Desire Disorder

Therapeutic Choices

Nonpharmacologic Choices

- Provide patient and partner with knowledge and understanding of sexual response cycle (see Figure 2). Explain the multiple reasons men and women have sex; desire is just one of them. Once sexual activity begins and arousal is experienced, desire can then co-occur.
- Screen for and treat mood disorders, especially depression.
- Counsel or refer the couple when their emotional intimacy is insufficient. Consider interpersonal factors such as:
  - poor communication of sexual and nonsexual needs and preferences
  - lack of stimuli
  - feeling unloved

- Address psychological factors that are inhibiting the effectiveness of sexual stimulation:
  - nonsexual stressors, distractions, e.g., the busyness of family life
  - sexual self-monitoring (concern regarding erection or orgasm)
  - low self-esteem, poor body image, insecurity, or difficulty with being vulnerable
  - feelings of shame over something in the past, or having a sexual secret
  - concern regarding female partner's pain (or less commonly his pain, e.g., with ejaculation)
  - feared negative outcome, e.g., partner's sexual dysfunction or lack of excitement
- Address biological factors (in addition to depression) that are limiting the effectiveness of stimulation:
  - medications (Table 3)
  - fatigue, e.g., chronic ill health, sleep disorder, shift work, disturbed nights
  - comorbid ED or partner dyspareunia (address primary problem)

Pharmacologic Choices

There are no approved pharmacologic treatments for HSDD that is not secondary to hormonal abnormality. Repeatedly low testosterone levels must be investigated as must high prolactin. **Testosterone** replacement restores sexual desire in younger men, but evidenced-based proof of its effectiveness in older men is scant.[39] Correction of high prolactin is expected to benefit low desire. **Sildenafil** may benefit SSRI-induced low sexual desire.[16]

Figure 2: **Model of Sexual Response Cycle**

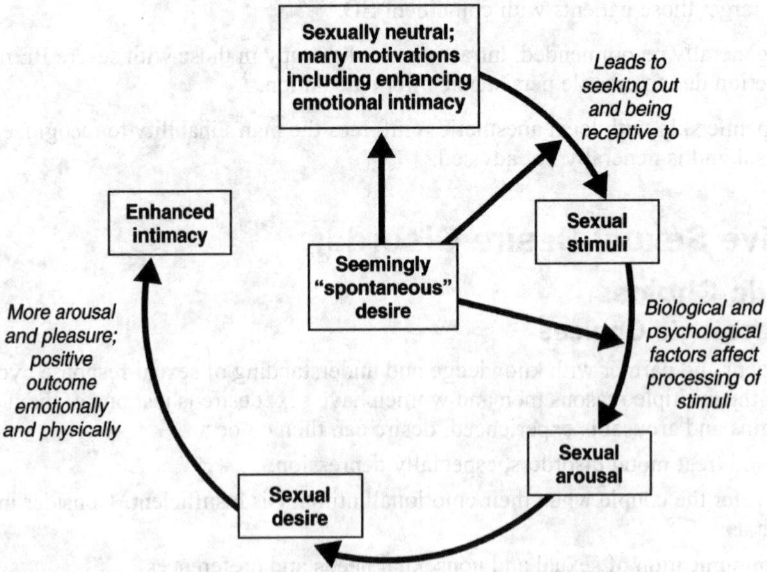

Therapeutic Tips

- ED and HSDD are couple entities. Interview the partner whenever possible. There may be reasons not to intervene (e.g., the man's desire for intercourse is low but he feels his partner expects/needs intercourse, when in reality she/he is pleased that intercourse is no longer possible, never enjoyed it, has chronic dyspareunia or prefers nonpenetrative sex).
- Sex is a biopsychosocial entity. If a patient's erections with self-stimulation are more firm and erect than with his partner, addressing the couple's interaction is more relevant than drug therapy. Prescribing alprostadil addresses only the erectile difficulty. PDE5 inhibitors are unlikely to be effective, given the minimal arousal.
- Plan follow-up, since "drug failures" are usually due to lack of sexual arousal, poor technique with intracavernosal therapy or low desire in the partner.
- Reinforce the contraindications to the use of nitrates and caution with alpha-blockers.
- Assess safety of resumption of sexual activity in cardiac patients prior to initiation of any therapy—this applies to both partners.
- Priapism is a urologic emergency most commonly caused by intracavernosal injections.
- For PE, the overall objective of the adaptation and sex therapy techniques (± medication) is to enable the man to focus his attention away from the act of intercourse and concentrate instead on his enjoyment of the total sexual experience, including the pleasure he gives to and receives from his sexual partner. The more he can become aware of and learn to enjoy lower states of arousal, the less anxious he will be and the slower his response becomes.

Table 6: **Drug Therapy for Erectile Dysfunction**

Class	Drug	Dose	Adverse Effects	Drug Interactions	Comments	Cost[a]
PDE_5 Inhibitors	*sildenafil* Viagra, generics	50–100 mg po 30–60 min before sexual activity. Maximum 100 mg per 24 h. Not for daily use. Start at 25 mg if patient is also using CYP3A4 inhibitors, >65 years or has renal/liver dysfunction	Headache, flushing, dyspepsia, nasal congestion, transient visual disturbances, dizziness, skin rash. Rare: priapism, permanent vision loss.	Contraindicated with nitrates (seek emergency care if chest pain present within 24–48 h of taking PDE5 inhibitor; not to be given for 5 days after stopping long-acting nitrates). May cause hypotension if used with nonselective alpha-blockers (e.g., doxazosin, prazosin). CYP3A4 inhibitors (e.g., cimetidine, clarithromycin, efavirenz, erythromycin, grapefruit juice, itraconazole, ketoconazole, ritonavir) can significantly decrease metabolism of the PDE5 inhibitor. CYP3A4 inducers (e.g., carbamazepine, phenobarbital, phenytoin, rifampin) may decrease efficacy of the PDE5 inhibitor.	Onset of action may be as early as 15 min. Duration of action may be up to 12 h. Efficacy dependent on mental arousal. Dyspepsia and transient visual disturbances (impaired blue/green discrimination, blurred vision or increased light sensitivity) >10% with doses of 100 mg. Use with caution in retinitis pigmentosa. High fat meal delays absorption.	$$
	tadalafil Cialis	Once-a-day dosing: 2.5–5 mg daily po On-demand dosing: 10–20 mg po 60 min before sexual activity. Maximum 20 mg every 36–48 h Start at 2.5–5 mg if patient is also using strong CYP3A4 inhibitors, >65 years of age or has renal/liver dysfunction	Headache, flushing, dyspepsia, nasal congestion, myalgia, back pain. Rare: visual disturbances, permanent vision loss.	See sildenafil.	Onset of action within 30–60 min. Efficacy dependent on mental arousal. Duration of effect up to 36 h. Once-a-day use is not recommended for those with severe renal impairment. Desirable in couples who want more freedom in timing their sexual activity. No delay in absorption after food. Not recommended in severe hepatic impairment.	Once-a-day: $ On-demand: $$

Class	Drug	Dose	Adverse Effects	Drug Interactions	Comments	Cost[a]
	vardenafil Levitra, Staxyn	Levitra (film-coated tablets): 10–20 mg po 30–60 min before sexual activity. Maximum 20 mg per 24 h. Staxyn (orally disintegrating tablets): 10 mg dissolved on tongue 45–90 min before sexual activity. Maximum 10 mg per 24 h. Not for daily use. Start with 5 mg film-coated tablets if patient is also using CYP3A4 inhibitors, >65 years of age or has liver dysfunction	Headache, flushing, dyspepsia, rhinitis, sinusitis, transient visual disturbances. Slight prolongation of QT_c interval.	See sildenafil. Do not use with quinidine, procainamide, amiodarone or sotalol due to increased risk of QT_c prolongation.	Onset of action may be as early as 10 min. Duration of action up to 12 h. Efficacy dependent on mental arousal. Fatty meals decrease maximum blood concentration. Do not use in men with congenital long QT syndrome. Orally disintegrating tablets and film-coated tablets are not bioequivalent.	$$
PGE_1 Analogues	*alprostadil (intracavernosal injection)* Caverject	Neurogenic ED: start with 1.25 µg. If needed, may increase to 2.5 µg then by 5 µg increments to a maximum of 60 µg. Vascular, psychogenic or mixed ED: start with 2.5 µg and titrate to response Severe vascular ED may require up to 40–60 µg Erection duration up to 1 h	Penile pain, hematoma, ecchymosis, penile fibrosis. Rare: priapism.	Increased risk of hypotension if combined with alcohol, antihypertensive agents or vasodilators.	Use 5–10 min prior to sexual activity. Do not use more than once daily or 3 times per week, at least 24 h between each dose. Caution regarding needle stick injury and risk of STI transmission. Stress strict sterile technique, especially if known risk of endocarditis. Stress one-time use of needle and syringe provided in Caverject kit. The initial dose is determined during self-injection teaching in the physician's office.	$$$
	alprostadil (intraurethral pellet) MUSE	250–1000 µg 10–30 min before sexual activity. Dose depends on venous anatomy rather than ED etiology. Onset of effect within 5–10 min	Penile pain, dizziness. Rare: syncope, priapism.	Additive hypotension with antihypertensives.	Do not use more than once per 24-h period. Monitor BP during in-office titration to detect asymptomatic hypotension.	$$$$

[a] Cost of 1 dose; includes drug cost only
Abbreviations: BP = blood pressure; ED = erectile dysfunction; STI = sexually transmitted infection
Legend: $ <$5 $$ $5–15 $$$ $15–25 $$$$ $25–35

Suggested Readings

Erectile Dysfunction

Bhasin S, Enzlin P, Coviello A et al. Sexual dysfunction in men and women with endocrine disorders. *Lancet* 2007;369(9561):597-611.

Hatzimouratidis K, Amar E, Eardley I et al. Guidelines on male sexual dysfunction: erectile dysfunction and premature ejaculation. *Eur Urol* 2010;57(5):804-14.

Jackson G, Boon N, Eardley I et al. Erectile dysfunction and coronary artery disease prediction: evidence-based guidance and consensus. *Int J Clin Pract* 2010;64(7):848-57.

Rees PM, Fowler CJ, Maas CP. Sexual function in men and women with menopause with neurological disorders. *Lancet* 2007;369(9560):512-25.

Premature Ejaculation

Basson R, Schultz WW. Sexual sequelae of general medical disorders. *Lancet* 2007;369(9559):409-24.

Leiblum SR, ed. *Principles and practice of sex therapy.* 4th ed. New York (NY): Guilford Press; 2007. p. 212-40.

Hypoactive Sexual Desire Disorder

DeRogatis L, Rosen RC, Goldstein I et al. Characterization of hypoactive sexual desire disorder (HSDD) in men. *J Sex Med* 2012;9(3):812-20.

Martin S, Atlantis E, Wilson D et al. Clinical and biopsychosocial determinants of sexual dysfunction in middle-aged and older Australian men. *J Sex Med* 2012;9(8):2093-103.

References

1. Basson R, Schultz WW. Sexual sequelae of general medical disorders. *Lancet* 2007;369(9559):409-24.
2. Jackson G, Boon N, Eardley I et al. Erectile dysfunction and coronary artery disease prediction: evidence-based guidance and consensus. *Int J Clin Pract* 2010;64(7):848-57.
3. Bohm M, Baumhakel M, Teo K et al. Erectile dysfunction predicts cardiovascular events in high-risk patients receiving telmisartan, ramipril, or both: The ONgoing Telmisartan Alone and in combination with Ramipril Global Endpoint Trial/Telmisartan Randomized AssessmeNt Study in ACE iNtolerant subjects with cardiovascular Disease (ONTARGET/TRANSCEND) Trials. *Circulation* 2010;121(12):1439-46.
4. Rastrelli G, Boddi V, Corona G et al. Impaired masturbation-induced erections: a new cardiovascular risk factor for male subjects with sexual dysfunction. *J Sex Med* 2013;10(4):1100-13.
5. El-Sakka AI. Erectile dysfunction, depression, and ischemic heart disease: does the existence of one component of this triad necessitate inquiring the other two? *J Sex Med* 2011;8(4):937-40.
6. Janssen E. Sexual arousal in men: a review and conceptual analysis. *Horm Behav* 2011;59(5):708-16.
7. Martin S, Atlantis E, Wilson D et al. Clinical and biopsychosocial determinants of sexual dysfunction in middle-aged and older Australian men. *J Sex Med* 2012;9(8):2093-103.
8. Do C, Huyghe E, Lapeyre-Mestre M et al. Statins and erectile dysfunction: results of a case/non-case study using the French Pharmacovigilance System Database. *Drug Saf* 2009;32(7):591-7.
9. Shiri R, Koskimaki J, Hakkinen J et al. Cardiovascular drug use and the incidence of erectile dysfunction. *Int J Impot Res* 2007;19(2):208-12.
10. Baumhäkel M, Schlimmer N, Kratz M et al. Cardiovascular risk, drugs and erectile dysfunction—a systematic analysis. *Int J Clin Pract* 2011;65(3):289-98.
11. Kostis JB, Jackson G, Rosen R et al. Sexual dysfunction and cardiac risk (the Second Princeton Consensus Conference). *Am J Cardiol* 2005;96(12B):85M-93M.
12. Gupta BP, Murad MH, Clifton MM et al. The effect of lifestyle modification and cardiovascular risk factor reduction on erectile dysfunction. *Arch Intern Med* 2011;171(20):1797-803.
13. Nehra A. Erectile dysfunction and cardiovascular disease: efficacy and safety of phosphodiesterase type 5 inhibitors in men with both conditions. *Mayo Clin Proc* 2009;84(2):139-48.
14. Tsertsvadze A, Fink HA, Yazdi F et al. Oral phosphodiesterase-5 inhibitors and hormonal treatment for erectile dysfunction: a systematic review and meta-analysis. *Ann Intern Med* 2009;151(9):650-61.
15. Hatzichristou D, Gambla M, Rubio-Aurioles E et al. Efficacy of tadalafil once daily in men with diabetes mellitus and erectile dysfunction. *Diabet Med* 2008;25(2):138-46.
16. Taylor MJ, Rudkin L, Bullemor-Day P et al. Strategies for managing sexual dysfunction induced by antidepressant medication. *Cochrane Database Syst Revi* 2013;5:CD003382.
17. Hamidi Madani A, Asadolahzade A, Mokhtari G et al. Assessment of the efficacy of combination therapy with folic acid and tadalafil for the management of erectile dysfunction in men with type 2 diabetes mellitus. *J Sex Med* 2013;10(4):1146-50.
18. Zinner N. Do food and dose timing affect the efficacy of sildenafil? A randomized placebo-controlled study. *J Sex Med* 2007;4(1):137-44.
19. Padma-Nathan H, Christ G, Adaikan G et al. Pharmacotherapy for erectile dysfunction. *J Sex Med* 2004;1(2):128-40.
20. Montorsi F, Padma-Nathan H, Buvat J et al. Earliest time to onset of action leading to successful intercourse with vardenafil determined in an at-home setting: a randomized, double-blind, placebo-controlled trial. *J Sex Med* 2004;1(2):168-78.
21. Doggrell SA. Comparison of clinical trials with sildenafil, vardenafil and tadalafil in erectile dysfunction. *Expert Opin Pharmacother* 2005;6(1):75-84.
22. Wright PJ. Comparison of phosphodiesterase type 5 (PDE5) inhibitors. *Int J Clin Pract* 2006;60(8):967-75.
23. Moore RA, Derry S, McQuay HJ. Indirect comparison of interventions using published randomised trials: systematic review of PDE-5 inhibitors for erectile dysfunction. *BMC Urol* 2005;5:18.

24. Berner MM, Kriston L, Harms A. Efficacy of PDE-5-inhibitors for erectile dysfunction. A comparative meta-analysis of fixed-dose regimen randomized controlled trials administering the International Index of Erectile Function in broad-spectrum populations. *Int J Impot Res* 2006;18(3):229-35.
25. Smith WB, McCaslin IR, Gokce A et al. PDE5 inhibitors: considerations for preference and long-term adherence. *Int J Clin Pract* 2013;67(8):768-80.
26. Giuliano F. Lower urinary tract symptoms and sexual dysfunction: a common approach. *BJU Int* 2008;101(Suppl 3):22-6.
27. Singh DV, Mete UK, Mandal AK et al. A comparative randomized prospective study to evaluate efficacy and safety of combination of tamsulosin and tadalafil vs. tamsulosin or tadalafil alone in patients with lower urinary tract symptoms due to benign prostatic hyperplasia. *J Sex Med* 2014;11(1):187-96.
28. Liguori G, Trombetta C, De Giorgi G et al. Efficacy and safety of combined oral therapy with tadalafil and alfuzosin: an integrated approach to the management of patients with lower urinary tract symptoms and erectile dysfunction. Preliminary report. *J Sex Med* 2009;6(2):544-52
29. Briganti A, Gallina A, Suardi N et al. Predicting erectile function recovery after bilateral nerve sparing radical prostatectomy: a proposal of a novel preoperative risk stratification. *J Sex Med* 2010;7(7):2521-31.
30. Montorsi F, Brock G, Lee J et al. Effect of nightly versus on-demand vardenafil on recovery of erectile function in men following bilateral nerve-sparing radical prostatectomy. *Eur Urol* 2008;54(4):924-31.
31. Porst H, Buvat J, Meuleman E et al. Intracavernous Alprostadil Alfadex--an effective and well tolerated treatment for erectile dysfunction. Results of a long-term European study. *Int J Impot Res* 1998;10(4):225-31.
32. Porst H. Transurethral alprostadil with MUSE (medicated urethral system for erection) vs intracavernous alprostadil--a comparative study in 103 patients with erectile dysfunction. *Int J Impot Res* 1997;9(4):187-92.
33. Waldinger MD, Zwinderman AH, Olivier B. Antidepressants and ejaculation: a double-blind, randomized, placebo-controlled, fixed-dose study with paroxetine, sertraline, and nefazodone. *J Clin Psychopharmacol* 2001;21(3):293-7.
34. Waldinger MD, Zwinderman AH, Schweitzer DH et al. Relevance of methodological design for the interpretation of efficacy of drug treatment of premature ejaculation: a systematic review and meta-analysis. *Int J Impot Res* 2004;16(4):369-81.
35. International Society for Sexual Medicine. *Quick reference guide to PE*. Version 1, October 2010. Available from: www.issm.info/images/uploads/issm_quick_reference_guide_to_pe.pdf. Accessed February 10, 2011.
36. McMahon CG, McMahon CN, Leow LJ et al. Efficacy of type-5 phosphodiesterase inhibitors in the drug treatment of premature ejaculation: a systematic review. *BJU Int* 2006;98(2):259-72.
37. Chen J, Keren-Paz G, Bar-Yosef Y et al. The role of phosphodiesterase type 5 inhibitors in the management of premature ejaculation: a critical analysis of basic science and clinical data. *Eur Urol* 2007;52(5):1331-9.
38. Aversa A, Francomano D, Bruzziches R et al. Is there a role for phosphodiesterase type-5 inhibitors in the treatment of premature ejaculation? *Int J Impot Res* 2011;23(1):17-23.
39. Makinen JI, Huhtaniemi I. Androgen replacement therapy in late-onset hypogonadism: current concepts and controversies—a mini-review. *Gerontology* 2011;57(3):193-202.

Chapter 75
Menopause

Amie J. Cullimore, BEd, MD, MSc, FRCSC

Natural menopause is defined as cessation of menses of 1 year's duration secondary to lack of estrogen production by the ovary. The average age of women experiencing menopause in Canada is 51, and this has been constant throughout the last few centuries.[1,2] Menopause may also be induced by medical or surgical intervention such as radiation or chemotherapy treatment or removal of the ovaries at time of hysterectomy. Perimenopause (a lay term) or the menopausal transition begins with an alteration in menstrual cycle length and ends with the final menstrual period (which is recognized as such only after 12 months of amenorrhea). Symptoms of the menopausal transition are frequently similar to that of menopause.

Vasomotor symptoms, commonly known as hot flashes and night sweats, are the most common presenting complaint of menopausal women. The frequency of bothersome hot flashes appears to commence about 2 years before the final menstrual period, with maximum symptoms occurring within the first 2 years after the last period. The frequency of hot flashes gradually decreases over 6 years.[1,3] However, some women experience hot flashes many years after menopause.

Other associated complaints of menopause, including vaginal symptoms such as dryness, itching, vaginitis and dyspareunia, generally persist or worsen with aging due to low estrogen levels. Women tend to report vaginal symptoms a few years after the last menstrual period. Unlike hot flashes, vaginal atrophy does not improve over time. Some women notice decreasing libido and an alteration in sexual function with the onset of menopause (see Chapter 73). The cause of this change is multifaceted.

Sleep disturbances (difficulty sleeping, fragmented sleep) and mood changes (depression, anxiety) have also been reported in the menopausal transition and may continue after menopause.

Goals of Therapy

- Reduce symptoms associated with declining estrogen levels, including vasomotor instability (hot flashes, hot flushes, night sweats), urogenital atrophy (vaginal dryness, dyspareunia) and mood-related changes (depression, anxiety, sleeplessness)
- Avoid potentially harmful effects of estrogen therapies including increased risk of endometrial and breast carcinoma, MI, stroke and venous thromboembolism (VTE)

Investigations

- Confirm cessation of menstrual period:
  - if duration of cessation of menses is greater than 1 year, ovarian failure is virtually certain
  - if ovarian function is uncertain, continued elevation of serum follicle-stimulating hormone (FSH) in excess of 40 IU/L on 2 occasions confirms ovarian failure
- Health maintenance screening:
  - initial evaluation should include blood pressure assessment, breast examination and cervical cytology
  - mammography is indicated for all women over 50 years of age, every 2–3 years.[4] Consider younger women for mammography if at higher risk of breast cancer, e.g., strong family history

  - screen women at high risk of cardiovascular disease or osteoporosis for dyslipidemia or bone mineral density, respectively
- Investigate any unexpected bleeding by means of endometrial sampling to rule out endometrial carcinoma
- Consider other diagnoses of vasomotor symptoms, e.g., hyperthyroidism, carcinoid syndrome, pheochromocytoma

Therapeutic Choices

Figure 1 summarizes the management of vasomotor symptoms in menopausal women.

Figure 1: Treatment of Vasomotor Symptoms

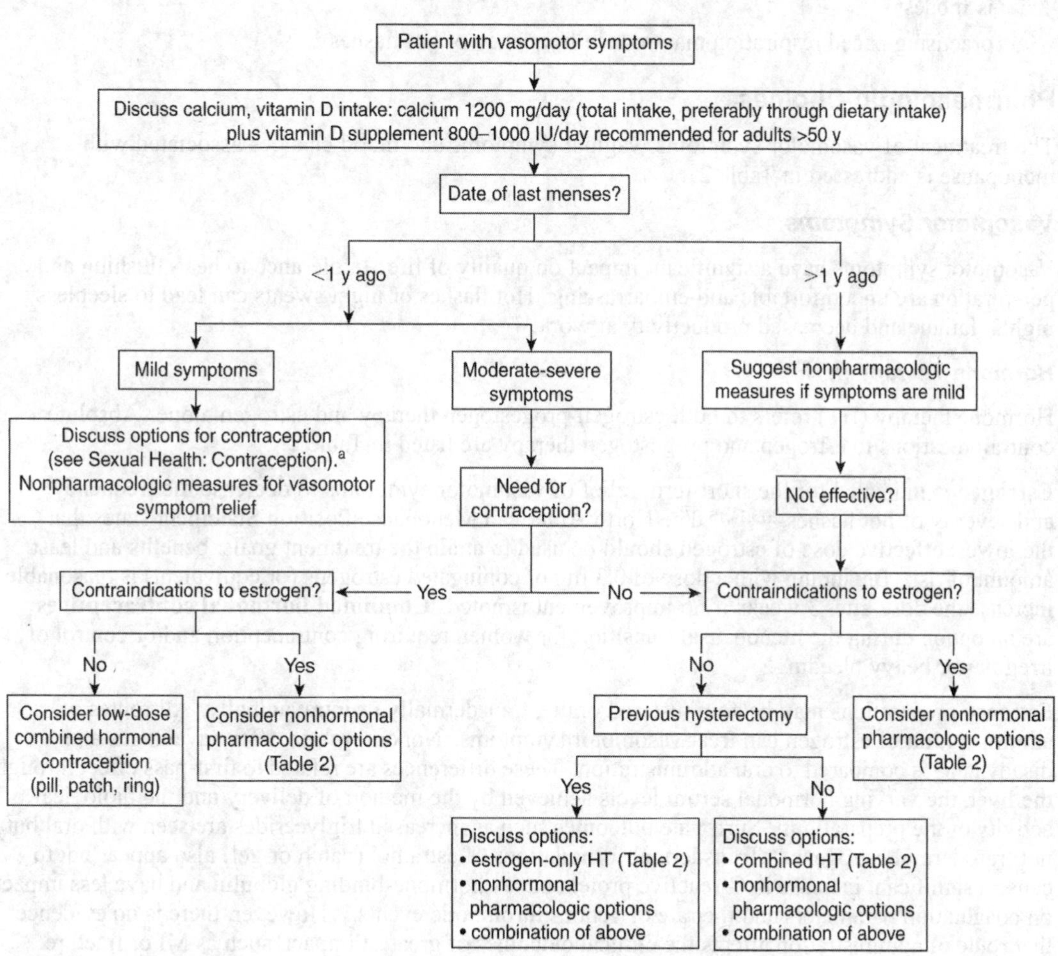

[a] See Chapter 70.
Abbreviations: HT = hormone therapy

Nonpharmacologic Choices

- Lifestyle modification may positively impact vasomotor symptoms.
  - passive smoke exposure and high body mass index (≥27 kg/m²) are associated with greater prevalence of hot flashes.[5]
  - dietary intervention via decreasing fat intake and increasing fruit, vegetables and whole grains along with weight loss may reduce vasomotor symptoms, as reported by the Women's Health Initiative (WHI) study.[6] However, only 10% of women reported moderate to severe vasomotor symptoms, and approximately 90% had mild or no hot flashes at baseline.
  - lowering the ambient temperature and reducing core body temperature (e.g., dressing in layers, using a fan, consuming cold drinks) may help reduce the intensity of hot flashes.
  - stretching improves hot flashes in overweight postmenopausal women.[7]
  - yoga may alleviate menopausal symptoms and improve quality of life but the improvement is modest.[8]
  - practising paced respiration may reduce frequency of hot flashes.[9]

Pharmacologic Choices

The treatment of vasomotor symptoms, vaginal symptoms and mood changes associated with menopause is addressed in Table 2.

Vasomotor Symptoms

Vasomotor symptoms have a significant impact on quality of life. Intolerance to heat, flushing and perspiration are uncomfortable and embarrassing. Hot flashes or night sweats can lead to sleepless nights, fatigue and decreased productivity at work.[12]

Hormone Therapy (HT)

Hormone therapy (HT) refers to both estrogen-progestogen therapy and estrogen alone. Absolute contraindications to estrogen and progestogen therapy are listed in Table 1.

Estrogen is indicated for the short-term relief of vasomotor symptoms to decrease the frequency and severity of hot flashes.[2,13,14,15] The North American Menopause Position Statement states that the lowest effective dose of estrogen should be used to attain the treatment goals, benefits and least amount of risk. Beginning with a dose of 0.3 mg of conjugated estrogens (or equivalent) is reasonable; increase the dose after 3 weeks if no improvement is noted. **Combined hormonal contraceptives** are an option during the menopausal transition for women requiring contraception and/or control of irregular or heavy bleeding.

Estrogen preparations may be administered orally, transdermally or intravaginally. All routes of administration of estrogen can treat vasomotor symptoms. Nonoral routes offer advantages and disadvantages compared to oral administration. These differences are related to first-pass effect through the liver, the varying hormonal serum levels achieved by the method of delivery and the biological activity of the preparation.[17] Surrogate outcomes such as increased triglycerides are seen with oral but not transdermal estrogens.[16] Transdermal formulations of estradiol (patch or gel) also appear not to cause a significant increase in C-reactive protein or sex hormone-binding globulin and have less impact on coagulation parameters and the rate of venous thrombotic events.[18] However, there is no evidence that route of administration affects the clinical outcomes of greatest impact, such as MI or fracture.

The effect of estrogen therapy on vasomotor symptoms is dose-related, with substantial relief seen within 4 weeks at standard doses (estradiol 1 mg or equivalent) and 8–12 weeks at low doses (conjugated estrogens 0.3 mg or equivalent).[19] Lower doses of estrogen are associated with a decreased incidence of irregular bleeding and breast tenderness compared to standard doses.[19]

Table 1: **Absolute Contraindications to Estrogen and Progestogen Therapy**

Hormone Therapy	Contraindications
Estrogen	Undiagnosed vaginal bleeding Active liver disease Active thromboembolic disease Known or suspected carcinoma of the breast or other estrogen-sensitive tumours Pregnancy **Note:** The risk of recurrence of breast cancer or thrombosis following estrogen therapy is unknown. Caution is recommended in women with cardiovascular disease. For all women, the risk vs. the benefit must be considered when prescribing estrogen therapy.
Progestogen	Undiagnosed vaginal bleeding Known or suspected carcinoma of the breast Pregnancy

In women without a uterus, estrogen **alone** should be used continuously throughout the month to reduce the risk of exacerbation of menopausal symptoms.

The term *progestogen* includes both natural progesterone and synthetic progestins. A **progestogen** is indicated in women with an intact uterus using systemic estrogen to reduce the risk of endometrial hyperplasia. The dose is the equivalent of **medroxyprogesterone acetate (MPA)** 5 mg daily for cyclical regimens or 2.5 mg daily for continuous regimens. Alternatively, a Cochrane review recommends a minimum dose of MPA 1.5 mg daily for continuous regimens.[20]

Consider progestins such as oral MPA and **megestrol acetate** as alternative treatments for hot flashes in symptomatic women who cannot or who do not want to use estrogen therapy. Do not recommend progesterone cream because it does not prevent endometrial hyperplasia when used in combination with estrogen therapy in women with an intact uterus.[21] It is currently unknown whether progestogen monotherapy increases the risk of breast cancer.[2]

The **levonorgestrel intrauterine system (IUS)** (Mirena) may be used in perimenopausal women requiring contraception who experience heavy bleeding. Although data are limited, the levonorgestrel IUS may also provide endometrial protection in perimenopausal women on estrogen therapy (not a Health Canada-approved indication).[22]

Continuous combined therapy with estrogen and a progestogen taken daily without a break is the most commonly prescribed regimen. This reduces the risk of bleeding and the risk of endometrial carcinoma. During the first year of use, unexpected spotting or light bleeding may occur.

Continuous estrogen with **cyclical** progestogen helps reduce the risk of endometrial hyperplasia or carcinoma in women with a uterus. In cyclic regimens, estrogen is taken continuously and a progestogen is taken from days 1–14 of the calendar month. A woman can expect a withdrawal bleed when the progestogen is stopped. This regimen is less favoured because of the induced bleeding.

There is no good evidence to suggest the best time to discontinue HT. The use of estrogen with or without progestogen for treatment of menopausal symptoms should be reviewed each year to determine if continued use is expected to result in more benefit than risk. Avoid the abrupt discontinuation of therapy by gradually reducing the dose and frequency. If the patient becomes symptomatic with lower doses, continue that dose until the vasomotor symptoms abate.[2]

Bioidentical Hormones

The term *bioidentical* describes a product that contains hormones (e.g., estrogen, progesterone) that are chemically the same as those produced by the human ovary.[23] Some bioidentical hormones are available as Health Canada-approved prescription products (see Table 2). However, there is concern regarding individually customized preparations compounded in pharmacies, with dosages prescribed based on salivary and blood testing of a woman's hormone levels. The US Food and Drug Administration states that there is no scientific basis for using saliva testing to adjust hormone levels.[24] These blood and salivary levels are not helpful as hormone levels fluctuate throughout the day. There may be increased risks to the women using these products; custom-compounded hormones have not been tested for efficacy or safety, and purity and standardization may be variable. Compounded progesterone dosing is difficult secondary to the differences in progesterone levels within saliva, blood and tissues. The North American Menopause Society recommends bioidentical hormone preparations be subject to the same rigor required for approved products, including providing patient inserts.[17]

Prevention of Cardiovascular Disease with Hormone Therapy (HT)

HT is not indicated for the primary or secondary prevention of cardiovascular disease.[2,25,26,27,28] Two randomized controlled trials have shown that estrogen-progestin treatment is ineffective for primary or secondary prevention of coronary artery disease.[29,30] However, reanalysis of the data from the WHI study suggests that increased risk of coronary artery disease was more likely in women who were ≥70 years old when they began HT. Women who started HT between the ages of 50 and 59 were less likely to die from coronary artery disease.[31] Evidence suggests that the younger women receiving estrogen had less calcified-plaque burden in the coronary arteries than women receiving placebo.[32] Nevertheless, a Cochrane systematic review of RCTs demonstrated that HT does not provide cardioprotection in postmenopausal women.[33] Prevention of coronary artery disease is best achieved by improving health, diet and fitness, and where necessary through risk reduction with drug therapy such as lipid-lowering agents and antihypertensives (see Chapter 37 and Chapter 39).

Prevention of Osteoporosis with Hormone Therapy (HT)

Current evidence indicates that the prevention of osteoporosis should be achieved through diet, exercise, calcium and vitamin D supplementation. Hormone therapy may be considered as a first-line treatment for osteoporosis in women who suffer from significant vasomotor symptoms and desire treatment for these symptoms.[10] Bisphosphonates or selective estrogen receptor modulators should be considered in women who do not have vasomotor symptoms (see Chapter 83).

Risks Associated with Hormone Therapy (HT)

In the estrogen-progestin arm of the WHI study, the risks of venous thromboembolism (VTE), MI, stroke and breast cancer outweighed the benefits of reduced fractures and reduced incidence of colorectal cancer after 5 years of treatment.

VTE risk was 3.6-fold higher with estrogen-progestin therapy (EPT) in the first year of use compared with placebo. Although the risk declined over time, the overall risk over 5 years remained significantly elevated (Hazard Ratio 2.11, 95% CI 1.26–3.55).[29] Thus, the WHI demonstrated an additional 18 VTEs per 10 000 women on EPT and 7 additional VTEs per 10 000 women on estrogen alone.[34] Additionally, the WHI demonstrated an overall CHD risk of 8 cases per 10 000 women per year on EPT and 3 cases per year for women on estrogen alone.[31] Reanalysis of the WHI has suggested that cardiac risk increases when the starting time of HT is further away from the onset of menopause and is also higher with increased age when starting HT.[31] In other words, older women starting HT and women who are further away from their final menstrual period appear to be at greater risk of a cardiac event compared to women who are younger and those who initiate HT closer to their menopause. A prospective cohort study of HT in recently postmenopausal women between the ages of 45 and 58 suggests that HT did not increase risk of mortality, MI, heart failure, breast cancer or stroke in this population.[35]

The WHI also demonstrated an increased risk of ischemic stroke in women on HT; there was no apparent increased risk of hemorrhagic stroke.[36,37] There were an additional 8 strokes per 10 000 women per year in the EPT group and an additional 11 strokes per 10 000 women (of any age) per year in the estrogen therapy group. For women aged 50–59 years, there were approximately 2 additional strokes per 10 000 woman-years.[38]

The risk of breast cancer with estrogen-progestogen use mirrors the increased risk with delaying menopause (the additional risk with each year of EPT is similar to the additional risk with each year older at menopause).[39] In the WHI study, the incidence of breast cancer was higher among EPT users than placebo users, rising to statistical significance after 5 years, but the absolute risk for individual users is small (38 cases in hormone users compared with 30 in placebo users per 10 000 women per annum, or 8 extra cases of breast cancer per 10 000 women using EPT therapy). However, there was no difference in breast cancer rates between women in the estrogen-alone arm (women with hysterectomy) and the placebo arm after an average use of 7.1 years. Interestingly, the French E3N observational study found that women using estrogen and micronized progesterone did not have a greater risk of breast cancer than women using estrogen alone. Women using estrogen and progestins, such as medroxyprogesterone acetate, were at greater risk of breast cancer, with a relative risk of 1.69 overall.[40]

In an 11-year follow up of women who received EPT in the WHI, there was a greater risk of invasive breast cancer compared to placebo (0.42% vs. 0.34% CI 1.07-1.46) and more node-positive breast cancers (23.7% vs. 16.2% CI 1.23-2.58).[41] In addition, more deaths directly attributable to breast cancer and more all-cause mortality after a breast cancer diagnosis were seen in women taking EPT compared to placebo.

Another analysis of data from the WHI has shown an increase in the risk of nephrolithiasis in women receiving HT.[42]

A recent study shows that systemic HT for more then ten years significantly increases the relative risk of acute pancreatitis (RR 2.44 CI 1.38–4.31).[43]

Nonhormonal Therapies

Not all women are candidates for HT or care to consider HT as a therapeutic option. A systematic review showed reduced frequency and severity of menopausal hot flashes in highly symptomatic women who used paroxetine, venlafaxine, clonidine and gabapentin.[44] Their use may be limited by side effects,[44] although SSRIs are better tolerated than other agents.[45]

Paroxetine controlled-release 12.5 mg decreased daily hot flash composite score by 62.2% compared to 37.8% with placebo after 6 weeks of treatment.[46] Doses of paroxetine as low as 7.5 mg/day have shown benefit.[47] However, paroxetine is associated with significant weight gain, a common problem in this patient population. Other SSRIs may also be effective. A phase III clinical trial showed a 50% reduction in hot flash scores with **fluoxetine** compared to 36% with placebo in women with a history of breast cancer experiencing ≥14 hot flashes per week.[48] In a meta-analysis, **escitalopram** demonstrated the most benefit among SSRIs.[45]

Venlafaxine 75 mg and 150 mg reduced hot flash scores by 61% compared to 27% with placebo in postmenopausal women after 4 weeks of treatment.[49] However, doses near 150 mg/day are associated with more noradrenergic adverse effects and may cause increased sweating. Usual doses for menopausal hot flashes are between 37.5 and 75 mg XR. The efficacy of **desvenlafaxine** is similar to that of venlafaxine (60–66% reduction in hot flashes from baseline compared to 47% with placebo); adverse effects (dizziness, nausea, headache) occur at similar rates as well.[50] Side effects may be minimized by increasing the dosage more gradually. Consider venlafaxine and escitalopram as first line in women experiencing hot flashes who have significant perimenopausal/menopausal mood and anxiety problems.[51,45]

Gabapentin 900 mg daily reduced hot flash frequency and severity by 54% compared to 31% with placebo after 12 weeks of treatment in postmenopausal women experiencing ≥7 hot flashes a day.[52] **Clonidine**, a centrally acting antihypertensive, and a combination product containing phenobarbital, ergotamine and belladonna (Bellergal Spacetabs), are indicated for the relief of hot flashes but are associated with side effects.[2]

Black cohosh and **red clover-derived isoflavones** may have a small effect or no effect on vasomotor symptoms.[44,53,54,55,56,57] Case reports link black cohosh to liver damage.[58,59] **Vitamin E** 800 IU daily has shown a small effect in decreasing hot flashes.[60]

There is insufficient evidence to support the use of acupuncture.[2,53,61]

Vaginal Symptoms

Intravaginal estrogen therapy (creams, vaginal tablets and/or estradiol-releasing ring) is used to treat symptoms of vaginal atrophy in postmenopausal women;[62] it may be considered in patients experiencing only vaginal symptoms.[2] In these women, intravaginal administration is preferred because it results in less systemic estrogen absorption (and therefore reduced endometrial stimulation, uterine bleeding and breast tenderness) compared to oral or transdermal formulations.[62] Some women who continue to have vaginal symptoms despite systemic hormone therapy will benefit from the addition of intravaginal estrogen.[63]

Women using systemic estrogen are prescribed a progestogen to reduce the risk of endometrial hyperplasia. However, when using recommended doses of intravaginal estrogen for ≤1 year, a progestogen is generally not indicated [Evidence: SORT C*].[62,64] The safety of intravaginal estrogen alone beyond one year has not been established. Women using intravaginal estrogen at higher than recommended doses, intervals >1 year or those at high risk of endometrial hyperplasia may be candidates for concomitant progestogen therapy. Risk factors for endometrial hyperplasia include late age at natural menopause (>52 years), nulliparity, obesity and diabetes mellitus. There is insufficient evidence to recommend one form of intravaginal estrogen (e.g., tablet or cream) over another.[62]

Intravaginal estrogen also reduces the incidence of recurrent urinary tract infections in postmenopausal women.[65] Urinary incontinence may be improved with intravaginal estrogen therapy, as indicated by a Cochrane systematic review of patients with stress and/or urge incontinence.[66] However, there was no evidence about whether improvement continued after intravaginal estrogen was discontinued. In women who received systemic estrogen, incontinence appeared to worsen compared to placebo. Other studies have suggested that intravaginal estrogen does not appear to act synergistically with antimuscarinics (tolterodine) to improve overactive bladder, a condition similar to urge incontinence.[67,68]

Vaginal moisturizers (Replens) improve vaginal dryness and dyspareunia when used continuously. Replens was shown to be equivalent to local hormone therapy for improvement of dyspareunia.[69] **Vaginal lubricants** can be used as needed (see Table 2).

Mood Changes

Women progressing through the menopausal transition may notice changes in mood resulting in anxiety and irritability, often compounded by sleeplessness. Women at greatest risk of development of depression include those with a previous history of depressive disorders, poor physical health and a long perimenopausal transition.[2] Treat mood disorders and anxiety with SSRIs. Add low-dose hormone therapy for those who do not respond to antidepressants alone.[70]

* SORT (Strength of Recommendation Taxonomy) is a rating system (A, B or C) that addresses the quality of available evidence. For more information consult **How to Use *Compendium of Therapeutic Choices*** on page xxv.

Therapeutic Tips

- Consider the needs and wants of each patient prior to recommending a course of therapy for menopausal symptoms. Each patient has a unique health history and risk profile that affects the relative benefit she will derive from hormone or nonhormonal therapies and how she makes decisions about life and health. Unswerving policy applied to all patients will likely fail to meet the individual needs of many.
- In recently menopausal women, very low doses of HT may be insufficient to relieve symptoms; reassess, and if necessary adjust doses after 1–2 weeks of therapy.
- Consider lifestyle choices either alone or in combination with HT, after assessing the individual's risks and benefits.
- Prescribe vaginal estrogen preparations if menopausal symptoms are vaginal only.
- Prescribe HT for patients who enter menopause prior to age 40, as premature ovarian failure is associated with an early rise in the incidence of cardiovascular disease and osteoporosis. Continue treatment until at least the age of 50, when most women reach natural menopause.[71]
- Both transdermal and low-dose oral estrogen may have lower risks of VTE and stroke than standard doses of oral estrogen; however, there are no randomized controlled trials to confirm these observations.[17]

Suggested Readings

North American Menopause Society. The 2012 hormone therapy position statement of The North American Menopause Society. *Menopause* 2012;19(3):257-71.

Reid RL, Blake J, Abramson B et al. Menopause and osteoporosis update 2009. *J Obstet Gynaecol Can* 2009;31(1 Suppl 1):S1-S52. Available from: www.sogc.org/guidelines/documents/menopause_JOGC-Jan_09.pdf.

Table 2: Drugs Used for the Management of Menopausal Symptoms

Class	Drug	Dose	Adverse Effects	Comments	Cost[a]
Alpha$_2$-Adrenergic Agonists	*clonidine* Dixarit, generics	0.05 mg BID	Dizziness, dry mouth, drowsiness, constipation.	Indicated for the treatment of vasomotor symptoms in patients who cannot or who do not want to take estrogens. Discontinue if no benefit after 2–4 weeks or if side effects. Monitor blood pressure with concomitant use of other antihypertensives.	$
Combined Estrogens and Progestins, oral	*estradiol-17β/ drospirenone* Angeliq	Patients with intact uterus: 1 tablet daily continuously (1 mg/1 mg)	Breakthrough bleeding/spotting, nausea, vomiting, bloating, chloasma, breast tenderness, mood changes, e.g., depression, headaches. Increased risk of VTE, CVD, breast cancer. Drospirenone-containing oral contraceptives show increased risk of VTE compared to other progestins.[11]	Amenorrhea or gradual reduction in menstrual blood flow occurs with continuous use. Risk of hyperkalemia in patients prone to increased K^+ (e.g., renal disease, concomitant ACEI, ARB, potassium-sparing diuretics, NSAIDs). Check K^+ after 1st cycle.	$$
	estradiol hemihydrate/ norethindrone acetate Activelle, Activelle LD	Patients with intact uterus: 1 tablet daily continuously (1 mg/0.5 mg or 0.5 mg/0.5 mg)	See estradiol-17β/ drospirenone.	Amenorrhea or gradual reduction in menstrual blood flow occurs with continuous use.	$$$
Combined Estrogens and Progestins, transdermal	*estradiol-17β/ levonorgestrel* Climara Pro	Patients with intact uterus: 1 patch applied once weekly (delivers 45 µg estradiol-17β and 15 µg levonorgestrel/day)	Breakthrough bleeding/spotting, nausea/vomiting, bloating, chloasma, breast tenderness, mood changes such as depression, headaches. Redness, skin irritation. Increased risk of VTE, CVD, breast cancer.	Avoids first-pass effect. Less effect on hepatic sex-hormone binding globulin synthesis than oral estrogens. May benefit women who report decreased sexual desire, smokers, women with malabsorption conditions and those with high triglyceride levels. Amenorrhea or gradual reduction in menstrual blood flow occurs with continuous use.	$$
	estradiol-17β/ norethindrone acetate Estalis	Patients with intact uterus: 1 patch applied twice weekly (delivers 50 µg estradiol-17β plus 140 µg *or* 250 µg norethindrone acetate/day)	See estradiol-17β/ levonorgestrel, transdermal.	See estradiol-17β/levonorgestrel, transdermal.	$$

Class	Drug	Dose	Adverse Effects	Comments	Cost[a]
Combined Estrogens and Progesterone, oral/transdermal	*estradiol-17β topical gel/progesterone* Estrogel Propak	Each package contains a metered-dose pump of estradiol-17β (Estrogel) and 30 capsules of micronized progesterone (Prometrium). See individual entries for possible dosing regimens.	Bloating, headache, nausea, chloasma, breast tenderness, breakthrough bleeding/spotting, irritability, weight gain, mood swings. Increased risk of VTE, CVD, breast cancer. Redness, skin irritation.	Topical estradiol-17β avoids first-pass effect. Less effect on hepatic sex-hormone binding globulin synthesis than oral estrogens. May benefit women who report decreased sexual desire, smokers, women with malabsorption conditions and those with high triglyceride levels. Topical estradiol-17β may be applied to abdomen or inner thighs (but not breasts). Not necessary to rotate application sites. Micronized progesterone contains peanut oil; avoid if peanut allergy.	$$$$
Ergot Combination Products	*ergotamine/belladonna alkaloids/phenobarbital* Bellergal Spacetabs	1 tablet each morning and evening Maximum: 16 tabs/week	Dizziness, dry mouth, drowsiness, constipation.	Indicated for the treatment of vasomotor symptoms in patients who cannot or who do not want to take estrogens. Avoid in combination with CYP3A4 inhibitors, e.g., erythromycin, clarithromycin, ritonavir, nelfinavir, ketoconazole, itraconazole.	$$$$$
Estrogens, oral	*conjugated estrogens* Premarin	0.3–1.25 mg daily	Bloating, headache, nausea, chloasma, breast tenderness, breakthrough bleeding/spotting. Increased risk of VTE, CVD, breast cancer.	Administer with a progestogen *in patients with intact uterus* to prevent endometrial hyperplasia or cancer. Consider vaginal estrogen for patients with vaginal symptoms only.	$
	estradiol-17β Estrace	0.5–2 mg daily	See conjugated estrogens.	See conjugated estrogens.	$
Estrogens, transdermal	*estradiol-17β, patch* Climara, Estradot, Oesclim, generics	Estradot, Oesclim, generics: 1 patch applied twice weekly Climara: 1 patch applied once weekly	See conjugated estrogens. Redness, skin irritation.	Avoids first-pass effect. Less effect on hepatic sex-hormone binding globulin synthesis than oral estrogens. May benefit women who report decreased sexual desire, smokers, women with malabsorption conditions and those with high triglyceride levels.	$
	estradiol-17β, topical gel Estrogel, Divigel	Estrogel: 0.75 mg estradiol per 1.25 g metered dose actuation. 0.75–1.5 mg (1–2 actuations) applied to arms daily Divigel (0.1%): 0.25, 0.5 and 1 mg estradiol per packet. Apply 1 packet daily to upper thigh	See conjugated estrogens. Redness, skin irritation.	Avoids first-pass effect. Less effect on hepatic sex-hormone binding globulin synthesis than oral estrogens. May benefit women who report decreased sexual desire, smokers, women with malabsorption conditions and those with high triglyceride levels. Estrogel: may also be applied to abdomen or inner thighs (but not breasts). Not necessary to rotate application sites. Divigel: alternate application site between left and right thigh. Application area should be 5 × 7 inches.	$$

(cont'd)

Table 2: **Drugs Used for the Management of Menopausal Symptoms** *(cont'd)*

Class	Drug	Dose	Adverse Effects	Comments	Cost[a]
Estrogens, vaginal	*conjugated estrogen vaginal cream* Premarin Vaginal Cream	0.625 mg CE/g: 0.3–1.25 mg CE (0.5–2 g cream) daily or 1–3 times weekly as directed, intravaginally or topically depending on the severity of condition	Local burning, irritation, vaginal leakage.	Indicated for the treatment of atrophic vaginitis and dyspareunia. Improves vaginal vascularity and lubrication. Administer cyclically, e.g., 3 weeks on and 1 week off, at the lowest dose for a short-term. Intermittent therapy may also be used. Absorbed systemically with higher doses, resulting in increased estrogen levels. With higher doses (e.g., daily use) in patients with an intact uterus, consider administering with a progestogen to prevent endometrial hyperplasia or cancer. Progestogens are generally not required with lower doses of vaginal estrogen.[10]	$
	estradiol-17β vaginal ring Estring	Insert 1 ring Q3 months vaginally Delivers 7.5 µg estradiol per 24 h at a sustained rate for up to 12 weeks	Spotting, discharge, genital pruritus.	Indicated for the treatment of atrophic vaginitis and dyspareunia. Improves vaginal vascularity and lubrication. Women may prefer the estrogen ring over vaginal tablets and cream likely due to comfort and ease of use.[62]	$$$$/ring
	estradiol-17β vaginal tablet Vagifem 10	Insert 10 µg vaginal tablet once daily vaginally for 2 weeks then twice weekly (3–4 day interval between doses)	Vaginal secretion, vaginal discomfort.	See estradiol-17β vaginal ring.	$$
	estrone vaginal cream Estragyn Vaginal Cream	2–4 g intravaginally daily or 2–3 times weekly	See conjugated estrogen vaginal cream.	See conjugated estrogen vaginal cream.	$
GABA Derivatives	*gabapentin* ❥ Neurontin, generics	300 mg TID. Start at 300 mg once daily, increase to TID over 3–7 days	Somnolence, dizziness.	*Not a Health Canada–approved indication.* For vasomotor symptoms in patients who cannot or who do not want to take estrogens. To discontinue, taper over a 1-week period.	$$
Lubricants, vaginal	*vaginal gels or jelly* K-Y Jelly, Gynemoistrin, Astroglide	Apply when needed		Provides rapid, short-term relief. Can be applied to penis and the opening of vagina to decrease discomfort in dyspareunia.	$

Class	Drug	Dose	Adverse Effects	Comments	Cost[a]
Moisturizers, vaginal	*polycarbophil gel* Replens	Apply 2–3 times weekly		Provides long-term relief (2–3 days) of vaginal dryness by changing fluid content of epithelium and lowering vaginal pH (longer duration of action than vaginal lubricants). Used on a continuous basis. Replens was equivalent to local hormone therapy for improvement of dyspareunia.[69]	$
Progestogens,[b] oral	*medroxyprogesterone acetate* Provera, generics	In combination with estrogen in patients with intact uterus: 5–10 mg daily cyclically *or* 2.5–5 mg daily continuously For prevention of hot flashes: 20 mg daily[2]	Bloating, irritability, weight gain, mood swings.	Progestogens normalize the endometrial response and decrease breakthrough bleeding; when given continuously, they prevent menstrual blood flow.	$
	megestrol acetate generics	For prevention of hot flashes: 20 mg daily[2]	See medroxyprogesterone acetate, oral.	See medroxyprogesterone acetate, oral. For symptomatic women who cannot or who do not want to use estrogen therapy.	$
	norethindrone Micronor	0.35–0.7 mg daily continuously	See medroxyprogesterone acetate, oral.	See medroxyprogesterone acetate, oral.	$$
	progesterone, micronized Prometrium	In combination with estrogen in patients with intact uterus: 200–300 mg QHS cyclically *or* 100–200 mg QHS continuously	See medroxyprogesterone acetate, oral. Drowsiness may occur.	Contains peanut oil; avoid if peanut allergy. Lack of evidence of effectiveness for vasomotor symptoms. Better side effect profile than medroxyprogesterone acetate and beneficial effect on sleep.	$$$$$
Progestins, intrauterine system	*levonorgestrel* Mirena	52 mg/IUS inserted once every 5 y	Bloating, irritability, weight gain and mood swings, to a lesser extent compared to medroxyprogesterone acetate.	See medroxyprogesterone acetate, oral.	$353/IUS
Serotonin-Norepinephrine Reuptake Inhibitors	*desvenlafaxine* ❥ Pristiq	50–100 mg daily	Gastrointestinal upset, dry mouth, drowsiness, nervousness, sexual dysfunction.	*Not a Health Canada-approved indication.* For vasomotor symptoms in patients who cannot or who do not want to take estrogens. Higher doses are not useful for the treatment of vasomotor symptoms and are associated with side effects.[44] Results may take 2–3 weeks. Taper gradually when stopping.	$$$$$

(cont'd)

Table 2: **Drugs Used for the Management of Menopausal Symptoms** *(cont'd)*

Class	Drug	Dose	Adverse Effects	Comments	Cost[a]
	venlafaxine (renal symbol) Effexor XR, generics	Start with 37.5 mg daily, increase to 75 mg daily after 1 week if necessary	See desvenlafaxine.	See desvenlafaxine.	$
Selective Serotonin Reuptake Inhibitors	*escitalopram* Cipralex	10–20 mg po daily	Nausea, dry mouth, sleep disturbance, somnolence, sweating, sexual dysfunction, increased risk of GI bleeding, dose-dependent QT_c prolongation.	See desvenlafaxine. Caution with other drugs that prolong the QT_c interval.	$$$
	fluoxetine Prozac, generics	20 mg po daily	Nausea, nervousness, anorexia, insomnia, sexual dysfunction, increase risk of GI bleeding.	See desvenlafaxine. Inhibitors of CYP2D6 (fluoxetine, paroxetine, sertraline) may decrease conversion of prodrug tamoxifen to its active metabolites. Avoid combination.	$
	paroxetine Paxil, Paxil CR, generics	12.5–25 mg po daily	Nausea, drowsiness, fatigue, sweating, constipation, dry mouth, dizziness, sexual dysfunction, increase risk of GI bleeding.	See desvenlafaxine. Inhibitors of CYP2D6 (fluoxetine, paroxetine, sertraline) may decrease conversion of prodrug tamoxifen to its active metabolites. Avoid combination.	$

[a] Cost of 30-day supply of usual dose unless otherwise specified; includes drug cost only.
[b] The term *progestogen* includes both natural progesterone and synthetic progestins.
(renal symbol) Dosage adjustment may be required in renal impairment; see Appendix I.
Abbreviations: ACEI = angiotensin-converting enzyme inhibitor; ARB = angiotensin receptor blocker; CE = conjugated estrogen; CVD = cardiovascular disease; CYP = cytochrome P450; IUS = intrauterine system; NSAID = nonsteroidal anti-inflammatory drug; VTE = venous thromboembolism
Legend: $ <$20 $$ $20–40 $$$ $40–60 $$$$ $60–80 $$$$$ $80–100

References

1. Guthrie JR, Dennerstein L, Taffe JR et al. The menopausal transition: a 9-year prospective population-based study. The Melbourne Women's Midlife Health Project. *Climacteric* 2004;7(4):375-89.
2. Belisle S, Blake J, Basson R et al. SOGC Clinical Practice Guideline. Canadian Consensus Conference on Menopause, 2006 update. *J Obstet Gynaecol Can* 2006;28(2 Suppl 1):S1-S112.
3. Kronenberg F. Hot flashes: epidemiology and physiology. *Ann N Y Acad Sci* 1990;592:52-86.
4. Canadian Task Force on Preventative Health Care. Recommendations on screening for breast cancer in average-risk women aged 40-74 years. *CMAJ* 2011;183(17):1991-2001.
5. Gold EB, Sternfeld B, Kelsey JL et al. Relation of demographic and lifestyle factors to symptoms in a multi-racial/ethnic population of women 40-55 years of age. *Am J Epidemiol* 2000;152(5):463-73.
6. Kroenke CH, Caan BJ, Stefanick ML et al. Effects of dietary intervention and weight change on vasomotor symptoms in the Women's Health Initiative. *Menopause* 2012;19(9):980-8.
7. Aiello EJ, Yasui Y, Tworoger SS et al. Effect of a yearlong, moderate-intensity exercise intervention on the occurrence and severity of menopause symptoms in postmenopausal women. *Menopause* 2004;11(4):382-8.
8. Reed SD, Guthrie KA, Newton KM et al. Menopausal quality of life: RCT of yoga, exercise and omega-3 supplements. *Am J Obstet Gynecol* 2014;210(3):244.e1-11.
9. Freedman RR, Woodward S. Behavioral treatment of menopausal hot flushes: evaluation by ambulatory monitoring. *Am J Obstet Gynecol* 1992;167(2):436-9.
10. Reid RL, Blake J, Abramson B et al. Menopause and osteoporosis update 2009. *J Obstet Gynaecol Can* 2009;31(1 Suppl 1):S1-S52. Available from: www.sogc.org/guidelines/documents/menopause_JOGC-Jan_09.pdf. Accessed March 25, 2011.
11. Gronich N, Lavi I, Rennert G. Higher risk of venous thrombosis associated with drospirenone-containing oral contraceptives: a population-based cohort study. *CMAJ* 2011;183(18):E1319-25.
12. Ohayon MM. Severe hot flashes associated with chronic insomnia. *Arch Intern Med* 2006;166(12):1262-8.
13. Nelson HD. Commonly used types of postmenopausal estrogen for treatment of hot flashes: scientific review. *JAMA* 2004;291(13):1610-20.
14. Brunner RL, Gass M, Aragaki A et al. Effects of conjugated equine estrogen on health-related quality of life in postmenopausal women with hysterectomy: results from the Women's Health Initiative Randomized Clinical Trial. *Arch Intern Med* 2005;165(17):1976-86.
15. Maclennan AH, Broadbent JL, Lester S et al. Oral oestrogen and combined oestrogen/progestogen therapy versus placebo for hot flushes. *Cochrane Database Syst Rev* 2004;(4):CD002978.
16. Sanada M, Tsuda M, Kodama I et al. Substitution of transdermal estradiol during oral estrogen-progestin therapy in postmenopausal women: effects on hypertriglyceridemia. *Menopause* 2004;11(3):331-6.
17. North American Menopause Society. The 2012 hormone therapy position statement of the North American Menopause Society. *Menopause* 2012;19(3):257-71.
18. Canonico M, Oger E, Plu-Bureau G et al. Hormone therapy and venous thromboembolism among postmenopausal women: impact of the route of estrogen administration and progestogens: the ESTHER study. *Circulation* 2007;115(7):840-5.
19. Ettinger B. Vasomotor symptom relief versus unwanted effects: role of estrogen dosage. *Am J Med* 2005;118(Suppl 12B):74-8.
20. Furness S, Roberts H, Marjoribanks J et al. Hormone therapy in postmenopausal women and risk of endometrial hyperplasia. *Cochrane Database Syst Rev* 2012;8:CD000402.
21. Vashisht A, Wadsworth F, Carey A et al. Bleeding profiles and effects on the endometrium for women using a novel combination of transdermal oestradiol and natural progesterone cream as part of a continuous combined hormone replacement regime. *BJOG* 2005;112(10):1402-6.
22. Varila E, Wahlstrom T, Rauramo I. A 5-year follow-up study on the use of a levonorgestrel intrauterine system in women receiving hormone replacement therapy. *Fertil Steril* 2001;76(5):969-73.
23. North American Menopause Society. *Bioidentical hormone therapy*. Mayfield Heights (OH): NAMS. Available from: www.menopause.org/publications/clinical-practice-materials/bioidentical-hormone-therapy. Accessed January 31, 2011.
24. U.S. Food and Drug Administration. *FDA takes action against compounded menopause hormone therapy drugs*. 2008. Available from: www.fda.gov/newsevents/newsroom/pressannouncements/2008/ucm116832.htm. Accessed November 27, 2012.
25. Mosca L, Banka CL, Benjamin EJ et al. Evidence-based guidelines for cardiovascular disease prevention in women: 2007 update. *Circulation* 2007;115(11):1481-501.
26. Farquhar CM, Marjoribanks J, Lethaby A et al. Long term hormone therapy for perimenopausal and postmenopausal women. *Cochrane Database Syst Rev* 2009;(2):CD004143.
27. Moyer VA; on behalf of the U.S. Preventive Services Task Force. Menopausal hormone therapy for the primary prevention of chronic conditions: U.S. Preventive Services Task Force recommendations. *Ann Intern Med* 2013;158(1):47-54.
28. Manson JE, Chleowski RT, Stefanick ML et al. Menopausal hormone therapy and health outcomes during the intervention and extended poststopping phases of the Women's Health Initiative randomized trials. *JAMA* 2013;310(13):1353-68.
29. Rossouw JE, Anderson GL, Prentice RL et al. Risks and benefits of estrogen plus progestin in healthy postmenopausal women: principal results from the Women's Health Initiative randomized controlled trial. *JAMA* 2002;288(3):321-33.
30. Hulley S, Grady D, Bush T et al. Randomized trial of estrogen plus progestin for secondary prevention of coronary heart disease in postmenopausal women. Heart and Estrogen/progestin Replacement Study (HERS) Research Group. *JAMA* 1998;280(7):605-13.
31. Rossouw JE, Prentice RL, Manson JE et al. Postmenopausal hormone therapy and risk of cardiovascular disease by age and years since menopause. *JAMA* 2007;297(13):1465-77.
32. Manson JE, Allison MA, Rossouw JE et al. Estrogen therapy and coronary-artery calcification. *N Engl J Med* 2007;356(25):2591-602.
33. Main C, Knight B, Moxham T et al. Hormone therapy for preventing cardiovascular disease in post-menopausal women. *Cochrane Database Syst Rev* 2013;4:CD002229.
34. Cushman M, Kuller LH, Prentice R et al. Estrogen plus progestin and risk of venous thrombosis. *JAMA* 2004;292(13):1573-80.
35. Scierbeck LL, Rejnmark L, Tofteng CL et al. Effect of hormone replacement therapy on cardiovascular events in recently postmenopausal women: randomised trial. *BMJ* 2012;345:e6409.
36. Wassertheil-Smoller S, Hendrix SL, Limacher M et al. Effect of estrogen plus progestin on stroke in post-menopausal women: the Women's Health Initiative: a randomized trial. *JAMA* 2003;289(20):2673-84.
37. Prentice RL, Manson JE, Langer RD et al. Benefits and risks of postmenopausal hormone therapy when it is initiated soon after menopause. *Am J Epidemiol* 2009;170(1):12-23.
38. Henderson VW, Lobo RA. Hormone therapy and the risk of stroke: perspectives 10 years after the Women's Health Initiative trials. *Climacteric* 2012;15(3):229-34.

39. Breast cancer and hormone replacement therapy: collaborative reanalysis of data from 51 epidemiological studies of 52,705 women with breast cancer and 108,411 women without breast cancer. Collaborative Group on Hormonal Factors in Breast Cancer. *Lancet* 1997;350(9084):1047-59.
40. Fournier A, Berrino F, Clavel-Chapelon F. Unequal risks for breast cancer associated with different hormone replacement therapies: results from the E3N cohort study. *Breast Cancer Res Treat* 2008;107(1):103-11.
41. Chlebowski, RT, Anderson GL, Gass M et al. Estrogen plus progestin and breast cancer incidence and mortality in postmenopausal women. *JAMA* 2010;304(15):1684-92.
42. Maalouf NM, Sato AH, Welch BJ et al. Postmenopausal hormone use and the risk of nephrolithiasis: results of the Women's Health Initiative hormone therapy trials. *Arch Intern Med* 2010;170(18):1678-85.
43. Oskarsson V, Orsini N, Sadr-Azodi O et al. Postmenopausal hormone replacement therapy and risk of acute pancreatitis: a prospective cohort study. *CMAJ* 2014;186(5):338-44.
44. Nelson HD, Vesco KK, Haney E et al. Nonhormonal therapies for menopausal hot flashes: systematic review and meta-analysis. *JAMA* 2006;295(17):2057-71.
45. Shams T, Firwana B, Habib F et al. SSRIs for hot flashes: a systematic review and meta-analysis of randomized trials. *J Gen Intern Med* 2014;29(1):204-13.
46. Stearns V, Beebe KL, Iyengar M et al. Paroxetine controlled release in the treatment of menopausal hot flashes: a randomized controlled trial. *JAMA* 2003;289(21):2827-34.
47. Simon JA, Portman DJ, Kaunitz AM et al. Low-dose paroxetine 7.5 mg for menopausal vasomotor symptoms: two randomized controlled trials. *Menopause* 2013;20(10):1027-35.
48. Loprinzi CL, Sloan JA, Perez EA et al. Phase III evaluation of fluoxetine for treatment of hot flashes. *J Clin Oncol* 2002;20(6):1578-83.
49. Loprinzi CL, Kugler JW, Sloan JA et al. Venlafaxine in management of hot flashes in survivors of breast cancer: a randomised controlled trial. *Lancet* 2000;356(9247):2059-63.
50. Archer DF, Dupont CM, Constantine GD et al. Desvenlafaxine for the treatment of vasomotor symptoms associated with menopause: a double-blind, randomized, placebo-controlled trial of efficacy and safety. *Am J Obstet Gynecol* 2009;200(3):238.e1-238.e10.
51. Carroll DG, Kelley KW. Use of antidepressants for management of hot flashes. *Pharmacotherapy* 2009;29(11):1357-74.
52. Guttuso T, Kurlan R, McDermott MP et al. Gabapentin's effects on hot flashes in postmenopausal women: a randomized controlled trial. *Obstet Gynecol* 2003;101(2):337-45.
53. Nedrow A, Miller J, Walker M et al. Complementary and alternative therapies for the management of menopause-related symptoms: a systematic evidence review. *Arch Intern Med* 2006;166(14):1453-65.
54. Newton KM, Reed SD, LaCroix AZ et al. Treatment of vasomotor symptoms of menopause with black cohosh, multibotanicals, soy, hormone therapy, or placebo: a randomized trial. *Ann Intern Med* 2006;145(12):869-79.
55. Uebelhack R, Blohmer JU, Graubaum HJ et al. Black cohosh and St. John's wort for climacteric complaints: a randomized trial. *Obstet Gynecol* 2006;107(2 Pt 1):247-55.
56. Pockaj BA, Gallagher JG, Loprinzi CL et al. Phase III double-blind, randomized, placebo-controlled crossover trial of black cohosh in the management of hot flashes: NCCTG Trial N01CC1. *J Clin Oncol* 2006;24(18):2836-41.
57. Tice JA, Ettinger B, Ensrud K et al. Phytoestrogen supplements for the treatment of hot flashes: the Isoflavone Clover Extract (ICE) Study: a randomized controlled trial. *JAMA* 2003;290(2):207-14.
58. Lynch CR, Folkers ME, Hutson WR. Fulminant hepatic failure associated with the use of black cohosh: a case report. *Liver Transpl* 2006;12(6):989-92.
59. Cohen SM, O'Connor AM, Hart J et al. Autoimmune hepatitis associated with the use of black cohosh: a case study. *Menopause* 2004;11(5):575-7.
60. Barton DL, Loprinzi CL, Quella SK et al. Prospective evaluation of vitamin E for hot flashes in breast cancer survivors. *J Clin Oncol* 1998;16(2):495-500.
61. Dodin S, Blanchet C, Marc I et al. Acupuncture for menopausal hot flushes. *Cochrane Database Syst Rev* 2013;7:CD007410.
62. Suckling J, Lethaby A, Kennedy R. Local oestrogen for vaginal atrophy in postmenopausal women. *Cochrane Database Syst Rev* 2006;(4):CD001500.
63. Johnston SL, Farrell SA, Bouchard C et al. The detection and management of vaginal atrophy. *J Obstet Gynaecol Can* 2004;26(5):503-15.
64. Management of symptomatic vulvovaginal atrophy: 2013 position statement of The North American Menopause Society. *Menopause* 2013;20(9):888-902.
65. Perrotta C, Aznar M, Mejia R et al. Oestrogens for preventing recurrent urinary tract infection in postmenopausal women. *Cochrane Database Syst Rev* 2008;(2):CD005131.
66. Cody JD, Jacobs ML, Richardson K et al. Oestrogen therapy for urinary incontinence in post-menopausal women. *Cochrane Database Syst Rev* 2012;10:CD001405.
67. Serati M, Salvatore S, Uccella S et al. Is there a synergistic effect of topical estrogens when administered with antimuscarinics in the treatment of symptomatic detrusor overactivity? *Eur Urol* 2009;55(3):713-9.
68. Tseng LH, Wang AC, Chang YL et al. Randomized comparison of tolterodine with vaginal estrogen cream versus tolterodine alone for the treatment of postmenopausal women with overactive bladder syndrome. *Neurourol Urodyn* 2009;28(1):47-51.
69. Nachtigall LE. Comparative study: Replens versus local estrogen in menopausal women. *Fertil Steril* 1994;61(1):178-80.
70. Cohen LS, Soares CN, Joffe H. Diagnosis and management of mood disorders during the menopausal transition. *Am J Med* 2005;118(Suppl 12B):93-7.
71. Writing Group for the British Menopause Society. Management of premature menopause. *J Br Menopause Soc* 2007;13(1):44-5.

Sexual Health

Chapter 76
Menorrhagia

Margaret Burnett, MD, FRCSC, FACOG

Abnormal uterine bleeding (AUB) includes, in women of childbearing age, any change in menses frequency or duration, amount of blood flow, or bleeding that occurs within cycles. AUB also includes unpredictable bleeding in postmenopausal women. This chapter will focus on menorrhagia.

Menorrhagia is AUB that is characterized by prolonged (>7 days) or excessive (>80 mL) menstrual blood flow[1] which interferes with quality of life and may result in iron-deficiency anemia. Recent definitions of menorrhagia focus on the woman's perception of the impact of abnormal bleeding on her quality of life.[2] Heavy menstrual bleeding is an important cause of absenteeism from work or school in women of childbearing age and poses a significant cost burden to the individual and to the healthcare system.[3] Thirty percent of women consider their menstrual bleeding to be excessive.[4]

Goals of Therapy

- To reduce the deleterious effects on women's health, well being and quality of life
- Target and treat the specific underlying causes of menorrhagia if present

Investigations

See Table 1 for possible causes of menorrhagia.

- The initial assessment of menorrhagia includes:
  - careful history regarding bleeding pattern, amount of blood loss, associated symptoms, personal and family history of bleeding disorders and risk factors for gynecologic malignancy
  - visual inspection of the vagina and cervix, bimanual examination, and general physical examination. Endometrial biopsy should be performed in women over the age of 40 and in those with risk factors for endometrial carcinoma[2]
  - basic laboratory investigations include a CBC, TSH, progesterone (day 21 of the cycle), follicle stimulating hormone (FSH), luteinizing hormone (LH), testosterone and dihydroepiandronstiendione (DHEA)
  - pelvic ultrasound, magnetic resonance imaging and/or hysteroscopy are helpful in the diagnosis of structural lesions
  - von Willebrandt's disease commonly presents as menorrhagia in adolescence.[2] Coagulation screening should be offered to these women and also considered when there is a family history of bleeding diatheses or a personal history of significant bleeding from nonuterine sites
- Women with menorrhagia may present with prolonged menses and/or heavy bleeding with flooding, large clots and symptoms of anemia. Etiologic factors include structural and functional causes. The rational treatment of menorrhagia necessitates a search for uterine abnormalities as well as for hormonal and hematologic conditions which may give rise to abnormal bleeding. If an underlying cause is suspected, directed therapy can be instituted. However, in many cases, a clear etiology is not readily identified. Most heavy uterine bleeding is not associated with any structural abnormality of the uterus. Irregular bleeding is frequently associated with anovulation, which results in excessive endometrial proliferation and potential endometrial hyperplasia. Abnormal endometrial factors may

be responsible for excessive bleeding in the presence of ovulatory cycles.[6] Symptomatic treatment should be offered to all women suffering from AUB regardless of etiology.

Table 1: **Etiology of Abnormal Bleeding: FIGO Classification[5]**

Structural Causes	Functional Causes
Polyps (endometrial or endocervical)	Coagulopathy (congenital or acquired)
Adenomyosis	Ovulatory dysfunction (polycystic ovarian syndrome, perimenopause, adolescence, hypothyroidism)
Leiomyomata	Iatrogenic (anticoagulants, hormones)
Malignancy	Endometrial factors
	Not otherwise classified

Abbreviations: FIGO = International Federation of Gynecology and Obstetrics

Therapeutic Choices

An algorithm for the management of menorrhagia is presented in Figure 1.

Nonpharmacologic Choices

Surgical Options

Pharmacologic therapy (medical management) is generally considered to be the first line of treatment for menorrhagia unless these therapies are contraindicated or undesired. Surgical options become an important consideration, particularly in those women who have completed childbearing and in those who have failed medical management. *Fibroid artery embolization* and *uterine myomectomy* may be considered for the treatment of menorrhagia related to leiomyomata. *Hysteroscopic resection* should be offered for definitive treatment of small submucous leiomyomata and endometrial polyps. *Endometrial ablation* is a highly effective minimally invasive procedure with 87–97% of women reporting reduction in bleeding.[7] The need for further operative intervention was 6–20% within 5 years with increased failure rates in young women undergoing this procedure. In women with normal uterine cavities, global ablation is preferable to hysteroscopic endometrial resection because of its safety, shorter operative time and greater efficacy.[2]

Hysterectomy is the ultimate treatment of menorrhagia and continues to be a cost-effective alternative for many women.[8] Furthermore, hysterectomy is associated with the highest degree of patient satisfaction and quality of life-years.[9] New technologies have facilitated options for minimally invasive hysterectomy including vaginal hysterectomy, laparoscopic-assisted vaginal hysterectomy, laparoscopic hysterectomy, robotic hysterectomy and mini-laparotomy. These techniques are continuing to evolve and information directing optimal patient selection for each technique is still incomplete. The type of hysterectomy depends on the presence or absence of uterine pathology, availability of specialized equipment, expertise of the surgeon, patient preference and surgical risk.

Pharmacologic Choices

Drug therapies for the management of menorrhagia are presented in Table 2.

Hormonal Therapies

Combined Hormonal Contraceptives

The mainstay of the treatment for menorrhagia has been the suppression of the pituitary ovarian axis using **combined hormonal contraceptives** containing **estrogen** and **progestin**. A variety of oral products as well as the transdermal patch and vaginal ring are available in Canada. These preparations act by suppressing FSH and inhibiting follicular development. As a result, ovarian estrogen secretion and endometrial proliferation are minimized. Most women are able to achieve good cycle control and a substantial reduction in menstrual blood loss with minimal side effects.[2]

Progestogen-only Contraceptives

The term *progestogen* includes both natural progesterone and synthetic progestins. In women unable to tolerate estrogen or in whom estrogen is contraindicated, **progestogen-only contraceptives** can be very useful in the treatment of menorrhagia.[10] If contraception is desired, the oral "mini pill" (norethindrone), injectable medroxyprogesterone acetate (DMPA) and levonorgestrel intrauterine system (LNG-IUS) are appropriate alternatives. These preparations act in a variety of ways by suppressing ovulation and antagonizing the proliferative effect of estrogen at the level of the endometrium. Uterine bleeding may be eliminated completely with continuous progestogen administration. Some women who do not require contraception prefer to use oral **medroxyprogesterone actetate** or **micronized progesterone** for at least 21 days per month. Luteal phase progesterone is a less effective option.[2] The progestogen-only preparations are inferior to the combined contraceptive products in their ability to produce regular menstrual cycles.[8]

The tolerability of systemic hormonal agents is somewhat limited by their progestogenic side effects such as weight gain and emotional lability. These quality of life concerns are minimized, if not eliminated, with the **levonorgestrel intrauterine system** (LNG-IUS). This device is more effective than other medical therapies in AUB[11,12] and is comparable to endometrial ablation in terms of patient satisfaction.[10,13] The LNG-IUS is indicated for first-line therapy in women of all ages with structurally normal uteri who are candidates for an intrauterine device.[8]

Gonadotropin-releasing Hormone (GnRH) Agonists

Suppression of the pituitary may be achieved using **gonadotropin-releasing hormone (GnRH) agonists**, such as **leuprolide**, **goserelin** and **nafarelin**. Follicular development does not occur because FSH is suppressed. As a result the endometrium does not proliferate and amenorrhea occurs. GnRH agonists are very effective in the short-term treatment of menorrhagia and also can be used to shrink leiomyomata.[14] Vasomotor symptoms are common side effects. Treatment beyond 6 months is not advisable without estrogen/progestogen add-back therapy to preserve bone health.[2]

Antifibrinolytics

Medications that inhibit fibrinolytic activity in the endometrium are useful in the treatment of both acute and chronic menorrhagia. Intermittent regular dosing of oral **tranxexamic acid** can be helpful for women with heavy periods who do not wish to use hormonal treatments.[15] The mechanism of action appears to be related to reversible inhibition of lysine-binding sites on plasminogen.

Nonsteroidal Anti-inflammatory Drugs (NSAIDs)

NSAIDs may decrease menstrual blood loss by inhibiting prostacyclin-mediated vasodilitation in the basalis layer of the endometrium. Regular dosing reduces blood flow through the spiral arteries and is an effective treatment for menorrhagia. Many women who wish to avoid exogenous hormones are happy to choose this method. It is particularly useful in women complaining of dysmenorrhea as well as menorrhagia. The use of NSAIDs is contraindicated in women with bleeding disorders. NSAIDs are superior to placebo but less effective than other medical therapies.[16]

Other

Progestin receptor modulators are a promising addition to the treatment of menorrhagia. **Ulipristal,** introduced in Canada in 2013, has been shown to be effective and well tolerated when used to reduce blood loss and size of uterine fibroids.[14] In women who are eligible for surgery, consider preoperative treatment with ulipristal 5–10 mg daily for up to 13 weeks [Evidence: SORT A*].[14,17] Maximum duration of use has yet to be determined. There is also some evidence that **mifepristone**, another progestin receptor modulator, reduces heavy menstrual bleeding associated with uterine fibroids.[18] Mifepristone is not available in Canada.

Menstrual cycle suppression and relief from menorrhagia may be achieved using **danazol** 100–400 mg daily. However, the potential for androgenic side effects makes this option unattractive to many women.[19]

Acute Menorrhagia

Acute menorrhagia involves life-threatening blood loss which requires immediate intervention to minimize patient morbidity and the need for blood transfusion.[2]

High doses of iv **conjugated estrogen** (25 mg initially, repeated in 3 hours) has been used to reduce blood loss in acute menorrhagia. It stimulates rapid proliferation of the endometrium, covering the exposed spiral arteries. Conjugated estrogen administration must be followed by progestogen or combined hormonal contraceptive administration in order to stabilize the endometrium and promote organized sloughing upon withdrawal.[1]

High-dose **progestogens** may be effective in the management of acute uterine bleeding.[20]

IV **tranexamic acid** 1000 mg Q6H can also be used in acute menorrhagia[2]

Therapeutic Tips

- Menorrhagia is common in the adolescent population. Long-acting reversible contraceptives (e.g., LNG-IUS) are first-line therapies in both sexually-active and non-sexually-active adolescents, with individualized counselling.[2]
- Acute menorrhagia can be medically managed with high-dose estrogen, tranexamic acid or high-dose progestogens once patient has been stabilized as required (e.g., iv fluids and blood products in case of hypovolemia).

* SORT (Strength of Recommendation Taxonomy) is a rating system (A, B or C) that addresses the quality of available evidence. For more information consult **How to Use *Compendium of Therapeutic Choices*** on page xxv.

Figure 1: **Management of Menorrhagia**

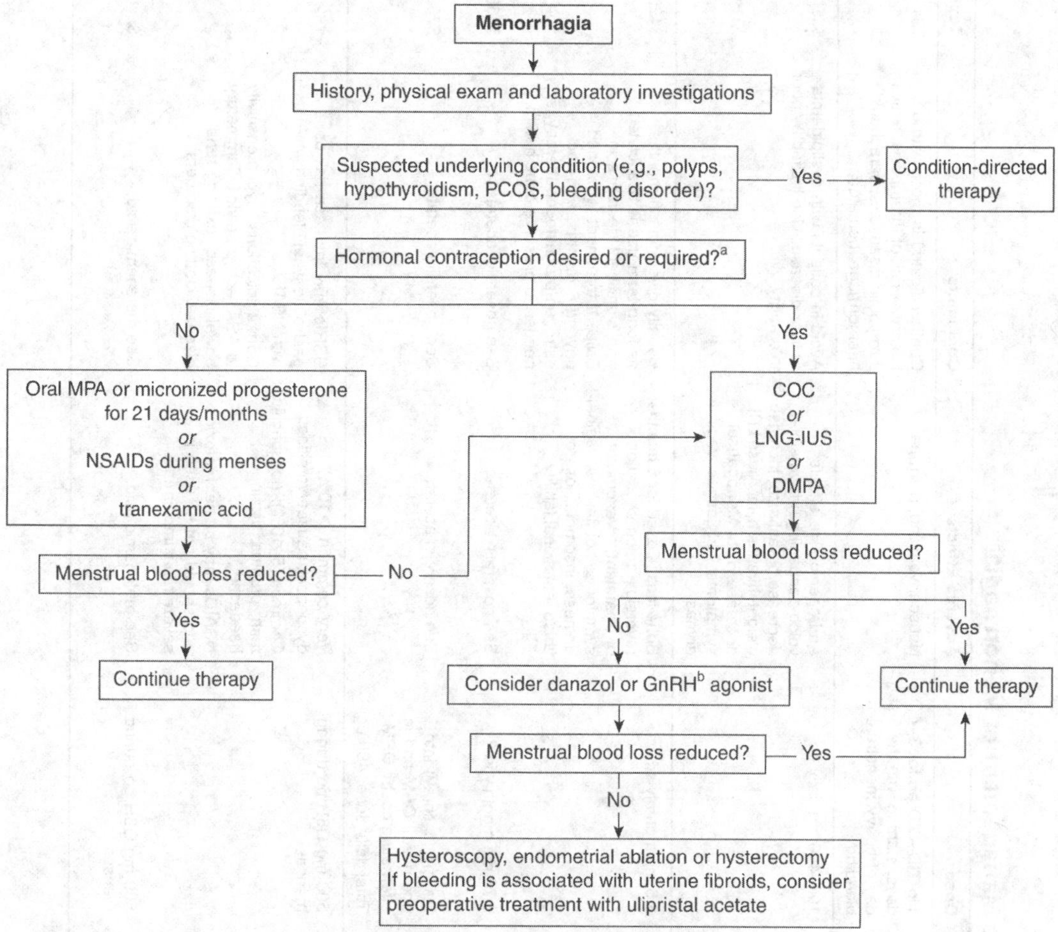

[a] Consider hormonal therapy as first-line treatment if menses are irregular or unpredictable in timing.
[b] Estrogen/progestogen add-back therapy is advisable for GnRH agonist treatment beyond 6 months.
Abbreviations: COC = combined oral contraceptive; DMPA = depot medroxyprogesterone acetate; GnRH = gonadotropin-releasing hormone; LNG-IUS = levonorgestrel-releasing intrauterine system; MPA = medroxyprogesterone acetate; PCOS = polycystic ovary syndrome

Table 2: **Pharmacologic Therapy for the Management of Menorrhagia**[a]

Class	Drug	Dose	Adverse Effects	Comments	Cost[b]
Antifibrinolytics	*tranexamic acid* Cyklokapron, generics	1 g TID–QID po for 3–4 days, starting with the first day of heavy menstrual bleeding	Nausea, vomiting, diarrhea.	Contraindicated in those with a history or risk of thrombosis, active thrombolic disease, subarachnoid haemorrhage, hematuria.	$$
Gonadotropin Inhibitors, pituitary	*danazol* Cyclomen	100–400 mg daily po	Androgenic side effects: voice deepening (irreversible), decrease breast size, increase weight, hirsutism, increase LDL, decrease HDL. Menopausal symptoms: hot flashes, vaginal dryness.	Avoid in patients with dyslipidemia or liver disease. Use limited by poor tolerability.	$$$
Gonadotropin-releasing Hormone Analogues	*goserelin acetate* Zoladex	3.6 mg monthly sc	Bone loss (if used for 6 months, reversible upon cessation of treatment). Vasomotor symptoms: hot flashes, vaginal dryness, insomnia, loss of libido, emotional lability.	Usually given for ≤6 months as long-term use is associated with significant decrease in BMD. If treatment is needed beyond 6 months, add-back estrogen-progestogen therapy is needed to preserve bone health.	$420/dose
	leuprolide acetate Lupron Depot	3.75 mg monthly im	See goserelin acetate.	See goserelin acetate.	$365/dose
	nafarelin acetate Synarel	200 µg (1 spray) into one nostril QAM and in alternating nostril QPM Total daily dose: 400 µg	See goserelin acetate.	See goserelin acetate.	$230
NSAIDs[c]	*mefenamic acid* Ponstan, generics	500 mg Q8H po during menses	Very common (>10%): dyspepsia, nausea/vomiting. Common (5–10%): nonspecific rash, pruritus, dizziness, headache. NSAIDs may be nephrotoxic and should not be used in severe renal impairment.	SSRIs may increase risk of gastrointestinal bleeding when used with NSAIDs. Contraindications: hypersensitivity to ASA, active pelvic inflammatory bowel disease, existing renal disease, clotting disorders.	$$
	naproxen Naprosyn, generics	500 mg Q8H po during menses	See mefenamic acid.	See mefenamic acid.	$

Class	Drug	Dose	Adverse Effects	Comments	Cost[b]
Progestogens[d], oral	*medroxyprogesterone acetate* Provera, generics	10 mg daily po for a minimum of 21 days per month	Bloating, irritability, weight gain, mood swings.	Progestogens normalize the endometrial response and decrease breakthrough bleeding; when given continuously, they prevent menstrual blood flow.	$
	norethindrone acetate Norlutate	5 mg daily po for a minimum of 21 days per month	See medroxyprogesterone acetate.	See medroxyprogesterone acetate.	$$
	progesterone, micronized Prometrium	300 mg QHS po for a minimum of 21 days per month	See medroxyprogesterone acetate.	Better side effect profile than medroxyprogesterone acetate. Contains peanut oil; avoid if peanut allergy.	$$$
Selective Progesterone Receptor Modulators	*ulipristal acetate* Fibristal	5–10 mg daily po × 13 weeks	Hot flashes, headache.	Indicated for the treatment of menorrhagia related to uterine fibroids.	$340–$700

[a] For dosing information on all forms of hormonal therapy including combined oral contraceptives, progestin-only products and LNG-IUS, see Chapter 70.
[b] Cost of 28-day supply unless otherwise specified; includes drug cost only.
[c] NSAIDs listed are examples. For a comprehensive listing of NSAIDs, see Chapter 82.
[d] The term *progestogen* includes both natural progesterone and synthetic progestins.
Abbreviations: BMD = bone mineral density; HDL = high-density lipoprotein cholesterol; LDL = low-density lipoprotein cholesterol
Legend: $ < $10 $$ $10–40 $$$ $40–140

Suggested Readings

Singh S, Best C, Dunn S et al. Abnormal uterine bleeding in pre-menopausal women. *J Obstet Gynaecol Can* 2013;35(5 Suppl 1):1-32. Available from: sogc.org/wp-content/uploads/2013/07/gui292CPG1305E.pdf.

Sweet MG, Schmidt-Dalton TA, Weiss PM et al. Evaluation and management of abnormal uterine bleeding in premenopausal women. *Am Fam Physician* 2012;85(1):35-43.

References

1. Mishell DR. Abnormal uterine bleeding. In: Stenchever MA et al. *Comprehensive gynecology*. 4th ed. St. Louis (MO): Mosby; 2001.
2. Singh S, Best C, Dunn S et al. Abnormal uterine bleeding in pre-menopausal women. *J Obstet Gynaecol Can* 2013;35(5 Suppl 1):1-32. Available from: sogc.org/wp-content/uploads/2013/07/gui292CPG1305E.pdf.
3. Jensen JT, Lefebvre P, Laliberté F et al. Cost burden and treatment patterns associated with management of heavy menstrual bleeding. *J Womens Health (Larchmt)* 2012;21(5):539-47.
4. Magon N, Chauhan M, Goel P et al. Levonorgestrel intrauterine system: current role in management of heavy menstrual bleeding. *J Midlife Health* 2013;4(1):8-15.
5. Munro MG, Critchley HO, Fraser IS. The FIGO classification of causes of abnormal uterine bleeding. *Int J Gynaecol Obstet* 2011;113(1):1-2.
6. Gleeson NC. Cyclic changes in endometrial tissue plasminogen activator and plasminogen activator inhibitor type 1 in women with normal menstruation and essential menorrhagia. *Am J Obstet Gynecol* 1994;171(1):178-83.
7. Lethaby A, Penninx J, Hickey M et al. Endometrial resection and ablation techniques for heavy menstrual bleeding. *Cochrane Database Syst Rev* 2013;8:CD001501.
8. Committee on Practice Bulletins—Gynecology. Practice bulletin no. 136: management of abnormal uterine bleeding associated with ovulatory dysfunction. *Obstet Gynecol* 2013;122(1):176-85.
9. Middleton LJ, Champaneria R, Daniels JP et al. Hysterectomy, endometrial destruction, and levonorgestrel releasing intrauterine system (Mirena) for heavy menstrual bleeding: systematic review and meta-analysis of data from individual patients. *BMJ* 2010;341:c3929.
10. Lethaby AE, Cooke I, Rees M. Progesterone or progestogen-releasing intrauterine systems for heavy menstrual bleeding. *Cochrane Database Syst Rev* 2005;(4):CD002126.
11. Gupta J, Kai J, Middleton L et al. Levonorgestrel intrauterine system versus medical therapy for menorrhagia. *N Engl J Med* 2013;368(2):128-37.
12. Matteson KA, Rahn DD, Wheeler TL et al. Nonsurgical management of heavy menstrual bleeding: a systematic review. *Obstet Gynecol* 2013;121(3):632-43.
13. Heliovaara-Peippo S, Hurskainen R, Teperi J et al. Quality of life and costs of levonorgestrel-releasing intrauterine system or hysterectomy in the treatment of menorrhagia: a 10-year randomized controlled trial. *Am J Obstet Gynecol* 2013;209(6):535.e1-535.e14.
14. Donnez J, Tomaszewski J, Vázquez F et al. Ulipristal acetate versus leuprolide acetate for uterine fibroids. *New Engl J Med* 2012;366(5):421-32.
15. Lethaby A, Farquhar C, Cooke I. Antifibrinolytics for heavy menstrual bleeding. *Cochrane Database Syst Rev* 2000;(4):CD000249.
16. Lethaby A, Duckitt K, Farquhar C. Non-steroidal anti-inflammatory drugs for heavy menstrual bleeding. *Cochrane Database Syst Rev* 2013;1:CD000400.
17. Donnez J, Tatarchuk TF, Bouchard P et al. Ulipristal acetate versus placebo for fibroid treatment before surgery. *New Engl J Med* 2012;366(5):409-20.
18. Tristan M, Orozco LJ, Steed A et al. Mifepristone for uterine fibroids. *Cochrane Database Syst Rev* 2012;8:CD007687.
19. Beaumont H, Augood C, Duckitt K et al. Danazol for heavy menstrual bleeding. *Cochrane Database Syst Rev* 2007;(3):CD001017.
20. Munro MG, Mainor N, Basu R et al. Oral medroxyprogesterone acetate and combination oral contraceptives for acute uterine bleeding: a randomized controlled trial.*Obstet Gynecol.* 2006;108(4):924-9

Chapter 77
Chronic Fatigue Syndrome

Kathleen Kerr, MD, Dip Env Health

Fatigue, usually short-lived, is common and is often related to some identified cause. Chronic fatigue syndrome (CFS), also known as myalgic encephalomyelitis or myalgic encephalopathy (ME), is characterized by persistent and unexplained fatigue resulting in severe impairment in daily function. It is defined by symptoms, disability and exclusion of medical and psychiatric conditions that could explain the fatigue.[1] CFS is also associated with chronic and episodic cardiovascular and autonomic dysfunction.[2] The prognosis for recovery for severely afflicted patients with ME/CFS is poor.[3]

CFS is found in all ages, races and socioeconomic groups and more women are affected than men.[4] In the Western world, the population prevalence is approximately 0.5% although a Canadian survey has reported a prevalence of 1.3%.[5]

In subsets of patients, ME/CFS may be associated with microbial infections, immune abnormalities, exposure to toxins, chemicals or pesticides and prior stressful events,[6] however, the precise underlying disease mechanisms remain to be clarified.[7] The common suspected infectious triggers are Epstein-Barr virus (EBV), enterovirus,[8] human cytomegalovirus (HCMV)[9] and human herpes virus-6 (HHV-6).[7]

A large body of evidence has found abnormalities in the central and autonomic nervous systems and activation of various parts of the immune system.[7] Several studies have found gene expression changes consistent with a state of chronic activation of the immune system[10,11,12,13] and mitochondrial dysfunction in cases of postinfectious fatigue caused by EBV.[14] Another study confirmed these findings while gene expression in patients with endogenous depression was similar to that in normal controls.[8]

Many of the symptoms experienced by some CFS patients strongly resemble the "sickness behaviour" (fever, malaise, pain, fatigue, poor concentration) that can be induced by the administration of pro-inflammatory cytokines.[9] Several studies, however, have found a shift from pro-inflammatory Th1 to Th2 cytokines, which is consistent with the hypothesis of viral triggers (e.g., EBV, HCMV).[15] A 2010 study found evidence of a group of murine leukemia virus (MLV)-related viruses in patients with CFS, supporting the argument that MLV-related viruses may be associated with CFS.[16] However, later data found no association between CFS and MLV-related viruses.[17] The finding of viral DNA sequences in persons with CFS or other diseases is not definitive proof that these viruses play a causative role in the development of CFS or that they may represent a threat to the blood supply. However, Canadian Blood Services has determined that any donor who has a medical history of CFS will be indefinitely deferred from donating blood.[18]

Goals of Therapy

- Provide a supportive environment where patients can safely discuss their illness and where the illness is validated
- Relieve symptoms as possible and according to patient preferences
- Educate and promote self-management, including exercise paced to avoid post-exertional malaise on one extreme and deconditioning on the other

Investigations

Diagnosis of CFS relies entirely on a combination of symptoms (not laboratory data) and on the exclusion of chronic active organic or psychiatric illnesses that can produce chronic fatigue (Figure 1). The Canadian consensus clinical diagnostic criteria[19] require the presence of specific symptoms (in particular, post-exertional malaise and cognitive difficulties) and differ from the US Centers for Disease Control consensus research case definition, which has 1 major and 4 of 8 minor criteria.[1] Although a diagnosis of CFS cannot be seriously entertained before 6 months of fatigue, clinical evaluation[5] should proceed in the interim to rule out other potentially treatable causes of fatigue. Well-controlled medical conditions do not preclude a diagnosis of CFS if the patient meets the criteria otherwise.

Figure 1: **Assessment of Chronic Fatigue Syndrome**[1,19]

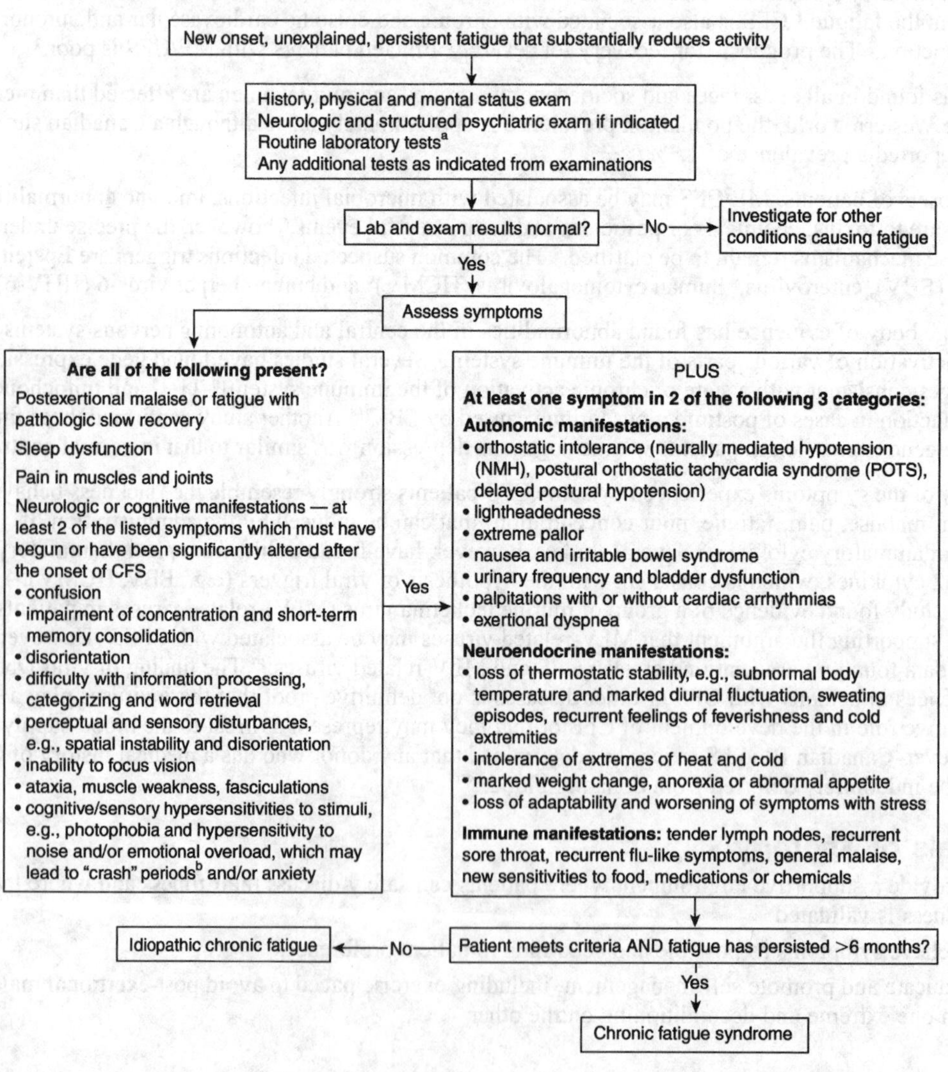
New onset, unexplained, persistent fatigue that substantially reduces activity
History, physical and mental status exam
Neurologic and structured psychiatric exam if indicated
Routine laboratory tests[a]
Any additional tests as indicated from examinations
Lab and exam results normal?
No
Investigate for other conditions causing fatigue
Yes
Assess symptoms
Are all of the following present?
Postexertional malaise or fatigue with pathologic slow recovery
Sleep dysfunction
Pain in muscles and joints
Neurologic or cognitive manifestations — at least 2 of the listed symptoms which must have begun or have been significantly altered after the onset of CFS
• confusion
• impairment of concentration and short-term memory consolidation
• disorientation
• difficulty with information processing, categorizing and word retrieval
• perceptual and sensory disturbances, e.g., spatial instability and disorientation
• inability to focus vision
• ataxia, muscle weakness, fasciculations
• cognitive/sensory hypersensitivities to stimuli, e.g., photophobia and hypersensitivity to noise and/or emotional overload, which may lead to "crash" periods[b] and/or anxiety
Yes
PLUS
At least one symptom in 2 of the following 3 categories:
Autonomic manifestations:
• orthostatic intolerance (neurally mediated hypotension (NMH), postural orthostatic tachycardia syndrome (POTS), delayed postural hypotension)
• lightheadedness
• extreme pallor
• nausea and irritable bowel syndrome
• urinary frequency and bladder dysfunction
• palpitations with or without cardiac arrhythmias
• exertional dyspnea
Neuroendocrine manifestations:
• loss of thermostatic stability, e.g., subnormal body temperature and marked diurnal fluctuation, sweating episodes, recurrent feelings of feverishness and cold extremities
• intolerance of extremes of heat and cold
• marked weight change, anorexia or abnormal appetite
• loss of adaptability and worsening of symptoms with stress
Immune manifestations: tender lymph nodes, recurrent sore throat, recurrent flu-like symptoms, general malaise, new sensitivities to food, medications or chemicals
Patient meets criteria AND fatigue has persisted >6 months?
No
Idiopathic chronic fatigue
Yes
Chronic fatigue syndrome

[a] Albumin, anti-tissue transglutaminase, calcium, CBC with differential, creatinine, electrolytes, ESR or CRP, fasting glucose, liver enzymes, phosphorus, total protein, TSH, urea, urinalysis.
[b] A temporary period of immobilizing physical and/or cognitive fatigue.

Neither viral titres nor neuro-imaging studies are required or helpful in routine clinical practice. However, most evidence suggests there is an underlying biological process in CFS with abnormal findings in the central and autonomic nervous systems and chronic activation of various parts of the immune system.[7]

Therapeutic Choices

There are no specific treatments for CFS. Patients benefit from receiving a positive diagnosis with reasonable explanations of their symptoms. Treatment should stress nonpharmacologic approaches, attempts at symptom control, a supportive environment and acknowledgment of suffering.

Nonpharmacologic Choices

Primarily, nonpharmacologic therapies should be utilized.

- Encourage a healthy balanced *diet* with adequate protein, fresh vegetables and fruit. Patients with CFS may need assistance with shopping and food preparation, and may need to purchase prepared foods. A multivitamin is generally recommended for people who do not have a balanced diet. Correct specific nutritional deficiencies or insufficiencies that occur due to fatigue affecting availability and preparation of balanced meals. Patients with orthostatic hypotension should include adequate amounts of salt in their diet.

  No specific diet or nutritional supplements have been proven to benefit this condition.
- Address *sleep* problems early as they may cause or worsen other symptoms such as fatigue, memory problems, headaches and joint pain. Refer for a sleep study if symptoms of sleep apnea, restless legs syndrome, sleep phase abnormalities or persistent/recurrent daytime sleeping are present. Encourage good sleep hygiene (see Chapter 8).
- *Graded exercise therapy* (see Table 1) and *activity pacing* may assist in improving fatigue and quality of life.

  Activity pacing may be a useful technique for patients with CFS.[20] It involves distributing activities throughout the day and dividing them into small, manageable tasks separated by rest breaks. Activities (e.g., laundry, shopping) should not make symptoms worse and patients should avoid "push-crash" cycles (doing too much at once causes them to feel worse; after resting they feel better and once again become active, only to again over-exert themselves). Patients able to stay within their personal *energy envelope* (expending only the energy that is available within their specific limits, thus avoiding over-exertion) had significant improvements in physical functioning and fatigue severity.[21] Health care professionals should help patients with ME/CFS maintain appropriate energy expenditures in coordination with personal energy reserves.
- A Cochrane review found that while *cognitive behavioural therapy* (CBT) reduced fatigue by the end of treatment compared to usual care. However, when evaluating the efficacy of CBT 1–7 months after treatment ended, results were inconsistent and the studies were heterogeneous, making it difficult to draw conclusions.[22] Another systematic review reached similar conclusions and noted the low quality of evidence for benefit, with very few studies reporting on acceptability of CBT and no studies examining side effects.[23] Some patients express a preference not to receive CBT and this preference should be respected.
- The benefit of adding nonpharmacologic therapies to standard care may exceed that of standard care alone. The PACE trial in the United Kingdom suggests that either CBT or graded exercise therapy (GET) when added to specialist medical care (standard care), is more effective and as safe as specialist medical care alone.[24] Activity pacing did not demonstrate similar results, although the lack of a standardized definition complicates evaluation.[25] Additionally, CBT and GET may be more cost-effective than specialist medical care alone,[26] but this analysis did not consider welfare benefits

due to lost work time. All groups, including those receiving CBT and GET, experienced an increase in welfare benefits received. Therefore, results should be interpreted cautiously.

Pharmacologic Choices

No definitive pharmacotherapy exists for ME/CFS. Patients may be managed with several medications, nonpharmacologic interventions and/or natural supplements as part of an individualized integrative treatment approach. One clinical trial found improvement on all outcome measures for 38 patients with ME/CFS and fibromyalgia who were treated with multiple combined interventions, compared to a placebo group.[27]

A systematic review of 70 studies of *complementary and alternative medicines* (CAM) for treating ME/CFS and fibromyalgia concluded with no definite treatment recommendations.[28] However, 86% of the trials showed some beneficial effects of the intervention and 74% also showed symptom-related improvement. Only 3 studies reported adverse effects (e.g., bruising, rashes, etc.) in conjunction with treatment. These findings suggest that alternative treatments appear to have few negative outcomes and may have beneficial effects for some patients. **L-carnitine**, oral **nicotinamide adenine dinucleotide** (NADH) and **magnesium** may be potentially effective supplements, but further investigation is needed.[28]

Current evidence does not support definitive conclusions about the efficacy of antidepressants or other psychotropic agents in the treatment of CFS.[29] Results of randomized, controlled trials have been inconsistent and much of the support for antidepressant use in CFS is derived from studies of fatigue associated with other unexplained symptoms or depression. **Tricyclic antidepressants** (TCAs) may induce sedation and orthostatic hypotension. Patients with CFS are prone to these effects because of their fatigue and frequent autonomic lability. TCA doses used in CFS research have been markedly lower than those used for depression.[29]

Stimulants are not recommended. One trial found no evidence that **modafinil** had any significant effects on self-rated physical or mental fatigue, health-related quality of life or mood.[30] Another trial of short-term **methylphenidate** use had a low rate of positive responders (about 20%).[31]

In the absence of specific diagnosed sleep disorders and if sleep hygiene is unsuccessful, a short-term trial of sedating **antihistamines** (e.g., diphenhydramine, doxylamine) or a prescription **hypnotic** in the smallest possible dose may be warranted. For more information, see Chapter 8.

Table 1: Graded Exercise Therapy[20]

Graded activity and exercise: start from a very low, basic level of exercise and/or activity and gradually increase it to a level where one can go about their daily life. The level of activity may not be the same as before the CFS diagnosis.

- People who have not been active for a long period of time and feel very weak should only do a basic activity (e.g., stretching, walking or biking for a few minutes). They should not feel tired after the activity. If the activity induces tiredness, it should be lessened.
- If symptoms of CFS get worse after adding activity, patient should return to the last level of activity where they felt comfortable.
- Lifting light weights and stretching can help some people with CFS feel better. Start with using body weight (e.g., raising arms) and gradually increase to wall push ups, modified chair dips and toe raises. Strengthening activity should precede aerobic activity.
- Very ill people who are housebound or bedbound can start with working on picking up and grasping objects. Activity should be increased until the person can handle activities of daily living, e.g., getting up, dressing, moving around the house, brushing teeth. Persons with CFS should not avoid these activities, but should go slowly when starting a new activity.

Adapted from: Centers for Disease Control and Prevention (US). *CFS toolkit and additional information for healthcare professionals.* Atlanta (GA): CDC.

Choices during Pregnancy and Breastfeeding

A case series involving 252 pregnancies has been published describing the effects of pregnancy on CFS symptoms and vice versa.[32] During pregnancy, there was no change in CFS symptoms in 41%, an improvement of symptoms in 30% and a worsening of symptoms in 29% of subjects. After pregnancy, there was no change in 30%, an improvement in 20%, and a worsening in 50% of patients. There was a significantly higher rate of spontaneous abortions, and a correspondingly lower rate of live births by vaginal delivery, a finding which could also be due to age or parity. Developmental delays or learning disabilities were significantly more frequent in children born from pregnancies that occurred after the onset of CFS. Larger, prospective controlled studies are needed to confirm these findings.

During pregnancy and breastfeeding, continue nonpharmacologic treatment measures that have been effective. If there is coexisting depression, the risk/benefit ratio may favour continuing treatment with antidepressants during pregnancy and afterwards (see Chapter 6). Medication for other conditions should be reevaluated and adjusted as clinically indicated to protect the fetus.

Therapeutic Tips

- Patients with CFS are often indoors a great deal and should take a daily vitamin D supplement appropriate for their age and gender.
- Avoid polypharmacy. Patients with CFS may see multiple care providers, and in a population-based case-control study, were significantly more likely to use antidepressants, sedatives, muscle relaxants and various nonprescription remedies.[33]
- Adverse effects of certain drugs may mimic the symptoms of CFS; evaluate patients carefully for potential drug-induced side effects and drug interactions.

Suggested Readings

Carruthers BM, Jain AK, De Meirleir KL et al. Myalgic encephalomyelitis/chronic fatigue syndrome: clinical working case definition, diagnostic and treatment protocols. *J Chronic Fatigue Syndr* 2003;11(1):7-115. Available from: www.cfids-cab.org/cfs-inform/CFS.case.def/carruthers.etal03.pdf.

Centers for Disease Control and Prevention (US). *CFS toolkit and additional information for healthcare professionals*. Atlanta (GA): CDC. Available from: www.cdc.gov/cfs/hcp.html.

Centers for Disease Control and Prevention (US). *Chronic fatigue syndrome (CFS)*. Atlanta (GA): CDC. Available from: www.cdc.gov/cfs/.

International Association for Chronic Fatigue Syndrome/Myalgic Encephalomyelitis (IACFS/ME). *Chronic fatigue syndrome/myalgic encephalomyelitis. A primer for clinical practitioners*. Chicago (IL): International Association for Chronic Fatigue Syndrome/Myalgic Encephalomyelitis (IACFS/ME); 2012.

Komaroff AL, Cho TA. Role of infection and neurologic dysfunction in chronic fatigue syndrome. *Semin Neurol* 2011;31(3):325-37.

References

1. Fukuda K, Straus SE, Hickie I et al. The chronic fatigue syndrome: a comprehensive approach to its definition and study. International Chronic Fatigue Syndrome Study Group. *Ann Intern Med* 1994;121(12):953-9.
2. Gerrity TR, Bates J, Bell DS et al. Chronic fatigue syndrome: what role does the autonomic nervous system play in the pathophysiology of this complex illness? *Neuroimmunomodulation* 2002-2003;10(3):134-41.
3. Jason LA, Benton MC, Valentine L et al. The economic impact of ME/CFS: individual and societal costs. *Dyn Med* 2008;7:6.
4. Reyes M, Nisenbaum R, Hoaglin DC et al. Prevalence and incidence of chronic fatigue syndrome in Wichita, Kansas. *Arch Intern Med* 2003;163(13):1530-6.
5. Lavergne MR, Cole DsC, Kerr K et al. Functional impairment in chronic fatigue syndrome, fibromyalgia, and multiple chemical sensitivity. *Can Fam Physician* 2010;56(2):e57-65.
6. Kerr JR, Mattey DL. Preexisting psychological stress predicts acute and chronic fatigue and arthritis following symptomatic parvovirus B19 infection. *Clin Infect Dis* 2008;46(9):e83-87.
7. Komaroff AL, Cho TA. Role of infection and neurologic dysfunction in chronic fatigue syndrome. *Semin Neurol* 2011;31(3):325-37.

8. Zhang L, Gough J, Christmas D et al. Microbial infections in eight genomic subtypes of chronic fatigue syndrome/myalgic encephalomyelitis. *J Clin Pathol* 2010;63(2):156-64.
9. Broderick G, Fuite J, Kreitz A et al. A formal analysis of cytokine networks in chronic fatigue syndrome. *Brain Behav Immun* 2010;24(7):1209-17.
10. Vernon SD, Shukla SK, Conradt J et al. Analysis of 16S rRNA gene sequences and circulating cell-free DNA from plasma of chronic fatigue syndrome and non-fatigued subjects. *BMC Microbiol* 2002;2:39.
11. Vernon SD, Whistler T, Aslakson E et al. Challenges for molecular profiling of chronic fatigue syndrome. *Pharmacogenomics* 2006;7(2):211-8.
12. Steinau M, Unger ER, Vernon SD et al. Differential-display PCR of peripheral blood for biomarker discovery in chronic fatigue syndrome. *J Mol Med* 2004;82(11):750-5.
13. Kaushik N, Fear D, Richards SC et al. Gene expression in peripheral blood mononuclear cells from patients with chronic fatigue syndrome. *J Clin Pathol* 2005;58(8):826-32.
14. Vernon SD, Whistler T, Cameron B et al. Preliminary evidence of mitochondrial dysfunction associated with post-infective fatigue after acute infection with Epstein Barr virus. *BMC Infect Dis* 2006;6:15.
15. Jason LA, Porter N, Herrington J et al. Kindling and oxidative stress as contributors to myalgic encephalomyelitis/chronic fatigue syndrome. *J Behav Neurosci Res* 2009;7(2):1-17.
16. Lo SC, Pripuzova N, Li B et al. Detection of MLV-related virus gene sequences in blood of patients with chronic fatigue syndrome and healthy blood donors. *Proc Natl Acad Sci U S A* 2010;107(36):15874-9.
17. Alter HJ, Mikovits JA, Switzer WM et al. A multicenter blinded analysis indicates no association between chronic fatigue syndrome/myalgic encephalomyelitis and either xenotropic murine leukemia virus-related virus or polytropic murine leukemia virus. *MBio* 2012;3(5). pii:e00266-12.
18. Canadian Blood Services. *Indefinite deferral for history of chronic fatigue syndrome*. Available from: www.blood.ca/centreapps/internet/uw_v502_mainengine.nsf/9749ca80b75a038585256aa20060d703/db5c4e0235b819cc85257705006e5452?OpenDocument. Accessed March 5, 2014.
19. Carruthers BM, Jain AK, De Meirleir KL et al. Myalgic encephalomyelitis/chronic fatigue syndrome: clinical working case definition, diagnostic and treatment protocols. *J Chronic Fatigue Syndr* 2003;11(1):7-115. Available from: www.cfids-cab.org/cfs-inform/CFS.case.def/carruthers.etal03.pdf. Accessed February 23, 2011.
20. Centers for Disease Control and Prevention (US). *CFS toolkit and additional information for healthcare professionals*. Atlanta (GA): CDC. Available from: www.cdc.gov/cfs/hcp.html. Accessed March 8, 2011.
21. Jason L, Benton M, Torres-Harding S et al. The impact of energy modulation on physical functioning and fatigue severity among patients with ME/CFS. *Patient Educ Couns* 2009;77(2):237-41.
22. Price JR, Mitchell E, Tidy E et al. Cognitive behaviour therapy for chronic fatigue syndrome in adults. *Cochrane Database Syst Rev* 2008;(3):CD001027.
23. Reid SF, Chalder T, Cleare A et al. Chronic fatigue syndrome. *Clin Evid (Online)* 2008;pii:1101.
24. White PD, Goldsmith KA, Johnson AL et al. Comparison of adaptive pacing therapy, cognitive behavior therapy, graded exercise therapy, and specialist medical care for chronic fatigue syndrome (PACE): a randomised trial. *Lancet* 2011;377(9768):823-36.
25. Goudsmit EM, Nijs J, Jason LA et al. Pacing as a strategy to improve energy management in myalgic encephalomyelitis/chronic fatigue syndrome: a consensus document. *Disabil Rehabil* 2012;34(13):1140-7.
26. McCrone P, Sharpe M, Chalder T et al. Adaptive pacing, cognitive behaviour therapy, graded exercise, and specialist medical care for chronic fatigue syndrome: a cost-effectiveness analysis. *PLoS One* 2012;7(8):e40808.
27. Teitelbaum JE, Bird B, Greenfield RM et al. Effective treatment of chronic fatigue syndrome and fibromyalgia: a randomized randomized, double-blind, placebo-controlled, intent-to-treat study. *J Chronic Fatigue Syndr* 2001;8(2):3-28.
28. Porter NS, Jason LA, Boulton A et al. Alternative medical interventions used in the treatment and management of myalgic encephalomyelitis/chronic fatigue syndrome and fibromyalgia. *J Altern Complement Med* 2010;16(3):235-49.
29. Pae CU, Marks DM, Patkar AA et al. Pharmacological treatment of chronic fatigue syndrome: focusing on the role of antidepressants. *Expert Opin Pharmacother* 2009;10(10):1561-70.
30. Randall DC, Cafferty FH, Shneerson JM et al. Chronic treatment with modafinil may not be beneficial in patients with chronic fatigue syndrome. *J Psychopharmacol* 2005;19(6):647-60.
31. Blockmans D, Persoons P, Van Houdenhove B et al. Does methylphenidate reduce the symptoms of chronic fatigue syndrome? *Am J Med* 2006;119(2):167.e23-30.
32. Schacterle RS, Komaroff AL. A comparison of pregnancies that occur before and after the onset of chronic fatigue syndrome. *Arch Intern Med* 2004;164(4):401-4.
33. Boneva RS, Lin JM, Maloney EM et al. Use of medications by people with chronic fatigue syndrome and healthy persons: a population-based study of fatiguing illness in Georgia. *Health Qual Life Outcomes* 2009;7:67.

Chapter 78
Fibromyalgia

Hillel M. Finestone, MDCM, FRCPC

Fibromyalgia is characterized by chronic widespread pain, increased tenderness at specific sites known as "tender points," unrefreshing sleep, fatigue and cognitive dysfunction not attributable to other disease states. Fibromyalgia affects 2–4% of the general population and of those affected, 80–90% are female. In general, symptom onset occurs between the ages of 30 and 60. Central and peripheral system changes in terms of hypothalamic–pituitary–adrenal axis dysfunction, central sensitization, wind-up (a progressive increase in sensitivity over time, i.e., lower stimuli result in increased pain), elevated excitatory neurotransmitters, vasoconstriction, ischemia and adrenergic receptor sensitivity have been described, although none have been identified as clear causative factors.

While the etiology of fibromyalgia is not entirely clear, associations with trauma, adverse life events, impaired mood (e.g., depression), anxiety, irritable bowel syndrome, irritable bladder syndrome, cold intolerance, paresthesias and other medical conditions have been described.[1] Accordingly, the diagnosis of fibromyalgia is an evolving one. See Figure 1 and Figure 3 for more information regarding associated conditions.

Goals of Therapy

- Reduce pain, fatigue, psychological distress and sleep problems
- Improve physical and emotional well-being, functioning and quality of life
- Address associated conditions on an individual basis
- Promote self-management via individual and group education

Investigations

Figure 1 presents suggested investigations and Figure 2, the tender point examination.

The American College of Rheumatologists has published provisional diagnostic criteria which provide a case definition for fibromyalgia (Figure 3) based on the widespread pain index (WPI) and the symptom severity (SS) scale.[2] The Canadian Rheumatology Association and Canadian Pain Society recently endorsed similar diagnostic criteria indicating that "examination for tender points is not required to confirm the diagnosis".[3] These criteria have not yet been widely adopted by physicians and there will likely be a need for further discussion in this regard. All clinicians seem to agree that the diagnosis, pathogenesis and treatment are complex and require greater understanding.

Therapeutic Choices

Nonpharmacologic Choices

Nonpharmacologic treatment of fibromyalgia should be first-line therapy, especially due to a lack of strong data to support the use of medications.

- Empathy and acknowledgment of suffering from health care providers is fundamental.
- A comprehensive, multidisciplinary program of education, self-management, nonpharmacologic pain reduction techniques, graded aerobic exercises, sleep hygiene, stress management and cognitive behavioural therapy is believed to be beneficial,[4] but a Cochrane review indicated too few

high-quality randomized controlled trials to support this common viewpoint.[5] A "person-centred" approach to care has been advocated.[6]

- Ongoing cognitive behavioural therapy (CBT) sessions are one component of the multidisciplinary treatment of fibromyalgia. CBT has been shown to improve the number of tender points, Visual Analogue Scale (VAS) pain scores, pain coping, pain behaviours, depression and physical function.[7]
- Supervised aerobic exercise, walking programs, pool exercises, graded exercise programs, strength training and tai chi can improve function, symptoms and well-being.[8,9,10,11,12]
- Nonpharmacologic pain reduction techniques include cold, heat, transcutaneous electrical nerve stimulation (TENS), massage and relaxation techniques such as biofeedback, meditation and hypnosis.[13] Electroacupuncture has also been shown to reduce pain and analgesic requirements in patients with fibromyalgia,[14] while another study concluded that acupuncture could not be recommended for fibromyalgia.[15] A Cochrane systematic review also found that electroacupuncture is probably more effective than acupuncture for pain and stiffness in fibromyalgia.[16]
- Patient education, e.g., the Arthritis Society's Arthritis Self-Management Program, can improve pain, sleep, fatigue, quality of life and the 6-minute walk test. Improvement can last at least 3–12 months.[4]
- Specific identification and subsequent therapy for a particular life event such as history of sexual,[17] physical or emotional abuse, deprivation, post-traumatic stress disorder or any other psychologically distressing event can be efficacious as part of the overall treatment approach, in the clinical experience of the author.

Figure 1: **Investigation of Diffuse Aches and Pains**

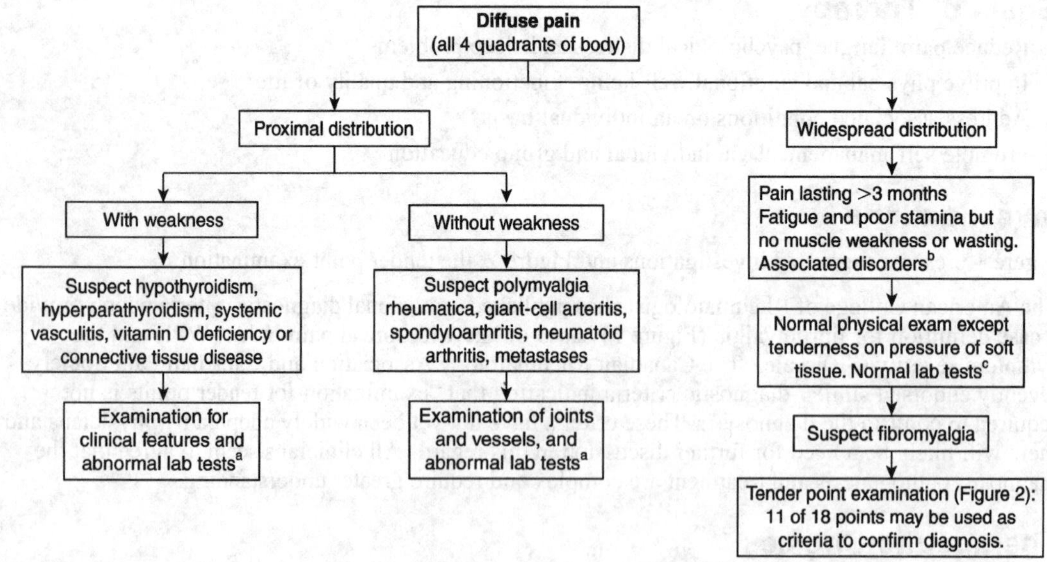

[a] AST, alkaline phosphatase, calcium, CBC, creatine kinase, creatinine, CRP, ESR, TSH and 25-hydroxyvitamin D.
[b] Associated disorders include mood disturbances, cognitive dysfunction, irritable bowel syndrome, irritable bladder syndrome, dizziness, cold intolerance, subjective swelling, paresthesiae, migraine, severe menstrual pain, myofascial facial pain, sexual dysfunction and temporomandibular joint syndrome.
[c] CBC, creatine kinase, ESR, CRP and TSH.

Abbreviations: AST = aspartate aminotransferase; CBC = complete blood count; CRP = C-reactive protein; ESR = erythrocyte sedimentation rate; TSH = thyroid-stimulating hormone

Figure 2: **Tender Point Examination**[a]

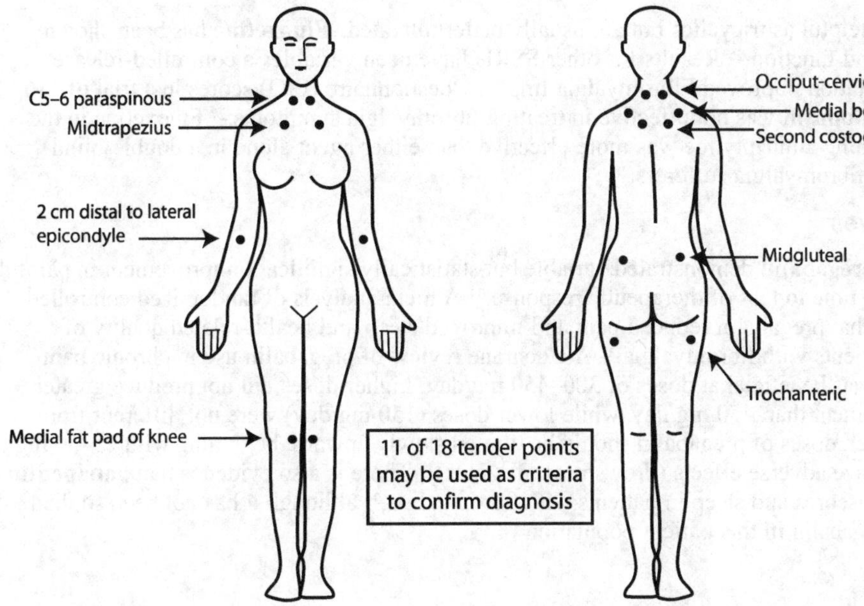

[a] Using thumb pressure sufficient to blanch fingernail.

Pharmacologic Choices (Table 1)

Because the etiology of fibromyalgia remains unknown, drug treatments are largely empiric. Studies have been of short duration and varying quality. Note, duloxetine and pregabalin are the only 2 prescription medications with official Health Canada indications for the treatment of fibromyalgia.

Antidepressants

A wide range of antidepressants may be useful in the management of fibromyalgia, including tricyclic antidepressants, selective serotonin reuptake inhibitors (SSRIs) and serotonin-norepinephrine reuptake inhibitors (SNRIs). They may be considered equally for initial therapy and are discussed below.[18,19]

Low doses of **tricyclic antidepressants** at bedtime (e.g., amitriptyline starting at 5 mg and progressing slowly, every 2–3 weeks, to a maximum of 50 mg) can improve sleep and reduce pain and fatigue.[20] Only short-term efficacy has been shown. A Cochrane review suggests that although it is an appropriate initial treatment, only a minority of patients will achieve satisfactory pain relief with amitriptyline.[21] If taken 1–2 hours before bedtime the effect will start at bedtime, and morning hangover will be lessened.

A "muscle relaxant" that is somewhat effective is **cyclobenzaprine**, perhaps because it too is a tricyclic molecule.[22]

The SNRI duloxetine provides a small but significant reduction in fibromyalgia pain but does not improve fatigue, quality of life or sleep disturbances [Evidence: SORT B*].[23] Duloxetine is generally well tolerated but some patients may discontinue its use due to nausea, dry mouth, constipation, or headache. Duloxetine may be considered as first-line drug therapy in fibromyalgia patients with

* SORT (Strength of Recommendation Taxonomy) is a rating system (A, B or C) that addresses the quality of available evidence. For information consult **How to Use *Compendium of Therapeutic Choices*** on page xxv.

concomitant depression. **Venlafaxine** has not been studied in patients with fibromyalgia. However, **milnacipran**, an SNRI not available in Canada, was shown to be beneficial in treating fibromyalgia symptoms.[24]

SSRIs are not as helpful as tricyclics but are usually better tolerated. **Fluoxetine** has been shown to improve pain and function.[25] Results for other SSRIs have been variable: a controlled-release **paroxetine** formulation improved Fibromyalgia Impact Questionnaire (FIQ) scores in a trial of 116 patients,[26] but **citalopram** was not effective in treating fibromyalgia symptoms.[27] Fluoxetine in the morning with evening amitriptyline was more effective than either agent alone in a double-blind controlled trial in fibromyalgia sufferers.[28]

GABA Derivatives

In clinical trials, **pregabalin** demonstrated variable but statistically significant improvement in painful symptoms[29,30] and time to loss of therapeutic response.[31] A meta-analysis of randomized controlled trials determined that pregabalin reduced pain and improved sleep and health-related quality of life indices for patients with fibromyalgia.[32] A Cochrane review of pregabalin use in chronic pain concluded that it was beneficial at doses of 300–450 mg/day; higher doses did not produce greater symptom improvement than 450 mg/day, while lower doses (150 mg/day) were not different from placebo.[33] However, doses of pregabalin should be titrated slowly upward, beginning with 25–50 mg at bedtime, to minimize adverse effects (drowsiness, dizziness). There is also evidence that **gabapentin** may improve pain scores and sleep in patients with fibromyalgia,[34] although it has not been studied as extensively as pregabalin in this patient population.

Other Drugs

Analgesics such as **acetaminophen** and **nonsteroidal anti-inflammatory drugs (NSAIDs)** may be tried but help very few patients. These drugs may not be useful for fibromyalgia because the pain is probably a result of central sensitization rather than peripheral pain or inflammation.

There is no good evidence to suggest that **opioid** analgesics (other than tramadol) are effective for the relief of pain in fibromyalgia.[35] Additionally, several fibromyalgia guidelines recommend against the use of opioids as part of therapy.[36] Of particular concern is the risk of opioid-induced hyperalgesia since fibromyalgia patients may already have central sensitization (hyperalgesia). Despite the lack of evidence and guidance, inappropriate and widespread use of opioids exists in this patient population.

Tramadol (with or without acetaminophen) has been reported to reduce pain and to improve health-related quality of life in individuals with fibromyalgia.[37,38,39,40] This effect, however, is likely due to the fact that it reduces reuptake of serotonin and norepinephrine[37,39] rather than to its narcotic action. The use of tramadol with serotonergic antidepressants may cause serotonin syndrome.

Sedatives may benefit those with severe sleep dysfunction but do not provide effective reduction of pain. Dependency and adverse effects are also concerns. **Zopiclone** might be useful intermittently but evidence is lacking.[41] Antidepressants with sedative properties, such as amitriptyline and trazodone, are commonly used in fibromyalgia patients to improve sleep.[42]

Human growth hormone improved symptoms in a placebo-controlled trial, although further investigation is required.[43] It may help only those with low growth hormone levels. Expense and availability limit its use.

Treatment of peripheral pain generators by local injection (e.g., usually **lidocaine** 1% with or without a depot form of **corticosteroid**) to myofascial trigger points may reduce the total pain burden and the perpetuation of central pain sensitization.[44]

Figure 3: **Preliminary Diagnostic Criteria for Fibromyalgia**

Widespread Pain Index (WPI)

Check the number of areas in which the patient has had pain over the last week.

Shoulder girdle	left ☐ right ☐	Hip (buttock, trochanter)	left ☐	right ☐	Upper back ☐		Abdomen ☐
Upper arm	left ☐ right ☐	Upper leg	left ☐	right ☐	Lower back ☐		Neck ☐
Lower arm	left ☐ right ☐	Lower leg	left ☐	right ☐	Chest ☐		
		Jaw	left ☐	right ☐			

Score will be between 0 and 19. **WPI =** ______

Symptom Severity (SS) Scale

A. Indicate the level of severity of each of the 3 symptoms listed below over the past week using the following scale:

0 = no problem
1 = slight or mild problems, generally mild or intermittent
2 = moderate, considerable problems, often present and/or at a moderate level
3 = severe: pervasive, continuous, life-disturbing problems

Fatigue ______ Waking unrefreshed ______ Cognitive symptoms ______ **= TOTAL A** ______

B. Considering somatic symptoms in general,[a] indicate whether the patient has:

0 = no symptoms; **1** = few symptoms; **2** = a moderate number of symptoms; **3** = a great deal of symptoms

= TOTAL B ______

Score (A + B) will be between 0 and 12. **SS SCALE SCORE =** ______

Criteria

A patient satisfies diagnostic criteria for fibromyalgia if the following 3 conditions are met:

1. Widespread pain index (WPI) ≥7 and symptom severity (SS) scale score ≥5 or WPI 3–6 and SS scale score ≥9.
2. Symptoms have been present at a similar level for at least 3 months.
3. The patient does not have a disorder that would otherwise explain the pain.

[a] Consider: muscle pain, irritable bowel syndrome, fatigue/tiredness, thinking or remembering problem, muscle weakness, headache, pain/cramps in the abdomen, numbness/tingling, dizziness, insomnia, depression, constipation, pain in the upper abdomen, nausea, nervousness, chest pain, blurred vision, fever, diarrhea, dry mouth, itching, wheezing, Raynaud's phenomenon, hives/welts, ringing in ears, vomiting, heartburn, oral ulcers, loss of or change in taste, seizures, dry eyes, shortness of breath, loss of appetite, rash, sun sensitivity, hearing difficulties, easy bruising, hair loss, frequent urination, painful urination, bladder spasms.

Adapted with permission from Wolfe F, Clauw D, Fitzcharles MA et al. The American College of Rheumatology preliminary diagnostic criteria for fibromyalgia and measurement of symptom severity. *Arthritis Care Res (Hoboken)* 2010;62(5):600-10.

Choices during Pregnancy and Breastfeeding

Fibromyalgia and Pregnancy/Postpartum Period

Before conception, women with fibromyalgia and comorbid myofascial face pain may have reduced fertility.[45]

There is little published evidence regarding the effects of pregnancy on women with fibromyalgia. Theoretically, elevated levels of cortisol and relaxin during pregnancy may ease symptoms in some patients. An analysis of 1178 women determined that fibromyalgia did not affect pregnancy outcomes or newborn health, but almost all patients reported worsening symptoms during pregnancy, especially during the last trimester.[46] Symptoms were worse postpartum in many patients (but eventually returned to previous levels); anxiety and depression also increased after delivery.

Management during Pregnancy and Postpartum Period

Nonpharmacologic approaches to pain control, stress management and energy conservation should be encouraged during pregnancy. A reminder that many fibromyalgia symptoms (generalized pain, fatigue, back pain, muscle weakness, depression and stiffness) are similar to those that also occur in healthy women during pregnancy may help women cope better. Adequate support is important throughout pregnancy and afterwards.

If nonpharmacologic options are insufficient to manage symptoms and drug treatment is deemed necessary, the following information may serve as a guide in making an informed decision. **Acetaminophen** is an appropriate analgesic for use in pregnancy. Short-term **NSAID** use may also be considered in the first and second trimester. However, their use in the third trimester may be of concern; because of antiprostaglandin effects, NSAIDs can increase risks of fetal and maternal bleeding and premature closure of the ductus arteriosus, and can also interfere with labour onset or duration.[47] The 2 most studied NSAIDs are **ibuprofen** and **naproxen**. Use of **tramadol** during pregnancy is not advised; neonatal withdrawal has been reported after long-term tramadol treatment in the pregnant mother.[48,49]

There is limited evidence on the effects of **gabapentin** or **pregabalin** in pregnancy or during breastfeeding. A preliminary study suggests gabapentin does not increase risk of major malformations, although it may be associated with other complications including low birth weight and preterm birth.[50] Until more information is available regarding their safety in pregnancy, use of gabapentin or pregabalin during pregnancy cannot be recommended.

If there is co-existing depression with fibromyalgia, the risk/benefit ratio may favour continuing treatment with antidepressants during pregnancy (see Chapter 6).

Tricyclic antidepressants, e.g., **amitriptyline** appear relatively safe during pregnancy. The SNRIs, e.g., **duloxetine**, while not associated with increased risk of congenital malformations, have been associated with short-term agitation, jitteriness and poor feeding in the neonate. Newborns exposed to **SSRIs** in utero had an increased incidence of preterm birth, low Apgar scores, increased admission to neonatal intensive care[51] and seizures; fetal death has been reported.[52] Maternal use of **fluoxetine** and other SSRIs has also been associated with neonatal persistent pulmonary hypertension[53] and septal heart defects.[54] Neonatal withdrawal syndrome may occur.[55]

Fibromyalgia and Breastfeeding

After delivery, lack of sleep and stress may aggravate fibromyalgia symptoms. Muscle pain, stiffness and fatigue may result in discomfort and interfere with the breastfeeding process. Proper positioning during feeding, feeding while lying down, use of pillows or other supports and adequate rest periods may assist breastfeeding by the mother with fibromyalgia. Referral to a lactation consultant may be useful.

Acetaminophen and **ibuprofen** are considered compatible with breastfeeding. Most other NSAIDs are also considered compatible; choose agents with shorter half-lives when possible. Small amounts of **tramadol** and its metabolites are excreted into breast milk, but published data of the effects on infants is lacking.[56]

Tricyclic antidepressants can cause sedation in the newborn if used in the antenatal period or during lactation. SSRIs and SNRIs are excreted into breast milk. Although some studies report no adverse effects from **fluoxetine** on breastfed infants,[57] poor weight gain, irritability, colic, vomiting, diarrhea, and/or decreased sleep have been noted in others.[58,59] The effects of **duloxetine**[60] on the infant are unknown. Until more data are available, **pregabalin** use is not advised for nursing mothers.[47]

A discussion of general principles on the use of medications in these special populations can be found in Appendix II and Appendix III. Other specialized reference sources are also provided in these appendices.

Therapeutic Tips

- The treatment of arthritis, hypothyroidism, peripheral neuropathy and other medical conditions may be complicated by concomitant fibromyalgia.
- Pharmacologic agents work best when combined with nonpharmacologic modalities, ideally as part of a multidisciplinary treatment program.[4]
- Patients may also require a combination of drugs with different mechanisms of action.
- It is important to document not only reduced pain but also improved function.
- In the experience of the author and other clinicians, patients with fibromyalgia may be unduly sensitive to drug side effects; a rational approach is to start medications at low doses and increase slowly by small increments.
- The initial improvement of fibromyalgia with pharmacotherapy fades with time. Patients may experience remission not necessarily attributed to any specific therapy. Conversely, there are subsets of patients who are intolerant of and/or unresponsive to all pharmacologic therapy.
- Sleep problems may need further study in a sleep disorder clinic.
- Concomitant mood disorders require higher doses of antidepressants than are used for fibromyalgia. For more information regarding antidepressants, see Chapter 6.
- Counselling the patient to recognize the roles of various social, psychological and/or environmental factors in the exacerbation or aggravation of his/her pain can lead to rewarding reductions in pain intensity. Emphasizing that the pain is "not in your head" but that life events and occurrences may be playing various roles in the syndrome's expression can be clinically beneficial.

Table 1: Drugs Used in Fibromyalgia

Class	Drug	Dose	Adverse Effects	Drug Interactions	Cost[a]
Analgesics	*acetaminophen*[c] Tylenol, Atasol Preparations, generics	325–1000 mg Q4H po Maximum dose 4 g/day	Hepatotoxicity with chronic high doses or in acute overdose.	Excessive alcohol intake may increase the risk of hepatotoxicity. Warfarin: increased anticoagulant effect particularly with use of >1.3 g/day for longer than 1 wk.	$
	tramadol extended-release Durela, Ralivia, Tridural, Zytram XL	Durela, Ralivia or Tridural: Start with 100 mg once daily po; may increase at weekly intervals to maximum 300 mg daily Zytram XL: Start with 150 mg once daily po; may increase at weekly intervals to maximum 400 mg daily	Somnolence, dizziness, flushing, constipation, nausea, pruritus, seizures, anaphylactoid reactions, dependence, withdrawal syndrome.	Possible increased risk of seizure with SSRIs, MAO inhibitors, tricyclic antidepressants and other tricyclic compounds, antipsychotics, amphetamines, linezolid, opioids or drugs that reduce the seizure threshold. Use with SSRIs or MAO inhibitors may also increase risk of serotonin syndrome. Use with CNS depressants may increase the risk of CNS and respiratory depression. Carbamazepine may increase the metabolism of tramadol. Also, tramadol may increase the risk of seizures in patients taking anticonvulsants.	$$$$
	tramadol with acetaminophen Tramacet, generics	Use lowest dose possible to achieve pain control. 1–2 tablets Q4–6H po PRN Maximum 8 tablets (300 mg tramadol + 2600 mg acetaminophen) daily	See tramadol extended-release.	See acetaminophen, tramadol extended-release.	$$$
GABA Derivatives	*gabapentin* Neurontin, generics	Starting dose: 100 mg QHS po. Titrate slowly as tolerated to 1200–2400 mg/day (in 2–3 divided doses).	Sedation, ataxia, tremor; less commonly, GI upset, peripheral edema, vision changes, weight gain.	Administration with aluminum/magnesium-containing antacids may decrease bioavailability. May have enhanced CNS depressant effects when coadministered with other CNS depressants.	$$
	pregabalin Lyrica, generics	Starting dose: 25–50 mg QHS po. Titrate slowly as tolerated to 300–450 mg/day (in 2 divided doses).	Sedation, dizziness, cognitive impairment, dry mouth, peripheral edema.	May have enhanced CNS depressant effects when coadministered with other CNS depressants. May cause peripheral edema/weight gain when coadministered with thiazolidinediones (pioglitazone, rosiglitazone).	$$

Class	Drug	Dose	Adverse Effects	Drug Interactions	Cost[a]
Nonsteroidal Anti-inflammatory Drugs[b]	*ibuprofen*[c] Advil, Motrin, generics	200–600 mg Q6H po	Peptic ulcer, dyspepsia, hypersensitivity, fluid retention, hypertension, renal toxicity.	Warfarin: increased anticoagulant effect. Antihypertensives: possible decreased in hypertensive effect. Lithium: may interfere with sodium/water balance. Monitor lithium levels when NSAID added. increased risk of GI bleeding when used with SSRIs.	$
Serotonin-Norepinephrine Reuptake Inhibitors	*duloxetine* Cymbalta	30–60 mg once daily po. Maximum: 120 mg/day (divided BID)	Nausea, headache, drowsiness, insomnia, dizziness, dry mouth. Do not use in patients with severe renal impairment (CrCl <30 mL/min).	Alcohol, CNS depressants. MAO inhibitors may cause serotonin syndrome (severe reaction—tremor, agitation, hypomania, hypertension). Tramadol may also increase risk of serotonin syndrome. Do not use with potent CYP1A2 inhibitors (e.g., ciprofloxacin, fluvoxamine, ketoconazole). CYP2D6 inhibitors (e.g., SSRIs) may increase duloxetine levels.	$$$$$
Selective Serotonin Reuptake Inhibitors	*fluoxetine*[c] Prozac, generics	10–20 mg QAM po (better efficacy in 1 trial when combined with amitriptyline in the evening)[28]	Nausea, dry mouth, somnolence, sweating, sexual dysfunction. increased risk of GI bleeding.	MAO inhibitors may cause severe reaction—tremor, agitation, hypomania, hypertension. Drugs that inhibit CYP enzymes (e.g., cimetidine, clarithromycin, erythromycin, fluconazole, indinavir, isoniazid, itraconazole, ketoconazole, quinidine, ritonavir) may increase SSRI levels. All SSRIs inhibit certain CYP isoenzymes and can decrease the clearance of other drugs (e.g., clozapine, methadone, mexiletine, phenytoin, pimozide, propafenone). Inducers of CYP enzymes (e.g., carbamazepine, phenobarbital, phenytoin, rifampin) can increase the clearance of SSRIs. increased risk of GI bleeding with NSAIDs.	$

(cont'd)

Table 1: **Drugs Used in Fibromyalgia** *(cont'd)*

Class	Drug	Dose	Adverse Effects	Drug Interactions	Cost[a]
Tricyclic Agents[b]	*amitriptyline*[c] Elavil, generics	5–50 mg 2–3 h before bedtime po (start low and titrate slowly)	Anticholinergic (dry mouth, blurred vision, constipation, urinary hesitancy, tachycardia, delirium), antihistaminergic (sedation, weight gain), orthostatic hypotension, lowered seizure threshold; sexual dysfunction.	Combination with MAO inhibitors may result in mania, excitation, hyperpyrexia; barbiturates, carbamazepine and rifampin may decrease effect; cimetidine and antipsychotics may increase effect and toxicity; possible interaction with antiarrhythmics (may lead to increased effect of either drug); may decrease antihypertensive effect of clonidine; may increase hypotensive effect of thiazides.	$
	cyclobenzaprine[c] generics	10 mg at bedtime po. May titrate to 40 mg/day taken in 2–4 divided doses. Lower doses (<5 mg) may also be effective.[61]	See amitriptyline.	See amitriptyline.	$

[a] Cost of 30-day supply of mean dose; includes drug cost only.
[b] Listed drugs are examples of medications in this class.
[c] Not a Health Canada-approved indication.
Dosage adjustment may be required in renal impairment; see Appendix I.
Abbreviations: CYP = cytochrome P450
Legend: $ <$25 $$ $25–50 $$$ $50–75 $$$$ $75–100 $$$$$ $100–125

Suggested Readings

Clauw DJ. Fibromyalgia: an overview. *Am J Med* 2009;122(12 Suppl):S3-S13.

Fitzcharles MA, Ste-Marie PA, Goldenberg DL et al. *2012 Canadian guidelines for the diagnosis and management of fibromyalgia syndrome*. Available from: fmguidelines.ca.

Fitzcharles MA, Ste-Marie PA, Pereira JX. Fibromyalgia: evolving concepts over the past 2 decades. *CMAJ* 2013 May 15. [Epub ahead of print].

Goldenberg MD, Burckhardt C, Crofford L. Management of fibromyalgia syndrome. *JAMA* 2004;292(19):2388-95.

Staud R. Pharmacological treatment of fibromyalgia syndrome: new developments. *Drugs* 2010;70(1):1-14.

Wolfe F, Clauw DJ, Fitzcharles MA et al. The American College of Rheumatology preliminary diagnostic criteria for fibromyalgia and measurement of symptom severity. *Arthritis Care Res (Hoboken)* 2010;62(5):600-10.

References

1. Abeles AM, Pillinger MH, Solitar BM et al. Narrative review: the pathophysiology of fibromyalgia. *Ann Intern Med* 2007;146(10):726-34.
2. Wolfe F, Clauw DJ, Fitzcharles MA et al. The American College of Rheumatology preliminary diagnostic criteria for fibromyalgia and measurement of symptom severity. *Arthritis Care Res (Hoboken)* 2010;62(5):600-10.
3. Fitzcharles MA, Ste-Marie PA, Pereira JX. Fibromyalgia: evolving concepts over the past 2 decades. *CMAJ* 2013 May 15. [Epub ahead of print].
4. Bennett RM. Multidisciplinary group programs to treat fibromyalgia patients. *Rheum Dis Clin North Am* 1996;22(2):351-67.
5. Karjalainen K, Malmivaara A, van Tulder M et al. Multidisciplinary rehabilitation for fibromyalgia and musculoskeletal pain in working age adults. *Cochrane Database Syst Rev* 2000;(2):CD001984.
6. Masi AT, White KP, Pilcher JJ. Person-centered approach to care, teaching, and research in fibromyalgia syndrome: justification from biopsychosocial perspective in populations. *Semin Arthritis Rheum* 2002;32(2):71-93.
7. Bennett R, Nelson D. Cognitive behavioral therapy for fibromyalgia. *Nat Clin Pract Rheumatol* 2006;2(8):416-24.
8. Busch AJ, Barber KA, Overend TJ et al. Exercise for treating fibromyalgia syndrome. *Cochrane Database Syst Rev* 2007;(4):CD003786.
9. Wang C, Schmid CH, Rones R et al. A randomized trial of tai chi for fibromyalgia. *N Engl J Med* 2010;363(8):743-54.
10. Mannerkorpi K. Exercise in fibromyalgia. *Curr Opin Rheumatol* 2005;17(2):190-4.
11. Rooks DS, Gautam S, Romeling M et al. Group exercise, education, and combination self-management in women with fibromyalgia: a randomized trial. *Arch Intern Med* 2007;167(20):2192-200.
12. Brosseau L, Wells GA, Tugwell P et al. Ottawa Panel evidence-based clinical practice guidelines for aerobic fitness exercises in the management of fibromyalgia: part 1. *Phys Ther* 2008;88(7):857-71.
13. Hassett AL, Gevirtz RN. Nonpharmacologic treatment for fibromyalgia: patient education, cognitive-behavioral therapy, relaxation techniques, and complementary and alternative medicine. *Rheum Dis Clin North Am* 2009;35(2):393-407.
14. Deluze C, Bosia L, Zirbs A et al. Electroacupuncture in fibromyalgia: results of a controlled trial. *BMJ* 1992;305(6864):1249-52.
15. Langhorst J, Klose P, Musial F et al. Efficacy of acupuncture in fibromyalgia syndrome—a systematic review with a meta-analysis of controlled clinical trials. *Rheumatology (Oxford)* 2010;49(4):778-88.
16. Deare JC, Zheng Z, Xue CC et al. Acupuncture for treating fibromyalgia. *Cochrane Database Syst Rev* 2013;5:CD007070.
17. Finestone HM, Stenn P, Davies F et al. Chronic pain and health care utilization in women with a history of childhood sexual abuse. *Child Abuse Negl* 2000;24(4):547-56.
18. Uceyler N, Hauser W, Sommer C. A systematic review on the effectiveness of treatment with antidepressants in fibromyalgia syndrome. *Arthritis Rheum* 2008;59(9):1279-98.
19. Hauser W, Bernardy K, Uceyler N et al. Treatment of fibromyalgia syndrome with antidepressants: a meta-analysis. *JAMA* 2009;301(2):198-209.
20. Arnold LM, Keck PE, Welge JA. Antidepressant treatment of fibromyalgia. A meta-analysis and review. *Psychosomatics* 2000;41(2):104-13.
21. Moore RA, Derry S, Aldington D et al. Amitriptyline for neuropathic pain and fibromyalgia in adults. *Cochrane Database Syst Rev* 2012;12:CD008242.
22. Tofferi JK, Jackson JL, O'Malley PG. Treatment of fibromyalgia with cyclobenzaprine: a meta-analysis. *Arthritis Rheum* 2004;51(1):9-13.
23. Hauser W, Urrutia G, Tort S et al. Serotonin and neoradrenaline reuptake inhibitors (SNRIs) for fibromyalgia syndrome. *Cochrane Database Syst Rev* 2013;1:CD010292.
24. Arnold LM, Gendreau RM, Palmer RH et al. Efficacy and safety of milnacipran 100 mg/day in patients with fibromyalgia: results of a randomized, double-blind, placebo-controlled trial. *Arthritis Rheum* 2010;62(9):2745-56.
25. Arnold LM, Hess EV, Hudson JI et al. A randomized, placebo-controlled, double-blind, flexible-dose study of fluoxetine in the treatment of women with fibromyalgia. *Am J Med* 2002;112(3):191-7.
26. Patkar AA, Masand PS, Krulewicz S et al. A randomized, controlled, trial of controlled release paroxetine in fibromyalgia. *Am J Med* 2007;120(5):448-54.
27. Norregaard J, Volkmann H, Danneskiold-Samsoe B. A randomized controlled trial of citalopram in the treatment of fibromyalgia. *Pain* 1995;61(3):445-9.
28. Goldenberg D, Mayskiy M, Mossey C et al. A randomized, double-blind crossover trial of fluoxetine and amitriptyline in the treatment of fibromyalgia. *Arthritis Rheum* 1996;39(11):1852-9.
29. Kim L, Lipton S, Deodhar A. Pregabalin for fibromyalgia: some relief but no cure. *Cleve Clin J Med* 2009;76(4):255-61. Erratum in: *Cleve Clin J Med* 2009;76(6):330.
30. Arnold LM, Russell IJ, Diri EW et al. A 14-week, randomized, double-blinded, placebo-controlled monotherapy trial of pregabalin in patients with fibromyalgia. *J Pain* 2008;9(9):792-805.

31. Crofford LJ, Mease PJ, Simpson SL et al. Fibromyalgia relapse evaluation and efficacy for durability of meaningful relief (FREEDOM): a 6-month, double-blind, placebo-controlled trial with pregabalin. *Pain* 2008;136(3):419-31.
32. Hauser W, Bernardy K, Uceyler N et al. Treatment of fibromyalgia syndrome with gabapentin and pregabalin—a meta-analysis of randomized controlled trials. *Pain* 2009;145(1-2):69-81.
33. Moore RA, Straube S, Wiffen PJ et al. Pregabalin for acute and chronic pain in adults. *Cochrane Database Syst Rev* 2009;(3):CD007076.
34. Arnold LM, Goldenberg DL, Stanford SB et al. Gabapentin in the treatment of fibromyalgia: a randomized, double-blind, placebo-controlled, multicenter trial. *Arthritis Rheum* 2007;56(4):1336-44.
35. Painter JT, Crofford LJ. Chronic opioid use in fibromyalgia syndrome: a clinical review. *J Clin Rheumatol* 2013;19(2):72-7.
36. Carville SF, Arendt-Nielsen S, Bliddal H et al. EULAR evidence-based recommendations for the management of fibromyalgia syndrome. *Ann Rheum Dis* 2008;67(4):536-41.
37. Biasi G, Manca S, Manganelli S et al. Tramadol in the fibromyalgia syndrome: a controlled clinical trial versus placebo. *Int J Clin Pharmacol Res* 1998;18(1):13-9.
38. Russell IJ, Kamin N, Bennett RM et al. Efficacy of tramadol in treatment of pain in fibromyalgia. *J Clin Rheumatol* 2000;6(5):250-7.
39. Bennett RM, Kamin M, Karim R et al. Tramadol and acetaminophen combination tablets in the treatment of fibromyalgia pain: a double-blind, randomized, placebo-controlled study. *Am J Med* 2003;114(7):537-45.
40. Bennett RM, Schein J, Kosinski MR et al. Impact of fibromyalgia pain on health-related quality of life before and after treatment with tramadol/acetaminophen. *Arthritis Rheum* 2005;53(4):519-27.
41. Gronblad M, Nykanen J, Konttinen Y et al. Effect of zopiclone on sleep quality, morning stiffness, widespread tenderness and pain and general discomfort in primary fibromyalgia patients. A double-blind randomized trial. *Clin Rheumatol* 1993;12(2):186-91.
42. Bossini L, Casolaro I, Koukouna D et al. Off-label uses of trazodone: a review. *Expert Opin Pharmacother* 2012;13(12):1707-17.
43. Bennett RM, Clark SC, Walczyk J. A randomized, double-blind, placebo-controlled study of growth hormone in the treatment of fibromyalgia. *Am J Med* 1998;104(3):227-31.
44. Borg-Stein J. Management of peripheral pain generators in fibromyalgia. *Rheum Dis Clin North Am* 2002;28(2):305-17.
45. Raphael KG, Marbach JJ. Comorbid fibromyalgia accounts for reduced fecundity in women with myofascial face pain. *Clin J Pain* 2000;16(1):29-36.
46. Ostensen M, Rugelsjoen A, Wigers SH. The effect of reproductive events and alterations of sex hormone levels on the symptoms of fibromyalgia. *Scand J Rheumatol* 1997;26(5):355-60.
47. Briggs GG, Freeman RK, Yaffe SJ. *Drugs in pregnancy and lactation: a reference guide to fetal and neonatal risk.* 9th ed. Philadelphia: Wolters Kluwer Health; Lippincott Williams & Wilkins; 2011.
48. Meyer FP, Rimasch H, Blaha B et al. Tramadol withdrawal in a neonate. *Eur J Clin Pharmacol* 1997;53(2):159-60.
49. Willaschek C, Wolter E, Buchhorn R. Tramadol withdrawal in a neonate after long-term analgesic treatment of the mother. *Eur J Clin Pharmacol* 2009;65(4):429-30.
50. Fujii H, Goel A, Bernard N et al. Pregnancy outcomes following gabapentin use: results of a prospective comparative cohort study. *Neurology* 2013;80(17):1565-70.
51. Lund N, Pedersen LH, Henriksen TB. Selective serotonin reuptake inhibitor exposure in utero and pregnancy outcomes. *Arch Pediatr Adolesc Med* 2009;163(10):949-54.
52. Wen SW, Yang Q, Garner P et al. Selective serotonin reuptake inhibitors and adverse pregnancy outcomes. *Am J Obstet Gynecol* 2006;194(4):961-6.
53. Chambers CD, Hernandez-Diaz S, Van Marter LJ et al. Selective serotonin-reuptake inhibitors and risk of persistent pulmonary hypertension of the newborn. *N Engl J Med* 2006;354(6):579-87.
54. Pedersen LH, Henriksen TB, Vestergaard M et al. Selective serotonin reuptake inhibitors in pregnancy and congenital malformations: population based cohort study. *BMJ* 2009;339:b3569.
55. Levinson-Castiel R, Merlob P, Linder N et al. Neonatal abstinence syndrome after in utero exposure to selective serotonin reuptake inhibitors in term infants. *Arch Pediatr Adolesc Med* 2006;160(2):173-6.
56. Ilett KF, Paech MJ, Page-Sharp M et al. Use of a sparse sampling study design to assess transfer of tramadol and its O-desmethyl metabolite into transitional breast milk. *Br J Clin Pharmacol* 2008;65(5):661-6.
57. Taddio A, Ito S, Koren G. Excretion of fluoxetine and its metabolite, norfluoxetine, in human breast milk. *J Clin Pharmacol* 1996;36(1):42-7.
58. Chambers CD, Anderson PO, Thomas RG et al. Weight gain in infants breastfed by mothers who take fluoxetine. *Pediatrics* 1999;104(5):e61.
59. Kristensen JH, Ilett KF, Hackett LP et al. Distribution and excretion of fluoxetine and norfluoxetine in human milk. *Br J Clin Pharmacol* 1999;48(4):521-7.
60. Lobo ED, Loghin C, Knadler MP et al. Pharmacokinetics of duloxetine in breast milk and plasma of healthy postpartum women. *Clin Pharmacokinet* 2008;47(2):103-9.
61. Moldofsky H, Harris HW, Archambault WT et al. Effects of bedtime very low dose cyclobenzaprine on symptoms and sleep physiology in patients with fibromyalgia syndrome: a double-blind randomized placebo-controlled study. *J Rheumatol* 2011;38(12):2653-63.

Chapter 79
Gout and Hyperuricemia

Suneil Kapur, MD, FRCPC and
Gunnar Kraag, MD, FRCPC

Gout is a disease in which monosodium urate monohydrate (MSU) crystals deposit in joints, soft tissues such as cartilage, tendon and bursa, or in renal tissues such as glomeruli, the interstitium and tubules. This can result in gouty arthritis, tophi, nephropathy or uric acid nephrolithiasis. Gouty arthritis is the most common cause of inflammatory arthritis in men older than 40 years of age. The mean age of onset is the fourth decade in males and the sixth decade in females. It is unusual for an attack to occur before age 30 in males and age 50 in females unless the patient has an inherited enzyme abnormality. The incidence and prevalence of gout is increasing, reflecting the fact that at-risk populations are increasing.

Studies have suggested an association between gout and metabolic syndrome,[1] as well as an increased risk of cardiovascular mortality in middle-aged men diagnosed with gout.[2] Studies have also shown that greater reduction of serum uric acid levels is associated with greater preservation of renal function.[3]

This chapter discusses the 4 stages of gouty arthritis: asymptomatic hyperuricemia, acute gouty arthritis, the intercritical period (prophylaxis of acute attacks and management of hyperuricemia) and chronic tophaceous gout.

Goals of Therapy

- Terminate the acute attack of arthritis
- Prevent recurrence
- Prevent or reverse complications
- Deal with associated disorders

The American College of Rheumatology (ACR) published the first guidelines for management of gout.[4,5] These guidelines provide a detailed set of recommendations for treating patients with gout and are incorporated into this chapter. They do not replace clinical judgement but provide viable therapeutic options.

Asymptomatic Hyperuricemia

Asymptomatic hyperuricemia refers to elevated serum urate levels (>360 μmol/L in females and 420 μmol/L in men) without any clinical manifestations.[6] During puberty, male serum urate levels increase by 60–120 μmol/L to levels of 240–360 μmol/L. These values remain sustained. Women develop increased urate levels after menopause, when values approach those of men. In 70% of patients with hyperuricemia, an underlying cause is discovered by history and physical examination.[6] Drugs and systemic conditions that may be associated with hyperuricemia are shown in Table 1. Hyperuricemia is not an indication for urate-lowering therapy. Most patients with hyperuricemia remain asymptomatic throughout life. Causes of uric acid overproduction should be assessed in certain patients, such as those with onset before the age of 25 and those with history of urolithiasis.[4]

This phase ends with the first attack of gouty arthritis or urolithiasis, typically after 20 years of sustained hyperuricemia. The annual incidence of acute arthritis is 0.1–0.5% among patients with a urate level between 420 and 540 µmol/L, and 5% when it is >540 µmol/L.[7] Similarly, the risk of nephrolithiasis increases with the serum urate level and the 24-hour urinary uric acid excretion.

Acute Gouty Arthritis

Investigations

History, physical and laboratory examinations:

- abrupt onset of excruciating pain and inflammation of joint during the night or early morning; patients cannot tolerate even light pressure such as a bed sheet on the affected joint
- most commonly affects joints of lower limb. There is a higher frequency of upper limb joint involvement in women compared to men[8]
- about 85% of first attacks are monoarticular; however, elderly patients often have a polyarticular presentation
- podagra (inflammation of first metatarsophalangeal [MTP] joint) is involved in >50% of first attacks. With time, >90% develop podagra. Other joints involved include, in decreasing order, insteps, ankles, heels, knees, wrists, interphalangeal joints and elbows
- predilection for damaged joints with osteoarthritis
- acute gouty bursitis may occur in prepatellar or olecranon bursa
- attacks often resolve spontaneously over 3–10 days
- precipitants of acute attacks include acute illness, surgery, trauma, alcohol, high purine diet and drugs (Table 1)
- presumptive diagnosis with triad of acute monoarthritis, hyperuricemia and dramatic response to **colchicine**
- definitive diagnosis requires identification of intracellular monosodium urate crystals in synovial fluid
- serum urate level can be difficult to interpret as a normal level does not necessarily rule out an acute gout attack.[9]

Table 1: Drugs and Conditions Associated with Hyperuricemia and Gout

Drugs	Conditions
Alcohol	Alcohol intake (excessive consumption)
Cyclosporine	Atherosclerosis
Cytotoxic chemotherapy	Chronic kidney, glomerular, interstitial renal disease
Diuretics (thiazide and loop)	Diabetes
Ethambutol	Hyperlipidemia
Interferon + ribavirin	Hypertension
Levodopa	Ischemic heart disease
Nicotinic acid (niacin)	Lead intoxication
Pyrazinamide	Metabolic syndrome
Salicylates, low-dose	Myeloproliferative disorders and some cancers
Tacrolimus	Obesity, dietary factors
Teriparatide	Urolithiasis history
	Rarely genetic or acquired causes of uric acid overproduction

Therapeutic Choices

Nonpharmacologic Choices

Topical ice application is an appropriate adjunctive therapy to one or more pharmacologic treatments for acute gouty arthritis.[5]

Pharmacologic Choices

Treatment of an acute gouty attack should be initiated as quickly as possible after onset (see Figure 1).

NSAIDs, **colchicine** or **oral corticosteroids** are appropriate first-line options in therapy of acute gout.[5] Treatment should be initiated within the first 24 hours of acute gout attack onset.

Traditionally, **colchicine** 0.6 mg was given each hour until there was control of inflammation, a total dose of 6 mg was reached or GI toxicity (nausea, vomiting, abdominal cramps or diarrhea) limited further use.[10] The current recommendation is to give 1.2 mg initially, then another 0.6 mg 1 hour later (for a total of 1.8 mg colchicine). This regimen is equally effective, with a much lower incidence of side effects [Evidence: SORT B*].[11] Colchicine is not recommended if the patient presents more than 36 hours after onset of symptoms [Evidence: SORT C*].[5]

NSAIDs including celecoxib are options for the therapy of acute gout.[5,12] They may become the first choice if colchicine is contraindicated but are also preferred by many clinicians. They are initiated at high doses then quickly reduced once improvement occurs (see Table 2). Adverse effects are more frequent in elderly patients with renal dysfunction. In patients at risk for ulcer complications (e.g., age >65, previous GI bleed or patients receiving anticoagulants or corticosteroids), celecoxib and/or cytoprotection with a proton pump inhibitor may be offered.[13]

Corticosteroids are a third option for acute gout therapy.[5,14] *Oral* corticosteroid options include high-dose prednisone, e.g., 0.5 mg/kg daily. With short-term use, tapering regimens are not usually necessary. The *intra-articular* injection of corticosteroids into a single joint at the time of diagnostic arthrocentesis is ideal therapy and usually results in rapid control of inflammation and symptoms. The intra-articular route may not be suitable for polyarticular joint involvement. Intra-articular, im or iv corticosteroids are particularly useful in patients unable to tolerate oral therapy.

Combination therapy is an appropriate option particularly when symptoms are severe, the attack is polyarticular or large joints are involved.[5] Combinations may include colchicine plus an NSAID, oral corticosteroids plus colchicine, or intra-articular corticosteroids plus an NSAID, oral corticosteroid or colchicine. Combination therapy may also be indicated in patients not responding to monotherapy.

Recombinant interleukin-1 beta (IL-1) receptor inhibitors such as **anakinra**[15] and **canakinumab**[16] inhibit the cytokine IL-1, which can contribute significantly to acute inflammation. These agents are not approved for use in gout but can be considered for off-label use in patients who are resistant to conventional therapy.[5]

Therapeutic Tips

- The earlier therapy is started, the more quickly the attack will be resolved.
- Do not stop or alter the dose of urate-lowering drugs during an acute attack, because symptoms may be exacerbated or prolonged.

* SORT (Strength of Recommendation Taxonomy) is a rating system (A, B or C) that addresses the quality of available evidence. For more information consult **How to Use *Compendium of Therapeutic Choices*** on page xxv.

Figure 1: **Treatment of Acute Gout**

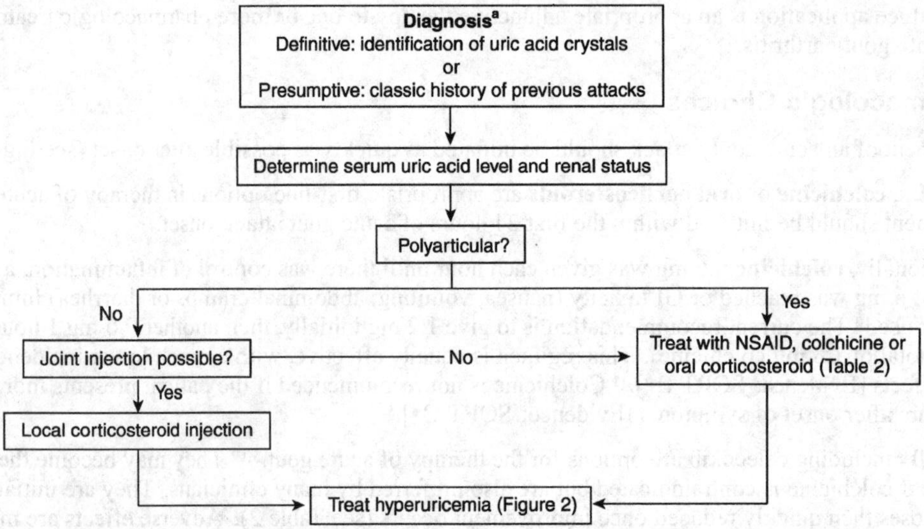

[a] Note: Do not stop or alter the dose of urate-lowering drugs during an acute attack.
Abbreviations: NSAID = nonsteroidal anti-inflammatory drug

Intercritical Period and Prophylaxis

The intercritical period is asymptomatic. Most patients have a second attack within 6–24 months of the first. Subsequent attacks are less explosive but more frequent, severe and enduring. These attacks are often polyarticular with upper extremity involvement and constitutional symptoms. Erosive radiographic changes and tophi may develop during the intercritical period, especially with frequent attacks of gouty arthritis. About 12–58% of patients have urate crystals in synovial fluid during this phase.[6] See Figure 2 for suggested management of hyperuricemia during the intercritical period.

Investigations

- History:
  - assess diet and lifestyle (Table 1)
  - assess comorbid conditions and intake of drugs that are associated with hyperuricemia (Table 1)
- Physical examination:
  - evaluate disease burden, including:
    - number of tophi
    - frequency and severity of gout attacks
- Laboratory tests:
  - complete blood count with differential
  - urinalysis
  - renal ultrasound
  - urine uric acid quantification
  - serum urate level

Figure 2: **Treatment of Hyperuricemia**

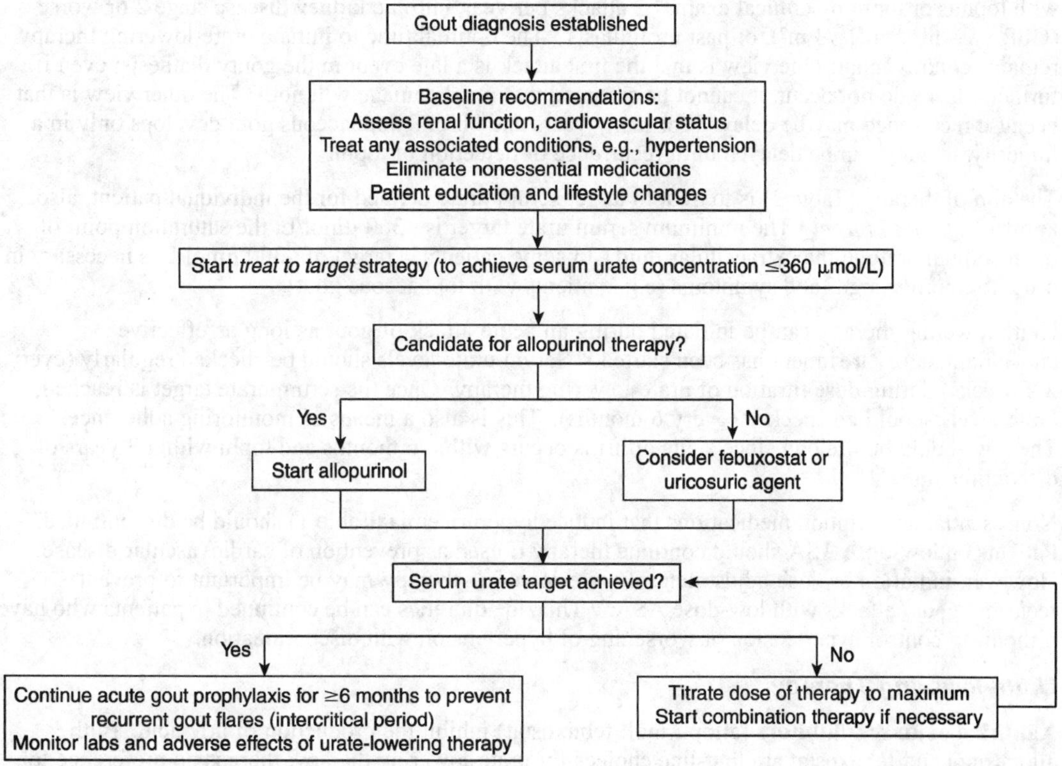

Therapeutic Choices

Nonpharmacologic Choices

There is a clear relationship between obesity (body mass index >30 kg/m^2) and gout. Obese patients should lose weight in order to achieve ideal body mass index. Encourage patients to exercise regularly, quit smoking, remain well hydrated and follow a healthy diet, as indicated below.[4] Such lifestyle changes can reduce serum urate by 10–18%.[17] The American College of Rheumatology recommends the following dietary guidelines:

- Avoid organ meats high in protein such as sweetbreads, liver, kidney
- Avoid foods and beverages high in fructose and corn syrup
- Avoid alcohol (particularly beer, but also wine and spirits) overuse, defined as >2 servings per day for a male or >1 serving per day for a female. Avoid any alcohol consumption during periods of frequent gout attacks or in poorly controlled gout
- Limit consumption of beef, lamb, pork and seafood with high purine content (sardines and shellfish)
- Limit consumption of table salt (including in sauces and gravies), table sugar and desserts
- Limit consumption of naturally sweet fruit juices, sweetened beverages
- Encourage low-fat or nonfat dairy products and vegetables

Pharmacologic Choices

Indications for pharmacologic urate-lowering therapy include established diagnosis of gouty arthritis with tophus or tophi by clinical exam, ≥2 attacks per year, chronic kidney disease stage 2 or worse (GFR ≤89 mL/min/1.73 m^2), or past urolithiasis.[4] The optimal time to initiate urate-lowering therapy remains controversial. One view is that the first attack is a late event in the gouty diathesis; even if further attacks do not occur, it cannot be assumed that renal damage will not.[18] The other view is that because recurrence may be delayed for many years and chronic tophaceous gout develops only in a minority, therapy can be delayed until recurrence or detection of tophi.

The aim of therapy (Table 2) is to treat to target serum urate defined for the individual patient, also known as *treat to target*.[4] The minimum serum urate target is <360 µmol/L, the saturation point of monosodium urate in the extracellular fluid.[6] In some patients, a target of <300 µmol/L is necessary in order to improve signs and symptoms (e.g., patients with tophaceous gout).

Urate-lowering therapy can be initiated during an acute attack of gout as long as effective anti-inflammatory treatment has been started.[19] Serum urate levels should be checked regularly (every 2–5 weeks) during dose titration of urate-lowering therapy. Once the serum urate target is reached, urate levels should be checked (every 6 months). This is also a means of monitoring adherence. Therapy should be lifelong since acute arthritis occurs within 6 months and tophi within 3 years of discontinuation.

Nonessential prescription medications that induce hyperuricemia (Table 1) should be discontinued. Patients on low-dose ASA should continue therapy if used as prevention of cardiovascular disease.[4] However, initiation or dose-adjustment of urate-lowering therapy may be important to prevent recurrent gouty attacks with low-dose ASA.[20] Thiazide diuretics can be continued in patients who have difficult-to-control hypertension or worsening of hypertension with discontinuation.

Urate-lowering Therapy

Xanthine oxidase inhibitors (allopurinol, febuxostat) inhibit the production of uric acid. Both allopurinol and febuxostat are first-line choices for urate-lowering therapy; there is no preference for one over the other.[4,21]

Full doses of **allopurinol** (300 mg per day) reduce serum urate concentrations to normal in 85% of patients with gout.[7] The starting dosage of allopurinol should not exceed 100 mg daily for any patient; if patients have stage 4 or worse chronic kidney disease (GFR ≤29 mL/min/1.73 m^2), the starting dose should be 50 mg daily. This strategy may help to reduce early gout flares during urate-lowering therapy and also to reduce severe hypersensitivity reactions. The dose should be titrated upward every 2–5 weeks to an appropriate maximum dose in order to achieve the target serum urate level (maximum dose is 800 mg daily). More than half of patients may require a dose of allopurinol greater than 300 mg daily. Doses this high may even be used in patients with renal impairment provided that they receive adequate education and regular monitoring for drug hypersensitivity and other adverse effects.

Rash is the most common side effect. Patients with mild reactions to allopurinol can be desensitized.[22] **Oxypurinol**, the metabolite of allopurinol, shares a 50% cross-reactivity with allopurinol, but it may be safer to desensitize with it.[23] It is currently unavailable in Canada.

The risk of allopurinol hypersensitivity syndrome (AHS) is about 1 in 1000 patients.[4] This can present with Stevens-Johnson syndrome, toxic epidermal necrolysis, or systemic diseases including rash, exfoliative dermatitis, fever, vasculitis, cytopenia, eosinophilia, and major end organ disease. The reported mortality rate is 20–25%. Risk factors for AHS include renal impairment, use of thiazide diuretics, high allopurinol starting dose, HLA-B*5801 genotype in persons of Korean descent with stage 3 or worse chronic kidney disease, or HLA-B*5801 in persons of Han Chinese or Thai descent.

Febuxostat, a newer xanthine oxidase inhibitor, is an option for patients with severe renal insufficiency because very small quantities are excreted renally compared with allopurinol. A study comparing febuxostat with allopurinol found that more patients achieved a serum uric acid level <360 µmol/L with febuxostat 80 mg per day than with allopurinol 300 mg per day; urate-lowering by febuxostat 40 mg per day was noninferior to allopurinol 300 mg per day.[24] The most commonly reported adverse reactions were liver function abnormalities, nausea, diarrhea, arthralgias and rash. Febuxostat is contraindicated in patients taking azathioprine or mercaptopurine due to the risk of severe toxicity from increased plasma concentrations of these drugs. Febuxostat is available as 80 mg only, which is also the maximum dose. The dose of febuxostat may be titrated up to 120 mg daily in patients who continue to have active disease with regular doses.

Probenecid is recommended as an alternative first-line urate-lowering therapy, although it is not currently available in Canada.[4] Other uricosuric agents that can be used include **fenofibrate**[25] or **losartan**.[26] Fenofibrate and losartan are not officially approved for gout prophylaxis and lack substantial evidence for this indication. Preliminary evidence suggests that either fenofibrate or losartan may provide a small decrease in uric acid levels when used as adjunctive therapy in patients with gout and dyslipidemia or hypertension.[27] While officially approved as a uricosuric, **sulfinpyrazone** is rarely used for treating gout. **Benzbromarone** is a uricosuric agent available through Health Canada's Special Access Programme; it may be used in patients not responsive to conventional uricosuric therapy.

It is important to accurately determine the creatinine clearance in order to select appropriate therapy. Uricosurics should not be used as first-line monotherapy in patients with creatinine clearance less than 50 mL per minute or with urolithiasis. Uricosurics are contraindicated in patients with elevated urine uric acid level (gross overproduction of uric acid). Patients should increase fluid intake and should be considered for urine alkalinization, i.e., potassium citrate.

If upward titration of the initial urate-lowering therapy (allopurinol or febuxostat) did not achieve target serum urate level or was not tolerated, substitute with another xanthine oxidase inhibitor. Combination therapy (xanthine oxidase inhibitor plus uricosuric agent) is appropriate if the serum urate target has not been achieved with monotherapy.

Uricases

Pegloticase, a recombinant pegylated uricase, is available in the United States for treatment of refractory hyperuricemia (not acute gout).[28] It is not yet available in Canada. **Rasburicase** is a uricolytic agent used only for treatment and prevention of hyperuricemia due to tumour lysis syndrome in cancer chemotherapy (see Chapter 127).

Prophylaxis of Acute Gout Flares during the Intercritical Period

Initiating any urate-lowering therapy may result in an increased incidence of acute gouty flares. Minimize the risk of acute attacks by protecting with a low-dose **NSAID** or **colchicine** when starting antihyperuricemic therapy.

In a study of patients prescribed allopurinol for chronic gouty arthritis, colchicine 0.6 mg twice daily was continued for 3 months after attaining a serum urate of <390 µmol/L.[29] This therapy effectively reduced the frequency and severity of acute gout flares and reduced the likelihood of recurrent flares. A lower dose of colchicine 0.6 mg once daily may also be effective.[5]

Fatalities have been reported in patients taking recommended doses of colchicine with concomitant medications that inhibit CYP3A4 or P-glycoprotein (P-gp), such as clarithromycin.[31] Reduce the dose or discontinue colchicine in patients with normal renal and hepatic function if treatment with a P-gp or a strong CYP3A4 inhibitor is required (see Table 2). Concomitant use of colchicine and P-gp or strong CYP3A4 inhibitors is contraindicated in patients with renal or hepatic impairment.

If there are contraindications to colchicine, substitute a low-dose NSAID (e.g., **naproxen** 250 mg twice daily). Although historically **indomethacin** use was common, there is no evidence that one NSAID is more effective than another. Use colchicine and NSAIDs with caution in elderly patients with renal and hepatic insufficiency.

If NSAIDs and colchicine are both contraindicated or ineffective, low-dose **prednisone** (<10 mg/day) is a second-line option.[5]

The ACR guidelines suggest the following options for duration of prophylaxis of acute gout flares during the intercritical period[5]:

- at least 6 months
- 3 months after achieving target serum urate and no tophi on exam
- 6 months after achieving target serum urate and 1 or more tophi on exam

Therapeutic Tips

- Do not treat asymptomatic hyperuricemia.
- Improve adherence by explaining the objectives of therapy, e.g., that antihyperuricemic drugs do not relieve pain and must be used continuously.
- A primary care physician should refer patients to a specialist in the following situations: unclear cause of hyperuricemia, unable to reach the target serum urate level, persistent symptoms or signs of gout, and multiple and/or serious adverse events from pharmacologic urate-lowering therapy.

Chronic Tophaceous Gout

This stage typically occurs 12 years from onset with a reported range of 3–42 years.[6] Only 2% of patients develop severe crippling disease. The strongest associated risk factor for developing tophi is the serum urate level.[6] Other factors include the frequency of attacks, duration of hyperuricemia and severity of renal disease. Common locations of tophi are the synovium, subchondral bone, digits of the hands and feet, olecranon bursa, Achilles tendon and helix of the ear. They can, however, occur anywhere including the conduction system of the heart. Tophi themselves are painless but they can lead to destruction of joints and deformities. Radiographic changes include paramarginal erosions with sclerotic margins and calcified tophi.[6] The optimal therapy for chronic tophaceous gout is prevention, through aggressive management of acute gout and correction of hyperuricemia. The aims of therapy are to control pain and inflammation, typically with NSAIDs, and to decrease serum uric acid levels. After several years of therapy, resorption of urate deposits will eventually lead to disappearance of tophi.

Table 2: Drug Therapy of Gout

Class	Drug	Dose	Adverse Effects	Drug Interactions	Comments	Cost[a]
Antimitotics	*colchicine* generics	Acute attack: 1.2 mg at first sign of flare, then 0.6 mg 1 h later Prophylaxis: 0.6–1.8 mg/day po	Common at higher doses: abdominal pain and cramps, diarrhea, nausea and vomiting. Rare: neuropathy, myopathy, bone marrow suppression.	May increase levels of HMG Co-A reductase inhibitors; monitor for statin myotoxicity (muscle pain, weakness). Decrease dose and monitor for colchicine toxicity (GI symptoms, fever, leukopenia) if also taking known inhibitors of CYP3A4 (e.g., antiretroviral drugs, clarithromycin, erythromycin, itraconazole, ketoconazole, verapamil) or P-gp (e.g., cyclosporine). Fatalities reported with clarithromycin which inhibits both CYP3A4 and P-gp.[31] Avoid grapefruit juice.	Reduce dosage, e.g., 0.6 mg daily or every 2nd day if elderly or renal impairment. Colchicine is contraindicated in patients with renal or hepatic impairment who are also taking CYP3A4 or P-gp inhibitors.	$$$$
Corticosteroids, intra-articular	*methylpred-nisolone acetate* Depo-Medrol, generics	Acute attack: Large joints: 20–80 mg intra-articularly Medium joints: 10–40 mg intra-articularly Small joints: 4–10 mg intra-articularly	Not usually significant after single intra-articular injection.			$
	triamcinolone acetonide Kenalog-10, Kenalog-40, generics	Acute attack: Large joints: 5–15 mg intra-articularly; maximum 40 mg Small joints: 2.5–5 mg intra-articularly; maximum 10 mg	See methylprednisolone acetate.			$$
	triamcinolone hexacetonide Aristospan	Acute attack: Large joints: 10–20 mg intra-articularly Small joints: 2–6 mg intra-articularly	See methylprednisolone acetate.			$$

(cont'd)

Table 2: **Drug Therapy of Gout** *(cont'd)*

Class	Drug	Dose	Adverse Effects	Drug Interactions	Comments	Cost[a]
Corticosteroids, systemic	*methylprednisolone sodium succinate* Solu-Medrol, generics	Acute attack: 0.5–2 mg/kg × 1 dose iv or im	Not usually significant after single injection.		Use when oral prednisone cannot be used.	$$
	prednisone generics	Acute attack: 0.5 mg/kg daily × 5 days po Effective dose range: 20–50 mg/day Prophylaxis: ≤10 mg/day	Except for GI disturbances and glucose intolerance, not usually significant with short-term use. Long-term effects are numerous.	Barbiturates, phenytoin and rifampin decrease corticosteroid effect.	Doses <20 mg/day may be ineffective. Simultaneous low-dose colchicine or NSAID helps prevent rebound when corticosteroid stopped.	$
Nonsteroidal Anti-inflammatory Drugs (NSAIDs)[b]	*celecoxib* Celebrex	Acute attack: 800 mg STAT po, then 400 mg on day 1, then 400 mg BID × 7 days po	For all NSAIDs: GI disturbances; headache is common with indomethacin. Other adverse effects are uncommon with short-term therapy but include fluid retention, hypertension, renal impairment, hypersensitivity. Celecoxib: patients with a history of heart attack, stroke, serious heart disease-related chest pain or serious heart disease such as HF should not use COX-2 inhibitors. Assess risk in patients with risk factors for heart attack and stroke.	Increased risk of bleeding with anticoagulants (e.g., warfarin) or antiplatelet agents (e.g., clopidogrel). Antihypertensives: may decrease antihypertensive effect. Lithium: may interfere with sodium/water balance. Monitor lithium levels when NSAID added. SSRIs: may increase risk of GI bleeding when used with NSAIDs.	There is no good evidence to suggest one NSAID is more efficacious than another. Suppositories may be used if oral route inadvisable. Contraindicated in patients with sulfa allergy.	~$55

Class	Drug	Dose	Adverse Effects	Drug Interactions	Comments	Cost[a]
	indomethacin generics	Acute attack: 75 mg STAT, then 50 mg Q6H × 2 days then 50 mg Q8H × 1 day then 25 mg Q8H × 1 day Prophylaxis: 25 mg BID po	For all NSAIDs: GI disturbances; headache is common with indomethacin. Other adverse effects are uncommon with short-term therapy but include fluid retention, hypertension, renal impairment, hypersensitivity.	Increased risk of bleeding with anticoagulants (e.g., warfarin) or antiplatelet agents (e.g., clopidogrel). Antihypertensives: may decrease antihypertensive effect. Lithium: may interfere with sodium/water balance. Monitor lithium levels when NSAID added. SSRIs: may increase risk of GI bleeding when used with NSAIDs.	There is no good evidence to suggest one NSAID is more efficacious than another. Suppositories may be used if oral route inadvisable.	$$
	naproxen Naprosyn, generics	Acute attack: 750 mg STAT, then 500 mg BID × 4–5 days po Prophylaxis: 250 mg BID	See indomethacin.	See indomethacin.	See indomethacin.	$
Uricosurics	*fenofibrate* Lipidil Micro, generics	200 mg daily po	Upper GI disturbances (nausea, abdominal pain, flatulence), myalgias, increases bile lithogenicity, increases CK, increases creatinine (not representative of renal function deterioration).	Caution when combining with statins. Monitor INR with concomitant warfarin use. Increases ezetimibe levels. Monitor for signs of cholelithiasis. Monitor renal function with concomitant cyclosporine use.	Not an approved use in Canada. Monitor CK, liver and renal function at 3, 6 and 12 months, then yearly. Contraindications: hepatic impairment, renal dysfunction, pre-existing gallbladder disease.	$$
	losartan Cozaar, generics	50 mg once daily po	Hypotension, hyperkalemia, renal insufficiency, angioedema (rare), headache, dizziness.	Diuretics: hypotension (monitor BP). Potassium-sparing diuretics and ACE inhibitors: hyperkalemia (monitor K+). Potassium: hyperkalemia (monitor K+). NSAIDs: may increase BP, fluid retention, renal failure. Lithium: lithium toxicity (monitor lithium levels).	Not an approved use in Canada. Monitor serum creatinine and potassium 7–14 days after initiation of therapy or dose changes.	$$

(cont'd)

Table 2: **Drug Therapy of Gout** *(cont'd)*

Class	Drug	Dose	Adverse Effects	Drug Interactions	Comments	Cost[a]
Xanthine Oxidase Inhibitors	*allopurinol* (renal symbol) Zyloprim, generics	Starting dose: 100 mg daily po Usual: 300 mg/day titrated to urate levels. Maximum: 800 mg/day Renal impairment: decrease maintenance dose to 100 mg/day if ClCr is 10–20 mL/min; 100 mg Q2–3 days if ClCr <10 mL/min	Skin rash, GI upset, hepatotoxicity, fever, severe hypersensitivity syndrome, xanthine stones (rare). May precipitate attack during initial phase of therapy.	Increases half-life of azathioprine and 6-mercaptopurine May increase toxicity of cyclophosphamide. Allopurinol inhibits hepatic metabolism of warfarin. Increased incidence of rashes when used with ampicillin or amoxicillin.	May need to increase dose or combine with uricosuric agents in chronic tophaceous gout. To prevent acute attacks on initiation of therapy, give prophylactic NSAID or colchicine for at least 6 months (see Prophylaxis of Acute Gout Flares during the Intercritical Period). Desensitization to allopurinol can be achieved in some patients, but sensitivity may recur.	$
	febuxostat Uloric	Starting dose: 40 mg daily po; may increase to 80 mg daily after 2 weeks if serum uric acid levels remain above 360 µmol/L	Nausea, arthralgia, skin rash (at higher dose). Increases hepatic aminotransferase levels. May precipitate attack during initial phase of therapy.	Azathioprine, mercaptopurine metabolism by xanthine oxidase may be decreased by febuxostat, resulting in significant toxicity. Do not use febuxostat with these drugs. Does not affect theophylline metabolism.[30] No dose adjustment necessary.	To prevent acute attacks on initiation of therapy, give prophylactic NSAID or colchicine for 2–3 weeks. May increase risk of stroke or MI compared with allopurinol.	~$55

[a] Cost of 30-day supply based on 70 kg body weight; includes drug cost only.
[b] Listed drugs are examples of medications in this class.
(renal symbol) Dosage adjustment may be required in renal impairment; see Appendix I.
Abbreviations: CYP = cytochrome P450; HF = heart failure; P-gp = P-glycoprotein
Legend: $ <$5 $$ $5–10 $$$ $10–15 $$$$ $15–20

Suggested Readings

Burns CM, Wortmann RL. Gout therapeutics: new drugs for an old disease. *Lancet* 2011;377(9760):165-77.

Khanna D, Fitzgerald JD, Khanna PP et al. 2012 American College of Rheumatology guidelines for management of gout. Part 1: systematic nonpharmacologic and pharmacologic therapeutic approaches to hyperuricemia. *Arthritis Care Res (Hoboken)* 2012;64(10):1431-46.

Khanna D, Khanna PP, Fitzgerald JD et al. 2012 American College of Rheumatology guidelines for management of gout. Part 2: therapy and antiinflammatory prophylaxis of acute gouty arthritis. *Arthritis Care Res (Hoboken)* 2012;64(10):1447-61.

Neogi T. Clinical practice. Gout. *N Engl J Med* 2011;364(5):443-52.

Sivera F, Andrés M, Carmona L et al. Multinational evidence-based recommendations for the diagnosis and management of gout: integrating systematic literature review and expert opinion of a broad panel of rheumatologists in the 3e initiative. *Ann Rheum Dis* 2014;73(2):328-35.

U.S. Food and Drug Administration. *Information for healthcare professionals: New safety information for colchicine (marketed as Colcrys)*. Available from: www.fda.gov/Drugs/DrugSafety/Post-marketDrug SafetyInformationforPatientsandProviders/DrugSafetyInformationfor HeathcareProfessionals/ucm174315.htm.

References

1. Choi HK, Ford ES, Li C et al. Prevalence of the metabolic syndrome in patients with gout: the Third National Health and Nutrition Examination Survey. *Arthritis Rheum* 2007;57(1):109-15.
2. Krishnan E, Svendsen K, Neaton JD et al. Long-term cardiovascular mortality among middle-aged men with gout. *Arch Intern Med* 2008;168(10):1104-10.
3. Whelton A et al. *Impact on renal function of quantitative serum uric acid reduction in gout patients*. Poster session presented at the American College of Rheumatology Annual Meeting; 2011 Nov 5-9; Chicago, IL.
4. Khanna D, Fitzgerald JD, Khanna PP et al. 2012 American College of Rheumatology guidelines for management of gout. Part 1: systematic nonpharmacologic and pharmacologic therapeutic approaches to hyperuricemia. *Arthritis Care Res (Hoboken)* 2012;64(10):1431-46.
5. Khanna D, Khanna PP, Fitzgerald JD et al. 2012 American College of Rheumatology guidelines for management of gout. Part 2: therapy and antiinflammatory prophylaxis of acute gouty arthritis. *Arthritis Care Res (Hoboken)* 2012;64(10):1447-61.
6. Wortmann RL. Gout and hyperuricemia. In: Firestein GS, Kelley WN, eds. *Kelley's textbook of rheumatology*. 8th ed. Philadelphia (PA): Saunders/Elsevier; 2009. p. 1481-524.
7. Emmerson BT. The management of gout. *N Engl J Med* 1996;334(7):445-51.
8. De Souza AW, Fernandes V, Ferrari AJ. Female gout: clinical and laboratory features. *J Rheumatol* 2005;32 (11):2186-8.
9. Schlesinger N, Norquist JM, Watson DJ. Serum urate during acute gout. *J Rheumatol* 2009;36(6):1287-9.
10. Schlesinger N, Schumacher R, Catton M et al. Colchicine for acute gout. *Cochrane Database Syst Rev* 2006;(4):CD006190.
11. Terkeltaub RA, Furst DE, Bennett K et al. High versus low dosing of oral colchicine for early acute gout flare: twenty-four-hour outcome of the first multicenter, randomized, double-blind, placebo-controlled, parallel-group, dose-comparison colchicine study. *Arthritis Rheum* 2010;62(4):1060-8.
12. Schumacher HR, Berger MA, Li-Yu J et al. Efficacy and tolerability of celecoxib in the treatment of acute gouty arthritis: a randomized controlled trial. *J Rheumatol* 2012;39(9):1859-66.
13. Lanza FL, Chan FK, Quigley EM et al. Guidelines for prevention of NSAID-related ulcer complications. *Am J Gastroenterol* 2009;104(3):728-38.
14. Janssens HJ, Lucassen PL, Van de Laar FA et al. Systemic corticosteroids for acute gout. *Cochrane Database Syst Rev* 2008;(2):CD005521.
15. So A, De Smedt T, Revaz S et al. Pilot study of IL-1 inhibition by anakinra in acute gout. *Arthritis Res Ther* 2007;9(2):R28.
16. So A, De Meulemeester M, Pikhlak A et al. Canakinumab for the treatment of acute flares in difficult-to-treat gouty arthritis: results of a multicenter, phase II, dose-ranging study. *Arthritis Rheum* 2010;62(10):3064-76.
17. Singh JA, Reddy SG, Kundukulam J. Risk factors for gout and prevention: a systematic review of the literature. *Curr Opin Rheumatol* 2011;23(2):192-202.
18. Fam AG. Should patients with interval gout be treated with urate lowering drugs? *J Rheumatol* 1995;22(9):1621-3.
19. Taylor TH, Mecchella JN, Larson RJ et al. Initiation of allopurinol at first medical contact for acute attacks of gout: a randomized clinical trial. *Am J Med* 2012;125(11):1126-34.e7.
20. Zhang Y, Neogi T, Chen C et al. Low-dose aspirin use and recurrent gout attacks. *Ann Rheum Dis*. 2014;73(2):385-90.
21. Tayar JH, Lopez-Olivo MA, Suarez-Almazor ME. Febuxostat for treating chronic gout. *Cochrane Database Syst Rev* 2012;11:CD008653.
22. Fam AG, Lewtas J, Stein J et al. Desensitization to allopurinol in patients with gout and cutaneous reactions. *Am J Med* 1992;93(3):299-302.
23. Earl JM, Saavedra M. Oxipurinol therapy in allopurinol-allergic patients. *Am Fam Physician* 1983;28(5):147-8.
24. Becker MA, Schumacher HR, Espinoza LR et al. The urate-lowering efficacy and safety of febuxostat in the treatment of the hyperuricemia of gout: the CONFIRMS trial. *Arthritis Res Ther* 2010;12(12):R63.
25. Feher MD, Hepburn AL, Hogarth MB et al. Fenofibrate enhances urate reduction in men treated with allopurinol for hyperuricaemia and gout. *Rheumatology (Oxford)* 2003;42(2):321-5.
26. Manolis AJ, Grossman E, Jelakovic B et al. Effects of losartan and candesartan monotherapy and losartan/hydrochlorothiazide combination therapy in patients with mild to moderate hypertension. Losartan Trial Investigators. *Clin Ther* 2000;22(10):1186-203.
27. Takahashi S, Moriwaki Y, Yamamoto T et al. Effects of combination treatment using anti-hyperuricaemic agents with fenofibrate and/or losartan on uric acid metabolism. *Ann Rheum Dis* 2003;62(6):572-5.
28. Anderson A, Singh JA. Pegloticase for chronic gout. *Cochrane Database Syst Rev* 2010;(3):CD008335.

29. Borstad GC, Bryant LR, Abel MP et al. Colchicine for prophylaxis of acute flares when initiating allopurinol for chronic gouty arthritis. *J Rheumatol* 2004;31(12):2429-32.
30. Tsai M, Wu JT, Gunawardhana L et al. The effects of xanthine oxidase inhibition by febuxostat on the pharmacokinetics of theophylline. *Int J Clin Pharmacol Ther* 2012;50(5):331-7.
31. Hung IF, Wu AK, Cheng VC et al. Fatal interaction between clarithromycin and colchicine in patients with renal insufficiency: a retrospective study. *Clin Infect Dis* 2005;41(3):291-300.

Chapter 80
Low Back Pain

Eldon Tunks, MD, FRCPC and
Paul Stacey, MD, MSc

This chapter summarizes the nonsurgical management of low back pain.

Goals of Therapy

Acute Low Back Pain

- Promote rapid/earlier recovery and reduce distress

Subacute/Recurrent Low Back Pain

- Assess appropriately and prevent chronicity
- Prevent or minimize work absence

Chronic Low Back Pain

- Promote or restore healthy behaviour, fitness and appropriate role functions by defining and treating medical and psychological factors associated with persistent/recurrent pain, according to evidence-based principles

Acute Low Back Pain

Acute: 0–30 days from onset (Figure 1).

Investigations

Clinical history, relevant physical examination and neurologic assessment. Identify "red flags" (Table 1).[1,2,3,4,5] When red flags are present, further investigation and/or referral for consultation are indicated. Arrange diagnostic imaging and laboratory tests consistent with bedside examination findings. Initial work up should consider common conditions, red flags and other possibilities (e.g., ankylosing spondylitis, lumbo-pelvic pain syndromes).

Sciatica refers to pain originating in the back and referred below the level of the knee. There are two subsets: sciatica with radiculopathy (demonstrable on neurologic exam, electromyogram, CT or MRI) and sciatica without radiculopathy, likely due to a referred pain mechanism.

Therapeutic Choices

Nonpharmacologic Choices

For acute or recurrent back pain without sciatica of <30 days, provide symptomatic relief, encourage the patient to continue or resume activity and work as soon as tolerated and educate the patient to expect early recovery. Avoid unnecessary bedrest for uncomplicated back pain as well as premature physical therapy. This approach results in the shortest duration of sick leave and pain and some improvement in ability to perform daily activity.[5,6,7,8,9]

Table 1: **"Red Flag" Symptoms/Signs in Assessment of Low Back Pain**

Condition	Red Flags in Patient with Low Back Pain	Investigations
Cancer	Age >50; previous cancer history; unexplained weight loss; failure to improve after 1 month of treatment[2]	Positive laboratory tests (including elevated ESR, reduced hematocrit)[2] and imaging showing erosion or blastic lesions
Cauda equina syndrome	Acute urinary retention or overflow incontinence; loss of anal sphincter tone/fecal incontinence; perineal numbness; change in sexual function; weakness of legs[1]	Emergency neurological assessment and MRI of lumbosacral spine
Epidural abscess	Intravenous drug abuse or sources of infection; local or radicular pain unrelieved by position change; fever, sensory loss, paraparesis or quadriparesis, bowel/bladder impairment	Emergency neurological examination, positive laboratory tests for source of infection; MRI of spinal cord, urine drug screen
Herniated nucleus pulposus	Positive SLR (leg pain at <60°); weak dorsiflexion of ankle (L4-5) or great toe (L5-S1 or L4-5); reduced ankle reflex (L5-S1); reduced light touch in L4, L5 or S1 dermatomes of foot/leg[1]	MRI of lumbar spine
Spinal fracture or compression fracture	Age >50, female gender, major trauma, pain and tenderness, and a distracting painful injury;[4] also consider a history of osteoporosis or corticosteroid use	Plain x-rays of the spine
Spinal osteomyelitis	Intravenous drug abuse; sources of infection (e.g., skin, teeth, urinary tract or indwelling catheter); fever; vertebral tenderness[3]	Positive laboratory tests for source of infection; urine drug screen, MRI of spine

Abbreviations: MRI = magnetic resonance imaging; SLR = straight leg raising

Although often used, especially by allied health professionals treating low back pain, the evidence for acupuncture efficacy is weak and contradictory.[10,11]

For acute back pain with sciatica, advise patients to continue activities according to tolerance. Physiotherapy offers slightly better functional status at 4 weeks' follow up compared to bed rest, with no difference in outcomes for pain. There is no advantage to bed rest in acute back pain with sciatica.[6,7]

Pharmacologic Choices

Drug therapies for the management of low back pain and neck pain are presented in Table 3.

For acute uncomplicated low back pain, **NSAIDs** are effective for pain relief, particularly during the first few weeks, but there is no evidence that one NSAID or COX-2 inhibitor (celecoxib) is more effective than another.[12] Celecoxib shows fewer GI side effects compared to traditional NSAIDs, and several NSAIDs (both COX-2 selective and nonselective NSAIDs) have been associated with increased cardiovascular risks in certain patient populations.[13] Vascular risk in particular is greater with celecoxib and diclofenac.[14] Therefore, when selecting an NSAID, consider tolerability, patient contraindications (risk of GI or cardiovascular adverse events, other contraindications to use) and cost.

There is moderate evidence that NSAIDs are not more effective than acetaminophen for back pain.[12] Given the greater safety profile compared to NSAIDs or COX-2 inhibitors, a trial of **acetaminophen** (e.g., 500 mg Q4H), is a reasonable option in acute uncomplicated back pain. Institute NSAID therapy in patients with acute uncomplicated back pain who fail to obtain relief with acetaminophen. NSAIDs may be considered first in patients with suspected facet joint syndrome or foraminal stenosis.

During the acute phase of low back pain, **muscle relaxants** may be effective for relief of pain and spasm during short-term use, but are more likely to cause adverse effects such as drowsiness and dizziness.[5,15] Muscle relaxants might include **benzodiazepines**, **cyclobenzaprine**, nonprescription preparations containing **methocarbamol** or **orphenadrine**, or the antispasticity drugs **baclofen** or **tizanidine**. A muscle relaxant may also be combined with an NSAID or COX-2 inhibitor for relief of pain and spasm in acute back pain.

Early use of strong opioids does not offer advantages in disability outcome, thus nonopioid options are preferable early on. A prospective study of patients with low back pain found slightly greater propensity for disability at 6 months for those taking opioids, compared to those not taking opioids.[16]

Not all types of back pain have the same mechanism. In soft tissue and hyperalgesic pain, agents with a central mechanism of action are preferred (e.g., baclofen, buprenorphine, GABA derivatives, tramadol). In prostaglandin-mediated pain, NSAIDs are preferred. When pain is severe and not responsive to other appropriate measures, opioids may be considered, beginning with acetaminophen with codeine.

The herbal medicines **devil's claw** (*harpagophytum procumbens*), **white willow bark** (*salix alba*) and topical **capsicum** (*capsicum frutescens*) have shown some efficacy in short-term trials, but there is no evidence that they are safe and useful for long-term use.[17]

Figure 1: Management of Low Back Pain

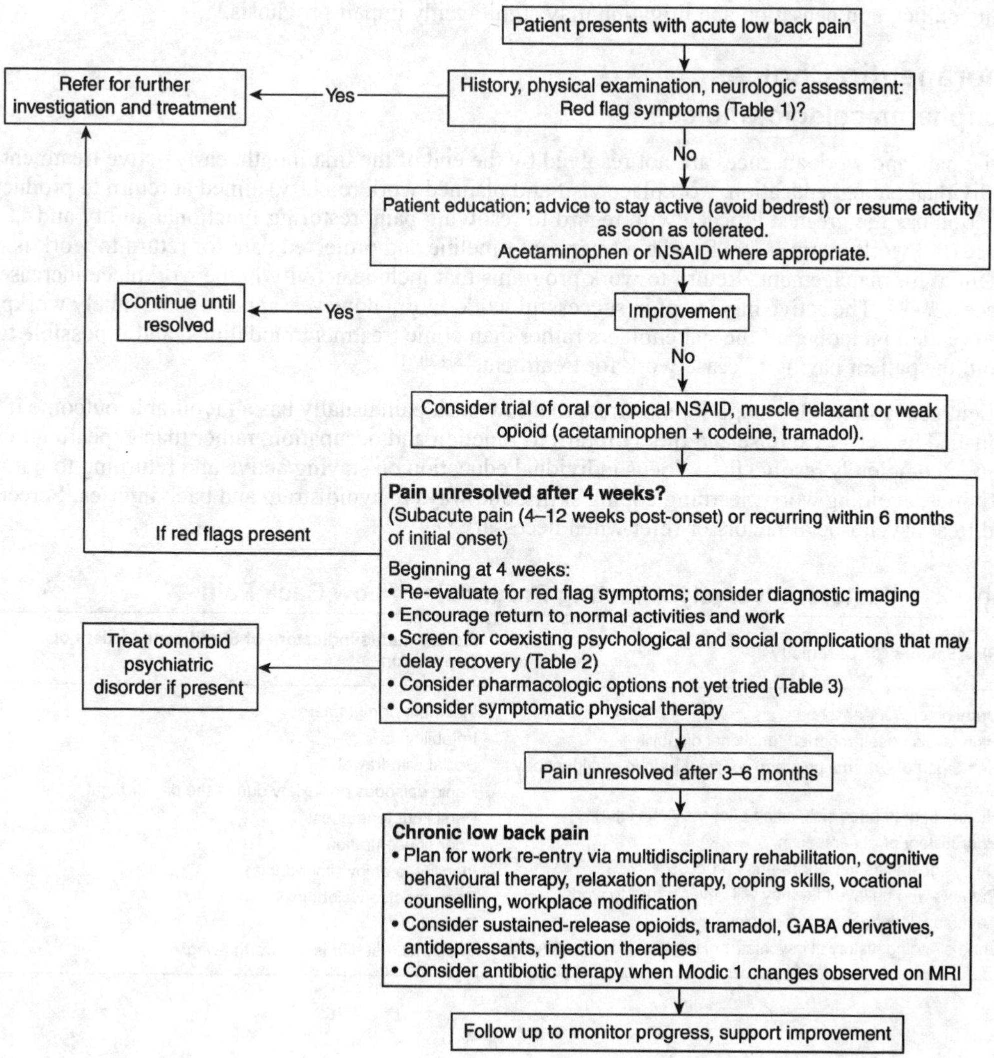

Subacute and Recurrent Low Back Pain

Subacute: 4–12 weeks post onset; recurrent: up to 6 months after onset (Figure 1).

Investigations

When there is persistent or recurrent pain and interference with vocational function, re-evaluate the patient.[5] When red flags are present (Table 1), imaging and consultation are recommended. After the first 4–6 weeks, in addition to imaging, electromyography may be helpful if there are clinical findings suggestive of nerve root involvement.

One of the strongest predictors of satisfactory adjustment is vocational status, and delay in work return significantly reduces the likelihood of ever returning.

For recurrent back pain or persistent back pain of 3–6 months, reassessment is advised. This should include screening for psychosocial complications (Table 2).[5,9,18] Although compensation or litigation alone has an indefinite effect on prognosis, where compensation levels are high or when the employee is in conflict, compensation and litigation may significantly impair prognosis.[18]

Therapeutic Choices

Nonpharmacologic Choices

If the pain and work absences are not resolved by the end of the first month, early active treatment (individual patient education, workplace visit and planned work re-entry) aimed at return to productive function has the greatest efficacy with regard to resolving pain, restoring functional ability and successful work return.[19,20,21] Setting a treatment timeline and projected date for return to work is essential for management. Return to work programs that include activity in the workplace increase success.[18,20,21] The active ingredient in successful work return, however, appears to be timely workplace intervention including all the stakeholders rather than clinic treatment modalities, and if possible to avoid the patient having to cease work for treatment.[7,8,9,20,21]

Patient education at this stage should stress that low back pain usually has a favourable outcome if it is managed by active exercise and timely return to function and occupation, rather than expecting the pain to completely resolve first. Focus individual education on staying active and returning to normal activities, avoiding worry, learning coping skills, and ways to avoid strain and back injuries. Screen for and treat psychosocial factors or refer when necessary.[9,18]

Table 2: **Factors Adversely Affecting Prognosis of Low Back Pain**

Risk Factors for Chronicity	Mental Status Indicators of Significant Anxiety or Depression
Duration of work absence	Insomnia or nightmares
High levels of self-reported functional disability	Irritability
Self-report of extreme pain and constant pain in multiple body areas	Social withdrawal
History of prolonged sick-listing after previous injuries	Panic episodes or anxiety during the day or night
Prior history of absenteeism	Persistent tearfulness
Delays/obstacles in work re-entry process	Poor concentration
Patients who believe that they will never return to work	Inability to enjoy (anhedonia)
Adversarial attitude toward employer	Poor appetite/weight loss
Long-standing history of psychiatric distress or maladjustment	Poor libido
	Thoughts that "life is not worth living"

There are many potential modalities of symptomatic physical therapy, e.g., ice, heat, laser, ultrasound, massage, manipulation, acupuncture, transcutaneous electrical nerve stimulation (TENS). Evidence for efficacy of any individual modality is presently inadequate, with the exception that active exercise and avoidance of unnecessary bedrest improve outcomes.[6,7] Combining modalities (e.g., massage plus exercise, or manipulation plus exercise) is more effective than single modality treatment.[22,23]

At approximately 3–6 months, the focus is on interrupting progress toward chronic pain. If there is marked functional disability associated with pain that is recurrent or persisting for 3 months or more, establish a coordinated program among the primary care provider, patient, employer and compensation agency. If the coordinated program is unsuccessful, identify possible psychological comorbidity and consider timely referral to a multidisciplinary chronic pain management clinic for intensive treatment.[5,18]

Pharmacologic Choices

Drug therapies for the management of low back pain and neck pain are presented in Table 3.

Chronic Low Back Pain

Chronic: ≥6 months post onset (Figure 1).

Investigations

Be aware of coexisting psychological and social complications since these are important obstacles to improvement or recovery (Table 2).

Therapeutic Choices

Nonpharmacologic Choices

Nonpharmacologic therapy is most effective with a combination of 2 or more modalities,[5,18] including:

- Active exercise
- "Back school" or patient education
- Functional restoration
- Physical conditioning programs[24]
- Yoga[25]
- Multidisciplinary rehabilitation[26]
- Relaxation therapy
- Cognitive and behavioral therapy (inconsistent evidence)[27,28]
- Psychosocial intervention and training in coping skills

For chronic low back pain, the goal of therapy is to regain function, which often translates into work re-entry. Efficacy for work return as a specific outcome is associated with conducting therapy if possible in the work setting or workplace visits, in the context of a planned work re-entry.[21] When combined in a multimodal package, nonpharmacologic options such as patient education, cognitive behavioral therapy and relaxation therapy are more effective for chronic low back pain if conducted in the context of workplace and work re-entry [Evidence: SORT B*].[20,21] Additionally, patients must be engaged in goal-setting and monitoring progress for optimal outcomes.[9,18] For pain management resources and links, see www.canadianpainsociety.ca/en/links.html.

* SORT (Strength of Recommendation Taxonomy) is a rating system (A, B or C) that addresses the quality of available evidence. For more information consult **How to Use *Compendium of Therapeutic Choices*** on page xxv.

There is a lack of evidence regarding whether patients who have failed treatment in a multidisciplinary rehabilitation program (or chronic pain management program) will benefit from a second attempt. After treatment failure, identify and address barriers that interfered with progress. These might include a psychiatric disorder (especially major depression, anxiety disorder or dysthymia), an attitudinal problem such as unwillingness to set goals for change, a substance or medication abuse problem, a previously undetected medical/surgical problem or obstacles to work re-entry within the job environment.

For chronic back pain, there is anecdotal but insufficient clinical trial evidence to recommend therapeutic ultrasound,[29] radiofrequency denervation of facet joints,[30] manual material handling intervention and assistive devices for preventing and treating back pain in workers,[31] insoles,[32] lumbar supports[33] or prolotherapy.[34] For *acupuncture* alone or combined with other therapies for chronic back pain, there is limited evidence of short-term relief of pain and functional impairment.[35]

Pharmacologic Choices

Drug therapies for the management of low back pain and neck pain are presented in Table 3.

Despite widespread use of many medications for the treatment of chronic low back pain, there is a lack of high-quality evidence. There is some support for **NSAID** use for chronic low back pain.[36]

Efficacy of antidepressants (e.g., bupropion, SSRIs, tricyclic antidepressants) has not been demonstrated for relief of chronic low back pain.[37] Nevertheless, chronic pain is often associated with comorbidities. When major depression or anxiety disorders are comorbid with chronic pain, psychotropic medications may be indicated for proper treatment, even though the pain itself will not necessarily be improved by these medications. **Duloxetine** is the only antidepressant approved for use in chronic low back pain but its place in therapy is undetermined. It may be a cost-effective option in the elderly, who are at an increased risk of GI and CV complications due to NSAIDs.[38]

Adequate evidence for muscle relaxants for chronic back pain is lacking.[36] Although there is no quality evidence, there is some clinical experience that the GABA derivatives **gabapentin** or **pregabalin** may sometimes be helpful for chronic low back pain associated with pain/tenderness in multiple areas.

There is limited evidence that **tramadol** with or without acetaminophen is more effective than placebo for uncomplicated chronic back pain.[39]

Some patients with persistent low back pain respond to **opioid analgesics**;[36] they may be used if other nonopioid and weak opioid analgesic options have proven inadequate for pain control and if there are no contraindications for their use. Physicians may prefer **acetaminophen with codeine** over strong opioids because of concerns about misuse. However codeine can also be misused, acetaminophen has a toxic effect on the liver with excessive use, and a significant minority of patients do not have effective analgesia from codeine due to impaired CYP2D6 function.[40] If used, acetaminophen with codeine should be only one part of a more comprehensive treatment plan.

If opioids are to be used in more than small doses and for a longer period of time, sustained-release preparations are preferable. Buprenorphine transdermal patch is useful in chronic back pain when there is significant central sensitization or myofascial pain. It is also well tolerated in the elderly and in cases of renal impairment, but approximately 20% of patients develop contact dermatitis under the transdermal patch.[41]

Consider strong opioid analgesics when pain is a significant barrier to function, is an unremitting source of distress, has not responded to other treatment options and if there are otherwise no significant psychological or medical contraindications. When prescribing opioids or other controlled substances, screen patients for risks of potential drug abuse and prescribe with appropriate precautions and follow-up.[42] If in doubt, obtain a consultation.

There is limited but encouraging evidence for the efficacy of **amoxicillin/clavulinate** for treatment of chronic low back pain associated with Modic 1 changes on MRI.[43] These changes are found in approximately 35–40% of patients and indicate vertebral bone edema that may be related to an infectious process.

Injection therapies for chronic low back pain, e.g., trigger point blocks with **local anesthetics** or **epidural steroids**, have not had statistically significant efficacy with regard to pain relief and work disability;[44,45] however, there is a tendency toward positive results with only minor side effects. Studies of facet joint injections with **corticosteroid**, with or without local anesthetic, have found conflicting evidence for relief compared to placebo. There is limited evidence for efficacy of trigger point blocks for short-term relief.[44] Injection therapy may be attempted in patients with low back pain, provided injections are well tolerated and accompanied by patient improvement for an adequate duration. Injection therapy should be accompanied by other proven rehabilitation therapies.

Choices during Pregnancy and Breastfeeding

Low Back Pain and Neck Pain in Pregnancy

More than 50% of pregnant women will experience back pain during pregnancy, usually in the lumbar and sacroiliac areas. Low back pain in pregnancy is more likely if there is a previous history of low back pain or overweight. Contributing factors include hormonal changes, anterior displacement of the centre of gravity which accentuates lumbar lordosis, and weight gain during pregnancy. Spondylolysis or the progression of spondylolisthesis may occur. There is a small risk of disk herniation during pregnancy; if imaging is necessary, noncontrast MRI could be performed.

Neck pain may also be exacerbated during pregnancy, especially if there is coexistent low back pain and weight gain.

Nonpharmacologic Choices

Since the majority of treatment of back and neck pain is nonpharmacologic, most of the recommendations remain applicable to the expectant mother. Ideally, a woman planning a pregnancy should address problems of weight and core fitness before conception. During pregnancy, a program of walking and modified exercise is recommended to strengthen abdominal and back muscles. Advice on exercise and body mechanics should be modified to be consistent with the stage of pregnancy.

Evidence suggests benefit from exercise, education, water-based exercise, multimodal physical therapies including manual therapy, and acupuncture.[46,47] However, the evidence for these treatments is limited in quantity and quality.

Transcutaneous electrical nerve stimulation (TENS) can be used over a limb during pregnancy but not over the low back or abdomen due to the possibility of precipitation of labour.

Pharmacologic Choices

If nonpharmacologic options are insufficient to manage back pain and drug treatment is deemed necessary, the following information may serve as a guide in making an informed decision.

Acetaminophen in therapeutic doses is an appropriate choice for analgesia in the pregnant woman. Short-term use of **NSAIDs** in the first or second trimester may be considered. Third-trimester use of NSAIDs should be avoided due to increased risk of oligohydramnios, premature closure of the ductus arteriosus and neonatal pulmonary hypertension.[48] Avoid use of topical diclofenac that is formulated in a dimethyl sulfoxide (DMSO) vehicle as the vehicle's safety in pregnancy is unknown.

Where possible, avoid **opioid** use during pregnancy; if not feasible, the lowest effective dose should be used for the shortest possible time, as high doses and use near term may result in adverse neonatal effects (opioid withdrawal syndrome, respiratory depression). Weaning from chronic opioid therapy, where feasible, should begin in the second trimester to reduce the risk of spontaneous abortion or preterm labour. Dose reductions of no more than 10% of the total dose per week are suggested.[49] The last 30% of dose reduction may require slower tapering, e.g., reducing by 5% of the total dose per week. Small amounts of immediate-release opioid may be required to treat transient symptoms of withdrawal during the final week of weaning.

Neonatal withdrawal has also been reported after long-term **tramadol** treatment in the pregnant mother.[50,51]

Tricyclic antidepressants are considered relatively safe in pregnancy,[48] but should generally not be used to treat chronic low back or neck pain during pregnancy as evidence regarding their efficacy is lacking.

Avoid use of **muscle relaxants** (baclofen, cyclobenzaprine, methocarbamol, orphenadrine) as there are insufficient data on their safe use during pregnancy. There is a possible risk of congenital malformations with **diazepam** use, and extended use in the pregnant mother has been associated with adverse effects in the neonate such as drug withdrawal and floppy infant syndrome.[48]

Insufficient data are available regarding the safe use of gabapentinoids (**gabapentin, pregabalin**) during pregnancy.

Lidocaine or **bupivacaine** may be used to inject trigger points for pain control. In pregnancy, the doses should be low, and lidocaine or bupivacaine should be avoided in the presence of fetal distress or anoxia—conditions that might occur during delivery.[52,53] **Normal saline** may be used for injection of trigger points as an alternative to lidocaine or other local anesthetics.

Low Back Pain and Neck Pain during Breastfeeding

In the postpartum and breastfeeding period, about one-third of women will continue to experience low back pain. Risk factors include the weight gain during pregnancy, lifting and carrying the infant and the ergonomics of how the mother carries and tends the infant.

Nonpharmacologic Choices

During the postpartum period, continue a program of walking and modified exercise to strengthen abdominal and back muscles. It is also important to institute appropriate diet and weight loss and to focus on good body mechanics when carrying and caring for the baby.

There is no contraindication to the use of TENS on the breastfeeding mother except while the infant is actually nursing.

Pharmacologic Choices

Acetaminophen in therapeutic doses is an appropriate choice for analgesia in the breastfeeding mother. **Ibuprofen** has also been used safely during breastfeeding. Short-term use of most other NSAIDs is generally considered compatible with breastfeeding;[54] choose agents with shorter half-lives where possible.

Opioid use by the breastfeeding mother can cause respiratory depression or lead to drug withdrawal syndrome in the newborn. A case of fatal morphine poisoning has been reported in an infant whose mother received **codeine** postpartum.[55] Since codeine is metabolized to morphine, high-dose or prolonged use of codeine products may lead to toxicity in the newborn. Mothers who are CYP2D6 ultrarapid metabolizers are at higher risk of excessive morphine levels in the breast milk.[56] To prevent possible accumulation of morphine in neonates, avoid codeine-containing products in breastfeeding mothers.[57]

Small amounts of **tramadol** and its metabolites are excreted into breast milk, but published data of the effects on infants are lacking.[58]

Tricyclic antidepressants can cause sedation in the newborn if used in the antenatal period or during breastfeeding.[54]

Diazepam accumulates in the newborn during breastfeeding and is associated with a risk of adverse effects in the infant.[48] There is no published information on the effects of most other nonbenzodiazepine muscle relaxants on the breastfed infant.

Limited data indicate that low levels of **gabapentin** appear in infant serum, but no apparent adverse effects to the baby have been reported.[59]

General Considerations

A discussion of general principles on the use of medications in these special populations can be found in Appendix II and Appendix III. Other specialized reference sources are also provided in these appendices.

Therapeutic Tips

- A significant minority of chronic pain sufferers have comorbid depression, anxiety or dysthymia (chronic depression/anxiety), often masked by the pain presentation. Key symptoms (Table 2) can reveal the underlying mood disorder. Comorbid mood disorders often respond to antidepressants, which can improve coping with pain.
- For back pain and chronic soft tissue pain, **tricyclic** or other types of **antidepressants** have equivocal efficacy, but may be useful for their antidepressant effect.[18]
- Some patients with back pain who have difficulty sleeping may benefit from a caffeine-free analgesic product.

Table 3: **Drugs Used in the Treatment of Back and Neck Pain**

Class	Drug	Dose	Adverse Effects	Drug Interactions	Comments	Cost[a]
Analgesics, nonopioid	*acetaminophen* Atasol Preparations, Tylenol, generics	325–650 mg Q4H po	Hepatotoxicity with acute overdose or chronic high doses.	Increased anticoagulant effect of warfarin may occur with use of >1.3 g/day acetaminophen for >1 wk.	Found in many combination products marketed for relief of pain, muscle spasms, cold and flu, menstrual symptoms, etc. Total intake **from all sources** not to exceed 4 g/day.	$
Benzodiazepines	*diazepam* Valium, generics	2–5 mg BID to QID po for acute pain	Drowsiness, cognitive impairment, drug dependence, falls, accumulation in the elderly and in presence of liver or kidney disease.	Potentiation of cognitive impairment when used with opioids. Potentiation of alcohol intoxication.	In acute pain, short-term use as muscle relaxant. Not recommended in the elderly.	$
GABA Derivatives	*gabapentin* Neurontin, generics	Initial: 300–400 mg/day po May increase at weekly intervals to a maximum of 3600 mg/day. Should be given in 3 divided doses.	Sedation, ataxia, tremor; less commonly, GI upset, peripheral edema, vision changes.	Administration with aluminum/magnesium-containing antacids may decrease bioavailability.	Not a Health-Canada approved indication. Do not discontinue treatment abruptly; taper dosage over at least 1 wk to avoid withdrawal effects.	$$$$
	pregabalin Lyrica, generics	Initial: 50–150 mg daily po in 2 divided doses. Increase dose weekly by 50–150 mg/day to a maximum of 600 mg/day	Sedation, ataxia, edema, diplopia, weight gain, dry mouth.	No significant known drug interactions.	BID dosing is an advantage over gabapentin.	$$$
Muscle Relaxants	*baclofen* Lioresal Oral, generics	Start with 5 mg TID po; increase gradually to maximum of 20 mg TID	Sedation, muscle weakness, nausea, dizziness. Very rare: hepatotoxicity.	Potential additive CNS depression with TCAs, opioids, benzodiazepines, antihypertensives.	Adjust dose gradually to minimize adverse effects or withdrawal symptoms. In acute pain, short-term use as muscle relaxant. Not recommended in the elderly.	$$

Class	Drug	Dose	Adverse Effects	Drug Interactions	Comments	Cost[a]
	cyclobenzaprine generics	5–10 mg TID po	Drowsiness, dry mouth, dizziness, fatigue, nausea, constipation.	May increase risk of CNS effects when used with opioids or other CNS depressants. Increased risk of seizures with tramadol. SSRIs and CYP1A2 inhibitors (quinolones, ketoconazole) may decrease clearance. Do not use with MAOIs.	Structurally similar to TCAs. Can be given as a single nighttime dose. In acute pain, short-term use as muscle relaxant. Not recommended in the elderly.	$
	methocarbamol Robaxin	1 g QID po	See cyclobenzaprine.	Combination with opioids or other CNS depressants may increase risk of CNS depression.	Also available in combinations with nonprescription analgesics, with or without codeine. In acute pain, short-term use as muscle relaxant. Not recommended in the elderly.	$$
	orphenadrine Norflex, Orfenace, generics	100–200 mg/day divided BID po	See cyclobenzaprine.		Can be given as a single nighttime dose. In acute pain, short-term use as muscle relaxant. Not recommended in the elderly.	$
	tizanidine Zanaflex, generics	Start with 2 mg BID po; increase to maximum of 4 mg TID	Sedation, dizziness, dry mouth, weakness, hypotension, hepatotoxicity (monitor liver function tests).	Increased hypotensive effect with antihypertensives. Decreased clearance with oral contraceptives or TCAs. Decreased clearance with CYP1A2 inhibitors such as cimetidine, ciprofloxacin, fluvoxamine, ketoconazole. May increase phenytoin levels.	Adjust dose gradually to minimize adverse effects or withdrawal symptoms (e.g., rebound hypertension). In acute pain, short-term use as muscle relaxant. Not recommended in the elderly.	$$

(cont'd)

Table 3: **Drugs Used in the Treatment of Back and Neck Pain** *(cont'd)*

Class	Drug	Dose	Adverse Effects	Drug Interactions	Comments	Cost[a]
Nonsteroidal Anti-inflammatory Drugs (NSAIDs), oral[b]	*celecoxib* Celebrex	100 mg BID or 200 mg once daily po	GI toxicity, CV effects. NSAIDs may be nephrotoxic and should be avoided in patients with severe renal impairment. See Chapter 82, Table 2 for more information.	See Chapter 82, Table 2 for more information.	No evidence that one NSAID is superior to another for back pain. See Chapter 82, Table 2 for a full listing of NSAIDs. Celecoxib is contraindicated in patients with sulfonamide allergy, although cross-reactivity between sulfonamide-antibiotics and other sulfonamide medications is uncommon.	$$
	ibuprofen Advil, Motrin IB, generics	600–1200 mg/day divided Q6–8H po	GI toxicity, CV effects. NSAIDs may be nephrotoxic and should be avoided in patients with severe renal impairment. See Chapter 82, Table 2 for more information.	See Chapter 82, Table 2 for more information.	No evidence that one NSAID is superior to another for back pain. See Chapter 82, Table 2 for a full listing of NSAIDs.	$
	naproxen Naprosyn, generics	500–1000 mg/day divided Q8–12H po	See ibuprofen.	See Chapter 82, Table 2 for more information.	See ibuprofen.	$
	naproxen sodium Aleve, Anaprox, Naprelan, generics	Aleve: 220 mg Q8–12H po Anaprox: 825–1375 mg/day divided Q6–12H po Naprelan: 750–1000 mg once daily po	See ibuprofen.	See Chapter 82, Table 2 for more information.	See ibuprofen.	$
	meloxicam Mobicox, generics	7.5–15 mg once daily po	See ibuprofen.	See Chapter 82, Table 2 for more information.	See ibuprofen.	$
Nonsteroidal Anti-inflammatory Drugs (NSAIDs), topical	*diclofenac diethylamine* Voltaren Emulgel	Apply to affected area TID–QID	Skin dryness or irritation, hypersensitivity. Serious GI toxicity has not been seen to date in clinical trials.		For external use only. Gel contains diclofenac diethylamine 1.16% w/w and is available without prescription.	$

Class	Drug	Dose	Adverse Effects	Drug Interactions	Comments	Cost[a]
Opioids, weak	*acetaminophen/ codeine 8, 15, 30 or 60 mg* Tylenol with codeine, Atasol with codeine, generics	1–2 tablets QID Maximum dose of acetaminophen from all sources: 4 g/day	Nausea and vomiting, constipation, sedation or drowsiness, confusion, urinary retention, dry mouth, allergic reactions, e.g., rash.	CNS depressants (e.g., sedatives, alcohol) may increase CNS depression. Potential enhancement of opioid effects with lidocaine. Avoid use with MAOIs because of enhanced CNS depressant effects. Avoid use of opioid antagonists. Be cautious of drugs that may precipitate withdrawal reactions.	Start low. Titrate dosage against pain gradually enough to manage adverse effects. Upper limits of clinically appropriate dosage of opioids have not been identified. Consider addition of stimulant laxative.	$
	buprenorphine transdermal BuTrans	Initial (may be used in opioid-naïve patients): 5 μg/h patch applied once weekly. Patch sites should not be reused for 3 weeks	Application site skin reactions, constipation, nausea, confusion in elderly patients; may precipitate withdrawal reactions if taking other strong opioids.	See acetaminophen with codeine. Concomitant use with potent CYP3A4 inhibitors, e.g., cimetidine, efavirenz, erythromycin, itraconazole, ketoconazole or ritonavir, may increase buprenorphine plasma concentrations.	See acetaminophen with codeine. Has opioid agonist-antagonist activity; partial agonist at mu receptor, antagonist at kappa and agonist activity at delta receptor. Do not use in patients <40 kg. Risk of discontinuation syndrome when stopping buprenorphine.	$$
	tramadol controlled-release ❥ Durela, Ralivia, Tridural, Zytram XL	Durela, Ralivia or Tridural: Start with 100 mg once daily po; may increase at weekly intervals to maximum 300 mg daily Zytram XL: Start with 150 mg once daily po; may increase at weekly intervals to maximum 400 mg daily	Respiratory depression, sedation, ataxia, constipation, seizures, nausea, orthostatic hypotension.	Do not use if MAOIs taken within past 14 days. Caution with drugs that decrease seizure threshold, e.g., SSRIs, TCAs, bupropion. Risk of serotonin syndrome with SSRIs. Increased sedation with other CNS depressants. Carbamazepine, bupropion may decrease analgesic effect of tramadol. Clearance may be decreased by CYP2D6 inhibitors, e.g., fluoxetine, paroxetine, quinidine, or by CYP3A4 inhibitors, e.g., erythromycin, itraconazole, ketoconazole.		$$$$

(cont'd)

Table 3: **Drugs Used in the Treatment of Back and Neck Pain** *(cont'd)*

Class	Drug	Dose	Adverse Effects	Drug Interactions	Comments	Cost[a]
	tramadol/ acetaminophen ➔ Tramacet, generics	1–2 tablets Q4–6H po Maximum: 8 tablets daily	See tramadol.	See tramadol.	37.5 mg tramadol + 325 mg acetaminophen per tablet. Maximum dose of acetaminophen from all sources: 4 g/day.	$$$$
Opioids, strong	*fentanyl transdermal* Duragesic MAT, generics	In opioid-tolerant patients taking at least 60 mg/day of oral morphine or equivalent, fentanyl 25 µg/h patch can be substituted for oral opioid. See conversion table in product monograph. Change patch Q72H	See acetaminophen with codeine. Similar to other opioids, possibly less constipation but more sweating.	See acetaminophen with codeine. Concomitant use with potent CYP3A4 inhibitors, e.g., cimetidine, efavirenz, erythromycin, itraconazole, ketoconazole or ritonavir, may increase fentanyl plasma concentrations.	See acetaminophen with codeine. Contraindicated in patients who are opioid-naïve. Some patients may require lower starting dose.	$$$$
	hydromorphone sustained-release Hydromorph Contin, Jurnista	Initial: Hydromorph Contin: 3 mg Q12H po Jurnista: 4 mg Q24H po	See acetaminophen with codeine.	See acetaminophen with codeine.	See acetaminophen with codeine. Jurnista: May be used in opioid-naïve patients but it is preferable to titrate with shorter-acting product, then convert to Q24H dose.	$$
	morphine sustained-release ➔ Kadian, M-Eslon, MS Contin, generics	Initial: M-Eslon, MS Contin: 15 mg Q12H po Kadian: 20–30 mg Q24H po	See acetaminophen with codeine.	See acetaminophen with codeine.	See acetaminophen with codeine. Kadian: Preferable to titrate with shorter-acting product, then convert to Q24H dose.	$-$$
	oxycodone sustained-release OxyNEO, generics	Initial: 10 mg Q12H po	See acetaminophen with codeine.	See acetaminophen with codeine.	See acetaminophen with codeine.	$$
Opioid/Opioid Antagonist Combination	*oxycodone/naloxone controlled release* Targin	Initial: 1 tablet Q12H po Maximum daily dose: 80 mg oxycodone + 40 mg naloxone	See acetaminophen with codeine. Naloxone decreases opioid-induced constipation. Severe withdrawal effects if given rectally.	See acetaminophen with codeine.	Patients previously on oxycodone sustained-release may be switched to equivalent dose, but single doses should not exceed 40 mg oxycodone + 20 mg naloxone. If higher doses are needed, supplement with a single-entity oxycodone sustained-release product.	$$$$

Class	Drug	Dose	Adverse Effects	Drug Interactions	Comments	Cost[a]
Serotonin-Norepinephrine Reuptake Inhibitors	*duloxetine* Cymbalta	30–60 mg once daily po Maximum: 120 mg/day (divided BID)	Nausea, headache, drowsiness, insomnia, dizziness, dry mouth. Do not use in patients with severe renal impairment (ClCr <30 mL/min).	Alcohol, CNS depressants. MAOIs may cause serotonin syndrome (severe reaction—tremor, agitation, hypomania, hypertension). Tramadol may also increase risk of serotonin syndrome. Do not use with potent CYP1A2 inhibitors (e.g., ciprofloxacin, fluvoxamine, ketoconazole). CYP2D6 inhibitors (e.g., SSRIs) may increase duloxetine levels.	May help with back pain associated with central sensitization, such as fibromyalgia or myofascial pain.	$$$$$

[a] Cost of 30-day supply or smallest available pack size, includes drug cost only.
[b] Listed drugs are examples of medications in this class.
Dosage adjustment may be required in renal impairment; see Appendix I
Abbreviations: CV = cardiovascular; CYP = cytochrome P450; DMSO = dimethyl sulfoxide; GABA = gamma-aminobutyric acid; TCA = tricyclic antidepressant
Legend: $ <$25 $-$$ <$25–50 $$ $25–50 $$$ $50–75 $$$$ $75-100 $$$$$ $100–125

Suggested Readings

Arthritis Research UK. *Practitioner-based complementary and alternative therapies for the treatment of rheumatoid arthritis, osteoarthritis, fibromyalgia and low back pain.* Available from: www.arthritisresearchuk.org/arthritis-information/complementary-and-alternative-medicines/complementary-and-alternative-therapies.aspx.

Casazza BA. Diagnosis and treatment of acute low back pain. *Am Fam Physician* 2012;85(4):343-50.

Chou R, Qaseem A, Snow V et al. Diagnosis and treatment of low back pain: a joint clinical practice guideline from the American College of Physicians and the American Pain Society. *Ann Intern Med* 2007;147(7):478-91.

Dagenais S, Tricco AC, Haldeman S. Synthesis of recommendations for the assessment and management of low back pain from recent clinical practice guidelines. *Spine J* 2010;10(6):514-29.

Toward Optimized Practice. *Guideline for the evidence-informed primary care management of low back pain.* Alberta (CA); 2011. Available from: nationalpaincentre.mcmaster.ca/documents/LowerBackPainGuidelineNov2011.pdf.

References

1. Deyo RA, Rainville J, Kent DL. What can the history and physical examination tell us about low back pain? *JAMA* 1992;268(6):760-5.
2. Henschke N, Maher CG, Refshauge KM. Screening for malignancy in low back pain patients: a systematic review. *Eur Spine J* 2007;16(10):1673-9.
3. Waldvogel FA, Papageorgiou PS. Osteomyelitis: the past decade. *N Engl J Med* 1980;303(7):360-70.
4. Henschke N, Maher CG, Refshauge KM. A systematic review identifies five "red flags" to screen for vertebral fracture in patients with low back pain. *J Clin Epidemiol* 2008;61(2):110-8.
5. Scientific approach to the assessment and management of activity-related spinal disorders. A monograph for clinicians. Report of the Quebec Task Force on Spinal Disorders. *Spine (Phila Pa 1976)* 1987;12(7 Suppl):S1-59.
6. Dahm KT, Brurberg KG, Jamtvedt G et al. Advice to rest in bed versus advice to stay active for acute low-back pain and sciatica. *Cochrane Database Syst Rev* 2010;(6):CD007612.
7. Philadelphia Panel. Philadelphia Panel evidence-based clinical practice guidelines on selected rehabilitation interventions for low back pain. *Phys Ther* 2001;81(10):1641-74.
8. NHS Centre for Reviews and Dissemination, University of York. Acute and chronic low back pain. *Eff Health Care* 2000;6(5):1-8. Available from: www.york.ac.uk/inst/crd/EHC/ehc65.pdf. Accessed July 10, 2013.
9. Carter JT, Birrell LN, eds. *Occupational health guidelines for the management of low back pain at work: principal recommendations.* London (GB): Faculty of Occupational Medicine of the Royal College of Physicians; 2000.
10. Lee JH, Choi TY, Lee MS et al. Acupuncture for acute low back pain: a systematic review. *Clin J Pain* 2013;29(2):172-85.
11. Vas J, Aranda JM, Modesto M et al. Acupuncture in patients with acute low back pain: a multicentre randomised controlled clinical trial. *Pain* 2012;153(9):1883-9.
12. Roelofs PD, Deyo RA, Koes BW et al. Non-steroidal anti-inflammatory drugs for low back pain. *Cochrane Database Syst Rev* 2008;(1):CD000396.
13. Trelle S, Reichenbach S, Wandel S et al. Cardiovascular safety of non-steroidal anti-inflammatory drugs: network meta-analysis. *BMJ* 2011;342:c7086.
14. Coxib and traditional NSAID Trialists' (CNT) Collaboration, Bhala N, Emberson J et al. Vascular and upper gastrointestinal effects of non-steroidal anti-inflammatory drugs: meta-analyses of individual participant data from randomised trials. *Lancet* 2013;382(9894):769-79.
15. van Tulder MW, Touray T, Furlan AD et al. Muscle relaxants for non-specific low back pain. *Cochrane Database Syst Rev* 2003;(2):CD004252.
16. Ashworth J, Green DJ, Dunn KM et al. Opioid use among low back pain patients in primary care: is opioid prescription associated with disability at 6-month follow-up? *Pain* 2013;(154):1038-44.
17. Gagnier JJ, van Tulder M, Berman B et al. Herbal medicine for low back pain. *Cochrane Database Syst Rev* 2006;(2):CD004504.
18. Tunks E et al. Natural history and efficacy of treatment of chronic pain arising from musculoskeletal injury. In: Sullivan T, ed. *Injury and the new world of work.* Vancouver (BC): UBC Press; 2000.
19. Engers A, Jellema P, Wensing M et al. Individual patient education for low back pain. *Cochrane Database Syst Rev* 2008;(1):CD004057.
20. Anema JR, Steenstra IA, Bongers PM et al. Multidisciplinary rehabilitation for subacute low back pain: graded activity or workplace intervention or both? A randomized controlled trial. *Spine (Phila Pa 1976)* 2007;32(3):291-8.
21. Loisel P, Abenhaim L, Durand P et al. A population-based, randomized clinical trial on back pain management. *Spine (Phila Pa 1976)* 1997;22(24):2911-8.
22. Walker BF, French SD, Grant W et al. A Cochrane review of combined chiropractic interventions for low-back pain. *Spine (Phila Pa 1976)* 2011;36(3):230-42.
23. Furlan AD, Imamura M, Dryden T et al. Massage for low-back pain. *Cochrane Database Syst Rev* 2008;(4):CD001929.
24. Schaafsma F, Schonstein E, Whelan KM et al. Physical conditioning programs for improving work outcomes in workers with back pain. *Cochrane Database Syst Rev* 2010;(1):CD001822.
25. Cramer H, Lauche R, Haller H et al. A systematic review and meta-analysis of yoga for low back pain. *Clin J Pain* 2013;29(5):450-60.
26. Jensen C, Jensen OK, Christiansen DH et al. One-year follow-up in employees sick-listed because of low back pain: randomized clinical trial comparing multidisciplinary and brief intervention. *Spine (Phila Pa 1976)* 2011;36(15):1180-9.
27. Henschke N, Ostelo RW, van Tulder MW et al. Behavioural treatment for chronic low-back pain. *Cochrane Database Syst Rev* 2010;(7):CD002014.
28. Williams AC, Eccleston C, Morley S. Psychological therapies for the management of chronic pain (excluding headache) in adults. *Cochrane Database Syst Rev* 2012;11:CD007407.

29. Licciardone JC, Minotti DE, Gatchel RJ et al. Osteopathic manual treatment and ultrasound therapy for chronic low back pain: a randomized controlled trial. *Ann Fam Med* 2013;11(2):122-9.
30. Niemisto L, Kalso E, Malmivaara A et al. Radiofrequency denervation for neck and back pain. A systematic review of randomized controlled trials. *Cochrane Database Syst Rev* 2003;(1):CD004058.
31. Verbeek JH, Martimo KP, Karppinen J et al. Manual material handling advice and assistive devices for preventing and treating back pain in workers. *Cochrane Database Syst Rev* 2011;(6):CD005958.
32. Sahar T, Cohen MJ, Ne'eman V et al. Insoles for prevention and treatment of back pain. *Cochrane Database Syst Rev* 2007;(4):CD005275.
33. van Duijvenbode IC, Jellema P, van Poppel MN et al. Lumbar supports for prevention and treatment of low back pain. *Cochrane Database Syst Rev* 2008;(2):CD001823.
34. Dagenais S, Yelland MJ, Del Mar C et al. Prolotherapy injections for chronic low-back pain. *Cochrane Database Syst Rev* 2007;(2):CD004059.
35. Furlan AD, van Tulder MW, Cherkin DC et al. Acupuncture and dry-needling for low back pain. *Cochrane Database Syst Rev* 2005;(1):CD001351.
36. Kuijpers T, van Middelkoop M, Rubinstein SM et al. A systematic review on the effectiveness of pharmacological interventions for chronic non-specific low-back pain. *Eur Spine J* 2011;20(1):40-50.
37. Urquhart DM, Hoving JL, Assendelft WW et al. Antidepressants for non-specific low back pain. *Cochrane Database Syst Rev* 2008;(1):CD001703.
38. Wielage R, Bansal M, Wilson K et al. Cost-effectiveness of duloxetine in chronic low back pain: a Quebec societal perspective. *Spine (Phila Pa 1976)* 2013;38(11):936-46.
39. Chaparro LE, Furlan AD, Deshpande A et al. Opioids compared to placebo or other treatments for chronic low-back pain. *Cochrane Database Syst Rev* 2013;(8):CD004959.
40. Zhou SF. Polymorphism of human cytochrome P450 2D6 and its clinical significance: part II. *Clin Pharmacokinet* 2009;48(12):761-804.
41. Likar R. Transdermal buprenorphine in the management of persistent pain—safety aspects. *Ther Clin Risk Manag* 2006;2(1):115-25.
42. National Opioid Use Guideline Group. *Canadian guideline for safe and effective use of opioids for chronic non-cancer pain.* Hamilton (ON): NOUGG; 2010. Available from: nationalpaincentre.mcmaster.ca/opioid/documents.html. Accessed July 10, 2013.
43. Albert HB, Sorensen JS, Christensen BS et al. Antibiotic treatment in patients with chronic low back pain and vertebral bone edema (Modic type 1 changes): a double-blind randomized clinical controlled trial of efficacy. *Eur Spine J* 2013;22(4):697-707.
44. Staal JB, de Bie R, de Vet HC et al. Injection therapy for subacute and chronic low-back pain. *Cochrane Database Syst Rev* 2008;(3):CD001824.
45. Mosshammer D, Mayer B, Joos S. Local anesthetics injection therapy for musculoskeletal disorders: a systematic review and meta-analysis. *Clin J Pain* 2013;29(6):540-50.
46. Pennick V, Liddle SD. Interventions for preventing and treating pelvic and back pain in pregnancy. *Cochrane Database Syst Rev* 2013;8:CD001139.
47. Waller B, Lambeck J, Daly D. Therapeutic aquatic exercise in the treatment of low back pain: a systematic review. *Clin Rehabil* 2009;23(1):3-14.
48. Briggs GG, Freeman RK, Yaffe SJ, eds. *Drugs in pregnancy and lactation: a reference guide to fetal and neonatal risk.* 9th ed. Philadephia (PA): Lippincott Williams & Wilkins; 2011.
49. Centre for Addiction and Mental Health; Motherisk. *Exposure to psychotropic medications and other substances during pregnancy and lactation: a handbook for health care providers*. 1st ed. Toronto (ON): CAMH; 2007. Available from: www.camh.net/Publications/Resources_for_Professionals/Pregnancy_Lactation/psychmed_preg_lact.pdf. Accessed April 4, 2011.
50. Meyer FP, Rimasch H, Blaha B et al. Tramadol withdrawal in a neonate. *Eur J Clin Pharmacol* 1997;53(2):159-60.
51. Willaschek C, Wolter E, Buchhorn R. Tramadol withdrawal in a neonate after long-term analgesic treatment of the mother. *Eur J Clin Pharmacol* 2009;65(4):429-30.
52. Joglar JA, Page RL. Antiarrhythmic drugs in pregnancy. *Curr Opin Cardiol* 2001;16(1):40-5.
53. Santos AC, Yun EM, Bobby PD et al. The effects of bupivacaine, L-nitro-L-arginine-methyl ester, and phenylephrine on cardiovascular adaptations to asphyxia in the preterm fetal lamb. *Anesth Analg* 1997;85(6):1299-306.
54. Sachs HC; Committee On Drugs. The transfer of drugs and therapeutics into human breast milk: an update on selected topics. *Pediatrics* 2013;132(3):e796-809.
55. Koren G, Cairns J, Chitayat D et al. Pharmacogenetics of morphine poisoning in a breastfed neonate of a codeine-prescribed mother. *Lancet* 2006;368(9536):704.
56. Madadi P, Koren G, Cairns J et al. Safety of codeine during breastfeeding: fatal morphine poisoning in the breastfed neonate of a mother prescribed codeine. *Can Fam Physician* 2007;53(1):33-5.
57. Health Canada. *Health Canada's review recommends codeine only be used in patients aged 12 and over*. Available from: healthycanadians.gc.ca/recall-alert-rappel-avis/hc-sc/2013/33915a-eng.php.
58. Ilett KF, Paech MJ, Page-Sharp M et al. Use of a sparse sampling study design to assess transfer of tramadol and its O-desmethyl metabolite into transitional breast milk. *Br J Clin Pharmacol* 2008;65(5):661-6.
59. Drugs and Lactation Database (LactMed). Bethesda (MD): U.S. National Library of Medicine. Available from: toxnet.nlm.nih.gov/cgi-bin/sis/htmlgen?LACT. Accessed April 4, 2011.

Chapter 81
Neck Pain and Whiplash

Eldon Tunks, MD, FRCPC and
Paul Stacey, MD, MSc

Neck pain is one of the most common conditions seen in primary practice,[1] and is one of the chief presenting symptoms of whiplash, resulting from motor vehicle collisions. Whiplash is defined as a hyperextension-hyperflexion mechanism of energy transfer to the neck which may cause bone or soft-tissue injuries.[2] This chapter will discuss the management of acute neck pain, including the common presentation of whiplash, in addition to the management of general subacute and chronic neck pain.

Goals of Therapy

Acute Phase

- Reduce distress
- Identify patients in need of urgent surgical intervention

1–4 Weeks

- Promote therapy to restore function
- Return to normal activities as soon as possible

Subacute Period (4–12 Weeks)

- Interrupt progress to chronicity
- Promote active therapy while encouraging return to work

Chronic Pain (6 Months or More)

- Multimodal therapy aimed at management of chronic pain/disability, with emphasis on restoring function and independence

Neck Pain: Acute Phase to 30 Days

Investigations

Acute Phase (Days 1–7)

- History and physical examination. Assess for "red flags" (Table 1); based on history, physical examination and laboratory findings, classify according to Whiplash-Associated Disorders (WAD) criteria (Table 2, Figure 1)[2] or according to Bone and Joint Decade 2000-2010 Task Force on Neck Pain and Its Associated Disorders (Table 3).[3]
- Decision to x-ray is based on history of severe trauma, impaired consciousness and neurologic signs and symptoms. However, neurologic findings may not be present or prominent with cervical fracture, so clinical judgment/experience and imaging are necessary when fracture is suspected.[2]

- When neurologic injury or cervical spine injury is a concern, please refer to the Canadian C-Spine Rule (Figure 2) and seek expert guidance.

Therapeutic Choices

Nonpharmacologic Choices

WAD-I to WAD-III (Bone and Joint Decade classification Grades I-III): Provide symptomatic relief as indicated, reassure and counsel to resume normal activity as soon as possible. Avoid immobilization or passive therapy, except in the case of acute cervical radiculopathy (see WAD-III below).[2]

Bone and Joint Decade classification Grade I or II neck pain: Patient education combined with urgent care improves acute whiplash outcome. However, educational interventions by themselves (advice to stay active, neck school, relaxation) have demonstrated only very weak efficacy in pain relief or functional improvement.[4] Collars and high health-care utilization may be associated with delayed recovery.[5]

WAD-III (Bone and Joint Decade classification Grade III): When dealing with acute cervical radiculopathy, there is evidence of benefit for treatment with rest and a semi-hard collar for 3–6 weeks.[6]

WAD-IV (Bone and Joint Decade classification Grade IV): Urgent referral and surgical management.[2,6]

There is considerable agreement among opinion leaders that initial management is most effective if patients are counselled to maintain activity or return to activity as soon as tolerated, avoiding collars, bedrest or immobilization and limiting or avoiding work absence.[2] However, most studies are of poor quality, and the evidence is conflicting.[7]

Table 1: **Possible Red Flags Associated with Neck Pain[2]**

• History of severe trauma	• Loss of reflexes	• Lower body sensory changes
• Impaired consciousness	• Sensory or motor deficits	• Loss of bowel or bladder function

Table 2: **Whiplash-Associated Disorders (WAD) Classification[2]**

WAD-I	neck pain, stiffness or tenderness, but no physical signs/limitations
WAD-II	pain and tenderness and reduced range
WAD-III	pain and neurologic signs; sensory or motor or reflex changes without fracture/instability
WAD-IV	fracture or dislocation

Table 3: **Bone and Joint Decade 2000-2010 Classification[3,a]**

Grade I	neck pain/associated disorders without indication of major structural pathology, and either minor interference or no interference with activities of daily living (ADL)
Grade II	no indication of major pathology, but major interference with ADL
Grade III	no indication of major pathology, but having neurologic signs (abnormal reflexes, weakness, sensory deficits)
Grade IV	signs/symptoms of major structural pathology (may include fracture, vertebral dislocation, spinal cord injury, infection, neoplasm, systemic inflammatory disease)

[a] This is applicable to all neck pain, not only WAD. Reference also recommends a separate dimension distinguishing presence of claim for reimbursement, or wage replacement, long-term disability, permanent disability or punitive damage.

If progress is not occurring as expected by the end of the first month, consider the possibility of psychosocial barriers or complications. Active exercise combined with psychosocial intervention results in reduced pain in the short term and accelerates return to work.[2] However, early multidisciplinary treatment (<4 weeks postinjury) has not been shown to be more effective than usual care.[8]

Pharmacologic Choices

Pharmacologic options to treat neck pain and whiplash are presented in Chapter 80, Table 3.

While **NSAIDs** are more effective for symptom relief than placebo during the first month of back pain,[9] there is a paucity of studies to evaluate efficacy of NSAIDs in acute neck pain and whiplash, even though in practice they are often recommended.[10] In back pain studies, there is no evidence that any one NSAID is more effective for reducing pain.[9] Consider individual patient contraindications and the risks associated with use of NSAIDs, such as history of GI or cardiovascular disease. **Acetaminophen**, **tramadol**, **codeine** or **muscle relaxants** are appropriate alternatives in the acute phase of neck pain.

A single high-quality study reported that iv **methylprednisolone** for acute whiplash of less than 8 hours' duration led to reduced pain at 1 week and reduced sick leave but not pain at 6 months.[11] Risks of high-dose corticosteroid therapy include immunosuppression and pulmonary infection.[12] This treatment option is not recommended until further studies become available.

Figure 1: **Early Management of Whiplash Disorder Based on WAD Classification**

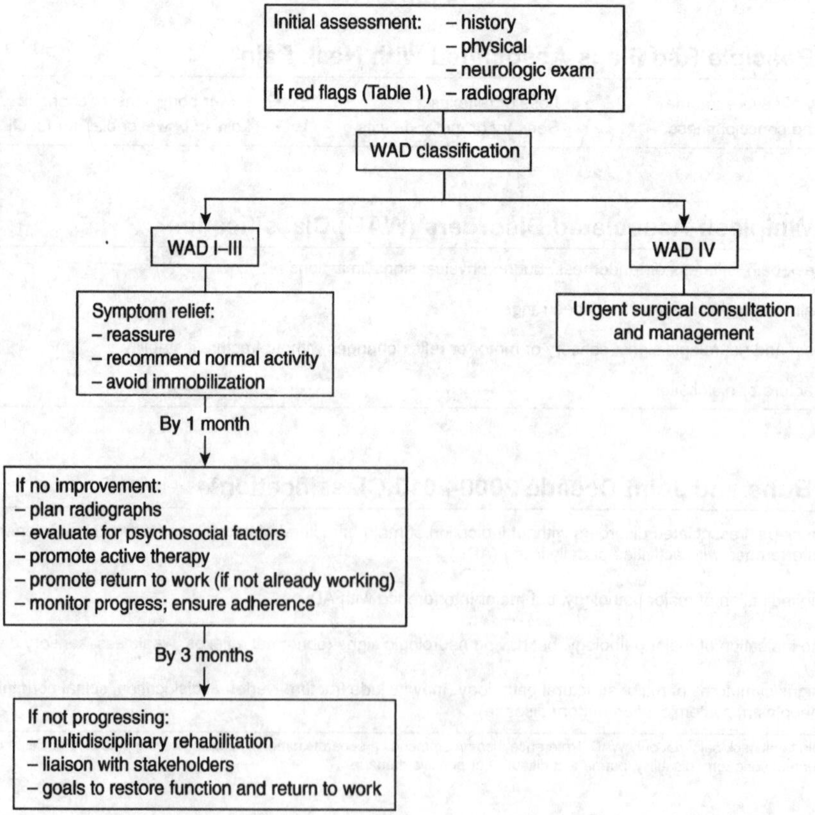

Figure 2: **Canadian C-Spine Rule**

For all alert and stable trauma patients where cervical spine injury is a concern

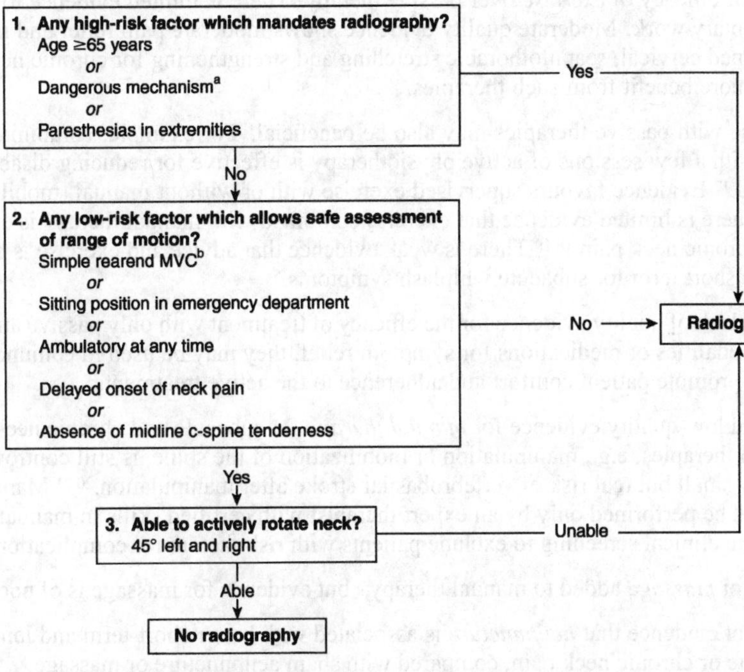

[a] Dangerous mechanism includes: fall from elevation ≥3 feet or 5 stairs; axial load to head; motor vehicle collision at high speed (>100 km/hr), rollover, ejection; motorized recreational vehicles; bicycle struck or collision.
[b] Simple rearend MVC (motor vehicle collision) excludes: pushed into oncoming traffic; hit by bus/large truck; rollover; hit by high speed vehicle.
Adapted with permission from: Canadian CT Head and C-Spine (CCC) Study Group. *CJEM* 2002;4(2):84-90.

Neck Pain: Subacute Period (4–12 Weeks)

Investigations

Order plain radiographs for neck pain lasting more than a few weeks, or more detailed studies if there is nerve root or spinal cord involvement or history of such injury.[13] For those not making progress in function, or suffering unexpected prolongation of pain, review to identify potential psychological risk factors (Table 4).

By this time, combined therapy is preferable: psychosocial, patient education and active exercise. Promote work re-entry, with modifications if appropriate, if there has been delay.

Table 4: **Identification of Psychological Risk Factors**[14,15]

Obvious psychological distress
Severe pain beyond what is expected
History of prior significant pain recurrences
Higher than expected functional impairment
Unexplained widespread pain
Pain and limitation not consistent with objective findings

Therapeutic Choices

Nonpharmacologic Choices

There is evidence of efficacy of *exercise* over passive therapy. There is limited evidence for taking breaks during sedentary work. Moderate quality evidence shows moderate pain relief and improved function for combined cervical, scapulothoracic stretching and strengthening for chronic neck pain.[16] Patients may feel more benefit from such therapies.

Combining exercise with passive therapies may also be beneficial. For example, combining psychoeducation with a few sessions of active physiotherapy is effective for reducing disability in the subacute period.[17] Evidence favours supervised exercise with or without manual (mobilization) therapy, although there is limited evidence that exercise combined with manual therapy is efficacious for subacute and chronic neck pain.[18,19] There is weak evidence that advice and exercise is better than advice alone in the short term for subacute whiplash symptoms.[5]

Although there is a lack of quality evidence for the efficacy of treatment with only passive and palliative physical therapy modalities or medications for symptom relief, they may be used in conjunction with active measures to promote patient comfort and adherence to the active treatments.

There is limited and low-quality evidence for *manual therapy* for subacute and chronic neck pain.[2,18] The role of manual therapies, e.g., manipulation or mobilization of the spine, is still controversial, partly due to a very small but real risk of vertebrobasilar stroke after manipulation.[20,21] Manipulation or mobilization should be performed only by an expert therapist with certified skills in manual therapy and with appropriate clinical screening to exclude patients with risk factors for complications.

There is evidence for *massage* added to manual therapy,[5] but evidence for massage is of poor quality.[22]

There is inconsistent evidence that *acupuncture* is associated with better short-term and long-term outcome in subacute or chronic neck pain, compared with sham acupuncture or massage.[5]

For neck pain Grade I and II, *patient education* focusing on self-efficacy, combined with usual medical care, appears promising. Weak and limited evidence exists that magnetic therapy or transcutaneous electrical nerve stimulation (TENS) is more effective in the short term than alternatives.[23]

Pharmacologic Choices

Pharmacologic options to treat neck pain and whiplash are presented in Chapter 80, Table 3. There is limited evidence supporting efficacy of muscle relaxants in subacute and chronic neck disorders.[5,10] (There is somewhat better evidence for efficacy in back pain.) In the absence of controlled studies, expert opinion is that if patients complain of high level of pain/tenderness in more than one area, **muscle relaxants** (cyclobenzaprine, baclofen, tizanidine, orphenadrine, methocarbamol), **tricyclic antidepressants**, **GABA derivatives** (gabapentin, pregabalin), or **tramadol** may be effective.

There is some evidence for intramuscular injection of **lidocaine** (block of trigger points) combined with stretching exercise for neck pain in the acute injury and in the subacute phase.[10] There is weak and contradictory evidence for efficacy of **NSAIDs** for subacute neck pain.[5,10]

Neck Pain: 3 months

If functional improvement and return to work/activity has not happened by this point, there is an increasing risk of chronic pain and poor function. Identify psychosocial and related risk factors that may impair progress. If work return (with or without modifications) is not successful, refer to multidisciplinary rehabilitation, in liaison with stakeholders, with the goal of return to work and function.

Chronic Neck Pain (≥ 6 Months)

Therapeutic Choices

With time there is increasing probability of associated psychological comorbidity.[14] Assess and treat comorbid depression, anxiety or adjustment problems. Refer to an appropriate specialist if indicated.

Nonpharmacologic Choices

For chronic musculoskeletal pain in general, there is limited evidence that intensive multimodal/multidisciplinary treatment programs (cognitive behavioural therapy with active exercise and psychosocial intervention, programs that include or simulate real-life work activities [work hardening] and planning for work re-entry) are effective for improving function and sense of well-being.[24] The active ingredient in successful work return, however, appears to be timely *workplace intervention* including all the stakeholders rather than clinic treatment modalities.[24,25]

Expert opinion is that multidisciplinary pain management should be recommended for chronic pain with impaired function and failure to improve or failure of work return. Evidence from the few available poor-quality studies is insufficient to estimate the efficacy of multidisciplinary biopsychosocial therapy for neck and shoulder pain.[26] The Bone and Joint Decade 2000-2010 Task Force found one nonrandomized study showing that multidisciplinary management of post-WAD pain was associated with quicker claim closure compared with usual care.[5] Another study did not find quicker recovery with referrals to fitness training, inpatient or outpatient rehabilitation plus usual care.[5]

In chronic pain, individual supervised active exercises (but not group exercise classes) can improve pain and function.[27,28] Otherwise, there is a lack of evidence of efficacy of individual physiotherapy modalities.

There is no evidence to support traction therapy for reducing neck pain or improving function in chronic neck disorders with or without radicular pain.[29] There is limited evidence that acupuncture provides short-term relief.[30]

Surgical Options

For neck pain with radicular symptoms, relatively rapid and substantial relief of pain and impairment is noted following surgical treatment of cervical radiculopathy in the 6–12 weeks after surgery, but there is absence of evidence for long-term outcomes. Anterior cervical plating seems to reduce kyphosis progression. It is not clear that complex open procedures including fusion, cage, or plate instrumentation, or fusion augmentation with bone morphogenic protein, provide superior outcomes versus simple cervical decompression alone. Limited evidence suggests possible favourable outcome with cervical disk arthroplasty for radicular symptoms, but long-term safety is unknown.[31]

Anterior cervical fusion or cervical disk arthroplasty for neck pain without radiculopathy or serious underlying pathology is not supported by evidence.[31]

Pharmacologic Choices

With respect to subacute widespread pain and tenderness, expert opinion is that **muscle relaxants, GABA derivatives** (gabapentin, pregabalin) and **tramadol** may be effective. There is limited published evidence that orphenadrine and acetaminophen are associated with greater pain reduction in the short term (8 days) in patients with subacute or chronic neck pain. There is weak and contradictory evidence for efficacy of **NSAIDs** for chronic neck pain.[5,10]

There is limited clinical trial evidence for the efficacy of **opioids** for chronic pain,[9,32] but there is expert acceptance of the use of opioids as one option.[32]

Although amitriptyline is widely used for soft tissue pain, neuralgia, headache and depression, **tricyclic antidepressants** have not been proven effective for mixed musculoskeletal and soft tissue pain relief.[24] Nevertheless, chronic pain is often associated with comorbidities. When major depression or anxiety disorders are comorbid with chronic pain, psychotropic medications may be an ingredient in proper treatment, though the pain itself will not necessarily be improved. For more information on the pharmacologic options to treat neck pain and whiplash, see Chapter 80, Table 3.

Interventional Options

Though it is becoming widely used for persistent pain, there is evidence that **botulinum toxin A** is not beneficial for pain and disability outcomes for subacute or chronic neck pain, compared with other treatments.[10,33]

Several low-quality studies suggest that local infiltration of anesthetic to muscle tissue (trigger/tender points) may afford short-term relief.[10] Support is lacking for the use of injection therapy alone for management of persistent neck pain/whiplash, and rehabilitation and work re-entry are recommended. There is limited and poor-quality evidence for treatment with epidural corticosteroid and lidocaine for chronic neck pain.[10]

Cervical zygapophyseal joint **corticosteroid** injection has been used for post-WAD of more than 3 months. A systematic review found that the evidence was inadequate; one RCT found that pain reduction after 5 months was not greater compared with placebo.[5]

A short course of epidural or selective root injection with corticosteroid may be associated with short-term symptomatic improvement of radicular symptoms but there is insufficient evidence to recommend radiofrequency neurotomy for suspected zygapophyseal (facet joint) pain. There is no evidence that cervical root or epidural injections decrease the rate of open surgery in seriously symptomatic radiculopathy.[31]

Choices during Pregnancy and Breastfeeding

For a brief discussion of therapeutic choices during pregnancy and breastfeeding for patients with low back or neck pain, see Chapter 80. A discussion of general principles on the use of medications in these special populations can be found in Appendix II and Appendix III. Other specialized reference sources are also provided in these appendices.

Therapeutic Tips

- Strong predictors of chronicity in neck pain problems include self-reported severe pain, pain in several body locations, pervasive functional impairment, a history of previous occurrences of whiplash/neck pain, female gender and older age. Identify these factors early and refer to intensive rehabilitation with cognitive behavioural therapy.

Suggested Readings

International Steering Committee. The Bone and Joint Decade 2000-2010 Task Force on Neck Pain and Its Associated Disorders. *Spine (Phila Pa 1976)* 2008;33(4 Suppl):S1-220.

Teasell RW, McClure JA, Walton D et al. A research synthesis of therapeutic interventions for whiplash-associated disorder: part 1–overview and summary. *Pain Res Manag* 2010;15(5):287-94.

References

1. Pace WD, Dickinson LM, Staton EW. Seasonal variation in diagnoses and visits to family physicians. *Ann Fam Med* 2004;2(5):411-7.
2. Spitzer WO, Skovron ML, Salmi LR et al. Scientific monograph of the Quebec Task Force on Whiplash-Associated Disorders: redefining "whiplash" and its management. *Spine (Phila Pa 1976)* 1995;20(8 Suppl):1S-73S.
3. Guzman J, Hurwitz EL, Carroll LJ et al. A new conceptual model of neck pain: linking onset, course, and care: the Bone and Joint Decade 2000-2010 Task Force on Neck Pain and Its Associated Disorders. *Spine (Phila Pa 1976)* 2008;33(4 Suppl):S14-23.
4. Gross A, Forget M, St George K et al. Patient education for neck pain. *Cochrane Database Syst Rev* 2012;3:CD005106.
5. Hurwitz EL, Carragee EJ, van der Velde G et al. Treatment of neck pain: noninvasive interventions: results of the Bone and Joint Decade 2000-2010 Task Force on Neck Pain and Its Associated Disorders. *Spine (Phila Pa 1976)* 2008;33(4 Suppl):S123-52.
6. Kuijper B, Tans JT, Beelen A et al. Cervical collar or physiotherapy versus wait and see policy for recent onset cervical radiculopathy: randomised trial. *BMJ* 2009;339:b3883.
7. Verhagen AP, Scholten-Peeters GG, van Wijngaarden S et al. Conservative treatments for whiplash. *Cochrane Database Syst Rev* 2007;(2):CD003338.
8. Jull G, Kenardy J, Hendrikz J et al. Management of acute whiplash: a randomized controlled trial of multidisciplinary stratified treatments. *Pain* 2013;154(9):1798-806.
9. Roelofs PD, Deyo RA, Koes BW et al. Non-steroidal anti-inflammatory drugs for low back pain. *Cochrane Database Syst Rev* 2008;(1):CD000396.
10. Peloso P, Gross A, Haines T et al. Medicinal and injection therapies for mechanical neck disorders. *Cochrane Database Syst Rev* 2007;(3):CD000319.
11. Pettersson K, Toolanen G. High-dose methylprednisolone prevents extensive sick leave after whiplash injury. A prospective, randomized, double-blind study. *Spine (Phila Pa 1976)* 1998;23(9):984-9.
12. Matsumoto T, Tamaki T, Kawakami M et al. Early complications of high-dose methylprednisolone sodium succinate treatment in the follow-up of acute cervical spinal cord injury. *Spine (Phila Pa 1976)* 2001;26(4):426-30.
13. Tsang I. Rheumatology: 12. Pain in the neck. *CMAJ* 2001;164(8):1182-7.
14. Tunks E et al. Natural history and efficacy of treatment of chronic pain arising from musculoskeletal injury. In: Sullivan T, ed. *Injury and the new world of work.* Vancouver (BC): UBC Press; 2000.
15. Borghouts JA, Koes BW, Bouter LM. The clinical course and prognostic factors of non-specific neck pain: a systematic review. *Pain* 1998;77(1):1-13.
16. Kay TM, Gross A, Goldsmith CH et al. Exercises for mechanical neck disorders. *Cochrane Database Syst Rev* 2012;8:CD004250.
17. Lamb SE, Williams MA, Williamson EM et al. Managing injuries of the neck trial (MINT): a randomised controlled trial of treatments for whiplash injuries. *Health Technol Assess* 2012;16(49):iii-iv,1-141.
18. Gross AR, Miller J, D'Sylva J et al. Manipulation or mobilisation for neck pain. *Cochrane Database Syst Rev* 2010;(1):CD004249.
19. Kay TM, Gross A, Goldsmith C et al. Exercises for mechanical neck disorders. *Cochrane Database Syst Rev* 2005;(3):CD004250.
20. Haynes MJ, Vincent K, Fischhoff C et al. Assessing the risk of stroke from neck manipulation: a systematic review. *Int J Clin Pract* 2012;66(10):940-7.
21. Cassidy JD, Boyle E, Cote P et al. Risk of vertebrobasilar stroke and chiropractic care: results of a population-based case-control and case-crossover study. *Spine (Phila Pa 1976)* 2008;33(4 Suppl):S176-83.
22. Patel KC, Gross A, Graham N et al. Massage for mechanical neck disorders. *Cochrane Database Syst Rev* 2012;(9):CD004871.
23. Kroeling P, Gross A, Goldsmith CH et al. Electrotherapy for neck pain. *Cochrane Database Syst Rev* 2009;(4):CD004251.
24. Loisel P, Abenhaim L, Durand P et al. A population-based, randomized clinical trial on back pain management. *Spine (Phila Pa 1976)* 1997;22(24):2911-8.
25. Anema JR, Steenstra IA, Bongers PM et al. Multidisciplinary rehabilitation for subacute low back pain: graded activity or workplace intervention or both? A randomized controlled trial. *Spine (Phila Pa 1976)* 2007;32(3):291-8.
26. Karjalainen K, Malmivaara A, van Tulder M et al. Multidisciplinary biopsychosocial rehabilitation for neck and shoulder pain among working age adults. *Cochrane Database Syst Rev* 2003;(2):CD002194.
27. Philadelphia Panel. Philadelphia Panel evidence-based clinical practice guidelines on selected rehabilitation interventions for neck pain. *Phys Ther* 2001;81(10):1701-17.
28. Bertozzi L, Gardenghi I, Turoni F et al. Effect of therapeutic exercise on pain and disability in the management of chronic nonspecific neck pain: systematic review and meta-analysis of randomized trials. *Phys Ther* 2013;93(8):1026-36.
29. Graham N, Gross A, Goldsmith CH et al. Mechanical traction for neck pain with or without radiculopathy. *Cochrane Database Syst Rev* 2008;(3):CD006408.
30. Trinh K, Graham N, Gross A et al. Acupuncture for neck disorders. *Cochrane Database Syst Rev* 2006;(3):CD004870.
31. Carragee EJ, Hurwitz EL, Cheng I et al. Treatment of neck pain: injections and surgical interventions: results of the Bone and Joint Decade 2000-2010 Task Force on Neck Pain and Its Associated Disorders. *Spine (Phila Pa 1976)* 2008;33(4 Suppl):S153-69.
32. McMaster University. National Opioid Use Guideline Group. *Canadian guideline for safe and effective use of opioids for chronic non-cancer pain.* Hamilton (ON): NOUGG; 2010. Available from: nationalpaincentre.mcmaster.ca/opioid/documents.html. Accessed March 28, 2011.
33. Langevin P, Peloso PM, Lowcock J et al. Botulinum toxin for subacute/chronic neck pain. *Cochrane Database Syst Rev* 2011;(7):CD008626.

Chapter 82
Osteoarthritis

Walter F. Kean, MB ChB (Glas), MD (Glas), FRCP (Edin Glas C)
Colin A. Kean, BSc and
Michael G. Hogan, MD, FRCSC

CPhA acknowledges the contribution of Dr. Paul Davis and Dr. Angela Juby as previous authors of this chapter.

Osteoarthritis (OA) and the related condition of cervical spine and lumbar spine facet joint pain are the most common musculoskeletal disorders worldwide,[1,2,3,4] and hip and knee OA ranked as the eleventh highest contributors to global disability.[5] OA is classified as primary or secondary. The latter is generally the result of an "insult" to the joint (e.g., trauma, congenital and post-trauma joint malalignment and joint infection). OA is often incorrectly referred to as a degenerative disorder, but is now recognized as a condition with definite biochemical and inflammatory changes within the cartilage matrix, the joint cavity and the joint capsule and support structures.[6,7] Patients with OA suffer mostly from pain, stiffness, discomfort and joint function impairment.

Goals of Therapy

- Alleviate or eliminate joint pain
- Improve or restore joint function and mobility
- Improve muscle strength to protect cartilage, ligaments and the joint capsule
- Prevent and reduce damage to joint cartilage, bone, ligaments, muscles and local nerves

All of the above goals may be achievable with appropriate early intervention.

Investigations

OA is most commonly identified by joint signs and symptoms and confirmed by diagnostic imaging if necessary.

- History:[8]
  - joint stiffness usually lasting <30 minutes, with joint pain and/or dysfunction on certain movements
  - absence of signs or symptoms of other types of inflammatory arthritis
  - secondary OA is related to other joint insults such as: a history of trauma, joint infection or other inflammatory arthropathy; genetic, biochemical or metabolic disease
- Physical examination:[8,9]
  - pain, stiffness and limitation of both passive and active movement of joint
  - crepitus, deformity, muscle atrophy, ligament tenderness in one or more of the affected joints
  - ligament and capsular laxity, muscle atrophy and joint deformity in later stages
  - primary OA is most frequently seen in the hands at the proximal and distal interphalangeal finger joints or the thumb base metacarpal-trapezio-scaphoid joints, in the cervical spine and lower lumbar facet joints, or in the hips, knees or great toe joints

- Imaging:
  - x-rays and diagnostic ultrasound may be of initial value to establish the presence and extent of joint structure damage. There is a discrepancy between the extent of imaging signs and the symptoms experienced by individuals suffering from OA: significant structural damage may not be accompanied with severe symptoms or minimal structural change can be associated with severe pain. Joint space narrowing, osteophyte formation, subchondral cysts (geodes) and bony sclerosis are the recognized radiological features of OA. Chondrocalcinosis (calcium pyrophosphate dehydrogenase [CPPD] deposition) may be seen in the joint cartilage areas of patients with some metabolic disorders which predispose to secondary OA
  - MRI has lower sensitivity than other more cost-effective radiographic diagnosis tools in detecting OA.[10] MRI my be useful when considering an associated soft tissue pathology, and when considering a rare differential diagnosis.[11] CT scan can be used if MRI is contraindicated
- Laboratory tests:
  - consider blood work for inflammatory markers (e.g., CBC, rheumatoid factor, ESR, CRP) if other inflammatory arthritides are suspected
  - joint fluid analyses are valuable primarily to exclude infection and less commonly to identify CPPD as a causative or contributory factor

Therapeutic Choices

A treatment algorithm for OA is presented in Figure 1.

See Suggested Readings for OA treatment guidelines by the American College of Rheumatology, European League Against Rheumatism and Osteoarthritis Research Society International. However, remember that guidelines are not intended to replace clinical judgement.

Prevention

Strategies for prevention or delay of disease involve advice on general health, exercise and nutrition, weight management and avoidance of repeated trauma to a potentially affected joint.

Knee malalignment valgus (knock knee) and knee varus (outward knee bending) are recognized as independent risk factors for development of knee OA.[12]

Nonpharmacologic Choices

Nonpharmacologic options are important in the management of OA and in improving the quality of life. Individuals with OA should be treated by a multidisciplinary team including occupational therapists, physiotherapists, social workers, pharmacists, family members and caregivers.

Patient Education

- Advise patients to attend educational sessions such as those offered by the Arthritis Society which are led by physiotherapists and occupational therapists across Canada.[13]

Physical Therapy

- Some patients may benefit from transcutaneous nerve stimulation (TENS).[14] However, the effectiveness of TENS has not been established.[15,16]
- Acupuncture around an affected joint may offer temporary relief but the effect may not be sustained or provide functional benefit, and a patient's response to acupuncture may depend on multiple variables including site of application and the acupuncturist's style of application.[17,18,19]

Figure 1: **Treatment of Osteoarthritis**[14,54]

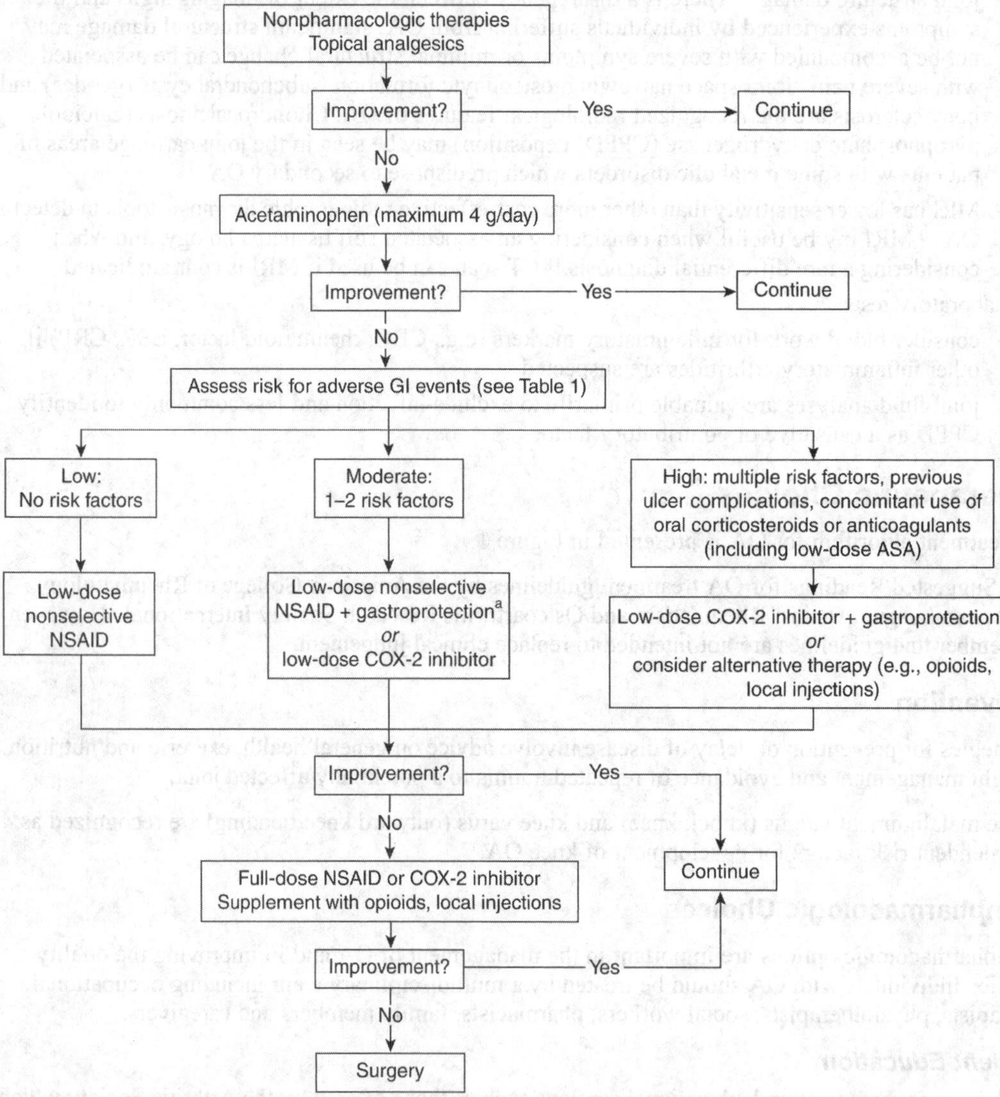

[a] Select either misoprostol or a proton pump inhibitor (see Chapter 60).
Abbreviations: COX-2 = cyclooxygenase-2; NSAID = nonsteroidal anti-inflammatory drug

Orthotics and Aids to Daily Living

- Orthotics that support the long and transverse arch of the foot may be of value in patients with flat arches and those with associated midfoot or ankle pronation or supination.[20] Orthotics can also be helpful in the management or prevention of great toe joint and midfoot OA.[21]
- Elastic supports may be beneficial to patients with elbow, knee or ankle OA pain and instability.
- Braces may be beneficial for patients awaiting surgery or for poor surgical candidates, but they are expensive and not well tolerated.[14,16,21,22]

- Splints can improve hand pain and function. Devices such as canes and walkers may be suggested for those with hip and knee OA.[14]

Exercise and Physiotherapy

- Introduction of exercise at home and structured exercise under the guidance of a physiotherapist are the key initial management strategies in OA.[23,24]
- In knee OA both resistance exercises and aerobic activities of different intensities were shown to effectively reduce pain and improve function. However, optimal exercise programs should have one aim and focus (i.e., improving aerobic capacity or quadriceps muscle strength).[24,25,26]
- Exercise programmes can also reduce pain and improve physical function in hip[27] and hand[28] OA.
- Yoga and Tai Chi may reduce pain and stiffness and improve physical function and quality of life for patients with OA.[23,29,30]

Weight Loss

- Obesity is one of the most important modifiable risk factors for knee OA.[11]
- Recent studies suggest that overweight patients with OA may significantly benefit from weight loss.[23,31,32]
- For more information on weight management, see Chapter 33.

Pharmacologic Choices

Standard pharmacological OA management involves a stepwise approach consisting of initial use of topical analgesics, followed by oral analgesics (e.g., acetaminophen, NSAIDs, opioids) and injectable agents.

Topical Analgesics

Topical analgesics offer an alternative to oral treatment, with the potential for a reduced risk of side effects.[33] These options may be especially useful in the elderly, who are at an increased risk of GI, renal, cardiovascular and other **NSAID** adverse effects. Topical NSAIDs have been shown to be superior to placebo and equal to oral NSAIDs in the treatment of OA.[34,35,36,37] The most common side effects are cutaneous reactions.

Topical **diclofenac** solution is as effective as oral NSAIDs for relief of hand and knee pain, and is associated with a lower incidence of GI bleeds compared to oral NSAIDs.[37] Begin NSAID therapy with topical rather than oral agents in persons ≥75 years [Evidence: SORT A*].[14,37] Monitor for serious adverse effects that may occur in the elderly, including GI upset and local irritation.[38]

Other topical analgesics (Table 3) can be used adjunctively with oral therapy, but evidence supporting their use is limited. They may be offered to those refusing systemic therapy. **Zucapsaicin** is approved only for adjunctive use with NSAIDs. **Capsaicin** has been shown to be superior to placebo for pain control in 2 small studies, but patients were permitted to use oral analgesics.[39,40] The burning sensation caused by capsicum derivatives is often not well tolerated. Preliminary studies indicate that **arnica** gel may be comparable to topical ibuprofen for relief of OA pain, but further confirmatory studies are required.[41] If patients experience pain, swelling or burning from topical analgesics, advise them to stop using the product and seek immediate medical attention.[42]

Simple Analgesics

Acetaminophen, a simple analgesic with weak anti-inflammatory properties, is recommended as the oral drug of first choice in the treatment of OA.[14,43] The maximum dose should not exceed 4000 mg

* SORT (Strength of Recommendation Taxonomy) is a rating system (A, B or C) that addresses the quality of available evidence. For more information consult **How to Use *Compendium of Therapeutic Choices*** on page xxv.

daily; special precaution should be taken for patients with liver dysfunction, those who consume large amounts of alcohol and those receiving concomitant opioids.[44] Doses greater than 2000 mg daily may exhibit GI toxicity, although more data are needed to confirm this potential adverse effect.[45]

Nonsteroidal Anti-inflammatory Drugs (NSAIDs)

NSAIDs are more effective analgesics than acetaminophen, but have a greater risk of GI toxicity.[45,46] Consider topical NSAIDs before initiating oral NSAID therapy, particularly in the elderly (see Topical Analgesics). If topical NSAIDs and acetaminophen are not sufficient, initiating low-dose NSAID therapy may be of benefit.[14] NSAID dosage can be adjusted upwards to control pain but precautions must be taken to minimize adverse effects. For more information regarding NSAID dosing, see Table 2.

Cardiovascular and Renal Risk

All NSAIDs demonstrate an increased risk of cardiovascular events (e.g., MI or stroke).[46,47,48,49] Patients with a history of cardiovascular disease require careful monitoring while using NSAIDs for OA. Studies indicate that **diclofenac**, **celecoxib**, and high-dose **ibuprofen**are particularly associated with an increased risk of cardiovascular events.[46,47,48,49] In contracts, naproxen has been found to have the lowest risk (among NSAIDs) for cardiovascular events and deaths.[46] All NSAIDs can increase blood pressure and worsen pre-existing hypertension; therefore, monitoring of blood pressure at baseline and periodically is advised.

All NSAIDs increase risk of edema, CHF and impaired renal function.[46,50] NSAIDs should be avoided in patients with severe renal impairment (ClCr <30 mL/min) and their prolonged use is not recommended in patients with mild to moderate renal impairment.

Gastrointestinal Risk

Although both nonselective NSAIDs and selective COX-2 inhibitors confer an increased risk of GI damage,[49] COX-2 inhibitors appear to be associated with a lower risk of endoscopic ulcers[51] and adverse GI outcomes compared to nonselective NSAIDs.[52] However, the reduction in GI adverse effects is modest and may not extend past 6 months.[49] Among the nonselective NSAIDs, evidence suggests that naproxen has a higher risk of GI adverse effects than ibuprofen.[46]

It has been shown that the combined use of a proton pump inhibitor (PPI) with a nonselective NSAID or a COX-2 inhibitor will significantly reduce the incidence and relapse of GI symptoms and ulcer formation.[51,53,54] If GI risk factors are present, an NSAID with a PPI is the drug regimen of choice for chronic OA management.[54] For more information on risk factors for GI toxicity, see Table 1 and Chapter 60.

Misoprostol 200 µg QID is effective in preventing NSAID-induced GI complications. However, misoprostol is not well tolerated.

Table 1: Risk Factors for Development of Upper GI Adverse Effects with NSAIDs[55]

Age ≥65
Comorbid medical conditions
High doses of NSAID
History of upper GI bleeding
Presence of *H. pylori* infection
Multiple NSAID use (including low-dose ASA)

Opioids

The use of opioids has potential value in terms of pain relief, but the side effect profile (constipation, dizziness, drowsiness and secondary dangers of falls and fractures) and potential for misuse preclude opioids as a first choice in OA management.[14]

Tramadol is an effective and relatively safe oral agent for relief of moderate to severe pain in OA.[56,57] Tramadol can be used in conjunction with or as an alternative to acetaminophen and/or NSAIDs. Tramadol has a less serious side effect potential than other opioids. The lack of pharmacokinetic differences in the elderly with either immediate-release or prolonged-release tramadol is a particular advantage of this drug.[58]

A Cochrane review of opioids for OA showed that the small to moderate beneficial effects of opioids other than tramadol are outweighed by significantly increased risks of adverse events.[59] Opioids other than tramadol should not be routinely used, even if OA pain is severe.

In selected cases of patients with moderate to severe pain, pain-related functional impairment, diminished quality of life due to pain or in patients with contraindications to NSAID use, chronic opioid use may be necessary; patients must be monitored at regular intervals. In certain circumstances, the American Geriatrics Society suggests that opioids may also be a safer option than NSAIDs in elderly patients.[60]

Antidepressants

Duloxetine, a serotonin-norepinephrine inhibitor (SNRI), demonstrated significantly greater improvement in OA knee pain compared with placebo.[61] Adverse effects leading to discontinuation of the drug included nausea and asthenia.

Although SNRIs exhibit antiplatelet properties, the combination of duloxetine and NSAIDs does not appear to be associated with an increased risk of bleeding-related events compared with NSAID used alone.[62]

Consider duloxetine if a patient with OA presents with concomitant depression and/or neuropathic pain.[11]

Glucosamine and Chondroitin

Endogenous **glucosamine** and **chondroitin** maintain the integrity of cartilage within a joint. Several systematic reviews and meta-analyses have failed to demonstrate the efficacy of exogenous glucosamine and chondroitin for relief of OA pain.[63,64,65] Results are difficult to interpret due to high levels of heterogeneity and differences in commercial formulations.[66] Accordingly, treatment guidelines do not recommend these supplements for the treatment of OA.[14]

Oral Corticosteroids

Preliminary studies have examined the use of oral **corticosteroids** for relief of acute OA pain.[67] However, corticosteroids are associated with significant side effects including loss of bone density and development of osteoporosis,[68] and may also increase the risk of joint osteonecrosis. Accordingly, oral corticosteroid use is not recommended for chronic OA pain.

Injectable Therapy

If nonpharmacologic, topical and oral options have been exhausted, injectable therapy may be considered.

Intra-articular corticosteroids are useful in patients with acutely inflamed painful joints but the effects typically last for 1–2 weeks,[69] though it can extend to 3–6 months in the authors' experience. Repeated intra-articular injections of corticosteroids should be administered no more often than 3–4 times per year in weight-bearing joints, because of the likelihood of producing a Charcot-type arthropathy.[70]

Hyaluronic acid injections have been shown to be marginally helpful in some patients with mild to moderate knee OA.[71] However, outcomes vary with different products and study designs.[71,72,73]

Platelet rich plasma (PRP) injections improve function from baseline in patients with knee OA and tend to be more effective than hyaluronic acid injections.[74,75] Multiple injections result in improvement after 6 months of therapy. Patients with mild to moderate OA with less degeneration tend to respond better to PRP injections.

Surgery

Arthroplasty is an option for patients with moderate to severe OA of the knee and hip with unremitting symptomatology despite adherence to conservative medical management. In the majority of patients, hip and knee arthroplasties result in improvement in both pain and functional status.[76] Possible complications include loosening of the prostheses (osteolysis) and postoperative infection.[77,78,79] Whether joint arthroplasty should be done early or late in the course of OA is heavily debated.

Athroscopic joint lavage and joint debridement are of questionable value.[80]

Therapeutic Tips

- Patients should receive only one **NSAID** at a time (with the exception of low-dose cardioprotective ASA). However, the advantages of COX-2 inhibitors (lower GI toxicity compared to nonselective NSAIDs) are negated when they are taken with low-dose ASA.[54]
- Dyspepsia with NSAIDs does not correlate with endoscopically proven ulcers or with serious upper GI complications. Patients treated with NSAIDs who complain of dyspepsia in the absence of risk factors (Table 1) can be switched to simple analgesics or offered a trial with a different class of NSAID, or the dyspepsia may be treated symptomatically.
- Making patients aware of the GI risks of NSAIDs has been shown to lower the incidence of acute GI bleeding.[81]
- For most patients, the use of nonpharmacologic measures combined with a flexible regimen of simple analgesics supplemented by anti-inflammatory medications provides adequate relief of symptoms and functional benefit.

  As many OA sufferers are elderly, always start with low doses, increasing slowly to therapeutic effect. Drug interactions are also a concern because many older patients are being treated for other conditions.
- Patients presenting with unstable angina or non-ST segment elevation MI (UA/NSTEMI) should discontinue use of nonselective NSAIDs or COX-2 inhibitors (except ASA) because of the increased cardiovascular risk associated with these agents.[82] An **opioid** analgesic such as morphine may be a suitable alternative for pain control in this setting.

Table 2: Oral Agents Used in Osteoarthritis

Class	Drug	Dose	Adverse Effects	Drug Interactions	Comments	Cost[a]
Analgesics	*acetaminophen* Tylenol, Atasol Preparations, generics	325–1000 mg Q4–6H SR: 650 mg Q8H Maximum: 4 g/day	Hepatotoxicity—see Comments.	Alcohol: increased risk of hepatotoxicity with excessive alcohol intake (>3 drinks/day). Warfarin: may increase anticoagulant effect of warfarin, particularly at doses >1.3 g/day for >1 wk.	May cause hepatic damage or failure if taken in excess or by patients with liver diseases.	$
	morphine MS-IR, Statex, generics	2.5–15 mg QID for immediate-release formulations	Sedation, nausea, vomiting, constipation.	Concurrent use of other sedating or constipating medications may increase these side effects. Lidocaine: potential enhancement of opioid effects.	Useful for short-term adjunctive therapy. May be poorly tolerated in the elderly.	$
	oxycodone Oxy-IR, generics	5–10 mg QID for immediate-release formulations	See morphine.	See morphine.	See morphine.	$
	tramadol controlled-release Durela, Ralivia, Tridural, Zytram XL	Durela, Ralivia or Tridural: start with 100 mg once daily; may increase at weekly intervals to maximum 300 mg daily Zytram XL: start with 150 mg once daily; may increase at weekly intervals to maximum 400 mg daily	Respiratory depression, sedation, ataxia, constipation, seizures, nausea, orthostatic hypotension.	Do not use if MAOIs taken within past 14 days. Caution with drugs that decrease seizure threshold, e.g., SSRIs, TCAs, bupropion. Risk of serotonin syndrome with SSRIs. Increased sedation with other CNS depressants. Carbamazepine, bupropion may decrease analgesic effect of tramadol. Clearance may be decreased by CYP2D6 inhibitors, e.g., fluoxetine, paroxetine, quinidine, or by CYP3A4 inhibitors, e.g., erythromycin, itraconazole, ketoconazole.		$$$

(cont'd)

Table 2: **Oral Agents Used in Osteoarthritis** *(cont'd)*

Class	Drug	Dose	Adverse Effects	Drug Interactions	Comments	Cost[a]
	tramadol/ acetaminophen Tramacet, generics	1–2 tablets Q4–6H Maximum: 8 tablets daily Maximum dose of acetaminophen from all sources: 4 g/day	See tramadol.	See tramadol.	37.5 mg tramadol + 325 mg acetaminophen per tablet.	$$$$
COX-2 Inhibitors	*celecoxib* Celebrex	100 mg BID or 200 mg once daily	Usual doses do not appear to have antiplatelet effects. Serious skin reactions have been reported. Patients with history of MI or stroke, serious heart disease–related chest pain or serious heart disease such as HF should not use COX-2 inhibitors. Assess overall risk in patients with risk factors for MI and stroke. GI: dyspepsia, epigastric pain, nausea/vomiting, diarrhea, gastric and duodenal ulcers, GI bleeding. Cardiovascular: MI, stroke, heart failure, fluid retention, hypertension. Nephrotoxicity may occur; avoid NSAIDs in patients with severe renal impairment (ClCr <30 mL/min). CNS: dizziness, drowsiness, headache, tinnitus, confusion (especially in the elderly); CNS effects may be dose related and respond to decreased dosage. Minor or serious skin rashes, pruritus.	Increased risk of bleeding with anticoagulants (e.g., warfarin) or antiplatelet drugs (e.g., clopidogrel). May decrease effect of antihypertensives. May decrease renal clearance of lithium; monitor lithium levels when NSAID added. Increased risk of GI bleeding when used with SSRIs.	Take with food. No NSAID has been shown to have superior efficacy; their tolerability may vary, especially in the elderly. Avoid NSAIDs, including COX-2 inhibitors, if history of peptic ulcer disease, cardiovascular risk factors, renal failure, heart failure or asthma. Celecoxib contraindicated if sulfonamide allergy.	$$

Class	Drug	Dose	Adverse Effects	Drug Interactions	Comments	Cost[a]
NSAIDs, acetic acid derivatives	*diclofenac* Voltaren, Voltaren SR, generics	Immediate-release: 25–50 mg BID–TID Sustained-release: 75 mg BID Maximum dose: 150 mg/day	GI: dyspepsia, epigastric pain, nausea/vomiting, diarrhea, gastric and duodenal ulcers, GI bleeding. Cardiovascular: MI, stroke, heart failure, fluid retention, hypertension. Nephrotoxicity may occur; avoid NSAIDs in patients with severe renal impairment (ClCr <30 mL/min). CNS: dizziness, drowsiness, headache, tinnitus, confusion (especially in the elderly); CNS effects may be dose related and respond to decreased dosage. Minor or serious skin rashes, pruritus.	Increased risk of bleeding with anticoagulants (e.g., warfarin) or antiplatelet drugs (e.g., clopidogrel). May decrease effect of antihypertensives. May decrease renal clearance of lithium; monitor lithium levels when NSAID added. Increased risk of GI bleeding when used with SSRIs.	Take with food. No NSAID has been shown to have superior efficacy; their tolerability may vary, especially in the elderly. Avoid NSAIDs, including COX-2 inhibitors, if history of peptic ulcer disease, cardiovascular risk factors, renal failure, heart failure or asthma.	$
	etodolac generics	200–300 mg BID	See diclofenac.	See diclofenac.	See diclofenac.	$$
	indomethacin generics	50–200 mg/day in 2 or 3 divided doses	See diclofenac. Headache is common (>10%).	See diclofenac.	See diclofenac. Not commonly used for OA.	$
	sulindac generics	150–200 mg BID	See diclofenac.	See diclofenac.	See diclofenac.	$
NSAIDs, naphthylalkanone derivatives	*nabumetone* ❥ generics	1000 mg once daily May increase up to 2000 mg daily given in 1–2 divided doses	See diclofenac.	See diclofenac.	See diclofenac.	$$
NSAIDs, oxicams	*piroxicam* generics	10–20 mg daily	See diclofenac.	See diclofenac.	See diclofenac.	$
	tenoxicam generics	20–40 mg daily	See diclofenac.	See diclofenac.	See diclofenac.	$$
	meloxicam Mobicox, generics	7.5–15 mg daily	See diclofenac.	See diclofenac.	See diclofenac.	$
NSAIDs, propionic acid derivatives	*flurbiprofen* generics	50–100 mg BID–TID	See diclofenac.	See diclofenac.	See diclofenac.	$

(cont'd)

Table 2: **Oral Agents Used in Osteoarthritis** *(cont'd)*

Class	Drug	Dose	Adverse Effects	Drug Interactions	Comments	Cost[a]
	ibuprofen Advil, Motrin, generics	200–600 mg Q6H–Q8H	See diclofenac.	See diclofenac.	See diclofenac. May decrease antiplatelet effect of ASA; give ibuprofen at least 30 minutes after or 8 h before ASA.	$
	ketoprofen generics	50–75 mg TID–QID	See diclofenac.	See diclofenac.	See diclofenac.	$
	naproxen Naprosyn, generics	250–500 mg BID	See diclofenac.	See diclofenac.	See diclofenac.	$
	naproxen sodium Aleve, Anaprox, generics	220–550 mg BID	See diclofenac.	See diclofenac.	See diclofenac. Nonprescription strength is 220 mg.	$
	naproxen sodium controlled-release Naprelan	750–1000 mg daily	See diclofenac.	See diclofenac.	See diclofenac.	$$
	tiaprofenic acid ❥ generics	200–300 mg BID	See diclofenac.	See diclofenac.	See diclofenac.	$
NSAIDs, salicylic acid derivatives	*ASA* Aspirin, Coated Aspirin, Entrophen, generics	325–650 mg Q4H	See diclofenac.	See diclofenac.	See diclofenac. Not commonly used for OA.	$
	diflunisal generics	250–500 mg BID	See diclofenac.	See diclofenac.	See diclofenac.	$
NSAID/Gastro-protection Combinations	*diclofenac/ misoprostol* Arthrotec, generics	1 tablet BID (contains 50 mg or 75 mg diclofenac + 200 μg misoprostol) Maximum: 150 mg/day diclofenac	See diclofenac. Misoprostol component increase risk of diarrhea.	See diclofenac.	See diclofenac. Contraindicated in pregnancy—misoprostol is an abortifacient.	$

Class	Drug	Dose	Adverse Effects	Drug Interactions	Comments	Cost[a]
	naproxen/ esomeprazole Vimovo	1 tablet BID (contains 375 mg or 500 mg naproxen + 20 mg esomeprazole)	See diclofenac.	See diclofenac. Esomeprazole may decrease efficacy of clopidogrel but clinical significance is uncertain.	See diclofenac.	$
Serotonin-Norepinephrine Reuptake Inhibitors	*duloxetine* Cymbalta	60 mg daily Maximum dose: 120 mg po daily	Nausea, constipation, diarrhea, dry mouth, asthenia, fatigue, dizziness, somnolence, headache, insomnia, decreased appetite, erectile dysfunction.	Do not use with potent CYP1A2 inhibitors (fluvoxamine, ciprofloxacin, ketoconazole) or monoamine oxidase inhibitors. Caution with other serotonergic drugs (dextromethorphan, trazodone, triptans).	May start with 30 mg/day and titrate to avoid adverse effects. Should not be abruptly discontinued. Avoid in severe hepatic or renal dysfunction.	$$$

[a] Cost of 1 week therapy; includes drug cost only.

Dosage adjustment may be required in renal impairment; see Appendix I.

Abbreviations: ClCr = creatinine clearance; COX-2 = cyclooxygenase-2; CYP = cytochrome P450; HF = heart failure; MI = myocardial infarction; OA = osteoarthritis; TCA = tricyclic antidepressant

Legend: $ <$10 $$ $10–20 $$$ $20–30 $$$$ $30–40

Table 3: Topical Agents Used in Osteoarthritis

Class	Drug	Dose	Adverse Effects	Drug Interactions	Comments	Cost[a]
Capsicum Derivatives	*capsaicin* Zostrix, Zostrix HP, generics	Apply TID–QID	Transient burning on application.		Marketed as a nonprescription natural health product. Avoid contact with eyes or open lesions.	$$
	zucapsaicin Zuacta	Apply TID to knee	See capsaicin.		Prescription product approved for adjunctive use with oral NSAIDs for severe pain in OA of knee for maximum of 3 months. Avoid contact with eyes or open lesions.	$$$$$
Nonsteroidal Anti-inflammatory Agents	*diclofenac diethylamine* Voltaren Emulgel	Apply QID	Skin dryness or irritation, hypersensitivity. Serious GI toxicity has not been seen to date in clinical trials.		Available without prescription as 1.16% gel.	$
	diclofenac sodium Pennsaid, generics	Apply QID	See diclofenac sodium.		For external use only. Approved for duration of ≤3 months (continuous or intermittent treatment). Available as 1.5% lotion; requires prescription.	$$$$
	methyl salicylate Rub A-535, others	Apply TID–QID	Skin irritation.	Warfarin: may increase anticoagulant effect.	Avoid in ASA-allergic patients. Avoid contact with eyes and mucous membranes.	$

[a] Cost of smallest available pack size; includes drug cost only.
Abbreviations: ASA = acetylsalicylic acid; GI = gastrointestinal; OA = osteoarthritis
Legend: $ <$10 $$ $10–20 $$$ $20–30 $$$$ $30–40 $$$$$ $40–50

Table 4: Intra-articular Agents Used in Osteoarthritis

Class	Drug	Dose	Adverse Effects	Comments	Cost[a]
Corticosteroids, intra-articular	*betamethasone acetate/betamethasone sodium phosphate* Celestone Soluspan	Large joints:[b] 1 mL (contains 3 mg betamethasone acetate + 3 mg betamethasone sodium phosphate) Medium joints:[c] 0.5–1 mL Small joints:[d] 0.25–0.5 mL	No clinically significant systemic effects.	Inexpensive, safe and effective therapy for individual joints (especially hips/knees). Maximum: 3 injections/joint/year. Minimize joint activity for 3 days following injection. Benefits last 4–6 wk.	$$$
	methylprednisolone acetate Depo-Medrol, generics	Large joints:[b] 20–80 mg Medium joints:[c] 10–40 mg Small joints:[d] 4–10 mg	See betamethasone.	See betamethasone.	$$
	triamcinolone acetonide Kenalog-10 Injection, Kenalog-40 Injection, generics	Large joints:[b] 5–40 mg Small joints:[d] 2.5–10 mg	See betamethasone.	See betamethasone.	$$
Viscosupple-mentation	*sodium hyaluronate* NeoVisc, SynVisc, SynVisc One, OrthoVisc, Durolane, Euflexxa, Ostenil	1 injection into the involved joint. May be given once only, or weekly × 3–5 wk depending on affected joint and product used.	No general systemic effect. Pseudogout. Pseudosepsis has been reported rarely in patients receiving Synvisc.		$90

[a] Cost of one injection; includes drug cost only.
[b] Large joints: hips, knees, shoulders, ankles.
[c] Medium joints: elbows, wrists.
[d] Small joints: metacarpophalangeal, interphalangeal, sternoclavicular, acromioclavicular.
Legend: $ <$5 $$ $5–10 $$$ $10–15

Suggested Readings

Fernandes L, Hagen KB, Bijlsma JW et al. EULAR recommendations for the non-pharmacological core management of hip and knee osteoarthritis. *Ann Rheum Dis* 2013;72(7):1125-35.

Hochberg MC, Altman RD, April KT et al. American College of Rheumatology 2012 recommendations for the use of nonpharmacologic and pharmacologic therapies in osteoarthritis of the hand, hip, and knee. *Arthritis Care Res* 2012;64(4):465-74.

Jordan KM, Arden NK, Doherty M et al. EULAR Recommendations 2003: an evidence based approach to the management of knee osteoarthritis: Report of a Task Force of the Standing Committee for International Clinical Studies Including Therapeutic Trials (ESCISIT). *Ann Rheum Dis* 2003;62(12):1145-55.

McAlindon TE, Bannuru RR, Sullivan MC et al. OARSI guidelines for the non-surgical management of knee osteoarthritis. *Osteoarthritis Cartilage* 2014;22(3):363-88.

Rostom A, Dube C, Jolicoeur E et al. Gastroduodenal ulcers associated with the use of non-steroidal anti-inflammatory drugs: a systematic review of preventive pharmacological interventions. Ottawa (ON): Canadian Coordinating Office for Health Technology Assessment. *Technology Overview* 2004;12. Available from: www.cadth.ca/media/pdf/261_gastro_ov_e.pdf.

References

1. Dieppe PA, Lohmander LS. Pathogenesis and management of pain in osteoarthritis. *Lancet* 2005;365(9463):965-73.
2. Buchanan WW, Kean WF. Osteoarthritis I: Epidemiological risk factors and historical considerations. *Inflammopharmacology* 2002;10(1):5-21.
3. Buchanan WW, Kean WF, Kean R. History and current status of osteoarthritis in the population. *Inflammopharmacology* 2003;11(4):301-16.
4. Altman RD. Classification of disease: osteoarthritis. *Semin Arthritis Rheum* 1991;20(6 Suppl 2):40-7.
5. Cross M, Smith E, Hoy D et al. The global burden of hip and knee osteoarthritis: estimates from the global burden of disease 2010 study. *Ann Rheum Dis* 2014 Feb 19. [Epub ahead of print.]
6. Adatia A, Rainsford KD, Kean WF. Osteoarthritis of the knee and hip. Part I: aetiology and pathogenesis as a basis for pharmacotherapy. *J Pharm Pharmacol* 2012;64(5):617-25.
7. Leung GJ, Rainsford KD, Kean WF. Osteoarthritis of the hand I: aetiology and pathogenesis, risk factors, investigations and diagnosis. *J Pharm Pharmacol* 2014;66(3):339-46.
8. Jvan Saase JL, van Romunde LK, Cats A et al. Epidemiology of osteoarthritis: Zoetermeer survey. Comparison of radiological osteoarthritis in a Dutch population with that of 10 other populations. *Ann Rheum Dis* 1989;48(4):271-80.
9. Buchanan WW, Kean WF. Osteoarthritis III: Radiological and clinical definition. *Inflammopharmacology* 2002;10(1-2):53-78.
10. Menashe L, Hirko K, Losina E et al. The diagnostic performance of MRI in osteoarthritis: a systematic review and meta-analysis. *Osteoarthritis Cartilage* 2012;20(1):13-21.
11. Bennell KL, Hunter DJ, Hinman RS. Management of osteoarthritis of the knee. *BMJ* 2012;345:e4934.
12. Tanamas S, Hanna FS, Cicuttini FM et al. Does knee malalignment increase the risk of development and progression of knee osteoarthritis? A systematic review. *Arthritis Rheum* 2009;61(4):459-67.
13. Superio-Cabuslay E, Ward MM, Lorig KR. Patient education interventions in osteoarthritis and rheumatoid arthritis: a meta-analytic comparison with nonsteroidal antiinflammatory drug treatment. *Arthritis Care Res* 1996;9(4):292-301.
14. Hochberg MC, Altman RD, April KT et al. American College of Rheumatology 2012 recommendations for the use of nonpharmacologic and pharmacologic therapies in osteoarthritis of the hand, hip, and knee. *Arthritis Care Res* 2012;64(4):465-74.
15. Rutjes AW, Nuesch E, Sterchi R et al. Transcutaneous electrostimulation for osteoarthritis of the knee. *Cochrane Database Syst Rev* 2009;(4):CD002823.
16. McAlindon TE, Bannuru RR, Sullivan MC et al. OARSI guidelines for the non-surgical management of knee osteoarthritis. *Osteoarthritis Cartilage* 2014;22(3):363-88.
17. Vas J, Mendez C, Perea-Milla E et al. Acupuncture as a complementary therapy to the pharmacological treatment of osteoarthritis of the knee: randomised controlled trial. *BMJ* 2004;329(7476):1216.
18. Berman BM, Lao L, Langenberg P et al. Effectiveness of acupuncture as adjunctive therapy in osteoarthritis of the knee: a randomized, controlled trial. *Ann Intern Med* 2004;141(12):901-10.
19. Suarez-Almazor ME, Looney C, Liu Y et al. A randomized controlled trial of acupuncture for osteoarthritis of the knee: effects of patient-provider communication. *Arthritis Care Res (Hoboken)* 2010;62(9):1229-36.
20. Kerrigan DC, Lelas JL, Goggins J et al. Effectiveness of a lateral-wedge insole on knee varus torque in patients with knee osteoarthritis. *Arch Phys Med Rehabil* 2002;83(7):889-93.
21. Raja K, Dewan N. Efficacy of knee braces and foot orthoses in conservative management of knee osteoarthritis: a systematic review. *Am J Phys Med Rehabil* 2011;90(3):247-62.
22. van Raaij TM, Reijman M, Brouwer RW et al. Medial knee osteoarthritis treated by insoles or braces: a randomized trial. *Clin Orthop Relat Res* 2010;468(7):1926-32.
23. Fernandes L, Hagen KB, Bijlsma JW et al. EULAR recommendations for the non-pharmacological core management of hip and knee osteoarthritis. *Ann Rheum Dis* 2013;72(2):1125-35.
24. Juhl C, Christensen R, Roos EM et al. Impact of exercise type and dose on pain and disability in knee osteoarthritis: a systematic review and meta-regression analysis of randomized controlled trials. *Arthritis Rheum* 2014;66(3):622-36.
25. Jansen MJ, Viechtbauer W, Lenssen AF et al. Strength training alone, exercise therapy alone, and exercise therapy with passive manual mobilisation each reduce pain and disability in people with knee osteoarthritis: a systematic review. *J Physiother* 2011;57(1):11-20.
26. Uthman OA, van der Windt DA, Jordan JL et al. Exercise for lower limb osteoarthritis: systematic review incorporating trial sequential analysis and network meta-analysis. *BMJ* 2013;347:f5555.

27. Fransen M, McConnell S, Hernandex-Molina G et al. Exercise for osteoarthritis of the hip. *Cochrane Database Syst Rev* 2014;4:CD007912.
28. Hennig T, Haehre L, Hornburg VT et al. Effect of home-based hand exercises in women with hand osteoarthritis: a randomised controlled trial. *Ann Rheum Dis* 2014 Mar 25. [Epub ahead of print.]
29. Lauche R, Langhorst J, Dobos G. A systematic review and meta-analysis of Tai Chi for osteoarthritis of the knee. *Complement Ther Med* 2013;21(4):396-406.
30. Yan JH, Gu WJ, Sun J et al. Efficacy of Tai Chi on pain, stiffness and function in patients with osteoarthritis: a meta-analysis. *PLoS One* 2013;8(4):e61672.
31. Messier SP, Mihalko SL, Legault C et al. Effects of intensive diet and exercise on knee joint loads, inflammation, and clinical outcomes among overweight and obese adults with knee osteoarthritis: the IDEA randomized clinical trial. *JAMA* 2013;310(12):1263-73.
32. Brosseau L, Wells GA, Tugwell P et al. Ottawa Panel evidence-based clinical practice guidelines for the management of osteoarthritis in adults who are obese or overweight. *Phys Ther* 2011;91(6):843-61.
33. Dromgoole SH. Topical nonsteroidal anti-inflammatory drugs in skin diseases and musculoskeletal disorders. In: Lewis AJ, Furst DE, eds. *Nonsteroidal anti-inflammatory drugs: mechanisms and clinical uses*. 2nd ed. New York: Marcel Dekker; 1994. p. 71-95.
34. Mason L, Moore RA, Edwards JE et al. Topical NSAIDs for acute pain: a meta-analysis. *BMC Fam Pract* 2004;5:10.
35. Mason L, Moore RA, Edwards JE et al. Topical NSAIDs for chronic musculoskeletal pain: systematic review and meta-analysis. *BMC Musculoskelet Disord* 2004;5:28.
36. Grace D, Rogers J, Skeith K et al. Topical diclofenac versus placebo: a double blind, randomized clinical trial in patients with osteoarthritis of the knee. *J Rheumatol* 1999;26(12):2659-83.
37. Derry S, Moore RA, Rabbie R. Topical NSAIDs for chronic musculoskeletal pain in adults. *Cochrane Database Syst Rev* 2012;9:CD007400.
38. Makris UE, Kohler MJ, Fraenkel L. Adverse effects of topical nonsteroidal antiinflammatory drugs in older adults with osteoarthritis: a systematic literature review. *J Rheumatol* 2010;37(6):1236-43.
39. Altman RD, Auen A, Holmburg CE et al. Capsaicin cream 0.025% as monotherapy for osteoarthritis: a double-blind study. *Semin Arthritis Rheum* 1994;23(6 Suppl 3):S25-33.
40. Deal CL, Schnitzer TJ, Lipstein E et al. Treatment of arthritis with topical capsaicin: a double-blind trial. *Clin Ther* 1991;13(3):383-95.
41. Cameron M, Chrubasik S. Topical herbal therapies for treating osteoarthritis. *Cochrane Database Syst Rev* 2013;5:CD010538.
42. U.S. Food and Drug Administration. *FDA Drug Safety Communication: Rare cases of serious burns with the use of over-the-counter topical muscle and joint pain relievers*. Available from: fda.gov/Drugs/DrugSafety/ucm318858.htm. Accessed January 24, 2014.
43. Jordan KM, Arden NK, Doherty M et al. EULAR Recommendations 2003: an evidence based approach to the management of knee osteoarthritis: Report of a Task Force of the Standing Committee for International Clinical Studies including Therapeutic Trials (ESCISIT). *Ann Rheum Dis* 2003;62(12):1145-55.
44. Graham GG, Davies MJ, Day RO et al. The modern pharmacology of paracetamol: therapeutic actions, mechanism of action, metabolism, toxicity and recent pharmacological findings. *Inflammopharmacology* 2013;21(3):201-32.
45. Gonzales-Perez A, Rodriguez LA. Upper gastrointestinal complications among users of paracetamol. *Basic Clin Pharmacol Toxicol* 2006;98(3):297-303.
46. Chou R, Helfand M, Peterson K et al. *Comparative effectiveness and safety of analgesics for osteoarthritis* [Internet]. Rockville (MD): Agency for Healthcare Research and Quality (US); 2006 Sep. (Comparative Effectiveness Reviews, No. 4).
47. Trelle S, Reichenbach S, Wandel S et al. Cardiovascular safety of non-steroidal anti-inflammatory drugs: network meta-analysis. *BMJ* 2011;342:c7086.
48. McGettigan P, Henry D. Cardiovascular risk with non-steroidal anti-inflammatory drugs: systematic review of population-based controlled observational studies. *PLoS Med* 2011;8(9):e1001098.
49. Coxib and traditional NSAID Trialists' (CNT) Collaboration. Vascular and upper gastrointestinal effects of non-steroidal anti-inflammatory drugs: meta-analyses of individual participant data from randomised trials. *Lancet* 2013;382(9894):769-79.
50. Kidney Disease: Improving Global Outcomes (KDIGO). KDIGO 2012 clinical practice guideline for the evaluation and management of chronic kidney disease. *Kidney Int Suppl* 2013;3(1):1-150. Available from: www.kdigo.org/clinical_practice_guidelines/ckd.php.
51. Rostom A, Dube C, Jolicoeur E et al. Gastroduodenal ulcers associated with the use of non-steroidal anti-inflammatory drugs: a systematic review of preventive pharmacological interventions. Ottawa (ON): Canadian Coordinating Office for Health Technology Assessment. *Technology Overview* 2004;12. Available from: www.cadth.ca/media/pdf/261_gastro_ov_e.pdf. Accessed April 5, 2011.
52. Chan FK, Lanas A, Scheiman J et al. Celecoxib versus omeprazole and diclofenac in patients with osteoarthritis and rheumatoid arthritis (CONDOR): a randomised trial. *Lancet* 2010;376(9736):173-9.
53. Hawkey CJ, Talley NJ, Scheiman JM et al. Maintenance treatment with esomeprazole following initial relief of non-steroidal anti-inflammatory drug-associated upper gastrointestinal symptoms: the NASA2 and SPACE2 studies. *Arthritis Res Ther* 2007;9(1):R17.
54. Lanza FL, Chan FK, Quigley EM et al. Guidelines for prevention of NSAID-related ulcer complications. *Am J Gastroenterol* 2009;104(3):728-38.
55. Laine L, Curtis SP, Cryer B et al. Risk factors for NSAID-associated upper GI clinical events in a long-term prospective study of 34 701 arthritis patients. *Aliment Pharmacol Ther* 2010;32(10):1240-8.
56. Kean WF, Bouchard S, Roderich Gossen E. Women with pain due to osteoarthritis: the efficacy and safety of a once-daily formulation of tramadol. *Pain Med* 2009;10(6):1001-11.
57. National Opioid Use Guideline Group. *Canadian guideline for safe and effective use of opioids for chronic non-cancer pain. Part B: Recommendations for practice*. April 30 2010. Available from: nationalpaincentre.mcmaster.ca/documents/opioid_guideline_part_b_v5_6.pdf.
58. Likar R., Wittels M, Molnar M et al: Pharmacokinetic and pharmacodynamic properties of tramadol IR and SR in elderly patients: a prospective, age-group-controlled study. *Clin Ther* 2006;28(12):2022-39.
59. Nuesch E, Rutjes AW, Husni E et al. Oral or transdermal opioids for osteoarthritis of the knee or hip. *Cochrane Database Syst Rev* 2009;(4):CD003115.
60. American Geriatrics Society Panel on Pharmacological Management of Persistent Pain in Older Persons. Pharmacological management of persistent pain in older persons. *J Am Geriatr Soc* 2009;57(8):1331-46.
61. Citrome L, Weiss-Citrome A. A systematic review of duloxetine for osteoarthritic pain: what is the number needed to treat, number needed to harm, and likelihood to be helped or harmed? *Postgrad Med* 2012;124(1):83-93.
62. Perahia DG, Bangs ME, Zhang Q et al. The risk of bleeding with duloxetine treatment in patients who use nonsteroidal anti-inflammatory drugs (NSAIDs): analysis of placebo-controlled trials and post-marketing adverse event reports. *Drug Healthc Patient Saf* 2013;5:211-9.
63. Wandel S, Juni P, Tendal B et al. Effects of glucosamine, chondroitin, or placebo in patients with osteoarthritis of hip or knee: network meta-analysis. *BMJ* 2010;341:c4675.

64. Samson DJ, Grant MD, Ratko TA et al. Treatment of primary and secondary osteoarthritis of the knee. *Evid Rep Technol Assess (Full Rep)* 2007;(157):1-157.
65. Reichenbach S, Sterchi R, Scherer M et al. Meta-analysis: chondroitin for osteoarthritis of the knee or hip. *Ann Intern Med* 2007;146(8):580-90.
66. Towheed TE, Maxwell L, Anastassiades TP et al. Glucosamine therapy for treating osteoarthritis. *Cochrane Database Syst Rev* 2005;(2):CD002946.
67. Abou-Raya A, Abou-Raya S, Khadrawi T et al. Effect of low-dose oral prednisolone on symptoms and systemic inflammation in older adults with moderate to severe knee osteoarthritis: a randomized placebo-controlled trial. *J Rheumatol* 2014;41(1):53-9.
68. Lane NE, Lukert B. The science and therapy of glucocorticoid-induced bone loss. *Endocrinol Metab Clin North Am* 1998;27(2):465-83.
69. Bellamy N, Campbell J, Robinson V et al. Intraarticular corticosteroid for treatment of osteoarthritis of the knee. *Cochrane Database Syst Rev* 2006;(2):CD005328.
70. Hochberg MC, Altman RD, Brandt KD et al. Guidelines for the medical management of osteoarthritis. Part II. Osteoarthritis of the knee. American College of Rheumatology. *Arthritis Rheum* 1995;38(11):1541-6.
71. Rutjes AW, Juni P, da Costa BR et al. Viscosupplementation for osteoarthritis of the knee: a systematic review and meta-analysis. *Ann Intern Med* 2012;157(3):180-91.
72. Arrich J, Piribauer F, Mad P et al. Intra-articular hyaluronic acid for the treatment of osteoarthritis of the knee: systematic review and meta-analysis. *CMAJ* 2005;172(8):1039-43.
73. Bellamy N, Campbell J, Robinson V et al. Viscosupplementation for the treatment of osteoarthritis of the knee. *Cochrane Database Syst Rev* 2006;(2):CD005321.
74. Chang KV, Hung CY, Aliwarga F et al. Comparative effectiveness of platelet-rich plasma injections for treating knee joint cartilage degenerative pathology: a systematic review and meta-analysis. *Arch Phys Med Rehabil* 2014;95(3):562-75.
75. Khosbin A, Leroux T, Wasserstein D et al. The efficacy of platelet-rich plasma in the treatment of symptomatic knee osteoarthritis: a systematic review with quantitative synthesis. *Arthroscopy* 2013;29(12):2037-48.
76. Hawker G, Wright J, Coyle P et al. Health-related quality of life after knee replacement. *J Bone Joint Surg Am* 1998;80(2):163-73.
77. Ross AC. Infected arthroplasties. *Curr Opin Rheumatol* 1991;3(4):628-33.
78. Wang J Zhu C, Cheng T et al. A systematic review and meta-analysis of antibiotic-impregnated bone cement use in primary total hip or knee arthroplasty. *PLos One* 2013;8(12):e82745.
79. Howie DW, Neale SD, Haynes DR et al. Periprosthetic osteolysis after total hip replacement: molecular pathology and clinical management. *Inflammopharmacology* 2013;21(6):389-96.
80. Reichenbach S, Rutjes AW, Nuesch E et al. Joint lavage for osteoarthritis of the knee. *Cochrane Database Syst Rev* 2010;(5):CD007320.
81. Wynne HA, Long A. Patient awareness of the adverse effects of non-steroidal anti-inflammatory drugs (NSAIDs). *Br J Clin Pharmacol* 1996;42(2):253-6.
82. Anderson JL, Adams CD, Antman EM et al. ACC/AHA 2007 Guidelines for the management of patients with unstable angina/non ST-elevation myocardial infarction: executive summary. *Circulation* 2007;116(7):803-77. Available from: circ.ahajournals.org/cgi/reprint/116/7/803. Accessed April 5, 2011.

Chapter 83
Osteoporosis

David A. Hanley, MD, FRCPC

Goals of Therapy

- Prevent fractures, disability and loss of independence
- Preserve or enhance bone mass

Investigations

Evidence-based clinical practice guidelines identify key predictors of osteoporosis-related fracture: age, history of previous fragility fracture, current corticosteroid use (>3 months' duration) and low bone mineral density.[1]

Table 1 lists risk factors used to select candidates for bone mineral density (BMD) testing.

Table 1: Risk Factors Prompting Assessment for Osteoporosis (Measurement of BMD)

Older Adults (≥50 y)	Younger Adults (<50 y)
• Age ≥65 y • Clinical risk factors for fracture (men age 50–64 y, menopausal women): - Vertebral compression fracture - Fragility fracture after age 40 - Prolonged use of corticosteroids[a] - Use of other high-risk medications, e.g., aromatase inhibitors, androgen deprivation therapy - Parent with hip fracture - Osteopenia identified on x-ray - Current smoking - High alcohol intake - Low body weight (<60 kg) or major weight loss (>10% of weight at age 25) - Rheumatoid arthritis - Other disorders strongly associated with osteoporosis	• Fragility fracture • Prolonged use of corticosteroids[a] • Use of other high risk medications, e.g., aromatase inhibitors, androgen deprivation therapy • Hypogonadism or premature menopause (<45 y) • Malabsorption syndrome • Primary hyperparathyroidism • Other disorders strongly associated with rapid bone loss or fracture

[a] Prednisone-equivalent dose ≥7.5 mg/day for at least 3 months (cumulative) in the previous year.
Adapted from 2010 clinical practice guidelines for the diagnosis and management of osteoporosis in Canada: summary. *CMAJ* 2010;182(17):1864-73 by permission of the publisher © 2010 Canadian Medical Association.

- History:
  - measured height loss of >6 cm since peak height as a young adult or >2 cm height loss within past year
  - history of falling
  - chronic or acute back pain
  - endocrine diseases: hyperthyroidism, hyperparathyroidism, hypogonadism, Cushing's syndrome; renal diseases, organ transplantation, GI disease (gastric surgery, malabsorption); chemotherapy for malignancy

- medications associated with increased risk of fractures: aromatase inhibitors, anticoagulants (unfractionated and low molecular weight heparins), antiretroviral therapy, cyclosporine, depot medroxyprogesterone acetate, corticosteroid therapy (at least 3 months' cumulative therapy in the previous year at a prednisone-equivalent dose ≥7.5 mg daily), loop diuretics, proton pump inhibitors (PPIs), SSRIs, thiazolidinediones. High doses of vitamin A are associated with increased risk of hip fracture so patients should not take double doses of multivitamins to try to increase their vitamin D intake[2]
- see Table 1 for other risk factors

- Physical examination:
  - kyphosis: <3 fingers' breadth between rib and pelvis
  - factors increasing risk of falling: muscle weakness (inability to rise from a chair), impaired visual acuity, poor balance, or disability causing a tendency to fall
- Laboratory investigations:
  - all should be normal: CBC, calcium, alkaline phosphatase (may be elevated in acute recovery from fracture), creatinine. Measure TSH if there is a clinical suspicion of thyroid disease. Serum protein electrophoresis if there is a suspicion of secondary causes of osteoporosis. Serum 25-OH vitamin D if the patient is at increased risk of deficiency (e.g., malabsorption syndromes, housebound, established osteoporosis requiring pharmacologic therapy). Measure after patient has been taking vitamin D supplements for 3 months.
  - markers of bone turnover are not appropriate for diagnosis or routine management[1]
- Diagnostic imaging:
  - x-rays are mainly used for detecting fractures.[1] If x-ray shows osteopenia (decreased bone mineral), confirm with a BMD measurement
  - bone scans can identify new fracture activity in patients with back pain and no obvious new fracture on x-ray
- BMD measurements:
  - BMD of the spine and hip by dual x-ray absorptiometry (DXA) is the preferred method of assessing bone mass and fracture risk, as well as monitoring response to therapy.[1] Other methods (e.g., heel ultrasound) are acceptable for assessing fracture risk if DXA is not available[3]
  - An estimated 10-year risk of osteoporotic fracture in women (Figure 1) and in men (Figure 2) which is reported as low (<10%), moderate (10–20%) or high (>20%), can be derived by combining age and epidemiologic data with DXA BMD measurements.[4] This risk stratification has been validated in 2 Canadian databases, and is now recommended as a guide to osteoporosis management. Risk categories are intended only for assessment of the as yet untreated patient.

    Pharmacologic therapy of osteoporosis is recommended for high-risk individuals and should be considered in individuals at moderate risk. A hip fracture or a vertebral fracture occurring after menopause or age 50 automatically places a patient in a high risk category irrespective of BMD, unless the fracture occurred due to a high trauma accident. Corticosteroid therapy or a fragility fracture at a site other than hip or spine moves a patient to a higher risk category than that indicated by BMD and age. Two such fractures place a patient in a high risk category. A fragility fracture is one that occurs with low trauma (e.g., a fall from a standing height or less). An individual in the "low risk" category is not likely to receive clinically meaningful fracture prevention benefit from pharmacologic therapy.
  - the WHO Collaborative Group has introduced a 10-year osteoporotic fracture risk assessment tool, FRAX (available at www.shef.ac.uk/FRAX/).[5] This tool uses a single femoral neck BMD measurement (or body mass index if BMD is not available) and a few risk factors to calculate a country-specific 10-year percentage risk of major osteoporotic fracture (forearm, humerus, spine, hip). CAROC (Canadian Association of Radiologists and Osteoporosis Canada Risk Assessment

tool), and a Canadian FRAX model have been developed and validated. Osteoporosis Canada recommends using the simpler CAROC tool (Figure 1 and Figure 2), as this is what most DXA centres are using to report BMD in Canada. However, FRAX can be used to determine a rough estimate of fracture risk.

Figure 1: Use of Bone Density and Age to Predict Fragility Fracture Risk in Women

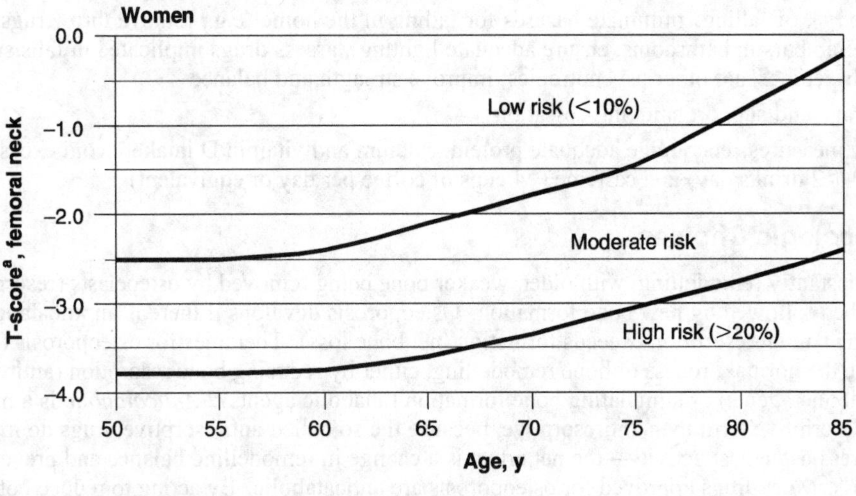

[a] T-score is calculated by comparing the BMD measurement of the patient to that of an average young adult of the same sex. A score ≥−1.0 is considered normal.

Reproduced from *CMAJ* 2010;182(17):1864-73 by permission of the publisher.

Figure 2: Use of Bone Density and Age to Predict Fragility Fracture Risk in Men

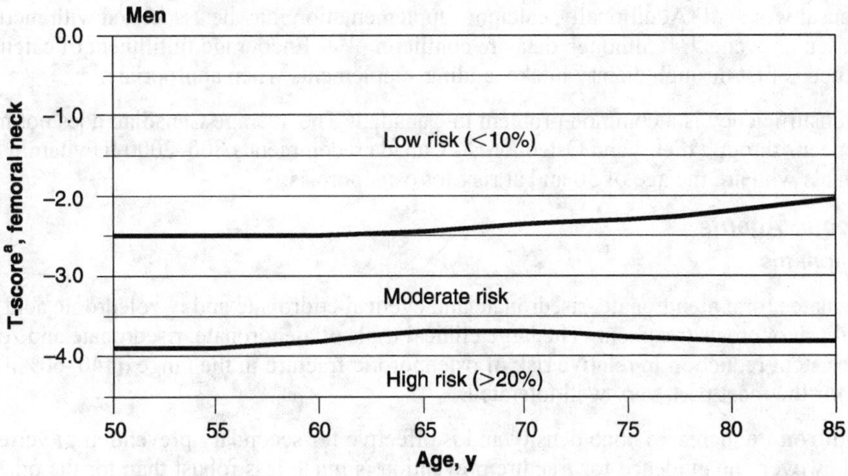

[a] T-score is calculated by comparing the BMD measurement of the patient to that of an average young adult of the same sex. A score ≥−1.0 is considered normal.

Reproduced from *CMAJ* 2010;182(17):1864-73 by permission of the publisher.

Therapeutic Choices

Osteoporosis therapy may be subdivided into *prevention* and *treatment* of established osteoporosis (Figure 3). Chronic corticosteroid therapy requires special attention for preventive intervention.[1]

Nonpharmacologic Choices

Recommended for everyone:

- Regular exercise (especially impact type)
- Reduce risk of falling: minimize hazards for falling in the home (e.g., remove throw rugs, install grab bars in bathrooms, ensure adequate lighting), assess drugs implicated in falls such as benzodiazepines and other psychotropics; improve strength and balance
- Encourage and support smoking cessation
- Dietary measures: encourage adequate protein, calcium and vitamin D intake, avoid excessive alcohol (>2 drinks/day) and caffeine (>4 cups of coffee per day or equivalent)

Pharmacologic Choices

Bone is constantly remodelling, with older, weaker bone being removed by osteoclasts (resorption), which is then followed by new bone formation. Osteoporosis develops if there is an imbalance in remodelling so that resorption exceeds formation (net bone loss). Therapies for osteoporosis (Table 2) manipulate the normal process of bone remodelling, either by reducing bone resorption (antiresorptive or anticatabolic agents) or stimulating bone formation (anabolic agents).[7] *Anticatabolic* is a more accurate descriptive term than antiresorptive, because the so-called antiresorptive drugs do more than suppress osteoclast activity—the net effect is a change in remodelling balance and prevention of bone loss. Most drugs approved for osteoporosis are anticatabolic. By acting to reduce both the depth and rate of bone resorption while bone formation proceeds normally, these agents cause an initial increase in bone mass. This increase eventually plateaus, as bone formation slows to match the reduced rate of resorption.[7]

In all age groups, adequate **calcium** and **vitamin D** preserves or enhances bone mass.[8] Calcium and vitamin D supplementation may prevent fractures in healthy postmenopausal women and older men.[9,10] However, data supporting a claim for fracture prevention are lacking in men under age 50 and premenopausal women.[11] Additionally, calcium supplementation may be associated with increased risk of cardiovascular events,[12,13] although data are conflicting.[14,15] Encourage fulfillment of calcium and vitamin D needs first through dietary intake, adding supplements when appropriate.

Vitamin D insufficiency is a common problem in Canada.[16] The average Canadian does not meet all vitamin D needs through diet,[11] and Osteoporosis Canada recommends 800–2000 IU vitamin D per day for individuals who are the age of 50 and at risk for osteoporosis.[17]

Anticatabolic Agents

Bisphosphonates

Bisphosphonates (oral alendronate, risedronate and cyclical etidronate and iv zoledronic acid) are the mainstay of osteoporosis treatment. The large clinical trials of alendronate, risedronate and zoledronate show a consistent reduction in relative risk of osteoporotic fracture in the range of 40–60%.[1] The drugs are, for the most part, very well tolerated.

Cyclical etidronate increases bone density and is effective for secondary prevention of vertebral fractures; however, the evidence for fracture prevention is much less robust than for the other bisphosphonates, with no clinical trials demonstrating prevention of nonvertebral fractures.[18] Safety and efficacy for up to 7 years of cyclical etidronate therapy has been demonstrated.[19] The dosage schedule of etidronate (only 14 days every 3 months, packaged with 76 days of elemental calcium 500 mg) and its lower cost are attractive to some patients.

Figure 3: Use of Bone Density, Risk Factors and Calculated 10-Year Fracture Risk in Osteoporosis Management

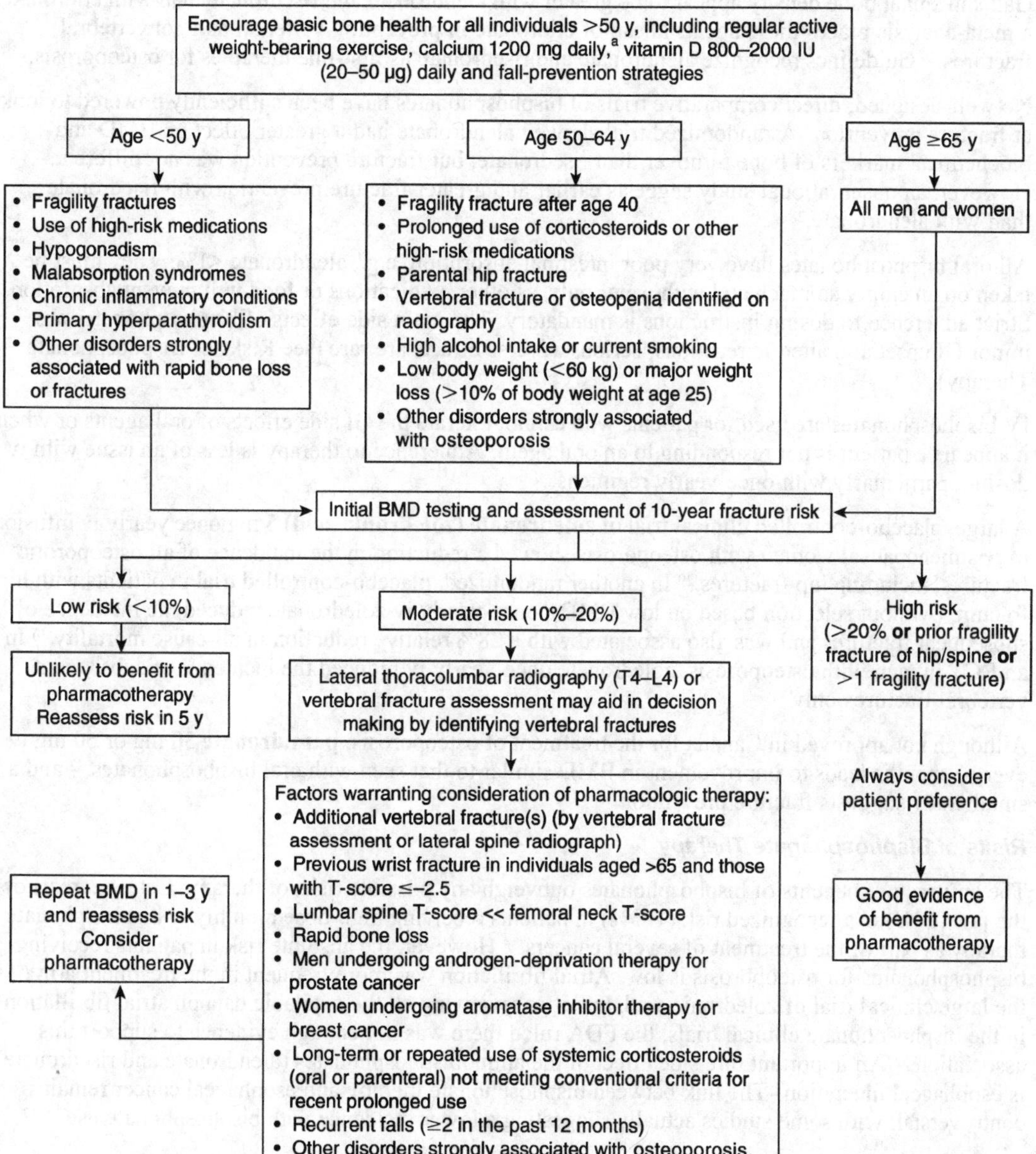
Encourage basic bone health for all individuals >50 y, including regular active weight-bearing exercise, calcium 1200 mg daily,[a] vitamin D 800–2000 IU (20–50 μg) daily and fall-prevention strategies
Age <50 y
Age 50–64 y
Age ≥65 y
• Fragility fractures
• Use of high-risk medications
• Hypogonadism
• Malabsorption syndromes
• Chronic inflammatory conditions
• Primary hyperparathyroidism
• Other disorders strongly associated with rapid bone loss or fractures
• Fragility fracture after age 40
• Prolonged use of corticosteroids or other high-risk medications
• Parental hip fracture
• Vertebral fracture or osteopenia identified on radiography
• High alcohol intake or current smoking
• Low body weight (<60 kg) or major weight loss (>10% of body weight at age 25)
• Other disorders strongly associated with osteoporosis
All men and women
Initial BMD testing and assessment of 10-year fracture risk
Low risk (<10%)
Moderate risk (10%–20%)
High risk (>20% or prior fragility fracture of hip/spine or >1 fragility fracture)
Unlikely to benefit from pharmacotherapy
Reassess risk in 5 y
Lateral thoracolumbar radiography (T4–L4) or vertebral fracture assessment may aid in decision making by identifying vertebral fractures
Factors warranting consideration of pharmacologic therapy:
• Additional vertebral fracture(s) (by vertebral fracture assessment or lateral spine radiograph)
• Previous wrist fracture in individuals aged >65 and those with T-score ≤–2.5
• Lumbar spine T-score << femoral neck T-score
• Rapid bone loss
• Men undergoing androgen-deprivation therapy for prostate cancer
• Women undergoing aromatase inhibitor therapy for breast cancer
• Long-term or repeated use of systemic corticosteroids (oral or parenteral) not meeting conventional criteria for recent prolonged use
• Recurrent falls (≥2 in the past 12 months)
• Other disorders strongly associated with osteoporosis, rapid bone loss or fractures
Repeat BMD in 1–3 y and reassess risk
Consider pharmacotherapy
Always consider patient preference
Good evidence of benefit from pharmacotherapy

[a] Encourage fulfillment of calcium needs first through dietary intake, adding supplements when appropriate.
Abbreviations: BMD = bone mineral density
Adapted from 2010 clinical practice guidelines for the diagnosis and management of osteoporosis in Canada: summary. *CMAJ* 2010;182(17):1864-73 by permission from the publisher.

Alendronate increases bone mass throughout the skeleton and reduces the risk of all fractures (including hip).[20,21,22] Although an observational study noted decreased efficacy of alendronate with concurrent use of PPIs,[23] this may have been due to the association of PPIs with fractures rather than a drug interaction with alendronate.

Risedronate, like alendronate, is associated with a reduced risk of all osteoporosis-associated fractures.[24,25]

Gains in spinal bone density appear to be greater with alendronate and risedronate than with etidronate; a meta-analysis places these agents ahead of etidronate in preventing vertebral and nonvertebral fractures.[26] Guidelines recognize alendronate and risedronate as first-line therapies for osteoporosis.[1]

No well-designed, direct comparative trials of bisphosphonates have been sufficiently powered to look at fracture prevention. A randomized trial showed alendronate had a greater effect on BMD and biochemical markers of bone turnover than risedronate, but fracture prevention was not different.[27] However, an observational study suggests earlier and greater fracture prevention with risedronate than with alendronate.[28]

All oral bisphosphonates have very poor intestinal absorption, e.g., alendronate <1%. They must be taken on an empty stomach and with water only, as other medications or food will prevent absorption. Strict adherence to dosing instructions is mandatory. The main side effects of bisphosphonates are minor GI upset and allergic reactions; serious adverse effects are rare (see Risks of Bisphosphonate Therapy).

IV bisphosphonates are used for patients who cannot tolerate the GI side effects of oral agents or when it appears a patient is not responding to an oral agent. Adherence to therapy is less of an issue with iv dosing, particularly with once-yearly regimens.

A large, placebo-controlled clinical trial of **zoledronate (zoledronic acid)** 5 mg once yearly iv infusion in postmenopausal women with osteoporosis showed a reduction in the incidence of all osteoporotic fractures, including hip fractures.[29] In another randomized, placebo-controlled trial in patients with hip fracture (without selection based on low BMD), once-yearly iv zoledronate reduced the incidence of subsequent fractures and was also associated with a 28% relative reduction in all-cause mortality.[30] In an RCT in men with osteoporosis, zoledronate once-yearly iv reduced the incidence of subsequent vertebral fractures only.[31]

Although not approved in Canada for the treatment of osteoporosis, **pamidronate** 30 mg or 60 mg iv every 3 months leads to improvement in BMD similar to that seen with oral bisphosphonates,[32] and a small study suggests fracture prevention.[33]

Risks of Bisphosphonate Therapy

The antifracture benefits of bisphosphonates outweigh any possible risks of therapy. Osteonecrosis of the jaw (ONJ) is a recognized risk (1–3%) in patients receiving high-dose monthly iv bisphosphonate therapy as part of the treatment of several cancers.[34] However, the absolute risk in patients receiving bisphosphonates for osteoporosis is low. Atrial fibrillation was more frequent in the treatment arm of the large clinical trial of zoledronic acid, but after reviewing all the available data on atrial fibrillation in the bisphosphonate clinical trials, the FDA ruled there was not enough evidence to support this association.[35] An important rare side effect of the aminobisphosphonates (alendronate and risedronate) is esophageal ulceration. The link between bisphosphonate therapy and esophageal cancer remains controversial, with some studies actually suggesting a lower incidence with bisphosphonate use.[36,37]

Case reports describe "atypical" femoral shaft fractures (AFSF) with some similarity to stress fractures, usually occurring as a spontaneous fracture in the subtrochanteric region of the femur, in patients treated for ≥2 years with bisphosphonates (mainly alendronate).[39] Two series of case reports have reported bone biopsies showing very low bone turnover.[38,39] Subtrochanteric osteoporotic fractures were also seen before bisphosphonates were available and one large cohort study suggests many or most are not different from osteoporotic fractures.[40] Undoubtedly, the association between bisphosphonate use and AFSFs is due in part to the fact that these drugs are used for the treatment of osteoporosis (confounding by indication). However, most osteoporosis experts believe the association of AFSFs with bisphosphonate therapy is indeed related to causation, although the mechanism has not been determined.[41]

Thirty to ninety percent of all AFSFs occur in bisphosphonate users.[42] Bisphosphonate use for 2–4 years is associated with 11 AFSFs per 100 000 patients per year, and the risk of AFSF increases with longer duration of use.[43] In contrast, the incidence of "typical" hip fracture is 750–4200 per 100 000 high-risk patients per year. Since bisphosphonate therapy reduces risk of hip fracture by 30–50%, the risk of causing an AFSF with bisphosphonate therapy is far outweighed by the number of hip fractures prevented in high-risk patients. Educate high-risk patients about the risk of AFSFs compared to the risk of no treatment. However, encourage lower-risk patients to stop bisphosphonate therapy after 5 years (see Bisphosphonate Drug Holidays).[44] If a patient is identified as having the beginning of an AFSF, stop the bisphosphonate and refer urgently to an orthopedic surgeon for consideration of fixation surgery to prevent a completed femoral shaft fracture. Alternatively, refer to a bone specialist for bone biopsy with histomorphometry.

If an atypical femoral shaft fracture (AFSF) is identified, do not restart bisphosphonate therapy. Consider an anabolic agent such as teriparatide to try to increase bone turnover and hasten repair [Evidence: SORT C *].[45,46] After the AFSF has healed, a referral to an osteoporosis specialist to reassess continuation of therapy may be appropriate. Alternatives to bisphosphonates, such as estrogen, raloxifene, teriparatide, denosumab or calcitonin may be considered. See warnings regarding calcitonin below.

Bisphosphonate Drug Holidays

Because of theoretical concerns about serious side effects, bisphosphonate *drug holidays*, i.e., stopping therapy for 1–3 years, have been suggested. The FLEX trial evaluated alendronate therapy past the 5-year mark of the Fracture Intervention Trial, randomizing patients to placebo versus continuing alendronate for another 5 years.[47] This study has been widely promoted as a rationale for offering patients a drug holiday after 5 years of alendronate therapy because patients in the placebo arm showed only a moderate decrease in BMD and no increase in nonvertebral fracture risk compared with those continuing alendronate over the second 5 years. However, the significantly increased risk of vertebral fractures in the placebo arm is notable; these fractures are not trivial, and are associated with increased mortality.[47] Also, bone biopsies from subjects who took alendronate for 10 years showed normal bone. The FLEX trial provides evidence of safety and further fracture protection in high-risk patients taking alendronate for 10 years.

Bisphosphonate "Drug Holiday" Recommendations:

- A 1- to 3-year drug holiday may be appropriate for low-risk patients who were prescribed alendronate for 5 years based solely on low BMD.[47]
- A 1- to 3-year drug holiday may be appropriate for low-risk patients who have been on zoledronic acid for 3 years and who do not have a history of a vertebral fracture.[48]
- A drug holiday of 1 year may be appropriate for low-risk patients on risedronate. Risedronate has a lower affinity to bone than alendronate.[49] BMD declined and bone turnover markers returned to placebo levels in the first year after risedronate was discontinued in one study (although fracture protection persisted in the year after discontinuation), suggesting an extended drug holiday may not be appropriate for patients treated with this agent.[50]

---

* SORT (Strength of Recommendation Taxonomy) is a rating system (A, B or C) that addresses the quality of available evidence. For more information consult **How to Use *Compendium of Therapeutic Choices*** on page xxv.

- Drug holidays are not recommended for high-risk patients (10-year fracture risk >20% or history of a previous fracture) as these individuals are at higher risk for recurrent fractures.[1]
- There is no clear evidence to guide when to end a drug holiday. Measure BMD after 2–3 years and recalculate the 10-year fracture risk (FRAX or CAROC). If the patient has lost BMD and is in a high-risk category, resume treatment for another 3–5 years.

RANK Ligand Inhibitors

Denosumab, the first biologic agent approved for the treatment of osteoporosis, is a human monoclonal antibody that binds receptor activator of nuclear factor-kappa B ligand (RANKL), thus preventing interaction with its receptor (RANK) on the surface of osteoclast precursors and osteoclasts. Inhibition of RANKL results in diminished osteoclast formation, function and survival, and the marked reduction in bone resorption increases cortical and trabecular bone mass and strength. In a large clinical trial, denosumab reduced the incidence of vertebral, nonvertebral and hip fractures in postmenopausal women with osteoporosis.[51] It may be used in postmenopausal women with a history of osteoporotic fracture, multiple risk factors for fracture or in those who have failed or are intolerant of other therapies.

Selective Estrogen Receptor Modulators

Raloxifene prevents postmenopausal bone loss,[52] increasing bone density by approximately 3% and reducing new vertebral fractures by 30–40% (NNT=16).[53,54] Raloxifene is an estrogen antagonist in breast and uterine tissue, but has estrogen-like activity in bone and lipid metabolism. Like estrogen, it causes a modestly increased risk of deep vein thrombosis and pulmonary embolism in postmenopausal women.[53] It also significantly reduces the relative risk of estrogen receptor-positive breast cancer by 76%.[55] Raloxifene is not associated with increased cardiovascular risk.[56]

Estrogen and Progesterone

Postmenopausal use of estrogen or estrogen/progesterone hormone therapy (HT) is no longer considered first choice for treatment of osteoporosis.[1,57] However, to prevent osteoporosis in women experiencing an early menopause (before age 45), HT should be taken until normal age of menopause.[1] For women entering menopause at the usual age, Canadian guidelines suggest HT should still be considered an option for women who wish to take an osteoporosis prevention therapy and who also wish to receive treatment for menopausal symptoms.[1] For the treatment of established osteoporosis in postmenopausal women over age 60, the Women's Health Initiative (WHI) studies showed HT is effective in preventing fractures but the reduction in hip and other fractures must be balanced against the increased risk of breast cancer and heart disease.[57] However, it should be noted that women participating in the WHI were at low risk for osteoporosis but had a high incidence of obesity and hypertension, increasing their risk of breast cancer and cardiovascular disease. The risk-benefit ratio may be different for postmenopausal women with osteoporosis, and the cardiovascular risk of HT was not seen in the women under age 60 in the WHI.[58]

Calcitonin

Salmon calcitonin nasal spray has been shown to prevent vertebral fractures, but because of weaker clinical trial data, it was regarded as a second-line therapy.[1] Additionally, a review by the European Medicines Agency (EMA) found that osteoporosis therapy with salmon calcitonin may be associated with a small increased risk of cancers.[59] The EMA has withdrawn calcitonin nasal spray from the European market, and more recently, Health Canada has recommended it be withdrawn from the Canadian market as well.[60] Injectable salmon calcitonin will continue to be available for the early treatment of hypercalcemia and a second-line therapy of Paget's disease of bone.

Calcitonin reduces pain associated with acute vertebral fractures.[61] Off-label use of injectable calcitonin could be considered for vertebral fracture pain in the short term, but the effective dose has not been standardized.

Anabolic Agents

Parathyroid Hormone and Analogues

Teriparatide, a parathyroid hormone (PTH) analogue, is an anabolic agent that demonstrates a steady gain in bone density and a 50% reduction in osteoporotic fractures (NNT=9).[54,62] It may also reduce pain associated with vertebral fractures.[1]

The major clinical trials of teriparatide were stopped at a median of 19 months of therapy because teratogenicity studies in rats given lifelong treatment with very high doses showed increased incidence of osteogenic sarcoma. This finding is not likely to be relevant to its use at a lower dose for a much shorter duration in humans. Additionally, several years of postmarketing surveillance has not detected any association between teriparatide therapy and osteosarcoma.[63] Teriparatide has been approved for 24 months' lifetime exposure.

After teriparatide therapy is completed, the gains in bone density are lost.[64] Treatment with a bisphosphonate or other anticatabolic agent is advised, as much of the increase in BMD may be lost during the first year after stopping the drug unless an anticatabolic is started.[65]

In a large placebo-controlled, 18-month clinical trial in patients at low risk of fracture, **recombinant human parathyroid hormone (PTH)** 100 µg daily sc significantly increased BMD and reduced the incidence of vertebral fractures.[66] This drug is approved for osteoporosis in Europe, but has not been introduced for osteoporosis therapy in North America.

Strontium Ranelate

Strontium ranelate is not available or approved for osteoporosis in Canada. However, some patients obtain strontium ranelate from Europe, or purchase other nonprescription strontium salts. Strontium replaces calcium in bone matrix and also appears to uncouple bone remodelling, causing a modest reduction in bone resorption in conjunction with a similarly modest increase in bone formation.[67] The dramatic increases in bone density are partly explained by the higher atomic weight of strontium compared to calcium, and partly by the positive bone balance. Clinical trials of strontium ranelate have shown similar effectiveness in fracture prevention to that seen with bisphosphonates.[67] Evidence for the efficacy of other strontium salts is lacking. Strontium ranelate 2 g orally is taken as powder mixed with water, once daily. Side effects appear to be infrequent, but in pooling the clinical trials, an increased incidence of venous thromboembolic events was noted in the subjects receiving strontium ranelate.[68] No effect of this drug on coagulation parameters has been identified, and the mechanism of this side effect remains unclear. Nervous system abnormalities (a variety of symptoms and disorders, including seizures and memory loss) were also reported slightly more frequently with strontium therapy. A serious systemic and skin reaction, "drug rash with eosinophilia systemic symptoms" (DRESS) is a rare complication of strontium ranelate therapy.[69]

Combination Therapy

Combining a bisphosphonate with other anticatabolic agents, e.g., estrogen[70,71] or raloxifene,[73] has additive or synergistic effects on BMD but no fracture benefit has been demonstrated.

Combining anticatabolic with anabolic therapy may seem an attractive approach, but results have been mixed. Giving a bisphosphonate concurrently with PTH or teriparatide may actually blunt the anabolic response.[72] However, combining teriparatide with either estrogen or raloxifene does not interfere with the anabolic action, and may enhance it.[74]

Therapeutic Tips

- A vertebral compression fracture, hip fracture or more than 1 fragility fracture after the age of 50 should be considered virtually diagnostic of osteoporosis irrespective of BMD testing. A single fragility fracture (e.g., wrist) in this age group should be considered a sign of osteoporosis until proven otherwise. Test these individuals with bone densitometry; they are still candidates for therapy if bone densitometry is not available.
- For the prevention of osteoporosis in early postmenopause, if estrogen deficiency symptoms also require treatment, **estrogen** or **estrogen/progesterone** remains a reasonable choice. If menopausal symptoms are not a problem, **raloxifene** is an alternative, with the potential added benefit of reducing breast cancer risk.
- For patients with established osteoporosis (e.g., a fragility fracture and bone density in the osteoporosis range), **bisphosphonates**, **denosumab**, **estrogen** and **teriparatide** are all considered first-line option. **Raloxifene** is also a first-line option but in the absence of nonvertebral fracture prevention data, consider it only after the other first-line therapies have been rejected for individuals at high risk of hip fracture (age >70 years with a prior fragility fracture history). Consider teriparatide first for severe cases characterized by more than one fragility fracture and a very low BMD.[75]
- For the prevention and treatment of *corticosteroid-induced osteoporosis*, **bisphosphonates** are the agents of choice.[1] **Teriparatide** is also approved for this indication and is first-line for a corticosteroid-treated individual with fractures and low BMD.
- Because of the absence of fracture prevention data, **calcitriol**, **androgens** and **sodium fluoride** are no longer considered appropriate alternative therapies.
- While women are more frequently affected by osteoporosis, vertebral deformities (which may represent vertebral fractures) occur almost as often in men as in women.[76] Hip fractures in men are also more likely to result in death or disability than those in women.
- Although higher body weight is associated with lower risk of fractures and greater BMD, increased abdominal fat mass in women may be associated with higher risk of fracture.[78,79]

Table 2: Drugs Used for the Management of Osteoporosis

Class	Drug	Dose	Adverse Effects	Comments	Cost[a]
Anabolic Agents	*teriparatide* Forteo	20 µg/day for 24 months sc (lifetime exposure)	Nausea, dizziness, leg cramps, hypercalcemia. Do not use in patients with higher baseline risk of osteosarcoma. Patients should be in a supine or sitting position during administration due to risk of orthostatic hypotension.	Limited data available concerning use in renal or hepatic impairment. Keep refrigerated.	~$920/ month
Bisphosphonates	*alendronate*[b] Fosamax, Apo-Alendronate, other generics	Prevention: 5 mg/day po Treatment: 10 mg/day or 70 mg once weekly po	Usually minimal: GI symptoms, altered taste, nighttime leg cramps. Rare: atypical fractures, ONJ (see Risks of Bisphosphonate Therapy), acute-phase reactions involving fever and lymphopenia, joint or muscle pain, skin reactions, ocular effects. Although available evidence does not prove a causal link between oral bisphosphonates and ONJ, advise patients to complete elective dental work if possible before starting therapy.[77] Safety in impaired renal function (ClCr <35 mL/min) is unknown.	Take on empty stomach—at least 30 min before the first food or drink (other than plain water) of the day or any other medication. Available as tablets and oral solution 70 mg/75 mL. Take with a full glass of water and do not lie down for 30 min after taking (to decrease risk of esophageal ulceration).	$
	etidronate[c] generics	400 mg/day × 14 days po Q3 months; then calcium alone × 76 days po	Usually minimal: GI symptoms, altered taste, nighttime leg cramps. Rarely reported: acute-phase reactions involving fever and lymphopenia, joint or muscle pain, skin reactions, ocular effects. Safety in impaired renal function (ClCr <35 mL/min) is unknown. ONJ has not been reported with cyclical etidronate (see Risks of Bisphosphonate Therapy).	Take on an empty stomach (at least 2 h before or after eating) with a full glass of water. To improve adherence, recommend that patients take at bedtime. Calcium supplements should be separated by at least 2 h (before or after etidronate).	$
	risedronate[b] Actonel, Actonel DR, generics	5 mg/day; or 35 mg once weekly po; or 150 mg once per month po	See alendronate.	Regular-release tablet should be taken on an empty stomach—at least 30 min before the first food or drink (other than plain water) of the day or any other medication. Delayed-release (DR) risedronate is taken with breakfast.	$

(cont'd)

Table 2: **Drugs Used for the Management of Osteoporosis** *(cont'd)*

Class	Drug	Dose	Adverse Effects	Comments	Cost[a]
	zoledronic acid[d] Aclasta, generics	5 mg once yearly iv; infuse over 15–30 min	10–20% of patients experience acute-phase reaction 24–72 h after infusion, lasting up to 3–4 days: fever and lymphopenia, joint or muscle pain, skin reactions, ocular effects. Hypocalcemia may occur. Rare: atrial fibrillation. Deterioration of renal function may occur following administration. To minimize risk, avoid in patients with ClCr <30 mL/min. ONJ has been reported in cancer patients on high-dose iv bisphosphonates and rarely with oral doses used for osteoporosis. Although available evidence does not prove a causal link, advise patients to complete elective dental work if possible before starting bisphosphonates.[77]	Product is packaged as 5 mg/100 mL ready-to-use infusion. Ensure patients are well hydrated (500 mL of water) prior to and following administration.	~$350 per dose
Bisphosphonate/ Nutritional Supplement Combinations	*alendronate/ vitamin D*[b] Fosavance, generics	alendronate 70 mg plus vitamin D 2800 IU or 5600 IU once weekly po	See alendronate. See vitamin D.	See alendronate. See vitamin D.	$
	etidronate/ calcium[c] generics	Cyclic: 400 mg/day × 14 days po then calcium 500 mg (as carbonate) on days 15 to 90 po	See etidronate. See calcium.	See etidronate. See calcium.	$$
Calcitonin Peptides	*calcitonin salmon, subcutaneous* Calcimar	20–100 IU daily for 2–4 weeks	Rarely associated with systemic effects such as nausea, vomiting, dizziness, flushing accompanied by a sensation of heat, polyuria and chills. Pain at site of injection, nausea, facial flushing, metallic taste, hypersensitivity (rare).	Not approved for osteoporosis but could be used for short term fracture pain management. Dose is not standardized.	$$$$$
Hormone Therapy (See Chapter 75)					

Class	Drug	Dose	Adverse Effects	Comments	Cost[a]
Nutritional Supplements	*calcium* Caltrate 600, Tums, generics	**Total intake** (from diet and supplements): <50 y: 1000 mg/day po >50 y: 1200 mg/day po	Constipation and nausea are the most common side effects. Other possible side effects include hypercalcemia, hypercalciuria, renal calcification and renal stones. There may be an increased risk of MI with high supplement doses.	Encourage fulfillment of calcium needs through dietary intake first. Calcium carbonate requires acidic medium for best absorption (take with or after meals); calcium citrate does not. May decrease absorption of bisphosphonates, ciprofloxacin, iron, levothyroxine, tetracycline. Separate administration by 2 h. Supplement doses >500 mg/day should be taken in divided doses.	$
	vitamin D various	800–2000 IU daily po [6]	Possible side effects are hypercalcemia, hypercalciuria, renal calcification and renal stones (usually at very high doses).	Increases calcium absorption. Many multivitamin supplements contain 400 IU vitamin D and are the most commonly used preparation. Vitamin D_3 (cholecalciferol) is preferred over vitamin D_2 (ergocalciferol).	$
RANK Ligand Inhibitors	*denosumab* Prolia	60 mg once every 6 months sc	Eczema, serious infections. Hypocalcemia in patients with impaired renal function. Osteonecrosis of the jaw was reported in trials using high doses (120 mg Q month) in oncology patients; risk is similar to bisphosphonates.	Keep refrigerated.	~$375 per dose
Selective Estrogen Receptor Modulators	*raloxifene* Evista, generics	60 mg/day po	Leg cramps, hot flashes especially in younger postmenopausal women. VTE risk similar to estrogen.	May aggravate hot flashes; should not be started until menopause is established.	$

[a] Cost of 30-day supply unless otherwise specified, includes drug cost only.
[b] Approved for prevention and treatment of postmenopausal osteoporosis and corticosteroid-induced osteoporosis (men and women), and treatment of osteoporosis in men.
[c] Cyclical use with calcium is approved for prevention and treatment of postmenopausal osteoporosis and prevention of corticosteroid-induced osteoporosis.
[d] Approved for prevention of osteoporosis in postmenopausal women with osteopenia, treatment of osteoporosis in men and postmenopausal women, prevention and treatment of corticosteroid-induced osteoporosis.

Dosage adjustment may be required in renal impairment; see Appendix I.

Abbreviations: ClCr = creatinine clearance; ONJ = osteonecrosis of the jaw; VTE = venous thromboembolism

Legend: $ <$15 $$ $15–30 $$$ $30–45 $$$$ $45–60 $$$$$ $60–75

Suggested Readings

Cranney A, Guyatt G, Griffith L et al. Meta-analyses of therapies for postmenopausal osteoporosis. IX: Summary of meta-analyses of therapies for postmenopausal osteoporosis. *Endocr Rev* 2002;23(4):570-8.

Khan AA, Sandor GK, Dore E et al. Bisphosphonate associated osteonecrosis of the jaw. *J Rheumatol* 2009;36(3):478-90.

McClung M, Harris ST, Miller PD et al. Bisphosphonate therapy for osteoporosis: benefits, risks, and drug holiday. *Am J Med* 2013;126(1):13-20.

Papaioannou A, Morin S, Cheung AM et al. 2010 clinical practice guidelines for the diagnosis and management of osteoporosis in Canada: summary. *CMAJ* 2010;182(17):1864-73.

Shane E, Burr D, Ebeling PR et al. Atypical subtrochanteric and diaphyseal femoral fractures: report of a task force of the American Society for Bone and Mineral Research. *J Bone Miner Res* 2010;25(11):2267-94.

References

1. Papaioannou A, Morin S, Cheung AM et al. 2010 clinical practice guidelines for the diagnosis and management of osteoporosis in Canada: summary. *CMAJ* 2010;182(17):1864-73.
2. Feskanich D, Singh V, Willett WC et al. Vitamin A intake and hip fractures among postmenopausal women. *JAMA* 2002;287(1):47-54.
3. Bauer DC, Gluer CC, Cauley JA et al. Broadband ultrasound attenuation predicts fractures strongly and independently of densitometry in older women. A prospective study. Study of Osteoporotic Fractures Research Group. *Arch Intern Med* 1997;157(6):629-34.
4. Siminoski K, Leslie WD, Frame H et al. Recommendations for bone mineral density reporting in Canada. *Can Assoc Radiol J* 2005;56(3):178-88.
5. Kanis JA, Oden A, Johansson H et al. FRAX and its applications to clinical practice. *Bone* 2009;44(5):734-43.
6. Hanley DA, Cranney A, Jones G et al. Vitamin D in adult health and disease: a review and guideline statement from Osteoporosis Canada (summary). *CMAJ* 2010;182(12):1315-9.
7. Riggs BL, Melton LJ. The prevention and treatment of osteoporosis. *N Engl J Med* 1992;327(9):620-7.
8. Heaney RP. The importance of calcium intake for lifelong skeletal health. *Calcif Tissue Int* 2002;70(2):70-3.
9. Chapuy MC, Arlot ME, Duboeuf F et al. Vitamin D3 and calcium to prevent hip fractures in the elderly women. *N Engl J Med* 1992;327(23):1637-42.
10. Avenell A, Mak JC, O'Connell D. Vitamin D and vitamin D analogues for preventing fractures in post-menopausal women and older men. *Cochrane Database Syst Rev* 2014;4:CD000227.
11. Ross AC, Taylor CL, Yaktine AL et al. *DRI dietary reference intakes for calcium and vitamin D*. Washington (DC): National Academies Press; 2011. Available from: www.nap.edu/openbook.php?record_id=13050.
12. Michaelsson K, Melhus H, Warensjo E et al. Long term calcium intake and rates of all cause and cardiovascular mortality: community based prospective longitudinal cohort study. *BMJ* 2013;346:f228.
13. Xiao Q, Murphy RA, Houston DK et al. Dietary and supplemental calcium intake and cardiovascular disease mortality: the National Institutes of Health-AARP Diet and Health Study. *JAMA Intern Med* 2013;173(8):639-46.
14. Wang L, Manson JE, Song Y et al. Systematic review: vitamin D and calcium supplementation in prevention of cardiovascular events. *Ann Intern Med* 2010;152(5):315-23.
15. Lewis JR, Calver J, Zhu K et al. Calcium supplementation and the risks of atherosclerotic vascular disease in older women: results of a 5-year RCT and a 4.5-year follow-up. *J Bone Miner Res* 2011;25(1):35-41.
16. Hanley DA, Davison KS. Vitamin D insufficiency in North America. *J Nutr* 2005;135(2):332-7.
17. Hanley DA, Cranney A, Jones G et al. Vitamin D in adult health and disease: a review and guideline statement from Osteoporosis Canada (summary). *CMAJ* 2010;182(12):1315-9.
18. Wells GA, Cranney A, Peterson J et al. Etidronate for the primary and secondary prevention of osteoporotic fractures in postmenopausal women. *Cochrane Database Syst Rev* 2008;(1):CD003376.
19. Miller PD, Watts NB, Licata AA et al. Cyclical etidronate in the treatment of postmenopausal osteoporosis: efficacy and safety after seven years of treatment. *Am J Med* 1997;103(6):468-76.
20. Black DM, Cummings SR, Karpf DB et al. Randomised trial of effect of alendronate on risk of fracture in women with existing vertebral fractures. Fracture Intervention Trial Research Group. *Lancet* 1996;348(9041):1535-41.
21. Black DM, Thompson DE, Bauer DC et al. Fracture risk reduction with alendronate in women with osteoporosis: the Fracture Intervention Trial. FIT Research Group. *J Clin Endocrinol Metab* 2000;85(11):4118-24.
22. Pols HA, Felsenberg D, Hanley DA et al. Multinational, placebo-controlled, randomized trial of the effects of alendronate on bone density and fracture risk in postmenopausal women with low bone mass: results of the FOSIT study. Fosamax International Trial Study Group. *Osteoporos Int* 1999;9(5):461-8.
23. Abrahamsen B, Eiken P, Eastell R. Proton pump inhibitor use and the antifracture efficacy of alendronate. *Arch Intern Med* 2011;171(11):998-1004.
24. Harris ST, Watts NB, Genant HK et al. Effects of risedronate treatment on vertebral and nonvertebral fractures in women with postmenopausal osteoporosis: a randomized controlled trial. Vertebral Efficacy With Risedronate Therapy (VERT) Study Group. *JAMA* 1999;282(14):1344-52.
25. McClung MR, Geusens P, Miller PD et al. Effect of risedronate on the risk of hip fracture in elderly women. Hip Intervention Program Study Group. *N Engl J Med* 2001;344(5):333-40.
26. Cranney A, Guyatt G, Griffith L et al. Meta-analyses of therapies for postmenopausal osteoporosis. IX: Summary of meta-analyses of therapies for postmenopausal osteoporosis. *Endocr Rev* 2002;23(4):570-8.
27. Rosen CJ, Hochberg MC, Bonnick SL et al. Treatment with once-weekly alendronate 70 mg compared with once-weekly risedronate 35 mg in women with postmenopausal osteoporosis: a randomized double-blind study. *J Bone Miner Res* 2005;20(1):141-51.

28. Silverman SL, Watts NB, Delmas PD et al. Effectiveness of bisphosphonates on nonvertebral and hip fractures in the first year of therapy: the risedronate and alendronate (REAL) cohort study. *Osteoporos Int* 2007;18(1):25-34.
29. Black DM, Delmas PD, Eastell R et al. Once-yearly zoledronic acid for treatment of postmenopausal osteoporosis. *N Engl J Med* 2007;356(18):1809-22.
30. Lyles KW, Colon-Emeric CS, Magaziner JS et al. Zoledronic acid and clinical fractures and mortality after hip fracture. *N Engl J Med* 2007;357(18):1799-809.
31. Boonen S, Reginster JY, Kaufman JM et al. Fracture risk and zoledronic acid therapy in men with osteoporosis. *N Engl J Med* 2012;367(18):1714-23.
32. Vis M, Bultink IE, Dijkmans BA et al. The effect of intravenous pamidronate versus oral alendronate on bone mineral density in patients with osteoporosis. *Osteoporos Int* 2005;16(11):1432-5.
33. Kim SH, Lim SK, Hahn JS. Effect of pamidronate on new vertebral fractures and bone mineral density in patients with malignant lymphoma receiving chemotherapy. *Am J Med* 2004;116(8):524-8.
34. Khan AA, Sandor GK, Dore E et al. Bisphosphonate associated osteonecrosis of the jaw. *J Rheumatol* 2009;36(3):478-90.
35. U.S. Food and Drug Administration. *Update of safety review follow-up to the October 1, 2007 early communication about the ongoing safety review of bisphosphonates*. Available from: www.fda.gov/Drugs/DrugSafety/PostmarketDrugSafetyInformationforPatientsand-Providers/DrugSafetyInformationforHeathcareProfessionals/ucm136201.htm.
36. Abrahamsen B. Bisphosphonate adverse effects, lessons from large databases. *Curr Opin Rheumatol* 2010;22(4):404-9.
37. Thosani N, Thosani SN, Kumar S et al. Reduced risk of colorectal cancer with use of oral bisphosphonates: a systematic review and meta-analysis. *J Clin Oncol* 2013;31(5):623-30.
38. Odvina CV, Zerwekh JE, Rao DS et al. Severely suppressed bone turnover: a potential complication of alendronate therapy. *J Clin Endocrinol Metab* 2005;90(3):1294-301.
39. Odvina CV, Levy S, Rao S et al. Unusual mid-shaft fractures during long term bisphosphonate therapy. *Clin Endocrinol (Oxf)* 2010;72(2):161-8.
40. Abrahamsen B, Eiken P, Eastell R. Subtrochanteric and diaphyseal femur fractures in patients treated with alendronate: a register-based national cohort study. *J Bone Miner Res* 2009;24(6):1095-102.
41. Gedmintas L, Solomon DH, Kim SC. Bisphophonates and risk of subtrochanteric, femoral shaft, and atypical femur fracture: a systematic review and meta-analysis. *J Bone Miner Res* 2013;28(8):1729-37.
42. Feldstein AC, Black D, Perrin N et al. Incidence and demography of femur fractures with and without atypical features. *J Bone Miner Res* 2012;27(5):977-86.
43. Dell RM, Adams AL, Greene DF et al. Incidence of atypical nontraumatic diaphyseal fractures of the femur. *J Bone Miner Res* 2012;27(12):2544-50.
44. McClung M, Harris ST, Miller PD et al. Bisphosphonate therapy for osteoporosis: benefits, risks, and drug holiday. *Am J Med* 2013;126(1):13-20.
45. Shane E, Burr D, Ebeling PR et al. Atypical subtrochanteric and diaphyseal femoral fractures: report of a task force of the American Society for Bone and Mineral Research. *J Bone Miner Res* 2010;25(11):2267-94.
46. Gomberg SJ, Wustrack RL, Napoli N et al. Teriparatide, vitamin D, and calcium healed bilateral subtrochanteric stress fractures in a postmenopausal woman with a 13-year history of continuous alendronate therapy. *J Clin Endocrinol Metab* 2011;96(6):1627-32.
47. Black DM, Schwartz AV, Ensrud KE et al. Effects of continuing or stopping alendronate after 5 years of treatment: the Fracture Intervention Trial Long-term Extension (FLEX): a randomized trial. *JAMA* 2006;296(24):2927-38.
48. Black DM, Reid IR, Boonen S et al. The effect of 3 versus 6 years of zoledronic acid treatment of osteoporosis: a randomized extension to the HORIZON-Pivotal Fracture Trial (PFT). *J Bone Miner Res* 2012;27(2):243-54.
49. Nancollas GH, Tang R, Phipps RJ et al. Novel insights into actions of bisphosphonates on bone: differences in interactions with hydroxyapatite. *Bone* 2006;38(5):617-27.
50. Watts NB, Chines A, Olszynski WP et al. Fracture risk remains reduced one year after discontinuation of risedronate. *Osteoporos Int* 2008;19(3):365-72.
51. Cummings SR, San Martin J, McClung MR et al. Denosumab for prevention of fractures in postmenopausal women with osteoporosis. *N Engl J Med* 2009;361(8):756-65.
52. Delmas PD, Bjarnason NH, Mitlak BH et al. Effects of raloxifene on bone mineral density, serum cholesterol concentrations, and uterine endometrium in postmenopausal women. *N Engl J Med* 1997;337(23):1641-7.
53. Ettinger B, Black DM, Mitlak BH et al. Reduction of vertebral fracture risk in postmenopausal women with osteoporosis treated with raloxifene: results from a 3-year randomized clinical trial. Multiple Outcomes of Raloxifene Evaluation (MORE) Investigators. *JAMA* 1999;282(7):637-45.
54. Ringe JD, Doherty JG. Absolute risk reduction in osteoporosis: assessing treatment efficacy by number needed to treat. *Rheumatol Int* 2010;30(7):863-9.
55. Cummings SR, Eckert S, Krueger KA et al. The effect of raloxifene on risk of breast cancer in postmenopausal women: results from the MORE randomized trial. Multiple Outcomes of Raloxifene Evaluation. *JAMA* 1999;281(23):2189-97.
56. Barrett-Connor E, Mosca L, Collins P et al. Effects of raloxifene on cardiovascular events and breast cancer in postmenopausal women. *N Engl J Med* 2006;355(2):125-37.
57. Rossouw JE, Anderson GL, Prentice RL et al. Risks and benefits of estrogen plus progestin in healthy postmenopausal women: principal results From the Women's Health Initiative randomized controlled trial. *JAMA* 2002;288(3):321-33.
58. Rossouw JE, Prentice RL, Manson JE et al. Postmenopausal hormone therapy and risk of cardiovascular disease by age and years since menopause. *JAMA* 2007;297(13):1465-77.
59. U.K. Medicines and Healthcare Products Regulatory Agency. *Class 2 drug alert (action within 48 hours): Miacalcic 200 IU nasal spray solution—Novartis Pharmaceuticals UK Ltd—EL 13(A)11*. Available from: www.mhra.gov.uk/Publications/Safetywarnings/Dru-gAlerts/CON257641.
60. Health Canada. *Synthetic calcitonin (salmon) nasal spray (NS)—Market withdrawal of all products, effective October 1st, 2013—For health professionals*. Available from: www.healthycanadians.gc.ca/recall-alert-rappel-avis/hc-sc/2013/34783a-eng.php.
61. Knopp JA, Diner BM, Blitz M et al. Calcitonin for treating acute pain of osteoporotic vertebral compression fractures: a systematic review of randomized, controlled trials. *Osteoporos Int* 2005;16(10):1281-90.
62. Neer RM, Arnaud CD, Zanchetta JR et al. Effect of parathyroid hormone (1-34) on fractures and bone mineral density in postmenopausal women with osteoporosis. *N Engl J Med* 2001;344(19):1434-41.

63. Andrews EB, Gilsenan AW, Midkiff K et al. The US postmarketing surveillance study of adult osteosarcoma and teriparatide: study design and findings from the first 7 years. *J Bone Miner Res* 2012;27(12):2429-37.
64. Leder BZ, Neer RM, Wyland JJ et al. Effects of teriparatide treatment and discontinuation in postmenopausal women and eugonadal men with osteoporosis. *J Clin Endocrinol Metab* 2009;94(8):2915-21.
65. Black DM, Bilezikian JP, Ensrud KE et al. One year of alendronate after one year of parathyroid hormone (1-84) for osteoporosis. *N Engl J Med* 2005;353(6):555-65.
66. Greenspan SL, Bone HG, Ettinger MP et al. Effect of recombinant human parathyroid hormone (1-84) on vertebral fracture and bone mineral density in postmenopausal women with osteoporosis: a randomized trial. *Ann Intern Med* 2007;146(5):326-39.
67. Reginster JY, Seeman E, De Vernejoul MC et al. Strontium ranelate reduces the risk of nonvertebral fractures in postmenopausal women with osteoporosis: Treatment of Peripheral Osteoporosis (TROPOS) study. *J Clin Endocrinol Metab* 2005;90(5):2816-22.
68. O'Donnell S, Cranney A, Wells GA et al. Strontium ranelate for preventing and treating postmenopausal osteoporosis. *Cochrane Database Syst Rev* 2006;(4):CD005326.
69. Jonville-Bera AP, Crickx B, Aaron L et al. Strontium ranelate-induced DRESS syndrome: first two case reports. *Allergy* 2009;64(4):658-9.
70. Lindsay R, Cosman F, Lobo RA et al. Addition of alendronate to ongoing hormone replacement therapy in the treatment of osteoporosis: a randomized, controlled clinical trial. *J Clin Endocrinol Metab* 1999;84(9):3076-81.
71. Wimalawansa SJ. A four-year randomized controlled trial of hormone replacement and bisphosphonate, alone or in combination, in women with postmenopausal osteoporosis. *Am J Med* 1998;104(3):219-26.
72. Cusano NE, Bilezikian JP. Combination anabolic and antiresorptive therapy for osteoporosis. *Endocrinol Metab Clin North Am* 2012;41(3):643-54.
73. Johnell O, Scheele WH, Lu Y et al. Additive effects of raloxifene and alendronate on bone density and biochemical markers of bone remodeling in postmenopausal women with osteoporosis. *J Clin Endocrinol Metab* 2002;87(3):985-92.
74. Deal C, Omizo M, Schwartz EN et al. Combination teriparatide and raloxifene therapy for postmenopausal osteoporosis: results from a 6-month double-blind placebo-controlled trial. *J Bone Miner Res* 2005;20(11):1905-11.
75. Hodsman A; Scientific Advisory Council of Osteoporosis Canada; Papaioannou A et al. Clinical practice guidelines for the use of parathyroid hormone in the treatment of osteoporosis. *CMAJ* 2006;175(1):48.
76. Khan AA, Hodsman AB, Papaioannou A et al. Management of osteoporosis in men: an update and case example. *CMAJ* 2007;176(3):345-8.
77. Shane E, Goldring S, Christakos S et al. Osteonecrosis of the jaw: more research needed. *J Bone Miner Res* 2006;21(10):1503-5.
78. Cohen A, Dempster DW, Recker RR et al. Abdominal fat is associated with lower bone formation and inferior bone quality in healthy premenopausal women: a transiliac bone biopsy study. *J Clin Endocrinol Metab* 2013;98(6):2562-72.
79. Yang S, Nguyen ND, Center JR et al. Association between abdominal obesity and fracture risk: a prospective study. *J Clin Endocrinol Metab* 2013;98(6):2478-83.

Chapter 84
Polymyalgia Rheumatica and Giant-Cell Arteritis

John G. Hanly, MD, MRCPI, FRCPC

Polymyalgia rheumatica (PMR) and giant-cell arteritis (GCA) are related conditions that affect older individuals and may reflect 2 ends of a spectrum of the same disease. PMR is characterized by aching and stiffness in the muscle groups of the neck, pectoral and pelvic girdles and thighs. The prevalence approaches 1% of people over the age of 50,[1,2] and the lifetime risk of developing the disease has been estimated at 2.4% for women and 1.7% for men.[3]

GCA is a chronic vasculitis of large and medium-sized arteries with a predominance for the cranial branches of the arteries originating from the aortic arch. Thus, headache, jaw claudication and visual loss are common presentations. GCA is less frequent than PMR and affects approximately 0.2% of people 50 years of age and older.[1,4]

Both conditions are twofold more frequent in women than in men. There is a clear association between PMR and GCA. Approximately 16–21% of patients with PMR will develop GCA concurrently or subsequent to the diagnosis of PMR;[1,2,5] conversely 40–60% of patients with GCA will develop symptoms of PMR. Although the etiology of both conditions is unknown, PMR is characterized pathologically by low grade synovitis of the proximal joints, while the hallmark of GCA is granulomatous inflammation with giant cells of affected arterial walls. Both conditions may be associated with systemic clinical manifestations.

Goals of Therapy

- Eliminate symptoms of musculoskeletal pain and stiffness and associated malaise
- Restore function
- Relieve symptoms due to GCA and prevent permanent visual loss
- Minimize the frequency and severity of corticosteroid toxicity

Investigations

The value of a thorough history and physical examination cannot be overemphasized. PMR and GCA are clinical diagnoses. Other than a positive temporal artery biopsy there are no laboratory tests that are specific for either disease.

The diagnostic approach is outlined in Table 1 and Figure 1.

History

Patients with PMR typically present with the following characteristics:

- Significant proximal muscle discomfort, especially around the shoulders, across the neck, and in the buttocks and thighs. The pain is generally severe and usually interferes with activities of daily living.
- Many patients describe an acute onset and can pinpoint the start of their symptoms to a specific day.
- Musculoskeletal morning stiffness lasting for hours is a prominent feature. Symptoms tend to worsen through the night, and movement during sleep causes discomfort severe enough to wake the patient.

- Systemic symptoms such as fever, malaise, anorexia and fatigue may be present in one-third of patients.[8]

Patients with GCA most frequently present with the following characteristics:

- Headache and scalp tenderness in the temporal or occipital areas, claudication of the jaw or tongue and partial or complete monocular visual loss which may affect the contralateral eye within 2 weeks even after starting corticosteroid therapy.
- Additional distinct clinical presentations may occur based upon the pattern of vascular involvement and the degree of systemic symptoms.[9] For example, involvement of large vessels such as the branches of the aortic arch, similar to that seen in Takayasu's arteritis, may occur in up to 15% of cases and is manifested by audible bruits and upper limb claudication. The treatment and outcome is comparable to GCA without large vessel involvement.[10]
- Systemic symptoms, including fever, occur in up to 50% of cases.
- A recognized late complication of GCA is a 17-fold increase in thoracic aortic aneurysm.[11]
- Patients who present with PMR should be questioned specifically about symptoms of GCA.

Physical Examination

Patients with suspected PMR:

- The physical findings in PMR are nonspecific and usually reveal a reduction in range of motion of the neck and shoulders.
- Large and small joint synovitis may be present but is unusual in locations distal to the wrist and ankle. Severe swelling with pitting edema over the dorsum of both hands and feet may also occur and forms a distinct clinical subset.[12,13]
- Proximal muscle tenderness may be present but muscle weakness, although difficult to assess due to pain, is not a predominant feature of PMR.

Patients with suspected GCA:

- Diminished or absent temporal artery pulsation and associated scalp tenderness, coupled with an appropriate history, is suggestive of GCA.
- Funduscopic findings related to GCA include optic neuritis with pallor and edema of the optic disc, cotton-wool patches and small hemorrhages.

Table 1: **Differential Diagnosis of Polymyalgia Rheumatica (PMR)**

Diagnosis	Features Differentiating Condition From PMR
Myositis	Muscle weakness on physical examination Elevated CPK Abnormalities on EMG and muscle biopsy
Fibromyalgia	Usually seen in younger patients Widespread pain and tenderness at a significant number of soft tissue sites not limited to the shoulders and hips Normal ESR and CRP
Rheumatoid Arthritis	Synovitis distal to the wrist and ankle Seropositivity for RF Consider anti-CCP antibodies if RF negative Inadequate response to low-dose prednisone therapy Radiographic erosions
Malignancy	No association between malignancy and PMR[6] or GCA[7], but some malignancies can mimic PMR. Investigate further as indicated by clinical exam and laboratory evaluation or if lack of response to conventional treatment.

Abbreviations: anti-CCP = anti-cyclic citrullinated peptide; CPK = creatine phosphokinase; CRP = C-reactive protein; EMG = electromyography; ESR = erythrocyte sedimentation rate; RF = rheumatoid factor

Laboratory Tests

Patients with suspected PMR:

- A rapid erythrocyte sedimentation rate (ESR) and elevated levels of C-reactive protein (CRP) are usually present. However, 5–6% of patients with PMR and GCA will have a normal ESR[14,15] although in the majority of such cases the CRP is elevated.[14]
- Anemia and/or thrombocytosis may also be found in patients presenting with PMR or GCA.
- A number of conditions must be considered in the differential diagnosis of PMR (Table 1) although GCA can usually be readily distinguished from other forms of vasculitis.

Patients with suspected GCA:

- See laboratory tests for PMR above.
- Temporal artery biopsy is indicated only if there is a clinical suspicion of GCA and is not routinely recommended in patients who present with isolated PMR. Due to patchy involvement of affected vessels, a normal biopsy does not exclude the diagnosis. Thus, even when up to 5 cm of bilateral temporal arteries are sampled, 9% of suspected cases have normal biopsies.[16,17,18,19] More recent studies have suggested that performing bilateral temporal artery biopsies increases the diagnostic yield by 1–12.7%.[20,21] Corticosteroid therapy should not be withheld while awaiting the result of a temporal artery biopsy. This biopsy can still show changes of arteritis when performed up to 4 weeks following the commencement of corticosteroid therapy.[22,23]

The diagnostic approach is outlined in Figure 1.

Figure 1: Diagnostic Approach in Patients with Suspected Polymyalgia Rheumatica (PMR) and Giant-Cell Arteritis (GCA)

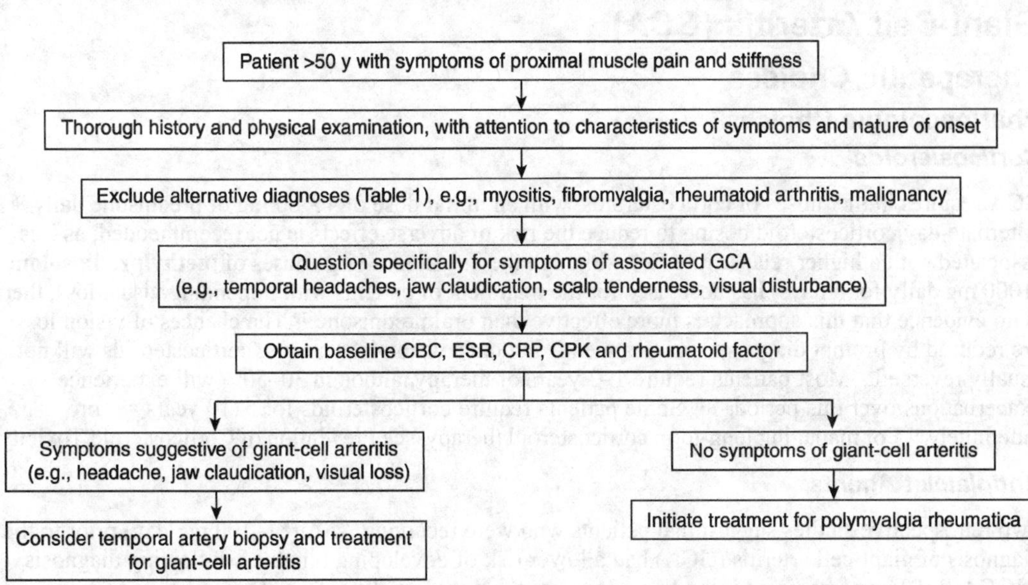

Abbreviations: CBC = complete blood count; CPK = creatine phosphokinase; CRP = C-reactive protein; ESR = erythrocyte sedimentation rate

Polymyalgia Rheumatica (PMR)

Therapeutic Choices

Pharmacologic Choices

Corticosteroids

Nonsteroidal anti-inflammatory drugs (NSAIDs) are generally ineffective or provide only partial improvement of symptoms in patients with PMR. Thus, systemic corticosteroids are the cornerstone of therapy. **Prednisone** 10–20 mg/day results in rapid and sustained clinical improvement[8] (Table 2). Substantial or complete resolution of symptoms occurs within days. In fact, the diagnosis of PMR should be reconsidered if symptoms fail to improve significantly after 1 week of corticosteroid therapy.[24] Most patients require 1–2 years of therapy, although 30–50% will experience exacerbations over this period.[25] Some patients require corticosteroids for 5–10 years[26] or indefinitely. For managing long-term corticosteroid therapy, see Prevention of Corticosteroid Toxicity.

Immunomodulators and Biologic Response Modifiers

Methotrexate and **azathioprine** have been used in the treatment of PMR primarily to minimize corticosteroid exposure. However, studies have yielded conflicting results.[27,28] Only 1 placebo-controlled study of methotrexate has shown benefit in patients with PMR.[29] These drugs should be considered only in patients with significant corticosteroid toxicity, those unable to wean below 7.5 mg of prednisone daily and/or in patients with frequent relapses.

The initial studies of biologic therapies such as **infliximab**[30] and **etanercept**[31,32] in steroid-resistant cases provided encouraging results, supported by a recent literature review.[33] However, controlled studies of infliximab did not confirm benefit in the treatment of either PMR or GCA.[34,35]

Giant-Cell Arteritis (GCA)

Therapeutic Choices

Pharmacologic Choices

Corticosteroids

GCA requires higher doses of corticosteroids, with an initial dose of 40–60 mg of prednisone daily.[36] Alternate-day corticosteroid dosing to reduce the risk of adverse effects is not recommended, as it is associated with a higher relapse rate.[37,38] Although the infusion of large doses of **methylprednisolone** (1000 mg daily for 3 days) has been used for the treatment of patients with impending visual loss, there is no evidence that this approach is more effective than oral prednisone.[39] The chances of vision loss are reduced by prompt diagnosis and treatment[20] but once vision loss occurs, corticosteroids will not usually reverse it. Most patients require 1–2 years of therapy, although 30–50% will experience exacerbations over this period.[25,40] Some patients require corticosteroids for 5–10 years[26,40] or indefinitely.[41] For managing long-term corticosteroid therapy, see Prevention of Corticosteroid Toxicity.

Antiplatelet Agents

Two retrospective studies suggest that patients who were receiving **ASA** (81–100 mg/day) prior to the diagnosis of giant-cell arteritis (GCA) had a lower risk of developing blindness following diagnosis of GCA.[42,43] Therefore, in addition to prednisone, consider low-dose ASA therapy immediately following diagnosis of GCA [Evidence: SORT C*].[36] Although there are no data to suggest a recommended duration of ASA therapy, it is reasonable to continue for 4–6 weeks until the clinical and

* SORT (Strength of Recommendation Taxonomy) is a rating system (A, B or C) that addresses the quality of available evidence. For more information consult **How to Use *Compendium of Therapeutic Choices*** on page xxv.

laboratory indicators of systemic inflammation have normalized and the risk of vision loss has abated. Cytoprotection with a **proton pump inhibitor** or **misoprostol** during concomitant prednisone and ASA therapy may reduce the risk of GI toxicity.[44]

Immunomodulators and Biologic Response Modifiers

Two out of 3 placebo-controlled studies[45,46,47] of **methotrexate** did not detect a statistically significant benefit in patients with GCA. However, a meta-analysis of the data from the same 3 studies found that adjunctive therapy with methotrexate lowered the risk of relapse and reduced exposure to corticosteroids.[48] These drugs should be considered only in patients with significant corticosteroid toxicity, those unable to wean below 7.5 mg of prednisone daily and/or in patients with frequent relapses.

A small controlled study of 17 patients suggested that the addition of **etanercept** in the treatment of patients with GCA resulted in lower cumulative doses of corticosteroids.[49] **Leflunomide**,[50] **rituximab**[50] and **tocilizumab**[50,51,52] may be considered in resistant cases. Consult a rheumatologist for initiation of an immunosuppressive or biologic agent.

Prevention of Corticosteroid Toxicity

Since corticosteroids are associated with significant side effects, the lowest dose of corticosteroid needed to control symptoms should be used for the shortest period of time possible in order to minimize toxicity. Treatment with prednisone doses greater than 7.5 mg daily for more than 3 months has been associated with significant bone loss. **Bisphosphonates** prevent the bone loss associated with corticosteroid use and should be prescribed in patients with PMR or GCA commencing corticosteroid therapy (see Chapter 83).[53] Weight-bearing exercise, calcium (1200 mg total intake daily, preferably through dietary intake) and vitamin D (800–2000 IU daily) also reduce the risk of osteoporosis and should be prescribed in conjunction with bisphosphonates.

Therapeutic Tips

- Prompt diagnosis and initiation of **corticosteroid** therapy is critical for the prevention of vision loss in patients with giant-cell arteritis. Treatment should not be delayed while awaiting a temporal artery biopsy which can still be positive up to 4 weeks after the initiation of corticosteroid therapy.
- Patients may report a transient increase in musculoskeletal symptoms after each corticosteroid dose reduction. These symptoms usually subside spontaneously over the ensuing week and do not necessarily represent a disease flare.
- The ESR and CRP usually parallel disease activity in patients with PMR and GCA. These tests can be used to confirm the clinical suspicion of a disease flare but should not be used in isolation to make treatment decisions.
- Reduction in shoulder range of motion may occur in some patients with PMR due to a localized rotator cuff tendonitis or capsulitis. This is more likely to occur when there has been a delay in diagnosis and initiation of therapy. A **local corticosteroid injection** (e.g., methylprednisolone acetate, triamcinolone hexacetonide) of the subacromial bursa or glenohumeral joint is often helpful.

Table 2: Drug Therapy of Polymyalgia Rheumatica and Giant-Cell Arteritis

Drug Class	Drug	Dose	Adverse Effects	Drug Interactions	Comments	Cost[a]
Antiplatelet Agents	*ASA* Aspirin, Coated Aspirin, Entrophen, generics	GCA: 81 mg daily po, starting immediately following diagnosis.	Gastritis, gastric/duodenal ulceration (rarely bronchospasm). Nausea, vomiting, GI hemorrhage, tinnitus, vertigo, hypersensitivity.	Increased risk of bleeding when coadministered with anticoagulants, corticosteroids, NSAIDs and SSRIs.	Not a Health Canada-approved indication. Cytoprotection with a proton pump inhibitor or misoprostol during concomitant prednisone and ASA therapy may reduce the risk of GI toxicity.	$
Cortico-steroids	*prednisone* generics	PMR: 15 mg daily po × 2 wk. Taper as follows: 12.5 mg daily po × 2 wk, 10 mg daily po × 4 wk, then decrease daily prednisone dose by 1 mg each month until completion GCA: 40–60 mg daily po × 4 wk. Taper as follows: decrease daily dose by 5 mg each wk until the dose is 10 mg daily. Then taper the daily dose more gradually by 1 mg each month until completion	Acne, glucose intolerance, weight gain, mood swings and agitation, cataracts, myopathy, hypertension, osteoporosis, aseptic necrosis of large joints, adrenal suppression, increased susceptibility to infection.	Barbiturates, phenytoin and rifampin decrease corticosteroid effect.	Avoid alternate-day corticosteroid dosing as it is associated with a higher rate of relapse.[37,38] Ensure regular clinical assessments to look for recurrence of the original symptoms while concurrently checking CBC, ESR and CRP during the prednisone taper. An isolated rise in ESR or CRP is usually not sufficient justification to increase the dose of corticosteroids. If a disease flare does occur, increase the dose of prednisone to the lowest level that was previously effective in controlling the disease. Maintain at that level for 1 month, then taper as before. Immunosuppressive agents may be required in some cases.	$

[a] Cost of 30-day supply; includes drug cost only.
Abbreviations: CBC = complete blood count; CRP = C-reactive protein; ESR = erythrocyte sedimentation rate; GCA = giant-cell arteritis; PMR = polymyalgia rheumatica
Legend: $ < $ 10

Suggested Readings

Cantini F, Niccoli L, Nannini C et al. Diagnosis and treatment of giant cell arteritis. *Drugs Aging* 2008;25(4):281-97.

Caylor TL, Perkins A. Recognition and management of polymyalgia rheumatica and giant cell arteritis. *Am Fam Physician* 2013;88(10):676-84.

Dasgupta B, Borg FA, Hassan N et al. BSR and BHPR guidelines for the management of giant cell arteritis. *Rheumatology (Oxford)* 2010;49(8):1594-7.

Dasgupta B, Borg FA, Hassan N et al. BSR and BHPR guidelines for the management of polymyalgia rheumatica. *Rheumatology (Oxford)* 2010;49(1):186-90.

Kermani TA, Warrington KJ. Polymyalgia rheumatica. *Lancet* 2013;281(9860):63-72.

References

1. Gonzalez-Gay MA, Vazquez-Rodriguez TR, Lopez-Diaz MJ et al. Epidemiology of giant cell arteritis and polymyalgia rheumatica. *Arthritis Rheum* 2009;61(10):1454-61.
2. Salvarani C, Gabriel SE, O'Fallon WM et al. Epidemiology of polymyalgia rheumatica in Olmsted County, Minnesota, 1970-1991. *Arthritis Rheum* 1995;38(3):369-73.
3. Crowson CS, Matteson EL, Myasoedova E et al. The lifetime risk of adult-onset rheumatoid arthritis and other inflammatory autoimmune rheumatic diseases. *Arthritis Rheum* 2011;63(3):633-9.
4. Salvarani C, Gabriel SE, O'Fallon WM et al. The incidence of giant cell arteritis in Olmsted County, Minnesota: apparent fluctuations in a cyclic pattern. *Ann Intern Med* 1995;123(3):192-4.
5. Franzen P, Sutinen S, von Knorring J. Giant cell arteritis and polymyalgia rheumatica in a region of Finland: an epidemiologic, clinical and pathologic study, 1984-1988. *J Rheumatol* 1992;19(2):273-6.
6. Myklebust G, Wilsgaard T, Jacobsen BK et al. No increased frequency of malignant neoplasms in polymyalgia rheumatica and temporal arteritis. A prospective longitudinal study of 398 cases and matched population controls. *J Rheumatol* 2002;29(10):2143-7.
7. Kermani TA, Schafer VS, Crowson CS et al. Malignancy risk in patients with giant cell arteritis: a population-based cohort study. *Arthritis Care Res (Hoboken)* 2010;62(2):149-54.
8. Salvarani C, Cantini F, Boiardi L et al. Polymyalgia rheumatica and giant-cell arteritis. *N Engl J Med* 2002;347(4):261-71.
9. Weyand CM, Goronzy JJ. Giant-cell arteritis and polymyalgia rheumatica. *Ann Intern Med* 2003;139(6):505-15.
10. Schmidt WA, Moll A, Seifert A et al. Prognosis of large-vessel giant cell arteritis. *Rheumatology (Oxford)* 2008;47(9):1406-8.
11. Evans JM, O'Fallon WM, Hunder GG. Increased incidence of aortic aneurysm and dissection in giant cell (temporal) arteritis. A population-based study. *Ann Intern Med* 1995;122(7):502-7.
12. Oide T, Ohara S, Oguchi K et al. Remitting seronegative symmetrical synovitis with pitting edema (RS3PE) syndrome in Nagano, Japan: clinical, radiological, and cytokine studies of 13 patients. *Clin Exp Rheumatol* 2004;22(1):91-8.
13. Queiro R. RS3PE syndrome: a clinical and immunogenetical study. *Rheumatol Int* 2004;24(2):103-5.
14. Cantini F, Salvarani C, Olivieri I et al. Erythrocyte sedimentation rate and C-reactive protein in the evaluation of disease activity and severity in polymyalgia rheumatica: a prospective follow-up study. *Semin Arthritis Rheum* 2000;30(1):17-24.
15. Salvarani C, Hunder GG. Giant cell arteritis with low erythrocyte sedimentation rate: frequency of occurrence in a population-based study. *Arthritis Rheum* 2001;45(2):140-5.
16. Hall S, Persellin S, Lie JT et al. The therapeutic impact of temporal artery biopsy. *Lancet* 1983;2(8361):1217-20.
17. Klein RG, Campbell RJ, Hunder GG et al. Skip lesions in temporal arteritis. *Mayo Clin Proc* 1976;51(8):504-10.
18. Gonzalez-Gay MA, Garcia-Porrua C, Llorca J et al. Biopsy-negative giant cell arteritis: clinical spectrum and predictive factors for positive temporal artery biopsy. *Semin Arthritis Rheum* 2001;30(4):249-56.
19. Hedges TR, Gieger GL, Albert DM. The clinical value of negative temporal artery biopsy specimens. *Arch Ophthalmol* 1983;101(8):1251-4.
20. Nordborg E, Nordborg C. Giant cell arteritis: strategies in diagnosis and treatment. *Curr Opin Rheumatol* 2004;16(1):25-30.
21. Breuer GS, Nesher G, Nesher R. Rate of discordant findings in bilateral temporal artery biopsy to diagnose giant cell arteritis. *J Rheumatol* 2009;36(4):794-6.
22. Achkar AA, Lie JT, Hunder GG et al. How does previous corticosteroid treatment affect the biopsy findings in giant cell (temporal) arteritis? *Ann Intern Med* 1994;120(12):987-92.
23. Ray-Chaudhuri N, Kine DA, Tijani SO et al. Effect of prior steroid treatment on temporal artery biopsy findings in giant cell arteritis. *Br J Ophthalmol* 2002;86(5):530-2.
24. Dasgupta B, Borg FA, Hassan N et al. BSR and BHPR guidelines for the management of polymyalgia rheumatica. *Rheumatology (Oxford)* 2010;49(1):186-90.
25. Salvarani C, Macchioni PL, Tartoni PL et al. Polymyalgia rheumatica and giant cell arteritis: a 5-year epidemiologic and clinical study in Reggio Emilia, Italy. *Clin Exp Rheumatol* 1987;5(3):205-15.
26. Bengtsson BA, Malmvall BE. Prognosis of giant cell arteritis including temporal arteritis and polymyalgia rheumatica. A follow-up study on ninety patients treated with corticosteroids. *Acta Med Scand* 1981;209(5):337-45.
27. De Silva M, Hazleman BL. Azathioprine in giant cell arteritis/polymyalgia rheumatica: a double-blind study. *Ann Rheum Dis* 1986;45(2):136-8.
28. Ferraccioli G, Salaffi F, De Vita S et al. Methotrexate in polymyalgia rheumatica: preliminary results of an open, randomized study. *J Rheumatol* 1996;23(4):624-8.
29. Caporali R, Cimmino MA, Ferraccioli G et al. Prednisone plus methotrexate for polymyalgia rheumatica: a randomized, double-blind, placebo-controlled trial. *Ann Intern Med* 2004;141(7):493-500.
30. Salvarani C, Cantini F, Niccoli L et al. Treatment of refractory polymyalgia rheumatica with infliximab: a pilot study. *J Rheumatol* 2003;30(4):760-3.
31. Tan AL, Holdsworth J, Pease C et al. Successful treatment of resistant giant cell arteritis with etanercept. *Ann Rheum Dis* 2003;62(4):373-4.
32. Catanoso MG, Macchioni P, Boiardi L et al. Treatment of refractory polymyalgia rheumatica with etanercept: an open pilot study. *Arthritis Rheum* 2007;57(8):1514-9.

33. Aikawa NE, Pereira RM, Lage L et al. Anti-TNF therapy for polymyalgia rheumatica: report of 99 cases and review of the literature. *Clin Rheumatol* 2012;31(3):575-9.
34. Salvarani C, Macchioni P, Manzini C et al. Infliximab plus prednisone or placebo plus prednisone for the initial treatment of polymyalgia rheumatica: a randomized trial. *Ann Intern Med* 2007;146(9):631-9.
35. Hoffman GS, Cid MC, Rendt-Zagar KE et al. Infliximab for maintenance of glucocorticosteroid-induced remission of giant cell arteritis: a randomized trial. *Ann Intern Med* 2007;146(9):621-30.
36. Dasgupta B, Borg FA, Hassan N et al. BSR and BHPR guidelines for the management of giant cell arteritis. *Rheumatology (Oxford)* 2010;49(8):1594-7.
37. Bengtsson BA, Malmvall BE. An alternate-day corticosteroid regimen in maintenance therapy of giant cell arteritis. *Acta Med Scand* 1981;209(5):347-50.
38. Hunder GG, Sheps SG, Allen GL et al. Daily and alternate-day corticosteroid regimens in treatment of giant cell arteritis: comparison in a prospective study. *Ann Intern Med* 1975;82(5):613-8.
39. Hayreh SS, Zimmerman B. Management of giant cell arteritis. Our 27-year clinical study: new light on old controversies. *Ophthalmologica* 2003;217(4):239-59.
40. Andersson R, Malmvall BE, Bengtsson BA. Long-term corticosteroid treatment in giant cell arteritis. *Acta Med Scand* 1986;220(5):465-9.
41. Gonzalez-Gay MA, Blanco R, Rodriguez-Valverde V et al. Permanent visual loss and cerebrovascular accidents in giant cell arteritis: predictors and response to treatment. *Arthritis Rheum* 1998;41(8):1497-504.
42. Nesher G, Berkun Y, Mates M et al. Low-dose aspirin and prevention of cranial ischemic complications in giant cell arteritis. *Arthritis Rheum* 2004;50(4):1332-7.
43. Lee MS, Smith SD, Galor A et al. Antiplatelet and anticoagulant therapy in patients with giant cell arteritis. *Arthritis Rheum* 2006;54(10):3306-9.
44. Lanza FL, Chan FK, Quigley EM et al. Guidelines for prevention of NSAID-related ulcer complications. *Am J Gastroenterol* 2009;104(3):728-38.
45. Hoffman GS, Cid MC, Hellmann DB et al. A multicenter, randomized, double-blind, placebo-controlled trial of adjuvant methotrexate treatment for giant cell arteritis. *Arthritis Rheum* 2002;46(5):1309-18.
46. Spiera RF, Mitnick HJ, Kupersmith M et al. A prospective, double-blind, randomized, placebo controlled trial of methotrexate in the treatment of giant cell arteritis (GCA). *Clin Exp Rheumatol* 2001;19(5):495-501.
47. Jover JA, Hernandez-Garcia C, Morado IC et al. Combined treatment of giant-cell arteritis with methotrexate and prednisone. a randomized, double-blind, placebo-controlled trial. *Ann Intern Med* 2001;134(2):106-14.
48. Mahr AD, Jover JA, Spiera RF et al. Adjunctive methotrexate for treatment of giant cell arteritis: an individual patient data meta-analysis. *Arthritis Rheum* 2007;56(8):2789-97.
49. Martínez-Taboada VM, Rodríguez-Valverde V, Carreno L et al. A double-blind placebo controlled trial of etanercept in patients with giant cell arteritis and corticosteroid side effects. *Ann Rheum Dis* 2008;67(5):625-30.
50. Unizony S, Stone JH, Stone JR. New treatment strategies in large-vessel vasculitis. *Curr Opin Rheumatol* 2013;25(1):3-9.
51. Isik M, Kilic L, Dogan I et al. Tocilizumab for giant cell arteritis: an amazing result. *Rheumatol Int* 2013;33(11):2961-2.
52. Unizony S, Arias-Urdaneta L, Miloslavksy E et al. Tocilizumab for the treatment of large-vessel vasculitis (giant cell arteritis, Takayasu arteritis) and polymyalgia rheumatica. *Arthritis Care Res (Hoboken)* 2012;64(11):1720-9.
53. Grossman JM, Gordon R, Ranganath VK et al. American College of Rheumatology 2010 recommendations for the prevention and treatment of glucocorticoid-induced osteoporosis. *Arthritis Care Res (Hoboken)* 2010;62(11):1515-26.

Chapter 85
Rheumatoid Arthritis

Glen Hazlewood, MD, FRCPC, PhD(c) and
Vivian P. Bykerk, MD, FRCPC

Rheumatoid arthritis (RA) is a systemic autoimmune disease manifesting primarily as a symmetric and erosive polyarthritis. It can cause pain, stiffness and fatigue as well as joint destruction resulting in disability and premature mortality and can be associated with systemic manifestations involving most internal organs. Patients with RA have an increased risk of cardiovascular disease and cardiovascular mortality.[1] The incidence of RA is 0.05% per year and prevalence is 1% of the adult population. Onset can occur at any age, including childhood, but most frequently starts at age 40–50. RA affects women 3 times more frequently than men.

Erosions will be seen on radiographs at the first visit in 20% of patients and will be present in up to 70% of patients at 1 year if left untreated. Rheumatologists recommend an early optimal approach to management.[2] This includes starting treatment with disease modifying anti-rheumatic drugs (DMARDs) as soon as the diagnosis of RA is made.[3] The diagnosis of rheumatoid arthritis may be difficult early on; new classification criteria have been developed to assist in an earlier diagnosis.[4,5] Any patient suspected of having RA should be referred promptly to a rheumatologist for assessment and institution of therapy.

Goals of Therapy

- To fully control signs and symptoms of the disease and to halt radiographic progression and joint damage
- The target of treatment is remission, or if not possible, at least low disease activity.[3,6] Remission can be defined using multiple composite disease activity measures. In general, remission means the absence of disease activity as assessed by a clinician (swollen and tender joints), patient (global assessment of disease activity) and labs (CRP and/or ESR).

Treatment should alleviate pain, stiffness and fatigue, prevent any further joint damage and destruction, maintain function and maximize quality of life.

Investigations

The diagnosis of RA should be considered in patients with joint swelling or inflammatory joint pain, although the differential diagnosis of joint swelling is broad.[7] To make a diagnosis of RA, objective joint swelling (by clinical exam or imaging) must be present. Patients with RA typically have multiple swollen joints, in a symmetric distribution, with involvement of the hands and feet. Early in the disease, however, typical features may be absent and radiographs of the hands and feet are usually normal. New classification criteria have been developed to assist in early diagnosis (see Table 1). Anyone suspected of having RA should be referred urgently to a rheumatologist for evaluation. For more information on evaluation of an RA patient, see Table 2.

Table 1: Classification Criteria for Rheumatoid Arthritis

Classification Criteria	Score
Add scores from categories A–D; a score of ≥6/10 is needed for a definite diagnosis of RA	
A. Joint involvement[a]	
1 large joint[b]	0
2–10 large joints	1
1–3 small joints[c]	2
4–10 small joints	3
>10 joints (at least 1 small joint)	5
B. Serology (at least 1 test result is needed for classification)[d]	
Negative RF and negative anti-CCP	0
Low-positive RF or low-positive anti-CCP	2
High-positive RF or high-positive anti-CCP	3
C. Acute-phase reactants (at least 1 test result is needed for classification)	
Normal CRP and normal ESR	0
Abnormal CRP or abnormal ESR	1
D. Duration of symptoms	
<6 weeks	0
≥6 weeks	1

[a] Joint involvement refers to any swollen or tender joint on examination, which may be confirmed by imaging evidence of synovitis.
[b] "Large joints" refers to shoulders, elbows, hips, knees, and ankles.
[c] "Small joints" refers to the metacarpophalangeal joints, proximal interphalangeal joints, second through fifth metatarsophalangeal joints, thumb interphalangeal joints, and wrists.
[d] Negative refers to IU values that are less than or equal to the upper limit of normal (ULN) for the laboratory and assay; low-positive refers to IU values that are higher than the ULN but ≤3 times the ULN for the laboratory and assay; high-positive refers to IU values that are >3 times the ULN for the laboratory and assay. Where rheumatoid factor (RF) information is only available as positive or negative, a positive result should be scored as low-positive for RF.
Abbreviations: Anti-CCP = antibody to cyclic citrullinated protein; CRP = C-reactive protein; ESR = erythrocyte sedimentation rate; RF = rheumatoid factor
Adapted from: Aletaha D et al. 2010 Rheumatoid arthritis classification criteria: an American College of Rheumatology/European League Against Rheumatism collaborative initiative. *Arthritis Rheum* 2010;62(9):2569-81.

Table 2: Baseline Evaluation of Disease Activity and Damage[8]

History	Severity of joint pain (0–10) Duration of morning stiffness (in minutes or hours) Physician and patient global assessment of disease activity Limitation of function
Physical examination	Number of actively inflamed/swollen joints Mechanical joint problems: loss of motion, crepitus, instability, malalignment and/or deformity Extra-articular manifestations: dry eyes, nodules, pulmonary findings, carpal tunnel syndrome
Investigations	Anti-CCP, CBC, CRP, ESR, RF, liver and renal blood panel Radiographs of hands and feet

Abbreviations: Anti-CCP = antibody to cyclic citrullinated protein; CBC = complete blood count; CRP = C-reactive protein; ESR = erythrocyte sedimentation rate; RF = rheumatoid factor
Adapted from: Guidelines for the management of rheumatoid arthritis: 2002 update. American College of Rheumatology Subcommittee on Rheumatoid Arthritis Guidelines. *Arthritis Rheum* 2002. Reprinted by permission of Wiley-Liss, Inc., a subsidiary of John Wiley & Sons Inc.

Therapeutic Choices

Nonpharmacologic Choices

RA is best treated using a multidisciplinary team approach that provides patient education, emotional and psychological support and physical rehabilitation. Advise patients regarding energy conservation, appropriate levels of activity and work roles, types of exercise, methods of pain modulation with heat and cold applications,[9] adjustments to activities of daily living and maintenance of joint range of motion and muscle strength. Studies have shown improvement in functional ability with dynamic exercise training, which increases aerobic capacity and muscle strength without increasing disease activity.[10] Periodically evaluate patients for splints, foot orthoses, proper footwear and surgery. There is insufficient evidence to support complementary or alternative therapies for the treatment of RA.[11]

Pharmacologic Choices

The diagnosis of RA should be confirmed by a rheumatologist who will start the patient on nonbiologic DMARD therapy (Figure 1, Table 4) as soon as the diagnosis is made. Before selecting an initial therapy consider severity of illness, prognostic factors,[3,12] presence of extra-articular features and comorbid conditions, potential adverse events, dosing intervals, routes of administration, monitoring requirements, patient preferences and costs. Most nonbiologic DMARDs reach maximum effect in 3–6 months.

Patients should be seen as frequently as every 1–3 months while their disease is active[3,6] (see Figure 2). Those with well controlled disease or in remission can be followed at longer intervals (6–12 months). Adjust therapy frequently until a patient reaches a target (remission or at least low disease activity), ideally by 3–6 months.[3,6] Consider major changes to DMARD therapy (adding or switching agents) if there is ongoing disease activity after 3 months of maximal therapy. Minor adjustments, including the judicious use of oral, im or intra-articular corticosteroids may occur more frequently. Also adjust therapy if the patient experiences repetitive flares, progressive joint damage or develops evidence of drug toxicity.

Traditional Disease-modifying Antirheumatic Drugs (DMARDs)

Methotrexate (MTX) is the reference DMARD and is an anchor drug in the treatment of RA.[3] It is usually the drug of first choice for treating RA. An adequate trial of MTX consists of a weekly dose of 20–25 mg (orally or parenterally) for at least 3 months. Discontinuation rates and side effects of MTX (GI adverse effects, liver dysfunction) can be reduced by concurrent use of folic acid (at least 5 mg/week).[13,14] Initial *combination* of MTX with hydroxychloroquine and/or sulfasalazine can also be used early for moderate to severe disease (swollen joint count ≥3 joints).

Monotherapy with **hydroxychloroquine** or **sulfasalazine** is sometimes used for early, very mild disease defined as <2 swollen joints in a setting of a negative or low titre rheumatoid factor (RF), normal erythrocyte sedimentation rate (ESR) and C-reactive protein (CRP) and absence of radiographic erosions in the hands or feet.

Leflunomide may be used in place of MTX for patients who have contraindications to MTX. A loading dose of leflunomide often causes significant diarrhea and is thus no longer recommended. There have been concerns that leflunomide may be associated with an increased risk of serious adverse events when compared to MTX. Reports of severe liver injury (49 cases, including 14 fatalities) resulted in the addition of a black box warning to the US labeling of leflunomide by the Food and Drug Administration in 2010.[15]

Rheumatologists often use combinations of DMARDs for the treatment of RA. In general, they prefer not to discontinue MTX even if the patient is an incomplete responder. There is evidence of efficacy using *combination therapy* with **MTX**, **hydroxychloroquine** and **sulfasalazine** ("triple therapy")[16] or **MTX** with **gold salts**,[17] **leflunomide**,[18] **azathioprine**[19] or **cyclosporine**.[20] MTX and leflunomide can be used together, but should be used with caution as the combination is associated with higher toxicity (GI and liver) and has not been shown to be superior to other DMARD combinations.

Oral and parenteral **gold, minocycline, D-penicillamine, azathioprine** and **cyclosporine** are now used less frequently and mostly in combination with other DMARDs. They could be used in patients who have failed MTX and who do not have access to biologic response modifiers.

Figure 1: Management of Rheumatoid Arthritis

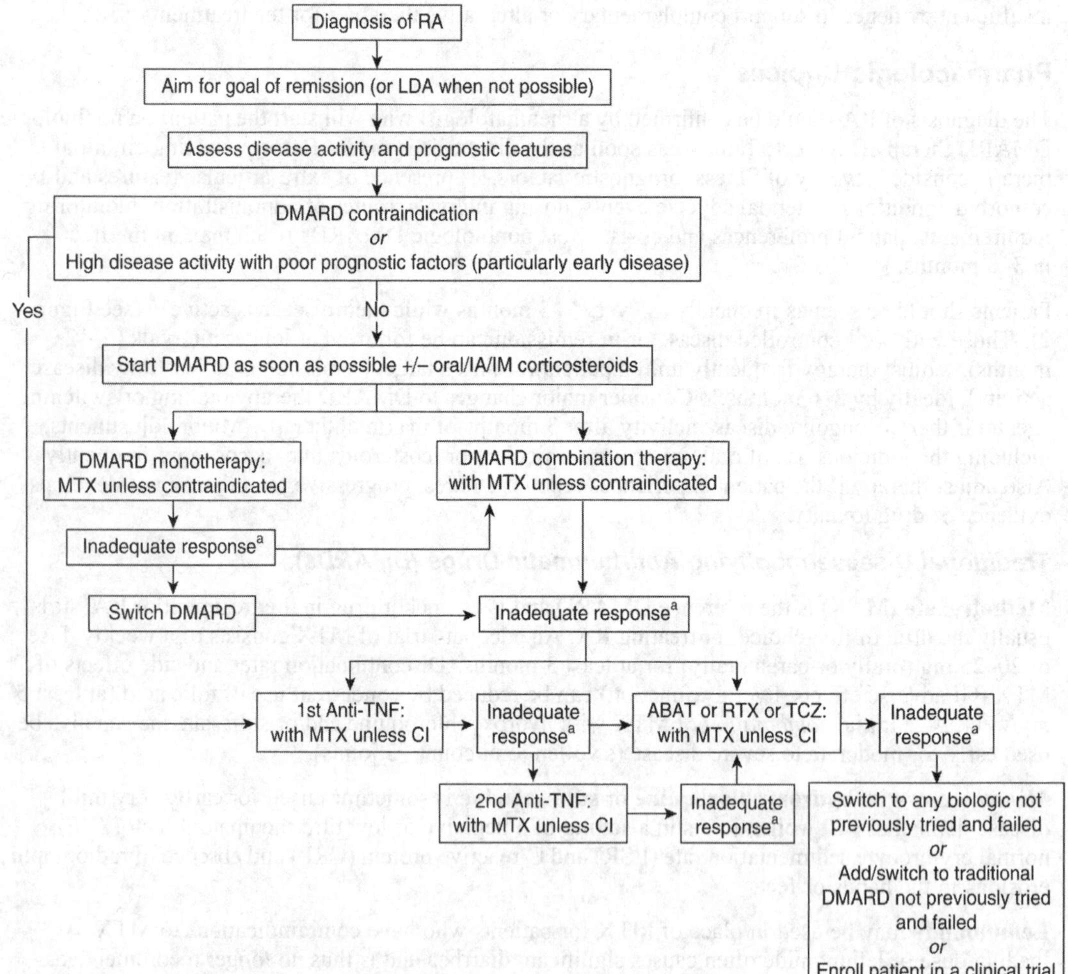

[a] Inadequate response: not reaching target by 3–6 months.

Abbreviations: ABAT = abatacept; Anti-TNF = tumour necrosis factor inhibitor; CI = contraindicated; DMARD = disease-modifying antirheumatic drug; IA = intra-articular; IM = intramuscular; LDA = low disease activity; MTX = methotrexate; RA = rheumatoid arthritis; RTX = rituximab; TCZ = tocilizumab

Adapted with permission from: Bykerk VP, Akhavan P, Hazlewood GS et al. Canadian Rheumatology Association recommendations for pharmacological management of rheumatoid arthritis with traditional and biologic disease-modifying antirheumatic drugs. *J Rheumatol* 2012;39(8):1559-82.

Figure 2: **Monitoring Rheumatoid Arthritis Activity**

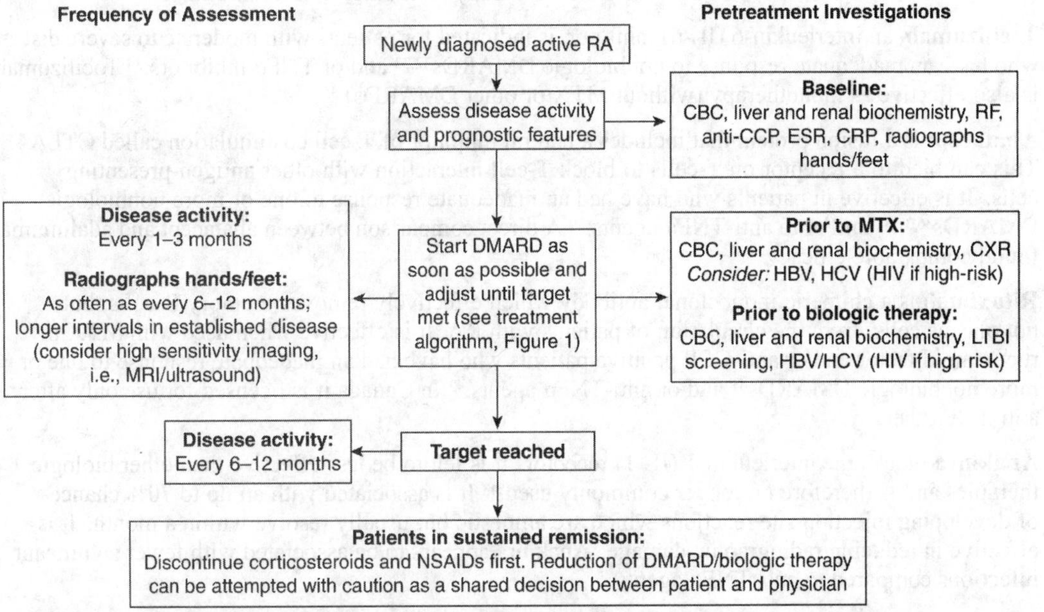

Abbreviations: Anti-CCP = antibody to cyclic citrullinated protein; CBC = complete blood count; CRP = C-reactive protein; CXR = chest x-ray; DMARD = disease-modifying antirheumatic drug; ESR = erythrocyte sedimentation rate; HBV/HCV = hepatitis B virus/C virus; HIV = human immunodeficiency virus; LTBI = latent tuberculosis infection; MTX = methotrexate; RA = rheumatoid arthritis; RF = rheumatoid factor
Adapted with permission from: Bykerk VP, Akhavan P, Hazlewood GS et al. Canadian Rheumatology Association recommendations for pharmacological management of rheumatoid arthritis with traditional and biologic disease-modifying antirheumatic drugs. *J Rheumatol* 2012;39(8):1559-82.

Biologic Response Modifiers (Biologic DMARDs)

Biologic response modifiers (Table 5) target key mediators of inflammatory synovitis and bone and cartilage destruction, e.g., tumour necrosis factor-alpha (TNFα) and others. These agents improve the signs and symptoms of active RA and reduce the radiologic progression of the disease.[21] In patients with a partial response to biologic therapy, maximizing the use of MTX or adding other nonbiologic DMARDs may provide additional benefits.

TNFα antagonists are currently the most commonly used first-line biologics, although other biologics may also be used. **Adalimumab, certolizumab, etanercept, golimumab** and **infliximab** are most effective when used with MTX or another DMARD.[22] All anti-TNFα agents are thought to have comparable efficacy leading to rapid improvement in signs and symptoms, as well as laboratory parameters of inflammation, usually within 8–12 weeks.[23] Patients with an inadequate response to anti-TNFα therapy may be switched to a different anti-TNFα agent or to a biologic with a different mechanism of action.

Infliximab, a chimeric mouse-human monoclonal antibody to TNFα, is approved only in combination with MTX in order to reduce the immune reaction to the murine component. In the case of inadequate response to infliximab, MTX doses should be maximized. Increasing the dose or decreasing the dosing interval of infliximab may be an option, although a randomized controlled trial did not show a benefit in dose escalation from 3 mg/kg to 5 mg/kg.[24]

Etanercept monotherapy is effective in early RA;[25] it is more effective in preventing radiographic damage when given with MTX.[26] SC etanercept is usually dosed at 50 mg once weekly[27] but may also be given as 25 mg twice weekly.[25]

Adalimumab,[28] **certolizumab**[29] and **golimumab**[30,31] also improve symptoms in patients with moderate to severe RA who are unresponsive to nonbiologic DMARD therapy alone. Golimumab has also been shown to be effective in patients who have failed therapy with other TNFα inhibitors.[30,31]

Tocilizumab, an interleukin-6 (IL-6) inhibitor, is indicated for patients with moderate to severe disease who have an inadequate response to nonbiologic DMARDs[32,33] and/or TNFα inhibitors.[34] Tocilizumab is also effective as monotherapy (without MTX or other DMARDs).[35]

Abatacept is a fusion protein that includes a natural inhibitor of T-cell costimulation called CTLA4. This can bind to a receptor on T-cells to block T-cell interaction with other antigen-presenting cells. It is effective in patients who have had an inadequate response to one or more nonbiologic DMARDs[36,37,38] and/or to anti-TNFα agents.[39] A direct comparison between abatacept and adalimumab found comparable efficacy.[40]

Rituximab is a chimeric monoclonal antibody which effectively removes memory B-cells, but not plasma cells, from the circulation of patients with RA. It is effective when used with MTX in rheumatoid factor and/or anti-CCP positive patients who have had an inadequate response to one or more nonbiologic DMARDs[41] and/or anti-TNFα agents.[42] In Canada it is licensed for use only after anti-TNFα therapy.

Anakinra blocks the interleukin-1 (IL-1) receptor. It is felt to be less effective than other biologic therapies and is therefore no longer commonly used.[43] It is associated with an up to 70% chance of developing injection site reactions which are amnestic but usually resolve within a month. It is effective in reducing radiographic damage. Anakinra appears to be associated with fewer significant infections compared to anti-TNFα agents.

Biologic agents should be discontinued during active infection and prior to surgery. The timing of withdrawal and reinstitution of therapy should be decided on an individual basis in discussion with the rheumatologist.

Safety of Biologic DMARDs

Biologic therapy is associated with a small increased risk of serious infections including zoster and opportunistic infections.[44,45] Although the humoral response to inactivated vaccines may be blunted due to biologic therapy, there is no convincing evidence that vaccine effectiveness is reduced.[46,47] Ideally, vaccinations should be up to date prior to initiating therapy, particularly in the case of live vaccines. If the patient has already commenced biologic therapy, most inactive vaccines are recommended, if indicated (e.g., influenza, pneumococcal) [Evidence: SORT B*].[46,47] Live vaccines are not recommended in patients taking biologic therapy due to risk of causing disseminated infection [Evidence: SORT C*].[46] For more information regarding specific vaccine recommendations, see Table 3 or the *Canadian Immunization Guide* (www.phac-aspc.gc.ca/publicat/cig-gci/index-eng.php).

The risk of tuberculosis (TB) is increased in patients on anti-TNF therapy, and is unknown with the other biologic agents.[22] An exception is rituximab, which does not appear to increase the risk of TB. Prior to starting biologic therapy, patients should be screened for latent tuberculosis by assessment of epidemiologic risk factors, chest x-ray and a Mantoux skin test. In patients who screen positive, exclude active TB and offer prophylactic therapy with **isoniazid**. Consider consultation with an infectious disease specialist if there is a concern about latent exposure to TB.

Long-term safety with respect to lymphoproliferative and other malignancies continues to be investigated.[48] Postmarketing reports indicate a possible increased risk of lymphomas and other malignancies in children and adolescents treated with TNF_α inhibitors.[49] However, long-term observational studies indicate that the risk of malignancy with the use of TNF_α antagonists remains

* SORT (Strength of Recommendation Taxonomy) is a rating system (A, B or C) that addresses the quality of available evidence. For more information consult **How to Use *Compendium of Therapeutic Choices*** on page xxv.

low.[22] Patients with RA not on biologic therapy are at increased risk of lymphoma compared to the general population. Long-term observational studies comparing RA patients on biologic therapy to RA patients not on biologic therapy have not found an increased risk for most cancers, although TNF_{α} inhibitors have been associated with an increased risk of nonmelanomatous and invasive melanomatous skin cancer.[50] Combination therapy with 2 biologic response modifiers is contraindicated due to increased risk of serious infections and malignancy.[51]

Table 3: **Recommendations for Vaccination in Patients with Rheumatoid Arthritis**

	Inactivated/Killed Vaccines			**Live Attenuated Vaccines**	
RA Therapy	**Influenza** (annual)	**Pneumococcal** (booster after 3–5 y)	**Hepatitis B**	**Herpes Zoster**	**Other**
Methotrexate[a]	Recommended	Recommended	High-risk patients[b]	>60 years	Caution
Leflunomide	Recommended	Recommended	High-risk patients[b]	>60 years	Caution
Sulfasalazine	Recommended	Recommended	High-risk patients[b]	>60 years	Caution
Biologics[c]	Recommended	Recommended	High-risk patients[b]	Avoid	Avoid

[a] Methotrexate ≤25 mg/week.
[b] High-risk groups include residents, travelers or close contact with individuals from hepatitis B endemic areas, illicit drug users, persons engaging in risky sexual behaviors/history of sexually transmitted infection, men who have sex with men, chronic liver disease, occupation exposures, frequent blood transfusions.
[c] B-cell depleting biologics, such as rituximab, may require specific timing recommendations regarding vaccine administration.[47]
Abbreviations: RA = rheumatoid arthritis
Adapted with permission from: Bombardier C, Hazlewood GS, Akhavan P et al. Canadian Rheumatology Association recommendations for the pharmacological management of rheumatoid arthritis with traditional and biologic disease-modifying antirheumatic drugs: part II safety. *J Rheumatol* 2012;39(8):1583-602.

Nonsteroidal Anti-inflammatory Drugs (NSAIDs)

NSAIDs have a role as an adjunct in relieving pain, but have no effect on underlying disease processes. Traditional NSAIDs (see Chapter 82, Table 2) are believed to be effective via their inhibition of cyclooxygenase (COX). Some adverse reactions of NSAIDs, including GI effects, may result from their inhibition of COX-1, whereas an increased risk of cardiovascular adverse events may be linked to the inhibition of COX-2. COX-2 inhibitors were specifically designed to access only the COX-2 enzyme. Their efficacy is similar to nonselective NSAIDs. Patients with heart disease should be on concurrent low-dose **ASA**, with appropriate gastroprotection if they are at risk of peptic ulcer disease.[52]

Corticosteroids

Corticosteroids rapidly reduce inflammation.[53] Chronic low doses of **prednisone** (≤10 mg/day) may have disease-modifying properties,[54] but are not recommended for routine use, due to concerns over long-term toxicity. Prednisone is the preferred oral preparation because of its moderate glucocorticoid potency, intermediate duration of action and low mineralocorticoid potency. Depot preparations are used as bridging therapy.[55] **Triamcinolone** should be reserved for deep intra-articular injections (thus lowering the propensity for lipoatrophy). Because of low systemic absorption and long action, depot preparations may be more effective for a longer period of time. All depot preparations of corticosteroids may cause atrophy after infiltration of superficial subcutaneous soft tissues, thus the shorter acting **methylprednisolone acetate** is recommended for small joints and tendon sheaths.

Corticosteroids are associated with a number of serious side effects including metabolic abnormalities (e.g., hyperglycemia, hypertension, muscle atrophy, truncal obesity), adrenal suppression, cataracts, infections and avascular necrosis. Corticosteroid use in RA patients has also been associated with an increased risk of MI.[56] In combination with NSAIDs, corticosteroids increase the risk of peptic ulcer disease. Moreover, corticosteroids will further aggravate osteoporosis and cardiovascular disease, conditions independently associated with RA.

Patients on prolonged corticosteroid steroid therapy should also take **calcium** (total intake of 1200 mg/day from diet and supplements, preferably from diet) and **vitamin D** supplementation 800–2000 IU/day as well as a bisphosphonate (e.g., **alendronate**, **risedronate**, **zoledronic acid**; see Chapter 83) to prevent the bone loss associated with corticosteroid use.[57,58] They should also be considered for prophylactic gastroprotective therapy and antiplatelet therapy with low-dose ASA.

Analgesia

RA is increasingly recognized as a chronic pain syndrome.[59] Many adjunctive medications and alternative therapies are being used. Although controlled trials supporting their effectiveness in RA are not available, some (including acetaminophen) are compatible with the medications used to treat RA and have fewer serious side effects than NSAIDs.

Opioids should be avoided if possible. There is limited direct evidence of their efficacy in patients with RA.[60] Avoid meperidine and pentazocine because of lack of proven efficacy, risk of accumulation and serious toxicity with prolonged use. Up to 10% of the population lacks the enzyme that converts codeine to morphine. Failure to respond to codeine warrants a trial with hydromorphone or morphine, opioids that do not require metabolic activation.

Choices during Pregnancy and Breastfeeding

Pregnancy itself has a favourable influence on disease activity, with 70–90% of women experiencing improvement while pregnant.[61] Medications can often be reduced or discontinued during pregnancy. Disease flares are common postpartum, with nearly all women experiencing an increase in disease activity by 4–6 months after delivery. The influence of breastfeeding on the risk of disease flare is uncertain.[62,63] Medications stopped during pregnancy are resumed postpartum, either immediately or after breastfeeding ceases.

- **Corticosteroids** remain the safest therapy during pregnancy and breastfeeding. In high doses they have been associated with low birth weight in humans and cleft palate in animal models, but there is no evidence in humans that prednisone or methylprednisolone is teratogenic.[57]
- Antifolate metabolic effects of **MTX** may cause open neural tube defects and other CNS abnormalities, facial anomalies and growth retardation, as well as other problems. MTX also has abortifacient properties.[64] MTX is contraindicated in pregnancy. Women of childbearing age should use reliable contraception while taking MTX. The drug should be stopped in both males and females at least 3 months before attempting conception, and folic acid supplementation should be given. However, recent small cohort studies showed no adverse pregnancy outcomes after preconceptional low-dose MTX exposure in males[65] or females.[66]
- Data relating to the use of **hydroxychloroquine** in pregnancy are scarce. Existing data do not indicate that the drug poses significant fetal risk.[64] Despite concerns regarding a potential risk of kernicterus, **sulfasalazine** has been used in pregnancy with relative safety.[64] Because sulfasalazine is a folic acid antagonist, folic acid supplementation should be ensured in women of reproductive age. Monitoring for hyperbilirubinemia is still recommended in fetuses exposed to sulfasalazine close to term.
- **NSAID** use in the third trimester may be of concern; because of antiprostaglandin effects, NSAIDs can increase risks of fetal and maternal bleeding and premature closure of the ductus arteriosus, and can also interfere with labour onset or duration. The 2 most studied NSAIDs are **ibuprofen** and **naproxen**.
- **Leflunomide** is known to be teratogenic and is contraindicated in pregnancy. Some experts consider it prudent to avoid the use of leflunomide in women of child-bearing potential. Women who wish to become pregnant or men who wish to father a child after taking leflunomide are advised to undergo a drug elimination protocol consisting of cholestyramine 8 g TID for 11 days, or activated charcoal 50 g QID for 11 days (not necessarily on consecutive days).[67] Plasma concentration of

leflunomide's active metabolite is then measured on 2 separate occasions at least 2 weeks apart to confirm levels below 0.02 mg/L.[67,68] Many laboratories do not perform this test; some manufacturers provide free measurement of these levels via an outside laboratory upon direct request from the physician. Following the second plasma level confirmation, an additional waiting period of 3 months before conception is recommended in men,[67] and some experts suggest a waiting period of 1–3 menstrual cycles in women.[68] Without the drug elimination protocol, it could take up to 2 years for plasma levels to drop to below 0.02 mg/L, due to interindividual variation in drug clearance.[67,68] In the case of unplanned pregnancy or any delay of menses or other suspicion of pregnancy while taking leflunomide, women should contact their physician immediately; rapid institution of the drug elimination protocol (outlined above) could reduce the risk to the fetus.[64,67]

- Data on the use of **anti-TNFα agents** in pregnancy are scarce; while there have been reports of congenital abnormalities,[69] their association with TNFα inhibitors has been questioned.[70] No controlled studies have shown an increased rate of adverse outcomes. Observational data suggest there are no adverse effects associated with conception and early pregnancy in women who use TNFα inhibitors.[71] It is recommended these be discontinued if possible during pregnancy. Insufficient data are available to ascertain their safety in breastfeeding.
- There are minimal to no human data for the use of **abatacept** and **tocilizumab** during pregnancy; caution dictates that these agents be stopped prior to conception. **Rituximab** has caused B-cell depletion in neonates in both animal studies and human case reports and should therefore be discontinued prior to pregnancy.[61]

Women who choose to breastfeed may use **corticosteroids**, **NSAIDs** (short-acting agents are preferred), **hydroxychloroquine** and **sulfasalazine** (except in infants with hyperbilirubinemia), as discussed above. **MTX** is secreted in low amounts into breast milk and is considered contraindicated. **Leflunomide** should also not be used, given the lack of data about excretion into breast milk. There are limited data for any of the biologic agents, so decisions should be made on a case-by-case basis, considering the importance of the medication to the mother.

A discussion of general principles on the use of medications in these special populations can be found in Appendix II and Appendix III. Other specialized reference sources are also provided in these appendices.

Therapeutic Tips

- Referral to a rheumatologist and prompt institution of therapy is essential. Early, aggressive treatment is linked to a positive outcome in RA.
- Only 30% of patients have a positive RF at initial presentation. A negative RF does not exclude the possibility of rheumatoid arthritis.
- Comorbidities, including infections, cardiovascular disease, lymphoma and osteoporosis are common in RA patients. Routine care should include screening for, prevention and treatment of these conditions.
- Fatigue is a common symptom in RA patients. Interventions such as physical activity and psychosocial intervention (e.g., self-help, coping strategies, talking therapies) have demonstrated benefit in some patients with persistent fatigue despite adequate disease control.[72]

Table 4: **Nonbiologic Disease-modifying Antirheumatic Drugs for Rheumatoid Arthritis**

Class	Drug	Dose	Adverse Effects	Monitoring[3,8,73]	Drug Interactions	Cost [a]
Aminosalicylates	*sulfasalazine* Salazopyrin, generics	Initial: 500 mg daily or BID po, increase by 500 mg weekly to a maintenance dose of 2–3 g daily po (in 2 divided doses)	Rash, marrow toxicity, GI intolerance. May cause sun sensitivity. Do not use if sulfa allergy or G-6-PD deficiency. Consider enteric coated tablets to reduce adverse GI effects.	Baseline CBC, LFTs, creatinine; CBC, LFTs Q3 months.	Sulfasalazine may decrease GI absorption of digoxin.	$
Antimalarial Agents	*hydroxychloroquine* Plaquenil, generics	200–400 mg daily po. Maximum: 6.5 mg/kg/day based on ideal body weight. Reduce dose if <60 kg	Nausea, cramps, diarrhea, rash, nightmares, hyperpigmentation. Rarely, if dosed too high for too long, corneal and retinal deposition can occur.	Baseline CBC, LFTs, creatinine Ophthalmologic exam required at baseline and annually after 5 years. If high risk, required annually from baseline. High risk: cumulative dose >1000 g, doses >6.5 mg/kg or 400 mg/day, treatment for greater than 5–7 years, liver or kidney disease, advanced age, obesity and pre-existing ophthalmologic disease.[74,75,76]	Avoid concomitant use of related drugs such as quinine.	$
Gold Preparations	*auranofin* Ridaura	6 mg daily po in 1–2 doses	Diarrhea, rash, pruritus, nausea, abdominal pain, stomatitis, cytopenia, proteinuria, nephrotoxicity.	Stop drug if no response observed after 4 months.		$$$$$
	sodium aurothiomalate Myochrysine	Initial: 10 mg first wk, 25 mg second wk, then 50 mg weekly for 20 wk im; then decrease to maintenance Maintenance: 50 mg Q2–6 wk im, usually monthly	Postdose reactions (arthralgias, flushing, hypotension). Stomatitis, pruritic dermatitis, cytopenia, proteinuria.	CBC, dipstick for urinary protein with every 1–2 injections. Hold if pruritus, mucosal ulcers, or >1+ proteinuria.		$

Class	Drug	Dose	Adverse Effects	Monitoring[3,8,73]	Drug Interactions	Cost [a]
Heavy Metal Antagonists	*penicillamine* Cuprimine	Initial: 125–250 mg once daily po, increase by 125–250 mg Q1–3 months Maintenance: 250–750 mg once daily po Doses >500 mg/day should be divided	Proteinuria, cytopenia, diarrhea, nausea, vomiting, taste alteration.	CBC, urine dipstick Q1–2 months.	Food: Since the effectiveness of penicillamine may be decreased by food, administer on an empty stomach at least 1 h before or 2 h after meals and at least 1 h apart from any other drug or milk.	$$$$$
Immunomodulators	*azathioprine* Imuran, generics	Initial: 50 mg daily po, may increase by 25–50 mg daily every 1–2 weeks (maximum dose 2.5 mg/kg/day) Maintenance: lowest tolerated dose, usually 50–150 mg/day (in 1–3 divided doses)	Hepatitis, drug fever, myelosuppression, immunosuppression, unconfirmed risk of malignancy.	Baseline CBC, LFTs and Q1–3 months.	Allopurinol may increase azathioprine toxicity; dosage adjustment may be necessary (one-quarter of regular dose).	$
	cyclosporine Neoral, Apo-Cyclosporine, other generics	Initial: 2.5 mg/kg/day po in 2 divided doses, increase every 1–2 wk Maintenance: 2.5–5 mg/kg/day (in 2 divided doses)	Renal toxicity, hypertension, hypertrichosis, cytopenia, gum hyperplasia.	Blood pressure monthly, periodic CBC, LFTs, electrolytes; monitor drug blood levels.	Metabolized by CYP450—many possible drug interactions (e.g., grapefruit, erythromycin, ketoconazole, rifampin).	$$$$$

(cont'd)

Table 4: **Nonbiologic Disease-modifying Antirheumatic Drugs for Rheumatoid Arthritis** *(cont'd)*

Class	Drug	Dose	Adverse Effects	Monitoring[3,8,73]	Drug Interactions	Cost[a]
	leflunomide ❥ Arava, generics	10–20 mg daily po	Nausea, diarrhea, anorexia, alopecia, hypertension, rash. May cause hepatic toxicity, cytopenias, profound anorexia and weight loss, pulmonary fibrosis, interstitial lung disease.	Baseline CBC, LFTs, creatinine, hepatitis B and C serology; CBC, LFTs, creatinine monthly × 3 months, then Q1–3 months, LFTs monthly if also on MTX.	Avoid alcohol because of possible increased risk of hepatotoxicity. Pregnancy is contraindicated while taking this medication. Washout procedure with cholestyramine 8 g TID × 11 days is recommended for serious toxicity or imminently planned pregnancy (see Choices during Pregnancy and Breastfeeding).	$$
	methotrexate ❥ Methotrexate Injection USP, Methotrexate (Pfizer), Methotrexate Tablets USP, Metoject, generics	Initial: 7.5–25 mg weekly po, sc or im; increase by 2.5–5 mg Q1–4 wk Maintenance: 7.5–25 mg weekly po, sc or im (single dose if tolerated, or in 2 divided doses Q12H) For doses >15 mg, divided doses are better absorbed	Nausea, malaise, flu-like aches, headache, oral ulcers, transient loose stools; rarely: bone marrow and liver toxicity, pneumonitis, immunosuppression, malignancy. Not to be used in patients with hepatitis B or C, renal insufficiency or lung disease.	Baseline CBC, LFTs, albumin, creatinine, hepatitis B and C serology, chest x-ray; monthly × 3 months, then Q1–3 months. Consider HIV screening in high-risk patients. LFTs monthly if also on leflunomide. Give folic acid 5 mg weekly to control minor adverse effects.	Alcohol restriction may minimize hepatotoxicity. NSAIDs or ASA may increase MTX serum concentrations minimally but this is not clinically significant; these can be combined at low doses. Penicillins (e.g., amoxicillin, cloxacillin, piperacillin) and sulfonamides (e.g., trimethoprim/sulfamethoxazole) may decrease MTX clearance.	$

[a] Cost of 4-week supply for maintenance dose based on 70 kg body weight; includes drug cost only.
❥ Dosage adjustment may be required in renal impairment; see Appendix I
Abbreviations: CBC = complete blood count; CYP450 = cytochrome P450; G-6-PD = glucose-6-phosphate dehydrogenase; LFT = liver function test; MTX = methotrexate
Legend: $ <$50 $$ $50–100 $$$ $100–150 $$$$ $150–200 $$$$$ $200–250

Table 5: **Biologic DMARDs (Biologic Response Modifiers) for Rheumatoid Arthritis**

Class	Drug	Dose	Adverse Effects	Monitoring[3,8,73]	Contraindications	Cost[a]
B-Cell Depletors	*rituximab* Rituxan	1 g × 2 doses 2 weeks apart iv. Infusions are given with 100 mg of methylprednisolone Premedicate with acetaminophen and an antihistamine (e.g., diphenhydramine) before infusion Doses can be repeated after 5–6 months. Indicated in patients who have failed an anti-TNFα agent	Mild to severe infusion reactions (very severe reactions resulting in death have been reported rarely). Rare: progressive multifocal leukoencephalopathy (PML).	Baseline CBC, LFTs, creatinine, hepatitis B and C serology. CD19 counts can be used to monitor B-cell levels.	Susceptibility to infection. Contraindicated in patients with known Type I hypersensitivity or anaphylactic reactions to murine proteins, Chinese Hamster Ovary (CHO) cell proteins or to any component of the product.	$9500
Interleukin-1 (IL-1) Inhibitors	*anakinra* ❥ Kineret	100 mg daily sc	Injection site reactions (70%).	Baseline CBC, LFTs, creatinine, hepatitis B and C serology.	Susceptibility to infection.	$
Interleukin-6 (IL-6) Inhibitors	*tocilizumab* Actemra	4 mg/kg Q4 wk iv, infused over 1 h; may increase to 8 mg/kg iv Q4 wk if response is inadequate	Infusion reactions (very severe reactions resulting in death have been reported rarely), serious infections, GI perforation, increased neutrophils, decreased platelets, increased lipids.	Baseline CBC, LFTs, creatinine, hepatitis B and C serology, PPD and chest x-ray to assess for latent TB. May consider screening for ANA. Monitor for neutropenia, thrombocytopenia and elevated aminotransferases 4–8 weeks after starting therapy. May increase CYP450 enzyme activity—monitor concurrent therapy with drugs metabolized by CYP450.	Active infection. Screen for latent/active TB before initiating therapy.	$

(cont'd)

Table 5: **Biologic DMARDs (Biologic Response Modifiers) for Rheumatoid Arthritis** *(cont'd)*

Class	Drug	Dose	Adverse Effects	Monitoring[3,8,73]	Contraindications	Cost[a]
T-Cell Costimulation Inhibitors	*abatacept* Orencia	Dosing for iv administration (initial infusion or loading dose): <60 kg: 500 mg iv initial infusion 60–100 kg: 750 mg iv initial infusion >100 kg: 1 g iv initial infusion After initial dosing, administer at 2 wk, 4 wk and then monthly Dosing for sc administration: 125 mg weekly starting within 24 hours of iv loading dose; the same weekly sc dose is recommended even if iv loading dose is not possible	IV: rare minor infusion reactions. SC: injection sites should be rotated and injections should never be given into areas where the skin is tender, bruised, red, or hard.	Baseline CBC, LFTs, creatinine, hepatitis B and C serology, PPD and chest x-ray to assess for latent TB. May consider screening for ANA.	Susceptibility to infection.	$$$
Tumour Necrosis Factor-alpha (TNFα) Inhibitors	*adalimumab* Humira	40 mg Q2 wk sc	Injection site reactions; infections (including TB and opportunistic organisms); new-onset psoriasis; increased risk of lymphoma (children and adolescents), leukemia and other malignancies; autoimmune phenomena.	Baseline CBC, LFTs, creatinine, hepatitis B and C serology, PPD and chest x-ray to assess for latent TB. May consider screening for ANA.	Susceptibility to or presence of serious and/or recurrent infection; SLE, demyelinating disease and heart failure are relative contraindications.	$
	certolizumab Cimzia	400 mg at weeks 0, 2 and 4, then 200 mg Q2 wk sc. May give 400 mg Q4 wk sc as maintenance dose	See adalimumab.	See adalimumab.	See adalimumab.	$
	etanercept Enbrel	25 mg twice weekly *or* 50 mg once weekly sc	See adalimumab.	See adalimumab.	See adalimumab.	$$

Class	Drug	Dose	Adverse Effects	Monitoring[3,8,73]	Contraindications	Cost[a]
	golimumab Simponi	50 mg once monthly on same date each month sc	See adalimumab.	See adalimumab.	See adalimumab.	$$
	infliximab Remicade	3–5 mg/kg iv at 0, 2 and 6 wk, and Q4–8 wk thereafter	Infections (including TB and opportunistic organisms), new-onset psoriasis, increased risk of lymphoma (children and adolescents), leukemia and other malignancies, autoimmune phenomena. Mild to severe infusion reactions (very severe reactions resulting in death have been reported rarely).	See adalimumab.	Contraindicated in patients with known Type I hypersensitivity or anaphylactic reactions to murine proteins; heart failure if using >5 mg/kg/infusion, demyelinating disease, susceptibility to or presence of serious and/or recurrent infection; SLE is a relative contraindication.	$$$$$

[a] Cost of 4-week supply based on 70 kg body weight; includes drug cost only.

Dosage adjustment may be required in renal impairment; see Appendix I

Abbreviations: ANA = antinuclear antibodies; CYP450 = cytochrome P450; DMARD = disease-modifying antirheumatic drug; LFT = liver function test; MTX = methotrexate; PPD = purified protein derivative; SLE = systemic lupus erythematosus; TB = tuberculosis; TNFα = tumour necrosis factor-alpha

Legend: $ $1000–1500 $$ $1500–2000 $$$ $2000–2500 $$$$ $2500–3000 $$$$$ $3000–3500

Suggested Readings

Bombardier C, Hazlewood GS, Akhavan P et al. Canadian Rheumatology Association recommendations for the pharmacological management of rheumatoid arthritis with traditional and biologic disease-modifying antirheumatic drugs: part II safety. *J Rheumatol* 2012;39(8):1583-602.

Bykerk VP, Akhavan P, Hazlewood GS et al. Canadian Rheumatology Association recommendations for pharmacological management of rheumatoid arthritis with traditional and biologic disease-modifying antirheumatic drugs. *J Rheumatol* 2011;39(8):1559-82.

Duru N, van der Goes M, Jacobs JW et al. EULAR evidence-based and consensus-based recommendations on the management of medium to high-dose corticosteroids therapy in rheumatic diseases. *Ann Rheum Dis* 2013;72(12):1905-13.

Singh JA, Furst DE, Bharat A et al. 2012 update of the 2008 American College of Rheumatology recommendations for the use of disease-modifying antirheumatic drugs and biologic agents in the treatment of rheumatoid arthritis. *Arthritis Care Res (Hoboken)* 2012;64(5):625-39.

van Assen S, Agmon-Levin N, Elkayam O et al. EULAR recommendations for vaccination in adult patients with autoimmune rheumatic diseases. *Ann Rheum Dis* 2011;70(3):414-22.

References

1. Meune C, Touze E, Trinquart L et al. Trends in cardiovascular mortality in patients with rheumatoid arthritis over 50 years: a systematic review and meta-analysis of cohort studies. *Rheumatology (Oxford)* 2009;48(10):1309-13.
2. Bykerk VP, Baron M, Boire G et al. Canadian consensus statement on early optimal therapy in early rheumatoid arthritis. *J Can Rheum Assoc* 2004;14(3):11-3. Available from: www.stacommunications.com/customcomm/Back-issue_pages/CRAJ/crajPDFs/fall2004e/11.pdf. Accessed April 5, 2011.
3. Bykerk VP, Akhavan P, Hazlewood GS et al. Canadian Rheumatology Association recommendations for pharmacological management of rheumatoid arthritis with traditional and biologic disease-modifying antirheumatic drugs. *J Rheumatol* 2012;39(8):1559-82.
4. Aletaha D, Neogi T, Silman AJ et al. 2010 Rheumatoid arthritis classification criteria: an American College of Rheumatology/European League Against Rheumatism collaborative initiative. *Arthritis Rheum* 2010;62(9):2569-81.
5. Radner H, Neogi T, Smolen JS et al. Performance of the 2010 ACR/EULAR classification criteria for rheumatoid arthritis: a systematic literature review. *Ann Rheum Dis* 2014;73(1):114-23.
6. Smolen JS, Aletaha D, Bijlsma JW et al. Treating rheumatoid arthritis to target: recommendations of an international task force. *Ann Rheum Dis* 2010;69(4):631-7.
7. Hazlewood G, Aletaha D, Carmona L et al. Algorithm for identification of undifferentiated peripheral inflammatory arthritis: a multinational collaboration through the 3e initiative. *J Rheumatol Suppl* 2011;87:54-8.
8. American College of Rheumatology Subcommittee on Rheumatoid Arthritis Guidelines. Guidelines for the management of rheumatoid arthritis: 2002 update. *Arthritis Rheum* 2002;46(2):328-46.
9. Bykerk VP, Keystone EC. What are the goals and principles of management in the early treatment of rheumatoid arthritis? *Best Pract Res Clin Rheumatol* 2005;19(1):147-61.
10. Hakkinen A. Effectiveness and safety of strength training in rheumatoid arthritis. *Curr Opin Rheumatol* 2004;6(2):132-7.
11. Macfarlane GJ, Paudyal P, Doherty M et al. A systematic review of evidence for the effectiveness of practitioner-based complementary and alternative therapies in the management of rheumatic diseases: rheumatoid arthritis. *Rheumatology (Oxford)* 2012;51(9):1707-13.
12. U.K. National Health Service. National Institute for Health and Clinical Excellence. *Rheumatoid arthritis: the management of rheumatoid arthritis in adults*. London (GB): NICE; 2009. Available from: www.nice.org.uk/nicemedia/pdf/CG79NICEGuideline.pdf. Accessed April 5, 2011.
13. Shea B, Swinden MV, Tanjong Ghogomu E et al. Folic acid and folinic acid for reducing side effects in patients receiving methotrexate for rheumatoid arthritis. *Cochrane Database Syst Rev* 2013;5:CD000951.
14. Visser K, Katchamart W, Loza E et al. Multinational evidence-based recommendations for the use of methotrexate in rheumatic disorders with a focus on rheumatoid arthritis: integrating systematic literature research and expert opinion of a broad international panel of rheumatologists in the 3E Initiative. *Ann Rheum Dis* 2009;68(7):1086-93.
15. U.S. Food and Drug Administration (FDA). *FDA Drug Safety Communication: New boxed warning for severe liver injury with arthritis drug Arava (leflunomide)*. Available from: www.fda.gov/Drugs/DrugSafety/PostmarketDrugSafetyInformationforPatientsand-Providers/ucm218679.htm. Accessed April 5, 2011.
16. O'Dell JR, Leff R, Paulsen G et al. Treatment of rheumatoid arthritis with methotrexate and hydroxychloroquine, methotrexate and sulfasalazine, or a combination of the three medications: results of a two-year, randomized, double-blind, placebo-controlled trial. *Arthritis Rheum* 2002;46(5):1164-70.
17. Lehman AJ, Esdaile JM, Klinkhoff AV et al. A 48-week, randomized, double-blind, double-observer, placebo-controlled multicenter trial of combination methotrexate and intramuscular gold therapy in rheumatoid arthritis: results of the METGO study. *Arthritis Rheum* 2005;52(5):1360-70.
18. Kremer JM, Genovese MC, Cannon GW et al. Concomitant leflunomide therapy in patients with active rheumatoid arthritis despite stable doses of methotrexate. A randomized, double-blind, placebo-controlled trial. *Ann Intern Med* 2002;137(9):726-33.
19. Willkens RF, Stablein D. Combination treatment of rheumatoid arthritis using azathioprine and methotrexate: a 48 week controlled clinical trial. *J Rheumatol Suppl* 1996;44:64-8.
20. Stein CM, Pincus T, Yocum D et al. Combination treatment of severe rheumatoid arthritis with cyclosporine and methotrexate for forty-eight weeks: an open-label extension study. The Methotrexate-Cyclosporine Combination Study Group. *Arthritis Rheum* 1997;40(10):1843-51.
21. Furst DE, Keystone EC, Fleischmann R et al. Updated consensus statement on biological agents for the treatment of rheumatic diseases, 2009. *Ann Rheum Dis* 2010;69(Suppl 1):i2-29.

22. Nam JL, Winthrop KL, van Vollenhoven RF et al. Current evidence for the management of rheumatoid arthritis with biological disease-modifying antirheumatic drugs: a systematic literature review informing the EULAR recommendations for the management of RA. *Ann Rheum Dis* 2010;69(6):976-86.
23. Greenberg JD, Reed G, Decktor D et al. A comparative effectiveness study of adalimumab, etanercept and infliximab in biologically nave and switched rheumatoid arthritis patients: results from the US CORRONA registry. *Ann Rheum Dis* 2012;71(7):1134-42.
24. Pavelka K, Jarosova K, Suchy D et al. Increasing the infliximab dose in rheumatoid arthritis patients: a randomised, double blind study failed to confirm its efficacy. *Ann Rheum Dis* 2009;68(8):1285-9.
25. Bathon JM, Martin RW, Fleischmann RM et al. A comparison of etanercept and methotrexate in patients with early rheumatoid arthritis. *N Engl J Med* 2000;343(22):1586-93.
26. Klareskog L, van der Heijde D, de Jager JP et al. Therapeutic effect of the combination of etanercept and methotrexate compared with each treatment alone in patients with rheumatoid arthritis: double-blind randomised controlled trial. *Lancet* 2004;363(9410):675-81.
27. Keystone EC, Schiff MH, Kremer JM et al. Once-weekly administration of 50 mg etanercept in patients with active rheumatoid arthritis: results of a multicenter, randomized, double-blind, placebo-controlled trial. *Arthritis Rheum* 2004;50(2):353-63.
28. Keystone EC, Kavanaugh AF, Sharp JT et al. Radiographic, clinical, and functional outcomes of treatment with adalimumab (a human anti-tumor necrosis factor monoclonal antibody) in patients with active rheumatoid arthritis receiving concomitant methotrexate therapy: a randomized, placebo-controlled, 52-week trial. *Arthritis Rheum* 2004;50(5):1400-11.
29. Smolen J, Landewe RB, Mease P et al. Efficacy and safety of certolizumab pegol plus methotrexate in active rheumatoid arthritis: the RAPID 2 study. A randomised controlled trial. *Ann Rheum Dis* 2009;68(6):797-804.
30. Smolen JS, Kay J, Doyle MK et al. Golimumab in patients with active rheumatoid arthritis after treatment with tumour necrosis factor alpha inhibitors (GO-AFTER study): a multicentre, randomised, double-blind, placebo-controlled, phase III trial. *Lancet* 2009;374(9685):210-21.
31. Keystone EC, Genovese MC, Klareskog L et al. Golimumab, a human antibody to tumour necrosis factor {alpha} given by monthly subcutaneous injections, in active rheumatoid arthritis despite methotrexate therapy: the GO-FORWARD Study. *Ann Rheum Dis* 2009;68(6):789-96.
32. Genovese MC, McKay JD, Nasonov EL et al. Interleukin-6 receptor inhibition with tocilizumab reduces disease activity in rheumatoid arthritis with inadequate response to disease-modifying antirheumatic drugs: the tocilizumab in combination with traditional disease-modifying antirheumatic drug therapy study. *Arthritis Rheum* 2008;58(10):2968-80.
33. Maini RN, Taylor PC, Szechinski J et al. Double-blind randomized controlled clinical trial of the interleukin-6 receptor antagonist, tocilizumab, in European patients with rheumatoid arthritis who had an incomplete response to methotrexate. *Arthritis Rheum* 2006;54(9):2817-29.
34. Emery P, Keystone E, Tony HP et al. IL-6 receptor inhibition with tocilizumab improves treatment outcomes in patients with rheumatoid arthritis refractory to anti-tumour necrosis factor biologicals: results from a 24-week multicentre randomised placebo-controlled trial. *Ann Rheum Dis* 2008;67(11):1516-23.
35. Gabay C, Emery P, van Vollenhoven R et al. Tocilizumab monotherapy versus adalimumab monotherapy for treatment of rheumatoid arthritis (ADACTA): a randomised, double-blind, controlled phase 4 trial. *Lancet* 2013;381(9877):1541-50.
36. Kremer JM, Genant HK, Moreland LW et al. Effects of abatacept in patients with methotrexate-resistant active rheumatoid arthritis: a randomized trial. *Ann Intern Med* 2006;144(12):865-76.
37. Kremer JM, Westhovens R, Leon M et al. Treatment of rheumatoid arthritis by selective inhibition of T-cell activation with fusion protein CTLA4Ig. *N Engl J Med* 2003;349(20):1907-15.
38. Schiff M, Keiserman M, Codding C et al. Efficacy and safety of abatacept or infliximab vs placebo in ATTEST: a phase III, multi-centre, randomised, double-blind, placebo-controlled study in patients with rheumatoid arthritis and an inadequate response to methotrexate. *Ann Rheum Dis* 2008;67(8):1096-103.
39. Genovese MC, Becker JC, Schiff M et al. Abatacept for rheumatoid arthritis refractory to tumor necrosis factor alpha inhibition. *N Engl J Med* 2005;353(11):1114-23.
40. Weinblatt ME, Schiff M, Valente R et al. Head-to-head comparison of subcutaneous abatacept versus adalimumab for rheumatoid arthritis: findings of a phase IIIb, multinational, prospective, randomized study. *Arthritis Rheum* 2013;65(1):28-38.
41. Emery P, Fleischmann R, Filipowicz-Sosnowska A et al. The efficacy and safety of rituximab in patients with active rheumatoid arthritis despite methotrexate treatment: results of a phase IIB randomized, double-blind, placebo-controlled, dose-ranging trial. *Arthritis Rheum* 2006;54(5):1390-400.
42. Cohen SB, Emery P, Greenwald MW et al. Rituximab for rheumatoid arthritis refractory to anti-tumor necrosis factor therapy: results of a multicenter, randomized, double-blind, placebo-controlled, phase III trial evaluating primary efficacy and safety at twenty-four weeks. *Arthritis Rheum* 2006;54(9):2793-806.
43. Singh JA, Christensen R, Wells GA et al. A network meta-analysis of randomized controlled trials of biologics for rheumatoid arthritis: a Cochrane overview. *CMAJ* 2009;181(11):787-96.
44. Sakai R, Komano Y, Tanaka M et al. Time-dependent increased risk for serious infection from continuous use of tumor necrosis factor antagonists over three years in patients with rheumatoid arthritis. *Arthritis Care Res (Hoboken)* 2012;64(8):1125-34.
45. Galloway JB, Mercer LK, Moseley A et al. Risk of skin and soft tissue infections (including shingles) in patients exposed to anti-tumour necrosis factor therapy: results from the British Society for Rheumatology Biologics Register. *Ann Rheum Dis* 2013;72(2):229-34.
46. Bombardier C, Hazlewood GS, Akhavan P et al. Canadian Rheumatology Association recommendations for the pharmacological management of rheumatoid arthritis with traditional and biologic disease-modifying antirheumatic drugs: part II safety. *J Rheumatol* 2012;39(8):1583-602.
47. van Assen S, Agmon-Levin N, Elkayam O et al. EULAR recommendations for vaccination in adult patients with autoimmune inflammatory rheumatic diseases. *Ann Rheum Dis* 2011;70(3):414-22.
48. Askling J, van Vollenhoven RF, Granath F et al. Cancer risk in patients with rheumatoid arthritis treated with anti-tumor necrosis factor alpha therapies: does the risk change with the time since start of treatment? *Arthritis Rheum* 2009;60(11):3180-9.
49. Health Canada. *Safety update on TNF blockers and risk of cancer in children and young adults*. Available from: healthycanadians.gc.ca/recall-alert-rappel-avis/hc-sc/2009/13327a-eng.php. Accessed April 5, 2011.
50. Raaschou P, Simard JF, Holmqvist M et al. Rheumatoid arthritis, anti-tumour necrosis factor therapy, and risk of malignant melanoma: nationwide population based prospective cohort study from Sweden. *BMJ* 2013;346:f1939.
51. Weinblatt M, Schiff M, Goldman A et al. Selective costimulation modulation using abatacept in patients with active rheumatoid arthritis while receiving etanercept: a randomised clinical trial. *Ann Rheum Dis* 2007;66(2):228-34.
52. Tannenbaum H, Bombardier C, Davis P et al. An evidence-based approach to prescribing nonsteroidal antiinflammatory drugs. Third Canadian Consensus Conference. *J Rheumatol* 2006;33(1):140-57.

53. Goekoop-Ruiterman YP, de Vries-Bouwstra JK, Allaart CF et al. Clinical and radiographic outcomes of four different treatment strategies in patients with early rheumatoid arthritis (the BeSt study): a randomized, controlled trial. *Arthritis Rheum* 2005;52(11):3381-90.
54. Kirwan JR. The effect of glucocorticoids on joint destruction in rheumatoid arthritis. The Arthritis and Rheumatism Council Low-Dose Glucocorticoid Study Group. *N Engl J Med* 1995;333(3):142-6.
55. Grigor C, Capell H, Stirling A et al. Effect of a treatment strategy of tight control for rheumatoid arthritis (the TICORA study): a single-blind randomised controlled trial. *Lancet* 2004;364(9430):263-9.
56. Aviña-Zubieta JA, Abrahamowicz M, De Vera MA et al. Immediate and past cumulative effects of oral glucocorticoids on the risk of acute myocardial infarction in rheumatoid arthritis: a population-based study. *Rheumatology (Oxford)* 2013;52(1):68-75.
57. Duru N, van der Goes MC, Jacobs JW et al. EULAR evidence-based and consensus-based recommendations on the management of medium to high-dose glucocorticoid therapy in rheumatic diseases. *Ann Rheum Dis* 2013;72(12):1905-13.
58. Grossman JM, Gordon R, Ranganath VK et al. American College of Rheumatology 2010 recommendations for the prevention and treatment of glucocorticoid-induced osteoporosis. *Arthritis Care Res (Hoboken)* 2010;62(11):1515-26.
59. American Pain Society. *Guideline for the management of pain in osteoarthritis, rheumatoid arthritis and juvenile chronic arthritis*. 2nd ed. Glenview (IL): American Pain Society; 2002.
60. Whittle SL, Richards BL, Husni E et al. Opioid therapy for treating rheumatoid arthritis pain. *Cochrane Database Syst Rev* 2011;(11):CD003113.
61. Ostensen M, Forger F. Management of RA medications in pregnant patients. *Nat Rev Rheumatol* 2009;5(7):382-90.
62. Jorgensen C, Picot MC, Bologna C et al. Oral contraception, parity, breast feeding, and severity of rheumatoid arthritis. *Ann Rheum Dis* 1996;55(2):94-8.
63. Liao KP, Alfredsson L, Karlson EW. Environmental influences on risk for rheumatoid arthritis. *Curr Opin Rheumatol* 2009;21(3):279-83.
64. Briggs GG, Freeman RK, Yaffe SJ, eds. *Drugs in pregnancy and lactation: a reference guide to fetal and neonatal risk*. 9th ed. Philadelphia (PA): Lippincott Williams & Wilkins; 2011.
65. Weber-Schoendorfer C, Hoeltzenbein M, Wacker E et al. No evidence for an increased risk of adverse pregnancy outcome after paternal low-dose methotrexate: an observational cohort study. *Rheumatology (Oxford)* 2014;53(4):757-63.
66. Weber-Schoendorfer C, Chambers C, Wacker E et al. Pregnancy outcome after methotrexate treatment for rheumatic disease prior to or during early pregnancy: a prospective multicenter cohort study. *Arthritis Rheumatol* 2014;66(5):1101-10.
67. *Arava product monograph*. Laval (QC): sanofi-aventis; May 2006.
68. Brent RL. Teratogen update: reproductive risks of leflunomide (Arava); a pyrimidine synthesis inhibitor: counseling women taking leflunomide before or during pregnancy and men taking leflunomide who are contemplating fathering a child. *Teratology* 2001;63(2):106-12.
69. Carter JD, Ladhani A, Ricca LR et al. A safety assessment of tumor necrosis factor antagonists during pregnancy: a review of the Food and Drug Administration database. *J Rheumatol* 2009;36(3):635-41.
70. Koren G, Inoue M. Do tumor necrosis factor inhibitors cause malformations in humans? *J Rheumatol* 2009;36(3):465-6.
71. Ali YM, Kuriya B, Orozco C et al. Can tumor necrosis factor inhibitors be safely used in pregnancy? *J Rheumatol* 2010;37(1):9-17.
72. Cramp F, Hewlett S, Almeida C et al. Non-pharmacological interventions for fatigue in rheumatoid arthritis. *Cochrane Database Syst Rev* 2013;8:CD008322.
73. Saag KG, Teng GG, Patkar NM et al. American College of Rheumatology 2008 recommendations for the use of nonbiologic and biologic disease-modifying antirheumatic drugs in rheumatoid arthritis. *Arthritis Rheum* 2008;59(6):762-84.
74. Marmor MF, Kellner U, Lai TY et al. Revised recommendations on screening for chloroquine and hydroxychloroquine retinopathy. *Ophthalmology* 2011;118(2):415-22.
75. Wolfe F, Marmor MF. Rates and predictors of hydroxycholoroquine retinal toxicity in patients with rheumatoid arthritis and systemic lupus erythematosus. *Arthritis Care Res (Hoboken)* 2010;62(6):775-84.
76. American College of Rheumatology. Position Statement. *Screening for hydroxychloroquine retinopathy*. August 2011. Available from: www.rheumatology.org/practice/clinical/position/hydroxyp2.pdf. Accessed December 4, 2013.

Chapter 86
Sports Injuries

Taryn-Lise Taylor, BKin, MSc, MD, CCFP, Dip Sport & Exercise Med

The majority of sports injuries encountered by physicians involve the soft tissues, including strains, sprains and contusions.

Goals of Therapy

- To reduce acute symptoms (pain, inflammation) and recurrences
- To correct contributing factors, e.g., malalignment, muscle weakness
- To return the athlete's weight-bearing capability, flexibility, range of motion, strength and proprioception to normal
- To enable the athlete to participate comfortably, safely and fully in all pre-injury activities

Therapeutic Choices

For management of specific injuries, see Table 1.

Nonpharmacologic Choices

Acute treatment is best summarized by the RICE protocol:

- **R**est the injured part.
- **I**ce: Wrap an ice bag, cold pack or package of frozen peas in a damp, thin cloth and apply to the injured area for 15–20 minutes at a time, at least QID for the first 48 hours (or longer if swelling continues).
- **C**ompress with an elastic bandage if there is swelling such as in an ankle sprain.
- **E**levation: Try to elevate the injured part above the heart.

Initial rehabilitation is directed toward allowing the injured tissues to heal. Aggravation of the injury must be avoided, but alternative activities should be encouraged (e.g., the runner with a stress fracture of the fibula should not run, but can swim or run in deep water). The next phase is directed toward restoring and improving range of motion, strength, endurance and proprioception. A progression toward full activity is then undertaken. Before the patient resumes activity, any factors that may have contributed to the injury (improper shoes, poor protective equipment) should be corrected, and sport-specific skills regained.

Pharmacologic Choices

Oral or topical **NSAIDs** (including COX-2 inhibitors) can decrease swelling and discomfort but should be used for short periods only (for more detailed information on specific drugs, see Chapter 14). In the elderly, **acetaminophen** should be considered for initial and ongoing treatment of persistent pain, particularly musculoskeletal pain. Elderly patients are more likely to experience adverse drug reactions; the benefits of NSAID therapy must be weighed against their potential risks (dyspepsia, GI bleeding, renal impairment, blood pressure elevation).

Intra-articular or peritendinous injection of **corticosteroids** such as **triamcinolone acetonide**, **methylprednisolone acetate** or **betamethasone** may be useful in treating specific injuries (see Table 1). These injections are used with some success but may have risks, especially following multiple injections or improper injection to a site (e.g., into the tendon). A systematic review of peritendinous corticosteroid injections suggested that while there is good evidence of short-term benefit (pain reduction) in treating tendinopathies, the effectiveness of therapy varied with the injury site and long-term outcomes were not beneficial (higher risk of recurrence).[7,35] See Chapter 82, Table 4 for more information on intra-articular corticosteroids.

Topical **nitroglycerin** patches effectively reduce pain associated with activities of daily living in patients with tendinopathies [Evidence: SORT A*].[4] Consider using one-quarter of a nitroglycerin 0.2 mg/h *matrix* patch (e.g., Nitro-Dur, Trinipatch) daily on the affected joint area, rotating the application site with each application. The most common side effect is headache, but patients may also experience skin rash, dizziness and hypotension. Use with caution in the elderly or patients taking antihypertensives, due to the increased risk of orthostatic hypotension. Coadministration of nitrates (including topical) and PDE5 inhibitors (sildenafil, tadalafil, vardenafil) is contraindicated.

Platelet-rich plasma (PRP), or autologous blood injections, supplement the inflamed tendon with natural growth factors to stimulate the healing process.[36] PRP injections may become a cost-effective alternative to surgery in resistant and chronic tendinopathies. PRP injections have been studied for the treatment of specific tendon injuries with mixed results (see Table 1).[37] Further randomized controlled trials are needed to assess the efficacy and safety of PRP injections before they become routine practice.

Choices during Pregnancy and Breastfeeding

The Society of Obstetricians and Gynaecologists of Canada (SOGC) and the Canadian Society for Exercise Physiology (CSEP) recommend that in uncomplicated pregnancies, women with or without a previously sedentary lifestyle should be encouraged to participate in aerobic and strength-conditioning exercises as part of a healthy lifestyle.[38] The American College of Obstetricians and Gynecologists (ACOG) recommends a clinical evaluation of each pregnant woman before recommending an exercise program, as there are both absolute (e.g., incompetent cervix, multiparity, heart disease, bleeding) and relative (e.g., intrauterine growth retardation, poorly controlled hypertension or diabetes) contraindications to exercise in pregnancy.[39]

Glycemic control in gestational diabetes is improved by exercise.[40] Participation in sports with a high risk of contact, falling or abdominal trauma should be avoided. Supine positions should be avoided, particularly after the first trimester, due to the potential for compression of the inferior vena cava by the gravid uterus, and the effect on the maternal cardiac output.[39] An increase in musculoskeletal injury rates during pregnancy has not been shown, despite increased ligamentous laxity found in pregnancy that is believed to be related to estrogen and relaxin. This is likely due to decreased participation in jumping, pivoting and contact activities in the later stages of pregnancy when this ligamentous laxity is greater.[41]

Moderate exercise during breastfeeding does not affect the quantity or composition of breast milk.[38]

The same principles of injury treatment apply to both nonpregnant and pregnant or breastfeeding athletes, with the following exceptions:

- **Acetaminophen** may be used if analgesia is required (see Chapter 14). Avoid NSAIDs, especially in the third trimester of pregnancy.
- Shock wave therapy is generally considered contraindicated in pregnant patients.

* SORT (Strength of Recommendation Taxonomy) is a rating system (A, B or C) that addresses the quality of available evidence. For more information consult **How to Use *Compendium of Therapeutic Choices*** on page xxv.

- If nonpharmacologic therapy and acetaminophen have been used without success, **injectable corticosteroids** may be considered in a pregnant patient. Small amounts of corticosteroid plus **lidocaine** injections appear to be safe in breastfeeding mothers but nonpharmacologic options remain the treatment of choice.

A discussion of general principles on the use of medications in these special populations can be found in Appendix II and Appendix III. Other specialized reference sources are also provided in these appendices.

Therapeutic Tips

- Therapeutic choices that are effective for acute pain related to sports injuries are not always effective for chronic pain (e.g., NSAIDs, corticosteroid injections). Use caution when prescribing these agents for longer than 6 weeks.
- Consider using topical rather than oral NSAIDs for patients who are elderly or have cardiovascular or GI disease.[42]

Table 1: Management of Specific Sports Injuries

Injury	Investigations	Therapeutic Choices
Supraspinatus Tendinosis (Rotator Cuff Disorders) Tendinosis, degenerative tears, acute tears (partial or full thickness), less commonly overuse inflammation (tendinopathy) of the rotator cuff muscles of the shoulder. These muscles act as movers (rotation, initial abduction) and stabilizers of the humeral head in the glenoid. Often results in subacromial impingement of supraspinatus (cuff muscle) and subacromial bursa.	**History:** Sudden pain if traumatic onset (e.g., fall), gradual onset of pain if tendinosis. Discomfort noted with shoulder movement (can vary with location of injury), especially reaching overhead. Often painful at night, difficult to find comfortable sleep position. Weakness if complete or significant partial tear. **Physical Examination:** Wasting may be noted posteriorly over scapula if full thickness tear. Pain on active ROM and resisted tests depending on injury type and location. Weakness is present with more significant tear. If subacromial impingement, often get "painful arc" in flexion or abduction, pain with Hawkins' test (pain when shoulder placed at 90° of flexion and internally rotated) and Neer's test (pain with pronated arm brought into full overhead elevation). Test for instability. **Imaging:** X-ray if concern of bony injury (acute trauma) or osteoarthritis. Ultrasound good at detecting rotator cuff tears. MRI good at detecting rotator cuff tears and other shoulder pathology (usually need MRI arthrogram or high field strength [3T] MRI if concern of labral tear). **Refer if:** X-rays show growth plate injuries in skeletally immature patients or fracture in patients >50 y.	Rest from aggravating activities. Ice may help if acute injury. **NSAIDs** (oral or topical) for acute pain. May need short-term analgesic medication, e.g., **acetaminophen** either alone or in a combination product containing a weak opioid (**codeine** or **tramadol**) for nighttime pain. Physiotherapy or home-based exercise program[1]: strengthening of scapular stabilizers, correction of impaired scapulohumeral rhythm, addressing soft tissue tightness followed by rotator cuff strengthening. Persistent impingement symptoms or bursitis may benefit from subacromial **corticosteroid** injection (e.g., **triamcinolone acetonide** 40 mg mixed with 2–3 mL **lidocaine** 1%) followed by resumption of exercise program.[2] Shock wave therapy by a physiotherapist may be considered, especially in calcific tendinopathy.[3] **Nitroglycerin transdermal patch** (one-quarter of a 0.2 mg/h patch) Q24H for 6–24 weeks directly over the site of injury enhances subjective and objective recovery of patients with supraspinatus tendinosis.[5,6] Consider surgical intervention to repair cuff if full thickness tear in younger, active person. If persistent pain and/or impingement despite above measures, consider debridement, acromioplasty, repair.
Lateral Epicondylosis ("Tennis Elbow") Tendinosis of the common extensor tendon at its origin at the lateral epicondyle. **Medial Epicondylosis ("Golfer's Elbow")** Tendinosis of the common flexor/pronator tendon at its origin at the medial epicondyle.	**History:** Pain at the lateral elbow or medial elbow usually due to overuse and/or faulty mechanics. **Physical Examination:** Tenderness just distal to the lateral or medial epicondyle, painful resisted wrist extension and painful grip (lateral epicondylosis), wrist flexion (medial epicondylosis). **X-rays:** Rarely required (only if any concern about bony pathology, may confirm calcific tendinopathy). **Refer if:** Neurologic symptoms, loss of ROM in elbow (further evaluation needed to rule out pathologies, e.g., osteochondritis dissecans of the capitellum, radial tunnel syndrome, posterior interosseous nerve compression).	Rest from aggravating activities; ice/ice massage; counter-force brace/band; stretching/strengthening of the wrist extensors.[7] **NSAIDs** (oral or topical) for initial pain and inflammation in first 4 weeks of condition. Physiotherapy:[8] acupuncture, mobilizations, soft tissue techniques, stretching. Strengthening exercises as improvement occurs. Correction of predisposing factors: in tennis—correct poor technique and biomechanics, especially backhand stroke, correct racquet grip size, string tension to maximum 50–55 lb, lighter racquet, avoid heavy-duty or wet balls. Suggest consultation with teaching professional/tennis instructor. Work/occupation activities important (e.g., ergonomic factors). Gradual return to activity. If above is unsuccessful, consider **corticosteroid injection** (e.g., **triamcinolone acetonide** 20 mg) to common extensor origin area at lateral epicondyle or common flexor origin at medial epicondyle. Consider applying **nitroglycerin transdermal patch** (one-quarter of a 0.2 mg/h patch) Q24H on elbow for 6–24 weeks.[9,10]

Injury	Investigations	Therapeutic Choices
		Consider referral to primary care sport medicine physician or orthopedic surgeon for PRP autologous blood injection at the site of the tendinosis; may reduce pain and improve function.[11,12,13] Consider referral to radiologist for sonographically guided percutaneous tenotomy (dry needling) at the site of tendinosis.[14] If still unsuccessful, consider surgery.
Patellofemoral Pain Syndrome ("Runner's Knee", chondromalacia patellae) Anterior knee pain resulting from patellofemoral articulation dysfunction.	**History:** Anterior knee pain, worse with prolonged flexion/sitting, running, stairs. **Physical Examination:** Impairments affecting the patellofemoral joint interface may be a consequence of an unbalanced muscle pull (weak VMO), muscle tightness (hamstring or iliotibial band), malalignment between the joint surfaces or excessive knee valgus, i.e., increased Q-angle. Both pes planus with pronation and pes cavus with supination can be predisposing factors. Pain with patellar pressure, painful quads setting, poor flexibility, medial quadriceps (VMO) weakness, lateral patellar tracking, poor control with single knee bends, pain with squat and stairs. **X-rays:** (including skyline view of patella) If trauma or bony pathology is a concern or to assess for patellofemoral arthritis or other conditions. **Refer if:** Patient develops joint effusion.	Relief of acute symptoms: Rest from aggravating activities (emphasize alternative activities); ice, both PRN and post-activity; **NSAIDs** (oral or topical) for acute pain. Corticosteroid injections should be avoided in both Achilles & patellar tendinopathy due to risk of tendon rupture.[15] Correction of contributing factors: foot overpronation—appropriate stability/motion control shoes with good medial arch and support. If severe, may require custom foot orthotic. Physiotherapy:[16] VMO strengthening, e.g., closed kinetic chain exercises; hip abductor and external rotator strengthening. Electrical muscle stimulation and/or biofeedback can assist. Improve flexibility: quadriceps, hamstrings, gastrocnemius, iliotibial band stretches may help (no firm evidence). Taping techniques to correct patellar malposition.[17] Correction of training errors: in runners, more gradual distance increases, fewer hills. Decrease jumping, squats; avoid resisted leg extensions to ≥90° flexion. Patellar stabilizing brace with supporting buttress and/or straps for use with activities. Surgery (lateral release of tight retinacula, patellar tendon transfer) is rarely required and should be a last resort.
Lower Leg Pain ("Shin Splints") (Tibial periostitis, medial tibial stress syndrome) Inflammation of the tibialis posterior at its origin or of the tibial periosteum.	**History:** Diffuse shin pain along the medial tibia, usually in inexperienced and/or inadequately stretched or strengthened athletes. **Physical Examination:** Tenderness, usually diffuse, at medial border of tibia and adjacent muscle. If localized bony tenderness, rule out stress fracture. If normal exam at rest, rule out exertional compartment syndrome. **X-rays** normal; may need bone scan to differentiate from stress fracture. **Refer if:** Possible exertional compartment syndrome. Lateral lower leg symptoms are less likely to be shin splints.	Rest from aggravating activities (e.g., running/impact).[18] Alternative activities: cycling, rowing, swimming, skating/roller blading, pool running. Ice/ice massage. **NSAIDs** (oral or topical) for acute pain. Muscle stretching and strengthening, dynamic flexibility. Physiotherapy/massage therapy. Lower legs may be taped or neoprene sleeve used to stabilize and take some load off the periosteum. Correction of predisposing anatomic factors (e.g., with foot orthotics) and training errors. Gradual return to running or activity.

(cont'd)

Table 1: **Management of Specific Sports Injuries** *(cont'd)*

Injury	Investigations	Therapeutic Choices
Stress Fractures of the Tibia or Fibula Result from repetitive subthreshold loading that, over time, exceeds the bone's intrinsic ability to repair itself.	**History:** Well-localized shin pain with pounding activities, e.g., running, jumping, marching. Early on, pain is typically mild and occurs toward the end of the inciting activity. There is often a recent change in training surface (density or topography). Intensive sustained muscular activity may result in bone strain and overload. This type of mechanism of injury is common in rowers, who are prone to stress fractures of the ribs. Night pain is a frequent complaint. **Physical Examination:** Point tenderness upon palpation or percussion of affected area. Loading the affected bone using specific maneuvers (such as the "hop test" or the "fulcrum test") may reproduce pain. Specific localized tenderness on palpation of the tibia may differentiate a stress fracture from shin splints (where pain is more diffuse along the medial tibia). **X-rays:** Usually negative until at least 2 weeks after onset; may see periosteal thickening. Bone scan will show discrete increased uptake at stress fracture site. CT scan or MRI can help to differentiate acute vs healing stress fracture. **Refer if:** Anterior midshaft tibial stress fractures ("the dreaded black line") which appear as a horizontal fissure extending into the cortex of the tibia on x-ray. They are slow to heal, often go on to nonunion and should be assessed by an orthopedic surgeon for possible immobilization or internal fixation.	Activity modification/restriction and rest; no pounding activities until pain-free and nontender at site (usually 8–12 weeks). May need short-term analgesic medication, e.g., **acetaminophen** either alone or in a combination product containing a weak opioid (**codeine** or **tramadol**). Alternative low-impact activities: cycling, swimming, pool running. Long Air Cast-type brace often provides more comfort and possibly earlier return to pounding activities.[19] Address muscle weakness/strength imbalances. Adjust for structural malalignments (e.g., lift for leg-length discrepancies) or biomechanical inefficiencies (e.g., orthotics for excessive subtalar pronation or pes cavus). Correction of training errors; avoid excessive volume or intensity or wearing worn-out running shoes. Runners should replace shoes every 500–800 km to ensure adequate midsole cushioning. Monitor for poor bone health, whether due to hormonal, dietary or pathological causes (e.g., osteoporosis, hyperparathyroidism, skeletal involvement from malignancy). Gradual/progressive return to activity when pain-free on walking and nontender at site permits progressively greater loading of the affected structure. Consider referral to a primary care sport medicine physician or an orthopedic surgeon for electromagnetic bone stimulation, which may be helpful if delayed healing or non-union.[20]
Ankle Sprain Partial or complete tear to ankle-stabilizing ligaments, most commonly lateral (anterior and posterior talofibular, calcaneofibular ligaments). **Grade I:** No laxity, weight bears without pain, minimal swelling **Grade II:** Swelling, painful weight bearing, possible slight laxity **Grade III:** Unstable, significant laxity, complete disruption of at least 2 ligaments	**History:** Acute inversion of ankle (eversion less common). **Physical Examination:** Tenderness (most marked over injured ligament), swelling, pain with passive inversion and plantar flexion, positive anterior drawer test and talar tilt in Grade III sprains. Note: Don't forget to check for associated injury more proximally in the leg. **X-rays:** Clinical decision rules for the use of x-rays in acute ankle sprains are outlined in the Ottawa Ankle Rules.[22] **Refer if:** Any suspicion of rupture of an Achilles or peroneal tendon (which require orthopedic referral).	**Grade I & II Sprains** Initial RICE protocol.[21] **NSAIDs** (oral or topical) for acute pain and inflammation. Gradually increase weight bearing; may use tape/brace as support. Initiate weight bearing as soon as pain and stability allow to facilitate healing and proprioception.[21] Early ROM exercises. Stretching in dorsiflexion and plantar flexion. Strengthening: ankle dorsiflexors, plantar flexors, progress to invertors and evertors. Proprioception/balance retraining. Progressive return to activity. **Grade III Sprains** Initial RICE protocol, activity restriction. **NSAIDs** for acute pain and inflammation. Removable cast brace for 3–6 weeks (allows for icing, physiotherapy); then stirrup-type ankle brace.[23] Once stable, follow protocol for Grade I and II sprains. Refer for orthopedic consultation if not improved after 6–8 weeks of conservative therapy, recurrent pain or instability, concern of syndesmotic involvement.

Injury	Investigations	Therapeutic Choices
Achilles Tendinitis Inflammation (tendinitis) or degenerative micro-tears (tendinosis) of Achilles tendon mainly occurring at insertion or distal part of tendon. In tendinitis, paratenon may also be inflamed.	**History:** Pain, often swelling, of distal Achilles tendon. May be acute—usually caused by rapid increase in training/activity (e.g., running, jumping), poor flexibility, excessive pronation or poor-fitting footwear. Chronic tendinosis occurs usually in those over 30. Aggravated by running, jumping, walking. Sore first few steps in morning. Beware history of sudden acute pain (and occasionally feeling of "pop"), which may indicate tear of Achilles tendon. **Physical Examination:** Occasional swelling of distal Achilles (monitor for bursitis). When chronic, may have nodule/thickening of tendon with tenderness on palpation. Pain with passive ankle dorsiflexion and resisted plantar flexion (especially in weight bearing, painful toe raises). May have pes planus with pronation or pes cavus. Thompson test normal if Achilles is intact (squeeze of calf should produce ankle plantar flexion against gravity). If test is not normal (no plantar flexion), suspect complete tear of Achilles tendon. **Imaging:** If concern of possible tear/rupture, ultrasound helpful. **Refer if:** Concern regarding complete tear, immediate orthopedic referral is needed.	Rest from aggravating activities (try bike as alternate). Ice/ice massage. **NSAIDs** (oral or topical) for initial pain and inflammation in first 4 weeks of condition. Heel lift (approximately one-quarter inch). Night splint (prevents plantar flexion of ankle so Achilles tendon remains stretched while sleeping, allowing healing to take place with foot in a functional position). Control of biomechanical factors by correcting malalignment with appropriate shoes, using appropriate training techniques and losing weight. Physiotherapy—progressive stretching and strengthening, eccentric exercise protocol (more effective for midsubstance Achilles tendinopathy) is associated with a faster recovery time.[24,25] Extracorporeal shock wave therapy may be considered (conflicting evidence).[26,27] Orthotics/arch supports if overpronates. Consider applying **nitroglycerin transdermal patch** on Achilles tendon area (one-quarter of a 0.2 mg/h patch) Q24H for 6–24 weeks.[28] Consider referral to radiologist for sonographically guided percutaneous tenotomy of tendinosis.[14] Consider PRP autologous blood injection at the site of the tendinosis; may reduce pain and improve function[29] (refer to primary care sport medicine physician or orthopedic surgeon). Corticosteroid injections should be avoided in both Achilles & patellar tendinopathy due to risk of tendon rupture.[15] Surgery rarely required for chronic tendinosis, but it is important to recognize complete tear.
Plantar Fasciitis Microtears of the plantar fascia and inflammation of the periosteum at its calcaneal origin (heel bone).	**History:** Pain at plantar aspect of calcaneus, worse with first steps of the day upon arising in the morning, getting up after a prolonged sit and with running or prolonged walking. **Physical Examination:** Tender at plantar fascial origin at the heel; may have pes planus with pronation or pes cavus. **X-rays:** Not usually needed, may show "spur" as a result of more chronic plantar fasciitis. **Refer if:** Severe bruising or swelling of the heel pad which indicates a greater concern for plantar fascia rupture or calcaneal stress fracture, and requires referral to a specialist.	Activity modification, rest from aggravating activities (e.g., bike or swim instead of run). **NSAIDs** (oral or topical) for initial pain and inflammation in first 4 weeks of condition. Footwear important: cushioning running shoe should be worn for all weight bearing. Custom foot orthotics, arch supports, heel pads or gel cups may be necessary. Ice or ice massage (roll foot on frozen water bottle). Plantar massage: roll foot on soup can/tennis ball before weight bearing in morning. Physiotherapy, including possible extracorporeal shock wave therapy.[30] Stretches: gastrocnemius, soleus, plantar fascia,[31] foot intrinsics. Night splint to prevent ankle plantar flexion while sleeping: decreases fascial shortening and morning pain.[32] **Corticosteroid** injection if not improving with above (e.g., **triamcinolone acetonide** 20 mg mixed with 0.5 mL **lidocaine** 1% to tender area). Consider referral to radiologist for sonographically guided percutaneous tenotomy.

(cont'd)

Table 1: **Management of Specific Sports Injuries** *(cont'd)*

Injury	Investigations	Therapeutic Choices
		Nitroglycerin transdermal patch (one-quarter of a 0.2 mg/h patch) Q24H on point of maximum tenderness at the plantar fascia insertion into the calcaneus for 6–24 weeks.[33] Consider referral to primary care sport medicine physician or orthopedic surgeon for PRP autologous blood injection at the site of the tendinosis to reduce pain and improve function.[34] Surgery rarely required.

Abbreviations: NSAID = nonsteroidal anti-inflammatory drug; PRP = platelet-rich plasma; RICE = rest, ice, compression, elevation; ROM = range of motion; VMO = vastus medialus obliquus

Suggested Readings

Brukner P, Khan K. *Clinical sports medicine*. 3rd ed. New York (NY): McGraw-Hill; 2007.

Childress MA, Beutler A. Management of chronic tendon injuries. *Am Fam Physician* 2013;87(7):486-90.

Crossley K, Bennell K, Green S et al. A systematic review of physical interventions for patellofemoral pain syndrome. *Clin J Sport Med* 2001;11(2):103-10.

De Smedt T, de Jong A, Van Leemput W et al. Lateral epicondylitis in tennis: update on aetiology, biomechanics and treatment. *Br J Sports Med* 2007;41(11):816-9.

Ellenbecker TS, Cools A. Rehabilitation of shoulder impingement syndrome and rotator cuff injuries: an evidence-based review. *Br J Sports Med* 2010;44(5):319-27.

Magnussen RA, Dunn WR, Thomson AB. Nonoperative treatment of midportion Achilles tendinopathy: a systematic review. *Clin J Sport Med* 2009;19(1):54-64.

References

1. Krischak G, Gebhard F, Reichel H et al. A prospective randomized controlled trial comparing occupational therapy with home-based exercises in conservative treatment of rotator cuff tears. *J Shoulder Elbow Surg* 2013;22(9):1173-9.
2. Koester MC, Dunn WR, Kuhn JE et al. The efficacy of subacromial corticosteroid injection in the treatment of rotator cuff disease: a systematic review. *J Am Acad Orthop Surg* 2007;15(1):3-11.
3. Loew M, Daecke W, Kusnierczak D et al. Shock-wave therapy is effective for chronic calcifying tendinitis of the shoulder. *J Bone Joint Surg Br* 1999;81(5):863-7.
4. Gambito ED, Gonzalez-Suarez CB, Oquiñena TI et al. Evidence on the effectiveness of topical nitroglycerin in the treatment of tendinopathies: a systematic review and meta-analysis. *Arch Phys Med Rehabil* 2010;91(8):1291-305.
5. Paoloni JA, Appleyard RC, Nelson J et al. Topical glyceryl trinitrate application in the treatment of chronic supraspinatus tendinopathy: a randomized, double-blinded, placebo-controlled clinical trial. *Am J Sports Med* 2005;33(6):806-13.
6. Cumpston M, Johnston RV, Wengier L et al. Topical glyceryl trinitrate for rotator cuff disease. *Cochrane Database Syst Rev* 2009;(3):CD006355.
7. Coombes BK, Bisset L, Vicenzino B. Efficacy and safety of corticosteroid injections and other injections for management of tendinopathy: a systematic review of randomised controlled trials. *Lancet* 2010;376(9754):1751-67.
8. Bisset L, Beller E, Jull G et al. Mobilisation with movement and exercise, corticosteroid injection, or wait and see for tennis elbow: randomized trial. *BMJ* 2006;333(7575):939.
9. Paoloni JA, Appleyard RC, Nelson J et al. Topical nitric oxide application in the treatment of chronic extensor tendinosis at the elbow: a randomized, double-blinded, placebo-controlled clinical trial. *Am J Sports Med* 2003;31(6):915-20.
10. Paoloni JA, Murrell GA, Burch RM et al. Randomised, double-blind, placebo-controlled clinical trial of a new topical glyceryl trinitrate patch for chronic lateral epicondylosis. *Br J Sports Med* 2009;43(4):299-302.
11. Peerbooms JC, Sluimer J, Bruijn DJ et al. Positive effect of an autologous platelet concentrate in lateral epicondylitis in a double-blind randomized controlled trial: platelet-rich plasma versus corticosteroid injection with a 1-year follow-up. *Am J Sports Med* 2010;38(2):255-62.
12. Gosens T, Peerbooms JC, van Laar W et al. Ongoing positive effect of platelet-rich plasma versus corticosteroid injection in lateral epicondylitis: a double-blind randomized controlled trial with 2-year follow-up. *Am J Sports Med* 2011;39(6):1200-8.
13. Mishra AK, Skrepnik NV, Edwards SG et al. Efficacy of platelet-rich plasma for chronic tennis elbow: a double-blind, prospective, multicenter, randomized controlled trial of 230 patients. *Am J Sports Med* 2014;42(2):463-71.
14. Housner JA, Jacobson JA, Misko R. Sonographically guided percutaneous needle tenotomy for the treatment of chronic tendinosis. *J Ultrasound Med* 2009;28(9):1187-92.
15. Brinks A, Koes BW, Volkers AC et al. Adverse effects of extra-articular corticosteroid injections: a systematic review. *BMC Musculoskelet Disord* 2010;11:206.
16. Warden SJ, Hinman RS, Watson MA et al. Patellar taping and bracing for the treatment of chronic knee pain: a systematic review and meta-analysis. *Arthritis Rheum* 2008;59(1):73-83.
17. McConnell J. The management of chondromalacia patellae: a long term solution. *Aust J Physiother* 1986;32(4):215-23.
18. Reshef N, Guelich DR. Medial tibial stress syndrome. *Clin Sports Med* 2012;31(2):273-90.
19. Swenson EJ, DeHaven KE, Sebastianelli WJ et al. The effect of a pneumatic leg brace on return to play in athletes with tibial stress fractures. *Am J Sports Med* 1997;25(3):322-8.
20. Gebauer D, Mayr E, Orthner E et al. Low-intensity pulsed ultrasound: effects on nonunions. *Ultrasound Med Biol* 2005;31(10):1391-402.
21. Kerkhoffs GM, van den Bekerom M, Elders LA et al. Diagnosis, treatment and prevention of ankle sprains: an evidence-based clinical guideline. *Br J Sports Med* 2012;46(12):854-60.
22. Stiell IG, Greenberg GH, McKnight RD et al. Decision rules for the use of radiography in acute ankle injuries. Refinement and prospective validation. *JAMA* 1993;269(9):1127-32.
23. Kemler E, van de Port I, Backx F et al. A systematic review on the treatment of acute ankle sprain: brace versus other functional treatment types. *Sports Med* 2011;41(3):185-97.
24. Wallmann H. Achilles tendinitis: eccentric exercise prescription. *ACSM's Health & Fitness Journal* 2000;4(1):7-16.
25. Alfredson H, Pietila T, Jonsson P et al. Heavy-load eccentric calf muscle training for the treatment of chronic Achilles tendinosis. *Am J Sports Med* 1998;26(3):360-6.
26. Costa ML, Shepstone L, Donell ST et al. Shock wave therapy for chronic Achilles tendon pain: a randomized placebo-controlled trial. *Clin Orthop Relat Res* 2005;440:199-204.
27. Rompe JD, Nafe B, Furia JP et al. Eccentric loading, shock-wave treatment, or a wait-and-see policy for tendinopathy of the main body of tendo Achillis: a randomized controlled trial. *Am J Sports Med* 2007;35(3):374-83.

28. Paoloni JA, Appleyard RC, Nelson J et al. Topical glyceryl trinitrate treatment of chronic noninsertional achilles tendinopathy. A randomized, double-blind, placebo-controlled trial. *J Bone Joint Surg Am* 2004;86-A:916-22.
29. de Vos RJ, Weir A, van Schie HT et al. Platelet-rich plasma injection for chronic Achilles tendinopathy: a randomized controlled trial. *JAMA* 2010;303(2):144-9.
30. Gerdesmeyer L, Frey C, Vester J et al. Radial extracorporeal shock wave therapy is safe and effective in the treatment of chronic recalcitrant plantar fasciitis: results of a confirmatory randomized placebo-controlled multicenter study. *Am J Sports Med* 2008;36(11):2100-9.
31. DiGiovanni BF, Nawoczenski DA, Lintal ME et al. Tissue-specific plantar fascia-stretching exercise enhances outcomes in patients with chronic heel pain. A prospective, randomized study. *J Bone Joint Surg Am* 2003;85-A(7):1270-7.
32. Batt ME, Tanji JL, Skattum N. Plantar fasciitis: a prospective randomized clinical trial of the tension night splint. *Clin J Sport Med* 1996;6(3):158-62.
33. Murrell GA. Using nitric oxide to treat tendinopathy. *Br J Sports Med* 2007;41(4):227-31.
34. Barrett SL, Erredge SE. Growth factors for chronic plantar fasciitis? *Podiatry Today* 2004;17(11):36-42.
35. Hart L. Corticosteroid and other injections in the management of tendinopathies: a review. *Clin J Sport Med* 2011;21(6):540-1.
36. Sanchez M, Anitua E, Orive G et al. Platelet-rich therapies in the treatment of orthopaedic sport injuries. *Sports Med* 2009;39(5):345-54.
37. Nguyen RT, Borg-Stein J, McInnis K. Applications of platelet-rich plasma in musculoskeletal and sports medicine: an evidence-based approach. *PM R* 2011;3(3):226-50.
38. Davies GA, Wolfe LA, Mottola MF et al. Joint SOGC/CSEP clinical practice guideline: exercise in pregnancy and the postpartum period. *Can J Appl Physiol* 2003;28(3):330-41.
39. ACOG Committee on Obstetric Practice. ACOG Committee opinion. Number 267, January 2002: exercise during pregnancy and the postpartum period. *Obstet Gynecol* 2002;99(1):171-3.
40. Dempsey JC, Butler CL, Sorensen TK et al. A case-control study of maternal recreational physical activity and risk of diabetes mellitus. *Diabetes Res Clin Pract* 2004;66(2):203-15.
41. Olson D, Sikka RS, Hayman J et al. Exercise in pregnancy. *Curr Sports Med Rep* 2009;8(3):147-53.
42. Mason L, Moore RA, Edwards JE et al. Topical NSAIDs for acute pain: a meta-analysis. *BMC Fam Pract* 2004;5:10.

Musculoskeletal Disorders

Chapter 87
Systemic Lupus Erythematosus

C. Douglas Smith, MD, FRCPC

Systemic lupus erythematosus (SLE) is a prototype autoimmune disease affecting 1 in 1000–2000 individuals, predominantly young women in their reproductive years. For research purposes, the American College of Rheumatology (ACR) developed criteria for the diagnosis of SLE in 1982 (see Table 1).[1] In 2012, the classification criteria were revised and expanded to improve clinical relevance and incorporate new knowledge regarding the immunology of SLE.[2] However, the original classification criteria are sufficient for the needs of primary care practitioners.

Table 1: **Criteria for the Diagnosis of SLE**[1]

Criteria[a]	Comments
Malar "butterfly" rash	Rashes occur in 70%, often photosensitive
Photosensitivity	Rash on sun exposure
Discoid rash	Plaques
Mucosal ulcers	
Arthritis	Occurs in up to 80%
Serositis, pleuritis/pericarditis	Occurs in up to 50%
Kidney involvement	Proteinuria >0.5 g/day or cellular casts, occurs in up to 40%
Central nervous system	Seizures, psychosis (15%) in the absence of drugs or metabolic causes
Hematologic	Antibodies to white blood cells (leukopenia), platelets (thrombocytopenia) and/or red blood cells (hemolytic anemia)
Immunologic	Antibodies to double stranded DNA (dsDNA), phospholipids (anticardiolipin, lupus anticoagulant) and/or Smith nuclear antigen (anti-Sm)
Antinuclear antibodies (ANA)	Abnormal titers of ANA in the absence of drugs known to be associated with drug-induced lupus (see Drug-induced Lupus Erythematosus, below)

[a] For diagnosis, at least 4 criteria of 11 criteria are required.

SLE is best viewed as a spectrum of diseases. Some individuals have mild disease with predominant involvement of the skin and/or joints, while others have more severe systemic disease. Loss of immunologic tolerance to nuclear antigens and the development of antibodies directed against self are key features of the disease.[3] These *autoantibodies* (produced by B cells and other immune cells) play a major role in the protean (widely variable) manifestations of the disease. Examples of autoantibodies include:

- antinuclear antibodies (ANA) in 90% of patients—highly sensitive but nonspecific
- antibodies to blood cells (red blood cells, white blood cells, platelets)
- antibodies to double stranded (native) DNA (dsDNA) in 60% of patients—highly specific, linked to disease activity (particularly to kidney involvement)
- antibodies to SSA/Ro and SSB/La in 33% of patients—linked to photosensitive rashes, dry eyes and neonatal complications

- antiphospholipid antibodies (anticardiolipin and lupus anticoagulant) in 33% of patients—linked to thrombosis and pregnancy complications

Goals of Therapy

- Treat SLE symptoms and prevent damage
- Control inflammation and autoimmune activation
- In severe disease: induce remission, followed by maintenance
- Prevent complications

Investigations

- History, physical examination
- Laboratory tests:
  - complete blood count (anemia, cytopenias)
  - kidneys: creatinine, albumin, urinalysis; if indicated, quantification of albumin/protein in urine, kidney biopsy
  - to confirm diagnosis: autoantibodies + tissue biopsy as indicated
  - to assess disease activity: anti-dsDNA antibodies (high in active disease) and levels of C3 and C4 complement (low in active disease)
  - if unexpected clots or pregnancy complications: antiphospholipid antibodies (anticardiolipin, lupus anticoagulant)

Therapeutic Choices

For an approach to the treatment of SLE, see Figure 1.

Nonpharmacologic Choices

- Patient education is a key component in supporting the goals of therapy
- Avoid prolonged sun exposure. Sun protection (both physical, e.g., protective hat and clothing, and use of **sunscreens with SPF ≥30**) is important for all patients since sun-induced skin changes can trigger rashes and disease flares
- Lifestyle modifications including a heart-healthy diet and adequate exercise
- Smoking cessation is important as smoking adds to the already increased vascular risk associated with SLE, and decreases the effectiveness of antimalarial drugs[9]
- Maintain immunizations including annual influenza vaccination (avoid live vaccines, particularly in individuals receiving corticosteroids or immunosuppressant drugs)

Pharmacologic Choices

To reduce the risk of osteoporosis, encourage adequate **calcium** intake (elemental Ca^{++}1200 mg daily total from all sources) and a **vitamin D** supplement (at least 1000 IU daily).

For drugs used in the treatment of SLE, see Table 2.

Topical Therapies

Rashes (occurring in 70% of patients) may be treated locally with **topical corticosteroids** or **calcineurin inhibitors** (e.g., **tacrolimus**, **pimecrolimus**).[10,11] For more information on these agents, see Chapter 89. More refractory skin disease may require systemic therapy, most often with antimalarial drugs.

Figure 1: Treatment of Systemic Lupus Erythematosus[4,5,6,7,8,15]

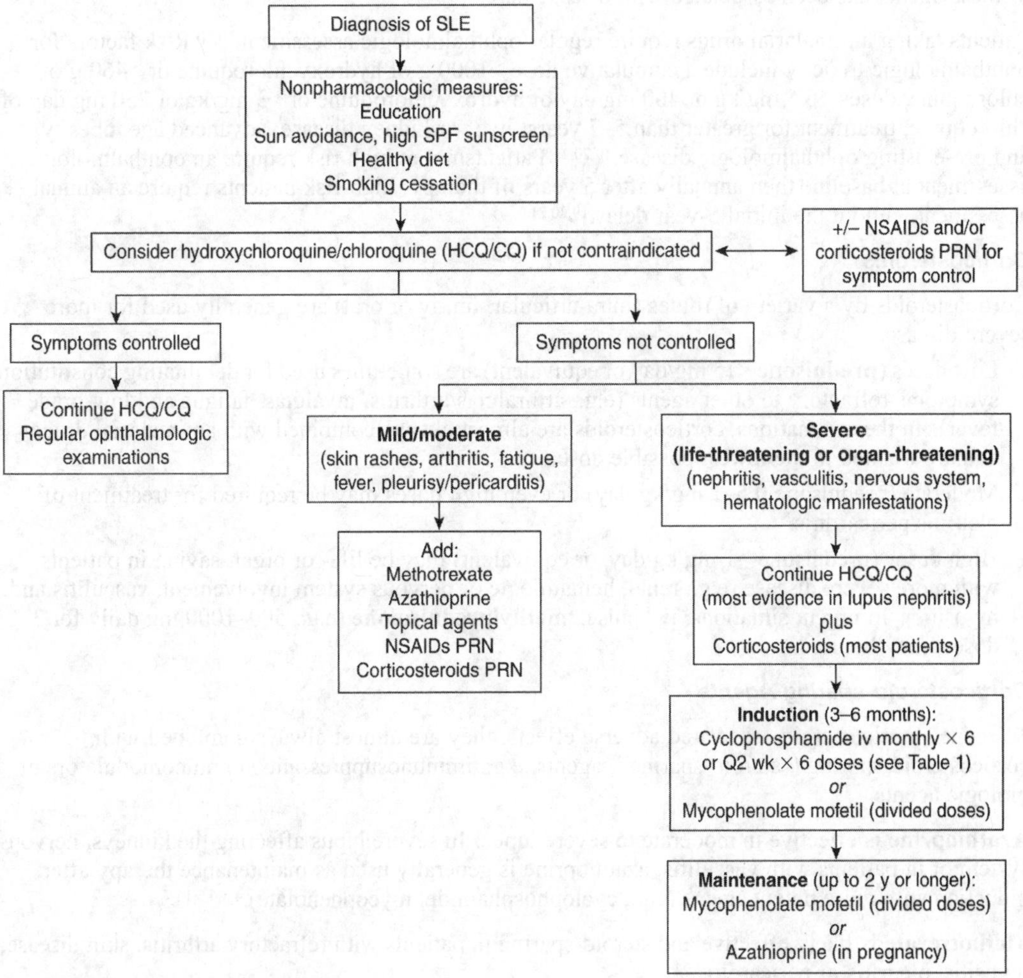

Abbreviations: CQ = chloroquine; HCQ = hydroxychloroquine; SLE = systemic lupus erythematosus; SPF = sun protection factor

Systemic Therapies

ASA and other **NSAIDs** are often used to treat joint pain (arthritis occurs in 80% of patients), as well as pleuritic chest pain in patients with pleuritis or pericarditis (about 50% of patients). High doses of NSAIDs (e.g., ibuprofen and sulindac) have been associated with the development of aseptic meningitis in some patients with SLE.[12] For more information about NSAIDs, see Chapter 82.

Low-dose ASA may be used to reduce the risk of MI and stroke, and may be used to reduce the risk of complications related to the presence of antiphospholipid antibodies.[13]

Antimalarials

Hydroxychloroquine or **chloroquine** is considered baseline therapy for the majority of patients with SLE.[14,15] They are particularly useful for the most common disease manifestations: photosensitive rashes, arthritis and fatigue. They are often used in combination with other agents, including corticosteroids and immunosuppressants. Early use of antimalarial drugs has been shown to reduce accrual of damage in patients with SLE.[16] Other relevant benefits ascribed to these agents include lipid- and glucose-lowering effects and reductions in blood clots.[15] In patients with stable disease, withdrawal of these agents has been associated with disease flares.[17,18]

Patients taking antimalarial drugs require regular ophthalmologic assessment.[19,20] Risk factors for ophthalmologic toxicity include a cumulative dose >1000 g of hydroxychloroquine or >460 g of chloroquine, doses >6.5 mg/kg or 400 mg/day of hydroxychloroquine or >3 mg/kg or 250 mg/day of chloroquine, treatment for greater than 5–7 years, liver or kidney disease, advanced age, obesity and pre-existing ophthalmologic disease.[19,20,21] Patients not at high risk require an ophthalmologic assessment at baseline then annually after 5 years of therapy; high-risk patients require an annual assessment without the initial 5-year delay.[19,20,21]

Corticosteroids

Corticosteroids by a variety of routes (intra-articular, im, iv or oral) are generally used for more severe disease.

- Low doses (**prednisone** <15 mg/day or equivalent) are sometimes used for debilitating constitutional symptoms refractory to other agents (e.g., arthralgias/arthritis, myalgias, fatigue and low-grade fever). In these situations, corticosteroids are almost always combined with antimalarial drugs and are weaned to the lowest possible dose.
- Moderate (prednisone 0.5–1 mg/kg/day) or even high doses may be required for treatment of pleuritis/pericarditis.
- High doses (prednisone ≥1 mg/kg/day, or equivalent) may be life- or organ-saving in patients with more severe disease (e.g., renal, hematologic or nervous system involvement, vasculitis and myositis). In urgent situations, iv "pulse" **methylprednisolone** (e.g., 500–1000 mg daily for 3 doses) may be used.

Corticosteroid-sparing Agents

To reduce corticosteroid-associated adverse effects, they are almost always combined with corticosteroid-sparing ("steroid-sparing") agents, e.g., immunosuppressants, immunomodulators or biologic agents.

Azathioprine is effective in moderate to severe lupus. In severe lupus affecting the kidneys, nervous system or in patients with vasculitis, azathioprine is generally used as maintenance therapy after induction with more potent agents (e.g., cyclophosphamide, mycophenolate).[4,5,6,7,15]

Methotrexate is likely effective and steroid-sparing in patients with refractory arthritis, skin disease, myositis, pleuritis or pericarditis.[22]

Cyclophosphamide is generally used as induction therapy and is combined with corticosteroids for treatment of severe lupus involving the kidneys or nervous system or in patients with vasculitis. It is usually given iv monthly for 6 doses, or a lower dose is given every 2 weeks for 3 months.[4,5,6,8] Guidelines recommend the low-dose regimen for white patients with Western or Southern European backgrounds.[15] In this patient population, the low-dose regimen showed fewer adverse effects and equivalent efficacy compared to the high-dose regimen.

Mycophenolate mofetil is equivalent to cyclophosphamide for induction therapy in proliferative lupus nephritis. It is preferred to cyclophosphamide in patients who wish to preserve their fertility, as high-dose cyclophosphamide is associated with permanent infertility. Evidence also suggests that mycophenolate is more effective than cyclophosphamide in patients with African or Hispanic backgrounds.[15] Additionally, mycophenolate demonstrated greater efficacy and equivalent safety to azathioprine for maintenance therapy in patients with nephritis.[23]

Leflunomide is occasionally used for refractory arthritis.[24]

Belimumab is the first agent of a new class of **biologic response modifiers**, the B-lymphocyte stimulator (BLyS)-specific inhibitors.[25,26,27,28,29] Belimumab is approved for use in combination with standard therapies to treat mild to moderate active autoantibody-positive SLE.[15] It has not been studied in severe disease. It should be reserved for patients who cannot tolerate or have failed traditional therapies. Other biologic response modifiers are being studied but are not currently approved for use in lupus. Selected examples include targeting B cells with **rituximab**[25,26,30,31] (useful in patients with severe refractory hematologic involvement) and targeting costimulation (CTLA-4) with **abatacept**.[32]

Thalidomide (initial dose 50–100 mg daily then reduced to the minimum effective dose) is highly effective for refractory skin disease[33] but its use is tightly restricted and long-term use remains problematic. A safer alternative for refractory skin disease may be **lenalidomide**.[34]

Drug-induced Lupus Erythematosus

Many drugs are capable of inducing a lupus-like illness.[35,36] Those definitively associated with lupus include chlorpromazine, hydralazine, isoniazid, methyldopa, minocycline, procainamide and quinidine. Antinuclear antibodies are universally seen. Antibodies to histones are present in 75% of cases but are also seen in 75–80% of patients with idiopathic lupus. Patients with idiopathic SLE form a number of other autoantibodies, including those against DNA, while those with drug-induced lupus generally do not. Antitumor necrosis factor-alpha therapy and interferon-alfa have been implicated in the development of drug-induced lupus. Subacute cutaneous lupus, including induction of autoantibodies to SSA/Ro and SSB/La, has been associated with a growing list of drugs including calcium channel blockers, hydrochlorothiazide, leflunomide, ranitidine and terbinafine.

Choices during Pregnancy and Breastfeeding

SLE and Pregnancy/Postpartum Period

The effect of pregnancy on SLE is variable. While some women may experience increased disease activity during pregnancy, the overall risk of flares is not greater than in nonpregnant patients. However, flares of renal disease activity (renal lupus nephritis) may occur, and during the postpartum period disease activity may increase due in part to hormonal fluctuations (increased prolactin, changes in estrogen and progesterone levels).

Pre-pregnancy Considerations

Pre-pregnancy assessment of disease activity, particularly renal function, is recommended at baseline and at least once per trimester during pregnancy. An active disease state prior to pregnancy is associated with high-activity lupus during pregnancy and negative outcomes (e.g., premature births, miscarriages).[37] Therefore, it is preferable that the patient be in remission for 6 months prior to conception.[38]

Patients on **methotrexate** and **mycophenolate** are counselled to avoid pregnancy. These medications should be stopped 3 months (methotrexate) or 6 weeks (mycophenolate) prior to attempting conception [Evidence: SORT C*].[15,39] However, recent small cohort studies showed no adverse pregnancy outcomes after preconceptional low-dose MTX exposure in males[40] or females[41].

Leflunomide is generally avoided in patients in whom future pregnancy is a possibility. If a pregnancy is desired, a "wash-out" regimen of **cholestyramine** 8 g TID or activated charcoal 50 g 4 times daily for 11 days (not necessarily on consecutive days) may be used to enhance leflunomide elimination following discontinuation.[42] For more information, see Chapter 85.

* SORT (Strength of Recommendation Taxonomy) is a rating system (A, B or C) that addresses the quality of available evidence. For more information consult **How to Use *Compendium of Therapeutic Choices*** on page xxv.

Cyclophosphamide may cause permanent infertility depending on the cumulative dose and the age of the patient.[39] A case-control study has shown that concomitant intake of synthetic gonadotropin releasing hormone (GnRH) may be effective in preserving fertility in women taking cyclophosphamide.[43]

Management during Pregnancy and Postpartum Period

Pregnant women with SLE are often co-managed with a high-risk pregnancy team. The presence of antiphospholipid antibodies (anticardiolipin, lupus anticoagulant) is associated with an increased risk of thrombosis and pregnancy complications (e.g., pregnancy losses, preeclampsia). Antibodies to SSA/Ro and SSB/La are associated with an increased risk of neonatal lupus, including congenital complete heart block.

ASA and **NSAIDs** are considered safe in the first 2 trimesters.[39] Their use in the third trimester may be of concern, because of antiprostaglandin effects, NSAIDs can increase risks of fetal and maternal bleeding and premature closure of the ductus arteriosus, and can also interfere with labour onset or duration. ASA can affect hemostasis in both the mother and fetus, leading to higher risk of hemorrhage. **Ibuprofen** is favoured because of its safe use historically; data concerning chronic use of other NSAIDs (celecoxib) during pregnancy are lacking.[44]

Hydroxychloroquine is considered safe in pregnancy.[14,45,46] Its use likely reduces flares and the need for more aggressive (and toxic) therapies.

Prednisone is generally considered safe but has been associated with a small increase in the risk of cleft palate.[47] Higher doses in pregnancy are associated with complications such as hypertension, preeclampsia and prematurity. Therefore, the dose of prednisone should be kept as low as possible.

Azathioprine is considered safe in pregnancy at doses ≤2 mg/kg.[15,48]

Methotrexate, mycophenolate and **cyclophosphamide** are teratogenic.[15,39] Although mycophenolate appears more effective in preventing flares of lupus nephritis, common practice would be to switch to azathioprine in those considering pregnancy and early data suggest this is safe.[49]

SLE and Breastfeeding

Although most **NSAIDs** have been shown to be present in breast milk, amounts are generally small and they are consequently considered to be safe for use by breastfeeding women. Ibuprofen might be preferred due to its short half-life.[44]

Hydroxychloroquine is considered safe in breastfeeding.[39,50]

Prednisone at doses ≥20 mg/day will appear in breast milk with potential to affect the infant.

Azathioprine is considered safe in and breastfeeding at doses ≤2 mg/kg.[51,52]

Methotrexate, mycophenolate and **cyclophosphamide** are not compatible with breastfeeding.[39]

General Considerations

Women on chronic corticosteroid therapy may be prescribed a bisphosphonate to prevent drug-induced osteoporosis. **Bisphosphonates** have demonstrated adverse effects (hypocalcemia, decreased fetal bone growth) in pregnancy.[53] While a small number of exposures reported in human pregnancies did not indicate skeletal or other abnormalities in the fetus,[54] the potential risks necessitate caution in prescribing bisphosphonates in women of childbearing age.

A discussion of general principles on the use of medications in these special populations can be found in Appendix II and Appendix III. Other specialized reference sources are also provided in these appendices.

Therapeutic Tips

- Evaluate the immunization status of the patient before initiating immunosuppressive therapy. Once immunosuppressed, live vaccines (e.g., measles, mumps and rubella, varicella) are generally not recommended.[55] Encourage keeping vaccinations up to date while on therapy, including influenza and pneumococcal (both inactivated vaccines).
- The increased risk of cardiovascular disease and stroke in SLE patients requires aggressive evaluation and management of other risk factors, particularly smoking, lipids and blood pressure.
- Patients with SLE are at increased risk for osteoporosis due to sun avoidance (thus, possible vitamin D insufficiency) and long-term corticosteroid use (see Chapter 83). Assess and treat patients as needed; **bisphosphonates** are recommended to prevent corticosteroid-induced osteoporosis in those taking oral corticosteroids (prednisone equivalent ≥7.5 mg/day) for >3 months.[56]
- Use **sulfamethoxazole/trimethoprim** with caution as it may induce disease flares and photosensitive rashes.
- **Estrogen** should be avoided in patients with a history of thrombosis and those who have antiphospholipid antibodies. Oral contraceptives have not been associated with increased risk of disease flare.[57] Hormone replacement therapy has been associated with increased risk of mild to moderate disease flares.[58]
- Patients with mild or inactive disease should be followed with clinical and laboratory assessment at 3–4 month intervals.

Table 2: **Drugs Used in SLE**

Class	Drug	Dose	Adverse Effects	Drug Interactions	Comments	Cost[a]
Antimalarials	*chloroquine* generics	250 mg daily po Maximum: 3.5 mg/kg/day based on ideal body weight	Nausea, cramps, diarrhea, rash, headache, skin deposition (hyperpigmentation). Rare retinal deposition and ocular toxicity (dose-related), myopathy.		Ophthalmologic assessment required Q1–5 years, depending on risk factors. See Systemic Therapies. To reduce the risk of retinal damage, do not exceed 3.5 mg/kg/day (based on ideal body weight).	$
	hydroxychloroquine sulfate Plaquenil, generics	200–400 mg daily po Maximum: 6.5 mg/kg/day based on ideal body weight	See chloroquine. Nightmares.	May increase digoxin levels, may increase effect of beta-blockers.	Ophthalmologic assessment required Q1–5 years, depending on risk factors. See Systemic Therapies. To reduce the risk of retinal damage, do not exceed 6.5 mg/kg/day (based on ideal body weight).	$
B-Cell Depletors	*rituximab* Rituxan	1 g iv × 2 doses, 2 weeks apart (with methylprednisolone 100 mg iv)	Mild to severe infusion reactions (very severe reactions resulting in death have been reported rarely). Rare: progressive multifocal leukoencephalopathy (PML).		Premedicate with acetaminophen and an antihistamine (e.g., diphenhydramine) before infusion. Monitor for hypersensitivity reactions.	$9500
B-Lymphocyte Stimulator-Specific Inhibitors	*belimumab* Benlysta	10 mg/kg infused over 1 h Q2 wk iv × 3 doses, then 10 mg/kg Q4 wk iv	Nausea, diarrhea, fever, anxiety, insomnia, depression, infusion reactions, hypersensitivity.		Premedicate with acetaminophen and an antihistamine (e.g., diphenhydramine) before infusion; monitor for hypersensitivity reactions. Safety and efficacy have not been evaluated in patients with severe active lupus nephritis or severe active central nervous system lupus.	~$1900 per dose[b]

Class	Drug	Dose	Adverse Effects	Drug Interactions	Comments	Cost[a]
Corticosteroids, oral	*prednisone* Winpred, generics	Low: Up to 15 mg/day po Moderate: 0.5 mg/kg/day po High: >1 mg/kg/day po	Acne, skin fragility, striae, GI upset, weight gain, glucose intolerance, mood swings, myopathy, glaucoma, cataracts, hypertension, osteoporosis, avascular necrosis, adrenal suppression, increased susceptibility to infections.	Increased risk of GI ulceration with NSAIDs.	Consider prophylaxis for drug-induced osteoporosis in patients taking ≥7.5 mg/day for >3 months (see Chapter 83).	$
Corticosteroids, injectable	*methylprednisolone sodium succinate* Solu-Medrol, generics	100 mg iv (with rituximab). "Pulse" dosing: 500–1000 mg daily iv × 3	See prednisone.			$
Immunomodulators	*azathioprine* Imuran, generics	2 mg/kg daily po	Nausea, vomiting, diarrhea, fever, malaise, hepatotoxicity, increased LFTs, leukopenia, thrombocytopenia, infection, myalgia.	Allopurinol may increase azathioprine toxicity; dosage adjustment may be necessary. Increased risk of infection with other immunosuppressants (leflunomide, mercaptopurine, tacrolimus).	Monitor CBC weekly × 1 month, twice monthly for months 2 and 3, monthly thereafter. LFTs and creatinine monthly.	$
	cyclophosphamide Procytox	First dose 500 mg/m² then 750–1000 mg/m² monthly iv × 6 doses; **or** 500 mg Q2 wk iv × 6 doses (in Caucasians)[6]	Nausea, vomiting, cytopenias, infertility, hemorrhagic cystitis, increased susceptibility to infections, malignancy potential.			$$
	leflunomide Arava, generics	10–20 mg daily po	Nausea, diarrhea, anorexia, weight loss, alopecia, rash, hypertension. May cause hepatotoxicity, cytopenias, pulmonary fibrosis, interstitial lung disease.	Decreased leflunomide levels with cholestyramine; increased risk of infection with live vaccines.	Avoid alcohol: possible increased risk of hepatotoxicity. Pregnancy is contraindicated while taking this medication. Wash-out procedure with cholestyramine 8 g TID × 11 days is recommended for serious toxicity or imminently planned pregnancy (see Chapter 85).	$$$$

(cont'd)

Table 2: **Drugs Used in SLE** *(cont'd)*

Class	Drug	Dose	Adverse Effects	Drug Interactions	Comments	Cost[a]
	methotrexate ❥ Methotrex-ateMethotrexate Injection USP, Methotrexate Tablets USP, Metoject, other generics	10–25 mg weekly po or sc	Nausea, malaise, headache, oral ulcers, alopecia, diarrhea, cytopenias, hepatotoxicity, pneumonitis.	Alcohol restriction may minimize hepatotoxicity. NSAIDs or ASA may increase MTX serum concentrations minimally but this is not clinically significant; these can be combined at low doses. Penicillins (e.g., amoxicillin, cloxacillin, piperacillin) and sulfonamides (e.g., sulfamethoxazole/trimethoprim) may decrease MTX clearance.	MTX is abortogenic/teratogenic.	$$
	mycophenolate mofetil Cellcept, Apo-Mycophenolate, other generics	Induction: 2–3 g daily po for 6 months; Maintenance: 1–2 g daily po	Anemia, leukopenia, thrombocytopenia, hyper/hypotension, edema, hyperglycemia, hypercholesteremia, hypokalemia, nausea, vomiting, diarrhea, abdominal pain, headache, dizziness, rash.	Antacids, iron, magnesium and cholestyramine decrease absorption. Decreased efficacy of oral contraceptives. Increased mycophenolate concentrations with probenecid.	Monitor CBC weekly × 1 month, twice monthly for months 2 and 3, monthly thereafter. LFTs and creatinine monthly. Mycophenolic acid is likely equivalent in efficacy in SLE to mycophenolate mofetil. Mycophenolic acid 1440–2160 mg = mycophenolate mofetil 2000–3000 mg.	$$$$

[a] Cost of 30-day supply, includes drug cost only.
[b] Based on 70 kg body weight.
❥ Dosage adjustment may be required in renal impairment; see Appendix I
Abbreviations: GI = gastrointestinal; LFT = liver function test; MTX = methotrexate; NSAID = nonsteroidal anti-inflammatory drug
Legend: $ <$20 $$ $20–40 $$$ $40–60 $$$$ $60–80

Suggested Readings

Bomback AS, Appel GB. Updates on the treatment of lupus nephritis. *J Am Soc Nephrol* 2010;21(12):2028-35.

Duru N, van der Goes MC, Jacobs JW et al. EULAR evidence-based and consensus-based recommendations on the management of medium to high-dose glucocorticoid therapy in rheumatic diseases. *Ann Rheum Dis* 2013;72(12):1905-13.

Hahn BH, McMahon MA, Wilkinson A et al. American College of Rheumatology guidelines for screening, treatment, and management of lupus nephritis. *Arthritis Care Res (Hoboken)* 2012;64(6):797-808.

Kuhn A, Ruland V, Bonsmann G. Cutaneous lupus erythematosus: update on therapeutic options part I. *J Am Acad Dermatol* 2011;65(6):e179-93.

Petri M, Orbai AM, Alarcon GS et al. Derivation and validation of the Systemic Lupus International Collaborating Clinics classification criteria for systemic lupus erythematosus. *Arthritis Rheum* 2012;64(8):2577-86.

References

1. Tan EM, Cohen AS, Fries JF et al. The 1982 revised criteria for the classification of systemic lupus erythematosus. *Arthritis Rheum* 1982;25(11):1271-7.
2. Petri M, Orbai AM, Alarcon GS et al. Derivation and validation of the Systemic Lupus International Collaborating Clinics classification criteria for systemic lupus erythematosus. *Arthritis Rheum* 2012;64(8):2577-86.
3. Rahman A, Isenberg DA. Systemic lupus erythematosus. *N Engl J Med* 2008;358(9):929-39.
4. Chan TM, Li FK, Tang CS et al. Efficacy of mycophenolate mofetil in patients with diffuse proliferative lupus nephritis. Hong Kong-Guangzhou Nephrology Study Group. *N Engl J Med* 2000;343(16):1156-62.
5. Contreras G, Pardo V, Leclercq B et al. Sequential therapies for proliferative lupus nephritis. *N Engl J Med* 2004;350(10):971-80.
6. Houssiau FA, Vasconcelos C, D'Cruz D et al. The 10-year follow-up data of the Euro-Lupus Nephritis Trial comparing low-dose and high-dose intravenous cyclophosphamide. *Ann Rheum Dis* 2010;69(1):61-4.
7. Ginzler EM, Appel GB, Dooley MA et al. Aspreva Lupus Management Study (ALMS): maintenance results [abstract]. *Arthritis Rheum* 2010;62(Suppl 10):2085.
8. Appel GB, Contreras G, Dooley MA et al. Mycophenolate mofetil versus cyclophosphamide for induction treatment of lupus nephritis. *J Am Soc Nephrol* 2009;20(5):1103-12.
9. Turchin I, Bernatsky S, Clarke AE et al. Cigarette smoking and cutaneous damage in systemic lupus erythematosus. *J Rheumatol* 2009;36(12):2691-3.
10. Kuhn A, Ruland V, Bonsmann G. Cutaneous lupus erythematosus: update on therapeutic options part I. *J Am Acad Dermatol* 2011;65(6):e179-93.
11. Kuhn A, Ruland V, Bonsmann G. Cutaneous lupus erythematosus: update on therapeutic options part II. *J Am Acad Dermatol* 2011;65(6):e195-213.
12. Rodríguez SC, Olguín AM, Miralles CP et al. Characteristics of meningitis caused by Ibuprofen: report of 2 cases with recurrent episodes and review of the literature. *Medicine (Baltimore)* 2006;85(4):214-20.
13. Wahl DG, Bounameaux H, de Moerloose P et al. Prophylactic antithrombotic therapy for patients with systemic lupus erythematosus with our without antiphospholipid antibodies: do the benefits outweigh the risks? A decision analysis. *Arch Intern Med* 2000;160(13):2042-8.
14. Ruiz-Irastorza G, Ramos-Casals M, Brito-Zeron P et al. Clinical efficacy and side effects of antimalarials in systemic lupus erythematosus: a systematic review. *Ann Rheum Dis* 2010;69(1):20-8.
15. Hahn BH, McMahon MA, Wilkinson A et al. American College of Rheumatology guidelines for screening, treatment, and management of lupus nephritis. *Arthritis Care Res (Hoboken)* 2012;64(6):797-808.
16. Akhavan PS, Su J, Lou W et al. The early protective effect of hydroxychloroquine on the risk of cumulative damage in patients with systemic lupus erythematosus. *J Rheumatol* 2013;40(6):831-41.
17. A randomized study of the effect of withdrawing hydroxychloroquine sulfate in systemic lupus erythematosus. Canadian Hydroxychloroquine Study Group. *N Engl J Med* 1991;324(3):150-4.
18. Tsakonas E, Joseph L, Esdaile JM et al. A long-term study of hydroxychloroquine withdrawal on exacerbations in systemic lupus erythematosus. The Canadian Hydroxychloroquine Study Group. *Lupus* 1998;7(2):80-5.
19. Marmor MF, Kellner U, Lai TY et al. Revised recommendations on screening for chloroquine and hydroxychloroquine retinopathy. *Ophthalmology* 2011;188(2):415-22.
20. American College of Rheumatology. Position Statement. *Screening for hydroxychloroquine retinopathy*. August 2011. Available from: www.rheumatology.org/practice/clinical/position/hydroxyp2.pdf. Accessed October 12, 2012.
21. Wolfe F, Marmor MF. Rate and predictors of hydroxychloroquine retinal toxicity in patients with rheumatoid arthritis and systemic lupus erythematosus. *Arthritis Care Res (Hoboken)* 2010;62(6):775-84.
22. Fortin PR, Abrahamowicz M, Ferland D et al. Steroid-sparing effects of methotrexate in systemic lupus erythematosus: a double-blind, randomized, placebo-controlled trial. *Arthritis Rheum* 2008;59(12):1796-804.
23. Dooley MA, Jayne D, Ginzler EM et al. Mycophenolate versus azathioprine as maintenance therapy for lupus nephritis. *N Engl J Med* 2011;365(20):1886-95.
24. Tam LS, Li EK, Wong CK et al. Double-blind, randomized, placebo-controlled pilot study of leflunomide in systemic lupus erythematosus. *Lupus* 2004;13(8):601-4.
25. Calero I, Sanz I. Targeting B cells for the treatment of SLE: the beginning of the end or the end of the beginning? *Discov Med* 2010;10(54):416-24.
26. Wallace DJ. Advances in drug therapy for systemic lupus erythematosus. *BMC Med* 2010;8:77.

27. Wallace DJ, Stohl W, Furie RA et al. A phase II, randomized, double-blind, placebo-controlled, dose-ranging study of belimumab in patients with active systemic lupus erythematosus. *Arthritis Rheum* 2009;61(9):1168-78.
28. Navarra SV, Guzman RM, Gallacher AE et al. Efficacy and safety of belimumab in patients with active systemic lupus erythematosus: a randomised, placebo-controlled, phase 3 trial. *Lancet* 2011;377(9767):721-31.
29. Furie R, Petri M, Zamani O et al. A phase III, randomized placebo-controlled study of belimumab, a monoclonal antibody that inhibits B lymphocyte stimulator, in patients with systemic lupus erythematosus. *Arthritis Rheum* 2011;63(12):3918-30.
30. Merrill JT, Neuwelt CM, Wallace DJ et al. Efficacy and safety of rituximab in moderately-to-severely active systemic lupus erythematosus: the randomized, double-blind, phase II/III systemic lupus erythematosus evaluation of rituximab trial. *Arthritis Rheum* 2010;62(1):222-33.
31. Terrier B, Amoura Z, Ravaud P et al. Safety and efficacy of rituximab in systemic lupus erythematosus: results from 136 patients from the French AutoImmunity and Rituximab registry. *Arthritis Rheum* 2010;62(8):2458-66.
32. Merrill JT, Burgos-Vargas R, Westhovens R et al. The efficacy and safety of abatacept in patients with non-life-threatening manifestations of systemic lupus erythematosus: results of a twelve-month, multicenter, exploratory, phase IIb, randomized, double-blind, placebo-controlled trial. *Arthritis Rheum* 2010;62(10):3077-87.
33. Duong DJ, Spigel GT, Moxley RT et al. American experience with low-dose thalidomide therapy for severe cutaneous lupus erythematosus. *Arch Dermatol* 1999;135(9):1079-87.
34. Cortes-Hernandez J, Avila G, Vilardell-Tarres M et al. Efficacy and safety of lenalidomide for refractory cutaneous lupus erythematosus. *Arthritis Res Ther* 2012;14(6):R265.
35. Katz U, Zandman-Goddard G. Drug-induced lupus: an update. *Autoimmun Rev* 2010;10(1):46-50.
36. Lowe G, Henderson CL, Grau RH et al. A systematic review of drug-induced subacute cutaneous lupus erythematosus. *Br J Dermatol* 2011;164(3):465-72.
37. Clowse ME, Magder LS, Witter F et al. The impact of increased lupus activity on obstetric outcomes. *Arthritis Rheum.* 2005 Feb;52(2):514-21
38. Mitchell K, Kaul M, Clowse ME. The management of rheumatic diseases in pregnancy. *Scand J Rheumatol* 2010;39(2):99-108.
39. Østensen M, Khamashta M, Lockshin M et al. Anti-inflammatory and immunosuppressive drugs and reproduction. *Arthritis Res Ther* 2006;8(3):209.
40. Weber-Schoendorfer C, Hoeltzenbein M, Wacker E et al. No evidence for an increased risk of adverse pregnancy outcome after paternal low-dose methotrexate: an observational cohort study. *Rheumatology (Oxford)* 2014;53(4):757-63.
41. Weber-Schoendorfer C, Chambers C, Wacker E et al. Pregnancy outcome after methotrexate treatment for rheumatic disease prior to or during early pregnancy: a prospective multicenter cohort study. *Arthritis Rheumatol* 2014;66(5):1101-10.
42. e-CPS. Ottawa (ON): Canadian Pharmacists Association; 2012. *Arava* [product monograph]. Available from: www.e-therapeutics.ca. Subscription required.
43. Somers EC, Marder W, Christman GM et al. Use of a gonadotropin-releasing hormone analog for protection against premature ovarian failure during cyclophosphamide therapy in women with severe lupus. *Arthritis Rheum* 2005;52(9):2761-7.
44. Reuvers M, Schaefer C. Analgesics and anti-inflammatory drugs. In: Schaefer C, Peters P, Miller, RK, eds. *Drugs during pregnancy and lactation: treatment options and risk assessment*. 2nd ed. London (GB): Elsevier; 2007. p. 29-49.
45. Clowse ME, Magder L, Witter F et al. Hydroxychloroquine in lupus pregnancy. *Arthritis Rheum* 2006;54(11):3640-7.
46. Buchanan NM, Toubi E, Khamashta MA et al. Hydroxychloroquine and lupus pregnancy: review of a series of 36 cases. *Ann Rheum Dis* 1996;55(7):486-8.
47. Park-Wyllie L, Mazzotta P, Pastuszak A et al. Birth defects after maternal exposure to corticosteroids: prospective cohort study and meta-analysis of epidemiological studies. *Teratology* 2000;62(6):385-92.
48. Polifka JE, Friendman JM. Teratogen update: azathioprine and 6-mercaptopurine. *Teratology* 2002;65(5):240-61.
49. Fischer-Betz R, Specker C, Brinks R et al. Low risk of renal flares and negative outcomes in women with lupus nephritis conceiving after switching from mycophenolate mofetil to azathioprine. *Rheumatology (Oxford)* 2013;52(6):1070-6.
50. American Academy of Pediatrics Committee on Drugs. Transfer of drugs and other chemicals into human milk. *Pediatrics* 2001;108(3):776-89.
51. Sau A, Clarke S, Bass J et al. Azathioprine and breastfeeding: is it safe? *BJOG* 2007;114(4):498-501.
52. Christensen LA, Dahlerup JF, Nielsen MJ et al. Azathioprine treatment during lactation. *Aliment Pharmacol Ther* 2008;28(10):1209-13.
53. Briggs GG, Freeman RK, Yaffe SJ, eds. *Drugs in pregnancy and lactation: a reference guide to fetal and neonatal risk.* 9th ed. Philadephia (PA): Lippincott Williams & Wilkins; 2011.
54. Djokanovic N, Klieger-Grossmann C, Koren G. Does treatment with bisphosphonates endanger the human pregnancy? *J Obstet Gynaecol Can* 2008;30(12):1146-8.
55. Public Health Agency of Canada. *Canadian immunization guide. Part 3: Vaccination of specific populations*. Available from: www.phac-aspc.gc.ca/publicat/cig-gci/p03-07-eng.php. Accessed January 17, 2014.
56. Papaioannou A, Morin S, Cheung AM et al. 2010 clinical practice guidelines for the diagnosis and management of osteoporosis in Canada: summary. *CMAJ* 2010;182(17):1864-73.
57. Culwell KR, Curtis KM, del Carmen Cravioto M. Safety of contraceptive method use among women with systemic lupus erythematosus: a systematic review. *Obstet Gynecol* 2009;114(2 Pt 1):341-53.
58. Buyon JP, Petri MA, Kim MY et al. The effect of combined estrogen and progesterone hormone replacement therapy on disease activity in systemic lupus erythematosus: a randomized trial. *Ann Intern Med* 2005;142(12 Pt 1):953-62.

Chapter 88
Acne

Duane Lichtenwald, MD, FRCPC

Acne vulgaris is the most common skin disorder, typically starting at puberty, increasing in severity until the late teens then slowly abating. There is a high degree of variability in the age of onset, distribution, severity and age of resolution. It often results in disfigurement, scarring and/or emotional distress. Even mild acne can cause major and sometimes permanent psychological disturbance.[1] Fortunately, acne can be safely and effectively treated.

The pathogenesis of acne is centred on the sebaceous gland. Hormonal changes alter sebum quality and production, which results in mild inflammation. This triggers comedones: sebaceous glands that have developed a keratin plug. If the plug is high in the duct, the keratin becomes oxidized, resulting in the appearance of a blackhead or open comedone. When the blockage is deeper, a flesh-coloured papule or closed comedone develops. As these lesions become overgrown with bacteria, cytokines are released, causing transformation into an inflammatory papule which may eventually develop a central pustule. If this inflammatory lesion ruptures below the dermis, an inflammatory cyst ensues. These are the lesions most likely to trigger scarring. Acne vulgaris is usually classified by the number, type and distribution of acne lesions.

Goals of Therapy

- Clear existing lesions
- Prevent new lesions
- Minimize scarring
- Minimize psychological impact

Investigations

- Usually not required
  - the diagnosis is a clinical one
- Culture and sensitivity of pustules
  - *Propionibacterium acnes*, a gram-positive anaerobe, is the prevalent organism
  - when patients are resistant to antibiotic therapy, perform cultures to identify gram-negative folliculitis and guide further therapy
- Hormonal investigations are indicated if there are other signs of hyperandrogenism such as:
  - hirsutism
  - infertility
  - irregular or infrequent menses
  - insulin resistance
  - middle-age onset in women

Therapeutic Choices

Nonpharmacologic Choices

The management of acne is primarily pharmacologic. Evidence is emerging that a low glycemic diet may be helpful in some cases but results of diet manipulation are mild, inconsistent and do not replace pharmacologic management.[2] Acne is not the result lack of or improper cleansing.[3] Modifying skin care regimens has minimal preventive effect. Picking, squeezing or excoriation of inflammatory lesions delays healing and promotes scarring, and therefore should be avoided. Sunlight and other sources of ultraviolet light can help but are rarely recommended in view of the risks of photodamage and carcinogenic effects. Various lasers, intense pulsed light, microdermabrasion, chemical peels and photodynamic therapy are all helpful in certain situations but are expensive, rarely insured, often painful and must be administered on an ongoing basis. They are rarely required for effective acne management. Laser treatments have a greater role in acne scar therapy.

Pharmacologic Choices

Information about pharmacologic choices for acne can be found in Figure 1.

Numerous pharmacologic agents can have some positive effect on acne. It can take 2–3 months to see significant improvement with the use of topical and/or systemic agents. In a patient who has achieved good control with a combination of topical and systemic therapy, consider withdrawal of the systemic agent and maintenance with topical therapy alone. If the topical therapy does not maintain control, the systemic agent can be resumed as maintenance.

Topical Agents

Information about topical agents for acne can be found in Table 1.

Benzoyl peroxide is antibacterial and mildly comedolytic. Its oxidation of bacterial proteins is not subject to bacterial resistance.[4] Benzoyl peroxide has the ability to prevent or eliminate *P. acnes* on the surface of the skin and in the sebaceous follicles.[5] It is a mild skin irritant and rare allergen. Formulations can bleach clothing. It is reasonable to initiate therapy with 2.5% products since limited evidence shows efficacy similar to 5% and 10% formulations but with less irritation [Evidence: SORT B*].[6,7,8]

Topical retinoids are the most powerful comedolytic agents, yet still take months to be effective. They are also effective for inflammatory lesions. **Tretinoin** is the most cost effective but also the most photosensitizing. **Adapalene** is the least irritating, **tazarotene** the most potent.[9] Topical retinoids (except when combined in a commercial product) are unstable in the presence of benzoyl peroxide and should be applied at a different time: usually benzoyl peroxide in the morning and retinoid at bedtime.

Of the **topical antibiotics**, **clindamycin** and **erythromycin** are the most commonly used.[10] Use in combination with benzoyl peroxide reduces the risk of bacterial resistance. They are mainly used in papulopustular acne to decrease skin colonization with *P. acnes*.

Glycolic acid (an alpha-hydroxy acid) is mildly comedolytic and can be used when topical retinoids are not tolerated. At higher concentrations, it is used for chemical peels which are a rapid but highly irritating method of clearing comedones.

Azelaic acid is comedolytic and antibacterial but does not promote resistant organisms. It is mildly irritating and can cause hypopigmentation.

* SORT (Strength of Recommendation Taxonomy) is a rating system (A, B or C) that addresses the quality of available evidence. For more information consult **How to Use *Compendium of Therapeutic Choices*** on page xxv.

Figure 1: **Management of Acne**

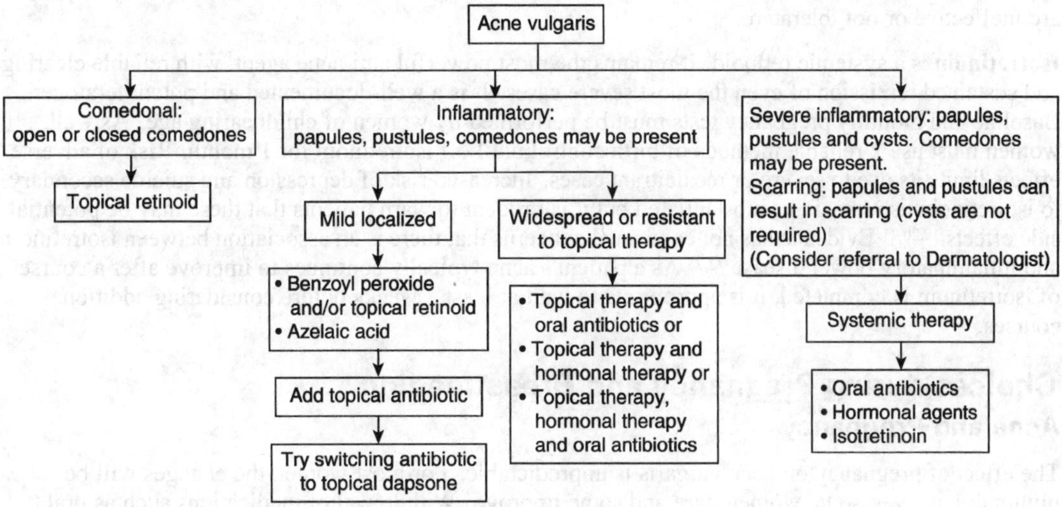

Salicylic acid is mildly comedolytic. Concentrations of 1–2% are tolerated but not as effective as topical retinoids. Higher concentrations are usually too irritating.

Dapsone, a synthetic sulfone, is an anti-inflammatory agent effective for acne when given orally, but is not used systemically due to the risk of serious side effects. A topical gel formulation of dapsone is effective for inflammatory acne,[11,12] thus far without the risks of systemic dapsone.[13]

Selection of topical agent(s) should be guided by identifying the type of acne lesions. If there are only comedones, a topical retinoid is appropriate. If there are only inflammatory lesions, benzoyl peroxide alone or benzoyl peroxide combined with a topical antibiotic is appropriate. The combination of a retinoid, benzoyl peroxide and a topical antibiotic can be used if there are both comedones and inflammatory lesions. Commercially prepared combination products can be useful when multiple topical agents are required (Table 1).

Systemic Agents

Information about systemic therapy for acne can be found in Table 2.

Consider systemic therapy when topical therapy has not been effective after 2–3 months, or has little chance of success (cystic acne).[10]

Tetracyclines, erythromycin and **trimethoprim** (alone or in combination with **sulfamethoxazole**) are effective systemic antibiotics.[14] Evidence regarding duration of use is lacking; recommendations are based on expert opinion. Allow at least 6 weeks to see if an antibiotic is effective. Bacterial resistance can be reduced by using oral antibiotics in combination with benzoyl peroxide.[10] When possible, limit duration of oral antibiotic therapy to 3 months while maintaining topical therapy. If acne relapses despite appropriate topical therapy, oral antibiotics may be required on a long-term suppressive basis or consideration given to alternative systemic therapy. The major concern regarding long-term oral antibiotic therapy remains bacterial resistance.[14]

Hormonal therapy for acne is an option for females. **Oral contraceptives** are effective for the treatment of acne[15] and several are indicated for this purpose in Canada (Table 2). Oral contraceptives with minimal androgenic effects (see Chapter 70) are especially useful in women with other signs of androgen excess. **Cyproterone acetate, drospirenone** and **spironolactone** are antiandrogens with good efficacy in acne management. There is a small risk of venous thromboembolic events with the use of any combined oral contraceptive.[16,17] This risk is slightly higher with those that contain cyproterone or drospirenone.[17,18] Therefore consider these agents when alternative oral contraceptives are ineffective or not tolerated.

Isotretinoin is a systemic retinoid. It remains the most powerful anti-acne agent, with reliable clearing and sustained remission of even the most severe cases. It is a well-documented and potent teratogen. Baseline and monthly pregnancy tests must be performed by women of childbearing age. As well, women must use 2 reliable methods of birth control until off isotretinoin for 1 month. Risk of adverse effects limits its use to severe or recalcitrant cases. Increased risk of depression and suicide secondary to isotretinoin use remain unsubstantiated but it is prudent to warn patients that these may be potential side effects.[19,20,21] Evidence has not confirmed concerns that there is an association between isotretinoin and inflammatory bowel disease.[22,23] As a patient's acne typically continues to improve after a course of isotretinoin is completed, it is appropriate to wait at least 8 weeks before considering additional courses.[24]

Choices during Pregnancy and Breastfeeding

Acne and Pregnancy

The effect of pregnancy on acne vulgaris is unpredictable. For most women the changes will be minimal; however, some women flare and some improve. Withdrawal of medications such as oral contraceptives and antibiotics can explain some flares.

Pre-pregnancy Considerations

Oral **isotretinoin** must be stopped at least 1 month prior to becoming pregnant.[25] After stopping oral contraceptives, women should avoid attempting to conceive until there has been at least 1 spontaneous menstrual cycle. A specific waiting period after stopping **spironolactone** has not been determined; however, the drug and its active metabolites should be cleared from the body within 1 week of discontinuation.[26]

Management during Pregnancy

Experience with topical use of **benzoyl peroxide** and **erythromycin** during pregnancy is extensive and both are generally considered safe.[27] Topical **clindamycin** is considered safe. **Glycolic acid** and **azelaic acid** have low systemic absorption and are unlikely to pose a risk to the fetus.[28,29] Although systemic absorption of topical **dapsone** appears to be very low, safety in pregnancy has not been established.[30] **Retinoids** are teratogens. Safety of topical retinoids (**adapalene**, **tretinoin** and **tazarotene**) has not been documented and their use remains contraindicated.[25] Oral **isotretinoin** is a well-documented teratogen and must be avoided in pregnancy. Proper use includes ensuring the woman is not pregnant prior to initiation, the use of 2 forms of birth control to prevent pregnancy and regular pregnancy tests.[32] **Erythromycin** (with the exception of the estolate salt) is safe to use and is the most commonly prescribed oral antibiotic for acne during pregnancy. **Tetracycline**, **doxycycline** and **minocycline** are contraindicated as second- and third-trimester exposure can cause dental staining and enamel hypoplasia in the baby and liver toxicity in the mother.[28,33,34] However, inadvertent exposure during the first few weeks of pregnancy is unlikely to cause harm.[33] Avoid **sulfamethoxazole/trimethoprim** as trimethoprim is associated with antifolate teratogenicity when administered in the first trimester and sulfonamides may increase risk of kernicterus in hyperbilirubinemic neonates if given after 32 weeks of pregnancy.[35] Hormonal therapy with **spironolactone** and **oral contraceptives** is contraindicated.[31]

Management during Breastfeeding

Topical antibiotics, **benzoyl peroxide**, **topical retinoids**, **azelaic acid** and **glycolic acid** have minimal systemic absorption and are compatible with breastfeeding.[28,29] Systemically administered dapsone is excreted into breast milk.[30] Although systemic absorption of topical **dapsone** is low and risk to a breastfeeding infant is expected to be minimal,[34] other topical medications have more evidence of safety. With the use of any topical medication, care should be taken to avoid direct contact of the infant's skin with treated areas of the mother. Minimal amounts of systemically administered **isotretinoin** are found in breast milk but its safety has not been documented and it remains contraindicated.[28] Oral **erythromycin** is generally considered compatible with breastfeeding though some data suggest increased risk of infantile pyloric stenosis in the early postnatal period.[28,36,37] **Sulfamethoxazole** poses a potential risk of hemolysis in glucose-6-phosphate dehydrogenase (G6PD)-deficient infants and can cause bilirubin displacement and kernicterus in stressed neonates and premature infants.[36,38] Long-term use of **trimethoprim** may interfere with folate metabolism in the infant. Although the short-term use of **tetracyclines** (<3 weeks) is not contraindicated during breastfeeding, daily use in acne is not recommended as the absorption of small amounts over a prolonged time could result in dental staining.[36] **Spironolactone** is compatible with breastfeeding as very minimal amounts are found in breast milk; decreased milk production is unlikely as spironolactone exerts only a mild diuretic effect.[36,38] See Chapter 70 for a discussion of oral contraceptive use while breastfeeding. Progestin-only products may worsen acne.

A discussion of general principles on the use of medications in these special populations can be found in Appendix II and Appendix III. Other specialized reference sources are also provided in these appendices.

Therapeutic Tips

- To prevent the development of new lesions, topical acne therapies should be applied as frequently as prescribed to the affected zones rather than to the lesions alone.
- Since many acne treatments are irritating, the skin-care regimen should be gentle; avoid astringents and abrasives.
- Initial irritation due to topical therapies (e.g., benzoyl peroxide, retinoids) can be minimized by starting with less frequent application (e.g., every 2 days) or shorter contact times (e.g., apply for 2 hours daily then wash off) and slowly increasing as tolerated.
- Topical antibiotic/benzoyl peroxide combinations have short shelf-lives: adhere to expiry dates.
- Each time an agent is added or changed, allow several weeks of treatment before assessing effectiveness.
- Acne is a disease that usually lasts years. Once control has been achieved, the treatment regimen may be simplified but some suppressive therapy will be required. The exception to this is **isotretinoin**, which can induce prolonged remission.

Table 1: **Topical Therapy for Acne**

Class	Drug	Dose	Adverse Effects	Comments	Cost[a]
Alpha-hydroxy Acids	*azelaic acid 15%* Finacea	Gel; apply BID	Irritating. Hypopigmentation.		$$
	glycolic acid 2%–15% Neostrata, Reversa, others	Gel, lotion, cream; apply up to BID	Irritating.	Available without prescription.	$
Antibiotics	*clindamycin 1%* Clindets (pledgets), Dalacin T Solution, generics	Apply BID	Rarely allergenic.	Avoid using as monotherapy to limit bacterial resistance.	Cream, Solution: $ Pledgets: $$
Combination Products	*adapalene 0.1%/benzoyl peroxide 2.5%* Tactuo	Gel; apply QHS	Photosensitivity. Mildly irritating. Rarely allergenic.	Bleaches clothing, towels, bedding.	$$$$
	clindamycin 1%/benzoyl peroxide 3% Clindoxyl ADV	Gel; apply QHS	Mildly irritating. Rarely allergenic.	Bleaches clothing, towels, bedding.	$$
	clindamycin 1%/benzoyl peroxide 5% BenzaClin, Clindoxyl	Gel; apply QHS	Mildly irritating. Rarely allergenic.	Bleaches clothing, towels, bedding.	$$
	erythromycin 3%/benzoyl peroxide 5% Benzamycin	Gel; apply BID	Mildly irritating. Rarely allergenic.	Bleaches clothing, towels, bedding.	$$$
	tretinoin 0.025%/clindamycin phosphate 1.2% Biacna	Gel; apply QHS	Photosensitivity. Irritating. Rarely allergenic.		$$$
	tretinoin 0.01%, 0.025% or 0.05%/erythromycin 4% Stievamycin Mild, Regular, Forte	Gel; apply QHS	Photosensitivity. Irritating. Rarely allergenic.		$$
Peroxides	*benzoyl peroxide 2.5%–10%* Benzagel, Panoxyl, Proactiv, others	Cream, lotion, gel; apply up to BID	Rarely allergenic.	Lower strengths may provide similar efficacy with less irritation.[6,7,8] Concentrations ≤5% available without a prescription. Bleaches clothing, towels, bedding.	$

Class	Drug	Dose	Adverse Effects	Comments	Cost[a]
Retinoid Analogues	*adapalene 0.1%, 0.3%* Differin, Differin XP	Cream, gel; once daily at HS	Less irritating and photosensitizing than tretinoin or tazarotene.		$$$
Retinoids	*tazarotene 0.05%, 0.1%* Tazorac Cream, Tazorac Gel	Cream, gel; once daily at HS to limit photosensitivity	Photosensitivity. Irritating.		$$
	tretinoin 0.01%, 0.025%, 0.05%, 0.1% Retin-A, Retin-A Micro, Stieva-A, Vitamin A Acid	Cream, gel; once daily at HS to limit photosensitivity	Photosensitivity. Irritating.		$
Sulfones	*dapsone 5%* Aczone	Gel; apply BID	Remote risk of hemolysis if G6PD-deficient.	Used for its anti-inflammatory (not antibacterial) effect. Not a sulfonamide; no cross-sensitivity in sulfa-allergic patients.[39]	$$$

[a] Cost of smallest available pack size; includes drug cost only.
Abbreviations: G6PD = glucose-6-phosphate dehydrogenase
Legend: $ < $25 $$ $25–50 $$$ $50–75 $$$$ $75–100

Table 2: Systemic Drug Therapy for Acne

Class	Drug	Dose	Adverse Effects	Drug Interactions	Cost[a]
Androgen Receptor Antagonists	*spironolactone* Aldactone, generics	25–200 mg/day po	Hyperkalemia, irregular menses, breast tenderness, nausea, headache.	May enhance the hyperkalemic effect of ACE inhibitors. Increased digoxin levels have been reported.	$
Antibiotics, diaminopyrimidines	*trimethoprim* generics	100–200 mg/day po	GI upset, very rare agranulocytosis or toxic epidermal necrolysis.	Increased phenytoin levels; increased myelosuppression with methotrexate.	$
Antibiotics, macrolides	*erythromycin* Eryc, generics	Initial: 500 mg BID po Maintenance: 250–1000 mg/day po	GI effects: nausea, vomiting, epigastric distress, diarrhea.	May increase blood levels of carbamazepine, cyclosporine, digitalis, ergotamine, theophylline, warfarin.	1 g/day base: $ EC caps: $$
Antibiotics, sulfonamide combinations	*sulfamethoxazole/trimethoprim* generics	2–4 regular-strength tabs/day divided BID po	GI upset, very rare agranulocytosis, toxic epidermal necrolysis or sulfonamide hypersensitivity syndrome.	Increased phenytoin levels, increased INR with warfarin, hypoglycemia with sulfonylureas, increased nephrotoxicity with cyclosporine.	$
Antibiotics, tetracyclines	*doxycycline* Vibramycin, generics	Initial: 100 mg/day po Maintenance: 100–200 mg/day po	GI effects; yeast overgrowth; photosensitivity; pseudotumor cerebri; contraindicated in children <8 y and pregnant women.	GI absorption impaired by aluminum, bismuth, iron and magnesium in drugs and foods. Separate doses by 2 h.	$$
	doxycycline modified release[b] Apprilon	40 mg/day po	See doxycycline. May cause less GI irritation than other tetracyclines. Used for anti-inflammatory properties: dose is subantimicrobial and may pose less risk of development of bacterial resistance.	See doxycycline.	$$$
	minocycline generics	Initial: 100 mg/day po Maintenance: 50–200 mg/day po	See doxycycline. Also dizziness; vertigo; cutaneous pigmentation; rarely LE-like syndrome; hepatic dysfunction.	See doxycycline.	$$

Class	Drug	Dose	Adverse Effects	Drug Interactions	Cost[a]
	tetracycline ❸ generics	Initial: 500 mg BID po Maintenance: 250–1000 mg/day po	See doxycycline.	See doxycycline.	$
Contraceptives, Oral	*EE 0.035 mg/cyproterone 2 mg* Diane-35, generics	1 tablet daily po × 21 days, off for 7 days and repeat cycle	Major: rare thromboembolism, stroke, retinal artery thrombosis, MI, benign liver tumor, cholelithiasis, hypertension. Common: breakthrough bleeding/spotting, amenorrhea, nausea/vomiting, weight gain, bloating, chloasma, breast tenderness, depression, headaches. Discontinue 3–4 cycles after acne resolved. Health Canada has prepared a Suggested prescriber/counselling checklist for Diane-35 and its generics[40] to facilitate documentation of discussion of risks.	Antibiotics: there is controversy as to whether a barrier method of birth control should also be used when women are using antibiotics and oral contraceptives. Patients with diarrhea or breakthrough bleeding may be at higher risk. Rifampin is the only antibiotic consistently shown to reduce estrogen levels.	$
	EE 0.03 mg/drospirenone 3 mg Yasmin, Zamine, Zarah	1 tablet daily po × 21 days, off 7 days and repeat cycle	See EE/cyproterone.	See EE/cyproterone.	$
	EE 0.02 mg/drospirenone 3 mg Yaz, MYA	1 tablet daily po (last 4 tablets of each 28-day pack are inert)	See EE/cyproterone.	See EE/cyproterone.	$
	EE 0.02 mg/drospirenone 3 mg/ levomefolate calcium 0.451 mg Yaz Plus	1 tablet daily po (last 4 tablets of each 28-day pack contain levomefolate calcium only)	See EE/cyproterone.	See EE/cyproterone.	$
	EE 0.02 mg/levonorgestrel 0.1 mg Alesse, Alysena, Aviane, ESME, Lutera	1 tablet daily po × 21 days, off for 7 days and repeat cycle	See EE/cyproterone.	See EE/cyproterone.	$

(cont'd)

Table 2: Systemic Drug Therapy for Acne *(cont'd)*

Class	Drug	Dose	Adverse Effects	Drug Interactions	Cost[a]
	EE 0.035 mg/norgestimate 0.18 mg × 7 days, 0.215 mg × 7 days, 0.25 mg × 7 days Tri-Cyclen	1 tablet daily po × 21 days, off 7 days and repeat cycle	See EE/cyproterone.	See EE/cyproterone.	$
Retinoids	*isotretinoin* Accutane, Clarus, Epuris	0.5–2 mg/kg/day po for 12–16 wk	Teratogenicity. Common: mucocutaneous dryness, myalgia, arthralgia, headache, photosensitivity. Uncommon–Rare: hypertriglyceridemia, mood disorder, possibly suicide ideation, pseudotumor cerebri. Very rare (possibly related): erythema multiforme, Stevens-Johnson syndrome, toxic epidermal necrolysis.	Tetracyclines: rare cases of benign intracranial hypertension (pseudotumor cerebri).	$$$

[a] Cost of 30-day supply of mean dose based on 70 kg body weight; includes drug cost only.
[b] Small studies with doxycycline 20 mg have shown it to be effective for acne.[41,42,43] Clinical experience with doxycycline 40 mg modified release has shown similar results.
Dosage adjustment may be required in renal impairment; see Appendix I.
Abbreviations: ACE = angiotensin-converting enzyme; EE = ethinyl estradiol; LE = lupus erythematosus
Legend: $ < $25 $$ $25–75 $$$ $75–125

Suggested Readings

Eichenfield LF, Krakowski AC, Piggott C et al. Evidence-based recommendations for the diagnosis and treatment of pediatric acne. *Pediatrics* 2013;131(Suppl 3):S163-86.

Nast D, Dreno B, Bettoli V et al. European evidence-based (S3) guidelines for the treatment of acne. *J Eur Acad Dermatol Venereol* 2012;26(Suppl 1):1-29.

Thiboutot D, Gollnick H, Bettoli V et al. New insights into the management of acne: an update from the Global Alliance to Improve Outcomes in Acne Group. *J Am Acad Dermatol* 2009;60(5 Suppl):S1-50.

Williams HC, Dellavalle RP, Garner S. Acne vulgaris. *Lancet* 2012;379(9813):361-72.

References

1. Magin P, Adams J, Heading G et al. Psychological sequelae of acne vulgaris: results of a qualitative study. *Can Fam Physician* 2006;52:978-9.
2. Burris J, Rietkerk W, Woolf K. Acne: the role of medical nutrition therapy. *J Acad Nutr Diet* 2013;113(3):416-30.
3. Leyden JJ. Therapy for acne vulgaris. *N Engl J Med* 1997;336(16):1156-62.
4. Hegemann L, Toso SM, Kitay K et al. Anti-inflammatory actions of benzoyl peroxide: effects on the generation of reactive oxygen species by leucocytes and the activity of protein kinase C and calmodulin. *Br J Dermatol* 1994;130(5):569-75.
5. Burkhart CG, Burkhart CN. Antibacterial properties of benzoyl peroxide in aerobic and anaerobic conditions. *Int J Dermatol* 2006;45(11):1373-4.
6. Mills OH, Kligman AM, Pochi P et al. Comparing 2.5%, 5%, and 10% benzoyl peroxide on inflammatory acne vulgaris. *Int J Dermatol* 1986;25(10):664-7.
7. Brandstetter AJ, Maibach HI. Topical dose justification: benzoyl peroxide concentrations. *J Dermatolog Treat* 2013;24(4):275-7.
8. Eichenfield LF, Krakowski AC, Piggott C et al. Evidence-based recommendations for the diagnosis and treatment of pediatric acne. *Pediatrics* 2013;131(Suppl 3):S163-86.
9. Kalita L. Tazarotene versus tretinoin or adapalene in the treatment of acne vulgaris. *J Am Acad Dermatol* 2000;43(2 Pt 3):S51-4.
10. Thiboutot D, Gollnick H, Bettoli V et al. New insights into the management of acne: an update from the Global Alliance to Improve Outcomes in Acne group. *Am Acad Dermatol* 2009;60(5 Suppl):S1-50.
11. Draelos ZD, Carter E, Maloney JM et al. Two randomized studies demonstrate the efficacy and safety of dapsone gel, 5% for the treatment of acne vulgaris. *J Am Acad Dermatol* 2007;56(3):439.e1-10.
12. Lucky AW, Maloney JM, Roberts J et al. Dapsone gel 5% for the treatment of acne vulgaris: safety and efficacy of long-term (1 year) treatment. *J Drugs Dermatol* 2007;6(10):981-7.
13. Piette WW, Taylor S, Pariser D et al. Hematologic safety of dapsone gel, 5%, for topical treatment of acne vulgaris. *Arch Dermatol* 2008;144(12):1564-70.
14. Strauss JS, Krowchuk DP, Leyden JJ et al. Guidelines of care for acne vulgaris management. *J Am Acad Dermatol* 2007;56(4):651-63.
15. Arowojolu AO, Gallo MF, Lopez LM et al. Combined oral contraceptive pills for treatment of acne. *Cochrane Database Syst Rev* 2012;7:CD004425.
16. Reid R; Society of Obstetricians and Gynaecologists of Canada. SOGC clinical practice guideline. No. 252, December 2010. Oral contraceptives and the risk of venous thromboembolism: an update. *J Obstet Gynaecol Can* 2010;32(12):1192-204.
17. Stegeman B, de Bastos M, Rosendaal F et al. Different combined oral contraceptives and the risk of venous thrombosis: systematic review and network meta-analysis. *BMJ* 2013;347:f5298.
18. de Bastos M, Stegeman BH, Rosendaal FR et al. Combined oral contraceptives: venous thrombosis. *Cochrane Database Syst Rev* 2014;3:CD010813.
19. Thiboutot D, Zaenglein A. Isotretinoin and affective disorders: thirty years later. *J Am Acad Dermatol* 2013;68(4):675-6.
20. Chia CY, Lane W, Chibnall J et al. Isotretinoin therapy and mood changes in adolescents with moderate to severe acne: a cohort study. *Arch Dermatol* 2005;141(5):557-60.
21. Sundtrom A, Alfredsson L, Sjolin-Forsberg G et al. Association of suicide attempts with acne and treatment with isotretinoin: retrospective Swedish cohort study. *BMJ* 2010;341:c5812.
22. Alhusayen RO, Juurlink DN, Mamdani MM et al. Isotretinoin use and the risk of inflammatory bowel disease: a population-based cohort study. *J Invest Dermatol* 2013;133(4):907-12.
23. Etminan M, Bird ST, Delaney JA et al. Isotretinoin and risk for inflammatory bowel disease: a nested case-control study and meta-analysis of published and unpublished data. *JAMA Dermatol* 2013;149(2):216-20.
24. e-CPS. Ottawa (ON): Canadian Pharmacists Association; 2013. Accutane Roche [product monograph]. Available from: www.e-therapeutics.ca. Accessed October 10, 2013. Subscription required.
25. Organization of Teratology Information Specialists (OTIS). Tucson (AZ): University of Arizona, OTIS National Office. Available from: www.otispregnancy.org. Accessed October 10, 2013.
26. UpToDate. *Spironolactone*. Waltham (MA): UpToDate. Available from: www.uptodate.com. Accessed October 10, 2013. Subscription required.
27. Akhavan A, Bershad S. Topical acne drugs: review of clinical properties, systemic exposure and safety. *Am J Clin Dermatol* 2003;4(7):473-92.
28. Leachman SA, Reed BR. The use of dermatologic drugs in pregnancy and lactation. *Dermatol Clin* 2006;24(2):167-97.
29. Bozzo P, Chua-Gocheco A, Einarson A. Safety of skin care products during pregnancy. *Can Fam Physician* 2011;57(6):665-7.
30. e-CPS. Ottawa (ON): Canadian Pharmacists Association; 2012. Aczone [product monograph]. Available from: www.e-therapeutics.ca. Accessed May 31, 2012. Subscription required.
31. Briggs GG, Freeman RK, Yaffe SJ. *Drugs in pregnancy and lactation: a reference guide to fetal and neonatal risk.* 9th ed. Philadelphia (PA): Wolter Kluwer Health; Lippincott Williams & Wilkins; 2011.
32. Rothman KF, Pochi PE. Use of oral and topical agents for acne in pregnancy. *J Am Acad Dermatol* 1988;19(3):431-42.
33. Zip C. A practical guide to dermatological drug use in pregnancy. *Skin Therapy Lett* 2006;11(4):1-4.
34. Hale EK, Pomeranz MK. Dermatologic agents during pregnancy and lactation: an update and clinical review. *Int J Dermatol* 2002;41(4):197-203.

35. Sivojelezova A, Einarson A, Shuhaiber S et al. Trimethoprim-sulfonamide combination therapy in early pregnancy. *Can Fam Physician* 2003;49:1085-6.
36. Hale TW. *Medications and mothers' milk: a manual of lactational pharmacology*. 15th ed. Amarillo (TX): Hale Publishing; 2012.
37. Sorenson HT, Skriver MV, Pedersen L et al. Risk of infantile hypertrophic pyloric stenosis after maternal postnatal use of macrolides. *Scand J Infect Dis* 2003;35(2):104-6.
38. Drugs and Lactation Database (LactMed). Bethesda (MD): U.S. National Library of Medicine. Available from: toxnet.nlm.nih.gov/cgi-bin/sis/htmlgen?LACT. Accessed October 17, 2013.
39. Webster GF. Is topical dapsone safe in glucose-6-phosphate dehydrogenase-deficient and sulfonamide-allergic patients? *J Drugs Dermatol* 2010;9(5):532-6.
40. Health Canada. *Suggested prescriber/counselling checklist for Diane-35 (cyproterone acetate/ethinyl estradiol) and its generics*. Available from: www.hc-sc.gc.ca/dhp-mps/alt_formats/pdf/medeff/advisories-avis/review-examen/checklist-verification-diane-35-eng.pdf. Accessed April 29, 2014.
41. Skidmore R, Kovach R, Walker C et al. Effects of subantimicrobial-dose doxycycline in the treatment of moderate acne. *Arch Dermatol* 2003;139(4):459-64.
42. Toossi P, Farshchian M, Malekzad F et al. Subantimicrobial-dose doxycycline in the treatment of moderate facial acne. *J Drugs Dermatol* 2008;7(12):1149-1152.
43. Parish LC, Parish JL, Routh HB et al. The treatment of acne vulgaris with low dosage doxycycline. *Acta Dermatovenerol Croat* 2005;13(3):156-9.

Chapter 89
Atopic Dermatitis

Miriam Weinstein, MD, FRCPC

Atopic dermatitis (AD), also known as *eczema*, is an inflammatory disorder of the skin with an onset usually in early childhood. Patients typically have flares of dermatitis that present as ill-defined patches of erythema, scale and excoriations. Significant pruritus and generalized dry skin are usually prominent features. Atopic dermatitis may be associated with other atopic conditions such as asthma, allergic rhinoconjunctivitis and food allergies. Although patients with atopic dermatitis are more likely to have food allergies, food ingestion as a causal factor in eczema flares is uncommon.

Goals of Therapy

Atopic dermatitis is a chronic, recurring condition without a cure, so the major focus is control of dermatitis, pruritus and dryness. Goals of therapy are:

- Relieve generalized dry skin and pruritus, particularly when they interfere with activities of daily living
- Treat patches of dermatitis to reduce inflammation and pruritus and reduce risk of secondary infection
- Prevent flare-ups caused by environmental irritants
- Promptly treat complications of atopic dermatitis such as secondary bacterial or viral infection

Investigations

- Physical exam may show 1 of 3 typical morphologic patterns:
  - facial and extensor dermatitis in infants
  - flexural and fold dermatitis in older children
  - prominence of facial and hand dermatitis in adults

Investigations are rarely required for the work-up of classic atopic dermatitis. Bacterial swabs showing moderate or heavy growth of organisms may suggest secondary bacterial infections in resistant patches of dermatitis. However, many patients with atopic dermatitis are colonized with *Staphylococcus aureus*, making swabs with minimal growth difficult to interpret.

Therapeutic Choices

An algorithm for the management of atopic dermatitis is presented in Figure 1.

Prevention

Maternal use of **probiotics** during pregnancy and maternal and/or infant use during breastfeeding may be helpful in reducing the development of atopic dermatitis in the child [Evidence: SORT B *].[1,2] However, there is not enough evidence to support the role of probiotics in the treatment of established atopic dermatitis.[3,4]

*SORT (Strength of Recommendation Taxonomy) is a rating system (A, B or C) that addresses the quality of available evidence. For more information consult **How to Use *Compendium of Therapeutic Choices*** on page xxv.

Figure 1: **Management of Atopic Dermatitis**

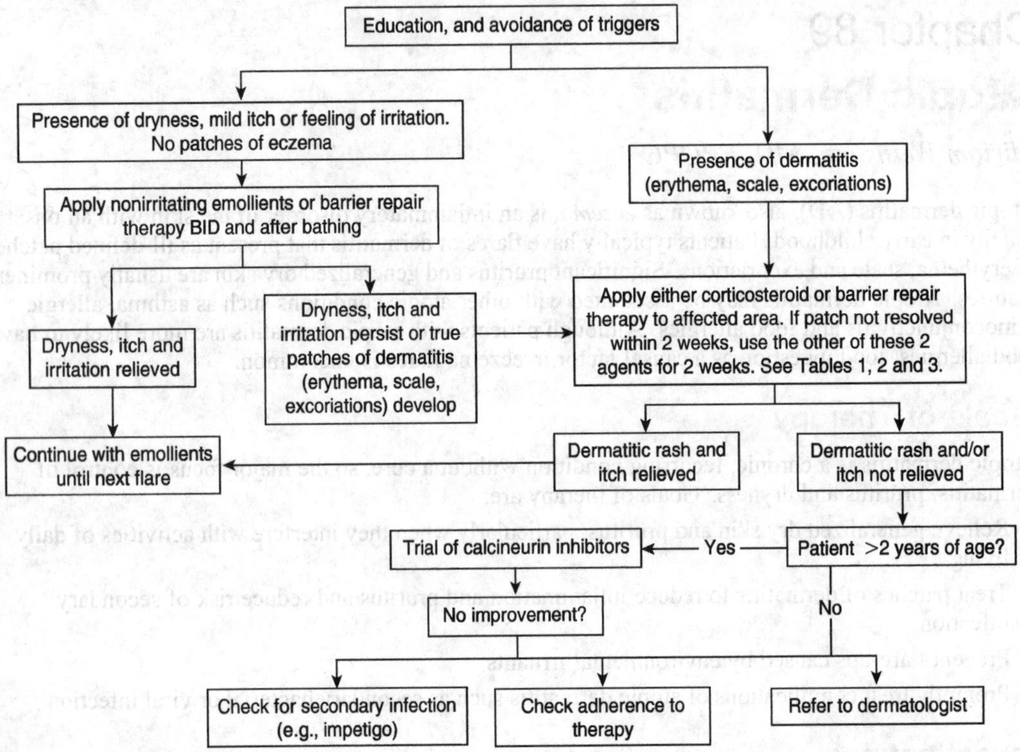

Nonpharmacologic Choices

Evidence suggests that disease-specific formal patient education programs, usually provided by a trained nurse, contribute to the success of treatment.[5]

Reducing environmental irritants is very useful; use nonirritating soaps and avoid perfumed products, wool and synthetic fibres, dry grass and leaves.

Patients with atopic dermatitis have abnormal barrier function, so they cannot maintain adequate hydration. Frequent use of lubricating skin **emollients** such as petrolatum helps seal in moisture. Emollients are first-line therapy for prevention of flares and treatment of minimal irritation and itch. Even when medication is required, emollients should be used at least twice daily. Remind patients to apply medicated treatments directly to the skin, not over emollients. Emollients should not contain fragrances or irritants (e.g., salicylic acid). Plain **petrolatum** jelly, while greasy, is highly effective, nonirritating and inexpensive.

Bathing, done properly, can help to hydrate the skin and protect the barrier. Bathing should be brief (5–10 minutes), the water warm (not hot) and the skin patted dry rather than rubbed aggressively. After bathing, apply emollients within 3 minutes of light drying.

Wet wraps (wet bandages applied over emollients or medication) are a useful second-line therapy but should be supervised by a physician experienced in this technique. Multiple different approaches are used and complications can occur. These include hypothermia, tissue maceration, infection and excessive absorption of medication.

Pharmacologic Choices

Topical **corticosteroids** affect several inflammatory pathways in the skin and work quickly and effectively. They are available in a wide variety of potencies and vehicles. The actual clinical potency of topical corticosteroids depends on the molecular structure and vehicle as well as the thickness and integrity of the skin. There is no formula to calculate the precise relationship between these factors. Some principles, however, can guide appropriate treatment selection (see Table 1 and Table 2). A systematic review of once-daily versus more frequent use of potent topical corticosteroids in atopic dermatitis found little difference between regimens with respect to clinical outcomes and adverse events.[6]

When prescribed and monitored by an experienced physician, topical corticosteroids are safe medications. Clinically significant adverse effects are rare and generally due to misuse.[7,8] Laboratory detection of adverse effects such as cutaneous atrophy and HPA axis suppression due to systemic absorption may not translate to clinical effects in the patient.[9,10,11,12,13,14] Regardless, in the setting of atopic dermatitis "steroid-phobia" is widespread[15] and many patients, particularly children, suffer with undertreated eczema due to exaggerated fears about corticosteroid side effects. Many health care providers automatically warn that these products should be used "sparingly", reinforcing this fear. This can lead to suboptimal therapy and result in the eczema being maintained in a chronic, active state. Inadequately treated eczema can lead to secondary infection and substantial sleep loss, and can significantly decrease quality of life [Evidence: SORT C*].[16] The negative effects of undertreatment outweigh the risk of adverse effects of corticosteroids. Ensure effective use of corticosteroids by choosing correct potency and vehicle (see Table 1 and Table 2) and using adequate quantities (see Table 3) for appropriate periods of time. Treatment should continue until rash and itch are resolved. This may be a few days or up to several weeks for each flare depending on the patient (see Figure 1). However, any eruption which does not improve significantly within 2 weeks, should be reassessed.

Table 1: Selection of Topical Corticosteroid by Body Area

Body Area	Skin Properties	Corticosteroid Potency
Face, intertriginous folds	Thin skin, more absorption	Low potency
Body and scalp	Medium thickness	Medium potency
Palms, soles	Thick skin	High potency

Table 2: Selection of Topical Therapy by Vehicle

Vehicle	Advantages	Disadvantages
Cream	Cosmetically elegant	Less absorption; additives can irritate
Lotion	Evaporates well, good for large areas, hairy areas	Alcohol base will sting/irritate open areas of eczema
Gel	Good for hairy areas, oily skin	Alcohol base will sting/irritate open areas of eczema
Ointment	Excellent penetration, offers emollient effect, little or no irritation	Cosmetically less acceptable, thick, greasy

* SORT (Strength of Recommendation Taxonomy) is a rating system (A, B or C) that addresses the quality of available evidence. For more information consult **How to Use *Compendium of Therapeutic Choices*** on page xxv.

Table 3: **Estimating Amount of Topical Therapy for One Application Using Fingertip Units (FTU)[a]**

Body Area to be Treated	Fingertip Units (FTUs) Required for One Application (by age group)[b]				
	3–6 Months	1–2 Years	3–5 Years	6–10 Years	Adults
Face and neck	1	1.5	1.5	2	2.5
1 Arm and hand	1	1.5	2	2.5	4
1 Leg and foot	1.5	2	3	4.5	8
Trunk (front)	1	2	3	3.5	7
Trunk (back, including buttocks)	1.5	3	3.5	5	7

Adapted from Patient.co.uk. *Fingertip units for topical steroids for eczema.* Available from: www.patient.co.uk/health/fingertip-units-for-topical-steroids.

[a] The fingertip unit is approximately 0.5 g, estimated to be the amount squeezed from a tube (with a standard 5 mm nozzle) from the fingertip to the first crease of an adult finger. Each 1 FTU should cover approximately 250 cm^2 of area (equal to approximately 2 adult hand prints with fingers together).[17]

[b] To calculate quantity to prescribe: (FTU for body area(s) involved × 0.5 g/FTU) × (# applications/day) × (# days of treatment). E.g., to treat a 10-yr old's trunk (front) once daily for 2 weeks: 3.5 FTU × 0.5 g/FTU × 1 application/day × 14 days = 24.5 g.

Calcineurin inhibitors, also referred to as topical immune modulators, are a newer class of medications designed to specifically block calcineurin. They provide a targeted, specific anti-inflammatory mechanism in contrast to the wide-ranging effects of corticosteroids. **Tacrolimus** and **pimecrolimus** are available in Canada. These products work more slowly than corticosteroids[18] and generally require twice-daily dosing. Evidence supports the short-term safety of these products.[19]

Concerns have been raised about the long-term safety of calcineurin inhibitors, particularly the risk of malignancy.[19] Currently, insufficient data exist to adequately support or refute this claim.[19,20] These agents can be useful in the treatment of atopic dermatitis but should be used only as indicated: in patients over 2 years of age, as second-line therapy and on an intermittent basis. Calcineurin inhibitors can be used as second-line agents for eczema of the face or folds if there is a concern about the amount or frequency of use of low-potency corticosteroids. These patients may continue to use corticosteroids elsewhere on the body while using calcineurin inhibitors on face or folds. Both pimecrolimus and tacrolimus significantly reduce eczema severity scores compared to placebo.[21] Tacrolimus 0.03% has demonstrated better efficacy than a mild corticosteroid,[22] and tacrolimus 0.1% has shown no difference compared with a mid-potency corticosteroid.[23] Pimecrolimus 1% was not as effective as betamethasone valerate 0.1% in patients with eczema of at least moderate severity, although it is indicated for patients with mild to moderate eczema.[24] Pimecrolimus has not been compared with low-potency topical corticosteroids as a treatment for mild eczema. Combining calcineurin inhibitors and topical corticosteroids does not appear to confer benefit over topical corticosteroids alone.[25]

Barrier repair therapies are new products developed in response to recognition of the contribution of a defective barrier to the etiology of atopic dermatitis.[26] Disrupted ceramide content is one aspect of barrier dysfunction, and restoring the correct balance of ceramides is a strategy employed by newer products. One study found that a ceramide-dominant product was equivalent to a mid-potency corticosteroid after 28 days.[27] However, another study found no difference in the management of mild-to-moderate eczema when comparing ceramide-dominant barrier repair therapy with another barrier repair therapy or a petrolatum-based moisturizer.[28]

Topical treatments for atopic dermatitis are addressed in Table 4.

There is no convincing evidence of the benefit of **dietary supplements** in eczema.[3]

Consider referral to a dermatologist for patients who fail to achieve good control of their eczema despite nonpharmacologic management (trigger avoidance, generous use of emollients) in combination with first- and second-line therapies such as topical corticosteroids or calcineurin inhibitors.

Other therapies such as systemic agents (e.g., **cyclosporine**, **methotrexate**, **azathioprine**) or ultraviolet (UV) light have been used in patients with extensive dermatitis, patients who have not responded to topical treatment and those who are unable to tolerate topical therapy. **Alitretinoin** is approved for severe chronic hand eczema in adults; referral to a dermatologist is recommended. *Oral* corticosteroids should not be routinely used in the treatment of atopic dermatitis, given their many side effects and the tendency for the eczema to rebound on withdrawal of corticosteroids.[29]

Flare Prevention

Evidence suggests the use of long-term intermittent topical corticosteroids or calcineurin inhibitors may help to keep atopic dermatitis in remission. Different regimens exist and generally involve application 2–3 times weekly. Duration of use has ranged from 16–40 weeks or longer, depending on the specific agent.[30,31,32,33,34] Use of tacrolimus twice weekly for flare prevention is an approved indication in Canada, while the other regimens remain off-label. A systematic review of proactive treatment suggests that both tacrolimus and topical corticosteroids (several potencies) aid in flare prevention when used twice weekly, and that a potent topical corticosteroid may be more efficacious in flare prevention than tacrolimus.[35] There is also evidence to support early intervention with calcineurin inhibitors at the first signs of a flare to prevent progression to a more serious episode.[36,37] This remains an off-label indication for these medications.

Secondary Infection

Secondary infection is common with atopic dermatitis. Treat obviously infected eczema with topical or oral antibiotics. Questions have arisen about the role of preventive strategies with topical antiseptics or prophylactic antibiotics. **Bleach baths** are a useful second-line therapy but should be supervised by a physician experienced in this technique. Complications can include irritation ranging from mild to severe if the dilution is incorrect. A systematic review examined 26 randomized controlled trials that used a variety of antistaphylococcal treatments in the management of atopic dermatitis, including oral antibiotics, antibacterial soaps, topical antibiotics or antiseptics, special textiles and combinations of topical corticosteroids with antibacterials. While reduction of *S. aureus* counts on the skin was reported with some interventions, no trials showed improvement in eczema control. The poor quality of many of the studies and low patient numbers make this evidence difficult to interpret.[38]

Choices during Pregnancy and Breastfeeding

Atopic Dermatitis and Pregnancy

Atopic dermatitis is the most common skin condition in pregnancy, although overall prevalence during pregnancy is unknown.[39] Sixty to 80% of affected pregnant patients develop symptoms for the first time during pregnancy, usually within the first 2 trimesters. One quarter of women with pre-existing atopic dermatitis will improve during pregnancy, but over half will experience worsening of the condition. Untreated atopic dermatitis can be extremely uncomfortable and carries the considerable risk of secondary infection. There is some evidence that maternal use of **probiotics** during pregnancy or maternal and/or infant use during breastfeeding may be helpful in reducing the development of atopic dermatitis in the child.[1,2]

Pre-pregnancy Management

Ideally, disease activity should be minimized prior to conception. Patients receiving systemic treatment may need to discontinue their medication well before conception; timing depends on the drugs involved. **Methotrexate** must be stopped at least 3 months prior to conception in women.[39,40] It is also recommended that men stop methotrexate 3 months prior to conception,[39,40] however a small cohort study showed no adverse pregnancy outcomes after paternal low-dose methotrexate exposure during time of conception.[41] Although no specific time period is recommended, **psoralens** with ultraviolet-A (UVA) should be stopped before attempting to conceive.

Management of Atopic Dermatitis during Pregnancy

Maximize nonpharmacologic approaches, such as use of emollients and avoidance of environmental irritants. There is no information available on the safety of barrier repair therapies in pregnancy but the ingredients (skin lipids) are not expected to pose a significant risk. **Topical corticosteroids** remain the main treatment option throughout pregnancy. Low- and mid-potency corticosteroids are preferred over potent or very potent agents.[39,42,43] If further treatment is needed, second-line choices include ultraviolet-B (UVB) therapy and **calcineurin inhibitors** (very low bioavailability when applied topically).[39] Systemic therapy with **cyclosporine** or **azathioprine** is considered only in the most severe cases after careful discussion, and requires close monitoring for both mother and baby in a hospital setting. **Methotrexate** is contraindicated during pregnancy.

Management of Atopic Dermatitis during Breastfeeding

Emollients and **topical corticosteroids** remain the main treatment options throughout breastfeeding. Though safety data are lacking for **ceramide**-based barrier repair therapies, there is no theoretical reason for concern. Risk to the baby via passage of topical corticosteroids into breast milk is unlikely since only extensive use of the most potent corticosteroids causes systemic effects in the mother. The topical corticosteroid with the lowest effective potency should be applied to the smallest area possible for the shortest possible time.[39,44,45] **Topical calcineurin inhibitors** appear to be poorly absorbed after topical administration and are second-line therapy.[39,44,45] Avoid direct contact of the infant with the mother's treated skin. UVB therapy is considered safe during breastfeeding.[39] Avoid **methotrexate** and **cyclosporine** during breastfeeding.

Up to 2% of mothers develop atopic dermatitis of the nipple or areola during breastfeeding.[39] Emollients and low-potency corticosteroids can be applied to the areola or nipple, and wiped off gently but thoroughly before nursing. To prevent ingestion by the infant, topical calcineurin inhibitors should not be applied to the nipple/areola.

A discussion of general principles on the use of medications in these special populations can be found in Appendix II and Appendix III. Other specialized reference sources are also provided in these appendices.

Therapeutic Tips

- Ointments are less irritating and penetrate better than creams or lotions. They are an excellent choice for atopic dermatitis but cosmetic acceptability and patient adherence are lower. Generally, the same corticosteroid molecule will be more potent in an ointment base than in cream or lotion.
- Education is a key part of therapy. Patients have to understand they have a chronic, recurring condition that can be controlled, not cured.
- Sweating, stress and overheating can all increase itching.
- Patches of dermatitis that are resistant to treatment despite good adherence to therapy may require a short course of a more potent corticosteroid.
- Pruritus in atopic dermatitis is not histamine-mediated and therefore does not respond well to histamine blockade. Nonsedating antihistamines are of little use in the pruritus of atopic dermatitis but may help associated allergic symptoms (e.g., allergic conjunctivitis). Potent, sedating antihistamines (e.g., diphenhydramine, hydroxyzine) taken 30–60 minutes prior to bedtime may provide some relief, possibly through central sedation.

Table 4: Topical Treatments for Atopic Dermatitis[a]

Class[b]	Drug	Dose	Adverse Effects	Comments	Cost[c]
Antibiotic/ Corticosteroid Combinations	*betamethasone valerate 0.1%/gentamicin 0.1%* Valisone-G	BID–TID	Striae, telangiectasia, atrophy, purpura. When used around the eye for longer periods of time, ocular side effects may rarely occur. Systemic effects include suppression of HPA axis although clinically relevant features are very rare.	For use in secondarily infected dermatitis. Caution: extensive use of gentamicin may lead to increased systemic absorption, especially in children.	$$$
	fusidic acid 2%/hydrocortisone 1% Fucidin H	TID	See betamethasone valerate/gentamicin.	For use in dermatitis with associated *S. aureus.*	$$$
Barrier Repair Products	*ceramides/cholesterol/free fatty acids* EpiCeram Skin Barrier Emulsion, others	BID	Mild burning or stinging lasting 10–15 min.	Do not apply within 4 h prior to radiation therapy.	$$
Calcineurin Inhibitors	*pimecrolimus cream* 1% Elidel	BID	Transient burning sensations, skin tingling, pruritus at site of application.	For use as a second-line agent until skin clears. Not for use in children <2 years of age or in patients who are immunocompromised. Apply a thin layer and avoid unnecessary UV exposure. Indicated for patients with mild to moderate atopic dermatitis.	$$$$
	tacrolimus ointment 0.03%, 0.1% Protopic	Pediatric (>2 years): 0.03% ointment BID Adult (≥16 years): 0.03% or 0.1% ointment BID	See pimecrolimus.	See pimecrolimus. Indicated for patients with moderate to severe atopic dermatitis.	$$$$
Corticosteroids, low-potency	*desonide* 0.05% Verdeso, generics	BID–TID	Striae, telangiectasia, atrophy, purpura. When used around the eye for longer periods of time, ocular side effects may rarely occur. Systemic effects include suppression of HPA axis although clinically relevant features are very rare.	Good for face, intertriginous areas. Safe and effective when used appropriately.	$
	hydrocortisone 1%, 2%, 2.5% Emo-Cort, Prevex HC, Topiderm, generics	BID–TID	See desonide.	See desonide.	$

(cont'd)

Table 4: **Topical Treatments for Atopic Dermatitis**[a] *(cont'd)*

Class[b]	Drug	Dose	Adverse Effects	Comments	Cost[c]
Corticosteroids, medium-potency	*betamethasone valerate* 0.05%, 0.1% Betaderm, Celestoderm V, Celestoderm V/2, Luxiq, Prevex B, generics	Daily–BID	See desonide.	Good for body areas. Safe and effective when used appropriately.	$
	clobetasone butyrate 0.05%[d] Spectro EczemaCare Medicated Cream	BID–TID	See desonide.	See betamethasone valerate.	$$
	diflucortolone valerate 0.1% Nerisone	Daily–BID	See desonide.	See betamethasone valerate.	$$
	fluocinolone acetonide 0.01% Derma-Smoothe/FS	BID–TID	See desonide.	See betamethasone valerate. Derma-Smoothe/FS product contains peanut oil but not peanut protein.	$
	hydrocortisone valerate 0.2% Hydroval	BID–TID	See desonide.	See betamethasone valerate.	$
	prednicarbate 0.1% Dermatop	BID	See desonide.	See betamethasone valerate.	$$
	triamcinolone acetonide 0.1%, 0.5% Aristocort Creams and Ointments, generics	BID	See desonide.	See betamethasone valerate.	0.1%: $ 0.5%: $$$
Corticosteroids, high-potency	*amcinonide* 0.1% Cyclocort, generics	BID–TID	See desonide.	Good for thick, lichenified plaques. Safe and effective when used appropriately.	$
	betamethasone dipropionate 0.05% Diprosone, generics	BID	See desonide.	See amcinonide. Glycol-based product is ultra potent. See betamethasone dipropionate glycol.	$
	desoximetasone 0.05%, 0.25% Topicort Preparations	BID	See desonide.	See amcinonide.	$$
	fluocinonide 0.05% Lidemol, Lidex, Lyderm, Tiamol, Topactin	BID–TID	See desonide.	See amcinonide.	$
	mometasone furoate 0.1% Elocom, generics	Daily	See desonide.	See amcinonide.	$
Corticosteroids, ultra-potent	*betamethasone dipropionate glycol* 0.05% Diprolene	BID	See desonide.	Good for palms and soles. Safe and effective when used appropriately.	$$

Class[b]	Drug	Dose	Adverse Effects	Comments	Cost[c]
	clobetasol propionate 0.05% Clobex Lotion, Dermovate, Olux-E, generics	BID	See desonide.	See betamethasone dipropionate glycol.	$
	halobetasol propionate 0.05% Ultravate	BID	See desonide.	See betamethasone dipropionate glycol.	$$$

[a] Few of the listed products are Health Canada-approved for use in the pediatric population but are often used in this population in practice.
[b] Different potency categories may be used by other authors. Vehicle also impacts potency categorization. These rankings are meant to serve as a guide only.
[c] Cost of 30 g or 30 mL for topical products; includes drug cost only.
[d] Clobetasone butyrate is available without a prescription.
Abbreviations: HPA = hypothalamic-pituitary-adrenal; UV = ultraviolet
Legend: $ < $10 $$ $10–25 $$$ $25–50 $$$$ $50–75

Suggested Readings

Arkwright PD, Motala C, Subramanian H et al. Management of difficult-to-treat atopic dermatitis. *J Allergy Clin Immonol Pract* 2013;1(2):142-51.

Lynde C, Barber K, Claveau J et al. Canadian practical guide for the treatment and management of atopic dermatitis. *J Cutan Med Surg* 2005;8(Suppl 5):1-9.

National Institute for Health and Clinical Evidence. NHS Evidence—Skin disorders. *2010 annual evidence update on atopic eczema.* September 13, 2010.

Ring J, Alomar A, Bieber T et al. Guidelines for treatment of atopic eczema (atopic dermatitis) part I. *J Eur Acad Dematol Venereol* 2012;26(8):1045-60.

Ring J, Alomar A, Bieber T et al. Guidelines for treatment of atopic eczema (atopic dermatitis) part II. *J Eur Acad Dematol Venereol* 2012;26(9):1176-93.

Sajic D, Asiniwasis R, Skotnicki-Grant S. A look at epidermal barrier function in atopic dermatitis: physiologic lipid replacement and the role of ceramides. *Skin Therapy Lett* 2012;17(7):6-9.

References

1. Rautava S, Kainonen E, Salminen S et al. Maternal probiotic supplementation during pregnancy and breast-feeding reduced the risk of eczema in the infant. *J Allergy Clin Immunol* 2012;130(6):1355-60.
2. Foolad N, Brezinski EA, Chase EP et al. Effect of nutrient supplementation on atopic dermatitis in children: a systematic review of probiotics, prebiotics, formula, and fatty acids. *JAMA Dermatol* 2013;149(3):350-5.
3. Bath-Hextall FJ, Jenkinson C, Humphreys R et al. Dietary supplements for established atopic eczema. *Cochrane Database Syst Rev* 2012;2:CD005205.
4. Boyle RJ, Bath-Hextall FJ, Leonardi-Bee J et al. Probiotics for treating eczema. *Cochrane Database Syst Rev* 2008;(4):CD006135.
5. Grillo M, Gassner L, Marshman G et al. Pediatric atopic eczema: the impact of an educational intervention. *Pediatr Dermatol* 2006;23(5):428-36.
6. Green C, Colquitt JL, Kirby J et al. Topical corticosteroids for atopic eczema: clinical and cost effectiveness of once-daily vs. more frequent use. *Br J Dermatol* 2005;152(1):130-41.
7. Gilbertson EO, Spellman MC, Piacquadio DJ et al. Super potent topical corticosteroid use associated with adrenal suppression: clinical considerations. *J Am Acad Dermatol* 1998;38(2 Pt 2):318-21.
8. Rogge FJ, Pacifico MD, Grobbelaar AO. Earlobe perforation after prolonged use of a topical corticosteroid. *J Plast Reconstr Aesthet Surg* 2007;60(1):100-1.
9. Kolbe L, Kligman AM, Schreiner V et al. Corticosteroid-induced atrophy and barrier impairment measured by non-invasive methods in human skin. *Skin Res Technol* 2001;7(2):73-7.
10. Zoller NN, Kippenberger S, Thaci D et al. Evaluation of beneficial and adverse effects of glucocorticoids on a newly developed full-thickness skin model. *Toxicol In Vitro* 2008;22(3):747-59.
11. Castela E, Archier E, Devaux S et al. Topical corticosteroids in plaque psoriasis: a systematic review of risk of adrenal axis suppression and skin atrophy. *J Eur Acad Dermatol Venereol* 2012;26(Suppl 3):47-51.
12. Levin E, Gupta R, Butler D et al. Topical steroid risk analysis: differentiating between physiologic and pathologic adrenal suppression. *J Dermatolog Treat* 2014;25(6):501-6.
13. Hong E, Smith S , Fischer G. Evaluation of the atrophogenic potential of topical corticosteroids in pediatric dermatology patients. *Pediatr Dermatolo* 2011;28(4):393-6.
14. Tan MH, Meador SL, Singer G et al. An open-label study of the safety and efficacy of limited application of fluticasone propionate ointment, 0.005%, in patients with atopic dermatitis of the face and intertriginous areas. *Int J Dermatol* 2002;41(11):804-9.
15. Charman CR, Morris AD, Williams HC. Topical corticosteroid phobia in patients with atopic eczema. *Br J Dermatol* 2000;142(5):931-6.
16. Hon KL, Pong NH, Poon TC et al. Quality of life and psychosocial issues are important outcome measures in eczema treatment. *J Dermatolog Treat* 2014 Feb 20. [Epub ahead of print].
17. Long CC, Mills CM, Finlay AY. A practical guide to topical therapy in children. *Br J Dermatol* 1998;138(2):293-6.
18. Luger TA, Lahfa M, Folster-Holst R et al. Long-term safety and tolerability of pimecrolimus cream 1% and topical corticosteroids in adults with moderate to severe atopic dermatitis. *J Dermatol Treat* 2004;15(3):169-78.
19. U.S. Food and Drug Administration. Pediatric Advisory Committee. Manthripragada A. *Addendum: Update on calcineurin inhibitor pediatric literature review. Tacrolimus (Protopic) and pimecrolimus (Elidel).* May 10, 2011. Available from: www.fda.gov/downloads/AdvisoryCommittees/CommitteesMeetingMaterials/PediatricAdvisoryCommittee/UCM255140.pdf. Accessed May 14, 2013.
20. Carr WW. Topical calcineurin inhibitors for atopic dermatitis: review and treatment recommendations. *Paediatr Drugs* 2013;15(4):303-10.
21. Iskedjian M, Piwko C, Shear NH et al. Topical calcineurin inhibitors in the treatment of atopic dermatitis: a meta-analysis of current evidence. *Am J Clin Dermatol* 2004;5(4):267-79.
22. Reitamo S, Harper J, Bos JD et al. 0.03% Tacrolimus ointment applied once or twice daily is more efficacious than 1% hydrocortisone acetate in children with moderate to severe atopic dermatitis: results of a randomized double-blind controlled trial. *Br J Dermatol* 2004;150(3):554-62.
23. Reitamo S, Rustin M, Ruzicka T et al. Efficacy and safety of tacrolimus ointment compared with that of hydrocortisone butyrate ointment in adult patients with atopic dermatitis. *J Allergy Clin Immunol* 2002;109(3):547-55.
24. Luger T, Van Leent EJ, Graeber M et al. SDZ ASM 981: an emerging safe and effective treatment for atopic dermatitis. *Br J Dermatol* 2001;144(4):788-94.
25. Spergel JM, Boguniewicz M, Paller AS et al. Addition of topical pimecrolimus to once-daily mid-potent steroid confers no short-term therapeutic benefit in the treatment of severe atopic dermatitis; a randomized controlled trial. *Br J Dermatol* 2007;157(2):378-81.
26. Danby SG, Cork MJ. A new understanding of atopic dermatitis: the role of epidermal barrier dysfunction and subclinical inflammation. *J Clin Dermatol* 2010;1(2):33-46. Available from: content.yudu.com/Library/A1p7hp/DermatologyVolumeIIs/resources/39.htm.

27. Sugarman JL, Parish LC. Efficacy of lipid-based barrier repair formulation in moderate-to-severe pediatric atopic dermatitis. *J Drugs Dermatol* 2009;8(12):1106-11.
28. Miller DW, Koch SB, Yentzer BA et al. An over-the-counter moisturizer is as clinically effective as, and more cost-effective than, prescription barrier creams in the treatment of children with mild-to-moderate atopic dermatitis: a randomized controlled trial. *J Drugs Dermatol* 2011;10(5):531-7.
29. Holten KB; American Academy of Dermatology. How should we care for atopic dermatitis? *J Fam Pract* 2005;54(5):426-7.
30. Breneman D, Fleischer AB, Abramovits W et al. Intermittent therapy for flare prevention and long-term disease control in stabilized atopic dermatitis: a randomized comparison of 3-times-weekly applications of tacrolimus ointment versus vehicle. *J Am Acad Dermatol* 2008;58(6):990-9.
31. Peserico A, Stadtler G, Sebastian M et al. Reduction of relapses of atopic dermatitis with methylprenisolone aceponate cream twice weekly in addition to maintenance treatment with emollient: a multicentre, randomized, double-blind, controlled study. *Br J Dermatol* 2008;158(4):801-7.
32. Berth-Jones J, Damstra RJ, Golsch S et al. Twice weekly fluticasone propionate added to emollient maintenance treatment to reduce risk of relapse in atopic dermatitis: randomised, double blind, parallel group study. *BMJ* 2003;326(7403):1367.
33. Wollenberg A, Reitamo S, Girolomoni G et al. Proactive treatment of atopic dermatitis in adults with 0.1% tacrolimus ointment. *Allergy* 2008;63(7):742-50.
34. Thaci D, Reitamo S, Gonzalez Ensenat MA et al. Proactive disease management with 0.03% tacrolimus ointment for children with atopic dermatitis: results of a randomized, multicentre, comparative study. *Br J Dermatol* 2008;159(6):1348-56.
35. Schmitt J, von Kobyletzki L, Svensson A et al. Efficacy and tolerability of proactive treatment with topical corticosteroids and calcineurin inhibitors for atopic eczema: systematic review and meta-analysis of randomized controlled trials. *Br J Dermatol* 2011;164(2):415-28.
36. Zuberbier T, Brautigam M. Long-term management of facial atopic eczema with pimecrolimus cream 1% in paediatric patients with mild to moderate disease. *J Eur Acad Dermatol Venereol* 2008;22(6):718-21.
37. Gollnick H, Kaufmann R, Stough D et al. Pimecrolimus cream 1% in the long-term management of adult atopic dermatitis: prevention of flare progression. A randomized controlled trial. *Br J Dermatol* 2008;158(5):1083-93.
38. Bath-Hextall FJ, Birnie AJ, Ravenscroft JC et al. Interventions to reduce Staphylococcus aureus in the management of atopic eczema: an updated Cochrane review. *Br J Dermatol* 2010;163(1):12-26.
39. Weatherhead S, Robson SC, Reynolds NJ. Eczema in pregnancy. *BMJ* 2007;335(7611):152-4.
40. Hospira. Methotrexate Tablets USP [product monograph]. In: *Compendium of pharmaceuticals and specialties: the Canadian drug reference for health professionals*. Ottawa (ON): CPhA; 2008.
41. Weber-Schoendorfer C, Hoeltzenbein M, Wacker E et al. No evidence for an increased risk of adverse pregnancy outcome after paternal low-dose methotrexate: an observational cohort study. *Rheumatology (Oxford)* 2014;53(4):757-63.
42. Lam J, Polifka J, Dohil M. Safety of dermatologic drugs used in pregnant patients with psoriasis and other inflammatory skin diseases. *J Am Acad Dermatol* 2008;59(2):295-315.
43. European Dermatology Forum. *Guidelines on steroids in pregnancy*. November 2010. Expiry date: 12/2013. Available from: www.euroderm.org/images/stories/guidelines/EDF-Guideline-on-Steroids-in-Pregnancy.pdf. Accessed May 14, 2013.
44. Drugs and Lactation Database (LactMed). Available from: toxnet.nlm.nih.gov/cgi-bin/sis/htmlgen?LACT. Accessed May 13, 2013.
45. Hale TW. *Medications and mothers' milk: a manual of lactational pharmacology*. 15th ed. Amarillo (TX): Hale Publishing; 2012.

Chapter 90
Bacterial Skin Infections

Peter Green, MD, FRCPC

This chapter addresses the following bacterial skin infections:

Impetigo: Superficial infection of skin primarily caused by *Staphylococcus aureus* and most often affecting young children. Two clinical forms include crusted or nonbullous (*S. aureus* and/or *Streptococcus pyogenes*) and bullous (*S. aureus*-mediated toxin).

Impetiginized: Secondary infection of the skin (most often involving *S. aureus*) resulting from the disrupted barrier function present in underlying inflammatory skin conditions such as atopic dermatitis and allergic contact dermatitis.

Folliculitis: Infection of skin and hair follicle to variable depths producing papules and pustules. Infectious causes include *S. aureus* (most common) and *Pseudomonas aeruginosa.* Noninfectious causes may be termed "pseudofolliculitis" and are induced by friction and/or occlusion.

Furuncle (boil): *S. aureus*-mediated infection of hair follicle with extension of suppurative material into dermis and subcutaneous tissue. Interconnecting multiple furuncles are termed **carbuncles**.

Cutaneous abscess: Deep cutaneous infection harbouring collections of pus that may be polymicrobial or *S. aureus* in origin and located independently of follicular structures.

Cellulitis: Acute onset infection of dermis and subcutaneous tissue characterized by poorly circumscribed bright red erythema, edema, warmth and tenderness caused by either *S. aureus* or beta-hemolytic streptococci in most patients. *Haemophilus influenzae* infection should be suspected in a child under 5 years presenting with facial cellulitis preceded by an upper respiratory tract prodrome, particularly if the child has not been immunized with Haemophilus influenzae B (HiB) vaccine.

Erysipelas: Acute onset infection of skin occurring most commonly on face and lower extremities. Distinguished from cellulitis by more superficial cutaneous involvement, prominent lymphatic involvement, higher risk of recurrence, sharply delineated margins, location, and by pathogen (most commonly *S. pyogenes*).

Necrotizing fasciitis: Limb and life-threatening mono- or polymicrobial infection with resultant tissue necrosis of skin, subcutaneous tissue, fascia and muscle.

Therapeutic Choices

Information on the management of bacterial skin infections can be found in Figure 1, Figure 2, Figure 3 and Figure 4.

Nonpharmacologic Choices

- For primary impetigo or secondarily impetiginized skin, use normal saline compresses for 10–15 minutes 2–3 times per day to expedite removal of crusts and promote healing.
- Address factors contributing to folliculitis in intertriginous areas by eliminating tight-fitting clothing and reducing friction, moisture and heat.
- Ruptured or inflamed epidermal inclusion cysts (often incorrectly called sebaceous cysts) may appear infected or may resemble an abscess given significant erythema and tenderness. Incision

with drainage of cystic contents combined with saline compresses is usually sufficient acute management. Oral antibiotics are reserved for patients with clear signs and symptoms of secondary cellulitis. Definitive treatment includes excision of cystic wall and contents, once inflammatory stage has subsided.

- Isolated uncomplicated abscesses may be treated with incision and drainage alone, even in the setting of methicillin-resistant *S. aureus* (MRSA) infection. Addition of antibiotics should be considered if the area involved is extensive, if there are associated signs and symptoms of cellulitis or if the patient has comorbidities that justify more aggressive treatment.[4]
- If necrotizing infection is suspected, obtain urgent surgical consultation for débridement.
- Use of graduated compression stockings should be considered after cellulitis or erysipelas affecting lower extremities, as nearly all patients will have significant lymphedema. Reducing edema may reduce recurrences of infection.[2]
- Various studies have examined measures to decrease colonization with *S. aureus* in patients with noninfected atopic dermatitis, including the use of "bleach baths."[5] A systematic review of these interventions did not find any evidence of clinical benefit.[6]

Pharmacologic Choices

Systemic Agents (Table 1)

Note that for invasive or life-threatening infections and those not responding to treatment, cultures must be used to guide specific pharmacologic therapy.

- **Penicillinase-resistant penicillins** are commonly used for uncomplicated bacterial skin infections because of their proven efficacy, familiarity and low cost. **First-generation cephalosporins** are also an excellent choice for uncomplicated skin and soft tissue bacterial infections caused by gram-positive organisms. First-generation cephalosporins are preferred over second- or third-generation cephalosporins because of their superior activity against gram-positive organisms.

Figure 1: **Management of Impetigo**[a]

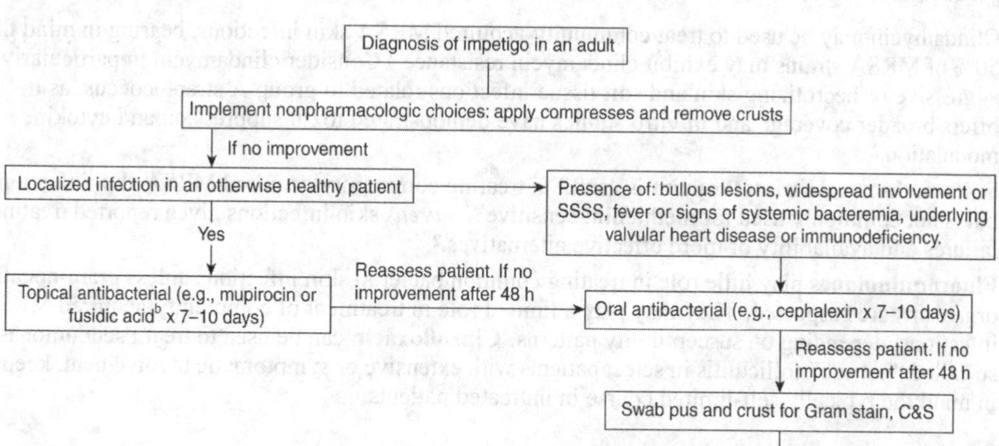

[a] If recurrent impetigo, consider nasal *S. aureus* carriage. Obtain nasal swab and eradicate with mupirocin or fucidin TID intranasally for 3 days.
[b] Fusidic acid and mupirocin are of similar efficacy, and are equally or more effective than oral treatment when disease is not extensive.[1]
Abbreviations: C&S = culture and sensitivity; SSSS = Staphylococcal scalded skin syndrome is suspected when a young child <5 y presents with scarlatiniform erythema accompanied by painful peeling and crusting of skin, most often localized to face and flexural areas (e.g., neck, axilla, groin).

Penicillin monotherapy should not be used for infections where *S. aureus* is suspected, given its resistance to penicillin. Where *S. pyogenes* is the suspected cause of infection (e.g., erysipelas), penicillin is the treatment of choice. In the setting of cellulitis, purulence or unexpected exudate warrants consideration of and coverage for community-acquired MRSA infection.[4]

Penicillin allergy is commonly reported. Administration of **cephalosporins** in these patients should be individualized based on the severity of the reaction to penicillin. Patients with immediate hypersensitivity reactions (e.g., anaphylaxis, bronchospasm, hives) should not receive cephalosporins. Patients with delayed hypersensitivity reactions (rash without hives) have a very low risk of experiencing anaphylaxis with cephalosporins (approximately 1%).[7,8,9]

There is evidence that patients with recurrent cellulitis may experience fewer recurrences over a 12-month period when receiving low-dose penicillin (250 mg BID). However, the protective effect is diminished with discontinuation of penicillin prophylaxis.[10]

Treat soft-tissue infections caused by human or animal bites (e.g., cat, dog) with **amoxicillin/clavulanate**. *Pasteurella multocida* is commonly present in animal bites, and resistance of this organism to cloxacillin, cephalosporins and clindamycin is documented. Second-line therapy with a combination of **clindamycin** plus one of **doxycycline**, **sulfamethoxazole/trimethoprim** or a **fluoroquinolone** can be considered when treatment with amoxicillin/clavulanate is not possible [Evidence: SORT B *].[2,11]

- Macrolide antibiotics (e.g., **erythromycin**) are indicated for gram-positive bacterial skin infections and are frequently used as alternatives to penicillin when patients are penicillin-allergic. Avoid erythromycin if *H. influenzae*-associated cellulitis is suspected, given resistance. Resistance of *S. pyogenes* to erythromycin is emerging.[2]

  Newer macrolide antibiotics (e.g., **azithromycin**, **clarithromycin**) offer more convenient dosing schedules but are more expensive. Both azithromycin and clarithromycin have better bioavailability than erythromycin and provide coverage for *H. influenzae*.
- **Clindamycin** is a reasonable agent for treating serious skin and soft tissue infections in penicillin-allergic patients, notwithstanding the increased risk of *Clostridium difficile* infection and pseudomembranous colitis.

  Clindamycin may be used to treat community-acquired MRSA skin infections, bearing in mind that 50% of MRSA strains may exhibit clindamycin resistance.[2] Consider clindamycin in particularly aggressive or necrotizing skin and soft tissue infections related to group A streptococcus, as it offers broader coverage and in vitro studies have demonstrated toxin suppression and cytokine modulation.[2]
- **Sulfamethoxazole/trimethoprim** is useful in treating community-acquired MRSA skin infections but is not commonly used for methicillin-sensitive *S. aureus* skin infections given reported treatment failures and availability of more effective alternatives.[2]
- **Fluoroquinolones** play little role in treating common bacterial skin infections unless gram-negative organisms are suspected. They may play a limited role in treatment of community-acquired MRSA infections, depending on susceptibility patterns. **Ciprofloxacin** can be used to treat Pseudomonas or so called "hot-tub" folliculitis in select patients with extensive or symptomatic involvement, keeping in mind the typically self-limited course in untreated patients.

---

*SORT (Strength of Recommendation Taxonomy) is a rating system (A, B or C) that addresses the quality of available evidence. For more information consult **How to Use *Compendium of Therapeutic Choices*** on page xxv.

Figure 2: Management of Folliculitis

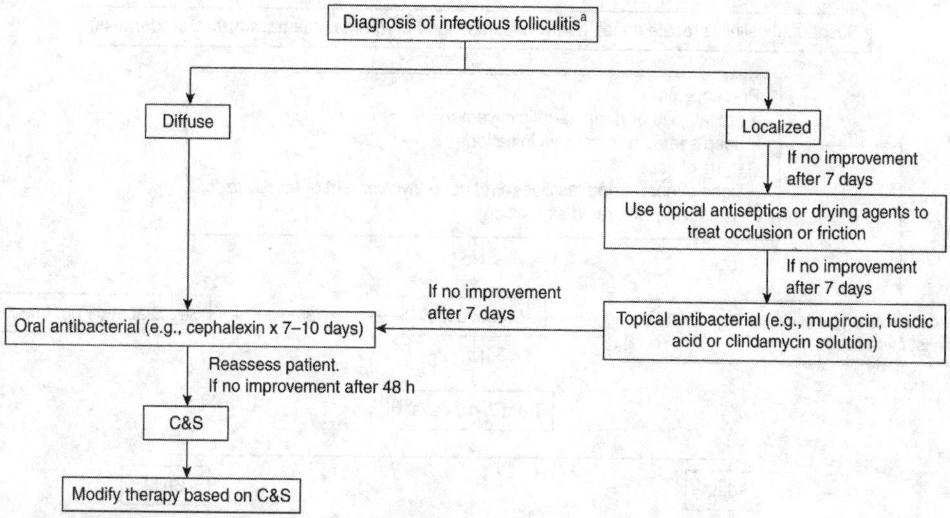

[a] Given the increasing prevalence of community-acquired MRSA skin infections, patients with risk factors who present with recurrent or persistent impetigo and furuncles should have cultures performed to determine antibiotic susceptibilities. Risk factors reported for community-acquired MRSA infection are: incarcerated prisoners, iv drug users, Native Americans, homosexual men, participants in contact sports and children.[2]

Abbreviations: C&S = culture and sensitivity

Figure 3: Management of Erysipelas

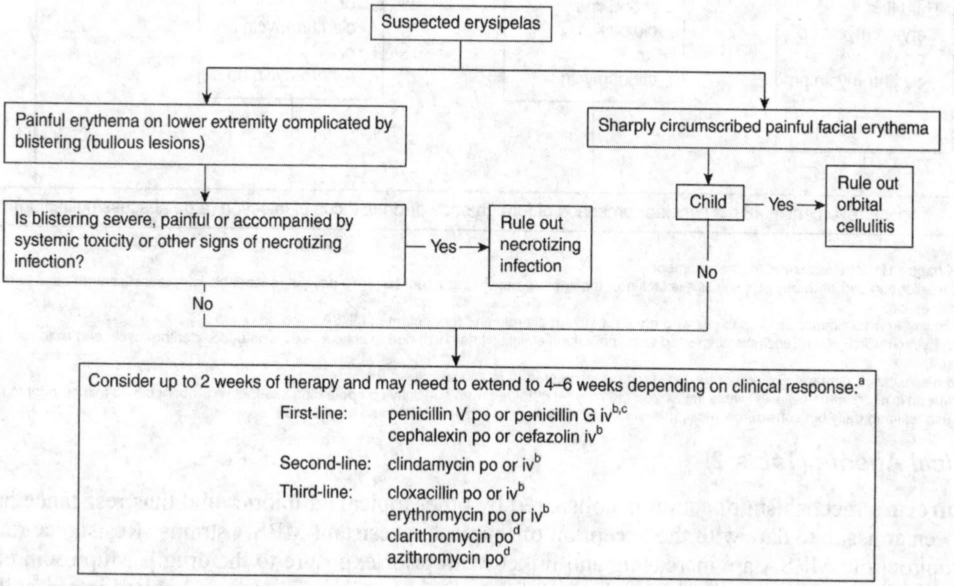

[a] Duration of treatment for erysipelas is usually longer than for cellulitis given lymphatic involvement and higher rate of recurrence.

[b] IV route to be used in severe cases: signs of systemic toxicity (e.g., heart rate >100, hypotension, fever); severe pain; rapid progression; blistering; comorbid conditions.[2]

[c] Vancomycin iv is recommended in patients who are beta-lactam allergic or who do not respond to therapy.

[d] Organisms resistant to erythromycin will also be resistant to clindamycin, clarithromycin and azithromycin.

Figure 4: **Management of Cellulitis**

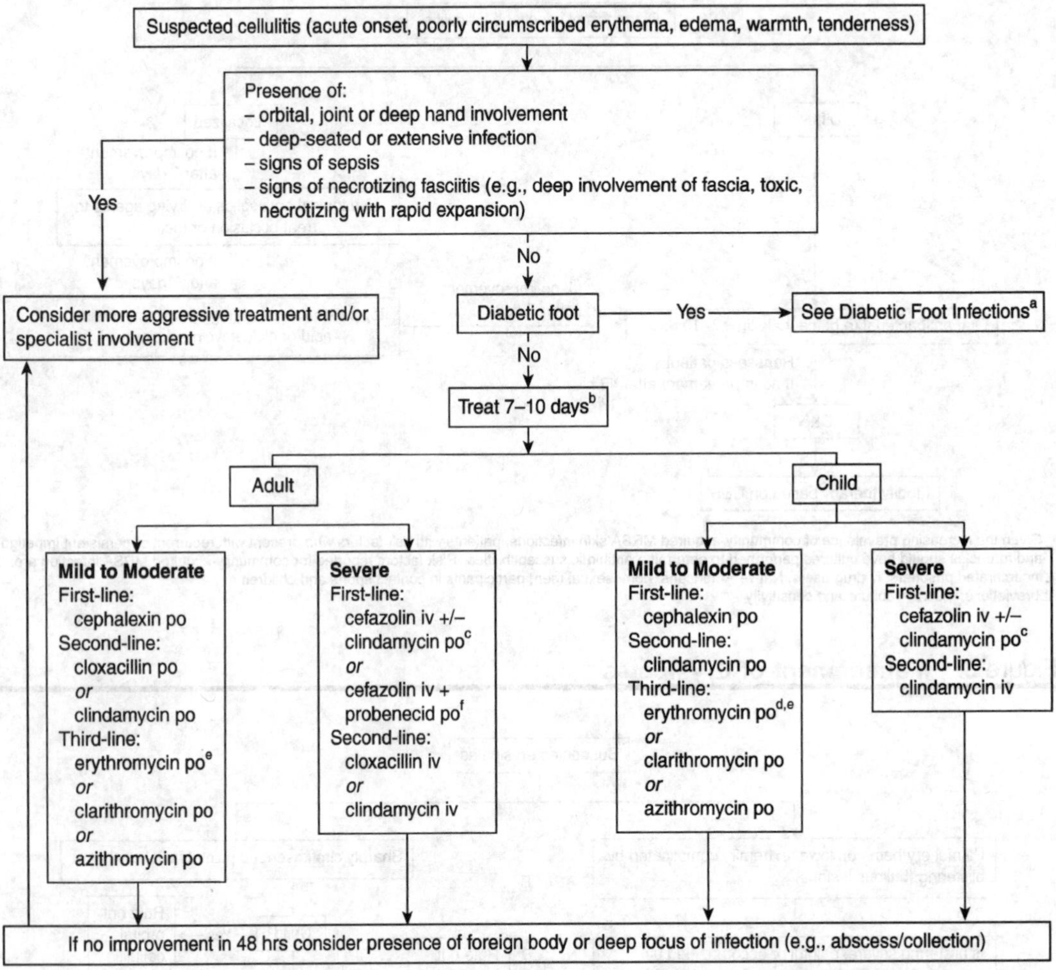

[a] See Chapter 111 for information on management.

[b] Evidence for duration of therapy for cellulitis is lacking,[3] though in practice, treatment for 7–10 days is reasonable with reassessment based on clinical response.

[c] Vancomycin iv is recommended in patients who are beta-lactam allergic and for confirmed MRSA infection.

[d] Avoid erythromycin if *H. influenzae* is suspected (e.g., periorbital cellulitis in a child) due to concerns of resistance: clarithromycin and azithromycin may be used.

[e] Avoid macrolides if *Group A Streptococcus* resistance is suspected or is a local issue.

[f] Probenecid is not commercially available in Canada but may be obtained from specialty compounding sites. Give probenecid 30 min po *prior* to cefazolin. May use regimen daily but consider increasing frequency to BID if not improving or if worse after 48 h.

Topical Agents (Table 2)

Mupirocin's mechanism of action is not shared by other topical antibiotics and thus resistance has not been an issue to date with the exception of mupirocin-resistant MRSA strains. Resistance rates to mupirocin in MRSA are increasing and linked with prior exposure to the drug.[12] Mupirocin is particularly useful for localized impetigo and folliculitis caused by *S. aureus*. Applied intranasally, it can be used to eradicate *S. aureus* nasal carriage.[12] See Figure 1.

Fusidic acid, like mupirocin, can be used to treat localized skin infections where oral therapy is not indicated. There are reports of increasing resistance of *S. aureus* to fusidic acid; therefore, it should only be used for appropriate indications and for brief, defined treatment courses.[13]

Numerous nonprescription proprietary preparations containing antibiotics with both gram-positive and gram-negative coverage are available (e.g., **bacitracin**, **gramicidin**, **polymyxin B**). These agents have limited efficacy for bacterial skin infections and are best used for prevention of infection and/or wound healing in minor cuts or abrasions.[12]

Silver sulfadiazine was previously believed to play a role in reducing microbes in wounds and burns. However, despite limitations in available evidence, there appears to be a risk of delayed wound healing associated with silver sulfadiazine, such that alternative wound regimens should be considered when feasible.[14]

Choices during Pregnancy and Breastfeeding

Skin Infections and Pregnancy/Postpartum Period

Indications and treatment principles for bacterial skin infections in pregnancy are similar to those for nonpregnant patients, with avoidance of oral antimicrobials known to have teratogenic risk. Pregnancy may exacerbate chronic folliculitis.

Pre-pregnancy Considerations

Women considering conception must discontinue potentially teratogenic antibiotics (e.g., tetracycline) if these are taken chronically to manage MRSA or folliculitis. Advise women with recurrent folliculitis of unknown origin to obtain bacterial swabs to rule out community-acquired MRSA, the presence of which would require appropriate counselling for management during pregnancy. Ensure skin therapy is optimized for patients with underlying skin disease (e.g., atopic dermatitis) who are prone to secondary skin infection.

Management during Pregnancy and Postpartum Period

Nonpharmacologic choices are important in preventing the spread of confirmed staphylococcal or MRSA skin infections in either the patient or a family member. General measures such as contact avoidance, not sharing personal items, avoiding contact with bandages or wounds of the infected individual and appropriate hand washing reduce risk of transmission. Nonprescription topical antibiotic combinations (e.g., **bacitracin**, **polymyxin B** and **gramicidin**) have been used for prevention of infection of minor cuts and abrasions for many years with no reports of congenital malformations.[15,16] There is little information available on safety in pregnancy of the topical antibiotics used for localized skin infections. **Mupirocin** is not expected to pose any risk to the fetus based on animal data and its very limited absorption with topical use.[17] The manufacturer states that there is some evidence that systemic **fusidic acid** crosses the placental barrier[18] but no reports of teratogenicity have been found. For confirmed bacterial infections requiring systemic antibacterial agents, **penicillins**, **cephalosporins**, **clindamycin** and **erythromycin** (with the exception of the estolate salt) can all be used safely during pregnancy.[16,19]

Management during Breastfeeding

Topical **mupirocin** for localized skin infections may be used safely during breastfeeding since very limited amounts are absorbed.[20,21] **Fusidic acid** is detectable in human milk after systemic use.[18] No information on safety of topical use by a breastfeeding mother is available; however, fusidic acid is used systemically in infants.[22] As a general precaution, direct skin-to-skin contact of the breastfeeding infant with the treated skin area of the mother should be avoided with topical use of any medication. If a breastfeeding mother develops cutaneous infection requiring oral antibiotics, **penicillins**,

cephalosporins and **erythromycin** may be used safely but may alter bowel flora of the infant and rarely may cause hypersensitivity.[19] With any wound, care should be taken to prevent contact with the nursing infant. Ensure the wound is covered and appropriate hand washing takes place after contact with potentially contaminated materials.

A discussion of general principles on the use of medications in these special populations can be found in Appendix II and Appendix III. Other specialized reference sources are also provided in these appendices.

Therapeutic Tips

- When assessing patients with atopic dermatitis, determine whether significant secondary infection due to *S. aureus* is present. This will manifest as crusting, weeping, painful fissured eczema or nonhealing erosions and crusts. Treating the secondary impetiginization is vital for providing symptom relief and control of the eczema.
- If a patient presents with symptoms and signs of a lower extremity cellulitis that is complicated by fluid-filled blisters and copious, clear, serous discharge, consider bullous erysipelas and ensure adequate coverage of *S. pyogenes*.
- Any limb cellulitis or serious soft tissue infection that manifests with blisters and/or necrosis, "dusky gray" appearance, severe pain, gas in soft tissue, numbness, exceptionally rapid spread or systemic toxicity should prompt urgent consideration and investigation for necrotizing fasciitis.
- In patients with recurrent painful, sterile abscesses and scarring in the axillae and groin, consider the possibility of hidradenitis suppurativa and refer for appropriate specialist care, e.g., dermatology or plastic surgery.
- Avoid prolonged use of topical antibacterials (>2 weeks) to prevent development of bacterial resistance.
- Given increasing reports of community-acquired MRSA, patients with recurrent impetigo or furuncles should have swabs to rule out MRSA, particularly if risk factors (Figure 2) are identified.[2] Similarly, presence of purulent drainage in the setting of cellulitis should prompt empiric treatment for MRSA.
- In patients receiving anti-TNF therapies, maintain increased vigilance for skin and soft tissue infections, a known complication of these agents.
- Avoid routine topical antibiotics in the management of chronic wounds such as venous stasis ulcers. Overuse may lead to resistance and possible allergic contact dermatitis.

Table 1: Antibiotics Used to Treat Bacterial Skin Infections

Class	Drug	Dose[a]	Adverse Effects[b]	Drug Interactions[b]	Cost[c]
Cephalosporins, first-generation	*cefadroxil* generics	Adults: 1 g daily po	Hypersensitivity reactions (ranging from minor rashes to anaphylactic shock), some cross-reactivity with penicillins. Nausea, vomiting, diarrhea.	Probenecid prolongs cephalosporin serum levels.	$
	cefazolin generics	Adults: 1 g Q8H iv Children: 50–100 mg/kg/day divided Q8H iv	See cefadroxil. Rash, increased AST and ALP, phlebitis.	See cefadroxil.	$$$
	cephalexin generics	Adults: 250–500 mg Q6H po Children: 25–50 mg/kg/day divided Q6H po	See cefadroxil.	See cefadroxil.	$
Fluoroquinolones	*ciprofloxacin* Cipro, generics	Adults: 500–750 mg BID po	Nausea, vomiting, diarrhea, abdominal pain, prolongation of QT_c interval, photosensitivity reactions, CNS stimulation, tendon inflammation or rupture.	Antacids and sucralfate decrease absorption of ciprofloxacin. Use cautiously with other drugs that cause QT_c prolongation. Inhibits cytochrome P450 enzyme system leading to many drug interactions (e.g., increased effects/toxicity of carbamazepine, cyclosporine).	$
Glycopeptides	*vancomycin* generics	Adults: 1 g Q12H iv Children: 40 mg/kg/day divided Q6H iv	Hypotension, flushing, red man syndrome, chills, drug fever, eosinophilia.	Increased toxicity with other nephrotoxic or ototoxic drugs.	~$900
Lincosamides	*clindamycin* Dalacin C, Dalacin C Flavored Granules, Dalacin-C Phosphate Sterile Solution, generics	Adults: 150–300 mg Q6H po or 450–600 mg Q8H iv Children: (>1 month) 10–30 mg/kg/day divided Q6H po	Diarrhea, *C. difficile* infection.[d]	Decreases effect of erythromycin.	po: $ iv: $$$$

(cont'd)

Table 1: Antibiotics Used to Treat Bacterial Skin Infections *(cont'd)*

Class	Drug	Dose[a]	Adverse Effects[b]	Drug Interactions[b]	Cost[c]
Macrolides	*azithromycin* Zithromax, Zmax SR, generics	Adults: 500 mg po on day 1, then 250 mg on days 2–5 (total 1.5 g) Children: 10 mg/kg/day on first day then 5 mg/kg po × 4 days	GI irritation (common), nausea and vomiting, diarrhea. Mild allergic reactions (serious reactions rare). QT_c interval prolongation	Appears less likely to cause interactions than other macrolides. Use cautiously with other drugs that cause QT_c prolongation.	$
	clarithromycin Biaxin, generics	Adults: 250–500 mg Q12H po Children: 15 mg/kg/day divided Q12H po	See azithromycin.	Inhibits cytochrome P450 enzyme system leading to many drug interactions (e.g., increased effects/toxicity of carbamazepine, cyclosporine). Use cautiously with other drugs that cause QT_c prolongation.	$
	erythromycin Eryc, generics	Adults: 250 mg Q6H po 500 mg Q6H iv Children: 30–50 mg/kg/day divided Q6H po	See azithromycin. Cholestatic jaundice with erythromycin estolate (rare).	See clarithromycin.	$
Penicillinase-resistant Penicillins	*cloxacillin* generics	Adults: 250–500 mg Q6H po Children: 25–50 mg/kg/day divided Q6H po	See penicillin V.	See penicillin V. Increases effect of warfarin.	$
Penicillin, Beta-lactamase Inhibitor Combinations	*amoxicillin/clavulanate* Clavulin, generics	Adults: 250–500 mg Q8H po Children: 40 mg/kg/day of amoxicillin divided Q8H po	See penicillin V.	See penicillin V.	$
Penicillins	*penicillin V* generics	Adults: 300 mg Q6H po Children: 25–50 mg/kg/day divided Q6–8H po	Hypersensitivity reactions (ranging from minor rashes to anaphylactic shock). Nausea, vomiting, diarrhea.	Probenecid prolongs penicillin serum levels. Increases methotrexate levels.	$

Class	Drug	Dose[a]	Adverse Effects[b]	Drug Interactions[b]	Cost[c]
	penicillin G ❥ Crystapen, generics	Adults: 2 million units Q4–6H iv	See penicillin V. Electrolyte imbalance possible with high-dose penicillin G Na^+ or K^+ (>10 million IU/day).	See penicillin V.	$$$
Sulfonamide Combinations	*sulfamethoxazole/ trimethoprim* ❥ generics	Adults: 1–2 DS tablets (800 mg/160 mg–1600/320 mg) BID po	Nausea, vomiting, diarrhea, rash, neutropenia, thrombocytopenia, anemia.	Increases phenytoin levels. Increases effect of warfarin. Hypoglycemia with sulfonylureas.	$

[a] Pediatric dose should not exceed recommended adult dose.
[b] Only select adverse effects/drug interactions are listed; consult product monograph for complete list.
[c] Cost of 7-day supply based on 20 kg body weight for cost of children's dose; includes drug cost only.
[d] Commonly associated with clindamycin but any antibiotic may cause this complication.
❥ Dosage adjustment may be required in renal impairment; see Appendix I.
Legend: $ <$30 $$ $30-60 $$$ $60-90 $$$$ $90–120

Table 2: Topical Antibacterials Used in Superficial Bacterial Skin Infections

Class	Drug	Dose	Antibacterial Spectrum	Adverse Effects	Cost[a]
Aminoglycosides	*framycetin* Sofra-Tulle dressing	BID–TID	*S. aureus*, *streptococci*, gram-negative organisms.	Allergic contact dermatitis, cross-reaction with neomycin.	$$$ (10 × 10 cm dressing, package of 10)
Antibacterial Combinations	*polymyxin B with gramicidin or bacitracin* Polysporin cream or ointment, generics	BID–TID	Gram-negative organisms.	Nephrotoxicity when used extensively, allergic contact dermatitis.	$[b]
Lincosamides	*clindamycin 1% topical solution* Dalacin T Topical Solution, generics	BID	Gram-positive cocci; anaerobic gram-positive and gram-negative organisms.	Local irritation. *C. difficile* infection reported (extremely rare).	$$ (30 mL bottle)
Miscellaneous Antibacterials	*bacitracin* Bacitracin, generics	BID–TID	Gram-positive organisms.	Allergic contact dermatitis, anaphylactic reactions following topical application (rare).	$[b]
	fusidic acid Fucidin Cream	BID–TID	Gram-positive organisms.	Allergic contact dermatitis (rare).	$$
	mupirocin Bactroban Ointment, generics	BID–TID	*S. aureus*, *S. epidermidis*, *S. pyogenes*, MRSA.	Stinging, allergic contact dermatitis (rare).	$$[b]
Sulfonamides	*silver sulfadiazine* Flamazine	BID–TID	*S. aureus*, gram-negative organisms, *Pseudomonas*.	Allergic contact dermatitis, leukopenia when applied to large area of burned skin. Possible delayed wound healing.[14]	$

[a] Cost of 15 g tube unless otherwise specified; includes drug cost only.
[b] Available without prescription; retail mark-up not included.
Legend: $ <$5 $$ $5–10 $$$ $10–15

Suggested Readings

Craft N, Lee P, Zipoli M et al. Superficial cutaneous infections and pyodermas. In: Goldsmith LA et al., eds. *Fitzpatrick's dermatology in general medicine*. 8th ed. New York (NY): McGraw-Hill; 2012. p. 2128-47.

Rajan S. Skin and soft-tissue infections: classifying and treating a spectrum. *Cleve Clin J Med* 2012;79(1):57-66.

Stevens DL, Bisno AL, Chambers HF et al. Practice guidelines for the diagnosis and management of skin and soft-tissue infections. *Clin Infect Dis* 2005;41(10):1373-406.

References

1. Koning S, van der Sande R, Verhagen AP et al. Interventions for impetigo. *Cochrane Database Syst Rev* 2012;1:CD003261.
2. Stevens DL, Bisno AL, Chambers HF et al. Practice guidelines for the diagnosis and management of skin and soft-tissue infections. *Clin Infect Dis* 2005;41(10):1373-406.
3. Kilburn SA, Featherstone P, Higgins B et al. Interventions for cellulitis and erysipelas. *Cochrane Database Syst Rev* 2010;(6):CD004299.
4. Liu C, Bayer A, Cosgrove SE et al Clinical practice guidelines by the Infectious Diseases Society of America for the treatment of methicillin-resistant Staphylococcus aureus infections in adults and children. *Clin Infect Dis* 2011;52(3):e18-55.
5. Huang JT, Abrams M, Tlougan B et al. Treatment of Staphylococcus aureus colonization in atopic dermatitis decreases disease severity. *Pediatrics* 2009;123(5):e808-14.
6. Bath-Hextall FJ, Birnie AJ, Ravenscroft JC et al. Interventions to reduce Staphylococcus aureus in the management of atopic eczema: an updated Cochrane review. *Br J Dermatol* 2010;163(1):12-26.
7. Campagna JD, Bond MC, Schabelman E et al. The use of cephalosporins in penicillin-allergic patients: a literature review. *J Emerg Med* 2012;42(5):612-20.
8. Daulat S, Solensky R, Earl HS et al. Safety of cephalosporin administration to patients with histories of penicillin allergy. *J Allergy Clin Immunol* 2004;113(6):1220-2.
9. Goodman EJ, Morgan MJ, Johnson PA et al. Cephalosporins can be given to penicillin-allergic patients who do not exhibit an anaphylactic response. *J Clin Anesth* 2001;13(8):561-4.
10. Thomas KS, Crook AM, Nunn AJ et al. Penicillin to prevent recurrent leg cellulitis. *N Engl J Med* 2013;368(18):1695-703.
11. Anti-infective Review Panel. *Anti-infective guidelines for community-acquired infections*. Toronto (ON): MUMS Guidelines Clearinghouse; 2012.
12. Motaparthis K, Hsu S. Topical antibacterial agents. In: Wolverton SE, ed. *Comprehensive dermatologic drug therapy*. 3rd ed. Philadelphia (PA): Saunders; 2013. p. 445-59.
13. Dobie D, Gray J. Fusidic acid resistance in Staphylococcus aureus. *Arch Dis Child* 2004;89(1):74-7.
14. Wasiak J, Cleland H, Campbell F et al. Dressings for superficial and partial thickness burns. *Cochrane Database Syst Rev* 2013;3:CD002106.
15. e-CPS. Ottawa (ON): Canadian Pharmacists Association; 2010. *Polysporin* [product monograph]. Available from: www.e-therapeutics.ca. Subscription required.
16. Lee K, Leachman S. Dermatologic drugs during pregnancy and lactation. In: Wolverton SE, ed. *Comprehensive dermatologic drug therapy*. 3rd ed. Philadelphia (PA): Saunders; 2013. p. 718-29.
17. Briggs GG, Freeman RK, Yaffe SJ. *Drugs in pregnancy and lactation: a reference guide to fetal and neonatal risk*. 9th ed. Philadelphia (PA): Wolters Kluwer Health; Lippincott Williams & Wilkins; 2011.
18. Leo Pharma. *Product monograph: Fucidin*. Ajax (ON): Leo Pharma; 1985.
19. Diav-Citrin O, Koren G. Drug use during pregnancy. In: Jovaisas B, ed. *Compendium of pharmaceuticals and specialties: Canada's trusted drug reference*. Ottawa (ON): CPhA; 2014. p. L10-3.
20. Drugs and Lactation Database (LactMed). *Mupirocin*. Bethesda (MD): National Library of Medicine. Available from: toxnet.nlm.nih.gov/. Accessed October 24, 2013.
21. Hale TW. *Medications and mothers' milk: a manual of lactational pharmacology*. 13th ed. Amarillo (TX): Hale Publishing; 2012.
22. Mandell GL, Douglas RG, Bennett JE et al., eds. *Mandell, Douglas and Bennett's principles and practice of infectious diseases*. 6th ed. Philadelphia (PA): Elsevier Churchill Livingstone; 2005.

Chapter 91
Burns

David Warren, MD, FRCPC

Goals of Therapy

- Provide early management of serious burns to reduce associated morbidity and mortality
- Ensure patients with severe and complicated burns are referred to appropriate specialized centres
- Optimize cosmetic results and minimize functional morbidity of burns
- Provide appropriate analgesia, burn wound management and follow-up

Investigations

- A thorough history of the burn injury with special attention to:
  - burning agent and its temperature and duration of exposure
  - circumstances of fire—open vs. enclosed space, explosion, fall, electrical or chemical exposure
  - past medical history, medications and status of tetanus immunization
- Physical examination:
  - general physical examination with attention initially to airway, breathing and circulation
  - head to toe examination to assess for other systemic or musculoskeletal injuries
  - presence of headache, irritability, nausea, confusion, agitation and uncoordination, which may indicate carbon monoxide poisoning
  - assess for pulmonary complications. Upper airway edema may occur from direct thermal injury, especially with steam. Smoke inhalation doubles the mortality risk of a burn from systemic and direct toxicant effects to the airway. Indicators include fire in an enclosed space, inhalation of noxious fumes, facial burns, pharyngeal burns, carbonaceous sputum, hoarseness, elevated carboxyhemoglobin >5% and abnormal pulmonary function. Pulmonary edema may be an early or late finding. Anticipate possible sudden cardiovascular collapse.
  - assess depth of wound (Table 1)
  - triage patients for inpatient, referral or outpatient care
  - assess the extent of the burn quantified as the percentage of total body surface area (BSA). The palm size of the victim is approximately 1% BSA, or estimate following the rule of nines (Figure 1)
  - some burns, due to their extent or potential morbidity, should be considered for referral to a burn centre or specialized care (Table 2). Transfer should be facilitated by contact between physicians. All pertinent documentation, tests, flow sheets and transfer records should accompany the patient
- Laboratory tests in moderate and severe burns:
  - CBC, electrolytes, glucose, BUN, creatinine, blood type and clotting studies
  - ethanol and drug toxicology if warranted
  - carboxyhemoglobin level and other toxins in suspected inhalation injuries
  - urinalysis: if urine positive for blood or if burn >30% BSA, measure urine myoglobin
  - arterial blood gas and chest radiograph; often normal early with findings 6–24 hours later

Table 1: **Burn Depth Classification**

Degree[1]	Class	Description	Example	Healing Time
First	Superficial	Involves epidermis: skin red and painful	Sunburn	7 days
Second	Superficial partial thickness	Epidermis and upper dermis: blisters, underlying skin red and moist, very painful	Scald with water	10–21 days
	Deep partial thickness	Epidermis and deep dermis: some hair follicle and sweat gland damage, blisters, broad epidermal skin loss, painful	Flame, oil	>14 days, some scarring
Third	Full thickness	Epidermis through dermis to subcutaneous fat: skin pale, painless, leathery	Flame, hot metal	Will not heal—results in scarring; surgery ± grafts

Figure 1: **Rule of Nines Estimation of Body Surface Area for Child and Adult**

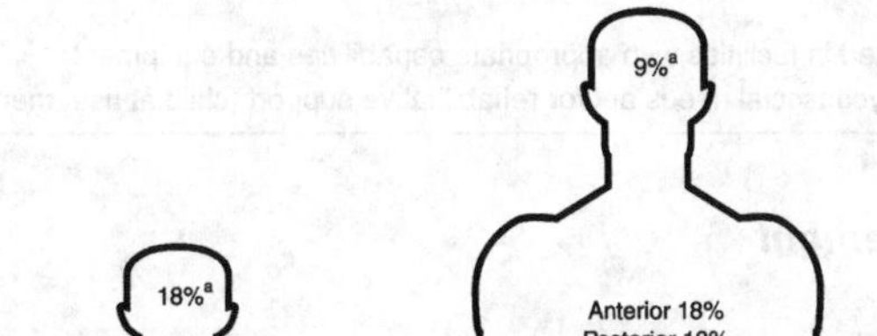

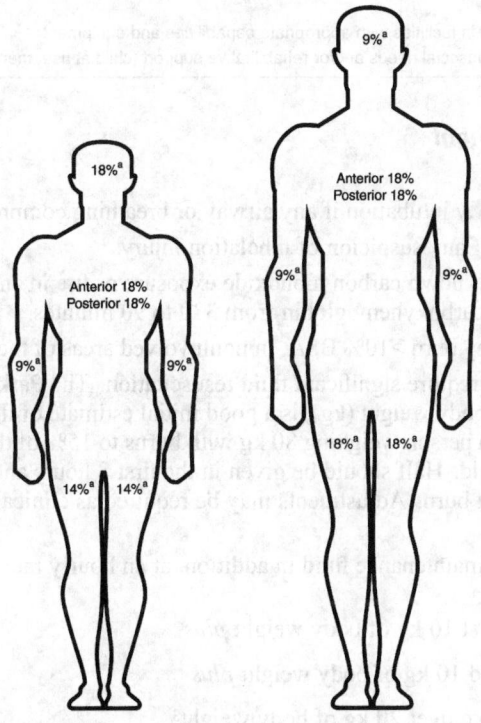

[a] Includes both anterior and posterior aspects.

Therapeutic Choices

Nonpharmacologic Choices

Initial First Aid Management

- Remove the victim from the source of injury, taking care to limit risk to rescuers in electrical and chemical burn injuries.
- Remove any burning clothing or hot material.

- Cool the burn appropriately by running lukewarm water over the area.
- Assess airway, breathing and circulation (ABC).
- In chemical exposures, copiously irrigate burn region with lukewarm water until testing demonstrates a normal tissue pH. Prolonged irrigation is often needed with alkali burns.
- Cover the exposed area with a clean cloth soaked in cool water. Avoid hypothermia in young infants and in extensive burns. Avoid putting ice or home remedies on burns.
- Cover with clean dry cloth on transport to hospital.

Table 2: **Criteria for Referral or Transfer to a Burn Centre**[2]

- Partial thickness burn >10% BSA if patient <10 y or >50 y
- Partial thickness burns >20% BSA in other age groups
- Partial and full thickness burns involving the face, eyes, ears, hands, feet, perineum or overlying major joints
- Full thickness burns >5% BSA
- Significant chemical or electrical burns
- Inhalation injuries
- Patients with pre-existing illness likely to complicate recovery
- Patients with concomitant trauma should be initially treated in an appropriate trauma setting and subsequently transferred to a burn centre
- Children should be treated in facilities with appropriate capabilities and equipment
- Patients with special psychosocial needs and/or rehabilitative support (child abuse, mental health needs, drug addiction)

Initial Medical Management

- Assess ABC.
- Consider the need for early intubation if any airway or breathing compromise.
- Use humidified oxygen if any suspicion of inhalation injury.
- Employ oxygen 100% if known carbon monoxide exposure or fire in an enclosed space. This will decrease the half-life of carboxyhemoglobin from 330 to 90 minutes.
- Establish iv access for any burn >10% BSA, in noninvolved areas of the upper body if possible.
- Major burns will always require significant fluid resuscitation. The Parkland formula, 4 mL × total burn surface area (%) × body weight (kg), is a good initial estimate of fluid requirements in the first 24 hours. For example, a person weighing 80 kg with burns to 15% of the body would require 4 mL × 15 × 80 = 4800 mL fluid. Half should be given in the first 8 hours and the remainder over the subsequent 16 hours post burn. Adjustments may be required as clinical assessment and urinary output indicate.
- Children should receive maintenance fluid in addition, at an hourly rate of:

    4 mL/kg for the first 10 kg of body weight *plus*

    2 mL/kg for second 10 kg of body weight *plus*

    1 mL/kg for each kg over 20 kg of body weight[3]

- Nasogastric tube drainage for ileus is likely in any major burn.
- Bladder catheterization to monitor appropriate urinary output, minimum 0.5 mL/kg/h (children <25 kg: 1 mL/kg/h).[4]
- Elevate any encircling limb burn and closely assess for neurovascular status. Assess chest burns for restriction of normal excursion and pulmonary compromise. Consider surgical escharotomy as required.

- Ensure adequate tetanus prophylaxis; 0.5 mL **tetanus toxoid** in previously immunized patient with additional 250 units **tetanus immune globulin** if *not* previously immunized.

Burn Wound Management

- Remove any attached clothing and loose tissue.
- Gently wash the burn surface with sterile water or normal saline.
- Débride open blisters and loose tissue.
- Use petroleum-based ointments such as **bacitracin/gramicidin/polymyxin B** to act as emulsifying agents to remove tar.[5]
- For information on the use of topical antibiotics in burn wound infections, see Pharmacologic Choices.

Dressings (Table 3)

Most commonly used are **semi-closed dressings** which permit ambulatory management while maintaining hygiene, limiting mobilization and preventing tampering with the wound. After cleansing the wound with saline irrigation or antiseptic solution apply the dressing, which consists of:

- an innermost dressing layer of porous mesh gauze impregnated with nonpetroleum-based water-soluble lubricant or antibiotic;
- a second layer of bulky, fluffed coarse mesh gauze to absorb exudate and protect the wound;
- an outer layer of semi-elastic coarse mesh, which provides moderate pressure to keep the dressing in place but should not be constrictive.

Change semi-closed dressings every other day, daily or twice daily depending on the wound, amount of exudate, antibiotic use and the patient.

Open therapy is often used on the head, neck and perineum, which are areas that are difficult to dress and prone to maceration.

Numerous commercially available dressing products are manufactured. They may provide benefits in specific burn indications, in ease of application and in suitability for home use. See Table 3.

Semisynthetic occlusive dressings (wound pads, hydrocolloids, polyurethane films) offer an alternative for flat partial thickness burns. Removal, cleansing and redressing are required if fluid collects beneath the dressing; otherwise, remove at 7–10 days.

Moisture retentive dressings (hydrogels, biosynthetic skin substitutes, antimicrobial silver-containing) are designed to lock exudates away from the wound, reducing maceration.[6,7] They can be used in mild and moderate thickness burns. Studies of effects on healing and infection prevention are limited, and no firm conclusions can be reached regarding the efficacy of specific dressings.[8] Use of these products includes the following steps in conjunction with the manufacturer's product-specific instructions:

- Cleanse and débride wound, moisten as directed if dry.
- Cover wound with dressing sheets, extending dressing beyond wound edges; trim as required.
- Cover dressing with sterile gauze.
- Cover may be removed periodically to inspect wound, but leave dressing in place for 3–14 days as per product directions.
- Trim dressing as it detaches; inspect frequently if any signs of infection.

Table 3: **Wound Dressings Used for the Treatment of Burns**

Class	Use	Comments	Cost[a]
Wound pads e.g., gauze and tulle	Minimal superficial wounds.	Pads applied directly to wound.	$
Hydrocolloid e.g., Comfeel, Duoderm, Nu-derm	Minimally exudative superficial wounds.	Gel facilitates autolytic debridement of wound.	$$
Polyurethane film e.g., Opsite, Tegaderm	Lightly exudative wounds.	Easy application. No antimicrobial coverage. Can be left in place for days if no underlying exudate.	$$
Hydrogel e.g., Intrasite, Soluge	Moderately exudative wounds.	Evidence of faster healing over routine dressings.[8] Available as amorphous gel or in sheet form.	$
Biosynthetic skin substitutes e.g., Biobrane	Large burns and skin graft donor sites.	Mimic function of skin. No improvement of healing over routine dressings.[8]	~$600/ box of 5
Antimicrobial, silver-containing e.g., Acticoat, Aquacel Ag, Mepilex Ag	Moderately exudative wounds.	Moisten dressing as directed. Fewer dressing changes: application for 3–14 days.	$$-$$$
Fibre e.g., Algenite, Biatain, Kaltostat, Melgisorb	Moderate to heavily exudative wounds.	May be washed off (less painful).	$$
Silicone-coated nylon e.g., Mepitel	Nonadherent dressing layer used as adjunct to assist dressing changes.	Decreases new tissue damage during dressing changes.	$$

[a] Cost of smallest available pack size; includes dressing cost only.
Legend: $ <$25 $$ $25–50 $$-$$$ $25–75 $$$ $50–75

Pharmacologic Choices

- Avoid prophylactic oral and parenteral antibiotics in all but exceptional circumstances to avoid development of resistant infections.
- **Topical antibiotics** have been routinely used for the initial management of burns,[4] although there is significant debate as to their efficacy in this setting.[9] There is no convincing evidence to support use of one topical antibiotic over another.[10] However, it may be prudent to avoid silver sulfadiazine if feasible, based on limited but consistent evidence that it is associated with poorer healing outcomes in superficial and partial thickness burns when compared to various types of dressings [Evidence: SORT B*].[8] Using sterile technique, apply topical antibiotic to approximately 2 mm thick twice daily, or as required if rubbed off. Cleanse the wound prior to reapplication. Information on various agents with specific indications and limitations can be found in Table 4. Choice of product is often based on cost and ease of use (petrolatum-based preparations spread more readily).
- A systematic review found inconclusive evidence of whether **aloe vera** gel or dressings improve outcomes for acute wounds including burns.[11]

Pain Management

- **Topical anesthetics** have been used to provide temporary pain relief. Evidence for efficacy is lacking. **Lidocaine** and **benzocaine** are common causes of contact dermatitis, while **pramoxine** has low sensitizing potential. There is a risk of systemic absorption and toxicity if local anesthetics are applied to blistered or large areas of skin.

* SORT (Strength of Recommendation Taxonomy) is a rating system (A, B or C) that addresses the quality of available evidence. For more information consult **How to Use *Compendium of Therapeutic Choices*** on page xxv.

- **NSAIDs** manage pain in minor burns and suppress the inflammatory response in major burns. Use standard doses for soft tissue injury given on a regular basis (e.g., **ibuprofen** 400 mg (10 mg/kg in children) every 4–6 hours).
- Potent analgesia with small aliquots of IV opioids (e.g., **morphine** 0.1–0.15 mg/kg iv or **fentanyl** 0.5–1 μg/kg iv), titrated to effect, is often required initially to manage pain related to burns. Avoid sc and im administration, as peripheral vasoconstriction and generalized interstitial edema inhibit absorption and can lead to overdose of the opioid as circulation improves.[12]
- Take care not to initially suppress the signs of other injuries with analgesia.
- Sedation and/or coanalgesia may be helpful in the follow-up stage of severe burn management after initial stabilization is achieved.
- Children especially require analgesia to manage their burns.
- Longer term and outpatient analgesia can be achieved with oral NSAIDs, and/or opioids as required.

Choices during Pregnancy and Breastfeeding

Burns and Pregnancy

In general, pregnancy does not negatively affect maternal outcomes following a minor burn injury.[13] Fetal outcomes correspond to maternal well-being.[14]

Management during Pregnancy

Any significant burn in a pregnant patient should be referred to an appropriate burn centre with obstetrical support as fluid management and oxygen delivery issues are considerable. Management of less severe burns (those not requiring transfer or referral) should be the same as for those who are not pregnant[13,14] with the additional consideration of the effect of any drugs used on the fetus.

Nonprescription topical antibiotics containing **bacitracin** have been used for many years with no reports of congenital malformations.[15,16] Very limited amounts of **mupirocin** are absorbed after topical use[17] and there are no reports of teratogenicity.[16] There is some evidence that systemic **fusidic acid** crosses the placental barrier[18] but there are no reports of teratogenicity.[16] Absorption of the sulfonamide portion of **silver sulfadiazine** may pose a potential risk of kernicterus in a premature or G6PD-deficient newborn if used near term.[16,19] There is no information available on the safety of **framycetin** in pregnancy. Avoid use of **povidone/iodine** during pregnancy since significant iodine absorption by the baby has been reported after maternal topical use.[19,20]

NSAIDs may be used for pain relief (avoid full anti-inflammatory doses in the 3rd trimester).[21] **Opioids** can generally be safely used in small amounts for short periods of time.[16]

Management during Breastfeeding

As a general precaution, direct skin to skin contact of the breastfeeding infant with the treated skin area of the mother should be avoided with topical use of any medication. **Bacitracin** is poorly absorbed after topical administration and oral ingestion, so is considered to present a low risk to a nursing infant.[22] Topical **mupirocin** may be safely used during breastfeeding as very limited amounts are absorbed.[16,23] **Fusidic acid** is detectable in human milk after systemic use.[18] No information on safety of topical use by a breastfeeding mother is available, however fusidic acid has been used systemically in infants.[24] The sulfadiazine portion of **silver sulfadiazine** is known to be excreted in human milk and exposure should be avoided in ill, stressed, premature, hyperbilirubinemic or G6PD-deficient infants.[19,23] There is limited information available regarding the use of **framycetin** by a nursing mother. **Povidone/iodine** application in a breastfeeding mother can increase breast milk iodine concentrations and interfere with thyroid function in the nursing infant. Avoid use on mucous membranes, prolonged contact time, repeated applications, and use on large surface areas to minimize this risk.[19,22,23]

NSAIDs may be used for pain relief as most are excreted in small amounts in breast milk and considered safe to use while breastfeeding. Most **opioids** are excreted in low amounts in breast milk and short-term use is considered safe while breastfeeding. Avoid **meperidine** as long-acting metabolites can accumulate in the baby.[23] **Codeine** use should be limited to 3–4 days and both mother and infant closely monitored for signs of toxicity.[25]

A discussion of general principles on the use of medications in these special populations can be found in Appendix II and Appendix III. Other specialized reference sources are also provided in these appendices.

Therapeutic Tips

- Avoid contamination of the wound; infection is the major threat to burn outcome.
- Advise patients regarding signs of infection; any evidence of infection should be reviewed quickly and treatment altered as appropriate.
- Outpatient follow-up schedule may be daily initially and extended as dressing requirements and healing progress.
- Electrical burns often have more extensive damage below the surface than is initially identified and should be followed appropriately.
- Moisturize healed burns and protect them from sun exposure with clothing or sunscreen.

Table 4: **Topical Anti-infectives for the Treatment of Burns**

Class	Drug	Application[a]	Limitations	Comments	Cost[b]
Antibiotics, topical	*bacitracin* generics	Daily–BID, open or semi-closed	Poor eschar penetration, moderate antibacterial spectrum. Risk of contact dermatitis.	Transparent, easy to apply, cosmetically acceptable.	$
	framycetin 1% Sofra-Tulle	Daily, semi-closed	Poor penetration, moderate antibacterial action.	Easy to use.	$$
	fusidic acid 2% Fucidin Cream	Daily–QID, open or semi-closed	Moderate antibacterial spectrum.	Development of resistance.	$$$$$
	mupirocin 2% Bactroban Ointment, generics	TID, open	Limited antimicrobial coverage.	Gram-positive coverage.	$$$
	silver sulfadiazine 1% Flamazine	BID–QID open or semi-closed	Only fair penetration, sulfonamide sensitivity (rash), leukopenia.	Broad antibacterial spectrum, limited applicability, multiple dressing changes, poorer wound healing than other dressings, questionable efficacy.[8]	$$
Antiseptics	*chlorhexidine ≤2%* Baxedin, Dexidin	Daily, open or semi-closed	Concern for wound healing at higher concentrations (>2%).	Broad antibacterial action.	$
	povidone/iodine 1% Betadine, generics	BID, open or semi-closed	Poor penetration, tissue staining, painful, iodine absorption.	Broad antibacterial action.	$

[a] Approximately 5 g per 1% BSA burn per application.
[b] Cost of 7-day supply based on 1% BSA burn; includes drug cost only.
Legend: $ < $10 $$ $10–25 $$$ $25–50 $$$$ $50–75 $$$-$$$$$ $25–100 $$$$$ $75–100

Suggested Readings

American College of Surgeons. Injuries due to burns and cold. In: *Advanced trauma life support*. 7th ed. Chicago (IL): American College of Surgeons; 2004. p. 231-42.

Benson A, Dickson WA, Boyce DE. Burns. *BMJ* 2006;332(7542):649-52.

Husspith J, Rayatt S. First aid treatment of minor burns. *BMJ* 2004;328(7454):1487-9.

Papini R. Management of burn injuries of various depths. *BMJ* 2004;329(7458):158-60.

Reed J, Pomerantz WJ. Emergency management of pediatric burns. *Pediatr Emerg Care* 2005;21(2):118-29.

References

1. Appendix B to hospital resources document. Guidelines for service standards and severity classifications in the treatment of burn injury. American Burn Association. *Bull Am Coll Surg* 1984;69(10):24-8.
2. Hospital and prehospital resources for optimal care of patients with burn injury: guidelines for development and operation of burn centers. American Burn Association. *J Burn Care Rehabil* 1990;11(2):98-104.
3. Hettiaratchy S, Papini R. Initial management of a major burn: II--assessment and resuscitation. *BMJ* 2004;329(7457):101-3.
4. Monafo WW. Initial management of burns. *N Engl J Med* 1996;335(21):1581-6.
5. Edlich RF et al. Thermal burns. In: Marx JA et al., eds. *Rosen's emergency medicine: concepts and clinical practice*. 5th ed. St. Louis (MO): Mosby; 2002.
6. Tredget EE, Shankowsky HA, Groeneveld A et al. A matched-pair, randomized study evaluating the efficacy and safety of Acticoat silver-coated dressing for the treatment of burn wounds. *J Burn Care Rehabil* 1998;19(6):531-7.
7. Bowler PG, Jones SA, Walker M et al. Microbicidal properties of a silver-containing hydrofiber dressing against a variety of burn wound pathogens. *J Burn Care Rehabil* 2004;25(2):192-6.
8. Wasiak J, Cleland H, Campbell F et al. Dressings for superficial and partial thickness burns. *Cochrane Database Syst Rev* 2013;3:CD002106.
9. Barajas-Nava LA, Lopez-Alcalde J, Roque i Figuls M et al. Antibiotic prophylaxis for preventing burn wound infection. *Cochrane Database Syst Rev* 2013;6:CD008738.
10. Rosanova MT, Stamboulian D, Lede R. Systematic review: which topical agent is more efficacious in the prevention of infections in burn patients? *Arch Argent Pediatr* 2012;110(4):298-303.
11. Dat AD, Poon F, Pham KB et al. Aloe vera for treating acute and chronic wounds. *Cochrane Database Syst Rev* 2012;2:CD008762.
12. Connor-Ballard PA. Understanding and managing burn pain: Part 2. *Am J Nurs* 2009;109(5):54-62.
13. Kennedy BB, Baird SM, Troiano NH. Burn injuries and pregnancy. *J Perinat Neonatal Nurs* 2008;22(1):21-30.
14. Polko LE, McMahon MJ. Burns in pregnancy. *Obstet Gynecol Surv* 1998;53(1):50-6.
15. e-CPS. Ottawa (ON): Canadian Pharmacists Association; 2010. Polysporin [product monograph]. Available from: www.e-therapeutics.ca. Subscription required.
16. Leachman SA, Reed BR. The use of dermatologic drugs in pregnancy and lactation. *Dermatol Clin* 2006;24(2):167-97.
17. *Bactroban monograph*. Mississauga (ON): Glaxo-Smith-Kline.
18. *Fucidin monograph*. Thornhill (ON): LEO Pharma Inc.
19. Briggs GG, Freeman RK, Yaffe SJ. *Drugs in pregnancy and lactation: a reference guide to fetal and neonatal risk*. 9th ed. Philadelphia (PA): Wolters Kluwer Health; Lippincott Williams & Wilkins; 2011.
20. Schaefer C, Peters P, Miller RK. *Drugs during pregnancy and lactation: treatment options and risk assessment*. 2nd ed. Boston (MA): Elsevier; 2007.
21. Diav-Citrin O, Koren G. Drug use during pregnancy. In: Repchinsky C, ed. *Therapeutic choices*. 6th ed. Ottawa (ON): Canadian Pharmacists Association; 2011.
22. Drugs and Lactation Database (LactMed). Bethesda (MD): U. S. National Library of Medicine. Available from: toxnet.nlm.nih.gov/cgi-bin/sis/htmlgen?LACT.
23. Hale TW. *Medications and mothers' milk: a manual of lactational pharmacology*. 15th ed. Amarillo (TX): Hale Publishing; 2012.
24. Mandell GL, Douglas RG, Bennett JE et al. *Mandell, Douglas, and Bennett's principles and practice of infectious diseases*. 6th ed. Philadelphia (PA): Elsevier Churchill Livingstone; 2005.
25. Koren G, Cairns J, Chitayat D et al. Pharmacogenetics of morphine poisoning in a breastfed neonate of a codeine-prescribed mother. *Lancet* 2006;368(9536):704.

Chapter 92
Fungal Nail Infections

Penny Miller, BSc(Pharm), MA

Onychomycosis (OM) is a fungal infection of the nails caused primarily by dermatophytes (*Epidermophyton*, *Microsporum* and *Trichophyton* genera), although yeasts and nondermatophyte molds can be implicated.[1] OM is commonly referred to as tinea unguium when dermatophytes are the causative agents, but up to 5% of OM cases involve the yeast *Candida albicans* which manifests in several forms typically involving the fingernails.[1,2,3]

OM affects about 6.5% of the Canadian population and can cause discomfort, pain and disfigurement resulting in functional limitations that impact quality of life.[1,4] Secondary bacterial infections and cellulitis may occur in patients with diabetes.[4] Treatment is prolonged and reinfection is common. OM is more prevalent in those >60 years of age,[3] and is associated with other medical conditions such as tinea pedis,[3,5] nail psoriasis or trauma, peripheral vascular insufficiency or immunosuppressed states (uncontrolled diabetes mellitus, HIV, immunosuppressive medications).[6,7]

OM is classified into 3 major subtypes. Distal and lateral subungual onychomycosis (DLSO) is the most common (90% of OM cases) and is characterized by nail thickening with white-yellowish discoloration and crumbling yellow debris;[2,8,9] onycholysis and separation of the nail plate from the nail bed usually occur.[4] Proximal subungual onychomycosis (up to 6% of OM cases) is characterized by white discoloration at the proximal nail fold beneath the nail bed;[3] the infecting dermatophyte enters through the proximal nail fold and penetrates the newly formed nail plate, then migrates distally.[10] This type of OM is most common in immunosuppressed patients and can be a marker for AIDS.[3,10] Superficial white onychomycosis (SWO; up to 7% of OM cases) more commonly affects children than adults and is characterized by chalky, white patches on the top surface of the nail plate because the dermatophyte invades the nail plate directly from above and does not involve the nail bed (the entire nail plate can be involved where the nail becomes roughened and crumbly).[3,10]

Goals of Therapy

- Achieve mycologic cure (eradication of the causative organism)
- Improve appearance of nail
- Prevent spread of fungal infection
- Prevent recurrences of fungal infection
- Prevent complications such as secondary bacterial infections

Investigations

OM is responsible for only 50–60% of cases of abnormal-appearing nails,[1] therefore it is essential to confirm the diagnosis of a fungal nail infection prior to initiating treatment (diseases mimicking OM are listed in Table 1).

Table 1: **Differential Diagnoses of Fungal Nail Infections**[7,12,13]

Differential Diagnosis to Consider	Clinical Features
Psoriasis	Symmetrical nail involvement. Nail pitting. Thick, silvery scales on elbows and knees. Terminal interphalangeal joint arthritis.
Eczema	Transverse ridges. Nail folds affected. History of eczema.
Onychogryphosis (senile)	Thickened, curved nail (claw-like) often seen in elderly persons with vascular insufficiency.
Trauma	Single nail affected, nail colour change is homogenous, nail shape is altered.
Lichen planus	Nails have prominent longitudinal ridges. Nail atrophy. Oral ulcers, itchy papules on wrists, shins and trunk.
Yellow-nail syndrome	Nails grow slowly, are yellow-green, thick and curved. Associated with defective lymphatic drainage in lungs causing pulmonary infections.
Drugs, e.g., tetracyclines, cancer chemotherapy	Onycholysis.
Malignant melanoma affecting the nail matrix or nail bed	Vertical pigmented bands form in the nail matrix (nail matrix melanoma) or red, brown or black nodule forms under the nail plate with ulceration and bleeding (subungual melanoma).
Squamous cell carcinoma	Papilloma or warty involvement of paronychia, erosions and scaling.
Bacterial paronychia	Acutely painful, red, swollen area of the nail fold or cuticle, which occurs suddenly in contrast to the slow onset seen with candidal paronychia. Bacterial paronychia is often also associated with pustules.

DLSO and SWO are diagnosed by potassium hydroxide (KOH) examination of scrapings from the nail bed. Hyphae may also be seen by examining scrapings from the white spots on the nail plate in SWO.[11] If KOH examination is negative, but there is strong suspicion that OM is present, nail culture (on Sabouraud's medium) or nail plate biopsy (with periodic acid-Schiff stain) with histopathologic examination should be performed. Proximal subungual OM is diagnosed by nail plate biopsy or partial/full nail removal with culture.

Infected fingernails are cultured to establish the causative organism since yeast is a significant cause of fingernail OM.

Therapeutic Choices

Figure 1 illustrates an approach to the treatment of OM. Consider treatment in patients with diabetes, prior cellulitis, venous insufficiency, nail pain or in those who wish to improve the cosmetic appearance of the affected nails. Management options for OM include chemical/mechanical debridement, topical antifungal agents, systemic antifungal agents and/or a combination of these. Inform patients that improvement will continue for months after the course of oral drug therapy is completed, but also that recurrences are common.

Nonpharmacologic Choices

Persons with OM should be treated for any associated tinea pedis. Nondrug treatments of OM include:

- Wear footwear and socks that minimize humidity
- Dry feet and interdigital spaces thoroughly after washing
- Use footwear to avoid fungal transmission from shared public spaces such as swimming pools
- Keep nails clean and cut short
- Avoid sharing nail clippers or footwear[10]

- Prevent further trauma to toenails; wearing nonrestrictive footwear or being fitted for orthotics may be helpful
- Wear rubber gloves to protect the fingernails if hands are immersed in water for long periods of time
- Apply emollients on cracked skin to reduce further entry points for fungus
- Control chronic health conditions, such as diabetes mellitus or peripheral vascular disease[5,8,11]

Figure 1: Management of Onychomycosis

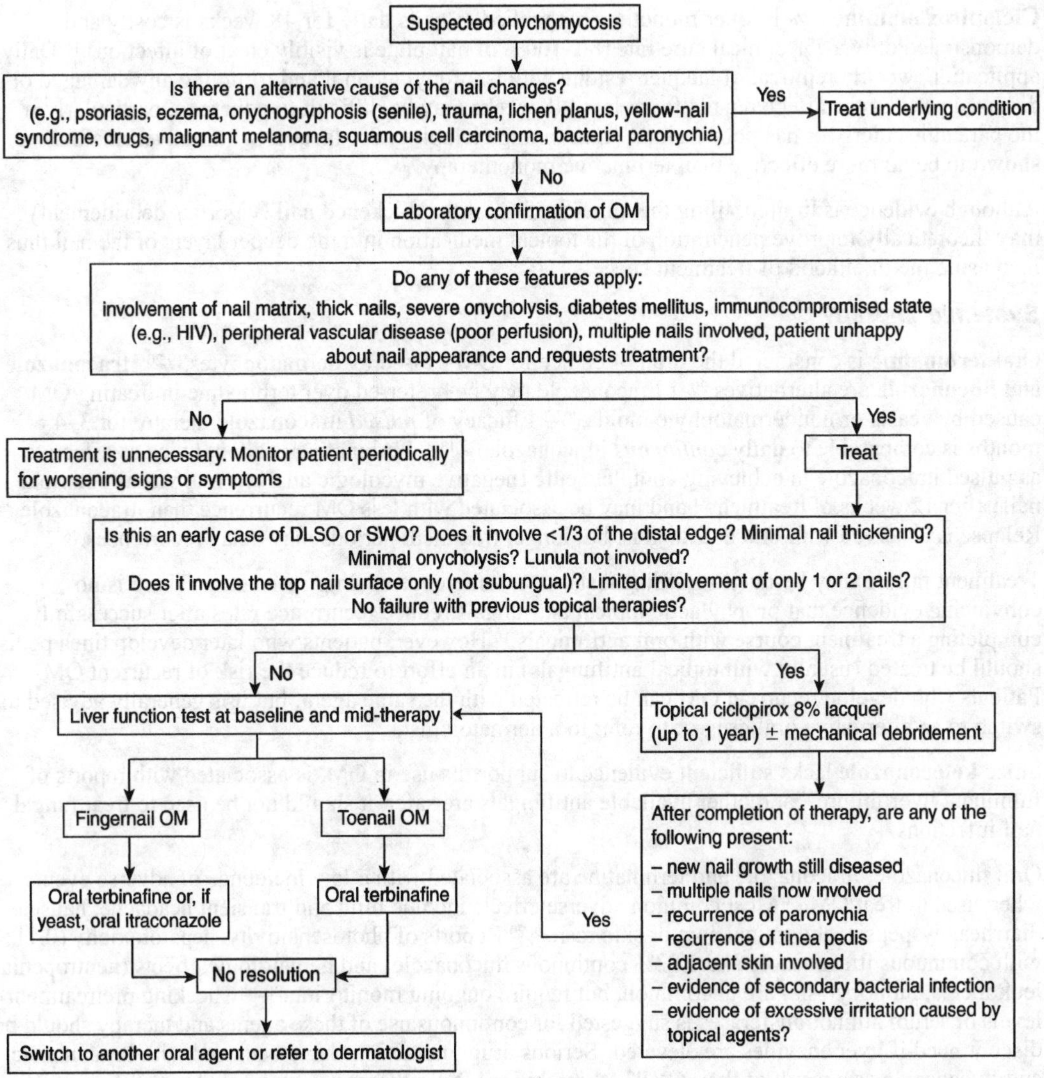

Abbreviations: DLSO = distal and lateral subungual onychomycosis; OM = onychomycosis; SWO = superficial white onychomycosis

Pharmacologic Choices

Topical and systemic agents used in the management of OM are described in Table 2.

Topical Therapy

Topical therapies are less effective than systemic agents and evidence suggests that cure rates are poor when compared to placebo.[12,13,14] Topical agents can be recommended only for very early, mild and limited cases of DLSO, SWO or when systemic therapy is contraindicated (Figure 1). Recurrence of infection is common upon discontinuation of treatment.[11] Cases with lunula involvement, subungual infections or onycholysis should not be treated topically.[15]

Ciclopirox olamine 8% lacquer monotherapy applied to nails daily for 48 weeks is costly and demonstrated only a 7% clinical cure rate (80–100% of nail plate is visibly clear of infection).[16] Daily application, weekly removal of lacquer residue with isopropyl alcohol and trimming any damaged or diseased parts of the affected nails for at least 48 weeks may be difficult to adhere to, particularly if the patient is elderly or has poor vision.[12] Combining ciclopirox 8% lacquer with oral terbinafine was shown to be no more effective than terbinafine monotherapy.[17]

Although evidence is limited, filing the upper surface of the thickened nail (vigorous débridement) may theoretically improve penetration of the topical medication into the deeper layers of the nail thus increasing the likelihood of treatment success.[15,18]

Systemic Therapy

Oral **terbinafine** is considered the drug of choice for OM caused by dermatophytes.[19,20] **Itraconazole** and **fluconazole** are alternatives.[20,21] Itraconazole may be preferred over terbinafine in treating OM caused by yeasts or nondermatophyte molds.[20,22] Efficacy of *pulsed* itraconazole therapy for 3–4 months is comparable to daily *continuous* itraconazole.[12,13,23] Terbinafine is about twice as effective as pulsed itraconazole in achieving complete cure (negative mycologic analysis and visually normal nail) after 12 weeks of treatment[24] and may be associated with less OM recurrence than itraconazole.[25] Relapse is observed with oral antifungals, but longer treatment periods may delay recurrences.[26]

Treatment failure may be due to misdiagnosis, poor adherence or drug resistance. There is no convincing evidence that prophylactic topical antifungals reduce recurrence rates after successfully completing a treatment course with oral antifungals.[19] However, patients who later develop tinea pedis should be treated (usually with topical antifungals) in an effort to reduce the risk of recurrent OM. Patients who develop recurrent OM can be retreated with the same agent, but it is generally advised to switch to an alternative oral drug or to refer to a dermatologist.

Since **ketoconazole** lacks sufficient evidence to support its use in OM, is associated with reports of fulminant liver failure[27] and other available antifungals are safer, it should not be used to treat fungal nail infections.

Oral fluconazole, itraconazole and terbinafine are associated with a low incidence of adverse events when used to treat OM.[28] Most common adverse effects include mild and transient headache, nausea, diarrhea, dyspepsia, abdominal pain or skin rash.[28,29] Reports of photosensitivity, hepatotoxicity (0.11% with continuous itraconazole and 1.22% continuous fluconazole) and hematologic effects (neutropenia, leukopenia, monocytosis) are uncommon, but require ongoing monitoring.[20,28] Checking pretreatment levels of serum aminotransferases is suggested for continuous use of these agents and therapy should be discontinued if liver enzymes are elevated. Serious drug interactions have occurred with itraconazole and fluconazole as a result of their CYP3A4 inhibition. Pulse therapy is associated with a lower risk of therapy discontinuation compared to continuous therapy.[28] Fluconazole may have a lower risk of treatment discontinuation compared with itraconazole or terbinafine.[28] The incidence of adverse events increases with higher doses of the antifungal agents.[28]

Chemical or Surgical Avulsion

In unresponsive cases, chemical or surgical nail avulsion combined with topical **ketoconazole 2%** cream or **ciclopirox 8%** lacquer applied under occlusion with polyethylene wrap may be directed by a podiatrist or dermatologist.[30] Risks associated with nail avulsion include pain, possible wound infection and scarring.

Device-based Therapy

Device-based therapeutic options (e.g., photodynamic therapy, iontophoresis and laser therapy) have been investigated for the treatment of OM in a few small trials with initial promising results. However, further evaluation and larger well-designed studies are needed to determine their long-term efficacy and place in therapy.[31,32]

Choices during Pregnancy and Breastfeeding

Choices during Pregnancy

Since fungal nail infections are generally nonurgent problems and require many months of systemic treatment, it is prudent to delay treatment until after pregnancy.[33] If drug treatment must be implemented, topical local therapy is preferred over oral systemic therapies.

Systemic antifungal agents in pregnancy have been insufficiently studied with regard to prenatal toxicity. In animal studies, teratogenic effects have been observed at very high doses of systemic antifungals. **Fluconazole**, used in high doses (>400 mg daily) for a prolonged period of time during the first trimester of pregnancy, may be associated with fetal malformations (craniofacial, skeletal and cardiac malformations), but more data are needed to confirm these observations.[34,35,36]

Although experience with **itraconazole** use in pregnancy is limited, prospective studies with first-trimester treatments for an average of 12 days and maximum of 90 days, revealed no increased rate of major malformations.[37,38] However, rates of spontaneous and induced abortion were higher in the exposed group. Larger studies are warranted to confirm these data.[37,38]

Animal reproduction studies with **terbinafine** do not suggest any embryotoxicity,[39] but human pregnancy data are lacking.

Choices during Breastfeeding

Systemic treatment of the mother with **itraconazole** or **terbinafine** should be avoided during breastfeeding since these drugs accumulate in breast milk.

It is not known whether **fluconazole** is compatible with breastfeeding when used for many weeks in the treatment of OM. Short-term (2–3 weeks) treatment with fluconazole is acceptable in nursing mothers for other conditions. The breastfed infant is expected to receive >15% of the maternal dose of fluconazole with a half-life in milk of 30 hours.

A discussion of general principles on the use of medications in these special populations can be found in Appendix II and Appendix III. Other specialized reference sources are also provided in these appendices.

Therapeutic Tips

- Not all cases of onychomycosis require drug treatment.
- Nail cultures are essential to confirm the diagnosis prior to initiating treatment.
- Oral antifungals should be used with caution in persons with liver impairment.
- Systemic treatment duration with a daily antifungal dosing regimen is usually 6 weeks for fingernails and 12 weeks for toenails.

- Improved outcomes may be achieved by combining systemic or topical antifungals with concomitant mechanical débridement of the nail.[15,16,40]
- Drug interactions can be significant with the azole antifungals, such as itraconazole and fluconazole.

Suggested Readings

Becker C, Bershow A. Lasers and photodynamic therapy in the treatment of onychomycosis: a review of the literature. *Dermatol Online J* 2013;19(9):19611.

Chang CH, Young-Xu Y, Kurth T et al. The safety of oral antifungal treatments for superficial dermatophytosis and onychomycosis: a meta-analysis. *Am J Med* 2007;120(9):791-8.

de Berker D. Clinical practice. Fungal nail disease. *N Engl J Med* 2009;360(20):2108-16.

de Sá DC, Lamas AP, Tosti A. Oral therapy for onychomycosis: an evidence-based review. *Am J Clin Dermatol* 2014;15(1):17-36.

U.K. National Institute for Health and Care Excellence. *Fungal nail infection*. 2013. Available from: cks.nice.org.uk/fungal-nail-infection.

Table 2: Antifungals for the Treatment of Onychomycosis

Class	Drug	Dose	Adverse Effects	Drug Interactions	Comments	Cost[a]
Allylamine Antifungals	*terbinafine* Lamisil, generics	Adults: 250 mg daily po Children: 10–20 kg: 62.5 mg daily po 20–40 kg: 125 mg daily po >40 kg: 250 mg daily po Duration: Fingernails: 6–12 wk Toenails: 12–24 wk	Gastrointestinal upset, headaches, minor rashes, sensory loss of smell or taste, hearing disturbances and rarely serious or fatal hepatotoxicity.	Cimetidine decreases and rifampicin increases systemic clearance of terbinafine. Terbinafine inhibits CYP2D6 enzymes and may decrease serum concentration of cyclosporine and formation of tamoxifen's active metabolites. May increase serum concentration of atomoxetine, bupropion, fluoxetine, paroxetine, tramadol and tricyclic antidepressants (monitor for toxicity). May decrease therapeutic effect of codeine.	76% mycologic cure rate.[41] Obtain baseline and mid-treatment serum aminotransferase level. More effective for dermatophyte OM (tinea unguium) with fewer serious side effects and drug interactions than itraconazole or fluconazole. Continuous terbinafine regimen is more effective than pulse regimen.	Adults: $$ Children: $
Azole Antifungals	*fluconazole* Diflucan, generics	Adults: 150–300 mg once weekly po Children: 3–6 mg/kg once weekly po Duration: Fingernails: 12–16 wk Toenails: 18–26 wk	Nausea, headache, pruritus, hepatotoxic reactions.	Inhibitor of CYP2C9, CYP2C19 and CYP3A4. Decreases serum concentration of clopidogrel's active metabolites and enhances the QT_c-prolonging effect of dronedarone, fluoroquinolones, macrolides, methadone, pimozide, quinine, tricyclic antidepressants and ziprasidone. Decreases metabolism of atorvastatin, benzodiazepines (monitor for increased toxic effects), calcium channel blockers, clarithromycin, colchicine, erythromycin, fentanyl, lovastatin, phenytoin, phosphodiesterase-5 inhibitors, simvastatin, solifenacin and sulfonylureas.	Alternative agent; less cost-effective than terbinafine or itraconazole. 48% mycologic cure rate.[41] Some evidence that treatment period for cure of toenail (and possibly fingernail) OM should be >6 months.[42]	$

(cont'd)

Table 2: **Antifungals for the Treatment of Onychomycosis** *(cont'd)*

Class	Drug	Dose	Adverse Effects	Drug Interactions	Comments	Cost[a]
	itraconazole Sporanox Capsules, Sporanox Oral Solution	**Pulsed dosing:** Adults: 200 mg BID po Children: <20 kg: 5 mg/kg daily po 20–40 kg: 100 mg daily po 40–50 kg: 200 mg daily po >50 kg: 200 mg BID po Duration: Fingernails: 1 wk/month × 2 Toenails: 1 wk/month × 3 **Continuous dosing:** Adults: 200 mg once daily po Duration: Fingernails: 6 wk Toenails: 12 wk	GI upset, headaches, minor rashes and, rarely, serious or fatal hepatotoxicity, heart failure.	Potent inhibitor of CYP3A4. Avoid use with or make appropriate dosage reductions to alfuzosin, atorvastatin, calcium channel blockers, clarithromycin, dronedarone, eplerenone, ergot derivatives, erythromycin, lovastatin, phosphodiesterase inhibitors, pimozide, quinidine, rivaroxaban, salmeterol, simvastatin, solifenacin and tamsulosin. Histamine-2 receptor antagonists and proton pump inhibitors increase gastric pH and decrease itraconazole's absorption.	Preferred initial agent for treatment of nondermatophyte OM. *Pulsed regimen:* 63% mycologic cure rate.[41] Preferred over continuous regimen. Drug interactions and side effects are less pronounced compared to continuous therapy. *Continuous regimen:* 59% mycologic cure rate.[41] Obtain baseline and mid-treatment serum aminotransferase levels.	Pulsed: Adults: $$$ Children: $ Continuous (Adults): $$$$$
Pyridones	*ciclopirox olamine 8% lacquer* Penlac, generics	Adults: apply daily to the affected nail, nail bed, undersurface of the nail plate and surrounding skin Duration: up to 48 weeks	Periungual erythema, erythema of the proximal nail fold and contact dermatitis.		30% mycologic cure rate.[16] Clean nail with alcohol weekly and remove infected growing part of nail periodically. Best for SWO or mild to moderate DLSO not involving the lunula. Filing nail surface may increase efficacy. No additional benefit if added to oral terbinafine.[17] Useful in patients who are poor candidates for oral therapy.	$$[b]

[a] Cost of 30-day supply for oral dose based on 30 kg body weight for cost of children's dose; includes drug cost only.
[b] Cost of 12 g for topical therapy.
Abbreviations: DLSO = distal and lateral subungual onychomycosis; OM = onychomycosis; SWO = superficial white onychomycosis
Legend: $ <$50 $$ $50–100 $$$ $100–150 $$$$ $150–200 $$$$$ $200–300

References

1. Roseeuw D. Achilles foot screening project: preliminary results of patients screened by dermatologists. *J Eur Acad Dermatol Venereol* 1999;12(Suppl 1):S6-9.
2. Foster KW, Ghannoum MA, Elewski BE. Epidemiologic surveillance of cutaneous fungal infection in the United States from 1999 to 2002. *J Am Acad Dermatol* 2004;50(5):748-52.
3. How should fungal nail infection be treated? *Drug Ther Bull* 2008;46(1):3-8.
4. Elewski BE. Onychomycosis. Treatment, quality of life, and economic issues. *Am J Clin Dermatol* 2000;1(1):19-26.
5. Roberts DT, Taylor WD, Boyle J. Guidelines for treatment of onychomycosis. *Br J Dermatol* 2003;148(3):402-10.
6. Gupta AK, Konnikov N, MacDonald P et al. Prevalence and epidemiology of toenail onychomycosis in diabetic subjects: a multicentre survey. *Br J Dermatol* 1998;139(4):665-71.
7. Burzykowski T, Molenberghs G, Abeck D et al. High prevalence of foot diseases in Europe: results of the Achilles Project. *Mycoses* 2003;46(11-12):496-505.
8. Gupta AK, Tu LQ. Onychomycosis therapies: strategies to improve efficacy. *Dermatol Clin* 2006;24(3):381-6.
9. Kyle AA, Dahl MV. Topical therapy for fungal infections. *Am J Clin Dermatol* 2004;5(6):443-51.
10. Gupta AK, Daniel CR. Onychomycosis: strategies to reduce failure and recurrence. *Cutis* 1998;62(4):189-91.
11. Scher RK, Baran R. Onychomycosis in clinical practice: factors contributing to recurrence. *Br J Dermatol* 2003;149(Suppl 65):5-9.
12. Crawford F, Hollis S. Topical treatments for fungal infections of the skin and nails of the foot. *Cochrane Database Syst Rev* 2007;(3):CD001434.
13. Ferrari J. Fungal toenail infections. *Clin Evid (Online)* 2008;pii:1715.
14. Crawford F, Hollis S. Topical treatments for fungal infections of the skin and nails of the foot. *Cochrane Database Syst Rev* 2007;(3):CD001434.
15. Gupta AK, Ryder JE, Chow M et al. Dermatophytosis: the management of fungal infections. *Skinmed* 2005;4(5):305-10.
16. Gupta AK, Fleckman P, Baran R. Ciclopirox nail lacquer topical solution 8% in the treatment of toenail onychomycosis. *J Am Acad Dermatol* 2000;43(4 Suppl):S70-80.
17. Gupta AK. Ciclopirox topical solution 8% combined with oral terbinafine to treat onychomycosis: a randomized, evaluator-blinded study. *J Drugs Dermatol* 2005;4(4):481-5.
18. Roberts DT, Evans EG. Subungual dermatophytoma complicating dermatophyte onychomycosis. *Br J Dermatol* 1998;138(1):189-90.
19. Piraccini BM, Sisti A, Tosti A. Long-term follow-up of toenail onychomycosis caused by dermatophytes after successful treatment with systemic antifungal agents. *J Am Acad Dermatol* 2010;62(3):411-4.
20. de Sá DC, Lamas AP, Tosti A. Oral therapy for onychomycosis: an evidence-based review. *Am J Clin Dermatol* 2014;15(1):17-36.
21. Meinhof W. Kinetics and spectrum of activity of oral antifungals: the therapeutic implications. *J Am Acad Dermatol* 1993;29(1):S37-41.
22. De Doncker PR, Scher RK, Baran RL et al. Itraconazole therapy is effective for pedal onychomycosis caused by some nondermatophyte molds and in mixed infection with dermatophytes and molds: a multicenter study with 36 patients. *J Am Acad Dermatol* 1997;36(2 Pt 1):173-7.
23. Crawford F, Young P, Godfrey C et al. Oral treatments for toenail onychomycosis: a systematic review. *Arch Dermatol* 2002;138(6):811-6.
24. Evans EG, Sigurgeirsson B. Double blind, randomised study of continuous terbinafine compared with intermittent itraconazole in treatment of toenail onychomycosis. The LION Study Group. *BMJ* 1999;318(7190):1031-5.
25. Piraccini BM, Sisti A, Tosti A. Long-term follow-up of toenail onychomycosis caused by dermatophytes after successful treatment with systemic antifungal agents. *J Am Acad Dermatol* 2010;62(3):411-4.
26. Sigurgeirsson B, Olafsson JH, Steinson JB et al. Long-term effectiveness of treatment with terbinafine vs itraconazole in onychomycosis: a 5-year blinded prospective follow-up study. *Arch Dermatol* 2002;138(3):353-7.
27. Health Canada. *Ketoconazole—risk of potentially fatal liver toxicity—for health professionals.* Available from: healthycanadians.gc.ca/recall-alert-rappel-avis/hc-sc/2013/34173a-eng.php.
28. Chang CH, Young-Xu Y, Kurth T et al. The safety of oral antifungal treatments for superficial dermatophytosis and onychomycosis: a meta-analysis. *Am J Med* 2007;120(9):791-8.
29. Elewski B, Tavakkol A. Safety and tolerability of oral antifungal agents in the treatment of fungal nail disease: a proven reality. *Ther Clin Risk Manag* 2005;1(4):299-306.
30. Baden HP. Treatment of distal onychomycosis with avulsion and topical antifungal agents under occlusion. *Arch Dermatol* 1994;130(5):558-9.
31. Ortiz AE, Avram MM, Wanner MA. A review of lasers and light for the treatment of onychomycosis. *Lasers Surg Med* 2014;46(2):117-24.
32. Gupta AK, Simpson FC. New therapeutic options for onychomycosis. *Expert Opin Pharmacother* 2012;13(8):1131-42.
33. Baran R, Hay RJ, Garduno JI. Review of antifungal therapy, part II: treatment rationale, including specific patient populations. *J Dermatolog Treat* 2008;19(3):168-75.
34. Lee BE, Feinberg M, Abraham JJ et al. Congenital malformations in an infant born to a woman treated with fluconazole. *Pediatr Infect Dis J* 1992;11(12):1062-4.
35. Pursley TJ, Blomquist IK, Abraham J et al. Fluconazole-induced congenital anomalies in three infants. *Clin Infect Dis* 1996;22(2):336-40.
36. Aleck KA, Bartley DL. Multiple malformation syndrome following fluconazole use in pregnancy: report of an additional patient. *Am J Med Genet* 1997;72(3):253-6.
37. Bar-Oz B, Moretti ME, Bishai R et al. Pregnancy outcome after in utero exposure to itraconazole: a prospective cohort study. *Am J Obstet Gynecol* 2000;183(3):617-20.
38. De Santis M, Di Gianantonio E, Cesari E et al. First-trimester itraconazole exposure and pregnancy outcome: a prospective cohort study of women contacting teratology information services in Italy. *Drug Saf* 2009;32(3):239-44.
39. Bechter R, Schmid BP. Teratogenicity in vitro—a comparative study of four antimycotic drugs using the whole-embryo culture system. *Toxicol In Vitro* 1987;1(1):11-5.
40. Potter LP, Mathias SD, Raut M et al. The impact of aggressive debridement used as an adjunct therapy with terbinafine on perceptions of patients undergoing treatment for toenail onychomycosis. *J Dermatolog Treat* 2007;18(1):46-52.
41. Gupta AK, Ryder JE, Johnson AM. Cumulative meta-analysis of systemic antifungal agents for the treatment of onychomycosis. *Br J Dermatol* 2004;150(3):537-44.
42. Gupta AK, Drummond-Main C, Paquet M. Evidence-based optimal fluconazole dosing regimen for onychomycosis treatment. *J Dermatolog Treat* 2013;24(1):75-80.

Chapter 93

Pressure Ulcers

Stephen R. Tan, MD, FRCPC

Goals of Therapy

- Recognize and modify risk factors for pressure ulcer formation
- Improve existing lesions that have the potential to heal
- Recognize and manage the complications of pressure ulcers
- Prevent recurrences in at-risk patients

Staging of Pressure Ulcers

Table 1 explains the staging criteria for pressure ulcers.

Table 1: Staging of Pressure Ulcers[1]

Stage I	Nonblanchable erythema of intact skin, usually over a bony prominence. In darker skin types, discolouration, warmth, edema or induration may be indicators. The area may be painful, firm, soft, warmer or cooler than adjacent skin.
Stage II	Partial-thickness skin loss involving the epidermis, dermis or both. Clinically, this presents as an abrasion, intact or ruptured blister or shallow erosion with a red-pink wound bed.
Stage III	Full-thickness ulceration. Subcutaneous fat may be visible, but bone, tendon or muscle is not exposed. Clinically, this presents as a deep crater that may have undermining of adjacent tissue.
Stage IV	Full-thickness ulceration with exposed bone, tendon, fascia, muscle or joint capsule. Often includes undermining and tunnelling.

Slough (yellow, tan, grey, green or brown) or eschar (tan, brown or black) may be present, and may cover the base of the ulcer. A pressure ulcer cannot be accurately staged until enough slough and/or eschar has been removed to expose the base of the wound.

Pressure ulcers do not necessarily progress in the order presented, nor do they heal by reverse staging.

Investigations

- Complete history:
  - assess for risk factors for pressure ulcers (Table 2). These affect pressure ulcer formation and the healing of existing ulcers.[2] Perform pressure ulcer risk assessment at the time of admission and reassess at regular intervals. In an acute care setting, reassess at least every 24 hours. In long-term care, assess weekly for 4 weeks, and then quarterly thereafter. Patients should also be reassessed whenever there is a change in their condition.[3] Early identification of at-risk patients allows for the implementation of interventions to attempt to prevent the development of pressure ulcers.[4] Modify care according to the individual risk factors present[3]
  - assess concurrent medical problems that may impair wound healing, including peripheral vascular disease, diabetes mellitus, immune deficiencies, collagen vascular diseases, malignancy, malnutrition, psychosis and depression[5]

- medication history: especially corticosteroids or immunosuppressives that impair wound healing. Also consider drugs that can decrease the level of consciousness/sensory perception, e.g., sedatives, analgesics

- Physical examination:
  - perform a head-to-toe skin exam, especially checking pressure points such as the sacrum, ischium, trochanters, heels, elbows, occiput and parts of the body in contact with devices that may apply pressure such as tape, tubes and restraints.[3,6,7] Assess skin daily in patients at risk for skin breakdown[6]
  - assess the pressure ulcer for location, depth, size, sinus tracts, undermining, tunnelling, exudate, necrotic tissue, odour, the presence or absence of granulation tissue and epithelialization and the condition of the peri-wound skin and wound edges (Table 1)[8,9,10]
  - stage the pressure ulcer[2] (Table 1)
  - vascular assessment, such as palpating pedal pulses, capillary refill, ankle/brachial pressure index and toe pressures, is recommended for lower extremity ulcers to assess for vascular compromise[8]
- Laboratory tests:
  - prealbumin[10] or albumin

Therapeutic Choices

Strategies for the management of pressure ulcers include risk/causative factor modification, local ulcer care and addressing complications if they arise. See also Figure 1.

Risk/Causative Factor Modification

Healing of pressure ulcers is unlikely unless the underlying causative factors are corrected. Management of these factors is likely more valuable in treating pressure ulcers than either topical or adjunctive therapies.[12]

Implement educational programs for the prevention of pressure ulcers. These should be structured, organized and directed at all levels of health care providers, patients, family and caregivers.[3,6,8]

Pressure: External pressure is concentrated over bony prominences.[6] If the external pressure applied to tissue is higher than the capillary closing pressure, there is occlusion of the blood vessels, decreased perfusion and tissue necrosis.[6] Pressure ulcers in subdermal tissues under bony prominences likely occur between 1 hour to 4–6 hours after sustained tissue loading.[13] If pressure is intermittently relieved, minimal skin changes occur.[9] Less pressure is required to create tissue ischemia in patients with impaired circulation secondary to disease process or injury, in patients receiving vasopressors and in patients with conditions resulting in impaired oxygenation or perfusion.[10] Pressure relief is the cornerstone of both prevention and treatment of pressure ulcers.

Table 2: **Select Risk/Causative Factors for Pressure Ulcers[9,11]**

Local	Systemic
Pressure, especially overlying bony prominences Dry skin Excessive moisture Friction Shearing Forces	Circulatory disturbance Malnutrition Prolonged immobilization, e.g., fractures, spinal cord injury, stroke, major surgery Sensory deficit Smoking

Figure 1: **Pressure Ulcer Therapy**

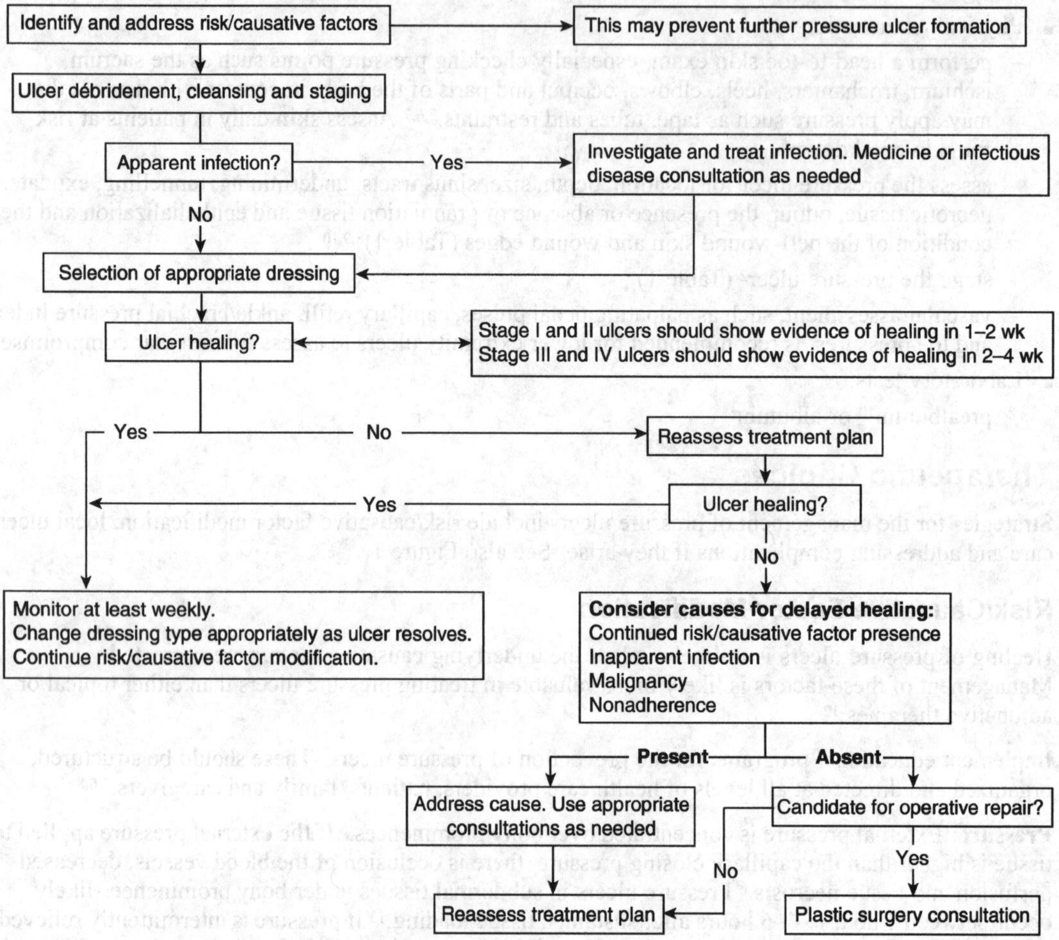

Strategies for pressure relief to *prevent* pressure ulcers include:

- Implement a written repositioning schedule to protect intact skin.[6,10]
- Encourage patients with enough mobility to shift position every 15 minutes.[3,6,14]
- Patients at risk of developing a pressure ulcer should not remain on a standard mattress.[6,8] Foam alternatives to the standard hospital mattress reduce the incidence of pressure ulcers in these patients.[15,16] Replace a standard mattress with one that has low interface pressure, such as high-density foam, to prevent pressure ulcers in patients at risk [Evidence: SORT B*].[6,8,15]
- If a specialized replacement mattress in not available, turn bedridden patients on standard mattresses every 2 hours.[3,17] Turn patients on any type of specialized pressure-reducing surface every 4 hours.[17]
- Avoid placing patients directly on bony prominences.[2,7] Positioning the patient in the 30° lateral side-lying position instead of directly over the trochanters allows for reduced pressure and improved circulation to the skin overlying the trochanters.[7,10] Repositioning patients every 3 hours at night

* SORT (Strength of Recommendation Taxonomy) is a rating system (A, B or C) that addresses the quality of available evidence. For more information consult **How to Use *Compendium of Therapeutic Choices*** on page xxv.

in the 30° tilt position has been shown to significantly reduce pressure ulcer development when compared to repositioning patients every 6 hours in the 90° lateral position.[18]

- Use soft pillows or foam wedges between bony prominences such as knees and ankles.[2,3,6]
- Manage pressure relief of the heels while the patient is in bed, independently of the support surface.[8] Suspend heels above the mattress with appropriate positioning methods or devices in at-risk patients.[17]
- Avoid using ring cushions (doughnuts) as these cause venous congestion and edema and are more likely to cause pressure ulcers than to prevent them.[3,6,7]
- Avoid positioning the patient directly onto medical devices such as tubes or drainage systems.[7]

Strategies for pressure relief to *treat* pressure ulcers include:

- Do not position patients in a way that puts pressure on the ulcer. Reposition the patient such that pressure is relieved or redistributed.[7]
- If the ulcer is on a sitting surface, use pressure-reducing devices for the seating surface.[6,7] Place the feet on a footstool or foot rest when the feet do not reach the floor. Limit the time the patient spends seated in a chair without pressure relief.[7]
- If a pillow is used to raise the heels above the mattress, place the pillow longitudinally underneath the calf with the heel suspended in air, allowing complete pressure offloading.[19] There may be difficulty in maintaining proper positioning of a pillow as patient movement and gravity may cause it to move and allow the heels to rest against the bed surface. Specialized heel-offloading devices are available and may be pillow-based, foam-based or air-based. These devices reduce friction and shear, and may stay in position better than pillows.[19] Any device used should be arranged such that the knee is in slight flexion and pressure is not placed on the Achilles tendon.[7] There is no evidence to recommend one support surface over another for heel pressure ulcers. Consider patient quality of life, intrusiveness of the device (such as noise or size), as well as ease of use, reliability and cost.[20]
- Pressure relief may be accomplished by using commercially available pressure-reducing surfaces.[9,21] Pressure-reducing surfaces may be static or dynamic. Static surfaces include mattresses or mattress overlays which are filled with air, water, gel, fluid, foam or a combination of these. Dynamic support surfaces include alternating-pressure mattresses, low-air-loss beds and air-fluidized mattresses.[2,22] A static support surface may be used if the patient can assume a variety of positions and does not bottom out the surface. A dynamic surface is recommended when the patient cannot assume a variety of positions without weight bearing on a pressure ulcer, if the patient fully compresses the static surface or the pressure ulcer does not show evidence of healing.[2,7] There is no conclusive evidence about the superiority of any support surface for the treatment of existing pressure ulcers.[23] However, specially designed products are generally more effective than standard mattresses for preventing and healing pressure ulcers.[22,24]

Shearing forces: Shearing occurs when 2 forces move in opposite directions.[25] Shearing forces diminish circulation and damage both tissue and blood vessel integrity.[10] Shearing occurs mainly in bed-bound patients utilizing the reclining feature of hospital beds.[25] When the head of a supine patient is raised more than 30°, shearing forces occur in the sacral and coccygeal areas.[9] Maintain the head of the bed at the lowest degree of elevation consistent with concurrent medical conditions and other restrictions.[3,6]

Friction: Friction occurs when a patient's skin rubs against another surface, causing tearing of the tissues.[25] Friction ulcers often occur over elbows and heels in bedridden patients as they use their elbows and heels to aid in movement.[10] Friction can be minimized by lifting rather than dragging a bedridden patient across bed sheets, keeping the bed free of particulate matter such as crumbs and by keeping sheets loose to avoid restricting movement. Lifting devices such as a trapeze bar or bed linen may be used to transfer or to change patient position.[3]

Excessive moisture: Maceration is softening of the skin when tissues become waterlogged due to excessive moisture.[25] A long-term moist environment may result from perspiration or fecal or urinary incontinence. Maceration leaves the skin more susceptible to tearing.[2,25] Fecal incontinence is a greater risk for skin breakdown than urinary incontinence, as the chemical irritation that results from the enzymes in stool is caustic to the skin.[2] Gently cleanse the skin and remove moisture at the time of soiling.[3,6] Moisture barrier creams, absorbent pads, dressings and incontinence briefs that wick moisture away from the skin may be used for incontinence and should be changed as they become saturated.[2,3,6,26] A bowel routine and intermittent or permanent catheterization may be considered.

Dry skin: There is an association between pressure ulcers and dry, flaky, scaling skin.[11,22] Well-moisturized skin retains its barrier properties and helps to prevent skin breakdown. Use moisturizers for dry skin and minimize contributing environmental factors such as low humidity and cold air.[3] Use nonsensitizing moisturizers with minimal alcohol content.[6]

Malnutrition: Although a causal relationship has not been established, nutritional parameters have been correlated with the development of pressure ulcers. Pressure ulcers may contribute to a worsening of nutritional status due to a chronic energy deficit: these patients have an increased resting energy expenditure and reduced energy intake.[27] Evidence suggests that improving nutritional status can help with pressure ulcer prevention and healing.[22,28] Early identification and treatment of protein malnutrition and other nutrient deficiencies are essential to optimize wound healing.[29] Regular monitoring of serial weight is a reliable, inexpensive and noninvasive method to determine whether a patient is in an anabolic, catabolic or stable state. Identification of an undesirable weight trend is an early indicator of risk, and allows for proactive intervention before malnutrition and impaired wound healing become severe.[2] Prealbumin is a more sensitive indicator of nutritional status than albumin. Albumin may be affected by hydration status and has a 21-day half-life, whereas prealbumin has a 2-day half-life and is more reflective of current nutritional status.[10] Ensure hydration through adequate fluid intake.[6] Encourage dietary intake or supplementation if an individual with a pressure ulcer is malnourished. A nutritional goal of 30 kcal/kg/day is recommended.[27] Malnourished patients with a high-protein diet have a higher frequency of ulcer healing and a greater decrease in ulcer size than patients with a low-protein diet.[8,30,31] Give vitamin and mineral supplements if deficiencies are suspected or confirmed.[8] A dietary consultation may be warranted to thoroughly assess patients who have a pressure ulcer or are at risk of developing one.[2,7,27]

Immobilization: Early mobilization is encouraged. A physiotherapy consultation may be valuable.

Sensory and circulatory compromise: Optimization of the treatment of contributing medical problems, such as diabetes, will assist in the healing of existing pressure ulcers and the prevention of new ones.

Smoking: Smoking causes vasoconstriction and relative tissue hypoxia, which may impair wound healing. Excessive smoking may also contribute to anorexia and ensuing malnutrition.[32]

Local Ulcer Care

Local ulcer care involves wound débridement, wound cleansing and appropriate dressing choices.

Wound Débridement

Removal of devitalized tissue and inflammatory agents is necessary to allow granulation tissue formation and subsequent re-epithelialization.[9,33] An exception is that stable, dry, adherent eschar on the heels serves as a natural cover, and should not be removed.[1] Prior to débridement of lower extremity ulcers, complete a vascular assessment (perform clinical assessment, palpate pedal pulses, check capillary refill, ankle/brachial pressure index and toe pressure) to rule out vascular compromise.[8]

Wound débridement may be accomplished in 4 ways:

- **Sharp débridement** with scissors or scalpel is indicated for thick adherent eschars, extensive devitalized tissue or urgent débridement in infected ulcers.[9] Use sterile instruments.[8] If there is bleeding during débridement, pressure should be applied with gauze until the bleeding is controlled. Electrocautery may also be used for hemostasis. A clean, dry dressing may be used for 6–24 hours, after which a moist dressing may be reinstated.[34] Algosteril, an absorptive **xerogel** type of dressing, also functions as a procoagulant and can be used to obtain hemostasis in oozing wounds.[35]
- **Autolytic débridement** involves synthetic dressings, especially **hydrocolloids** and **hydrogels**, to cover a wound and allow devitalized tissue to self-digest with wound fluid enzymes. Autolytic débridement may be appropriate for patients who cannot tolerate other methods and have uninfected wounds.[9] Wounds must be frequently and effectively cleansed to wash out partially degraded tissue fragments at each dressing change.[33] If wound fluid remains in prolonged contact with intact skin, maceration and further skin impairment may occur. Peri-wound skin protection is vital; use skin sealants or barrier ointments to protect the surrounding intact skin.[10]
- **Mechanical débridement** may be performed in several ways, including wet-to-dry dressings, hydrotherapy or wound irrigation at moderate pressures. Wet-to-dry dressings adhere to eschar and remove the eschar when the dry dressing is removed. They should be used only for débridement and then immediately discontinued. Hydrotherapy and wound irrigation are useful for softening and mechanically removing eschar and debris.[9] Proper irrigation pressure may be obtained using a 35 mL syringe with a 19-gauge angiocatheter or a single-use 100 mL saline squeeze bottle.[8,9]
- **Enzymatic débridement** is performed by applying enzyme-impregnated dressings to wounds.[35] This method may be used in long-term care facilities and in home care on uninfected ulcers.[9]

Wound Cleansing

Wound cleansing uses noncytotoxic fluids to reduce the bacterial burden and to remove devitalized tissue, metabolic wastes and topical agents that can delay wound healing.[8]

- Wounds should be cleansed at initial examination and at each dressing change.
- Irrigation with normal saline may be used to clean most ulcers. Ringer's lactate, sterile water or noncytotoxic wound cleansers may also be used. The fluid used for cleansing should be warmed to at least room temperature. To reduce surface bacteria and tissue trauma, gently irrigate the wound with 100–150 mL of solution.[8] Following irrigation, the surrounding skin should be gently patted dry to facilitate optimal adherence of the dressing.[34] Care must be taken to avoid maceration and to avoid spreading bacteria to other skin sites.
- Cleansing of the wound bed should be done with minimal chemical and mechanical trauma. Antiseptic agents, hydrogen peroxide and skin cleansers are toxic to wound tissue and should not be used.[8,34]
- Whirlpool treatment may be helpful for ulcers with thick exudate, slough and necrotic tissue, but is inappropriate for clean wounds.[5] Discontinue whirlpool treatment when the ulcer is clean.

Choice of Dressings

Wound Dressing categories are shown in Table 3. Wound dressing choices for ulcer stages are outlined in Figure 2.

- Select dressings by evaluating the current status of the ulcer, while considering cost, ease of use, nursing time requirements and patient comfort. The goal is to choose a dressing that will:
  - keep the ulcer bed continuously moist but not macerated[8,36]
  - be absorbent enough to control exudate without desiccating the ulcer bed[8,36]
  - keep the surrounding skin intact and dry[8]
  - provide thermal insulation and wound temperature stability[8]

- protect the wound, particularly in areas at risk of urine or fecal contamination[6,8,9]
- maintain its integrity and not leave fibres or foreign substances within the wound[8]
- not cause trauma to the wound bed on removal[8]

- No single dressing is consistently superior to other dressings.[37] Comparisons between advanced dressings do not demonstrate significant differences in healing rates.[37]
- When compared to conventional gauze dressings, **hydrocolloid** dressings are more efficacious when treating pressure ulcers, with increased healing rates and reduced healing times.[37] One trial suggests that sequential treatment with **calcium alginate** dressings for 4 weeks for débridement, followed by hydrocolloid dressings for 4 weeks to promote tissue granulation, will accelerate the healing of grade III and IV pressure ulcers.[38]
- As wounds heal, the dressing needs may change and the wound care plan should be re-evaluated. Monitor the ulcer at every dressing change and reassess at least once per week.[5] Tracings or colour photos may be helpful for record keeping.[9]
- When applying the dressing:
  - dead space should be eliminated by loosely filling all cavities. Tissue must not be overpacked, as this may increase intra-wound pressure and cause additional tissue damage[2,9]
  - optimal secondary dressings should cover about 3 cm of intact, dry skin around the ulcer[34]
  - dressings should not exert tension on the skin, as the resulting shearing forces increase the risk of further tissue breakdown[34]
  - change dressing when drainage has seeped out from beneath it, indicating that the bacterial barrier has been compromised[34]
- The frequency of dressing changes must be individually determined. For uncomplicated wounds, change occlusive dressings every 3–7 days, as this minimally disturbs healing tissue between dressing changes. If there are other factors, such as an underlying infection or excessive exudate, the dressing changes should be more frequent.

Other therapy

Negative pressure wound therapy (NPWT) is a technology that promotes wound healing by draining and removing infectious material or other fluids through continuous and/or intermittent (5 minutes on/2 minutes off) negative pressure.[39]

- NPWT applies subatmospheric pressure to the wound bed via a computerized therapy unit attached to a reticulated foam dressing placed in the wound and secured with an adhesive drape.[39,40] This application causes mechanical stress on tissue and the wound is drawn closed. While the degree of pressure to the wounded tissue is small, all areas of the wound work together in an effort to close towards the centre point.[39]
- The wound should be large enough for adequate contact between the foam dressing and the wound bed, and for safe removal of the foam.[39]
- Overall nursing time may be reduced, as fewer dressing changes are required.[40]
- The role of NPWT with pressure ulcers is evolving, with some trials suggesting quicker closure and resolution of wounds, while others suggest no benefit.[12,39,41] NPWT may be considered for Stage III or IV pressure ulcers, particularly if the wound has inadequate or poor granulation tissue or heavy exudate.[39] Early initiation of NPWT was associated with a shorter length of stay for patients receiving home care for Stage III or Stage IV pressure ulcers.[41] NPWT may be beneficial if pressure ulcers are not healing with other modalities.
- NPWT may be associated with bleeding or infections. Bleeding may occur in patients receiving anticoagulant therapy and during the removal of dressings that adhere to tissue. Infection may occur

with retention of dressing pieces in the wound. NPWT is contraindicated in pressure ulcers with necrotic tissue and eschar present, untreated osteomyelitis and exposed vasculature or nerves.[42]

Complications

Infection: All Stage II–IV ulcers are colonized with bacteria. In most cases, adequate cleansing and débridement prevent colonization from progressing to clinical infection, and healing will still occur.[9]

Inapparent infection may occur, with increased bacterial burden and the usual signs of infection absent. Consider a 2-week trial of **topical antibiotics** for clean pressure ulcers that are not healing or are continuing to produce excessive exudate after 2–4 weeks of optimal patient care.[9] Choice of antibiotic should be determined by ulcer location and wound cultures. Contact dermatitis, bacterial resistance and systemic absorption may occur with topical antibiotics.

Table 3: Classification of Wound Dressings[26,35]

Dressing	Dressing Characteristics	Wound Types
Transparent film dressings Bioclusive, Opsite, TegaDerm	Semi-permeable, highly flexible dressings that reduce evaporative water loss, provide good antibacterial barriers and reduce shearing forces.	Superficial wounds, abrasions and partial-thickness wounds.
Gauze dressings Adherent: 4×4 gauze Non-adherent: Release, Telfa	These dressings débride, but are painful upon removal unless moistened first. Must be secured in place.	Partial- or full-thickness wounds with necrotic debris or covered with antibiotic ointment.
Hydrocolloid dressings Comfeel, DuoDerm, Restore	Available as composite sheets with a hydrophilic polymer and a water-impermeable vapour-transmitting backing or in paste form. They are occlusive and provide an excellent barrier. Wound exudate is absorbed and a gel is formed that expands into the wound cavity. Promote autolytic débridement. Usually require less frequent changes.	Both partial- and full-thickness wounds, especially superficial wounds.
Hydrogel dressings DuoDerm gel, Intrasite gel, Normlgel, Nu-Gel	Three-dimensional networks of hydrophilic polymers made from gelatin and polysaccharides. Absorb exudate with medium capacity and provide cooling and pain relief. Promote autolytic débridement and granulation. Can both absorb fluid and hydrate desiccated eschars.	Full-thickness wounds with or without undermining.
Xerogel dressings Algosteril, Aquacel, Kaltostat	Dry dressings with high absorptive capacity that change into a gel-like substance upon contact with wound exudate. After the exudate is absorbed, xerogels act similarly to hydrogels in facilitating moist wound healing. Alginates (xerogels with hemostatic properties) are also procoagulants and can be used to obtain hemostasis in oozing wounds.	Full-thickness wounds with slough, with or without undermining.
Foam dressings Allevyn, Cutinova, Mepilex	Polymeric dressings that maximize absorbency and vapour permeability to provide optimal exudate handling. May be combined with a water-impermeable but vapour-transmitting backing to allow vapour loss. When the exudate contacts the backing, evaporative loss facilitates exudate control. Expansion of the foam as it absorbs exudate creates gentle pressure on the wound, possibly reducing wound edema.	Full-thickness wounds with exudate. Can be used around wound drains and tubes or over incisions.
Enzymatic dressings Collagenase	Enzymatic dressings apply topical débriding agents to devitalized tissue on the wound surface. A clean moist dressing should be applied over the ulcer after enzyme application.	Wounds with eschar.

Figure 2: Dressing Choices for Pressure Ulcers

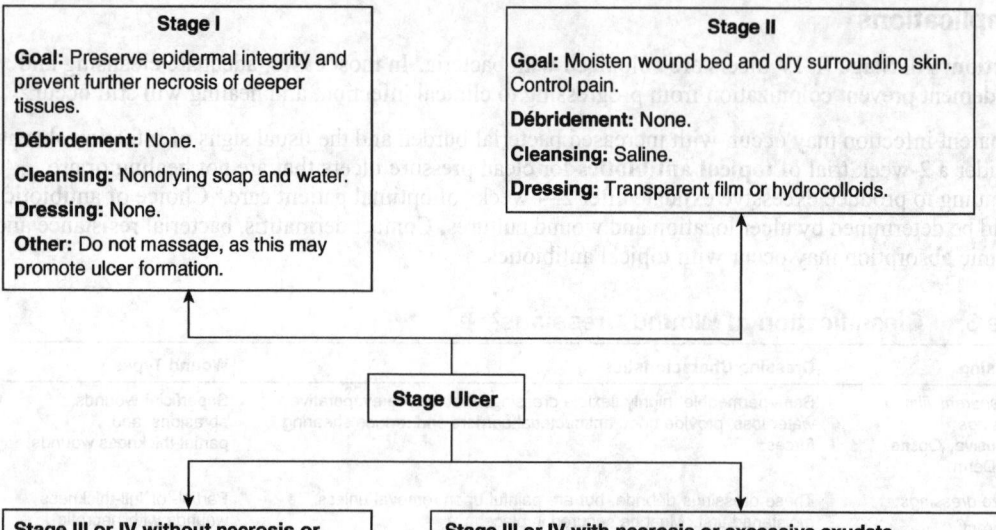

Stage Ulcer

Stage I

Goal: Preserve epidermal integrity and prevent further necrosis of deeper tissues.

Débridement: None.

Cleansing: Nondrying soap and water.

Dressing: None.

Other: Do not massage, as this may promote ulcer formation.

Stage II

Goal: Moisten wound bed and dry surrounding skin. Control pain.

Débridement: None.

Cleansing: Saline.

Dressing: Transparent film or hydrocolloids.

Stage III or IV without necrosis or excessive exudate

Goal: Moisten wound bed and dry surrounding skin.

Débridement: Autolytic with occlusive dressings.

Cleansing: Saline irrigation (35 mL syringe with 19-gauge angiocatheter).

Dressing:

1. If very shallow, use hydrocolloids or hydrogel wafers.
2. If dead space present, lightly fill with hydrogels. Apply hydrocolloid dressing over wound filler.
3. If no signs of healing are seen after several weeks of appropriate care, consider referral for negative pressure wound therapy.

At all stages: Search for and address risk/causative factors. Especially relieve local pressure and optimize systemic condition.

Stage III or IV with necrosis or excessive exudate

Goal: Débride necrotic material, minimize damage to granulating tissue, keep surrounding skin intact and dry.

Débridement:

1. Infection (advancing cellulitis, bacteremia or sepsis)—sharp débridement.
2. Eschars—soften with an occlusive dressing then use sharp débridement.
3. Slough—use mechanical wet-to-dry saline dressings, enzymatic, or autolytic débridement. Switch once slough resolved. Whirlpool baths may be used.

Cleansing: Saline irrigation (35 mL syringe with 19-gauge angiocatheter).

Dressing:

1. If mechanical débridement is appropriate, use wet-to-dry saline-soaked gauze. Loosely fill dead space and undermined area. Do not moisten before removal.
2. After sharp débridement with bleeding, dry dressing or xerogel with hemostatic properties for 6–24 h. Moisten any dry dressings before removal.
3. If excessive exudate, use xerogels or foams. Protect surrounding skin with barrier ointment.
4. If malodorous or purulent exudate, use topical antibacterial agents. If cellulitis, use systemic antibacterials.
5. If no signs of healing are seen after several weeks of appropriate care, consider referral for negative pressure wound therapy.
6. Once necrosis is no longer present, stop débridement and refer to **Stage III and IV without necrosis or excessive exudate.**

Infected pressure ulcers may lead to cellulitis, bacteremia, sepsis or osteomyelitis.[9] Surrounding erythema or swelling greater than 2 cm may indicate cellulitis. If a sterile probe can be inserted to bone, the patient should be considered to have osteomyelitis until proven otherwise,[43] and appropriate **systemic antibiotic therapy** instituted.[9] Quantification of bacterial levels in wound tissue may be accomplished by culture swab, tissue biopsy or needle aspiration. Proper swabbing technique is imperative. Thoroughly cleanse the wound with normal saline, superficially débride to access the deepest wound compartment and swab the culturette in the part of the wound with the most visible signs of infection.[10] Swab the wound bed, not eschar, slough, exudates or edges.[8] Consider an internal medicine or infectious disease consult.

Malignancy: Squamous cell carcinoma has been reported in pressure ulcers, and malignancy should be considered in nonhealing ulcers.[9] If a malignancy is suspected, obtain a dermatology or plastic surgery consultation.

Sinus tracts: Sinus tracts may occur even in superficial pressure ulcers and may contribute to abscess formation or osteomyelitis.[9] If a sinus tract is suspected, consider a plastic surgery consultation.

Pain: Assess patients for pain related to the pressure ulcer or its treatment; pain may decrease mobility and activity.[6] Monitor the level of pain on an ongoing basis.[6,8] Pain relief may be appropriate at certain times, such as before dressing changes.[44] If necessary, administer analgesics prior to wound examination or manipulation.[10,44] Oral analgesics may be used if necessary. Potential topical medications include the **lidocaine** 5% patch or **eutectic mixture of local anesthetics** (EMLA), consisting of lidocaine 2.5% and prilocaine 2.5%.[44] If pain continues to be an issue, consider the pain-reducing properties of various dressings. **Hydrogels** and **hydrocolloids** are both associated with decreased pain.[10]

Therapeutic Tips

- Conduct a weekly reassessment to gauge wound progress and the treatment plan's effectiveness.[8]
- Stage I and II pressure ulcers should show evidence of healing within 1–2 weeks, and Stage III and IV pressure ulcers should show evidence of healing within 2–4 weeks. If no progress is seen, consider the presence of complications and re-evaluate the treatment plan.[5]
- In general, Stage I, II and III pressure ulcers are more likely to heal with local therapy. Stage IV pressure ulcers, especially over ischial tuberosities, often require surgical intervention.[32]
- Pressure-redistribution foam mattresses significantly reduce pressure ulcer incidence, and should be used in patients at risk for pressure ulcers. The overall cost increase from improving preventive measures is minimal compared to the cost avoidance associated with reducing or delaying pressure ulcers.[16]
- Continually assess patients for adequate pain management throughout the treatment of the pressure ulcer. Nonpharmacologic methods to reduce pain at dressing changes include identifying what the patient recognizes as pain triggers and as pain-alleviating factors. Involve the patient in the dressing change if possible, including allowing the patient to remove the dressing themselves. Encourage slow, rhythmic breathing throughout the procedure, and offer the patient the option of a "time-out" during the dressing change.[44]
- When undergoing NPWT, patients may experience pain during dressing changes. Unless medically contraindicated, lidocaine 1% solution may be introduced down the tubing or injected into the foam dressing before a dressing change. Set the pump no higher than 50 mm Hg during this procedure. Wait 15–20 minutes before removing the dressing.[39]
- Consider caregiver time and associated labour costs when selecting a dressing. Caregiver labour costs can exceed the cost of supplies in wound management. For example, continuously moistened saline gauze is inexpensive, but can consume up to 10 times more nursing time than more expensive occlusive dressings such as hydrocolloids or transparent film.[36]

- Caregiver labour costs also vary with repositioning schedule and the position used. Repositioning patients to the 30° tilt position every 3 hours at night requires fewer nurses and takes less time than repositioning patients to the 90° lateral position every 6 hours.[18] This intervention reduces both labour costs and the incidence of pressure ulcers.[18]
- The early recognition and correction of risk factors will expedite the healing of existing pressure ulcers and may prevent the formation of new pressure ulcers. Specialized support surfaces and dressings do not replace the need for vigilant nursing care. Consider incorporating pressure ulcer risk-factor monitoring and prevention into regular nursing procedures to cue nurses to implement preventive measures.[10]

Suggested Readings

Grey JE, Harding KG, Enoch S. Pressure ulcers. *BMJ* 2006;332(7539):472-5.

National Pressure Ulcer Advisory Panel, European Pressure Ulcer Advisory Panel. Pressure ulcer prevention recommendations. In: *Prevention and treatment of pressure ulcers: clinical practice guideline*. Washington (DC): National Pressure Ulcer Advisory Panel; 2009. p. 21-50.

Reddy M, Gill SS, Kalkar SR et al. Treatment of pressure ulcers: a systematic review. *JAMA* 2008;300(22):2647-62.

Reddy M, Gill SS, Rochon PA. Preventing pressure ulcers: a systematic review. *JAMA* 2006;296(8):974-84.

Registered Nurses' Association of Ontario. *Assessment & management of Stage I to IV pressure ulcers*. Toronto (ON): RNAO; revised March 2007. Available from: rnao.ca/sites/rnao-ca/files/Assessment__Management_of_Stage_I_to_IV_Pressure_Ulcers.pdf.

References

1. National Pressure Ulcer Advisory Panel. *Pressure ulcer stages/categories*. Washington (DC): NPUAP; 2007. Available from: www.npuap.org/resources/educational-and-clinical-resources/npuap-pressure-ulcer-stagescategories/. Accessed July 23, 2013.
2. Keast DH, Parslow N, Houghton PE et al. Best practice recommendations for the prevention and treatment of pressure ulcers: update 2006. *Wound Care Canada* 2006;4(1):31-43.
3. National Pressure Ulcer Advisory Panel. *Pressure ulcer prevention points*. Washington (DC): NPUAP; 2006. Available from: www.npuap.org/wp-content/uploads/2012/03/PU_Prev_Points.pdf. Accessed May 28, 2013.
4. Shukla VK, Shukla D, Singh A et al. Risk assessment for pressure ulcer: a hospital-based study. *J Wound Ostomy Continence Nurs* 2008;35(4):407-11.
5. van Rijswijk L, Braden BJ. Pressure ulcer patient and wound assessment: an AHCPR clinical practice guideline update. *Ostomy Wound Manage* 1999;45(1A Suppl):56S-67S.
6. Registered Nurses' Association of Ontario. *Risk assessment & prevention of pressure ulcers*. Toronto (ON): RNAO; revised March 2005. Available from: rnao.ca/sites/rnao-ca/files/Risk_Assessment_and_Prevention_of_Pressure_Ulcers.pdf. Accessed July 4, 2013.
7. National Pressure Ulcer Advisory Panel, European Pressure Ulcer Advisory Panel. Pressure ulcer prevention recommendations. In: *Prevention and treatment of pressure ulcers: clinical practice guideline*. Washington (DC): National Pressure Ulcer Advisory Panel; 2009. p. 21-50. Available from: www.guideline.gov/content.aspx?id=24492.
8. Registered Nurses' Association of Ontario. *Assessment & management of Stage I to IV pressure ulcers*. Toronto (ON): RNAO; revised March 2007. Available from: rnao.ca/sites/rnao-ca/files/Assessment__Management_of_Stage_I_to_IV_Pressure_Ulcers.pdf. Accessed May 28, 2013.
9. Kanj LF, Wilking SV, Phillips TJ. Pressure ulcers. *J Am Acad Dermatol* 1998;38(4):517-36.
10. Arnold MC. Pressure ulcer prevention and management: the current evidence for care. *AACN Clin Issues* 2003;14(4):411-28.
11. Guralnik JM, Harris TB, White LR et al. Occurrence and predictors of pressure sores in the National Health and Nutrition Examination survey follow-up. *J Am Geriatr Soc* 1988;36(9):807-12.
12. Reddy M, Gill SS, Kalkar SR et al. Treatment of pressure ulcers: a systematic review. *JAMA* 2008;300(22):2647-62.
13. Gefen A. How much time does it take to get a pressure ulcer? Integrated evidence from human, animal, and in vitro studies. *Ostomy Wound Manage* 2008;54(10):26-8, 30-5.
14. Grey JE, Harding KG, Enoch S. Pressure ulcers. *BMJ* 2006;332(7539):472-5.
15. McInnes E, Jammali-Blasi A, Bell-Syer SE et al. Support surfaces for pressure ulcer prevention. *Cochrane Database Syst Rev* 2011;(4):CD001735.
16. Pham B, Stern A, Chen W et al. Preventing pressure ulcers in long-term care: a cost-effectiveness analysis. *Arch Intern Med* 2011;171(20):1839-47.
17. Krapfl LA, Gray M. Does regular repositioning prevent pressure ulcers? *J Wound Ostomy Continence Nurs* 2008;35(6):571-7.
18. Moore Z, Cowan S, Posnett J. An economic analysis of repositioning for the prevention of pressure ulcers. *J Clin Nurse* 2013;22(15-16):2354-60.
19. Fowler E, Scott-Williams S, McGuire JB. Practice recommendations for preventing heel pressure ulcers. *Ostomy Wound Manage* 2008;54(10):42-8, 50-2, 54-7.
20. McGinnis E, Stubbs N. Pressure-relieving devices for treating heel pressure ulcers. *Cochrane Database Syst Rev* 2011;(9):CD005485.
21. Wysocki AB. Decubitus ulcers. In: Freedberg IM et al., eds. *Fitzpatrick's dermatology in general medicine*. 5th ed. New York (NY): McGraw-Hill; 1999.
22. Reddy M, Gill SS, Rochon PA. Preventing pressure ulcers: a systematic review. *JAMA* 2006;296(8):974-84.
23. McInnes E, Dumville JC, Jammali-Blasi A et al. Support surfaces for treating pressure ulcers. *Cochrane Database Syst Rev* 2011;(12):CD009490.
24. Cullum N, Nelson EA, Flemming K et al. Systematic reviews of wound care management: (5) beds; (6) compression; (7) laser therapy, therapeutic ultrasound, electrotherapy and electromagnetic therapy. *Health Technol Assess* 2001;5(9):1-221.
25. Blagg MK. Preventing pressure ulcers: proper equipment and monitoring can minimize pressure sores. *Rehab Manag* 2009;22(9):20-2.
26. Bergstrom NI. Strategies for preventing pressure ulcers. *Clin Geriatr Med* 1997;13(3):437-54.
27. Cereda E, Klersy C, Rondanelli M et al. Energy balance in patients with pressure ulcers: a systematic review and meta-analysis of observational studies. *J Am Diet Assoc* 2011;111(12):1868-76.
28. Thomas DR. Improving outcome of pressure ulcers with nutritional interventions: a review of the evidence. *Nutrition* 2001;17(2):121-5.
29. Doley J. Nutrition management of pressure ulcers. *Nutr Clin Pract* 2010;25(1):50-60.
30. Cannon BC, Cannon JP. Management of pressure ulcers. *Am J Health Syst Pharm* 2004;61(18):1895-905.
31. Lyder CH. Pressure ulcer prevention and management. *Annu Rev Nurs Res* 2002;20:35-61.
32. Staas WE, LaMantia JG. Decubitus ulcers and rehabilitation medicine. *Int J Dermatol* 1982;21(8):437-44.
33. Rodeheaver GT. Pressure ulcer debridement and cleansing: a review of current literature. *Ostomy Wound Manage* 1999;45(1A Suppl):80S-85S.

34. Goode PS, Thomas DR. Pressure ulcers. Local wound care. *Clin Geriatr Med* 1997;13(3):543-52.
35. Ladin DA. Understanding dressings. *Clin Plast Surg* 1998;25(3):433-41.
36. Ovington LG. Dressings and ajunctive therapies: AHCPR guidelines revisited. *Ostomy Wound Manage* 1999;45(1A Suppl):94S-106S.
37. Bouza C, Saz Z, Munoz A et al. Efficacy of advanced dressings in the treatment of pressure ulcers: a systematic review. *J Wound Care* 2005;14(5):193-9.
38. Belmin J, Meaume S, Rabus MT et al. Sequential treatment with calcium alginate dressings and hydrocolloid dressings accelerates pressure ulcer healing in older subjects: a multicenter randomized trial of sequential versus nonsequential treatment with hydrocolloid dressings alone. *J Am Geriatr Soc* 2002;50(2):269-74.
39. Gupta S, Baharestani M, Baranoski S et al. Guidelines for managing pressure ulcers with negative pressure wound therapy. *Adv Skin Wound Care* 2004;17(Suppl 2):1-16.
40. Banwell PE, Teot L. Topical negative pressure (TNP): the evolution of a novel wound therapy. *J Wound Care* 2003;12(1):22-8.
41. Baharestani MM, Houliston-Otto DB, Barnes S. Early versus late initiation of negative pressure wound therapy: examining the impact on home care length of stay. *Ostomy Wound Manage* 2008;54(11):48-53.
42. U.S. Food and Drug Administration. FDA Safety Communication. *Update on serious complications associated with Negative Pressure Wound Therapy systems*. Available from: www.fda.gov/MedicalDevices/Safety/AlertsandNotices/ucm244211.htm#summary. Accessed May 29, 2013.
43. Grayson ML, Gibbons GW, Balogh K et al. Probing to bone in infected pedal ulcers. A clinical sign of underlying osteomyelitis in diabetic patients. *JAMA* 1995;273(9):721-3.
44. Local approaches to the pain of pressure ulcers. *Ostomy Wound Manage* 2005;51(1):20, 22.

Chapter 94
Pruritus

Jerry K.L. Tan, MD, FRCPC

Goals of Therapy

- Determine cause of pruritus (Table 1)
- Rule out underlying systemic disease (found in about 20% of pruritic patients without skin disorders)[1] (Figure 1)
- Individualize management of pruritus to maximize effectiveness while minimizing risk of side effects

Investigations

- History should include:
  - location, duration, severity, temporal features (constant or waxing/waning) and aggravating/relieving factors of pruritus
  - association of itching with visible skin rash
  - history of renal, hepatic, hematopoietic, lymphoreticular or endocrine disease
  - skin care, including cleansing routine (harsh soaps, bubble bath preparations and hot tubs can dry and irritate the skin) and topical agents applied to the skin
  - unintended weight loss, fever/chills, night sweats
  - prescription, nonprescription and illicit drug use, particularly opioids
- Physical examination should focus on presence of skin rash, dryness, burrows, excoriations, dermatographism (urtication on stroking the skin), abnormal skin pigmentation (sallowness, jaundice, purple-red discoloration of skin), lymphadenopathy, hepatosplenomegaly
- Laboratory investigations are indicated only if a primary dermatologic cause for pruritus has been excluded and include CBC with differential, fasting serum glucose, liver function tests (including bilirubin), renal function tests, thyroid function tests, chest x-ray, HIV testing
- Depending on the index of suspicion, further investigations may be required to identify underlying systemic disease (Figure 1)

Therapeutic Choices

Information on therapeutic choices can be found in Figure 1.

Nonpharmacologic Choices

- **Skin hydration:** Dry skin due to low ambient humidity or harsh soaps frequently exacerbates pruritus and can be improved with use of gentle cleansers and moisturizers. As most soaps are alkaline and can strip natural moisturizers from the skin, the use of synthetic detergents (such as Spectrogel or Cetaphil cleanser, which have a neutral or slightly acidic pH) or moisturizing gentle soaps with neutral pH can be useful. Helpful measures include avoiding hot water, hot tubs and dry saunas and ensuring adequate indoor humidity.

Colloidal oatmeal bath preparations or adding 4 tablespoons of **baking soda** (sodium bicarbonate) to the bath can be soothing. Bathing is therapeutic for dry skin if water can be entrapped within the skin. A daily tepid bath or shower for 5–10 minutes hydrates the skin. Hydration can be retained by immediate application of moisturizers (e.g., fragrance-free **mineral oil** or moisturizing cream) in the shower stall, after drying the skin. Moisturizers help repair the skin barrier and prevent ingress of irritants. Ointment-based moisturizers are more occlusive and help to retain moisture more effectively but creams are lighter and more cosmetically acceptable.

- **Minimize friction and irritation to the skin.** Gentle towel drying and applying moisturizers and topical medications by dabbing rather than rubbing can help minimize further irritation. Clothing should be soft and loose, and preferably made from cotton. Avoid woolen and synthetic fabrics as well as rough, exposed seams or interfacing. Rinse out detergents thoroughly during laundering, and avoid antistatic agents in the dryer. Use fragrance-free products for laundry, skin cleansing and personal care.
- **Minimize scratching.** Pruritus produces a powerful stimulus to scratch. This scratch-itch cycle is self-perpetuating. Cool compresses can be applied for 20 minutes 4–6 times daily for acute localized itch. A covering of light clothing over the itchy area decreases nonintentional scratching. Fingernails should be kept short.
- **Avoid aggravating factors.** Examples include excessive exercise, high environmental temperature and humidity, hot or prolonged showers or baths, spicy foods, caffeine and alcohol. Patients should maintain a flare diary to identify triggering factors.
- **Ensure adequate sleep.** Pruritus is frequently worse at night, though the reason for this is not completely understood.[2] Moisturizer/emollient or antipruritic topical lotion applied just before bedtime, use of light bedclothes, cool ambient temperature, sleeping without blankets, and a use of sedating antihistamine may be helpful.[2] See Pharmacologic Choices.

Pharmacologic Choices

Topical therapy is the first choice for treatment of mild or localized itch. Systemic therapy is generally reserved for severe and generalized itch that has not responded to topical therapy.[3]

Topical Antipruritics

There is inadequate evidence to support use of **topical antihistamines** (e.g., **diphenhydramine**) for relief of pruritus.[4] Topical diphenhydramine can also cause allergic contact dermatitis.

Menthol 0.25–3% or **camphor** 0.25–0.5% in a light, nonperfumed lotion are commonly used in dermatological practice. They are applied PRN up to TID. Menthol may be preferred as it is less toxic if systemically absorbed.[5,6] These agents elicit a cooling sensation on the skin, which reduces the sensation of itch. Patients reporting reduction in itching with application of cool compresses may benefit from topical therapies containing these agents.[3,5]

Pramoxine hydrochloride 1% is a topical anesthetic with low sensitizing potential that may provide short-term relief.[7,8] Avoid topical benzocaine and other "caine" topical anesthetics as they can sensitize the skin.

Crotamiton, a scabicide and antipruritic, may also be used for its nonspecific antipruritic properties.

Calamine may be useful. Its astringent properties are helpful in blistering conditions, such as chickenpox and acute contact dermatitis, but will dry the skin excessively with long-term use.

Topical corticosteroids are useful and appropriate only if the pruritus is caused by an inflammatory skin condition, which typically presents as visible redness along with symptoms of itch and/or tenderness. Urgent referral to a dermatologist is recommended if there is an extensive area of involvement, presence of erosions or blisters or an adverse impact on quality of life. Choice of topical corticosteroid is based on factors such as location and extent of the eruption, severity and type of inflammation, age of the patient and anticipated duration of use. They are not recommended for chronic, generalized pruritus or for long periods of time.[3] **Topical immune modulators** such as **tacrolimus** or **pimecrolimus** may be useful in pruritus due to a variety of conditions[9] (see Chapter 89).

Capsaicin blocks transmission of itch along peripheral nerves and has been shown to have a beneficial effect in pruritus of various origins.[9] It can cause a transient burning sensation on initial application.

Table 1: **Physical Appearance and Management of Pruritic Skin Diseases**

Physical Appearance	Skin Disease	Management
Urticarial (hives)	Urticaria	Avoid precipitants; antihistamines
	Dermatographism	Avoid precipitants; antihistamines
	Drug eruption	Discontinue drug; symptomatic therapy, antihistamines, topical corticosteroids
Dermatitic (eczematous)	Atopic dermatitis (see Chapter 89)	Mild topical corticosteroids; topical calcineurin inhibitors; hydrate skin; avoid skin irritants
	Xerosis	Hydrate skin
	Contact dermatitis	Avoid precipitants; topical corticosteroids
Dermatitic with burrows	Scabies (see Chapter 97)	Topical permethrin Treat household contacts
Papular (inflamed, elevated bumps)	Drug eruption	Discontinue drug, symptomatic therapy, antihistamines, topical corticosteroids
	Swimmer's itch	Symptomatic therapy, antihistamines
	Insect bites	Symptomatic therapy, antihistamines, topical corticosteroids
	Viral exanthem	Symptomatic therapy
Papulosquamous (scaly, inflamed, elevated bumps)	Lichen planus	Topical or oral corticosteroids, phototherapy
	Lichen simplex chronicus	Moisturization; occlude to prevent scratching; topical corticosteroids
Pustular	Folliculitis (see Chapter 90)	Minimize friction to hair follicles; topical antimicrobials
	Miliaria (heat rash)	Keep skin cool; talcum powder
Nodular	Nodular scabies	Topical permethrin; treat household contacts (see Chapter 97)
	Prurigo nodularis	Occlude to prevent scratching; topical corticosteroids
Vesiculobullous (blistering)	Dermatitis herpetiformis	Gluten-free diet; dapsone
	Bullous pemphigoid	Oral corticosteroids, immunosuppressive agents
	Varicella	Symptomatic; acyclovir or other antivirals
Pigmented macules or papulonodules (flat or elevated orange/brown marks which urticate with rubbing)	Urticaria pigmentosa (mastocytosis)	Antihistamines; avoid ASA, opioids; avoid rubbing the marks

Figure 1: **Management of Pruritus**

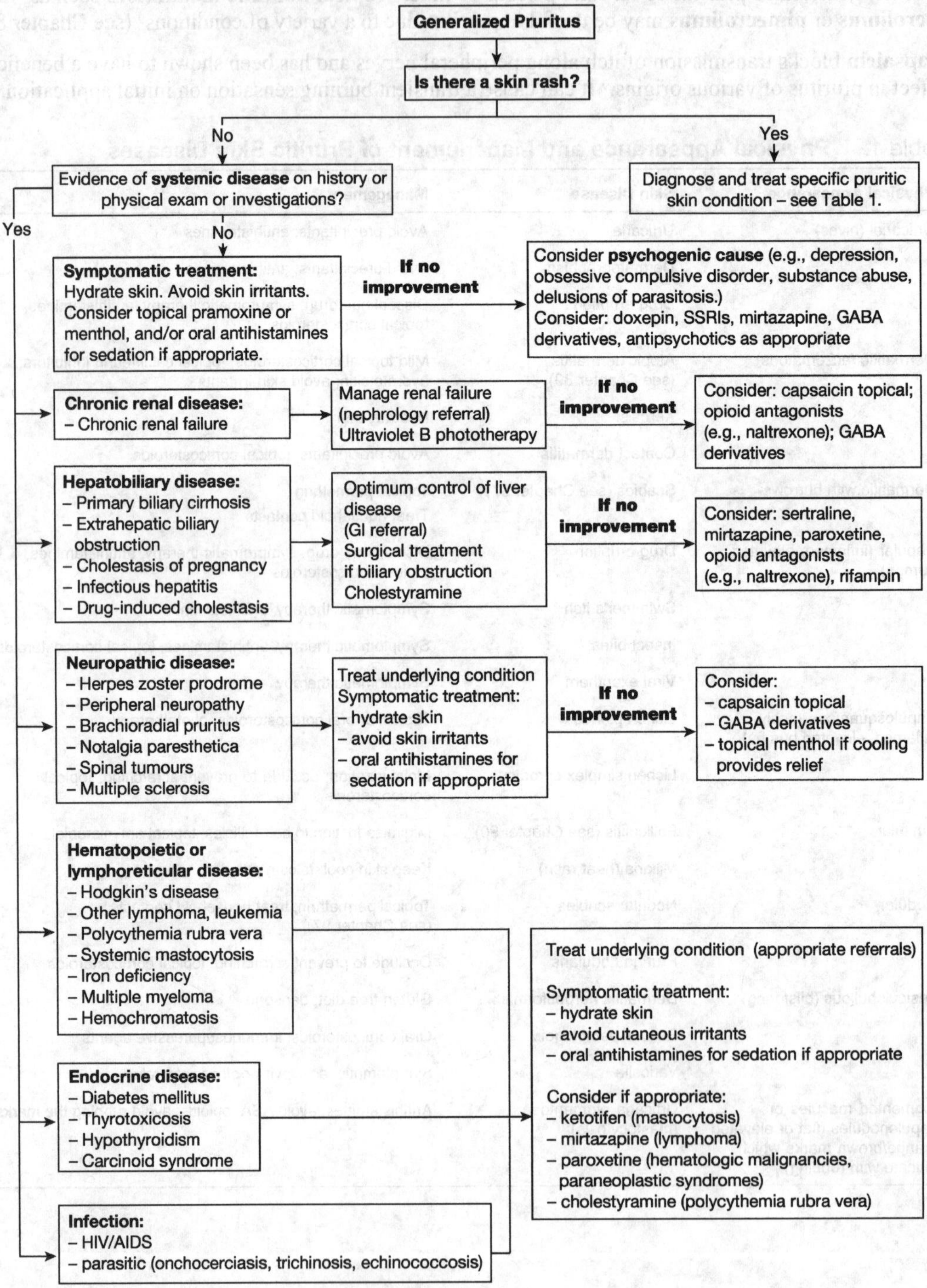

Systemic Therapy

Antihistamines

With the exception of urticaria, antihistamines have little direct effect on other conditions associated with pruritus; however, **first-generation antihistamines** have a sedative effect, which can be useful at night to facilitate sleep.[2]

In the specific case of urticaria, histamine 1 (H_1) blockers are the agents of choice. Antihistamines are more effective at preventing histamine release than combating the effects of previously released histamine.[10] Therefore, in chronic urticaria, administer antihistamines on a regular basis rather than intermittently when itch is most severe.[10,11] **Second-generation (nonsedating) antihistamines** are usually preferred because they have less adverse effects. Some recommend up to 4 times the normal dose of a nonsedating antihistamine in refractory cases of chronic urticaria.[12] Caution regarding sedation may be indicated in this situation.[10] Although good evidence to support the practice is lacking, it may be reasonable to switch to or add on an antihistamine from a different chemical class in patients whose response is inadequate. However, theoretically multiple H_1 antihistamines (from the same or different classes) may not offer additional clinical benefit due to competition for the same (saturated) histamine receptors.[13] First-generation agents such as **hydroxyzine** cause sedation which can be useful at bedtime, though there are concerns that patients suffer significant impairment of daytime performance without subjective awareness of drowsiness[10] and that anticholinergic side effects can be problematic, particularly in the elderly. Histamine 2 (H_2) receptors are not directly involved in itch.[14] Evidence is insufficient regarding whether the addition of H_2 receptor antagonists is useful to reduce itching from urticaria when the sole use of H_1 antihistamines is inadequate.[13,15] See Chapter 50 for more information on dosage, adverse effects and drug interactions of the various classes of antihistamines.

Other Systemic Pharmacologic Treatments

The evolving understanding of the pathophysiology of pruritus has led to many different therapies being tried. Many of those listed below have limited available evidence or results have not been confirmed with large, randomized trials.

Doxepin, a tricyclic antidepressant with potent antihistaminic properties, is useful in some cases of chronic urticaria.[16] It may also be helpful in those patients with psychogenic causes of pruritus.[17] **Mirtazapine**, a dual action antidepressant with potent antihistaminic and serotonergic effects, has also been shown to be effective in pruritus with various underlying etiologies.[3,18] In a small (n=72) open label study, the SSRIs **paroxetine** and **fluvoxamine** reduced chronic itch in patients with atopic dermatitis, systemic lymphoma and solid carcinoma.[19] Additionally, a randomized double-blind cross-over study in palliative care patients (n=26) showed paroxetine reduced itch after 2–3 days of treatment in patients with severe pruritus associated with nondermatologic etiologies including drug-induced (nonopioid), paraneoplastic syndromes and cholestasis.[20] **Sertraline** reduced itch in patients with pruritus associated with cholestatic liver disease in a small (n=12), randomized double-blind, placebo-controlled trial.[21]

Gabapentin and **pregabalin** may act to inhibit central itch pathways, as they are structural congeners of the neurotransmitter gamma-butyric acid (GABA). There is evidence that they may reduce uremic itch.[22,23] They may also be useful for neuropathic and psychogenic pruritus and in those with intractable pruritus from systemic causes.[9]

An imbalance of the endogenous opioid pathways that contribute to itch is thought to play a role in the pathophysiology of pruritus. Itch is induced by μ-receptor agonists and κ-receptor antagonists. Correspondingly, reduction in itch can be mediated by μ-receptor antagonists and κ-receptor agonists. **Naltrexone** (μ-receptor antagonist) has been reported to improve pruritus in patients with end-stage renal disease, atopic dermatitis, cholestasis and burns.[24,25,26,27] In a small (n=5) open-label case series **butorphanol** (κ-receptor agonist and mixed μ-receptor agonist-antagonist) produced marked improvement in patients with intractable pruritus.[28]

Ketotifen, a selective H_1 antihistamine that also stabilizes mast cells and inhibits mediator release, is used primarily in asthma prophylaxis but small studies have shown some benefit in urticaria[29] and mastocytosis.[30]

Cholestyramine and **colestipol resins** are effective for pruritus related to cholestatic liver disease[31] (see Chapter 57). These agents have also been used successfully in uremic pruritus and polycythemia rubra vera.[14]

Rifampin has been reported to be helpful for treatment of pruritus due to chronic cholestasis due to its ability to lower hepatocyte bile salt concentrations.[23]

Serotonin antagonists (e.g., **ondansetron**) have been used in some cases of pruritus of renal or hepatic origin,[32,33] however a systematic review found negligible benefit.[34]

Montelukast, a leukotriene receptor antagonist, may be an effective adjunct to standard antihistamines for a minority of patients with chronic idiopathic urticaria, particularly those with severe disease.[35]

Aprepitant, a substance p antagonist may be effective in refractory pruritus and in severe pruritus due to biologic cancer treatments.[36]

The use of **systemic corticosteroids** for pruritus is indicated only when there is associated cutaneous inflammation for which more specific treatments are inadequate or delayed in onset. In view of the potential for serious adverse effects, such an option requires careful consideration.

Phototherapy

Phototherapy with ultraviolet B (UVB) wavelength (290–320 nm) is an effective treatment for uremic pruritus. A course of 8–10 treatments usually results in symptomatic improvement. Maintenance therapy may be administered as required. UVB phototherapy is often effective for pruritus of other etiologies, particularly primary inflammatory conditions of the skin.[16]

Choices during Pregnancy and Breastfeeding

Pregnancy and Pruritus

There are a number of pruritic conditions specific to pregnancy which should always be considered when evaluating a pregnant patient with pruritus: pruritic urticarial papules and plaques of pregnancy, prurigo of pregnancy, pemphigoid gestationis, intrahepatic cholestasis of pregnancy and pruritic folliculitis of pregnancy. The assessment and management of these conditions is outside the scope of this chapter. With respect to possible changes in pre-existing pruritus during pregnancy, there is no consistent prognostic pattern as it depends on how the underlying cause is affected by the pregnancy.

Management of Pruritus during Pregnancy

General nonpharmacologic measures including avoidance of triggers and adequate skin moisturization are important for all patients with pruritus. **Colloidal oatmeal** baths and **calamine** lotion are generally considered safe during pregnancy.[37] There are no reports of teratogenicity with topical use of **menthol** or **camphor**. Systemic absorption is minimal.[38] Specialized sources suggest that limited topical use during pregnancy is not expected to pose significant risks to the fetus.[39,40,41] The **local anesthetics** lidocaine and prilocaine are generally considered safe for use on small areas for short periods of time (e.g., to facilitate skin biopsy or dental procedures) since their absorption is low[42] but there is no information on safety of other dermatologic uses during pregnancy and these agents can cause skin sensitization. There is no information available about the safety of the less skin-sensitizing anesthetic **pramoxine**. However, since its systemic absorption is low it does not appear to pose a significant risk to the fetus.[39] There have been no reports of teratogenicity due to topical use of **crotamiton** during pregnancy. Systemic absorption after dermal application is low[40] and it has been recommended as a second-line option for treatment of scabies during pregnancy.[41] **Topical corticosteroids** are useful if pruritus is caused by an inflammatory skin condition. Except in the case of extensive use of the most potent agents, systemic absorption of topical corticosteroids is low and poses no known risk to the baby.[43,44] Topical **capsaicin** use is not recommended due to lack of information on safety in pregnancy.[41] Oral antihistamines are helpful in the specific case of urticaria. **Cetirizine** and **loratadine** are the nonsedating second-generation antihistamines of choice during pregnancy. **Fexofenadine** and **desloratadine** are safe alternatives.[45] If the sedative side effect of a first-generation antihistamine is desired to improve sleep in patients with pruritus of any etiology, **chlorpheniramine**, **diphenhydramine** and **hydroxyzine** have the most evidence of safety in pregnancy.[41,45]

Management of Pruritus during Breastfeeding

Maximize nonpharmacologic measures (e.g., use of moisturizers and avoidance of triggers). As a general precaution care should be taken to avoid contact of the infant's skin with any topically treated areas of the mother's skin. **Colloidal oatmeal** baths and use of **calamine** lotion are considered safe while breastfeeding. Due to low systemic absorption, maternal use of topical **menthol** or **camphor** is unlikely to result in significant exposure to the infant via breast milk.[41] Topical use of the local anesthetic **lidocaine** can cause skin sensitization in the mother but should not pose any risk to a breastfed baby as even systemic use results in low excretion into breast milk and poor absorption in the infant.[46] Due to insignificant systemic absorption, there is not expected to be any excretion of **pramoxine** (a local anesthetic with low sensitizing potential) into breast milk and therefore no risk to the infant during maternal use.[39] There are no reports of adverse effects on breastfed infants whose mothers used topical **crotamiton** but its safety has not been studied. Some experts recommend crotamiton as second-line therapy for scabies in breastfeeding women due to its low absorption.[41] Risk to the baby via passage of **topical corticosteroids** into breast milk is unlikely since only extensive use of the most potent corticosteroids causes systemic effects in the mother. The lowest effective potency topical corticosteroid should be applied to the smallest area possible for the shortest possible time.[46] If applied to the areola/nipple area, wipe off prior to nursing. There is no information on the safety of topical **capsaicin** in breastfeeding though exposure of the infant to significant quantities via breast milk is unlikely.[41] Use of oral second-generation antihistamines (**cetirizine**, **desloratadine, fexofenadine, loratadine**) for urticaria in breastfeeding women should not pose any risk to the baby.[46] Occasional small doses of first-generation antihistamines (**chlorpheniramine**, **diphenhydramine**, **hydroxyzine**) should not adversely affect a breastfed infant, but larger doses or prolonged use may lead to drowsiness in the infant or decrease in the milk supply.[46]

A discussion of general principles on the use of medications in these special populations can be found in Appendix II and Appendix III. Other specialized reference sources are also provided in these appendices.

Therapeutic Tips

- Dry skin leads to dermatitis which can exacerbate other causes of pruritus. Use gentle cleansers (e.g., synthetic detergents) rather than soap to avoid drying skin further. Avoid hot water showers as this leads to greater risk of irritation. Use moisturizers to repair disruptions in skin barrier and improve dryness.
- Avoid topical corticosteroids and immune modulators in the absence of clinically evident skin inflammation.
- Always check for burrows to evaluate for the possibility of scabies.
- Test for dermatographism or pressure sensitivity (urticarial lesion appears in site of superficial scratch on skin) because this common cause of pruritus can be suppressed with antihistamines

[Evidence: SORT B *].[12] Consider regular daily use of nonsedating antihistamine with periodic tapering to determine ongoing need.

- Careful follow-up is required. The itching of scabies, urticaria and drug eruptions may precede onset of skin manifestations. Likewise, declarative symptoms of a systemic disease may eventually develop in a patient with pruritus.
- Topical agents may be kept in a refrigerator because the physical cooling enhances their antipruritic effect.

* SORT (Strength of Recommendation Taxonomy) is a rating system (A, B or C) that addresses the quality of available evidence. For more information consult **How to Use *Compendium of Therapeutic Choices*** on page xxv.

Table 2: Pharmacologic Therapy of Pruritus

Class	Drug	Dose	Adverse Effects	Comments	Cost[a]
Antihistamines, Oral	*hydroxyzine* Atarax, generics	25–75 mg TID–QID po	Dizziness, drowsiness, fatigue, rash, dry mouth, blurred vision. Occasionally may cause paradoxical excitation in children.	Indicated only in urticaria (histamine-mediated). Often used for sedative properties in other types of pruritus. Liquid form available.	$$
Antihistamines, Other	See Chapter 50, Table 2			Indicated only in urticaria (histamine-mediated). Often used for sedative properties in other types of pruritus.	
Astringents	*calamine lotion* generics	Apply once daily–QID PRN topically	Skin irritation.	Use only on moist lesions, otherwise too drying.	$
Bath Emollients	*colloidal oatmeal* Aveeno Bath Preparations, generics	Added to warm (not hot) bath water as needed—soak for 10–15 min			$
Counterirritants	*menthol*[b]	0.25–3% in moisturizing cream, ointment or lotion base. Apply PRN up to TID, topically	Skin irritation (burning, redness) at higher concentrations.	Lower concentration products preferred. Do not apply to large areas of skin or open wounds.	$$$
	camphor[b]	0.25–0.5% in moisturizing cream, ointment or lotion base. Apply PRN up to TID, topically	Skin irritation (burning, redness) at higher concentrations. Absorbed through intact and broken skin. Excessive topical use can result in systemic toxicity (including nausea, vomiting, headache, dizziness, tremors, seizures).	Lower concentration products preferred. Do not apply to large areas of skin or open wounds. Young children may be more susceptible to adverse effects associated with even minor systemic absorption of camphor (including via topical use and inhalation); the American Academy of Pediatrics recommends that camphor not be used in children.	$$$
Local Anesthetics	*pramoxine*[c] Aveeno Anti-Itch	1% lotion. Apply up to TID–QID PRN topically	Contact dermatitis, burning, stinging.	Do not apply to large areas of skin or open wounds.	$

(cont'd)

Table 2: Pharmacologic Therapy of Pruritus *(cont'd)*

Class	Drug	Dose	Adverse Effects	Comments	Cost[a]
Scabicides and Antipruritics	*crotamiton* Eurax	10% cream. Apply PRN topically	Local irritation, warm sensation.		$$$
Topical Corticosteroids	See Chapter 89, Table 3			Indicated only for pruritus due to cutaneous inflammation (visible redness, itch and/or tenderness).	

[a] Cost of 50 g or 50 mL for topical products and 10-day supply for oral doses; includes drug cost and estimate of compounding fees for extemporaneously compounded preparations where applicable.
[b] Extemporaneously compounded preparations can be used.
[c] Usually available as a combination product. Aveeno Anti-Itch also contains calamine.
Dosage adjustment may be required in renal impairment; see Appendix I
Legend: $ < $5 $$ $5–15 $$$ $15–25

Suggested Readings

Etter L, Myers SA. Pruritus in systemic disease: mechanisms and management. *Dermatol Clin* 2002;20(3):459-72.

Moses S. Pruritus. *Am Fam Physician* 2003;68(6)1135-42.

Patel T, Yosipovitch G. The management of chronic pruritus in the elderly. *Skin Therapy Lett* 2010;15(8):5-9.

Patel T, Yosipovitch G. Therapy of pruritus. *Expert Opin Pharmacother* 2010;11(10):1673-82.

Xander C, Meerpohl JJ, Glandi D et al. Pharmacological interventions for pruritus in adult palliative care patients. *Cochrane Database of Syst Rev* 2013;6:CD008320.

References

1. Kantor GR, Lookingbill DP. Generalized pruritus and systemic disease. *J Am Acad Dermatol* 1983;9(3):375-82.
2. Patel T, Ishiuji Y, Yosipovitch G. Nocturnal itch: why do we itch at night? *Acta Derm Venereol* 2007;87(4):295-8.
3. Patel T, Yosipovitch G. Therapy of pruritus. *Expert Opin Pharmacother* 2010;11(10):1673-82.
4. Eschler DC, Klein PA. An evidence-based review of the efficacy of topical antihistamines in the relief of pruritus. *J Drugs Dermatol* 2010;9(8):992-7.
5. Patel T, Ishiuji Y, Yosipovitch G. Menthol: a refreshing look at this ancient compound. *J Am Acad Dermatol* 2007;57(5):873-8.
6. Camphor revisited: focus on toxicity. Committee on Drugs. American Academy of Pediatrics. *Pediatrics* 1994;94(1):127-8. (Reaffirmed May 2009).
7. Yosipovitch G, Maibach HI. Effect of topical pramoxine on experimentally induced pruritus in humans. *J Am Acad Dermatol* 1997;37(2 Pt 1):278-80.
8. Young TA, Patel TS, Camacho F et al. A pramoxine-based anti-itch lotion is more effective than a control lotion for the treatment of uremic pruritus in adult hemodialysis patients. *J Dermatolog Treat* 2009;20(2):76-81.
9. Weisshaar E, Szepietowski JC, Darsow U et al. European guideline on chronic pruritus. *Acta Derm Venereol* 2012;92(5):563-81.
10. Wallace DV, Dykewicz MS, Bernstein DI et al. The diagnosis and management of rhinitis: an updated practice parameter. *J Allergy Clin Immunol* 2008;122(2 Suppl):S1-84.
11. Mattila MJ, Paakkari I. Variations among non-sedating antihistamines: are there real differences? *Eur J Clin Pharmacol* 1999;55(2):85-93.
12. Zuberbier T, Asero R, Bindslev-Jensen C et al. EAACI/GA(2)LEN/EDF/WAO guideline: management of urticaria. *Allergy* 2009;64(10):1427-43.
13. Ortonne JP. Chronic urticaria: a comparison of management guidelines. *Expert Opin Pharmacother* 2011;12(17):2683-93.
14. Denman ST. A review of pruritus. *J Am Acad Dermatol* 1986;14(3):375-92.
15. Fedorowicz Z, van Zuuren EJ, Hu N. Histamine H2-receptor antagonists for urticaria. *Cochrane Database Syst Rev* 2012;3:CD008596.
16. Greaves MW. Recent advances in pathophysiology and current management of itch. *Ann Acad Med Singapore* 2007;36(9):788-92.
17. Patel T, Yosipovitch G. The management of chronic pruritus in the elderly. *Skin Therapy Lett* 2010;15(8):5-9.
18. Demierre MF, Taverna J. Mirtazapine and gabapentin for reducing pruritus in cutaneous T-cell lymphoma. *J Am Acad Dermatol* 2006;55(3):543-4.
19. Stander S, Bockenholt B, Schurmeyer-Horst F et al. Treatment of chronic pruritus with the selective serotonin re-uptake inhbitors paroxetine and fluvoxamine: results of an open-labelled, two-arm proof of concept study. *Acta Derm Venereol* 2009;89(1):45-51.
20. Zylicz Z, Krajnik M, Sorge AA et al. Paroxetine in the treatment of severe non-dermatological pruritus: a randomized, controlled trial. *J Pain Symptom Manage* 2003;26(6):1105-12.
21. Mayo MJ, Handem I, Saldana S et al. Sertraline as a first-line treatment for cholestatic pruritus. *Hepatology* 2007;45(3):666-74.
22. Manenti L, Tansinda P, Vaglio A. Uraemic pruritus: clinical characteristics, pathophysiology and treatment. *Drugs* 2009;69(3):251-63.
23. Xander C, Meerpohl JJ, Glandi D et al. Pharmacological interventions for pruritus in adult palliative care patients. *Cochrane Database of Syst Rev* 2013;6:CD008320.
24. Peer G, Kivity S, Agami O et al. Randomised crossover trial of naltrexone in uraemic pruritus. *Lancet* 1996;348(9041):1552-4.
25. Malekzad F, Arbabi M, Mohtasham N et al. Efficacy of oral naltrexone on pruritus in atopic eczema: a double-blind, placebo-controlled study. *J Eur Acad Dermatol Venereol* 2009;23(8):948-50.
26. Mansour-Ghanaei F, Taheri A, Froutan H et al. Effect of oral naltrexone on pruritus in cholestatic patients. *World J Gastroenterol* 2006;12(7):1125-8.
27. Jung SI, Seo CH, Jang K et al. Efficacy of naltrexone in the treatment of chronic refractory itching in burn patients: preliminary report of an open trial. *J Burn Care Res* 2009;30(2):257-60.
28. Dawn AG, Yosipovitch G. Butorphanol for treatment of intractable pruritus. *J Am Acad Dermatol* 2006;54(3):527-31.
29. Kamide R, Niimura M, Ueda H et al. Clinical evaluation of ketotifen for chronic urticaria: multicenter double-blind comparative study with clemastine. *Ann Allergy* 1989;62(4):322-5.
30. Povoa P, Ducla-Soares J, Fernandes A et al. A case of systemic mastocytosis; therapeutic efficacy of ketotifen. *J Intern Med* 1991;229(5):475-7.
31. Kremer AE, Beuers U, Oude-Elferink RP et al. Pathogenesis and treatment of pruritus in cholestasis. *Drugs* 2008;68(15):2163-82.
32. Frigon C, Desparmet J. Ondansetron treatment in a child presenting with chronic intractable pruritus. *Pain Res Manag* 2006;11(4):245-7.
33. Mela M, Mancuso A, Burroughs AK. Review article: pruritus in cholestatic and other liver diseases. *Aliment Pharmacol Ther* 2003;17(7):857-70.
34. To TH, Clark K, Lam L et al. The role of ondansetron in the management of cholestatic or uremic pruritus—a systematic review. *J Pain Symptom Manage* 2012;44(5):725-30.
35. Kosnik M, Subic T. Add-on montelukast in antihistamine-resistant chronic idiopathic urticaria. *Respir Med* 2011;105(Suppl 1):S84-8.
36. Santini D, Vincenzi B, Guida FM et al. Aprepitant for management of severe pruritus related to biological cancer treatments: a pilot study. *Lancet Oncol* 2012;13(10):1020-4.
37. American Pregnancy Association. *Skin changes during pregnancy*. Available from: www.americanpregnancy.org/pregnancyhealth/skin-changes.html. Accessed November 18, 2013.

38. Martin D, Valdez J, Boren J et al. Dermal absorption of camphor, menthol, and methyl salicylate in humans. *J Clin Pharmacol* 2004;44(10):1151-7.
39. Briggs GG, Freeman RK, Yaffe SJ. *Drugs in pregnancy and lactation: a reference guide to fetal and neonatal risk*. 9th ed. Philadelphia (PA): Wolters Kluwer Health; Lippincott Williams & Wilkins; 2011.
40. Schaefer C, Peters P, Miller R. *Drugs during pregnancy and lactation: treatment options and risk assessment*. 2nd ed. Boston (MA): Elsevier Academic Press; 2007.
41. Ferreira E, Martin B, Morin C. *Grossesse et allaitement: guide thérapeutique*. 2nd ed. Montréal (QC): CHU Sainte Justine; 2013.
42. Lee K, Leachman S. Dermatologic drugs during pregnancy and lactation. In: Wolverton SE. *Comprehensive dermatologic drug therapy*. 3rd ed. Edinburgh (GB): Saunders/Elsevier; 2013.
43. Lam J, Polifka JE, Dohil MA. Safety of dermatologic drugs used in pregnant patients with psoriasis and other inflammatory skin diseases. *J Am Acad Dermatol* 2008;59(2):295-315.
44. Weatherhead S, Robson SC, Reynolds NJ. Eczema in pregnancy. *BMJ* 2007;335(7611):152-4.
45. Moretti ME. Pregnancy and breastfeeding: nonprescription therapy for common conditions. In: *Therapeutic choices for minor ailments*. 1st ed. Ottawa (ON): Canadian Pharmacists Association; 2013. p. 982-7.
46. Drugs and Lactation Database (LactMed). Bethesda (MD): U.S. National Library of Medicine. Available from: toxnet.nlm.nih.gov/cgi-bin/sis/htmlgen?LACT. Accessed November 18, 2013.

Skin Disorders

Chapter 95
Psoriasis

Richard G. B. Langley, MD, FRCPC

Psoriasis is a chronic immunologically mediated skin disease with markedly increased epidermal cellular turnover. Up to one-third of patients may develop psoriatic arthritis. In addition, a number of comorbidities have been recognized to occur with psoriasis (e.g., cardiovascular disease, hypertension, diabetes, obesity, inflammatory bowel disease, depression, anxiety, alcoholism). Before making therapeutic choices, it is essential to rule out other conditions that affect the same areas of the body and to establish the correct diagnosis. A regional approach is provided since patients often present with a skin problem affecting their scalp, face, hands and feet, body, fold areas or nails.

Goals of Therapy

- Improve the signs and symptoms of psoriasis and the patient's quality of life
- Provide psoriasis control for the longest periods possible
- Identify patients with more severe forms of disease or psoriatic arthritis, for appropriate management and/or referral

The management of psoriasis affecting all areas of the body is illustrated in Figure 1.

Figure 1: Management of Psoriasis[4,6,25]

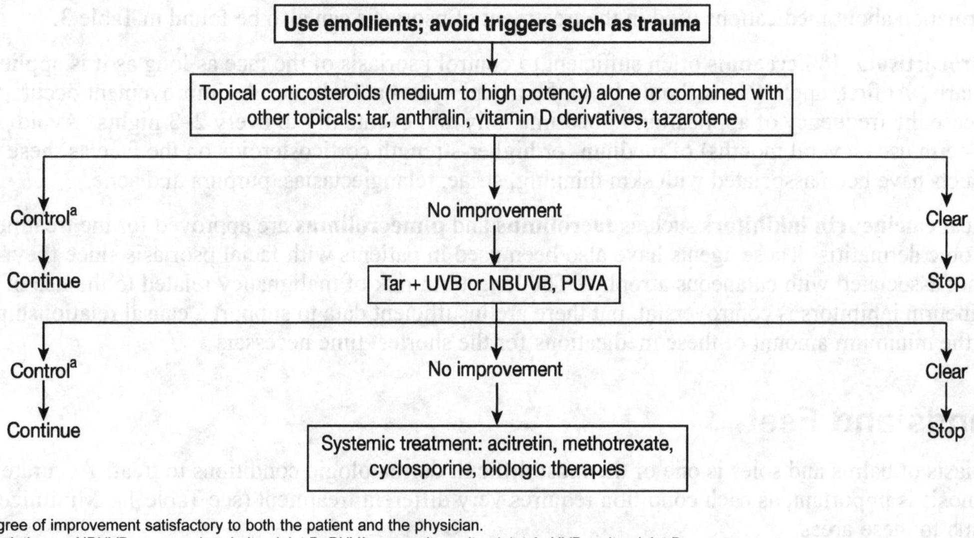

[a] Degree of improvement satisfactory to both the patient and the physician.
Abbreviations: NBUVB = narrow-band ultraviolet B; PUVA = psoralens ultraviolet A; UVB = ultraviolet B

Scalp

Seborrheic dermatitis can mimic psoriasis; however, distinct patterns and morphology help to distinguish these conditions. In psoriasis the scale is usually thicker and more adherent than in seborrheic dermatitis, and there are often signs of psoriasis on the knees, elbows or sacral area. Typical nail changes and arthritis may accompany psoriasis.

Pharmacologic Choices

Information about medications used in the treatment of psoriasis can also be found in Table 3.

In scalp psoriasis, removal of the scales is important. This can be done with **oil-based products** with or without **salicylic acid**, **calcipotriol scalp solution**, and/or a medium-strength **corticosteroid** such as **betamethasone** left on the scalp overnight. For more resistant cases, higher-potency topical corticosteroids may be useful as well as **tar-based shampoos** which can be used in the morning to wash off the oil and scales. Tar shampoos are most effective if used daily; however, if adherence to daily use is an issue, application every 2–3 days is better than not at all. New formulations of many scalp products (gel, solution, foam) are easier to use and may increase patient acceptance and adherence.

Face

On the face, the nature of the scale helps to differentiate among the possible diagnoses:

- Psoriasis—sharply demarcated, silvery scale
- Seborrheic dermatitis—greasy, brownish-yellow scale typically involving eyebrows and perinasal area
- Discoid lupus erythematosus—adherent, carpet-tack scale with scarring
- Tinea of face—little or no scale except at the margins (central clearing)

Pharmacologic Choices

Information about medications used in the treatment of psoriasis can also be found in Table 3.

Hydrocortisone 1% cream is often sufficient to control psoriasis of the face as long as it is applied regularly. At first, applications should be in the morning and at bedtime. As improvement occurs, decrease the frequency of application to bedtime only and eventually to every 2–3 nights. Avoid long-term use (several months) of medium- or higher-strength corticosteroids on the face as these products have been associated with skin thinning, striae, telangiectasias, purpura and acne.

Topical **calcineurin inhibitors** such as **tacrolimus** and **pimecrolimus** are approved for the treatment of atopic dermatitis. These agents have also been used in patients with facial psoriasis since they are not associated with cutaneous atrophy.[1] The long-term risk of malignancy related to the use of calcineurin inhibitors is controversial, but there are insufficient data to support a causal relationship.[2,3] Use the minimum amount of these medications for the shortest time necessary.

Hands and Feet

Psoriasis of palms and soles is one of the most difficult dermatologic conditions to treat. Accurate diagnosis is important, as each condition requires very different treatment (see Table 1). Minimize trauma to these areas.

Table 1: **Differential Diagnosis of Psoriasis of the Hands and Feet**

Characteristics	Psoriasis	Tinea[a]	Eczema
Lesion	Well-defined scaling, hyperkeratosis and/or pustules	Scaling and vesicles (central clearing)	Poorly defined scaling, vesicles, pustules with crusting
	Maceration between all toes	Maceration between 4th and 5th toes	Maceration between all toes
Site	Weight-bearing areas of soles	Instep area	Weight-bearing area
	Bilateral hands and feet	Asymmetrical	Symmetrical
	Pits of nails or yellow discolouration and lifting of the nail plate (onycholysis)	Asymmetrical nail changes	Nonspecific nail changes
	Psoriasis elsewhere	Tinea cruris	Eczema elsewhere, personal or family history of atopy
Response to topical therapy			
Tar	++	–	+
Topical corticosteroids	+	–	++
Antifungals	–	++	–

[a] A potassium hydroxide scraping or a fungal culture can help to confirm the diagnosis.

Pharmacologic Choices

Topical Therapy (Table 3)

One choice is frequent lubrication with **petrolatum** as well as use of medium- to high-potency **corticosteroid ointment** with or without added **salicylic acid**. Ointments are the most effective delivery system since they increase permeability in areas that are dry and scaly. Lotions can be used in thinner-skinned areas. Creams are cosmetically more acceptable and can be used in areas involved in movement.

Phototherapy

Phototherapy includes UVB with **tar, anthralin, calcipotriol** or **tazarotene**. This treatment is best guided by a dermatologist. Some centres have added Narrow-Band UVB (NBUVB; 311–313 nm) to their phototherapy modalities. These newer lamps may obviate the need for topical or systemic treatments. Phototherapy is also advancing with the use of excimer laser (308 nm) for resistant localized psoriatic plaques.[4,5,6]

Systemic Therapy

Information about systemic medications used in the treatment of psoriasis can also be found in Table 4.

Acitretin (an oral retinoid) 10–75 mg daily, **methotrexate** 7.5–22.5 mg once a week or **cyclosporine** for short periods at a starting dose of 2.5–5 mg/kg/day have been used in the treatment of moderate to severe psoriasis (Figure 1).

Body and Extremities

Classic psoriasis with nonpruritic, silvery scaling plaques affecting the elbows, knees and sacral areas is usually easy to diagnose. A family history of psoriasis may be present. Tinea versicolor has a fine orange-brown scale with areas of hypopigmentation and is usually limited to the upper thorax. Pityriasis rosea presents with a "herald" patch and approximately a week later with an acute eruption of oval pink lesions with a fine collarette of central scale and rarely affects elbows and knees. Eczematous dermatitis is itchy and often crusty, lichenified and excoriated. Tinea corporis has an active periphery with a clear centre and a positive potassium hydroxide (KOH) examination for fungal elements, and/or a positive fungal culture.

Pharmacologic Choices

Information about medications used in the treatment of psoriasis can also be found in Table 3 and Table 4.

Choosing appropriate therapy from a number of effective topical and systemic agents can be challenging. Topical agents such as medium-high potency **corticosteroids**, **vitamin D derivatives**, **tazarotene**, **tar** and **anthralin** are used alone or in combination (Figure 1).

Phototherapy is typically used only if common local treatments with corticosteroids, vitamin D derivatives (calcipotriol, calcitriol), tazarotene, tars or anthralin are ineffective on their own. It is also highly effective for guttate psoriasis. If required, consult a dermatologist who is familiar with phototherapy and the various systemic therapies (see Table 4). The tars used with UVB are either **crude coal tar** 2% or **coal tar distillate** 10% with or without **salicylic acid**. UVA therapy following topical or systemic administration of the photosensitizing agent **psoralens** (PUVA) is used less frequently than in the past due to concerns about long-term adverse effects and because of the increasing use of NBUVB therapy.

Fold Areas

In these areas, the diagnosis can be difficult (see Table 2), but the treatment will usually include a topical corticosteroid.

Pharmacologic Choices

Information about medications used in the treatment of psoriasis can also be found in Table 3.

In most cases, daily to twice-daily applications of **hydrocortisone 1% cream** with or without an antimonilial/antifungal agent such as **ketoconazole** (to combat possible fungal infection in warm, moist skin folds), will dramatically improve the eruption with little or no adverse effects.

Topical **calcineurin inhibitors** such as **tacrolimus** and **pimecrolimus** are approved for the treatment of atopic dermatitis. These agents have also been used in patients with psoriasis of the fold areas.[1] See Face: Pharmacologic Choices.

Table 2: **Differential Diagnosis of Psoriasis in Fold Areas**

Psoriasis	Tinea	Eczema	Moniliasis
Bright red, well-defined	Scaling at edge	Very itchy	Satellite papules and pustules
KOH-negative	KOH-positive	KOH-negative	KOH-positive
Psoriasis elsewhere	Maceration between 4th and 5th toes	Eczema elsewhere	Affects fold areas mainly

Abbreviations: KOH = potassium hydroxide stain, which is diagnostic for fungi

Nails

Psoriatic nail changes can be difficult to differentiate from fungal infection of the nails. Both cause yellowish-white discolouration of the distal nail plate but psoriasis produces small "ice pick" pits of the nail.

Pharmacologic Choices

Information about systemic medications used in the treatment of nail psoriasis can also be found in Table 4.

Most topical therapeutic measures are unsatisfactory. **Corticosteroid** injections to the nail matrix may be effective, but are painful and seldom tolerated. Systemic therapy is often required for patients with psoriatic nail changes. It is advisable to keep the nails short to decrease the risk of nail separation caused by trauma. Discourage aggressive manicures.

Severe or Resistant Psoriasis

Pharmacologic Choices

- Combining **oral retinoids** and phototherapy gives better results in severe psoriasis than using each treatment separately.[1]
- **Biologic response modifiers** are alternatives for patients with moderate to severe psoriasis.[7] **Adalimumab**, **etanercept**, **infliximab** and **ustekinumab** are approved in Canada for the treatment of psoriasis. See Table 4.
- Emerging therapies pending approval in Canada include **apremilast**, **tofacitinib** and new interleukin-17 and tumor necrosis factor alpha inhibitors.
- **Intralesional corticosteroid injections** (e.g., **triamcinolone**) are used occasionally for very resistant psoriatic plaques.

Choices during Pregnancy and Breastfeeding

Psoriasis and Pregnancy

Psoriasis often improves during pregnancy. In one study, 76% of patients reported either improvement or no change in their condition, whereas only 23% of patients reported worsening of their psoriasis during pregnancy.[8] The effect of psoriasis on pregnancy outcomes is unclear: studies have shown both adverse effects[9] and no effect.[10]

Pre-pregnancy Considerations

Methotrexate must be stopped at least 3 months prior to conception in women.[11] It is also recommended that men stop methotrexate 3 months prior to conception,[11] however, a small cohort study showed no adverse pregnancy outcomes after paternal low-dose methotrexate exposure during time of conception.[12] It is recommended that women taking **acitretin** avoid pregnancy for 3 years after cessation of therapy due to the extremely long half-life of the teratogenic metabolite etretinate, produced when alcohol is consumed while on acitretin.[13,14] There is no standard waiting period before conception following treatment with acitretin in males. Small studies indicate that there does not appear to be any risk of developmental toxicity due to paternal exposure.[15,16]

Management of Psoriasis during Pregnancy

Many clinicians recommend that patients discontinue all unnecessary therapies during pregnancy, particularly if the disease is relatively mild. For patients with moderate to severe disease this may not be practical. If treatment is required topical therapy is preferred. **Topical corticosteroids** are safe to use since systemic absorption (with the exception of extensive use of the most potent agents) is very low.[17,18] **Anthralin** and **tar** products have measurable levels of systemic absorption but no adverse fetal effects have been reported.[1] Due to lack of evidence of safety and concerns of potential mutagenic effects, some recommend avoiding these products during pregnancy,[19] while others feel they are likely safe during the second and third trimesters.[1,20] There is no theoretical reason for concern with the use during pregnancy of topical **salicylic acid** in the concentrations used for psoriasis.[19] Safety of topical vitamin D derivatives (**calcitriol**, **calcipotriol**) has not been established. Systemic absorption of topical **calcipotriol** is only 6% and unlikely to have significant effects.[1] Systemic **retinoids** are known teratogens. Safety of the topical retinoid **tazarotene** has not been documented and it is not recommended for use in pregnancy.[21] Avoid **psoralens UVA (PUVA)** therapy in pregnancy due to known mutagenicity, though there is no evidence of teratogenicity. UVB phototherapy is considered the safest treatment for widespread psoriasis during pregnancy that is not controlled with topical therapy.[1,17] **Cyclosporine** does not seem to be associated with adverse outcomes in transplant patients; reserve its use for severe cases and maintain at the minimal effective dose.[11,17] Limited available evidence suggests that **adalimumab**, **etanercept** and **infliximab** do not pose a major teratogenic risk.[22] Published information about use of **ustekinumab** during pregnancy is too scant to assess risk.[13]

Management of Psoriasis during Breastfeeding

As a general precaution, avoid direct contact of the infant's skin with any area of the mother's skin that has been treated with topical therapy. Avoid **coal tar** due to risk of absorption by the infant via skin-skin or skin-mouth contact.[23] Due to variability of systemic absorption of topical **salicylic acid** it is not recommended while breastfeeding.[24] Risk to the baby via passage of **topical corticosteroids** into breast milk is unlikely since only extensive use of the most potent agents causes systemic effects in the mother.[23,24] No information on safety of the vitamin D derivatives (**calcitriol**, **calcipotriol**) is available, though the very low systemic absorption of **calcipotriol** is unlikely to pose any risk to the nursing infant.[23] Systemic absorption of **tazarotene** after topical use is minimal; the risk to a nursing infant via breast milk is considered low, though caution is recommended if used over large surface areas.[24] Avoid **psoralens UVA (PUVA)** in nursing mothers if possible. UVB phototherapy is a safe option for resistant or widespread disease.[1] Although excretion of **acitretin** and **methotrexate** into breast milk is low, avoid these medications while breastfeeding due to their inherent toxicity.[24] Limited information indicates that excretion of **cyclosporine** into breast milk is generally low and adverse effects would not be expected, though close follow-up and monitoring of serum levels in the infant have been suggested.[23] Due to their large molecular weight it is unlikely that the any of the biologic therapies (**adalimumab**, **etanercept**, **infliximab**, **ustekinumab**) are excreted into breast milk in significant amounts.[23,24]

A discussion of general principles on the use of medications in these special populations can be found in Appendix II and Appendix III. Other specialized reference sources are also provided in these appendices.

Therapeutic Tips

- Changing the base of the topical corticosteroid from cream to ointment may be helpful if response is not adequate, particularly for thick, hyperkeratotic lesions.
- Combining topical corticosteroids with other topical agents (e.g., vitamin D derivatives) may be helpful when corticosteroids alone have failed.
- Customize the treatment to the patient. A number of factors need to be considered when opting for one treatment versus another, and the patient must be an equal partner in the decision process.
  - Consider affordability of prescribed medication. This may be especially important when considering the use of a biologic agent.

  - Poor adherence to topical therapy can be problematic. This is due to the complexity of the regimen, inconvenience and time constraints, and whether the topicals are cosmetically acceptable (e.g., tar has an odour and anthralin stains). Understanding the reasons for patient nonadherence and making appropriate changes may be helpful.
  - Phototherapy sessions require considerable patient commitment (3–5 sessions per week).
  - Side effects of systemic therapies can be severe and must be understood by the patient.
  - Consider the risk-benefit profile of systemic agents. In general, the risks of biologic therapies are low, and the benefit is high.
  - Question the diagnosis if there is no relief of disease within 1–2 months of optimal therapy.
- Length of remission is longer with phototherapy but there still is no definitive cure for psoriasis.
- The continued care of the patient by the family physician should be the foundation on which occasional evaluations by the dermatologist can be added as needed.

Table 3: **Topical Psoriasis Therapies**

Class	Drug	Dose	Adverse Effects	Comments	Cost[a]
Anthracene Derivatives	*anthralin*[c]	Once daily	Irritating to surrounding normal skin. Stains skin and fabrics.	Indicated: plaques. Contraindicated: folds. Can be combined with UVB. Effective, economical.	$$
Corticosteroids, low-potency	For information on available topical corticosteroids see Chapter 89, Table 3.			Hydrocortisone is recommended for psoriasis of the flexures or face.	
Corticosteroids, mid-potency	For information on available topical corticosteroids see Chapter 89, Table 3.			Mid-potency topical corticosteroids can be used to treat plaques of psoriasis on the trunk and extremities.	
Corticosteroids, high-potency	For information on available topical corticosteroids see Chapter 89, Table 3.			Stronger corticosteroids may be necessary for short-term intervals on the palms and the soles.	
Corticosteroids (for use on the scalp)[b]	*betamethasone dipropionate 0.05%* Diprolene, Diprosone, generics	Once daily–BID	Burning/irritation at application site, pruritus, dryness, atrophy.	Topical corticosteroid potency: very potent (glycol base); potent (lotion).	$
	betamethasone valerate 0.1% lotion Valisone Scalp Lotion, generics	BID–TID	See betamethasone dipropionate.	Topical corticosteroid potency: moderate.	$
	betamethasone valerate 0.12% foam Luxiq	BID	See betamethasone dipropionate.	Topical corticosteroid potency: moderate.	$$
	clobetasol propionate 0.05% Clobex Lotion, Clobex Shampoo, Clobex Spray, generics	Shampoo: once daily Spray: BID Lotion: once daily–BID	See betamethasone dipropionate.	Topical corticosteroid potency: very potent.	Lotion: $ Shampoo/ Spray: $$$
	hydrocortisone 2.5% Emo-Cort	BID–TID	See betamethasone dipropionate.	Topical corticosteroid potency: weak.	$
	mometasone furoate 0.1% Elocom, generics	Once daily	See betamethasone dipropionate.	Topical corticosteroid potency: potent.	$

Class	Drug	Dose	Adverse Effects	Comments	Cost[a]
Corticosteroid/ Keratolytic Combinations	*betamethasone/salicylic acid* Diprosalic, generics	Once daily–BID	Corticosteroid: burning, itching, irritation, acneiform eruptions, skin atrophy, striae. Keratolytic: erythema, scaling, local irritation.	See Keratolytic Agents.	$
Keratolytic Agents	*salicylic acid*[c] 3–10%	Lotion, cream, gel: once or twice daily Shampoo: once or twice weekly	Erythema, scaling, local irritation. Prolonged use over large areas may result in salicylate toxicity, especially in children.	Indicated: for keratolytic effect to flatten thick, scaly psoriatic plaques. Also for hyperkeratosis of palms and soles.	$
Retinoids	*tazarotene* *0.05%, 0.1%* Tazorac Cream, Tazorac Gel	Once daily	Skin irritation.	Indicated: body. Contraindicated: face and folds.	$$$
Tars	*coal tar* Liquor Carbonis Detergens, Targel, others	Once daily	Dermatitis, folliculitis, photosensitivity. Malodorous, stains skin and hair.	Indicated: plaques. Contraindicated: folds. Can be combined with UVB. Effective, economical.	$
Vitamin D Derivatives	*calcipotriol* Dovonex	BID	Skin irritation.	Indicated: body. Contraindicated: face and folds.	$$
	calcitriol Silkis	BID	Skin irritation.	Indicated: body (mild to moderate plaque type involving ≤35% body surface area). Contraindicated: face and folds.	$$$
Vitamin D Derivative/ Corticosteroid Combinations	*calcipotriol/ betamethasone* Ointment: Dovobet Scalp Gel: Dovobet	Ointment: once daily Scalp Gel: once daily at bedtime. Wash out in morning.	Skin irritation.	Indicated: body (ointment), scalp (gel). Contraindicated: face and folds. Manufacturers recommend use for 4 weeks only but is often used for longer periods.	$$$$

[a] Cost of 50 g or 50 mL; includes drug cost only.
[b] Different potency categories may be used by other authors. Vehicles also impacts potency. These rankings are meant to serve as a guide only.
[c] Extemporaneously compounded preparations can be used.
Abbreviations: UVB = ultraviolet B
Legend: $ < $25 $$ $25–50 $$$ $50–75 $$$$ $75–100

Table 4: Systemic Psoriasis Therapies

Class	Drug	Dose	Adverse Effects	Drug Interactions	Comments	Cost[a]
Biologic Response Modifiers	*adalimumab* Humira	80 mg sc followed by 40 mg sc every 2 wk starting 1 wk after the initial dose	Injection site reactions, serious infections, neurologic events and malignancies.	Possible increased risk of serious infection with concomitant use of immunosuppressives. Live vaccines should not be given concurrently. MTX reduces adalimumab clearance (29% for single dose MTX, 44% for multiple doses MTX).	Indicated: chronic moderate to severe psoriasis, psoriatic arthritis.	~$20 000 for 1 y
	etanercept Enbrel	Initial: 50 mg sc twice weekly for 3 months Maintenance: 50 mg sc weekly	Injection site reactions, infections, autoimmune phenomena, worsening heart failure. Not to be used in patients with demyelinating disease. May increase risk of malignancy.	Possible increased risk of serious infection with concomitant use of immunosuppressives. Live vaccines should not be administered during therapy. Sulfasalazine: decrease in mean white blood cell counts.	Indicated: chronic moderate to severe plaque psoriasis, psoriatic arthritis.	~$21 000 for 1 y
	infliximab Remicade	5 mg/kg iv infusion at 0, 2 and 6 wk and then every 8 wk thereafter If adequate response not achieved by wk 14, discontinue	Infections, allergic reactions, infusion reactions, hepatobiliary events, demyelinating disorders and lymphoma.	Possible increased risk of serious infection with concomitant use of immunosuppressives. Live vaccines should not be given concurrently.	Indicated: chronic moderate to severe plaque psoriasis, psoriatic arthritis.	~$13 000 for 14 wk
	ustekinumab Stelara	45 mg sc at wk 0 and 4, then every 12 wk thereafter (patients >100 kg may require 90 mg per dose)	Nasopharyngitis, upper respiratory tract infection, headache, infections, malignancy.	Possible increased risk of serious infection with concomitant use of immunosuppressives. Live vaccines should not be given concurrently.	Indicated: chronic moderate to severe plaque psoriasis.	~$21 000 for 1 y
Immunosuppressives	*methotrexate* ❥ Methotrexate, Methotrexate Tablets, Methotrexate Injection, Metoject, other generics	7.5–22.5 mg weekly po/sc/im	Bone marrow suppression, hepatotoxicity, gastrointestinal effects, pulmonary toxicity, blood dyscrasias.	Ethanol and acitretin may increase the risk of MTX-induced liver injury. Cholestyramine and colestipol may bind MTX in the gut. Trimethoprim may increase bone marrow suppression.	Indicated: moderate to severe psoriasis; psoriatic arthritis. Contraindicated: liver disease. Use in conjunction with folic acid.	$

Class	Drug	Dose	Adverse Effects	Drug Interactions	Comments	Cost[a]
	cyclosporine Neoral, Apo-Cyclosporine, other generics	2.5–5 mg/kg/day po	Hypertension, hyperlipidemia, renal dysfunction, tremor, headache, hypertrichosis.	Metabolized by cytochrome P450: many possible drug interactions (e.g., erythromycin, ketoconazole, rifampin, St. John's wort).	Indicated: moderate to severe psoriasis.	$$$–$$$$
Retinoids	*acitretin* Soriatane	10–75 mg/day po	Arthralgia, myalgia, alopecia, dry lips and mucosa, hyperlipidemia, hepatotoxicity.	Ethanol increases the risk of conversion of acitretin to etretinate, which is also a major teratogen and can remain in the body for years. Women of child-bearing potential taking acitretin must abstain from alcohol during treatment and for 2 months afterwards to allow for clearance of acitretin. Risk of MTX-induced liver injury may be increased with acitretin. "Minipill" progestin-only contraceptives may not be effective in patients taking acitretin. Avoid this combination. Combination with tetracycline leads to higher risk of increased intracranial pressure. Caution with concomitant use of vitamin A doses beyond recommended dietary allowances.	Indicated: moderate to severe psoriasis. Contraindicated in pregnancy. In women of child-bearing potential effective contraception must begin 1 month before beginning therapy with acitretin and continue for at least 3 y after discontinuation; in consultation with the physician.	$$–$$$

[a] Cost of 30-day supply unless otherwise specified; based on 70 kg body weight; includes drug cost only.
Dosage adjustment may be required in renal impairment; see Appendix I.
Abbreviations: MTX = methotrexate; TNF = tumour necrosis factor
Legend: $ < $100 $$ $100-200 $$-$$$ $100–300 $$$ $200–300 $$$-$$$$ $200–400 $$$$ $300–400

Suggested Readings

Canadian Psoriasis Guidelines Committee. *Canadian guidelines for the management of plaque psoriasis*. 1st ed. Ottawa (ON): Canadian Dermatology Association; 2009. Available from: www.dermatology.ca/wp-content/uploads/2012/01/cdnpsoriasisguidelines.pdf.

Guenther L, Langley RG, Shear NH et al. Integrating biologic agents into management of moderate-to-severe psoriasis: a consensus of the Canadian Psoriasis Expert Panel. *J Cutan Med Surg* 2004;8(5):321-37.

Langley RG. *Psoriasis*. 2nd ed. Toronto (ON): Key Porter Books; 2010.

Lui H. Phototherapy of psoriasis: update with practical pearls. *J Cutan Med Surg* 2002;6(3 Suppl):17-21.

Menter A, Gottlieb A, Feldman SR et al. Guidelines of care for the management of psoriasis and psoriatic arthritis: section 1. Overview of psoriasis and guidelines of care for the treatment of psoriasis with biologics. *J Am Acad Dermatol* 2008;58(5):826-50.

Menter A, Griffiths CE. Current and future management of psoriasis. *Lancet* 2007;370(9583):272-84.

Schon MP, Boehncke WH. Psoriasis. *N Engl J Med* 2005;352(18):1899-912.

References

1. Canadian Psoriasis Guidelines Committee. *Canadian guidelines for the management of plaque psoriasis*. 1st ed. Ottawa (ON): Canadian Dermatology Association; 2009. Available from: www.dermatology.ca/wp-content/uploads/2012/01/cdnpsoriasisguidelines.pdf. Accessed May 28, 2014.
2. U.S. Food and Drug Administration. Pediatric Advisory Committee. Manthripragada A. *Addendum: Update on calcineurin inhibitor pediatric literature review. Tacrolimus (Protopic) and pimecrolimus (Elidel)*. May 10, 2011. Available from: www.fda.gov/downloads/AdvisoryCommittees/CommitteesMeetingMaterials/PediatricAdvisoryCommittee/UCM255140.pdf. Accessed May 14, 2013.
3. Carr WW. Topical calcineurin inhibitors for atopic dermatitis: review and treatment recommendations. *Paediatr Drugs* 2013;15(4):303-10.
4. Tremblay JF, Bissonnette R. Topical agents for the treatment of psoriasis, past, present and future. *J Cutan Med Surg* 2002;6(3 Suppl):8-11
5. Lui H. Phototherapy of psoriasis: update with practical pearls. *J Cutan Med Surg* 2002;6(3 Suppl):17-21.
6. Lebwohl M, Ali S. Treatment of psoriasis. Part 1. Topical therapy and phototherapy. *J Am Acad Dermatol* 2001;45(4):487-98.
7. Kipnis CD, Myers WA, Opeola M et al. Biologic treatments for psoriasis. *J Am Acad Dermatol* 2005;52(4):671-82.
8. Murase JE, Chan KK, Garite TJ et al. Hormonal effect on psoriasis in pregnancy and post partum. *Arch Dermatol* 2005;141(5):601-6.
9. Ben-David G, Sheiner E, Hallak M et al. Pregnancy outcome in women with psoriasis. *J Reprod Med* 2008;53(3):183-7.
10. Seeger JD, Lanza LL,West WA et al. Pregnancy and pregnancy outcome among women with inflammatory skin diseases. *Dermatology* 2007;214(1):32-9.
11. Ferreira E, Martin B, Morin C. *Grossesse et allaitement: guide thérapeutique*. 2nd ed. Montréal (QC): CHU Sainte Justine; 2013.
12. Weber-Schoendorfer C, Hoeltzenbein M, Wacker E et al. No evidence for an increased risk of adverse pregnancy outcome after paternal low-dose methotrexate: an observational cohort study. *Rheumatology (Oxford)* 2014;53(4):757-63.
13. Briggs G, Freeman RK, Yaffe S. *Drugs in pregnancy and lactation: a reference guide to fetal and neonatal risk*. 9th ed. Philadelphia (PA): Wolters Kluwer Health; Lippincott Williams & Wilkins; 2011.
14. UK Teratology Information Service (UKTIS). *Use of acitretin/etretinate in pregnancy*. October 2012. Available from: www.uktis.org/docs/Acitretin.pdf#search="acitretin". Accessed May 14, 2014.
15. e-CPS. Ottawa (ON): Canadian Pharmacists Association; 2013. Soriatane [product monograph]. Available from: www.e-therapeutics.ca. Accessed May 14, 2014. Subscription required.
16. Geiger JM, Walker M. Is there a reproductive safety risk in male patients treated with acitretin (neotigason/soriatane)? *Dermatology* 2002;205(2):105-7.
17. Al Hammadi A, Al-Haddab M, Sasseville D. Dermatologic treatment during pregnancy: practical overview. *J Cutan Med Surg* 2006;10(4):183-92.
18. Oren D, Nulman I, Makhija M et al. Using corticosteroids during pregnancy. Are topical, inhaled, or systemic agents associated with risk? *Can Fam Physician* 2004;50:1083-5.
19. Schaefer C, Peters P, Miller RK, eds. *Drugs during pregnancy and lactation: treatment options and risk assessment*. 2nd ed. Boston (MA): Elsevier Academic Press; 2007.
20. Weatherhead S, Robson SC, Reynolds NJ. Management of psoriasis in pregnancy. *BMJ* 2007;334(7605):1218-20.
21. Organization of Teratology Information Specialists (OTIS). Tucson (AZ): University of Arizona, OTIS National Office. Available from: www.otispregnancy.org. Accessed April 12, 2011.
22. Diav-Citrin O, Otcheretianski-Volodarsky A, Shechtman S et al. Pregnancy outcome following gestational exposure to TNF-alpha-inhibitors: a prospective, comparative, observational study. *Reprod Toxicol* 2014;43:78-84.
23. Drugs and Lactation Database (LactMed). Bethesda (MD): U.S. National Library of Medicine. Available from: toxnet.nlm.nih.gov/cgi-bin/sis/htmlgen?LACT. Accessed April 12, 2011.
24. Hale TW. *Medications and mothers' milk: a manual of lactational pharmacology*. 15th ed. Amarillo (TX): Hale Publishing; 2012.
25. Lebwohl M, Ali S. Treatment of psoriasis. Part 2. Systemic therapies. *J Am Acad Dermatol* 2001;45(5):649-61.

Chapter 96
Rosacea

W. Stuart Maddin, MD, FRCPC

Rosacea is the fifth most common diagnosis made by dermatologists. It is estimated that 5% of Americans suffer from rosacea.[1] A genetic predisposition is commonly found in those of Celtic and North European descent with fair skin.[2] It is seen in women 2–3 times more often than in men.

Rosacea is a chronic and progressive cutaneous vascular disorder and is often misdiagnosed as adult acne. More than 50% of patients with rosacea suffer eye involvement characterized by irritation, dryness, blepharitis and conjunctivitis. See Table 1 for classification of rosacea.

The traditional explanation is that damage to dermal connective tissue such as that caused by sun exposure may initiate rosacea. However, there is some evidence that the prevalence of papulopustular rosacea is not significantly related to photodamage or UV exposure.[5] Further larger-scale research is needed to confirm the role of UV exposure in rosacea. The facial skin of rosacea patients has also been shown to exhibit elevated levels of both the antimicrobial peptide cathelicidin and the stratum corneum tryptic enzyme (SCTE). The overproduction of these 2 inflammatory proteins is responsible for the increased production of a third protein (immune system peptide) which triggers the symptoms associated with rosacea.[6] Additionally, a meta-analysis reported a significant association between infestation with *Demodex folliculoriium* and the development of rosacea.[7] These new understandings have the potential to modify the way clinicians view the disease and influence the future development of drugs to treat rosacea.

Table 1: Subtypes of Rosacea[a,3,4]

Type of Rosacea	Clinical Features
Erythematotelangiectatic	1. Mild: flushing, faint erythema and occasionally telangiectatic 2. Moderate: frequent flushing, moderate persistent erythema, distinct telangiectasia 3. Severe: frequent severe flushing, pronounced and persistent erythema, many prominent telangiectasias
Papulopustular	1. Mild: few papules or pustules, mild erythema 2. Moderate: scattered papules or pustules, moderate erythema 3. Severe: many papules or pustules, pronounced erythema, plaques or edema may be present
Phymatous	1. Mild: slight puffiness of nose, patulous follicular orifices 2. Moderate: bulbous nasal swelling, dilated open follicular orifices, hypertrophy of sebaceous glands and change in nasal contour 3. Severe: marked nasal swelling, large dilated follicles, distortion of nasal contour with nodular component
Ocular	1. Mild: mild itch, dryness, fine scaling and erythema of lid margins and conjunctival injection 2. Moderate: burning, stinging, crusting of lid margins with erythema/edema, conjunctival hyperemia, chalazion 3. Severe: pain, photosensitivity or blurred vision, loss of lashes, severe conjunctival injection corneal changes with potential loss of vision

[a] The National Rosacea Society Expert Committee on the classification and staging of Rosacea lists 4 subtypes of rosacea (as above). They consider granulomatous rosacea a "variant" and rosacea fulminans, steroid-induced acneiform eruption and perioral dermatitis separate entities. This chapter does not address these conditions.

Table 2: **Triggers That Can Worsen Rosacea**

Sunlight
Heat
Hot beverages
Spicy foods, vinegar
Alcohol
Application of topical corticosteroids to the face
Use of astringents
Emotional stress

Goals of Therapy

- Increase awareness of triggers of outbreaks of cutaneous rosacea, and how to avoid these triggers
- Make the patient aware of signs and symptoms of ocular rosacea and how they can be managed
- Reduce the number and severity of recurrences of cutaneous and ocular rosacea
- Prevent the development of rhinophyma (nose enlargement) with aggressive early treatment
- Reduce or obliterate broken small diameter linear blood vessels that are most often found on the sides of the nose and cheeks. Treating vascular lesions, flushing and redness can restore a more even skin tone to the face.

Investigations

- Establish the diagnosis:
  - family history
  - later onset than acne (late 20s to 40s)
  - history of recurrent bouts of papules and pustules, inappropriate flushing and/or persistent redness of the face
  - history of eye irritation, blepharitis, dry eyes or recurrent styes
  - flare-up of rosacea following sun exposure
- Physical examination:
  - presence of papules or pustules along with erythema of the central face; absence of comedones
  - presence of telangiectasia
  - evidence of conjunctivitis, blepharitis, stye formation or complaint of dry eyes
  - rhinophyma (not common)
- Differential diagnosis:
  - acne vulgaris, perioral dermatitis, seborrheic dermatitis, photosensitivity reactions or discoid lupus erythematosus

Therapeutic Choices

Management of rosacea is presented in Figure 1.

Nonpharmacologic Choices

- Advise patients how to avoid triggers that can worsen rosacea (Table 2).
- Protect skin from the sun with the use of proper clothing, hat and regular use of an effective sunscreen (see Chapter 98). The sun and other climatic influences, such as intense cold or harsh winds may cause an exacerbation.

- Avoid hot beverages, soups, spices, vinegar and undiluted liquor. Dietary factors may precipitate flushing.
- Scalpel, electrosurgery or laser therapy: telangiectasia and persistent erythema may significantly improve after 1–3 laser treatments. The energy from a laser is targeted at the contents of the blood vessels that form the lesion, selectively destroying the lesion while minimizing the damage sustained by adjacent tissues. For rhinophyma, worthwhile options include the use of a scalpel to shave the nose, or an electric loop or carbon dioxide laser to sculpt the nose to more normal proportions.

Table 3: Treatment of Rosacea

	Treatment Method		
Type of Rosacea	**Topical**	**Systemic**	**Physical**
Erythematotelangiectatic	Metronidazole Azelaic acid Brimonidine	Tetracycline, minocycline or doxycycline Erythromycin Isotretinoin	Lasers Intense pulsed light Cosmetic camouflage
Papulopustular	Clindamycin Erythromycin Metronidazole Azelaic acid	Tetracycline, minocycline or doxycycline	
Phymatous		To combat lymphedema: prednisone, isotretinoin	To combat rhinophyma: shave or debulk
Ocular	Ophthalmic antibiotic ointment Artificial tears	Tetracycline, minocycline or doxycycline	Lasers Intense pulsed light Maintain eyelid hygiene

Figure 1: Treatment of Rosacea

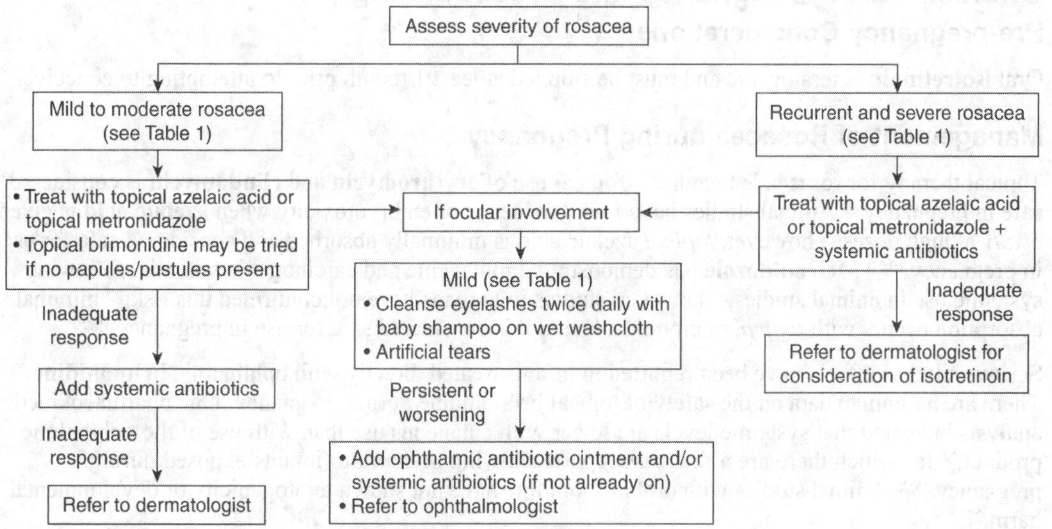

Pharmacologic Choices

Table 3 provides a summary of treatment of the subtypes of rosacea. Also see Table 4 and Table 5.

Mild to moderate rosacea: start with **topical metronidazole** or **azelaic acid**.[8] Treatment duration will depend upon the severity of symptoms, but improvement can generally be expected in 2–4 weeks. Counsel patients that topical treatment may need to be continued indefinitely: relapse is to be expected upon discontinuation. Reassess patients and institute oral antibiotics if the response to topical agents alone is inadequate.

Topical **brimonidine** gel appears to be safe and effective for treatment of the facial redness associated with rosacea, presumably acting by constricting dilated blood vessels. Effects can last up to 12 hours. It is not indicated for the treatment of inflammatory lesions (papules and pustules) of rosacea.[9,10]

Recurrent and severe rosacea: in addition to stressing the avoidance of triggers (see Table 2) an initial therapeutic approach commonly consists of an oral antibiotic (to quickly gain control of symptoms) in combination with a topical agent (to reduce redness and inflammation). The rationale for the use of antibiotics in the treatment of rosacea resides with their anti-inflammatory benefits, rather than their antimicrobial properties. Do not hesitate to use oral antibiotics such as **tetracycline**, **doxycycline**, **minocycline** or **erythromycin** for up to 6 months. Low-dose (subantimicrobial) doxycycline is now available and appears to be safe and effective.[11]

The use of low-dose **isotretinoin** is an effective and useful option for the management of patients with treatment-resistant rosacea.[12,13] Isotretinoin can also be used to treat persistent facial edema (Morbihan's disease), which may accompany rosacea.[14]

Mild ocular involvement (Table 1) can be managed with good eyelid hygiene and use of artificial tears (Figure 1). There is little scientific evidence available to guide treatment of moderate to severe ocular rosacea. Experts recommend use of ophthalmic antibiotic ointment applied to the lid margins/eyelashes and/or use of oral **doxycycline**, **minocycline** or **tetracycline** for several weeks. When symptoms subside, stop topical and oral antibiotics and maintain lid hygiene and artificial tears.[4,15] Patients with persistent or severe ocular involvement should be referred to an ophthalmologist.[4]

Choices during Pregnancy and Breastfeeding

Pre-pregnancy Considerations

Oral **isotretinoin** is teratogenic and must be stopped at least 1 month prior to attempting to conceive.[16]

Management of Rosacea during Pregnancy

Topical therapy for rosacea is favoured. Topical use of **erythromycin** and **clindamycin** is considered safe in pregnancy.[17] Animal studies have found evidence of embryotoxicity when **azelaic acid** is given *orally* at high doses,[18] however, *topical* azelaic acid is minimally absorbed and considered safe for use in pregnancy.[19,20] **Metronidazole** has demonstrated mutagenic and carcinogenic potential following systemic use in animal studies,[21] however, studies in humans have not confirmed this risk;[22] minimal absorption occurs with *topical* metronidazole and it is considered safe for use in pregnancy.[19,20]

Serious adverse effects have been reported in infants treated directly with ophthalmic **brimonidine**.[23] There are no human data on the safety of topical brimonidine during pregnancy. One pharmacokinetic analysis indicated that systemic levels are lower with cutaneous use than with use of the ophthalmic product,[24] for which there are a few case reports showing no harm to infants exposed during pregnancy.[25,26] Animal studies with oral brimonidine have not shown teratogenicity or developmental harm.[27]

Oral **tetracycline**, **doxycycline** and **minocycline** are associated with tooth staining (when taken after the first trimester), decreased bony growth and maternal liver toxicity. However, inadvertent exposure in the first few weeks of pregnancy is extremely unlikely to be harmful.[17,20,28] Oral use of **erythromycin** is considered safe during pregnancy. One study reported a possible increased risk of cardiovascular malformations with its use in early pregnancy.[29,30] The estolate salt of erythromycin should be avoided during pregnancy as it has been linked to hepatotoxicity in pregnant patients.[31] Oral **isotretinoin** is teratogenic. Pregnancy must be avoided one month before, during and one month after therapy. Women taking isotretinoin must adhere to the manufacturers' pregnancy prevention programs, and close supervision by the treating physician is necessary.

Management of Rosacea during Breastfeeding

Topical **erythromycin**, **clindamycin**, **azelaic acid** and **metronidazole** are all considered safe to use while breastfeeding due to limited systemic absorption and/or low excretion into breast milk.[19,20,32] Care should be taken to avoid direct contact of the infant's skin with treated areas of the mother.

Serious adverse effects have been reported in infants treated directly with ophthalmic **brimonidine**.[23] There are no human data on the safety of topical brimonidine during breastfeeding. One pharmacokinetic analysis indicated that systemic levels are lower with cutaneous use than with use of the ophthalmic product,[24] for which there are a few case reports showing no harm to nursing infants during maternal use.[25,26]

Tetracycline, **doxycyline** and **minocycline** are excreted into breast milk in low concentrations. Tooth discoloration and impaired bone growth could theoretically occur in breastfed infants whose mothers are being treated with these agents. Studies have shown this to be a remote risk as serum levels in exposed infants were found to be undetectable, and short term use of tetracycline, doxycyline or minocycline is considered compatible with breastfeeding.[28,34] However, as a theoretical precaution, prolonged or repeated courses (as may be the case in the treatment of rosacea) should be avoided while breastfeeding.[34] Oral **erythromycin** is excreted into breast milk in low amounts and is considered to be compatible with breastfeeding, though some data suggest an increased risk of infantile pyloric stenosis in the early postnatal period in infants exposed to erythromycin via breast milk.[35] The safety of oral **isotretinoin** during breastfeeding has not been documented and it is not recommended.[36]

A discussion of general principles on the use of medications in these special populations can be found in Appendix II and Appendix III. Other specialized reference sources are also provided in these appendices.

Therapeutic Tips

- Sun protection is very important.
- Recommend the use of a green-tinted foundation, which works well for camouflaging the erythema of rosacea.
- Avoid topical corticosteroids; they can precipitate or worsen rosacea by adding to the dermal dystrophy that characterizes the disorder.
- When evaluating patients with cutaneous rosacea, inquire about ocular symptoms and examine the eyelids. This is especially important in patients with mild disease who are more likely to be treated with topical treatment alone.
- Counsel patients with particularly intense erythema that following successful treatment, posterythema-revealed telangiectasia (PERT) may become apparent. This prevents worries that the therapy "produced" the telangiectasia.
- Pulsed dye laser and other laser systems (e.g., variable pulse width laser) can be very effective for telangiectasia. These procedures should be performed by skilled practitioners.

Table 4: Topical Treatment of Rosacea

Class	Drug	Dose	Adverse Effects	Comments	Cost[a]
Alpha$_2$-adrenergic Agonist	*brimonidine tartrate* Onreltea	0.33% gel applied once daily Small pea-sized amount to each of the 5 areas of the face (i.e., forehead, chin, nose, each cheek) avoiding the eyes and eyelids, lips, mouth or inside of the nose.	Erythema, flushing, skin burning sensation, contact dermatitis, headache.	May start to reduce redness within 30 min with peak effect at 3 h. Wash hands immediately after applying.	$110
Dicarboxylic Acids	*azelaic acid* Finacea	15% gel applied BID	Initial mild, transient burning, tingling or stinging, pruritus, scaling, xerosis, erythema, contact dermatitis.	Can be used for initial therapy or for long-term maintenance.	$$
Nitroimidazoles	*metronidazole* 0.75%: MetroCream, MetroGel, MetroLotion 1%: Noritate	0.75% gel or cream, or 1% cream, gel or lotion applied as thin film daily or BID × 9 wk, then as needed	Local irritation.	Treatment of choice. If discontinued, relapse can occur. May need up to 12 wk therapy to show pronounced improvement. Can be used in combination with oral tetracyclines. There does not appear to be any significant difference in efficacy among varying strengths and vehicles.[8]	$$

[a] Cost of smallest available pack size, unless otherwise specified; includes drug cost only.
Legend: $ < $25 $$ $25–35

Table 5: Oral Drugs for the Treatment of Rosacea

Class	Drug	Dose	Adverse Effects	Drug Interactions	Comments	Cost[a]
Macrolides	*erythromycin* Eryc, generics	0.5–1 g/day divided BID × 6–8 wk	GI effects; hepatotoxicity, especially with the estolate; candidiasis.	May increase blood levels of theophylline, cyclosporine, carbamazepine, warfarin, digitalis, ergotamine, methylprednisolone.	May be taken with food.	$$
Retinoids	*isotretinoin* Accutane, Clarus, Epuris	0.3–1 mg/kg/day × 4–5 months	Teratogenicity (major concern); cheilitis, dry skin; mucocutaneous effects, myalgia; psychiatric events.	Note: no adverse interaction known between retinoids and oral contraceptives. Tetracyclines: rare cases of benign intracranial hemorrhage (pseudotumor cerebri).	For recalcitrant cases.[37] Provides worthwhile benefit, but not consistently. Uncertain if permanent remission can be induced. Requires at least **2 types** of contraception when used in females of childbearing age.	$$$$ [b]
Tetracyclines	*doxycycline* Vibramycin, generics	100 mg daily × 12 wk	See tetracycline. Photosensitivity may occur.	Serum concentrations of doxycycline may be reduced by carbamazepine, chronic alcohol ingestion, phenobarbital and phenytoin. Methotrexate concentrations may be increased by doxycycline.	No food restriction required. Useful for improving ocular rosacea. Recurrences of rosacea do occur after treatment is discontinued.	$
	doxycycline modified-release Apprilon	40 mg daily × 12 wk	See tetracycline. Also mild-moderate headache, nasopharyngitis.	See doxycycline.	To be taken on an empty stomach. Useful for improving ocular rosacea. Recurrences of rosacea do occur after treatment is discontinued.	$$$$

(cont'd)

Table 5: **Oral Drugs for the Treatment of Rosacea** *(cont'd)*

Class	Drug	Dose	Adverse Effects	Drug Interactions	Comments	Cost[a]
	minocycline generics	50–100 mg daily × 6–8 wk	See tetracycline. Also dizziness; vertigo; abnormal cutaneous pigmentation; rarely lupus-like syndrome; hepatic dysfunction.	Oral iron preparations and antacids containing aluminum, calcium, magnesium may impair GI absorption of minocycline.	Can be tried if tetracycline fails after 4–6 wk trial with good adherence to therapy. No food restriction required. Recurrences of rosacea do occur after treatment is discontinued.	$$
	tetracycline ◖ generics	500 mg BID × 2 wk, then 500 mg daily until rosacea controlled, then 250 mg daily × 3–4 wk	GI effects; yeast overgrowth; photosensitivity; may increase risk of azotemia; pseudotumor cerebri; contraindicated in pregnant women.	GI absorption of tetracycline may be impaired by iron, bismuth, aluminum, calcium, magnesium, in drugs and foods (e.g., dairy products). Separate doses by 2 h.	Lowest cost; used in combination with topical metronidazole. Not to be taken with milk or milk products. Recurrences of rosacea do occur after treatment is discontinued.	$

[a] Cost of 30-day supply; includes drug cost only.
[b] Cost based on 70 kg body weight.
◖ Dosage adjustment may be required in renal impairment; see Appendix I.
Legend: $ < $20 $$ $20–40 $$$ $40–60 $$$$ $60–80

Suggested Readings

Baldwin HE. Diagnosis and treatment of rosacea: state of the art. *J Drugs Dermatol* 2012;11(6):725-30.

Elewski BE, Draelos Z, Dreno B et al. Rosacea—global diversity and optimized outcome: proposed international consensus from the Rosacea International Expert Group. *J Eur Acad Dermatol Venereol* 2011;25(2):188-200.

Nally JB, Berson DS. Topical therapies for rosacea. *J Drugs Dermatol* 2006;5(1):23-6.

Powell FC. Clinical practice. Rosacea. *N Engl J Med* 2005;352(8):793-803.

van Zuuren EJ, Kramer S, Carter B et al. Interventions for rosacea. *Cochrane Database Syst Rev* 2011;(3):CD003262.

References

1. National Rosacea Society. Rosacea diagnosis now more common. *Rosacea Review* Winter 1999. Available from: www.rosacea.org/rr/1999/winter/article_2.php. Accessed October 17, 2013.
2. Crawford GH, Pelle MT, James WD. Rosacea: I. Etiology, pathogenesis and subtype classification. *J Am Acad Dermatol* 2004;51(3):327-41.
3. Wilkin J, Dahl M, Detmar M et al. Standard classification of rosacea: report of the National Rosacea Society Expert Committee on the Classification and Staging of Rosacea. *J Am Acad Dermatol* 2002;46(4):584-7.
4. Powell FC. Clinical practice. Rosacea. *N Engl J Med* 2005;352(8):793-803.
5. McAleer MA, Fitzpatrick P, Powell FC. Papulopustular rosacea: prevalence and relationship to photodamage. *J Am Acad Dermatol* 2010;63(1):33-9.
6. Yamasaki K, Di Nardo A, Bardan A et al. Increased serine protease activity and cathelicidin promote skin inflammation in rosacea. *Nat Med* 2007;13(8):975-80.
7. Zhao YE, Wu LP, Peng Y et al. Retrospective analysis of association between Demodex infestation and rosacea. *Arch Dermatol* 2010;146(8):896-902.
8. van Zuuren EJ, Kramer S, Carter B et al. Interventions for rosacea. *Cochrane Database Syst Rev* 2011;(3):CD003262.
9. Fowler J, Jackson M, Moore A et al. Efficacy and safety of once-daily topical brimonidine tartrate gel 0.5% for the treatment of moderate to severe facial erythema of rosacea: results of two randomized, double-blind, and vehicle-controlled pivotal studies. *J Drugs Dermatol* 2013;12(6):650-6.
10. Moore A, Kempers S, Murakawa G et al. Long-term safety and efficacy of once-daily topical brimonidine tartrate gel 0.5% for the treatment of moderate to severe facial erythema of rosacea: results of a 1-year open-label study. *J Drugs Dermatol* 2014;13(1):56-61.
11. Del Rosso JQ, Webster GF, Jackson M et al. Two randomized phase III clinical trials evaluating anti-inflammatory dose doxycycline (40-mg doxycycline, USP capsules) administered once daily for treatment of rosacea. *J Am Acad Dermatol* 2007;56(5):791-802.
12. Erdogan FG, Yurtsever P, Aksoy D et al. Efficacy of low-dose isotretinoin in patients with treatment-resistant rosacea. *Arch Dermatol* 1998;134(7):884-5.
13. Park H, Del Rosso JQ. Use of oral isotretinoin in the management of rosacea. *J Clin Aesthet Dermatol* 2011;4(9):54-61.
14. Mazzatenta C, Giorgino G, Rubegni P et al. Solid persistent facial oedema (Morbihan's disease) following rosacea, successfully treated with isotretinoin and ketotifen. *Br J Dermatol* 1997;137(6):1020-1.
15. Odom R, Dahl M, Dover J et al. Standard management options for rosacea, part 2: options according to subtype. *Cutis* 2009;84(2):97-104.
16. Organization of Teratology Information Specialists. *Isotretinoin (Accutane) and pregnancy*. August 2010. Available from: www.otispregnancy.org/files/isotretinoin.pdf. Accessed October 17, 2013.
17. Zip C. A practical guide to dermatological drugs use in pregnancy. *Skin Therapy Lett* 2006;11(4):1-4.
18. e-CPS. Ottawa (ON): Canadian Pharmacists Association; 2010. Finacea [product monograph]. Available from: www.e-therapeutics.ca. Accessed March 18, 2014. Subscription required.
19. Akhavan A, Bershad S. Topical acne drugs: review of clinical properties, systemic exposure, and safety. *Am J Clin Dermatol* 2003;4(7):473-92.
20. Leachman SA, Reed BR. The use of dermatologic drugs in pregnancy and lactation. *Dermatol Clin* 2006;24(2):167-97.
21. *Flagyl (metronidazole)* [product monograph]. sanofi-aventis Canada; 2013.
22. Organization of Teratology Information Specialists. *Metronidazole (Flagyl) and pregnancy*. July 2010. Available from: www.otispregnancy.org/files/metronidazole.pdf. Accessed October 17, 2013.
23. e-CPS. Ottawa (ON): Canadian Pharmacists Association; 2013. Alphagan [product monograph]. Available from: www.e-therapeutics.ca. Accessed April 22, 2014. Subscription required.
24. Benkali K, Leoni M, Rony F et al. Comparative pharmacokinetics and bioavailability of brimonidine following ocular administration and dermal application of brimonidine tartrate ophthalmic solution and gel in subjects with moderate to severe facial erythema of rosacea. *Br J Dermatol* 2014 Feb 7. [Epub ahead of print].
25. Johnson SM, Martinez M, Freedman S. Management of glaucoma in pregnancy and lactation. *Surv Ophthalmol* 2001;45(5):449-54.
26. Madadi P, Koren G, Freeman DJ et al. Timolol concentrations in breast milk of a woman treated for glaucoma: calculation of neonatal exposure. *J Glaucoma* 2008;17(4):329-31.
27. Health Canada. Drugs and Health Products. *Onreltea* [product monograph]. Thornhill (ON): Galderma; 2014. Available from: webprod5.hc-sc.gc.ca/dpd-bdpp/info.do?code=90580⟨=eng. Accessed April 24, 2014.
28. Posner AC, Prigot A, Konicoff NG. Further observations on the use of tetracycline hydrochloride in prophylaxis and treatment of obstetric infections. In: *Antibiotics annual 1954-55*. New York (NY): Medical Encyclopedia; 1955. p. 5948.
29. Kallen BA, Otterblad Olausson P. Maternal drug use in early pregnancy and infant cardiovascular defect. *Reprod Toxicol* 2003;17(3):255-61.
30. Kallen BA, Otterblad Olausson P, Danielsson BR. Is erythromycin therapy teratogenic in humans? *Reprod Toxicol* 2005;20(2):209-14.
31. Briggs GG, Freeman RK, Yaffe SJ. *Drugs in pregnancy and lactation: a reference guide to fetal and neonatal risk*. 9th ed. Philadelphia (PA): Wolters Kluwer Health; Lippincott Williams & Wilkins; 2011.
32. Zip C. Common sense dermatological drug suggestions for women who are breast-feeding. *Skin Therapy Lett* 2002;7(3):5-7.
33. Drugs and Lactation Database (LactMed). *Brimonidine*. Bethesda (MD): U.S. National Library of Medicine; 2013. Available from: toxnet.nlm.nih.gov. Accessed April 17, 2014.

34. Drugs and Lactation Database (LactMed). *Tetracycline*. Bethesda (MD): U.S. National Library of Medicine; 2013. Available from: toxnet.nlm.nih.gov. Accessed March 18, 2014.
35. Sorenson HT, Skriver MV, Pedersin L et al. Risk of infantile hypertrophic pyloric stenosis after maternal postnatal use of macrolides. *Scand J Infect Dis* 2003;35(2):104-6.
36. Hale TW. *Medications and mothers' milk: a manual of lactational pharmacology*. 15th ed. Amarillo (TX): Hale Publishing; 2012.
37. Ortonne JP. Oral isotretinoin treatment policy. Do we all agree? *Dermatology* 1997;195(Suppl 1):34-7.

Chapter 97
Scabies and Lice

Sandra Knowles, BScPhm and
Neil H. Shear, MD, FRCPC

Scabies and lice are common infestations that cause significant discomfort and are associated with large outbreaks in institutions (e.g., long-term care facilities, schools, prisons).

Goals of Therapy

- Eradicate causative organisms and eggs
- Control symptoms (pruritus) and prevent complications (secondary bacterial infection)
- Prevent spread to contacts

Investigations

Table 1 addresses the clinical features of lice and scabies.

- History of exposure and itching
- Physical examination for identification of organisms (or evidence of organisms such as eggs or nits)[1]

Table 1: Clinical Features of Scabies and Lice

Type	Organism	Mode of Transmission	Clinical Features	Diagnosis	Differential Diagnosis
Pediculosis capitis (head lice)	*Pediculus humanus capitis*	Head-to-head contact; sharing personal items such as combs, brushes, hats.	Pruritic scalp with red papules around ears, face and neck.	Detection of lice, eggs or nits close to scalp.	Dandruff, hair casts, hairspray droplets.
Pediculosis corporis (body lice)	*Pediculus humanus corporis*	Via clothing and bedding; poor hygiene.	Pruritus and skin reactions (usually in the flanks, in the axillae and around the waist and neck); lives in seams of clothing not on the body.	Detection of lice, eggs or nits in the seams of clothing.	Seborrheic dermatitis, flea or insect bites, eczema, folliculitis.
Pediculosis pubis (pubic lice)	*Phthirus pubis*	Sexual contact; may be associated with other sexually transmitted diseases.	Pruritus in the anogenital area; may also be found on facial hair (including eyelashes) and rarely the scalp.	Detection of lice, eggs or nits in the pubic hair.	Seborrheic dermatitis, folliculitis, dermatophytosis.
Scabies	*Sarcoptes scabiei*	Skin-to-skin contact (also via bedding, furniture).	Intense pruritus and an erythematous, papular eruption on skin; lesions most commonly located on finger webs, wrists, waist, areolae and genitals.	Mite visualized as a pinpoint at the end of a burrow; also detection of mites, eggs or feces in skin scrapings.	Impetigo, seborrheic dermatitis, atopic dermatitis.

Therapeutic Choices

Management of scabies or lice is presented in Figure 1.

Nonpharmacologic Choices

- **Nit removal:** Although time-consuming and tedious, lice and nits should be mechanically removed after pharmacologic treatment.[1,2] Lice are commonly found behind the ears and at the nape of the neck. Because of increased resistance to various pharmacologic treatments, nit removal is becoming increasingly important. However, wet combing alone, which involves combing wet hair with a specially designed comb every 3–4 days for 2 weeks, produces poor results. There are a variety of louse or nit combs available (e.g., LiceMeister developed by the National Pediculosis Association).[3] Another method of nit removal is wrapping hair in a **vinegar**-soaked towel for 30–60 minutes.[2]
- **Treatment of room:** Indirect spread through contact with personal belongings of an infested individual may occur rarely.[2] Laundering pillowcases, sheets, nightclothes, towels, personal articles (e.g., hats, shared helmets, headphones, headbands) and stuffed animals on the hot water cycle (at least 50°C/122°F) of a residential washing machine kills all lice and nits.[4] Alternatively, items that cannot be washed can be dry cleaned or sealed in a plastic bag for 2 weeks. Vacuum the patient's room. Head lice usually do not survive for more than 48 hours when separated from a person.[2] Treatment of clothing and bed linen (machine washing in hot water or putting in a hermetically sealed bag for several days) is recommended for patients with crusted scabies.[5]
- **Combs and brushes:** soak in a disinfectant solution (e.g., Lysol 2% for 1 hour, or rubbing alcohol for 10–20 minutes[6]) or in hot water (at least 50°C for 5–10 minutes).
- Identify and examine potential human contacts to prevent a cycle of reinfection. For head lice, only those contacts with live lice or nits within 1 cm of the scalp should be treated. Pets do not transmit human lice and should not be treated. *All* contacts of a person with scabies, even if asymptomatic, require treatment.[7] This includes sexual and close personal or household contacts within the preceding month.
- Hot air (e.g., LouseBuster, wall-mounted dryer) has also been found to kill lice, although it has not been compared directly to standard chemical shampoos.[8]

Figure 1: **Management of Scabies or Lice**

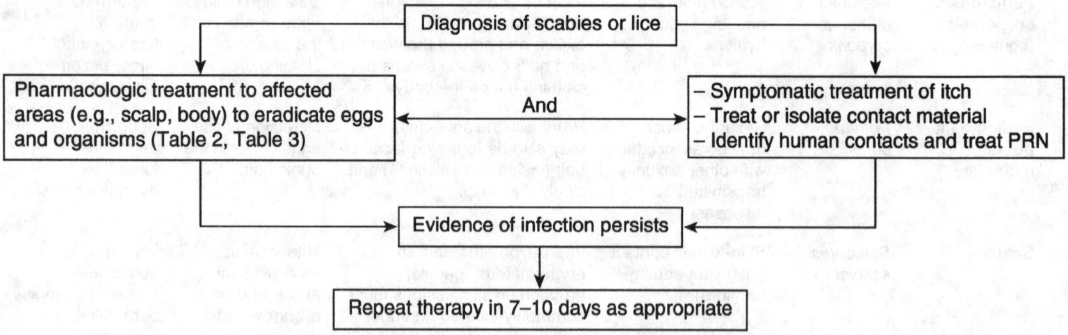

Pharmacologic Choices

- **Head Lice:** The following products are effective with minimal side effects: **permethrin 1%**,[9] **pyrethrins/piperonyl butoxide**,[10] **isopropyl myristate 50%/cyclomethicone 50%**[11,12] and **dimeticone** (dimethicone) [Evidence: SORT B*].[13,14] Permethrin and pyrethrins/piperonyl butoxide are neurotoxic to lice. Isopropyl myristate/cyclomethicone acts physically, causing disruption of the wax layer that covers the cuticle of the louse exoskeleton leading to death via dehydration.[15] Dimeticones are synthetic silicone oils with low surface tension which can coat most surfaces, thus killing head lice by physically blocking spiracles and trachae.[16] Most treatments are not considered reliably ovicidal. Although dimeticone has been shown to be 100% ovicidal in some studies,[13] many patients are not fully adherent with application, and re-treatment in 7–10 days is recommended for all products (see Table 2).[17,18] Although **lindane** is effective for head lice and pubic lice, there is some concern about possible neurotoxicity and bone marrow suppression following percutaneous absorption.[17,19] Lindane is currently not available in Canada.

  Treatment failure of head lice may be due to resistance to topical agents with a neurotoxic mode of action, including permethrin and pyrethrin/piperonyl butoxide.[20] In contrast, resistance to those products with a physical mode of action (**isopropyl myristate 50%/cyclomethicone 50%** and **dimeticone**) is unlikely to develop. Other explanations for treatment failure include misdiagnosis, lack of adherence or re-infestation. Treatment with **permethrin** may fail if hair is not thoroughly soaked. Two bottles are often needed for thick or long hair. In cases of resistance, switching to a different pharmacologic class may be helpful, although resistance to permethrin may cross over to pyrethrins and other pyrethroids.[18] The following have been advocated: **permethrin** 5% cream applied to scalp and left on for several hours or overnight;[1] oral **sulfamethoxazole/trimethoprim** in combination with permethrin 1%;[7] topical **crotamiton** 10% applied to scalp and left on for 24 hours in adults;[2] oral **ivermectin** 200 µg/kg (available through the Health Canada Special Access Programme), repeated in 10 days[18] or an alternative regimen of 400 µg/kg repeated in 7 days.[21] Topical ivermectin 0.5% (not available in Canada) is effective for treatment of head lice.[22]

  Unconventional Treatment of Head Lice: An uncontrolled study showed that **Cetaphil cleanser** ("Nuvo" lotion) was effective in treatment of lice; the lotion, which is applied to the scalp and allowed to dry in place, suffocates the lice.[23] Other unconventional treatments include hot air,[8] hair styling gels and mayonnaise. One study examined 6 home remedies including vinegar, isopropyl alcohol, olive oil, mayonnaise, melted butter and petroleum jelly. The authors found that only application of **petroleum jelly** caused significant louse mortality but no treatment prevented lice from laying eggs.[24] Various alternative therapies including **acetomicellar complex** (SH-206) and naturally occurring substances (e.g., **tea tree oil**, other essential oils, herbal remedies) have been advocated for the treatment of head lice. However, there is no published evidence to suggest that any of these are consistently effective.[18]
- **Pubic lice:** Treatment with **permethrin** 1% cream rinse or **pyrethins with piperonyl butoxide** is recommended (see Table 2). Alternatively, oral **ivermectin** 250 µg/kg repeated in 2 weeks can be used.[25]
- **Body Lice:** Pediculicides are generally unnecessary for patients with body lice, although oral **ivermectin** (12 mg × 3 doses administered weekly) is effective.[26] Nonpharmacologic measures, such as bathing and laundering of infested clothing and linens in hot water, are usually sufficient.
- **Scabies**: The drug of choice for treatment of scabies is **permethrin 5%**.[5,27] Other treatments include **crotamiton** and **sulfur** (see Table 3). Oral **ivermectin** 200 µg/kg orally repeated in 2 weeks is an alternative regimen.[25]

---

* SORT (Strength of Recommendation Taxonomy) is a rating system (A, B or C) that addresses the quality of available evidence. For more information consult **How to Use *Compendium of Therapeutic Choices*** on page xxv.

In patients with scabies, *itching* can persist for weeks after mites are eradicated. Medium-potency **topical corticosteroids** (e.g., betamethasone valerate 0.1% cream), intensive use of emollients[7] and oral antihistamines[28] can be helpful (see Chapter 94). Insufficient treatment of itch and fear of infestation may cause patients with scabies to overuse scabicides, resulting in skin irritation and unnecessary repeated therapy.

Crusted scabies can be treated with oral **ivermectin** 200 µg/kg on days 1, 2, 8, 9 and 15.[25] Additional treatment on days 22 and 29 might be required for severe cases. Oral ivermectin should be combined with topical **permethrin** 5% (full body application to be repeated daily for 7 days then twice weekly until cure).[25]

Choices during Pregnancy and Breastfeeding

Management of Scabies and Lice in Pregnant Women

- The Centers for Disease Control and Prevention (CDC) recommends **permethrin** or **pyrethrins/piperonyl butoxide** for the treatment of pubic lice in pregnant women.[25] Although not specifically stated, these agents should also be used if other areas of a pregnant woman, such as the head, are infested with lice. Cutaneous absorption of **isopropyl myristate/cyclomethicone** is unknown and there is no information on its safety during pregnancy. **Dimeticone** is not absorbed topically but there are no data on use in pregnancy.[29]
- For pregnant women with scabies, **permethrin** is considered the drug of choice.[30] **Sulfur** and **crotamiton** are considered possible second line choices in pregnancy due to their limited cutaneous absorption and low risk of toxicity.[29]
- **Ivermectin** is generally not recommended in pregnancy as safety data are very limited. No major teratogenic effects have been documented in humans. Animal studies have shown teratogenic effects at or near doses producing maternal toxicity.[29]

Management of Scabies and Lice in Breastfeeding Women

- The Centers for Disease Control and Prevention (CDC) recommends **permethrin** or **pyrethrins/piperonyl butoxide** for the treatment of pubic lice in breastfeeding women.[25] Although not specifically stated, these agents should also be used if other areas of a breastfeeding woman, such as the head, are infested with lice. Cutaneous absorption of **isopropyl myristate/cyclomethicone** is unknown and there is no information on its safety during breastfeeding. **Dimeticone** is not absorbed topically but there are no data on use in breastfeeding.[29]
- For breastfeeding women with scabies, **permethrin** is considered the drug of choice. **Sulfur** and **crotamiton** are considered possible second-line choices while breastfeeding due to their limited cutaneous absorption and low risk of toxicity.[29]
- Limited data indicate that **ivermectin** is poorly excreted into breast milk.[31]

A discussion of general principles on the use of medications in these special populations can be found in Appendix II and Appendix III. Other specialized reference sources are also provided in these appendices.

Therapeutic Tips

- **White petrolatum** (e.g., Vaseline) can be applied to *eyelashes* 2–4 times daily for 10 days.[18] Removal of lice and nits with forceps or tweezers prior to application is recommended.

Table 2: Drugs Used to Treat Lice

Class	Drug[a]	Directions	Adverse Effects	Comments	Cost[b]
Pediculicides	*dimeticone 50%* NYDA	Spray carefully all over dry hair. Massage in until hair is completely wetted with solution. Leave solution on hair. After 30 minutes, comb the hair with a lice comb. Allow the solution to dry on the hair for at least 8 hours and then wash. Repeat after 8–10 days.	May cause local irritation.	Not recommended for infants or children younger than 2 y. Resistance to product is unlikely as it has a physical mode of action. No data on safety during pregnancy and breastfeeding.	$$$
	isopropyl myristate 50%/ cyclomethicone 50% Resultz	Head Lice: Apply to dry hair and scalp (30–60 mL for short hair, 60–90 mL for shoulder-length hair, 90–120 mL for long hair). Allow product to remain on hair and scalp for 10 min. Rinse off with warm water. Repeat in 7 days.	May cause local irritation. If contact with eyes, immediately flush well with water.	Not recommended for infants or children younger than 2 y. Resistance to product is unlikely as it has a physical mode of action. No data on safety during pregnancy and breastfeeding.	$$
	permethrin 1% Nix Creme Rinse, Kwellada-P Creme Rinse	Head Lice: Wash hair with conditioner-free shampoo, rinse with water and towel dry. Apply permethrin to saturate the hair and scalp (½–1 bottle for adults and children with long hair); leave on for 10 min then rinse. May repeat after 7 days if live lice are observed. Pubic Lice: Thoroughly saturate the pubic hair: leave on for 10 min then rinse. May repeat after 7 days if live lice are observed.	May temporarily exacerbate the pruritus, erythema and scalp edema of lice infestation. Burning/stinging, tingling, numbness or scalp discomfort are usually mild and transient.	Drug of choice for most patients. Contraindicated in patients with chrysanthemum allergy. Permethrin resistance may result in treatment failure. Do not use to treat pubic lice of the eyelashes or eyebrows. Recommended during pregnancy and breastfeeding.[25]	$
	pyrethrins/piperonyl butoxide R&C Shampoo, R&C II Spray, Pronto Lice Killing Shampoo, generics	Head Lice/Pubic Lice Shampoo: Apply to thoroughly saturate dry hair and massage scalp/skin; leave on for 10 min. Add a little water; work the shampoo into the hair and skin to form a lather. Rinse thoroughly. Repeat treatment in 7 days. Aerosol: Saturate area (5–10 squirts); wash off after 30 min.	Few adverse effects, although contact dermatitis and eye irritation have been reported.	Contraindicated in patients allergic to ragweed, chrysanthemums or other pyrethrin products. Do not use to treat pubic lice of the eyelashes or eyebrows. Recommended during pregnancy and breastfeeding.[25]	$

[a] Lindane is an effective pediculicide however there are concerns about neurotoxicity and bone marrow suppression after percutaneous absorption. Lindane is currently not available in Canada.
[b] Cost of 1 unit (tube or bottle) of product; includes drug cost only. NB: All products are available without prescription; retail mark-ups may vary.
Legend: $ <$10 $$ $10–20 $$$ $20–30

Table 3: Drugs Used to Treat Scabies

Class	Drug[a]	Directions	Adverse Effects	Comments	Cost[b]
Scabicides	*crotamiton 10%* Eurax cream	Massage into all skin areas, from the neck down to the soles of the feet; every bit of skin must be treated, including the fingernails, waist and genitalia. Repeat in 24 h; wash off 48 h after last application.	Local irritation.	Less effective than permethrin. Multiple applications recommended.[28] Not recommended for patients with exudative or vesicular dermatitis. Possible second-line treatment during pregnancy and breastfeeding.[29]	$$
	permethrin 5%[c] Nix Dermal Cream, Kwellada-P Lotion	Massage into all skin areas, from the neck down to the soles of the feet; every bit of skin must be treated, including the fingernails, waist and genitalia; leave on for 8–14 h without interruption, then wash off (shower may be the best way).	Pruritus, edema and erythema.	Drug of choice for scabies.[5,27] Contraindicated in patients allergic to chrysanthemums. Second administration 1 wk after first often routinely prescribed.[7] Recommended during pregnancy and breastfeeding.[25]	Cream: $$ Lotion: $$$
	sulfur 5–10%[d]	Apply to all skin areas[e] at bedtime daily for 5–7 days.	Local irritation or dermatitis with repeated applications.	Not popular because it is malodorous, requires multiple applications and stains clothing. Limited study data to support use. Extemporaneously compounded. May be used for small children. Possible second-line treatment during pregnancy and breastfeeding.[29]	$

[a] Lindane is an effective scabicide however there are concerns about neurotoxicity and bone marrow suppression after percutaneous absorption. Lindane is currently not available in Canada.
[b] Cost of smallest available pack size; includes drug cost only. NB: All products are available without prescription; retail mark-ups may vary.
[c] Lower strengths are not effective as scabicides.
[d] Extemporaneously compounded preparations can be used.
[e] As for permethrin.
Legend: $ <$10 $$ $10–20 $$$ $20–30

Suggested Readings

Burgess IF. Head lice. *Clin Evid (Online)* 2011;2011. pii:1703.

Canadian Agency for Drugs and Technologies in Health. *Lindane and other treatments for lice and scabies: a review of clinical effectiveness and safety*. 11 June 2010. Available from: www.cadth.ca/media/pdf/l0186_treatments_for_lice_scabies_htis-2.pdf.

Frankowski BL, Bocchini JA; Council on School Health and Committee on Infectious Diseases. Head lice. *Pediatrics* 2010;126(2):392-403.

Head lice infestations: a clinical update. *Paediatr Child Health* 2008;13(8):692-704.

Mounsey KE, McCarthy JS. Treatment and control of scabies. *Curr Opin Infect Dis* 2013;26(2):133-9.

References

1. Hill N, Moor G, Cameron MM et al. Single blind, randomised, comparative study of the Bug Buster kit and over the counter pediculicide treatments against head lice in the United Kingdom. *BMJ* 2005;331(7513):384-7.
2. Frankowski BL, Bocchini JA; Council on School Health and Committee on Infectious Diseases. Head lice. *Pediatrics* 2010;126(2):392-403.
3. Speare R, Canyon DV, Cahill C et al. Comparative efficacy of two nit combs in removing head lice (Pediculus humanus var. capitis) and their eggs. *Int J Dermatol* 2007;46(12):1275-8.
4. Chosidow O, Giraudeau B. Topical ivermectin—a step toward making head lice dead lice? *N Engl J Med* 2012;367(18):1750-2.
5. Heukelbach J, Feldmeier H. Scabies. *Lancet* 2006;367(9524):1767-74.
6. Scheinfeld N. Sklice (ivermectin) lotion for the treatment of head lice. *Skinmed* 2013;11(3):171-2.
7. Chosidow O. Clinical practices. Scabies. *N Engl J Med* 2006;354(16):1718-27.
8. Goates BM, Atkin JS, Wilding KG et al. An effective nonchemical treatment for head lice: a lot of hot air. *Pediatrics* 2006;118(5):1962-70.
9. Taplin D, Meinking TL, Castillero PM et al. Permethrin 1% creme rinse for the treatment of Pediculus humanus var capitis infestation. *Pediatr Dermatol* 1986;3(4):344-8.
10. Burgess IF, Brown CM, Burgess NA. Synergized pyrethrin mousse, a new approach to head lice eradication: efficacy in field and laboratory studies. *Clin Ther* 1994;16(1):57-64.
11. Kaul N, Palma KG, Silagy SS et al. North American efficacy and safety of a novel pediculicide rinse, isopropyl myristate 50% (Resultz). *J Cutan Med Surg* 2007;11(5):161-7.
12. Burgess IF. Randomised, controlled, parallel group clinical trials to evaluate the efficacy of isopropyl myristate/cyclomethicone solution against head lice. *Pharma J* 2008;280:371-5.
13. Heukelbach J, Sonnberg S, Becher H et al. Ovicidal efficacy of high concentration dimeticone: a new era of head lice treatment. *J Am Acad Dermatol* 2011;64(4):e61-2.
14. Burgess IF, Brunton ER, Burgess NA. Single application of 4% dimeticone liquid gel versus two applications of 1% permethrin creme rinse for treatment of head louse infestation: a randomised controlled trial. *BMC Dermatol* 2013;13:5.
15. Barnett E, Palma KG, Clayton B et al. Effectiveness of isopropyl myristate/cyclomethicone D5 solution of removing cuticular hydrocarbons from human head lice (Pediculus humanus capitis). *BMC Dermatol* 2012;12:15.
16. Heukelbach J, Oliveira FA, Richter J et al. Dimeticone-based pediculicides: a physical approach to eradicate head lice. *Open Dermatol J* 2010;4:77-81.
17. Burgess IF. Head lice. *Clin Evid (Online)* 2011;2011. pii:1703.
18. Ko CJ, Elston DM. Pediculosis. *J Am Acad Dermatol* 2004;50(1):1-12.
19. Nolan K, Kamrath J, Levitt J. Lindane toxicity: a comprehensive review of the medical literature. *Pediatr Dermatol* 2012;29(2):141-6.
20. Marcoux D, Palma KG, Kaul N et al. Pyrethroid pediculicide resistance of head lice in Canada evaluated by serial invasive signal amplification reaction. *J Cutan Med Surg* 2010;14(3):115-8.
21. Chosidow O, Giraudeau B, Cottrell J et al. Oral ivermectin versus malathion lotion for difficult-to-treat head lice. *N Engl J Med* 2010;362(10):896-905.
22. Pariser DM, Meinking TL, Bell M et al. Topical 0.5% ivermectin lotion for treatment of head lice. *N Engl J Med* 2012;367(18):1687-93.
23. Pearlman DL. A simple treatment for head lice: dry-on, suffocation-based pediculicide. *Pediatrics* 2004;114(3):e275-9.
24. Takano-Lee M, Edman JD, Mullens BA et al. Home remedies to control head lice: assessment of home remedies to control the human head louse, Pediculus humanus capitis (Anoplura: Pediculidae). *J Pediatr Nurs* 2004;19(6):393-8.
25. Workowski KA, Berman S; Centers for Disease Control and Prevention (CDC). Sexually transmitted diseases treatment guidelines, 2010. *MMWR Recomm Rep* 2010;59(RR-12):1-110.
26. Foucault C, Ranque S, Badiaga S et al. Oral ivermectin in the treatment of body lice. *J Infect Dis* 2006;193(3):474-6.
27. Strong M, Johnstone PW. Interventions for treating scabies. *Cochrane Database Syst Rev* 2007;(3):CD000320.
28. Mounsey KE, McCarthy JS. Treatment and control of scabies. *Curr Opin Infect Dis* 2013;26(2):133-9.
29. Ferreira E, Martin B, Morin C. *Grossesse et allaitement: guide thérapeutique*. 2nd ed. Montreal (QC): CHU Sainte-Justine; 2013.
30. Public Health Agency of Canada. Ectoparasitic infestations (pubic lice, scabies). In: *Canadian guidelines on sexually transmitted infections*. Ottawa (ON): PHAC; modified 2013. Available from: www.phac-aspc.gc.ca/std-mts/sti-its/cgsti-ldcits/section-5-3-eng.php. Accessed September 1, 2013.
31. Drugs and Lactation Database (LactMed). Bethesda (MD): U.S. National Library of Medicine. Available from: toxnet.nlm.nih.gov/cgi-bin/sis/htmlgen?LACT. Accessed February 24, 2014.

Skin Disorders

Chapter 98
Sunburn

Lyn Guenther, MD, FRCPC

Sunburn is caused by acute excessive exposure to ultraviolet (UV) radiation. It is characterized by erythema, with onset 2–6 hours after exposure to a threshold dose of UV radiation; it peaks at 15–36 hours and regresses by 72–120 hours. Erythema resulting from sun bed UVA exposure starts immediately, peaks at 8 hours and regresses by 24–48 hours. Edema, pain and pruritus may be present. Blistering in severe cases may take a week or more to resolve. Nausea, abdominal cramping, fever, chills, weakness, malaise and headache may also occur. Desquamation with resolution results from cellular injury and death.

Any person, regardless of skin colour, will burn with large doses of UV radiation. Blue or green-eyed, lighter-skinned individuals, who tan poorly and freckle, will burn more readily. The trunk, neck and head burn at a lower dose of UV radiation than the upper limbs, which burn more readily than the lower limbs. This may be due to the differences in thickness of the epidermis and/or stratum corneum on different areas of the body.[1]

Sun exposure in children is approximately thrice that of adults.[2] According to a Canadian survey, adolescents and young adults have the highest incidence of sunburn.[3] One U.S. study estimated the incidence of sunburn in the previous year as 34% for adults, 58% for young adults (18–29 y) and 69% for adolescents (11–18 y). Men experience more sunburns and use fewer sun protective measures than women.[3,4] There is evidence that high-risk young adult females do not follow through with appropriate sun protection despite being aware of their high-risk of skin cancer, and that they still believe tanning is beneficial. This suggests that psychosocial interventions are needed to assist these high-risk individuals in exerting more control over their sun protection behaviour.[5]

Sunburns are common in tanning salons. In fact, sunburns are more common in sun bed users than non-users.[6]

Characteristics of Ultraviolet Radiation

- UV radiation (UVR) accounts for approximately 5% of terrestrial solar radiation. UV light that causes skin injury is classified by wavelength. UVA is divided into UVA 1 (340–400 nm) which has a longer wavelength, and UVA 2 (320–340 nm). UVA is responsible for phototoxicity, photoaging, immunosuppression and skin cancer. It also accounts for ~95% of radiation found in artificial tanning beds. It penetrates the skin more deeply than UVB and is responsible for most phototoxic reactions to drugs.
- UVB (290–320 nm) is the primary cause of sunburn from sunlight. It does not penetrate glass. It can also cause immunosuppression and skin cancer.[7]

A 1% decrease in ozone results in a 1.5% increase in UVB, leading to a 2–6% increase in basal and squamous cell cancers and a 0.3–2% increase in melanomas.[8] Radiation effects are enhanced by reflective surfaces (e.g., sand, snow, cement and water). Up to 80% of UV radiation penetrates clouds. Increased humidity decreases the threshold for erythema from UV radiation. The UV index forecasts the intensity of UV rays (Table 1). Sun protection should be used if the UV index is 3 or higher.[9]

Table 1: **UV Index and Risk of Sunburn**

UV index	Risk	Estimated time for fair-skinned person to burn
0–2	Minimal	1 h
3–4	Low	<20 min
5–6	Moderate	<15 min
7–9	High	<10 min
≥10	Extreme	<5 min

Prevention of Sunburn

Prevention is critical since repeated sun exposure and sunburns are associated with skin cancer and premature skin aging. UV exposure has been linked to 90% of nonmelanoma skin cancers and 65% of melanomas.[10] Two blistering sunburns during childhood can double the risk of melanoma later in life.[10] UV radiation can also suppress the immune system and habitual exposure can cause cataracts.

Nonpharmacologic Choices

- Cosmetic tanning should be avoided. Pigmentation does not occur without damage/death of epidermal cells.
- Self-tanners contain dihydroxyacetone (DHA) which causes staining of the skin after it reacts with amino acids in the stratum corneum. Self-tanners are safe to use, but do not provide sufficient photoprotection; sunscreens are still required on UV-exposed skin.[11]
- Tanning salons should be avoided as they significantly increase the risk of both melanoma[12] and nonmelanoma[13] skin cancer. The World Health Organization (WHO) recognizes the direct link between artificial tanning and cancer.[14]
- Avoid outdoor activities at peak UV irradiance times (10 a.m. to 4 p.m. when your shadow is shorter than you; when the UV index is high or extreme).
- Choose shady areas for outdoor activities if possible.
- Umbrellas may reduce UV radiation by about 70%; however, they do not protect against reflected radiation.
- Seek shade from trees. Forests provide a sun protection factor (SPF) of 6–100 and single trees 2–50.[15,16]
- Wear protective clothing (pants, long-sleeved shirts, gloves) and sunglasses. Loosely woven, white or wet clothing offers less protection. Women's hosiery provides minimal protection.
- Protect the face, ears and neck by wearing wide-brimmed hats (at least 7.5 cm) of tightly woven fabric (not straw). Regular use could decrease the lifetime risk of skin cancer by 40%.[17]
- Minimize sun exposure while taking phototoxic medications or using certain local agents (Table 2), which can interact with UV/visible light to cause a dose-related increased risk of sunburn.
- Avoid alcohol as it may increase risk of excessive sun exposure.[18] There is also some preliminary evidence that alcohol increases the risk of sunburn by decreasing antioxidants in the skin that may play a role in neutralizing free radicals generated by exposure to UV light, and that this effect may be mitigated by the concomitant ingestion of antioxidant-containing fruit juice.[19]

Table 2: **Medications That May Cause Phototoxic Reactions**[a]

Antimicrobials
- antimalarials
  - chloroquine
  - quinine
- azole antifungals
  - itraconazole
  - voriconazole
- ceftazidime
- pyrazinamide
- quinolones
  - ciprofloxacin
  - norfloxacin
  - ofloxacin
- sulfonamides
- tetracyclines
  - doxycycline
  - tetracycline
- trimethoprim

Antineoplastics
- dacarbazine
- EGF inhibitors
  - cetuximab
  - erlotinib
  - gefitinib
  - lapatinib
  - panitumumab
- 5-fluorouracil
- paclitaxel
- vemurafenib
- vinblastine

Diuretics
- furosemide
- hydrochlorothiazide

HMG-CoA Reductase Inhibitors

NSAIDs
- diclofenac
- ibuprofen
- indomethacin
- ketoprofen
- naproxen
- piroxicam
- sulindac
- tiaprofenic acid

Psychiatric Medications
- alprazolam
- chlordiazepoxide
- chlorpromazine
- desipramine
- fluphenazine
- imipramine
- perphenazine
- prochlorperazine
- trifluoperazine

Retinoids, systemic
- acitretin
- alitretinoin
- isotretinoin

Retinoids, topical[b]
- adapalene
- tazarotene
- tretinoin

Others
- amiodarone
- coal tar derivatives, topical
- diltiazem
- eculizumab
- fluorescein, topical
- methoxsalen
- rose bengal, topical
- quinidine
- sulfites
- sulfonylureas
- tolbutamide
- verteporfin

[a] Phototoxic reactions are dose related sunburn-like reactions which can potentially occur in all people with sufficient light exposure and a high enough dose of the drug. In contrast, photoallergic reactions are delayed hypersensitivity reactions after light exposure and only occur in a small percentage of individuals. In contrast to phototoxic reactions, photoallergic reactions may extend beyond the area exposed to light. Radiation in the UVA range causes most drug-related phototoxic reactions.

[b] After continued use due to thinning of the stratum corneum.

Abbreviations: EGF = epidermal growth factor

Pharmacologic Choices

No sunscreen offers complete protection from the sun. Sunscreens should be adjunctive rather than the primary means of protection. In Canada, it is estimated that in 2013 there were approximately 81 700 new cases of nonmelanoma skin cancer with 420 deaths,[20] and 6000 new cases of melanoma with 1050 deaths.[21] Regular sunscreen use for the first 18 years could decrease the lifetime risk of skin cancer by about 80%.[22] Daily sunscreen use for 4.5 years decreased the incidence of squamous cell cancer[23] and has also been shown to reduce new primary melanomas by 50% and invasive melanomas by 73%.[24] Sunscreens can also prevent UV-induced immunosuppression[25] and skin aging.[26]

Sunscreens

Inorganic (Physical) Sunscreens

Titanium dioxide, zinc oxide, kaolin, talc (magnesium silicate), ferric chloride and **melanin** protect against UVA and UVB. These agents are photostable and reflect and scatter UV and visible light. They protect against UV and visible-light-induced photosensitivity. Microfine zinc oxide provides better UVA protection than titanium dioxide since it protects from UVB to UVA 1 (290–400 nm), while microfine titanium dioxide protects from UVB to UVA 2 (290–340 nm) only.[27] Physical sunscreens are generally thicker and less cosmetically elegant, and may rub off easily or melt with the sun's heat. Although they pose less risk of sensitization, their occlusive effect may cause miliaria ("heat rash", "prickly heat") and folliculitis. Micronized titanium dioxide and zinc oxide are relatively transparent to visible light and more cosmetically acceptable.

Organic (Chemical) Sunscreens (Table 3)

Commercial products usually contain more than 1 active ingredient in order to provide broader protection and photostability. They should be applied 15 minutes before UV exposure to allow active ingredients to bind to the skin.

Table 3: **Organic (Chemical) Sunscreens[a]**

Class	Active Ingredients	Comments
UVB Absorbers		
Benzimidazoles	*ensulizole (2-phenylbenzimidazole-5-sulfonic acid, Eusolex 232, Parsol HS)*	UVB protection. Minimal UVA protection. Photostable. Rarely causes sensitization.
Benzylidene camphor derivative	*enzacamene (4-methylbenzylidene camphor, MBC, Eusolex 6300, Parsol 5000)*	Maximum absorption at 300 nm. Photostabilizes dibenzoylmethanes. Not available in the United States.
Cinnamates	*cinoxate (2-ethoxyethyl p-methoxycinnamate)*	Does not adhere well to skin; easily removed by sweating and swimming. Cross-sensitivity with balsam of Peru, benzyl and methyl cinnamate, cinnamic alcohol, cinnamic aldehyde, cinnamon oil, cocoa leaves.
	octinoxate (octyl methoxycinnamate, 2-ethylhexylmethoxycinnamate, EMC, OMC, Escalol 557, Parsol MCX)	Does not adhere well to skin; easily removed by sweating and swimming. Cross-sensitivity with balsam of Peru, benzyl and methyl cinnamate, cinnamic alcohol, cinnamic aldehyde, cinnamon oil, cocoa leaves. Photostabilizes dibenzoylmethanes.
	octocrylene (2-ethylhexyl-2-cyano-3,3 diphenyl acrylate, OCR Eusolex)	See octinoxate.
Para-aminobenzoic acid (PABA) esters	*p-aminobenzoic acid (octyl dimethyl PABA)*	Adheres well to skin. May cause contact/photocontact dermatitis. Cross-sensitivity with ester anesthetics, sulfonamides, sulfonylurea hypoglycemics, thiazides.
Salicylates	*homosalate (homomenthyl salicylate, HMS)*	Does not adhere well to skin; easily removed by perspiration or swimming. Rarely causes contact dermatitis. Photostabilizes dibenzoylmethanes.
	octisalate (octyl salicylate, 2-ethylhexyl salicylate, Escalol 587)	See homosalate.
	triethanolamine salicylate (trolamine salicylate)	Does not adhere well to skin; easily removed by perspiration or swimming. Rarely causes contact dermatitis.
UVA Absorbers		
Anthranilates	*meradimate (menthyl anthranilate, menthyl-2-aminobenzoate)*	Incomplete UVA protection. Rarely causes sensitization.
Benzophenones	*dioxybenzone (benzophenone-8)*	Broad-spectrum UVB/UVA 2 protection May cause contact urticaria/contact dermatitis. Photostable.

(cont'd)

Table 3: **Organic (Chemical) Sunscreens**[a] *(cont'd)*

Class	Active Ingredients	Comments
	oxybenzone (benzophenone-3, Escalol 567, Eusolex 4360)	Broad-spectrum UVB/UVA 2 protection. May cause contact/photocontact dermatitis. Photostable. Photostabilizes dibenzoylmethanes.
	sulisobenzone (benzophenone-4, 2-hydroxy-4-methoxybenzophenone-5-sulfonic acid)	Broad-spectrum UVB/UVA 2 protection. May cause contact urticaria/contact dermatitis. Photostable.
Benzotriazole based	*bisoctrizole (methylene-bis-benzotriazolyl-tetramethylbutylphenol, Tinosorb M)*	UVB + UVA protection with peaks at 305 and 360 nm. Has organic and inorganic properties. Microfine particles (100–200 nm) in aqueous dispersion that absorb, scatter and reflect UV. Photostable. Not available in the United States.
Benzylidene camphor derivative	*ecamsule (terephthalylidene dicamphor sulfonic acid, Mexoryl SX)*	Maximum absorption at 345 nm. Water soluble. Photostable.
Dibenzoylmethanes	*avobenzone (t-butylmethoxy-dibenzoylmethane, Eusolex 9020, Parsol 1789)*	Broad UVA absorption with peak at UVA 1 (357 nm). Better protection against UVA than anthranilates, benzophenones and benzylidene camphor derivatives. Photodegradable. May cause contact and photocontact dermatitis.
Hydroxybenzotriazole based	*drometriazole trisiloxane (silatriazole, Mexoryl XL)*	UVA + UVB protection with peaks at 303 and 344 nm. Oil soluble. Photostable. Not available in the United States.
Hydroxyphenyl-triazine based	*bemotrizinol (anizotriazine, bis-ethylhexyloxyphenol methoxyphenyl triazine, Tinosorb S)*	UVB + UVA protection with peaks at 310 and 343 nm. Photostable. Not available in United States.

[a] For a listing of Canadian Dermatology Association-recognized sunscreens, see www.dermatology.ca/programs-resources/programs/recognized-products.

Sunscreen Labelling

Sunscreens should be used to protect the skin and not to prolong sun exposure. They should be "broad spectrum" meaning contain recognized ingredients that protect against both UVA and UVB. Sunscreens should have a *sun protection factor* (SPF) of at least 15 and preferably 30. SPF is defined as the least amount of energy needed to produce erythema (primarily UVB) with sunscreen, divided by the least amount of energy needed to produce erythema without sunscreen. Health Canada states that products with a critical wavelength (that at which the sunscreen is still able to block 90% of UVA rays) of at least 370 nm may use the designation "Broad Spectrum". The higher the critical wavelength, the greater the UVA protection.[28,29]

Sunscreens with the "broad spectrum" designation and SPF ≥15 may use the following statement: "If used as directed with other sun protection measures, decreases the risk of skin cancer and early skin aging caused by the sun". Sunscreens with an SPF <15 or critical wavelength <370 nm must use the following statement: "This product has been shown only to help prevent sunburn, *not* skin cancer or early skin aging".[28]

Water-resistant products may only be labelled as "Water/Sweat Resistant [40 minutes]" or "Water/Sweat Resistant [80 minutes]".[28,29]

Sunscreen Application

The SPF of sunscreens is measured under ideal laboratory conditions and may be considerably lower when applied thinly and used outdoors. Topical sunscreens should be applied generously (2 mg/cm^2) to all exposed surfaces including lips, tops of ears and tops of feet. Approximately 30 mL is needed for full coverage of the average adult body. Sunscreen effectiveness is dramatically reduced when under-applied. A second application shortly after the first increases the amount of sunscreen applied and may result in protection closer to that stated on the sunscreen product.[30]

Sunscreens should be applied liberally 15 minutes before sun exposure and reapplied at least every 2 hours. Water-resistant/sweat-resistant products should be used if swimming/sweating and reapplied after 40 or 80 minutes (as indicated on the label) of swimming/sweating. All sunscreens should be reapplied after washing or towel drying. Products applied to the lips should be reapplied after eating or drinking. Although sunscreens can prevent sunburn, many biological effects (e.g., immunosuppression, carcinogenicity) can occur before the UV erythema threshold is reached. Encourage outdoor workers and fair-skinned individuals to apply sunscreen as part of their daily routine.

Sunscreens are available in a number of different formulations including creams, lotions, gels, sprays and sticks. Sprays can be useful for hard to reach areas such as the back and creams can be helpful for individuals with dry skin. Although gels are preferable for individuals with oily skin and/or acne, they are often removed with swimming and sweat.[31] Sticks are good for small areas such as the lips and nose and tend not to drip with sweating, which minimizes eye irritation when used on the face.

Concurrent application of sunscreen with the insect repellent n,n-diethyl-meta-toluamide (DEET) may lower SPF but the efficacy of DEET appears to be maintained.[32] If application of DEET is delayed after the sunscreen has been applied, the sunscreen product maintains more of its original SPF.

Vitamin D

The Institute of Medicine of the National Academies updated Dietary Reference Intakes for Calcium and Vitamin D[33] concludes that the impact of sunscreen use on vitamin D synthesis needs to be clarified by further studies. Although vitamin D production is dependent on UVB exposure, "real world" application of sunscreen may not actually be affecting vitamin D production significantly. The Institute of Medicine of the National Academies based its vitamin D dietary intake recommendations on an assumption of minimal sun exposure, and recommends the same daily intake irrespective of sunscreen use.[33] Further information on vitamin D requirements and supplementation can be found in Appendix IV.

Safety of Sunscreens

A nonprofit research organization (the Environmental Working Group) has published concerns regarding the safety of some sunscreen ingredients.[34] They list oxybenzone as being a potential "hormone disruptor"; however, a study in humans failed to find any effect on follicle-stimulating hormone or luteinizing hormone levels.[35] The same group reports concerns regarding the safety of the antioxidant retinyl palmitate (a form of vitamin A) with respect to a significantly shorter time to tumour formation in mice exposed to this compound;[34] however, a critical review based on in vitro, animal and human studies did not find convincing evidence that retinyl palmitate was photocarcinogenic and commented that retinoids can in fact prevent skin cancer.[36] Addition of antioxidants to sunscreen may help prevent skin damage induced by free radicals in the presence of UV light.[37]

Metal oxide nanoparticles are smaller than micronized ones, appear transparent on the skin and provide excellent protection against sunburn. Theoretical concerns about possible adverse effects due to absorption of these particles have been dismissed as there is evidence that only negligible amounts if any are absorbed percutaneously.[38,39,40,41]

Sunscreen and Infants

For infants <6 months of age, avoid sun exposure whenever possible. Seek or create shade using items such as stroller hoods/covers and umbrellas. Dress the infant in wide-brimmed hats and lightweight, loose-fitting clothing that covers the arms and legs. In the exceptional case where sun exposure is unavoidable despite these measures, a broad-spectrum SPF 30 sunscreen for babies can be applied to the small exposed areas (e.g., face, back of hands) [Evidence: SORT C*].[42,43,44] To date, no data show toxicity from absorption of sunscreen ingredients in infants.[45] Inorganic (physical) sunscreens containing zinc oxide and/or titanium oxide are minimally absorbed and less likely to cause sensitization.[46] Children 6 months of age or older should follow the same sun protection as advised for adults.

Other Potential Protective Agents

Other agents showing some promise as photoprotectants include oral beta-carotene supplements,[47] topical antioxidant solutions containing vitamins C and E,[47,48] oral Polypodium leucotomos (a natural fern leaf extract), oral and topical green tea polyphenols and chocolate rich in flavanols;[47] however, there is insufficient evidence to recommend them at the present time.

Treatment of Sunburn

- Assess for and treat heat exhaustion or heat stroke if present (see Chapter 27).
- Since most sunburns are superficial and resolve over a few days to a week, treatment is symptomatic.
- Blisters may require dressings and wound care (see Chapter 91). Blisters should not be unroofed since the overlying skin protects against secondary infection.
- Severe sunburns may require admission to a burn unit if there is extensive denudation of skin and fluid and electrolyte loss.[49] (See Chapter 91.)
- Counsel patients presenting with sunburn regarding the risks associated with sunburn and the importance of using photoprotection appropriately.

Nonpharmacologic Choices

Cool baths or **wet compresses** with tap water or saline for 20 minutes 4–6 times a day provide some relief. **Fluids** should be replenished with nonalcoholic beverages.

Pharmacologic Choices

Calamine lotion and **colloidal oatmeal** may be soothing.

Moisturizers help with dryness and peeling.

Simple analgesics (e.g., **acetaminophen**, **ibuprofen**) may provide pain relief.

Pramoxine hydrochloride 1% is a topical anesthetic with low sensitizing potential[50] that may provide short-term relief. Avoid topical benzocaine and other "caine" topical anesthetics as they can sensitize the skin.[51]

Topical **diclofenac gel** applied 6 and 10 hours after irradiation decreased pain, erythema and edema in studies conducted by the manufacturer.[52]

Evidence of the effectiveness of **aloe vera** in treating sunburn is limited and conflicting.[53,54] A systematic review looking at its use in acute and chronic wounds including burns was inconclusive.[55]

* SORT (Strength of Recommendation Taxonomy) is a rating system (A, B or C) that addresses the quality of available evidence. For more information consult **How to Use *Compendium of Therapeutic Choices*** on page xxv.

Studies of the treatment of sunburn with **topical corticosteroids** have shown mixed results.[56,57,58,59] As it is unclear if there is any benefit and sunburn is a self-limiting condition, they are not generally recommended.[60,61,62]

Small studies have examined whether experimentally induced UV erythema and epidermal injury may be suppressed by oral **NSAIDs**[58,63] but the evidence is not convincing and they are not routinely recommended except as simple analgesics for sunburn pain.

Opioids such as fentanyl and morphine may be required to relieve the pain associated with severe sunburn.

Choices during Pregnancy and Breastfeeding

Sun Protection during Pregnancy and Breastfeeding

As for all patients, nonpharmacologic measures to prevent sun-induced skin damage (e.g., seeking shade, protective clothing, minimizing sun exposure) should be the first choice in pregnant or breastfeeding women. The systemic absorption of all sunscreens is very small, particularly the physical sunscreens zinc and titanium dioxide.[64] Chemical and physical sunscreens are considered safe to use during pregnancy and breastfeeding. As a general precaution, care should be taken to avoid contact of a nursing infant's skin with any treated area of the mother's skin.

Treatment of Sunburn while Pregnant or Breastfeeding

Sunburn can be safely soothed with **calamine lotion** and/or **colloidal oatmeal** baths while pregnant or breastfeeding. **Acetaminophen** is safe to use for pain relief. Oral **ibuprofen** or **topical diclofenac** gel[52] may also provide pain relief. These medications are considered safe to use in pregnancy though full anti-inflammatory doses should be avoided in the 3rd trimester due to the risk of oligohydramnios and premature closure of the ductus arteriosus.[65] Oral ibuprofen and topical diclofenac are also considered safe to use while breastfeeding.[66]

A discussion of general principles on the use of medications in these special populations can be found in Appendix II and Appendix III. Other specialized reference sources are also provided in these appendices.

Therapeutic Tips

- Systemic corticosteroids have little effect in treating sunburn and may increase the risk of secondary infection.
- Consider possibility of a phototoxic drug reaction (see Table 2).
- After a sunburn, the skin should not be exposed to the sun for at least a week.
- Scarring rarely occurs unless there is secondary infection.

Suggested Readings

Bissonnette R, Claveau J, Gupta AK. Ultraviolet A radiation and the need for protection. *J Cutan Med Surg* 2006;10(Suppl 1):1-7.

Driscoll MS, Wagner RF. Clinical management of the acute sunburn reaction. *Cutis* 2000;66(1):53-8.

Jansen R, Osterwalder U, Wang SQ et al. Photoprotection: part II. Sunscreen: development, efficacy, and controversies. *J Am Acad Dermatol* 2013;69(6):867.e1-14.

Kutlubay Z, Sevim A, Engin B et al. Photodermatoses, including phototoxic and photoallergic reactions (internal and external). *Clin Dermatol* 2014;32(1):73-9.

Rivers JK, Bang B, Marcoux D. Ultraviolet radiation exposure: public health concerns. *J Cutan Med Surg* 2006;10(Suppl 1):8-13.

References

1. Waterston K, Naysmith L, Rees JL. Variation in skin thickness may explain some of the within-person variation in ultraviolet radiation-induced erythema at different body sites. *J Invest Dermatol* 2005;124(5):1078.
2. Stern RS. Proportion of lifetime UV dose received by age 18, what Stern et al actually said in 1986. *J Invest Dermatol* 2005;124(5):1079-80.
3. Lovato C, Shoveller J, Rivers J. *National survey on sun & protective behaviours. Final report.* Vancouver (BC): Institute of Health Promotion Research, UBC; 1998.
4. Buller DB, Cokkinides V, Hall HI et al. Prevalence of sunburn, sun protection, and indoor tanning behaviors among Americans: review from national surveys and case studies of 3 states. *J Am Acad Dermatol* 2011;65(5 Suppl):S114-23.
5. Heckman CJ, Darlow S, Cohen-Filipic J et al. Psychosocial correlates of sunburn among young adult women. *Int J Environ Res Public Health* 2012;9(6):2241-51.
6. Thieden E, Philipsen PA, Sandby-Moller J et al. Sunburn related to UV radiation exposure, age, sex, occupation, and sun bed use based on time-stamped personal dosimetry and sun behavior diaries. *Arch Dermatol* 2005;141(4):482-8.
7. Schwarz T. The dark and the sunny sides of UVR-induced immunosuppression: photoimmunology revisited. *J Invest Dermatol* 2010;130(1):49-54.
8. Coldiron BM. Thinning of the ozone layer: facts and consequences. *J Am Acad Dermatol* 1992;27(5 Pt 1):653-62.
9. Cancer Council Australia. *Preventing skin cancer*. Available from: www.cancer.org.au/preventing-cancer/sun-protection/preventing-skin-cancer. Accessed December 27, 2013.
10. Geller AC, Cantor M, Miller DR et al. The Environmental Protection Agency's National SunWise School Program: sun protection education in US schools (1999-2000). *J Am Acad Dermatol* 2002;46(5):683-9.
11. Gordon D, Guenther L. Tanning behaviour of London-area youth. *J Cutan Med Surg* 2009;13(1):22-32.
12. Boniol M, Autier P, Boyle P et al. Cutaneous melanoma attributable to sunbed use: systematic review and meta-analysis. *BMJ* 2012;345:e4757.
13. Wehner MR, Shive ML, Chren MM et al. Indoor tanning and non-melanoma skin cancer: systematic review and meta-analysis. *BMJ* 2012;345:e5909.
14. World Health Organization. *The World Health Organization recommends that no person under 18 should use a sunbed.* Geneva (CH): WHO; March 17, 2005. Available from: www.who.int/mediacentre/news/notes/2005/np07/en/. Accessed February 11, 2014.
15. Grant RH, Heisler GM, Gao W. Estimation of pedestrian level UV exposure under trees. *Photochem Photobiol* 2002;74(4):369-76.
16. Diffey BL, Diffey JL. Sun protection with trees. *Br J Dermatol* 2002;147(2):397-9.
17. Marks R. Photoprotection and prevention of melanoma. *Eur J Dermatol* 1999;9(5):406-12.
18. Mukamal KJ. Alcohol consumption and self-reported sunburn: a cross-sectional, population-based survey. *J Am Acad Dermatol* 2006;55(4):584-9.
19. Darvin ME, Sterry W, Lademann J et al. Alcohol consumption decreases the protection efficiency of the antioxidant network and increases the risk of sunburn in human skin. *Skin Pharmacol Physiol* 2013;26(1):45-51.
20. Canadian Cancer Society. *Non-melanoma skin cancer statistics*. Available from: www.cancer.ca/en/cancer-information/cancer-type/skin-non-melanoma/statistics/?region=on#ixzz2ohfpixPS. Accessed December 27, 2013.
21. Canadian Cancer Society. *Melanoma statistics*. Available from: www.cancer.ca/en/cancer-information/cancer-type/skin-melanoma/statistics/?region=on#ixzz2ohdDwael. Accessed December 27, 2013.
22. Stern RS, Weinstein MC, Baker SG. Risk reduction for nonmelanoma skin cancer with childhood sunscreen use. *Arch Dermatol* 1986;122(5):537-45.
23. Green A, Williams G, Neale R et al. Daily sunscreen application and betacarotene supplementation in prevention of basal-cell and squamous-cell carcinomas of the skin: a randomised controlled trial. *Lancet* 1999;354(9180):723-9.
24. Green AC, Williams GM, Logan V et al. Reduced melanoma after regular sunscreen use: randomized trial follow-up. *J Clin Oncol* 2011;29(3):257-63.
25. Baron ED, Stevens SR. Sunscreens and immune protection. *Br J Dermatol* 2002;146(6):933-7.
26. Hughes MC, Williams GM, Baker P et al. Sunscreen and prevention of skin aging: a randomized trial. *Ann Intern Med* 2013;158(11):781-90.
27. Hexsel CL, Bangert SD, Hebert AA et al. Current sunscreen issues: 2007 Food and Drug Administration sunscreen labelling recommendations and combination sunscreen/insect repellent products. *J Am Acad Dermatol* 2008;59(2):316-23.
28. Health Canada. *Sunscreen monograph*. July 2013. Available from: webprod.hc-sc.gc.ca/nhpid-bdipsn/atReq.do?atid=sunscreen-ecransolaire⟨=eng. Accessed February 11, 2014.
29. U.S. Department of Health and Human Services. Food and Drug Administration. Labeling and effectiveness testing; sunscreen drug products for over-the-counter human use. 21 CFR Parts 201 and 310. *Federal Register* 2011;76(117):35620-65. Available from: www.gpo.gov/fdsys/pkg/FR-2011-06-17/pdf/2011-14766.pdf. Accessed February 11, 2014.
30. Teramura T, Mizuno M, Asano H et al. Relationship between sun-protection factor and application thickness in high-performance sunscreen: double application of sunscreen is recommended. *Clin Exp Dermatol* 2012;37(8):904-8.
31. Sambandan DR, Ratner D. Sunscreens: an overview and update. *J Am Acad Dermatol* 2011;64(4):748-58.

32. Murphy ME, Montemarano AD, Debboun M et al. The effect of sunscreen on the efficacy of insect repellent: a clinical trial. *J Am Acad Dermatol* 2000;43(2 Pt 1):219-22.
33. Institute of Medicine of the National Academies. *Dietary reference intakes for calcium and vitamin D.* Available from: www.iom.edu/Reports/2010/Dietary-Reference-Intakes-for-Calcium-and-Vitamin-D.aspx. Accessed February 11, 2014.
34. Environmental Working Group. *EWG's 2013 guide to safer sunscreens.* Available from: www.ewg.org/2013sunscreen. Accessed August 8, 2013.
35. Janjua NR, Mogensen B, Andersson AM et al. Systemic absorption of the sunscreens benzophenone-3, octyl-methoxycinnamate, and 3-(4-methyl-benzylidene) camphor after whole-body topical application and reproductive hormone levels in humans. *J Invest Dermatol* 2004;123(1):57-61.
36. Wang SQ, Dusza SW, Lim HW. Safety of retinyl palmitate in sunscreens: a critical analysis. *J Am Acad Dermatol* 2010;63(5):903-6.
37. Murray JC, Burch JA, Streilein RD et al. A topical antioxidant solution containing vitamins C and E stabilized by ferulic acid provides protection for human skin against damage caused by ultraviolet irradiation. *J Am Acad Dermatol* 2008;59(3):418-25.
38. Gulson B, McCall M, Korsch M et al. Small amounts of zinc from zinc oxide particles in sunscreens applied outdoors are absorbed through human skin. *Toxicol Sci* 2010;118(1):140-9.
39. Osmond MJ, McCall MJ. Zinc oxide nanoparticles in modern sunscreens: an analysis of potential exposure and hazard. *Nanotoxicology* 2010;4(1):15-41.
40. European Commission. Scientific Committee on Consumer Safety. *Opinion on zinc oxide (nano form): Colipa S 76.* September 2012. Available from: ec.europa.eu/health/scientific_committees/consumer_safety/docs/sccs_o_103.pdf. Accessed July 25, 2013.
41. Canadian Dermatology Association. *Position statement on the use of nanoparticles in sunscreens and cosmetics.* Available from: www.dermatology.ca/wp-content/uploads/2012/01/Position-statement-nanoparticles2011EN.pdf. Accessed August 8, 2013.
42. Environment Canada. *Sun protection for babies.* Available from: www.ec.gc.ca/uv/default.asp?lang=En&n=2B3B8766-1. Accessed February 11, 2014.
43. Cancer Council Australia. Position Statement. *Sun protection and infants (0-12 months).* Available from: wiki.cancer.org.au/prevention/Position_statement_-_Sun_protection_and_infants_%280-12_months%29. Accessed March 26, 2014.
44. American Academy of Pediatrics. *Sunburn: treatment and prevention.* Available from: www.healthychildren.org/English/safety-prevention/at-play/Pages/Sunburn-Treatment-And-Prevention.aspx. Accessed March 26, 2014.
45. Balk SJ; Council on Environmental Health; Section on Dermatology. Ultraviolet radiation: a hazard to children and adolescents. *Pediatrics* 2011;127(3):e791-817.
46. Paller AS, Hawk JL, Honig P et al. New insights about infant and toddler skin: implications for sun protection. *Pediatrics* 2011;128(1):92-102.
47. Jansen R, Wang SQ, Burnett M et al. Photoprotection: part 1. Photoprotection by naturally occurring, physical, and systemic agents. *J Am Acad Dermatol* 2013;69(6):853.e1-12.
48. Aguilera J, de Gálvez MV, Sánchez C et al. Changes in photoinduced cutaneous erythema with topical application of a combination of vitamins C and E before and after UV exposure. *J Dermatol Sci* 2012;66(3):216-20.
49. Mah L, Di Giovine P, Quinn L et al. Paediatric sunburn: the experience of an Australian paediatric burns unit. *J Paediatr Child Health* 2013;49(8):654-7.
50. Rietschel TL, Fowler JF, Fisher AA. *Fisher's contact dermatitis.* 6th ed. Hamilton (ON): BC Decker; 2008. p. 244.
51. Spring S, Pratt M, Chaplin A. Contact dermatitis to topical medicaments: a retrospective chart review from the Ottawa Hospital Patch Test Clinic. *Dermatitis* 2012;23(5):210-3.
52. Kienzler JL, Magnette J, Queille-Roussel C et al. Diclofenac-Na gel is effective in reducing the pain and inflammation associated with exposure to ultraviolet light - results of two clinical studies. *Skin Pharmacol Physiol* 2005;18(3):144-52.
53. Puvabanditsin P, Vongtongsri R. Efficacy of aloe vera cream in prevention and treatment of sunburn and suntan. *J Med Assoc Thai* 2005;88(Suppl 4):S173-6.
54. Reuter J, Jocher A, Stump J et al. Investigation of the anti-inflammatory potential of Aloe vera gel (97.5%) in the ultraviolet erythema test. *Skin Pharmacol Physiol* 2008;21(2):106-10.
55. Dat AD, Poon F, Pham KB et al. Aloe vera for treating acute and chronic wounds. *Cochrane Database Syst Rev* 2012;2:CD008762.
56. Russo PM, Scneiderman LJ. Effect of topical corticosteroids on symptoms of clinical sunburn. *J Fam Pract* 1978;7(6):1129-32.
57. Duteil L, Queille-Roussel C, Lorenz B et al. A randomized, controlled study of the safety and efficacy of topical corticosteroid treatments of sunburn in healthy volunteers. *Clin Exp Dermatol* 2002;27(4):314-8.
58. Hughes GS, Francom SF, Means LK et al. Synergistic effects of oral nonsteroidal drugs and topical corticosteroids in the therapy of sunburn in humans. *Dermatology* 1992;184(1):54-8.
59. Faurschou A, Wulf HC. Topical corticosteroids in the treatment of acute sunburn: a randomized, double-blind clinical trial. *Arch Dermatol* 2008;144(5):620-4.
60. Land V, Small L. The evidence on how to best treat sunburn in children: a common treatment dilemma. *Dermatol Nurs* 2009;21(3):126, 133-7.
61. PatientPlus. *Sunburn.* Available from: www.patient.co.uk/doctor/Sunburn.htm. Accessed February 10, 2014.
62. Han A, Maibach HI. Management of acute sunburn. *Am J Clin Dermatol* 2004;5(1):39-47.
63. Rodriguez-Burford C, Tu JH, Mercurio M et al. Selective cyclooxygenase-2 inhibition produces heterogeneous erythema response to ultraviolet irradiation. *J Invest Dermatol* 2005;125(6):1317-20.
64. Newman MD, Stotland M, Ellis JI. The safety of nanosized particles in titanium dioxide- and zinc oxide-based sunscreens. *J Am Acad Dermatol* 2009;61(4):685-92.
65. Diav-Citrin O, Koren G. Drug use during pregnancy. In: *Compendium of pharmaceuticals and specialties: Canada's trusted drug reference.* Ottawa (ON): CPhA; 2014.
66. Brochet MS, Ito S. Drug use during breastfeeding. In: *Compendium of pharmaceuticals and specialties: Canada's trusted drug reference.* Ottawa (ON): CPhA; 2014.

Blood Disorders

Chapter 99
Common Anemias

Wendy Lim, MD, FRCPC

Anemia is most commonly defined as a reduction in hemoglobin (Hb) concentration that is more than 2 standard deviations below the mean, adjusted for sex and age. A reduction in hematocrit (Hct) or red blood cell (RBC) count can also be used to define anemia. Typically, based on these normal ranges a Hb of <135 g/L defines anemia in men an Hb <120 g/L defines anemia in women. It is notable that these normal ranges may not be applicable for all patients. Examples include patients living at high altitude, who have values higher than those living at sea level,[1] and patients who smoke or are exposed to carbon monoxide, who have higher Hct values than nonsmokers.[2] African-Americans have Hb values 5–10 g/L lower than comparable Caucasian populations.[3] The presence of anemia is associated with an increased risk of hospitalization and death in community-dwelling older adults.[4] In this review, anemias responsive to pharmacologic therapy will be discussed. These include anemias due to iron, vitamin B_{12} or folate deficiency, or anemias responding to erythropoietin therapy.

Goals of Therapy

- Alleviate the signs and symptoms of anemia
- Determine and address the underlying cause(s) of the anemia
- Restore normal or adequate Hb level
  - improve quality of life[5]
  - prolong survival[6]

Investigations

- Signs and symptoms of anemia occur when the oxygen-carrying capacity of the blood is unable to meet the oxygen requirements of body tissues (Figure 1).[4]
- Underlying cause(s) for anemia are variable and include obvious or occult blood loss, hemolysis, inherited defects in hemoglobin (e.g., thalassemias) or the RBC membrane (e.g., G-6-PD deficiency), suppression of the bone marrow (e.g., due to medications including cytotoxic agents, antiretrovirals and folate antagonists or infectious causes), alcohol use, deficiencies in dietary intake (e.g., iron, folate or vitamin B_{12} deficiency), deficiencies of erythropoietin from chronic kidney disease or comorbid conditions (e.g., hypothyroidism, hypogonadism). Primary diseases affecting the bone marrow (e.g., leukemia, myelodysplastic syndrome, aplastic anemia) or infiltrative diseases (e.g., cancer, sarcoidosis) can also result in anemia.
- A history detailing bleeding symptoms, family history of anemia, medication use, diet, alcohol intake, comorbid conditions, GI symptoms and menorrhagia is warranted. On physical examination, seek signs and symptoms that point to the etiology of the anemia (e.g., glossitis and koilonychia in iron deficiency, paresthesia in vitamin B_{12} deficiency).
- Diagnostic algorithms in Figure 2, Figure 3 and Figure 4 are given as guidelines and are based on the traditional classification of anemia according to red cell size, as reflected in the mean cell volume (MCV).[7]
- All pregnant women should be screened for anemia.[8] In addition, postmenopausal women and adult men presenting with anemia should be screened for GI blood loss as well as celiac disease.

- The screening test for iron deficiency anemia is a ferritin level, which can be influenced by presence of inflammation, infection, obesity[9] and other conditions and must be interpreted in the correct context. Iron-deficiency anemia is typically defined as a ferritin level <30 ng/mL. However, in a state of chronic inflammation, the definition changes to <50 ng/mL.[8]
- The serum folate level is prone to short-term fluctuations and may be misleading. The red blood cell (RBC) folate level reflects time-averaged folate availability and is a more reliable indicator of tissue folate adequacy.[10]
- There is significant intra- and interindividual variation in serum cobalamin (vitamin B_{12}) levels, so patients with macrocytosis and borderline cobalamin levels (as defined by the local laboratory) need further assessment.[11] Cobalamin levels drop during pregnancy without other evidence of deficiency.[12]

Iron-deficiency Anemia

Pathophysiology

Iron-deficiency anemia (a microcytic anemia characterized by small RBCs) is the most common nutritional disorder, accounts for nearly half of all anemia cases, and is most prevalent among preschool children and women. Iron deficiency anemia is present in 1–2% of adults; iron deficiency without anemia occurs in up to 11% of women and 4% of men.[13] The most common cause of iron deficiency is blood loss, which can be overt or occult. Blood loss through the GI tract is the most common cause of occult blood loss in men and in postmenopausal women. Women who are menstruating may develop iron deficiency. Decreased iron absorption due to disorders such as celiac disease or autoimmune atrophic gastritis may also result in iron deficiency. Less common causes include hemolysis, patients undergoing gastric bypass surgery for morbid obesity and patients with congenital iron deficiency.

Figure 1: Evaluation of Anemia

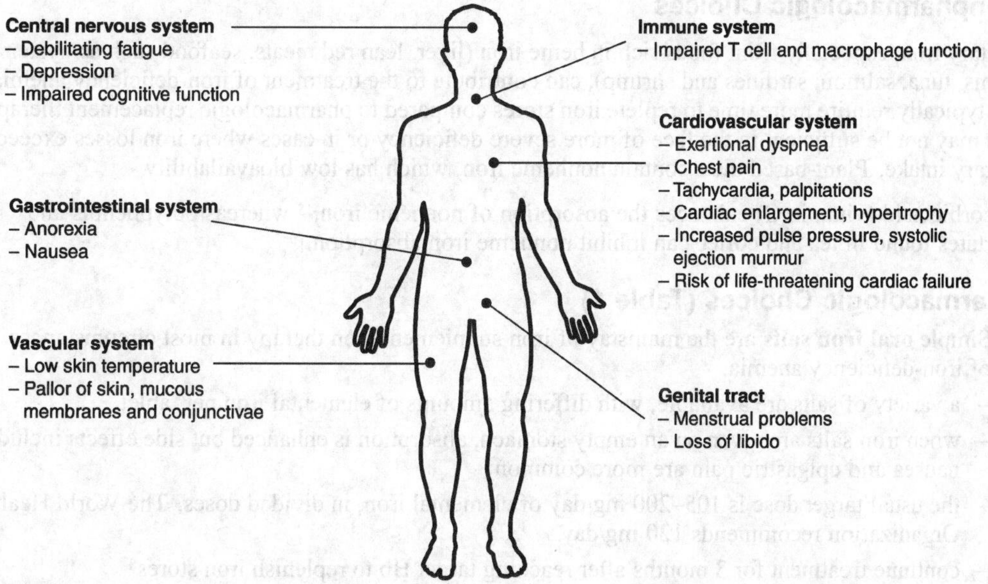

Signs and symptoms of anemia occur when the oxygen-carrying capacity of the blood is unable to meet the oxygen requirements of body tissues. Modified from Ludwig H, Fritz E. Anemia in cancer patients. *Semin Oncol* 1998;25(3 Suppl 7):2-6. Copyright 1998, with permission from Elsevier Inc.

Figure 2: **Diagnostic Algorithm for Microcytic Anemia**

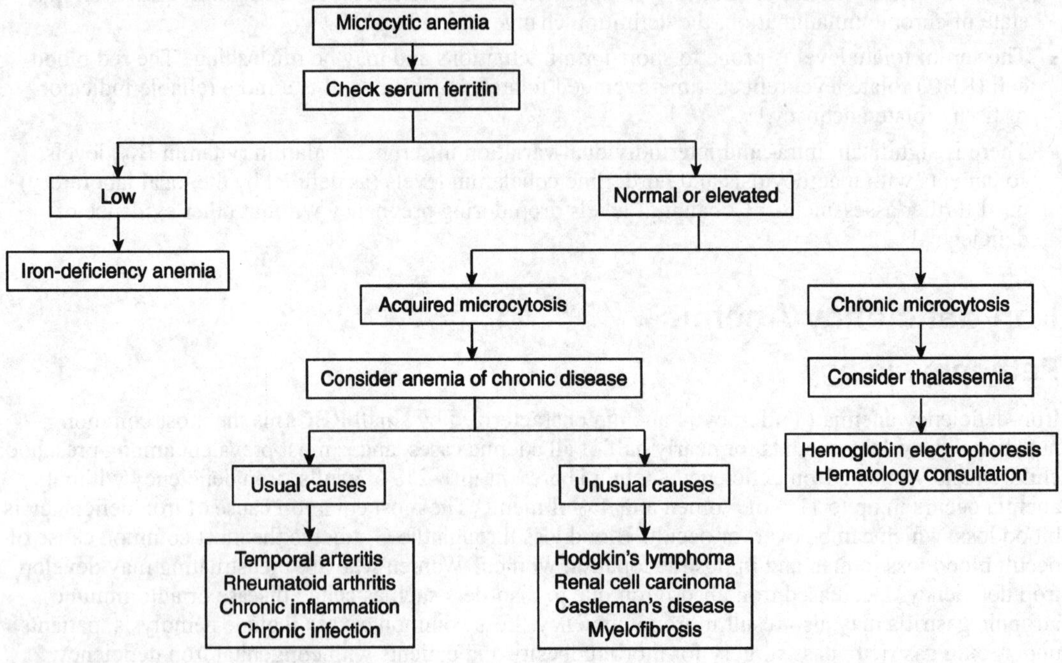

Adapted with permission from: Tefferi A, Hanson CA, Inwards DJ. How to interpret and pursue an abnormal complete blood cell count in adults. *Mayo Clin Proc* 2005;80(7):923-36.

Therapeutic Choices

Nonpharmacologic Choices

Dietary iron, especially from foods rich in heme iron (liver, lean red meats, seafood such as oysters, clams, tuna, salmon, sardines and shrimp), can contribute to the treatment of iron-deficiency anemia, but typically require more time to replete iron stores compared to pharmacologic replacement therapy,[14] and may not be sufficient in the face of more severe deficiency or in cases where iron losses exceed dietary intake. Plant-based diets contain nonheme iron, which has low bioavailability.

Ascorbic acid (vitamin C) enhances the absorption of nonheme iron,[15] whereas polyphenols and phytates found in tea and coffee can inhibit nonheme iron absorption.[16]

Pharmacologic Choices (Table 1)

- Simple **oral iron salts** are the mainstay of iron supplementation therapy in most circumstances of iron-deficiency anemia.
  - a variety of salts are available, with differing amounts of elemental iron per tablet
  - when iron salts are given on an empty stomach, absorption is enhanced but side effects including nausea and epigastric pain are more common
  - the usual target dose is 105–200 mg/day of elemental iron, in divided doses. The World Health Organization recommends 120 mg/day.
  - continue treatment for 3 months after reaching target Hb to replenish iron stores[8]

- **Parenteral iron** is reserved for patients with malabsorption or true intolerance to oral iron therapy, or where ongoing losses exceed the capacity of the GI tract to absorb oral iron. Although newer formulations are safer and better tolerated than older preparations, a low risk of anaphylaxis remains.[17]
  - parenteral iron may result in a more rapid rise in Hb compared to oral iron salts,[18] but requires administration in a hospital or outpatient clinic
  - parenteral iron may reduce the need for red blood cell transfusion,[19] but may also increase the risk of infection[19]

A reticulocyte response should be evident within 1 week of beginning iron therapy, with subsequent improvement in the Hb of about 10 g/L every 7–10 days.

Choices during Pregnancy and Breastfeeding

It is recommended that pregnant women meet the dietary requirements of iron through diet and/or supplements to prevent the development of iron deficiency during pregnancy and postpartum. During pregnancy, iron requirements increase due to expansion of maternal red cell mass and growth of the fetus and placenta. All pregnant women should be screened for anemia.

Treatment of iron deficiency in pregnant women is the same as in the nonpregnant woman. There are no reported teratogenic effects of iron supplementation on the fetus. Iron normally passes into breast milk where it is an important source of dietary iron for the developing infant. The amount of iron in breast milk is generally not influenced significantly by maternal iron status.

In pregnant women, 20 mg/day of elemental iron started at 20 weeks' gestation is sufficient to prevent iron deficiency,[20] and may also reduce the risk of low birth weight in the infant.[21,22]

- Simple oral **iron salts** are the mainstay of iron supplementation therapy in most pregnant women.
  - pregnant women who experience nausea and GI symptoms during pregnancy and find the GI side effects of oral iron intolerable can attempt to take lower doses of iron and/or take the iron with meals
  - another option for women who do not tolerate daily iron is intermittent iron supplementation. Limited data suggest intermittent iron supplementation (taken once, twice, or three times weekly on nonconsecutive days) in pregnant women is as effective in preventing iron deficiency and is associated with fewer side effects (constipation and nausea) compared to daily regimens [Evidence: SORT B*].[23]
- **Parenteral iron** is reserved for pregnant women with malabsorption or true intolerance to oral iron therapy, or where ongoing losses exceed the capacity of the GI tract to absorb oral iron resulting in severe anemia.

A discussion of general principles on the use of medications in these special populations can be found in Appendix II and Appendix III. Other specialized reference sources are also provided in these appendices.

Therapeutic Tips

- Assess the underlying cause of anemia.
- The most common cause of microcytic anemia in North America is iron deficiency. Occult GI bleeding should be ruled out, particularly since iron deficiency can be the first presentation of a GI malignancy (see Suggested Readings). Other causes must be ruled out before menorrhagia is accepted as the sole cause of iron deficiency.[24]

* SORT (Strength of Recommendation Taxonomy) is a rating system (A, B or C) that addresses the quality of available evidence. For more information consult **How to Use *Compendium of Therapeutic Choices*** on page xxv.

- If there is no obvious GI blood loss, consider screening patients for celiac disease, which results in decreased absorption of iron from the GI tract.
- Pregnant women can develop a decrease in Hb levels that is physiologic; however, iron deficiency is a common cause of anemia in this population and must be ruled out.
- If the Hb fails to respond as anticipated, consider that there may be:
  - ongoing blood loss
  - use of other medications that impair iron absorption (Table 1)
  - a different or concurrent cause of anemia and/or an impaired erythropoietic response
  - adherence issues
- GI side effects are the most common reasons for nonadherence.
  - use a graduated approach to iron dosing. One suggested method is to begin with a single tablet taken after a meal. On a weekly basis, as tolerance permits, add another tablet until the patient is taking 1 dose with each meal. Thereafter, gradually shift the timing of the doses to beginning of meals
  - small oral doses may be adequate in patients who are susceptible to GI upset. In the elderly, daily doses of elemental iron as low as 15–50 mg are effective in the treatment of iron deficiency anemia[17]
  - intermittent iron given once, twice or three times weekly on nonconsecutive days may decrease side effects in nonanemic pregnant women[23]
  - iron contained in enteric-coated tablets is poorly absorbed. These products should be avoided
- There is no specific duration for iron supplementation. If an underlying cause of anemia is identified and treated, iron supplementation can be continued until iron stores are replenished. Some clinicians recommend continuing treatment for 3 months after the target Hb has been reached. If an underlying cause cannot be identified or cannot be definitively treated, it may be reasonable to educate the patient on signs and symptoms of anemia and to routinely screen for recurrence of anemia through blood testing.

Megaloblastic Anemia

Pathophysiology

Megaloblastic anemias arise because of impaired DNA synthesis caused by deficiencies of vitamin B_{12} (cobalamin) or folate (folic acid), or due to impaired DNA and RNA metabolism (drugs, myelodysplasia). Megaloblastic anemias are a subset of macrocytic anemias (anemia associated with increased red cell size). Megaloblastic anemias are characterized by hypersegmented neutrophils on the peripheral blood film.

Patients with vitamin B_{12} deficiency may present with anemia/macrocytic RBCs or pancytopenia and may have neurologic complications including dementia, weakness, sensory neuropathy and paresthesias (subacute combined degeneration of the spinal cord). Folic acid supplementation may partially alleviate and mask the hematologic effects of cobalamin deficiency, but does nothing to slow the progression of the neurologic lesion. Patients with low-normal or even normal serum vitamin B_{12} values may be deficient and respond to vitamin B_{12} replacement.[25]

The clinical manifestations of megaloblastosis may be subtle in older adults and may precede the development of anemia. A high index of suspicion is warranted.[26]

Figure 3: **Diagnostic Algorithm for Normocytic Anemia**

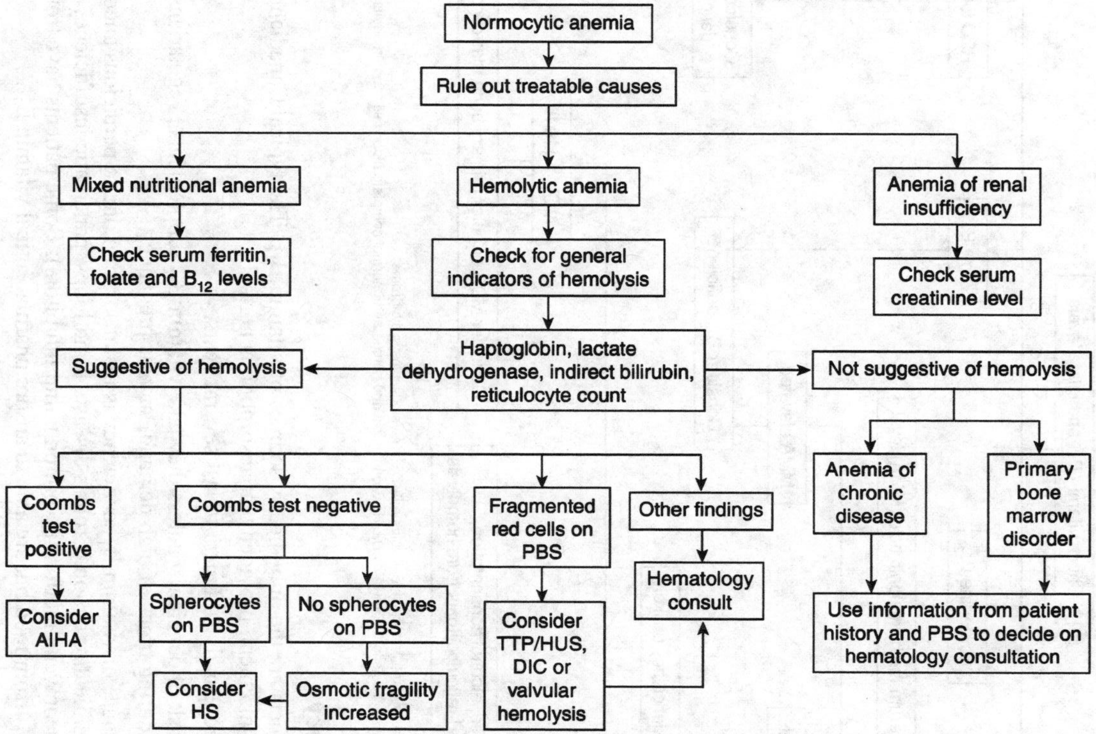

Abbreviations: AIHA = autoimmune hemolytic anemia; DIC = disseminated intravascular coagulation; HS = hereditary spherocytosis; PBS = peripheral blood smear; TTP/HUS = thrombotic thrombocytopenic purpura/hemolytic uremic syndrome

Adapted with permission from: Tefferi A, Hanson CA, Inwards DJ. How to interpret and pursue an abnormal complete blood cell count in adults. *Mayo Clin Proc* 2005;80(7):923-36.

Figure 4: **Diagnostic Algorithm for Macrocytic Anemia**

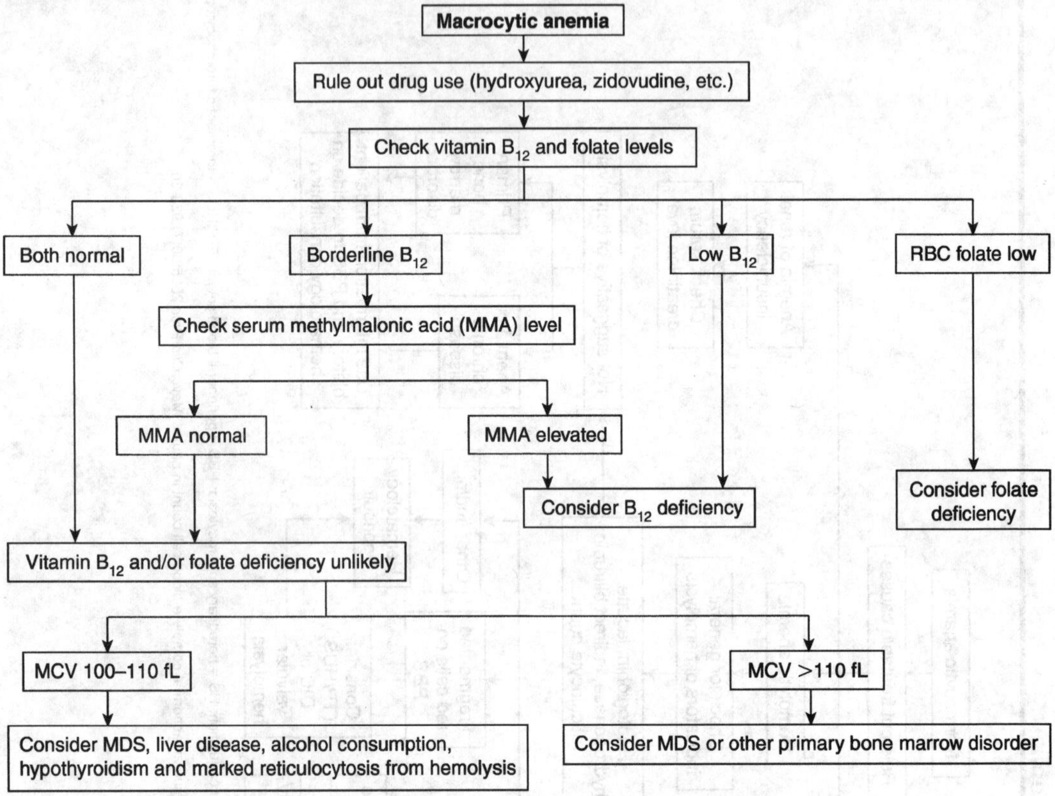

Abbreviations: fL = femtolitre; 10^{-15} litres; MCV = mean cell volume; MDS = myelodysplastic syndrome
Adapted with permission from: Tefferi A, Hanson CA, Inwards DJ. How to interpret and pursue an abnormal complete blood cell count in adults. *Mayo Clin Proc* 2005;80(7):923-36.

Vitamin B_{12} Deficiency

- Meat and dairy products are the only dietary sources of vitamin B_{12}. The typical Canadian diet exceeds the daily requirement, provided that absorption is normal.
- Vitamin B_{12} stores are usually sufficient to last several years.
- Strict vegans are at risk of deficiency unless they take vitamin B_{12} supplements. Vegetarians may be at risk of deficiency during times of high demand, such as pregnancy.
- The most common cause of vitamin B_{12} deficiency is malabsorption due to pernicious anemia, gastrectomy, gastritis, ileal resection, Crohn's disease, blind loops, pancreatic insufficiency and certain drugs (e.g., neomycin, metformin, proton pump inhibitors). Some patients have trouble absorbing vitamin B_{12} from food but are able to absorb pharmaceutical vitamin B_{12}.

Folate Deficiency

- Folate is a water-soluble B vitamin that occurs naturally in food (e.g., leafy green vegetables, liver, legumes). Folic acid is the synthetic form of folate that is found in vitamin supplements and is added to fortified foods.
- Dietary deficiency and alcoholism are the most common causes of folate deficiency.

- Although folate is plentiful in a variety of foods it is labile and easily destroyed by exposure to light and during cooking.
- Alcohol inhibits folate absorption and interferes with its enterohepatic cycle.
- Folate deficiency can develop within a few months of adopting a folate-deficient diet and even more quickly in the setting of increased alcohol intake.
- Increased folate requirements are seen in pregnancy, hemolytic anemia and therapy with certain drugs (e.g., methotrexate, phenytoin, trimethoprim).

Therapeutic Choices

Nonpharmacologic Choices

Restoring normal dietary intake of vitamin B_{12} and folate may be sufficient to completely reverse megaloblastosis. However, patients with neurologic deficits due to vitamin B_{12} deficiency should be treated pharmacologically to maximize the likelihood of full neurologic recovery.

Abstinence from alcohol may be necessary.

Pharmacologic Choices (Table 1)

Vitamin B_{12}

- Vitamin B_{12} deficiency is treated with either **cyanocobalamin** or **hydroxocobalamin (hydroxycobalamin)**. The daily requirement is 6–9 µg. Cobalamin replacement for treatment of pernicious anemia is in doses of 1000 µg. Doses greater than 100 µg/day exceed the physiologic binding capacity, but the excess is not toxic and is readily excreted by the kidneys. For this reason there is a tendency to give more rather than less cobalamin, especially in patients with neurologic deficits.
- Vitamin B_{12} has traditionally been given parenterally because deficiency is most often due to malabsorption, and most cases of malabsorption are attributable to pernicious anemia with its lack of intrinsic factor.
- High-dose oral vitamin B_{12} therapy is effective,[27] feasible[28,29] and cost-effective,[30] but patient adherence and the need for more attentive monitoring[31] are limitations.
- A suggested approach is to:
  - administer parenteral vitamin B_{12} until all neurologic symptoms and hematologic abnormalities resolve
  - provide maintenance therapy by the route that best fits the patient's circumstances. If oral vitamin B_{12} is used, follow up with the patient to monitor Hb and ensure adherence.
- Where dietary deficiency is clearly the cause of the vitamin B_{12} deficiency and the patient has no neurologic deficits, oral supplementation is adequate.
- It is important that patients with vitamin B_{12} deficiency are not treated with folic acid alone because this would improve hematologic parameters with potential worsening of neurologic symptoms, which may become permanent.

Folic Acid

- Folate deficiency is treated with folic acid. The daily requirement for disease prevention is 200 µg. Folate replacement is used in doses of 1–5 mg daily.
- Folic acid should be given only for confirmed folate deficiency, pregnancy or in situations of increased demand, such as hemolysis.
- Prophylaxis with **folic acid** before and during pregnancy is strongly recommended for the prevention of neural tube defects (see Appendix IV for specific dosing recommendations).

- The oral route is sufficient to correct folate deficiency, even in patients with malabsorption syndromes.
- It is important to ensure that patients do not have concomitant vitamin B_{12} deficiency before folic acid replacement is started, since folate does not treat the neurologic manifestations of vitamin B_{12} deficiency.

Choices during Pregnancy and Breastfeeding

It is recommended that pregnant women meet the dietary requirements of vitamin B_{12} and supplement with folic acid during pregnancy. With the exception of strict vegans, some vegetarians and patients with malabsorption (pernicious anemia), vitamin B_{12} is maintained at sufficient levels during pregnancy and does not typically require supplementation. However, due to the recognized association between folate deficiency and fetal neural tube defects, folic acid supplementation is universally recommended during pregnancy. There are no teratogenic effects of either vitamin B_{12} or folic acid during pregnancy. Most authorities recommend that pregnant women take a multivitamin containing folic acid during pregnancy and breastfeeding. Maternal or pregnancy multivitamins typically contain higher doses of folic acid than regular multivitamins. Both vitamin B_{12} and folate pass into breast milk but are compatible with breastfeeding.

- **Vitamin B_{12}** supplementation is reserved for pregnant women with malabsorptive conditions such as pernicious anemia, or women who are strict vegans. Women who are vegetarians may become deficient during pregnancy due to increased demand. Supplementation is done in an identical manner to nonpregnant women.
- **Folate** supplementation is universally recommended. This can be done in the form of a pregnancy multivitamin that contains increased doses of folic acid, or individual folic acid supplements.

A discussion of general principles on the use of medications in these special populations can be found in Appendix II and Appendix III. Other specialized reference sources are also provided in these appendices.

Therapeutic Tips

- A reticulocyte response should be evident within 3–4 days of beginning vitamin B_{12} or folic acid therapy, with improvement in the Hb level by about day 10. Full resolution of the anemia should occur within about 2 months.
- The rapid production of new hematopoietic cells leads to a potentially dramatic shift of potassium from extracellular to intracellular compartments, which may cause profound hypokalemia.
  - older patients on diuretic therapy for heart failure are at particular risk
  - in at-risk patients, obtain a baseline potassium level and give potassium supplementation in patients with low or borderline potassium levels. Monitor potassium levels carefully in the first few days of therapy and adjust supplementation accordingly.
- If the Hb fails to respond as anticipated, consider that there may be:
  - a different or concurrent cause of anemia and/or an impaired erythropoietic response
    - concomitant iron deficiency may show itself with an MCV that shifts from the macrocytic to the microcytic range
  - adherence issues, particularly in patients using oral supplements.
- Neurologic deficits may take 6 months or more to resolve; some severe deficits may persist.

Anemias Responsive to Pharmacologic Stimulation of Erythropoiesis

Pathophysiology

Most patients with nutritional anemias (iron, vitamin B_{12} or folate deficiency), hemolysis or bleeding have elevated levels of endogenous erythropoietin. However, there are a number of situations in which pharmacologic stimulation of red cell production using erythropoiesis stimulating agents (ESAs) is beneficial including:

- Chronic renal failure
- HIV-infected patients receiving antiretroviral therapy[32]
- Chronic hepatitis C patients receiving ribavirin[33]
- Patients receiving chemotherapy for nonhematologic cancers[34,35]
- Surgery patients[34]
- Low-risk myelodysplasia[36]

Other clinical applications are beyond the scope of this discussion.[37,38]

Investigations

Selection of patients for ESA therapy is determined in part by baseline endogenous erythropoietin levels (approximately 3–30 IU/L in healthy individuals). In most patients, Hb should be <100 g/L in order to qualify for ESA therapy.

For example:

- A zidovudine-treated HIV patient is unlikely to respond if the baseline erythropoietin level is >500 IU/L
- A chemotherapy-treated cancer patient is unlikely to respond if the baseline erythropoietin level is >200 IU/L

It is important to ensure an adequate iron supply in conjunction with erythropoietin use.

Therapeutic Choices

Pharmacologic Choices (Table 2)

The choice of agent and dosage regimen varies according to the clinical situation. Both available agents in Canada may be given by iv or sc injection. **Epoetin alfa** is a recombinant human erythropoietin with a relatively short half-life that is typically given at least 3 times per week. It may also be administered daily in the preoperative surgical setting where a more rapid rise is desired. **Darbepoetin alfa** is a synthetic erythropoietin analogue with a longer half-life that is typically given weekly or biweekly, and monthly in some patients.

Although ESAs have improved quality of life in patients with anemia due to chronic renal failure,[39] they did not improve quality of life or fatigue in patients with anemia due to AIDS or cancer.[40,41] Additionally, the use of ESAs increases the risk of serious cardiovascular events when dosed to achieve a normal Hb.[42] Clinicians should carefully weigh the risks and benefits of ESAs before initiating their use. If ESAs are initiated, target Hb should be <100–120 g/L depending on the indication, and Hb should be monitored at least monthly.[43]

Choices during Pregnancy and Breastfeeding

There are no adequate and well-controlled studies using ESAs in pregnant women. Use of ESAs in pregnancy does not seem to present a major risk to the fetus.[44] Worsening of hypertension or thrombosis are serious potential risks. However, anemia and frequent blood transfusions also presents risks to the fetus. In these situations, ESAs should be given only if the potential benefits justify the potential risk to the fetus. Adequate iron supplementation is particularly important in this setting if ESAs are used.

ESAs have been used in infants with no serious adverse effects.[44] It is not known whether ESAs pass into breast milk; exercise caution in breastfeeding women.

A discussion of general principles on the use of medications in these special populations can be found in Appendix II and Appendix III. Other specialized reference sources are also provided in these appendices.

Therapeutic Tips

- ESAs have significant potential for toxicity and adverse consequences so they should be used judiciously in patients who would otherwise require transfusion support.
- Doses are titrated to achieve a gradual improvement in anemia, without overshooting the target Hb.
- Rapid and/or excessive correction of anemia may provoke hypertension and seizures in susceptible individuals; erythrocytosis may predispose patients to thrombotic complications. Monitor blood pressure 3 times per week initially, and after each dose thereafter.
- ESAs have been associated with the development of pure red cell aplasia (PRCA), a potentially devastating complication in which neutralizing antibodies to the exogenous protein cross-react with endogenous erythropoietin, resulting in profound anemia. Changes in the formulation and handling of these proteins have greatly reduced the risk of PRCA.[6] Nevertheless, the possibility of PRCA should be considered if a patient becomes refractory to therapy.

Table 1: **Drugs for the Treatment of Iron-deficiency and Megaloblastic Anemias**

Class	Drug	Dose	Adverse Effects	Comments	Cost[a]
Iron Supplements, oral	*ferrous fumarate* Palafer, generics	105–200 mg elemental iron daily in 3 divided doses (100 mg elemental iron/ 300 mg ferrous fumarate)	GI: nausea, dyspepsia, constipation and/or diarrhea. Ameliorated by stepwise initiation of therapy (see text).	There is no evidence that one preparation is more effective than another. Avoid enteric-coated preparations. Vitamin C enhances absorption of nonheme iron. Absorption is decreased by food and certain drugs: antacids, calcium carbonate, cholestyramine, levodopa, methyldopa, penicillamine, quinolones, sodium bicarbonate, tetracyclines. Separate administration by ~2 h.	$$
	ferrous gluconate generics	105–200 mg elemental iron daily in 3 divided doses (35 mg elemental iron/ 300 mg ferrous gluconate)	See ferrous fumarate.	See ferrous fumarate.	$
	ferrous sulfate Fer-In-Sol, generics	105–200 mg elemental iron daily in 3 divided doses (60 mg elemental iron/ 300 mg ferrous sulfate)	See ferrous fumarate.	See ferrous fumarate.	$
	polysaccharide-iron complex FeraMAX, Polyride-Fe	105–200 mg elemental iron daily (150 mg elemental iron per capsule)	See ferrous fumarate.	See ferrous fumarate.	$$
Iron Supplements, parenteral	*ferumoxytol* Feraheme	Chronic kidney disease: 510 mg iv then repeat once 2–8 days later Administered as a rapid iv infusion	Hypersensitivity reaction (rare). Chest pain, dizziness, hypotension, infusion site reaction.	Test dose not required; observe for 30 min post-dose. Good safety profile expected, but not yet established.	$$$$$

(cont'd)

Table 1: **Drugs for the Treatment of Iron-deficiency and Megaloblastic Anemias** *(cont'd)*

Class	Drug	Dose	Adverse Effects	Comments	Cost[a]
	iron dextran DexIron, Infufer	Total dose infusion: iv dose calculated to restore iron deficit in red cell mass and iron stores In chronic dialysis patients: 100 mg 1–3 times weekly iv × 10 doses or until replete; adjust as able to maintain adequate iron availability Administered as slow iv infusion DexIron: maximum rate 50 mg/min (1 mL/min) Infufer: maximum rate 3–4 mL/min	Anaphylaxis (rare). Anaphylactoid reactions, hypotension (avoid rapid iv infusion). Fever, chills, headache, myalgia, arthralgia, urticaria, dizziness. May have delayed onset, 24–48 h after iv infusion and 3–4 days after im administration.	Consult prescribing information for dose calculation, dilution and administration details. 0.9% NaCl is the preferred infusion solution. D5W causes more local irritation and phlebitis. Give a 25 mg test dose 1 h before the initial dose, with epinephrine available. Side effects are more common with larger doses and in underweight patients.	$$$$
	iron sucrose Venofer	Chronic dialysis patients: 100 mg 1–3 times weekly iv until replete; adjust as able to maintain adequate iron availability Administered as iv infusion or slow injection	See iron dextran.	Test doses are not recommended by the manufacturer. Incidence of life-threatening adverse effects is lower than with iron dextran.	$$$$
	sodium ferric gluconate Ferrlecit	Chronic dialysis patients: 125 mg 1–3 times weekly iv × 8 doses; adjust as able to maintain adequate iron availability Administered as iv infusion over 1 h or slow iv injection (maximum rate of 12.5 mg/min)	See iron dextran.	Test doses are no longer recommended by the manufacturer. Incidence of life-threatening adverse effects is lower than with iron dextran.	$$$$$

Class	Drug	Dose	Adverse Effects	Comments	Cost[a]
Vitamins	*folic acid (folate)* generics	1–5 mg daily po	Occasional allergic reactions—rash, pruritus, flushing, bronchospasm.	Available for iv use in patients who are fasting. Empiric supplementation of folate in patients who are at risk of B_{12} deficiency and not receiving B_{12} is not recommended. 5 mg daily po × 10–12 weeks is recommended for pregnant women with a history of a pregnancy with neural tube defect (NTD) or increased risk due to a 1st degree relative with NTD, women belonging to a high-risk ethnic group (e.g., Sikh, Celtic, northern Chinese), or those with certain medical conditions (e.g., type I diabetes, therapy with valproic acid or carbamazepine, BMI >35 kg/m^2, malabsorption disorders).	$
	vitamin B_{12} (cyanocobalamin, hydroxocobalamin) generics	Pernicious anemia/other chronic malabsorption disorders: 100 µg daily sc/im × 1 week; 200 µg weekly sc/im until Hb normalizes Life-long maintenance: 100 µg monthly sc/im *or* 500–2000 µg daily po Vitamin B_{12} deficiency: 30 µg daily sc/im × 5–10 days Life-long maintenance: 100–200 µg monthly sc/im *or* 250 µg daily po	Occasional peripheral vascular thrombosis, rash, pruritus, headache, nausea and vomiting, diarrhea. Occasional heart failure. Possibility of profound hypokalemia due to intracellular potassium shift.	Oral absorption is reduced by anticonvulsants, colchicine, metformin, neomycin and omeprazole. Consider baseline measurement and potassium supplementation if levels are low or borderline; serial monitoring of potassium levels may be warranted. Folate supplementation may mask hematologic findings of B_{12} deficiency, without halting progression of the neurologic deficits. Vitamin B_{12} should be given parenterally in patients with documented malabsorption or in patients who are nonadherent to oral therapy.	$$

[a] Cost of 30-day supply; includes drug cost only.
Legend: $ < $5 $$ $5–25 $$$ $25–175 $$$$ $175–325 $$$$$ $325–475

Table 2: **Erythropoiesis-Stimulating Agents**

Class	Drug	Dose	Adverse Effects	Comments	Cost[a]
Erythropoietics	*darbepoetin alfa* Aranesp	**Chronic renal failure:** 0.45 µg/kg weekly sc/iv, then: increase by 25% monthly if no response. Decrease by 25% as Hb approaches 120/L **Cancer chemotherapy (endogenous erythropoietin level ≤200 IU/L):** 2.25 µg/kg weekly sc/iv If inadequate response after 6 weeks, increase to 4.5 µg/kg weekly sc/iv	Hypertension, hypotension, headache, thrombosis, nausea, vomiting, diarrhea, constipation, arthralgia, myalgia, chest pain, arrhythmia, edema, dyspnea, cough.	May be able to shift to biweekly or monthly dosing in some patients. Target Hb ≤120 g/L with increase limited to 10 g/L per 2 weeks. If excessive response, decrease dose by 40%. If still excessive, hold dose until Hb falls.	$285/100 µg
	epoetin alfa Eprex	**Chronic renal failure:** Initial: 50–100 IU/kg 3 times weekly sc/iv, then: increase by 25% every 4–8 weeks to maximum 300 IU/kg/dose to achieve Hb of 120 g/L As Hb approaches 120 g/L, decrease dose by 25% **HIV, on antiretrovirals (endogenous erythropoietin level ≤500 IU/L):** Initial: 100 IU/kg 3 times weekly sc/iv, then: increase by 50 IU/kg/dose every 4–8 weeks to maximum 300 IU/kg/dose **Cancer chemotherapy (endogenous erythropoietin level ≤200 IU/L):** Initial: 50 IU/kg 3 times weekly sc/iv, or 40 000 IU weekly sc/iv, then: increase by 50 IU/kg/dose every 8 weeks to maximum 300 IU/kg/dose **Chronic hepatitis C, on ribavirin:** 40 000 IU weekly sc/iv **Surgery:** 600 IU/kg sc/iv 21, 14 and 7 days before surgery and then on the day of surgery	Hypertension, headache, seizures, thrombosis, nausea, vomiting, diarrhea, arthralgia, chest pain, edema, cough. Increases risk of deep venous thrombosis and other thrombotic complications in spine surgery patients. Pure red cell aplasia (rare).	Usually given by sc injection. May be given iv if access already established. Do not exceed target Hb. If no response to the maximum dose after 8 weeks, discontinue. If Hb increased by more than 10 g/L/2 weeks, decrease dose by 25%. Target Hb ≤120 g/L. In patients with renal failure, achievement of higher Hb targets is not associated with better outcomes.[45,46,47] Survival was worse in patients treated to higher Hb targets (>120 g/L) with erythropoietin as compared with placebo in patients with head and neck cancer and in those with breast cancer.[48,49]	$150/10 000 IU

[a] Cost per dose; includes drug cost only.

Suggested Readings

Kwong JC, Carr D, Dhalla IA et al. Oral vitamin B12 therapy in the primary care setting: a qualitative and quantitative study of patient perspectives. *BMC Fam Pract* 2005;6(1):8.

Macdougall IC, Eckardt KU. Novel strategies for stimulating erythropoiesis and potential new treatments for anaemia. *Lancet* 2006;368(9539):947-53.

Manning-Dimmitt LL, Dimmitt SG, Wilson GR. Diagnosis of gastrointestinal bleeding in adults. *Am Fam Physician* 2005;71(7):1339-46.

Nilsson M, Norberg B, Hultdin J et al. Medical intelligence in Sweden. Vitamin B12: oral compared with parenteral? *Postgrad Med J* 2005;81(953):191-3.

Short MW, Domagalski JE. Iron deficiency anemia: evaluation and management. *Am Fam Physician* 2013;87(2):98-104.

Tefferi A, Hanson CA, Inwards DJ. How to interpret and pursue an abnormal complete blood cell count in adults. *Mayo Clin Proc* 2005;80(7):923-36.

References

1. Ruiz-Arguelles GJ. Altitude above sea level as a variable for definition of anemia. *Blood* 2006;108(6):2131.
2. Nordenberg D, Yip R, Binkin NJ. The effect of cigarette smoking on hemoglobin levels and anemia screening. *JAMA* 1990;264(12):1556-9.
3. Beutler E, Waalen J. The definition of anemia: what is the lower limit of normal of the blood hemoglobin concentration? *Blood* 2006;107(5):1747-50.
4. Culleton BF, Manns BJ, Zhang J et al. Impact of anemia on hospitalization and mortality in older adults. *Blood* 2006;107(10):3841-6.
5. Ross SD, Fahrbach K, Frame D et al. The effect of anemia treatment on selected health-related quality-of-life domains: a systematic review. *Clin Ther* 2003;25(6):1786-805.
6. Macdougall IC, Eckardt KU. Novel strategies for stimulating erythropoiesis and potential new treatments for anaemia. *Lancet* 2006;368(9539):947-53.
7. Tefferi A, Hanson CA, Inwards DJ. How to interpret and pursue an abnormal complete blood cell count in adults. *Mayo Clin Proc* 2005;80(7):923-36.
8. Short MW, Domagalski JE. Iron deficiency anemia: evaluation and management. *Am Fam Physician* 2013;87(2):98-104.
9. Gartner A, Berger J, Bour A et al. Assessment of iron deficiency in the context of the obesity epidemic: importance of correcting serum ferritin concentrations for inflammation. *Am J Clin Nutr* 2013;98(3):821-6.
10. Galloway M, Rushworth L. Red cell or serum folate? Results from the National Pathology Alliance benchmarking review. *J Clin Pathol* 2003;56(12):924-6.
11. Solomon LR. Cobalamin-responsive disorders in the ambulatory care setting: unreliability of cobalamin, methylmalonic acid, and homocysteine testing. *Blood* 2005;105(3):978-85.
12. Metz J, McGrath K, Bennett M et al. Biochemical indices of vitamin B12 nutrition in pregnant patients with subnormal serum vitamin B12 levels. *Am J Hematol* 1995;48(4):251-5.
13. Looker AC, Dallman PR, Carroll MD et al. Prevalence of iron deficiency in the United States. *JAMA* 1997;277(12):973-6.
14. Patterson AJ, Brown WJ, Roberts DC et al. Dietary treatment of iron deficiency in women of childbearing age. *Am J Clin Nutr* 2001;74(5):650-6.
15. Hunt JR, Mullen LM, Lykken GI et al. Ascorbic acid: effect on ongoing iron absorption and status in iron-depleted young women. *Am J Clin Nutr* 1990;51(4):649-55.
16. Zijp IM, Korver O, Tijburg LB. Effect of tea and other dietary factors on iron absorption. *Crit Rev Food Sci Nutr* 2000;40(5):371-98.
17. Rimon E, Kagansky N, Kagansky M et al. Are we giving too much iron? Low-dose iron therapy is effective in octogenarians. *Am J Med* 2005;118(10):1142-7.
18. Bhandal N, Russell R. Intravenous versus oral iron therapy for postpartum anaemia. *BJOG* 2006;113(11):1248-52.
19. Litton E, Xiao J, Ho KM. Safety and efficacy of intravenous iron therapy in reducing requirement for allogeneic blood transfusion: systematic review and meta-analysis of randomised clinical trials. *BMJ* 2013;347:f4822.
20. Makrides M, Crowther CA, Gibson RA et al. Efficacy and tolerability of low-dose iron supplements during pregnancy: a randomized controlled trial. *Am J Clin Nutr* 2003;78(1):145-53.
21. Peña-Rosas JP, De-Regil LM, Dowswell T et al. Daily oral iron supplementation during pregnancy. *Cochrane Database Syst Rev* 2012;12:CD004736.
22. Haider BA, Olofin I, Wang M et al. Anaemia, prenatal iron use, and risk of adverse pregnancy outcomes: systematic review and meta-analysis. *BMJ* 2013;346:f3443.
23. Pena-Rosas JP, De-Regil LM, Dowswell T et al. Intermittent oral iron supplement during pregnancy. *Cochrane Database Syst Rev* 2012;7:CD009997.
24. Green BT, Rockey DC. Gastrointestinal endoscopic evaluation of premenopausal women with iron deficiency anemia. *J Clin Gastroenterol* 2004;38(2):104-9.
25. Naurath HJ, Joosten E, Riezler R et al. Effects of vitamin B12, folate, and vitamin B6 supplements in elderly people with normal serum vitamin concentrations. *Lancet* 1995;346(8967):85-9.
26. Dharmarajan TS, Adiga GU, Norkus EP. Vitamin B12 deficiency. Recognizing subtle symptoms in older adults. *Geriatrics* 2003;58(3):30-4,37-8.
27. Vidal-Alaball J, Butler CC, Cannings-John R et al. Oral vitamin B12 versus intramuscular vitamin B12 for vitamin B12 deficiency. *Cochrane Database Syst Rev* 2005;(3):CD004655.
28. Kwong JC, Carr D, Dhalla IA et al. Oral vitamin B12 therapy in the primary care setting: a qualitative and quantitative study of patient perspectives. *BMC Fam Pract* 2005;6(1):8.

29. Nilsson M, Norberg B, Hultdin J et al. Medical intelligence in Sweden. Vitamin B12: oral compared with parenteral? *Postgrad Med J* 2005;81(953):191-3.
30. van Walraven C, Austin P, Naylor CD. Vitamin B12 injections versus oral supplements. How much money could be saved by switching from injections to pills? *Can Fam Physician* 2001;47:79-86.
31. Solomon LR. Oral vitamin B12 therapy: a cautionary note. *Blood* 2004;103(7):2863.
32. Henry DH, Volberding PA, Leitz G. Epoetin alfa for treatment of anemia in HIV-infected patients: past, present, and future. *J Acquir Immune Defic Syndr* 2004;37(2):1221-7.
33. Sherman M, Cohen L, Cooper MA et al. Clinical recommendations for the use of recombinant human erythropoietin in patients with hepatitis C virus being treated with ribavirin. *Can J Gastroenterol* 2006;20(7):479-85.
34. Epoetins and darbepoetin alfa in malignant disease. *Drug Ther Bull* 2004;42(3):21-3.
35. Bokemeyer C, Oechsle K, Hartmann JT. Anaemia in cancer patients: pathophysiology, incidence and treatment. *Eur J Clin Invest* 2005;35(Suppl 3):26-31.
36. Rizzo JD, Brouwers M, Hurley P et al. American Society of Clinical Oncology/American Society of Hematology clinical practice guideline update on the use of epoetin and darbepoetin in adult patients with cancer. *J Oncol Pract* 2010;6(6):317-20.
37. Corwin HL. The role of erythropoietin therapy in the critically ill. *Transfus Med Rev* 2006;20(1):27-33.
38. Henry DH, Bowers P, Romano MT et al. Epoetin alfa. Clinical evolution of a pleiotropic cytokine. *Arch Intern Med* 2004;164(3):262-76.
39. Cody J, Daly C, Campbell M et al. Recombinant human erythropoietin for chronic renal failure anaemia in pre-dialysis patients. *Cochrane Database Syst Rev* 2005;(3):CD003266.
40. Marti-Carvajal AJ, Sola I, Pena-Marti GE et al. Treatment for anemia in people with AIDS. *Cochrane Database Syst Rev* 2011;(10):CD004776.
41. Tonia T, Mettler A, Robert N et al. Erythropoietin or darbepoetin for patients with cancer. *Cochrane Database Syst Rev* 2012;12:CD003407.
42. U.S. Food and Drug Administration. *FDA modifies dosing recommendations for erythropoiesis-stimulating agents*. Available from: www.fda.gov/NewsEvents/Newsroom/PressAnnouncements/ucm260670.htm. Accessed August 6, 2013.
43. National Kidney Foundation. KDOQI Guidelines. *KDOQI clinical practice guidelines and clinical practice recommendations for anemia in chronic kidney disease (2006)*. Available from: www.kidney.org/professionals/kdoqi/guidelines_anemia/. Accessed August 6, 2013.
44. Briggs GG, Freeman RK, Yaffe SJ. *Drugs in pregnancy and lactation: a reference guide to fetal and neonatal risk*. 9th ed. Philadelphia (PA): Wolters Kluwer Health; Lippincott Williams & Wilkins; 2011.
45. Drueke TB, Locatelli F, Clyne N et al. Normalization of hemoglobin level in patients with chronic kidney disease and anemia. *N Engl J Med* 2006;355(20):2071-84.
46. Phrommintikul A, Haas SJ, Elsik M et al. Mortality and target haemoglobin concentrations in anaemic patients with chronic kidney disease treated with erythropoietin: a meta-analysis. *Lancet* 2007;369(9559):381-8.
47. Singh AK, Szczech L, Tang KL et al. Correction of anemia with epoetin alfa in chronic kidney disease. *N Engl J Med* 2006;355(20):2085-98.
48. Henke M, Laszig R, Rube C et al. Erythropoietin to treat head and neck cancer patients with anaemia undergoing radiotherapy: randomised, double-blind, placebo-controlled trial. *Lancet* 2003;362(9392):1255-60.
49. Leyland-Jones B, Semiglazov V, Pawlicki M et al. Maintaining normal hemoglobin levels with epoetin alfa in mainly nonanemic patients with metastatic breast cancer receiving first-line chemotherapy: a survival study. *J Clin Oncol* 2005;23(25):5960-72.

Chapter 100
Chronic Kidney Disease

Lori Wazny, BSc (Pharm), PharmD and
Louise Moist, BScPhm, MSc, MD, FRCPC

Chronic kidney disease (CKD) is estimated to affect approximately 2 million Canadians.[1] It often coexists with cardiovascular disease and diabetes and is recognized as a risk factor for all-cause mortality and cardiovascular disease.[2]

Kidney function is described using the glomerular filtration rate (GFR) or creatinine clearance. Estimates of GFR (eGFR) are calculated and reported using the MDRD formula which includes age, sex and creatinine, with a correction for black race.[3] Alternatively, an estimated creatinine clearance can be calculated using the Cockcroft-Gault equation (see Appendix I) or measured using a 24-hour urine collection. Both equations have limitations, especially at the extremes of age and kidney dysfunction, but are more reliable than serum creatinine alone. The eGFRs used to characterize the stages of CKD are listed in Table 1.

CKD is now defined as the presence of kidney damage for a period greater than 3 months. An estimated or measured GFR of less than 60 mL/min/1.73 m^2 is considered abnormal for all adults. A value of more than 60 mL/min/1.73 m^2 is considered abnormal if it is accompanied by abnormalities of urine sediment or of imaging tests, or if the patient has had a kidney biopsy with abnormalities.

Until recently CKD was thought to be progressive, with the patient experiencing a decline in function over time and ultimately requiring dialysis. With the development of new interventions and prevention strategies, patients with CKD, particularly those without proteinuria, may have little progression of their kidney disease. However, they remain at high risk for cardiovascular events and death.[5]

This chapter summaries the management of patients up to, but not including, the introduction of dialysis.

Goals of Therapy

- Slow the progression of CKD
- Manage reversible cardiovascular risk factors
- Treat the complications of CKD

Table 1: KDIGO Stages of Chronic Kidney Disease[4]

KDIGO Stage	GFR (mL/min/1.73 m^2)	Description
G1	>90	Normal or high
G2	60–89	Mildly decreased
G3a	45–59	Mildly to moderately decreased
G3b	30–44	Moderately to severely decreased
G4	15–29	Severely decreased
G5	<15	Kidney failure (add 'D' if treated by dialysis)

Abbreviations: GFR = glomerular filtration rate; KDIGO = Kidney Disease: Improving Global Outcomes

Investigations

- History:
  - Many causes of CKD are hereditary, genetic or associated with other conditions, so a patient and family history is very important. Risk factors for CKD are listed in Table 2. Patients with risk factors, especially cardiovascular disease and diabetes mellitus, should be screened for CKD.[6]

Table 2: **Risk Factors for Chronic Kidney Disease[4]**

• Atherosclerotic vascular disease	• History of acute kidney injury
• Autoimmune diseases, such as lupus, rheumatoid arthritis, connective tissue disease and vasculitis	• Hypertension
• Chronic urinary tract obstruction from prostatic enlargement, neurogenic bladder, kidney stones	• Multiple myeloma
• Chronic viral infections, such as Hepatitis B and C, HIV	• Pregnancy complications including edema, hypertension, proteinuria
• Diabetes mellitus	• Recurrent pyelonephritis
• Family history of kidney disease	• Reduced nephron mass (e.g., congenital single kidney, post nephrectomy, scarring from reflux nephropathy)
• First Nations people	• Use of known nephrotoxic drugs (e.g., acetaminophen, NSAIDs including COX-2 inhibitors, lithium, cyclosporine, tacrolimus, contrast dyes)
• Hereditary polycystic kidney disease	

- Physical exam:
  - general appearance: in advanced stages of CKD patients develop cachexia or loss of muscle mass. Advanced uremia is often accompanied by a sallow, grayish complexion and so-called "uremic fetor" which is secondary to breakdown of urea in saliva to ammonia
  - weight: measure at each visit to assess fluid and nutritional status. Large changes are usually associated with fluid gains or loss
  - vitals: lying and standing blood pressures, pulse, jugular venous pressure and the presence of edema
  - abdominal exam: palpation for enlarged, cystic kidneys, and auscultation for renal artery bruits at a position approximately 2 cm above and 2 cm lateral to the umbilicus. Among patients with known hypertension, a bruit audible in both systole and diastole is moderately specific for renal artery stenosis[7]
- Laboratory investigations:
  - urine tests (Table 3, Table 4)
    - urinalysis: standard urinalysis is recommended as part of the yearly adult assessment to screen for hematuria (Figure 1) and should be done in the following patients:
      - any patient at risk for CKD (see Table 2)
      - abnormal creatinine
      - patients with diabetes at the time of diagnosis and yearly thereafter
      - patients with hypertension
    - urine albumin to creatinine ratio (ACR) or urine protein to creatinine ratio (PCR): these tests detect small amounts of proteinuria (<300 mg) not detected by the urinalysis. The level of proteinuria is used to risk stratify patients for cardiovascular and kidney events. Note that urine dipsticks (an alternate test for protein loss) are affected by hydration status
    - 24-hour urine collection: to measure creatinine clearance or confirm the amount of proteinuria
  - blood tests (Table 4)
    - CBC, Na, K, Cl, HCO_3, urea, creatinine (calculated eGFR), fasting lipid profile. If diabetes present add HbA_{1c}. At Stage G3b or higher add albumin, calcium, phosphorus, parathyroid hormone, serum iron, TIBC, ferritin.

- imaging
  - renal ultrasound in patients who have an increased creatinine, proteinuria or abnormal urine sediment to determine renal size and look for anatomic abnormalities, such as a solitary or polycystic kidney
  - abdominal ultrasound: consider if the eGFR <60 mL/min/1.73 m^2

Refer the following patients to a nephrologist:[8]

- acute kidney failure
- eGFR <30 mL/min/1.73 m^2
- progressive loss of kidney function
- persistent significant proteinuria (present on 2 out of 3 samples)
  - on dipstick *or* quantified PCR >100 mg/mmol *or* quantified ACR >60 mg/mmol
- inability to achieve treatment targets or other difficulties in the management of the CKD patient

Table 3: Categories of Albuminuria and Tests Used to Quantify Them[4]

	Albuminuria Category		
Urine Test	**A1 (normoalbuminuria)**	**A2 (microalbuminuria)**	**A3 (macroalbuminuria)[a]**
AER (mg/24h)[b]	<30	30–300	>300
PER (mg/24h)[b]	<150	150–500	>500
ACR (mg/mmol)	<3	3–30	>30
PCR (mg/mmol)	<15	15–50	>50
Protein reagent strip	Negative to trace	Trace to +	+ or greater

[a] Includes nephrotic syndrome (defined as albumin excretion >2200 mg/24h or protein excretion >3000 mg/24h).
[b] Requires a 24-hour urine collection.
Abbreviations: ACR = albumin to creatinine ratio; AER = albumin excretion rate; PCR = protein to creatinine ratio; PER = protein excretion rate

Table 4: Recommended Frequency of Blood and Urine Screening Tests in Chronic Kidney Disease[4]

	Testing Frequency (months)[a]		
KDIGO Stage	**A1 albuminuria**	**A2 albuminuria**	**A3 albuminuria**
G1	12	12	6
G2	12	12	6
G3a	12	6	4
G3b	6	4	4
G4	4	4	2–3
G5	1–3	1–3	1–3

[a] See text for suggested blood tests. Urine tests include ACR (or PCR if indicated) and standard urinalysis. Urine culture and sensitivity only if urine tract infection suspected.
Abbreviations: ACR = albumin to creatinine ratio; KDIGO = Kidney Disease: Improving Global Outcomes; PCR = protein to creatinine ratio

Figure 1: **Stepwise Investigation of Hematuria**

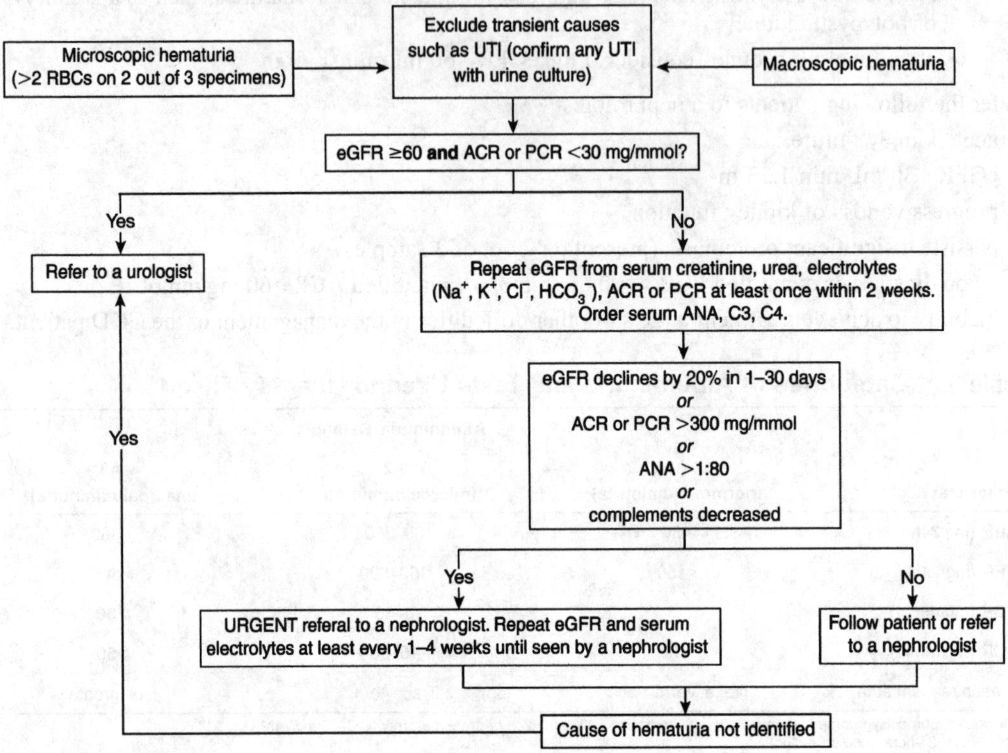

Abbreviations: ACR = albumin to creatinine ratio; ANA = antinuclear antibody; C3 = complement C3; C4 = complement C4; PCR = protein to creatinine ratio; RBC = red blood cell; UTI = urinary tract infection
Adapted with permission from the Manitoba Renal Program www.kidneyhealth.ca website.

For patients with a new finding of eGFR between 30 and 60 mL/min/1.73 m², the physician should determine the stability of the patient's eGFR and repeat test within 2–4 weeks, and then in 3–6 months.[1] Consider reversible causes, such as intercurrent illness, volume depletion, medications (NSAIDs, aminoglycosides, iv contrast dye) and obstruction. If the eGFR remains between 30 and 60 mL/min/1.73 m² consider referral to a nephrologist.

Figure 2 and Figure 3 outline the management guidelines for diabetic and nondiabetic CKD.

Therapeutic Choices

Nonpharmacologic Choices[1,4]

Encourage patients to exercise for 30–60 minutes 4–7 days per week to reduce the possibility of becoming hypertensive or to lower blood pressure in those with hypertension.

Encourage smoking cessation to slow progression of CKD and to reduce the risk of cardiovascular disease (see Chapter 13).

Alcohol intake should be limited to 2 drinks or less per day and should not exceed 14 standard drinks per week for men and 9 standard drinks per week for women so as not to increase blood pressure.

Figure 2: Management of Diabetic Chronic Kidney Disease

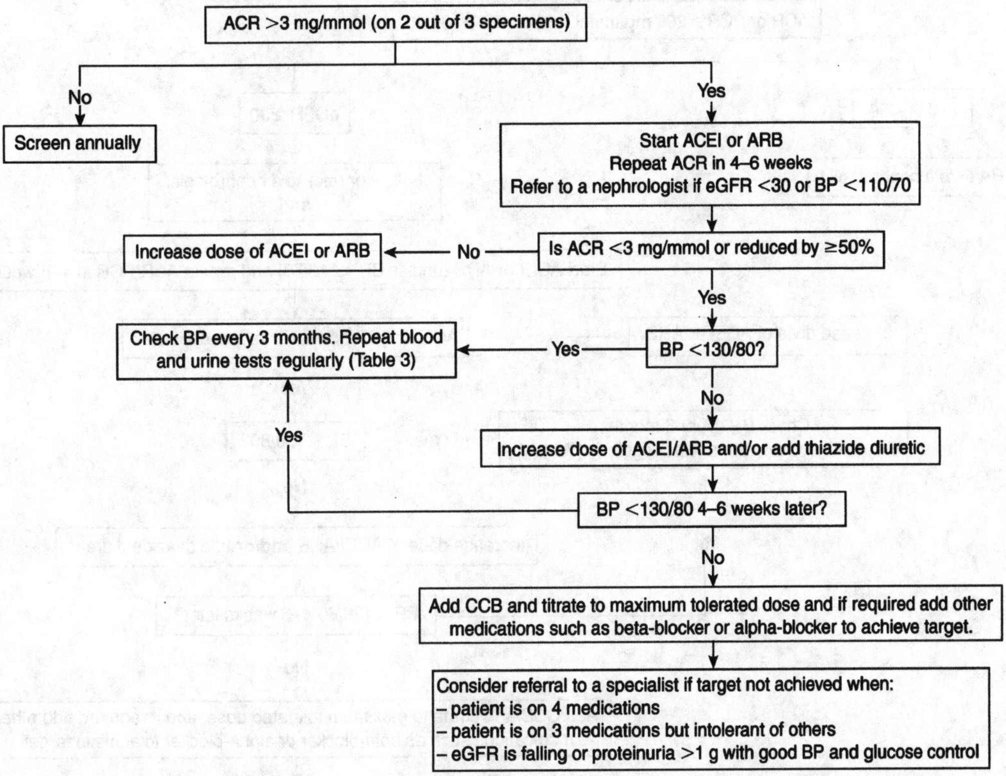

Abbreviations: ACR = albumin to creatinine ratio; ACEI = angiotensin converting enzyme inhibitor; ARB = angiotensin receptor blocker; BP = blood pressure; CCB = calcium channel blocker
Adapted with permission from the Manitoba Renal Program www.kidneyhealth.ca website.

Patients with CKD and hypertension should follow a low sodium diet: <90 mmol/day Na, or 2 g Na or 5 g NaCl/day.

If serum potassium >5 mmol/L, first consider medications that can be discontinued, such as potassium supplements and potassium-sparing diuretics. If these medications are not present, advise dietary potassium restriction. Note that ACE inhibitors (ACEIs), ARBs and aldosterone antagonists may also contribute to the hyperkalemia; continue these agents if being used to decrease proteinuria and restrict dietary potassium instead (see Chapter 105).

Dietary protein intake has been the focus of several trials. However, there is a lack of convincing evidence that a long-term protein restricted diet (<0.7 g/kg/day) delays the progression of CKD. Referral to a dietitian to provide a diet that is protein-controlled (0.8–1 g/kg/day) is recommended.

Encourage weight loss if obese (BMI >30 kg/m^2) or overweight (BMI 25–29 kg/m^2) to lower the risk of CVD.

Figure 3: **Management of Nondiabetic Chronic Kidney Disease**

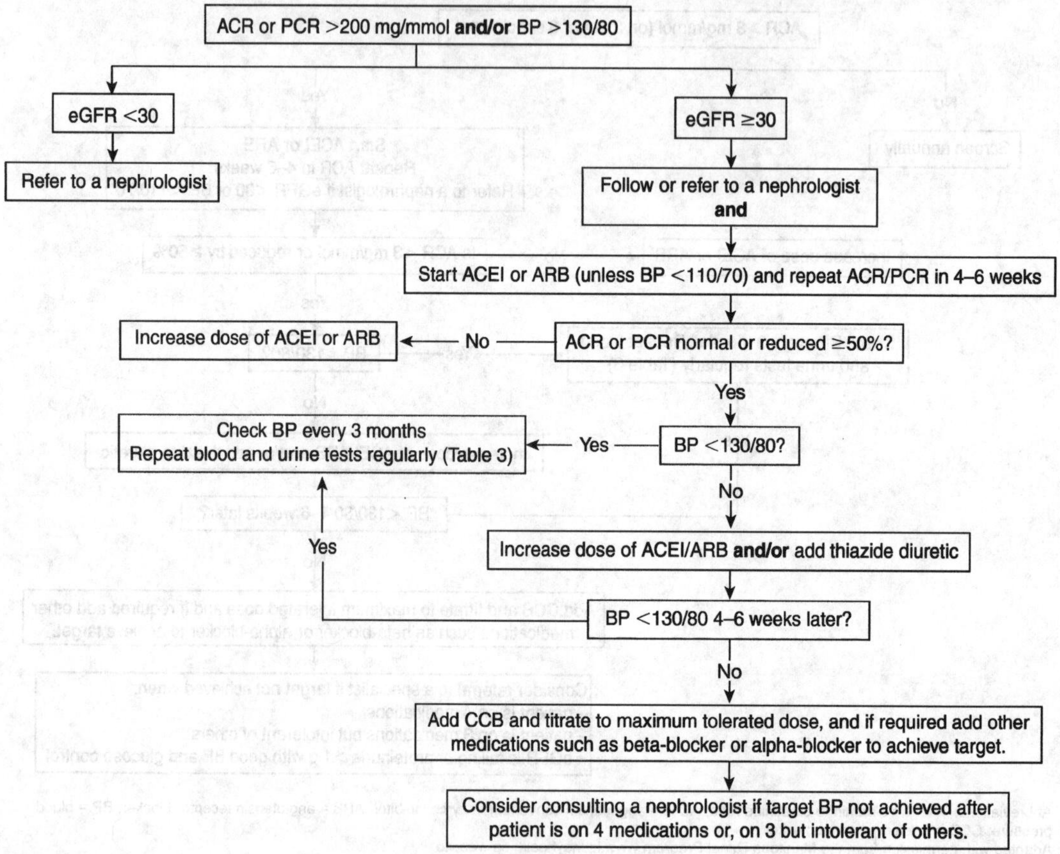

Abbreviations: ACEI = angiotensin converting enzyme inhibitor; ACR = albumin to creatinine ratio; ARB = angiotensin receptor blocker; CCB = calcium channel blocker; PCR = protein to creatinine ratio
Adapted with permission from the Manitoba Renal Program www.kidneyhealth.ca website.

Pharmacologic Choices

Antihypertensives

Encourage patients with hypertension to purchase a BP cuff for home monitoring, with review of these measurements at the medical follow-up. The blood pressure target in adult patients with an ACR <3 mg/mmol is ≤140/90 mm Hg. In adult patients with an ACR >3 mg/mmol, the blood pressure target is ≤130/80 mm Hg.[9] Table 5 presents guidelines on the choice of antihypertensive agent in CKD.

ACE Inhibitors and Angiotensin Receptor Blockers

ACEIs and ARBs are the preferred agents for certain types of CKD (Table 5) because they have the following class effects:[10]

- Reduction of blood pressure and intraglomerular pressure: in controlled trials, the beneficial effect of ACEIs and ARBs on the progression of CKD is greater than would be expected based on their antihypertensive effects alone.

- Reduction of proteinuria: ACEIs and ARBs reduce proteinuria more than any other antihypertensive even when the effect of blood pressure reduction on urinary protein excretion has been taken into account.
- Other mechanisms: ACEIs and ARBs reduce intraglomerular pressure, alter the function of mesangial cells and interfere with angiotensin-mediated generation of free radical formation, which also help slow the progression of CKD.

Increase the ACEI or ARB dose in patients whose BP is above target, and in patients with elevated proteinuria, even if BP is within target (Figure 2, Figure 3). Moderate to high doses of ACEIs and ARBs have been associated with beneficial effects on slowing progression of CKD. Begin with low doses and increase at 4–6 week intervals while monitoring for side effects and hypotension.

Measure eGFR and serum K^+ prior to and 1–2 weeks after initiating or increasing the dose of ACEI or ARB. Repeat ACR or PCR in 4–6 weeks.[10] Suggestions for monitoring and modifying ACEI and ARB therapy are provided in Table 6.

ACEIs/ARBs are contraindicated in pregnancy. Counsel premenopausal females on appropriate contraception (see Chapter 70).

Hold ACEI/ARB if patient has severe vomiting, diarrhea or volume depletion.[11]

Table 5: Choices of Antihypertensive Medication in Chronic Kidney Disease[9,10]

Clinical Condition	Antihypertensive
Proteinuric CKD (ACR ≥3 mg/mmol)	ACEI or ARB[a] The combination of an ACEI plus ARB is not recommended
Nonproteinuric CKD (ACR <3 mg/mmol)	Choose agents based on current hypertension guidelines (see Chapter 39). The combination of an ACEI plus ARB is not recommended

[a] See Figure 2 and Figure 3 for additional therapy options.
Abbreviations: ACEI = angiotensin converting enzyme inhibitor; ACR = albumin to creatinine ratio; ARB = angiotensin receptor blocker; CKD = chronic kidney disease

Table 6: Monitoring ACEI and ARB Therapy in Chronic Kidney Disease[10]

Test	Monitoring Frequency	Action
eGFR	If eGFR ≥60 mL/min, repeat in 4–12 weeks If eGFR 30–59 mL/min, repeat in 2–4 weeks If eGFR <30 mL/min, repeat in ≤2 weeks	Dosage adjustment is based on change in eGFR since previous test. eGFR decreased by 0–15%: no dose change eGFR decreased by 15–30%: no dose change, but repeat eGFR in 10–14 days eGFR decreased by 30–50%: reduce dose and repeat eGFR every 5–7 days until GFR within 30% of baseline eGFR decreased by >50%: discontinue ACEI or ARB and repeat eGFR every 5–7 days until eGFR is within 15% of baseline value
K^+	If eGFR ≥60 mL/min, repeat in 4–12 weeks If eGFR 30–59 mL/min, repeat in 2–4 weeks If eGFR <30 mL/min, repeat in ≤2 weeks	If K^+ 5–6 mmol/L advise dietary potassium restriction If K^+ 6–6.5 mmol/L prescribe loop diuretic if tolerated ± cation exchange resin

Abbreviations: eGFR = estimated glomerular filtration rate; K+ = serum potassium

Diabetic Chronic Kidney Disease

Follow the Canadian Diabetes Association guidelines for glycemic targets (see Chapter 32). Discontinue **metformin** when ClCr or eGFR <30 mL/min/1.73 m^2 due to an increased risk of lactic acidosis.[12] Metformin should also be discontinued when there are acute decreases in kidney function or illnesses/procedures that could lead to acute kidney injury (e.g., nausea/vomiting, dehydration, administration of iv contrast dye) or cause hypoxia (e.g., cardiac or respiratory failure) as these are also risk factors for lactic acidosis.[1]

Patients with CKD are at higher risk of developing hypoglycemia because the ability of the kidney to metabolize insulin is impaired. Patients with eGFR <30 mL/min/1.73 m^2 should be taught how to recognize and treat hypoglycemia. **Gliclazide** is the preferred sulfonylurea because, with a shorter half-life and no renally excreted active metabolite, it causes less hypoglycemia.[1] Doses of insulin and some oral diabetes medications may need to be reduced as CKD progresses (Table 7).

Table 7: **Diabetes Medications That Require Dosing Adjustment in Chronic Kidney Disease[13,14]**

Drug	Concern	Stage G3 CKD	Stage G4 CKD	Stage G5 CKD/Dialysis
Acarbose	No data for patients with creatinine >177 µmol/L	May use	Avoid	Avoid
Chlorpropamide	Decreased drug clearance leading to prolonged hypoglycemia	Reduce dose to 100 mg/day. Avoid if ClCr <50 mL/min	Avoid; gliclazide is preferred	Avoid; gliclazide is preferred
Exenatide	Decreased clearance and increased side effects in CKD stages 4–5	May use	Not recommended	Not recommended
Glyburide	Accumulation of renally excreted active metabolite leading to prolonged hypoglycemia	Use with caution	Avoid; gliclazide is preferred	Avoid; gliclazide is preferred
Liraglutide	Gastrointestinal effects: nausea, vomiting, diarrhea	May use	Not recommended	Not recommended
Metformin	Risk of lactic acidosis	Use with caution	Contraindicated	Contraindicated
Nateglinide	Decreased clearance of drug and active metabolites	Use with caution	Use with caution	Avoid if possible
Saxagliptin	Decreased clearance	Reduce dose to 2.5 mg/day	Reduce dose to 2.5 mg/day	Reduce dose to 2.5 mg/day
Sitagliptin	Decreased clearance when ClCr <50 mL/min. Risk of pancreatitis	Reduce dose to 50 mg/day	Reduce dose to 25 mg/day	Reduce dose to 25 mg/day

Cardiovascular Risk Reduction for Patients with Chronic Kidney Disease

Both a reduced eGFR[5] and proteinuria confer substantial increases in cardiovascular risk and death. A secondary analysis of the Multiple Risk Factor Intervention Trial found that the presence of microalbuminuria is associated with a 2.5-fold greater risk of cardiovascular events, even after controlling for other cardiovascular risk factors.[15] Additionally, the prognosis associated with a given level of eGFR varies substantially based on the presence and severity of proteinuria. In fact, patients with heavy proteinuria, but without overtly abnormal eGFR, appear to have worse clinical outcomes than those with moderately reduced eGFR without proteinuria.[2]

If a patient with CKD is >50 years old, treatment with a low-dose statin or statin/ezetimibe combination is recommended irrespective of LDL level [Evidence: SORT A*].[16,17] Suggested doses for these drugs are presented in Table 8. In an 18–49-year-old patient with CKD, statin treatment is suggested if one or more of the following is present: known coronary disease (MI or coronary revascularization), diabetes mellitus, prior ischemic stroke or estimated 10-year incidence of coronary death or nonfatal MI >10% [Evidence: SORT C*].[18]

In adults with CKD and hypertriglyceridemia, therapeutic lifestyle changes are suggested. Treatment with fibrates is not recommended.[18]

Table 8: Suggested Daily Doses of Lipid-lowering Agents in Chronic Kidney Disease[18]

Atorvastatin	20 mg	Pravastatin	40 mg	Simvastatin	40 mg
Fluvastatin	80 mg	Rosuvastatin	10 mg	Simvastatin/Ezetimibe	20 mg/10 mg

No randomized controlled trials have examined the safety or efficacy of **ASA** for primary or secondary prevention of atherosclerotic events in patients with CKD. Based on decreased mortality in observational studies, ASA therapy is recommended following MI in patients with CKD.[4,19,20]

Drug Therapy Adjustment in Patients with Chronic Kidney Disease

Dosage adjustment of drugs in renal impairment is described in Appendix I.

Very few drugs are absolutely contraindicated in patients with CKD. However, medications that are generally avoided in patients with stages G4–G5 CKD are listed in Table 9.

Table 9: Medications to be Avoided in Stage G4–G5 Chronic Kidney Disease

Medication	Complication
Apixaban	Increased risk of bleeding with ClCr <25 mL/min.
Baclofen	Increased neurotoxicity even at very low doses.[21]
Dabigatran	Increased risk of bleeding with ClCr <30 mL/min. In patients with ClCr 15–29 mL/min, 75 mg BID is suggested, but safety has not been established.
Magnesium-containing medications, e.g., antacids, laxatives	Magnesium accumulation.
Meperidine (pethidine)	Accumulation of an active metabolite that can lead to seizures.
Metformin	Risk of lactic acidosis with ClCr <30 mL/min.
NSAIDs, COX-2 inhibitors and other nephrotoxins	Increased risk of acute kidney injury.
Phosphorus-containing products (e.g., Fleet Phospho-soda)	Deaths due to hyperphosphatemia and resulting hypocalcemia have been reported and these products can also cause acute phosphate nephropathy.[22,23]
Potassium-sparing diuretics and herbals, such as alfalfa, dandelion, noni juice	Risk of hyperkalemia.[24]
Rivaroxaban	Increased risk of bleeding with ClCr <30 mL/min.
Sotalol	Risk of accumulation and torsades de pointes.[25]
Vitamin A	Risk of accumulation secondary to decreased renal catabolism and increased serum levels of retinol-binding protein.[26]
Vitamin C	Limit to no more than 60–100 mg/day as the metabolite (oxalate) can result in kidney stones and deposits of calcium oxalate in soft tissues.[26]

* SORT (Strength of Recommendation Taxonomy) is a rating system (A, B or C) that addresses the quality of available evidence. For more information consult **How to Use *Compendium of Therapeutic Choices*** on page xxv.

Complications of Chronic Kidney Disease

Complications are seen in Stages G3–G5 CKD. These complications include:

Hyperkalemia: refer to Chapter 105.

Metabolic acidosis: treat with **sodium bicarbonate** tablets or **Shohl's solution** (citric acid/sodium citrate). Start at 0.5 mmol/kg/day in 2–3 divided doses and titrate to achieve a CO_2 level ≥22 mmol/L.[4] Monitor closely since some patients will experience fluid retention and heart failure.

Anemia: Detailed clinical practice guidelines are provided by Kidney Disease: Improving Global Outcomes.[27] See also Chapter 99.

Mineral metabolism:

- Start therapy with a calcium-containing phosphate binder (**calcium carbonate** or **calcium citrate**) if a low phosphate diet (800–1000 mg phosphate/day) fails to control hyperphosphatemia and if hypercalcemia is not present.[1]
- If hypercalcemia develops, reduce the dose of calcium-containing phosphate binders. If hyperphosphatemia is still present, the patient may be changed to a non-calcium-containing phosphate binder, such as **lanthanum**, **sevelamer carbonate** or **sevelamer hydrochloride**. The carbonate salt of sevelamer may help to neutralize uremia-induced metabolic acidosis.
- If serum intact parathyroid hormone (PTH) is >53 pmol/L, consider starting a vitamin D analogue, such as **alfacalcidol** or **calcitriol**. These analogues are required since the kidney is less able to activate other forms of vitamin D. Reduce the dose or discontinue therapy if hypercalcemia or hyperphosphatemia develops or if PTH levels are <10.6 pmol/L.[1] **Cinacalcet** may also be considered as a second-line agent to reduce PTH in patients receiving dialysis, but this drug is very expensive and not often covered by medication insurance plans. This drug is not recommended for use in predialysis CKD patients due to an increased incidence of hypocalcemia.[28]

Therapeutic Tips

- Screen individuals at risk for CKD annually with a history and physical exam including BP assessment, calculation of eGFR or ClCr from serum creatinine, urinalysis and spot urine for albumin/creatinine (ACR) or protein/creatinine (PCR) ratio.
- The use of once-daily ACEI or ARB is preferred to enhance patient adherence and prevent fluctuations in daily blood pressure.
- Start ACEIs or ARBs at moderate doses in those patients with normal GFR and titrate up to the maximally tolerated dose.

Table 10: **Drugs Used to Treat Chronic Kidney Disease**

Class	Drug	Adult Dose	Adverse Effects	Drug Interactions	Cost[a]
Bicarbonate Supplements	*sodium bicarbonate* generics	Start at 0.5 mmol/kg/day in 2–3 divided doses and titrate to achieve an HCO_3^- level ≥22 mmol/L 325 mg tablet = 3.8 mmol bicarbonate 500 mg tablet = 5.8 mmol bicarbonate	Bloating, flatulence, increased Na^+ absorption.	Reduced absorption of medications requiring an acidic gastric pH (e.g., atazanavir, calcium carbonate, iron tablets, itraconazole, ketoconazole).	$
	Shohl's solution (citric acid/sodium citrate) Dicitrate Solution, generics	1 mmol bicarbonate/mL Start at 0.5 mmol/kg/day in 2–3 divided doses and titrate to achieve an HCO_3^- level ≥22 mmol/L	See sodium bicarbonate.	See sodium bicarbonate.	$
Calcimimetics	*cinacalcet* Sensipar	Start at 30 mg po daily. Titrate every 2–4 wk to PTH <53 pmol/L	Diarrhea, nausea, vomiting, hypocalcemia, hypophosphatemia. Not for use in predialysis CKD.	Cinacalcet strongly inhibits CYP2D6 and can increase levels of metoprolol, flecainide, vinblastine, thioridazine and most tricyclic antidepressants.	~$350
Phosphate Binders	*calcium carbonate* Caltrate, Tums, generics	Start at 250–500 mg elemental Ca^{++}/day TID po with meals. Titrate to achieve a PO_4 level in the normal range Calcium carbonate is 40% elemental calcium	Constipation and nausea are the most common. Others: hypercalcemia.	Oral iron salts, fluoroquinolones, tetracyclines and levothyroxine: absorption reduced. Give 2 h before or 4 h after calcium. H_2-blockers (e.g., ranitidine), proton pump inhibitors and sodium bicarbonate increase gastric pH and reduce dissolution and phosphate binding of calcium carbonate.	$
	calcium citrate Osteocit, generics	Start at 300–900 mg elemental Ca^{++} (1–3 tablets) TID po with meals. Titrate to achieve a PO_4 level in the normal range	See calcium carbonate.	See calcium carbonate. Less dependent on acidic gastric pH for dissolution. May increase absorption of aluminum from aluminum-containing antacids.	$
	lanthanum carbonate Fosrenol	Start at 250–500 mg TID po with meals. May be used in combination with other PO_4 binders	Nausea, diarrhea, flatulence. Potential for accumulation of lanthanum due to GI absorption, but long-term clinical consequences unknown.	Reduced absorption of levothyroxine and mycophenolate mofetil. Administer lanthanum 2 h after these drugs.	$$$

(cont'd)

Table 10: **Drugs Used to Treat Chronic Kidney Disease** *(cont'd)*

Class	Drug	Adult Dose	Adverse Effects	Drug Interactions	Cost[a]
	sevelamer carbonate Renvela	800–2400 mg (1–3 tablets) TID po with meals. May be used in combination with other PO_4 binders	Heartburn, bloating, gas.	Cholesterol-lowering drugs may need to be reduced as sevelamer can lower LDL cholesterol by an average of 30%. Reduced absorption of ciprofloxacin, levothyroxine and mycophenolate mofetil. Administer sevelamer 2 h after these drugs.	$$$$$
	sevelamer hydrochloride Renagel	800–2400 mg (1–3 tablets) TID po with meals. May be used in combination with other PO_4 binders	See sevelamer carbonate. If used alone in patients with nondialysis CKD, monitor CO_2 levels as can worsen uremic metabolic acidosis.	See sevelamer carbonate.	$$$$$
Vitamin D Analogues	*alfacalcidol* One-Alpha	Start at 0.25 µg po every other day or daily. Titrate to PTH <53 pmol/L	Hypercalcemia, hyperphosphatemia.	Phenytoin, carbamazepine, phenobarbital, thiazide diuretics may reduce levels of alfacalcidol.	$
	calcitriol Rocaltrol	Start at 0.25 mg po every other day or daily. Titrate to PTH <53 pmol/L	Hypercalcemia, hyperphosphatemia.	Phenytoin, carbamazepine, phenobarbital, thiazide diuretics may reduce levels of calcitriol.	$

[a] Cost of 30-day supply of usual dose of drug, based on 70 kg weight; includes drug cost only.
Abbreviations: HCO_3^- = bicarbonate; PO_4 = phosphate; PTH = parathyroid hormone
Legend: $ <$40 $$ $40–80 $$$ $80–120 $$$$ $120–160 $$$$$ $160–200

Suggested Readings

Kidney Disease: Improving Global Outcomes (KDIGO). KDIGO 2012 clinical practice guideline for the evaluation and management of chronic kidney disease. *Kidney Int Suppl* 2013;3(1):1-150. Available from: www.kdigo.org/clinical_practice_guidelines/ckd.php.

Kidney Disease: Improving Global Outcomes (KDIGO). KDIGO clinical practice guideline for the management of blood pressure in chronic kidney disease. *Kidney Int Suppl* 2012;2(5):337-414. Available from: www.kdigo.org/clinical_practice_guidelines/bp.php.

Matzke GR, Aronoff GR, Atkinson AJ et al. Drug dosing consideration in patients with acute and chronic kidney disease—a clinical update from Kidney Disease: Improving Global Outcomes (KDIGO). *Kidney Int* 2011;80(11):1122-37.

References

1. Levin A, Hemmelgarn B, Culleton B et al. Guidelines for the management of chronic kidney disease. *CMAJ* 2008;179(11):1154-62.
2. Hemmelgarn BR, Manns BJ, Lloyd A et al. Relation between kidney function, proteinuria, and adverse outcomes. *JAMA* 2010;303(5):423-9.
3. Levey AS, Berg RL, Gassman JJ et al. Creatinine filtration, secretion and excretion during progressive renal disease. Modification of Diet in Renal Disease (MDRD) Study Group. *Kidney Int Suppl* 1989;27:S73-80.
4. Kidney Disease: Improving Global Outcomes (KDIGO). KDIGO 2012 clinical practice guideline for the evaluation and management of chronic kidney disease. *Kidney Int Suppl* 2013;3(1):1-150. Available from: www.kdigo.org/clinical_practice_guidelines/ckd.php.
5. Go AS, Chertow GM, Fan D et al. Chronic kidney disease and the risks of death, cardiovascular events, and hospitalization. *N Engl J Med* 2004;351(13):1296-305.
6. Fink HA, Ishani A, Taylor BC et al. Screening for, monitoring, and treatment of chronic kidney disease stages 1 to 3: a systematic review for the U.S. Preventive Services Task Force and for an American College of Physicians Clinical Practice Guideline. *Ann Intern Med* 2012;156(8):570-81.
7. Krijnen P, Steyerberg EW, Postma CT et al. Validation of a prediction rule for renal artery stenosis. *J Hypertens* 2005;23(8):1583-8.
8. Mendelssohn DC, Barrett BJ, Brownscombe LM et al. Elevated levels of serum creatinine: recommendations for management and referral. *CMAJ* 1999;161(4):413-7.
9. Kidney Disease: Improving Global Outcomes (KDIGO). KDIGO clinical practice guideline for the management of blood pressure in chronic kidney disease. *Kidney Int Suppl* 2012;2(5):337-414. Available from: www.kdigo.org/clinical_practice_guidelines/bp.php.
10. Kidney Disease Outcomes Quality Initiative (K/DOQI). K/DOQI clinical practice guidelines on hypertension and antihypertensive agents in chronic kidney disease. *Am J Kidney Dis* 2004;43(5 Suppl 1):S1-290.
11. Schoolwerth AC, Sica DA, Ballermann BJ et al. Renal considerations in angiotensin converting enzyme inhibitor therapy: a statement for healthcare professionals from the Council on the Kidney in Cardiovascular Disease and the Council for High Blood Pressure Research of the American Heart Association. *Circulation* 2001;104(16):1985-91.
12. Harper W, Clement M, Goldenberg R et al. Canadian Diabetes Association 2013 clinical practice guidelines for the prevention and management of diabetes in Canada: Pharmacologic management of type 2 diabetes. *Can J Diabetes* 2013;37(Suppl 1):S61-8. Available from: guidelines.diabetes.ca/App_Themes/CDACPG/resources/cpg_2013_full_en.pdf. Accessed November 19, 2013.
13. Lubowsky ND, Siegel R, Pittas AG. Management of glycemia in patients with diabetes mellitus and CKD. *Am J Kidney Dis* 2007;50(5):865-79.
14. Nowicki M, Rychlik I, Haller H et al. Long-term treatment with the dipeptidyl peptidase-4 inhibitor saxagliptin in patients with type 2 diabetes mellitus and renal impairment: a randomised controlled 52-week efficacy and safety study. *Int J Clin Pract* 2011;65(12):1230-9.
15. Keane WF. Proteinuria: its clinical importance and role in progressive renal disease. *Am J Kidney Dis* 2000;35(4 Suppl 1):S97-105.
16. Palmer SC, Craig JC, Navaneethan SD et al. Benefits and harms of statin therapy for persons with chronic kidney disease: a systematic review and meta-analysis. *Ann Intern Med* 2012;157(4):263-75.
17. Baigent C, Landray MJ, Reith C et al. The effects of lowering LDL cholesterol with simvastatin plus ezetimibe in patients with chronic kidney disease (Study of Heart and Renal Protection): a randomised placebo-controlled trial. *Lancet* 2011;377(9784):2181-92.
18. Kidney Disease: Improving Global Outcomes (KDIGO). Lipid Work Group. KDIGO 2013 clinical practice guideline for lipid management in chronic kidney disease. *Kidney Int Suppl* 2013;3(3):259-305. Available from: kdigo.org/home/guidelines/lipids/.
19. D Beattie JN, Soman SS, Sandberg KR et al. Determinants of mortality after myocardial infarction in patients with advanced renal dysfunction. *Am J Kidney Dis* 2001;37(6):1191-200.
20. McCullough PA, Sandberg KR, Borzak S et al. Benefits of aspirin and beta-blockade after myocardial infarction in patients with chronic kidney disease. *Am Heart J* 2002;144(2):226-32.
21. Chen KS, Bullard MJ, Chien YY et al. Baclofen in patients with severely impaired renal function. *Ann Pharmacother* 1997;31(11):1315-20.
22. Piccoli GB, Vigotti FN, Consiglio V et al. Quiz page. Severe hypocalcemia caused by intravascular calcium phosphate precipitation after sodium phosphate-containing bowel preparation. *Am J Kidney Dis* 2010;55(2):A35-7.
23. U.S. Food and Drug Administration. FDA Alert. *Oral Sodium Phosphate (OSP) products for bowel cleansing (marketed as Visicol and OsmoPrep, and oral sodium phosphate products available without a prescription)*. Available from: www.fda.gov/Drugs/DrugSafety/PostmarketDrugSafetyInformationforPatientsandProviders/ucm103354.htm. Accessed December 6, 2011.
24. Isnard Bagnis C, Deray G, Baumelou A et al. Herbs and the kidney. *Am J Kidney Dis* 2004;44(1):1-11.
25. Dancey D, Wulffhart Z, McEwan P. Sotalol-induced torsades de pointes in patients with renal failure. *Can J Cardiol* 1997;13(1):55-8.
26. Rocco MV, Ikizler TA. Nutrition. In: Daugirdas JT, Blake PG, Ing TS, eds. *Handbook of dialysis*. 4th ed. Philadelphia (PA): Wolters Kluwer/Lippincott Williams & Wilkins; 2007. p. 462-81.
27. Kidney Disease: Improving Global Outcomes (KDIGO). Anemia Work Group. KDIGO clinical practice guideline for anemia in chronic kidney disease. *Kidney Int Suppl* 2012;2(4):279-335. Available from: www.kdigo.org/clinical_practice_guidelines/pdf/KDIGO-Anemia%20GL.pdf.
28. Health Canada. *Health Canada endorsed important safety information on Sensipar (cinacalcet hydrochloride)—for health professionals*. Available from: www.healthycanadians.gc.ca/recall-alert-rappel-avis/hc-sc/2007/14477a-eng.php. Accessed December 6, 2011.

Chapter 101
Dehydration in Children

Gary I. Joubert, MD, FRCPC

Newborns and young children have a much higher water content than adolescents and adults (Table 1) and are more prone to water, sodium (Na^+) and potassium (K^+) loss during illness.

Table 1: Percentage of Body Water by Age Group

Age	% Body Water
Newborn (≤1 month)	75–80
Infant (1 month–1y)	70–75
Child (1–12 y)	60–70
Adolescent/adult	55–60

Goals of Therapy

- Treat shock/impending shock
- Treat dehydration using an appropriate fluid and route
- Treat electrolyte imbalances
- Prevent complications (seizures or edema)
- Provide education to family members to help prevent recurrence

Investigations

- Thorough history with attention to:
  - underlying cause(s): vomiting and/or diarrhea or other excessive fluid loss
  - frequency and amount of loss
  - frequency and amount of urinary output
- Physical examination including:[1] heart rate, respiratory rate, blood pressure, temperature, oxygen saturation and capillary refill
- Laboratory tests: serum Na^+, K^+, Cl^-, urea, creatinine, glucose and bicarbonate (HCO_3^-), blood gases and urinalysis as indicated clinically

The assessment of dehydration in infants and children is challenging (Table 2) because children are able to maintain adequate blood pressure despite moderate to severe dehydration.

Therapeutic Choices

Pharmacologic Choices

Intravenous Rehydration Therapy

Treatment of dehydration involves replacing fluid deficits, then maintaining normal hydration.

Shock occurs when adequate tissue perfusion cannot be maintained. The systolic blood pressure at which this happens varies with age: neonates, <60 mm Hg; 1 month to 1 year, <70 mm Hg; children

>1 year, <70 mm Hg + (age in years × 2). Shock often presents in children as an increased capillary refill time and an elevated heart rate (Table 2). It must be treated aggressively using isotonic saline (NaCl 0.9%).

The calculation of the fluid deficit for a given degree of dehydration can be based on historical or objective information (e.g., predehydration and present dehydrated weight). When the predehydration weight is known:

Deficit litres (L) = predehydration weight (kg) – present weight (kg).

For children ≥1 year, predehydration body weight can be estimated by:

Body weight (kg) = 3 × age (y) + 7. This gives an estimated weight at or about the 50th percentile for age and can be used for children up to 10 years of age.[2]

Maintenance fluid (Table 3, Table 4) is the amount of fluid required to maintain normal hydration. Maintenance fluids are linked to caloric requirements and take into account insensible losses.

Dehydration is classified into 3 types depending on serum Na^+ concentration (Table 5).

Table 2: **Estimation of Dehydration**

	Severity of Dehydration		
Assessment Parameter	**Mild**	**Moderate**	**Severe**
Weight loss—Infants (under 1 y)	5%	10%	15%
Weight loss—Children (≥1 y)	3–4%	6–8%	10%
History	Decreased fluid intake Decreased urine output Normal activity	Decreased fluid intake Markedly decreased urine output Listless, acute weight loss	Markedly decreased fluid intake Anuria Obtunded Longer duration of illness
Pulse	Normal	Slightly increased	Rapid
Blood pressure	Normal	Normal to orthostatic hypotension, >10 mm Hg change	Orthostatic hypotension to shock
Behaviour	Normal	Irritable	Hyperirritable to lethargic
Thirst	Slight	Moderate	Intense
Mucous membranes[b]	Normal	Dry	Parched
Tears	Present	Decreased	Absent, sunken eyes
Anterior fontanelle (<3 months)	Normal	Normal to sunken	Sunken
External jugular vein[a]	Visible when supine	Not visible except with supraclavicular pressure	Not visible even with supraclavicular pressure
Skin (less useful in children >2 y[b])	Capillary refill <2 s	Slowed capillary refill (2–4 s), decreased turgor	Significantly delayed capillary refill (>4 s) and tenting; skin cool, acrocyanotic or mottled
Urine specific gravity	>1.020	>1.020, oliguria	Oliguria (<1 mL/kg/hour) or anuria
Lab values	Normal urea and creatinine	Increased urea and creatinine	Increased^{+++} urea and creatinine, increased Hb, low glucose

[a] This may not be a reliable sign in young children.
[b] These signs are less prominent in patients who have hypernatremia.

Table 3: Maintenance Intravenous Fluid and Electrolyte Requirements in Children

Body Weight	Daily Fluid Requirement Method	Hourly Rate Method
≤10 kg	100 mL/kg	4 mL/kg
11–20 kg	1000 mL + 50 mL for each kg over 10 kg	40 mL/h + 2 mL/h for each kg over 10 kg
>20 kg	1500 mL + 20 mL for each kg over 20 kg	60 mL/h + 1 mL/h for each kg over 20 kg
Daily Electrolytes:		
Sodium: 2.5–3 mmol/100 mL fluid. Potassium: 2–2.5 mmol/100 mL fluid		

Table 4: Sample Calculation of Maintenance Intravenous Fluid and Electrolyte Requirements

Using information for a **15 kg** child from Table 3, first estimate the fluid requirements as either an hourly or daily amount. Next, estimate basic electrolyte requirements.

	For the first 10 kg body weight	For the next 5 kg body weight	Total
Hourly Fluid Rate Method	40 mL/h	5 kg × 2 mL/kg/h = 10 mL/h	50 mL/h
Daily Fluid Rate Method	1000 mL/day	5 kg × 50 mL/kg/day = 250 mL/day	1250 mL/day

Electrolytes: (using the daily fluid values)

Na^+ 1250 mL × 3 mmol/100 mL = 37.5 mmol (37.5 mmol/1250 mL or 30 mmol/L)

K^+ 1250 mL × 2 mmol/100 mL = 25 mmol (25 mmol/1250 mL or 20 mmol/L)
(administration of large amounts of potassium may not be tolerated, so estimate requirements using the low end of the range)

Commercially available solutions that would ensure adequate sodium replacement are NaCl 0.45% or 0.9%, with or without dextrose.

Table 5: Types of Dehydration

Type of Dehydration (percentage of cases)	Serum Na^+ (mmol/L)	Serum Osmolality (mOsm/kg)
Isonatremic (80%)	130–150	Normal: 280–295 mOsm/kg Equal water and salt loss
Hypernatremic (15%)	>150	Elevated: 295 mOsm/kg Water loss > salt loss
Hyponatremic (5%)	<130	Serum osmolality may be normal, elevated or reduced Must determine subgroup (see text)

Isonatremic dehydration (Figure 1, Table 6) is the most common form of dehydration, with loss of both K^+ and Na^+. K^+ can be added to the iv mixture following establishment of urinary output. K^+ administration should not normally exceed 4 mmol/kg/day.[3] Higher K^+ concentrations can be used in life-threatening hypokalemia.

Hypernatremic dehydration usually develops slowly and is corrected slowly to prevent cerebral edema and seizures. Shock is treated aggressively by administering iv NaCl 0.9% until urinary output is re-established, then NaCl 0.45% + D5W is used to correct dehydration states and restore Na^+ to normal levels.

The goal of therapy is to reduce serum Na^+ by 10–15 mmol/L/day and to restore hydration to normal in no less than 48 hours. If the serum concentration drops rapidly (>10–15 mmol/day or >1 mmol every 2 hours), change the iv solution to NaCl 0.9% + D5W.

Hyponatremic dehydration is classified into 3 subgroups:

- excessive water
- Na^+ depletion
- factitious lowering of serum Na^+ concentration due to increased glucose, electrolytes, lipids and proteins

Symptomatic hyponatremia is usually related to the degree of serum Na^+ depletion. Children with serum Na^+ >120 mmol/L rarely demonstrate any clinical manifestations. When serum Na^+ drops below 120 mmol/L, neurologic manifestations (e.g., seizures) are common. Children who are symptomatic require aggressive replacement using hypertonic saline (NaCl 3%) to achieve a serum Na^+ >125 mmol/L. In general, 2–4 mL/kg of NaCl 3% is given at a rate of 1–3 mL/kg/hour. Serum sodium will increase by approximately 5 mmol/L for every 6 mL/kg of NaCl 3%.

Figure 1: Management of Isonatremic Dehydration

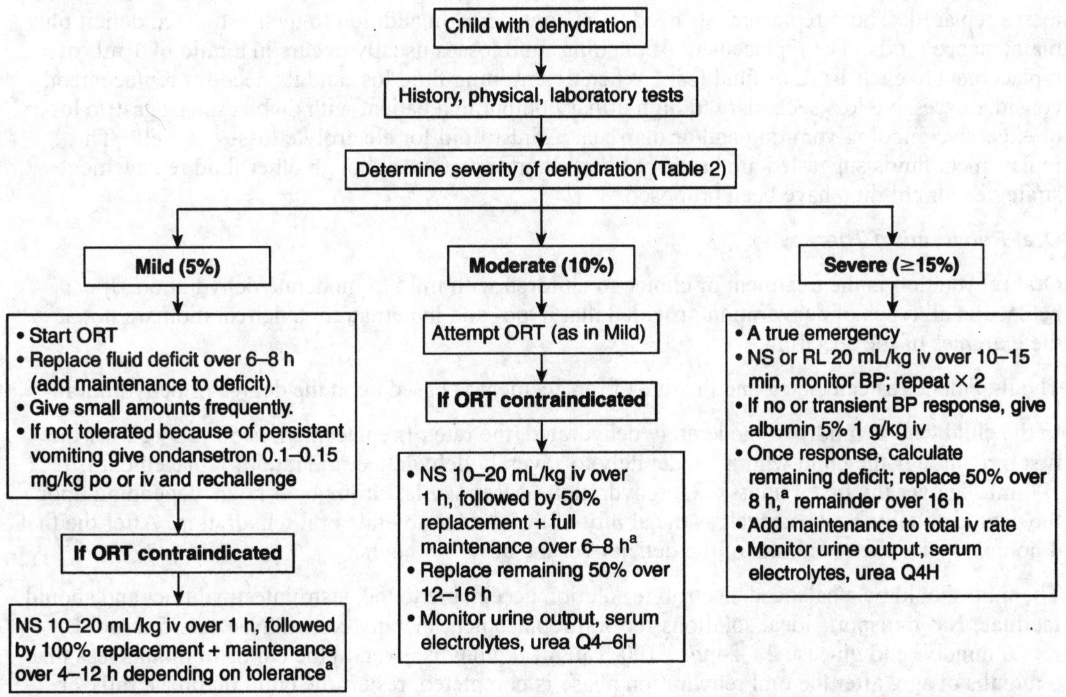

[a] Replacement therapy after bolus should contain at least 50–60 mmol/L Na^+ plus a source of glucose (e.g., D5W) plus appropriate K^+. Consider NaCl 0.45% (Na^+ 77 mmol/L) + D5W (5 g glucose/100 mL) + appropriate K^+. K^+ should not exceed 4 mmol/kg/day and replenishment should be done gradually over 2 days. **If no urine output, do not give K^+.**

Abbreviations: BP = blood pressure; NS = normal saline, 0.9% NaCl; ORT = oral rehydration therapy; RL = Ringer's lactate

Table 6: **Sample Calculation for Initial Management of Isonatremic Dehydration**

Fluid	Total fluid replacement equals *deficit* replacement plus *maintenance*. Fluid deficit in 10% dehydration is 100 mL/kg; in 5% dehydration 50 mL/kg *Example:* For a 15 kg child who has 10% isonatremic dehydration: Deficit replacement calculation = 15 kg × 100 mL/kg = 1500 mL Need to replace 50% or 750 mL over first 8 h at a rate of *94 mL/h* Maintenance = 50 mL/h (using calculation from Table 4) Total = *144 mL/h* (94 mL/h + 50 mL/h) for first 8 h Reduce to 100 mL/h for next 16 h (replace remaining deficit of 750 mL + maintenance over 16 h [47 mL/h + 50 mL/h ≈ 100 mL/h]). Reduce to maintenance rate as tolerated after this time.
Electrolytes	Na^+ loss would be approximately 120 mmol (8–10 mmol/kg/day) and K^+ loss would be approximately 120 mmol (8–10 mmol/kg/day).
Solution Choice	Using NaCl 0.45% + D5W at the above rates will replace the Na^+ loss in 13h. K^+ replacement should not exceed 4 mmol/kg/day (60 mmol per day in this example). Replacement of K^+ will require 2 days.[8]

Serum Na^+ deficit can be calculated as follows:

Na^+ deficit (mmol) = [Na^+ desired – Na^+ actual (mmol/L)] × body weight (kg) × total body water (L/kg)

After initial elevation of Na^+ to >125 mmol/L, the remaining deficit can be replaced over 24–48 hours.

Remember that children who are dehydrated and have ongoing fluid losses need to have those fluid losses replaced. Those replacements need to be considered in addition to their estimated deficit plus maintenance fluids. The replacement of ongoing fluid losses usually occurs in a ratio of 1 mL of replacement to each 1 mL of fluid lost.[4] When determining fluid loss and its need for replacement, consider excessive loss secondary to high urinary output in a patient with diabetes, nasogastric losses, or excessive ongoing vomiting and/or diarrhea. Adjust fluid for electrolyte losses as well.[5] The replacement fluids suggested are based on the author's practice, although other fluid replacement strategies for children have been proposed.[6,7]

Oral Rehydration Therapy

Oral rehydration is the treatment of choice in children with mild to moderate dehydration. It can be used in all types of dehydration provided that hypo- and hypernatremic dehydration are not at the extremes of the spectrum.

The fluid deficit is calculated and the rate of replacement is based upon the degree of dehydration.

In the child who is mildly to moderately dehydrated, the rate of replacement is 50 mL/kg over the first 4 hours; for the child who is moderately to severely dehydrated, the rate of replacement is 100 mL/kg over the first 4 hours. The rehydration phase may last from 4–12 hours depending upon the degree of dehydration as well as the ability of the child to tolerate oral rehydration. After the first 4 hours, replace the remainder of the deficit over the next 6–8 hours.

The fluid should be a balanced electrolyte solution acceptable to the gastrointestinal tract and should facilitate Na^+ transport. Ideal solutions for oral replacement therapy contain Na^+ 45–75 mmol/L, K^+ 20 mmol/L and glucose 20–24 g/L; 100–150 mL/kg/day is given to the child. In infants less than 6 months of age, after the oral rehydration phase is completed, restart the child on breast milk or half-strength formula.[8]

Commercially available preparations (Table 7) may be used to rehydrate the child with observation in an ambulatory/emergency room setting or at home.

Table 7: **Oral Rehydration Solutions**

Product	Composition				
	Dextrose g/L	K^+ mmol/L	Na^+ mmol/L	Cl^- mmol/L	Cost[a]
Gastrolyte	17.8	20	60	60	$
Hydralyte Electrolyte Maintenance Solution	16	20	45	45	$$
Pedialyte	25	20	45	35	$$
Pediatric Electrolyte	20	20	45	35	$$

[a] Cost per litre; includes drug cost only.
Legend: $ < $5 $$ $5–10

Children who have been started on iv replacement therapy can be switched to oral replacement therapy at any point. It is important to ensure that no contraindications (shock or impending shock, high diarrheal purge rates, intractable vomiting, altered sensorium) are present.

In the child failing oral replacement therapy secondary to vomiting, oral replacement solutions may be delivered via nasogastric tube.

The use of **ondansetron** can decrease vomiting and increase the rate of oral rehydration tolerance in patients with gastroenteritis and significant vomiting.[9,10] When compared to placebo, ondansetron 0.1–0.15 mg/kg resulted in a significant decrease in vomiting. Ondansetron increases oral rehydration therapy success and hence discharge from emergency departments without the need for iv fluid intervention. Ondansetron can be administered orally or iv if the patient is intolerant of the oral preparation. IV doses of 0.1–0.15 mg/kg are administered with a fluid challenge commencing 20 minutes after administration.

Therapeutic Tips

- Absolute indications for admission to hospital are:
  - shock
  - hypo/hypernatremia
  - intractable vomiting/diarrhea
  - altered sensorium
- Possible indications for admission to hospital are:
  - serum HCO_3 <15 mmol/L at onset of therapy
  - poor response to oral replacement therapy and ongoing requirement for iv therapy
- Clinical signs of dehydration are often not present until at least 5% of a child's body weight is lost.
- Depending on the clinical situation, consider measuring serum electrolytes before, at the time of and after starting iv fluids.

Suggested Readings

Bailey B, Gravel J, Goldman RD et al. External validation of the clinical dehydration scale for children with acute gastroenteritis. *Acad Emerg Med* 2010;17(6):583-8.

Choong K, Kho ME, Menon K et al. Hypotonic versus isotonic saline in hospitalised children: a systematic review. *Arch Dis Child* 2006;91(10):828-35.

Duke T, Molyneux EM. Intravenous fluids for seriously ill children: time to reconsider. *Lancet* 2003;362(9392):1320-3.

Moritz ML, Ayus JC. Prevention of hospital-acquired hyponatremia: a case for using isotonic saline. *Pediatrics* 2003;111(2):227-30.

Powell CV, Priestley SJ, Young S et al. Randomized clinical trial of rapid versus 24-hour rehydration for children with acute gastroenteritis. *Pediatrics* 2011;128(4):e771-8.

Steiner MJ, DeWalt DA, Byerley JS. Is this child dehydrated? *JAMA* 2004;291(22):2746-54.

References

1. Cairns J. Dehydration secondary to gastroenteritis. *Paediatr Child Health* 2001;6(2):69.
2. Luscombe M, Owens B. Weight estimation in resuscitation: is the current formula still valid? *Arch Dis Child* 2007;92(5):412-5.
3. Kallen RJ. The management of diarrheal dehydration in infants using parenteral fluids. *Pediatr Clin North Am* 1990;37(2):265-86.
4. Rice HE, Caty MG, Glick PL. Fluid therapy for the pediatric surgical patient. *Pediatr Clin North Am* 1998;45(4):719-27.
5. Boineau FG, Lewy JE. Estimation of parenteral fluid requirements. *Pediatr Clin North Am* 1990;37(2):257-64.
6. Duke T, Molyneux EM. Intravenous fluids for seriously ill children: time to reconsider. *Lancet* 2003;362(9392):1320-3.
7. Moritz ML, Ayus JC. Prevention of hospital-acquired hyponatremia: a case for using isotonic saline. *Pediatrics* 2003;111(2):227-30.
8. Casteel HB, Fiedorek SC. Oral rehydration therapy. *Pediatr Clin North Am* 1990;37(2):295-311.
9. Freedman SB, Adler M, Seshadri R et al. Oral ondansetron for gastroenteritis in a pediatric emergency department. *N Engl J Med* 2006;354(16):1698-705.
10. Cheng A. Emergency department use of oral ondansetron for acute gastroenteritis-related vomiting in infants and children. *Paediatr Child Health* 2011;16(3):177-82.

Fluid and Electrolyte Disorders

Chapter 102
Edema

Tammy M. Keough-Ryan, MD, MSc, FRCPC

Edema is a sign of an underlying disorder that should be investigated and identified. The underlying disorder should be treated prior to or concurrently with initiation of directed therapy for the edema. Edema is caused by an imbalance of fluid homeostasis that leads to increased extracellular fluid volume. Therapy must be individualized.

Peripheral edema is swelling in a dependent area that is visible on physical examination. Palpation can differentiate pitting (indentation left when pressure applied) from nonpitting edema. *Anasarca* is gross, generalized edema.

Common conditions that are associated with edema include heart failure (HF), liver failure including hepatic cirrhosis and renal failure including nephrotic syndrome. The main focus of this chapter is peripheral edema. For edema associated with specific conditions, see Chapter 38 and Chapter 57.

Goals of Therapy

- Decrease fluid overload
- Improve patient comfort and quality of life
- Identify and manage diuretic resistance

Investigations

- History:
  - conditions associated with edema:
    - general conditions: renal dysfunction, HF, liver dysfunction, pregnancy, hypothyroidism (myxedema)
    - localized conditions: lymphatic or venous obstruction, infection
  - salt intake
  - drugs that may cause or exacerbate edema, e.g., NSAIDs, calcium channel blockers, corticosteroids, thiazolidinediones or drugs that may interact with diuretic agents, limiting their effectiveness
- Physical exam:
  - generalized edema
  - localized edema:
    - pitting or nonpitting—for nonpitting edema, consider lymphatic obstruction or myxedema
    - symmetric or asymmetric—for asymmetric edema, consider lymphedema from lymphatic obstruction, deep vein thrombosis (DVT) or infection
  - location of edema:
    - diffuse edema in anasarca
    - dependent edema: legs if patient ambulatory, sacrum if patient recumbent
  - weight, blood pressure, heart rate, respiratory rate

  - signs of fluid overload: jugular venous pulsation (JVP) elevation (or distention), pulmonary edema, ascites
- Laboratory investigations:
  - serum electrolytes (including Na^+, K^+, Cl^-, HCO_3^-, Ca^{++}, Mg^{++}), uric acid, urea, creatinine
  - urinalysis
  - liver function tests
  - chest x-ray
  - other: TSH, glucose and lipids, albumin, 24-hour urine collection to quantify proteinuria and sodium if symptoms/signs are suggestive of primary or secondary renal disorder

Therapeutic Choices

Figure 1 suggests a strategy for the management of edema.

Nonpharmacologic Choices

- Sodium: decrease sodium intake to <88 mmol/day (2 g Na^+ or 5 g NaCl).[1,2]
- Fluid: decrease fluid intake based on individual patient assessment of volume and disease state.
- Posture: supine position improves cardiac output; elevate legs.
- Stockings: consider supportive compression stockings.
- Paracentesis for ascites under direction of a specialist.
- Ultrafiltration therapy: if renal insufficiency is significant, consider referral to a specialist for this therapy.

Pharmacologic Choices

Consider if nonpharmacologic actions do not significantly reduce the symptoms related to the edema, and treatment of the underlying disorder has been implemented.

Diuretic Therapy

Peripheral edema, in the absence of respiratory or cardiac compromise (shortness of breath, decreased functional capacity, chest pain), is not life threatening and fluid removal must be slow. The maximum recommended rate of weight loss is 1 kg/day if significant peripheral edema is present.[2,3,4] Diuretics (Table 1) are not effective if lymphatic or venous drainage obstruction is the underlying problem. Diuretics should not be prescribed in pregnancy (see Choices during Pregnancy and Breastfeeding).

Diuretics decrease sodium reabsorption at various sites in the nephron by interfering with carrier proteins or channels.[3,5] Diuretics increase sodium and water losses; this decreases extracellular fluid volume and improves the edema. Closely monitor for electrolyte imbalances (K^+, Cl^-, Ca^{++}, Mg^{++}, HCO_3^-) and prerenal azotemia (urea, creatinine) to identify and respond to significant alterations.

Loop Diuretics

The loop diuretics, **furosemide, ethacrynic acid, bumetanide** and **torsemide** (not available in Canada) are potent diuretic agents that act in the loop of Henle in the nephron. The onset and duration of action are short. Loop diuretics are particularly useful in the presence of moderate to severe renal insufficiency (ClCr ≤50 mL/min). If there is no response with the maximum dose, switching to an alternative loop diuretic will not improve efficacy.[6]

Figure 1: **Management of Edema**

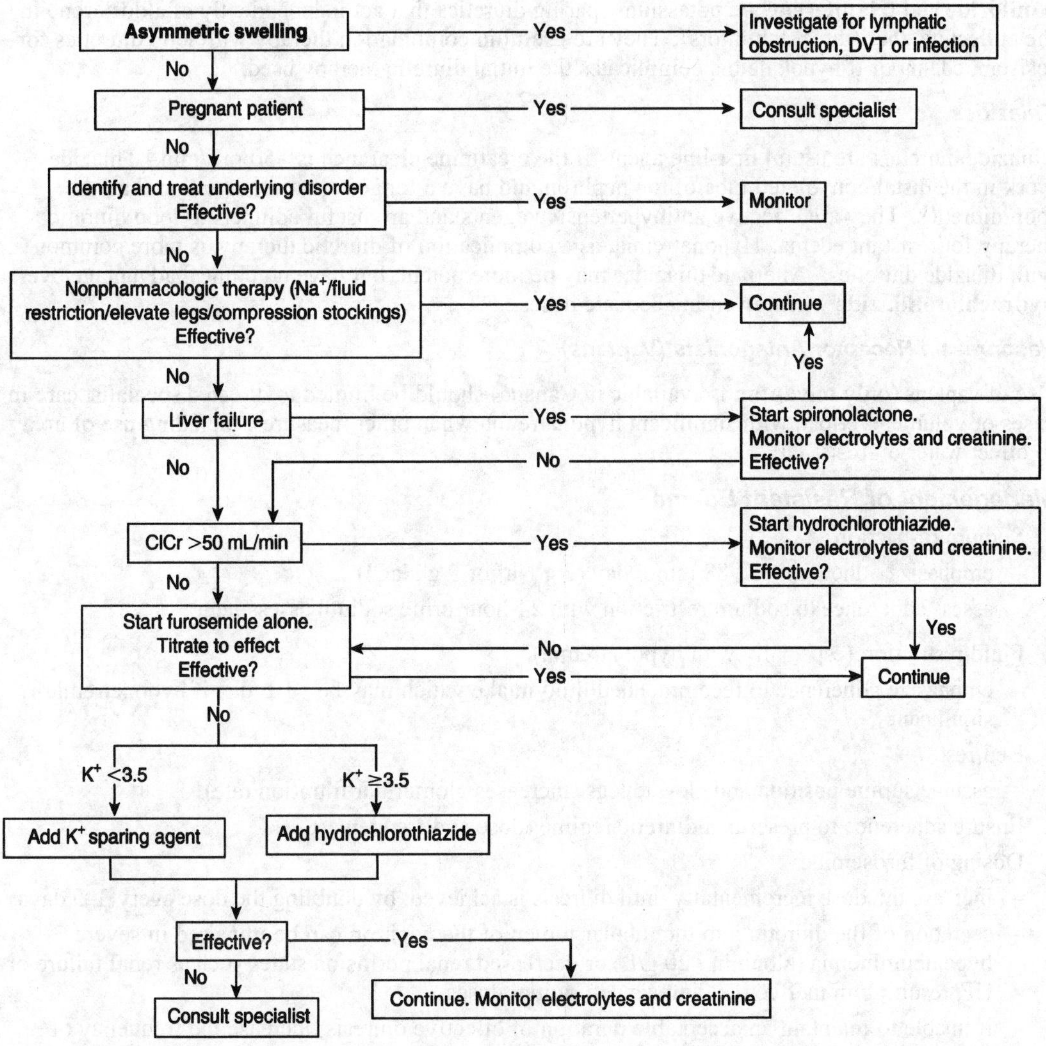

Bumetanide and torsemide have no clear advantages over furosemide despite differing sites of metabolism and increased and more predictable bioavailability. Torsemide has a longer half-life, so once daily dosing may be used. Ethacrynic acid is reserved for use in patients with sulfa allergy that contraindicates the use of the other loop diuretics. There are reports of ototoxicity with all the loop diuretics including ethacrynic acid.[3,4,5]

Potassium-sparing Diuretics

Spironolactone and **eplerenone** are aldosterone receptor antagonists. Spironolactone is the first-line agent in patients with hepatic disease in whom secondary hyperaldosteronism leads to sodium and water retention. Spironolactone and eplerenone can be effective adjunctive therapy for NYHA Class II to IV HF (see Chapter 38) associated with high aldosterone levels. Eplerenone is a more selective antagonist for aldosterone with a low affinity for progesterone and androgen receptors. This may limit the side effects of gynecomastia and erectile dysfunction.[7,8,9]

Amiloride and **triamterene** are potassium-sparing diuretics that act independently of aldosterone in the collecting duct (direct inhibitors). They are useful in combination therapy with loop diuretics for resistant edema or if hypokalemia complicates the initial diuretic therapy used.[5]

Thiazides

Thiazide diuretics are useful first-line agents if the creatinine clearance is >50 mL/min.[5] Thiazides work in the distal convoluted tube of the nephron and have a longer duration of action than the loop diuretics. They are effective antihypertensive agents and are useful adjuncts to loop diuretic therapy for resistant edema. Hyponatremia, as a complication of diuretic therapy, is more common with thiazide diuretics.[2] Alternate thiazides may be more potent, but have no clinical advantage over **hydrochlorothiazide** when given in adequate doses.[5,10]

Vasopressin Receptor Antagonists (Vaptans)

Use of vaptans (only **tolvaptan** is available in Canada) should be limited to directed specialist care in cases of volume overload with significant hyponatremia when other measures, including use of urea to effect water diuresis, fail.

Management of Resistant Edema

- Sodium restriction
  - emphasize adherence to ≤88 mmol/day (2 g Na^+ or 5 g NaCl)
  - assess adherence to sodium restriction with 24-hour urine sodium assessment
- Fluid restriction (especially with hyponatremia)
  - emphasize adherence to recommended fluid intake which may be ≤1 L/day if hyponatremia significant
- Bed rest
  - assume supine position and elevate legs (increases glomerular filtration rate)
- Ensure adherence to prescribed diuretic regime (dose and frequency)
- Dosing of furosemide
  - increase the dose incrementally until diuresis is achieved, by doubling the dose every 3–5 days
  - secretion of the diuretic into the tubular lumen of the nephron can be impaired in severe hypoalbuminemia (albumin <20 g/L) or decreased renal perfusion states such as renal failure or HF, resulting in ineffective diuresis with initial doses
  - if unable to maintain an acceptable duration of effective diuresis, increase the frequency of dosing to 2–3 times per day
  - double the dose if switching from iv to oral route
  - consider intravenous dosing if the GI tract is edematous or in decreased cardiac output states that can lead to impaired absorption of oral drug
  - consider continuous iv infusion
  - monitor clinical status carefully, including weight, to ensure daily weight loss does not exceed 1 kg
  - monitor for and manage electrolyte disturbances and prerenal azotemia

Combination Diuretic Therapy

- Adding a **thiazide** to a **loop diuretic** adds blockade at a distal site of sodium reabsorption to improve diuresis. If the thiazide is given orally with iv furosemide, administer 30–60 minutes prior to the loop diuretic. If both diuretics are taken orally, administer at the same time.
- **Potassium-sparing agents** can be added to further block sodium reabsorption, particularly if the patient is hypokalemic. As life-threatening hyperkalemia can result, exercise caution and monitor electrolytes frequently if the patient has renal failure, diabetes mellitus or is taking any of the following medications: ACE inhibitors, angiotensin receptor blockers, beta-blockers, cyclosporine, NSAIDs, pentamidine, tacrolimus or trimethoprim.
- **Aldosterone antagonists** are effective adjunctive agents in the presence of neurohumoral activation, e.g., hepatic disease, HF or nephrotic syndrome.
- **Carbonic anhydrase inhibitors** such as **acetazolamide** may occasionally be added on the advice of a specialist if diuresis is ineffective using a combination of other diuretic agents or if diuresis is complicated by metabolic alkalosis.
- If all above measures fail, a specialist may consider other options such as ultrafiltration in renal failure or paracentesis in cirrhosis.

Idiopathic Edema

This condition occurs most often in postpubertal, young to middle-aged, obese females. It is a diagnosis of exclusion when physical exam and laboratory investigations fail to define an underlying cause (cardiac, hepatic or renal) for edema. In 80% of cases, the edema is orthostatic, that is, the edema develops in the standing position and is more evident at the end of the day. The edema usually presents in the lower extremities but can also present in the face, hands and breasts, particularly in the morning. This can be demonstrated by weight gains of 0.7–1 kg/day from morning to evening weight.[11] An altered homeostatic response to an upright position promotes the retention of sodium and water.

- Consider nonpharmacologic measures such as restriction of sodium and fluid intake, recumbent position, avoidance of prolonged periods of standing and use of supportive compression stockings.
- Consider discontinuation of diuretic therapy.
- Reassess fluid-restricted diet if rebound edema persists when diuretics are stopped. Sodium retention due to neurohormonal adaptation may persist for 1–3 weeks before spontaneous induction of diuresis.
- Consider intermittent daily diuretic use only when nonpharmacologic measures fail.

Choices during Pregnancy and Breastfeeding

Patients who are pregnant should be referred to a specialist. Diuretics are usually not recommended so as to avoid intravascular contraction and potential negative effects on placental perfusion. For breastfeeding mothers, **hydrochlorothiazide** and **spironolactone** can be used since their excretion in breast milk is very low and no adverse effects have been documented in babies. However, intense diuresis should be avoided as, in theory, diuretics may compromise milk production by depleting intravascular volume.

A discussion of general principles on the use of medications in these special populations can be found in Appendix II and Appendix III. Other specialized reference sources are also provided in these appendices.

Therapeutic Tips

- Investigate unilateral edema for venous obstruction or infection.
- Refer pregnant or breastfeeding patients to a specialist.

- Monitor electrolytes and renal function closely when initiating diuretic therapy, increasing the dose or using combination therapy, and/or when the patient is clinically unwell.
- Avoid using potassium-sparing agents for patients with renal failure, but if they are used follow potassium levels closely as these agents may cause life-threatening hyperkalemia.
- Avoid using fixed combination products as dosing is more difficult to titrate or decrease if changes in volume status occur.
- Identify overdiuresis in patients by monitoring for clinical signs of weakness or hypotension and/or laboratory evidence of prerenal azotemia, hypokalemia and/or metabolic alkalosis. Consider holding diuretics and antihypertensives, using gentle hydration, and/or referral of these patients to a specialist.

Table 1: Diuretic Agents for Treatment of Edema

Class	Drug	Dose	Adverse Effects	Drug Interactions	Comments	Cost[a]
Loop Diuretics	*bumetanide* Burinex	0.5–2 mg po as a single dose; maximum daily dose 10 mg If diuretic response not adequate with 1 mg, a 2nd and 3rd dose may be given at 4- to 5-h intervals May give BID. Evening dose appears to have a greater diuretic effect than morning dose Maintenance: lowest effective daily dose Impaired hepatic function: use minimum effective dose; maximum daily dose 5 mg	Volume depletion. Electrolyte disturbances: hypochloremia, hypokalemia (evident during first 1–2 wk), hyponatremia, hyperuricemia (usually asymptomatic). Azotemia, increase in serum creatinine. Hyperglycemia. Dizziness, hypotension. Acute interstitial nephritis. Ototoxicity. Myalgias (common with high doses of bumetanide). Allergy (sulfa).	Aminoglycosides, cisplatin: increased ototoxicity. Thiazide diuretics: increased diuresis and electrolyte abnormalities; monitor for dehydration and electrolyte abnormalities when used in combination. Digoxin: hypokalemia and hypomagnesemia may lead to arrhythmias Lithium: reduced renal clearance of lithium resulting in lithium toxicity; monitor lithium levels and adjust dose as needed. NSAIDs: increased risk of renal failure secondary to reduced renal blood flow resulting from prostaglandin inhibition; monitor for reduced diuretic and natriuretic response.	Diuresis within 30–60 min following oral administration. Monitor electrolytes, urea, creatinine and daily weight. Bumetanide 1 mg produces a diuretic response similar to furosemide 40 mg in healthy patients; in renal failure, bumetanide 2 mg produces a diuretic response similar to furosemide 40 mg. Caution in patients with sulfa allergy. Contraindications: hepatic coma, states of severe electrolyte depletion.	$$$$$
	ethacrynic acid Edecrin	Initial: 50 mg po as single dose after a meal Titrate gradually in increments of 25–50 mg daily until desired response; may require up to 200 mg BID in severe, refractory cases of edema Maintenance: lowest effective daily dose When adding to another diuretic, start low (25 mg daily) and titrate as necessary	See bumetanide. May be associated with severe ototoxicity. Can be used in sulfa-allergic patients.	See bumetanide.	May be considered in individuals with sulfonamide hypersensitivity or in cases of severe, refractory edema. Onset of diuresis: po 30 min; iv 5 min. Duration of action: po 6–8 h; iv 2 h. Monitor electrolytes, urea, creatinine and daily weight. Similar in potency to furosemide. IV route used when oral intake is not viable or in urgent situations such as pulmonary edema.	$$

(cont'd)

Table 1: **Diuretic Agents for Treatment of Edema** *(cont'd)*

Class	Drug	Dose	Adverse Effects	Drug Interactions	Comments	Cost[a]
	furosemide Lasix, generics	Initial: 20–80 mg po as a single dose preferably in a.m. If desired response not achieved, increase by 20–40 mg Q6–8H; maximum single dose dependent on disease state and renal function; increase dose if initial dose fails to produce adequate increase in urinary output within 4–6 h IV dose: 20–40 mg as a single injection, may repeat Q2H. If no response, may increase dose in 20 mg increments Continuous infusion: 3–20 mg/h titrated to response Maintenance: lowest effective dose taken daily, BID or intermittently on alternate days Severe edema: can use 250–500 mg tablet po under direction of a specialist	See bumetanide.	See bumetanide.	Half-life: 1.5–2 h and prolonged in kidney insufficiency. Extent and rate of absorption varies between patients depending on concomitant disease states. Effectiveness diminishes in the presence of gut wall edema. Onset of diuresis: po 30–60 min; iv 5 min. Duration of action: po 4–8 h, iv 2 h. Monitor electrolytes, urea, creatinine and daily weight. Furosemide 500 mg tablet: for patients with ClCr 5–20 mL/min who have not responded to conventional doses. May use in combination with thiazides for synergy. Caution in patients with sulfa allergy.	$
Potassium-sparing Diuretics	*amiloride* Midamor	Initial: 5 mg daily po; increase to 10 mg daily if necessary If persistent hypokalemia, may increase to 15 mg, then 20 mg daily with careful monitoring of electrolytes ClCr 10–50 mL/min: administer 50% of normal dose	Hyperkalemia—common if used as monotherapy; incidence greater in patients with renal impairment, elderly and in diabetes. Headache, impotence. Hyponatremia, hypochloremia when used in combination with other diuretics.	ACEI and ARBs: Increased K^+ levels; monitor renal function and potassium levels when used in combination, especially in patients with renal impairment and type 2 diabetes mellitus; adjust dose as needed. Potassium preparations: Increased K^+; avoid combination unless documented hypokalemia; monitor K^+ levels. Tacrolimus, cyclosporine: Increased K^+ levels. NSAIDs: may negate the diuretic effect and increase risk of NSAID-induced renal dysfunction.	Contraindications: significant renal function impairment, hyperkalemia.	$

Class	Drug	Dose	Adverse Effects	Drug Interactions	Comments	Cost[a]
	eplerenone Inspra	Initial: 25 mg daily po or every 2 days Maximum: 50 mg daily po If ClCr 30–50 mL/min maximum dose is 25 mg daily Continue initial dose for ≥7 days, then titrate accordingly If adequate diuresis has not occurred, add a 2nd diuretic that acts proximally in nephron for additive effect.	Hyperkalemia, dehydration, dizziness, diarrhea, nausea.	See amiloride. Avoid combining with strong inhibitors/inducers of CYP3A4 (e.g., clarithromycin, carbamazepine, ketoconazole, phenytoin).	Avoid if ClCr <30 mL/min	$$$$$
	spironolactone Aldactone, generics	Initial: 25 mg daily po Increase by 25–50 mg Q5 days to a maximum of 200 mg daily If adequate diuresis has not occurred, add a 2nd diuretic which acts proximally in nephron for additive effects ClCr 10–50 mL/min: administer Q12–24H ClCr <10 mL/min: avoid	See amiloride. Gynecomastia.	See amiloride. Digoxin: Increased plasma levels due to reduced renal tubular secretion; spironolactone may interfere with digoxin radioimmunoassay, resulting in falsely increased digoxin levels. Salicylates: may result in sodium retention; monitor sodium levels and blood pressure. Mitotane: antagonism of mitotane activity; avoid combination.	See amiloride.	$
Thiazide Diuretics	*chlorthalidone* generics	50–100 mg once daily po; can be given every other day Maintain on lowest effective dose Ineffective as monotherapy in patients with ClCr <50 mL/min When adding to another diuretic, start low and titrate as necessary	Usually well tolerated. Orthostatic hypotension. Electrolyte abnormalities: hyperuricemia (usually asymptomatic), hyponatremia (common), hypochloremia, hypokalemia (evident during first 1–2 wk). Headache, vertigo, dizziness, asthenia, muscle cramps. Volume depletion. Acute interstitial nephritis. Thiazides can exacerbate gout.	Loop diuretics: Increased diuresis and electrolyte abnormalities; monitor for dehydration and electrolyte abnormalities when used in combination. Digoxin: hypokalemia and hypomagnesemia may lead to arrhythmias. Antidiabetic medications: thiazides may increase blood sugar—seen at higher doses. Monitor blood glucose and adjust dose of antidiabetic medications as necessary. Lithium: Reduced renal clearance of lithium resulting in toxicity; monitor lithium levels and adjust dose as needed. NSAIDs: may negate the diuretic effect; increased risk of NSAID-induced renal dysfunction.	Half-life: 24–55 h. Onset: 2–6 h, persists for 24–72 h. Contraindications: severe renal or hepatic failure, hypercalcemia, refractory hypokalemia or hyponatremia, symptomatic hyperuricemia.	$

(cont'd)

Table 1: **Diuretic Agents for Treatment of Edema** *(cont'd)*

Class	Drug	Dose	Adverse Effects	Drug Interactions	Comments	Cost[a]
	hydrochlorothiazide generics	Initial: 25–100 mg daily po or divided BID or TID Can also be given on alternate days Ineffective as monotherapy in patients with ClCr <50 mL/min When adding to a loop diuretic, start low and titrate as necessary	See chlorthalidone. Increased fasting blood glucose may be dose-related as not seen with doses <12.5 mg.	See chlorthalidone.	Half-life: 2.5 h, prolonged in renal insufficiency. Onset: 2 h with duration of 6–12 h. Used in combination with furosemide for synergistic effect.	$
	indapamide Lozide, generics	Initial: 2.5 mg once daily po; may increase to 5 mg daily if no response within 1 wk When adding to a loop diuretic, start low and titrate as necessary Ineffective as monotherapy in patients with ClCr <50 mL/min	See chlorthalidone.	See chlorthalidone.	Half-life: 15–25 h. Take with food or milk to decrease GI side effects. Monitor electrolytes in patients who may be at increased risk of hypokalemia, e.g., patients on digoxin, patients with cardiac arrhythmias. Contraindications: progressive and severe oliguria, hepatic coma.	$
	metolazone Zaroxolyn	Single daily dose is recommended; start low and titrate 2.5–20 mg daily po Ineffective as monotherapy in patients with ClCr <50 mL/min	See chlorthalidone.	See chlorthalidone.	Diuresis and saluresis begin within 1 h and persist for 12–24 h, depending on dose. May be given for a limited time period initially. May be given indefinitely to patients who remain volume expanded, based on target weight. Contraindications: hepatic coma, sulfa allergy.	$-$$

[a] Cost of 30-day supply; includes drug cost only.

Dosage adjustment may be required in renal impairment; see Appendix I

Abbreviations: ACEI = ACE inhibitor; ARB = angiotensin receptor blocker; GFR = glomerular filtration rate; NSAID = nonsteroidal anti-inflammatory drug

Legend: $ < $20 $-$$ < $20–40 $$ $20–40 $$$ $40–60 $$$$ $60–80 $$$$$ $80–100

Suggested Readings

Brater DC. Pharmacology of diuretics. *Am J Med Sci* 2000;319(1):38-50.

Brater DC. Update in diuretic therapy: clinical pharmacology. *Semin Nephrol* 2011;31(6):483-94.

O'Brien JG, Chennubhotla SA, Chennubhotla RV. Treatment of edema. *Am Fam Physician* 2005;71(11):2111-7.

Palmer BF. Metabolic complications associated with use of diuretics. *Semin Nephrol* 2011;30(6):542-52.

Trayes KP, Studdiford JS, Pickle S et al. Edema: diagnosis and management. *Am Fam Physician* 2013;88(2):102-10.

References

1. Dasgupta K, Quinn RR, Zarnke KB et al. The 2014 Canadian Hypertension Education Program (CHEP) recommendations for blood pressure measurement, diagnosis, assessment of risk, prevention and treatment of hypertension. *Can J Cardiol* 2014;30(5):485-501.
2. Leung W, Wong F. Medical management of ascites. *Expert Opin Pharmacother* 2011;12(8):1269-83.
3. Basraon J, Deedwani PC. Diuretics in heart failure. *Med Clin North Am* 2012;96(5):933-42.
4. Yancy CW, Jessup M, Bozkurt B et al. 2013 ACCF/AHA guideline for the management of heart failure: executive summary: a report of the American College of Cardiology Foundation/American Heart Association Task Force on practice guidelines. *Circulation* 2013;128(16):1810-52.
5. Wile D. Diuretics: a review. *Ann Clin Biochem* 2012;49(Pt 5):419-31.
6. Brater DC. Update in diuretic therapy: clinical pharmacology. *Semin Nephrol* 2011;31(6): 483-94.
7. Liou IW. Management of end-stage liver disease. *Med Clin North Am* 2014;98(1):119-52.
8. Watanabe M, Krum H. Eplerenone for the treatment of cardiovascular disorders. *Expert Rev Cardiovasc Ther* 2012;10(7):831-8.
9. Dhillon S. Eplerenone: a review of its use in patients with chronic systolic heart failure and mild symptoms. *Drugs* 2013;73(13):1451-62.
10. Karadsheh F, Weir MR. Thiazide and thiazide-like diuretics: an opportunity to reduce blood pressure in patients with advanced kidney disease. *Curr Hypertens Rep* 2012;14(5):416-20.
11. Streeten DH. Idiopathic edema. Pathogenesis, clinical features, and treatment. *Endocrinol Metab Clin North Am* 1995;24(3):531-47.

Chapter 103
Hypercalcemia

Walter Watral, BScPharm, PharmD

Goals of Therapy

- Normalize serum calcium levels
  - enhance renal excretion of calcium
  - inhibit accelerated calcium resorption from bone
  - decrease intestinal calcium absorption
- Correct extracellular fluid (ECF) volume contraction and dehydration
- Alleviate signs and symptoms of hypercalcemia
- Diagnose and treat underlying disorder

Investigations

- History and physical examination,[1,2] with special attention to:
  - onset and duration of symptoms (anorexia, constipation, nausea, vomiting, altered mental status, drowsiness, malaise, polydipsia, polyuria, bone pain and muscle weakness are symptoms usually associated with acute hypercalcemia)
  - chronic hypercalcemia is usually asymptomatic
- Laboratory evaluation:[2,3]
  - serum ionized calcium (preferred where available) or serum calcium and albumin. Corrected Ca^{++} value (mmol/L) = (0.02 × [40 − measured albumin g/L]) + measured Ca^{++}
  - serum intact parathyroid hormone (PTH). Perform this test before giving bisphosphonates as they can alter serum PTH levels.[4]
  - serum parathyroid hormone-related peptide (PTHrP) if PTH low
  - 24-hour urine collection to measure calcium to creatinine ratio (if familial hypocalciuric hypercalcemia or milk-alkali syndrome is suspected)
  - serum phosphate, alkaline phosphatase, total protein, serum creatinine and urea

Therapeutic Choices

- Aggressiveness of initial interventions depends on the rapidity of onset and severity of the hypercalcemia (see Table 1).
- Definitive therapy for long-term control of hypercalcemia requires diagnosis and treatment of the underlying condition (see Figure 1).

Nonpharmacologic Choices

Mobilize

Hypercalcemia is exacerbated by immobilization. Ambulation helps to reduce bone resorption and normalize serum calcium.[3,4]

Diet

Dietary changes rarely correct hypercalcemia. Patients with sarcoidosis and other granulomatous causes of hypercalcemia or those who have vitamin D-mediated hypercalcemia may benefit from dietary calcium restriction. Limit the use of vitamin D supplements, calcium supplements or calcium-containing antacids in all patients.[3,4]

Hemodialysis

If it is available and can be instituted promptly, hemodialysis (zero or low-calcium bath) provides rapid correction of severe hypercalcemia. It is of particular value in those with severe hypercalcemia and severe renal impairment or heart failure who could not safely tolerate hydration.[3,4]

Table 1: **Using the Duration of Hypercalcemia, Parathyroid Hormone and Parathyroid Hormone-related Peptide Level to Suggest a Diagnosis**

Duration of Hypercalcemia	PTH	PTHrP	Most Likely Diagnosis
Acute or Chronic	High	–	• Primary hyperparathyroidism • Familial hypocalciuric hypercalcemia possible if urine calcium/creatinine ratio <0.02
Acute	Low	High	• Malignancy (perform a more complete clinical evaluation)
Chronic	Low	Low	• Adrenal insufficiency • Drug-induced (e.g., androgens, antiestrogens, derivatives and analogues of vitamin A, estrogens, excess vitamin A or D, ingestion of >3 g elemental calcium per day, lithium, parenteral nutrition, progestins, thiazide diuretics) • Familial disorders • Granulomatous diseases • Hyperthyroidism or milk-alkali syndrome

Abbreviations: PTH = parathyroid hormone; PTHrP = parathyroid hormone-related peptide

Figure 1: **Management of Hypercalcemia**

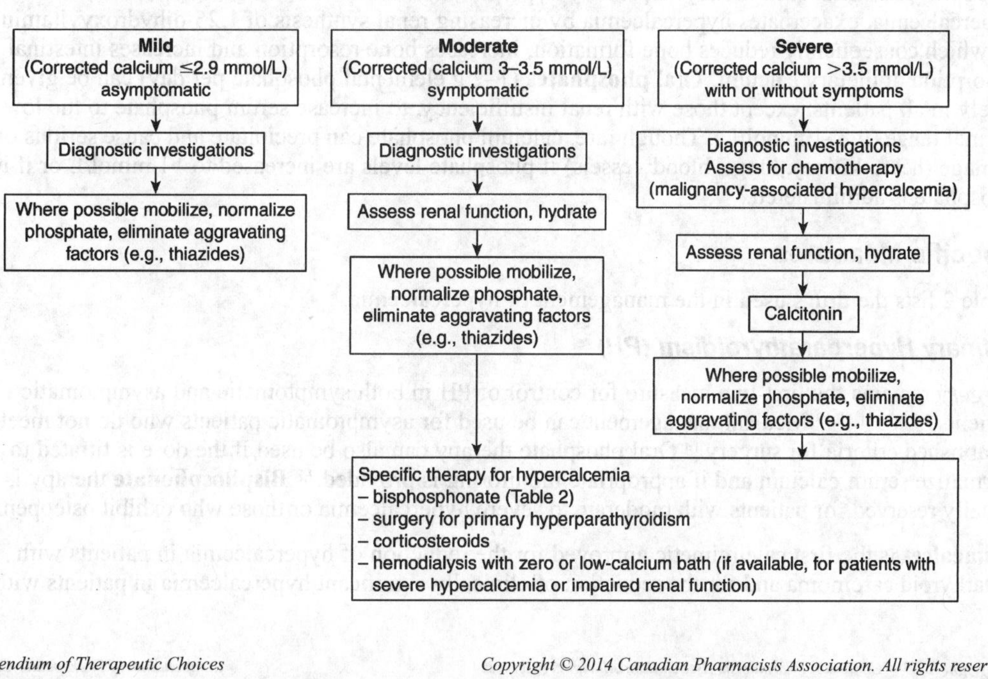

Pharmacologic Choices

General Measures

Stop Offending Agents

If possible, discontinue offending agents (see drug-induced causes in Table 1) and replace with agents that do not exacerbate hypercalcemia.

Fluid Replacement

Patients with hypercalcemia are often dehydrated as a result of a renal water-concentrating defect induced by hypercalcemia and by decreased fluid intake resulting from nausea and vomiting. Expansion of intravascular volume enhances renal calcium clearance. Hydration alone usually reduces serum calcium by ≤0.6 mmol/L. This effect is present only during hydration.[2,3,4] Serum magnesium and potassium may also decrease and should be monitored and replaced as needed.

Patients with mild to moderate asymptomatic hypercalcemia should drink 3 L per day of noncaffeinated beverages to achieve and maintain euvolemia. Patients with moderate to severe symptomatic hypercalcemia should receive **normal saline** (0.9% NaCl) intravenously, typically at 250–500 mL/hour, if safe to do so, until euvolemic, and then reduce the infusion rate to maintain normal intravascular volume. Volume correction may require 2–3 L of fluid within the first 8 hours. Patients with a significant volume deficit may need 3–5 L of fluid in the first 24 hours and 2–3 L per 24 hours thereafter until a good urine output (≥0.5–1 mL/kg/hour) has been established.[5,6,7,8] Renal dysfunction is common among hypercalcemic patients. Careful monitoring of hydration is essential, especially in elderly patients and those with pre-existing renal insufficiency or left ventricular systolic dysfunction as fluid overload can develop. Refer to Figure 1 for further information on the management of mild, moderate and severe hypercalcemia.

Use a loop diuretic (**furosemide**, **ethacrynic acid**) to treat fluid overload and heart failure, as needed, but only after volume depletion is corrected. Thiazide diuretics are contraindicated because they impair calcium excretion.[9,10]

Normalize Serum Phosphate

Hypophosphatemia, seen mostly in primary hyperparathyroidism and malignancy-associated hypercalcemia, exacerbates hypercalcemia by increasing renal synthesis of 1,25-dihydroxyvitamin D, which consequently reduces bone formation, increases bone resorption and increases intestinal absorption of dietary calcium. Oral **phosphates** (1–2 g elemental phosphate per day) can be given safely in all patients, except those with renal insufficiency, to increase serum phosphate to the low normal range (0.8–1 mmol/L). Though rare, calcium phosphate can precipitate and cause serious organ damage (heart, kidney, lungs, blood vessels) if phosphate levels are increased to >1 mmol/L or if iv phosphate is administered.[2]

Specific Measures

Table 2 lists the drugs used in the management of hypercalcemia.

Primary Hyperparathyroidism (PH)

Surgery remains the first-line measure for control of PH in both symptomatic and asymptomatic patients.[1,5,8,10,11,12,13] Medical management can be used for asymptomatic patients who do not meet established criteria for surgery.[14] Oral phosphate therapy can also be used if the dose is titrated to normalize serum calcium and if appropriate monitoring is provided.[7,8] **Bisphosphonate** therapy is usually reserved for patients with moderate to severe hypercalcemia or those who exhibit osteopenia.[11]

Cinacalcet is the first calcimimetic approved for the reduction of hypercalcemia in patients with parathyroid carcinoma and for the reduction of clinically significant hypercalcemia in patients with

PH for whom parathyroidectomy is not clinically appropriate or is contraindicated.[15,16,17,18] Cinacalcet is also indicated for treatment of secondary hyperparathyroidism in patients with chronic kidney disease on dialysis.

Malignancy

Antineoplastic therapy aimed at the underlying malignancy is the key to long-term calcium control, although not all patients are candidates. **Bisphosphonates** are first-line drugs if effective antineoplastic therapy is not available or appropriate, if the patient has severe hypercalcemia (>3.5 mmol/L with or without symptoms) or if the patient has multiple myeloma, breast or lung cancer. For acute management, parenteral **pamidronate**, **clodronate** or **zoledronic acid** may be used.[19,20] Two-hour iv infusion of pamidronate and clodronate is convenient for outpatient therapy (Table 2). Additionally, clodronate can be administered by a subcutaneous infusion, useful in the palliative setting.[21] Zoledronic acid can be infused over 15 minutes in most patients.[22] Response to treatment with an iv bisphosphonate is generally seen within 24–48 hours so they are usually given in conjunction with saline or calcitonin. For patients who respond, serum calcium levels can be maintained at acceptable levels for up to 5 weeks before retreatment is required.[20,23,24] Patients with multiple myeloma benefit from reduced bone pain, decreased skeletal morbidity and prevention of hypercalcemia recurrence with prolonged therapy.[19] There is insufficient evidence to recommend the use of other bisphosphonates (e.g., alendronate, risedronate) for serum calcium control.[25] **Calcitonin** rapidly reduces serum calcium levels in severe hypercalcemia, however, the response tends to abate within 48 hours.[21]

Denosumab, a monoclonal antibody that binds to the bone resorption mediator RANKL, is being investigated as a treatment option for patients with persistent or relapsed hypercalcemia of malignancy despite recent bisphosphonate treatment.[26]

Granulomatous Diseases

Excess production of 1,25-dihydroxyvitamin D is characteristic of granulomatous diseases (e.g., sarcoidosis). Therapy includes restricting vitamin D and calcium intake and avoiding excessive exposure to sunlight. Corticosteroids may be used in acutely ill patients.[7,11]

Therapeutic Tips

- Overly aggressive use of loop diuretics can aggravate hypercalcemia by depleting extracellular fluid volume. Routine prescription of a loop diuretic with hydration therapy is discouraged.[27]
- To reduce serum calcium rapidly (within 6–12 hours) in severe hypercalcemia of malignancy, use **calcitonin** *plus hydration*. Serum calcium usually declines 0.8 mmol/L at 12–24 hours following combined therapy. To augment and prolong serum calcium control, use definitive therapy, e.g., antineoplastic therapy, for the underlying cause. Until antineoplastic therapy takes effect, or if it is not an option, use a **bisphosphonate** when dehydration is corrected and adequate urine output is achieved—preferably within 24 hours of hypercalcemia diagnosis.
- Premedication with **acetaminophen** 650 mg can prevent bisphosphonate-induced fever in patients with hypercalcemia of malignancy.
- Adjunctive corticosteroid therapy, e.g., **prednisone** 40–100 mg/day or equivalent for up to 1 week, is useful in patients with lymphoma, myeloma, lymphoid leukemia and breast cancer, in situations where hypercalcemic flares are caused by hormonal treatment.

Table 2: Drugs Used for the Treatment of Hypercalcemia

Class	Drug	Dose	Adverse Effects	Comments	Cost[a]
Antiparathyroid Hormones	*calcitonin salmon* Calcimar	Initial: 4 IU/kg Q12H sc or im If unsatisfactory response after 1–2 days, may increase to 8 IU/kg Q12H. May increase to a maximum of 8 IU/kg Q6H	Nausea, vomiting (dose dependent), flushing of face and hands. Hypersensitivity reaction.	Used for rapid early effect, i.e., within 6 h. Duration: 1–4 days. Tachyphylaxis develops in 2–7 days; combining with corticosteroids may increase efficacy and reduce tachyphylaxis. Use with bisphosphonate lowers serum Ca^{++} levels more rapidly than with either agent alone. Perform skin test to rule out systemic sensitivity; if marked erythema and/or wheal formation does not occur within 15 min after administration, therapy can begin.	$60/200 IU vial
Bisphosphonates	*clodronate, iv* Bonefos	**Treatment:** Establish and maintain adequate hydration. Single infusion: 1500 mg iv over 4 h diluted in 500 mL of NS or D5W Multiple infusion: 300 mg iv over 2–6 h diluted in 500 mL of NS or D5W Do not dilute with calcium-containing solutions or give as bolus injections.	Mild infusion site toxicity, vomiting. Osteonecrosis of the jaw. (See Comments.) Fatal acute renal failure reported from infusion <2 h.	Onset: 2 days; maximal effect: 6 days. Duration of normocalcemia: variable, 2–3 wk in hypercalcemia of malignancy. Monitor renal function (serum creatinine and/or urea), evaluate within 1 wk after infusion and just prior to next scheduled dose. Osteonecrosis of the jaw: regular dental exam, especially prior to therapy or within 3 months if possible, as well as good oral hygiene.	$70/300 mg vial
	clodronate, oral Bonefos, Clasteon	**Maintenance:** 1600–2400 mg po given once daily or divided BID (2 h AC or 2 h PC) Maximum daily dose is 3200 mg. Ensure adequate fluid rehydration.	Nausea, vomiting, anorexia, diarrhea, muscle cramps. Osteonecrosis of the jaw. (See Comments.)	Concomitant intake of oral iron, calcium, magnesium, aluminum, e.g., antacids, may prevent absorption of oral clodronate. Do not take with or within 1 h before or after food or milk. Reintroduce iv clodronate if elevated serum Ca^{++} present during oral clodronate treatment. Osteonecrosis of the jaw: regular dental exam, especially prior to therapy or within 3 months if possible, as well as good oral hygiene.	$1.30/400 mg capsule

Class	Drug	Dose	Adverse Effects	Comments	Cost[a]
	pamidronate Aredia, generics	**Tumor-induced hypercalcemia:** Adequate hydration with normal saline necessary before treatment. 30–90 mg iv depending on serum Ca^{++}. Consult product monograph for details Not to exceed 90 mg in 250 mL administered over 2–4 h Total dose can be given as a single infusion or divided into smaller infusions given over a period of 2–4 consecutive days. Do not dilute with calcium-containing solutions or give as bolus injections.	Local infusion site reactions, febrile reaction within 24–48 h of infusion—may be accompanied by malaise, rigor, fatigue and flushes.[28] Rare: posterior uveitis.[29] Osteonecrosis of the jaw. (See Comments.)	Onset: 4–72 h; reduction in Ca^{++} levels seen in 24–48 h; maximum lowering occurs in 3–7 days. Duration: 3–4 wk. Repeat infusion if Ca^{++} level does not fall within 7 days or if hypercalcemia recurs. Monitor renal function (serum creatinine and/or urea), evaluate within 1 wk after infusion and just prior to next scheduled dose. Case reports of safe and effective use, without dosage modification, in patients on hemodialysis. Osteonecrosis of the jaw: regular dental exam, especially prior to therapy or within 3 months if possible, as well as good oral hygiene.	$275/90 mg vial
	zoledronic acid Aclasta, Zometa Concentrate, generics	**Tumor-induced hypercalcemia:** Establish and maintain adequate hydration. 4 mg in patients with albumin-corrected serum Ca^{++} ≥3 mmol/L given as a single dose iv infusion over 15 min[20] Retreatment: 8 mg as a single dose over 15 min, in patients demonstrating complete or partial response without normalization of Ca^{++} levels. Use only in patients who can tolerate standard rehydration procedures (3–5 L fluids and >400 mmoL of NaCl per day) Do not dilute with calcium-containing solutions or give as bolus injections.	Febrile reactions, nausea, vomiting, flu-like syndrome, local infusion site reactions, mild hypomagnesemia, hypokalemia and hypophosphatemia.[28] Osteonecrosis of the jaw. (See Comments.) Renal function deterioration reported with infusion <15 min.	Onset: 24–48 h. Duration: 4–5 wk. Monitor renal function, evaluate within 1 wk after infusion and just prior to next scheduled dose. Osteonecrosis of the jaw: regular dental exam, especially prior to therapy or within 3 months if possible, as well as good oral hygiene.	$420/4 mg vial

(cont'd)

Table 2: **Drugs Used for the Treatment of Hypercalcemia** *(cont'd)*

Class	Drug	Dose	Adverse Effects	Comments	Cost[a]
Calcimimetics	*cinacalcet* Sensipar	**Dialysis Patients:** Initial: 30 mg once daily po; titrate every 2–4 wk to a maximum dose of 180 mg once daily to achieve a target PTH level **Primary Hyperparathyroidism:** Initial: 30 mg BID po; titrate every 2–4 wk to 60 mg, then 90 mg BID to reduce serum Ca^{++} levels Moderate to severe hepatic impairment increases drug concentrations by approximately 2- to 4-fold; dosage modification may be required	Nausea, vomiting, diarrhea, myalgia, hypocalcemia.	Inhibits CYP2D6; dose adjustments may be required for concomitant CYP2D6-metabolized drugs with narrow therapeutic index, e.g., tricyclic antidepressants, flecainide. Increases the sensitivity of the Ca^{++}-sensing receptor to circulating serum Ca^{++}, thereby reducing the secretion of PTH. Onset: PTH level reduced within 2–6 h after a dose. Food increases bioavailability. Monitor serum Ca^{++}, serum PO_4 and PTH.	$22/60 mg tablet
Corticosteroids, systemic	*dexamethasone* Dexasone, generics	8 mg BID po for 5–10 days		Slow onset. Potential for diabetes mellitus, osteoporosis, increased susceptibility to infection.	$12.50 for 40 tabs of 4 mg
	hydrocortisone sodium succinate Solu-Cortef, generics	200–300 mg daily iv for 3–5 days		See dexamethasone.	$6/500 mg vial
	prednisone generics	40–60 mg daily po for 5–10 days		See dexamethasone.	$3 for 100 tabs of 5 mg
Crystalloids	*sodium chloride 0.9% (normal saline, NS)* generics	Initial: 200–300 mL/h iv Dependent on concomitant disease states and extent of hypercalcemia		Onset: 24–48 h. Can be given ± other electrolytes. Contraindications: renal insufficiency, heart failure.	$9/1000 mL bag
Diuretics, loop	*furosemide* ❥ generics	Initial: 40–80 mg iv Q1–4H after volume expansion	Electrolyte abnormalities, e.g., hypokalemia, orthostatic hypotension.	Given following aggressive rehydration restoring intravascular volume. Prevents fluid overload and inhibits calcium reabsorption in the distal renal tubule.	$4/40 mg vial

[a] Drug cost only.
Abbreviations: D5W = dextrose 5% in water; NS = normal saline; PTH = parathyroid hormone
❥ Dosage adjustment may be required in renal impairment; see Appendix I

Suggested Readings

Ariyan CE, Sosa JA. Assessment and management of patients with abnormal calcium. *Crit Care Med* 2004;32(4 Suppl):S146-54.

Gasser RW. Clinical aspects of primary hyperparathyroidism: clinical manifestations, diagnosis, and therapy. *Wien Med Wochenschr* 2013;163(17-18):397-402.

Jacob TP, Bilezikian JP. Clinical review: Rare causes of hypercalcemia. *J Clin Endocrinol Metab* 2005;90(11):6316-22.

Reagan P, Pani A, Rosner MH. Approach to diagnosis and treatment of hypercalcemia in a patient with malignancy. *Am J Kidney Dis* 2014;63(1):141-7.

References

1. Carroll MF, Schade DS. A practical approach to hypercalcemia. *Am Fam Physician* 2003;67(9):1959-66.
2. Reagan P, Pani A, Rosner MH. Approach to diagnosis and treatment of hypercalcemia in a patient with malignancy. *Am J Kidney Dis* 2014;63(1):141-7.
3. Shepard MM, Smith JW. Hypercalcemia. *Am J Med Sci* 2007;334(5):381-5.
4. Crowley R, Gittoes N. How to approach hypercalcaemia. *Clin Med* 2013;13(3):287-90.
5. Ralston SH, Coleman R, Fraser WD et al. Medical management of hypercalcemia. *Calcif Tissue Int* 2004;74(1):1-11.
6. Lumachi F, Brunello A, Roma A et al. Cancer-induced hypercalcemia. *Anticancer Res* 2009;29(5):1551-5.
7. Makras P, Papapoulos SE. Medical treatment of hypercalcaemia. *Hormones (Athens)* 2009;8(2):83-95.
8. Bilezikian JP. Clinical review 51: Management of hypercalcemia. *J Clin Endocrinol Metab* 1993;77(6):1445-9.
9. Gasser RW. Clinical aspects of primary hyperparathyroidism: clinical manifestations, diagnosis, and therapy. *Wien Med Wochenschr* 2013;163(17-18):397-402.
10. Silverberg SJ, Walker MD, Bilezikian JP. Asymptomatic primary hyperparathyroidism. *J Clin Densitom* 2013;16(1):14-21.
11. Dowthwaite SA, Young JE, Pasternak JD et al. Surgical management of primary hyperparathyroidism. *J Clin Densitom* 2013;16(1):48-53.
12. Khan AA. Medical management of primary hyperparathyroidism. *J Clin Densitom* 2013;16(1):60-3.
13. Marcocci C, Cetani F. Clinical practice. Primary hyperparathyroidism. *N Engl J Med* 2011;365(25):2389-97.
14. Bilezikian JP, Khan AA, Potts JT et al. Guidelines for the management of asymptomatic primary hyperparathyroidism: summary statement from the third international workshop. *J Clin Endocrinol Metab* 2009;94(2):335-9.
15. Silverberg SJ, Rubin MR, Faiman C et al. Cinacalcet hydrochloride reduces the serum calcium concentration in inoperable parathyroid carcinoma. *J Clin Endocrinol Metab* 2007;92(10):3803-8.
16. Peacock M, Bilezikian JP, Klassen PS et al. Cinacalcet hydrochloride maintains long-term normocalcemia in patients with primary hyperparathyroidism. *J Clin Endocrinol Metab* 2005;90(1):135-41.
17. Peacock M, Bilezikian JP, Bolognese MA et al. Cinacalcet HCl reduces hypercalcemia in primary hyperparathyroidism across a wide spectrum of disease severity. *J Clin Endocrinol Metab* 2011;96(1):E9-E18.
18. Yousaf F, Charytan C. Review of cinacalcet hydrochloride in the management of secondary hyperparathyroidism. *Ren Fail* 2014;36(1):131-8.
19. Lacy MQ, Dispenzieri A, Gertz MA. Mayo Clinic consensus statement for the use of bisphosphonates in multiple myeloma. *Mayo Clin Proc* 2006;81(3):1047-53.
20. Major P, Lortholary A, Hon J et al. Zoledronic acid is superior to pamidronate in the treatment of hypercalcemia of malignancy: a pooled analysis of two randomized, controlled clinical trials. *J Clin Oncol* 2001;19(2):558-67.
21. Berenson JR. Treatment of hypercalcemia of malignancy with bisphosphonates. *Semin Oncol* 2002;29(6 Suppl 21):12-8.
22. Berenson J, Hirschberg R. Safety and convenience of a 15-minute infusion of zoledronic acid. *Oncologist* 2004;9(3):319-29.
23. Watters J, Gerrand G, Dodwell D. The management of malignant hypercalcaemia. *Drugs* 1996;52(6):837-48.
24. Perry CM, Figgitt DP. Zoledronic acid: a review of its use in patients with advanced cancer. *Drugs* 2004;64(11):1197-211.
25. Lteif AN, Zimmerman D. Bisphosphonates for treatment of childhood hypercalcemia. *Pediatrics* 1998;102(4 Pt 1):990-3.
26. Hu MI, Glezerman I, Leboulleux S et al. Denosumab for patients with persistent or relapsed hypercalcemia of malignancy despite recent bisphosphonate treatment. *J Natl Cancer Inst* 2013;105(18):1417-20.
27. LeGrand SB, Leskuski D, Zama I. Narrative review: furosemide for hypercalcemia: an unproven yet common practice. *Ann Intern Med* 2008;149(4):259-63.
28. Woo SB, Hellstein JW, Kalmar JR. Narrative [corrected] review: bisphosphonates and osteonecrosis of the jaws. *Ann Intern Med* 2006;144(10):753-61.
29. Haverbeke G, Pertile G, Claes C et al. Posterior uveitis: an under-recognized adverse effect of pamidronate: 2 case reports. *Bull Soc Belge Ophtalmol* 2003;(290):71-6.

Chapter 104
Hypovolemia

Peter J. McLeod, MD, FRCPC, FACP

Hypovolemia is a generic term encompassing volume depletion and dehydration.[1] Volume depletion is the loss of salt and water from the intravascular space, and is more frequently associated with hypotension and tachycardia than is dehydration. Dehydration, such as from excess sweating, implies loss of water from both extracellular (intravascular and interstitial) and intracellular spaces and leads to elevated plasma Na^+ and osmolality.

Goals of Therapy

- Restore normal volume to relieve symptoms and prevent organ damage

Investigations

- History:
  - symptoms of hypovolemia include thirst, fatigue and postural lightheadedness
  - causes of hypovolemia include: hemorrhage; volume losses from GI tract, kidneys, skin, respiratory tract; fluid sequestration or third-space losses
- Physical exam:
  - determine the presence and severity of hypovolemia
  - pulse: heart rate (HR) increase of more than 30 beats/min after 1 minute of standing from recumbent position is the most accurate sign of volume depletion.[1] Supine tachycardia is insensitive
  - blood pressure: postural decline of systolic pressure of more than 20 mm Hg suggests volume depletion.[1] Severe volume loss may lead to persistently low blood pressure, even while supine
  - Dry axillae support the diagnosis of hypovolemia.[1] Moist mucous membranes and axillae argue against hypovolemia. Abnormal skin turgor, prolonged capillary refill time and decreased eyeball tension are late signs and are insensitive in adults[2]
- Laboratory tests:
  - blood: in hypovolemia, hematocrit and albumin concentrations increase and urea increases disproportionately to creatinine. Sodium concentration may be normal, low or high and is dependent on the type and amount of fluid consumed by the patient in response to thirst.
  - urine: hypovolemia is suggested if urine volume is <0.5 mL/kg/h, if Na^+ is <20 mmol/L or if osmolality is >450 mOsm/kg.[3] Urine specific gravity (SG) is less accurate but SG >1.015 suggests concentrated urine and may indicate hypovolemia

Therapeutic Choices

Therapy is designed to restore volume while replacing ongoing losses (Figure 1). Concurrent fluid and electrolyte disorders will influence choice of fluid used (Table 1). The severity of hypovolemia is expressed as a percentage of total body weight, assuming each litre of fluid lost weighs 1 kg.

Figure 1: **Management of Suspected Hypovolemia**

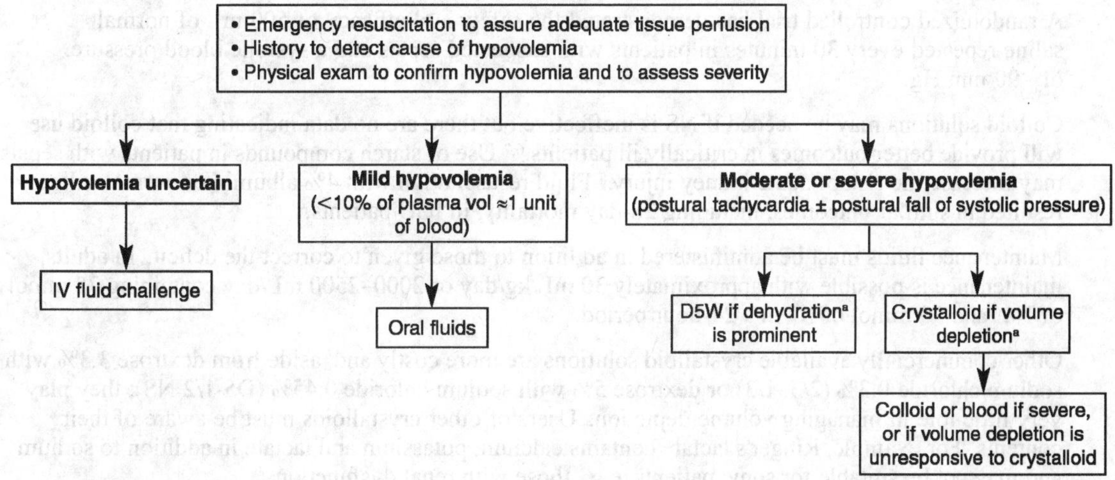

[a] Dehydration refers to loss of intracellular water leading to elevated plasma sodium and osmolality. Patients with dehydration may or may not have hypotension and tachycardia. Volume depletion results from loss of salt and water from the extracellular space. Volume-depleted patients exhibit circulatory instability.

- *Hypovolemia suspected but uncertain:* consider an IV fluid challenge of 250–500 mL of normal saline over 30 minutes. Closely monitor HR and BP to determine if low cardiac output is due to hypovolemia.
- *Mild hypovolemia* (<5% of body weight): oral therapy is usually adequate. Water, juices, soft drinks or soup broth with extra salt or a commercially available electrolyte solution (see Chapter 101) may be used.[4] Rice-based oral solutions have proven effective for diarrheal conditions in developing countries.
- *Moderate* (5–10% of body weight) *or severe* (>10% of body weight) *hypovolemia* or inability to ingest oral fluids: IV therapy is required and 4 types of solutions are used:
  - **dextrose 5% in water** (D5W) distributes throughout total body water and is useful for intracellular volume loss (dehydration). It is a poor plasma volume expander as very little remains in the intravascular space; therefore, it is not useful for managing acute hypotension or tachycardia.
  - **sodium chloride 0.9%** (normal saline or NS) is the fluid of choice for initial treatment of acute hypotension and tachycardia associated with volume depletion. Like other crystalloid solutions, it distributes to extracellular fluid. For every litre infused, about 250 mL remains in the intravascular space and the remainder goes to the interstitial space.[4]
  - **colloid solutions**, including albumin, gelatins (not available in Canada) and starch compounds, are better intravascular volume expanders than NS because they remain in the intravascular space longer than crystalloids. Their cost is high, and the duration of benefit is relatively short; their use as the primary fluid is not justified in most hypovolemic states.
  - **blood** is an excellent intravascular expander. Packed red blood cells with normal saline is indicated for hemorrhagic hypovolemia.

Determining Fluid Requirements

There is no precise formula since disease, age, source and rate of fluid loss influence fluid requirements. In severe and less severe hypovolemia with obvious hemodynamic compromise, begin with at least

1 L of NS over 30 minutes and a second litre over the next hour. Closely monitor HR, BP and jugular venous pressure, watching for improvement or fluid overload. In less severe hypovolemia, give 250–500 mL/hour of NS. Continue fluid administration until treatment goals are achieved. A randomized controlled trial has demonstrated the safety and efficacy of 500 mL of normal saline repeated every 30 minutes in patients with suspected sepsis and a systolic blood pressure of <90 mm Hg.[5]

Colloid solutions may be needed if NS is ineffective but there are no data indicating that colloid use will provide better outcomes in critically ill patients.[6,7] Use of starch compounds in patients with sepsis may increase the risk of acute kidney injury.[8] Fluid resuscitation with 4% albumin or normal saline resulted in similar outcomes, including 28-day mortality, in ICU patients.[9]

Maintenance fluids must be administered in addition to those given to correct the deficit. In adults, maintenance is possible with approximately 30 mL/kg/day or 2000–2500 mL/day containing 75 mmol of Na^+ and 50 mmol of K^+ in a 24-hour period.

Other commercially available crystalloid solutions are more costly and, aside from dextrose 3.3% with sodium chloride 0.3% (2/3–1/3) or dextrose 5% with sodium chloride 0.45% (D5-1/2 NS), they play very little role in managing volume depletion. Users of other crystalloids must be aware of their contents. For example, Ringer's lactate contains calcium, potassium and lactate in addition to sodium and may not be suitable for some patients, e.g., those with renal dysfunction.

Therapeutic Tips

- If presence of hypovolemia is uncertain, consider a fluid challenge.
- Normal saline is the fluid of first choice for patients with hypotension and tachycardia associated with volume depletion. Dextrose in water is a poor plasma volume expander.
- Additional potassium may be required for fluid loss associated with diarrhea, vomiting or over-diuresis.
- Colloid solutions are usually reserved as second-line plasma volume expanders; burns and other volume losses containing protein may require additional colloid.

Table 1: **Intravenous Solutions for Hypovolemia**

Class	Drug	Use	Adverse Effects	Comments
Crystalloids	*sodium chloride 0.9%, normal saline or NS (Na$^+$ 154 mmol/L)* generics	Initial treatment of hypovolemia.	Fluid overload; peripheral edema. Dilutional coagulopathy. Hyperchloremic metabolic acidosis with infusion of large amounts of NS (usually >3 L). Hypernatremia.	IV solutions with Na$^+$ concentrations that approximate normal serum Na$^+$ cause more intravascular and interstitial expansion than do D5W solutions.
	Ringer's lactate (Na$^+$ 130 mmol/L) Lactated Ringer's Injection, generics	Initial treatment of hypovolemia.	Fluid overload; peripheral edema. Dilutional coagulopathy. Hyponatremia. May aggravate pre-existing hyperkalemia.	Contains Ca^{++} 1.4 mmol/L, K^+ 4 mmol/L, Cl^- 109 mmol/L, lactate 28 mmol/L.
	dextrose 5% with sodium chloride 0.9%, D5W-NS (Na$^+$ 154 mmol/L) generics	Hypovolemia and dehydration.	See sodium chloride 0.9%.	See sodium chloride 0.9%. Compared to NS or Ringer's lactate, D5W results in comparatively small changes in plasma volume because it distributes throughout the total body water space, including the intracellular space.
	dextrose 5% in water, D5W generics	Dehydration; poor plasma volume expander.		Water is distributed to both intracellular fluid and extracellular fluid after dextrose metabolism.
	sodium chloride 0.45%, half-normal saline or 1/2 NS (Na$^+$ 77 mmol/L) generics	Maintenance fluids.	See sodium chloride 0.9%.	See sodium chloride 0.9%.
	dextrose 3.3% with sodium chloride 0.3%, 2/3–1/3 (Na$^+$ 51 mmol/L) generics	Maintenance fluids.	See sodium chloride 0.9%.	See sodium chloride 0.9%.
	dextrose 5% with sodium chloride 0.45%, D5W-1/2NS (Na$^+$ 77 mmol/L) generics	Maintenance fluids.	See sodium chloride 0.9%.	See sodium chloride 0.9%.

(cont'd)

Table 1: **Intravenous Solutions for Hypovolemia** *(cont'd)*

Class	Drug	Use	Adverse Effects	Comments
Colloids	*albumin* Alburex, Plasbumin-5, Plasbumin-25, generics	Volume expander, useful for hypoproteinemic hypovolemia. Used to replace or in conjunction with crystalloids. Volume remains within the extracellular compartment. Contraindicated in patients at risk of circulatory overload such as those with history of HF, renal insufficiency or stabilized chronic anemia.	Rare: anaphylactoid/anaphylaxis. Fluid overload.	Albumin 5% is iso-oncotic (does not pull fluid into the intravascular space) with normal plasma; IV infusion will expand circulating blood volume by an amount approximately equal to the amount infused; does not aggravate tissue dehydration; concomitant use of crystalloids may be necessary to maintain fluid balance. Albumin 25% is used in situations of oncotic deficit, e.g., blood loss due to surgery or trauma; may be used when treatment of shock has been delayed. IV infusion will expand plasma volume 3–4 times the volume infused. May be used in patients with clinical evidence of both edema and hypovolemia, i.e., is normally hydrated or interstitial edema is present. May be used in combination with crystalloids.
	blood	Packed cells with saline indicated for hemorrhage.	Fluid overload.	Replaces or increases oxygen-carrying capacity but only if not stored for >3–5 days.
	dextrans generics	Volume expander.	Aggravation of bleeding; interfere with blood coagulation. Anaphylaxis with higher molecular weight solutions.	Not used as plasma expanders as frequently as albumin and starch compounds.
	hetastarch 6% in lactated electrolyte Hextend	Volume expander.	Bleeding, fluid overload, pruritus. Macroamylase formation may lead to incorrect diagnosis of pancreatitis because of possibility of increase in blood amylase. Rare: anaphylactoid reaction.	Hetastarch exhibits comparable plasma expansion with respect to 5% albumin solution. Contraindicated in patients at risk of circulatory overload such as those with history of HF, renal insufficiency or stabilized chronic anemia.
	hydroxyethyl starch (tetrastarch) 6% in isotonic electrolyte or normal saline, respectively Volulyte, Voluven	Volume expander.	See hetastarch.	See hetastarch.

Suggested Readings

Brenner BM, Rector FC, eds. *Brenner and Rector's the kidney*. 6th ed. Philadelphia (PA): Saunders; 2000.

Halperin ML, Goldstein MB. *Fluid, electrolyte, and acid-base physiology a problem-based approach*. 2nd ed. Philadelphia (PA): Saunders; 1994.

Maxwell MH, Kleeman CR, Narins RG. *Maxwell & Kleeman's clinical disorders of fluid and electrolyte metabolism*. 5th ed. New York (NY): McGraw-Hill, Health Professions Division; 1994.

McGee S, Abernethy WB, Simel DL. The rational clinical examination. Is this patient hypovolemic? *JAMA* 1999;281(11):1022-9.

References

1. McGee S, Abernethy WB, Simel DL. The rational clinical examination. Is this patient hypovolemic? *JAMA* 1999;281(11):1022-9.
2. Webb AR. Recognizing hypovolaemia. *Minerva Anesthesiol* 2001;67(4):185-9.
3. Sterns RH. Renal function and disorders of water and sodium balance. In: *Scientific American medicine*. New York (NY): WebMD Professional Publishing; 2002.
4. Boldt J. Volume replacement in the surgical patient--does the type of solution make a difference? *Br J Anaesth* 2000;84(6):783-93.
5. Rivers E, Nguyen B, Havstad S et al. Early goal-directed therapy in the treatment of severe sepsis and septic shock. *N Engl J Med* 2001;345(19):1368-77.
6. Webb AR. The appropriate role of colloids in managing fluid imbalance: a critical review of recent meta-analytic findings. *Crit Care* 2000;4(Suppl 2):S26-32.
7. Perel P, Roberts I, Ker K. Colloids versus crystalloids for fluid resuscitation in critically ill patients. *Cochrane Database Syst Rev* 2013;2:CD000567.
8. Dart AB, Mutter TC, Ruth CA et al. Hydroxyethyl starch (HES) versus other fluid therapies: effects on kidney function. *Cochrane Database Syst Rev* 2010;(1):CD007594.
9. Finfer S, Bellomo R, Boyce N et al. A comparison of albumin and saline for fluid resuscitation in the intensive care unit. *N Engl J Med* 2004;350(22):2247-56.

Chapter 105
Potassium Disturbances

Jean Ethier, MD, FRCPC

Potassium, the major intracellular cation in the human body, is found in abundance in fruits (e.g., tomatoes, cucumbers), vegetables (e.g., leafy greens) and meats. The average dietary daily intake is 100 mEq. Normal potassium concentration is 3.5–5 mmol/L.

Hypokalemia, defined as a plasma potassium concentration of less than 3.5 mmol/L, can be mild (3–3.5 mmol/L), moderate (2.5–3 mmol/L) or severe (<2.5 mmol/L). *Hyperkalemia*, defined as a plasma concentration of greater than 5 mmol/L, can be mild (5–6 mmol/L), moderate (6.1–6.5 mmol/L) or severe (>6.5 mmol/L). Hypokalemia and hyperkalemia are associated with potentially fatal cardiac arrhythmias.

Goals of Therapy

- Prevent life-threatening cardiac arrhythmias and improve neuromuscular conductivity
- Re-establish normal body stores of potassium (K^+) and prevent undue losses or accumulations
- Identify and correct underlying causes

Investigations

- History with attention to possible etiology (see Table 1)
- Physical examination to assess cardiac rhythm, paresis, muscle weakness, paresthesias, blood pressure (consider hyperaldosteronism in the presence of hypokalemia and high blood pressure)
- ECG when clinically necessary
- Laboratory tests may be useful in assessing hypokalemia or hyperkalemia, if not already evident:
  - urea, creatinine, Na^+, K^+, Cl^-, glucose
  - arterial or venous blood gases or total CO_2
  - spot urine for Na^+, K^+, Cl^- and osmolality to calculate the transtubular K^+ concentration gradient (TTKG) and the potassium-creatinine ratio and, in select cases, 24-hour urine collection for Na^+, K^+ and creatinine
  - aldosterone, cortisol, renin, screening tests for adrenal disease, TSH for thyrotoxicosis, renal artery imaging in select cases
  - magnesium in refractory hypokalemia, especially when patient is at risk for hypomagnesemia, e.g., diarrhea or taking cisplatin, diuretics or proton pump inhibitor
  - rule out pseudohyperkalemia (possible with thrombocytosis, severe leukocytosis, in vitro hemolysis or forearm contraction)[1]

Table 1: **Causes of Potassium Disturbances**

Hyperkalemia	Hypokalemia
Drug-induced: ACE inhibitors, aliskiren, aminocaproic acid, angiotensin II receptor blockers (ARBs), beta-blockers, cyclosporine, digoxin overdose, drospirenone, heparin, K^+ supplements, K^+-sparing diuretics, ketoconazole, NSAIDs, penicillin G potassium, pentamidine, succinylcholine, tacrolimus, trimethoprim or TMP/SMX (high-dose or in susceptible patients, i.e., elderly, renal failure), some herbal and nutritional supplements (e.g., alfalfa, nettle) especially in the presence of renal failure	Diarrhea, vomiting Inadequate dietary intake Drug-induced: aminoglycosides, amphotericin B, antipseudomonal penicillins, $beta_2$-agonists, caffeine, foscarnet, insulin, laxatives, licorice, long-term corticosteroid therapy, loop and thiazide diuretics, theophylline, tocolytic agents Familial history (Bartter's or Gitelman's syndrome) Mineralocorticoid excess (e.g., primary aldosteronism)
Renal failure, diabetes, adrenal insufficiency, hyporeninemic hypoaldosteronism	Renovascular disease Metabolic alkalosis
Familial history of hyperkalemia	Osmotic diuresis (diabetes)
Acidosis	Hypomagnesemia
Crush injury, trauma, hemolysis, tumor lysis, massive transfusions	Increased sweat loss Dialysis/plasmapheresis

Abbreviations: ACE = angiotensin converting enzyme; TMP/SMX = trimethoprim/sulfamethoxazole

Hyperkalemia

Therapeutic Choices

Nonpharmacologic Choices

- Stop K^+ supplements and/or drugs inducing hyperkalemia (see Table 1). If necessary, resume K^+ supplements at a reduced dose once the hyperkalemia is resolved.
- Reduce dietary K^+ intake to ≤60 mmol/day.

In mild hyperkalemia (plasma K^+ 5–6 mmol/L) these measures are usually sufficient. Increasing K^+ level, ongoing K^+ load or renal failure require further measures, e.g., hemodialysis.

Pharmacologic Choices

Do not rely only on the plasma K^+ or ECG to determine the urgency of treatment. Changes in the ECG have an uncertain diagnostic and prognostic significance. Cardiac toxicity depends not only on the level of plasma K^+ but also on the rate of increase, chronicity of hyperkalemia, levels of other electrolytes (hypocalcemia, hyponatremia and acidosis increase cardiotoxicity) and cardiac irritability. Consider all these factors.

In severe hyperkalemia (K^+>6.5 mmol/L) or when significant or advanced ECG changes are present (loss of P waves or widening of QRS complexes), *continuous cardiac monitoring* should accompany treatment. Give **iv calcium** promptly and begin **insulin**. Initiate K^+ removal simultaneously (Figure 1, Table 2).

In less severe situations, K^+ removal with or without redistribution agents (e.g., insulin) may be sufficient. Estimate renal function and ongoing gain of K^+ in extracellular fluid. Initiate treatment early and more aggressively when renal failure is present or there is rapid and severe input of K^+ (e.g., rhabdomyolysis, tumor lysis syndrome) than when there is slow or no input (e.g., hyperkalemia induced by K^+-sparing diuretics).

Membrane Antagonists

Calcium gluconate or **calcium chloride** antagonize the adverse cardiac effects of K^+ and should be used in the presence of ECG changes or a high risk of cardiotoxicity since they are fast acting. Calcium iv has a rapid onset but relatively short duration of action and should be administered simultaneously with other treatments.

Redistribution Agents

These agents act for a longer period than membrane antagonists. Stimulation of insulin and beta receptors as well as correcting acidosis facilitates the reuptake of K^+ into cells.

Insulin should be the first choice since it is the most effective and reliable agent. Insulin must be administered iv.[2] **Glucose** (40–50 g per 10 units insulin) is given to avoid hypoglycemia, but avoid bolus administration because an acute increase in plasma tonicity can induce a rise in plasma K^+. Expect a 1–1.5 mmol/L fall in plasma K^+ in 60 minutes.

Sodium bicarbonate ($NaHCO_3$) is usually reserved for hyperkalemia associated with significant metabolic acidosis. It has a synergistic effect with insulin in the presence of mild acidosis.[3] In the absence of low serum bicarbonate concentration or pH, sodium bicarbonate has a smaller effect.[4] To avoid an acute increase in plasma K^+ induced by an osmolality change, hypertonic $NaHCO_3$ solutions should not be used.[5] The correction of acidosis in hypocalcemic patients may induce tetany. Insulin administration is faster, more reliable and more effective than sodium bicarbonate.[2]

Figure 1: **Management of Hyperkalemia**

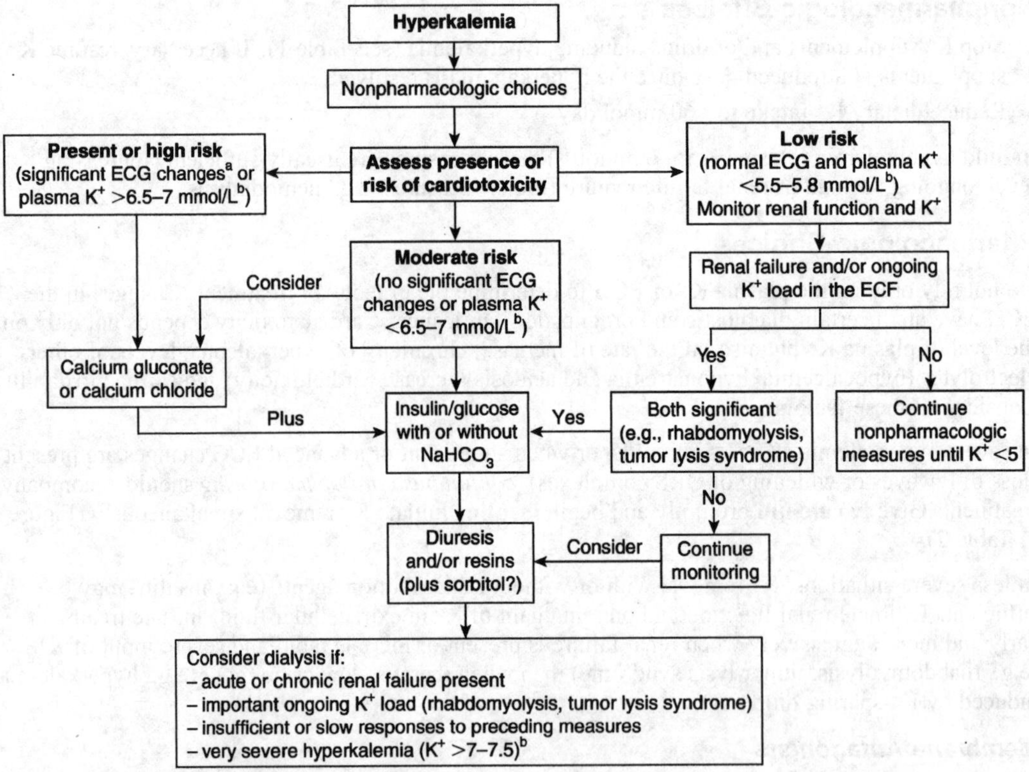

[a] Loss of P waves, widening of QRS complexes or more severe changes are considered significant. Isolated peaked T waves may not be significant. Note that ECG changes have uncertain prognostic significance.
[b] Plasma potassium level is given as a guide; therapy should not rely on the plasma level alone, but consider all other risk factors for cardiotoxicity (see text).
Abbreviations: ECF = extracellular fluid

The $beta_2$-agonist **salbutamol** is effective in lowering plasma K^+ [Evidence: SORT C*].[6] Concurrent administration of insulin and salbutamol has a synergistic effect.[7] High doses of nebulized salbutamol have an effect similar to iv salbutamol;[8] however, up to 50% of patients with chronic renal failure are resistant to this therapy.[9] Administration using a metered-dose inhaler and spacer is also effective.[10] Reserve salbutamol for patients at low risk of coronary artery disease or for life-threatening situations when other therapies have failed, because it is arrhythmogenic and has the potential to exacerbate angina.

Potassium Removal

In patients with volume contraction and oliguria (prerenal disease), volume repletion should be implemented to quickly improve renal K^+ excretion.

The administration of **loop diuretics** in patients with sufficient renal function can significantly increase renal K^+ excretion. Provide enough fluid with the diuretic to avoid volume contraction.

If large amounts of K^+ must be removed rapidly, hemodialysis is the technique of choice. Because time is required to prepare the equipment and to insert a catheter, other treatments must be initiated while preparing for dialysis. Peritoneal dialysis is far less efficient in acutely reducing plasma K^+.

Cation-exchange resins (sodium polystyrene sulfonate, calcium polystyrene sulfonate) promote the exchange of Na^+ and Ca^{++} for K^+, respectively, in the bowel; they also bind calcium and magnesium. Despite their theoretical value and their widespread clinical use with apparent efficacy, the K^+-lowering effect of single-dose resin-cathartic therapy is subject to debate.[6,11,12,13] The addition of resins does not seem to increase bowel K^+ removal above the effect of the diarrhea induced by the simultaneous administration of osmotic or secretory cathartics.[14] Because cation-exchange resins are constipating, it is suggested that they are given with a **laxative**.

Resins have serious side effects. The Na^+ released in exchange for K^+ may lead to volume overload. Rectal ulceration or colonic necrosis has been described when sodium polystyrene sulfonate mixed in **sorbitol** is given orally or by enema.[15] Necrosis may be caused by sorbitol rather than by resins.[16,17] The duration of drug contact with the mucosa may be a risk factor. A cleansing enema (sodium-free) is recommended to reduce this risk. Do not use sorbitol when the resin is administered by enema, especially in postoperative patients.

Given the potential problems with cation-exchange resins some recommend trying all other alternatives for managing hyperkalemia first.[12] Others feel that resins should continue to be used when indicated, preferably administered in water.[13] Resins in sorbitol should not be used in the immediate postsurgical period, or in patients with compromised gastrointestinal function.[13]

Therapeutic Tips

- Focus the treatment of chronic hyperkalemia on the cause or pathophysiological mechanism (Table 1). The treatments are similar to those used in acute hyperkalemia (diuretics, $NaHCO_3$, resins).
- The mineralocorticoid 9-alpha-**fludrocortisone** may be used in patients with hypoaldosteronism or renal resistance to mineralocorticoids.
- Closely monitor K^+ after introducing or changing the dose of any medication that could induce hyperkalemia such as ACE inhibitors, aliskiren, ARB, K^+-sparing diuretics, in particular in patients at risk of hyperkalemia, e.g., renal failure, elderly, cardiac insufficiency. Monitoring is even more important when a combination of these medications is prescribed (ACE inhibitor + ARB + spironolactone). In this case measure K^+ 3 and 7 days after the introduction of these medications

* SORT (Strength of Recommendation Taxonomy) is a rating system (A, B or C) that addresses the quality of available evidence. For more information consult **How to Use *Compendium of Therapeutic Choices*** on page xxv.

and after any change in the dose.[18] In addition, measure creatinine and K^+ at least monthly for 3 months[19] and, if stable, every 3 months thereafter.

Hypokalemia

Therapeutic Choices

Nonpharmacologic Choices

- If clinically appropriate reduce or stop medication leading to K^+ loss.
- Determine and treat the etiology (Table 1).
- If the deficit is mild (plasma K^+ 3–3.5 mmol/L) and there are no ongoing losses or clinical conditions warranting prompt treatment, dietary intake of potassium-rich foods should be adequate. If there are still unusual losses, K^+ supplements or K^+-sparing diuretics will be needed.

Pharmacologic Choices

The appropriate pharmacologic approach is determined by:

- Relative urgency for treatment.
- The estimated total body deficit for an adult with plasma K^+ of 3 mmol/L is approximately 200–400 mmol and for plasma K^+ of 2 mmol/L, approximately 500–700 mmol. *Note:* The true deficit will be larger with an extracellular shift of K^+ (e.g., acidosis or insulin deficit) and smaller with an intracellular shift of K^+, (e.g., periodic paralysis or hyperadrenergic state).
- Ongoing losses must be added to the deficit when replacement therapy is planned. Renal losses can be estimated based on urine K^+ levels and the volume excreted per hour.
- In the presence of renal failure the treatment should be more cautious.

Potassium Salts

In most cases **potassium chloride** (KCl) is the salt of choice (Table 3), and oral administration is the preferred route. If there is no paralytic ileus or suspected absorption problem, oral administration of KCl can rapidly increase plasma K^+ (40–60 mmol of a liquid preparation will increase plasma K^+ by 1–1.5 mmol/L).

Reserve **potassium bicarbonate** or **potassium citrate** for hypokalemic patients with metabolic acidosis (e.g., renal tubular acidosis, diarrhea). **Potassium phosphate** is used when severe hypophosphatemia is present.

Reserve iv administration of K^+ for patients requiring urgent treatment (e.g., respiratory muscle weakness, cardiac arrhythmias especially if digitalis is present, hepatic encephalopathy) or those unable to take oral supplements (e.g., postsurgery, paralytic ileus). To avoid sclerosis, iv K^+ should be administered via a large peripheral vein at a maximum concentration of 40–60 mmol/L. Administer higher concentrations via a central line with the catheter positioned away from the right atrium or ventricle. In patients with severe hypokalemia, administer K^+ in a dextrose-free solution to avoid stimulating insulin secretion and subsequent intracellular K^+ shift.[20] Administering K^+ iv rather than po is more likely to result in hyperkalemia. Thrombophlebitis and pain at site of injection are other risks.

The *rate of administration* depends on the urgency to treat (Table 3). Protocols for the treatment of hypokalemia in the hospital setting have been proposed.[21,22]

Potassium-sparing Diuretics

If renal K^+ losses are involved in the pathogenesis of hypokalemia (e.g., hyperaldosteronism, concomitant use of other diuretics), K^+-sparing diuretics (Table 4) may be used to decrease these losses; they also prevent or decrease magnesium losses. **Amiloride**, **spironolactone** and **triamterene** (triamterene is available only in combination with hydrochlorothiazide in Canada) are equally effective but differ in side effects. Use spironolactone in patients with primary or secondary hyperaldosteronism. The most frequent and serious side effect is hyperkalemia.

Avoid K^+-sparing diuretics in patients with renal or adrenal insufficiency, the elderly, patients with diabetes and patients taking other drugs that may increase plasma K^+ (Table 1).

Therapeutic Tips

- Avoid the use of K^+ supplements and K^+-sparing diuretics together as the risk of hyperkalemia is greatly increased. Combined use may be required temporarily at the beginning of replacement therapy if renal K^+ losses are very high; however, frequent monitoring of plasma K^+ is mandatory, and one of the drugs should be stopped when plasma K^+ reaches 3–3.5 mmol/L.
- Treat hypomagnesemia if present.

Table 2: **Drugs Used in the Treatment of Hyperkalemia**

Class	Drug	Dose	Comments
Beta$_2$-adrenergic Agonists	*salbutamol* Ventolin HFA, Ventolin Nebules P.F., generics	10–20 mg by nebulizer 1200 µg by pMDI with spacer Onset: 30 min Duration of action: 2–4 h	Reserved for life-threatening cases when other treatments have failed; risk of arrhythmia or angina; variable response.
Cation-exchange Resins	*sodium polystyrene sulfonate* Kayexalate, Solystat, generics	**Oral:** 15–60 g in 50–100 mL of 20% sorbitol Q4–6H PRN; usual dose: 30 g. Do not mix with orange juice or other fruit juices with high potassium content Onset: 1–2 h **Rectal:** 30–50 g in 100–200 mL of water or 10% dextrose Q4–6H PRN; retain at least 30–60 min Onset: 30–60 min Duration of action: 4–6 h	Effectiveness seriously questioned. Laxative alone might be as effective. Constipating; risk of bowel ulceration or necrosis. Cleansing enema before pr use recommended. Cleansing enema after pr use to be given after evacuation of the resins or after retention for 1–6 h. Available as powder and rectal suspension. Sodium overload may be a concern.
	calcium polystyrene sulfonate Resonium Calcium	**Oral:** 15 g 3 or 4 times daily. May mix resin into a paste with sweetened vehicle. Do not mix with orange juice or other fruit juices with high potassium content **Rectal:** 30 g in 100 mL methylcellulose 2% plus 100 mL of water as a daily retention enema; if possible, enema should be retained for 9 h	See sodium polystyrene sulfonate. Use if sodium overload is a concern. Avoid concomitant administration of sorbitol with calcium polystyrene sulfonate as use has been associated with colonic necrosis and intestinal obstruction.
Diuretics	*furosemide* ❥ Lasix, generics	40–250 mg po/iv depending on renal function Onset: 30–60 min Duration of action: to end of increased diuresis (about 4–6 h)	Risk of volume depletion; transient ototoxicity with high-dose furosemide.
Electrolytes	*calcium gluconate 10%* generics	10 mL iv over 2–5 min; may repeat once after 5 min (depending on ECG) Onset: 1–3 min Duration of action: 30–60 min	Continuous ECG monitoring required; infuse more slowly in patients taking digoxin because of increased risk of digoxin toxicity; incompatible with $NaHCO_3$-containing solutions (precipitation). 1 g calcium gluconate = 93 mg elemental calcium = 4.6 mEq elemental calcium = 2.3 mmol elemental calcium.
	calcium chloride generics	5–10 mL iv over 2–5 min; may repeat once after 5 min (depending on ECG) Onset: 1–3 min Duration of action: 30–60 min	Continuous ECG monitoring required; infuse more slowly in patients taking digoxin because of increased risk of digoxin toxicity; incompatible with $NaHCO_3$-containing solutions (precipitation). Recommended in cardiac arrest in the presence of hyperkalemia or hypocalcemia or magnesium toxicity. May cause tissue necrosis if extravasation occurs. 1 g calcium chloride = 270 mg elemental calcium = 14 mEq elemental calcium = 7 mmol elemental calcium.

Class	Drug	Dose	Comments
	sodium bicarbonate	50–100 mmol iv over 5 min; repeat Q10–15 min (depending on ECG) Onset: variable, within 1 h Duration of action: 2 h	Variable response; risk of tetany if hypocalcemia present (give calcium first); watch for Na^+ overload. Can induce bicarbonaturia with an incease in renal K^+ excretion. Hypertonic $NaHCO_3$ solutions should not be used.
Insulin	*insulin, regular with glucose*	Bolus: 5–10 units iv with dextrose 25–50 g over 5 min. If less urgent, infuse 10 units insulin in 500 mL dextrose 10% at the rate of 50–100 mL/h Onset: 30 min Duration of action: 4–6 h	The most reliable medication for redistribution of K^+. Risk of hypoglycemia. Avoid bolus administration of glucose because acute increase in plasma tonicity can increase K^+ in plasma.

Dosage adjustment may be required in renal impairment; see Appendix I.
Abbreviations: $NaHCO_3$ = sodium bicarbonate; pMDI = pressurized metered dose inhaler

Table 3: Potassium Supplements Used in the Management of Hypokalemia

Class	Drug	Indications	Dose	Adverse Effects	Comments	Cost[a]
Potassium Supplements, intravenous	*potassium salts, intravenous* generics	**Urgent (immediate treatment required):** Severe hypokalemia (plasma K^+ <2.5 mmol/L) Symptomatic hypokalemia (respiratory muscle weakness or paresis, paralysis) Cardiac arrhythmia or conduction disturbances **Less urgent (prompt treatment required):** Plasma K^+ = 2.5–3 mmol/L Hypokalemia with digitalis toxicity, myocardial infarction or ischemia Hypokalemia with diabetic ketoacidosis (risk of insulin-induced life-threatening hypokalemia) Hypokalemia with hepatic insufficiency (risk of hepatic encephalopathy)	**Urgent (immediate treatment required):** 20–40 mmol iv in the first hour with continuous ECG monitoring and frequent serum K^+ measurements to adjust further rate of administration. When plasma K^+ = 3 mmol/L, correct the remaining deficit more slowly. **Less urgent (prompt treatment required):** 10–20 mmol iv over 1 hour (increase serum K^+ by 0.25–0.5 mmol/L)[23,24] with ECG monitoring if >10 mmol/h. Should be repeated according to resulting serum K^+. Correct the remaining deficit more slowly.	Sclerosis: Administer via a large peripheral vein at a maximum concentration of 40–60 mmol/L. Cardiac arrhythmias and other effects if infusion too rapid.	Doses >40 mmol/h have been given in life-threatening hypokalemia.[25] Potassium (20–40 mmol) can be diluted in 100 mL NaCl 0.9% if administered via a central vein. A maximum concentration of 10 mmol in 100 mL NaCl 0.9% can be administered in a large peripheral vein; however, it could induce pain and sclerosis of the vein. Measure serum K+ frequently when a large dose is administered. Measure each time after the administration of 20–40 mmol.	$$
Potassium Supplements, oral	*potassium chloride, oral liquid or powder* K-10 (20 mEq K^+/15 mL), generics	**Not urgent:** Plasma K^+ >3–3.5 mmol/L	Initially, 40–60 mmol/day po (divided 2–4 times daily), is usually sufficient	Unpleasant taste, aftertaste, nausea, heartburn.	Salt of choice, especially in alkalotic patients. Rapid absorption, good bioavailability. Avoid use with potassium-sparing diuretics because of increased risk of severe hyperkalemia. If combination therapy is required, frequent monitoring (at least every day) of plasma K^+ is mandatory; discontinue one of the drugs when plasma K^+ reaches 3–3.5 mmol/L. Salt substitutes also contain potassium chloride.	$–$$

Class	Drug	Indications	Dose	Adverse Effects	Comments	Cost[a]
	potassium chloride, oral wax matrix tablet Slow-K (8 mEq K^+/tab), generics	**Not urgent:** Plasma K^+ >3–3.5 mmol/L	Initially, 40–60 mmol/day po (divided doses), is usually sufficient	GI symptoms, though less frequent than with liquid, GI ulceration (rare).	See potassium chloride, oral liquid or powder. Avoid in patients with delayed GI transit or impaired esophageal or intestinal motility. Empty wax matrix may appear in stool.	$
	potassium chloride, oral micro-encapsulated K-Dur (20 mEq K^+/tab), generics Micro-K Extencaps (8 mEq K^+/cap)	**Not urgent:** Plasma K^+ >3–3.5 mmol/L	Initially, 40–60 mmol/day po (divided doses), is usually sufficient	May be less ulceration than with wax matrix.	See potassium chloride, oral liquid or powder. Avoid in patients with delayed GI transit or impaired esophageal or intestinal motility.	$
	potassium citrate, oral effervescent tablets K-Lyte (25 mEq K^+/tab)	**Not urgent:** Plasma K^+ >3–3.5 mmol/L	Initially, 40–60 mmol/day po (divided doses), is usually sufficient	See potassium chloride, oral liquid or powder.	Avoid use with potassium-sparing diuretics because of increased risk of severe hyperkalemia. If combination therapy is required, frequent monitoring of plasma K^+ is mandatory; discontinue one of the drugs when plasma K^+ reaches 3–3.5 mmol/L. Useful for patients with metabolic acidosis. More convenient for transport. Useful for hypokalemia secondary to thiazides given for kidney stones. Increases urinary citrate excretion.	$$
	potassium citrate, oral tablets K-Citra	**Not urgent:** Plasma K^+ >3–3.5 mmol/L	Initially, 40–60 mmol/day po (divided doses), is usually sufficient	See potassium chloride, oral liquid or powder.	See potassium citrate, oral effervescent tablets. Also contains 10 mEq of bicarbonate per 5 mL of oral solution.	$
	potassium gluconate, oral liquid generics	**Not urgent:** Plasma K^+ >3–3.5 mmol/L	Initially, 40–60 mmol/day po (divided doses), is usually sufficient	See potassium chloride, oral liquid or powder.	See potassium chloride, oral liquid or powder. Useful in patients with acidosis.	$

[a] Cost of 30-day supply of a 20 mmol/day dose; includes drug cost only.

Dosage adjustment may be required in renal impairment; see Appendix I.

Legend: $ <$10 $-$$ <$10–20 $$ $10–20

Table 4: Potassium-sparing Diuretics Used in the Management of Hypokalemia

Class	Drug	Dose	Adverse Effects	Drug Interactions	Cost[a]
Diuretics, potassium-sparing	*spironolactone* Aldactone, generics	25–200 mg/day po (in single or divided doses). Up to 400 mg/day in patients with hyperaldosteronism	Hyperkalemia, gynecomastia, androgen-like side effects, breast tenderness, gastrointestinal symptoms.	Avoid NSAIDs, ACE inhibitors, aliskiren, angiotensin II receptor blockers, K^+ supplements: may cause severe hyperkalemia.	$
	amiloride Midamor, generics	5–20 mg/day po	Hyperkalemia, muscle cramps, headaches, gastrointestinal symptoms (rare).	See spironolactone.	$–$$

[a] Cost of 30-day supply; includes drug cost only.

Dosage adjustment may be required in renal impairment; see Appendix I.

Abbreviations: ACE = angiotensin converting enzyme; NSAID = nonsteroidal anti-inflammatory agent

Legend: $ <$20 $-$$ <$20–40 $$ $20–40

Suggested Readings

Cohn JN, Kowey PR, Whelton PK et al. New guidelines for potassium replacement in clinical practice: a contemporary review by the National Council on Potassium in Clinical Practice. *Arch Intern Med* 2000;160(16):2429-36.

Perazella MA. Drug-induced hyperkalemia: old culprits and new offenders. *Am J Med* 2000;109(4):307-14.

Rastegar A, Soleimani M. Hypokalaemia and hyperkalaemia. *Postgrad Med J* 2001;77(914):759-64.

References

1. Smellie WS. Spurious hyperkalaemia. *BMJ* 2007;334(7595):693-5.
2. Blumberg A, Weidmann P, Shaw S et al. Effect of various therapeutic approaches on plasma potassium and major regulating factors in terminal renal failure. *Am J Med* 1988;85(4):507-12.
3. Kim HJ. Combined effect of bicarbonate and insulin with glucose in acute therapy of hyperkalemia in end-stage renal disease patients. *Nephron* 1996;72(3):476-82.
4. Blumberg A, Weidmann P, Ferrari P. Effect of prolonged bicarbonate administration on plasma potassium in terminal renal failure. *Kidney Int* 1992;41(2):369-74.
5. Conte G, Dal Canton A, Imperatore P et al. Acute increase in plasma osmolality as a cause of hyperkalemia in patients with renal failure. *Kidney Int* 1990;38(2):301-7.
6. Mahoney BA, Smith WA, Lo DS et al. Emergency interventions for hyperkalaemia. *Cochrane Database Syst Rev* 2005;(2):CD003235.
7. Allon M, Copkney C. Albuterol and insulin for treatment of hyperkalemia in hemodialysis patients. *Kidney Int* 1990;38(5):869-72.
8. Allon M, Dunlay R, Copkney C. Nebulized albuterol for acute hyperkalemia in patients on hemodialysis. *Ann Intern Med* 1989;110(6):426-9.
9. Sterns RH, Spital A. Disorders of internal potassium balance. *Semin Nephrol* 1987;7(4):399-415.
10. Mandelberg A, Krupnik Z, Houri S et al. Salbutamol metered-dose inhaler with spacer for hyperkalemia: how fast? how safe? *Chest* 1999;115(3):617-22.
11. Kamel KS, Wei C. Controversial issues in the treatment of hyperkalaemia. *Nephrol Dial Transplant* 2003;18(11):2215-8.
12. Sterns RH, Rojas M, Bernstein P et al. Ion-exchange resins for the treatment of hyperkalemia: are they safe and effective? *J Am Soc Nephrol* 2010;21(5):733-5.
13. Watson M, Abbott KC, Yuan CM. Damned if you do, damned if you don't: potassium binding resins in hyperkalemia. *Clin J Am Soc Nephrol* 2010;5(10):1723-6.
14. Gruy-Kapral C, Emmett M, Santa Ana CA et al. Effect of single dose resin-cathartic therapy on serum potassium concentration in patients with end-stage renal disease. *J Am Soc Nephrol* 1998;9(10):1924-30.
15. Harel Z, Harel S, Shah PS et al. Gastrointestinal adverse events with sodium polystyrene sulfonate (Kayexalate) use: a systematic review. *Am J Med* 2013;126(3):264.e9-24.
16. Lillemoe KD, Romolo JL, Hamilton SR et al. Intestinal necrosis due to sodium polystyrene (Kayexalate) in sorbitol enemas: clinical and experimental support for the hypothesis. *Surgery* 1987;101(3):267-72.
17. Romolo JL, Williams GM. Effect of kayexalate and sorbitol on colon of normal and uremic rats. *Surg Forum* 1979;30:369-70.
18. Palmer BF. Managing hyperkalemia caused by inhibitors of the renin-angiotensin-aldosterone system. *N Engl J Med* 2004;351(6):585-92.
19. Writing Committee Members, Yancy CW, Jessup M et al. 2013 ACCF/AHA guideline for the management of heart failure: a report of the American College of Cardiology Foundation/American Heart Association Task Force on practice guidelines. *Circulation* 2013;128(16):e240-319.
20. Kunin AS, Surawicz B, Sims EA. Decrease in serum potassium concentrations and appearance of cardiac arrhythmias during infusion of potassium with glucose in potassium-depleted patients. *N Engl J Med* 1962;266:228-33.
21. Chapman SA, Kaufenberg AJ, Anderson P et al. Safety and effectiveness of a modification diet in renal disease equation-based potassium replacement protocol. *Ann Pharmacother* 2009;43(3):436-43.
22. Todd SR, Sucher JF, Moore LJ et al. A multidisciplinary protocol improves electrolyte replacement and its effectiveness. *Am J Surg* 2009;198(6):911-5.
23. Hamill RJ, Robinson LM, Wexler HR et al. Efficacy and safety of potassium infusion therapy in hypokalemic critically ill patients. *Crit Care Med* 1991;19(5):694-9.
24. Kruse JA, Carlson RW. Rapid correction of hypokalemia using concentrated intravenous potassium chloride infusions. *Arch Intern Med* 1990;150(3):613-7.
25. Gennari FJ. Hypokalemia. *N Engl J Med* 1998;339(7):451-8.

Infectious Diseases

Chapter 106

Acute Bronchitis

Cindy Marshall, MD, CCFP, FCFP

Cough is one of the most common presenting symptoms in family practice. When present for <3 weeks, with or without sputum production, it is consistent with the diagnosis of acute bronchitis.[1,2] Acute bronchitis should be differentiated from the common cold, acute exacerbation of chronic bronchitis, asthma and community-acquired pneumonia.[3] A nonbacterial cause is present in >90% of uncomplicated acute bronchitis (Table 1).[4] Acute bronchitis is generally self-limited and symptoms usually resolve in 10–14 days, but cough can last for up to 8 weeks.[1,5]

Table 1: **Etiologic Agents in Acute Bronchitis**[3,6,7,8]

Etiology of Bronchitis	Frequency of Causation	Comments
Viral	>90 %	Most common viral isolates in acute bronchitis based on age (in order of prevalence): <1 y—RSV, parainfluenza, coronavirus 1–10 y—parainfluenza, enterovirus, RSV >10 y—influenza, RSV, parainfluenza (less commonly adenovirus, coronavirus, rhinovirus)
Noninfectious	Not well studied	Includes chemical and fume inhalational exposures
Bacterial	5–10%	The only isolates shown to cause acute bacterial bronchitis are *Chlamydophila pneumoniae*, *Mycoplasma pneumoniae*, *Bordetella pertussis* and *Bordetella parapertussis*. There is no evidence that *Streptococcus pneumoniae*, *Haemophilus influenzae* or *Moraxella catarrhalis* cause acute bronchitis in adults in the absence of underlying lung disease.

Abbreviations: RSV = respiratory syncytial virus

Goals of Therapy

- Rule out serious illness, e.g., acute exacerbation of COPD, asthma exacerbation, pertussis, pneumonia
- Minimize symptoms
- Limit the unnecessary use of antibiotics

Investigations

For the recommended approach to a patient presenting with acute cough (<3 weeks) see Figure 1.

- History:
  - primary symptom is cough, which may or may not be productive. Prolonged cough (>3 weeks) can occur in up to 50% of cases due to viral infections.[6] Green sputum production is a function of peroxidase release from leukocytes, hence it implies only inflammation, not necessarily infection[6,7]
  - in children, the infection of the tracheobronchial tree may result in prolonged cough; consider diagnosis of reactive airways, not acute bronchitis (see Chapter 52). Consider a diagnosis of pertussis, especially in children, when a history of spasmodic cough is elicited, a known outbreak exists in the area or there has been prior travel in an outbreak area[4]

- other symptoms may include wheezing, tachypnea, respiratory distress and hypoxemia
- consider alternative diagnoses if symptoms persist longer than 3 weeks[1,3,6]
- obtain vaccination history, travel history, use of cigarettes, underlying pulmonary disease and comorbidities

- Physical exam is key to diagnosis:
  - absence of tachycardia (heart rate >100 beats/min), tachypnea (adults, >24 breaths/min), fever (oral temperature of >38°C) and localized chest findings suggest acute bronchitis and obviate the need for chest x-ray.[2] Abnormal breath sounds and oral temperature >38°C are the best clinical predictors of pneumonia in adults.[9] Some analyses have found physicians can be highly accurate in excluding pneumonia in adults based on history and physical exam alone (negative predictive value 96–100%).[10,11]
  - Clinical predictors of pneumonia in children include fever and tachypnea (2–12 months, >60 breaths/min; 1–5 years, >40 breaths/min; >5 years, >20 breaths/min) but these are not always present.[12]
- Objective measurements:
  - no role for routine chest x-ray, viral culture, serologic assays, sputum culture or Gram stain, or pulmonary function testing/spirometry[2,3,6]

Therapeutic Choices

See Figure 1 for the recommended management of acute bronchitis.

Nonpharmacologic Choices

The nonpharmacologic approach is the mainstay of management.

- Patient education regarding the pathophysiology of acute bronchitis.
- Avoidance of tobacco and other pulmonary irritants.
- Limit risk of inoculation and transmission by employing strict hand-washing techniques and covering the cough.[6]
- Increased humidity may help reduce cough.[6]
- Increased fluids may prevent dehydration in children[8] but there is no evidence to recommend in adults.[13]

Pharmacologic Choices

Therapeutic options for the symptomatic management of acute bronchitis are presented in Table 2.

Analgesics

Antipyretics or analgesics, such as **acetaminophen** or **ibuprofen**, may be used for symptomatic relief of fever or chest discomfort.[1] The use of NSAIDs in patients with uncomplicated acute bronchitis is not superior to placebo in reducing the number of days of cough.[4,14] In children, recommend only in the presence of fever.[8]

Antitussives and Nonprescription Cough and Cold Products

Antitussives (**codeine**, **dextromethorphan**, **hydrocodone**) may provide short-term symptom relief (based on use in chronic bronchitis) but do not shorten the duration of illness.[1,2] A Cochrane review concluded there is no good evidence for the use of nonprescription medications in the treatment of acute cough in adults and children as the studies are of varying quality with conflicting results.[15] Higher-quality studies are needed in this area.

Figure 1: **Management of Acute Bronchitis**

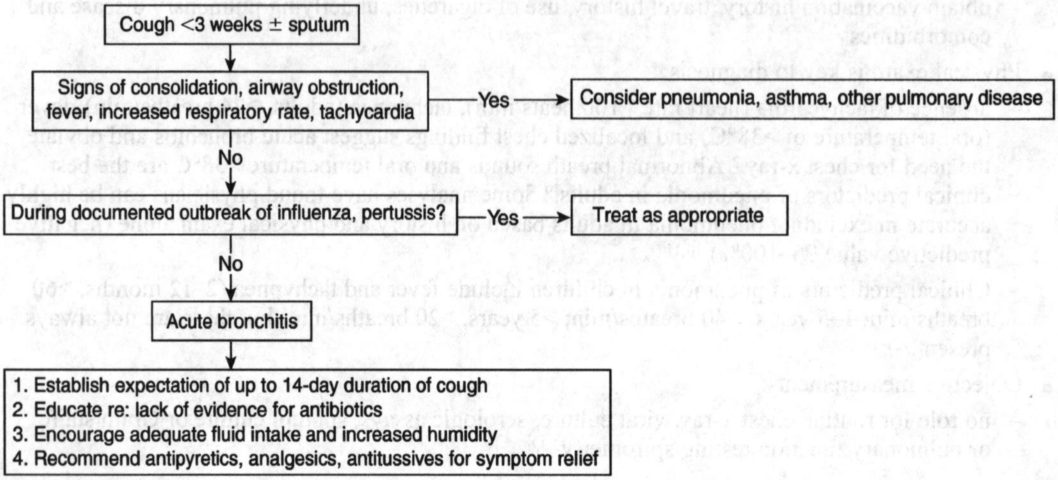
Cough <3 weeks ± sputum
Signs of consolidation, airway obstruction, fever, increased respiratory rate, tachycardia
Yes
Consider pneumonia, asthma, other pulmonary disease
No
During documented outbreak of influenza, pertussis?
Yes
Treat as appropriate
No
Acute bronchitis
1. Establish expectation of up to 14-day duration of cough
2. Educate re: lack of evidence for antibiotics
3. Encourage adequate fluid intake and increased humidity
4. Recommend antipyretics, analgesics, antitussives for symptom relief

Bronchodilators

Beta$_2$-agonists (e.g., **salbutamol**, **fenoterol**) are not recommended for the routine treatment of acute bronchitis [Evidence: SORT A*],[16] but they may reduce cough in patients experiencing bronchial hyper-responsiveness, wheeze or FEV$_1$ <80% of predicted value [Evidence: SORT B*].[16] This potential benefit must be weighed against common adverse effects such as tremor and nervousness. Studies in the pediatric population did not demonstrate any improvement in cough; however trials excluded children with airflow obstruction.[16]

Corticosteroids

There is no available evidence to support the use of **inhaled** or **oral corticosteroids** in the management of acute bronchitis.[4]

Antibiotics

Routine antibiotic treatment in uncomplicated acute bronchitis is not recommended [Evidence: SORT B*].[2,4,17,18] Antibiotic treatment does not have a consistent impact on the severity of illness or the prevention of potential complications (e.g., pneumonia).[6,17] A Cochrane systematic review assessed 17 trials involving almost 4000 patients.[17] Overall, patients taking antibiotics showed a modest benefit if any, compared to placebo. Evidence suggests antibiotics may reduce the duration of cough by half a day.[17] However, this marginal benefit is offset by the potential for adverse reactions to antibiotics and an increase in antibiotic resistance, for treatment of a self-limiting illness.[17] In otherwise healthy patients, the use of antibiotics is not recommended even when a bacterial cause is suspected.[19]

Natural Health Products

Pelargonium sidoides (Umckaloabo, South African geranium) is a herbal remedy that, according to some low quality RCTs, may be effective in relieving symptoms in acute bronchitis.[20] The preparation appears to be generally well tolerated, although allergic skin reactions, GI upset and liver toxicity have been reported.

* SORT (Strength of Recommendation Taxonomy) is a rating system (A, B or C) that addresses the quality of available evidence. For more information consult **How to Use *Compendium of Therapeutic Choices*** on page xxv.

There is some evidence that a **North American ginseng** extract taken prophylactically may reduce the duration of the common cold but there is insufficient evidence that it reduces the incidence or severity.[21] No studies have evaluated the effect of the extract on acute bronchitis (see Chapter 56).

Two small RCTs have shown the use of **honey** in children may be better than diphenhydramine or no treatment in the symptomatic relief of cough, but no better than dextromethorphan.[22] Because of the risk of botulism, honey should be pasteurized and given only to immunocompetent children over the age of 1 year.

There is insufficient evidence to recommend **Chinese herbal medicine** for the treatment of acute bronchitis.[23]

Choices during Pregnancy and Breastfeeding

During pregnancy and breastfeeding, symptomatic management of acute bronchitis can be achieved via supportive measures similar to those used in the nonpregnant patient. Fever and discomfort can be managed safely with **acetaminophen**.[24] **NSAIDs** are not recommended in late pregnancy due to the risk of premature closure of the ductus arteriosus.[25] If needed, cough may be controlled with **dextromethorphan**[26,27] or **opioids**; however, opioids should be used cautiously near term. Extreme caution is recommended with the use of **codeine** in breastfeeding mothers due to the risk of CNS and respiratory depression in the infant.[28] Inhaled **beta$_2$-agonists** are considered safe during pregnancy and breastfeeding but side effects need to be weighed against minimal symptomatic benefit.[29]

A discussion of general principles on the use of medications in these special populations can be found in Appendix II and Appendix III. Other specialized reference sources are also provided in these appendices.

Therapeutic Tips

- Treatment is only supportive in the vast majority of cases of acute bronchitis.
- Patient satisfaction does not depend on receiving an antibiotic; it is related to the quality of communication between the primary care provider and the patient.[1,4,7,30]
- Educate patients regarding the lack of evidence for the use of antibiotics in most circumstances. It is helpful to review the concerns of increased antibiotic resistance, possible side effects of antibiotic use and the cost of unnecessary treatment.[31] Providing a related patient information handout may also reduce antibiotic use. Use of a decision support tool (print or electronic) has been shown to reduce antibiotic overuse.[32]
- Referring to acute bronchitis as a "chest cold" may help patients understand that their cough is due to a virus and that antibiotics are not necessary.
- Set the patient's expectations of a 10- to 14-day duration of cough.[4] Most patients feel much better within the first week.[33]
- Mucolytic and expectorant preparations have failed to show any significant benefit in the management of acute bronchitis.[3]
- Annual influenza vaccine is recommended in high-risk groups. See Chapter 116.
- If the patient has unresolved symptoms in 2–3 weeks from onset of symptoms, consider follow-up.
- In those presenting with frequent or prolonged bouts of bronchitis consider asthma, COPD, bronchiectasis or medication effects (ACE inhibitor-induced cough).

Table 2: Drugs for the Symptomatic Management of Acute Bronchitis

Class	Drug	Dose	Adverse Effects	Drug Interactions	Comments	Cost[a]
Analgesics/ Antipyretics	*acetaminophen* Atasol, Tempra, Tylenol, generics	Adults and children >12 y: 325–650 mg Q4–6H PRN po; maximum 4000 mg/day Children: 10–15 mg/kg Q4–6H PRN po; maximum 65 mg/kg/day or adult dose whichever is less	Well tolerated (rare GI upset, less than salicylates).	May enhance anticoagulant effect of warfarin, particularly with doses of >1.3 g/day for >1 wk	Use with caution in patients with hepatic impairment. Severe hepatic damage can occur with overdose.	$[b]
	ibuprofen Advil, Motrin, Motrin (Children's),Motrin Liquid Gels, generics	Adults: 300–400 mg TID–QID PRN po; maximum 2400 mg/day Children: 5–10 mg/kg Q6–8H PRN po; maximum 40 mg/kg/day or adult dose whichever is less	Primarily GI (nausea, epigastric pain, heartburn).	ASA/anticoagulants may increase risk of bleeding.	Contraindicated in patients with active peptic ulcer disease or inflammatory bowel disease. Contraindicated in patients who have a history of or are at risk of ASA/NSAID intolerance (asthma, anaphylaxis, urticaria, angioedema, rhinitis).	$[b]
Antitussives	*codeine* ❥ (many products contain additional ingredients): CoActifed, Dimetapp-C, Dimetane Expectorant-C, Robitussin AC, generics	Immediate-release: Adults and children >12 y: 10–20 mg Q4–6H PRN po; maximum 120 mg/day	Sedation, nausea/vomiting, constipation.	Additive sedation with other CNS depressants; use with caution. Inhibitors of CYP2D6 (e.g., amiodarone, cimetidine, fluoxetine, moclobemide, paroxetine, quinidine) may antagonize codeine's effect.	Use with caution in elderly or debilitated patients. Genetic polymorphisms cause some individuals to more rapidly metabolize codeine to its active form (morphine), resulting in potentially toxic levels. Conversely, others may not produce enough morphine for efficacy. Avoid in breastfeeding women because of risk of toxicity in the infant.[28] Some products available without prescription.	$
	dextromethorphan ❥ Benylin DM, Robitussin DM, generics	Adults and children >12 y: 30 mg Q6–8H PRN po; maximum 120 mg/day Children 6–12 y: 15 mg Q6–8H po; maximum 60 mg/day	Rare but can cause nausea, drowsiness, dizziness.	Caution with CNS depressants (can potentiate effects). Do not use with monoamine oxidase inhibitor (MAOI) or for 2 wk after stopping MAOI. SSRIs may enhance adverse effects of dextromethorphan.	Not recommended in patients with asthma or children <6 years.	$[b]

Class	Drug	Dose	Adverse Effects	Drug Interactions	Comments	Cost[a]
	hydrocodone ☛ Hycodan, generics	Adults and children >12 y: 5 mg Q4–6H PRN po; may increase to 10 mg/dose; maximum 30 mg/day Children 6–12 y: 2.5 mg Q4–6H PRN po; maximum 15 mg/day	Lightheadedness, dizziness, sedation, nausea and vomiting, constipation.	Additive sedation and risk of respiratory depression with other CNS depressants; use with caution.	Caution in the elderly and debilitated.	$
Beta$_2$-adrenergic Agonists, short-acting	*salbutamol* Airomir, Ventolin Diskus, Ventolin HFA, generics	**Diskus (200 µg/inhalation):** Adults and children ≥4 y: 1 inhalation TID–QID PRN; maximum 800 µg/day **MDI:** Adults and children ≥4 y: 1–2 puffs (100– 200 µg) QID PRN Maximum (adults and children ≥12 y: 800 µg/day Maximum (children <12 y: 400 µg/day	Tremor, restlessness, palpitations, dizziness, headache, nausea.	Caution with other sympathomimetic agents.	Contraindicated in patients with arrhythmias or hypertrophic obstructive cardiomyopathy. No evidence for use in acute bronchitis unless airflow obstruction is present. Caution with ischemic heart disease, vascular disease and hypertension.	Diskus: $$$ MDI: $$
	terbutaline Bricanyl Turbuhaler	Adults and children ≥6 y: 1 inhalation (0.5 mg/inhalation) QID PRN; maximum 6 inhalations/day	See salbutamol.	See salbutamol.	See salbutamol.	$$$

[a] Costs are per day for oral medications and per unit for inhaled medications; includes drug cost only.
[b] Available without prescription.
☛ Dosage adjustment may be required in renal impairment; see Appendix I.
Abbreviations: CNS = central nervous system; GI = gastrointestinal; MDI = metered dose inhaler; NSAID = nonsteroidal anti-inflammatory drug; SSRI = selective serotonin reuptake inhibitor
Legend: $ < $5 $$ $5–10 $$$ $10–15

Suggested Readings

Albert RH. Diagnosis and treatment of acute bronchitis. *Am Fam Physician* 2010;82(11):1345-50.

Alberta Clinical Practice Guidelines Working Group. *Guideline for the management of acute bronchitis, 2008 update*. Edmonton (AB): Toward Optimized Practice (TOP) Program, Alberta Medical Association; 2008. Available from: www.topalbertadoctors.org.

Irwin RS, Baumann MH, Bolser DC et al. Diagnosis and management of cough: ACCP evidence-based clinical practice guidelines. *Chest* 2006;129(1 Suppl):1S-292S.

Michigan Quality Improvement Consortium. *Management of uncomplicated acute bronchitis in adults*. Southfield (MI): Michigan Quality Improvement Consortium; May 2014. Available from: mqic.org/pdf/mqic_management_of_uncomplicated_acute_bronchitis_in_adults_cpg.pdf.

Wenzel RP, Fowler AA. Clinical practice: acute bronchitis. *N Engl J Med* 2006;355(20):2125-30.

Worrall G. Acute cough in adults. *Can Fam Physician* 2011;57(1):48-51.

References

1. Snow V, Mottur-Pilson C, Gonzales R et al. Principles of appropriate antibiotic use for treatment of acute bronchitis in adults. *Ann Intern Med* 2001;134(6):518-20.
2. Braman SS. Chronic cough due to acute bronchitis: ACCP evidence-based clinical practice guidelines. *Chest* 2006;129(1 Suppl):95S-103S.
3. Irwin RS, Baumann MH, Bolser DC et al. Diagnosis and management of cough executive summary: ACCP evidence-based clinical practice guidelines. *Chest* 2006;129(1 Suppl):1S-23S.
4. Alberta Clinical Practice Guidelines Working Group. *Guideline for the management of acute bronchitis, 2008 update*. Edmonton (AB): Toward Optimized Practice (TOP) Program, Alberta Medical Association; 2008. Available from: www.topalbertadoctors.org. Accessed February 22, 2011.
5. Centers for Disease Control and Prevention. *Get smart: know when antibiotics work. Bronchitis (chest cold)*. September 2013. Available from: www.cdc.gov/getsmart/antibiotic-use/URI/bronchitis.html. Accessed March 17, 2014.
6. Gonzales R, Bartlett JG, Besser RE et al. Principles of appropriate antibiotic use for treatment of uncomplicated acute bronchitis: background. *Ann Emerg Med* 2001;37(6):720-7.
7. Albert RH. Diagnosis and treatment of acute bronchitis. *Am Fam Physician* 2010;82(11):1345-50.
8. Fleming DM, Elliott AJ. The management of acute bronchitis in children. *Expert Opin Pharmacother* 2007;8(4):415-26.
9. Evertsen J, Baumgardner DJ, Regnery A et al. Diagnosis and management of pneumonia and bronchitis in outpatient primary care practices. *Prim Care Respir J* 2010;19(3):237-41.
10. Blaeuer SR, Bally K, Tschudi P et al. Acute cough illness in general practice — predictive value of clinical judgement and accuracy of requesting chest x-rays. *Praxis (Bern 1994)* 2013;102(21):1287-92.
11. van Vugt SF, Verheij TJ, de Jong PA et al. Diagnosing pneumonia in patients with acute cough: clinical judgment compared to chest radiography. *Eur Respir J* 2013;42(4):1076-82.
12. McIntosh K. Community-acquired pneumonia in children. *N Engl J Med* 2002;346(6):429-37.
13. Guppy MP, Mickan SM, Del Mar CB et al. Advising patients to increase fluid intake for treatment of acute respiratory infections. *Cochrane Database Syst Rev* 2011;(2):CD004419.
14. Llor C, Moragas A, Bayona C et al. Efficacy of anti-inflammatory or antibiotic treatment in patients with non-complicated acute bronchitis and discolored sputum: a randomized placebo controlled trial. *BMJ* 2013;347:f5762.
15. Smith SM, Schroeder K, Fahey T. Over-the-counter (OTC) medications for acute cough in children and adults in ambulatory settings. *Cochrane Database Syst Rev* 2012;8:CD001831.
16. Becker LA, Hom J, Villasis-Keever M et al. Beta2-agonists for acute bronchitis. *Cochrane Database Syst Rev* 2011;(7):CD001726.
17. Smith SM, Fahey T, Smucny J et al. Antibiotics for acute bronchitis. *Cochrane Database Syst Rev* 2014;3:CD000245.
18. National Institute for Health and Care Excellence. *Prescribing of antibiotics for self-limiting respiratory tract infections in adults and children in primary care*. Manchester (GB): NICE; 2008. Available from: www.nice.org.uk/cg69. Accessed April 16, 2013.
19. Blush RR. Acute bronchitis: evaluation and management. *Nurse Pract* 2013;38(10):14-20.
20. Timmer A, Gunther J, Motschall E et al. Pelargonium sidoides extract for treating acute respiratory tract infections. *Cochrane Database Syst Rev* 2013;10:CD006323.
21. Seida JK, Durec T, Kuhle S. North American (Panax quinquefolius) and Asian Ginseng (Panax ginseng) preparations for prevention of the common cold in healthy adults: a systematic review. *Evid Based Complement Alternat Med* 2011;2011:282151.
22. Oduwole O, Meremikwu MM, Oyo-Ita A et al. Honey for acute cough in children. *Cochrane Database Syst Rev* 2012;3:CD007094.
23. Jiang L, Li K, Wu T. Chinese medicinal herbs for acute bronchitis. *Cochrane Database Syst Rev* 2012;2:CD004560.
24. Erebara A, Bozzo P, Einarson A et al. Treating the common cold during pregnancy. *Can Fam Physician* 2008;54(5):687-9.
25. Koren G, Florescu A, Costei AM et al. Nonsteroidal antiinflammatory drugs during third trimester and the risk of premature closure of the ductus arteriosus: a meta-analysis. *Ann Pharmacother* 2006;40(5):824-9.
26. Martinez-Frias ML, Rodriguez-Pinilla E. Epidemiologic analysis of prenatal exposure to cough medicines containing dextromethorphan: no evidence of human teratogenicity. *Teratology* 2001;63(1):38-41.
27. Einarson A, Lyszkiewicz D, Koren G. The safety of dextromethorphan in pregnancy: results of a controlled study. *Chest* 2001;119(2):466-9.
28. Madadi P, Koren G, Cairns J et al. Safety of codeine during breastfeeding: fatal morphine poisoning in the breastfed neonate of a mother prescribed codeine. *Can Fam Physician* 2007;53(1):33-5.
29. Schatz M, Zeiger RS, Harden K et al. The safety of asthma and allergy medications during pregnancy. *J Allergy Clin Immunol* 1997;100(3):301-6.
30. Phillips TG, Hickner J. Calling acute bronchitis a chest cold may improve patient satisfaction with appropriate antibiotic use. *J Am Board Fam Pract* 2005;18(6):459-63.
31. Colgan R, Powers JH. Appropriate antimicrobial prescribing: approaches that limit antibiotic resistance. *Am Fam Physician* 2001;64(6):999-1004.

32. Gonzales R, Anderer T, McCulloch CE et al. A cluster randomized trial of decision support strategies for reducing antibiotic use in acute bronchitis. *JAMA Intern Med* 2013;173(4):267-73.
33. Snow V, Mottur-Pilson C, Gonzales R et al. Principles of appropriate antibiotic use for treatment of nonspecific upper respiratory tract infections in adults. *Ann Intern Med* 2001;134(6):487-9.

Chapter 107
Acute Osteomyelitis

Simon Dobson, MD, FRCPC

Goals of Therapy

- Cure the acute infection
- Minimize morbidity, e.g., loss of limb function
- Prevent recurrence and progression to chronic osteomyelitis

Investigations

- History:
  - duration of symptoms: fever, pain, redness, swelling, limping or other loss of function or movement
  - any recent surgery, trauma or penetrating wound
  - vascular insufficiency
  - neuropathic ulcer of the diabetic foot. For further discussion of diabetic foot infections, see Chapter 111
- Examination:
  - tenderness over affected bone (often exquisite)[1]
  - range of movement in affected limb (any suggestion of septic arthritis?)
- Laboratory tests:
  - complete blood count and acute-phase reactants (erythrocyte sedimentation rate, C-reactive protein) as baseline[2]
  - blood culture before starting antibacterials (positive in 30–60%)
- Aspiration:
  - an organism can be obtained in up to 80% of cases of acute hematogenous osteomyelitis. This may become an increasingly important test as resistant organisms such as community-acquired methicillin-resistant *Staphylococcus aureus* (CA-MRSA) play a greater role in acute osteomyelitis.[3,4] Early consultation with an orthopedic surgeon is recommended
  - culture of superficial ulcer or draining sinus may be unreliable due to the possible presence of colonizing organisms. In addition, some true pathogens may be sufficiently fastidious that recovery from superficial culture is difficult (e.g., anaerobes). The best specimen is bone or periosteal aspirate, obtained surgically or by percutaneous biopsy through unaffected skin[5]
- Imaging:
  - x-ray may be normal initially; changes (e.g., periosteal reaction) are not evident for at least 10 days after onset
  - rarefaction of bone visible only when 50% loss of bone density (early in neonates, later in older children and adults)
  - rarefaction of bone may be due to an adjacent chronic inflammatory lesion, which must be distinguished from lytic lesions of osteomyelitis

  - x-ray does not rule out osteomyelitis diagnosis in a person with a diabetic foot infection. Chronic osteopathy may be present and may complicate radiographic interpretation. For more information see Chapter 111
- Magnetic resonance imaging (MRI) is a highly sensitive modality of imaging especially when it is necessary to define the location and extent of infection and extraosseous complications such as periosteal abscesses.[6] It has the advantage of assessing bone, joint and soft tissue simultaneously while also sparing the patient ionizing radiation.[7] However, where there are limits to the accessibility of MRI, its use in the investigation of acute presentation is not routine.
- Bone scan:
  - imaging using technetium 99^{m}-labelled methylene diphosphonate has improved early diagnosis. Early "blood pool images" should be taken, as well as later bone uptake images, to help differentiate cellulitis from bone infection
  - a negative bone scan does not rule out osteomyelitis.[8] In neonates an x-ray may be more reliable.[9] Other causes of enhanced bone turnover (e.g., fracture or tumor) will also give a positive result
  - in the neuropathic foot, small stress fractures may be difficult to detect clinically or radiographically, but still show uptake on the bone scan. Vascular insufficiency may attenuate changes on the bone scan
  - *Note*: If the clinical findings suggest osteomyelitis, do not delay treatment while waiting for a bone scan to be performed

Therapeutic Choices

Figure 1 outlines the management of acute osteomyelitis.

Nonpharmacologic Choices

Surgical Drainage

Antibacterials do not penetrate well into collections of pus or into bone in which blood supply is compromised by infection. Surgical decompression and exploration may be necessary when there has been a delay in presentation or diagnosis, when pus has been found on aspiration or when there is x-ray evidence of bone destruction. For early disease the role of immediate surgery has been controversial.[1,8] However, if swelling, pain, tenderness and fever do not resolve within days after starting antibacterials, consider surgical exploration, especially if initial empiric therapy did not cover MRSA. Suspicion of osteomyelitis secondary to a penetrating injury (e.g., to the calcaneus) requires bone exploration, débridement and culture. Osteomyelitis associated with diabetic foot infection (see Chapter 111) often requires surgical débridement. This should be aggressive and may involve amputation of the infected bone.

Pharmacologic Choices

Antibacterials

While cultures are pending, start empiric iv antibacterial therapy, based on the most likely infecting organism (Table 1) and on the prevalence in your geographical location of CA-MRSA as a cause of invasive staphylococcal infections.[10] A definitive choice can be made once the organism and sensitivities are identified (Table 2). The role of adjunctive antibacterials such as **fusidic acid** or **rifampin** has not been studied systematically. They cannot be used alone for staphylococcal infections because resistance develops rapidly.

Figure 1: Management of Acute Osteomyelitis

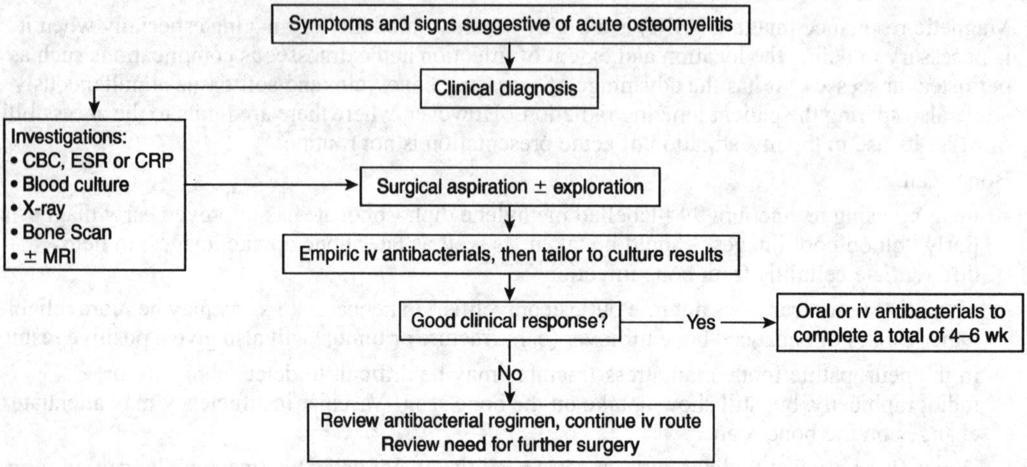

Abbreviations: CBC = complete blood count; CRP = C-reactive protein; ESR = erythrocyte sedimentation rate

Table 1: Initial Empiric Antibacterial Therapy for Acute Osteomyelitis[a]

Source	Characteristics	Usual Causative Organisms	Empiric IV Antibacterials
Hematogenous Osteomyelitis	Most common type Predominant in children Bloodborne bacteria lodge in bone as nidus of infection Possible in any bone but usually in long bones: femur 36%, tibia 33%, humerus 10% Vertebral osteomyelitis not uncommon in adults. Predisposing factors are iv drug abuse, trauma, other source of infection, e.g., urinary tract In neonates, septic arthritis often coexists	**Neonates:** group B streptococci, gram-negative enterics, *S. aureus* **Children:** *S. aureus* (MSSA & MRSA[b]), group A streptococci Rare: *H. influenzae*,[c] *S. pneumoniae*, gram-negative enterics, *K. kingae* (children <3 years) **Adults:** *S. aureus*, gram-negative enterics	**Neonates:** if MRSA unlikely, cloxacillin[d] + cefotaxime (to cover gram-negative enteric bacilli); if MRSA possible, vancomycin + cefotaxime or ceftriaxone **Children:** if MRSA unlikely, cloxacillin[d] or cefazolin; if MRSA possible, vancomycin. Replace cefazolin with cefotaxime if not immunized against *H. influenzae* **Adults:** cloxacillin[d] or cefazolin
Spread from Contiguous Sites[b,e]	Spread from head/neck	*S. aureus*, anaerobes, gram-negative organisms, mixed infection	**Adults:** clindamycin ± gentamicin
	Spread from soft tissue infection	*S. aureus*, streptococci	**Adults:** cloxacillin or cefazolin
	Spread from genitourinary system	gram-negative enteric bacilli	**Adults:** fluoroquinolone or extended-spectrum beta-lactam (extended-spectrum penicillin, carbapenem, 3rd generation cephalosporin)
Penetrating Trauma	Example: puncture wound of foot	*P. aeruginosa*, *S. aureus*	**Children:** cloxacillin[d] + ceftazidime + gentamicin **Adults:** fluoroquinolone

[a] The site and origin of infection and organism responsible are largely related to age.
[b] MRSA is increasing in importance as a cause of acute osteomyelitis.
[c] *H. influenzae* is of decreasing importance due to success of immunization.
[d] A semisynthetic, penicillinase-resistant penicillin (e.g., cloxacillin) provides coverage against *S. aureus* and streptococci.
[e] Common in elderly; predisposing factors include surgery, soft tissue infection.
Abbreviations: MRSA = methicillin-resistant *S. aureus*; MSSA = methicillin-sensitive *S. aureus*

Table 2: **Definitive Antibacterial Therapy for Acute Osteomyelitis**

Organism	Initial IV Antibacterials	Oral Antibacterials (for completion of course)
MSSA	Cloxacillin, cefazolin or clindamycin	Cloxacillin, cephalexin, clindamycin or amoxicillin/clavulanate
MRSA	Vancomycin	CA-MRSA may be sensitive to clindamycin as an oral agent; otherwise use home iv therapy[a]
Streptococcus group A	Penicillin	Penicillin, amoxicillin or clindamycin
Streptococcus group B	Penicillin	In neonates, oral antibacterials are not appropriate
Enteric gram-negative bacilli	Cefotaxime	In neonates, oral antibacterials are not appropriate Adults: fluoroquinolone
K. kingae	Cefazolin	Susceptible to most beta-lactams
P. aeruginosa	Ceftazidime + Gentamicin	Adults: ciprofloxacin (if susceptible) No suitable oral drug available for children. However, oral ciprofloxacin is sometimes used in children after careful consideration and discussion of potential risks with child's parents/guardians

[a] The microbiology laboratory must do a test (usually a "D" test) of inducible clindamycin resistance in MRSA.
Abbreviations: CA-MRSA = community-acquired methicillin-resistant *S. aureus*; MRSA = methicillin-resistant *S. aureus*; MSSA = methicillin-sensitive *S. aureus*

Duration of Antibacterial Therapy

Duration of antibacterial therapy should be a minimum of 4 weeks; many authorities recommend 6 weeks.[11] More severe initial presentation, extensive bone involvement, and slow resolution of systemic and local signs indicate a 6-week course. In osteomyelitis following penetrating injury, 10–14 days of treatment is sufficient if adequate débridement has been performed. As home iv therapy programs have become more accessible to patients, this is an option for shortening hospital stay. The type of home iv pumps used in a particular program may limit specific treatment options, especially regarding dosing intervals. Choice of antibacterial therapy should not be compromised for the convenience of the local home iv program.

Shorter regimens of sequential iv-oral antibacterial therapy explored in a Finnish trial suggest a total treatment course of 20 days.[12] However, with the rise of CA-MRSA, an argument can be made that the longer, more conservative treatment courses are still appropriate in the North American setting.[10]

Sequential IV-Oral Antibacterial Therapy

Since a long course is required, a switch from the iv to oral route has many advantages including shortened hospital stay and reduced complications from iv cannulae.[13] In children, continue iv antibacterials until the patient is systemically better, the temperature is normal and local signs of inflammation and tenderness are improved. This may take several days. Step-down oral antibacterial therapy may also be appropriate for adults.[14]

Switching to oral therapy can be undertaken with the following provisos:

- Patient is beyond neonatal age group and can be expected to attend for regular review.
- No underlying immunodeficiency present.
- The dose of oral antibacterial is larger than that usually used for minor infections (Table 3).
- Adherence is vital. For children, the taste of the oral antibacterial is an important factor. **Cloxacillin** liquid preparations are unpalatable; **cephalexin** has a more acceptable taste.
- If no organism was isolated but the patient has recovered well on the empiric iv regimen, a switch to a comparable oral antibacterial therapy can still be made. Recurrence of symptoms while on oral

step-down therapy demands immediate reassessment and resumption of iv antibacterials. Home iv therapy is recommended when oral step-down is not appropriate.

- Some infectious disease specialists suggest obtaining blood for serum inhibitory concentration testing in order to assess the bioavailability of some drugs, particularly oral **beta-lactams**.

Follow-up

Success of treatment is judged by careful follow-up of systemic signs (fever and well-being, local signs of decreasing inflammation and tenderness and return of full function). Erythrocyte sedimentation rate gradually returns to normal over several weeks. The C-reactive protein returns to normal in a matter of days.

Therapeutic Tips

- The consequences of treating osteomyelitis empirically with what turns out to be the wrong antibiotic can be dire. In an era of increasing incidence of CA-MRSA, persuading a surgeon to obtain pus by aspirating the bone at the time of presentation allows an accurate microbiologic diagnosis and tailored antibiotic therapy.
- Home iv therapy or oral step-down therapy can be appropriate for many patients, reducing hospital stay and still assuring cure.

Table 3: **Antibacterials Used for the Treatment of Acute Osteomyelitis**[a]

Class	Antibacterial	Dose	Adverse Effects	Drug Interactions	Cost[b]
Aminoglycosides	*gentamicin* generics	Children: 6–7.5 mg/kg/day divided Q8H iv Adults: 5–7 mg/kg/day divided Q8H iv or once daily if renal function permits	Nephrotoxicity usually reversible; risk increases with dose and duration of therapy; ototoxicity often irreversible.	Increased toxicity with other nephrotoxic or ototoxic drugs; increased effects of anesthetic agents.	Pediatric: $ Adult: $$
Carbapenems	*imipenem/cilastatin* Primaxin, generics	Adults: 500 mg Q6H iv	Caution in beta-lactam sensitivity; risk of seizures if dose exceeded in renal failure.	Carbapenems may decrease valproic acid levels. Seizures have been reported with concurrent use of imipenem and ganciclovir.	$$$$
	meropenem Merrem, Meropenem for Injection	Adults: 500 mg Q6H iv	See imipenem/cilastatin.	Carbapenems may decrease valproic acid levels.	$$$$
Cephalosporins	*cefazolin* generics	Children: 100 mg/kg/day divided Q8H iv; maximum 6 g/day Adults: 2 g Q8H iv	GI effects, especially diarrhea.	Increased nephrotoxic effects of aminoglycosides; increased INR with warfarin.	Pediatric: $ Adult: $$
	cefotaxime Claforan	Children: 150 mg/kg/day divided Q8H iv; maximum 12 g/day Adults: 2 g Q4–8H iv	Phlebitis, hypersensitivity, positive Coombs' test.	See cefazolin.	Pediatric: $$ Adult: $$$$
	ceftazidime Fortaz, generics	Children: 150 mg/kg/day divided Q8H iv; maximum 6 g/day Adults: 2 g Q8H iv	Phlebitis, eosinophilia, positive Coombs' test, elevated aspartate transaminase, superinfections.	See cefazolin.	Pediatric: $$$ Adult: $$$$$
	ceftriaxone generics	Children: 75 mg/kg/day divided Q12–24H iv; maximum 4 g/day Adults: 1–2 g/day divided Q12–24H iv; maximum 4 g/day	See ceftazidime.	See cefazolin. Do not reconstitute or mix with calcium-containing solutions. Contraindicated in neonates if a calcium-containing iv solution is or will be required during care. Do not administer simultaneously with calcium-containing iv solutions via a Y-site. Administration may be done sequentially provided the infusion lines are thoroughly flushed between infusions.	$

(cont'd)

Table 3: **Antibacterials Used for the Treatment of Acute Osteomyelitis**[a] *(cont'd)*

Class	Antibacterial	Dose	Adverse Effects	Drug Interactions	Cost[b]
	cephalexin generics	Pediatric: 100–150 mg/kg/day divided Q6H po; maximum 4 g/day Adults: 1–4 g/day divided Q6H po	GI effects, rash, eosinophilia, leukopenia, positive Coombs' test, elevated aspartate transaminase.	See cefazolin.	$
Fluoroquinolones	*ciprofloxacin* Cipro, generics	Adults: 400 mg Q12H iv or 750 mg Q12H po Children (off-label): 30 mg/kg/day divided Q12H po; maximum 1500 mg/day po	Abdominal pain, nausea, vomiting, rash, dizziness, headache, drowsiness, diarrhea.	Absorption decreased by antacids, iron salts, magnesium sucralfate; decreased theophylline and caffeine elimination.	iv: $$ po: $
	moxifloxacin Avelox	Adults: 400 mg Q24H po/iv	See ciprofloxacin. Cases of severe liver injury including liver failure have been reported.	Absorption decreased by antacids, iron salts, magnesium sucralfate.	iv: $$ po: $
Glycopeptides	*vancomycin* generics	Children: 40 mg/kg/day divided Q6H iv; maximum 4 g/day prior to therapeutic drug monitoring Adults: 1 g Q12H iv	Hypotension, flushing, red man syndrome, chills, drug fever, eosinophilia.	Increased toxicity with other nephrotoxic or ototoxic drugs. Target serum trough levels to 15–20 mg/L.	Pediatric: $$ Adult: $$$$$
Lincosamides	*clindamycin* Dalacin C, Dalacin C Flavored Granules, Dalacin C Phosphate Sterile Solution, generics	Children: 40 mg/kg/day divided Q6H iv or 30 mg/kg/day divided Q8H po; maximum 2 g/day Adults: 600 mg Q6H iv/po	Rash, neutropenia, elevated aspartate transaminase and alkaline phosphatase, pseudomembranous colitis.	Decreased absorption with aluminum salts; increased effects of anesthetic agents.	iv: $$ po: $
Penicillins	*amoxicillin* generics	Children: 100 mg/kg/day, divided Q8H po; maximum 4 g/day Adults: 0.5–1 g Q8H po	GI effects, rash, eosinophilia.	Tetracyclines decrease the effectiveness of penicillins; increased methotrexate serum levels; some penicillins can inactivate aminoglycosides if mixed.	$
	amoxicillin/ clavulanate Clavulin, generics	Children: (amoxicillin) 100 mg/kg/day divided Q8H po; maximum 1750 mg/day, given as amoxicillin 40 mg/mL + clavulanate 5.7 mg/mL suspension (7:1 ratio) Adults: (amoxicillin) 500 mg Q8H po or 875 mg Q12H po	GI effects, diarrhea.	See amoxicillin.	$
	cloxacillin generics	Children: 200 mg/kg/day iv or 150–200 mg/kg/day po divided Q6H; maximum 6 g/day Adults: 2 g Q4H iv	Rash, eosinophilia, GI effects.	See amoxicillin.	Pediatric: $ Adult: $$

Class	Antibacterial	Dose	Adverse Effects	Drug Interactions	Cost[b]
	penicillin G ❥ Crystapen, generics	Children: 200 000 units/kg/day divided Q4–6H iv; maximum 24 million units/day Adults: 12–24 million units/day divided Q4–6H iv	GI effects, hypersensitivity, rash, drug fever, positive Coombs' test. Monitor K+ and Na+ when using high-dose parenteral penicillin G.	See amoxicillin.	Pediatric: $ Adult: $
	penicillin V ❥ generics	Children: 100 mg/kg/day divided Q6H po; maximum 3 g/day Adults: 0.75–1 g QID po	GI effects, hypersensitivity, rash, drug fever, positive Coombs' test.	See amoxicillin.	$

[a] Therapy is initiated with iv antibacterials. Patients can be stepped down to oral antibacterials under certain conditions.
[b] Cost per day (pediatric dosage based on 20 kg and adult based on 70 kg body weights); includes drug cost only.
❥ Dosage adjustment may be required in renal impairment; see Appendix I.
Legend: $ < $25 $$ $25–50 $$$ $50–75 $$$$ $75–100 $$$$$ $100–125

Suggested Readings

Hatzenbuehler J, Pulling TJ. Diagnosis and management of osteomyelitis. *Am Fam Physician* 2011;84(9):1027-33.

Kram BL, Raasch RH. Osteomyelitis/septic arthritis. In: Alldredge BK, Corelli RL, Ernst ME et al., eds. *Applied therapeutics: the clinical use of drugs*. 10th ed. Philadelphia (PA): Wolters Kluwer Health/Lippincott Williams & Wilkins; 2013. p. 1648-60.

Lew DP, Waldvogel FA. Osteomyelitis. *Lancet* 2004;364(9431):369-79.

Peltola H, Paakkönen M. Acute osteomyelitis in children. *N Engl J Med* 2014;370(4):352-60.

References

1. Nade S. Acute haematogenous osteomyelitis in infancy and childhood. *J Bone Joint Surg Br* 1983;65(2):109-19.
2. Unkila-Kallio L, Kallio MJ, Eskola J et al. Serum C-reactive protein, erythrocyte sedimentation rate, and white blood cell count in acute hematogenous osteomyelitis of children. *Pediatrics* 1994;93(1):59-62.
3. Kaplan SL. Community-acquired methicillin-resistant Staphylococcus aureus infections in children. *Semin Pediatr Infect Dis* 2006;17(3):113-9.
4. Arnold SR, Elias D, Buckingham SC et al. Changing patterns of acute hematogenous osteomyelitis and septic arthritis: emergence of community-associated methicillin-resistant Staphylococcus aureus. *J Pediatr Orthop* 2006;26(6):703-8.
5. Caputo GM, Cavanagh PR, Ulbrecht JS et al. Assessment and management of foot disease in patients with diabetes. *N Engl J Med* 1994;331(13):854-60.
6. Browne LP, Mason EO, Kaplan SL et al. Optimal imaging strategy for community-acquired Staphylococcus aureus musculoskeletal infections in children. *Pediatr Radiol* 2008;38(8):841-7.
7. Guillerman RP. Osteomyelitis and beyond. *Pediatr Radiol* 2013;43(Suppl 1):S193-203.
8. Lew DP, Waldvogel FA. Osteomyelitis. *N Engl J Med* 1997;336(14):999-1007.
9. Overturf GD. Bacterial infections of the bones and joints. In: Remington JS, Klein JO, Wilson CB et al., eds. *Infectious diseases of the fetus and newborn infant*. 7th ed. Philadelphia (PA): Elsevier; 2011. p. 296-310.
10. Kaplan SL. Acute hematogenous osteomyelitis in children: differences in clinical manifestations and management. *Pediatr Infect Dis J* 2010;29(12):1128-9.
11. Lazzarini L, Lipsky BA, Mader JT. Antibiotic treatment of osteomyelitis: what have we learned from 30 years of clinical trials? *Int J Infect Dis* 2005;9(3):127-38.
12. Peltola H, Paakkonen M, Kallio P et al. Short- versus long-term antimicrobial treatment for acute hematogenous osteomyelitis of childhood: prospective, randomized trial on 131 culture-positive cases. *Pediatr Infect Dis J* 2010;29(12):1123-8.
13. Lew DP, Waldvogel FA. Osteomyelitis. *Lancet* 2004;364(9431):369-79.
14. Daver NG, Shelburne SA, Atmar RL et al. Oral step-down therapy is comparable to intravenous therapy for Staphylococcus aureus osteomyelitis. *J Infect* 2007;54(6):539-44.

Chapter 108
Acute Otitis Media in Childhood

Joseph V. Vayalumkal, MD, FRCPC

One of the most frequently encountered situations in primary care is the irritable child with a history of 2–3 days of fever, runny nose and cough. Most children with this clinical presentation have viral infections that do not require antibiotics; however, some will have signs of acute otitis media (AOM) evident on physical examination and may benefit from antibiotic therapy.

AOM can be caused by both viral and bacterial pathogens.[1] It is often preceded by a viral upper respiratory tract infection which may alter respiratory tract defences by disturbing the epithelium and impairing mucociliary clearance. This may subsequently lead to eustachian tube dysfunction.[2,3] The combination of events allows bacterial pathogens colonizing the nasopharynx to invade the middle ear and cause acute infection. An investigation of the microbiology of acute otitis media reported that bacteria were isolated in 92% of middle ear effusions while viruses were isolated in 70%. Coinfection was noted in 66% of patients.[4]

A number of prevention strategies for AOM have been assessed. Most strategies involve vaccination against AOM pathogens (see Therapeutic Tips) but risk factor modification has also been studied.[5,6,7,8,9] Exposure to tobacco smoke and exposure to other children (e.g., daycare) are associated with higher risk of AOM in childhood.[6,8,9] Breastfeeding is protective against respiratory tract colonization and is associated with lower rates of acute otitis media in childhood.[7]

Goals of Therapy

- Relieve symptoms (fever, irritability, pain)
- Sterilize the middle ear
- Prevent complications, e.g., mastoiditis, intracranial infection, facial paralysis
- Avoid inappropriate therapy which may lead to the emergence of resistant pathogens and adverse drug effects such as antibiotic-associated diarrhea

Investigations

- History:
  - fever
  - nonspecific symptoms of viral upper respiratory tract infection such as cough and coryza
  - otalgia is a common manifestation and may be the best clue to the diagnosis; however, ear pain is not always easily communicated by infants and toddlers (disturbed sleep, irritability, tugging the ear or rubbing the head may suggest otalgia in young children)
- Physical examination:
  - focus on the head and neck region to rule out other causes of pain referred to the ear such as mastoiditis or dental abscess
  - proper visual inspection of the tympanic membrane may require the following: child to be restrained by parents, proper lighting, removal of cerumen obscuring proper view
  - assess for signs of middle ear effusion and middle ear inflammation

- four key features of the tympanic membrane should be evaluated: *colour*, *position*, *translucency* and *mobility*. A red, displaced/bulging, opaque and immobile tympanic membrane indicates acute otitis media
- Referral:
  - for treatment failures or recurrences unresponsive to therapy, consider referral to an ENT specialist who can obtain middle ear fluid for culture to identify the pathogen involved and its antibiotic susceptibility profile
  - refer children who have frequent, recurrent episodes (≥3 episodes in 6 months or ≥4 episodes in 12 months) to an ENT specialist for consideration of myringotomy and tympanostomy tubes
  - children with recurrent episodes of AOM should also have audiology assessment to determine any conductive hearing loss

Therapeutic Choices

An approach to management of AOM based on risk factors is presented in Figure 1.

Figure 1: Management of Acute Otitis Media Using a Risk Factor–based Approach

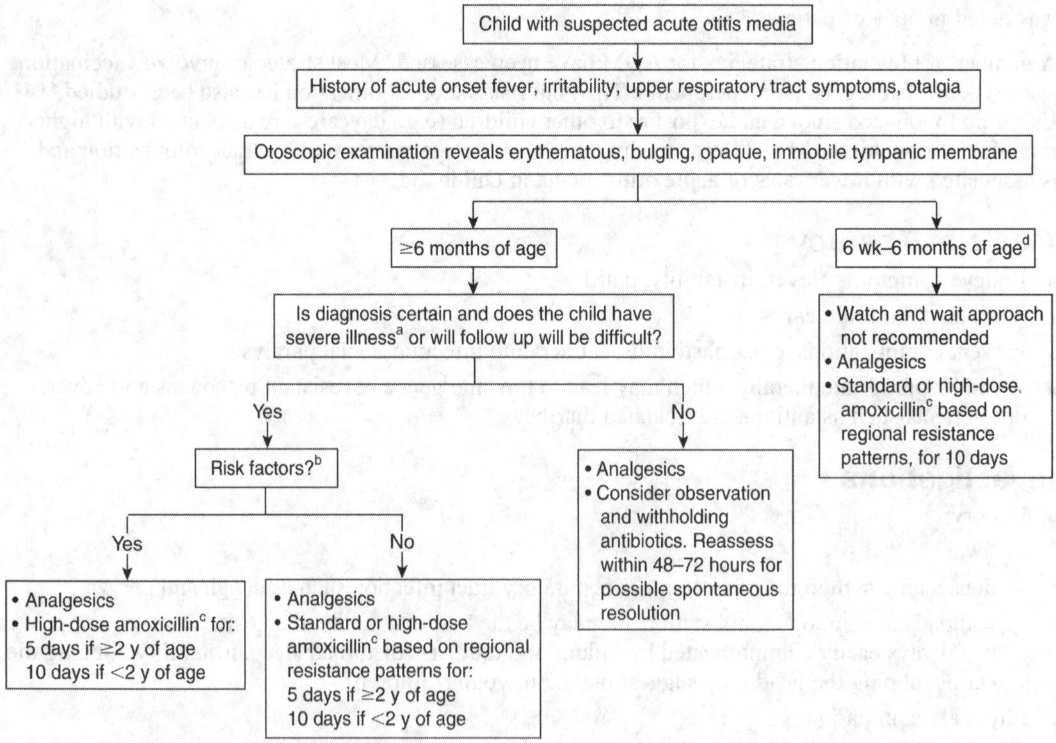

[a] Toxic appearance, temperature ≥39°C, severe otalgia.
[b] Risk factors for drug-resistant organisms: recent antibiotic use, daycare attendance, recent episode of AOM, treatment failure or early recurrence.
[c] If treatment failure or recurrence within 1 month, consider alternative agents and repeated course of treatment or referral for tympanocentesis.
[d] If <6 weeks old refer to emergency department. Infants >6 weeks of age require very careful assessment; other occult sources of infection should be considered as a cause of fever.

Nonpharmacologic Choices

The strategy of watchful waiting has been recommended in many clinical practice guidelines for clinical situations in which the child is over 2 years of age, illness is mild and uncomplicated, and a parent/caregiver can easily access the physician for communication/re-evaluation.[10,11,12,13,14] Canadian guidelines[15] suggest a watchful waiting approach for the first 48–72 hours in children over 6 months of age, provided they have:

- nonsevere illness (fever <39ºC, mild otalgia)
- uncomplicated AOM
- no craniofacial anomalies, immunodeficiencies, cardiac or pulmonary disease, Down syndrome or history of complicated AOM
- parents capable of recognizing worsening illness with ready access to medical care.

Pharmacologic Choices

Analgesics

Provide adequate analgesia in the early stages of infection. In most cases, **acetaminophen** 10–15 mg/kg every 4–6 hours or **ibuprofen** 10 mg/kg every 6–8 hours is sufficient to control the ear pain.

Antibiotics (Table 1, Table 2)

The primary bacterial pathogens involved in acute otitis media are *Streptococcus pneumoniae*, *Haemophilus influenzae* and *Moraxella catarrhalis*. Clinical observations suggest that spontaneous resolution rates of acute otitis media caused by these 3 pathogens are 20%, 50% and 75%, respectively.[16] Therefore, a wait and see approach (or "watchful waiting"; see Nonpharmacologic Choices) has been proposed for a subset of patients,[10] which may lead to reduced number of antibiotic prescriptions.[17,18] Furthermore, with the introduction of pneumococcal conjugate vaccine the epidemiology of acute otitis media is changing. Specifically, pneumococcal serotypes included in the vaccine have decreased in frequency while other serotypes have increased. Also, the proportion of cases due to *S. pneumoniae* has decreased while those due to *H. influenzae* have increased. Overall, vaccination may be contributing to a decreased incidence of AOM.[19,20,21,22,23]

Antibiotic resistance is common among these 3 pathogens; therefore, choosing appropriate therapy depends on understanding the mechanisms of resistance involved. *S. pneumoniae* resistance to penicillin is a result of alteration of penicillin-binding cell wall proteins, leading to decreased drug affinity. Doubling the dose of amoxicillin raises the drug concentration in the middle ear to allow effective killing of penicillin-resistant strains. For *H. influenzae* and *M. catarrhalis,* beta-lactamase production confers resistance to amoxicillin and therefore adding a beta-lactamase inhibitor such as clavulanate allows the antibiotic to work effectively.

Amoxicillin is considered first-line therapy in the treatment of AOM, however the appropriate dose is controversial [Evidence: SORT C*].[10,24,25,26,27] *Standard-dose* amoxicillin (40 mg/kg/day) was considered first-line therapy in patients without risk factors for antibiotic resistance (recent antibiotic use, daycare attendance, recent episode of acute otitis media, treatment failure or early recurrence). However, the Canadian Pediatric Society suggests that *high-dose* amoxicillin (75–90 mg/kg/day) be used in all patients irrespective of risk factors for antibiotic resistance as it is not possible to definitively identify those with resistant *S. pneumoniae*.[15] Comparative antimicrobial studies have not been able to demonstrate clear superiority of one antibiotic (including standard- vs. high-dose amoxicillin) over another, with the possible exception of amoxicillin over azithromycin.[24,25] Furthermore, it is not clear

* SORT (Strength of Recommendation Taxonomy) is a rating system (A, B or C) that addresses the quality of available evidence. For more information consult **How to Use *Compendium of Therapeutic Choices*** on page xxv.

whether in vitro resistance is directly related to clinical failures for various infections caused by *S. pneumoniae*.[26] In addition, US data indicate that 83% and 87% of *S. pneumoniae* isolates are susceptible to standard- and high-dose amoxicillin, respectively.[10] Based on a lack of evidence indicating superiority of high-dose amoxicillin, standard-dose amoxicillin is still a reasonable first-line option for AOM in children without risk factors for resistance, keeping in mind local resistance patterns.[27]

Amoxicillin/clavulanate (with high-dose amoxicillin) possesses the added benefit of stability against beta-lactamases, produced by some strains of *H. influenzae* and most strains of *M. catarrhalis*. Amoxicillin/clavulanate is effective against most penicillin-resistant *S. pneumoniae*. Randomized, placebo-controlled studies show that children with properly diagnosed acute otitis media benefit from treatment with amoxicillin/clavulanate although diarrhea was noted as a common side effect.[28,29]

All other treatment options for acute otitis media are less favourable than amoxicillin or amoxicillin/clavulanate. Rates of resistance to other antibiotic classes such as cephalosporins and macrolides are on the rise.[30,31,32] However, in situations of treatment failures and penicillin allergy these antibiotic classes are alternatives.[10,11,12,33,34] It is important to differentiate between those patients who have true type I hypersensitivity (anaphylactic) reactions and those who experience a nonspecific adverse effect to the antibiotic. In general, parents and patients overestimate the true frequency of allergic reactions.[35,36] Cephalosporins can be used for patients who have previously experienced a non-type I hypersensitivity reaction to penicillins.

Cefuroxime axetil and **cefprozil** are second-generation cephalosporins with reasonable activity against *H. influenzae* and *M. catarrhalis* because they are less susceptible than amoxicillin to the action of beta-lactamases. However, cephalosporins are less effective than high-dose amoxicillin against penicillin-resistant strains of *S. pneumoniae*. They can be used as second-line agents.

Ceftriaxone is the most effective of the cephalosporins against otitis media pathogens but is not used routinely because it is administered iv or im daily for 3 days.[37]

Reserve **azithromycin** and **clarithromycin** for patients with type I hypersensitivity reactions to beta-lactam antibiotics due to increased rates of treatment failure with macrolides.[38]

Clindamycin is an alternative agent that can be used for patients with type I hypersensitivity reactions to beta-lactam antibiotics, but it does not cover *H. influenzae* or *M. catarrhalis*.

Therapeutic Tips

- Use of **vaccines** for influenza and *S. pneumoniae* may have a beneficial impact on the incidence of acute otitis media and therefore should be encouraged for eligible patients.[5,23,39,40,41,42] (See Table 3.)
- Most children will have middle ear effusions after completion of therapy. There is no need to treat an abnormal-appearing tympanic membrane in an asymptomatic child. If middle ear effusion persists over 3 months, arrange an audiology assessment to evaluate hearing.
- Nasal and oral **decongestants** alone or in combination with an **antihistamine** have not shown efficacy in resolving symptoms and infection or preventing complications and are not recommended for the management of acute otitis media.[1,43]

Table 1: Antibiotic Treatment Recommendations for Acute Otitis Media[10]

Characteristics	Therapeutic Tips	First Choice[a]	Treatment Failure Noted on Day 3[a]	Treatment Failure Noted on Day 10–28[a,b]
Age <6 weeks	Investigate for bacteremia; AOM often due to gram-negative bacteria	Refer to nearest emergency department for further assessment; symptoms such as fever may be related to sepsis in this age group	N/A	N/A
Age 6 weeks to 6 months	Treat most cases of AOM with antibiotic for 10 days	Standard-dose amoxicillin *or* High-dose (HD) amoxicillin	HD amoxicillin/clavulanate *or* cefprozil *or* cefuroxime axetil *or* ceftriaxone im/iv × 3 days Consider tympanocentesis	HD amoxicillin/clavulanate × 10 days *or* cefprozil × 10 days *or* cefuroxime axetil × 10 days *or* ceftriaxone im/iv × 3 days Consider tympanocentesis
Age ≥6 months, no risk factors (no frequent bouts of AOM and no antibiotics in previous 3 months)	Consider deferring treatment to see if AOM resolves in 48–72 h only if follow up can be ensured and if antibacterial therapy can be initiated if symptoms worsen <2 years: treat for 10 days ≥2 years: treat for 5 days[c,10]	Standard-dose amoxicillin *or* HD amoxicillin	HD amoxicillin/clavulanate *or* cefprozil *or* cefuroxime axetil *or* ceftriaxone im/iv × 3 days Consider tympanocentesis	HD amoxicillin/clavulanate × 10 days *or* cefprozil × 10 days *or* cefuroxime axetil × 10 days *or* ceftriaxone im/iv × 3 days Consider tympanocentesis
Age ≥6 months, with risk factors (received antibiotics in previous 3 months)	Consider deferring treatment to see if AOM resolves in 48–72 h only if follow up can be ensured and if antibacterial therapy can be initiated if symptoms worsen <2 years: treat for 10 days ≥2 years: treat for 5 days[c,10]	HD amoxicillin	HD amoxicillin/clavulanate *or* cefprozil *or* cefuroxime axetil *or* ceftriaxone im/iv × 3 days Consider tympanocentesis	HD amoxicillin/clavulanate × 10 days *or* cefprozil × 10 days *or* cefuroxime axetil × 10 days *or* ceftriaxone im/iv × 3 days Consider tympanocentesis
Any age Frequent bouts of AOM	Verify AOM Treat AOM episode for ≥10 days Consider conjugated pneumococcal vaccine if <5 years Give influenza vaccine yearly, all ages	HD amoxicillin/clavulanate	Ceftriaxone im/iv × 3 days Consider tympanocentesis	HD amoxicillin/clavulanate × 10 days *or* cefprozil × 10 days *or* cefuroxime axetil × 10 days *or* ceftriaxone im/iv × 3 days Consider tympanocentesis
Allergy to penicillin	Verify true anaphylactic-type allergy: hives; swollen lips, mouth, or throat; wheezing; hypotension; vomiting and diarrhea. Consider penicillin skin testing	Clarithromycin *or* azithromycin	Clindamycin May consider levofloxacin after consultation with an infectious disease specialist Consider tympanocentesis	Clindamycin May consider levofloxacin after consultation with an infectious disease specialist Consider tympanocentesis

[a] Unless otherwise specified, see Therapeutic Tips column for recommended duration of therapy. For dosage of antibiotics see Table 2.
[b] Choose an agent not previously used for the same infection.
[c] If the child has experienced treatment failure after 5 days of therapy, then subsequent treatment for the episode should be for 10 days.
Abbreviations: AOM = acute otitis media; HD = high-dose; N/A = not applicable

Table 2: Antibiotics for Acute Otitis Media

Class	Drug	Dose[a]	Adverse Effects	Comments	Cost[b]
Cephalosporins	*cefprozil* Cefzil, generics	30 mg/kg/day (maximum 1 g/day) po divided BID	Low incidence of diarrhea or GI upset.	Most children like the taste of the liquid formulation and it is well absorbed.	$
	ceftriaxone generics	50 mg/kg (maximum 1 g) Q24H im/iv × 3 days	Pain at injection site when administered im.	Second- or third-line agent. May be diluted with lidocaine 1% **plain** to a final concentration of 300 mg/mL to minimize pain at injection site when given im **only**. Do not reconstitute or mix with calcium-containing solutions.	$$$
	cefuroxime axetil Ceftin, generics	30 mg/kg/day (maximum 1 g/day) po divided BID	See cefprozil.		$$$
Lincosamides	*clindamycin* Dalacin C, Dalacin C Flavored Granules, Dalacin C Phosphate Sterile Solution, generics	30 mg/kg/day (maximum 1.8 g/day) po/iv divided TID–QID For severe infections may increase to 40 mg/kg/day (maximum 2.7 g/day) iv divided TID–QID	Nausea, vomiting, diarrhea (common), esophagitis, rash, *Clostridium difficile*-associated diarrhea.	Reserve for cases of true anaphylactic-type beta-lactam allergy and/or treatment failure. Clindamycin suspension has an unpleasant taste. If the dose prescribed is a multiple of a capsule strength (150 mg), capsules can be opened and mixed with a soft solid, e.g., apple sauce, pudding, chocolate sauce.	Caps: $ Oral susp: $$$ iv: $120
Macrolides	*azithromycin* Zithromax, generics	**5-day treatment:** Day 1: 10 mg/kg (maximum 500 mg) once daily po Days 2–5: 5 mg/kg (maximum 250 mg) once daily **3-day treatment:** 10 mg/kg (maximum 500 mg) once daily po	Low incidence of diarrhea or GI upset.	Most children like the taste of the suspension. Pneumococci with decreased susceptibility to penicillins and cephalosporins are sometimes resistant to azithromycin. Short course may improve adherence. Use if true anaphylactic-type beta-lactam allergy.	$$
	clarithromycin Biaxin, generics	15 mg/kg/day (maximum 1000 mg/day) po divided BID Because it sometimes has a bitter aftertaste, the suspension should be taken with food and/or juice	Diarrhea or vomiting (15%).	Pneumococci with decreased susceptibility to penicillins and cephalosporins are sometimes resistant to clarithromycin. Use if true anaphylactic-type beta-lactam allergy.	$$$

Class	Drug	Dose[a]	Adverse Effects	Comments	Cost[b]
Penicillins	*amoxicillin* ➧ generics	**Standard dose:** 40 mg/kg/day po divided BID–TID **High dose:** 75–90 mg/kg/day po divided BID–TID Maximum: 4 g/day Reserve standard-dose amoxicillin for the limited number of children at low risk of being infected with drug-resistant bacteria (no daycare, no antibiotic in the prior 3-month period)	Excellent safety profile. Occasionally causes mild diarrhea. Maculopapular rash occurs uncommonly but is difficult to distinguish from a concomitant viral exanthem.	**Drug of choice.** Most active agent against pneumococci with decreased susceptibility to penicillins and cephalosporins. For pneumococci with decreased susceptibility to penicillins and cephalosporins, amoxicillin is more active than cephalosporins.	$
	amoxicillin/ clavulanate ➧ Clavulin, generics	75–90 mg/kg/day po amoxicillin divided BID–TID Maximum: 4 g/day amoxicillin Best given as 2 simultaneous prescriptions to minimize the risk of diarrhea: one prescription of amoxicillin 40 mg/kg/day *plus* one prescription of 7:1 formulation amoxicillin/clavulanate liquid (Clavulin-200 or Clavulin-400) 40 mg/kg/day of the amoxicillin component Alternatively, one of the 7:1 formulations of amoxicillin/clavulanate liquid (Clavulin-200 or Clavulin-400) can be given at a dose of 80 mg/kg/day of the amoxicillin component, but may cause more diarrhea. Some patients will tolerate these high-dose regimens better if daily dose is divided TID rather than BID	Excellent safety profile. Diarrhea occurs frequently.	Avoid the original formulations of amoxicillin/clavulanate (Clavulin-125F and Clavulin-250F) in the high-dose protocol because the higher content of clavulanate increases the incidence of diarrhea. To avoid confusion when prescribing high-dose regimens, confirm intention on the prescription (e.g., write **"high-dose amoxicillin intended"** at the bottom). Active against most bacteria likely to cause acute otitis media.	$$

[a] Duration of treatment is 5 days for children over 2 years and 10 days if under 2 years; exceptions are ceftriaxone and azithromycin.
[b] Cost of 10-day supply based on 20 kg body weight, except 5-day supply for azithromycin, 3-day supply for ceftriaxone; includes drug cost only.
➧ Dosage adjustment may be required in renal impairment; see Appendix I.
Legend: $ < $15 $$ $15–30 $$$ $30–45 $$$$ $45–60

Table 3: **Vaccines for Prevention of Acute Otitis Media**

Class	Drug	Dose[44]	Comments	Cost[a]
Vaccines, bacterial	*pneumococcal vaccine, 10-valent conjugate* Synflorix	2–6 months: 4 doses im at 2, 4, 6 and 12–15 months. Alternatively, a 3-dose schedule may be considered; doses are given at 2, 4 and 11–12 months 7–11 months: 2 doses im given 1 month apart *plus* a booster given after the 1st birthday and at least 2 months after the second dose 12–59 months:[b] 2 doses im given 2 months apart		$$$$
	pneumococcal vaccine, 13-valent conjugate Prevnar 13	2–6 months: 4 doses im at 2, 4, 6 and 12–15 months 7–11 months: 2 doses im given 4 wk apart *plus* a booster given after the 1st birthday and at least 2 months after the second dose 12–23 months: 2 doses im given 2 months apart 24–59 months: 1 dose im	NACI recommends the 13-valent conjugate vaccine as the vaccine of choice for routine childhood immunization.[44]	$$$$
Vaccines, viral	*influenza vaccine, inactivated* Agriflu, Fluviral, Vaxigrip	≥6 months: 0.5 mL im Children 6 months–<9 y who have not previously received influenza vaccine should receive a second dose ≥4 wk after the first dose	Contraindicated in persons with history of anaphylactic reaction to a previous dose. May now be used in persons with an allergy to eggs based on an assessment of risk of a severe allergic reaction. For detailed information see the *Canadian Immunization Guide*.[44]	$
	influenza vaccine, live attenuated FluMist	≥2 y: 0.2 mL intranasally given as 1 spray (0.1 mL) per nostril Children 2–<9 y who have not previously received influenza vaccine should receive a second dose ≥4 wk after the first dose	Contraindicated in children receiving ASA therapy or those with severe asthma, immune-compromising conditions or a history of anaphylactic reaction to a previous dose or to eggs.[44]	$

[a] Cost of 1 dose; includes drug cost only.
[b] A booster dose may be needed in children 12–23 months of age to provide optimal protection, particularly if they are at high risk of pneumococcal infection.
Legend: $ < $25 $$ $25–50 $$$ $50–75 $$$$ $75–100

Suggested Readings

Forgie S, Zhanel G, Robinson J. Management of acute otitis media. *Paediatr Child Health* 2009;14(7):457-64.

Lieberthal AS, Carroll AE, Chonmaitree T et al. The diagnosis and management of acute otitis media. *Pediatrics* 2013;131(3):e964-99.

Neff MJ; American Academy of Pediatrics; American Academy of Family Physicians. AAP, AAFP release guideline on diagnosis and management of acute otitis media. *Am Fam Physician* 2004;69(11):2713-5.

Rovers MM, Glasziou P, Appelman CL et al. Antibiotics for acute otitis media: a meta-analysis with individual patient data. *Lancet* 2006;368(9545):1429-35.

Rovers MM, Glasziou P, Appelman CL et al. Predictors of pain and/or fever at 3 to 7 days for children with acute otitis media not treated initially with antibiotics: a meta-analysis of individual patient data. *Pediatrics* 2007;119(3):579-85.

References

1. Chonmaitree T. Acute otitis media is not a pure bacterial disease. *Clin Infect Dis* 2006;43(11):1423-5.
2. Faden H, Stanievich J, Brodsky L et al. Changes in nasopharyngeal flora during otitis media of childhood. *Pediatr Infect Dis J* 1990;9(9):623-6.
3. Sanyal MA, Henderson FW, Stempel EC et al. Effect of upper respiratory tract infection on eustachian tube ventilatory function in the preschool child. *J Pediatr* 1980;97(1):11-5.
4. Ruohola A, Meurman O, Nikkari S et al. Microbiology of acute otitis media in children with tympanostomy tubes: prevalences of bacteria and viruses. *Clin Infect Dis* 2006;43(11):1417-22.
5. Klein JO, Chonmaitree T, Loosmore S et al. Otitis media: a preventable disease? Proceedings of an international symposium organized by the Marcel Merieux Foundation, Veyrier-du-Lac, France, February 13 to 16, 2000. *Pediatr Infect Dis J* 2001;20(5):473-81.
6. Adair-Bischoff CE, Sauve RS. Environmental tobacco smoke and middle ear disease in preschool-age children. *Arch Pediatr Adolesc Med* 1998;152(2):127-33.
7. Duffy LC, Faden H, Wasielewski R et al. Exclusive breastfeeding protects against bacterial colonization and day care exposure to otitis media. *Pediatrics* 1997;100(4):E7.
8. Paradise JL, Rockette HE, Colborn DK et al. Otitis media in 2253 Pittsburgh-area infants: prevalence and risk factors during the first two years of life. *Pediatrics* 1997;99(3):318-33.
9. Greenberg D, Givon-Lavi N, Broides A et al. The contribution of smoking and exposure to tobacco smoke to Streptococcus pneumoniae and Haemophilus influenzae carriage in children and their mothers. *Clin Infect Dis* 2006;42(7):897-903.
10. Lieberthal AS, Carroll AE, Chonmaitree T et al. The diagnosis and management of acute otitis media. *Pediatrics* 2013;131(3):e964-99.
11. Alberta Medical Association. *Guideline for the diagnosis and treatment of acute otitis media.* Edmonton (AB): Toward Optimized Practice, Alberta Medical Association; 2008. Available from: www.topalbertadoctors.org/download/366/AOM_guideline.pdf. Accessed October 7, 2011.
12. British Columbia Medical Association, Guidelines and Protocols Advisory Committee. *Acute otitis media (AOM).* Victoria (BC): BCMA; 2004. Available from: www.bcguidelines.ca/gpac/pdf/otitaom.pdf. Accessed October 7, 2011.
13. Hoberman A, Marchant CD, Kaplan SL et al. Treatment of acute otitis media consensus recommendations. *Clin Pediatr (Phila)* 2002;41(6):373-90.
14. Scottish Intercollegiate Guidelines Network. *Diagnosis and management of childhood otitis media in primary care: a national clinical guideline.* Edinburgh (GB): Royal College of Physicians; 2003. Available from: www.sign.ac.uk/pdf/sign66.pdf. Accessed October 7, 2011.
15. Forgie S, Zhanel G, Robinson J. Management of acute otitis media. *Paediatr Child Health* 2009;14(7):457-64.
16. Klein JO. Microbiologic efficacy of antibacterial drugs for acute otitis media. *Pediatr Infect Dis J* 1993;12(12):973-5.
17. Rovers MM, Glasziou P, Appelman CL et al. Antibiotics for acute otitis media: a meta-analysis with individual patient data. *Lancet* 2006;368(9545):1429-35.
18. Spiro DM, Tay KY, Arnold DH et al. Wait-and-see prescription for the treatment of acute otitis media: a randomized controlled trial. *JAMA* 2006;296(10):1235-41.
19. Casey JR, Pichichero ME. Changes in frequency and pathogens causing acute otitis media in 1995-2003. *Pediatr Infect Dis J* 2004;23(9):824-8.
20. Leibovitz E, Jacobs MR, Dagan R. Haemophilus influenzae: a significant pathogen in acute otitis media. *Pediatr Infect Dis J* 2004;23(12):1142-52.
21. Coker TR, Chan LS, Newberry SJ et al. Diagnosis, microbial epidemiology, and antibiotic treatment of acute otitis media in children: a systematic review. *JAMA* 2010;304(19):2161-9.
22. Casey JR, Adlowitz DG, Pichichero ME. New patterns in the otopathogens causing acute otitis media six to eight years after introduction of pneumococcal conjugate vaccine. *Pediatr Infect Dis J* 2010;29(4):304-9.
23. Taylor S, Marchisio P, Vergison A et al. Impact of pneumococcal conjugate vaccination on otitis media: a systematic review. *Clin Infect Dis* 2012;54(12):1765-73.
24. Shekelle PG, Takata G, Newberry SJ et al. Management of acute otitis media: update. Evidence Report/Technology Assessment No. 198. (Prepared by the Southern California Evidence-based Practice Center under Contract No. 290 2007 10056 I). Rockville, MD: Agency for Healthcare Research and Quality. November 2010. Available from: www.ahrq.gov/research/findings/evidence-based-reports/otitisup-evidence-report.pdf. Accessed May 28, 2013.
25. Courter JD, Baker WL, Nowak KS et al. Increased clinical failures when treating acute otitis media with macrolides: a meta-analysis. *Ann Pharmacother* 2010;44(3):471-8.
26. Lynch JP, Zhanel GG. Streptococcus pneumoniae: does antimicrobial resistance matter? *Semin Respir Crit Care Med* 2009;30(2):210-38.
27. Garbutt J, St. Geme JW 3rd, May A et al. Developing community-specific recommendations for first-line treatment of acute otitis media: is high-dose amoxicillin necesaary? *Pediatrics* 2004;114(2):342-7.

28. Hoberman A, Paradise JL, Rockette HE et al. Treatment of acute otitis media in children under 2 years of age. *N Engl J Med* 2011;364(2):105-15.
29. Tahtinen PA, Laine MK, Huovinen P et al. A placebo-controlled trial of antimicrobial treatment for acute otitis media. *N Engl J Med* 2011;364(2):116-26.
30. Doern GV, Pfaller MA, Kugler K et al. Prevalence of antimicrobial resistance among respiratory tract isolates of Streptococcus pneumoniae in North America: 1997 results from the SENTRY antimicrobial surveillance program. *Clin Infect Dis* 1998;27(4):764-70.
31. Jacobs MR, Bajaksouzian S, Zilles A et al. Susceptibilities of Streptococcus pneumoniae and Haemophilus influenzae to 10 oral antimicrobial agents based on pharmacodynamic parameters: 1997 U.S. Surveillance study. *Antimicrob Agents Chemother* 1999;43(8):1901-8.
32. Jacobs MR. Increasing antibiotic resistance among otitis media pathogens and their susceptibility to oral agents based on pharmacodynamic parameters. *Pediatr Infect Dis J* 2000;19(5 Suppl):S47-55.
33. Brook I. Use of oral cephalosporins in the treatment of acute otitis media in children. *Int J Antimicrob Agents* 2004;24(1):18-23.
34. Dunne MW, Latiolais T, Lewis B et al. Randomized, double-blind study of the clinical efficacy of 3 days of azithromycin compared with co-amoxiclav for the treatment of acute otitis media. *J Antimicrob Chemother* 2003;52(3):469-72.
35. Langley JM, Halperin SA, Bortolussi R. History of penicillin allergy and referral for skin testing: evaluation of a pediatric penicillin allergy testing program. *Clin Invest Med* 2002;25(5):181-4.
36. Langley J, Halperin S. Allergy to antibiotics in children: perception versus reality. *Paediatr Child Health* 2002;7(4):233-7.
37. Leibovitz E, Piglansky L, Raiz S et al. Bacteriologic and clinical efficacy of one day vs. three day intramuscular ceftriaxone for treatment of nonresponsive acute otitis media in children. *Pediatr Infect Dis J* 2000;19(11):1040-5.
38. Courter JD, Baker WL, Nowak KS et al. Increased clinical failures when treating acute otitis media with macrolides: a meta-analysis. *Ann Pharmacother* 2010;44(3):471-8.
39. Eskola J, Kilpi T, Palmu A et al. Efficacy of a pneumococcal conjugate vaccine against acute otitis media. *N Engl J Med* 2001;344(6):403-9.
40. Jenson HB, Baltimore RS. Impact of pneumococcal and influenza vaccines on otitis media. *Curr Opin Pediatr* 2004;16(1):58-60.
41. Ozgur SK, Beyazova U, Kemaloglu YK et al. Effectiveness of inactivated influenza vaccine for prevention of otitis media in children. *Pediatr Infect Dis J* 2006;25(5):401-4.
42. Clements DA, Langdon L, Bland C et al. Influenza A vaccine decreases the incidence of otitis media in 6- to 30-month-old children in day care. *Arch Pediatr Adolesc Med* 1995;149(10):1113-7.
43. Coleman C, Moore M. Decongestants and antihistamines for acute otitis media in children. *Cochrane Database Syst Rev* 2008;(3):CD001727.
44. National Advisory Committee on Immunization (NACI). Public Health Agency of Canada. *Canadian immunization guide*. Evergreen ed. Available from: www.phac-aspc.gc.ca/publicat/cig-gci/index-eng.php. Accessed April 24, 2013.

Chapter 109
Bacterial Meningitis

Alana Rosenthal, MD, FRCPC

Meningitis is described as inflammation of the cranial and spinal leptomeninges. *Bacterial meningitis* is characterized by bacterial invasion of the cranial and spinal leptomeninges. It most often develops following bacteremia but can also occur via extension from surrounding structures (e.g., mastoiditis, sinusitis) or direct inoculation during neurosurgery or open head trauma. The causative pathogens in bacterial meningitis depend on age and specific host and environmental factors (Table 1, Table 2).

Table 1: Bacterial Meningitis: Probable Pathogens and Empiric Therapy Based on Age

Age Group	Bacteria	Empiric Antibacterial Regimen
Infants <6 wk	Group B streptococcus *Escherichia coli* *Listeria monocytogenes* Other *Enterobacteriaceae* *Streptococcus pneumoniae* (rare) *Neisseria meningitidis* (rare)	Ampicillin + cefotaxime[a] Add gentamicin if early neonatal meningitis suspected given synergy for Group B streptococcal infections
Infants 6 wk–3 months	*S. pneumoniae* (pneumococcus) *N. meningitidis* (meningococcus) Group B streptococcus *Haemophilus influenzae* type b[b] *E. coli* (rare) *L. monocytogenes* (rare) Other *Enterobacteriaceae* (rare)	Ceftriaxone or cefotaxime + Ampicillin + Vancomycin[c]
Infants >3 months, children and adults	*S. pneumoniae* *N. meningitidis* *H. influenzae* type b[b]	Ceftriaxone or cefotaxime + Vancomycin[c]
Adults >50 y or alcoholics	*E. coli* *S. pneumoniae* *N. meningitidis* *L. monocytogenes*[d]	Ceftriaxone or cefotaxime + Ampicillin + Vancomycin[c]

[a] Cefotaxime is preferred over ceftriaxone in neonates because of the theoretical risk of displacement of bilirubin from albumin and possible subsequent hyperbilirubinemia.
[b] *H. influenzae* type b is rare since implementation of universal vaccination.
[c] Vancomycin is included in the initial antibacterial regimen due to increasing prevalence of resistant *S. pneumoniae*.
[d] *L. monocytogenes* is also associated with meningitis in pregnancy.

- There is still significant mortality and morbidity associated with bacterial meningitis. Acute complications may include but are not limited to:
  - subdural effusion or empyema
  - brain abscess
  - cerebritis or ventriculitis
  - venous sinus thrombosis

- seizures
- CNS infarction, resulting in hemiparesis, quadriparesis or spinal cord infarction
- brain herniation
- shock and/or disseminated intravascular coagulopathy
- diabetes insipidus and/or SIADH

- Neurologic *sequelae* may include but are not limited to:
  - sensorineural hearing loss
  - visual problems including cortical blindness
  - ataxia
  - hydrocephalus
  - behavioural difficulties
  - intellectual deficits
  - epilepsy

Table 2: **Bacterial Meningitis: Probable Pathogens and Empiric Therapy Based on Specific Host and Environmental Factors**

Risk Factor	Bacteria	Empiric Antibacterials
Cerebrospinal fluid leak, basilar skull fracture	*S. pneumoniae* *Streptococcus pyogenes* *H. influenzae* type b	Ceftriaxone or cefotaxime + Vancomycin
Penetrating head trauma/neurosurgery[a]	*Staphylococcus* spp. *Streptococcus* spp. *E. coli* *Klebsiella* spp. *Pseudomonas aeruginosa*	3rd generation cephalosporin[b] + Vancomycin[a]
Ventriculoperitoneal shunt	*Staphylococcus epidermidis* *Staphylococcus aureus* *S. pneumoniae* *N. meningitidis* *H. influenzae* type b Aerobic gram-negative bacilli (including *P. aeruginosa*) *Propionibacterium acnes*	3rd generation cephalosporin[b] + Vancomycin
Humoral immune deficiency states e.g., agammaglobulinemia	*S. pneumoniae* *N. meningitidis* *H. influenzae* type b	Ceftriaxone or cefotaxime + Vancomycin
Cellular immune deficiency states e.g., chemotherapy, HIV	*S. pneumoniae* *N. meningitidis* *L. monocytogenes* *H. influenzae* type b	Ceftriaxone or cefotaxime + Ampicillin + Vancomycin
Asplenia (anatomic or functional)	*S. pneumoniae* *N. meningitidis* *Salmonella* spp. *H. influenzae* type b	Ceftriaxone or cefotaxime + Vancomycin

[a] Consider adding anaerobic and antifungal coverage if the wound is contaminated.
[b] Ceftazidime is the cephalosporin of choice if there is a high suspicion of *P. aeruginosa* infection. If cephalosporin-resistant *P. aeruginosa* is suspected, use meropenem instead.

Goals of Therapy

- Eradicate bacteria from the CNS
- Decrease mortality
- Manage and minimize acute and chronic complications including permanent neurologic damage

Investigations

Clinical Presentation

- The clinical presentation varies and is related to age and developmental stage. Onset may be acute or insidious.
  - *infants* may present with only a change in temperature (fever *or* hypothermia). Other signs are usually nonspecific and may include inconsolable crying, irritability, lethargy, seizures, poor feeding, vomiting, diarrhea, jaundice and/or a bulging anterior fontanelle. Signs of meningeal irritation such as a stiff neck are often absent, and therefore in infants clinicians should have a low threshold for suspecting meningitis. A fever in a baby <6 weeks of age warrants examination and culture of the cerebrospinal fluid (CSF) in all circumstances.
  - in *children and adults*, symptoms usually include fever, severe headache, stiff neck or back pain and/or photophobia. Patients often report feeling systemically unwell with associated vomiting. Neurologic signs may include loss of balance, seizures, disorientation, confusion, altered level of consciousness, stiff neck, positive Kernig's and Brudzinski's signs, cranial nerve palsies and/or other signs of increased intracranial pressure, e.g., papilledema. Signs of cerebral infarction may also be present.
  - patients of any age can present in septic shock. Other physical exam findings may include petechia or purpura, which are usually suggestive of meningococcal meningitis but can also be seen with *S. pneumoniae* and other bacterial pathogens.

Laboratory Investigations

Cerebral Spinal Fluid (CSF)

- Examination of the CSF is essential for making the diagnosis and is warranted whenever meningitis is suspected. Lumbar puncture (LP) is contraindicated in the presence of increased intracranial pressure (ICP), papilledema, focal neurologic signs, deteriorating Glasgow Coma Score, shock, infection at the LP site and bleeding disorders.[1] Brain imaging may or may not be helpful in excluding increased ICP prior to lumbar puncture. If raised ICP is strongly suspected clinically, then the LP should be deferred. *Do not delay empiric antibacterial therapy* if an LP cannot be performed at the time of presentation.
- In patients with a ventriculoperitoneal shunt, CSF may be obtained by tapping the shunt percutaneously, although strict sterile technique is mandatory.
- Examine the CSF for cell count and differential, culture and sensitivity, and glucose and protein concentrations. Findings consistent with bacterial meningitis include:
  - elevated CSF WBC count with a predominance of neutrophils is usually present; however, *initially* the CSF WBC count may be considerably less elevated. It is often not possible to differentiate bacterial from viral or other types of meningitis based purely on the CSF WBC
  - reduced CSF glucose (CSF-serum ratio <0.6 for infants and <0.4 for those over 2 months of age)[2]
  - normal or elevated CSF protein (range varies according to age)
  - CSF Gram stain is positive in up to 80–90% of hematogenously acquired meningitis,[3] but this varies according to the causative pathogen.[4]
- Culture is the gold standard for diagnosis but may not be positive, particularly in those previously treated with antibacterials.

- In the setting of negative Gram stain and culture with significant CSF pleocytosis, consult an infectious diseases expert to determine the utility of PCR and/or latex agglutination on the CSF
  - PCR for *N. meningitidis* is performed routinely in some institutions
  - the use of PCR for other bacteria looks promising
  - latex agglutination of the CSF in meningitis has poor sensitivity and specificity but some experts find it useful in certain situations[5,6]
- An elevated CSF lactate level (>4 mmol/L) may be present in postoperative neurosurgical patients with bacterial meningitis.[7]
- A repeat LP is indicated in the following situations:
  - failure to improve clinically
  - immunocompromised patients
  - cephalosporin-resistant pneumococcal meningitis
  - meningitis caused by enteric gram-negative bacilli or other unusual pathogens
  - patients who received corticosteroids for prevention of complications due to meningitis (because corticosteroids may temporarily mask treatment failure)
- Consider a repeat LP in all neonatal meningitis caused by Group B streptococcus (GBS).

Blood

- Complete blood count and differential; culture and sensitivity. Draw a blood glucose level at or near the time of the CSF glucose to enable comparison of the 2 values.

Imaging

- Imaging studies (CT or MRI of the head) are not routinely required but are indicated for those individuals with focal neurologic signs, clinical evidence of brain herniation, decreased/fluctuating level of consciousness, clinical deterioration, or persistent fever. In addition, some evidence suggests that CT scans should be done prior to LP in those with underlying neurologic conditions, immunodeficiency states or in individuals >60 years of age.[8]

Therapeutic Choices

Pharmacologic Choices

Antibacterial Therapy

- Choice of empiric antibacterial therapy is based on the most likely causative organisms, host factors such as patient age (Table 1, Table 2) and local antimicrobial resistance patterns.
- Initiate antimicrobial therapy without delay; each hour of delaying antibiotic administration has been shown to increase the risk of an unfavourable outcome (mortality or disability) by 30% in adults with bacterial meningitis.[9]
- Re-evaluate and modify antibacterial therapy when results of the CSF Gram stain, culture and then sensitivity become available (Table 3).
- The duration of therapy depends on host factors and the causative pathogen. General guidelines for duration of therapy for some common pathogens are shown in Table 3.
- Doses, most common adverse effects and drug interactions are shown in Table 4.
- Due to the increasing incidence of penicillin-resistant pneumococci and meningococci in Canada, **penicillin G** is no longer appropriate as empiric therapy.
- Use **vancomycin** and high-dose **ceftriaxone** or **cefotaxime** as empiric therapy for presumed pneumococcal meningitis in all individuals >6 weeks of age. If an infant <6 weeks of age has a Gram stain suggestive of pneumococcal meningitis, use vancomycin and cefotaxime pending sensitivity results.[15]

- For penicillin and cephalosporin-resistant pneumococci, the use of **cephalosporins** alone, even in high doses, may be inadequate. The addition of **vancomycin** ± **rifampin** to high-dose cephalosporins appears to enhance bacterial eradication in the CSF.[16,17]
- **Imipenem** is not recommended for the treatment of bacterial meningitis because it is thought to increase the risk of seizures more than other beta-lactams, although the real risk is unclear.[18]

Table 3: Antibacterial Regimens for Specific Pathogens in Uncomplicated Bacterial Meningitis

Pathogen	First-line	Alternative	Duration of Therapy[a]
S. pneumoniae (penicillin-susceptible)	Penicillin G	Ceftriaxone or cefotaxime	10–14 days
S. pneumoniae (intermediate- or high-level resistance to penicillin, sensitive to cephalosporins)	Cefotaxime or ceftriaxone Consult infectious diseases specialist	Meropenem Consult infectious diseases specialist	10–14 days
S. pneumoniae (intermediate- or high-level resistance to penicillin and third-generation cephalosporins)	Cefotaxime or ceftriaxone + Vancomycin ± Rifampin Consult infectious diseases specialist	Meropenem Consult infectious diseases specialist	10–14 days
N. meningitidis (penicillin-sensitive)	Penicillin G	Cefotaxime or ceftriaxone	5–7 days
N. meningitidis (penicillin-resistant)	Cefotaxime or ceftriaxone[b]		5–7 days
H. influenzae type b (ampicillin-susceptible)	Ampicillin	Cefotaxime or ceftriaxone	7–10 days
H. influenzae type b (ampicillin-resistant)	Ceftriaxone or cefotaxime		7–10 days
Group B streptococcus	Penicillin + Gentamicin for synergy[c]	Ampicillin or cefotaxime	14–21 days
L. monocytogenes	Ampicillin + Gentamicin for synergy[c]	Sulfamethoxazole/trimethoprim	At least 21 days
Enterobacteriaceae[d]	Ceftriaxone or cefotaxime[e] ± Gentamicin[f]	Meropenem[1]	21 days (Gentamicin for first 7–14 days)[1]

[a] These are general guidelines only; some cases may require a longer duration of therapy.
[b] Superiority over high-dose penicillin has not been proven.
[c] The addition of gentamicin provides in vitro and in vivo synergy. Gentamicin therapy should be continued for 3–7 days, but may be longer in the case of delayed sterilization of the CSF.
[d] Therapy may be different depending on suspected pathogen and susceptibilities.
[e] Ampicillin can be used if organism is susceptible.
[f] Pediatric guidelines recommend addition of gentamicin; recommended in adults only when organism is *P. aeruginosa*.

Adjunctive Corticosteroids

The rationale behind adjunctive therapy with **dexamethasone** is that it will decrease the inflammatory response in the CNS, thereby limiting neurologic sequelae.

A theoretical concern regarding the use of dexamethasone in meningitis is the potential for delayed sterilization of the CSF (due to altered CSF drug penetration) in individuals treated with **vancomycin** for resistant *S. pneumoniae*. There are no large clinical studies to answer this question. Strongly consider the addition of **rifampin** to the antibacterial regimen if resistant pneumococci are isolated in a patient who has received dexamethasone.[4,19]

The effect of dexamethasone on long-term cognitive function remains unclear. Therefore, careful follow up of these patients is required.

Children

A meta-analysis of randomized controlled trials in children performed between 1988 and 1996 showed a beneficial effect of adjunctive dexamethasone therapy in reducing severe hearing loss in children with *H. influenzae* type b meningitis. In meningitis caused by *S. pneumoniae*, the use of dexamethasone showed a trend toward protection against hearing loss. If dexamethasone was given before or at the time of antibacterial administration, the benefit became significant.[20]

The use of adjunctive dexamethasone in children >6 weeks of age with community-acquired bacterial meningitis may be considered after weighing the potential benefits and risks. Consultation with an infectious diseases specialist is warranted. The recommended dose for children is 0.6 mg/kg/day in 4 divided doses for 2–4 days.[15] This should be initiated either before or with the first dose of antibacterials.

Adults

A systematic review of adjunctive corticosteroid therapy in adults with acute bacterial meningitis showed an overall trend toward lower mortality.[21] In the subgroup analysis, there was a significant decrease in mortality in *S. pneumoniae* meningitis. In high income countries, corticosteroids reduced hearing loss and short-term neurologic sequelae. This same benefit was not seen in resource-poor countries. For adults, the use of adjunctive dexamethasone is initially recommended in cases of community-acquired bacterial meningitis.

The dose for adults has been variable in published studies. Dexamethasone 10 mg every 6 hours for 4 days has been used.[22] Practice guidelines from the Infectious Diseases Society of America recommend 0.15 mg/kg every 6 hours for 2–4 days, commencing either before or with the first dose of antibacterials.[4]

Prevention

Vaccines

- With the implementation in Canada of universal infant immunization programs with conjugated *H. influenzae* type b, *S. pneumoniae* and *N. meningitidis* vaccines, the rates of bacterial meningitis have decreased significantly. There is also evidence of the development of herd immunity (protection of unvaccinated individuals extending from immunization of a majority of the population).
- The conjugated vaccine against *H. influenzae* type b has led to the virtual disappearance of meningitis due to this pathogen. The conjugated pneumococcal vaccine is >95% effective in preventing invasive disease caused by the seven serotypes included in the 7-valent vaccine, and preliminary data suggest a further reduction in meningitis due to the additional serotypes included in the 13-valent vaccine which is now in use.[23,24]
- The conjugated meningococcal vaccine against *N. meningitidis* type C has a reported efficacy of >90% against invasive infection.[25] Quadrivalent conjugate meningococcal vaccines against

N. meningitidis types A,C,W,Y-135 are also available for use in individuals over the age of 2 years. A vaccine against *N. meningitidis* type B is now available for individuals 2 months to 17 years of age.

- In individuals >2 years of age, polysaccharide vaccines are safe and efficacious for the prevention of invasive pneumococcal and meningococcal infections. Certain high-risk individuals may benefit from receiving both conjugated and polysaccharide vaccines; consult the *Canadian Immunization Guide*.[26]
- Vaccination to prevent meningitis is recommended in Canada for certain high-risk individuals as well. These recommendations are outlined in the *Canadian Immunization Guide*.[26]

Intrapartum Prophylaxis

- The administration of intrapartum antibacterials to prevent mother-to-child transmission significantly reduces the incidence of early-onset invasive neonatal GBS infections.[27]

Postexposure Prophylaxis

- Those in close contact (as defined in the corresponding references[10,11,28]) with individuals who have meningitis caused by either *H. influenzae* type b or *N. meningitidis* are at increased risk of developing infection. Postexposure prophylaxis is recommended for close contacts only, to reduce the risk of transmission.
- The regimen following exposure to *H. influenzae* type b is **rifampin** 20 mg/kg (maximum dose 600 mg) orally once daily for 4 days. The dose for infants <1 month of age is not established; consultation with an infectious diseases specialist is recommended. Rifampin is contraindicated in pregnant women; therefore, prophylaxis is not recommended.
- Following exposure to *N. meningitidis*, the prophylactic regimen for infants <1 month is **rifampin** 5 mg/kg Q12H po for 2 days.[28] Children ≥1 month should receive rifampin 10 mg/kg (maximum 600 mg) Q12H po for 2 days. Alternatively, **ceftriaxone** can be given as a single dose of 125 mg im in those 1 month to <15 years old, and 250 mg im in those ≥15 years.[10] **Ciprofloxacin** 20 mg/kg (maximum 500 mg) can be administered orally to patients ≥1 month old as a single dose. Ceftriaxone is the drug of choice for pregnant women.
- In cases of meningitis involving either *N. meningitidis* or *H. influenzae*, the index patient should also receive prophylaxis prior to discharge to eradicate bacterial carriage, unless cefotaxime or ceftriaxone was used for treatment.

Therapeutic Tips

- In the case of empiric antimicrobial therapy consisting of **vancomycin** and a **cephalosporin**, give the cephalosporin first to ensure initial broad coverage and penetration into the CSF.
- With ventriculoperitoneal shunt-associated meningitis, successful treatment should include removal of the shunt with insertion of an external ventricular drain in addition to antimicrobial therapy.

Table 4: **Intravenous Antibacterial Therapy for Bacterial Meningitis**[4,10,11,12,13]

Class	Antibacterial	Dose	Adverse Effects	Comments	Cost[a]
Aminoglycosides	*gentamicin* ❥ generics	**Neonates ≤7 days:** <1.2 kg: 2.5 mg/kg Q18–24H **Neonates >7 days and older children:** 1.2–2 kg: 2.5 mg/kg Q12H >2 kg: 2.5 mg/kg Q8H **Adults and adolescents:** 1–2 mg/kg Q8H	Nephrotoxicity: Increased risk with higher dose and duration. Ototoxicity. Levels should be closely monitored to reduce incidence of toxicity.	Enhanced toxicity with use of amphotericin B, magnesium, cephalosporins, penicillins, loop diuretics, vancomycin, cisplatin, cyclosporin and indomethacin. Aminoglycosides are used for synergy and should always be used in conjunction with a bactericidal drug.	$
Carbapenems	*meropenem* ❥ Merrem, Meropenem for Injection	**Neonates:** 80 mg/kg/day divided Q12H **Infants >4 weeks and children:** 120 mg/kg/day divided Q8H **Adults:** 6 g/day divided Q8H	Diarrhea, nausea, hypersensitivity reactions, rarely seizures.	Meropenem may decrease valproic acid levels. Risk of seizure increased in the presence of poor renal function; caution is advised.	$$$$$
Cephalosporins	*cefotaxime* ❥ Claforan	**Neonates ≤7 days:** <2 kg: 100 mg/kg/day divided Q12H ≥2 kg: 100–150 mg/kg/day divided Q8H **Neonates >7 days:** 1.2–2 kg: 150 mg/kg/day divided Q8H >2 kg: 150–200 mg/kg/day divided Q6–8H **6 wk–12 y:** 300 mg/kg/day divided Q6H[b] **>12 y:** 2 g Q4–6H Maximum: 12 g/day	Hypersensitivity, phlebitis, diarrhea, pseudomembranous colitis, transient elevation in liver enzymes; leukopenia; neutropenia, eosinophilia; thrombocytopenia. Seizures, nephrotoxicity with large doses.		$$$$
	ceftazidime ❥ Fortaz, generics	**Neonates ≤7 days:** <2 kg: 100 mg/kg/day divided Q12H ≥2 kg: 100–150 mg/kg/day divided Q8–12H **Infants >7 days and children:** 150 mg/kg/day divided Q8H **Adults:** 2 g Q8H Maximum: 6 g/day	See cefotaxime.	Preferred cephalosporin for *P. aeruginosa* infection.	$$$$$

Class	Antibacterial	Dose	Adverse Effects	Comments	Cost[a]
	ceftriaxone generics	**Infants and children:** 100 mg/kg Q12H × 3 doses, then Q24H **Adults:** 2 g Q12–24H Maximum: 4 g/day	See cefotaxime.	Contraindicated in neonates. Do not reconstitute or mix with calcium-containing solutions as an insoluble precipitate may form. Do not administer simultaneously with calcium-containing iv solutions via a Y-site. Administration may be done sequentially provided the infusion lines are thoroughly flushed between infusions.	$$
Glycopeptides	*vancomycin* ❥ generics	**Neonates:**[c] >2 kg or PCA >37 weeks: 22.5 mg/kg/dose Q12H **Infants >4 weeks and children:** 60 mg/kg/day divided Q6H Maximum: 1 g/dose or 4 g/day prior to therapeutic drug monitoring **Adults:**15–20 mg/kg Q8–12H	Flushing, hypotension with rapid iv infusion; phlebitis.	May cause ototoxicity, nephrotoxicity if receiving other drugs with these effects. Adjust dose to achieve serum trough levels of 15–20 µg/mL in adults.[14] While more studies are needed to confirm appropriate trough levels in infants and children, it is reasonable to consider trough levels of 15–20 µg/mL for serious infections in this population.	$$$$$
Penicillins	*penicillin G* ❥ Crystapen, generics	**Neonates ≤7 days:** GBS: 450 000 units/kg/day divided Q8H **Neonates >7 days:** GBS: 450 000–500 000 units/kg/day divided Q4–6H **Older infants and children:** 400 000 units/kg/day divided Q4–6H Maximum: 24 million units/day **Adults:** 20–24 million units/day divided Q4–6H	Rash, hypersensitivity, drug fever, hemolytic anemia, interstitial nephritis, seizures (with high doses).	Tetracycline may decrease effectiveness of penicillins.	$

(cont'd)

Table 4: **Intravenous Antibacterial Therapy for Bacterial Meningitis**[4,10,11,12,13] *(cont'd)*

Class	Antibacterial	Dose	Adverse Effects	Comments	Cost[a]
	ampicillin ➔ generics	**Neonates ≤7 days:** ≤2 kg: 100 mg/kg/day divided Q12H >2 kg: 150 mg/kg/day divided Q8H GBS: 200 mg/kg/day divided Q8H **Neonates >7 days:** <1.2 kg: 100 mg/kg/day divided Q12H 1.2–2 kg: 150 mg/kg/day divided Q8H >2 kg: 200 mg/kg/day divided Q6H GBS: 300–400 mg/kg/day divided Q4–6H **Older infants and children:** 200 mg/kg/day divided Q4–6H GBS: 400 mg/kg/day divided Q4–6H **Adults:** 2 g Q4H Maximum: 12 g/day	Rash, hypersensitivity, diarrhea, vomiting, drug fever, seizures (with high doses).	Increased incidence of rash with concurrent use of allopurinol.	$$
Sulfonamide Combinations	*sulfamethoxazole/ trimethoprim* ➔ Septra Injection	**Infants ≥2 months, children and adults:** 10–20 mg/kg/day (based on trimethoprim component) divided Q6–12H Maximum (children): 320 mg/day trimethoprim component Maximum (adults): 960 mg/day trimethoprim component	Nausea, vomiting, hypersensitivity reactions (may be severe), myelosuppression, hyperkalemia (with higher doses).	Contraindicated in neonates due to risk of kernicterus in the newborn. Use with caution in patients with G6PD deficiency. May increase effect of phenytoin, sulfonylureas and warfarin. Enhanced bone marrow suppression with methotrexate.	$$$

[a] Cost per day based on 70 kg body weight; includes drug cost only.
[b] Use high-dose cefotaxime for presumed resistant pneumococcal meningitis. Dose can be decreased to 200 mg/kg/day divided Q6H once it is known that the organism is susceptible to cephalosporins.
[c] Various algorithms for neonatal vancomycin dosing exist (including preterm infants). Consult the formulary at your institution.

➔ Dosage adjustment may be required in renal impairment; see Appendix I.
Abbreviations: GBS = group B streptococcus; PCA = postconceptional age
Legend: $ < $30 $$ $30–60 $$$ $60–90 $$$$ $90–120 $$$$$ $120–150

Suggested Readings

Brouwer MC, Tunkel AR, van de Beek D. Epidemiology, diagnosis, and antimicrobial treatment of acute bacterial meningitis. *Clin Microbiol Rev* 2010;23(3):467-92.

Le Saux N; Canadian Paediatric Society, Infectious Diseases and Immunization Committee. Guidelines for the management of suspected and confirmed bacterial meningitis in Canadian children older than one month of age. *Paediatr Child Health* 2014;19(3):141-52.

Public Health Agency of Canada. National Advisory Committee on Immunization. *Canadian immunization guide*. Evergreen ed. Available from: www.phac-aspc.gc.ca/publicat/cig-gci/index-eng.php.

Straus SE, Thorpe KE, Holroyd-Leduc J. How do I perform a lumbar puncture and analyze the results to diagnose bacterial meningitis? *JAMA* 2006;296(16):2012-22.

Tunkel AR, Hartman BJ, Kaplan SL et al. Practice guidelines for the management of bacterial meningitis. *Clin Infect Dis* 2004;39(9):1267-84.

References

1. Schaad UB. Management of bacterial meningitis in childhood. *Rev Med Microbiol* 1997;8(3):171.
2. Straus SE, Thorpe KE, Holroyd-Leduc J. How do I perform a lumbar puncture and analyze the results to diagnose bacterial meningitis? *JAMA* 2006;296(16):2012-22.
3. Saez-Llorens X et al. Acute bacterial meningitis beyond the newborn period. In: Long SS et al., eds. *Principles and practice of pediatric infectious diseases*. 2nd ed. New York (NY): Churchill Livingstone; 2003.
4. Tunkel AR, Hartman BJ, Kaplan SL et al. Practice guidelines for the management of bacterial meningitis. *Clin Infect Dis* 2004;39(9):1267-84.
5. Maxson S, Lewno MJ, Schutze GE. Clinical usefulness of cerebrospinal fluid bacterial antigen studies. *J Pediatr* 1994;125(2):235-8.
6. Tarafdar K, Rao S, Recco RA et al. Lack of sensitivity of the latex agglutination test to detect bacterial antigen in the cerebrospinal fluid of patients with culture-negative meningitis. *Clin Infect Dis* 2001;33(3):406-8.
7. Leib SL, Boscacci R, Gratzl O et al. Predictive value of cerebrospinal fluid (CSF) lactate level versus CSF/blood glucose ratio for the diagnosis of bacterial meningitis following neurosurgery. *Clin Infect Dis* 1999;29(1):69-74.
8. Hasbum R, Abrahams J, Jekel J et al. Computed tomography of the head before lumbar puncture in adults with suspected meningitis. *N Engl J Med* 2001;345(24):1727-33.
9. Køster-Rasmussen R, Korshin A, Meyer CN. Antibiotic treatment delay and outcome in acute bacterial meningitis. *J Infect* 2008;57(6):449-54.
10. American Academy of Pediatrics. Meningococcal infections. In: Pickering LK, ed. *2012 Red book: report of the Committee on Infectious Diseases*. 29th ed. Elk Grove Village (IL): American Academy of Pediatrics; 2012.
11. American Academy of Pediatrics. Haemophilus influenzae infections. In: Pickering LK, ed. *2012 Red book: report of the Committee on Infectious Diseases*. 29th ed. Elk Grove Village (IL): American Academy of Pediatrics; 2012.
12. Taketomo CK. *Pediatric dosage handbook: including neonatal dosing, drug administration & extemporaneous preparations*. 9th ed. Hudson (OH): Lexi-Comp; 2002.
13. Wubbel L, McCracken GH. Management of bacterial meningitis: 1998. *Pediatr Rev* 1998;19(3):78-84.
14. Liu C, Bayer A, Cosgrove SE et al. Clinical practice guidelines by the infectious diseases society of America for the treatment of methicillin-resistant Staphylococcus aureus infections in adults and children: executive summary. *Clin Infect Dis* 2011;52(3):285-92.
15. Le Saux N; Canadian Paediatric Society, Infectious Diseases and Immunization Committee. Guidelines for the management of suspected and confirmed bacterial meningitis in Canadian children older than one month of age. *Paediatr Child Health* 2014;19(3):141-52.
16. Doit C, Barre J, Cohen R et al. Bactericidal activity against intermediately cephalosporin-resistant Streptococcus pneumoniae in cerebrospinal fluid of children with bacterial meningitis treated with high doses of cefotaxime and vancomycin. *Antimicrob Agents Chemother* 1997;41(9):2050-2.
17. Klugman KP, Friedland IR, Bradley JS. Bactericidal activity against cephalosporin-resistant Streptococcus pneumoniae in cerebrospinal fluid of children with acute bacterial meningitis. *Antimicrob Agents Chemother* 1995;39(9):1988-92.
18. Hoffman J, Trimble J, Brophy GM. Safety of imipenem/cilastatin in neurocritical care patients. *Neurocrit Care* 2009;10(3):403-7.
19. van de Beek D, de Gans J, Tunkel AR et al. Community-acquired bacterial meningitis in adults. *N Engl J Med* 2006;354(1):44-53.
20. McIntyre PB, Berkey CS, King SM et al. Dexamethasone as adjunctive therapy in bacterial meningitis. A meta-analysis of randomized clinical trials since 1988. *JAMA* 1997;278(11):925-31.
21. Brouwer MC, McIntyre P, Prasad K et al. Corticosteroids for acute bacterial meningitis. *Cochrane Database Syst Rev* 2013;6:CD004405.
22. de Gans J, van de Beek D et al. Dexamethasone in adults with bacterial meningitis. *N Engl J Med* 2002;347(20):1549-56.
23. Black S, Shinefield H, Fireman B et al. Efficacy, safety and immunogenicity of heptavalent pneumococcal conjugate vaccine in children. Northern California Kaiser Permanente Vaccine Study Center Group. *Pediatr Infect Dis J* 2000;19(3):187-95.
24. Kaplan SL, Barson WJ, Lin PL et al. Early trends for invasive pneumococcal infections in children after the introduction of the 13-valent pneumococcal conjugate vaccine. *Pediatr Infect Dis J* 2013;32(3):203-7.
25. Balmer P, Borrow R, Miller E. Impact of meningococcal C conjugate vaccine in the UK. *J Med Microbiol* 2002;51(9):717-22.
26. Public Health Agency of Canada. National Advisory Committee on Immunization. *Canadian immunization guide*. Evergreen ed. Available from: www.phac-aspc.gc.ca/publicat/cig-gci/index-eng.php.
27. Verani JR, McGee L, Schrag SJ et al. Prevention of perinatal group B streptococcal disease—revised guidelines from CDC, 2010. *MMWR Recomm Rep* 2010;59(RR-10):1-36.
28. Public Health Agency of Canada. Guidelines for the prevention and control of meningococcal disease. *Can Commun Dis Rep* 2005;31(ACS-1):1-21. Available from: www.phac-aspc.gc.ca/publicat/ccdr-rmtc/05vol31/31s1/index-eng.php.

Infectious Diseases

Chapter 110
Community-acquired Pneumonia

Mark Loeb, MD, MSc, FRCPC

Community-acquired pneumonia (CAP) is a common and serious illness. The very young and the very old, smokers and those with cardiopulmonary conditions, alcohol dependence or immunosuppression are at highest risk. While most cases (about 80%) are treated at home, the mortality rate among those requiring hospitalization is 8–10% and up to 40% for those requiring treatment in an intensive care unit (ICU).[1] In general, the clinical presentation of CAP does not allow for an etiologic diagnosis. Many microorganisms cause CAP (Table 1). *Mycobacterium tuberculosis* is an uncommon and often forgotten cause of pneumonia. Consider *M. tuberculosis* particularly in those with pneumonia who are born outside Canada, have HIV or other immune deficiencies and those who are residents of long-term care facilities. Also consider tuberculosis in patients who do not respond to treatment. See Chapter 124.

Each microbe can result in an illness that spans the spectrum from mild to life-threatening disease. *Streptococcus pneumoniae* accounts for about 50% of all cases of CAP that require hospital admission.[1]

Goals of Therapy

- Assess severity of pneumonia. The pneumonia-specific severity of illness score guides the appropriate location for treatment, i.e., home, hospital ward or ICU (Table 2). Alternatively, consider the functional status of the patient in the week or two prior to admission. For patients who are fully functional, walking with assistance, wheelchair bound and bedridden, the mortality rate is 4%, 5.6%, 20% and 25%, respectively[3]
- Eradicate infecting pathogen
- Relieve symptoms such as cough, pleuritic chest pain, sputum production and/or dyspnea
- Promptly recognize and treat complications such as metastatic infection (meningitis, purulent pericarditis, endocarditis, osteomyelitis), empyema, cavitation, pneumothorax, parapneumonic effusion, septic shock, syndrome of inappropriate antidiuretic hormone (SIADH), delirium, deep vein thrombosis in bedridden patients, respiratory failure and/or worsening of comorbid conditions (ischemic heart disease, diabetes mellitus, COPD)
- Provide compassionate end-of-life care if this emerges

Table 1: Pathogens in Community-acquired Pneumonia

Streptococcus pneumoniae	*Mycobacterium tuberculosis* (uncommon)
Mycoplasma pneumoniae	Respiratory viruses[a]
Haemophilus influenzae	Mixed or polymicrobial etiology (e.g., viral *plus* bacterial)
Chlamydophila pneumoniae	Fungi (uncommon)
Moraxella catarrhalis	Aspiration[b]
Legionella spp.	
Gram-negative bacilli (e.g., *Escherichia coli*, *Klebsiella* spp., *Enterobacter* spp., *Serratia* spp., *Pseudomonas aeruginosa*)	

[a] Influenza A and B, adenovirus, parainfluenza, respiratory syncytial virus, human metapneumovirus. Respiratory viruses account for about 15% of CAP cases.[2]

[b] Polymicrobial; etiology depends on state of oral hygiene (e.g., periodontal disease—anaerobes; edentulous state—viridans streptococci) and age (aerobic gram-negative bacilli in elderly persons, especially those in long-term care facilities).

Investigations

- History and physical examination with particular attention to:
  - symptoms: cough, shortness of breath, pleuritic chest pain, hemoptysis, sputum production, fever, chills, myalgia, headache, arthralgia, confusion (new onset may be common in the elderly)

    Check patients with ongoing fever (oral temperature >37.5°C) for empyema. Perform drainage early. Drug fever should be kept in mind and the diagnosis reconsidered if the patient is not improving.
  - history of recent travel and other risk factors for pneumonia such as tobacco smoking, excessive alcohol ingestion, hobbies such as exploring old caves, removal of wild rodent excrement (associated with hantavirus), recent loss of consciousness or comorbid illnesses. Some of these risk factors may influence recovery
  - physical findings: general appearance, e.g., respiratory distress, well or chronically ill or acutely ill. Crackles, wheezes, findings of consolidation of pulmonary tissue (dullness to percussion, increased tactile and vocal fremitus, bronchial breathing, whispered pectoriloquy), pleural friction rub, altered mental status
- Objective measurements:
  - vital signs: respiratory rate ≥30 breaths/minute is the most sensitive and specific sign of severe pneumonia in adults; ≥25 for patients who are <50 years of age
  - oxygenation status: measure oxygen saturation in all patients with CAP presenting to the emergency department. If oxygen saturation <92% in a COPD patient, perform arterial blood gas
  - chest radiograph: posterior-anterior and lateral views. Consider a CT scan of the chest in those who have a negative chest radiograph when pneumonia is clinically suspected
- Laboratory tests for hospitalized patients:
  - electrolytes, glucose, urea, creatinine, CBC and differential white blood cell count
  - consider blood cultures in critically ill patients: 2 samples drawn at separate sites. Anaerobic culture is generally not necessary
  - sputum for Gram stain and culture if a good quality specimen can be obtained. Confirm sputum sample is from the lower respiratory tract (<10 squamous epithelial cells/low-power field). Special requests such as culture for *M. tuberculosis*, *Legionella*, fungi such as *Blastomyces dermatiditis* or *Cryptococcus* are dictated by the clinical setting. Consult a microbiologist
  - urine for *Legionella* antigen if high clinical suspicion for Legionnaires' disease or for patients who require ICU admission because of progressive pneumonia. If available, use polymerase chain reaction test on sputum or other respiratory secretions that can amplify DNA of all *Legionella* species
  - consider rapid or culture tests for influenza during influenza season
  - consider serologic studies as dictated by clinical setting, e.g., suspected *Mycoplasma pneumoniae* pneumonia. Obtain an acute or a 10- to 14-day convalescent phase serum sample. If Legionnaires' disease is suspected, collect a convalescent phase sample 6 weeks following acute phase serum sample. Hantavirus infection and Q fever (*Coxiella burnetii*) are best diagnosed serologically
  - if a pleural effusion is >1 cm on a decubitus chest film with the affected side down, aspirate and send for pH, culture (aerobes, anaerobes, *M. tuberculosis*), white cell count, LDH and protein. A pH <7.2 suggests the need for prompt drainage to avoid loculation and fibrotic pleural disease
  - for patients admitted to hospital and who undergo bronchoalveolar lavage in addition to routine testing samples, some laboratories have the capacity to use nucleic acid amplification tests to detect nucleic acid of *Legionella* spp., *M. pneumoniae*, Influenza A and B, respiratory syncytial virus, adenovirus, human metapneumovirus, parainfluenza viruses, coronaviruses, rhinoviruses

Therapeutic Choices

Pharmacologic Choices

Successful management of pneumonia (Figure 1) is based on an accurate assessment of illness severity (Table 2) and selection of the most appropriate site for treatment.[4]

Figure 1: Initial Management of Community-acquired Pneumonia (CAP)

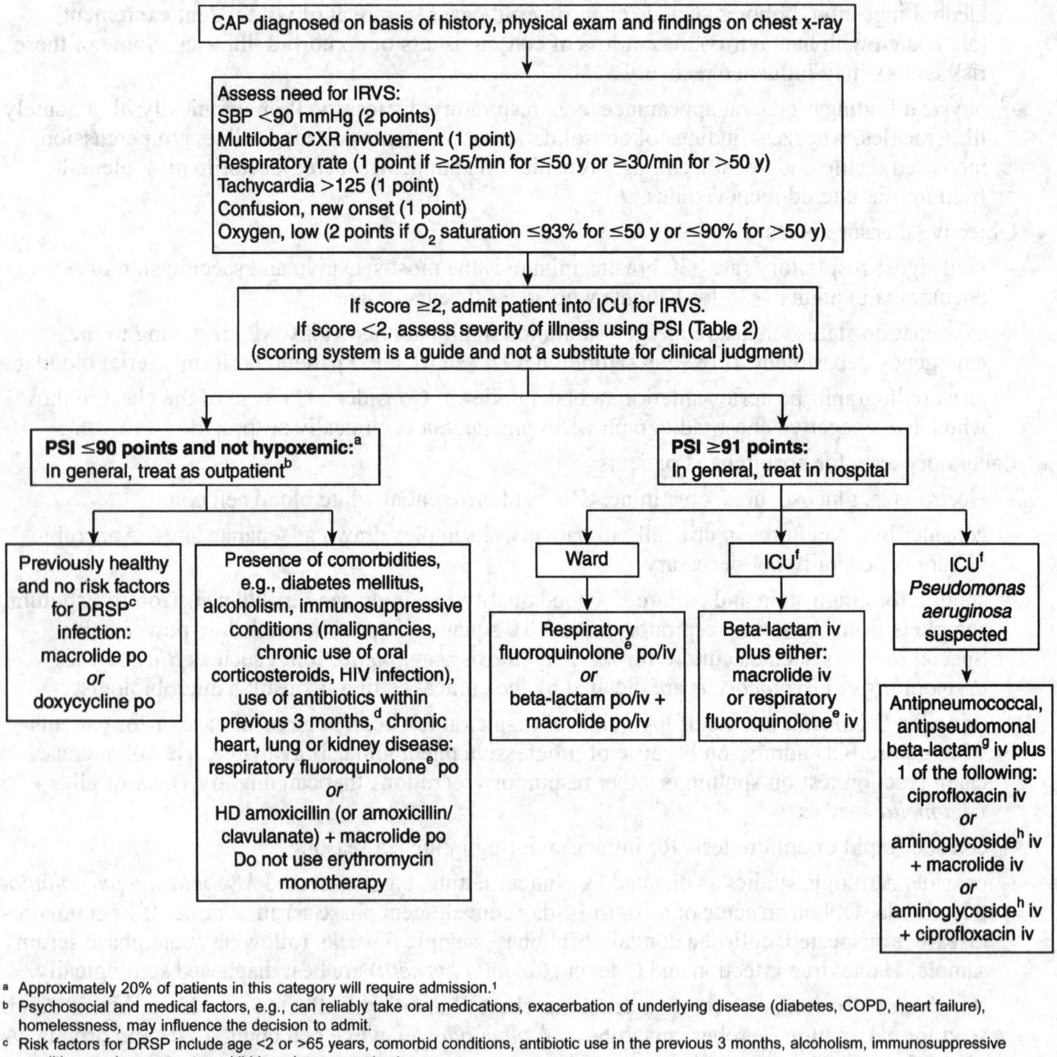

[a] Approximately 20% of patients in this category will require admission.[1]

[b] Psychosocial and medical factors, e.g., can reliably take oral medications, exacerbation of underlying disease (diabetes, COPD, heart failure), homelessness, may influence the decision to admit.

[c] Risk factors for DRSP include age <2 or >65 years, comorbid conditions, antibiotic use in the previous 3 months, alcoholism, immunosuppressive conditions and exposure to a child in a daycare centre.[4]

[d] For patients who have received an antibiotic within the past 3 months, use another class of antibiotics.

[e] Respiratory fluoroquinolone: levofloxacin, moxifloxacin. For hospitalized patients, the dose of levofloxacin is 750 mg once daily for 5 days.

[f] Absolute indications for admittance into ICU: a) septic shock requiring vasopressors; b) acute respiratory failure requiring endotracheal intubation and mechanical ventilation.

[g] Cefepime, imipenem, meropenem, piperacillin/tazobactam.

[h] For patients who have received a fluoroquinolone within the past 3 months choose an aminoglycoside-containing regimen.

Abbreviations: CXR = chest x-ray; DRSP = drug-resistant *S. pneumoniae*; HD = high-dose; ICU = intensive care unit; IRVS = intensive respiratory or vasopressor support; PSI = pneumonia-specific severity of illness

Assessment of Illness Severity

The **Pneumonia-specific Severity of Illness (PSI)** score is designed to predict 30-day mortality rates among patients with CAP and is a validated tool for determining the need for admitting patients to hospital.[5,6] If the score is **≤90**, treat as outpatient. Some patients in this category may require hospital admission (see Figure 1). If the PSI score is **≥91**, treat in hospital. However, physician judgment is paramount in the assessment of any patient and should always override any scoring system.

The CURB-65 tool predicts risk of death and assigns 1 point for each of the following: new onset confusion, urea >7 mmol/L, respiratory rate ≥30 breaths/min, systolic blood pressure <90 mm Hg or diastolic blood pressure ≤60 mm Hg and age ≥65 years. Scores will range from 0.6% (0 points) to 57% (5 points).[7,8,9]

SMRT-CO is a tool that accurately predicts which patients with CAP are likely to require intensive respiratory or vasopressor support (IRVS).[10] At initial patient assessment, it measures the systolic blood pressure (<90 mmHg), multilobular chest radiography involvement, respiratory rate (≥25 breaths/minute for those ≤50 years and ≥30 for those >50 years), tachycardia (≥125 bpm), confusion and oxygenation. SMRT-CO scores ≥2, increase the likelihood of the patient requiring IRVS (see Figure 1). SMART-COP includes the above assessments plus measurements of serum albumin and pH.[10]

Table 2: **Pneumonia-specific Severity of Illness (PSI) Score**

Category	Patient Characteristics	Points Assigned
Demographic factors	Male	age (years)
	Female	age (years) minus 10
	Nursing home resident	10
Comorbid illness	Neoplastic disease	30
	Liver disease	20
	Heart failure	10
	Cerebrovascular disease	10
	Renal disease	10
Physical examination findings	Altered mental status	20
	Respiratory rate ≥30 breaths/min	20
	Systolic blood pressure <90 mm Hg	20
	Temperature <35°C or ≥40°C	15
	Pulse ≥125 beats/min	10
Laboratory findings	Arterial pH <7.35	30
	Blood urea nitrogen >11 mmol/L	20
	Sodium <130 mmol/L	20
	Glucose ≥14 mmol/L	10
	Hematocrit <30%	10
	Partial pressure of arterial oxygen <60 mm Hg	10
	Pleural effusion	10

Reproduced with permission from Fine MJ, Auble TE, Yealy DM et al. A prediction rule to identify low-risk patients with community-acquired pneumonia. *N Engl J Med* 1997;336(4):243-50.

Empiric Therapy

Initial empiric antibiotic therapy (Figure 1) is based on the likely causative pathogen after considering specific risk factors for each patient (e.g., COPD, smoking). Once the etiology is established (Table 3), tailor the antibiotic and/or antifungal therapy paying heed to local susceptibility patterns of bacteria (e.g., *S. pneumoniae*) and local epidemiologic patterns (e.g., outbreaks or endemic foci of Legionella species and dimorphic fungi such as Histoplasma). Antibiotics used in the treatment of CAP are described in Table 4.

Duration of Antibiotic Therapy

For patients who are well enough to be treated on an ambulatory basis, a minimum of 5 days of antibiotic therapy is required.[4] Patients who are hospitalized and who respond to treatment within 48 hours can be treated with 10 days of antibiotics.[1] Specific etiologies may require longer treatment such as 21 days for severe Legionnaires' disease, 14 days for bacteremic aerobic gram-negative bacilli pneumonia and up to 21 days for pneumonia caused by *Pseudomonas aeruginosa*.[1] Empyema requires drainage and treatment for 14 days or longer. Prolonged therapy is necessary when a lung abscess complicates pneumonia. Antibiotics are given intravenously until the patient has been afebrile for 72 hours and then orally until the cavity has closed, a process that may take 12–16 weeks.

Table 3: **Antibiotic Therapy for Community-acquired Pneumonia caused by Specific Pathogens[4]**

Organism	Recommended Antibiotics
Streptococcus pneumoniae	**Penicillin nonresistant (MIC <2 mg/L)** *Initial therapy:* penicillin G, amoxicillin. *Alternatives:* macrolide, **po** cephalosporins (cefprozil, cefuroxime), **iv** cephalosporins (cefuroxime, ceftriaxone, cefotaxime), clindamycin, doxycycline, respiratory fluoroquinolones[a] **Penicillin resistant (MIC ≥2 mg/L)** *Initial therapy:* cefotaxime, ceftriaxone, po or iv respiratory fluoroquinolone[a] *Alternatives:* vancomycin, linezolid, high-dose amoxicillin (3 g/day for penicillin MIC ≤4 mg/L)
Haemophilus influenzae	2nd or 3rd generation cephalosporin or amoxicillin/clavulanate, fluoroquinolones, doxycycline, azithromycin, clarithromycin. Amoxicillin monotherapy if non-beta-lactamase producing.
Staphylococcus aureus	Methicillin-susceptible: cloxacillin, cefazolin, clindamycin Methicillin-resistant: vancomycin, linezolid, tigecycline
***Legionella* species** (*Legionnaires' disease*)	Fluoroquinolones or azithromycin, doxycycline (alternative)
Mycoplasma pneumoniae, Chlamydophila pneumoniae	Macrolides or tetracyclines, fluoroquinolones (alternative)
Coxiella burnetii (Q fever)	Doxycycline, fluoroquinolones, macrolides (alternative—although some strains may be resistant)
Aerobic gram-negative bacilli (e.g., *Escherichia coli*, *Enterobacter* spp., *Klebsiella* spp., *Serratia* spp, *Proteus* spp.)	3rd generation cephalosporin, carbapenem[b] (some *Enterobacter* spp. and uncommon strains of *E. coli* and *Klebsiella* spp. produce cephalosporinases and initial therapy should be with piperacillin/tazobactam)
Pseudomonas aeruginosa	Antipseudomonal beta-lactam[c] *plus* ciprofloxacin or aminoglycoside; or aminoglycoside *plus* ciprofloxacin (alternative)

[a] Respiratory fluoroquinolones: levofloxacin, moxifloxacin.
[b] Carbapenem: ertapenem, imipenem/cilastatin, meropenem.
[c] Antipseudomonal beta-lactam: aztreonam, cefepime, ceftazidime, imipenem, meropenem, piperacillin, ticarcillin.

Aspiration Pneumonia

Aspiration pneumonia denotes 2 distinct clinical entities. The first is *aspiration pneumonitis*, which is aspiration of gastric contents (usually sterile as long as there is gastric acid present) into the lungs with a resultant inflammatory response. The second is pneumonia resulting from the aspiration of oropharyngeal flora into the lung with resultant bacterial infection. Risk factors for aspiration include altered level of consciousness, incompetent gastroesophageal junction, elevated intragastric pressure or volume, impaired swallowing mechanisms secondary to neurologic diseases and interference of glottic closure due to neuromuscular diseases.[11]

Generally, younger patients aspirate due to altered level of consciousness (seizures, drugs, alcohol) and older patients aspirate due to neurologic diseases that affect the swallowing mechanism. Patients with aspiration pneumonia require admission to ICU more commonly than those with CAP due to other causes.[12]

Aspiration pneumonitis does not require antibiotic therapy. Patients with aspiration pneumonia who have poor dental hygiene or putrid sputum or who are alcoholics (anaerobic infection suspected), should be treated with **metronidazole**, **clindamycin**, **beta-lactam/beta-lactamase inhibitor** combinations, **carbapenems** and **fluoroquinolones** with established anaerobic activity (e.g., **moxifloxacin**). Treat patients without these specific risk factors for anaerobic infection with standard antibiotics (Figure 1).

Methicillin-resistant Staphylococcus aureus (MRSA) Pneumonia[13]

MRSA, an uncommon yet emerging cause of CAP, accounts for 1–5% of cases. MRSA pneumonia is more common in patients with severe pneumonia who require treatment in an ICU and among residents in long-term care facilities. *S. aureus*, both methicillin-sensitive (MSSA) and MRSA, is about the third most frequent cause of bacteremic pneumonia in the community. *S. aureus* pneumonia has classically been described as a secondary bacterial pathogen in the setting of a primary influenza virus upper respiratory tract infection.[14,15,16] In the setting of bacteremic *S. aureus* pneumonia, exclude endocarditis (often right sided), especially if multiple rounded opacities are present on the chest radiograph (septic emboli). More recently, community-acquired MRSA infections have been caused by strains producing the Panton-Valentine leukocidin (PVL), known to be associated with tissue necrosis. To date, PVL *S. aureus* infections including pneumonia have been more common in young patients.[17,18] **Vancomycin** and **linezolid** are effective choices.[19]

Tigecycline is a glycylcycline, broad-spectrum, intravenous antibiotic that demonstrated noninferiority compared to levofloxacin in clinical trials of CAP.[20] In a murine model of *M. pneumoniae* pneumonia, tigecycline significantly improved lung histologic inflammation and reduced pulmonary cytokines and chemokines.[21] It does have MRSA activity but its role in the treatment of MRSA pneumonia is still unclear.[22] However, an increase in mortality has been observed when tigecycline was used for certain severe infections including hospital-acquired pneumonia (HAP).[23,24] Because of a lack of data, tigecycline is not indicated in severe CAP.

Do not use **daptomycin** in MRSA or any other pneumonia as it is inactivated by pulmonary surfactant.[25]

There is insufficient evidence on which to base firm recommendations for the treatment of severe PVL-producing MRSA pneumonia. In seriously ill patients, consider blocking toxin production by using **clindamycin** in combination with an anti-MRSA agent.

Influenza Pneumonia

The 2009-2010 pandemic of H1N1 (pH1N1) was associated with increased morbidity in younger patients, particularly those aged 20–30 years. Groups at high risk for complications included the morbidly obese, pregnant women, and aboriginal persons.[26] Studies from autopsy specimens of deaths from pH1N1 revealed that bacteria (*S. pneumonia*, Group A Streptococcus, and *S. aureus*) were present in over 55% of cases of which *S. aureus* was a secondary pathogen in 40% and pneumococcus in 35% of cases.[27,28]

Current recommendations for treatment of Influenza A or B virus infection include the neuramidase inhibitors **oseltamivir** and **zanamivir**.[29] **Amantadine** is no longer recommended because of viral resistance (see Chapter 116). The appropriate treatment will vary from year to year depending on the susceptibilities of the season's circulating strains. Unlike uncomplicated influenza, treatment may be initiated in hospitalized patients with influenza pneumonia even after 48 hours of the onset of symptoms.[4] The major concern is bacterial superinfection and this has to be treated immediately.

Prevention of Community-acquired Pneumonia

Smoking Cessation

Encourage smoking cessation (see Chapter 13). Tobacco smoking is associated with a two-fold increase in risk for invasive pneumococcal pneumonia.[30] It is likely that cessation of tobacco smoking will reduce the rate of pneumonia, but there are no data from clinical trials. Nevertheless, this recommendation is likely to have many benefits, including slowing the age-related decline in lung function and reducing the risk of lung cancer.

Vaccines

Influenza Vaccine

Annual influenza vaccination is recommended for those at high risk of complications from influenza and anyone >6 months who wants to avoid developing influenza.[31] Previous studies have reported that immunization of the elderly reduces the rate of admission to hospital for both pneumonia and heart failure;[32] hospitalized patients with CAP demonstrated improved survival from prior vaccination;[33] and immunization of health care workers against influenza reduces the mortality rate due to influenza in patients.[34] Although these studies demonstrated benefit, later evidence suggested that the beneficial effects of influenza vaccine may have been overestimated because of a "healthy user effect"; a 51% reduction in mortality with influenza vaccination was observed in patients who developed CAP outside the influenza season.[35] Until newer vaccine formulations are introduced and proven to be effective (e.g., higher dosages) current recommendations should be followed. Cluster randomized trial data suggest that immunizing healthcare workers reduces morbidity and mortality in patients,[36,37,38,39] although a Cochrane review concluded otherwise.[40] See Chapter 116.

Pneumococcal Vaccine

Two types of pneumococcal vaccines are available in Canada—polysaccharide and conjugate (polysaccharide conjugated to a protein carrier to enhance immunogenicity). A 23-valent capsular **polysaccharide vaccine (PNEU-P-23)** contains the most common capsular polysaccharide types of *S. pneumoniae* that cause bacteremic pneumonia.[41] While evidence of effectiveness has been mixed, a Cochrane review showed that pneumococcal polysaccharide vaccines are effective in preventing pneumococcal bacteremia and pneumococcal pneumonia; however, the evidence for preventing all-cause pneumonia is weak.[42] In patients admitted to hospital with CAP, prior PNEU-P-23 vaccination reduced mortality and ICU admission.[43]

Conjugate pneumococcal vaccines are used in the routine immunization of children, which has resulted in a reduction in but not elimination of invasive pneumococcal disease among adults because of herd immunity.[44] A 13-valent polysaccharide-protein **conjugate vaccine (PNEU-C-13)** is approved for adults ≥50 years of age though there is no clear evidence that it is more effective than PNEU-P-23.[45] However, based on improved immunogenicity over PNEU-P-23 seen in some studies and an increased risk of invasive pneumococcal disease in immunocompromised persons, Canadian recommendations are to provide PNEU-C-13 to immunocompromised adults, followed by immunization with PNEU-P-23 [Evidence: SORT C*].[45] See Table 5 for indications and schedules for the recommended pneumococcal vaccines.

Prevention of Aspiration Pneumonia

For patients at risk of aspiration, the "chin down" posture may reduce the occurrence of aspiration both before and during the swallow, however definitive evidence is lacking.[46] This posture results in a posterior shift of the anterior pharyngeal structures, narrowing the laryngeal entrance while widening the angle of the epiglottis to the anterior tracheal wall. The end result is protection of the airway. Cleaning of the teeth and gingiva by caregivers after each meal reduced the latency time of the swallowing reflex and increased substance P in the saliva of patients with dysphagia due to cerebrovascular disease.[47] Substance P stimulates the neural pathways to improve the swallowing reflex. Elevation of the head of the bed is also helpful in preventing aspiration pneumonia.

Choices during Pregnancy and Breastfeeding

Community-acquired Pneumonia (CAP) and Pregnancy

CAP in pregnancy is not uncommon, accounting for about 4% of antepartum hospitalizations for nonobstetric complications.[48] It is believed that CAP poses a disproportionate burden of illness in pregnant women and should be promptly diagnosed and treated.[49] If left untreated, pneumonia in pregnancy can cause life-threatening disease to the mother and adverse effects to the infant (e.g., preterm birth, low birth weight).

Management of CAP in Pregnant Women

Clinical presentation of CAP is similar to nonpregnant patients. Perform a chest radiograph in patients for whom CAP is suspected. In healthy pregnant women with no recent antibiotic exposure, use of **azithromycin** or **erythromycin** (except the estolate salt) is recommended.[4] One small study (n=122) suggests a possible increased risk of spontaneous abortion with the use of **clarithromycin**, but this has not been confirmed with additional studies and may have been due to confounding factors.[50] Treat women with severe CAP with a **beta-lactam** and **macrolide**.[4] **Amoxicillin** or **amoxicillin/clavulanate** are preferred beta-lactams; alternatives include **ceftriaxone** and **cefuroxime**. Ideally, local macrolide and beta-lactam resistance rates should be available to tailor the regimen. In settings with high beta-lactam and macrolide resistance, **fluoroquinolones** are preferred; their risk of teratogenicity is low. If community-acquired MRSA is suspected, add **vancomycin** to the chosen regimen. If *Pseudomonas* is isolated, use an antipseudomonal beta-lactam such as **piperacillin/tazobactam** or **cefepime** plus an **aminoglycoside** and **azithromycin**.[4] In most women there will be clinical improvement within 48–72 hours, and therapy should not be changed in the first 72 hours unless there is marked clinical deterioration.[49] Fever should resolve in 2–4 days and cough after 7–10 days. Radiologic abnormalities may persist for up to 6 weeks, so continued hospitalization is not required to await radiologic improvement. Therapy is recommended for a minimum of 5 days for uncomplicated CAP. Treatment failures may be encountered in up to 15% of cases; choose a broad-spectrum regimen or more specific treatment if the infecting agent is identified.

Management of CAP in Breastfeeding Women

The antimicrobials recommended in pregnancy (above), including those for MRSA, are considered compatible with breastfeeding.[51,52]

* SORT (Strength of Recommendation Taxonomy) is a rating system (A, B or C) that addresses the quality of available evidence. For more information consult **How to Use *Compendium of Therapeutic Choices*** on page xxv.

Prevention of CAP in Pregnant and Breastfeeding Women

Pregnant women should be immunized against influenza because of the high risk for complications. Pneumococcal 23-valent polysaccharide conjugate vaccine is recommended for pregnant women with conditions placing them at higher risk of pneumococcal disease, i.e., immunosuppression, cigarette smoking, alcoholism, diabetes, cardiac, pulmonary or renal disease or asplenia (e.g., sickle-cell disease). Primary prevention strategies such as handwashing and limiting contact with sick individuals reduce the risk of respiratory infections.

A discussion of general principles on the use of medications in these special populations can be found in Appendix II and Appendix III. Other specialized reference sources are also provided in these appendices.

Therapeutic Tips

- Administer an agent from a different therapeutic class if the patient has received antibiotics within the 3 months prior to diagnosis of CAP.
- Because of its lowered activity against *H. influenzae*, **erythromycin** *monotherapy* is not routinely recommended in patients with COPD.
- In the outpatient setting, the superiority of one agent over another is difficult to define because most of the randomized, controlled trials are noninferiority studies conducted for licensing purposes. Despite the recommendation from various guidelines for empiric coverage of atypical pathogens in hospitalized patients, there is no evidence that regimens which include atypical coverage result in better outcomes than those that do not.[53]
- Switch patients from intravenous to oral antibiotics when the following criteria are met:[4,54,55] GI tract is functioning normally (e.g., no vomiting, diarrhea or disorder compromising GI absorption); hemodynamically stable; 2 temperature readings are normal (oral temperature <37.5°C) over a period of 16 hours in previously febrile patients; normalized white blood cell count; subjective improvement in cough and shortness of breath; able to consume oral medications. If blood cultures are positive, the duration of intravenous therapy is dictated by the organism recovered from the blood. Use of clinical pathways that emphasize early antibiotic switch and early mobilization may reduce lengths of hospital stay.[56]
- Discharge the patient when the following criteria are met in addition to those above: absence of complications from the pneumonia (e.g., empyema); absence of complications from comorbid illnesses (e.g., MI); absence of complications from treatment (e.g., severe adverse drug reactions); physiological stability as indicated by an oxygen saturation of ≥92% while breathing room air for those who do not have COPD (for patients with COPD, a return to baseline status is desirable), pulse rate of <100 beats/minute and respiratory rate ≤24 breaths/minute.[4]
- Evidence from one randomized, controlled trial suggests that early mobilization during management of CAP can reduce length of stay.[57]
- Prevent recurrent pneumonia in patients ≥65 years and in those suffering from recurrent episodes. A checklist that includes identification of causes of aspiration and measures to prevent recurrent aspiration may be useful.
- Review pneumococcal and influenza vaccine status and immunize if indicated.
- Consider follow-up chest radiographs for *all patients over age 50*, particularly if a smoker. One to two per cent of all patients with CAP will have lung cancer and in half of these the cancer is not diagnosed on the initial radiograph.[58,59] Do the follow-up chest radiograph 6–12 weeks after presentation. If the pneumonic opacity is still present, further investigation such as bronchoscopy may be warranted.

Table 4: **Anti-infectives for the Treatment of Pneumonia**

Drug Class	Drug	Dose	Adverse Effects	Comments	Cost[a]
Aminoglycosides	*gentamicin* generics	Conventional dosing: 1.5 mg/kg DBW[b] Q8H iv Extended-interval dosing: 4–7 mg/kg DBW[b] once daily iv	Nephrotoxicity, ototoxicity.	Aminoglycosides do not penetrate pulmonary tissue very well. Exhibits concentration-dependent bacterial killing and postantibiotic effect. Coadministration of vancomycin or loop diuretics may increase risk of nephrotoxicity and ototoxicity, respectively. Coadministration of penicillins in vivo or in iv bags and syringes may result in aminoglycoside inactivation.	$
	tobramycin generics	Conventional dosing: 1.5 mg/kg DBW[b] Q8H iv Extended-interval dosing: 4–7 mg/kg DBW[b] once daily iv	See gentamicin.	See gentamicin.	$
Carbapenems	*ertapenem* Invanz	1 g daily iv	Anaphylaxis, increased seizure risk (compromised renal function, CNS disorders, e.g., history of seizures), diarrhea, headache.	Indicated for *S. pneumoniae* (penicillin-susceptible strain only), *H. influenzae* (beta-lactamase negative strain only) or *M. catarrhalis*.	$$
	imipenem/cilastatin Primaxin, generics	500 mg Q6H iv	Hypotension, nausea with rapid infusion; seizure activity with high serum levels.	Antipseudomonal. For patients with risk factors for *P. aeruginosa*.	$$$
	meropenem Merrem, Meropenem for Injection	1 g Q8H iv	Hypotension, nausea with rapid infusion; less likely than imipenem to cause seizures.	Antipseudomonal. For patients with risk factors for *P. aeruginosa*.	$$$$
Cephalosporins, first-generation	*cefazolin* generics	1–2 g Q8H iv	Anaphylaxis, rash, GI upset, renal and hepatic dysfunction, phlebitis at site of injection.	Alternative choice in methicillin-sensitive *S. aureus* pneumonia.	$
Cephalosporins, second-generation	*cefaclor* Ceclor, generics	250 mg TID po	Anaphylaxis, rash, GI upset, renal and hepatic dysfunction.		$
	cefprozil Cefzil, generics	500 mg BID po	See cefaclor.		$

(cont'd)

Table 4: **Anti-infectives for the Treatment of Pneumonia** *(cont'd)*

Drug Class	Drug	Dose	Adverse Effects	Comments	Cost[a]
	cefuroxime axetil Ceftin, generics	500 mg BID po	See cefaclor.	Do not use for treatment of penicillin-resistant *S. pneumoniae.*	$
	cefuroxime sodium generics	750 mg Q8H iv	See cefazolin.	Do not use for treatment of penicillin-resistant *S. pneumoniae.*	$$
Cephalosporins, third-generation	*cefotaxime* Claforan	1–2 g Q8H iv	See cefazolin.	Can be used in hepatobiliary disease.	$$
	ceftazidime Fortaz, generics	1–2 g Q8H iv	See cefazolin.		$$$–$$$$
	ceftriaxone generics	1–2 g Q24H iv	See cefazolin.	Do not reconstitute or mix with calcium-containing solutions. Do not administer simultaneously with calcium-containing iv solutions via a Y-site. Administration may be done sequentially provided the infusion lines are thoroughly flushed between infusions.	$
Cephalosporins, fourth-generation	*cefepime* Maxipime, generics	1–2 g Q12H iv	See cefazolin. Risk of seizures particularly in those with renal dysfunction.	Antipseudomonal; for patients with risk factors for *P. aeruginosa*.	$$
Fluoro-quinolones	*ciprofloxacin* Cipro, generics	Oral: 500–750 mg BID IV: 400 mg Q12H	Gastrointestinal upset, headache, dizziness, photosensitivity, hepatitis. Cartilage toxicity: *avoid in children.*	Ciprofloxacin is *not* a first-line agent for CAP. Available as an oral suspension. Incidence of ciprofloxacin-resistant (MIC ≥4 mg/L) *S. pneumoniae* isolates in Canada in 2012 was 2.2%.[60] Concomitant antacids, metal cations, sucralfate decrease absorption of fluoroquinolones. Ciprofloxacin may decrease theophylline or cyclosporine elimination; may prolong the INR if given with warfarin.	Oral: $ iv: $$

Drug Class	Drug	Dose	Adverse Effects	Comments	Cost[a]
	levofloxacin ◗ Levaquin, generics	Oral: 500 mg Q24H × 10 days *or* 750 mg Q24H × 5 days IV: 500 mg once daily	See ciprofloxacin.	Levofloxacin 750 mg daily for 5 days is equivalent to 500 mg daily for 10 days.[61] An alternative to β-lactam/macrolide combination for patients on hospital wards. Can switch from iv to po therapy while maintaining serum levels. Concomitant antacids, metal cations, sucralfate decrease absorption of fluoroquinolones. May increase warfarin effect. Avoid in patients on Class Ia or III antiarrhythmics or with prolonged QT_c interval. Cases of severe liver injury including liver failure have been reported.	Oral: $ iv: $$
	moxifloxacin Avelox	400 mg Q24H po/iv	See ciprofloxacin.	An alternative to beta-lactam/macrolide combination for patients on hospital wards. Can switch from iv to po therapy while maintaining serum levels. Concomitant antacids, metal cations, sucralfate decrease absorption of fluoroquinolones. Avoid in patients on Class Ia or III antiarrhythmics or with prolonged QT_c interval. Cases of severe liver injury including liver failure have been reported.	Oral: $ iv: $$
Glycopeptides	*vancomycin* ◗ generics	1 g Q12H iv	Infusion-related adverse effects occur with shorter infusion times: intense flushing (red man or red neck syndrome), hypotension. Nephrotoxicity, ototoxicity.	For MRSA-pneumonia. Coadministration with aminoglycosides may increase risk of nephrotoxicity.	$$$$
Glycylcyclines	*tigecycline* Tygacil	100 mg iv then 50 mg Q12H	Nausea, vomiting, diarrhea, acute pancreatitis (rare).	Contraindicated if hypersensitivity with tetracyclines as it is structurally related. Not indicated for severe CAP or hospital-acquired pneumonia (HAP). Lower cure rates and higher mortality have been seen when used for HAP.	$$$$$
Lincosamides	*clindamycin* Dalacin C, Dalacin C Flavored Granules, Dalacin C Phosphate Solution Sterile, generics	Oral: 300–450 mg Q6H IV: 600 mg Q8H	Abdominal pain, nausea, vomiting, diarrhea, *C. difficile* colitis.	Incidence of clindamycin-resistant *S. pneumoniae* isolates in Canada in 2012 was 9.6%.[60] For suspected aspiration; provides oral anaerobic coverage.	$

(cont'd)

Table 4: **Anti-infectives for the Treatment of Pneumonia** *(cont'd)*

Drug Class	Drug	Dose	Adverse Effects	Comments	Cost[a]
Macrolides	*azithromycin* Z-PAK, Zithromax, Zmax SR, generics	Oral: 500 mg 1st day then 250 mg × 4 days *or* 500 mg daily × 3 days IV: 500 mg daily × 7–10 days Zmax SR: 2 g po once; indicated for mild CAP only	Better tolerated than erythromycin. Gastrointestinal upset, rash, cholestatic hepatitis, QT_c interval prolongation.	Oral azithromycin given daily × 5 days is equivalent to oral erythromycin QID × 10 days. A 5-day course of azithromycin is adequate for mild to moderate CAP. Azithromycin more active than clarithromycin for *H. influenzae*. Use cautiously with other drugs that cause QT_c prolongation.	$
	clarithromycin ❥ Biaxin, Biaxin XL, generics	Regular-release: 500 mg BID po Extended-release: 1000 mg once daily po	Better tolerated than erythromycin. Gastrointestinal upset, rash, cholestatic hepatitis, QT_c interval prolongation. May increase the risk of cardiovascular events that last beyond the period of clarithromycin therapy.[62]	Coadministration with pimozide is contraindicated. Rifampin: decreased macrolide concentrations. May increase warfarin effect; increased concentrations of substrates of CYP3A4 (potent inhibitor), e.g., atorvastatin, carbamazepine, digoxin, lovastatin, simvastatin. Use cautiously with other drugs that cause QT_c prolongation.	$
	erythromycin Eryc, generics	500 mg QID po	Gastrointestinal upset, rash, cholestatic hepatitis, QT_c interval prolongation.	See clarithromycin.	$
Nitroimidazoles	*metronidazole* Flagyl, generics	500 mgQ8H po/iv	Vertigo, headache, ataxia, gastrointestinal upset, taste alterations.	For suspected aspiration pneumonia; provides anaerobic coverage. Not to be used as monotherapy. Concomitant intake of ethanol may lead to a disulfiram-like reaction; avoid alcohol for at least 24 h after last dose of metronidazole.	$
Oxazolidinones	*linezolid* Zyvoxam	600 mg Q12H po/iv	Gastrointestinal upset, headache, dose- and time-dependent bone marrow suppression, peripheral neuropathy, optic neuritis (rare).	Suitable choice for MRSA-pneumonia.[19,63] Monitor complete blood count at least weekly for myelosuppression particularly if given for over 2 wk. Increased risk of serotonin toxicity with concomitant serotonergic drugs, e.g., selective serotonin reuptake inhibitors.[64,65]	$$$$$
Penicillins	*penicillin V potassium* ❥ generics	300 mg TID–QID po	Hypersensitivity reactions, rash, gastrointestinal upset, interstitial nephritis.		$
	penicillin G ❥ Crystapen, generics	2 million U Q4H iv	See penicillin V.		$

Drug Class	Drug	Dose	Adverse Effects	Comments	Cost[a]
	amoxicillin generics	500 mg TID po High-dose: 1 g TID po	See penicillin V.	Consider high-dose amoxicillin if patient presents with drug-resistant *S. pneumoniae* risk factors.	$
	amoxicillin/clavulanate Clavulin, generics	500/125 mg TID *or* 875/125 mg BID po	See penicillin V.	Consider high-dose amoxicillin/clavulanate if patient presents with drug-resistant *S. pneumoniae* risk factors.	$
	ampicillin generics	1 g Q6H iv	See penicillin V.		$
	cloxacillin generics	1–2 g Q6H iv	See penicillin V.		$
	piperacillin generics	3 g Q4H iv *or* 4 g Q6H iv	See penicillin V.		$$$
	piperacillin/ tazobactam Tazocin, Piperacillin/Tazobactam for Injection, other generics	3 g/0.375 g Q6H iv	See penicillin V.	Antipseudomonal; for patients with risk factors for *P. aeruginosa*.	$$$
	ticarcillin/clavulanate Timentin	>60 kg: 3.1 g Q4–6H iv <60 kg: 200–300 mg/kg/day divided Q4–6H iv	Hypersensitivity, gastrointestinal upset.		$$
Rifamycins	*rifampin* Rifadin, Rofact	300 mg BID po	Rash (petechial rash may suggest thrombocytopenia), orange discolouration of body fluids (contact lens staining), GI upset, liver toxicity, hematologic effects (e.g., thrombocytopenia).	*Should never be used as a single agent for CAP.* May be used as adjunctive therapy in *Legionella* or *S. aureus* pneumonia. Induction of CYP isozymes resulting in many potential interactions (e.g., may decrease levels of cyclosporine, tacrolimus, sirolimus, phenytoin, warfarin and oral contraceptives). Adjust dose of affected drug when rifampin is initiated or discontinued.	$

(cont'd)

Table 4: **Anti-infectives for the Treatment of Pneumonia** *(cont'd)*

Drug Class	Drug	Dose	Adverse Effects	Comments	Cost[a]
Tetracyclines	*doxycycline* Vibramycin, generics	100 mg BID po 1st day then 100 mg daily	Gastrointestinal upset, photosensitivity.	Iron or antacids may decrease doxycycline absorption. Alcohol, barbiturates, phenytoin, rifampin, carbamazepine may decrease doxycycline levels.	$
Antivirals	*oseltamivir* ❸ Tamiflu	75 mg BID po × 5 days	Nausea, vomiting, headache.		$
	zanamivir Relenza	10 mg (2 inhalations) BID × 5 days	Bronchospasm has been reported, especially in patients with respiratory disease. Headache, dizziness, cough.	Do not use in patients with asthma or COPD due to risk of serious bronchospasm.	$$

[a] Cost of oral and iv medications is per 1-day supply based on 6-foot male; cost of inhaled agents is per unit; includes drug cost only.

[b] In obese patients (>30% ideal body weight [IBW]), use dosing body weight (DBW) instead of total body weight (TBW) to prevent overdosing. DBW = IBW + 0.4(TBW – IBW) where IBW (kg; males) = 50 + (2.3 × height in inches over 5 feet). IBW (kg; females) = 45.5 + (2.3 × height in inches over 5 feet).

❸ Dosage adjustment may be required in renal impairment; see Appendix I.

Legend: $ < $25 $$ $25–50 $$$ $50–100 $$$-$$$$ $50–150 $$$$ $100–150 $$$$$ $150–200

Table 5: Pneumococcal Vaccines for Preventing Community-acquired Pneumonia

Class	Vaccine	Indications	Dose[41]	Comments	Cost[a]
Pneumococcal vaccines, conjugate	*pneumococcal 13-valent conjugate vaccine (PNEU-C-13)* Prevnar 13	Routine infant immunization	For dose schedule in children, see Table 3 in Chapter 108		$95
		Adult hematopoietic stem cell transplant (HSCT) recipients	3 doses (0.5 mL/dose) im administered 4 wk apart, starting 3–9 months after transplant	Persons who are eligible for both conjugate and polysaccharide vaccines should receive conjugate vaccine first. However, those who have already received PNEU-P-23 may still receive PNEU-C-13, in which case administer at least 1 y after PNEU-P-23. No role for booster dose.	
		Adults with HIV infection and other immunocompromising conditions	0.5 mL im once	See HSCT recipients.	
Pneumococcal vaccines, polysaccharide	*pneumococcal 23–valent polysaccharide vaccine (PNEU-P-23)* Pneumovax 23	Recommended for children ≥24 months and adults with conditions that increase risk of invasive pneumococcal disease (IPD),[b] adults ≥65 y, residents of long-term care facilities, persons with alcoholism, smokers, homeless persons and illicit drug users	Single 0.5 mL dose im/sc Give 8 wk after last dose of conjugate vaccine (if eligible for both). In HSCT recipients, give 6–12 months after last dose of conjugate vaccine A booster dose recommended in those with asplenia, sickle cell disease, hepatic cirrhosis, chronic kidney disease or nephrotic syndrome, HIV infection, immunosuppression: • after 5 y if ≥11 y of age when initially immunized • after 3 y if ≤10 y of age at time of initial immunization	Persons who are eligible for both conjugate and polysaccharide vaccines should receive conjugate vaccine first.	$20

[a] Cost of 1 dose; includes vaccine cost only.
[b] Conditions increasing risk of invasive pneumococcal disease: chronic cerebral spinal fluid leak, chronic neurologic condition that may impair clearance of secretions, cochlear implants, chronic cardiac or pulmonary disease, diabetes mellitus, chronic kidney disease, nephrotic syndrome, chronic liver disease (including hepatic cirrhosis due to any cause), asthma that required medical care in the preceding 12 months, sickle cell disease or other hemoglobinopathies, congenital immunodeficiencies, anatomic or functional asplenia, immunocompromising therapy, HIV infection, hematopoietic stem cell transplant recipient, malignant neoplasms, solid organ or islet transplant candidate or recipient.
Abbreviations: HSCT = hematopoietic stem cell transplant

Suggested Readings

Almirall J, Gonzalez CA, Balanzo X et al. Proportion of community-acquired pneumonia cases attributable to tobacco smoking. *Chest* 1999;116(2):375-9.

Mandell LA, Wunderink RG, Anzueto A et al. Infectious Diseases Society of America/American Thoracic Society consensus guidelines on the management of community-acquired pneumonia in adults. *Clin Infect Dis* 2007;44(Suppl 2):S27-72.

References

1. Marrie T, Campbell G, Walker D et al. Pneumonia. In: Kasper DL et al. *Harrison's principles of internal medicine*. 16th ed. New York (NY): McGraw-Hill; 2005. p. 1528-41.
2. Johnstone J, Majumdar SR, Fox JD et al. Viral infection in adults hospitalized with community-acquired pneumonia: prevalence, pathogens and presentation. *Chest* 2008;134(6):1141-8.
3. Marrie TJ, Wu L. Factors influencing in-hospital mortality in community-acquired pneumonia: a prospective study of patients not initially admitted to the ICU. *Chest* 2005;127(4):1260-70.
4. Mandell LA, Wunderink RG, Anzueto A et al. Infectious Diseases Society of America/American Thoracic Society consensus guidelines on the management of community-acquired pneumonia in adults. *Clin Infect Dis* 2007;44(Suppl 2):S27-72.
5. Lin CC, Lee CH, Chen CZ et al. Value of the pneumonia severity index in assessment of community-acquired pneumonia. *J Formos Med Assoc* 2005;104(3):164-7.
6. Renaud B, Coma E, Labarere J et al. Routine use of the Pneumonia Severity Index for guiding the site-of-treatment decision of patients with pneumonia in the emergency department: a multicenter, prospective, observational, controlled cohort study. *Clin Infect Dis* 2007;44(1):41-9.
7. Lim WS, Macfarlane JT, Boswell TC et al. Study of community acquired pneumonia aetiology (SCAPA) in adults admitted to hospital: implications for management guidelines. *Thorax* 2001;56(4):296-301.
8. Lim WS, Baudouin SV, George RC et al. BTS guidelines for the management of community acquired pneumonia in adults: update 2009. *Thorax* 2009;64(Suppl 3):iii1-55.
9. Aujesky D, Auble TE, Yealy DM et al. Prospective comparison of three validated prediction rules for prognosis in community-acquired pneumonia. *Am J Med* 2005;118(4):384-92.
10. Charles PG, Wolfe R, Whitby M et al. SMART-COP: a tool for predicting the need for intensive respiratory or vasopressor support in community-acquired pneumonia. *Clin Infect Dis* 2008;47(3):375-84.
11. Marik PE. Aspiration pneumonitis and aspiration pneumonia. *N Eng J Med* 2001;344(9):665-71.
12. Reza Shariatzadeh M, Huang JQ, Marrie TJ. Differences in the features of aspiration pneumonia according to site of acquisition: community or continuing care facility. *J Am Geriatr Soc* 2006;54(2):296-302.
13. Soderquist B, Berglund C, Stralin K. Community-acquired pneumonia and bacteremia caused by an unusual methicillin-resistant Staphylococcus aureus (MRSA) strain with sequence type 36, staphylococcal cassette chromosome mec type IV and Panton-Valentine leukocidin genes. *Eur J Clin Microbiol Infect Dis* 2006;25(9):604-6.
14. Adam H, McGeer A, Simor A. Fatal case of post-influenza, community-associated MRSA pneumonia in an Ontario teenager with subsequent familial transmission. *Can Commun Dis Rep* 2007;33(4):45-8.
15. Frazee BW, Salz TO, Lambert L et al. Fatal community-associated methicillin-resistant Staphylococcus aureus pneumonia in an immunocompetent young adult. *Ann Emerg Med* 2005;46(5):401-4.
16. Hageman JC, Uyeki TM, Francis JS et al. Severe community-acquired pneumonia due to Staphylococcus aureus, 2003-04 influenza season. *Emerg Infect Dis* 2006;12(6):894-9.
17. Gillet Y, Issartel B, Vanhems P et al. Association between Staphylococcus aureus strains carrying gene for Panton-Valentine leukocidin and highly lethal necrotising pneumonia in young immunocompetent patients. *Lancet* 2002;359(9308):753-9.
18. Francis JS, Doherty MC, Lopatin U et al. Severe community-onset pneumonia in healthy adults caused by methicillin-resistant Staphylococcus aureus carrying the Panton-Valentine leukocidin genes. *Clin Infect Dis* 2005;40(1):100-7.
19. Barton M, Hawkes M, Moore D et al. Guidelines for the prevention and management of community-associated methicillin-resistant Staphylococcus aureus: a perspective for Canadian health care practitioners. *Can J Infect Dis Med Microbiol* 2006;17(Suppl C):4C-24C.
20. McKeage K, Keating GM. Tigecycline: in community-acquired pneumonia. *Drugs* 2008;68(18):2633-44.
21. Salvatore CM, Techasaensiri C, Tagliabue C et al. Tigecycline therapy significantly reduces inflammatory pulmonary cytokines and chemokines in a murine model of Mycoplasma pneumoniae pneumonia. *Antimicrob Agents Chemother* 2009;53(4):1546-51.
22. Tverdek FP, Crank CW, Segreti J. Antibiotic therapy of methicillin-resistant Staphylococcus aureus in critical care. *Crit Care Clin* 2008;24(2):249-60.
23. U.S. Food and Drug Administration. *FDA Safety Communication: Increased risk of death with Tygacil (tigecycline) compared to other antibiotics used to treat similar infections*. Available from: www.fda.gov/Drugs/DrugSafety/ucm224370.htm. Accessed December 4, 2013.
24. U.S. Food and Drug Administration. *FDA Safety Communication: FDA warns of increased risk of death with IV antibacterial Tygacil (tigecycline) and approves new boxed warning*. Available from: www.fda.gov/drugs/drugsafety/ucm369580.htm.
25. Silverman JA, Mortin LI, Vanpraagh AD et al. Inhibition of daptomycin by pulmonary surfactant: in vitro modeling and clinical impact. *J Infect Dis* 2005;191(12):2149-52.
26. Kumar A, Zarychanski R, Pinto R et al. Critically ill patients with 2009 influenza A (H1N1) infection in Canada. *JAMA* 2009;302(17):1872-9.
27. Gill JR, Sheng ZM, Ely SF et al. Pulmonary pathologic findings of fatal 2009 pandemic influenza A/H1N1 viral infections. *Arch Pathol Lab Med* 2010;134(2):235-43.
28. Morens DM, Taubenberger JK, Fauci AS. Predominant role of bacterial pneumonia as a cause of death in pandemic influenza: implications for pandemic influenza preparedness. *J Infect Dis* 2008;198(7):962-70.
29. Aoki FY, Allen UD, Stiver HG et al. The use of antiviral drugs for influenza: guidance for practitioners 2012/2013. *Can J Infect Dis Med Microbiol* 2012;23(4):e79-e92. Available from: www.ammi.ca/media/48038/14791_aoki_final.pdf.pdf. Accessed September 26, 2013.
30. Nuorti JP, Butler JC, Farley MM et al. Cigarette smoking and invasive pneumococcal disease. Active Bacterial Core Surveillance Team. *N Engl J Med* 2000;342(10):681-9.

31. National Advisory Committee on Immunization (NACI). An Advisory Committee Statement (ACS). Statement on seasonal influenza vaccine for 2012-2013. *Can Commun Dis Rep* 2012;38(ACS-2). Available from: www.phac-aspc.gc.ca/publicat/ccdr-rmtc/12vol38/acs-dcc-2/index-eng.php. Accessed September 26, 2013.
32. Nichol KL, Nordin J, Mullooly J et al. Influenza vaccination and reduction in hospitalizations for cardiac disease and stroke among the elderly. *N Engl J Med* 2003;348(14):1322-32.
33. Spaude KA, Abrutyn E, Kirchner C et al. Influenza vaccination and risk of mortality among adults hospitalized with community-acquired pneumonia. *Arch Intern Med* 2007;167(1):53-9.
34. Carman WF, Elder AG, Wallace LA et al. Effects of influenza vaccination of health-care workers on mortality of elderly people in long-term care: a randomised controlled trial. *Lancet* 2000;355(9198):93-7.
35. Eurich DT, Marrie TJ, Johnstone J et al. Mortality reduction with influenza vaccine in patients with pneumonia outside "flu" season: pleiotropic benefits or residual confounding? *Am J Respir Crit Care Med* 2008;178(5):527-33.
36. Potter J, Stott DJ, Roberts MA et al. Influenza vaccination of health care workers in long-term care hospitals reduces the mortality of elderly patients. *J Infect Dis* 1997;175(1):1-6.
37. Carman WF, Elder AG, Wallace LA et al. Effects of influenza vaccination of health-care workers on mortality of elderly people in long-term care: a randomized controlled trial. *Lancet* 2000;355(9198):93-7.
38. Hayward AC, Harling R, Wetten S et al. Effectiveness of an influenza vaccine programme for care home staff to prevent death, morbidity, and health service use among residents: cluster randomized controlled trial. *BMJ* 2006;333(7581):1241.
39. Lemaitre M, Meret T, Rothan-Tondeur M et al. Effect of influenza vaccination of nursing home staff on mortality of residents: a cluster-randomized trial. *J Am Geriatr Soc* 2009;57(9):1580-6.
40. Thomas RE, Jefferson T, Lasserson TJ. Influenza vaccination for healthcare workers who care for people aged 60 or older living in long-term care institutions. *Cochrane Database Syst Rev* 2013;7:CD005187.
41. National Advisory Committee on Immunization (NACI). Public Health Agency of Canada. *Canadian immunization guide*. Evergreen ed. Available from: www.phac-aspc.gc.ca/publicat/cig-gci/index-eng.php. Accessed September 26, 2013.
42. Moberley S, Holden J, Tatham DP et al. Vaccines for preventing pneumococcal infection in adults. *Cochrane Database Syst Rev* 2013;1:CD000422.
43. Johnstone J, Marrie TJ, Eurich DT et al. Effect of pneumococcal vaccination in hospitalized adults with community-acquired pneumonia. *Arch Intern Med* 2007;167(18):1938-43.
44. Lexau CA, Lynfield R, Danila R et al. Changing epidemiology of invasive pneumococcal disease among older adults in the era of pediatric pneumococcal conjugate vaccine. *JAMA* 2005;294(16):2043-51.
45. National Advisory Committee on Immunization (NACI). An Advisory Committee Statement (ACS). Statement on the use of conjugate pneumococcal vaccine—13 valent in adults (Pneu-C-13). *Can Commun Dis Rep* 2013;39(ACS-5). Available from: www.phac-aspc.gc.ca/publicat/ccdr-rmtc/13vol39/acs-dcc-5/index-eng.php.
46. Robbins J, Gensler G, Hind J et al. Comparison of 2 interventions for liquid aspiration on pneumonia incidence: a randomized trial. *Ann Intern Med* 2008;148(7):509-18.
47. Yoshino A, Ebihara T, Ebihara S et al. Daily oral care and risk factors for pneumonia among elderly nursing home patients. *JAMA* 2001;286(18):2235-6.
48. Gazmararian JA, Petersen R, Jamieson DJ et al. Hospitalizations during pregnancy among managed care enrollees. *Obstet Gynecol* 2002;100(1):94-100.
49. Sheffield JS, Cunnington FG. Community-acquired pneumonia in pregnancy. *Obstet Gynecol* 2009;114(4):915-22.
50. Einarson A, Phillips E, Mawji F et al. A prospective controlled multicentre study of clarithromycin in pregnancy. *Am J Perinatol* 1998;15(9):523-5.
51. American Academy of Pediatrics Committee on Drugs. Transfer of drugs and other chemicals into human milk. *Pediatrics* 2001;108(3):776-89.
52. Mitrano JA, Spooner LM, Belliveau P. Excretion of antimicrobials used to treat methicillin-resistant Staphylococcus aureus infections during lactation: safety in breastfeeding infants. *Pharmacotherapy* 2009;29(9):1103-9.
53. Eliakim-Raz N, Robenshtok E, Shefet D et al. Empiric antibiotic coverage of atypical pathogens for community acquired pneumonia in hospitalized adults. *Cochrane Database Syst Rev* 2012;9:CD004418.
54. Ramirez JA, Srinath L, Ahkee S et al. Early switch from intravenous to oral cephalosporins in the treatment of hospitalized patients with community-acquired pneumonia. *Arch Intern Med* 1995;155(12):1273-6.
55. Oosterheert JJ, Bonten MJ, Schneider MM et al. Effectiveness of early switch from intravenous to oral antibiotics in severe community acquired pneumonia: multicentre randomised trial. *BMJ* 2006;333(7580):1193.
56. Carratalà J, Garcia-Vidal C, Ortega L et al. Effect of a 3-step critical pathway to reduce duration of intravenous antibiotic therapy and length of stay in community-acquired pneumonia: a randomized controlled trial. *Arch Intern Med* 2012;172(12):922-8.
57. Mundy LM, Leet TL, Darst K et al. Early mobilization of patients hospitalized with community-acquired pneumonia. *Chest* 2003;124(3):883-9.
58. Alberta Medical Association. *Diagnosis and management of community-acquired pneumonia: adult.* Edmonton (AB): Toward Optimized Practice; 2008. Available from: www.topalbertadoctors.org/cpgs.php?sid=15&cpg_cats=59. Accessed September 26, 2013.
59. Tang KL, Eurich DT, Minhas-Sandhu JK et al. Incidence, correlates, and chest radiographic yield of new lung cancer diagnosis in 3398 patients with pneumonia. *Arch Intern Med* 2011;171(13):1193-8.
60. Canadian Antimicrobial Resistance Alliance. *2012 National antimicrobial susceptibility testing results: Streptococcus pneumoniae*. Available from: www.can-r.com/. Accessed May 15, 2014.
61. Dunbar LM, Wunderink RG, Habib MP et al. High-dose, short-course levofloxacin for community-acquired pneumonia: a new treatment paradigm. *Clin Infect Dis* 2003;37(6):752-60.
62. Schembri S, Williamson PA, Short PM et al. Cardiovascular events after clarithromycin use in lower respiratory tract infections: analysis of two prospective cohort studies. *BMJ* 2013;346:f1235.
63. Wunderink RG, Rello J, Cammarata SK et al. Linezolid vs vancomycin: analysis of two double-blind studies of patients with methicillin-resistant Staphylococcus aureus nosocomial pneumonia. *Chest* 2003;124(5):1789-97.
64. Lawrence KR, Adra M, Gillman PK. Serotonin toxicity associated with the use of linezolid: a review of postmarketing data. *Clin Infect Dis* 2006;42(11):1578-83.
65. Clark DB, Andrus MR, Byrd DC. Drug interactions between linezolid and selective serotonin reuptake inhibitors: case report involving sertraline and review of the literature. *Pharmacotherapy* 2006;26(2):269-76.

Chapter 111
Diabetic Foot Infections

John M. A. Embil, BSc(Hon), MD, FRCPC, FACP and
Elly Trepman, MD

Patients with diabetes may develop neuropathy and associated loss of protective sensation. As a result, they may develop a foot ulcer or traumatic wound that may be complicated by a severe, limb-threatening or life-threatening infection.[1,2] Furthermore, impaired arterial blood supply from peripheral vascular disease in the patient with diabetes may impair healing of ulcers and infections. Treatment morbidity and sequelae, including foot deformity and amputation, may impair function and quality of life.[3,4] Consensus guidelines may assist clinicians in evaluation and treatment of diabetic foot problems.[2,5,6]

Goals of Therapy

- Cure the acute or chronic infection
- Heal wounds (diabetic foot ulcers, traumatic wounds)
- Restore limb function for activities of daily living with appropriate footwear and orthoses
- Prevent recurrence

Investigations

Patients with diabetes should have regular foot screening (see Prevention of Diabetic Foot Infections and Figure 1). In the case of a suspected diabetic foot infection appropriate investigations include:[5,6]

- Past history:
  - duration of diabetes
  - complications of diabetes including ophthalmopathy, nephropathy, neuropathy and vasculopathy
  - previous or current foot ulcers, infection, Charcot arthropathy, gangrene, trauma, amputations, surgery
- History:
  - known or perceived trauma (blunt or penetrating)
  - fever, chills, rigors
  - new or different pain in a limb
  - swelling of limb
  - change in footwear
  - recent antimicrobial therapy
  - recent aggravation of glycemic control
  - presence and duration of a skin ulcer; any recent change such as new or increased drainage and odour
- Physical examination:
  - discolouration (red, pink, blue, white, black), lymphangitis
  - increased warmth or coldness
  - swelling, joint stiffness

- malodorous foot
- corns, calluses
- ulcer, skin crack or traumatic wound (location, size, depth, vascularity, drainage or pus, probe for palpable or exposed bone)
- nail problems (ingrown toenail, onychomycosis)
- web spaces between toes (cracks, maceration, ulcer or drainage)
- deformity of toes, foot or ankle
- pedal pulses, capillary refill and assessment of other pulses or evidence of arterial obstruction
- neuropathy (assessed with the inability to perceive the 10 g Semmes-Weinstein monofilament)
- footwear inspection (rough edges and seams; shoe size and fit; foreign body in the shoe or penetrating through the sole; blood stains, odour or pressure; wear pattern on sole)

■ Radiographic investigations:
- plain radiography of the foot and ankle may show soft tissue swelling, gas in soft tissues, vascular calcification and bony changes (lytic changes/erosions in bone, osteopenia, periosteal elevation, fracture, or sequestrum) or may be normal in early stages. Radiography is a simple, cost effective technique for following response to treatment for osteomyelitis

■ Other diagnostic imaging:[7]
- bone scintigraphy may be abnormal with bone infection, fracture or Charcot arthropathy, and may be difficult to interpret in the setting of overlying skin and soft tissue infection
- gallium scintigraphy or indium-labelled white blood cell scan sometimes may distinguish between fracture and infection
- magnetic resonance imaging with or without gadolinium enhancement may show bony changes or abscess, but availability is frequently limited
- ultrasonography may demonstrate abscess or non-radio-opaque foreign bodies
- computed tomography may show bony changes or abscess

■ Laboratory studies:
- complete blood count and differential
- blood cultures (if systemic involvement is suspected)
- erythrocyte sedimentation rate and C-reactive protein (to follow course of treatment)
- fasting blood glucose (aggravation of glycemic control may be a sign of sepsis)
- electrolytes, renal and liver function tests (baseline toxicity parameters for antimicrobial therapy)
- superficial swab for culture (with pathogen identification and antimicrobial sensitivities) of ulcer or traumatic wound (including drainage) frequently demonstrate superficial contamination or colonization of the wound and may not correlate with deep wound or bone culture.[8] Superficial specimens are generally discouraged, and the results must be interpreted with caution.
- tissue (deep soft tissue and bone) biopsy and culture (with pathogen identification and antimicrobial sensitivities) provide a more accurate representation of the actual pathogens than superficial swab culture, and are more useful in guiding antimicrobial therapy[8]
- aspiration of joint (if septic arthritis is suspected) and submission of the joint fluid specimen for cell count, crystal analysis and culture

■ Vascular studies:
- ankle-brachial index (ABI)—less than 0.8 may indicate delayed wound healing potential; less than 0.5 may indicate inadequate arterial inflow and very poor chance of healing, and vascular consultation may be indicated to assess for vascular reconstruction or amputation
- Doppler arterial waveforms

- toe blood pressures (pressure less than 40 mm Hg may indicate poor healing potential)

Table 1 summarizes the differential diagnosis of diabetic foot problems.

Therapeutic Choices

Optimal treatment of diabetic foot infections includes drainage and débridement, proper wound care to promote healing, appropriate antimicrobial therapy, surgery as indicated and correction of metabolic irregularities (glucose control). Treatment choices are guided by the severity of infection. Noninfected wounds do not need to be treated with topical or systemic antibiotics. Figure 2 outlines the recommended approach to a suspected diabetic foot infection.

Nonpharmacologic Choices

Surgery

There are various situations when surgical interventions are appropriate:[1]

- Incision and drainage of abscess with submission of purulent material for culture.
- Irrigation and débridement of infected wounds with submission of purulent material for culture.
- Amputation of gangrenous tissue (toes, forefoot), attempting to salvage remaining healthy foot for functional activities of daily living.
- Amputation proximal to the foot: acute (rapidly progressive, life-threatening infection) or chronic (limb dysfunction from chronic infection or deformity).
- Further surgery to improve healing potential (ostectomy, wound coverage procedures, bony reconstruction, vascular reconstruction).

Figure 1: **Primary Care Screening Evaluation of Diabetic Foot**

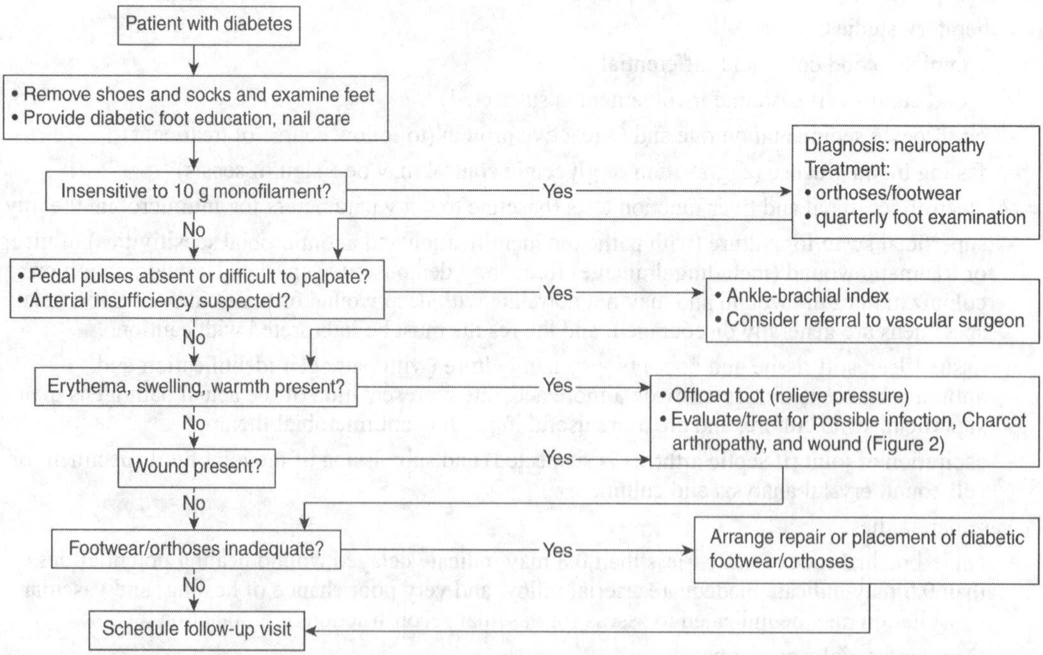

Table 1: Differential Diagnosis of Diabetic Foot Infection

Differential Diagnosis	Characteristics	Most Likely Pathogen
Infectious[a]		
Abscess	Erythema, swelling, fluctuance MRI or ultrasonography may show a cavity Pus may be aspirated from abscess cavity	*Staphylococcus aureus* (MSSA or MRSA)
Cellulitis	Erythema without raised borders, swelling, with or without fluctuance	*S. aureus* (MSSA or MRSA) and β-hemolytic streptococci (group A or B most common)
Erysipelas	Erythema with raised borders, swelling, with or without fluctuance	*Streptococcus pyogenes* (group A streptococcus)
Lymphangitis	Erythematous streaking following the distribution of the lymphatics, not raised	*S. aureus* (MSSA or MRSA) and β-hemolytic streptococci (group A or B most common)
Macerated foot	Tissues are excessively moist and macerated from soaking the foot	*Pseudomonas aeruginosa* may be the predominant pathogen in conjunction with other microorganisms
Osteomyelitis	Palpation of bone at base of ulcer Radiographic changes may be noted (periosteal elevation, bone destruction, sequestrum) but may be absent in the early stages	*S. aureus* (MSSA or MRSA) is the most common pathogen, but may also be caused by less virulent organisms (e.g., coagulase-negative staphylococci)
Septic arthritis	Erythema, swelling, stiffness, fluctuance at joint, malalignment of foot distal to involved joint.	*S. aureus* (MSSA or MRSA) is the most common pathogen
Septic foot	Necrotic, foul-smelling foot, with extensive areas of nonviable tissue Gas may be seen in the soft tissues	Polymicrobial process involving gram-positive bacteria, including enterococci Gram-negative bacteria and anaerobic bacteria
Suppurative tenosynovitis	Erythema, swelling, fluctuance along tendon; pain with tendon motion MRI or ultrasonography may show fluid in tendon sheath Pus may be aspirated from tendon sheath	*S. aureus* (MSSA or MRSA) and β-hemolytic streptococci (group A or B most common), but may be polymicrobial including gram-negative bacteria
Systemic sepsis	Fever, chills, rigors, shock, changes in mental status, impaired glycemic control, blood cultures that may yield bacteria	Can be caused by any organism arising from a foot infection
Noninfectious		
Charcot arthropathy	Erythema, swelling, increased warmth; erythema may decrease with elevation of foot Radiographic changes of fracture and dislocation may be noted several weeks after onset	NA
Crystalline arthropathy	Erythema, swelling, fluctuance and tenderness of joint Joint fluid analysis may show crystals consistent with pseudogout (calcium pyrophosphate) or gout (uric acid)	NA
Fracture, dislocation	Erythema and swelling may be present Radiographic findings of fracture or dislocation	NA
Ischemia, gangrene	Discolouration (pale, dusky or black), dependent rubor, coldness to touch, prolonged or absent capillary refill, absent peripheral pulses; decreased ankle-brachial index, toe blood pressures and tissue oxygen level	NA

[a] All infections may present with or without fever, chills, rigors, localized pain, swelling, erythema, leukocytosis, elevated erythrocyte sedimentation rate, elevated C-reactive protein, and aggravation of glycemic control.

Abbreviations: MRSA = methicillin-resistant *S. aureus*; MSSA = methicillin-sensitive *S. aureus*; MRI = magnetic resonance imaging; NA = not applicable

Figure 2: **Evaluation and Initial Treatment of Diabetic Foot Infections**

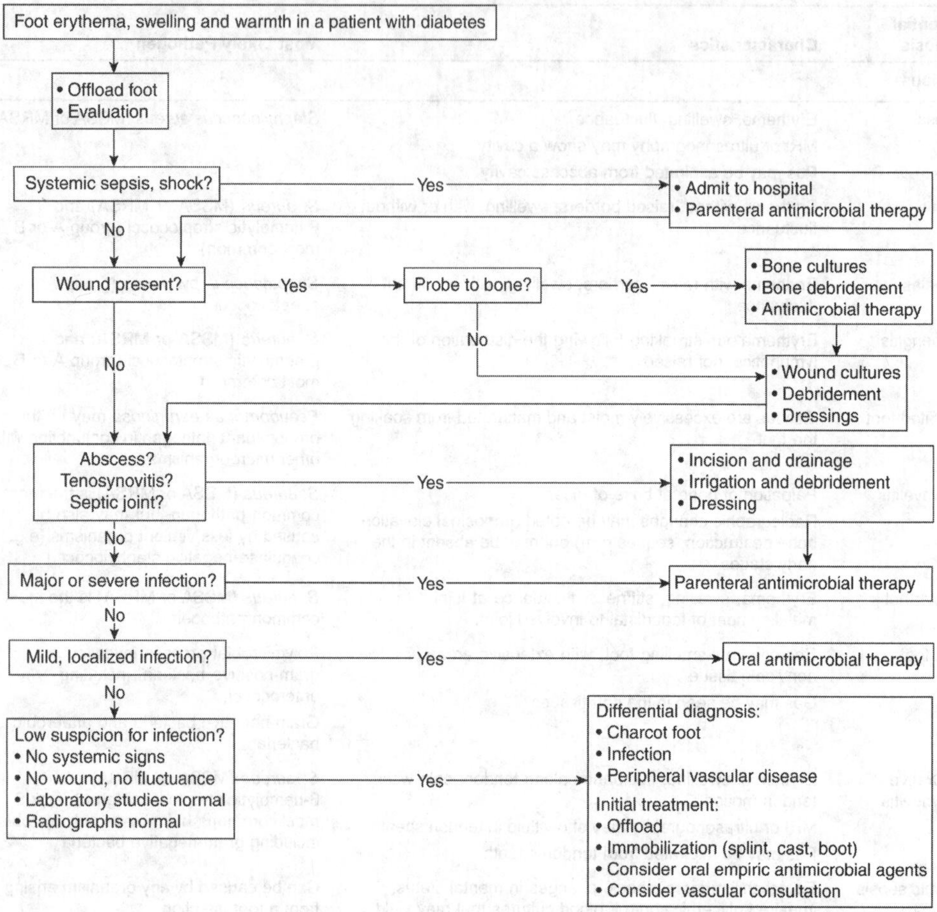

Wound Care

Proper wound care is essential regardless of the presence of infection. Continue wound healing measures until the wound is healed even if infection is cleared. *Débridement* removes necrotic debris. *Paring of calluses* removes hyperkeratotic tissue, which could otherwise serve as an impediment to healing or, if excessive, could increase plantar pressure beneath the callus, and undermine and destroy the soft tissues.

There are many dressing choices; dressings that provide a moist environment for wound healing are the most desirable. Saline-moistened gauze or hydroactive gel dressings provide a moist wound healing environment and assist in débridement. However, there are limited data to support the use of any specific dressing,[9,10,11,12] including those that are antimicrobial-based.[13,14,15,16] If the wound is excessively moist and becoming macerated, a dressing such as a hydrofibre or an alginate will absorb exudate; if the wound has necrotic debris at its base, a debriding dressing such as saline-moistened gauze may be beneficial. See Chapter 93 for a description of various dressings.

Pressure relief (offloading the wound) with orthoses (braces, removable walker boots or ankle/foot orthoses), crutches or casts may promote wound healing.[17]

Pharmacologic Choices

Antimicrobial Therapy

Factors contributing to choice of antimicrobial agents include:

- Culture and antimicrobial susceptibility data pending (empiric therapy) or available (culture-directed therapy)
- Severity of infection
- Local epidemiology and antimicrobial resistance profiles
- Antibiotic use in the past month (if so, select regimen with broader coverage, e.g., to include gram-negative bacilli if not already covered)
- Cost and availability of agents
- Frequency of dosing
- Bioavailability of oral antimicrobials
- Patient residence (ease of access to medical care for antimicrobial administration, toxicity screening and follow-up evaluation)
- Availability of home iv therapy program[18]
- Likelihood of adherence to treatment

There is a paucity of data to allow recommendation of one antimicrobial agent over another.[2] Initial therapy is usually empiric and based on the severity of infection (see Table 2). Empiric therapy for early infections should target *Staphylococcus aureus* and the β-hemolytic streptococci; however, use the local epidemiology of methicillin-resistant *S. aureus* (MRSA) to guide decision making about empiric therapy.[19]

Patients who present with well-established infections, including necrotic tissue or foul-smelling discharge, should receive empiric therapy that also targets gram-negative and anaerobic pathogens, particularly if the patient has been soaking the foot.[2] If necrotic tissue is present and/or deep infection such as an abscess is suspected or confirmed, arrange a surgical opinion because antimicrobial therapy alone is unlikely to resolve the situation.

Oral therapy is usually sufficient for patients with mild and localized infections.[20] In patients with more extensive infections which may be associated with systemic manifestations, iv therapy is indicated.

Duration of antimicrobial therapy is usually guided by response to therapy. For superficial and limited infections, a 7- to 14-day course of oral antimicrobial agents may be sufficient. If the infection is slow to improve or if it recurs, evaluate for other processes such as undrained abscess, foreign body, osteomyelitis or septic arthritis.

Treatment of osteomyelitis is more complex because of bone involvement, and surgery is considered in the decision-making process. Potentially beneficial treatment options include either a prolonged course of oral therapy lasting months, guided by clinical, laboratory (ESR, CRP) and plain radiographic follow-up evaluation, or a 6-week course of parenteral therapy.[18,20,21] Follow-up evaluation with clinical examination and radiography may indicate that the 6-week course of parenteral therapy is sufficient or that it should be extended or followed with a prolonged course of oral therapy. Regardless of the route of antimicrobial administration, if clinical improvement is not observed (resolution of erythema, edema, heat, draining sinus; coverage of bone with soft tissue) and there is persisting plain radiographic evidence of osteomyelitis without improvement, consult an infectious disease specialist and a surgeon knowledgeable in the treatment of the diabetic foot.

For additional information regarding acute osteomyelitis, see Chapter 107.

Table 2: **Empiric Therapy for Infection in the Diabetic Foot**

Infection Severity	Antimicrobial Agent[a,b,c]
Localized infections: Neither limb- nor life-threatening Usually associated with cellulitis surrounding an ulcer Purulent debris may be present at the base of the ulcer Usual organisms: aerobic gram-positive cocci (*S. aureus* and β-hemolytic streptococci) Frequently treated with outpatient oral antimicrobial therapy	**Oral Preferred** • Amoxicillin/clavulanic acid • Cephalexin • Clindamycin • Cloxacillin • Doxycycline • SMX/TMP
More extensive infections: Includes more severe infections, including more extensive cellulitis, plantar abscess and deep space infections The choice of oral vs. parenteral therapy should be guided by the extent of the infection and the patient's overall clinical status Initial antimicrobial therapy against staphylococci, streptococci, anaerobes and common *Enterobacteriaceae* species Empiric treatment targeting *P. aeruginosa* is generally unnecessary unless risk factors present (e.g., history of foot soaking, severe or chronic infection) Patients who are not toxic may be treated with débridement and oral antimicrobial therapy Patients who are ill or toxic despite moderate local signs are treated as having a severe infection • limb- or life-threatening • frequently polymicrobial • immediate hospitalization, early surgical débridement and parenteral antimicrobial therapy • if MRSA is present or suspected, consider addition of vancomycin or linezolid	**Oral Options** • Amoxicillin/clavulanic acid • Ciprofloxacin or levofloxacin *plus* clindamycin or metronidazole • Moxifloxacin • SMX/TMP *plus* clindamycin or metronidazole **Parenteral Options** • 1st, 2nd or 3rd generation cephalosporin *plus* metronidazole • Carbapenem • Clindamycin *plus* 3rd generation cephalosporin • Piperacillin/tazobactam
Osteomyelitis: Treat with iv therapy or long-term oral antimicrobial therapy using agents that are well absorbed from the GI tract and have good distribution to bone and tissue Surgical débridement indicated to remove necrotic debris, abscess or sequestrum Therapy should be based on culture results whenever possible If MRSA is present or suspected, consider addition of vancomycin or linezolid	**Oral Options** • Amoxicillin/clavulanic acid • Cephalexin • Clindamycin • Cloxacillin • Doxycycline • Ciprofloxacin or levofloxacin *plus* clindamycin or metronidazole • Linezolid • Moxifloxacin • SMX/TMP • SMX/TMP *plus* clindamycin or metronidazole **Parenteral Options** • Carbapenem • Clindamycin po/iv or metronidazole *plus* 3rd generation cephalosporin • Piperacillin/tazobactam

[a] The agents suggested in this section are for empiric therapy prior to the availability of final culture and susceptibility results. Knowledge of local epidemiology and antimicrobial resistance profiles must also guide therapeutic choices.

[b] Many of the agents identified in this table do not have Health Canada approval specifically for treatment of diabetic foot infections including osteomyelitis, but may have an indication for the treatment of skin and soft tissue infections or antimicrobial activity against typical pathogens encountered in osteomyelitis of the diabetic foot.

[c] Duration of therapy is based on clinical response. However, typical treatment courses for skin and soft tissue infections range from 7 (mild) to 21 (severe) days, and the treatment of osteomyelitis may require 4–6 weeks of parenteral or several months of oral antimicrobial therapy. Whenever possible it is desirable to switch to oral antimicrobial therapy to avoid complications from parenteral administration.

Abbreviations: MRSA = methicillin-resistant *S. aureus*; SMX/TMP = sulfamethoxazole/trimethoprim

Modified and used with permission from Embil JM, Trepman E. Diabetic foot infections. In: *Principles and practice of hospital medicine*. New York: McGraw-Hill; 2011.

Prevention of Diabetic Foot Infections

Prevention of diabetic foot infections involves local and systemic factors. Interventions include care of the feet, callus paring, glucose control and treatment of medical comorbidities, including smoking cessation. Correcting glucose control may not only help prevent progression of diabetic complications but may also aid the resolution of any existing infection and promote wound healing.[22]

Advise patients with diabetes who have peripheral neuropathy to inspect the feet and shoes daily, have a foot examination by a health care provider at least 4 times per year, avoid walking barefoot and to use appropriately fitted footwear with soft protective insoles.[23] Advise patients to have regular nail care (cutting nails straight across) and to avoid the application of heat or chemicals to the feet. Individuals who smoke should be encouraged to stop (see Chapter 13).

Allow noninfected lesions to heal, to prevent infection. An open lesion on the foot of a person with diabetes does not require antibacterial treatment unless it is clinically infected (erythema, edema, purulent discharge, new or intensified pain, systemic signs). The use of antimicrobial agents for clinically uninfected wounds could lead to adverse outcomes such as allergic reactions, antibiotic-associated diarrhea, *Clostridium difficile*-associated disease, taste perversion and painful peripheral neuropathy (with metronidazole). See Nonpharmacologic Choices: Wound Care.

Consult with a surgeon who has experience in foot and ankle surgery if corrective surgery for treatment of morphologic abnormalities is being considered.

Diabetic foot clinics may provide coordinated care for persons with diabetes and foot-related complications.

Therapeutic Tips

- Examine an ulcer using an instrument such as a forceps. If bone is palpated at the base of a diabetic foot or ankle ulcer, osteomyelitis is present unless proven otherwise.
- Foot baths are not recommended because they may lead to maceration of the skin.[5]
- In the absence of a previous history of foot ulcer or open wound or current systemic signs of infection, a red, warm, swollen foot may be a sign of early Charcot arthropathy.[24,25]
- Biopsy or aspiration of joints in Charcot arthropathy could create risk of iatrogenic infection; if systemic signs of infection (fever, chills, rigors, or dysglycemia) are absent, consider risk-benefit of invasive tests that could introduce infection.

Table 3: **Commonly Used Antibiotics for Treating Diabetic Foot Infections**

Class	Drug	Adult Dose[a]	Adverse Effects[b]	Comments	Cost[c]
Carbapenems[d]	*ertapenem* Invanz	1 g Q24H iv	Loose stools, hypersensitivity reactions.	Very broad spectrum agent targeting gram-positive, gram-negative and anaerobic bacteria, but is not effective against MRSA, enterococci or *Pseudomonas* spp.	$$
	imipenem/cilastatin Primaxin, generics	500–1000 mg Q6H iv	See ertapenem.	Very broad spectrum agent targeting gram-positive, gram-negative (including *Pseudomonas* spp.) and anaerobic bacteria, but is not effective against MRSA.	$$–$$$
	meropenem Merrem, Meropenem for Injection	500 mg–1 g Q8H iv	See ertapenem.	See imipenem/cilastatin.	$$–$$$
Cephalosporins, first-generation[d]	*cefazolin* generics	2 g Q8H iv	Loose stools, hypersensitivity reactions.	Effective against gram-positive and some gram-negative bacteria but is not effective against MRSA, anaerobes or *Pseudomonas* spp.	$
	cephalexin generics	500 mg Q6H po	See cefazolin.	See cefazolin.	$
Cephalosporins, second-generation[d]	*cefoxitin* generics	2 g Q8H iv	See cefazolin.	Effective against many gram-negative bacteria except *Pseudomonas* spp. Also effective against MSSA, streptococci and anaerobic bacteria.	$$$
	cefuroxime generics	750 mg–1.5 g Q8H iv	See cefazolin.	Antimicrobial spectrum similar to cefoxitin but does not possess activity against anaerobic bacteria.	$$$
Cephalosporins, third-generation[d]	*ceftazidime* Fortaz, generics	1–2 g Q8H iv	See cefazolin.	Effective against gram-negative bacteria including *Pseudomonas* spp. Limited activity against gram-positive bacteria.	$$–$$$
	ceftriaxone generics	1–2 g Q24H iv	See cefazolin.	Effective against gram-negative bacteria excluding *Pseudomonas* spp. Poor activity against *S. aureus*.	$

Class	Drug	Adult Dose[a]	Adverse Effects[b]	Comments	Cost[c]
Fluoroquinolones	*ciprofloxacin* Cipro, generics	500–750 mg Q12H po; or 400 mg Q12H iv	Photosensitivity; avoid in pregnant or breastfeeding women, and children <16 y as joint cartilage abnormalities have been reported in studies of young animals. Achilles tendon rupture has been reported.	Effective against gram-negative bacteria including *Pseudomonas* spp. May be effective against some strains of MRSA, but is not usually considered a choice for gram-positive bacteria. No antianaerobic activity. Ciprofloxacin is the preferred fluoroquinolone for *P. aeruginosa* infections.	$
	levofloxacin Levaquin, generics	500–750 mg Q24H po/iv	See ciprofloxacin.	See ciprofloxacin. No antianaerobic activity.	po: $ iv: $$
	moxifloxacin Avelox	400 mg Q24H po/iv	See ciprofloxacin.	See ciprofloxacin. Possesses antianaerobic activity.	$
Glycopeptides	*vancomycin* generics	1 g Q12H iv	If infused over <1 hour, “red man” syndrome may occur due to release of histamine. Rare reports of nephro- and ototoxicity, usually in those in whom aminoglycosides were co-administered.	Effective exclusively against gram-positive bacteria including MRSA, and must be administered parenterally. To guide dosing, levels must be monitored.	$$$
Lincosamides	*clindamycin* Dalacin C, Dalacin C Phosphate Sterile Solution, generics	300–450 mg Q6H po or 600–900 mg Q8H iv	High propensity for diarrhea, particularly *C. difficile*.	Effective exclusively against gram-positive bacteria (including some strains of MRSA) and anaerobes. Increasing clindamycin resistance seen in CA-MRSA and HA-MRSA; consider local resistance rates.	$
Nitroimidazoles	*metronidazole* generics	500 mg Q8H po/iv	Metallic taste. May cause painful peripheral neuropathy (incidence increases with cumulative dose of 30–40 g).	Effective exclusively against anaerobic bacteria. May cause a disulfiram-like reaction when taken with alcohol.	$
Oxazolidinones	*linezolid* Zyvoxam	600 mg Q12H po/iv	May cause reversible myelosuppression (anemia, neutropenia and thrombocytopaenia) if used for more than 2 weeks (monitor complete blood counts). Other complications include peripheral neuropathy, optic neuropathy and lactic acidosis, which have been observed after 4 weeks of therapy.	Effective exclusively against gram-positive aerobic bacteria, including MRSA. Does not have an indication for osteomyelitis. Linezolid is an inhibitor of monoamine oxidase and can lead to hypertension in persons consuming foods rich in tyramine. Avoid in those taking SSRIs.	po: $$$$ iv: $$$$$
Penicillins	*amoxicillin/ clavulanate* Clavulin, generics	500/125 mg Q8H po or 875/125 mg Q12H po	Loose stools, hypersensitivity reactions.	Effective against gram-positive, anaerobic and some gram-negative bacteria but is not effective against MRSA or *Pseudomonas* spp.	$

(cont'd)

Table 3: Commonly Used Antibiotics for Treating Diabetic Foot Infections (cont'd)

Class	Drug	Adult Dose[a]	Adverse Effects[b]	Comments	Cost[c]
	cloxacillin generics	500 mg Q6H po or 2 g Q6H iv	Dyspepsia, loose stools, hypersensitivity reactions.	Effective against gram-positive bacteria only but is not effective against MRSA or anaerobes.	$
	piperacillin/ tazobactam ◗ Tazocin, Piperacillin/Tazobactam for Injection, other generics	3.375 g Q6H or 4.5 g Q8H iv	Loose stools, hypersensitivity reactions.	Broad spectrum including antipseudomonal activity, gram-positives and anaerobes. Not effective against MRSA. Ideal as empiric therapy but once results of culture available, streamline therapy accordingly.	$$
Sulfonamide Combinations	*sulfamethoxazole/ trimethoprim* ◗ generics	800/160 mg (1 DS tablet or 2 regular-strength tablets) Q12H po	Nausea and dyspepsia are most common adverse effects. Photosensitivity and skin reactions (e.g., Stevens-Johnson syndrome and toxic epidermal necrolysis) can occur.	Effective against staphylococci (including MRSA) and gram-negative bacteria (excluding *Pseudomonas* spp).	$
Tetracyclines	*doxycycline* Vibramycin, generics	100 mg Q12H po	Nausea, dyspepsia, photosensitivity.	Effective exclusively against gram-positive aerobic bacteria, including some strains of MRSA.	$

[a] The usual adult dose is shown in the table. Consider renal function and age when prescribing any antibiotic.
[b] All antibiotics can cause antibiotic-associated diarrhea, taste perversion and oral and vaginal candidiasis, and predispose to *Clostridium difficile*-associated diarrhea.
[c] Cost per day: includes drug cost only.
[d] Individuals who have had an IgE-mediated sensitivity reaction (angioedema, immediate urticaria) with a penicillin must not receive a cephalosporin or carbapenem due to potential cross-reactivity. Persons who have had a measles-like rash with a penicillin may receive a cephalosporin with caution.

◗ Dosage adjustment may be required in renal impairment; see Appendix I.
Abbreviations: CA-MRSA = community-acquired MRSA; DS = double strength; HA-MRSA = healthcare-associated MRSA; MRSA = methicillin-resistant *S. aureus*; MSSA = methicillin-sensitive *S. aureus*; SSRI = serotonin selective reuptake inhibitor
Legend: $ <$50 $-$$ <$50–100 $$ $50–100 $$-$$$ $50–150 $$$ $100–150 $$$$ $150–200 $$$$$ $200–250

Suggested Readings

Lipsky BA, Berendt AR, Cornia PB et al. 2012 Infectious Diseases Society of America clinical practice guideline for the diagnosis and treatment of diabetic foot infections. *Clin Infect Dis* 2012;54(12):e132-73.

References

1. Shields NN. The diabetic foot and ankle. In: Trepman E, Arangio GA, eds. *Instructional course lectures: foot and ankle.* Rosemont (IL): American Academy of Orthopaedic Surgeons; 2009. p. 2-80.
2. Lipsky BA, Berendt AR, Cornia PB et al. 2012 Infectious Diseases Society of America clinical practice guideline for the diagnosis and treatment of diabetic foot infections. *Clin Infect Dis* 2012;54(12):e132-73.
3. Goodridge D, Trepman E, Sloan J et al. Quality of life of adults with unhealed and healed diabetic foot ulcers. *Foot Ankle Int* 2006;27(4):274-80.
4. Sochocki MP, Verity S, Atherton PJ et al. Health related quality of life in patients with Charcot arthropathy of the foot and ankle. *Foot Ankle Surg* 2008;14(1):11-5.
5. Apelqvist J, Bakker K, van Houtum WH et al. Practical guidelines on the management and prevention of the diabetic foot: based upon the International Consensus on the Diabetic Foot (2007) Prepared by the International Working Group on the Diabetic Foot. *Diabetes Metab Res Rev* 2008;24(Suppl 1):S181-7.
6. Pinzur MS, Slovenkai MP, Trepman E et al. Guidelines for diabetic foot care: recommendations endorsed by the Diabetes Committee of the American Orthopaedic Foot and Ankle Society. *Foot Ankle Int* 2005;26(1):113-9.
7. Sella EJ. Current concepts review: diagnostic imaging of the diabetic foot. *Foot Ankle Int* 2009;30(6):568-76.
8. Embil JM, Trepman E. Microbiological evaluation of diabetic foot osteomyelitis. *Clin Infect Dis* 2006;42(1):63-5.
9. Dumville JC, O'Meara S, Deshpande S et al. Hydrogel dressings for healing diabetic foot ulcers. *Cochrane Database Syst Rev* 2013;7:CD009101.
10. Dumville JC, Deshpande S, O'Meara S et al. Foam dressings for healing diabetic foot ulcers. *Cochrane Database Syst Rev* 2013;6:CD009111.
11. Dumville JC, O'Meara S, Deshpande S et al. Alginate dressings for healing diabetic foot ulcers. *Cochrane Database Syst Rev* 2013;6:CD009110.
12. Dumville JC, Deshpande S, O'Meara S et al. Hydrocolloid dressings for healing diabetic foot ulcers. *Cochrane Database Syst Rev* 2013;8:CD009099.
13. Vermeulen H, van Hattem JM, Storm-Versloot MN et al. Topical silver for treating infected wounds. *Cochrane Database Syst Rev* 2007;(1):CD005486.
14. Bergin SM, Wraight P. Silver based wound dressings and topical agents for treating diabetic foot ulcers. *Cochrane Database Syst Rev* 2006;(1):CD005082.
15. Canadian Agency for Drugs and Technologies in Health. Health Technology Assessment. *Silver dressings for the treatment of patients with infected wounds: a review of clinical and cost-effectiveness.* July 7 2010. Available from: www.cadth.ca/media/pdf/l0193_silver_dressings_htis-2.pdf. Accessed April 6, 2011.
16. Storm-Versloot MN, Vos CG, Ubbink DT et al. Topical silver for preventing wound infection. *Cochrane Database Syst Rev* 2010;(3):CD006478.
17. Lewis J, Lipp A. Pressure-relieving interventions for treating diabetic foot ulcers. *Cochrane Database Syst Rev* 2013;1:CD002302.
18. Embil JM, Choudhri SH, Germaine G et al. Community Intravenous Therapy Program and a treatment plan for foot infections in persons with diabetes: a clinical perspective. *Can J Infect Dis* 2000;11(Suppl A):49A-56A.
19. Lagacé-Wiens PR, Ormiston D, Nicolle LE et al. The diabetic foot clinic: not a significant source for acquisition of methicillin-resistant Staphylococcus aureus. *Am J Infect Control* 2009;37(7):587-9.
20. Embil JM, Rose G, Trepman E et al. Oral antimicrobial therapy for diabetic foot osteomyelitis. *Foot Ankle Int* 2006;27(10):771-9.
21. Byren I, Peters EJ, Hoey C et al. Pharmacotherapy of diabetic foot osteomyelitis. *Expert Opin Pharmacother* 2009;10(18):3033-47.
22. Bowering K, Ekoe JM, Kalla TP. Foot care. In: Canadian Diabetes Association 2008 clinical practice guidelines for the prevention and management of diabetes in Canada. *Can J Diabetes* 2008;32(Suppl 1):S143-6.
23. Trepman E, Bracilovic A, Lamborn KK et al. Diabetic foot care: multilingual translation of a patient education leaflet. *Foot Ankle Int* 2005;26(1):64-107.
24. Trepman E, Nihal A, Pinzur MS. Current concepts review: Charcot neuroarthropathy of the foot and ankle. *Foot Ankle Int* 2005;26(1):46-63.
25. Embil JM, Trepman E. A case of diabetic Charcot arthropathy of the foot and ankle. *Nat Rev Endocrinol* 2009;5(10):577-81.

Chapter 112
Herpesvirus Infections

Gerald A. Evans, MD, FRCPC

This chapter addresses treatment of herpes simplex virus (HSV) and varicella-zoster virus (VZV) infections in immunocompetent and immunocompromised patients.

In immunocompromised patients, HSV and VZV infections may be more severe and resolve less rapidly than in immunocompetent hosts. The recommended antivirals are the same in both types of patients; however, dosage regimens may be different.

Herpes Simplex Virus

The characteristics of some herpesvirus infections, such as recurrent genital or orolabial herpes simplex virus infection, differ depending on whether they are caused by HSV type 1 or type 2. However, knowledge of HSV type is not of practical value in guiding selection of drug therapy since both are similarly susceptible to available drugs. Drug choices can be based on the nature and severity of the disease and evidence from controlled clinical trials. Although data are lacking, there is a general consensus that the available antiviral drugs are pharmacologically similar and likely to have similar efficacy at comparable doses.

Orolabial HSV Infection

Goals of Therapy

- Improve symptoms. Pharmacologic treatment does not appear to reduce the likelihood of future outbreaks; therefore, reduced transmission is not considered a primary goal of therapy.

Pharmacologic Choices

Primary HSV Gingivostomatitis

Primary HSV gingivostomatitis is more commonly seen in children. If the child can swallow, treat mild to moderate gingivostomatitis with **acyclovir** oral suspension to accelerate resolution of oral signs and symptoms and fever, and reduce the duration of viral shedding (Table 1).[1,2] Acyclovir is well tolerated. If the severity of disease precludes ingestion of medication, iv acyclovir in pediatric doses analogous to those which are effective and safe in adults with primary genital herpes (Table 1) can be inferred to be appropriate treatment, although no published data support this recommendation.

Recurrent Orolabial Herpes

Recurrent orolabial herpes ("cold sores") can be treated in immunocompetent adults with oral antivirals (**acyclovir**, **famciclovir** and **valacyclovir**) for 1–5 days (Table 1).[3,4,5] Topical antiviral creams are considerably less effective than oral antivirals, require frequent applications and carry a risk of self-inoculation. Provide patients with prescriptions for oral antivirals to enable them to self-initiate therapy at the onset of symptoms.

Oral acyclovir initiated within 1 hour of onset may reduce the duration of pain by approximately 1 day compared with placebo. No other disease parameters, such as time to healing and duration of virus shedding, are expected to improve.[3]

Valacyclovir is approved for 1-day treatment of cold sores in patients 12 years of age or older.[4] Valacyclovir self-initiated an average of 2 hours after the earliest symptom of tingling, itching or burning may reduce the duration of an episode by about 1 day compared with placebo.[5] Valacyclovir is well tolerated.

Famciclovir started within 1 hour of onset of cold sore prodromal symptoms improved a number of lesional symptoms and signs,[6] reduced the duration of pain and tenderness and the median time to healing. Median times to normal skin were 4.5–5.7 days with treatment compared to 7 days with placebo. Famciclovir is well tolerated.

Acyclovir 5% cream self-initiated within 1 hour of the onset of a recurrent episode (Table 1) may reduce the duration of pain by about 1/2 day compared with placebo; however, acyclovir cream is not expected to prevent progression to vesicles, ulcers and/or crusts.[7] Topical acyclovir *ointment* may not be as effective.[8,9] Therefore, these agents are not generally recommended.

For healthy persons with recurrent cold sores (>6 times per year) daily ingestion of oral antivirals can suppress recurrences during therapy of up to 4 months (Table 1).[10,11,12] However, once therapy is discontinued cold sores tend to recur. The effectiveness of these regimens for periods >4 months is unknown.

For individuals in whom orolabial herpes is reactivated by exposure to sunlight, oral acyclovir begun 12 hours prior to sun exposure with frequent **sunscreen** use prevents attacks (Table 1). Prophylaxis is continued for the duration of sun exposure.[13]

Anogenital HSV Infection

Goals of Therapy

- Improve symptoms
- Prevent transmission or acquisition of infection

Pharmacologic Choices

Before embarking on any long-term pharmacologic treatments, it should be emphasized that the diagnosis of genital HSV is sometimes clinically difficult, recurrent ulcers may have other etiologies and proof of the diagnosis by culture is often necessary.

Primary Episodes of Genital Herpes

First episodes of genital herpes in otherwise healthy individuals may range from inapparent to severe. Treatment is effective if initiated up to 7 days after onset.[14] Use iv **acyclovir** for severe cases (Table 2).[15] Oral acyclovir is also effective.[16] IV treatment is approximately 25% more effective than oral treatment overall with improved resolution of local and systemic symptoms and decreased time to healing but no difference in viral shedding.[14] **Famciclovir** and **valacyclovir** have comparable efficacy and tolerability to that of oral acyclovir (Table 2).[17,18] The simplicity of famciclovir and valacyclovir dosing regimens is an advantage over acyclovir when choosing an agent.

Genital Herpes and HIV

In HIV-infected patients, first episodes of genital HSV infection may be more severe and prolonged than in non-HIV infected patients.[19] Although data from controlled trials are lacking, iv and oral regimens recommended for immunocompetent patients are likely to be effective in HIV-infected patients. However, some experts recommend higher doses and longer duration of therapy than that used in HIV-negative patients (e.g., oral **acyclovir** 400 mg 3–5 times daily, continued until healing is complete).[20,21]

Treat recurrent genital herpes in HIV-infected patients with **acyclovir** 200–400 mg 5 times per day, **famciclovir** 500 mg BID or **valacyclovir** 1000 mg BID for 5–7 days. Controlled trials have shown that **famciclovir** 500 mg BID for 7 days is as effective as acyclovir 400 mg 5 times per day for 7 days.[22] **Valacyclovir** 1000 mg BID for 5 days was as effective as acyclovir 200 mg 5 times daily for 5 days.[23] Shorter 1- and 3-day courses have not been tested in HIV-infected patients.

In patients with frequently recurring episodes of genital herpes complicating HIV infection, valacyclovir 500 mg BID reduced recurrences by 20% compared with 1000 mg daily.[24] Famciclovir 500 mg BID reduced recurrences by 69% compared with placebo.[25] However, oral acyclovir does not seem to reduce transmission of HSV-2 from HIV-1/HSV-2 coinfected individuals to their partners.[26] All regimens are well tolerated.

There is a significant risk that drug-resistant HSV mutants will be selected by suppressive therapy in HIV-infected patients, especially among those who are severely immunocompromised.[27] Accordingly, it is important that optimal antiretroviral therapy be coadministered if appropriate. If refractory mucocutaneous HSV infection appears, consultation with an infectious diseases expert is advised.

Recurrent Genital Herpes

Recurrent genital herpes in immunocompetent patients is treated with oral **acyclovir**, **famciclovir** or **valacyclovir** (Table 2).[28,29,30] When initiated within the first 12 hours after symptom onset, these agents may reduce median times to pain relief and lesion healing by 1–2 days.

Shorter courses of therapy (1–3 days) initiated within hours of symptom onset appear to be as effective as 5-day treatments for episodes of recurrent genital herpes in healthy individuals (Table 2).[28,31,32,33]

For individuals with frequently recurring disease (≥6 episodes per year), *suppressive* therapy with oral acyclovir, famciclovir or valacyclovir for 3–6 months is more effective than *episodic* therapy (Table 2).[34,35,36,37,38] Valacyclovir, 500 or 1000 mg, is the only treatment approved for once-daily dosing. Compared with famciclovir, valacyclovir may exert greater suppression of genital herpes and associated HSV shedding.[39] Transmission of symptomatic genital herpes disease was reduced by 77% with valacyclovir 500 mg daily in a placebo-controlled trial in monogamous couples discordant for genital herpes infection who also were counselled on safer sex and offered condoms at each visit.[40] Transmission of infection as well as asymptomatic seroconversion was reduced by 50%.

Although suppressive treatment with antivirals significantly reduces HSV-2 transmission, these agents (at standard or higher doses) do not eliminate viral shedding completely.[41] Therefore, encourage HSV-2 infected patients to also use condoms and adopt safe sex practices even if they are receiving suppressive antivirals.

The safety of all the drugs has been demonstrated in placebo-controlled trials up to 1 year and in the case of acyclovir, an uncontrolled study suggested it is safe for up to 5 years.[42] Interrupt suppression periodically to evaluate the need for continued treatment. One strategy is to stop every 3–6 months and to await 2 recurrences. A second 3- to 6-months course would be appropriate only if these 2 recurrences are close together (≤2 months apart). This strategy can be continued indefinitely.[43]

Herpes Proctitis

Herpes proctitis refers to the inflammation of the rectal mucosa caused by HSV infection. It can be acquired by anal intercourse or through oral-anal contact.[44] Symptoms include anorectal pain and mucopurulent or bloody rectal discharge.[44] Treat herpes proctitis with a 10-day course of **acyclovir** (Table 2). If initiated within 12 days of onset, healing time for first-episode is reduced from 14 to 5 days.[45]

Eczema Herpeticum

Eczema herpeticum is an uncommon HSV infection of eczematous skin that can cause extensive disease (fever, malaise, lymphadenopathy), presumably arising from autoinoculation from a cold sore or asymptomatic viral shedding in saliva. Complications include keratoconjunctivitis, viremia and multiorgan involvement with meningitis and encephalitis.

Pharmacologic Choices

Table 3 details the antivirals used for the management of herpesvirus infections of the skin.

Acyclovir is expected to significantly shorten disease duration and may be life saving (Table 3).[46,47] In severe cases, iv acyclovir is recommended (Table 3).[48]

There are no published trials supporting the effectiveness and safety of valacyclovir and famciclovir in eczema herpeticum.[48]

Encephalitis

Herpes simplex encephalitis (HSE) is characterized by acute onset of fever plus focal neurologic symptoms and signs (behavioural changes, speech disturbances and, less frequently, seizures). A brain abscess/cerebritis is the principal differential diagnostic possibility and antibiotic therapy should be included in the initial treatments prescribed, preferably with the help of an infectious diseases consultant.

During therapy, diagnostic testing to demonstrate focal unilateral frontotemporal encephalitis (e.g., MRI, CT), EEG changes and HSV etiology (by detection of HSV DNA in CSF) should be rapidly undertaken. Viral culture of CSF for HSV is uniformly negative. Acute phase serum will contain no HSV antibody in 1 out of 3 patients. A rise in antibody titre demonstrated in a convalescent phase serum sample indicates primary HSV infection.[49]

Goals of Therapy

- Prevent death
- Prevent permanent neurologic sequelae

Pharmacologic Choices

Initiate parenteral **acyclovir** as soon as the diagnosis of HSE is considered (Table 4).[50] The dose is infused iv over at least 60 minutes to prevent obstructive nephropathy caused by formation of acyclovir crystals in the renal tubular lumen. Because acyclovir is eliminated exclusively through the kidneys, extend dosing intervals in the setting of renal dysfunction (see Appendix I). Duration of treatment is usually 21 days. Rarely, relapse with virologically confirmed recrudescence occurs, necessitating prolonged therapy for 10–14 more days.

Valacyclovir and famciclovir have not been evaluated as treatment for HSE.

Aseptic Meningitis, including Recurrent (Mollaret's) Lymphocytic Meningitis

HSV-2 is an important cause of aseptic meningitis with or without the presence of mucocutaneous lesions, comprising up to 20% of cases. Recurrent lymphocytic meningitis is chiefly caused by HSV-2 and is estimated to occur in 20–30% of cases following primary HSV meningitis.

Goals of Therapy

- Ameliorate symptoms
- Prevent recurrent episodes

Pharmacologic Choices

Antiviral treatment of acute HSV-2 aseptic meningitis has not been assessed in clinical trials. However, administration of 1 g oral **valacyclovir** 3 times daily for 7 days is commonly used particularly in the setting of a primary genital herpes episode. Suppressive therapy with valacyclovir is ineffective in preventing recurrent meningitis in patients at high risk (e.g., following an acute episode of HSV-2 meningitis).

Keratoconjunctivitis

HSV can cause keratitis and/or conjunctivitis and uveitis. Because of the risk of visual impairment and the potential difficulty in distinguishing HSV conjunctivitis from bacterial infection, consultation with an ophthalmologist is strongly advised if HSV infection is suspected. Consult with an ophthalmologist for all HSV eye infections, except typical dendritic keratitis.

Goals of Therapy

- Ameliorate symptoms
- Prevent corneal injury with vision impairment

Pharmacologic Choices

Topical **trifluridine** (Viroptic) is more effective than topical **idoxuridine** (not available in Canada) for the treatment of keratoconjunctivitis.[51] The use of oral **acyclovir** in combination with 1 or 2 topical antivirals may not be better than topical antiviral therapy alone (Table 5).[51]

The role of oral acyclovir monotherapy remains unclear. However, oral acyclovir therapy for 12 months was shown to reduce the rate of recurrent stromal keratitis (the most common serious form of HSV ocular disease) in immunocompetent patients.[52]

Varicella-Zoster Virus

Chickenpox

Goals of Therapy

- Accelerate healing of skin lesions
- Prevent complications, e.g., pneumonia, encephalitis

Nonpharmacologic Choices

- Individuals who do not have a history of chickenpox should avoid patients with chickenpox. Varicella-zoster virus (VZV) can be transmitted through the air and by direct contact from skin lesions. A person is infectious from 2 days prior to the development of the rash until the last lesion has crusted.
- Closely crop finger nails and use astringent soaks to avoid secondary bacterial infection associated with scratching pruritic skin lesions.

Pharmacologic Choices

Antivirals

Table 3 details the antivirals used for the management of herpesvirus infections of the skin.

In healthy children, adolescents and adults, **acyclovir** therapy reduces the number of lesions, total time to crusting and duration of fever, if initiated within 24 hours of rash onset (Table 3).[53,54,55] However, the American Academy of Pediatrics does not recommend routine use of acyclovir in healthy children.[56] Consider acyclovir prophylaxis in healthy patients who are at increased risk of moderate to severe varicella such as those ≥12 years, patients with chronic cutaneous or pulmonary disorders, patients receiving long-term salicylate treatment and in those receiving short or intermittent courses of oral or inhaled corticosteroids.

Rare complications such as varicella pneumonia are more common in adults than in children. Lesions in the distal nares are associated with corneal involvement, and should prompt increased vigilance for this complication. It is not known whether acyclovir prevents complications or whether **famciclovir** or **valacyclovir** is as effective as acyclovir in the treatment of chickenpox.

In immunocompromised patients, treat chickenpox even if >24 hours have elapsed since the rash began. Data regarding antiviral efficacy in immunocompromised patients are lacking.

Vaccines

Varicella virus vaccine is a live attenuated virus vaccine (Table 6). Two doses of varicella virus vaccine is recommended in healthy patients ≥12 months old.[57] Vaccinate all susceptible adults.

Acute Herpes Zoster (Shingles)

Goals of Therapy

- Stop viral replication
- Accelerate healing of skin lesions
- Relieve acute neuritis
- Prevent postherpetic neuralgia (see Chapter 21)
- Prevent viral dissemination and VZV-related mortality in immunocompromised patients

Nonpharmacologic Choices

- Keep rash clean and dry to reduce risk of bacterial superinfection.[58]
- Prevent transmission of the virus to another person:
  - keep the fluid-filled blisters and rash covered.
  - wash hands often.
  - do not touch or scratch the rash.
- Avoid use of topical antibiotics and dressing with adhesives as these may cause irritation and delay rash healing.[58]
- Use sterile wet dressings to relieve discomfort in some patients.

Pharmacologic Choices

Antivirals

Systemic antiviral nucleoside analogues (**acyclovir, famciclovir, valacyclovir**), initiated within 72 hours of rash onset, reduce the duration of viral shedding, acute pain and the appearance of new lesions (Figure 1, Table 3).[58,59,60,61] Increasing age (patients <50 years of age rarely develop postherpetic neuralgia),[62] severe pain and extensive disease correlate with an increased risk of postherpetic neuralgia.[58,62,63] Oral acyclovir does not significantly reduce the risk of postherpetic neuralgia and the effect of the other nucleoside analogues on this sequela is not known.[64] Topical antivirals are not effective in the treatment of herpes zoster.[58] To prevent ocular complications, treat patients with ocular zoster even if the rash has been present for up to 7 days. Promptly refer patients with ocular complications to an ophthalmologist. Famciclovir and valacyclovir may improve patient adherence because they can be given less frequently (e.g., TID dosing).

Patients with severe immunosuppression (such as hematopoietic stem-cell transplant recipients or patients with lymphoproliferative malignancies) are at highest risk for VZV dissemination and visceral organ involvement. Disseminated infection is defined as a widespread rash (>20 skin lesions) affecting 3 or more dermatomes or spreading beyond the primarily affected and adjacent dermatome. Visceral dissemination most often involves the CNS (e.g., cerebellar ataxia, encephalitis, transverse myelitis) or the lungs (e.g., viral pneumonitis). The drug of choice for treating dissemination in immunocompromised patients is acyclovir 10–15 mg/kg iv every 8 hours. When the infection is under control, switch therapy to an oral antiviral drug until healing is complete or for a minimum of 10–14 days (whichever is longer) to reduce the risk of disease relapse.

Corticosteroids, Analgesics and Opioids

Prevention of postherpetic neuralgia using antiviral therapy is not absolute. **Analgesics**, **opioids**, **gabapentin**, **pregabalin** and **corticosteroids** may be used in the treatment of acute pain related to herpes zoster.[58] Corticosteroid therapy improves quality of life (resolution of acute neuritis, uninterrupted sleep and return to normal activity) but does not accelerate healing or reduce the incidence of postherpetic neuralgia compared to acyclovir alone.[65] The risk of immunosuppression with corticosteroids may hinder their use in high-risk patients (e.g., elderly, patients with diabetes, hypertension, GI ulcers). Therefore, limit use of corticosteroids to healthy patients with moderate-to-severe pain. For information on postherpetic neuralgia, see Chapter 21.

Figure 1: **Management of Herpes Zoster**

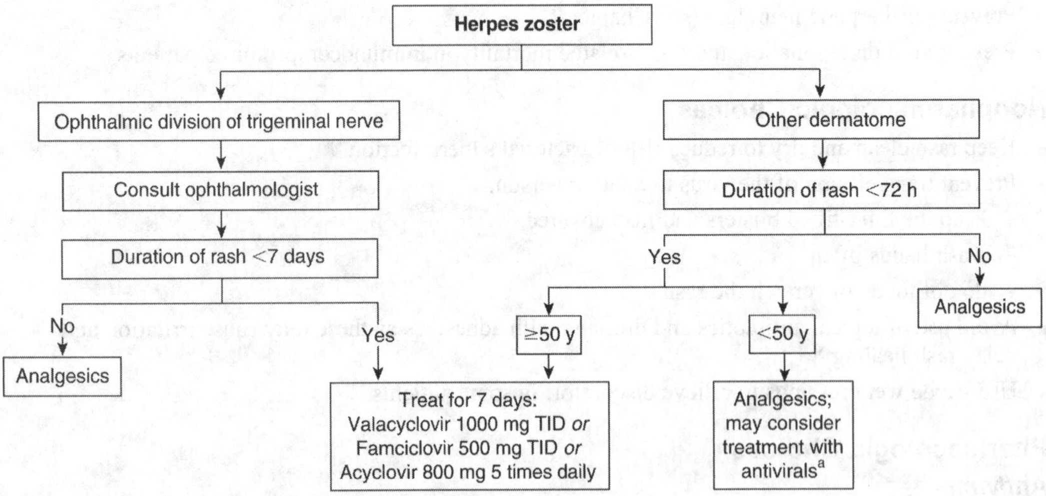

[a] Patients <50 years of age with severe acute pain associated with an acute episode of zoster may benefit from antivirals, but this lacks firm evidence from randomized clinical trials in this population. Antivirals pose a low risk of adverse events.

Vaccines

The live, attenuated **varicella zoster vaccine** (Zostavax), containing approximately 15 times more virus than varicella virus (chickenpox) vaccine, is well tolerated and effective in reducing the incidence of shingles and postherpetic neuralgia [Evidence: SORT A*].[66] It is recommended for persons ≥60 years of age but may be used in adults ≥50 years (Table 6).[67,68] The zoster vaccine may be cost-effective as a public health measure in Canada when administered to patients at approximately 65 years of age.[69] Over 3 years, zoster vaccine prevents 1 case of herpes zoster for every 60 patients vaccinated, and 1 case of postherpetic neuralgia for every 360 patients vaccinated.[70] The vaccine has unclear long-term safety and effectiveness in immunocompromised patients or those with previous episodes of shingles.[70]

Choices during Pregnancy and Breastfeeding

Genital herpes in the pregnant woman may result in neonatal herpes, a serious and potentially fatal infection.[71] Transmission occurs at parturition and is greater if the maternal infection is acquired late in pregnancy than if the mother had been infected prior to becoming pregnant.[72]

The **guanine nucleoside analogues** have been used extensively in pregnant women with genital herpes suggesting a lack of toxicity to either the fetus or mother. Recent published data from a population-based historical cohort study of almost 1 million live-born infants in Denmark from 1996 to 2008 demonstrated no association between multiple categories of birth defects and exposure to **acyclovir**, **famciclovir** or **valacyclovir**.[73] Acyclovir, taken daily beginning at 36 weeks' gestation, reduces recurrences, asymptomatic shedding and the need for Caesarean section, because herpetic lesions are less commonly observed in labour. Doses of acyclovir 200 mg QID to 400 mg TID are effective and safe.[74] In managing genital herpes in a pregnant woman, consultation with an infectious diseases specialist is recommended.

Avoid the varicella virus vaccine in pregnancy.[57]

Acyclovir appears in breast milk in small concentrations both after acyclovir and valacyclovir administration to the mother.[75,76] Exposure to the nursing infant is <2% of the maternal dose or of a therapeutic dose administered to an infant to treat active herpes infections. On this basis the risk of exposure during breastfeeding is not considered to be clinically meaningful.

A discussion of general principles on the use of medications in these special populations can be found in Appendix II and Appendix III. Other specialized reference sources are also provided in these appendices.

Therapeutic Tips

- For orolabial and genital herpes virus infections, provide patients with prescriptions enabling them to self-initiate therapy at the onset of recurrent symptoms.
- For patients with mild to moderate pain secondary to herpes zoster, a constant level of analgesia may be more beneficial than PRN dosing.
- **Famciclovir** 125 mg BID is recommended for treating recurrences of genital herpes whereas famciclovir 250 mg BID is recommended for prevention and suppression of recurrences. Assess most appropriate dose case by case.

* SORT (Strength of Recommendation Taxonomy) is a rating system (A, B or C) that addresses the quality of available evidence. For more information consult **How to Use *Compendium of Therapeutic Choices*** on page xxv.

Table 1: **Antivirals for Orolabial and Mouth HSV Infections**

Class	Drug	Indication/Dose	Adverse Effects	Cost[a]
Nucleoside Analogues	*acyclovir* (kidney symbol) Zovirax Cream, Zovirax Oral, generics	**HSV gingivostomatitis in children:** 15 mg/kg 5 times daily po × 7 days *or* 600 mg/m^2 QID po × 10 days 250 mg/m^2 Q8H iv × 5–10 days **Recurrent orolabial HSV:** *Treatment, oral:* 400 mg 5 times daily × 5 days *Treatment, topical:* Start within 1 h of onset of signs or symptoms. Apply the cream 5 times daily during waking hours × 4 days. *Prophylaxis:* 400 mg BID po 12 h prior to sun exposure × duration of exposure *Suppression:* 200 mg QID po or 400 mg BID po for up to 4 months	Not different from placebo.	HSV gingivostomatitis in children: po[b]: $$$$$ iv[c]: $135/day Recurrent orolabial HSV: Treatment, po[b]: $ Treatment, topical cream: $$$$$ Prophylaxis[b]: $$$/30-day supply Suppression[b]: $$$/30-day supply
	famciclovir (kidney symbol) Famvir, generics	**Recurrent orolabial HSV:** *Treatment:* 750 mg BID po × 1 day *or* 1500 mg po as a single dose	See acyclovir.	$
	valacyclovir (kidney symbol) Valtrex, generics	**Recurrent orolabial HSV:** *Treatment:* 2 g BID po × 1 day *Suppression:* 500 mg once daily po × 4 months	See acyclovir.	Treatment: $ Suppression: $$/30-day supply
Nucleoside Analogue/ Corticosteroid Combinations	*acyclovir/hydrocortisone* Xerese	**Recurrent orolabial HSV:** *Treatment, topical:* Start immediately after the onset of signs or symptoms. Apply the cream 5 times daily during waking hours × 5 days.	Cheilitis, skin reactions at application site, swelling of the lips	$$$

[a] Cost per course of treatment unless otherwise specified; includes drug cost only.
[b] Cost of po acyclovir for adults is based on using 800 mg tablets.
[c] Based on 20 kg body weight for children and 70 kg for adults.
(kidney symbol) Dosage adjustment may be required in renal impairment; see Appendix I.
Legend: $ <$15 $$ $15–30 $$$ $30–45 $$$$ $45–60 $$$$$ $60–75

Table 2: Antivirals for Anogenital HSV Infections

Class	Drug	Dose	Adverse Effects	Cost[a]
Nucleoside Analogues	*acyclovir* Zovirax, generics	**Genital HSV infection, first episode:** 200 mg 5 times daily po × 5–10 days 5 mg/kg Q8H iv × 5–10 days **Recurrent genital HSV infection:** *Treatment:* 200 mg 5 times daily po × 5–7 days *or* 800 mg TID po × 2 days *Suppression:* 200 mg po up to 5 times daily *or* 400 mg BID po *or* 800 mg once daily po × 3–6 months **HSV proctitis:** 400 mg 5 times daily po × 10 days	Not different from placebo.	Genital HSV infection, first episode: po[b]: $$ iv[c]: $400/day Recurrent genital HSV infection: Treatment[b]: $ Suppression[b]: $$$/30-day supply HSV proctitis[b]: $$$
	famciclovir Famvir, generics	**Genital HSV infection, first episode:** 250 mg TID po × 10 days **Recurrent genital HSV infection:** *Treatment:* 125 mg BID po × 5 days *or* 1000 mg BID po × 1 day *Suppression:* 250 mg BID po × 3–6 months	See acyclovir.	Genital HSV infection, first episode: $$ Recurrent genital HSV infection: Treatment: $ Suppression: $$$$/30-day supply
	valacyclovir Valtrex, generics	**Genital HSV infection, first episode:** 1000 mg BID po × 10 days **Recurrent genital HSV infection:** *Treatment:* 500 mg BID po × 3–5 days *Suppression:* ≤9 recurrences per y: 500 mg once daily po × 3–6 months >9 recurrences per y: 1000 mg once daily po × 3–6 months **Reduction in genital HSV infection transmission:** 500 mg once daily po	See acyclovir.	Genital HSV infection, first episode: $$$ Recurrent genital HSV infection: Treatment: $ Suppression: $$/30-day supply Reduction in genital HSV infection transmission: $$/30-day supply

[a] Cost per course of treatment unless otherwise specified; includes drug cost only.
[b] Cost of po acyclovir is based on using 800 mg tablets.
[c] Based on 20 kg body weight for children and 70 kg for adults.
Dosage adjustment may be required in renal impairment; see Appendix I.
Legend: $ <$15 $$ $15–30 $$$ $30–45 $$$$ $45–60

Table 3: Antivirals for Herpesvirus Infections of the Skin

Class	Drug	Indication/Dose	Adverse Effects	Cost[a]
Nucleoside Analogues	*acyclovir* Zovirax, generics	**Chickenpox:** Children: 5–7 years: 20 mg/kg QID po × 5–7 days 8–12 years: 15 mg/kg QID po × 5–7 days 13–16 years: 10 mg/kg QID po × 5–7 days Adults: 800 mg 5 times daily po × 5 days *or* 10 mg/kg Q8H iv × 5 days **Eczema herpeticum:** 200 mg 5 times daily po × 5 days 5–10 mg/kg Q8H iv × 7 days in patients >12 years 750 mg/m² TID iv × 7 days in patients <12 years **Herpes zoster:** 800 mg 5 times daily po × 7 days	Not different from placebo.	Chickenpox: po: Children: $$$$–$$$$$ Adults[b]: $$ iv[c]: ~$700/day Eczema herpeticum: po: $$ iv:[c] Children: ~$275/day Adults: $400–700/day Herpes zoster: $$$
	famciclovir Famvir, generics	**Herpes zoster:** 500 mg TID po × 7 days	See acyclovir.	$$$
	valacyclovir Valtrex, generics	**Herpes zoster:** 1000 mg TID po × 7 days	See acyclovir.	$$$

[a] Cost per course of treatment unless otherwise specified; includes drug cost only.
[b] Cost of po acyclovir for adults is based on using 800 mg tablets.
[c] Based on 20 kg body weight for children and 70 kg for adults.
Dosage adjustment may be required in renal impairment; see Appendix I.
Legend: $ <$15 $$ $15–30 $$$ $30–45 $$$$ $45–60 $$$$-$$$$$ $45–75 $$$$$ $60–75

Table 4: Antivirals for Herpes Simplex Virus Encephalitis

Class	Drug	Dose	Adverse Effects	Cost[a]
Nucleoside Analogues	*acyclovir* (renal symbol) Zovirax, generics	10 mg/kg Q8H iv × 21 days	Injection site reactions, nausea, vomiting, nephrotoxicity, headache.	Children: ~$275/day Adults: ~$700/day

[a] Based on 20 kg body weight for children and 70 kg for adults. Includes drug cost only.

(renal symbol) Dosage adjustment may be required in renal impairment; see Appendix I.

Table 5: **Antivirals for HSV Keratoconjunctivitis**

Class	Drug	Indication/Dose	Adverse Effects	Cost[a]
Nucleoside Analogues	*acyclovir* (renal symbol) Zovirax, generics	**Suppression of recurrent keratoconjunctivitis:** 400 mg BID po up to 12 months	Not different from placebo.	$$/30-day supply
	trifluridine Viroptic 1% solution, generics	*Treatment:* 1 drop Q2H onto cornea while awake (maximum 9 drops/day) until complete re-epithelialization of cornea, then decrease to 1 drop Q4H while awake (maximum 5 drops/day) × 7 days post re-epithelialization of the cornea Store under refrigeration	Burning, stinging.	$/7.5 mL

[a] Cost per course of treatment unless otherwise specified; includes drug cost only.

(renal symbol) Dosage adjustment may be required in renal impairment; see Appendix I.

Legend: $ <$25 $$ $25–50

Table 6: Vaccines for Prevention of Varicella Virus Infection and Acute Herpes Zoster

Class	Drug	Dose	Comments	Cost[a]
Vaccines, viral	*varicella virus vaccine, live attenuated* Varilrix, Varivax III	≥12 months of age: 2 doses sc[57]	Avoid in pregnancy.[57] Common side effects: local pain, swelling, redness. A rash, resembling varicella zoster virus infection, may occur, although it is generally minor and self-limited. The need for booster doses is unclear, and still under study. Do not administer the vaccine to immunocompromised patients (especially those with T-cell immunodeficiency).	$75
	zoster virus vaccine, live attenuated Zostavax, Zostavax II	≥60 y: 1 dose sc Can be considered for those ≥50 years of age.	See varicella virus vaccine, live attenuated. Not recommended in pediatric patients. Can be co-administered (using a different site) with pneumococcal vaccine. Zostavax must be stored frozen. Zostavax II must be refrigerated. Can be given at least one year following the last episode of herpes zoster. The need for revaccination has not been established and duration of protection is unknown beyond 5 years.	$180

[a] Cost of 1 dose; includes drug cost only.

Suggested Readings

American Academy of Pediatrics. Varicella-zoster infections. In: Pickering LK, ed. *Red Book: 2009 report of the Committee on Infectious Diseases*. 28th ed. Elk Grove Village (IL): American Academy of Pediatrics; 2009. p. 714-27.

Aoki FY. Contemporary antiviral drug regimens for the prevention and treatment of orolabial and anogenital herpes simplex virus infection in the normal host: four approved indications and 13 off-label uses. *Can J Infect Dis* 2003;14(1):17-27.

Aoki FY. Genital herpes simplex virus (HSV) infections. In: *Canadian guidelines on sexually transmitted infections*. Ottawa (ON): Public Health Agency of Canada; 2008. Available from: origin.phac-aspc.gc.ca/std-mts/sti-its/pdf/sti-its-eng.pdf.

Cernik C, Gallina K, Brodell RT. The treatment of herpes simplex infections: an evidence-based review. *Arch Intern Med* 2008;168(11):1137-44.

Hyndiuk RA, Tabbara KF, eds. *Infections of the eye*. Boston (MA): Little, Brown; 1986.

References

1. Amir J, Harel L, Smetana Z et al. Treatment of herpes simplex gingivostomatitis with aciclovir in children: a randomized, double blind, placebo controlled study. *BMJ* 1997;314(7097):1800-3.
2. Aoki FY et al. Acyclovir suspension for the treatment of acute HSV gingivostomatitis in children: a placebo-controlled, double-blind trial [abstract]. *33rd Interscience Conference on Antimicrobial Agents and Chemotherapy*; 1993 Oct 17-20; New Orleans (LA).
3. Spruance SL, Stewart JC, Rowe NH et al. Treatment of recurrent herpes simplex labialis with oral acyclovir. *J Infect Dis* 1990;161(2):185-90.
4. Valacyclovir (Valtrex) for herpes labialis. *Med Lett Drugs Ther* 2002;44(1143):95-6.
5. Spruance SL, Jones TM, Blatter MM et al. High dose, short-duration, early valacyclovir therapy for episodic treatment of cold sores: results of two randomized, placebo-controlled, multicenter studies. *Antimicrob Agents Chemother* 2003;47(3):1072-80.
6. Bodsworth N. Single-dose, patient-initiated famciclovir for episodic treatment of herpes labialis; expert opinions in new herpes data [abstract]. *Update from recent international congresses at 12th Annual Meeting of the IHMF*; 2005 Oct 28-30; Lisbon (PO).
7. Spruance SL, Nett R, Marbury R et al. Acyclovir cream for treatment of herpes simplex labialis: results of two randomized, double-blind, vehicle-controlled, multicenter clinical trials. *Antimicrob Agents Chemother* 2002;46(7):2238-43.
8. Worrall G. Topical Acyclovir for Recurrent Herpes Labialis in Primary Care: Critical appraisal. *Can Fam Physician* 1991;37:92-8.
9. Worrall G. Acyclovir in recurrent herpes labialis. *BMJ* 1996;312(7022):6.
10. Rooney JF, Straus SE, Mannix ML et al. Oral acyclovir to suppress frequently recurrent herpes labialis. A double-blind, placebo-controlled trial. *Ann Intern Med* 1993;118(4):268-72.
11. Meyrick Thomas RH, Dodd HJ, Yeo JM et al. Oral acyclovir in the suppression of recurrent non-genital herpes simplex virus infection. *Br J Dermatol* 1985;113(6):731-5.
12. Baker DA et al. Valacyclovir effective for suppression of recurrent HSV-1 herpes labialis [abstract]. *40th Interscience Conference on Antimicrobial Agents and Chemotherapy*; 2000 Sep 17-20; Toronto (ON).
13. Spruance SL, Hamill ML, Hoge WS et al. Acyclovir prevents reactivation of herpes simplex labialis in skiers. *JAMA* 1988;260(11):1597-9.
14. Corey L, Benedetti J, Critchlow C et al. Treatment of primary first-episode genital herpes simplex virus infections with acyclovir: results of topical, intravenous and oral therapy. *J Antimicrob Chemother* 1983;12(Suppl B):79-88.
15. Corey L, Fife KH, Benedetti JK et al. Intravenous acyclovir for the treatment of primary genital herpes. *Ann Int Med* 1983;98(6):914-21.
16. Mertz GJ, Critchlow CW, Benedetti J et al. Double-blind, placebo-controlled trial of oral acyclovir in first-episode genital herpes simplex virus infection. *JAMA* 1984;252(9):1147-51.
17. Loveless M, Sacks SL, Harris JR. Famciclovir in the management of first-episode genital herpes. *Infect Dis Clin Prac* 1997;6(Suppl 1):S12-S16.
18. Fife KH, Barbarash RA, Rudolph T et al. Valaciclovir versus acyclovir in the treatment of first-episode genital herpes infection. Results of an international, multicenter, double-blind, randomized clinical trial. The Valaciclovir International Herpes Simplex Virus Study Group. *Sex Transm Dis* 1997;24(8):481-6.
19. Maier JA, Bergman A, Ross MG. Acquired immunodeficiency syndrome manifested by chronic primary genital herpes. *Am J Obstet Gynecol* 1986;155(4):756-8.
20. Strick LB, Wald A, Celum C. Management of herpes simplex virus type 2 infection in HIV type-1 infected persons. *Clin Infect Dis* 2006;43(3):347-56.
21. Drew WL, Stempien MJ, Kheraj M et al. Management of herpesvirus infections (cytomegalovirus, herpes simplex virus and varicella-zoster virus). In: Sande MA, Volberding PA, eds. *The medical management of AIDS*. 6th ed. Philadelphia (PA): Saunders; 1999. p. 444.
22. Romanowski B, Aoki FY, Martel AY et al. Efficacy and safety of famciclovir for treating mucocutaneous herpes simplex infection in HIV-infected individuals. Collaborative Famciclovir HIV Study Group. *AIDS* 2000;14(9):1211-7.
23. Schacker T. The International Valaciclovir HSV Study Group. Valaciclovir as acute treatment for recurrent anogenital herpes in immunocompromised (HIV positive) individuals [abstract]. *International Society for Sexually Transmitted Diseases Research*; Denver (CO); 1999.
24. Warren T, Harris J, Brennan CA. Efficacy and safety of valacyclovir for the suppression and episodic treatment of herpes simplex virus in patients with HIV. *Clin Infect Dis* 2004;39(Suppl 5):S258-66.
25. Schacker T, Hu HL, Koelle DM et al. Famciclovir for the suppression of symptomatic and asymptomatic herpes simplex virus reactivation in HIV-infected persons. A double-blind, placebo-controlled trial. *Ann Intern Med* 1998;128(1):21-8.
26. Mujugira A, Magaret AS, Celum C et al. Daily acyclovir to decrease herpes simplex virus type 2 (HSV-2) transmission from HSV-2/HIV-1 coinfected persons: a randomized controlled trial. *J Infect Dis* 2013;208(9):1366-74.
27. Levin MJ, Bacon TH, Leary JJ. Resistance of herpes simplex virus infections to nucleoside analogues in HIV-infected patients. *Clin Infect Dis* 2004;39(Suppl 5):S248-57.

28. Tyring SK, Douglas JM, Corey L et al. A randomized, placebo-controlled comparison of oral valacyclovir and acyclovir in immunocompetent patients with recurrent genital herpes infections. The Valaciclovir International Study Group. *Arch Dermatol* 1998;134(2):185-91.
29. Sacks SL, Aoki FY, Diaz-Mitoma F et al. Patient-initiated, twice-daily oral famciclovir for early recurrent genital herpes. A randomized, double-blind multicenter trial. Canadian Famciclovir Study Group. *JAMA* 1996;276(1):44-9.
30. Spruance SL, Tyring SK, DeGregorio B et al. A large-scale, placebo-controlled, dose-ranging trial of peroral valaciclovir for episodic treatment of recurrent herpes genitalis. Valaciclovir HSV Study Group. *Arch Intern Med* 1996;156(15):1729-35.
31. Wald A, Carrell D, Remington M et al. Two-day regimen of acyclovir for treatment of recurrent genital herpes simplex virus type 2 infection. *Clin Infect Dis* 2002;34(7):944-8.
32. Leone PA, Trottier S, Miller JM. Valacyclovir for episodic treatment of genital herpes: a shorter 3-day treatment course compared with 5-day treatment. *Clin Infect Dis* 2002;34(7):958-62.
33. Aoki FY, Tyring S, Diaz-Mitoma F et al. Single-day, patient-initiated famciclovir therapy for recurrent genital herpes: a randomized, double-blind, placebo-controlled trial. *Clin Infect Dis* 2006;42(1):8-13.
34. Douglas JM, Critchlow C, Benedetti J et al. A double-blind study of oral acyclovir for suppression of recurrences of genital herpes simplex virus infection. *N Engl J Med* 1984;310(24):1551-6.
35. Mertz GJ, Jones CC, Mills J et al. Long-term acyclovir suppression of frequently recurring genital herpes simplex virus infection. A multicenter double-blind trial. *JAMA* 1988;260(2):201-6.
36. Mostow SR, Mayfield JL, Marr JJ et al. Suppression of recurrent genital herpes by single daily dosages of acyclovir. *Am J Med* 1988;85(2A):30-3.
37. Mertz GJ, Loveless MO, Levin MJ et al. Oral famciclovir for suppression of recurrent genital herpes simplex virus infection in women. A multicenter, double-blind, placebo-controlled trial. Collaborative Famciclovir Genital Herpes Research Group. *Arch Intern Med* 1997;157(3):343-9.
38. Reitano M, Tyring S, Lang W et al. Valaciclovir for the suppression of recurrent genital herpes simplex virus infection: a large-scale dose range-finding study. International Valaciclovir HSV Study Group. *J Infect Dis* 1998;178(3):603-10.
39. Wald A, Selke S, Warren T et al. Comparative efficacy of famciclovir and valacyclovir for suppression of recurrent genital herpes and viral shedding. *Sex Trans Dis* 2006;33(9):529-33.
40. Corey L, Wald A, Patel R et al. Once-daily valacyclovir to reduce the risk of transmission of genital herpes. *N Engl J Med* 2004;350(1):11-20.
41. Johnston C, Saracino M, Kuntz S et al. Standard-dose and high-dose daily antiviral therapy for short episodes of genital HSV-2 reactivation: three randomised, open-label, cross-over trials. *Lancet* 2012;379(9816):641-7.
42. Goldberg LH, Kaufman R, Kurtz TO et al. Long-term suppression of recurrent genital herpes with acyclovir. A 5-year benchmark. Acyclovir Study Group. *Arch Dermatol* 1993;129(5):582-7.
43. Aoki FY. Contemporary antiviral drug regimens for the prevention and treatment of orolabial and anogenital herpes simplex virus infection in the normal host: four approved indications and 13 off-label uses. *Can J Infect Dis* 2003;14(1):17-27.
44. Rompalo AM. Diagnosis and treatment of sexually acquired proctitis and proctocolitis: An update. *Clin Infect Dis* 1999;28(Suppl 1):S84-S90.
45. Rompalo AM, Mertz GJ, Davis LG et al. Oral acyclovir for treatment of first-episode herpes simplex virus proctitis. *JAMA* 1988;259(19):2879-81.
46. Niimura M, Nishikawa T. Treatment of eczema herpeticum with oral acyclovir. *Am J Med* 1988;85(2A):49-52.
47. Sanderson IR, Brueton LA, Savage MO et al. Eczema herpeticum: a potentially fatal disease. *Br Med J (Clin Res Ed)* 1987;294(6573):693-4.
48. Wollenberg A, Wetzel S, Burgdorf WH et al. Viral infections in atopic dermatitis: pathogenic aspects and clinical management. *J Allergy Clin Immunol* 2003;112(4):667-74.
49. Whitley RJ, Lakeman F. Herpes simplex virus infection of the central nervous system: therapeutic and diagnostic considerations. *Clin Infect Dis* 1999;20(2):414-20.
50. Whitley RJ, Alford CA, Hirsch MS et al. Vidarabine versus acyclovir therapy in herpes simplex encephalitis. *N Eng J Med* 1986;314(3):144-9.
51. Wilhelmus KR. Antiviral treatment and other therapeutic interventions for herpes simplex virus epithelial keratitis. *Cochrane Database Syst Rev* 2010;(12):CD002898.
52. Acyclovir for the prevention of recurrent herpes simplex virus eye disease. Herpetic Eye Disease Study Group. *N Engl J Med* 1998;339(5):300-6.
53. Dunkle LM, Arvin AM, Whitley RJ et al. A controlled trial of acyclovir for chickenpox in normal children. *N Engl J Med* 1991;325(22):1539-44.
54. Balfour HH, Rothart HA, Feldman S et al. Acyclovir treatment of varicella in otherwise healthy adolescents. The Collaborative Acyclovir Varicella Study Group. *J Pediatr* 1992;120(4 Pt 1):627-33.
55. Wallace MR, Bowler WA, Murray NB et al. Treatment of adult varicella with oral acyclovir. A randomized, placebo-controlled trial. *Ann Intern Med* 1992;117(5):358-63.
56. American Academy of Pediatrics. Varicella-zoster infections. In: Pickering LK, Baker CJ, Long SS et al., eds. *Red Book: 2006 report of the Committee on Infectious Diseases*. 27th ed. Elk Grove Village (IL): American Academy of Pediatrics; 2006. p. 711-25.
57. Advisory Committee Statement (ACS). National Advisory Committee on Immunization (NACI). Varicella vaccination two-doses recommendations. *Can Commun Dis Rep* 2010;36(ACS-8). Available from: www.phac-aspc.gc.ca/publicat/ccdr-rmtc/10vol36/acs-8/index-eng.php#pg7. Accessed March 14, 2011.
58. Dworkin RH, Johnson RW, Breuer J et al. Recommendations for the management of herpes zoster. *Clin Infect Dis* 2007;44:(Suppl 1):S1-26.
59. Beutner KR, Friedman DJ, Forszpaniak C et al. Valacyclovir compared with acyclovir for improved therapy for herpes zoster in immunocompetent adults. *Antimicrob Agents Chemother* 1995;39(7):1546-53.
60. Degreef H. Famciclovir, a new oral anti herpes drug: results of the first controlled clinical study demonstrating its efficacy and safety in the treatment of uncomplicated herpes zoster in immunocompetent patients. *Int J Antimicrob Agents* 1994;4(4):241-6.
61. Wood, MJ, Kay R, Dworkin RH et al. Oral acyclovir accelerates pain resolution in herpes zoster: a meta-analysis of placebo-controlled trials. *Clin Infect Dis* 1996;22(2):341-7.
62. Choo PW, Galil K, Donahue JG et al. Risk factors for postherpetic neuralgia. *Arch Intern Med* 1997;157(11):1217-24.
63. Whitley RJ, Weiss HL, Soong SJ et al. Herpes zoster: risk categories for persistent pain. *J Inf Dis* 1999;179(1):9-15.
64. Chen N, Li Q, Yang J et al. Antiviral treatment for preventing postherpetic neuralgia. *Cochrane Database Syst Rev* 2014;(2):CD006866.
65. Whitley RJ, Weiss H, Gnann JW et al. Acyclovir with and without prednisone for the treatment of herpes zoster. A randomized, placebo-controlled trial. The National Institute of Allergy and Infectious Diseases Collaborative Antiviral Study Group. *Ann Int Med* 1996;125(5):376-83.

66. Gagliardi AM, Gomes Silva BN, Torloni MR et al. Vaccines for preventing herpes zoster in older adults. *Cochrane Database Syst Rev* 2012;(10):CD008858.
67. e-CPS. Ottawa (ON): Canadian Pharmacists Association. *Zostavax* [product monograph]. Available from: www.e-therapeutics.ca. Subscription required.
68. Advisory Committee Statement (ACS). National Advisory Committee on Immunization (NACI). *Update on the use of herpes zoster vaccine*. Ottawa (ON): Public Health Agency of Canada; 2014. Available from: publications.gc.ca/collections/collection_2014/aspc-phac/HP40-92-2014-eng.pdf.
69. Drolet M, Oxman MN, Levin MJ et al. Vaccination against herpes zoster in developed countries: state of the evidence. *Hum Vaccin Immunother* 2013;9(5):1177-84.
70. Oxman MN, Levin MJ, Johnson GR et al. A vaccine to prevent herpes zoster and post-herpetic neuralgia in older adults. *N Engl J Med* 2005;352(22):2271-84.
71. Brown ZA, Wald A, Morrow RA et al. Effect of serologic status and cesarean delivery on transmission rates of herpes simplex virus from mother to infant. *JAMA* 2003;289(2):203-9.
72. Nahmias AJ, Josey WE, Naib ZM et al. Perinatal risk associated with maternal genital herpes simplex virus infection. *Am J Obstet Gynecol* 1971;110(6):825-37.
73. Pasternak B, Hviid A. Use of acyclovir, valacyclovir, and famciclovir in the first trimester of pregnancy and the risk of birth defects. *JAMA* 2010;304(8):859-66.
74. Aoki FY. Genital herpes simplex virus (HSV) infections. In: *Canadian guidelines on sexually transmitted infections*. Evergreen ed. Ottawa (ON): Public Health Agency of Canada; 2008. Available from: www.phac-aspc.gc.ca/std-mts/sti-its/cgsti-ldcits/index-eng.php. Accessed March 14, 2011.
75. Taddio A, Klein J, Koren G. Acyclovir excretion in human breast milk. *Ann Pharmacother* 1994;28(5):585-7.
76. Sheffield JS, Fish DN, Hollier LM et al. Acyclovir concentrations in human breast milk after valaciclovir administration. *Am J Obstet Gynecol* 2002;186(1):100-2.

Chapter 113
HIV Infection

Marianne Harris, MD, CCFP
Valentina Montessori, MD, FRCPC and
Julio S.G. Montaner, MD, DSc (hon), FRCPC, FCCP, FACP, FRSC, OBC

Human immunodeficiency virus (HIV) is a chronic viral infection that, left untreated, ultimately leads to death from opportunistic infections and/or specific cancers associated with acquired immunodeficiency syndrome (AIDS). However, since the advent and availability of highly active combination antiretroviral therapy (cART) in the mid-1990's, the prognosis has shifted dramatically.[1,2,3] The primary goal of therapy, to preserve the health of the infected individual, is readily achievable with current cART, and in most cases HIV can be considered a chronic manageable condition. The benefits of cART are maximized when it is given continuously, starting as early as possible in the course of HIV infection, to avert damage to the immune system and irreversible organ damage caused by chronic inflammation.[4,5,6,7]

More recently it has become apparent that widespread use of cART can also have significant benefits at the population level, by preventing new HIV infections.[8,9] In conjunction with education and other prevention strategies, expanded use of cART in the "treatment as prevention" model has the potential to significantly impact the HIV epidemic. Early diagnosis is critical to achieving the proven benefits of early HIV treatment at both the individual and societal levels. This highlights the need to expand HIV testing and incorporate it as part of standard health care for all sexually active adults.

Goals of Therapy

- Prolong survival
- Slow disease progression
- Improve quality of life
- Decrease viral replication
- Prevent/reverse immunologic impairment
- Delay/prevent the emergence of drug-resistant strains of HIV
- Prevent transmission of HIV

Investigations

- Clinical history:
  - risk behaviours, social support, need for counselling and/or support regarding disclosure
  - establish date of infection if possible based on a review of past sexual contacts, period of needle sharing, receipt of blood or blood products, availability of a previous negative test or a history of possible seroconversion illness (e.g., mononucleosis-like or severe flu-like illness) shortly after a high-risk exposure
  - general indicators: anorexia, weight loss, fatigue or malaise, lymphadenopathy
  - symptoms of opportunistic infections, e.g., fever, night sweats, cough, dyspnea, diarrhea, headache or skin rashes

- travel history
- sexual history, HIV status of regular partner(s)

- Past medical history:
  - sexually transmitted infections (including syphilis, gonorrhea, chlamydia, granuloma inguinale, lymphogranuloma venereum, herpes simplex, genital warts, pubic lice)
  - past history or exposure to tuberculosis (TB), hepatitis A, B or C, varicella
  - conditions that may compromise future drug therapy, e.g., kidney dysfunction, peripheral neuropathy, liver disease, pancreatitis, cardiovascular disease, diabetes, osteoporosis, mental health diagnoses, substance use
  - allergies
  - immunization history
  - prescription and non-prescription medications, including complementary and alternative therapies and supplements
  - tobacco smoking history
- Physical examination:
  - focus on signs of immune dysfunction and indications of opportunistic disease
  - direct specific attention to examination of the mental status, skin, visual fields, ocular fundi, oral cavity, lymph nodes, abdomen, rectal and genital exam (including cervical Pap smear in women)
- Laboratory investigations:
  - HIV antibody test
  - plasma HIV RNA level (viral load), used in conjunction with the CD4+ T-lymphocyte count (CD4 count), is the best prognostic marker for progression to AIDS and survival in untreated patients.[10] Plasma viral load ranges vary according to the test employed. There is no "safe" level. The most commonly used plasma HIV-1 RNA assay has a quantitation limit of 40 copies/mL
  - CD4 count and percentage are useful in determining where a patient lies in the continuum of HIV disease and the need for specific intervention (Table 1). Knowledge of the CD4 count can also help to narrow the differential diagnosis in a symptomatic HIV-infected patient. In adults, a CD4 count of 430–1360 cells/µL (0.43–1.36 Giga/Litre or G/L) is considered normal in most laboratories
  - HIV drug resistance should be assessed in all patients at baseline (as soon as possible after HIV is diagnosed) and in cases of confirmed viral load rebound to >200 copies/mL while on treatment
  - screen all patients for the presence of the HLA-B*5701 allele at baseline, especially before starting or restarting **abacavir**.[11,12,13] A positive test result should be recorded in the patient's chart as an abacavir allergy
  - perform a tropism assay to determine the chemokine receptor status (CCR5, CXCR4 or dual-mixed tropic) if considering use of the CCR5 inhibitor **maraviroc**.
  - CBC, differential and platelet count
  - liver (AST, ALT, bilirubin, INR) and renal (creatinine, estimated glomerular filtration rate (eGFR), serum phosphate, urinalysis, urine albumin to creatinine ratio (UACR) or urine protein to creatinine ratio (UPCR)) profiles
  - metabolic profiles (fasting glucose and lipids—total cholesterol, LDL, HDL, triglycerides; apolipoprotein B if triglycerides elelvated)
  - hepatitis A, hepatitis B, hepatitis C, syphilis and Toxoplasma serologies
  - cultures, NAATs (nucleic acid amplification tests) and smears for sexually transmitted infections (gonorrhea and Chlamydia) as indicated

- TB skin test, sputum cultures and smears for mycobacteria as indicated
- cervical pap for women
- chest x-ray

Therapeutic Choices

Nonpharmacologic Choices

Management recommendations for persons with HIV infection are included in Table 1.

Pharmacologic Choices

Antiretroviral Therapy

Durability of the treatment effect is related to the prevention of drug resistance and this is achieved only with intense suppression of viral replication. Long-term nonprogression of disease can be expected if the plasma viral load is maintained below the level of detection on a long-term basis. However, due to recent changes in viral load testing methodology, the clinical significance of a viral load result between 40 and 200 copies/mL is uncertain.[12,13] Therefore, the goal of plasma viral load suppression is <40 copies/mL (for polymerase chain reaction assays) or <75 copies/mL (for branched DNA tests), whereas the inability to maintain HIV RNA levels <200 copies/mL (measured by either test) is considered virologic failure.[12,13]

Combination antiretroviral therapy (cART) is the standard of care and is defined as a combination of at least 3 active antiretroviral drugs.[12,13] cART regimens recommended for first-line therapy consist of 2 **nucleoside (or nucleotide) reverse transcriptase inhibitors** (N[t]RTIs) plus either a **non-nucleoside reverse transcriptase inhibitor** (NNRTI), a **ritonavir-boosted protease inhibitor** (PI) or an **integrase inhibitor** (see Table 2). Other classes of drugs (**fusion inhibitors** and **entry inhibitors**) are reserved for use in treatment-experienced patients with limited options due to drug resistance, contraindications or intolerable adverse events. See Table 3 for a full list of available antiretroviral medications.

Table 1: Management of Patients with HIV Infection

CD4 Count (cells/µL)	Action
At all levels	• General counselling (safer sex, nutrition, need for follow up, importance of adherence) • History and physical examination at least annually • Start antiretroviral therapy when patient is ready • Plasma viral load and CD4 count every 3–4 months; can be decreased to every 6–12 months if on stable antiretroviral therapy with viral load <40 copies/mL, CD4 >350 cells/µL and good adherence for >1 year; increase monitoring if symptomatic or diagnosed with AIDS • Pneumococcal vaccine; hepatitis A and B vaccines if appropriate serology; update diphtheria, tetanus and pertussis (Td/TdaP) vaccines as needed; annual influenza vaccinations; measles/mumps/rubella (MMR) and Varicella vaccines if CD4 >200 cells/µL • Tuberculin skin test and isoniazid treatment of latent tuberculosis infection if indicated
<200	• Start prophylaxis for *Pneumocystis jirovecii* pneumonia (PCP) if not starting antiretroviral therapy imminently
<100	• Start toxoplasmosis prophylaxis if seropositive and not on sulfamethoxazole/trimethoprim for PCP prophylaxis
<50	• Consider *Mycobacterium avium* complex (MAC) prophylaxis after ruling out active MAC infection

Table 2: **Options for First-line Antiretroviral Therapy Regimens**

Regimen	Comments
2 N[t]RTIs + NNRTI	Once-daily dosing, lower pill burden. May not be effective in the presence of primary NNRTI resistance. Adverse effects: rash, CNS effects (efavirenz), hepatotoxicity.
2 N[t]RTIs + PI + low-dose ritonavir	Once- or twice-daily dosing. Drug interactions more likely. Adverse effects: GI intolerance, lipid abnormalities, hepatotoxicity.
2 N[t]RTIs + integrase inhibitor	Once- or twice-daily dosing.

Abbreviations: CNS = central nervous system; GI = gastrointestinal; NNRTI = non-nucleoside reverse transcriptase inhibitor; N[t]RTI = nucleoside [or nucleotide] reverse transcriptase inhibitor; PI = protease inhibitor

Preferred N[t]RTI options are **emtricitabine/tenofovir** (available as a fixed-dose combination), **lamivudine/tenofovir** or **abacavir/lamivudine** (only for patients who are HLA-B*5701 negative; available as a fixed-dose combination). Preferred options for the third drug in the regimen are:

- NNRTIs: **efavirenz** (available as a fixed-dose combination with emtricitabine/tenofovir)
- PIs: **atazanavir/ritonavir** or **darunavir/ritonavir**
- Integrase inhibitors: **dolutegravir**, **elvitegravir/cobicistat** (only for patients with ClCr >70 mL/min; available only as a fixed-dose combination with emtricitabine/tenofovir), or **raltegravir**.

Effective control of HIV infection with cART reduces the incidence of opportunistic infections and certain cancers, and prolongs life.[1,2,3] It also decreases infectivity and lowers the risk of HIV transmission from pregnant women to their infants, between drug-using partners and among sexual contacts.[9,14,15] Long-term treatment with cART may be associated with metabolic complications and reduced bone mineral density;[16,17] however, these effects are offset by the demonstrated improvement in survival and significantly reduced rates of major cardiovascular, hepatic and renal events associated with continuous antiretroviral therapy.[7]

Antiretroviral therapy is recommended in all patients, with the possible exception of those consistently maintaining both a CD4 count >500 cells/μL and a viral load <1000 copies/mL while off therapy. Initiation of antiretroviral therapy should be considered more urgently in symptomatic patients, those with a history of an AIDS-defining illness, and in asymptomatic patients with CD4 <500 cells/μL.[12,13] Analysis of a large, long-term observational cohort has shown a reduction in the risk of disease progression or death when cART is initiated in patients with CD4 counts between 351 and 450 cells/μL as compared to 251–350 cells/μL.[4] Similarly, another large cohort study demonstrated reduced mortality among patients starting cART with a CD4 of 350–500 cells/μL as compared to those who deferred treatment until their CD4 fell below the 350 cells/μL threshold.[5] Evidence from cohort studies for a possible benefit of initiating cART in individuals with CD4 >500 cells/μL is conflicting;[4,5] however, such individuals are at increased risk for non-AIDS-associated cancers, coronary artery disease, hepatic and renal disease and other conditions, possibly due to uncontrolled viral replication and chronic immune activation.[6,7] Therefore, cART initiation is appropriate irrespective of current CD4 cell count particularly in patients with HIV-associated nephropathy, hepatitis coinfection, HIV-uninfected sexual partners and those at high risk for cardiovascular disease.[12,13]

When selecting the antiretroviral regimen, use agents with additive antiviral effects and avoid those with additive toxicities. Also consider issues of cross-resistance, adherence, convenience and cost (Table 3). Nonadherence to therapy promotes the emergence of drug-resistant HIV strains and is the most important remaining challenge in the management of HIV infection.[18,19] Counselling and support are critical to ensure ongoing adherence.[20]

Drug interactions are an important consideration whenever starting or stopping antiretrovirals or other drugs.[12,13] In addition to toxicity, reduced serum drug levels can be an important consequence.

Suboptimal antiretroviral levels not only reduce efficacy but may also promote resistance. All PIs and NNRTIs are metabolized by the CYP450 enzyme system and consequently are associated with many drug interactions. N[t]RTIs are not metabolized by CYP450 but other interactions can occur.

A confirmed rebound in plasma viral load implies treatment failure or nonadherence. If adherence is confirmed, drug resistance testing should be performed and the cART regimen should be changed to a new 3-drug regimen, avoiding cross-resistance with previous treatments.[12,13]

If a patient experiences unmanageable drug toxicity, simultaneous cessation of *all* medications is recommended if necessary prior to starting a new cART regimen. Avoid decreasing the dosage or stopping only 1 or 2 medications, as this can promote the development of resistance.[12,13,21]

In the past, planned treatment interruptions ("drug holidays") were proposed as a strategy to reduce long-term toxicity and treatment cost for patients. However, the risk of opportunistic infections and death was higher in patients randomized to episodic treatment interruptions based on CD4 count as compared with continuous cART in the SMART study.[7] For this reason, treatment interruptions are not recommended [Evidence: SORT B*].[12,13]

Postexposure Prophylaxis

For recommendations on occupational HIV postexposure prophylaxis (PEP), visit www.jstor.org/stable/10.1086/672271. Recommendations for nonoccupational PEP can be found at www.hivguidelines.org/clinical-guidelines/adults/hiv-prophylaxis-following-non-occupational-exposure/.

Choices during Pregnancy and Breastfeeding

HIV Infection and Pregnancy

Optimal management of HIV in pregnancy requires consultation with a physician with expertise in this area. Considerations during pregnancy should include optimal therapy of the pregnant woman, results of resistance testing, risk of mother-to-child-transmission of HIV, changes in pharmacokinetics of antiretrovirals during pregnancy and possible teratogenic and other effects of cART on the developing fetus.[22,23,24] All pregnant women should be offered cART with a discussion of its risks and benefits.[12,13]

Choices during Pregnancy

Among the antiretrovirals, **zidovudine (AZT)** has been most extensively used in pregnancy and should be included in a treatment regimen unless contraindicated.[14,22,23,24] The cART regimen should include **AZT** and **lamivudine (3TC)** as the preferred **NRTI** backbone plus a **ritonavir-boosted PI**, either once-daily **atazanavir/ritonavir** or twice daily **lopinavir/ritonavir**. Doses of the PI should be increased during the third trimester because of the increased volume of distribution of pregnancy.[24] Conflicting evidence suggests PIs may be associated with a small increased risk of preterm delivery (<37 weeks gestation) without an observed increase in infant hospitalizations or death.[25]

If AZT/3TC is contraindicated or not tolerated, **abacavir** plus 3TC is an alternative NRTI backbone, if the mother's HLA-B*5701 test is negative. Because animal data suggest the potential for fetal bone toxicity with **tenofovir**, this agent is considered an alternative N[t]RTI in pregnancy, except in women coinfected with chronic hepatitis B infection where it is considered first line.[24]

Alternative third agents include **darunavir/ritonavir** or **efavirenz**. The latter agent should be avoided during the first trimester because of demonstrated teratogenicity in nonhuman primates. Nevirapine

* SORT (Strength of Recommendation Taxonomy) is a rating system (A, B or C) that addresses the quality of available evidence.
For more information consult **How to Use *Compendium of Therapeutic Choices*** on page xxv.

should not be initiated during pregnancy if a suitable alternative is available, because of the increased risk of life-threatening hepatotoxicity observed in this setting.[24]

Data on the use of **raltegravir** in pregnancy are limited, but it may be considered when preferred or alternative agents cannot be used. Use of other antiretroviral agents should be considered on an individual basis, in consultation with an expert in the management of HIV during pregnancy.[24]

Choices during Breastfeeding

Breastfeeding by HIV-positive women is contraindicated in the developed world due to the risk of HIV transmission to the child and ready availability of infant formula. Therefore, HIV treatment recommendations for the breastfeeding mother are the same as for the general HIV-infected population.

A discussion of general principles on the use of medications in these special populations can be found in Appendix II and Appendix III. Other specialized reference sources are also provided in these appendices.

Therapeutic Tips

- Consider cART for all HIV-infected patients irrespective of their CD4 cell count. Initiation of treatment should be considered more urgent in pregnant women, in patients with symptomatic HIV infection, in asymptomatic patients with CD4 cell counts <500 cells/μL, and in the presence of certain concomitant medical conditions.
- Poor adherence is the most critical determinant of therapeutic failure. Ensure patient readiness before starting cART. Assess regimen tolerability and adherence on an ongoing basis and provide education and support as necessary.
- The target of therapy is to maintain a plasma viral load consistently below the detectable threshold (usually 40 copies/mL with current assays). However, nonquantifiable plasma viral levels do not imply cure, eradication or a reason for complacency with safer sex practices or similar safety measures.
- If the plasma viral load rebounds to >200 copies/mL despite ongoing cART, consider nonadherence and viral drug resistance as the most likely causes. Also consider drug interactions that may result in suboptimal therapeutic responses even in an adherent patient.
- The variability of the plasma viral load assays is approximately 0.3 to 0.5 $\log_{10}$ copies/mL. Hence, in untreated patients, changes in plasma viral load of <0.3 to 0.5 $\log_{10}$ are usually not regarded as clinically significant.[26]
- Intercurrent illnesses or vaccinations can transiently but substantially increase plasma viral load in patients not receiving cART.[27]
- CD4 counts show diurnal variation, from lowest in the morning to highest in the evening.[28] Fluctuations of up to 30% may occur, which are not attributable to a change in disease status. Overall, it is important to monitor the trends in CD4 counts over time rather than making treatment decisions based on a single reading.
- As the immune system recovers with cART, patients may experience new or worsening symptoms of opportunistic infections. For more information, see Immune Reconstitution Inflammatory Syndrome in Chapter 118.

Table 3: Antiretroviral Medications for HIV Therapy

Class	Drug	Standard Dose	Adverse Effects	Drug Interactions[a]	Comments	Cost[b]
Nucleoside Reverse Transcriptase Inhibitors (NRTI)	*abacavir* Ziagen	600 mg once daily po *or* 300 mg BID po	Hypersensitivity reactions in patients with a genetic predisposition (can be severe).[c]	Low potential for drug interactions.	Screen patients for the presence of HLA-B*5701 before starting; do not use if patient is positive for HLA-B*5701.[c] Monitor closely early on for hypersensitivity reaction.	$$
	didanosine (ddI) Videx EC	<60 kg: 250 mg once daily po ≥60 kg: 400 mg once daily po	GI intolerance, pancreatitis, increased uric acid and lactic acid, reversible peripheral neuropathy, hepatic steatosis.	Tenofovir, cimetidine, ganciclovir increase ddI levels. Contraindicated with allopurinol, pentamidine or ribavirin. Increased risk of toxicity with dapsone, stavudine, vinca alkaloids.	Avoid combined use of ddI and stavudine or tenofovir. When used with tipranavir separate doses by at least 2 h.	$
	lamivudine (3TC) 3TC, generics	150 mg BID po *or* 300 mg once daily po	Minimal toxicity, generally well tolerated.	Low potential for drug interactions.	Avoid combined use of 3TC and emtricitabine (similar resistance profiles).	$
	stavudine (d4T) Zerit	<60 kg: 30 mg BID po ≥60 kg: 40 mg BID po	Reversible peripheral neuropathy, increased lactic acid, hepatic steatosis, pancreatitis, lipoatrophy, dyslipidemia.	Pharmacologic antagonism with zidovudine. Increased toxicity with dapsone, didanosine, vinca alkaloids.	Avoid combined use of d4T and didanosine, pentamidine, ribavirin or zidovudine.	$$
	zidovudine (AZT) Retrovir, generics	300 mg BID po *or* 200 mg TID po	Nausea, headache, malaise, fatigue, rash, myositis, myocarditis, anemia, leukopenia, hepatic steatosis, elevated liver enzymes, lactic acid and CK. Long-term use associated with peripheral lipoatrophy.	Additive hemotoxicity with other agents, e.g., anemia with dapsone, foscarnet, ganciclovir, petamidine, ribavirin. Pharmacologic antagonism with stavudine. Fluconazole, methadone, probenicid and valproic acid increase AZT levels.	Avoid combined use of AZT and ribavirin or stavudine.	$

(cont'd)

Table 3: Antiretroviral Medications for HIV Therapy *(cont'd)*

Class	Drug	Standard Dose	Adverse Effects	Drug Interactions[a]	Comments	Cost[b]
Nucleotide Reverse Transcriptase Inhibitors (NtRTI)	*tenofovir (TDF)* ◗ Viread	300 mg once daily po	Renal toxicity; monitor renal function, urinalysis and serum phosphorus. Decreased bone mineral density and increased osteoporotic fractures; caution in postmenopausal women and in patients with established or high risk of osteoporosis.[29,30]	TDF increases ddI levels. TDF decreases atazanavir levels, therefore administer only in combination with ritonavir. Atazanavir increases TDF levels.	Avoid combined use of TDF and didanosine or nephrotoxic drugs.	$$
Non-nucleoside Reverse Transcriptase Inhibitors (NNRTI)	*delavirdine* Rescriptor	400 mg TID po *or* 600 mg BID po	Rash, headache, increased liver enzymes.	Do not administer with alprazolam, carbamazepine, ergot derivatives, ginkgo biloba, midazolam,[d] phenobarbital, phenytoin, pimozide, rifabutin, rifampin, St. John's wort and triazolam. Inhibits metabolism of atorvastatin, lovastatin, maraviroc and simvastatin. Increases levels of some benzodiazepines.	Inferior efficacy and higher pill burden compared to first-line options.	$
	efavirenz (EFV) Sustiva, generics	600 mg once daily po	CNS toxicity (e.g., sleep disturbance, abnormal dreams, depressed mood), rash, increased liver enzymes. Avoid in patients with a history of anxiety, depression or psychosis. Contraindicated in 1st trimester of pregnancy (teratogenic in animals). Avoid in women of child-bearing potential.	Do not administer with boceprevir, ergot derivatives, midazolam,[d] pimozide, rifabutin, simeprevir and triazolam. Induces metabolism of maraviroc. St. John's wort decreases EFV levels. EFV decreases telaprevir levels; increase telaprevir dose. EFV decreases methadone and posaconazole levels. Voriconazole: EFV levels increased and voriconazole levels decreased when used together; dosage adjustments needed.	Should be taken without food.	$

Class	Drug	Standard Dose	Adverse Effects	Drug Interactions[a]	Comments	Cost[b]
	etravirine Intelence	200 mg BID po	Rash, nausea. Rare reports of severe skin reactions (Stevens-Johnson syndrome, toxic epidermal necrolysis and erythema multiforme), hypersensitivity reactions (may include hepatotoxicity or hepatic failure).	Do not administer with carbamazepine, ginkgo biloba, phenobarbital, phenytoin, rifampin, St. John's wort. Rifabutin not recommended if etravirine coadministered with a ritonavir-boosted PI due to decreased etravirine levels. Ritonavir-boosted tipranavir decreases etravirine exposure (avoid combined use). Etravirine increases fosamprenavir exposure and decreases atazanavir exposure (avoid combined use). Induces metabolism of maraviroc. Decreased clarithromycin levels; consider alternative for MAC prophylaxis and treatment.	May be effective against NNRTI-resistant HIV. Should be taken with food.	$$$
	nevirapine (NVP) Viramune, Viramune XR, generics	200 mg once daily po for 2 wk then either: 200 mg BID po (immediate-release) *or* 400 mg once daily po (extended-release)	Rash (rare severe allergic reactions). Increased liver enzymes (rare cases of fatal hepatitis). Not recommended in liver disease or if the baseline CD4 count is >250 cells/μL in women or >400 cells/μL in men.	Do not administer with ginkgo biloba, itraconazole, ketoconazole, rifampin, simeprevir, St. John's wort. Decreases clarithromycin levels; consider alternative for MAC prophylaxis and treatment. Fluconazole significantly increases NVP levels increasing the risk of hepatotoxicity.		$

(cont'd)

Table 3: **Antiretroviral Medications for HIV Therapy** *(cont'd)*

Class	Drug	Standard Dose	Adverse Effects	Drug Interactions[a]	Comments	Cost[b]
	rilpivirine (RPV) Edurant	Treatment-naïve: 25 mg once daily	Most common adverse effects: depression, insomnia, rash, headache. Early benign increase in serum creatinine (first 2–4 weeks, then stable).	Contraindicated with carbamazepine, dexamethasone, other NNRTIs, phenobarbital, phenytoin, proton pump inhibitors, rifamycins, St. John's wort. RPV absorption is acid-dependent; stagger administration of antacids (2 h before or 4 h after RPV) or H_2-antagonists (12 h before or 4 h after RPV). Clarithromycin, ketoconazole and PIs may increase levels of rilpivirine. Rilpivirine decreases ketoconazole levels.	Use only if HIV RNA levels ≤100 000 copies/mL at the time of rilpivirine initiation. Should be taken with a meal.	$$
Protease Inhibitors (PI)	*atazanavir* Reyataz	Treatment-experienced or with tenofovir: 300 mg (+ RTV 100 mg) once daily po Treatment-naïve: 400 mg once daily *or* 300 mg (+ RTV 100 mg) once daily po	Benign hyperbilirubinemia in patients with a genetic predisposition.[e] Less common: nephrolithiasis,[33,34] possible renal dysfunction,[35] rash. All PIs may be associated with PR interval prologation.[36]	PIs are not recommended in combination with boceprevir, ergot alkaloids, fluticasone, lovastatin, midazolam,[d] rifampin, salmeterol, sildenafil when used for pulmonary arterial hypertension, simeprevir, simvastatin, St. John's wort or triazolam. If used with rifabutin, monitor rifabutin drug levels and consider dose reduction of rifabutin. All PIs except ritonavir-boosted tipranavir inhibit metabolism of maraviroc. Use caution when administering PIs with other PR-prolonging drugs, e.g., antiarrhythmics, beta-blockers, calcium channel blockers, digoxin. Do not use ritonavir-boosted atazanavir with etravirine.	Should be taken with food (at least 340 kCal).	$$$

Class	Drug	Standard Dose	Adverse Effects	Drug Interactions[a]	Comments	Cost[b]
	darunavir Prezista	Treatment-naïve: 800 mg (+ RTV 100 mg) once daily po *or* 600 mg (+ RTV 100 mg) BID po Treatment-experienced (with PI resistance): 600 mg (+ RTV 100 mg) BID po	Diarrhea, nausea, headache, rash (possible cross-sensitivity with sulfonamides), hyperlipidemia. Drug-induced hepatotoxicity, in some cases fatal, has been reported rarely with darunavir in combination with ritonavir. All PIs may be associated with PR interval prolongation.[36]	See atazanavir. Do not use ritonavir-boosted darunavir with telaprevir.	Approved for use only with ritonavir (do not use as a sole PI). Should be taken with food.	$$$
	fosamprenavir Telzir	Treatment-naïve: 700 mg (+ RTV 100 mg) BID po *or* 1400 mg (+ RTV 200 mg) once daily po Treatment-experienced (with PI resistance): 700 mg (+ RTV 100 mg) BID po	Rash, GI upset, hyperlipidemia. Possible increased risk of cardiovascular events.[37] All PIs may be associated with PR interval prolongation.[36]	See atazanavir. Do not use ritonavir-boosted fosamprenavir with delavirdine, etravirine, telaprevir or antiarrhythmics (e.g., amiodarone, lidocaine, quinidine).	Approved for use only with ritonavir (do not use as a sole PI).	$$
	indinavir Crixivan	800 mg Q8H po *or* 800 mg (+ RTV 100 or 200 mg) Q12H po	Nephrolithiasis, chronic interstitial nephritis, liver enzyme elevations, hyperlipidemia. Possible increased risk of cardiovascular events.[37,38] All PIs may be associated with PR interval prolongation.[36]	See atazanavir.	Avoid because of adverse effects and safety concerns. Adequate fluid intake recommended (at least 1.5 L/day) to reduce risk of nephrolithiasis. Take on an empty stomach especially if not taken with RTV. Must be taken in 8 hour intervals if not taken with RTV.	$$

(cont'd)

Table 3: **Antiretroviral Medications for HIV Therapy** *(cont'd)*

Class	Drug	Standard Dose	Adverse Effects	Drug Interactions[a]	Comments	Cost[b]
	lopinavir/ritonavir Kaletra	Treatment-naïve: 400/100 mg BID po *or* 800/200 mg once daily po Treatment-experienced: 400/100 mg BID po With EFV or NVP: 400/100 mg, 500/125 mg *or* 600/150 mg BID po	GI upset, liver enzyme elevations, hyperlipidemia, QT_c and PR interval prolongation. Possible increased risk of renal dysfunction[35] and cardiovascular events.[37,38]	See atazanavir. Efavirenz, nevirapine decrease levels of lopinavir. Do not use with telaprevir. Use caution when administered with other medications that prolong the QT_c interval (e.g., azoles, fluoroquinolones, macrolides, methadone, quetiapine).	Once daily lopinavir/ritonavir not recommended in pregnancy or with PI resistance; use twice daily regimen. Use with caution because of potential QT_c prolongation.	$$$
	nelfinavir Viracept	1250 mg BID po *or* 750 mg TID po	Diarrhea, hyperlipidemia. All PIs may be associated with PR interval prolongation.[36]	See atazanavir.	Not boosted by ritonavir to a significant extent. Less potent that ritonvir-boosted PIs.	$$
	ritonavir (RTV) Norvir	600 mg BID po (sole PI) As a PK booster, see atazanavir, darunavir, fosamprenavir, indinavir, saquinavir and tipranavir	GI upset, diarrhea, circumoral paresthesia, liver enzyme elevations, hyperlipidemia. All PIs may be associated with PR interval prolongation.[36]	See atazanavir.	As a PK booster, low-dose RTV is a component of many regimens. Avoid use as a sole PI because of adverse effects.	$$
	saquinavir Invirase	1000 mg (+ RTV 100 mg) BID po	Increased liver enzymes, GI upset, headache, QT_c and PR interval prolongation, hyperlipidemia.	See atazanavir. Use caution when administered with other medications that prolong the QT_c interval (e.g., azoles, fluoroquinolones, macrolides, methadone, quetiapine). Saquinavir contraindicated with trazodone.	Avoid unboosted saquinavir: inferior efficacy. Use with caution because of potential QT_c prolongation.	$$
	tipranavir Aptivus	500 mg (+ RTV 200 mg) BID po	Hepatotoxicity, rash (possible cross-sensitivity with sulfonamides), hyperlipidemia. Intracranial hemorrhage (rare). All PIs may be associated with PR interval prolongation.[36]	See atazanavir. Do not use tipranavir with etravirine.	Reserve for treatment-experienced patients with limited options. Approved for use only with ritonavir; do not use as a sole PI. When used with ddI separate doses by at least 2 h.	$$$$

Class	Drug	Standard Dose	Adverse Effects	Drug Interactions[a]	Comments	Cost[b]
Entry Inhibitors	*maraviroc* Celsentri	300 mg BID po with NRTIs, tipranavir/RTV, NVP and/or other drugs that are not strong inhibitors or inducers of CYP3A4 150 mg BID po with strong CYP3A4 inhibitors including PIs (except tipranavir/RTV), delavirdine 600 mg BID po with strong CYP3A4 inducers including EFV, etravirine See Drug Interactions	Few; generally well-tolerated.	Decreased levels with CYP3A4 inducers: EFV, etravirine, rifampin. Increased levels with CYP3A4 inhibitors: PIs (except RTV-boosted tipranavir), itraconazole, ketoconazole, clarithromycin, telithromycin.	Tropism test required prior to treatment: effective only in patients with CCR5 tropic HIV (not CXCR4 or mixed-tropic virus).	$$$$
Fusion Inhibitors	*enfuvirtide (T20)* Fuzeon	90 mg BID sc	Most patients experience injection site reactions (may be severe). Hypersensitivity reactions (<1%).	Does not interact with CYP isozymes.	Reserve for treatment-experienced patients with limited options.	~$2550
Integrase Inhibitors	*dolutegravir* Tivicay	50 mg once daily po Treatment-experienced and integrase resistant: 50 mg BID po	Early benign increase in serum creatinine (first 2–4 weeks, then stable).	Should be taken 2 h before or 6 h after medications containing polyvalent cations (e.g., aluminum, calcium, iron, or magnesium) including cation-containing antacids or laxatives, sucralfate, oral iron or calcium supplements, and buffered medications. Avoid use with carbamazepine, nevirapine, phenobarbital, phenytoin, nevirapine, St. John's wort. Dosage adjustment may be required with fosamprenavir, NNRTIs, rifampin, tipranavir.		$$
	raltegravir Isentress	400 mg BID po	Rare severe, life-threatening skin and hypersensitivity reactions.	Not an inhibitor or inducer of CYP isozymes. Rifampin decreases raltegravir levels by inducing glucuronidation. Increase raltegravir dose to 800 mg BID when coadministered with rifampin.		$$$

(cont'd)

Table 3: **Antiretroviral Medications for HIV Therapy** *(cont'd)*

Class	Drug	Standard Dose	Adverse Effects	Drug Interactions[a]	Comments	Cost[b]
Combination Antiretrovirals, Lamivudine-based	*abacavir/ lamivudine* Kivexa	600 mg/300 mg once daily po	See abacavir.	See abacavir.	See abacavir. Renal impairment: combination products are not recommended. Use individual products and adjust each agent accordingly.	$$$
	abacavir/ lamivudine/ zidovudine Trizivir	300 mg/150 mg/300 mg BID po	See abacavir. See zidovudine.	See zidovudine.	See abacavir. Renal impairment: combination products are not recommended. Use individual products and adjust each agent accordingly.	$$$$
	lamivudine/ zidovudine Combivir, generics	150 mg/300 mg BID po	See zidovudine.	See zidovudine.	Renal impairment: combination products are not recommended. Use individual products and adjust each agent accordingly.	$
Combination Antiretrovirals, Emtricitabine/ Tenofovir-based	*efavirenz/ emtricitabine/ tenofovir* Atripla	600 mg/200 mg/300 mg once daily po	See efavirenz. See tenofovir.	See efavirenz. Avoid combined use of emtricitabine and lamivudine (similar resistance profiles). See tenofovir.	Should be taken without food. Renal impairment: combination products are not recommended. Emtricitabine is not available as a single entity product.	$$$$$
	elvitegravir/ cobicistat/ emtricitabine/ tenofovir Stribild	150 mg/150 mg/200 mg/ 300 mg once daily po	Diarrhea, headache. Early benign increase in serum creatinine (first 2–4 weeks, then stable). See tenofovir.	Many interactions. Do not use with other antiretrovirals or adefovir, alfuzosin, ergot derivatives, lovastatin, midazolam, pimozide, rifamycins, simvastatin, St. John's wort, triazolam. Should be separated by at least 2 hours from antacids containing aluminum, calcium or magnesium.	Renal impairment: combination products are not recommended. Cobicistat, elvitegravir and emtricitabine are not available as single entity products. Do not use if pretreatment ClCr <70 mL/min. Cobicistat has no antiviral activity but is a CYP3A inhibitor used to boost elvitegravir. Should be taken with food.	$$$$$

Class	Drug	Standard Dose	Adverse Effects	Drug Interactions[a]	Comments	Cost[b]
	emtricitabine/ rilpivirine/ tenofovir ❥ Complera	200 mg/25 mg/300 mg once daily po	See rilpivirine. See tenofovir.	See rilpivirine. See tenofovir.	Renal impairment: combination products are not recommended. Emtricitabine is not available as a single entity product. Should be taken with food (390 kCal).	$$$$$
	emtricitabine/ tenofovir ❥ Truvada	200 mg/300 mg once daily po	See tenofovir.	Avoid combined use of emtricitabine and lamivudine (similar resistance profiles). See tenofovir.	Renal impairment: combination products are not recommended. Emtricitabine is not available as a single entity product.	$$$

[a] Many drug interactions occur among antiretroviral drugs. Those listed here are limited to more significant or relevant interactions. Always consult a reputable drug interaction reference (e.g., www.hivclinic.ca/main/drugs_interact.html) or the product monograph for more information.

[b] Cost of 30-day supply; includes drug cost only.

[c] Patients with the HLA-B*5701 allele, present in 5–8% of white patients but rare in patients of African and Asian descent, are predisposed to allergic reactions.[11] A positive test result for the allele should be recorded as an allergy to abacavir in the patient's chart.

[d] May use a single dose of parenteral midazolam with caution for monitored medical procedures.

[e] Patients with a particular polymorphism in the multidrug resistance gene 1 have higher plasma levels of atazanavir and higher bilirubin levels during atazanavir therapy than those without this polymorphism. The risk of severe hyperbilirubinemia during atazanavir therapy is further increased by the presence of distinct variants in the gene coding for UDP-glucuronosyltransferase (UGT1A).[31,32]

❥ Dosage adjustment may be required in renal impairment; see Appendix I.

Abbreviations: AZT = zidovudine; CK = creatine kinase; CCR5 = chemokine receptor 5; ClCr = creatinine clearance; CNS = central nervous system; CYP = cytochrome P450; d4T = stavudine; ddI = didanosine; EFV = efavirenz; MAC = *Mycobacterium avium* complex; NNRTI = non-nucleoside reverse transcriptase inhibitor; NRTI = nucleoside reverse transcriptase inhibitor; NVP = nevirapine; PI = protease inhibitor; PK = pharmacokinetic; RPV = rilpivirine; RTV = ritonavir

Legend: $ < $300 $$ $300–600 $$$ $600–900 $$$$ $900–1200 $$$$$ $1200–1500

Suggested Readings

Aberg JA, Gallent JE, Ghanem KG et al. Primary care guidelines for the management of persons infected with HIV: 2013 update by the HIV medicine association of the infectious diseases society of America. *Clin Infect Dis* 2014;58(1):e1-34.

Cohen MS, Chen YQ, McCauley M et al. Prevention of HIV-1 with early antiretroviral therapy. *N Engl J Med* 2011;365(6):493-505.

Montaner JS, Hogg R, Wood E et al. The case for expanding access to highly active antiretroviral therapy to curb the growth of the HIV epidemic. *Lancet* 2006;368(9534):531-6.

Montaner JS, Lima VD, Harrigan PR et al. Expansion of HAART coverage is associated with sustained decreases in HIV/AIDS morbidity, mortality, and HIV transmission: the "HIV Treatment as Prevention" experience in a Canadian setting. *PloS One* 2014;9(2):e87872.

New York State Department of Health AIDS Institute, Office of the Medical Director. *Primary care approach to the HIV-infected patient*. April 2011. Available from: www.hivguidelines.org/clinical-guidelines/adults/primary-care-approach-to-the-hiv-infected-patient/.

Panel on Antiretroviral Guidelines for Adults and Adolescents. *Guidelines for the use of antiretroviral agents in HIV-1 infected adults and adolescents*. Department of Health and Human Services; 2014. Available from: www.aidsinfo.nih.gov/ContentFiles/AdultandAdolescentGL.pdf.

Samji H, Cescon A, Hogg RS et al. Closing the gap: increases in life expectancy among treated HIV-positive individuals in the United States and Canada. *PLoS One* 2013;8(12):e81355.

Thompson MA, Aberg JA, Hoy JF et al. Antiretroviral treatment of adult HIV infection: 2012 recommendations of the International Antiviral Society-USA panel. *JAMA* 2012;308(4):387-402.

Thompson MA, Mugavero MJ, Amico KR et al. Guidelines for improving entry into and retention in care and antiretroviral adherence for persons with HIV: evidence-based recommendations from an International Association of Physicians in AIDS Care Panel. *Ann Intern Med* 2012;156(11):817-33.

Strategies for Management of Antiretroviral Therapy (SMART) Study Group, El-Sadr WM, Lundgren J et al. CD4+ count-guided interruption of antiretroviral treatment. *N Engl J Med* 2006;355(22):2283-96.

References

1. Palella FJ, Delaney KM, Moorman AC et al. Declining morbidity and mortality among patients with advanced human immunodeficiency virus infection. HIV Outpatient Study Investigators. *N Engl J Med* 1998;338(13):853-60.
2. Antiretroviral Therapy Cohort Collaboration. Life expectancy of individuals on combination antiretroviral therapy in high-income countries: a collaborative analysis of 14 cohort studies. *Lancet* 2008;372(9635):293-9.
3. Samji H, Cescon A, Hogg RS et al. Closing the gap: increases in life expectancy among treated HIV-positive individuals in the United States and Canada. *PLoS One* 2013;8(12):e81355.
4. When To Start Consortium, Sterne JA, May M et al. Timing of initiation of antiretroviral therapy in AIDS-free HIV-1-infected patients: a collaborative analysis of 18 HIV cohort studies. *Lancet* 2009;373(9672):1352-63.
5. Kitahata MM, Gange SJ, Abraham AG et al. Effect of early versus deferred antiretroviral therapy for HIV on survival. *N Engl J Med* 2009;360(18):1815-26.
6. Deeks SG, Phillips AN. HIV infection, antiretroviral treatment, ageing, and non-AIDS related morbidity. *BMJ* 2009;338:a3172.
7. Strategies for Management of Antiretroviral Therapy (SMART) Study Group, El-Sadr WM, Lundgren J et al. CD4+ count-guided interruption of antiretroviral treatment. *N Engl J Med* 2006;355(22):2283-96.
8. Montaner JS, Hogg R, Wood E et al. The case for expanding access to highly active antiretroviral therapy to curb the growth of the HIV epidemic. *Lancet* 2006;368(9534):531-6.
9. Cohen MS, Chen YQ, McCauley M et al. Prevention of HIV-1 with early antiretroviral therapy. *N Engl J Med* 2011;365(6):493-505.
10. Mellors JW, Kingsley LA, Rinaldo CR et al. Quantitation of HIV-1 RNA in plasma predicts outcome after seroconversion. *Ann Intern Med* 1995;122(8):573-9.
11. Mallal S, Phillips E, Carosi G et al. HLA-B*5701 screening for hypersensitivity to abacavir. *N Engl J Med* 2008;358(6):568-79.
12. Thompson MA, Aberg JA, Hoy JF et al. Antiretroviral treatment of adult HIV infection: 2012 recommendations of the International Antiviral Society-USA panel. *JAMA* 2012;308(4):387-402.
13. Panel on Antiretroviral Guidelines for Adults and Adolescents. *Guidelines for the use of antiretroviral agents in HIV-1 infected adults and adolescents*. Department of Health and Human Services; 2014. Available from: www.aidsinfo.nih.gov/ContentFiles/AdultandAdolescentGL.pdf. Accessed June 5, 2014.
14. Connor EM, Sperling RS, Gelber R et al. Reduction of maternal-infant transmission of human immunodeficiency virus type 1 with zidovudine treatment. Pediatric AIDS Clinical Trials Group Protocol 076 Study Group. *N Engl J Med* 1994;331(18):1173-80.
15. Wood E, Kerr T, Marshall BD et al. Longitudinal community plasma HIV-1 RNA concentrations and incidence of HIV-1 among injecting drug users: prospective cohort study. *Br Med J* 2009;338:b1649.
16. Morse CG, Kovacs JA. Metabolic and skeletal complications of HIV infection: the price of success. *JAMA* 2006;296(7):844-54.
17. Grund B, Peng G, Gilbert CL et al. Continuous antiretroviral therapy decreases bone mineral density. *AIDS* 2009;23(12):1519-29.

18. Condra JH, Schleif WA, Blahy OM et al. In vivo emergence of HIV-1 variants resistant to multiple protease inhibitors. *Nature* 1995;374(6522):569-71.
19. Descamps D, Flandre P, Calvez V et al. Mechanisms of virologic failure in previously untreated HIV-infected patients from a trial of induction-maintenance therapy. Trilege (Agence Nationale de Recherches sur le SIDA 072) Study Team). *JAMA* 2000;283(2):205-11.
20. Thompson MA, Mugavero MJ, Amico KR et al. Guidelines for improving entry into and retention in care and antiretroviral adherence for persons with HIV: evidence-based recommendations from an International Association of Physicians in AIDS Care Panel. *Ann Intern Med* 2012;156(11):817-33.
21. Vanhove GF, Schapiro JM, Winters MA et al. Patient compliance and drug failure in protease inhibitor monotherapy. *JAMA* 1996;276(24):1955-6.
22. Anderson BL, Cu-Uvin S. Pregnancy and optimal care of HIV-infected patients. *Clin Infect Dis* 2009;48(4):449-55.
23. Panel on Treatment of HIV-Infected Pregnant Women and Prevention of Perinatal Transmission. *Recommendations for use of antiretroviral drugs in pregnant HIV-1-infected women for maternal health and interventions to reduce perinatal HIV transmission in the United States.* Available from: aidsinfo.nih.gov/contentfiles/PerinatalGL.pdf. Accessed June 5, 2014.
24. Money D, Tullock K, Boucoiran I et al. *British Columbia guidelines for the care of HIV positive pregnant women and interventions to reduce perinatal transmission.* July 23, 2013. Available from: www.cfenet.ubc.ca/sites/default/files/uploads/docs/guidelines/BC_HIV_in_pregnancy_guidelines.pdf. Accessed December 18, 2013.
25. Powis KM, Kitch D, Ogwu A et al. Increased preterm delivery among HIV-infected women randomized to protease versus nucleoside reverse transcriptase inhibitor-based HAART during pregnancy. *J Infect Dis* 2011;204(4):506-14.
26. Raboud JM, Montaner JS, Conway B et al. Variation in plasma RNA levels, CD4 cell counts, and p24 antigen levels in clinically stable men with human immunodeficiency virus infection. *J Infect Dis* 1996;174(1):191-4.
27. Staprans SI, Hamilton BL, Follansbee SE et al. Activation of virus replication after vaccination of HIV-1-infected individuals. *J Exp Med* 1995;182(6):1727-37.
28. Raboud JM, Haley L, Montaner JS et al. Quantification of the variation due to laboratory and physiologic sources in CD4 lymphocyte counts of clinically stable HIV-infected individuals. *J Acquir Immune Defic Syndr Hum Retrovirol* 1995;10(Suppl 2):S67-73.
29. McComsey GA, Kitch D, Daar ES et al. Bone mineral density and fractures in antiretroviral-nave persons randomized to receive abacavir-lamivudine or tenofovir disoproxil fumarate-emtricitabine along with efavirenz or atazanavir-ritonavir: AIDS Clinical Trials Group A5224s, a substudy of ACTG A5202. *J Infect Dis* 2011;203(12):1791-801.
30. Bedimo R, Maalouf NM, Zhang S et al. Osteoporotic fracture risk associated with cumulative exposure to tenofovir and other antiretroviral agents. *AIDS* 2012;26(7):825-31.
31. Lankisch TO, Moebius U, Wehmeier M et al. Gilbert's disease and atazanavir: from phenotype to UDP-glucuronosyltransferase haplotype. *Hepatology* 2006;44(5):1324-32.
32. Rodriguez-Novoa S, Martin-Carbonero L, Barreiro P et al. Genetic factors influencing atazanavir plasma concentrations and the risk of severe hyperbilirubinemia. *AIDS* 2007;21(1):41-6.
33. Chan-Tack KM, Truffa MM, Struble KA et al. Atazanavir-associated nephrolithiasis: cases from the US Food and Drug Administration's Adverse Event Reporting System. *AIDS* 2007;21(9):1215-8.
34. Rockwood N, Mandalia S, Bower M et al. Ritonavir-boosted atazanavir exposure is associated with an increased rate of renal stones compared with efavirenz, ritonavir-boosted lopinavir and ritonavir-boosted darunavir. *AIDS* 2011;25(13):1671-3.
35. Ryom L, Mocroft A, Kirk O et al. Association between antiretroviral exposure and renal impairment among HIV-positive persons with normal baseline renal function: the D:A:D study. *J Infect Dis* 2013;207(9):1359-69.
36. Soliman EZ, Lundgren JD, Roediger MP et al. Boosted protease inhibitors and the electrocardiographic measures of QT and PR durations. *AIDS* 2011;25(3):367-77.
37. Lang S, Mary-Krause M, Cotte L et al. Impact of individual antiretroviral drugs on the risk of myocardial infarction in human immunodeficiency virus-infected patients: a case-control study nested within the French Hospital Database on HIV ANRS cohort CO4. *Arch Intern Med* 2010;170(14):1228-38.
38. Worm SW, Sabin C, Weber R et al. Risk of myocardial infarction in patients with HIV infection exposed to specific individual antiretroviral drugs from the 3 major drug classes: the data collection on adverse events of anti-HIV drugs (D:A:D) study. *J Infect Dis* 2010;201(3):318-30.

Chapter 114
Infections in the Cancer Patient

Coleman Rotstein, MD, FRCPC, FACP, FIDSA

Infections are a significant cause of morbidity and mortality in cancer patients despite progress in their recognition, therapy and prevention. The ever expanding armamentarium of antineoplastic chemotherapeutic agents, radiation therapy and immunotherapy has improved survival in cancer patients, but simultaneously has rendered them more susceptible to infections because of prolonged immune dysfunction.

Goals of Therapy

- Decrease morbidity associated with infection
- Minimize risk of death from infection
- Enhance the supportive care and quality of life of cancer patients by using prophylactic measures to prevent infection while being cognizant of the possibility of the emergence of resistant organisms
- Utilize outpatient antibiotic management appropriately to facilitate care, to prevent or reduce length of hospital stay and to enhance the quality of life for cancer patients

Investigations

- Thorough history with attention to:
  - the nature of the malignancy and associated defects in host defenses, e.g., neutropenia, B-cell and/or T-cell dysfunction
  - the effects on host defenses of cytotoxic, myelosuppressive or immunosuppressive therapy to treat the patient's cancer; note day of onset of fever relative to the first day of the most recent cycle of chemotherapy
  - neutropenia (severity and expected duration)
  - iatrogenic procedures performed on the patient, e.g., splenectomy, placement of venous access devices or other surgical procedures
  - whether the nature of the malignancy suggests obstruction of natural body passages, e.g., bronchus, bowel, ureter, biliary tree
  - CNS dysfunction
  - occupational and travel history, and exposure to animals
- Complete physical examination with particular attention to venous access sites, wounds, skin, mouth, pharynx, sinuses, rectum and other possible sites of infection; note any localizing signs of possible infection, e.g., weakness of an extremity indicating a CNS infection
- Laboratory tests:
  - CBC and differential to assess the total neutrophil count
  - biochemical profile with attention to renal and liver function
  - at least 2 sets of blood cultures: ensure blood cultures are done from peripheral site as well as all lumens of venous access devices
  - culture of any other suspected site of infection, e.g., urine, skin, sputum

- radiographic studies appropriate for suspected sites of infection, e.g., chest x-ray or CT scan of the chest for pneumonia, CT scan of the abdomen for an intra-abdominal focus of infection, CT scan or MRI of the head for encephalitis or cerebral abscess
- stool for *Clostridium difficile* and other potential pathogens (e.g., *Salmonella* spp., *Shigella* spp., *Campylobacter* spp., viruses and protozoa) if diarrhea is present
- serological or quantitative tests (serology, antigen or nucleic acid amplification tests for cytomegalovirus, *Cryptococcus* spp., Epstein-Barr virus, hepatitis and *Toxoplasma* spp.) if indicated
- when appropriate, biopsy for pathology and culture of skin lesions suspected to be infectious

Therapeutic Choices

Nonpharmacologic Choices

Environmental precautions are important to prevent infection in cancer patients.

- Standard infection control measures, especially handwashing, are of particular importance in immunocompromised patients.
- Special air handling, including high-efficiency particulate filtration rooms are mandatory for profoundly neutropenic patients at high risk for filamentous fungal infections.
- Use specialized infection control procedures (contact precautions) for patients colonized with multi-drug resistant organisms, e.g., methicillin-resistant *Staphylococcus aureus* (MRSA), vancomycin-resistant enterococci (VRE), extended spectrum beta-lactamase (ESBL)-producing *Enterobacteriaceae* and carbapenem-resistant *Enterobacteriaceae*.
- Use droplet or air-borne precautions as required for respiratory viral illnesses.
- Neutropenic patients should avoid ingesting raw fruits and vegetables; avoid fresh flowers and plants in the patient's room.

Pharmacologic Choices

Antimicrobials (antibacterials, antifungals and antivirals) used to treat infections in cancer patients are presented in Table 1.

Antibacterial Therapy

- Although neoplasms can cause fevers in cancer patients, seek an infectious etiology in all cases of elevated temperature. *Fever* is defined as a single oral temperature ≥38.3°C or a temperature of ≥38°C for ≥1-hour period in the absence of obvious environmental causes.[1]
- Most infections are caused by microorganisms that have colonized the patient at or near the site of infection, e.g., the skin, oropharynx, genitourinary tract, GI tract or lungs.
- Bacteria are the principal pathogens causing infections in cancer patients, representing >60% of initially documented episodes of infection.
- The choice of antibacterial agents in febrile cancer patients is predicated on the neutrophil count, the patient's clinical status, the site of infection and local microorganism susceptibilities, with particular attention to prevalent multi-drug resistant organisms such as MRSA, VRE, ESBL-producing organisms and carbapenem-resistant organisms (Figure 1). *Neutropenia* is defined as a neutrophil count $\leq 0.5 \times 10^9$/L. A more profound degree of neutropenia ($<0.1 \times 10^9$/L) confers a much greater risk of developing more severe infection. In addition, the risk of infection is directly related to the duration of neutropenia. Lower risk of infection is present in patients with neutropenia of ≤7 days whereas higher risk patients are those with neutropenia >7 days' duration. Because of the high risk of life-threatening bacterial infection and the inability to reliably distinguish patients with bacterial infection from noninfected patients at presentation (particularly in neutropenic patients), initiate prompt empiric iv antibiotic therapy to cover the potential pathogens.[1]

- In selecting the initial antibiotic regimen and the site of care (the inpatient or outpatient setting), consider concurrent comorbid medical illnesses (e.g., heart failure, renal disease, liver disease, bleeding disorders), the control of the cancer and presence of serious medical complications.[2,3,4,5] Outpatient antibiotic therapy may be employed not only for nonneutropenic patients, but also for low-risk neutropenic patients who do not have the aforementioned medical conditions or uncontrolled cancer (Figure 2). Broad spectrum antibiotic therapy that ensures adequate coverage for both gram-positive and gram-negative organisms is necessary for febrile neutropenic patients.
- **Vancomycin** may be incorporated into the initial therapeutic regimen for patients with suspected venous access catheter-related infection, positive blood cultures for gram-positive bacteria in groups or chains, severe mucositis, known colonization with MRSA, hypotension or other evidence of cardiovascular impairment.[1] Alternatively, vancomycin may be added later to the initial broad spectrum regimen once susceptibility testing has been completed. Vancomycin should be discontinued if the infecting organism is subsequently shown to be susceptible to other antibiotics or if no vancomycin-susceptible organism is recovered.
- **Linezolid** or **daptomycin** may be required for MRSA or VRE infections.
- **Metronidazole** or **clindamycin** may be used as part of the initial antibiotic regimen for presumed anaerobic infection related to the GI tract or skin provided that antianaerobic activity is not already included in the initially selected regimen (e.g., beta-lactam/beta-lactamase inhibitor combination or a carbapenem).
- In neutropenic patients with a suspected bacterial infection, continue antibacterial therapy until they are no longer neutropenic (neutrophils $\geq 0.5 \times 10^9$/L) and are afebrile for ≥48 hours. For patients with microbiologically or clinically documented infection, continue broad spectrum antibacterial therapy for a minimum of 10–14 days and until patients are afebrile and no longer neutropenic (neutrophils $\geq 0.5 \times 10^9$/L).
- In nonneutropenic cancer patients with a suspected bacterial infection, continue antibiotic therapy for approximately 7 days and until the patient is afebrile for ≥48 hours. Alternatively, switch from iv antibiotic therapy to oral therapy to complete an appropriate course of therapy directed towards the site that is infected.
- In patients who are persistently febrile and neutropenic after 4–7 days of appropriate antibacterial therapy reassess and consider antifungal therapy as outlined below.

Antifungal Therapy

- Nonneutropenic patients who develop oral and or esophageal candidiasis may be treated with a topical agent such as **nystatin** or systemic oral agents such as **fluconazole, itraconazole, posaconazole** or **voriconazole**. Patients with extensive lesions may require parenteral therapy with **fluconazole**, an **amphotericin B** formulation, **caspofungin**, **micafungin** or **voriconazole**.
- Parenteral antifungal therapy should be initiated for documented invasive or disseminated fungal infection in nonneutropenic and neutropenic cancer patients.
- Treatment of a proven, probable or possible invasive fungal infection in a neutropenic patient requires parenteral antifungal therapy with **amphotericin B**, **caspofungin** or **voriconazole**. **Caspofungin** or **voriconazole** (for invasive aspergillosis) may be preferred in patients with renal dysfunction.[1]
- The **lipid-based preparations of amphotericin B** have equivalent efficacy but produce less nephrotoxicity and infusion reactions than conventional amphotericin B. They may be used as salvage therapy for patients with fungal infections that fail to respond to amphotericin B or for patients with amphotericin B toxicity or intolerance.[6]
- **Caspofungin**, **micafungin** or **anidulafungin** may effectively treat candidemia in neutropenic or nonneutropenic patients.[7,8]

- **Itraconazole**, which is available only in an oral formulation, has enhanced activity against *Aspergillus* spp. compared to fluconazole and is an alternative for oral step-down therapy after parenteral treatment for invasive aspergillosis.
- **Voriconazole**, available both in iv and oral formulations, conferred superior efficacy and survival compared to **amphotericin B** for primary therapy of invasive aspergillosis,[9] and has better activity against infections caused by *Scedosporium* spp. and *Fusarium* spp.
- **Voriconazole** (alone or in combination with **anidulafungin** or **caspofungin**) or a lipid-based formulation of **amphotericin B** may be used in the treatment of documented invasive aspergillosis.[10,11,12]
- **Posaconazole** may be used for refractory invasive fungal infections or in patients intolerant to other medications.[13]

Figure 1: Approach to Fever in Cancer Patients

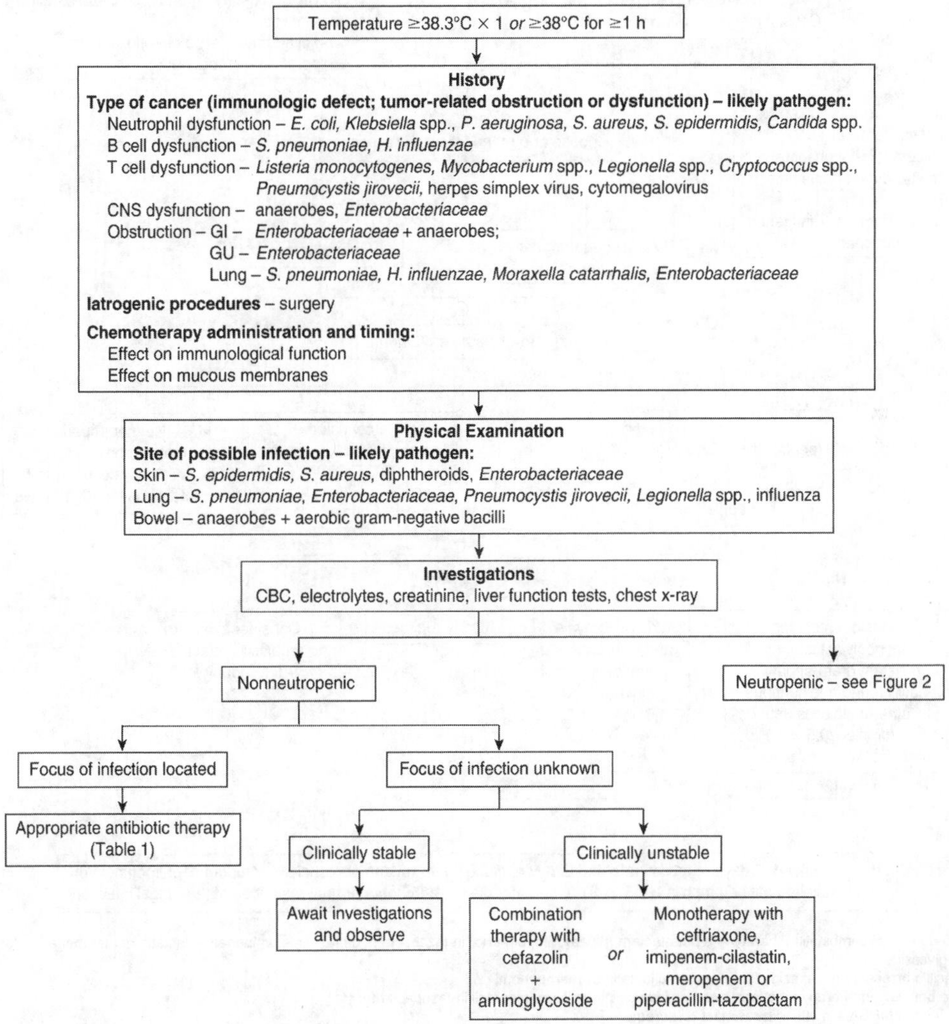

Abbreviations: CBC = complete blood count; CNS = central nervous system; GI = gastrointestinal; GU = genitourinary

Figure 2: **Management of Infection in Febrile Neutropenic Cancer Patients**

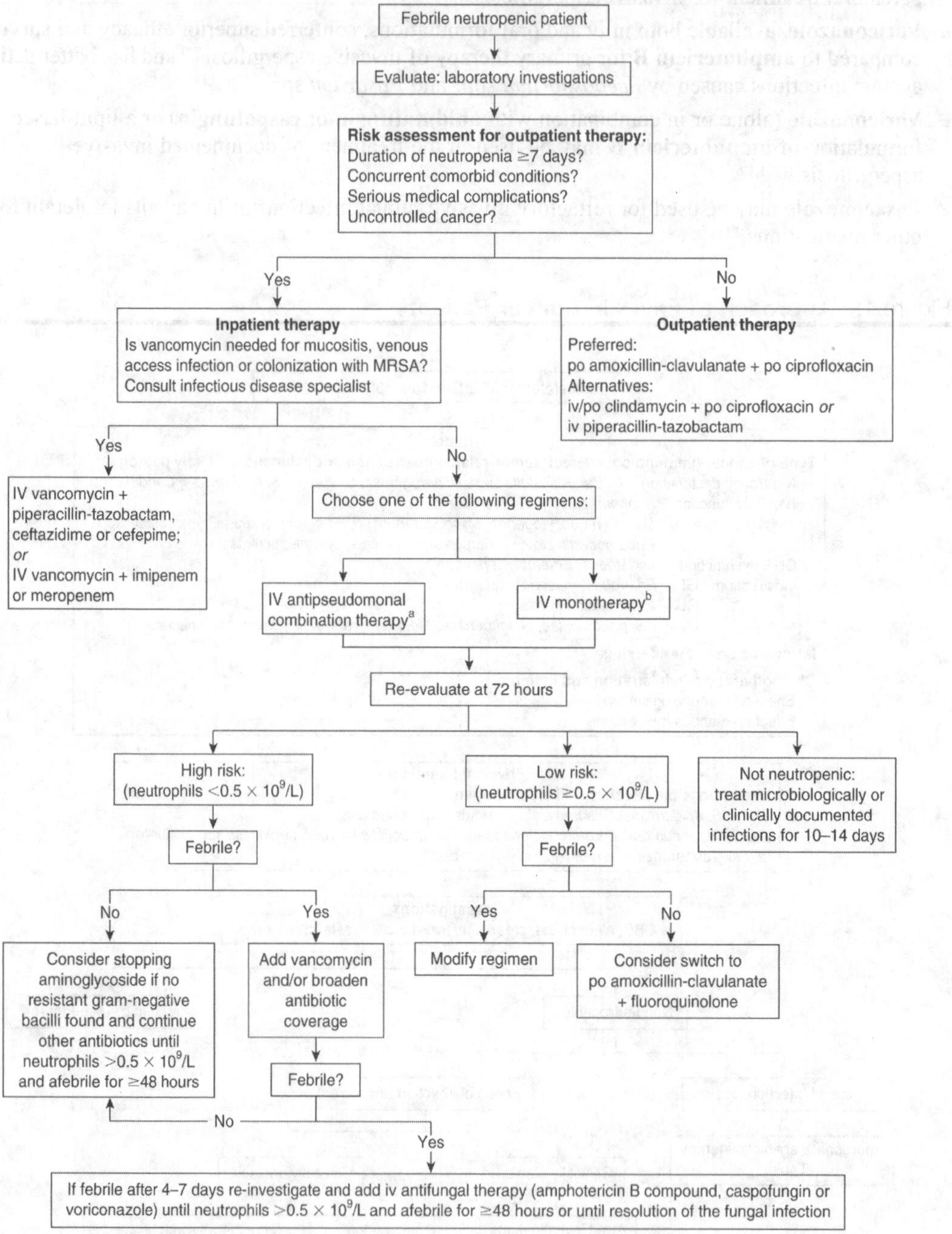

[a] Antipseudomonal combination therapy = a beta-lactam (piperacillin, piperacillin-tazobactam, ceftazidime, imipenem-cilastatin *or* meropenem) plus an aminoglycoside.
[b] Piperacillin-tazobactam, ceftazidime, imipenem-cilastatin *or* meropenem.
[c] Double beta-lactam therapy = ceftazidime plus *either* piperacillin *or* piperacillin-tazobactam.
Abbreviations: MRSA = methicillin-resistant *S. aureus*

Antiviral Therapy

- There is no indication for the empiric use of antiviral drugs in the treatment of cancer patients without evidence of viral disease.[1]
- **Neuraminidase inhibitors**, such as oseltamivir, are the mainstay of therapy for susceptible influenza virus causing respiratory tract infections in cancer patients.
- Skin or mucous membrane lesions due to herpes simplex virus or varicella-zoster virus may be treated with oral or iv **acyclovir**. Oral **famciclovir** or **valacyclovir** are better absorbed from the GI tract than acyclovir, and are alternatives.[14]
- IV **foscarnet** is available through Health Canada's Special Access Programme for acyclovir-resistant herpesvirus infections.
- Cytomegalovirus infection in bone marrow transplant recipients may be treated with **ganciclovir** iv, or with **valganciclovir** when oral therapy is desirable.

Supportive Care Measures

- **Granulocyte (G-CSF)** and **granulocyte-macrophage (GM-CSF) colony-stimulating factors** may decrease the incidence and duration of neutropenia after chemotherapy. They are not routinely recommended as adjunctive treatment of febrile neutropenia. However, they may be considered for patients who remain profoundly neutropenic and have failed to respond to appropriate antimicrobial therapy for documented infection such as pneumonia, severe cellulitis or sinusitis.[1,15] Once neutrophil counts reach $\geq 0.5 \times 10^9$/L, colony-stimulating factor support should be discontinued.

Prevention of Infection in Cancer Patients

- For cancer patients with pronounced T cell dysfunction, prophylaxis with oral **sulfamethoxazole/trimethoprim** is recommended to prevent *Pneumocystis jirovecii* pneumonia. Alternative prophylactic agents are inhaled **pentamidine** and **dapsone**.
- Strategies designed to prevent bacterial infection in profoundly neutropenic cancer patients, such as those with acute leukemia, focus on eliminating indigenous microflora and preventing acquisition of new potential pathogens. Potential antimicrobial regimens are **fluoroquinolones**, **sulfamethoxazole/trimethoprim** or orally nonabsorbable antibiotics (**gentamicin**, **vancomycin** and **nystatin**). **Ciprofloxacin** or **levofloxacin** significantly decrease febrile morbidity, bacterial infections and mortality for patients with acute leukemia and those undergoing bone marrow transplantation.[16] Prophylaxis during the expected period of neutropenia in the first month of chemotherapy in patients with solid tumors or lymphoma (levofloxacin 500 mg for 7 days) also reduces the rate of febrile episodes.[17] There may be a predilection for gram-positive infection when ciprofloxacin is used prophylactically. This may be overcome by adding another antibiotic with good activity against gram-positive organisms (e.g., a penicillin or a macrolide);[18] however, this practice is not currently recommended in international guidelines.[1]
- Antifungal prophylaxis with oral **fluconazole** prevents invasive fungal infection in allogeneic bone marrow transplant recipients and in patients with acute leukemia who are undergoing remission-induction chemotherapy.[19,20] **Itraconazole** prophylaxis may be preferred for individuals at greater risk of developing invasive aspergillosis.

  Posaconazole is as effective as fluconazole in preventing all invasive fungal infections, but is superior for prevention of invasive aspergillosis in hematopoietic stem-cell transplant recipients with graft-versus-host disease.[21] In patients with acute leukemia who are undergoing chemotherapy, posaconazole is more effective than both fluconazole and itraconazole for prevention of invasive fungal infections.[22,23]

  Micafungin is effective as prophylaxis in hematopoietic stem-cell transplant recipients.[24]
- If **fluconazole** has been used prophylactically, it should not be used empirically or for documented fungal infections in neutropenic cancer patients. For these situations, a parenteral

amphotericin B formulation[1] or **caspofungin**[10] are the drugs of choice. However, **voriconazole** is the drug of choice for invasive aspergillosis.

Vaccination of Cancer Patients

- Cancer patients are considered to be immunocompromised and as a result should not receive live vaccines during periods of immunosuppression.[25,26]
- Live vaccines should be administered ≥4 weeks prior to immunosuppression.
- The magnitude and duration of immune response to vaccinations may be diminished in immunosuppressed cancer patients.

Therapeutic Tips

- Avoid **aminoglycosides** in patients with impaired renal function, particularly those receiving treatment with other nephrotoxic drugs such as cisplatin, cyclosporine or amphotericin B.
- In deciding on cost-effective empiric therapy, drug acquisition costs by themselves are of limited value. Also consider the relative effectiveness, side effect profile and overall resource consumption of the available treatments.
- Monotherapy with an iv broad-spectrum antipseudomonal beta-lactam (**ceftazidime, imipenem/cilastatin, meropenem** or **piperacillin/tazobactam**) is suitable for the treatment of febrile neutropenic episodes. A 2007 meta-analysis found **cefepime** monotherapy may be associated with higher all-cause mortality compared to other beta-lactams;[27] however a subsequent meta-analysis found no association with increased mortality.[28]
- Combination therapy for febrile neutropenia with a **beta-lactam** and an **aminoglycoside** is associated with more adverse events (e.g., a higher incidence of nephrotoxicity, ototoxicity) than monotherapy with a beta-lactam.
- Identification of low-risk patients appropriate for outpatient antibiotic management may enhance the patient's quality of life and reduce costs.

Suggested Readings

Bow EJ, Evans G, Fuller J et al. Canadian clinical practice guidelines for invasive candidiasis in adults. *Can J Infect Dis Med Microbiol* 2010;21(4):e122-50.

Freifeld AG, Bow EJ, Sepkowitz KA et al. Clinical practice guideline for the use of antimicrobial agents in neutropenic patients with cancer: 2010 update by the Infectious Diseases Society of America. *Clin Infect Dis* 2011;52(4):427-31.

Paul M, Dickstein Y, Schlesinger A et al. Beta-lactam versus beta-lactam-aminoglycoside combination therapy in cancer patients with neutropenia. *Cochrane Database Syst Rev* 2013;6:CD003038.

Rotstein C, Laverdiere M, Marciniak A et al. An economic evaluation of voriconazole versus amphotericin B for the treatment of invasive aspergillosis in Canada. *Can J Infect Dis Med Microbiol* 2004;15(5):277-84.

Yu DT, Seger DL, Peterson JF et al. Fluconazole for empiric antifungal therapy in cancer patients with fever and neutropenia. *BMC Infect Dis* 2006;6:173.

Table 1: Drugs Used to Treat Infections in Cancer Patients

Class[a]	Drug	Dose	Adverse Effects	Drug Interactions	Cost[b]
Aminoglycosides	*amikacin* generics	15–20 mg/kg once daily iv (extended- interval regimen)[c]	Ototoxicity (auditory and/or vestibular), nephrotoxicity, neuromuscular paralysis (rare).	Synergistic or additive toxicity if used with vancomycin and/or platinum-derived antineoplastics, amphotericin B and/or other nephrotoxic/ototoxic drugs.	$$
	gentamicin generics	5–7 mg/kg once daily iv (extended-interval regimen)[c]	See amikacin.	See amikacin.	$
	tobramycin generics	5–7 mg/kg once daily iv (extended-interval regimen)[c]	See amikacin.	See amikacin.	$
Carbapenems	*imipenem/cilastatin* Primaxin, generics	500 mg Q6H iv	Diarrhea, hypersensitivity reactions, neutropenia, hemolytic anemia, thrombocytopenia. Associated with seizures especially with high doses (1 g Q6H) and in patients with renal dysfunction.	Carbapenems may decrease valproic acid levels. Seizures have been reported with concurrent use of imipenem and ganciclovir.	$$$
	meropenem Merrem, Meropenem for Injection	1 g Q8H iv	Diarrhea, nausea, hypersensitivity reactions, neutropenia, hemolytic anemia, thrombocytopenia.	Carbapenems may decrease valproic acid levels.	$$$
Cephalosporins	*cefepime* Maxipime, generics	2 g Q8H iv	Rash, diarrhea, GI upset, headache, hypersensitivity reactions, hematologic reactions. Risk of seizures particularly in those with renal dysfunction.	May enhance anticoagulant effect of warfarin.	$$
	ceftazidime Fortaz, generics	2 g Q8H iv	Rash, diarrhea, GI upset, headache, hypersensitivity reactions, hematologic reactions.	See cefepime.	$$$
	ceftriaxone generics	1–2 g once daily iv	See ceftazidime. Pseudocholelithiasis.	See cefepime. Do not reconstitute or mix with calcium-containing solutions. Do not administer simultaneously with calcium-containing iv solutions via a Y-site. Administration may be done sequentially provided the infusion lines are thoroughly flushed between infusions.	$

(cont'd)

Table 1: **Drugs Used to Treat Infections in Cancer Patients** *(cont'd)*

Class[a]	Drug	Dose	Adverse Effects	Drug Interactions	Cost[b]
Cyclic Lipopeptides	*daptomycin* Cubicin	4–6 mg/kg once daily iv	Headache, rash, elevated creatine kinase, constipation.	Possible increased risk of myopathy when used concurrently with HMG-CoA reductase inhibitors.	$$$$
Fluoroquinolones	*ciprofloxacin* Cipro, generics	500 or 750 mg BID po 400 mg Q12H iv	GI upset, rash, CNS toxicity.	Warfarin: increases INR. Binds with antacids, iron, sucralfate.	$
	levofloxacin Levaquin, generics	500 mg once daily po/iv	Nausea, diarrhea, headache, insomnia, dizziness. Cases of severe liver injury including liver failure have been reported. QT_c prolongation.	Binds with antacids, metal cations, sucralfate. Avoid in patients on Class Ia or III antiarrhythmics or with prolonged QT_c interval.	$
	moxifloxacin Avelox	400 mg once daily po/iv	See levofloxacin.	Binds with antacids, metal cations, sucralfate. Avoid in patients on Class Ia or III antiarrhythmics or with prolonged QT_c interval.	$
	ofloxacin generics	400 mg BID po	Nausea, vomiting, rash, headache insomnia, dizziness.	Warfarin: increases INR. Binds with antacids, metal cations, sucralfate.	$
Glycopeptides	*vancomycin* generics	15 mg/kg Q12H iv	Shock after rapid iv infusion (<1 h), fever, chills, phlebitis, "red-neck" syndrome, tingling and flushing of head, neck, chest, rash, transient leukopenia or eosinophilia, ototoxicity.	Nephrotoxicity may be enhanced if given with aminoglycosides or other nephrotoxins.	$$$
Lincosamides	*clindamycin* Dalacin C Phosphate Sterile Solution, generics	600 mg Q8H iv	Diarrhea, minor reversible increase in liver aminotransferases, reversible neutropenia, thrombocytopenia, pseudomembranous colitis.	May enhance action of neuromuscular blocking agents.	$
Macrolides	*azithromycin* Zithromax, generics	500 mg once daily iv	GI upset, QT_c interval prolongation.	May increase bioavailability of digoxin, warfarin. Less likely than other macrolides to cause interactions.	$
	erythromycin Erythrocin, generics	1 g Q6H iv	Abdominal pain, nausea, vomiting, diarrhea, QT_c interval prolongation, thrombophlebitis, transient hearing loss with high doses.	May increase bioavailability of digoxin, warfarin. Inhibitor of CYP3A4 enzymes therefore many potential interactions (e.g., carbamazepine, cyclosporine, lovastatin, methylprednisolone, simvastatin, theophylline).	$$$

Class[a]	Drug	Dose	Adverse Effects	Drug Interactions	Cost[b]
Nitroimidazoles	*metronidazole* generics	500 mg Q8–12H iv	GI upset, reversible neutropenia, seizures, peripheral neuropathy (rare), rash, metallic taste.	Disulfiram-like reaction with alcohol. Potentiation of warfarin effects and other oral coumarin-type anticoagulants.	$
Oxazolidinones	*linezolid* Zyvoxam	600 mg Q12H po/iv	Thrombocytopenia, anemia, leukopenia, peripheral neuropathy.	May potentiate the pressor effect of adrenergic agents. Possible serotonin syndrome when used with SSRIs or MAOIs.	$$$$
Penicillins	*amoxicillin/clavulanate* Clavulin, generics	One 500/125 mg tablet TID po *or* One 875/125 mg tablet BID po	Diarrhea, rash, hypersensitivity reactions, interstitial nephritis, neutropenia, hemolytic anemia; thrombocytopenia.	May increase serum levels of methotrexate. May enhance anticoagulant effect of warfarin.	$
	piperacillin generics	4 g Q6H iv	See amoxicillin/clavulanate.	See amoxicillin/clavulanate.	$$
	piperacillin/tazobactam Tazocin, Piperacillin/Tazobactam for Injection, other generics	3.375–4.5 g Q6–8H iv	See amoxicillin/clavulanate.	See amoxicillin/clavulanate.	$$
Sulfonamide Combinations	*sulfamethoxazole/ trimethoprim* Septra Injection, generics	trimethoprim 20 mg/kg/day and sulfamethoxazole 100 mg/kg/day divided QID po/iv	Nausea, vomiting, diarrhea; hypersensitivity reactions, leukopenia, thrombocytopenia, hepatitis (rare).	May increase effect of phenytoin, warfarin. Enhances toxicity of methotrexate.	po: $ iv: $$$
Antifungals, echinocandins	*anidulafungin* Eraxis	200 mg loading dose iv, then 100 mg daily iv	Diarrhea, hypokalemia, elevated liver function tests, rash.	No clinically significant interactions.	$$$$
	caspofungin Cancidas	70 mg loading dose iv, then 50 mg daily iv	Fever, nausea, vomiting, phlebitis at the injection site, diarrhea.	Increased liver function tests with cyclosporine. Carbamazepine, dexamethasone, efavirenz, nelfinavir, phenytoin, rifampin decrease caspofungin levels. Caspofungin decreases levels of tacrolimus.	$$$$
	micafungin Mycamine	50 mg daily iv as prophylaxis 150 mg daily iv for treatment of esophageal candidiasis	Headache, rash, nausea, vomiting, phlebitis at the injection site.	Micafungin increases serum levels of nifedipine and sirolimus.	$$$$
Antifungals, polyenes	*amphotericin B* Fungizone	0.3–1.5 mg/kg Q24H iv	Rigors, renal dysfunction (azotemia), headache, hypokalemia, phlebitis, thrombocytopenia, anemia, leukopenia (rare), hypotension.	Increased risk of azotemia when used with other nephrotoxic drugs.	$$

(cont'd)

Table 1: **Drugs Used to Treat Infections in Cancer Patients** *(cont'd)*

Class[a]	Drug	Dose	Adverse Effects	Drug Interactions	Cost[b]
	amphotericin B lipid preparations Abelcet, AmBisome	3–5 mg/kg Q24H iv	Less nephrotoxicity than with amphotericin B.		$$$$$
	nystatin, generics	3.6 million units Q4H po	Nausea, vomiting, diarrhea.		$
Antifungals, triazoles	*fluconazole* Diflucan, generics	100–400 mg Q24H po 100–400 mg Q24H iv	Nausea, headache, skin rash, abdominal pain, vomiting, diarrhea.	May cause hepatotoxicity if used with other potentially hepatotoxic drugs. Coumarin-like drugs, cyclosporine, phenytoin, sulfonylureas may require dosage adjustment (monitor).	$
	itraconazole Sporanox Sporanox Oral Solution	100–200 mg daily–BID po	Nausea, rash, headache, reversible increase in hepatic enzymes.	Coumarin-like drugs, cyclosporine, digoxin, phenytoin, sulfonylureas may require dosage adjustment (monitor). Didanosine, H_2-antagonists, phenytoin, rifampin may decrease itraconazole levels; itraconazole increases levels of statins.	$
	posaconazole Posanol	Prophylaxis: 200 mg TID po Refractory invasive fungal infections: 400 mg BID po	Nausea, vomiting, fever, diarrhea, dry mouth, abdominal pain, headache.	Cyclosporine, midazolam, sirolimus, statins, tacrolimus and vinca alkaloids require dose adjustments (monitor). Cimetidine, phenytoin, rifabutin may decrease posaconazole levels.	$$$$
	voriconazole Vfend, generics	200 mg BID po; 4–6 mg/kg Q12H iv	Visual disturbances, nausea, vomiting, rash, increased hepatic enzymes.	Coumarin-like drugs, cyclosporine, sulfonylureas may require dosage adjustment (monitor); barbiturates, carbamazepine, phenytoin and rifampin may decrease voriconazole levels.	po:$$ iv: $$$$$
Antivirals, guanine nucleoside analogues	*acyclovir* generics	5–10 mg/kg Q8H iv	Phlebitis, rash, hypotension, headache, nausea, tremors, confusion, seizures (1%), renal dysfunction.	Probenecid decreases renal clearance; may increase theophylline levels.	$$$$$
	famciclovir Famvir, generics	500 mg TID po	Headache, nausea, pruritus.	Probenecid decreases renal clearance.	$
	ganciclovir Cytovene	Induction: 5 mg/kg Q12H iv Maintenance: 6 mg/kg Q24H iv	Leukopenia, nausea, headache, behavioural changes.	Avoid use with zidovudine (increased hematologic toxicity).	$$
	valacyclovir Valtrex, generics	1 g TID po	Headache, nausea.	Probenecid decreases renal clearance.	$

Class[a]	Drug	Dose	Adverse Effects	Drug Interactions	Cost[b]
	valganciclovir ❥ Valcyte, generics	900 mg daily po	See ganciclovir.	Prodrug of ganciclovir. See ganciclovir.	$$
Antivirals, neuraminidase inhibitors	*oseltamivir* ❥ Tamiflu	75 mg Q12H po	Nausea, vomiting, diarrhea, abdominal pain.		$

[a] In this table, antibacterial agents are presented first followed by antifungals and antivirals, each in alphabetical order.
[b] Cost of 1-day supply based on 50 kg body weight; includes drug cost only.
[c] The extended interval regimen (high-dose, once-daily administration) is thought to be associated with less toxicity. However, for patients with uncertain or impaired renal function some clinicians prefer to use the conventional dosing method (daily dose divided Q8H) because of more experience with this regimen in this population. Whichever regimen is used, serum levels and renal function should be monitored and the dose and/or interval should be adjusted accordingly.

❥ Dosage adjustment may be required in renal impairment; see Appendix I.
Legend: $ < $25 $$ $25–75 $$$ $75–150 $$$$ $150–225 $$$$$ $225–300

References

1. Freifeld AG, Bow EJ, Sepkowitz KA et al. Clinical practice guideline for the use of antimicrobial agents in neutropenic patients with cancer: 2010 update by the Infectious Diseases Society of America. *Clin Infect Dis* 2011;52(4):427-31.
2. Talcott JA, Siegel RD, Finberg R et al. Risk assessment in cancer patients with fever and neutropenia: a prospective, two-center validation of a prediction rule. *J Clin Oncol* 1992;10(2):316-22.
3. Talcott JA, Whalen A, Clark J et al. Home antibiotic therapy for low-risk cancer patients with fever and neutropenia: a pilot study of 30 patients based on a validated prediction rule. *J Clin Oncol* 1994;12(1):107-14.
4. Klastersky J, Paesmans M, Rubenstein EB et al. The Multinational Association for Supportive Care in Cancer risk index: a multinational scoring system for identifying low-risk febrile neutropenic cancer patients. *J Clin Oncol* 2000;18(16):3038-51.
5. Paul M, Yahav D, Fraser A et al. Empirical antibiotic monotherapy for febrile neutropenia: systematic review and meta-analysis of randomized controlled trials. *J Antimicrob Chemother* 2006;57(2):176-89.
6. Walsh TJ, Finberg RW, Arndt C et al. Liposomal amphotericin B for empirical therapy in patients with persistent fever and neutropenia. National Institute of Allergy and Infectious Diseases Mycoses Study Group. *N Engl J Med* 1999;340(10):764-71.
7. Pappas PG, Kauffman CA, Andes D et al. Clinical practice guidelines for the management of candidiasis: 2009 update by the Infectious Diseases Society of America. *Clin Infect Dis* 2009;48(5):503-35.
8. Bow EJ, Evans G, Fuller J et al. Canadian clinical practice guidelines for invasive candidiasis in adults. *Can J Infect Dis Med Microbiol* 2010;21(4):e122-50.
9. Herbrecht R, Denning DW, Patterson TF et al. Voriconazole versus amphotericin B for primary therapy of invasive aspergillosis. *N Engl J Med* 2002;347(6):408-15.
10. Walsh TJ, Teppler H, Donowitz GR et al. Caspofungin versus liposomal amphotericin B for empirical antifungal therapy in patients with persistent fever and neutropenia. *N Engl J Med* 2004;351(14):1391-402.
11. Marr KA, Boeckh M, Carter RA et al. Combination antifungal therapy for invasive aspergillosis. *Clin Infect Dis* 2004;39(6):797-802.
12. Marr KA, Schlamm H, Rottinghaus ST et al. A randomized, double-blind study of combination antifungal therapy with voriconazole and anidulafungin versus voriconazole monotherapy for invasive aspergillosis [poster]. *Proceedings of the 22nd European Congress of Clinical Microbiology and Infection Diseases*; 2012 Mar 31-Apr 3; London, UK. Abstract LB2812.
13. Walsh TJ, Raad I, Ratterson JF et al. Treatment of invasive aspergillosis with posaconazole in patients who are refractory or intolerant of conventional therapy: an externally controlled trial. *Clin Infect Dis* 2007;44(1):2-12.
14. Drugs for non-HIV viral infections. *Med Lett Drugs Ther* 2002;44(1123):9-16.
15. Smith TJ, Khatcheressian J, Lyman GH et al. 2006 update of recommendations for the use of white blood cell growth factors: an evidence-based clinical practice guideline. *J Clin Oncol* 2006;24(19):3187-205.
16. Leibovici L, Paul M, Cullen M et al. Antibiotic prophylaxis in neutropenic patients: new evidence, practical decisions. *Cancer* 2006;107(8):1743-51.
17. Cullen M, Steven N, Billingham L et al. Antibacterial prophylaxis for solid tumors and lymphomas. *N Engl J Med* 2005;353(14):988-98.
18. Rotstein C, Mandell LA, Goldberg N. Fluoroquinolone prophylaxis for profoundly neutropenic cancer patients: a meta-analysis. *Curr Oncol* 1997;4(Suppl 2):S2-S7.
19. Rotstein C, Bow EJ, Laverdiere M et al. Randomized placebo-controlled trial of fluconazole prophylaxis for neutropenic cancer patients: benefit based on purpose and intensity of cytotoxic therapy. *Clin Infect Dis* 1999;28(2):331-40.
20. Bow EJ, Laverdiere M, Lussier N et al. Antifungal prophylaxis for severely neutropenic chemotherapy recipients: a meta analysis of randomized-controlled clinical trials. *Cancer* 2002;94(12):3230-46.
21. Ullmann AJ, Lipton JH, Vesole DH et al. Posaconazole versus fluconazole or itraconazole prophylaxis in severe graft-versus-host disease. *N Engl J Med* 2007;356(4):335-47.
22. Cornely OA, Maertens J, Winston DJ et al. Posaconazole vs. fluconazole or itraconazole prophylaxis in patients with neutropenia. *N Engl J Med* 2007;356(4):348-59.
23. Pechlivanoglou P, Le HH, Daenen S et al. Mixed treatment comparison of prophylaxis against invasive fungal infections in neutropenic patients receiving therapy for haematological malignancies: a systematic review. *J Antimicrob Chemother* 2014;69(1):1-11.
24. van Burik JA, Ratanatharathorn V, Stepan DE et al. Micafungin versus fluconazole for prophylaxis against fungal infections during neutropenia in patients undergoing hematopoietic stem cell transplantation. *Clin Infect Dis* 2004;39(10):1407-16.
25. National Advisory Committee on Immunization (NACI). Public Health Agency of Canada. Part 3. Vaccination of specific populations. In: *Canadian immunization guide.* Evergreen ed. Available from: www.phac-aspc.gc.ca/publicat/cig-gci/p03-eng.php. Accessed January 2, 2014.
26. Rubin LG, Levin MJ, Ljungman P et al. 2013 IDSA clinical practice guideline for vaccination of the immunocompromised host. *Clin Infect Dis* 2014;58(3):e44-e100.
27. Paul M, Yahav D, Bivas A et al. Anti-pseudomonal beta-lactams for the initial, empirical treatment of febrile neutropenia: comparison of beta-lactams. *Cochrane Database Syst Rev* 2010;(11):CD005197.
28. Kim PW, Wu YT, Cooper C et al. Meta-analysis of a possible signal of increased mortality associated with cefepime use. *Clin Infect Dis* 2010;51(4):381-9.

Chapter 115
Infective Endocarditis—Management and Prevention

Alfred Gin, BScPharm, PharmD, FCSHP

Infective endocarditis (IE) is a life-threatening infection of the cardiac endothelium associated with significant morbidity and mortality. IE occurs as a result of a combination of injury or trauma to the cardiac endothelial surface (e.g., turbulent blood flow, intravenous catheter or foreign particulate matter), fibrin deposition and bacterial adherence. IE may involve the heart valves and surrounding tissues on either the left or right side of the heart although bilateral involvement has been described. Metastatic infection to extracardiac sites may occur. Complications include heart failure, periannular abscess, mycotic aneurysm and glomerulonephritis. Emboli to extracardiac sites such as the brain, lung or kidney may also occur.

Goals of Therapy

- Reduce morbidity and mortality associated with IE
- Eradicate infection
- Stabilize or normalize patient hemodynamics via pharmacologic, surgical and supportive interventions as necessary
- Avoid or minimize drug toxicity
- Prevent IE in patients with cardiovascular conditions at risk of severe outcome

Investigations

The modified Duke criteria are widely accepted as the gold standard for determining the likelihood of IE.[1,2] It classifies IE cases as definite, probable or rejected based on pathologic, clinical, laboratory and radiologic findings (see Table 1 and Table 2).[1,2] Due to the heterogeneous nature of IE, use clinical judgment in conjunction with the modified Duke criteria.[2]

- Systematic history and physical examination:
  - *history*: conduct a thorough history to document signs and symptoms, time course of illness and potential risk factors (e.g., recent dental or surgical procedures, dental health, cardiac disease or malformation, history of cardiac surgery or valve replacement, prior history of IE, intravenous drug use, placement or manipulation of any intravascular device)
  - *medication history*: conduct a thorough medication review. Assess patients receiving oral anticoagulation to determine anticoagulation need (e.g., temporarily stopping anticoagulants) if IE is suspected or documented. Note whether patient is taking any antibiotics that may interfere with culture results. Document drug allergies including antibiotic-related
  - *symptoms*: fever, chills, weakness, dyspnea, pleuritic chest pain, anorexia, weight loss, fatigue, malaise, arthralgia, night sweats, skin lesions, nausea/vomiting, headache, abdominal pain, back pain
  - *physical findings*: general appearance (e.g., respiratory distress, acute or chronic illness). Signs of IE stigmata include splinter hemorrhages, Janeway's lesions, Osler's nodes, buccal or mucosal surface petechiae, clubbing, Roth's spots, loss of visual acuity, conjunctival petechiae, cardiac murmurs, heart failure, pulmonary edema, pleuritic chest rub, neurologic deficits, splenomegaly

- Laboratory investigations:
  - CBC and differential, electrolytes, glucose, urea, creatinine, liver function tests, erythrocyte sedimentation rate, C-reactive protein
  - blood cultures prior to initiation of antibiotic therapy to identify the pathogen, antibiotic sensitivities and to determine antibiotic management. Take at least 3 blood cultures from different venipuncture sites over a 24-hour period.[3] Alternatively, at least 3 blood cultures taken 1 hour apart has also been recommended.[4] Ensure sufficient blood volume to improve detection. Repeat blood cultures during antibiotic therapy to confirm clearance of bacteremia
  - urinalysis to detect abnormalities such as hematuria, proteinuria or pyuria.
  - culture-negative blood cultures may require serologic and/or molecular diagnostics to identify difficult to grow pathogens such as *Coxiella burnetii*. Consultation with an infectious diseases specialist is encouraged
- Diagnostic:
  - baseline ECG and chest radiograph
  - echocardiography in all patients with suspected or documented IE. Transthoracic echocardiography (TTE) is commonly available and performed initially especially in patients with low suspicion or risk of IE.[1] Transesophageal echocardiography (TEE) is more sensitive than TTE for detecting small extension into tissue surrounding the valve or for assessing prosthetic heart valves.[1] TEE may be used in high risk patients (e.g., *S. aureus* bacteremia) or those with moderate to high suspicion of IE. Repeat or follow-up echocardiography may be used to assess response to antimicrobial therapy, disease progression or need for surgery
- Consider consultations with an infectious diseases specialist and/or cardiothoracic surgeon

Treatment of Infective Endocarditis

Therapeutic Choices

Nonpharmacologic Choices

Surgical Intervention

Surgery is indicated for patients with life-threatening heart failure secondary to valvular damage (regurgitation or stenosis) due to IE.[1,5] Other indications for surgical intervention include persistent emboli, embolic complication, large vegetation (>10 mm), failure of adequate antimicrobial treatment to control infection, severe valvular failure (abscess, dehiscence, perforation or rupture) or evidence of extension into surrounding cardiac tissues or relapsing infection.[1,5] The timing for the surgery should be done in consultation with the cardiothoracic surgeon.

Pharmacologic Choices (Table 9)

Pathogens and Considerations for Treatment

The gram-positive bacteria staphylococci, streptococci and enterococci account for the majority of pathogens causing IE.[6] Other bacterial pathogens include gram-negative bacteria. Selection of an antibiotic regimen is based on patient risk factors and adherence, left versus right-sided IE, native versus prosthetic valve, cultures and antibiotic sensitivities and likelihood of antibiotic resistance. Prosthetic valve involvement or disseminated infection (e.g., vertebral osteomyelitis, abscesses or septic arthritis) require a longer duration of treatment.

Table 1: Definition of Infective Endocarditis According to the Modified Duke Criteria[2]

Diagnosis	Criteria
Definite infective endocarditis	Pathological criteria • Microorganisms demonstrated by culture or histological examination of a vegetation, a vegetation that has embolized, or an intracardiac abscess specimen; or pathological lesions; vegetation or intracardiac abscess confirmed by histological examination showing active endocarditis Clinical criteria • 2 major criteria; or • 1 major criterion and 3 minor criteria; or • 5 minor criteria
Possible infective endocarditis	1 major criterion and 1 minor criterion; or 3 minor criteria
Rejected diagnosis of infective endocarditis	Firm alternative diagnosis explaining evidence of IE; or Resolution of IE syndrome with antibiotic therapy for ≤4 days; or No pathological evidence of IE at surgery or autopsy, with antibiotic therapy for ≤4 days; or Does not meet criteria for possible IE as above

Table 2: Definition of Terms Used in the Modified Duke Criteria for the Diagnosis of Infective Endocarditis[2]

Terms	Definition
Major criteria	Blood culture positive for IE • Typical microorganisms consistent with IE from 2 separate blood cultures: Viridans streptococci, *Streptococcus bovis*, HACEK group, *Staphylococcus aureus*; or community-acquired enterococci in the absence of a primary focus; or • Microorganisms consistent with IE from persistently positive blood cultures defined as follows: At least 2 positive cultures of blood samples drawn >12 h apart; or all of 3 or a majority of ≥4 separate cultures of blood (with first and last sample drawn at least 1 h apart) • Single positive blood culture for *Coxiella burnetii* or anti-phase 1 IgG antibody titer >1:800 Evidence of endocardial involvement Echocardiogram positive for IE (TEE recommended for patients with prosthetic valves, rated at least "possible IE" by clinical criteria, or complicated IE (paravalvular abscess); TTE as first test in other patients) defined as follows: • oscillating intracardiac mass on valve or supporting structures, in the path of regurgitant jets, or on implanted material in the absence of an alternative anatomic explanation; or abscess; or new partial dehiscence of prosthetic valve New valvular regurgitation (worsening or changing or pre-existing murmur not sufficient)
Minor criteria	Predisposition, predisposing heart condition or intravenous drug use Fever, temperature >38°C Vascular phenomena, major arterial emboli, septic pulmonary infarcts, mycotic aneurysm, intracranial hemorrhage, conjunctival hemorrhages and Janeway's lesions Immunologic phenomena: glomerulonephritis, Osler's nodes, Roth's spots and rheumatoid factor Microbiological evidence: positive blood culture but does not meet a major criterion as noted above[a] or serological evidence of active infection with organism consistent with IE Echocardiographic minor criteria eliminated

[a] Excludes single positive cultures for coagulase-negative staphylococci and organisms that do not cause endocarditis.
Abbreviations: IE = infective endocarditis; TEE = transesophageal echocardiography; TTE = transthoracic echocardiography

Staphylococci (Table 3)

S. aureus, including methicillin-sensitive (MSSA) and methicillin-resistant (MRSA) strains, or coagulase-negative staphylococci (e.g., *S. epidermidis*, *S. lugdunensis*) may occur in both native and prosthetic valve IE and together account for approximately 40% of cases of IE. IE involving a prosthetic valve requires a longer duration of treatment. For MSSA, use **cloxacillin** or **cefazolin** for primary treatment. Although **gentamicin** may be added for 3–5 days, the benefit of short-course aminoglycoside has been questioned for MSSA IE.[7,8,9,10] In patients with right-sided uncomplicated MSSA IE (no renal impairment, no extracardiac metastatic infection), a 2-week course may be used.[1] **Vancomycin** is the agent of choice for the treatment of MRSA IE and in patients with a type-1 hypersensitivity reaction to beta-lactams. For MSSA IE, use beta-lactams preferentially over vancomycin. In patients with a beta-lactam type-1 hypersensitivity reaction, consider beta-lactam desensitization. **Daptomycin** may be used to treat MSSA or MRSA right-sided IE in select patients only.

Streptococci (Table 4)

Alpha-hemolytic or viridans streptococci account for 20% of IE cases.[6] Viridans streptococci include *S. sanguis*, *S. oralis* (*mitis*), *S. salivarius*, *S. mutans*, and *Gemella morbillorum* (formerly called *S. morbillorum*), *S. anginosus* group (*S. intermedius*, *anginosus*, and *constellatus*) and *S. bovis* group (includes *S. gallolyticus* spp, *S. infantarius* spp).[1] Other viridans streptococci include *Abiotrophia defectiva* and *Granulicatella* species. Most streptococci are sensitive to penicillin, however, tolerance or resistance to penicillin has been reported.[1,11] Depending on the penicillin susceptibility, monotherapy with IV **penicillin G** or **ceftriaxone** is recommended. In select patients, **gentamicin** may be added in combination with **penicillin** or **ceftriaxone** to shorten the duration of treatment to 2 weeks. In cases of intermediate penicillin-sensitive streptococci, **gentamicin** must be added for the first 2 weeks of a 4-week treatment course. Prosthetic valve IE is treated for 6 weeks. IE due to *A. defectiva*, *Granulicatella* species, *Gemella* species or viridans streptococci with MIC >0.5 µg/mL may be difficult to treat and should be treated with antibiotic regimens used for enterococcal IE (see Table 5).

Table 3: **Treatment of Staphylococcal Native or Prosthetic Valve Endocarditis[1]**

Suggested Regimen	Duration	Comments
Staphylococci—No Prosthetic Material		
Methicillin-sensitive:		
Cloxacillin or cefazolin	6 weeks	May use 2 weeks' treatment if the IE is *uncomplicated*[a] and right-sided only.
+/- gentamicin	First 3–5 days	
Methicillin-resistant:		
Vancomycin	6 weeks	
Staphylococci—Prosthetic Valve		
Methicillin-sensitive:		
Cloxacillin + rifampin	≥6 weeks	Cefazolin may be used in place of cloxacillin.
+ gentamicin	First 2 weeks	
Methicillin-resistant:		
Vancomycin + rifampin	≥6 weeks	
+ gentamicin	First 2 weeks	

[a] No renal impairment or metastatic infection.

Table 4: **Treatment of Viridans Group Streptococci and *S. bovis* Endocarditis**[1]

Suggested Regimen(s)	Duration	Comments
Viridans Group Streptococci and *S. bovis* Sensitive to Penicillin[a]—Native Valve		
Penicillin G or ceftriaxone	4 weeks	Consider avoiding gentamicin-containing regimen in elderly patients or those at risk of aminoglycoside toxicity. Do *not* use short course treatment (2 weeks) in IE cases with cardiac or extra-cardiac abscesses.
or		
Penicillin G or ceftriaxone + gentamicin	2 weeks	
or		
Vancomycin	4 weeks	Vancomycin reserved for patients unable to tolerate beta-lactam antibiotics.
Viridans Group Streptococci and *S. bovis* Relatively Resistant to Penicillin[b]—Native Valve		
Penicillin G or ceftriaxone + gentamicin (for first 2 weeks only)	4 weeks	Treat penicillin-resistant strains (MIC >0.5 µg/mL) with regimens recommended for enterococcal endocarditis.
or		
Vancomycin	4 weeks	Vancomycin reserved for patients unable to tolerate beta-lactam antibiotics.
Viridans Group Streptococci and *S. bovis*—Prosthetic Valve		
Penicillin G or ceftriaxone	6 weeks	
If penicillin MIC ≤0.12: +/- gentamicin	First 2 weeks	
If penicillin MIC >0.12: + gentamicin	6 weeks	
or		
Vancomycin	6 weeks	Vancomycin reserved for patients unable to tolerate beta-lactam antibiotics.

[a] Sensitive to penicillin = MIC ≤0.12 µg/mL.
[b] Relatively resistant to penicillin in the context of IE = MIC >0.12–≤0.5 µg/mL.
Abbreviations: IE = infective endocarditis; MIC = minimum inhibitory concentration

Enterococci (Table 5)

Enterococci (e.g., *E. faecalis*, *E. faecium*) account for approximately 10% of IE cases.[6] Choice and duration of the antibiotic regimen depends on the enterococcal species and its susceptibility to **penicillin**, **gentamicin** or **vancomycin**. Patients with enterococcal IE generally require 4–6 weeks of concomitant beta-lactam and aminoglycoside therapy. In beta-lactam-allergic patients vancomycin is the agent of choice. Vancomycin-resistant enterococcal endocarditis is uncommon. For IE caused by enterococci resistant to penicillin, aminoglycosides and vancomycin, a minimum of 8 weeks of therapy is recommended. Depending on the enterococcal species, combination **beta-lactam** therapy, **linezolid** or **dalfopristin/quinupristin** is recommended (see Table 5). Management of multidrug-resistant enterococcal IE may be difficult and is not clearly defined. Various combination regimens including those with linezolid or **daptomycin** have been suggested although clinical data remain limited.[12]

Gentamicin peak and trough concentrations are suggested to be maintained at 3–4 mg/L and <1 mg/L respectively.[1,13,14] Concerns with nephrotoxicity and lack of additional efficacy with higher peak levels have led clinicians to recommend these lower gentamicin peak concentrations.[15]

Table 5: **Treatment of Enterococci in Native or Prosthetic Valve Endocarditis**[1]

Regimen(s)	Duration	Comments
Sensitive to Penicillin, Gentamicin and Vancomycin		
Ampicillin or penicillin G + gentamicin	4–6 weeks	
or		
Vancomycin + gentamicin	6 weeks	Vancomycin reserved for patients unable to tolerate beta-lactam antibiotics.
Sensitive to Penicillin, Streptomycin and Vancomycin and Resistant to Gentamicin		
Ampicillin or penicillin G + streptomycin	4–6 weeks	*Native valve:* 4-week therapy recommended for patients with symptoms of illness <3 months; 6-week therapy recommended for patients with symptoms >3 months.
or		*Prosthetic valve:* 6-week minimum therapy recommended. Vancomycin reserved for patients unable to tolerate beta-lactam antibiotics.
Vancomycin + streptomycin	6 weeks	
Sensitive to Aminoglycosides and Vancomycin, Resistant to Penicillin		
Vancomycin + gentamicin	6 weeks	
Resistant to Aminoglycosides, Penicillin and Vancomycin		
E. faecium Linezolid *or* dalfopristin/quinupristin	≥8 weeks	Optimal treatment not defined.
E. faecalis Imipenem/cilastatin *or* ceftriaxone + ampicillin	≥8 weeks	

Gram-negative Bacteria

IE due to gram-negative bacteria may account for 2% of cases.[6] Identification of the gram-negative pathogen and susceptibility to antibiotics is important in determining the antibiotic regimen and course. Gram-negative bacteria may be divided into HACEK and non-HACEK group bacteria. HACEK group organisms are fastidious, slow growing, gram-negative bacilli accounting for approximately 1–2% of IE. HACEK group pathogens include *Haemophilus* species (e.g., *H. parainfluenzae*, *H. aphrophilus*), *Aggregatibacter* (formerly *Actinobacillus*) *actinomycetemcomitans*, *Cardiobacterium hominis*, *Eikenella corrodens* and *Kingella* species.[1]

Due to concerns with beta-lactamase production among HACEK strains, ampicillin is *not* recommended for treatment of HACEK IE. Third-generation or higher **cephalosporins** may be used to treat HACEK IE. In patients with beta-lactam allergies, fluoroquinolones (**ciprofloxacin, levofloxacin** or **moxifloxacin**) are alternatives.

Culture-negative IE

Blood cultures may remain negative in 8% of cases despite radiologic and clinical evidence of IE. Reasons for this may include difficult-to-grow pathogens (e.g., *Coxiella burnetii* or *Bartonella* spp.), nonbacterial or unusual pathogens and administration of antibiotic therapy prior to blood cultures. Conduct a thorough review of the patient host factors (e.g., immunosuppression, burn), comorbidities (e.g., diabetes), history of intravenous drug use, animal or insect exposure, indwelling devices, prior surgical procedures, etc., to search for possible etiologic causes of culture-negative IE. Staining techniques may be used to identify potential pathogens.[16] Molecular diagnostics may be used to identify pathogens such as *Coxiella burnetii*, *Bartonella* or *Chlamydia* species.[1] Select antibiotic therapy based on the most likely pathogen after a review of available patient data. Consult with an infectious diseases specialist and clinical microbiologist.

Outpatient Parenteral Antimicrobial Therapy of IE

Although outpatient parenteral antimicrobial therapy (OPAT) has been used to treat IE, consider stringent entry criteria and close patient follow-up for patients receiving OPAT.[17,18] In uncomplicated IE patients, OPAT may be used to complete a 4- to 6-week total treatment course providing proper patient assessment and follow-up is conducted. In general, eligible patients should have received an initial 2 weeks of iv antibiotic therapy administered as an inpatient before initiation of OPAT.[17,18] Monitor patients for clinical response, complications and adverse drug effects from antibiotic therapy (e.g., resulting from prolonged aminoglycoside therapy).

Prevention of Infective Endocarditis

Concerns about bacteremia and severity of IE led to a consensus among experts over the past 50 years to recommend antibiotic prophylaxis for patients with risk factors undergoing procedures known to cause bacteremia.[19,20,21,22] Assumptions were made that antibiotic prophylaxis would prevent IE in patients undergoing dental, GI and genitourinary tract procedures. However, there is an absence of randomized controlled trials documenting the efficacy of antibiotic prophylaxis in preventing IE. Most cases of IE cannot be attributed to invasive procedures. Systematic reviews did not find supportive data.[23,24] The benefit of widespread antibiotic prophylaxis to prevent IE is small.[25] As a result, revised recommendations limit antibiotic prophylaxis to patients with underlying cardiac conditions at highest risk of adverse outcome from IE (see Table 6).[21,22] Population-based studies evaluating the incidence of IE before and after revised guidelines found the rates of IE unchanged.[26,27,28] Prescriptions in the U.K. for prophylactic antibiotics decreased after publication of the new guidelines.[26] Cumulatively, this suggests limiting the indications for IE antibiotic prophylaxis to high-risk patients has not led to an increase in the prevalence of IE.

Antibiotic prophylaxis is directed against alpha-hemolytic (viridans) streptococci for patients with underlying cardiac conditions at highest risk of adverse outcomes undergoing procedures outlined in Table 7. Administer the antibiotic to provide effective serum concentrations at the time of the anticipated bacteremia and for a few hours thereafter.

Table 6: Cardiac Conditions Associated with Highest Risk of Adverse Outcomes from Infective Endocarditis[21]

Prosthetic cardiac valve, or prosthetic material used for cardiac valve repair
Previous infective endocarditis
Congenital heart disease (CHD)[a]
• Unrepaired cyanotic congenital heart disease, including those with palliative shunts and conduits
• Completely repaired congenital heart disease with prosthetic material or device, whether placed by surgery or catheter intervention, during the first 6 months after the procedure[b]
• Repaired congenital heart disease with residual defects at the site or adjacent to the site of a prosthetic patch or prosthetic device (which inhibit endothelialization)
Cardiac transplantation recipients with cardiac valvular disease

[a] Except for the conditions above, antibiotic prophylaxis is no longer recommended for any other forms of CHD.
[b] Prophylaxis is reasonable because endothelialization of prosthetic material occurs within 6 months following the procedure.
Reprinted with permission *Circulation* 2007;116(15):1736-54. ©2007 American Heart Association, Inc.

Table 7: Dental or Surgical Procedures for which Endocarditis Prophylaxis is Reasonable for Patients with Cardiac Conditions Identified in Table 6[a,21]

Prophylaxis is reasonable with:

- All dental procedures that involve **manipulation of gingival tissue or the periapical region of teeth or perforation of the oral mucosa**

  The following dental procedures and events do **not** need prophylaxis: routine anesthetic injections through noninfected tissue, taking dental radiographs, placement of removable prosthodontic or orthodontic appliances, adjustment of orthodontic appliances, placement of orthodontic brackets, shedding of deciduous teeth and bleeding from trauma to the lips or oral mucosa
- Procedures on respiratory tract involving **incision or biopsy of respiratory mucosa** (such as tonsillectomy or adenoidectomy)

  Use the agents recommended in Table 8. For known *S. aureus* infections, use an antistaphylococcal penicillin (e.g., cloxacillin) or cephalosporin (e.g., cephalexin); use vancomycin in patients unable to take beta-lactam antibiotics or if the strain is methicillin-resistant
- Procedures in patients with **infected skin, skin structures or musculoskeletal tissue**

  Use the agents recommended in Table 8. For patients who cannot take beta-lactam antibiotics or those with known or suspected methicillin-resistant staphylococcus infection, use vancomycin or clindamycin

[a] Antibiotic prophylaxis solely to prevent IE is no longer recommended for genitourinary or gastrointestinal tract procedures.

If the antibiotic is inadvertently not administered before the procedure, the dose may be administered up to 2 hours after the procedure. This should be reserved only for those patients who did not receive a dose prior to the procedure.

If the patient is already taking an antibiotic that would be used for endocarditis prophylaxis, select an agent from a different class, to avoid encountering resistant strains [Evidence: SORT C*].[21] Alternatively, delay the procedure until 10 days or more after completion of the antibiotic course, to allow the bacterial flora to return to its usual state [Evidence: SORT C*].[21]

Therapeutic Tips

- Intravenous therapy is the route of choice for antimicrobial administration.
- When considering the duration of treatment in IE patients with an initial positive blood culture, count the required duration of treatment from the first day the blood culture is negative.[1]
- Due to an association with colon cancer, patients with *S. bovis* IE or positive blood cultures should undergo a colonoscopy to investigate for presence of malignancy.[29,30]

Suggested Readings

Baddour LM, Wilson WR, Bayer AS et al. Infective endocarditis: diagnosis, antimicrobial therapy, and management of complications: a statement for healthcare professionals from the Committee on Rheumatic Fever, Endocarditis, and Kawasaki Disease, Council on Cardiovascular Disease in the Young, and the Councils on Clinical Cardiology, Stroke, and Cardiovascular Surgery and Anesthesia, American Heart Association: endorsed by the Infectious Diseases Society of America. *Circulation* 2005;111(23):e394-434.

Wilson W, Taubert KA, Gewitz M et al. Prevention of infective endocarditis: guidelines from the American Heart Association: a guideline from the American Heart Association Rheumatic Fever, Endocarditis, and Kawasaki Disease Committee, Council on Cardiovascular Disease in the Young, and the Council on Clinical Cardiology, Council on Cardiovascular Surgery and Anesthesia, and the Quality of Care and Outcomes Research Interdisciplinary Working Group. *Circulation* 2007;116(15):1736-54.

* SORT (Strength of Recommendation Taxonomy) is a rating system (A, B or C) that addresses the quality of available evidence. For more information consult **How to Use *Compendium of Therapeutic Choices*** on page xxv.

Table 8: **Antibiotic Regimens for Endocarditis Prophylaxis in Dental Procedures**[a,21]

Drug	Adult Dose[b]	Pediatric Dose[b,c]
Standard Regimen		
Amoxicillin	2 g po	50 mg/kg
Unable to Take Oral Medications		
Ampicillin *or*	2 g im[d] or iv	50 mg/kg im[d] or iv
Cefazolin *or*	1 g im[d] or iv	50 mg/kg im[d] or iv
Ceftriaxone	1 g im[d] or iv	50 mg/kg im[d] or iv
Allergic to Penicillins		
Cephalexin[e,f] *or*	2 g po	50 mg/kg
Clindamycin *or*	600 mg po	20 mg/kg
Azithromycin *or*	500 mg po	15 mg/kg
Clarithromycin	500 mg po	15 mg/kg
Allergic to Penicillins and Unable to Take Oral Medications		
Cefazolin[f] *or*	1 g im[d] or iv	50 mg/kg im[d] or iv
Ceftriaxone[f] *or*	1 g im[d] or iv	50 mg/kg im[d] or iv
Clindamycin	600 mg im[d] or iv	20 mg/kg im[d] or iv

[a] See Table 6 and Table 7.
[b] Administered 30–60 min prior to procedure.
[c] Pediatric dose should not exceed adult dose.
[d] Avoid im injections in anticoagulated patients.
[e] Or other first- or second-generation oral cephalosporin in equivalent adult or pediatric dosage.
[f] Cephalosporins should not be used in an individual with a history of anaphylaxis, angioedema or urticaria with penicillins or ampicillin.
Source: American Heart Association, Inc.

Table 9: Intravenous Therapy for Infective Endocarditis

Class	Drug	Dose	Adverse Effects	Drug Interactions	Comments	Cost[a]
Aminoglycosides	*gentamicin* generics	1 mg/kg Q8H iv *or* 3 mg/kg once daily iv/im (for viridans streptococci and *S. bovis*)	Nephrotoxicity, ototoxicity.	Enhanced effects with concomitant nephrotoxins or ototoxins (e.g., amphotericin B, vancomycin). Increased risk of respiratory depression with neuromuscular blocking agents.	Toxicity risk may increase with prolonged administration and/or concomitant nephrotoxins or ototoxins. Monitor renal function and serum gentamicin concentrations especially for prolonged courses. Consider maintaining gentamicin trough concentrations ≤1 mg/L to minimize risk of nephrotoxicity. For enterococcal IE only, gentamicin peak and trough levels of 3–4 mg/L and 1 mg/L respectively, may be considered.	$
	streptomycin generics	7.5 mg/kg Q12H iv/im	Nephrotoxicity, ototoxicity.	See gentamicin.	Serum concentration assay not commonly available. Toxicity risk may increase with prolonged administration and/or concomitant nephrotoxins or ototoxins.	$$$
Carbapenems	*imipenem/cilastatin* Primaxin, generics	500 mg Q6H iv	Phlebitis, rash, hypersensitivity, drug fever, nausea, vomiting diarrhea; seizure (high dose).	May reduce valproic acid levels. Seizures have been reported with concurrent use of imipenem and ganciclovir.		$$$
Cephalosporins	*cefazolin* generics	2 g Q8H iv	Rash, hypersensitivity, drug fever, diarrhea.	Possible increased INR with warfarin.		$
	ceftriaxone generics	2 g Q24H iv (see Comments)	Rash, hypersensitivity, drug fever, diarrhea, eosinophilia, thrombocytosis, elevated AST and/or ALT.	See cefazolin. Ceftriaxone binds with iv calcium salts to form an insoluble precipitate.	2 g Q12H for vancomycin-resistant *E. faecalis* IE combined with ampicillin.	$
Glycopeptides	*vancomycin* generics	15 mg/kg Q12H iv (see Comments)	Thrombophlebitis, rash, fever, anemia, nephrotoxicity, otoxicity, red man syndrome.	Increased incidence of nephrotoxicity when used with aminoglycosides.	Monitor vancomycin troughs to maintain concentrations between 15–20 μg/mL for *S. aureus* IE[31] (may require >30 mg/kg/day dosing); nephrotoxicity and ototoxicity have been reported with higher dosages.	$$$$

Class	Drug	Dose	Adverse Effects	Drug Interactions	Comments	Cost[a]
Lipopeptides	*daptomycin* Cubicin	6 mg/kg Q24H iv	Diarrhea, nausea, vomiting, constipation, thrombophlebitis, injection site pain/reaction, anemia, creatinine kinase elevation; myalgia, rhabdomyolysis.	Consider avoiding concomitant HMG-CoA reductase inhibitor administration as a precaution as daptomycin may increase its levels.	Monitor creatinine kinase weekly at minimum, especially in patients with renal impairment and/or HMG-CoA reductase co-administration.	$$$$$
Oxazolidi-nones	*linezolid* Zyvoxam	600 mg Q12H iv	Diarrhea, nausea, vomiting, myelosuppression (e.g., anemia, thrombocytopenia).	MAO inhibitor therefore use caution; evaluate concomitant agents for potential interaction. Avoid tyramine-rich foods.		$$$$$
Penicillins	*penicillin G* Crystapen, generics	12–18 million units per day divided Q4–6H iv *or* 24 million units per day divided Q4–6H iv	Rash, hypersensitivity, drug fever, interstitial nephritis, seizure (high dose).	May increase serum levels of methotrexate. May enhance anticoagulant effect of warfarin.	Use 24 million units per day for viridans streptococci and *S. bovis* in a prosthetic valve IE.	$
	ampicillin generics	2 g Q4H iv	See penicillin G.	See penicillin G.		$$
	cloxacillin generics	2 g Q4H iv	See penicillin G.	See penicillin G.		$$
Rifamycins	*rifampin* Rifadin, Rofact, generics	300 mg Q8H iv/po	Rash, orange discolouration of body fluids (e.g., contact lens staining), nausea, vomiting, hepatic toxicity, thrombocytopenia.	Potent inducer of multiple substrates—evaluate when coadministered with other drugs (e.g., may reduce levels of cyclosporine, tacrolimus, sirolimus, phenytoin, warfarin and oral contraceptives).	Use only in combination with other antibiotics.	iv: [b] po: $
Strep-togramins	*quinupristin/ dalfopristin*	7.5 mg/kg Q8H iv	Diarrhea, nausea, vomiting, thrombophlebitis, injection site pain/reaction, conjugated hyperbilirubinemia.	CYP3A4 inhibitor therefore use caution; evaluate concomitant agents for potential interaction (e.g., increased levels of calcium channel blockers, carbamazepine, cyclosporine, tacrolimus, statins).		[b]

[a] Cost per day based on 70 kg body weight; includes drug cost only.
[b] Available through Health Canada's Special Access Programme.
Dosage adjustment may be required in renal impairment; see Appendix I.
Abbreviations: IE = infective endocarditis; MAO = monoamine oxidase inhibitor
Legend: $ < $40 $$ $40–80 $$$ $80–120 $$$$ $120–160 $$$$$ $160–200

References

1. Baddour LM, Wilson WR, Bayer AS et al. Infective endocarditis: diagnosis, antimicrobial therapy, and management of complications: a statement for healthcare professionals from the Committee on Rheumatic Fever, Endocarditis, and Kawasaki Disease, Council on Cardiovascular Disease in the Young, and the Councils on Clinical Cardiology, Stroke, and Cardiovascular Surgery and Anesthesia, American Heart Association: endorsed by the Infectious Diseases Society of America. *Circulation* 2005;111(23):e394-434.
2. Li JS, Sexton DJ, Mick N et al. Proposed modifications to the Duke criteria for the diagnosis of infective endocarditis. *Clin Infect Dis* 2000;30(4):633-8.
3. Haldar SM, O'Gara PT. Infective endocarditis: diagnosis and management. *Nat Clin Pract Cardiovasc Med* 2006;3(6):310-7.
4. Horstkotte D, Follath F, Gutschik E et al. Guidelines on prevention, diagnosis and treatment of infective endocarditis executive summary; the Task Force on Infective Endocarditis of the European Society of Cardiology. *Eur Heart J* 2004;25(3):267-76.
5. Bonow RO, Carabello BA, Kanu C et al. ACC/AHA 2006 guidelines for the management of patients with valvular heart disease: a report of the American College of Cardiology/American Heart Association Task Force on Practice Guidelines (writing committee to revise the 1998 Guidelines for the Management of Patients With Valvular Heart Disease): developed in collaboration with the Society of Cardiovascular Anesthesiologists: endorsed by the Society for Cardiovascular Angiography and Interventions and the Society of Thoracic Surgeons. *Circulation* 2006;114(5):e84-231.
6. Fowler VG, Miro JM, Hoen B et al. Staphylococcus aureus endocarditis: a consequence of medical progress. *JAMA* 2005;293(24):3012-21.
7. Falagas ME, Matthaiou DK, Bliziotis IA. The role of aminoglycosides in combination with a beta-lactam for the treatment of bacterial endocarditis: a meta-analysis of comparative trials. *J Antimicrob Chemother* 2006;57(4):639-47.
8. Paul M, Leibovici L. Combination antimicrobial treatment versus monotherapy: the contribution of meta-analyses. *Infect Dis Clin North Am* 2009;23(2):277-93.
9. Ribera E, Gomez-Jimenez J, Cortes E et al. Effectiveness of cloxacillin with and without gentamicin in short-term therapy for right-sided Staphylococcus aureus endocarditis. A randomized, controlled trial. *Ann Intern Med* 1996;125(12):969-74.
10. Cosgrove SE, Vigliani GA, Fowler VG et al. Initial low-dose gentamicin for Staphylococcus aureus bacteremia and endocarditis is nephrotoxic. *Clin Infect Dis* 2009;48(6):713-21.
11. Knoll B, Tleyjeh IM, Steckelberg JM et al. Infective endocarditis due to penicillin-resistant viridans group streptococci. *Clin Infect Dis* 2007;44(12):1585-92.
12. Arias CA, Contreras GA, Murray BE. Management of multi-drug resistant enterococcal infections. *Clin Microbiol Infect* 2010;16(6):555-62.
13. Wilson WR, Karchmer AW, Dajani AS et al. Antibiotic treatment of adults with infective endocarditis due to streptococci, enterococci, staphylococci, and HACEK microorganisms. American Heart Association. *JAMA* 1995;274(21):1706-13.
14. Bisno AL, Dismukes WE, Durack DT et al. Antimicrobial treatment of infective endocarditis due to viridans streptococci, enterococci, and staphylococci. *JAMA* 1989;261(10):1471-7.
15. Geraci JE. The antibiotic therapy of bacterial endocarditis: therapeutic data on 172 patients seen from 1951 through 1957: additional observations on short-term therapy (two weeks) for penicillin-sensitive streptococcal endocarditis. *Med Clin North Am* 1958;42(4):1101-40.
16. Houpikian P, Raoult D. Diagnostic methods. Current best practices and guidelines for identification of difficult-to-culture pathogens in infective endocarditis. *Cardiol Clin* 2003;21(2):207-17.
17. Andrews MM, von Reyn CF. Patient selection criteria and management guidelines for outpatient parenteral antibiotic therapy for native valve infective endocarditis. *Clin Infect Dis* 2001;33(2):203-9.
18. Tice AD. Safety of outpatient parenteral antimicrobial therapy for endocarditis. *Clin Infect Dis* 2002;34(3):419-20.
19. Elliott TS, Foweraker J, Gould FK et al. Guidelines for the antibiotic treatment of endocarditis in adults: report of the Working Party of the British Society for Antimicrobial Chemotherapy. *J Antimicrob Chemother* 2004;54(6):971-81.
20. Embil JM, Chan KL. The American Heart Association 2007 endocarditis prophylaxis guidelines: a compromise between science and common sense. *Can J Cardiol* 2008;24(9):673-5.
21. Wilson W, Taubert KA, Gewitz M et al. Prevention of infective endocarditis: guidelines from the American Heart Association: a guideline from the American Heart Association Rheumatic Fever, Endocarditis, and Kawasaki Disease Committee, Council on Cardiovascular Disease in the Young, and the Council on Clinical Cardiology, Council on Cardiovascular Surgery and Anesthesia, and the Quality of Care and Outcomes Research Interdisciplinary Working Group. *Circulation* 2007;116(15):1736-54.
22. Stokes T, Richey R, Wray D. Prophylaxis against infective endocarditis: summary of NICE guidance. *Heart* 2008;94(7):930-1.
23. Oliver R, Roberts GJ, Hooper L et al. Antibiotics for the prophylaxis of bacterial endocarditis in dentistry. *Cochrane Database Syst Rev* 2008;(4):CD003813.
24. Van der Meer JT, Van Wijk W, Thompson J et al. Efficacy of antibiotic prophylaxis for prevention of native-valve endocarditis. *Lancet* 1992;339(8786):135-9.
25. Duval X, Alla F, Hoen B et al. Estimated risk of endocarditis in adults with predisposing cardiac conditions undergoing dental procedures with or without antibiotic prophylaxis. *Clin Infect Dis* 2006;42(12):e102-7.
26. Thornhill MH, Dayer MJ, Forde JM et al. Impact of the NICE guideline recommending cessation of antibiotic prophylaxis for prevention of infective endocarditis: before and after study. *BMJ* 2011;342:d2392.
27. Duval X, Delahaye F, Alla F et al. Temporal trends in infective endocarditis in the context of prophylaxis guideline modifications: three successive population-based surveys. *J Am Coll Cardiol* 2012;59(22):1968-76.
28. Desimone DC, Tleyjeh IM, Correa de Sa DD et al. Incidence of infective endocarditis caused by viridans group streptococci before and after publication of the 2007 American Heart Association's endocarditis prevention guidelines. *Circulation* 2012;126(1):60-4.
29. Gupta A, Madani R, Mukhtar H. Streptococcus bovis endocarditis, a silent sign for colonic tumour. *Colorectal Dis* 2010;12(3):164-71.
30. Boleij A, van Gelder MM, Swinkels DW et al. Clinical importance of Streptococcus gallolyticus infection among colorectal cancer patients: systematic review and meta-analysis. *Clin Infect Dis* 2011;53(9):870-8.
31. Rybak M, Lomaestro B, Rotschafer JC et al. Therapeutic monitoring of vancomycin in adult patients: a consensus review of the American Society of Health-System Pharmacists, the Infectious Diseases Society of America, and the Society of Infectious Diseases Pharmacists. *Am J Health Syst Pharm* 2009;66(1):82-98.

Chapter 116
Influenza

Susan K. Bowles, PharmD, MSc, FCCP and
Robert Strang, MD, MHSc, FRCPC

Influenza is an acute viral illness of the respiratory tract caused by influenza A or influenza B viruses. Illness may be mild to severe and can be a major cause of morbidity and mortality. A typical influenza season in Canada runs from mid-October to the end of April.

Influenza-like illness (ILI) is a term often used in public health surveillance programs for influenza, which refers to any acute illness having symptoms typical of influenza. Adenovirus, parainfluenza or respiratory syncytial virus may cause similar symptoms.

Influenza-like illness[1] is defined as an acute onset of respiratory illness with fever, cough and one or more of: sore throat, arthralgia, myalgia or extreme exhaustion/weakness. Gastrointestinal symptoms may be present in children <5 years. Fever may not be prominent in children <5 years or adults ≥65 years.

Investigations

- History with particular attention to symptoms and onset of symptoms is the key to appropriate use of antiviral agents:
  - healthy adolescents and adults: when influenza is known to be circulating in the community or the individual has returned from a travel area where influenza is known to be circulating, abrupt onset of fever of 38.5°C or greater and dry cough is likely to be influenza.[2,3] The predictive value of these symptoms is considerably lower in the very young or the elderly
  - young children: can present with either a nonspecific febrile illness or with a respiratory illness resembling croup, bronchitis and occasionally bronchiolitis.[4] GI symptoms (nausea, vomiting, diarrhea) may also be present in children <5 years
  - older adults: fever may not be prominent.[4,5] When influenza is known to be circulating in the community or the individual has returned from a travel area where influenza is known to be circulating, have a high index of suspicion for influenza if older patients present with ≥2 symptoms of sore throat, arthralgia, myalgia or prostration;[5] this is particularly true of elderly residents of long-term care facilities
- Laboratory testing:
  - beyond formal surveillance programs, widespread laboratory testing in the community is not necessary or practical, but it is important to differentiate between influenza and other respiratory viruses in the event of an outbreak of ILI in the long-term care setting or other institutional settings, including schools
  - as a general guideline, nasopharyngeal swabs from ill long-term care residents should be sent for laboratory testing in the event of ≥2 cases of ILI within a 72-hour period.[6] Obtain swabs from the initial cases as well as the next 3–5 individuals presenting with ILI. Public health officials should also be notified
  - contact the lab to obtain instructions on specimen collection, storage and transport.

– based on recommendations from the Canadian Public Health Laboratory Network, collect specimens within 5 days of onset of symptoms but preferably within 48 hours. Sampling beyond 5 days may be considered in patients with persisting or worsening symptoms regardless of age, in young children or the elderly and in the immunocompromised.[7]

Prevention

Goals of Therapy

- Prevent influenza illness from occurring, especially in individuals at high risk of developing serious influenza-related complications, e.g., pneumonia, exacerbation of cardiac or respiratory disease, death
- Decrease influenza-related symptoms, hospitalizations and deaths

Therapeutic Choices

Nonpharmacologic Choices

General measures to prevent acquisition of influenza include:

- wash hands often; use hand sanitizer if water and soap are not available.
- cough/sneeze into tissues (or into a sleeve if tissues are not available) and throw all used tissues into the garbage.
- if flu symptoms are present, stay home from work or school and do not visit hospitals, nursing homes or individuals at high risk of influenza-related complications.

In the event of a cluster of ILI in the nursing home or other long-term care setting, implement the following to reduce the potential of influenza spreading from ill to well residents (Figure 1):

- promote and enhance proper hand washing by staff, ambulatory residents and visitors.
- confine ill residents to their rooms until their acute symptoms have resolved.
- enhance environmental controls, e.g., more frequent cleaning.
- if possible, ill residents should be cared for only by staff who have received their annual influenza immunization.
- if possible, ill residents should be cared for by separate staff members who are not looking after well residents. If this is not possible, provide care for well individuals first, with strict hand washing between each patient.
- limit gatherings or activities where residents from different areas of the facility come into contact with each other.
- limit visitors when possible and exclude visits from all individuals with ILI.
- staff with symptoms of ILI should not work until their acute symptoms have resolved.

Pharmacologic Choices (Table 2)

Influenza Vaccine[8]

October to mid-November is the usual recommended time for influenza immunization in the Northern Hemisphere. Annual influenza vaccination of individuals at high risk of influenza-related complications (Table 1) remains the primary strategy for the reduction of influenza-related morbidity and mortality, in both community and long-term care settings. In addition, annual vaccination of individuals who have significant contact with individuals at high risk of influenza-related complications (Table 1) or who provide essential community services is recommended. In 2012, the National Advisory Committee on Immunization (NACI) increased the age range of healthy children considered to be at high risk of complications from ≤23 months to ≤59 months.[8]

Figure 1: **Prevention and Control of Influenza in the Long-term Care Setting**

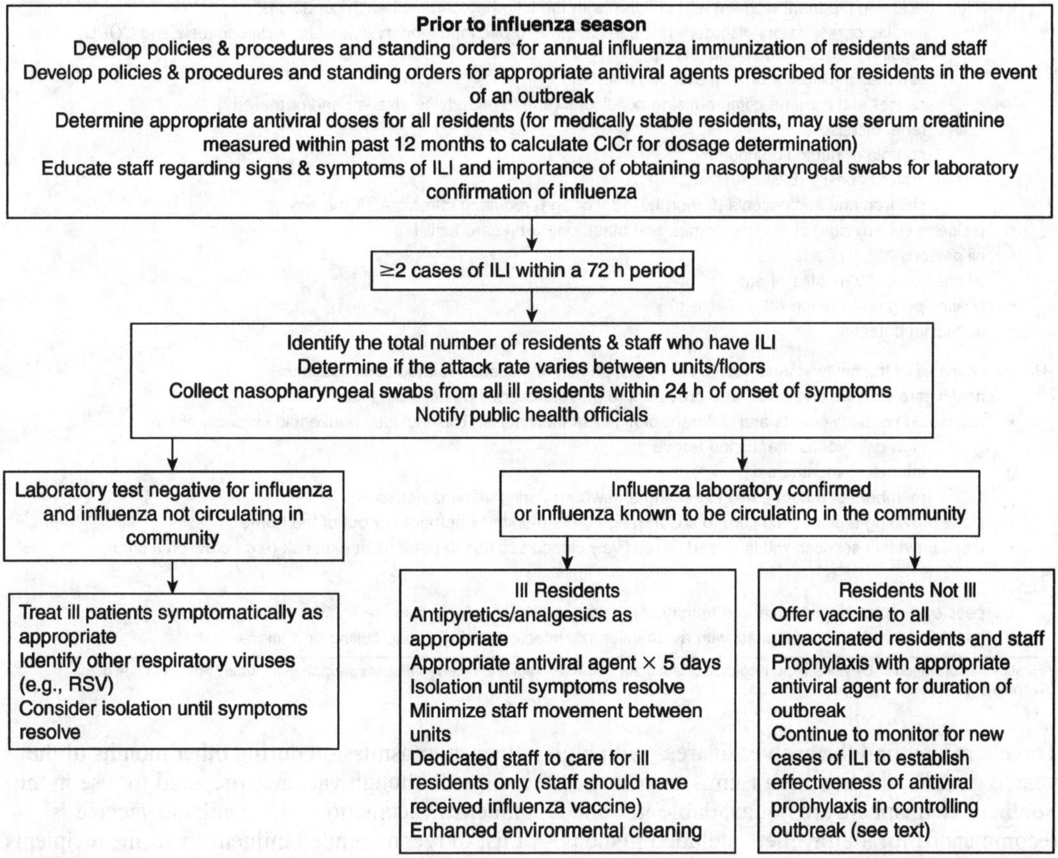
Prior to influenza season
Develop policies & procedures and standing orders for annual influenza immunization of residents and staff
Develop policies & procedures and standing orders for appropriate antiviral agents prescribed for residents in the event of an outbreak
Determine appropriate antiviral doses for all residents (for medically stable residents, may use serum creatinine measured within past 12 months to calculate ClCr for dosage determination)
Educate staff regarding signs & symptoms of ILI and importance of obtaining nasopharyngeal swabs for laboratory confirmation of influenza
≥2 cases of ILI within a 72 h period
Identify the total number of residents & staff who have ILI
Determine if the attack rate varies between units/floors
Collect nasopharyngeal swabs from all ill residents within 24 h of onset of symptoms
Notify public health officials
Laboratory test negative for influenza and influenza not circulating in community
Influenza laboratory confirmed or influenza known to be circulating in the community
Treat ill patients symptomatically as appropriate
Identify other respiratory viruses (e.g., RSV)
Consider isolation until symptoms resolve
Ill Residents
Antipyretics/analgesics as appropriate
Appropriate antiviral agent × 5 days
Isolation until symptoms resolve
Minimize staff movement between units
Dedicated staff to care for ill residents only (staff should have received influenza vaccine)
Enhanced environmental cleaning
Residents Not Ill
Offer vaccine to all unvaccinated residents and staff
Prophylaxis with appropriate antiviral agent for duration of outbreak
Continue to monitor for new cases of ILI to establish effectiveness of antiviral prophylaxis in controlling outbreak (see text)

Adapted with permission from Gomolin IH, Kathpalia RK. Influenza. How to prevent and control nursing home outbreaks. *Geriatrics* 2002;57(1):30. Geriatrics is a copyrighted publication of Advanstar Communications Inc. All rights reserved.
Abbreviations: ILI = influenza-like illness; RSV = respiratory syncytial virus

Significant illness and societal costs also occur with seasonal influenza in people who may not be considered at high risk of complications (healthy people aged 6–64 years). Therefore, NACI also encourages influenza vaccine for all Canadians. See Table 2 for a description of available influenza vaccines in Canada.

Recommendations regarding influenza vaccination in egg-allergic individuals were revised in the 2011–2012 season.[9] Egg-allergic individuals may be vaccinated against influenza using a trivalent inactivated vaccine (Table 2) based on a risk assessment. Those with mild reactions (e.g., hives or GI upset) or who tolerate eggs in baked goods may receive intramuscular or intradermal vaccinations in regular immunization settings but should be observed for 15–30 minutes.[8] Persons reporting more severe reactions (e.g., anaphylaxis) should be immunized in a setting where appropriate expertise and equipment are available to manage potential severe respiratory or cardiovascular symptoms. These individuals should always be observed for a period of 30 minutes.[8] Due to a lack of data, the live attenuated intranasal influenza vaccine should not be administered to persons with a documented egg allergy.[8,9]

Table 1: **Recommended Recipients of Seasonal Influenza Immunization**[a,8]

Persons at high risk for influenza-related complications
• adults (including pregnant women) and children with the following chronic health conditions:
- cardiac or respiratory disorders (includes asthma, bronchopulmonary dysplasia, cystic fibrosis and COPD) requiring regular medical follow-up
- diabetes mellitus or other metabolic disorder
- cancer and immune compromising conditions (due to underlying disease and/or therapy)
- renal disease
- anemia or hemoglobinopathy
- morbid obesity (BMI ≥40)
- children and adolescents (6 months–18 y of age) requiring chronic ASA therapy
• residents (of any age) of nursing homes and other long-term care facilities
• all persons ≥65 y of age
• all children 6–59 months of age
• healthy pregnant women (all trimesters)
• aboriginal persons
Persons capable of transmitting influenza to those at high risk of influenza-related complications
• health care workers and other care providers (e.g., volunteers, housekeeping staff)
• household contacts (adults and children) of high risk individuals. This includes household contacts of:
- high-risk groups mentioned above
- infants <6 months old
- members of a household expecting a newborn during influenza season
• those providing regular child care to children age 0–59 months, whether in or out of the home
• those providing services within closed or relatively closed settings to persons at high risk (e.g., crew on a ship)
Other
• people who provide essential community services, e.g., police officers and fire fighters
• people who are in direct contact with avian influenza-infected poultry during culling operations

[a] Healthy persons aged 5–64 years without contraindication are also encouraged to receive influenza vaccine even if they are not in one of the recommended recipient groups.

Travellers may find themselves in areas with high influenza transmission during other months of the year, e.g., Asia, the Southern Hemisphere and cruise ships. Although vaccines prepared for use in the Southern Hemisphere are not available in Canada, influenza vaccination with available vaccine is recommended for all travellers included in the NACI list of recommended influenza vaccine recipients (Table 1) due to increased risk of influenza-related complications.[8] NACI also encourages influenza immunization for all Canadians ≥6 months of age, which also applies to travellers.[8]

Antiviral Agents

Chemoprophylaxis with antiviral agents have their greatest utility in the long-term care environment (see Figure 1).[10] When an influenza outbreak is identified in a long-term care setting, give antiviral prophylaxis as soon as possible to all residents who are not yet ill, regardless of their vaccination status, as well as to nonimmunized health care providers.

Monitoring of antiviral resistance of circulating influenza viruses has been incorporated into national surveillance. **Amantadine** has exhibited high levels of resistance and is therefore no longer recommended for prophylaxis.[10,11] Some resistance has been documented against the neuraminidase inhibitors, **oseltamivir** and **zanamivir** but is reported at <1%.[11]

Oseltamivir is the first-line agent during outbreaks of influenza A (if expected to be sensitive) or influenza B. When using zanamivir as chemoprophylaxis, clinicians should be aware of the potential risk of bronchospasm in persons with pre-existing severe respiratory disease, and potential difficulty experienced by some frail elderly patients in using the inhaler device.

In a long-term care setting, continue surveillance for new cases of ILI to establish effectiveness of antiviral prophylaxis in controlling an influenza outbreak once postexposure prophylaxis is initiated in a facility. Regardless of the agent used, reports of drug specific-resistant strains of influenza A during outbreak situations demand change in therapy.

If cases of laboratory-confirmed influenza continue to occur more than 96 hours after initiation of antiviral prophylaxis, consider antiviral prophylaxis failure.[12] Contact the local Medical Officer of Health for assistance.

Treatment

Goals of Therapy

- Relieve influenza symptoms
- Reduce duration of influenza infection
- Reduce the potential for influenza-related complications
- Decrease influenza-related hospitalizations and deaths

Therapeutic Choices

Pharmacologic Choices

Analgesics/Antipyretic Agents

Use **acetaminophen** or **ibuprofen** for relief of fever, headache and myalgias. To avoid overdose, caution patients about the concurrent use of cough and cold products that contain acetaminophen or ibuprofen. Cough and cold products contain other ingredients such as antihistamines, which may not be needed.

Children and adolescents less than 18 years of age should *not* take **ASA** due to the associated risk of Reye's syndrome.

Antiviral Agents

The use of antiviral agents for treatment of influenza in healthy children and adults is controversial. However, they can be considered for treatment when influenza is either laboratory confirmed or strongly suspected based on symptoms and known local circulation. The use of antiviral agents for treatment of influenza in the community setting is illustrated in Figure 2.

The usual duration of influenza symptoms is 4–7 days. Studies in otherwise healthy adults and children demonstrated that **neuraminidase inhibitors** reduce the duration of symptoms by about 1 day.[13,14] Early treatment with **oseltamivir** may reduce influenza-related complications (need for antibiotics, hospitalizations, asthma exacerbations) in children ≤2 years of age,[10] as well as adults and children >2 years at high-risk of complications.[10,15,16,17,18,19]

Treatment with any antiviral agent is best initiated within 48 hours after the onset of symptoms.[10] However, treatment can be considered beyond 48 hours in the following circumstances: the illness is serious enough to require hospitalization, the illness is progressive, severe or complicated, regardless of previous health status or the individual belongs to a group at high-risk for severe disease.[10,20]

In the community setting, the duration of treatment for both adults and children is 5 days.[10] Five days is an adequate treatment period and it minimizes the risk of resistance.

Choices during Pregnancy and Breastfeeding

Influenza and Pregnancy

Several studies demonstrate an increased risk of influenza-related complications not only in those with comorbidities but also healthy pregnant women.[21,22,23] The risk appears to be the greatest during the third trimester.[21,24,25] Immunization of the mother appears to extend protection to infants following birth,[26] possibly via maternal-infant transfer of antibodies.[27]

Management

Prevention is the best strategy to reduce maternal morbidity associated with seasonal influenza. Immunization with seasonal trivalent influenza vaccine appears to be both safe and effective in all stages of pregnancy.[28,29] Until safety data are available do not use the live attenuated influenza vaccine in pregnant women; it may be used in breastfeeding women.[8]

While data are limited, both **oseltamivir** and **zanamivir** appear to be safe in pregnancy and during breastfeeding in preclinical and observational reports.[30,31,32] As such, early treatment with oseltamivir is recommended for pregnant women.[10] Oseltamivir is recommended over zanamivir as more safety data are available and its systemic absorption is expected to result in more consistent delivery to virus-infected respiratory tissues, especially in the later stages of pregnancy when distribution of inhaled zanamivir may be impacted by the gravid uterus.[10,32]

A discussion of general principles on the use of medications in these special populations can be found in Appendix II and Appendix III. Other specialized reference sources are also provided in these appendices.

Figure 2: **Treatment of Mild, Uncomplicated Influenza-like Illness in the Community**[10]

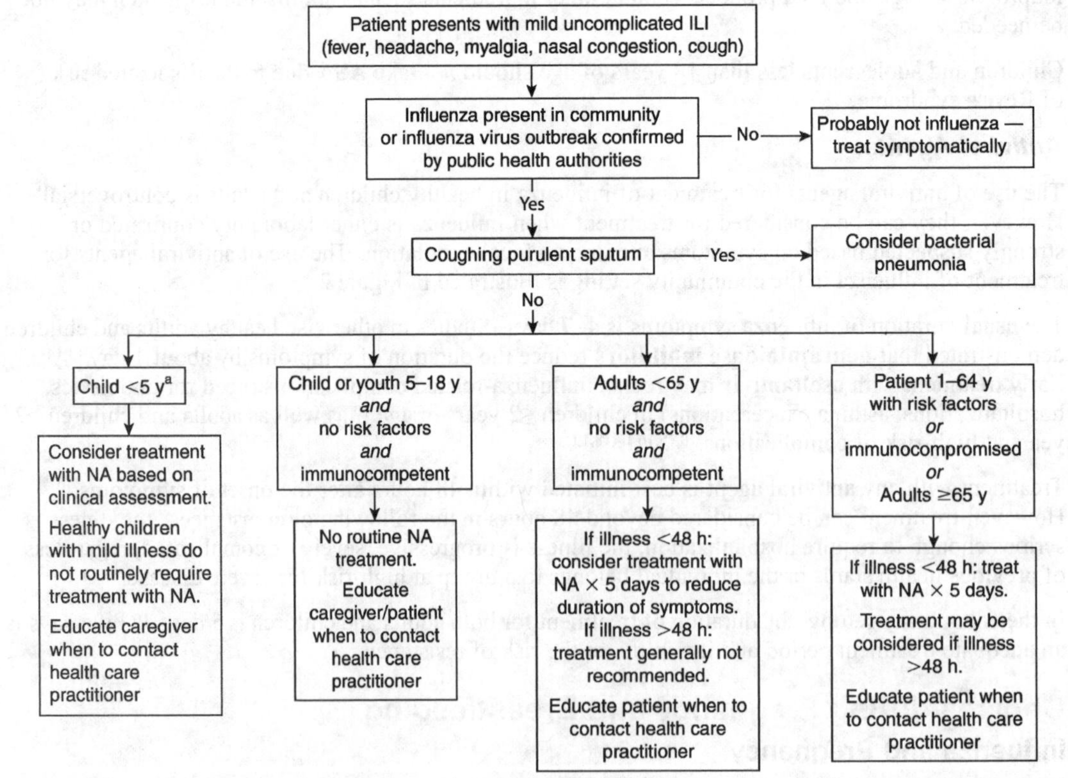

[a] Neuraminidase inhibitors are not approved by Health Canada for use in children <1 year of age.
Abbreviations: ILI = influenza-like illness; NA = neuraminidase inhibitor

Therapeutic Tips

- Antivirals are not substitutes for the influenza vaccine for prevention of influenza.
- Influenza surveillance information can be obtained from the FluWatch program from the Public Health Agency of Canada (www.phac-aspc.gc.ca/fluwatch/index-eng.php). Contact local Public Health authorities to determine if influenza is circulating in a specific community and if so, whether it is influenza A or B.
- Rapid identification of influenza in the long-term care setting allows timely implementation of control measures, thereby reducing influenza-related morbidity and mortality. Therefore, each facility should have a surveillance program in place to identify ILI, and policies and procedures regarding laboratory testing for ill residents. Staff should be familiar with the case definition of ILI.

Suggested Readings

Aoki FY, Allen UD, Stiver HG et al. The use of antiviral drugs for influenza: a foundation document for practitioners. *Can J Infect Dis Med Microbiol* 2013;24(Suppl C):1C-15C. Available from: www.ammi.ca/guidelines.

National Advisory Committee on Immunization (NACI). Statement on seasonal influenza vaccine for 2013-2014. An Advisory Committee Statement (ACS). *Can Commun Dis Rep* 2013;39(ACS-4):1-37. Available from: www.phac-aspc.gc.ca/publicat/ccdr-rmtc/13vol39/acs-dcc-4/index-eng.php.

Public Health Agency of Canada. FluWatch. *Definitions for the 2013-2014 season.* Ottawa (ON): PHAC; 2013. Available from: www.phac-aspc.gc.ca/fluwatch/13-14/def13-14-eng.php.

Zaman K, Roy E, Arifeen SE et al. Effectiveness of maternal influenza immunization in mothers and infants. *N Engl J Med* 2008;359(15):1555-64.

Table 2: Drugs Used for the Prevention and Treatment of Influenza[8]

Class	Drug	Dose	Adverse Effects	Comments	Cost[a]
Antivirals, neuraminidase inhibitors	*oseltamivir* Tamiflu	**Treatment:**[10] **Adults:** 75 mg BID po × 5 days ClCr >30–60 mL/min: 75 mg once daily or 30 mg BID po × 5 days ClCr 10–30 mL/min: 30 mg once daily po × 5 days ClCr <10 mL/min: single 75 mg dose po Low-flux HD: 30 mg po after each dialysis session; stop after 5 days High-flux HD: 75 mg po after each dialysis session; stop after 5 days CAPD dialysis: single 30 mg dose po prior to dialysis CRRT high-flux dialysis: 30 mg daily or 75 mg Q48H po × 5 days **Treatment: Children:**[33,34] ≥1 y and ≤15 kg: 30 mg BID po × 5 days >15–23 kg: 45 mg BID po × 5 days >23–40 kg: 60 mg BID po × 5 days >40 kg: 75 mg BID po × 5 days **Prevention:** **Adults and children ≥13 y:** 75 mg once daily po ClCr >30–60 mL/min: 75 mg Q48H or 30 mg once daily po ClCr 10–30 mL/min: 30 mg Q48H po **Prevention: Children:**[33,34] ≥1 y and ≤15 kg: 30 mg once daily po >15–23 kg: 45 mg once daily po >23–40 kg: 60 mg once daily po >40 kg: 75 mg once daily po Duration of prophylaxis is variable and is used for the duration of the outbreak	Nausea, vomiting, headache.	Effective for treatment and prevention of influenza A and B. Treatment is best initiated within 48 h of symptom onset but may be started after 48 h if the illness is severe enough to require hospitalization, the illness is progressive, severe or complicated irrespective of previous health status, or the individual belongs to a high-risk group for severe disease.[10] Available as 30, 45 and 75 mg capsules. Also available as a suspension of 6 mg/mL. If oral suspension is not available the capsules may be opened and mixed with sweetened liquid, such as regular or sugar-free chocolate syrup.	$$-$$$
	zanamivir	**Treatment for ≥7 y:** 10 mg (2 inhalations) BID × 5 days	Bronchospasm has been reported, especially in patients with respiratory disease.	Effective for treatment and prophylaxis against influenza A and B.	$$$

Class	Drug	Dose	Adverse Effects	Comments	Cost[a]
	Relenza	**Prevention for ≥7 y:** Household setting: 10 mg (2 inhalations) daily × 10 days	Headache, dizziness, gastrointestinal upset, cough.	Treatment is best initiated within 48 h of symptom onset but may be started after 48 h if the illness is severe enough to require hospitalization, the illness is progressive, severe or complicated irrespective of previous health status, or the individual belongs to a high-risk group for severe disease.[10] Do not use in patients with asthma or COPD due to risk of serious bronchospasm. Should not be reconstituted and used for nebulization.	
Vaccines, viral	*influenza vaccine, trivalent, inactivated (TIV)* Agriflu, Fluviral, Influvac, Vaxigrip	**All persons ≥6 months:** 0.5 mL im Children 6 months to 8 y who have not previously received influenza vaccine should receive a second dose (0.5 mL) ≥4 weeks after the first dose **Influvac is approved for use in ≥18 y only**	Common: soreness at injection site. Less common: mild flu-like symptoms (myalgias, malaise, low-grade fever). Oculorespiratory syndrome (ORS; bilateral red eyes, breathing symptoms or facial swelling): not considered an allergic reaction.[35] People who had mild or moderate cases of ORS, or severe ORS without lower respiratory symptoms can be reimmunized.[8] Consult the local Medical Officer of Health for advice on more severe reactions.	Acetaminophen after vaccination may help minimize soreness and mild flu-like symptoms. Contraindicated in persons with history of anaphylactic reaction to a previous dose. May be used in persons with an allergy to eggs after a risk assessment. If history of mild reaction to eggs vaccinate in a regular immunization setting; if history of severe reaction consider vaccinating in a specialized setting.[8] Delay vaccination in adults with an acute febrile illness. Vaccine can be given to those with mild upper respiratory tract illness. Can be used in pregnant and nursing women.[8] Case reports of elevated theophylline blood levels following immunization and modified INR (increased or decreased) in patients taking warfarin. Monitor following vaccination.	$[b]
	influenza vaccine, trivalent,inac-tivated (TIV), adjuvanted Fluad	**≥65 y:** 0.5 mL im as a single dose	Common: Injection site reactions (pain, redness) more common than nonadjuvanted influenza vaccine but still considered mild. Less common: mild flu-like symptoms (headache, myalgias, malaise).	Not indicated for persons <65 years of age. Adjuvanted with squalene-based oil-in-water emulsion, MF59. May induce higher immunogenicity than nonadjuvanted influenza vaccines, however, data on comparative efficacy is lacking. Contraindicated in persons with history of anaphylactic reaction to a previous dose. May be used in persons with an allergy to eggs after a risk assessment. If history of mild reaction to eggs vaccinate in a regular immunization setting; if history of severe reaction consider vaccinating in a specialized setting.[8]	$[b]

(cont'd)

Table 2: Drugs Used for the Prevention and Treatment of Influenza[8] *(cont'd)*

Class	Drug	Dose	Adverse Effects	Comments	Cost[a]
	influenza vaccine, trivalent, inactivated (TIV), intradermal Intanza	**18–59 y:** 0.1 mL of 9 µg/strain intradermally **≥60 y:** 0.1 mL of 15 µg/strain intradermally	Common: redness and soreness at intradermal injection site. Less common: mild flu-like symptoms (headache, myalgias, malaise).	Not indicated for children or adolescents <18 y of age. Can be used in pregnant and nursing women.[8] Contraindicated in persons with history of anaphylactic reaction to a previous dose. May be used in persons with an allergy to eggs after a risk assessment. If history of mild reaction to eggs vaccinate in a regular immunization setting; if history of severe reaction consider vaccinating in a specialized setting.[8]	$[b]
	influenza vaccine, trivalent, live attenuated (LAIV) FluMist	**2–59 y:** 0.2 mL intranasally given as 1 spray (0.1 mL) per nostril. Children 2–8 y who have not previously received influenza vaccine should receive a second dose ≥4 wk after the first dose	Nasal congestion, rhinorrhea. Increased incidence of wheezing when administered to children <24 mo of age. This was not observed in older children and adults.	Not indicated for children <2 y or adults >59 y. Preferred vaccine for healthy children 2–18 years of age according to the National Advisory Committee on Immunization. Contraindicated in persons with history of anaphylactic reaction to a previous influenza vaccination or to eggs at this time. Do not use in pregnant women, severely immunocompromised individuals, persons with medically-attended wheezing in the prior 7 days or severe asthma (current use of oral or high-dose inhaled corticosteroid or active wheezing) and those <18 y who use ASA regularly.	$[b]

[a] Cost of course of adult treatment; includes drug cost only.
[b] Public funding of vaccines and eligible recipients varies by province/territory. Check local public health unit for funding status in your area.
Dosage adjustment may be required in renal dysfunction; see Appendix I.
Abbreviations: CAPD = continuous ambulatory peritoneal dialysis; ClCr = creatinine clearance; COPD = chronic obstructive pulmonary disease; CRRT = chronic renal replacement therapy; HD = hemodialysis
Legend: $ < $15 $$ $15–30 $$-$$$ $15–45 $$$ $30–45

References

1. Public Health Agency of Canada. FluWatch. *Definitions for the 2013-2014 season.* Ottawa (ON): PHAC; 2013. Available from: www.phac-aspc.gc.ca/fluwatch/13-14/def13-14-eng.php. Accessed October 11, 2013.
2. Boivin G, Hardy I, Tellier G et al. Predicting influenza infections during epidemics with use of a clinical case definition. *Clin Infect Dis* 2000;31(5):1166-9.
3. Monto AS, Gravenstein S, Elliott M et al. Clinical signs and symptoms predicting influenza infection. *Arch Intern Med* 2000;160(21):3243-7.
4. Cox NJ, Subbarao K. Influenza. *Lancet* 1999;354(9186):1277-82.
5. Govaert TM, Dinant GJ, Aretz K et al. The predictive value of influenza symptomatology in elderly people. *Fam Pract* 1998;15(1):16-22.
6. Gomolin IH, Leib HB, Arden NH et al. Control of influenza outbreaks in the nursing home: guidelines for diagnosis and management. *J Am Geriatr Soc* 1995;43(1):71-4.
7. Canadian Public Health Laboratory Network. *Guidance for laboratory testing for detection and characterization of human influenza virus for the 2010-2011 respiratory virus season.*
8. National Advisory Committee on Immunization (NACI). An Advisory Committee Statement (ACS). Statement on seasonal influenza vaccine for 2013-2014. *Can Commun Dis Rep* 2013;39(ACS-4):1-37. Available from: www.phac-aspc.gc.ca/publicat/ccdr-rmtc/13vol39/acs-dcc-4/index-eng.php. Accessed October 16, 2013.
9. National Advisory Committee on Immunization (NACI). Statement on seasonal influenza vaccine for 2011-2012. An Advisory Committee Statement (ACS). *Can Commun Dis Rep* 2011;37(ACS-5):1-55. Available from: www.phac-aspc.gc.ca/publicat/ccdr-rmtc/11vol37/acs-dcc-5/index-eng.php. Accessed October 3, 2012.
10. Aoki FY, Allen UD, Stiver HG et al. The use of antiviral drugs for influenza: a foundation document for practitioners. *Can J Infect Dis Med Microbiol* 2013;24(Suppl C):1C-15C. Available from: http://www.ammi.ca/guidelines. Accessed December 18, 2013.
11. Public Health Agency of Canada. *FluWatch report: August 11 to August 24, 2013 (Weeks 33 & 34). Antiviral resistance*. Available from: www.phac-aspc.gc.ca/fluwatch/12-13/w34_13/index-eng.php#t3. Accessed October 14, 2013.
12. Bowles SK, Lee W, Simor AE et al. Use of oseltamivir during influenza outbreaks in Ontario nursing homes, 1999-2000. *J Am Geriatr Soc* 2002;50(4):608-16.
13. Jefferson T, Jones MA, Doshi P et al. Neuraminidase inhibitors for preventing and treating influenza in healthy adults and children. *Cochrane Database Syst Rev* 2012;1:CD008965.
14. Wang K, Shun-Shin M, Gill P et al. Neuraminidase inhibitors for preventing and treating influenza in children (published trials only). *Cochrane Database Syst Rev* 2012;4:CD002744.
15. Piedra PA, Schulman KL, Blumentals WA. Effects of oseltamivir on influenza-related complications in children with chronic medical conditions. *Pediatrics* 2009;124(1):170-8.
16. Orzeck EA, Shi N, Blumentals WA. Oseltamivir and the risk of influenza-related complications and hospitalizations in patients with diabetes. *Clin Ther* 2007;29(10):2246-55.
17. Kaiser L, Wat C, Mills T et al. Impact of oseltamivir treatment on influenza-related lower respiratory tract complications and hospitalizations. *Arch Intern Med* 2003;163(14):1667-72.
18. Machado CM, Boas LS, Mendes AV et al. Use of oseltamivir to control influenza complications after bone marrow transplantation. *Bone Marrow Transplant* 2004;34(2):111-4.
19. Aoki FY, Macleod MD, Paggiaro P et al. Early administration of oral oseltamivir increases the benefits of influenza treatment. *J Antimicrob Chemother* 2003;51(1):123-9.
20. Louie JK, Yang S, Acosta M et al. Treatment with neuraminidase inhibitors for critically ill patients with influenza A (H1N1)pdm09. *Clin Infect Dis* 2012;55(9):1198-204.
21. Dodds L, McNeil SA, Fell DB et al. Impact of influenza exposure on rates of hospital admissions and physician visits because of respiratory illness among pregnant women. *CMAJ* 2007;176(4):463-8.
22. Schanzer DL, Langley JM, Tam TW. Influenza-attributed hospitalization rates among pregnant women in Canada 1994-2000. *J Obstet Gynaecol Can* 2007;29(8):622-9.
23. Tuyishime JD, De Wals P, Moutquin JM et al. Influenza-like illness during pregnancy: results from a study in the eastern townships, province of Quebec. *J Obstet Gynaecol Can* 2003;25(12):1020-5.
24. Hartert TV, Neuzil KM, Shintani AK et al. Maternal morbidity and perinatal outcomes among pregnant women with respiratory hospitalizations during influenza season. *Am J Obstet Gynecol* 2003;189(6):1705-12.
25. Neuzil KM, Reed GW, Mitchel EF et al. Impact of influenza on acute cardiopulmonary hospitalizations in pregnant women. *Am J Epidemiol* 1998;148(1):1094-102.
26. Zaman K, Roy E, Arifeen SE et al. Effectiveness of maternal influenza immunization in mothers and infants. *N Engl J Med* 2008;359(15):1555-64.
27. Steinhoff MC, Omer SB, Roy E et al. Influenza immunization in pregnancy—antibody responses in mothers and infants. *N Engl J Med* 2010;362(17):1644-6.
28. MacDonald NE, Riley LE, Steinhoff MC. Influenza immunization in pregnancy. *Obstet Gynecol* 2009;114(2 Pt 1):365-8.
29. Munoz FM, Greisinger AJ, Wehmanen OA et al. Safety of influenza vaccination during pregnancy. *Am J Obstet Gynecol* 2005;192(4):1098-106.
30. Greer LG, Sheffield JS, Rogers VL et al. Maternal and neonatal outcomes after antepartum treatment of influenza with antiviral medications. *Obstet Gynecol* 2010;115(4):711-6.
31. Donner B, Niranjan V, Hoffman G. Safety of oseltamivir in pregnancy: a review of preclinical and clinical data. *Drug Saf* 2010;33(8):631-42.
32. Tanaka T, Nakajima K, Murashima A et al. Safety of neuraminidase inhibitors against novel influenza A (H1N1) in pregnant and breastfeeding women. *CMAJ* 2009;18(1-2):55-8.
33. Oo C, Barrett J, Hill G et al. Pharmacokinetics and dosage recommendations for an oseltamivir oral suspension for the treatment of influenza in children. *Paediatr Drugs* 2001;3(3):229-36.
34. Oo C, Hill G, Dorr A et al. Pharmacokinetics of anti-influenza prodrug oseltamivir in children aged 1-5 years. *Eur J Clin Pharmacol* 2003;59(5-6):411-5.
35. Oculo-respiratory syndrome following influenza vaccination: review of post-marketing surveillance through four influenza seasons in Canada. *Can Commun Dis Rep* 2005;31(21):217-25.

Chapter 117
Malaria Prevention

Courtney Thompson, MD, FRCPC and
Jay Keystone, MSc (CTM), MD, FRCPC

Malaria results in >1 million deaths worldwide each year. The risk of malaria for travellers is *greatest* in sub-Saharan Africa and Oceania, *intermediate* on the Indian subcontinent and Haiti and *lowest* in Southeast Asia and Latin America. There is regional and seasonal variation of risk within these areas. Each year in Canada 300–400 cases of malaria are reported along with several deaths. Since malaria is a potentially fatal disease, it is of utmost importance that travellers take appropriate measures to prevent this infection.

Goals of Therapy

- Assess risk of acquisition of malaria
- Provide safe and effective chemoprophylaxis

Therapeutic Choices

Nonpharmacologic Choices

Malaria transmission by the anopheline mosquito mainly occurs between dusk and dawn. The following measures optimize protection during this time:

- Use **insect repellents** containing **diethyltoluamide** (DEET) before outdoor activity during the main hours of malarial transmission. DEET has been rarely associated with neurologic side effects in children exposed to high concentrations (>35%) and prolonged use. The American Academy of Pediatrics now supports the use of DEET 30% in children as young as 2 months of age.[1]
- In standard formulations, DEET 30% is effective for 4–6 hours. Citronella is usually effective for <1 hour.[2,3]
- Use *bed nets*, preferably impregnated with **permethrin.**[4]
- Use *mosquito coils*, *aerosolized insecticides* or *electrically operated insecticide generators* containing **pyrethroids**.
- Wear clothes covering exposed skin, weather permitting. Permethrin-impregnated clothing adds an additional measure of protection. Sleep in an air-conditioned or screened room if possible.

Pharmacologic Choices

Figure 1 presents pharmacologic choices for malaria prevention.

Principles of Chemoprophylaxis

Determinants of acquisition risk include malaria endemicity, season, altitude, degree of rural travel and preventive measures for mosquito bites. Additional considerations in choosing chemoprophylaxis include antimalarial drug resistance, side effects, concurrent medications and illnesses, contraindications, pregnancy, age and allergies. In theory, all travellers to an endemic area require prophylaxis. However, in parts of Europe, and recently among some North American travel medicine practitioners, prophylaxis recommendations vary according to the degree of risk within a country. For example, personal protection measures alone may be recommended in low-risk areas such as many large urban centres of India. Official national information sources such as the Public Health Agency of Canada and the Centers for Disease Control and Prevention do not usually recommend this approach. Consult an up-to-date source (e.g., Centers for Disease Control and Prevention at wwwnc.cdc.gov/travel/ or Public Health Agency of Canada at www.phac-aspc.gc.ca/tmp-pmv/index-eng.php) about the location and extent of drug-resistant *Plasmodium* species when counselling patients about malaria chemoprophylaxis, as recommendations may change periodically (Figure 1, Table 1).

In Canada, **chloroquine** is recommended for prevention of malaria in areas where the parasite is still sensitive to this drug (Central America [except Panama], Haiti and parts of the Dominican Republic and Middle East).[5] In areas where chloroquine-resistant *P. falciparum* malaria exists, **mefloquine** (except in areas of mefloquine resistance), **doxycycline** or **atovaquone/proguanil** are the drugs of choice.[5] **Primaquine** is an effective alternative (see discussion below). Do not recommend the combination of chloroquine and proguanil because it has limited efficacy in areas with chloroquine-resistant *P. falciparum*.[5] Drugs that are effective in chloroquine-resistant areas may also be used in chloroquine-sensitive areas. Physicians without experience and expertise in malaria chemoprophylaxis should consider referring patients to a well-recognized travel medicine clinic. Listings of travel medicine clinics can be obtained from www.phac-aspc.gc.ca/tmp-pmv/travel/clinic-eng.php.

Figure 1: Malaria Prophylaxis

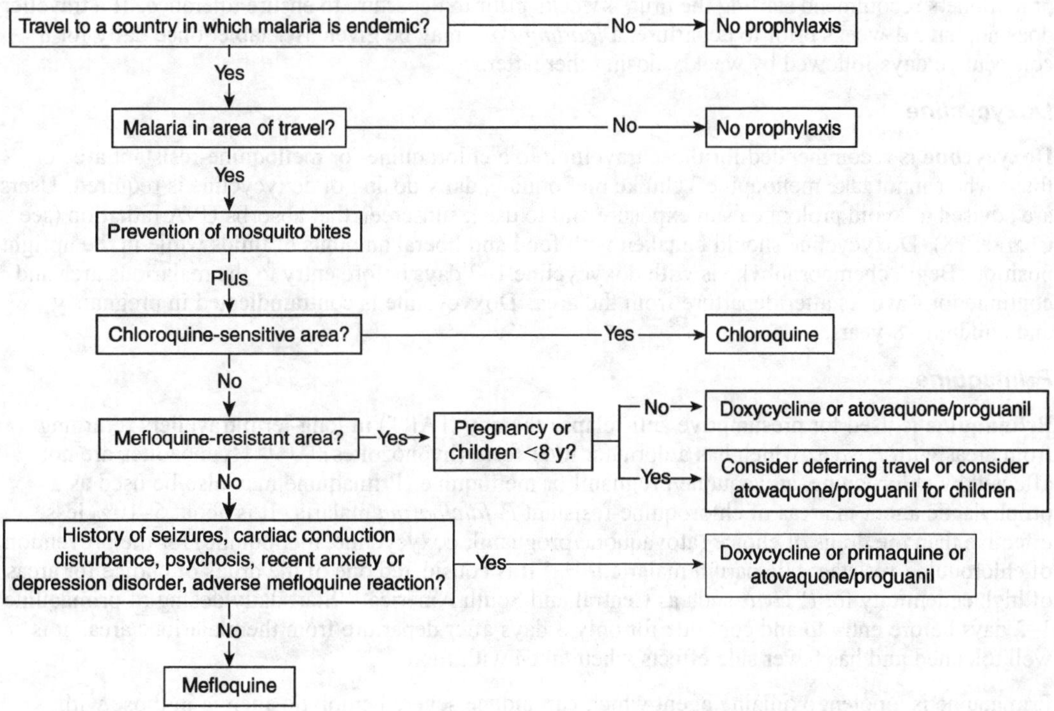

Chloroquine and Hydroxychloroquine

Chloroquine is suitable for travellers of all ages and for pregnant women. **Hydroxychloroquine** is an acceptable alternative to chloroquine and shares a similar side effect profile. Both should be started 1–2 weeks before travelling to and continued until 4 weeks after leaving a malarious area. These agents are well tolerated; however, they may worsen psoriasis and rarely may cause seizures and psychosis. Avoid in travellers with a history of epilepsy or generalized psoriasis. Stomach upset may be reduced by taking with food.

Mefloquine

Mefloquine is used to prevent malaria in travellers going to areas reporting chloroquine-resistant *P. falciparum*.[6,7,8] Do not recommend mefloquine in areas of high resistance such as the Thai-Cambodian and Thai-Myanmar borders, Eastern Myanmar, Western Cambodia and South/Central Vietnam.[6,7,8] Severe neuropsychiatric reactions (seizures and psychosis) occur rarely in patients who use the drug at appropriate prophylactic doses.[9,10] In clinical trials, side effects of mefloquine severe enough to require discontinuation occurred in about 5% of users. Less severe but disabling neuropsychological side effects (e.g., anxiety, nightmares, depression, irritability) are more common, particularly in women.[9,10,11] Other adverse effects (e.g., dizziness, loss of balance or tinnitus) can occur at any time during drug use, and can last for months to years after the drug is stopped or can be permanent.[12] Mefloquine is contraindicated in those with a history of seizures, psychosis, depression or a recent anxiety disorder. Mefloquine should be started 1–2 weeks before travelling to and continued until 4 weeks after leaving a malarious area. Since most adverse events occur during the first 3 doses, many practitioners recommend starting the drug 4 weeks prior to departure to ensure tolerance. If a traveller does not have 4 weeks prior to departure, a *loading dose* may be given as 1 tablet once daily for 3 consecutive days followed by weekly dosing thereafter.

Doxycycline

Doxycycline is recommended for those travelling to a chloroquine- or mefloquine-resistant area or those who cannot take mefloquine.[7] Unlike mefloquine, daily dosing of doxycycline is required. Users are advised to avoid prolonged sun exposure and to use a sunscreen that absorbs UVA radiation (see Chapter 98). Doxycycline should be taken with food and liberal amounts of fluids while in the upright position. Begin chemoprophylaxis with doxycycline 1–2 days before entry to the malarious area and continue for 4 weeks after departure from the area. Doxycycline is contraindicated in pregnancy and children <8 years.

Primaquine

Primaquine is used for presumptive anti-relapse therapy (PART) in long-term travellers returning from areas with *P. vivax* which has a dormant liver form (hypnozoites).[13,14,15] Hypnozoites are not affected by chloroquine, atovaquone/proguanil or mefloquine. Primaquine may also be used as a prophylactic agent in areas of chloroquine-resistant *P. falciparum* malaria. It is about 5–10% less effective than the drugs of choice (atovaquone/proguanil, doxycycline, mefloquine) for the prevention of chloroquine-resistant falciparum malaria.[13,14,15] It is considered one of the drugs of choice for areas of high endemicity for *P. vivax* such as Central and South America.[16] Start daily dosing of primaquine 1–2 days before entry to and continue for only 3 days after departure from the malarious area. It is well tolerated and has fewer side effects when taken with food.

Primaquine is a potent oxidizing agent which can induce severe hemolytic anemia in those with glucose-6-phosphate dehydrogenase (G6PD) deficiency. In risk groups for this enzyme deficiency (Blacks, Mediterraneans, Asians and Southeast Asians), a G6PD level is mandatory before primaquine is used. The drug is contraindicated in pregnancy.

Atovaquone/Proguanil

Atovaquone/proguanil is useful for malaria prophylaxis in areas resistant to chloroquine and mefloquine.[17] Atovaquone/proguanil should be taken daily with food, starting 1–2 days before entry to a malarious area and discontinued 1 week after departure from the area, making it particularly suitable for last-minute travellers or those going on short trips.[17] Compared to mefloquine, atovaquone/proguanil is more expensive but causes significantly less neuropsychiatric adverse effects [Evidence: SORT A*].[18,19] The drug is not recommended in pregnancy, severe renal impairment or when breastfeeding a child <5 kg.[20,21]

Malaria Prophylaxis in Children

For children planning to visit malarious areas, effective protection against mosquitoes and appropriate chemoprophylaxis is strongly recommended. **Doxycycline** is contraindicated in children <8 years old or <11 kg. In chloroquine-sensitive areas, **chloroquine** is recommended for young children. In chloroquine-resistant areas, **mefloquine** can be used in children >5 kg. **Atovaquone/proguanil** in pediatric dosage form is safe and effective for children weighing >5 kg. **Azithromycin** is safe in young children but its effectiveness is suboptimal. Although there are no data on the safety or efficacy of chemoprophylaxis for children <5 kg who travel to mefloquine-resistant areas, travel medicine practitioners recommend atovaquone/proguanil or mefloquine for children <5 kg based on a risk-benefit assessment.

Choices during Pregnancy and Breastfeeding

Malaria Prophylaxis during Pregnancy

Pregnant women are more susceptible to malaria (anopheline mosquitoes are more attracted to pregnant than nonpregnant women) and once infected exhibit higher morbidity and mortality rates than the nonpregnant population.[22] Malaria in pregnancy is associated with an increased risk of low birth weight, maternal anemia and fetal death. In addition, premature labour may result from fever causing uterine contractions.[23] The risk of adverse effects from malaria is highest in those with falciparum malaria and in women who have not been exposed to malaria before. Adverse events associated with *P. vivax* malaria tend to be less severe. Since the consequences of malaria in pregnancy are potentially very serious, women who wish to travel to malarious areas need to consider both the risk of malaria and potential adverse effects of chemoprophylaxis. However, even the best personal protection measures, including chemoprophylaxis, are not always effective.

Avoidance and prevention of bites, particularly between dusk and dawn, requires the application of insect repellents to exposed skin and, weather permitting, wearing of long-sleeved shirts and trousers. Although **DEET** crosses the placenta, DEET-containing repellents are highly recommended because of their demonstrated efficacy and safety in the 2nd and 3rd trimesters of pregnancy.[24] However, more information is required on the safety of DEET in the 1st trimester of pregnancy. In addition, pyrethroid derivatives such as **permethrin** can be safely used to impregnate bed nets and clothing.

Chloroquine has a long history of safe use during pregnancy and is recommended for prophylaxis in the few areas of the world where malaria is still sensitive to chloroquine. When used, start chloroquine 1–2 weeks before travel and continue for 4 weeks after leaving a malarious area. Although there are case reports of stillbirths and spontaneous abortions associated with **mefloquine** use,[25] causality has not been determined. Mefloquine remains the drug of choice for pregnant women who require malaria prophylaxis in a chloroquine-resistant area.[26] Seizures and psychosis due to mefloquine are rare during prophylaxis but anxiety, nightmares, depression and irritability are more common. Consequently, mefloquine is contraindicated in those with a history of seizures, psychosis, depression or a recent

* SORT (Strength of Recommendation Taxonomy) is a rating system (A, B or C) that addresses the quality of available evidence. For more information consult **How to Use *Compendium of Therapeutic Choices*** on page xxv.

anxiety disorder. **Azithromycin** is safe in pregnant women but its effectiveness is suboptimal. There is no safe and effective chemoprophylaxis for pregnant women who travel to mefloquine-resistant areas. **Doxycycline**, **primaquine** and **atovaquone/proguanil** are contraindicated in pregnancy. For women who are contemplating pregnancy soon after travel to a chloroquine-resistant area, it is advisable to wait long enough (depending on the half-life of the antimalarial used) before conceiving. See the CDC website wwwnc.cdc.gov/travel/yellowbook/2014/chapter-8-advising-travelers-with-specific-needs/pregnant-travelers.

Malaria Prophylaxis during Breastfeeding

Nursing mothers may use **DEET**-containing mosquito repellents on exposed skin. No adverse effects have been reported among breastfed infants whose mothers use DEET.

There is little evidence-based information on malaria chemoprophylaxis in breastfeeding travellers. Breastfed children do not receive sufficient drug in breast milk to protect them from malaria and must receive chemoprophylaxis regardless of age. Both **chloroquine** and **hydroxychloroquine** may be used safely during breastfeeding. Although no neuropsychiatric adverse effects have been reported in breastfed infants whose mothers are taking **mefloquine**, it is prudent to discontinue breastfeeding if significant change in sleep or behaviour is suspected in the child. However, such changes may be due to travel itself. There are no data regarding the excretion of **atovaquone/proguanil** in breast milk in humans. According to the American Academy of Pediatrics no untoward effects have been found in infants of breastfeeding women using tetracyclines, suggesting that **doxycycline** should be safe. No data are available on the use of **primaquine** during breastfeeding or the excretion of primaquine in breast milk. Primaquine is contraindicated during breastfeeding unless normal G6PD activities have been documented in both the mother and the infant.

A discussion of general principles on the use of medications in these special populations can be found in Appendix II and Appendix III. Other specialized reference sources are also provided in these appendices.

Therapeutic Tips

- **Mefloquine** is not favoured as a prophylactic agent by some physicians in the United Kingdom and in developing countries. Travellers may be advised by physicians and travellers from these areas that they are taking a dangerous drug. In general, such advice should be accepted politely and ignored.
- No currently available regimen of malaria chemoprophylaxis is ideal and completely effective. Adhering to the chemoprophylaxis regimen helps reduce the risk of malaria acquisition. Drug-resistant malaria continues to spread.
- Remind travellers in writing to continue taking their antimalarials even after their return from an endemic region. All travellers in whom fever develops within 1 year (particularly within 3 months) of return from a malaria-endemic area must be considered to have malaria, regardless of chemoprophylaxis. Consider this a medical emergency. Request thick and thin blood films or a rapid diagnostic test to rule out malaria. If negative, repeat them twice over 48 hours.
- In sub-Saharan Africa, the rate of false-positive blood films for malaria is at least 40%.[27] Warn travellers in this area that if they are taking an appropriate antimalarial regularly and are diagnosed with "malaria," they should follow the advice of local practitioners, but not stop their chemoprophylaxis.
- Advise travellers to buy their full supply of medications before departure. The sale of poor-quality and counterfeit antimalarials is rampant in the developing world.[28]

Table 1: Drugs Used for Malaria Chemoprophylaxis

Class	Drug	Dose	Adverse Effects	Comments	Cost[a]
Antimalarials, combination	*atovaquone/ proguanil* Malarone, Malarone Pediatric, generics	Start 1 day prior to exposure, continue *daily* while in the malarial region and for 1 wk after leaving the endemic area Administer with a meal **Children:**[36] Use Malarone Pediatric (62.5 mg/25 mg) 5–8 kg: ½ pediatric tablet once daily po 9–10 kg: ¾ pediatric tablet once daily po 11–20 kg: 1 pediatric tablet once daily po 21–30 kg: 2 pediatric tablets once daily po 31–40 kg: 3 pediatric tablets once daily po >40 kg: Adult dose **Adults:** 250 mg/100 mg daily po (use Malarone 250 mg/100 mg) ClCr <30 mL/min: avoid	Common: GI upset, headache.	Used in regions of chloroquine-resistant *P. falciparum*; can be used for prevention of multidrug-resistant *P. falciparum.* Acts on pre-erythrocytic hepatic phase of malaria but it does not prevent the hypnozoite formation by *P. ovale* or *P. vivax*. Not recommended in pregnancy. Contraindicated in patients with renal insufficiency.	$$$$$
Quinoline Derivatives	*chloroquine phosphate* ❥ generics	Each tablet contains chloroquine phosphate 250 mg (equivalent to chloroquine base 155 mg) Start 1–2 wk prior to exposure and continue *weekly* for 4 wk after leaving the endemic area A loading dose of 1000 mg phosphate salt can be used in adults or 16 mg/kg phosphate salt can be given to children in 2 divided doses 6 h apart if chloroquine is not initiated 1–2 wk prior to exposure **Children:**[29] 8 mg/kg phosphate salt (5 mg/kg base) once/wk po to a maximum of 500 mg phosphate salt (310 mg base) **Adults:** 500 mg phosphate salt (310 mg base or 2 tablets) once/wk po Adjust dose when ClCr <10 mL/min	Common: nonallergic pruritus in African Canadians, vomiting, headache, bitter taste. Uncommon: hair depigmentation, skin eruptions, myopathy, reversible corneal opacity, partial alopecia, blood dyscrasias. Rare: nail and mucous membrane discolouration, nerve deafness, photophobia, retinopathy, myopathy.	Safe to use in pregnancy. Retinal toxicity a concern with continuous use of chloroquine, i.e., cumulative dose >100 g chloroquine base. Screen for retinal changes every 6–12 months if taking chloroquine for >5 y.[30,31] No pediatric formulation is available in Canada and drug has an exceptionally bitter taste. Crushed tablets can be difficult to manipulate and store. The powder must be mixed with a very sweet food. Alternatively, a compounding pharmacist can prepare a flavoured suspension.	$

(cont'd)

Table 1: **Drugs Used for Malaria Chemoprophylaxis** *(cont'd)*

Class	Drug	Dose	Adverse Effects	Comments	Cost[a]
	hydroxychloroquine sulfate Plaquenil, generics	Each tablet contains hydroxychloroquine sulfate 200 mg (equivalent to hydroxychloroquine base 155 mg) Start 1–2 wk prior to exposure and continue *weekly* for 4 wk after leaving the endemic area An oral loading dose of 800 mg sulfate salt can be used in adults or 13 mg/kg sulfate salt can be given to children in 2 divided doses 6 h apart if hydroxychloroquine is not initiated 2 wk prior to exposure **Children:** 6.5 mg/kg sulfate salt (5 mg/kg base) once/wk po. Maximum: 400 mg sulfate salt (310 mg base) once/wk po **Adults:** 400 mg sulfate salt (310 mg base) once/wk po	See chloroquine.	See chloroquine. Each dose should be taken with a meal or a glass of milk.	$
	mefloquine generics	Each tablet contains mefloquine base 250 mg (equivalent to mefloquine hydrochloride 274 mg) Start 1 wk prior to exposure, *weekly* during the stay in the region and weekly for 4 wk after leaving the endemic area. Administer with a meal and with at least 240 mL of water. **Children:** 5–9 kg: 31.25 mg base (⅛ tablet) once/wk po 10–19 kg: 62.5 mg base (¼ tablet) once/wk po 20–29 kg: 125 mg base (½ tablet) once/wk po 30–45 kg: 187.5 mg base (¾ tablet) once/wk po >45 kg: adult dose **Adults:** 250 mg base (1 tablet) once/wk po Loading dose: 250 mg base *daily* po for 3 days, then 250 mg base *weekly* thereafter.	Common: GI upset, dizziness, nausea, vomiting, diarrhea, headaches, sinus bradycardia, nightmares, insomnia, mood alteration, anxiety, irritability. Uncommon: hair loss, skin rash. Rare: seizures, psychosis, thrombotic-thrombocytopenia purpura.[32]	Used in regions of chloroquine-resistant *P. falciparum*; does not prevent mefloquine-resistant *P. falciparum*. Contraindicated in patients with seizure disorders, active depression, recent history of depression episodes, anxiety disorders. Loading dose confers quicker attainment of steady state (4 days as opposed to 7–9 wk). Loading dose is associated with an increased risk of depression. When possible, mefloquine may be started 4 wk prior to departure since 70% of severe adverse reactions occur within the first 3 doses. Considered drug of choice for pregnant women who require malaria prophylaxis in a chloroquine-resistant area.	$$

Class	Drug	Dose	Adverse Effects	Comments	Cost[a]
	primaquine phosphate Primaquine	Each tablet contains primaquine base 15 mg (equivalent to primaquine phosphate 26.3 mg) Start 1 day prior to exposure, continue *daily* while in the malarial region and for 3 days after leaving the endemic area Administer with food **Children (>9 y):** Prophylaxis: 0.5 mg base/kg/day po. Maximum: 30 mg base (2 tablets) daily po Post-exposure: 0.5 mg base/kg/day po × 14 days. Maximum: 30 mg base (2 tablets) daily po **Adults:** Prophylaxis: 30 mg base (2 tablets) daily po; <60 kg: 0.5 mg base/kg/day po. Maximum: 30 mg base or 2 tablets daily po[33] Post-exposure: 30 mg base (2 tablets) daily po × 14 days	Common: hemolysis with glucose-6-phosphate dehydrogenase deficiency. Uncommon: GI upset (take with food). Rare: methemoglobinemia.	Used in regions of chloroquine-resistant *P. falciparum*. Determine glucose-6-phosphate dehydrogenase deficiency in all individuals prior to administration. Contraindicated in pregnancy because of unknown glucose-6-phosphate dehydrogenase status of infant and subsequent risk of hemolysis. Methemoglobinemia has been precipitated in HIV-infected patients who are being treated or are on prophylactic therapy for *P. jirovecii* pneumonia, especially if taken with dapsone.[33,34,35]	$
Tetracyclines	*doxycycline* Vibramycin, generics	Start 1 day prior to exposure, continue *daily* while in the malarial region and for 4 wk after leaving the endemic area Administer with food and plenty of water. Important not to recline after administration. **Children: ≥8 y:** 2 mg/kg/day po. Maximum: 100 mg/day **Adults:** 100 mg daily po	Common: GI upset, photosensitivity, staining of teeth in children and fetuses, *candida vaginitis* (use fluconazole for self-treatment). Uncommon: azotemia in renal disease, enterocolitis. Rare: allergic reactions, blood dyscrasias, esophageal ulcerations.	Used in regions of chloroquine-resistant *P. falciparum*; can be used for prevention of multidrug-resistant *P. falciparum*. Contraindicated in pregnancy and children <8 y. Because of the increased risk of photosensitivity, use sunscreens to block UV radiation.	$$

[a] Cost of adult dosage for 1 week of travel; includes drug cost only.

Dosage adjustment may be required in renal impairment; see Appendix I.

Legend: $ <$15 $$ $15–30 $$$ $30–45 $$$$ $45–60 $$$$$ $60–75

Suggested Readings

Amet S, Zimner-Rapuch S, Launay-Vacher V et al. Malaria prophylaxis in patients with renal impairment: a review. *Drug Saf* 2013;36(2):83-91.

Chen LH, Zeind C, Mackell S et al. Breastfeeding travelers: precautions and recommendations. *J Travel Med* 2010;17(1):32-47.

Fischer PR, Bialek R. Prevention of malaria in children. *Clin Infect Dis* 2002;34(4):493-8.

Genton B, D'Acremont V. Malaria prevention in travelers. *Infect Dis Clin North Am* 2012;26(3):637-54.

Heppner DG. The malaria vaccine—status quo 2013. *Travel Med Infect Dis* 2013;11(1):2-7.

Johnson BA, Kalra MG. Prevention of malaria in travelers. *Am Fam Physician* 2012;85(10):973-7.

Royal College of Obstetricians and Gynaecologists (RCOG). *The prevention of malaria in pregnancy.* London (GB): RCOG; 2010. Available from: www.guideline.gov/content.aspx?id=25671.

References

1. American Academy of Pediatrics. *Summer safety tips*. Elk Grove Village (IL): AAP; 2013. Available from: www.aap.org/en-us/about-the-aap/aap-press-room/news-features-and-safety-tips/Pages/Summer-Safety-Tips.aspx. Accessed November 15, 2013.
2. Fradin MS, Day JF. Comparative efficacy of insect repellents against mosquito bites. *N Engl J Med* 2002;347(1):13-8.
3. Hill DR, Ericsson CD, Pearson RD et al. The practice of travel medicine: guidelines by the Infectious Diseases Society of America. *Clin Infect Dis* 2006;43(12):1499-539.
4. Nevill CG, Some ES, Mung'ala VO et al. Insecticide-treated bednets reduce mortality and severe morbidity from malaria among children on the Kenyan coast. *Trop Med Int Health* 1996;1(2):139-46.
5. Kain KC, Shanks GD, Keystone JS. Malaria chemoprophylaxis in the age of drug resistance. I. Currently recommended drug regimens. *Clin Infect Dis* 2001;33(2):226-34.
6. Nosten F, ter KF, Maelankiri L et al. Mefloquine prophylaxis prevents malaria during pregnancy: a double-blind, placebo-controlled study. *J Infect Dis* 1994;169(3):595-603.
7. Ohrt C, Richie TL, Widjaja H et al. Mefloquine compared with doxycycline for the prophylaxis of malaria in Indonesian soldiers. A randomized, double-blind, placebo-controlled trial. *Ann Intern Med* 1997;126(12):963-72.
8. Overbosch D, Schilthuis H, Bienzle U et al. Atovaquone-proguanil versus mefloquine for malaria prophylaxis in nonimmune travelers: results from a randomized, double-blind study. *Clin Infect Dis* 2001;33(7):1015-21.
9. Taylor WR, White NJ. Antimalarial drug toxicity: a review. *Drug Saf* 2004;27(1):25-61.
10. Palmer KJ, Holliday SM, Brogden RN. Mefloquine. A review of its antimalarial activity, pharmacokinetic properties and therapeutic efficacy. *Drugs* 1993;45(3):430-75.
11. van Riemsdijk MM, Sturkenboom MC, Ditters JM et al. Low body mass index is associated with an increased risk of neuropsychiatric adverse events and concentration impairment in women on mefloquine. *Br J Clin Pharmacol* 2004;57(4):506-12.
12. U.S. Food and Drug Administration. *Mefloquine hydrochloride: Drug safety communication—Label changes due to risk of serious psychiatric and nerve side effects*. Available from: www.fda.gov/Safety/MedWatch/SafetyInformation/SafetyAlertsforHumanMedicalProducts/ucm362887.htm.
13. Baird JK, Lacy MD, Basri H et al. Randomized, parallel placebo-controlled trial of primaquine for malaria prophylaxis in Papua, Indonesia. *Clin Infect Dis* 2001;33(12):1990-7.
14. Soto J, Toledo J, Rodriquez M et al. Primaquine prophylaxis against malaria in nonimmune Colombian soldiers: efficacy and toxicity. A randomized, double-blind, placebo-controlled trial. *Ann Intern Med* 1998;129(3):241-4.
15. Weiss WR, Oloo AJ, Johnson A et al. Daily primaquine is effective for prophylaxis against falciparum malaria in Kenya: comparison with mefloquine, doxycycline, and chloroquine plus proguanil. *J Infect Dis* 1995;171(6):1569-75.
16. Arguin PM, Tan KR. Chapter 3: Infectious diseases related to travel. Malaria. In: Centers for Disease Control and Prevention. *Travelers' health: Yellow book*. Available from: wwwnc.cdc.gov/travel/yellowbook/2014/chapter-3-infectious-diseases-related-to-travel/malaria. Accessed November 15, 2013.
17. Public Health Agency of Canada. 8. Drugs for the prevention and treatment of malaria. In: *Canadian recommendations for the prevention and treatment of malaria among international travellers*. Available from: www.phac-aspc.gc.ca/publicat/ccdr-rmtc/09vol35/35s1/page8-eng.php. Accessed December 5, 2014.
18. U.S. National Library of Medicine. PubMed Health. Drugs for preventing malaria in travellers. *Cochrane Database Syst Rev* 2009;(4):CD006491. [Plain language summaries].
19. Kato T, Okuda J, Ide D et al. Questionnaire-based analysis of atovaquone-proguanil compared with mefloquine in the chemoprophylaxis of malaria in non-immune Japanese travelers. *J Infect Chemother* 2013;19(1):20-3.
20. Public Health Agency of Canada. 5. Prevention in special hosts. In: *Canadian recommendations for the prevention and treatment of malaria among international travellers*. Available from: www.phac-aspc.gc.ca/publicat/ccdr-rmtc/09vol35/35s1/page5-eng.php. Accessed December 5, 2014.
21. U.S. Centers for Disease Control and Prevention. *Choosing a drug to prevent malaria*. Available from: www.cdc.gov/malaria/travelers/drugs.html. Accessed December 5, 2014.
22. McGready R, Ashley EA, Nosten F. Malaria and the pregnant traveller. *Travel Med Infect Dis* 2004;2(3-4):127-42.
23. Luxemburger C, McGready R, Kham A et al. Effects of malaria during pregnancy on infant mortality in an area of low malaria transmission. *Am J Epidemiol* 2001;154(5):459-65.
24. McGready R, Hamilton KA, Simpson JA et al. Safety of the insect repellent N,N-diethyl-M-toluamide (DEET) in pregnancy. *Am J Trop Med Hyg* 2001;65(4):285-9.
25. Vanhauwere B, Maradit H, Kerr L. Post-marketing surveillance of prophylactic mefloquine (Lariam) use in pregnancy. *Am J Trop Med Hyg* 1998;58(1):17-21.
26. Irvine MH, Einarson A, Bozzo P. Prophylactic use of antimalarials during pregnancy. *Can Fam Physician* 2011;57(11):1279-81.

27. Reyburn H, Mbatia R, Drakeley C et al. Overdiagnosis of malaria in patients with severe febrile illness in Tanzania: a prospective study. *BMJ* 2004;329(7476):1212.
28. Dondorp AM, Newton PN, Mayxay M et al. Fake antimalarials in Southeast Asia are a major impediment to malaria control: multinational cross-sectional survey on the prevalence of fake antimalarials. *Trop Med Int Health* 2004;9(12):1241-6.
29. Chiodini PL, Field VK, Hill DR et al. *Guidelines for malaria prevention in travellers from the UK*. London (GB): Public Health England; August 2013. Available from: www.hpa.org.uk/web/HPAwebFile/HPAweb_C/1203496943523. Accessed November 15, 2013.
30. Chen LH, Wilson ME, Schlagenhauf P. Prevention of malaria in long-term travelers. *JAMA* 2006;296(18):2234-44.
31. Hughes C, Tucker R, Bannister B et al. Malaria prophylaxis for long-term travellers. *Commun Dis Public Health* 2003;6(3):200-8.
32. Fiaccadori E, Maggiore U, Rotelli C et al. Thrombotic-thrombocytopenic purpura following malaria prophylaxis with mefloquine. *J Antimicrob Chemother* 2006;57(1):160-1.
33. Hill DR, Baird JK, Parise ME et al. Primaquine: report from CDC expert meeting on malaria chemoprophylaxis I. *Am J Trop Med Hyg* 2006;75(3):402-15.
34. Sin DD, Shafran SD. Dapsone- and primaquine-induced methemoglobinemia in HIV-infected individuals. *J Acquir Immune Defic Syndr Hum Retrovirol* 1996;12(5):477-81.
35. Kantor GS. Primaquine-induced methemoglobinemia during treatment of Pneumocystis carinii pneumonia. *N Engl J Med* 1992;327(20):1461.
36. Boggild AK, Parise ME, Lewis LS et al. Atovaquone-proguanil: report from the CDC expert meeting on malaria chemoprophylaxis (II). *Am J Trop Med Hyg* 2007;76(2):208-23.

Chapter 118
Opportunistic Infections in HIV-positive Patients

Lise Bondy, BSc, MD, FRCPC and
Sharon Walmsley, MSc, MD, FRCPC

CPhA acknowledges the contribution of Dr. Edward Ralph as a previous author of this chapter.

Opportunistic infections are a major cause of mortality and morbidity in HIV-positive patients and may be the first evidence of immunodeficiency leading to the diagnosis of HIV (human immunodeficiency virus) or acquired immunodeficiency syndrome (AIDS). Susceptibility to specific opportunistic infections increases as the CD4 (helper T-cell) count declines. This relationship is very useful in the differential diagnosis of various infectious syndromes, especially at CD4 counts <200/µL.[1]

Goals of Therapy

- Prevent specific infections
- Treat established opportunistic infections
- Reduce drug burden by discontinuing chemoprophylactic regimens and maintenance therapy when appropriate
- Initiate antiretroviral therapy at the appropriate time and minimize drug interactions during treatment of opportunistic infections

Investigations

The initial investigations will be predicated on whether the patient is symptomatic. If a patient is asymptomatic, the following tests establish a baseline for determining the susceptibility to reactivation of various opportunistic infections.[2] In general, latent infections can reactivate as the CD4 count declines.

- Complete blood count
- Lymphocyte flow cytometry—CD4 count and percentage, CD4/CD8 ratio
- HIV viral load and genotypic resistance test
- Tuberculin skin test (consider a 2-step test), or interferon gamma release assay (used in some settings but reliability in HIV unclear). Either test may not perform as well in those with advanced HIV disease; in this setting consider repeating the test after CD4 improves with antiretroviral therapy or consider empiric prophylaxis in individuals from high-risk endemic areas
- Hepatitis A, B and C virus serology
- Herpes virus serology: varicella-zoster virus (VZV), cytomegalovirus (CMV)
- Toxoplasma serology
- Syphilis serology (screening test)
- Chest x-ray
- Pap test (cervical ± anal if available)

- Baseline biochemistry profile (prior to initiating drug therapy):
  - albumin
  - alkaline phosphatase
  - aminotransferases
  - bilirubin
  - urea
  - serum creatinine, creatinine clearance
  - serum electrolytes
  - serum amylase
  - creatine kinase
  - lactate dehydrogenase
  - lipid profile (fasting)
  - fasting blood glucose/HbA_{1C}
  - urinalysis
- Glucose-6-phosphate dehydrogenase—in members of at-risk groups prior to treatment with oxidant medications (sulfonamides or dapsone)

If a patient has symptoms of a specific opportunistic infection, order appropriate investigations.

Therapeutic Choices

Nonpharmacologic Choices

Advise patients with HIV infection and immunosuppression that their risk of infections can be reduced by following good hygienic practices.

- Ensure thorough hand washing after contact with potentially contaminated substances (diapers, soil, uncooked meat and produce) or handling pets and their feces
- Avoid raw or uncooked meat and eggs, e.g., Caesar salad
- Drink from treated water sources only
- Avoid handling sick animals or pet (especially cat) litter
- Avoid cat scratches and do not allow cats to lick wounds
- Avoid contact with reptiles
- Take appropriate precautions when travelling to countries with poor sanitary standards

Pharmacologic Choices

Preventive interventions are outlined in Table 1.

Consider starting antiretroviral therapy (ART) concurrently with therapy for opportunistic infections, with the possible exception of cryptococcal meningitis, to improve immune function.[1] Early ART initiation after cryptococcal meningitis decreases survival; delay starting ART for 2–10 weeks after initiation of cryptococcal therapy.[1] In cases of advanced disease (CD4 <50 cells/µL), ART may need to be initiated earlier, but would require monitoring for immune reconstitution syndrome and aggressive treatment if it occurs. See also Immune Reconstitution Inflammatory Syndromes and Chapter 113.

In patients who are not receiving ART at the time of TB therapy initiation and whose CD4 count is <50 cells/µL, ART should be initiated within 2 weeks of therapy; if the CD4 count is >50 cells/µL ART should be initiated within 8 weeks.[1] In the setting of other opportunistic infections, such as *P. jirovecii* pneumonia, early initiation of ART is associated with increased survival.

Table 1: **Preventive Interventions for HIV-positive Patients**[1,3]

Indications	Condition	Prophylactic Therapy[a]
Independent of CD4 count	Routine immunizations	Update all vaccines (no live vaccines with the possible exception of MMR and varicella vaccines if CD4 ≥200/μL)
	CA-MRSA	Higher rates in men who have sex with men (MSM) and intravenous drug users. Consider screening swabs in patients with recurrent skin and soft tissue infections. For patients with recurrent MRSA infections consider offering decolonization
	Hepatitis	Hepatitis A vaccine for nonimmune individuals Hepatitis B vaccine for nonimmune individuals. Consider 40 μg dose (dialysis dose or double adult dose depending on preparation used) as vaccine less immunogenic in HIV-positive patients Perform postimmunization serologic testing for hepatitis B. Repeat vaccination series if anti-HBs titre of >10 IU/L not achieved
	Herpes simplex, frequent oral or genital outbreaks	Suppressive therapy with acyclovir, famciclovir or valacyclovir (Table 5)
	Human papillomavirus (HPV)[b]	Cervical Pap smear twice in the first year after diagnosis of HIV infection, then annually if the results are normal. Refer women with atypical squamous cells for colposcopy HPV vaccine in men 9–26 years and women 9–45 years. May be considered in MSM ≥27 years Use of HPV vaccine in older adults with HIV controversial
	Influenza	Annual influenza immunization with inactivated vaccine preparation; live-attenuated influenza vaccine contraindicated
	Meningococcal disease	Meningococcal conjugate vaccine (Men ACYW-135)—consider in all HIV-infected patients, especially MSM and travellers to endemic or outbreak regions Give 2 doses at least 8 weeks apart and a booster dose every 5 years
	Pneumococcal infection	Conjugate pneumococcal vaccine 13-valent as the first dose, followed by at least 8 weeks later by the 23-valent polysaccharide pneumococcal vaccine. Repeat the 23-valent polysaccharide vaccine once after 5 years
	Sexually transmitted infections (STIs)	Patients on antiretroviral therapy can become infected with STIs including resistant HIV strains. Condom use is recommended for oral, anal and vaginal intercourse Screen all patients at baseline for chlamydia, gonorrhea and syphilis. Female patients should be screened for trichomoniasis Lymphogranuloma venereum, caused by *Chlamydia trachomatis* serotypes L1, L2 and L3, has emerged as a cause of proctitis and/or femoral or inguinal lymphadenopathy in MSM. Diagnosis is based on a compatible clinical syndrome in combination with serology, nucleic acid amplification testing or chlamydial culture Periodic follow-up screening for STIs depending on patient's risk behaviours. Syphilis screening recommended at least yearly for MSM
	Travel	Consultation with a travel medicine provider 4–6 weeks before travel is advised HIV-positive individuals are at higher risk of developing severe malaria. Effective chemoprophylaxis and personal protection measures are essential. Prophylaxis with atovaquone and proguanil may be less effective in patients taking efavirenz-containing ART due to a drug interaction
	Varicella	Postexposure prophylaxis with IVIG for nonimmune patients Immunization with 2 doses of varicella vaccine administered 3 months apart may be considered if CD4 cell count ≥200/μL and percentage ≥15% Risks and benefits of live vaccine should be discussed with patient's HIV specialist

(cont'd)

Table 1: **Preventive Interventions for HIV-positive Patients**[1,3] *(cont'd)*

Indications	Condition	Prophylactic Therapy[a]
Positive PPD (≥5 mm) or IGRA, independent of CD4 count	*Mycobacterium tuberculosis*	The preferred prophylactic therapy is isoniazid + pyridoxine for 9 months (Table 9) Rifampin for 4 months is an alternative[c]
CD4 <200 cells/µL or thrush	*Pneumocystis jirovecii* pneumonia (PCP)	The preferred prophylactic therapy is SMX/TMP (Table 10) Alternatives include dapsone, atovaquone or monthly inhaled pentamidine (Table 10)
CD4 <100 cells/µL and positive *T. gondii* serology	*Toxoplasma gondii* encephalitis	The preferred prophylactic therapy is SMX/TMP (Table 10) Atovaquone is an alternative (Table 10)
CD4 <50 cells/µL	*Mycobacterium avium* complex	The preferred prophylactic therapy is a macrolide (azithromycin once weekly or clarithromycin twice daily) (Table 9) Rifabutin is an alternative (Table 9)
	Cytomegalovirus	Prophylaxis is not cost effective. The focus of therapy is restoration of the immune system
	Fungal infections	Fluconazole may be used for persons with recurrent thrush or prior esophageal candidiasis (Table 6)

[a] For many vaccines, suppression of HIV RNA by antiretroviral therapy is recognized as a factor to increased immunogenicity. In some settings it may be prudent to delay or repeat immunization once this has occurred.
[b] Only the quadrivalent HPV vaccine is indicated in males.
[c] Rifampin significantly alters the pharmacokinetics of many drugs including antiretroviral agents and its use is contraindicated with some drugs. Therefore, the regimen must be carefully reviewed, and modified if necessary, before starting and stopping rifampin therapy.
Abbreviations: Anti-HBs = antibody to hepatitis B surface; ART = antiretroviral therapy; CA-MRSA = community-acquired methicillin-resistant *S. aureus*; HPV = human papillomavirus; IGRA = interferon-gamma release assay; IVIG = iv immune globulin; MSM = men who have sex with men; PPD = purified protein derivative; SMX/TMP = sulfamethoxazole/trimethoprim

Clinical Syndromes

Respiratory Tract Syndromes

Most upper respiratory tract symptoms are caused by viruses, but bacterial superinfections (otitis media, sinusitis) are more common in HIV-infected patients and require antibiotic treatment. Community-acquired pneumonia in patients with CD4 counts >200/µL can be treated in the same manner as for a patient without HIV infection (see Chapter 110). As the CD4 count declines to <200/µL, *Pneumocystis jirovecii* (formerly *P. carinii*) becomes an increasingly important pathogen. At counts <100/µL, *Mycobacterium avium* complex (MAC), CMV, *Cryptococcus neoformans* and *Aspergillus* spp. are more frequently isolated. Empiric treatment for *P. jirovecii* is often started in patients in whom the diagnosis is suspected (fever, dyspnea, chest x-ray findings). Bronchoscopy with bronchoalveolar lavage or induced sputum is often required to confirm the diagnosis and may reveal the presence of other opportunistic pathogens.

Painful Mouth and Swallowing

Oral candidiasis is very common and occurs more frequently with CD4 counts <200/µL. Diagnosis is based on clinical appearance (white curdy lesions on the buccal mucosa that scrape off) and not on the basis of isolation of *Candida* from the oral mucosa. Treatment with azole antifungal agents is usually very effective, but with prolonged use and repeated courses, especially in those with low CD4 counts, resistance can develop. Discrete painful ulcerative lesions are usually caused by herpes simplex virus (HSV), CMV or aphthous ulcers. The same pathogens can cause odynophagia, but empiric treatment for candidiasis is instituted. Failure to respond after a week's treatment necessitates endoscopy with cultures and biopsy.

Central Nervous System Symptoms

HIV-infected patients are at increased risk for opportunistic infections of the CNS, especially as their CD4 counts decline to <200/µL. At CD4 counts >200/µL suspect the usual bacterial, mycobacterial (*M. tuberculosis*) and viral causes. Unusual causes of CNS infection, especially *C. neoformans* (meningitis) and *T. gondii* (focal lesions) are disproportionately more common as the CD4 count falls to <200/µL (Figure 1). Progressive multifocal leukoencephalopathy (PML) is an opportunistic infection caused by JC virus that can occur even at CD4 counts above 200/µL and for which there is no effective prophylaxis or treatment. HIV or CMV encephalopathy are also recognized in those with advanced HIV infection.

Fever of Unknown Origin

Patients with low CD4 counts may present with fever and flu-like symptoms but no specific focal symptoms to suggest a source. Possible infectious causes to be investigated include hepatitis viruses, sinusitis, MAC, *M. tuberculosis,* bartonellosis, CMV disease, *P. jirovecii* pneumonia (negative chest x-ray) and HIV viremia (Figure 1).

Figure 1: Management of Fever and Neurologic Complaints in HIV-positive Patients

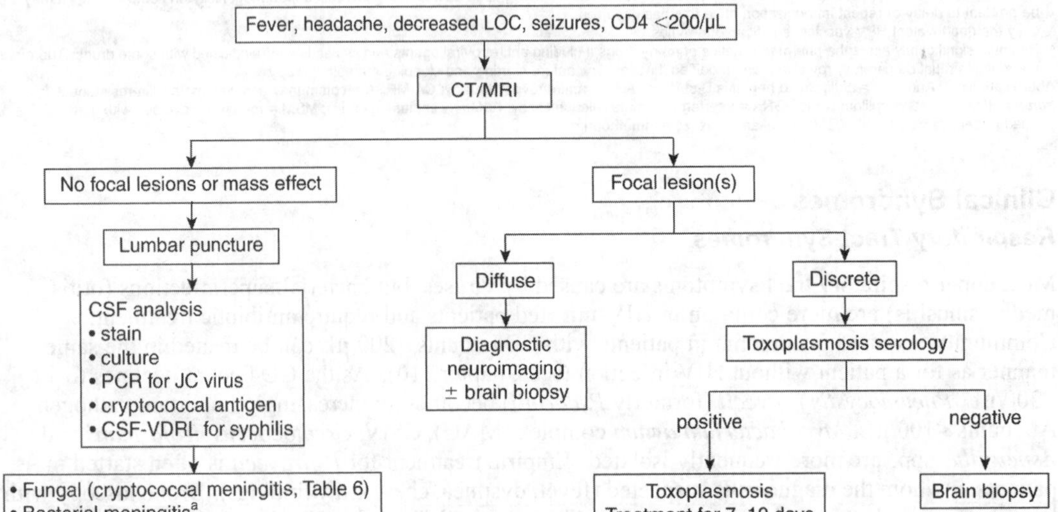

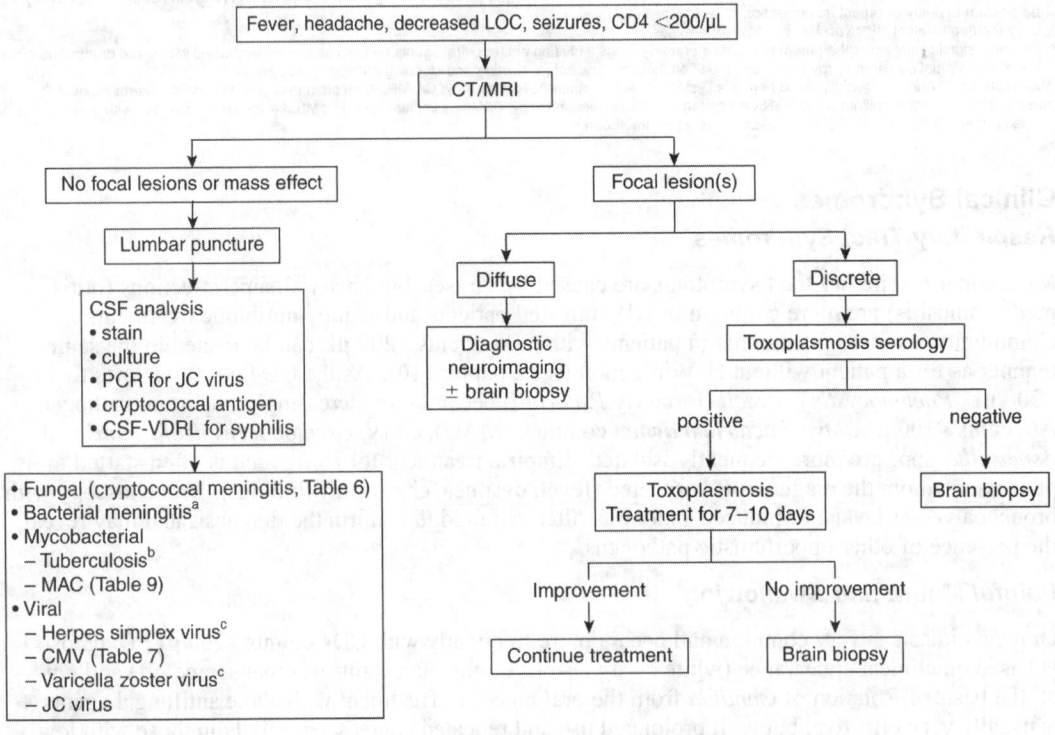

a See Chapter 109.
b See Chapter 124.
c See Chapter 112.

Abbreviations: CMV = cytomegalovirus; CSF = cerebrospinal fluid; CT = computed tomography; LOC = level of consciousness; MAC = *Mycobacterium avium* complex; MRI = magnetic resonance imaging; PCR = polymerase chain reaction; VDRL = Venereal Disease Research Laboratory

Diarrhea

Diarrhea is a very common symptom in HIV-positive patients, and infectious causes must be distinguished from noninfectious causes including adverse drug effects. Acute bacterial gastroenteritis caused by the usual enteric bacterial pathogens may be more severe, may result in bacteremia and may require prolonged antibiotic treatment. Long-term antibiotic prophylaxis and hospitalization are risk factors for *C. difficile* infection, especially in patients with low CD4 counts. Chronic diarrheal syndromes in patients with CD4 counts <150/µL may be associated with MAC or parasitic infections including giardiasis, cryptosporidiosis, cyclosporiasis, isosporiasis and microsporidiosis. Patients (in particular men who have sex with men) may be colonized with the nonpathogenic amoeba *Entamoeba dispar*. Standard stool examinations for ova and parasites cannot differentiate this harmless commensal from the pathogenic *Entamoeba histolytica*. Polymerase chain reaction or enzyme immunoassay should be performed on a separate, fresh, unpreserved stool specimen to differentiate these organisms.

Immune Reconstitution Inflammatory Syndromes

Patients initiating antiretroviral therapy, especially those with low initial CD4 counts, may experience worsening of opportunistic infections usually within 1–3 months as their CD4 count improves, despite appropriate antimicrobial treatment.[4,5] The opportunistic infections most frequently encountered in this setting are mycobacterial (tuberculosis or MAC), cryptococcal and viral (herpes simplex virus, cytomegalovirus, varicella-zoster virus, progressive multifocal leukoencephalopathy) although any opportunistic infection, as well as autoimmune conditions and malignancies, may be exacerbated by immune reconstitution. This phenomenon has been attributed to an enhanced inflammatory response at the site of infection and is usually self-limited. Both combination antiretroviral therapy and antimicrobial treatment are usually continued with the judicious use of **NSAIDs** and **steroids** in select individuals.

Discontinuation of Prophylaxis

Prophylaxis for some infections can be discontinued as the immune system recovers during antiretroviral therapy (Table 2).[6,7,8,9,10]

Table 2: Criteria for Discontinuing Prophylaxis of Opportunistic Infections in HIV-positive Patients[1]

Pathogen	Type of Prophylaxis	Criteria for Discontinuing
P. jirovecii	Primary and secondary	CD4 >200 cells/µL × ≥3 months
T. gondii	Primary	CD4 >200 cells/µL × ≥3 months
	Secondary	CD4 >200 cells/µL × ≥6 months
M. avium complex	Primary	CD4 >100 cells/µL × ≥3 months
	Secondary	CD4 >100 cells/µL × ≥6 months
CMV retinitis	Secondary	CD4 >100 cells/µL × ≥3–6 months No active disease Regular ophthalmic examination
C. neoformans	Secondary	CD4 >100–200 cells/µL × ≥6 months Suppressed viral load in response to antiretroviral therapy

Management of Specific HIV-associated Infections[1,2]

Bartonellosis

Both *Bartonella henselae* and *B. quintana* can cause disseminated infection with lesions of bacillary angiomatosis in patients with CD4 counts <50 cells/µL. Risk factors include cat scratches or contact with cats who have fleas. Diagnosis is made on tissue biopsy, serologic testing or blood cultures. Preferred therapy is **doxycycline**; alternative agents include **clarithromycin** or **azithromycin** (see Table 4).

Candida Species

The frequency of mucosal infection increases as the CD4 count decreases. Esophageal candidiasis is usually a later manifestation, but can occur in the absence of oral or vaginal disease. Severe discomfort or esophageal disease requires systemic therapy (see Table 6).

For *oral thrush*, topical therapy can be used initially. For example, use **nystatin** suspension (swish and swallow) or use **miconazole** or **clotrimazole** vaginal tablets/suppositories as oral lozenges (see Table 6). For *vaginal candidiasis*, topical azole antifungal creams or tablets/suppositories are first-line therapy (see Table 6). **Fluconazole** is the first-line oral systemic agent. **Itraconazole** and **ketoconazole** are alternative oral agents. Higher doses of fluconazole are used for esophageal disease with tapering of the dose when symptoms improve. **Amphotericin B** suspension is an alternative for less advanced disease. IV amphotericin B, **caspofungin** or **micafungin** are used in patients who do not respond to oral therapy. Lipid-based preparations of amphotericin B are less toxic but more expensive than the conventional formulation.

Cryptococcus neoformans

C. neoformans is a major cause of meningitis in the later stages of HIV infection (10% of AIDS patients). The diagnosis requires culture of the organism or detection of cryptococcal antigen in blood or CSF.

Induction therapy usually involves 2–6 weeks of iv **amphotericin B** with or without **flucytosine**, then completion of a minimum 8-week course of oral or iv **fluconazole** 400 mg/day (see Table 6). *Maintenance therapy* consists of daily oral fluconazole for at least 12 months. Note that echinocandins such as caspofungin do not have activity against *C. neoformans*.

Cytomegalovirus (CMV)

CMV usually occurs in patients with CD4 counts <50 cells/µL. Retinitis with visual disturbances is the most common manifestation; however, enteritis, colitis, pneumonitis, encephalitis, myelitis and/or neuritis can also occur. The prognosis is poor without therapy. Ganciclovir-resistant strains of CMV have emerged and these strains may be cross-resistant to cidofovir and foscarnet.

Induction therapy involves oral **valganciclovir** (a prodrug of ganciclovir), or iv **ganciclovir**, or iv **foscarnet** for 14–21 days (see Table 7). *Maintenance therapy* involves daily administration of oral valganciclovir, iv foscarnet or iv **cidofovir**. Note that foscarnet and cidofovir are not licensed in Canada, can be difficult to obtain (available through the Special Access Programme) and are expensive and quite toxic.

Intestinal Protozoa

Intestinal protozoa can cause persistent profuse watery diarrhea in patients with CD4 counts <150 cells/µL. *Cryptosporidium* and microsporidia (protists related to fungi) can also involve the biliary tract. In addition, microsporidia can cause disseminated infection. These organisms may be foodborne, waterborne (the spores are often resistant to chlorination), zoonotic or transmitted person to person. The mainstay of diagnosis is based on microscopic identification of oocysts or spores in stool samples. The laboratory should be notified that the patient is HIV-positive as these organisms require special stains to be visualized and may be missed on routine ova and parasite examination.

The only consistently effective therapy is immune reconstitution with ART. Patients should be treated supportively with rehydration and electrolyte replacement, and antimotility agents may provide symptomatic relief. Adjunctive therapies with variable success include **nitazoxanide** and **paromomycin** for cryptosporidiosis, **sulfamethoxazole/trimethoprim** for *Cyclospora* and *Isospora*, and **albendazole** for certain species of microsporidia (see Table 8).

Mycobacterium avium Complex

MAC occurs in patients with CD4 counts <100 cells/μL. Symptoms include fever, weight loss, fatigue, night sweats alone or with diarrhea, anemia, lymphadenopathy and/or hepatitis. The diagnosis is made primarily by mycobacterial blood culture or biopsy and culture of involved tissue.

Multidrug regimens are used to treat MAC (see Table 9), the basis of which is an oral macrolide (**clarithromycin** or **azithromycin**) plus **ethambutol**. Additional drugs such as **rifabutin** (or **rifampin**), **ciprofloxacin** or **levofloxacin**, or **amikacin** may also be used depending on the circumstances. Duration of induction therapy is 2–4 months, followed by maintenance therapy. *Maintenance therapy* consisting of clarithromycin (or azithromycin) plus ethambutol with or without rifabutin is continued for life unless a patient has sustained immune recovery on combination ART.

Pneumocystis jirovecii

P. jirovecci (formerly *P. carinii*) is the primary cause of pneumonia in patients with CD4 counts <200 cells/μL. *P. jirovecii* pneumonia (PCP) commonly presents as a persistent fever with progressive shortness of breath and cough, often with a normal chest x-ray. The organism cannot be cultured. Definitive diagnosis requires histopathologic examination of induced sputum, bronchoalveolar lavage or lung biopsy.

Standard therapy is 21 days of oral or iv **sulfamethoxazole/trimethoprim** (SMX/TMP, cotrimoxazole) (see Table 10). For severe disease, iv **pentamidine** may be given for 21 days. Oral **dapsone** plus trimethoprim is better tolerated than SMX/TMP, but is suitable only for mild or moderate disease (there is no iv formulation). Other alternatives include oral **atovaquone** (for mild to moderate cases) and **clindamycin** plus **primaquine**. In patients with severe PCP, the addition of oral **prednisone** decreases morbidity and the side effects of SMX/TMP (rash, hyperkalemia). Patients with paO_2 <70 mm Hg on room air or an alveolar-arterial O_2 gradient >35 mm Hg should receive adjunctive prednisone 40 mg twice daily for 5 days, then 20 mg twice daily for 5 days, then 20 mg daily to complete 21 days of treatment.

Toxoplasma gondii

Up to 50% of HIV-positive patients with antibodies to this parasite will develop toxoplasma encephalitis when their CD4 cell count decreases to <200 cells/μL. Patients most commonly present with a fever and focal neurologic signs. A CT scan with contrast or MRI usually reveals multiple intracranial-enhancing lesions.

Treat patients empirically. A marked clinical response usually occurs within 7 days; if there is no response, refer to a specialty centre. Standard therapy has traditionally been **pyrimethamine** plus **leucovorin** and **sulfadiazine** given for 4–8 weeks followed by chronic maintenance therapy. Sulfadiazine is frequently not available and the manufacture of pyrimethamine has been discontinued. First-line therapy in Canada is now oral or iv high-dose **SMX/TMP** (see Table 10). Alternatives include atovaquone with or without sulfadiazine. Patients with perilesional edema require **dexamethasone**.

Choices during Pregnancy and Breastfeeding

Prevention and Management of Opportunistic Infections

Prior to a planned pregnancy and during pregnancy, treat the patient with combination ART to ensure an undetectable viral load. This will prevent many of the serious opportunistic infections.

During pregnancy **SMX/TMP** can be given to prevent PCP and toxoplasmosis, although risk versus benefit needs to be assessed in the first trimester.[1] Initiate treatment for PCP with SMX/TMP in any trimester (see Table 3). Preferred agents for MAC and mucocutaneous candidiasis are **azithromycin** and **topical antifungal** drugs respectively. For less common opportunistic infections, consult a reference such as the Guidelines for Prevention and Treatment of Opportunistic Infections in HIV-Infected Adults and Adolescents[1] for specific regimens approved for use in pregnancy.

In the postpartum period, the usual preventive and therapeutic regimens can be reintroduced since breastfeeding is contraindicated because of possible transmission of HIV to the child.

A discussion of general principles on the use of medications in these special populations can be found in Appendix II and Appendix III. Other specialized reference sources are also provided in these appendices.

Therapeutic Tips

- All practitioners caring for patients who are HIV-positive should be aware of and participate in preventive interventions.
- Treatment of opportunistic infections requires specialized expertise and should be done in centres experienced with the management of HIV-infected patients.
- Consult with pharmacists when using therapy for opportunistic infections in combination with ART, given the potential for drug interactions.

Table 3: Preferred Agents during Pregnancy[1]

Type of Infection	Prevention	Treatment
PCP	SMX/TMP[a]	SMX/TMP[a]
MAC	1st choice: Azithromycin 2nd choice: Azithromycin + ethambutol	Azithromycin + ethambutol ± rifampin[b]
Toxoplasma encephalitis	SMX/TMP[a]	Referral
Mucocutaneous candidiasis	None	Topical antifungals
CMV	None	Valganciclovir

[a] Monitor neonate for hyperbilirubinemia and kernicterus.
[b] If rifampin is given during the last few weeks of pregnancy vitamin K is indicated to prevent postnatal hemorrhage in the mother and neonate.
Abbreviations: CMV = cytomegalovirus; MAC = *Mycobacterium avium* complex; PCP = *Pneumocystis jirovecii* pneumonia; SMX/TMP = sulfamethoxazole/trimethoprim

Table 4: Drugs for Treatment of Bartonellosis

Class	Drug	Adult Dose	Adverse Effects	Comments	Cost[a]
Macrolide Antibiotics	*azithromycin* Zithromax, generics	***Bartonella* infection (alt):** 500 mg/day po × 3 months	GI upset, QT_c prolongation.	Not for use in CNS infections or endocarditis. May increase effect of digoxin, warfarin, theophylline. Use cautiously with other drugs that cause QT_c prolongation.	$$
	clarithromycin Biaxin, generics	***Bartonella* infection (alt):** 500 mg BID po × 3 months	GI upset, abnormal taste, QT_c prolongation.	Not for use in CNS infections or endocarditis. Substrate and inhibitor of CYP3A4 (many potential interactions, e.g., carbamazepine, digoxin, warfarin). Protease inhibitors may decrease clearance of clarithromycin. Use cautiously with other drugs that cause QT_c prolongation.	$
Tetracycline Antibiotics	*doxycycline* Vibramycin, generics	***Bartonella* infection (1st choice):** 100 mg BID po/iv × 3 months	Photosensitivity, GI upset, rash, esophagitis.	For endocarditis treatment should be combined with gentamicin or rifampin.	$

[a] Cost per day based on dosages in this table for a 50 kg person; includes drug cost only.

Dosage adjustment may be required in renal impairment; see Appendix I.

Abbreviations: Alt = alternative therapy; CYP = cytochrome P450

Legend: $ < $2 $$ $2–4

Table 5: Drugs for Suppression of Frequent Oral or Genital Outbreaks of Herpes Simplex Virus

Class	Drug	Adult Dose	Adverse Effects	Comments	Cost[a]
Guanine Nucleoside Analogue Antiviral Agents	*acyclovir* Zovirax Oral, generics	200 mg TID or 400 mg BID po	Nausea, headache.	Increased CNS adverse effects when taken with AZT or probenecid. May impair renal excretion of tenofovir.	$$
	famciclovir Famvir, generics	500 mg BID po	See acyclovir.	Prodrug of penciclovir.	$$
	valacyclovir Valtrex, generics	500 mg BID or 1000 mg once daily po	See acyclovir.	Prodrug of acyclovir. See acyclovir.	$

[a] Cost per day based on dosages in this table for a 50 kg person; includes drug cost only.

Dosage adjustment may be required in renal impairment; see Appendix I.

Abbreviations: AZT = zidovudine

Legend: $ < $2 $$ $2–4

Table 6: **Drugs for Prophylaxis and Treatment of *Candida* spp and *Cryptococcus neoformans* Infections**

Class	Drug	Indication and Adult Dose	Adverse Effects	Comments	Cost[a]
Azole Antifungal Agents, systemic	*fluconazole* ❥ Diflucan, generics	**Prophylaxis for frequent recurrence of oral or esophageal candidiasis:** 100–200 mg/day po or 400 mg/wk po **Oral, esophageal or severe vaginal candidiasis:** 100–200 mg/day po × 7–14 days for oral or vaginal lesions; up to 400 mg/day po or iv × 14–21 days for esophageal lesions ***C. neoformans* consolidation therapy:** 400 mg/day po or iv to complete at least 8 weeks of therapy after amphotericin B induction or until CSF sterile ***C. neoformans* maintenance therapy:** 200 mg/day po for at least 1 year	Gastrointestinal, rash, elevated aminotransferase levels.	Inhibits CYP2C9, 2C19 and 3A4 (many potential interactions, e.g., citalopram, cyclosporine, fentanyl, phenytoin, sulfonylureas, tacrolimus and warfarin, some benzodiazepines and HMG-CoA reductase inhibitors). Rifampin decreases fluconazole levels.	po: $ iv: $
	itraconazole Sporanox Capsules, Sporanox Oral Solution	**Oral, esophageal or vaginal candidiasis:** 200 mg/day po × 7–14 days for oral or vaginal lesions, × 14–21 days for esophageal lesions	Gastrointestinal, rash, headache, edema, hypokalemia.	Absorption requires gastric acid: Decreased absorption with antacids, H_2-blockers, PPIs. Absorption improved with oral solution. Inhibits CYP3A4 (many potential interactions, e.g., cyclosporine, digoxin, efavirenz, fentanyl, tacrolimus, warfarin and some benzodiazepines and HMG-CoA reductase inhibitors). Carbamazepine, phenytoin and rifampin decrease itraconazole levels.	$
	ketoconazole generics	**Oral, esophageal or vaginal candidiasis:** 200–400 mg once daily or BID po	Gastrointestinal, elevated aminotransferase levels, hepatotoxicity.	See itraconazole. Used less frequently as safer alternatives exist (e.g., fluconazole).	$
	voriconazole Vfend, generics	**Invasive aspergillosis, candidemia, disseminated candidiasis:** 6 mg/kg Q12H iv × 2 doses then 4 mg/kg Q12H or 400 mg Q12H po × 2 doses then 200 mg Q12H po (>40 kg BW) or 100 mg Q12H po (<40 kg BW)	Hepatotoxicity, visual disturbances.	Inhibits CYP3A4 (many potential interactions, e.g., cyclosporine, digoxin, efavirenz, fentanyl, tacrolimus, warfarin and some benzodiazepines and HMG-CoA reductase inhibitors). Only use oral therapy in patients with ClCr <50 mL/min because of nephrotoxic vehicle in iv formulation.	po: $$ iv: $$$$$

Class	Drug	Indication and Adult Dose	Adverse Effects	Comments	Cost[a]
Azole Antifungal Agents, topical	*clotrimazole* Canesten Vaginal, generics	**Oral candidiasis:** 200 mg vaginal tab sucked 5 times daily × 7–14 days **Topical therapy for vulvovaginal candidiasis:** 1% cream nightly × 6 nights; or 2% cream and 200 mg vaginal tablet nightly × 3 nights	Local irritation.		$
	miconazole Monistat, generics	**Oral candidiasis:** 100 mg vaginal tab sucked 5 times daily × 7–14 days **Topical therapy for vulvovaginal candidiasis:** 2% cream and/or 100 mg vaginal ovule nightly × 7 nights; or 4% cream and/or 400 mg vaginal ovule nightly × 3 nights	Local irritation.		$
	terconazole Terazol, generics	**Topical therapy for vulvovaginal candidiasis:** 0.4% cream nightly × 7 nights; or 0.8% cream and/or 80 mg vaginal ovule nightly × 3 nights	Local irritation.		$
Echinocandin Antifungal Agents	*caspofungin* Cancidas	**Esophageal candidiasis treatment (alt):** 50 mg/day iv × 14 days	Headache, fever, elevated aminotransferase levels.	Rifampin and NNRTIs may decrease caspofungin levels.	$$$$
	micafungin Mycamine	**Esophageal candidiasis:** 150 mg/day iv × 15 days	See caspofungin.		$$$$$
Polyene Antifungal Agents	*amphotericin B* Fungizone	**Esophageal candidiasis treatment:** 0.3–0.5 mg/kg/day iv × 2–3 wk then weekly after symptoms resolve ***C. neoformans*** **induction therapy:** 0.7 mg/kg/day iv × 2–6 wk ± flucytosine	**IV:** infusion reactions (fever, chills, nausea), hypotension, nephrotoxicity, electrolyte disturbances, anemia, myelosuppression.	Increased risk of nephrotoxicity with other nephrotoxic drugs. Increases hemotoxicity of AZT. Consider use of a liposomal preparation to reduce the incidence of nephrotoxicity.	iv: $$ po:[b]
	amphotericin B lipid preparations Abelcet, AmBisome	AmBisome: 3–5 mg/kg/day iv Abelcet: 5 mg/kg/day iv	See amphotericin B.	Lipid preparations are better tolerated than standard amphotericin B.	~$640

(cont'd)

Table 6: **Drugs for Prophylaxis and Treatment of *Candida* spp and *Cryptococcus neoformans* Infections** *(cont'd)*

Class	Drug	Indication and Adult Dose	Adverse Effects	Comments	Cost[a]
	nystatin generics	**Oral candidiasis treatment:** 500 000 U po suspension QID swish and swallow; or 100 000 U vaginal tab sucked QID	Gastrointestinal, local irritation.		$
Pyrimidine Antifungal Agents	*flucytosine* ❥ Ancotil	***C. neoformans* induction therapy:** 100–150 mg/kg/day Q6H po × 2 wk + amphotericin B iv	Gastrointestinal, neurological, myelosuppression (especially with high serum levels).	Amphotericin-induced nephrotoxicity predisposes patients to adverse effects. Increased myelosuppression with other myelosuppressive agents (e.g. AZT, ganciclovir).	[b]

[a] Cost per day based on dosages in this table for 50 kg person; includes drug cost only.
[b] Available through Special Access Programme, Therapeutic Products Directorate, Health Canada.
❥ Dosage adjustment may be required in renal impairment; see Appendix I.
Abbreviations: Alt = alternative therapy; AZT = zidovudine; BW = body weight; CSF = cerebrospinal fluid; CYP = cytochrome P450; NNRTI = non-nucleoside reverse transcriptase inhibitor; PPI = proton pump inhibitor
Legend: $ < $50 $$ $50–100 $$$ $100–200 $$$$ $200–250 $$$$$ $250–300

Table 7: Drugs for Prophylaxis and Treatment of Cytomegalovirus Infections

Class	Drug	Indication and Adult Dose	Adverse Effects	Comments	Cost[a]
Cytidine Nucleotide Analogue Antiviral Agents	*cidofovir* Vistide	**CMV treatment (alt):** 5 mg/kg iv once weekly × 2 wk, then Q2 wk Hydrate with NS. Give probenecid 2 g 3 h before, and 1 g 2 h and 8 h after each infusion	GI upset, myelosuppression, ocular hypotony, nephrotoxicity.	Avoid other nephrotoxins (additive nephrotoxicity). Carcinogenic and teratogenic in animal studies, however maternal benefit may outweigh risks.[11]	b
Guanine Nucleoside Analogue Antiviral Agents	*ganciclovir* Cytovene	**CMV treatment:** 5 mg/kg Q12H iv × 14–21 days **CMV maintenance:** 5 mg/kg daily iv or 6 mg/kg iv 5–7 times per wk	Fever, GI upset, headache, confusion, pruritus, neuropathy, myelosuppression.	Increases AZT levels and hemotoxicity. Decreases renal excretion of tenofovir. G-CSF can be used for neutropenia; ganciclovir-resistant strains of CMV have emerged.	~$25
	valganciclovir Valcyte	**CMV treatment:** 900 mg BID po × 21 days **CMV maintenance:** 900 mg/day po	See ganciclovir.	Prodrug of ganciclovir. See ganciclovir.	~$36
Inorganic Pyrophosphate Analogue Antiviral Agents	*foscarnet* Foscavir	**CMV induction (alt):** 60 mg/kg Q8H iv or 90 mg/kg Q12H × 14–21 days **CMV maintenance (alt):** 90–120 mg/kg daily iv. Give 500 mL NS before and after each infusion	GI upset, fever, headache, electrolyte disturbances (may cause tetany, seizures), nephrotoxicity, anemia.	Prehydrate to decrease risk of nephrotoxicity. Avoid other nephrotoxins (additive nephrotoxicity). More difficult to administer and more toxic than ganciclovir, but may prolong survival. Ciprofloxacin increases seizure potential.	b

[a] Cost per day based on maintenance dosages in this table for 50 kg person; includes drug cost only.
[b] Available through Special Access Programme, Therapeutic Products Directorate, Health Canada.
Dosage adjustment may be required in renal impairment; see Appendix I.
Abbreviations: Alt = alternative therapy; AZT = zidovudine; CMV = cytomegalovirus; G-CSF = granulocyte colony-stimulating factor; NS = normal saline

Table 8: **Drugs for Treatment of Intestinal Protozoa**

Class	Drug	Indication and Adult Dose	Adverse Effects	Comments	Cost[a]
Aminogycosides	*paromomycin* Humatin	**Cryptosporidiosis treatment (adjunct with optimal ART):** 500 mg QID po × 14–21 days	Gastrointestinal.	Off-label use. To be used in conjunction with optimized ART; not effective without immune restoration.	~$25
Antiparasitics	*albendazole* Zentel	**Microsporidiosis treatment for species other than *Enterocytozoon bienuesi* and *Vittaforma corneae* (adjunct):** 400 mg BID po until CD4 >200 cells/μL for >6 months on ART	Bone marrow suppression, gastrointestinal, headache, hepatotoxicity, hypersensitivity reaction, reversible alopecia.	For intestinal and disseminated infections (not ocular).	b
	nitazoxanide Alinia	**Cryptosporidiosis treatment (adjunct with optimal ART):** 500–1000 mg BID po × 14 days **Cyclosporiasis treatment (alt):** 500 mg BID po × 7 days	Gastrointestinal.	Cryptosporidiosis: to be used in conjunction with optimized ART; not effective without immune restoration.	b
Sulfonamide Combinations	*sulfamethoxazole/ trimethoprim* (renal-dose symbol) Septra Injection, generics	**Cyclosporiasis (1st choice):**[12] 1 DS tab QID po × 10 days, then 1 DS tab M/W/F for maintenance until CD4 >200 cells/μL for >6 months **Isosporiasis treatment (adjunct):** 1 DS tab QID po/iv × 10 days, then 1 DS tab M/W/F until CD4 >200 cells/μL for >6 months and no evidence of *Isospora belli* infection	Adverse reactions are common. Nausea, vomiting and fever, hypersensitivity reactions (may be severe), myelosuppression, hyperkalemia with high treatment) doses.	Use with caution in patients with G6PD deficiency, or impaired renal or hepatic function. May increase therapeutic effect of sulfonylureas and warfarin. Increased hemotoxicity with AZT and methotrexate.	$1

[a] Cost per day based on dosages in this table for 50 kg person; includes drug cost only.
[b] Available through Special Access Programme, Therapeutic Products Directorate, Health Canada.
(renal-dose symbol) Dosage adjustment may be required in renal impairment; see Appendix I.
Abbreviations: Alt = alternative therapy; ART = antiretroviral therapy; AZT = zidovudine; DS = double strength; G6PD = glucose-6-phosphate dehydrogenase

Table 9: **Drugs for Prophylaxis and Treatment of *Mycobacterium avium* complex Infections and for Prophylaxis of *Mycobacterium tuberculosis* Infections**

Class	Drug	Indication and Adult Dose	Adverse Effects	Comments	Cost[a]
Aminoglycoside Antibiotics	*amikacin* generics	**MAC treatment:** 10–15 mg/kg/day iv × 2–4 months as an optional component in a regimen containing a macrolide + ethambutol	Nephrotoxicity, ototoxicity (auditory and vestibular).	Increased nephrotoxicity with other nephrotoxic drugs. Monitor renal, auditory and vestibular function.	$48-72
Anti-mycobacterial Agents	*ethambutol* Etibi, generics	**MAC treatment:**15 mg/kg/day po × 2–4 months + clarithromycin or azithromycin ± 1–3 additional drugs (amikacin, ciprofloxacin or levofloxacin, rifabutin or rifampin) **MAC maintenance:** 15 mg/kg/day po + clarithromycin or azithromycin ± rifabutin	GI upset, headache, confusion, peripheral neuritis, optic neuritis, rash, pruritus.	Absorption decreased by aluminum salts (separate administration). Patient should have regular eye exams and be advised to report any changes in vision.	$
	isoniazid generics	**TB prophylaxis (1st choice):** 300 mg/day po or 900 mg twice weekly × 9 months with pyridoxine 50 mg/day	GI upset, hepatotoxicity, peripheral neuropathy.	Absorption decreased by antacids (administer separately). Inhibits metabolism of carbamazepine, phenytoin and theophylline.	$
Fluoroquinolone Antibiotics	*ciprofloxacin* Cipro, generics	**MAC treatment:** 500–750 mg BID po × 2–4 months as an optional component in a regimen containing a macrolide + ethambutol	Headache, GI upset, tendon rupture (rare).	Absorption decreased by antacids, calcium and iron (separate administration). Inhibits CYP1A2 and 3A4 (many potential interactions).	$
	levofloxacin Levaquin, generics	**MAC treatment:** 500 mg/day po × 2–4 months as an optional component in a regimen containing a macrolide + ethambutol	See ciprofloxacin.	Absorption decreased by antacids, calcium and iron (separate administration). Inhibits CYP1A2 (many potential interactions).	$
Macrolide Antibiotics	*azithromycin* Zithromax, generics	**MAC prophylaxis (1st choice):** 1200 mg once weekly po **MAC treatment:** 500 mg/day po + ethambutol ± 1–3 additional drugs (amikacin, ciprofloxacin or levofloxacin, rifabutin or rifampin) × 2–4 months **MAC maintenance (alt):** 500 mg/day po + ethambutol ± rifabutin	GI upset, QT_c prolongation.	Interchangeable with clarithromycin for MAC therapy. May increase effect of digoxin, warfarin, theophylline.	$

(cont'd)

Table 9: **Drugs for Prophylaxis and Treatment of *Mycobacterium avium* complex Infections and for Prophylaxis of *Mycobacterium tuberculosis* Infections** *(cont'd)*

Class	Drug	Indication and Adult Dose	Adverse Effects	Comments	Cost[a]
	clarithromycin Biaxin, generics	**MAC prophylaxis (1st choice):** 500 mg BID po **MAC treatment:** 500 mg BID po + ethambutol ± 1–3 additional drugs (amikacin, ciprofloxacin or levofloxacin, rifabutin or rifampin) × 2–4 months **MAC maintenance (1st choice):** 500 mg BID po + ethambutol ± rifabutin	GI upset, abnormal taste, QT_c prolongation.	Interchangeable with azithromycin for MAC therapy. Substrate and inhibitor of CYP3A4 (many potential interactions, e.g., carbamazepine, digoxin, warfarin). PIs may decrease clearance of clarithromycin. Use cautiously with other drugs that cause QT_c prolongation.	$
Rifamycin Antibiotics	*rifabutin* Mycobutin	**MAC prophylaxis (alt):** 300 mg/day po **MAC treatment:** 300 mg/day po × 2–4 months as an optional component in a regimen containing a macrolide + ethambutol	GI upset, rash, pruritus, myelosuppression. Uveitis at doses >300 mg/day. Hepatotoxicity is rare.	Substrate of CYP1A2 and 3A4; induces 3A4 (many potential interactions). Clinically significant drug interactions with PIs and NNRTIs: do not use in combination with ritonavir, saquinavir, lopinavir/ritonavir. Discolours body fluids and feces.	$$
	rifampin Rifadin, Rofact	**MAC treatment:** 600 mg/day po × 2–4 months as an optional component in a regimen containing a macrolide + ethambutol **TB prophylaxis (alt):** 600 mg/day po × 4–6 months	Rash, pruritus, hepatitis (rare).	Broad-based induction of CYP isozymes (many potential interactions). Clinically significant drug interactions with many PIs and NNRTIs. Induces metabolism of AZT. Discolours body fluids and feces.	$

[a] Cost per day based on dosages in this table for 50 kg person; includes drug cost only.

Dosage adjustment may be required in renal impairment; see Appendix I.

Abbreviations: Alt = alternative therapy; AZT = zidovudine; CYP = cytochrome P450; MAC = *Mycobacterium avium* complex; NNRTI = non-nucleoside reverse transcriptase inhibitor; PI = protease inhibitor; TB = tuberculosis

Legend: $ < $5 $$ $5–10

Table 10: **Drugs for Prophylaxis and Treatment of *Pneumocystis jirovecii* and *Toxoplasma gondii* Infections**

Class	Drug	Indication and Adult Dose	Adverse Effects	Comments	Cost[a]
Antiprotozoal Agents	*atovaquone* Mepron	**PCP prophylaxis (alt):** 1500 mg/day po **PCP treatment (alt):** 750 mg BID po × 21 days ***T. gondii* prophylaxis (alt):** 1500 mg daily po ***T. gondii* treatment (alt):** 1500 mg BID po ± sulfadiazine × 6–8 wk ***T. gondii* maintenance (alt):** 750–1500 mg BID po ± sulfadiazine	Gastrointestinal, headache, rash.	Less effective than SMX/TMP for treatment of mild-moderate PCP. High fat meal increases absorption. Increased absorption with liquid formulation. Clearance increased by rifabutin, rifampin.	$$$$
	pentamidine generics	**PCP prophylaxis (alt):** aerosol 300 mg/month **PCP treatment (alt for severe):** 4 mg/kg/day iv × 21 days	**Aerosol:** chest pain, rash, wheezing. **Injection:** anemia, arrhythmias, dysglycemia, hypotension, nephrotoxicity, myelosuppression, pancreatitis.	Aerosolized pentamidine is better tolerated but less effective than iv for PCP treatment. Give aerosol by Respirgard inhaler. Infuse over 1 h while monitoring BP. Caution with other drugs that cause QT_c prolongation. Increased nephrotoxicity with other nephrotoxic drugs.	$135/ 300 mg vial
	primaquine Primaquine, generics	**PCP treatment (alt):** 15–30 mg/day po + clindamycin × 21 days	Gastrointestinal, hemolytic anemia, methemoglobinemia.		$
Corticosteroids	*dexamethasone* Dexasone, generics	**Adjunctive *T. gondii* treatment:** 4 mg Q6H po/iv	Gastrointestinal upset, hyperglycemia.	Used only when evidence of midline shift or increased intracranial pressure observed.	$$
	prednisone generics	**Adjunctive PCP treatment:** 40 mg BID × 5 days, then 20 mg BID × 5 days, then 20 mg daily to complete 21 days of treatment	See dexamethasone.	Used if paO_2 <70 mm Hg on room air or an alveolar-arterial O_2 gradient >35 mm Hg.	$
Lincosamides	*clindamycin* Dalacin C, Dalacin C Flavored Granules, Dalacin C Phosphate Solution Sterile, generics	**PCP treatment (alt):** 300–450 mg Q6–8H po or 600–900 mg Q8H iv + primaquine × 21 days	Nausea, vomiting, diarrhea, esophagitis, rash.		po: $ iv: $$$$$

(cont'd)

Table 10: Drugs for Prophylaxis and Treatment of *Pneumocystis jirovecii* and *Toxoplasma gondii* Infections *(cont'd)*

Class	Drug	Indication and Adult Dose	Adverse Effects	Comments	Cost[a]
Sulfonamide Antibiotics	*sulfadiazine*	***T. gondii* treatment (alt):** 1 g (if ≤60 kg) or 1.5 g (if >60 kg) Q6H po + atovaquone × 6–8 wk ***T. gondii* maintenance (alt):** 2–4 g daily in 2–4 divided doses po + atovaquone	Nausea, vomiting and fever, hypersensitivity reactions (may be severe), myelosuppression.	Use with caution in patients with G6PD deficiency, or impaired renal or hepatic function. May increase therapeutic effect of sulfonylureas and warfarin. Increased hemotoxicity with AZT.	[b]
Sulfonamide Combinations	*sulfamethoxazole/ trimethoprim* Septra Injection, generics	**PCP, *T. gondii* prophylaxis (1st choice):** 1 DS tab/day (800/160 mg) is preferred; 1 SS tab/day (400/80 mg) or 1 DS tab M/W/F are alternatives **PCP treatment (1st choice):** 15–20 mg/kg/day (TMP) iv or po (divided Q6–8H) × 21 days ***T. gondii* treatment (1st choice):** 5–10 mg/kg (TMP) BID iv or po × 6–8 weeks ***T. gondii* maintenance (1st choice):** 1 DS tab BID po	Adverse reactions are common, often requiring alternative agents. Nausea, vomiting and fever, hypersensitivity reactions (may be severe), myelosuppression, hyperkalemia with high (treatment) doses.	Use with caution in patients with G6PD deficiency, or impaired renal or hepatic function. May increase therapeutic effect of sulfonylureas and warfarin. Increased hemotoxicity with AZT.	po: $ iv: $$$
Sulfone Antibiotics	*dapsone* Dapsone, generics	**PCP prophylaxis (alt):** 100 mg/day po **PCP treatment (alt):** 100 mg/day po + TMP 15–20 mg/kg/day po × 21 days	Hypersensitivity reactions (may be severe), myelosuppression, hemolytic anemia, methe-moglobinemia (more common in G6PD deficiency).	Better tolerated than SMX/TMP. Clearance increased by rifampin. Excretion decreased by probenecid. TMP + dapsone results in increased toxicity of both drugs. Increased hemotoxicity with AZT, pyrimethamine, primaquine, TMP.	$

[a] Cost per day based on dosages in this table for 50 kg person; includes drug cost only.
[b] Available through Special Access Programme, Therapeutic Products Directorate, Health Canada.
Dosage adjustment may be required in renal impairment; see Appendix I.
Abbreviations: Alt = alternative therapy; AZT = zidovudine; BP = blood pressure; CYP = cytochrome P450; DS = double strength; G6PD = glucose-6-phosphate dehydrogenase; PCP = *Pneumocystis jirovecii* pneumonia; SMX/TMP = sulfamethoxazole/trimethoprim; SS = single strength; TMP = trimethoprim
Legend: $ < $5 $$ $5–10 $$$ $10–20 $$$$ $20–30 $$$$$ $30–40

Suggested Readings

Aberg JA, Gallant JE, Ghanem KG et al. Primary care guidelines for the management of persons infected with HIV: 2013 update by the HIV Medicine Association of the Infectious Diseases Society of America. *Clin Infect Dis* 2014;58(1):e1-e34.

Drug Interaction Tables: antiretroviral interactions [database on the Internet]. Toronto (ON): Immunodeficiency Clinic, Toronto General Hospital. Available from: www.hivclinic.ca/main/drugs_interact.html.

Lipman M, Breen R. Immune reconstitution inflammatory syndrome in HIV. *Curr Opin Infect Dis* 2006;19(1):20-5.

Panel on Opportunistic Infections in HIV-Infected Adults and Adolescents. *Guidelines for the prevention and treatment of opportunistic infections in HIV-infected adults and adolescents: recommendations from the Centers for Disease Control and Prevention, the National Institutes of Health, and the HIV Medicine Association of the Infectious Diseases Society of America.* Updated 2013. Available from: aidsinfo.nih.gov/contentfiles/lvguidelines/adult_oi.pdf.

References

1. Panel on Opportunistic Infections in HIV-Infected Adults and Adolescents. *Guidelines for the prevention and treatment of opportunistic infections in HIV-infected adults and adolescents: recommendations from the Centers for Disease Control and Prevention, the National Institutes of Health, and the HIV Medicine Association of the Infectious Diseases Society of America.* Updated 2013. Available from: aidsinfo.nih.gov/contentfiles/lvguidelines/adult_oi.pdf. Accessed October 2013.
2. Saag MS, Chambers HF, Eliopoulos GM et al. *The Sanford guide to HIV/AIDS therapy 2013.* 21st ed. Sperryville (VA): Antimicrobial Therapy; 2013.
3. National Advisory Committee on Immunization (NACI). Public Health Agency of Canada. *Canadian immunization guide.* Evergreen ed. Available from: www.phac-aspc.gc.ca/publicat/cig-gci/index-eng.php. Accessed January 17, 2014.
4. Battegay M, Nuesch R, Hirschel B et al. Immunological recovery and antiretroviral therapy in HIV-1 infection. *Lancet Infect Dis* 2006;6(5):280-7.
5. Lawn SD, Bekker LG, Miller RF. Immune reconstitution disease associated with mycobacterial infections in HIV-infected individuals receiving antiretrovirals. *Lancet Infect Dis* 2005;5(6):361-73.
6. Aberg JA, Williams PL, Liu T et al. A study of discontinuing maintenance therapy in human immunodeficiency virus-infected subjects with disseminated Mycobacterium avium complex: AIDS Clinical Trial Group 393 Study Team. *J Infect Dis* 2003;187(7):1046-52.
7. Ledergerber B, Mocroft A, Reiss P et al. Discontinuation of secondary prophylaxis against Pneumocystis carinii pneumonia in patients with HIV infection who have a response to antiretroviral therapy. Eight European Study Groups. *N Engl J Med* 2001;344(3):168-74.
8. Lopez Bernaldo de Quiros JC, Miro JM, Pena JM et al. A randomized trial of the discontinuation of primary and secondary prophylaxis against Pneumocystis carinii pneumonia after highly active antiretroviral therapy in patients with HIV infection. Grupo de Estudio del SIDA 04/98. *N Engl J Med* 2001;344(3):159-67.
9. Miro JM, Lopez JC, Podzamczer D et al. Discontinuation of primary and secondary Toxoplasma gondii prophylaxis is safe in HIV-infected patients after immunological restoration with highly active antiretroviral therapy: results of an open, randomized, multicenter clinical trial. *Clin Infect Dis* 2006;43(1):79-89.
10. Vibhagool A, Sungkanuparph S, Mootsikapun P et al. Discontinuation of secondary prophylaxis for cryptococcal meningitis in human immunodeficiency virus-infected patients treated with highly active antiretroviral therapy: a prospective, multicenter, randomized study. *Clin Infect Dis* 2003;36(10):1329-31.
11. Briggs GG, Freeman RK, Yaffe SJ. *Drugs in pregnancy and lactation: a reference guide to fetal and neonatal risk.* 9th ed. Philadelphia (PA): Lippincott Williams & Wilkins; 2011.
12. Pape JW, Verdier RI, Boncy M et al. Cyclospora infection in adults infected with HIV. Clinical manifestations, treatment, and prophylaxis. *Ann Intern Med* 1994;121(9):654-7.

Chapter 119
Sepsis and Septic Shock

Steven C. Reynolds, MD, FRCPC and
Harinderpal Brar, MD, FRCPC

Goals of Therapy

- Recognize sepsis early (Table 1)
- Promptly initiate goal-directed resuscitative efforts to restore tissue perfusion within the first 6 hours
- Eradicate causative pathogens (administer appropriate antibiotics within the first hour of recognizing sepsis)
- Establish source control (eliminate potential sources of infection) within the first 12 hours if possible through measures such as:
  - débridement of infected necrotic tissue
  - drainage of abscesses
  - removal of potentially infected devices or foreign bodies
- Restore intravascular fluid volume
- Reduce oxygen demand
- Manage complications, e.g., acute renal failure, acute respiratory distress syndrome, disseminated intravascular coagulation, multiple organ dysfunction syndrome
- Prevent nosocomial infections
- Prevent progression from sepsis to full septic shock

Investigations

- Thorough history with special attention to underlying disease, precipitating event and possible sites of infection
- Physical examination to determine the site and extent of infection, assess end-organ dysfunction and identify evidence of disseminated intravascular coagulation or disseminated infection (e.g., skin rash, purpura, ecthyma gangrenosum, subcutaneous nodules)
- Clinical monitoring of vital signs, urine output, weight, level of consciousness and total fluids in and out
- Laboratory monitoring:
  - CBC and differential
  - arterial blood gases
  - plasma lactate
  - electrolytes, acid-base status
  - urea and serum creatinine
  - liver function tests
  - serum magnesium, phosphate and ionized calcium
  - chest x-ray, ECG
  - coagulation status

- stool for occult blood
- Gram stain and cultures of: blood drawn from 2 separate sites (peripheral and central lines), urine, sputum and other body sites as appropriate
- imaging studies to search for the focus of infection

- Note: the cardinal signs of infection, fever and leukocytosis, may not be present in sepsis
- Additional investigations may be necessary to monitor cardiopulmonary status. Informal transthoracic echocardiograms are increasingly being performed by the bedside intensivist.[5] Pulmonary artery catheters provide dynamic information on cardiac output but their routine use is not warranted[6,7]
- Give serious consideration to insertion of a central venous catheter (CVC) into the superior vena cava for the measurement of central venous oxygen saturation and central venous pressure in all patients with suspected sepsis. This facilitates rapid and appropriate resuscitation efforts. Furthermore, a CVC should be placed into the superior vena cava in all patients not responsive to initial fluid resuscitation or those who have ongoing hemodynamic instability

Classification of Sepsis and Septic Shock

Categorize patients into 1 of 3 syndromes (Table 1).

Therapeutic Choices

Figure 1 summarizes the essential resuscitation and infection control activities in severe sepsis and septic shock.

Resuscitation and Monitoring

Meticulous monitoring of the patient's circulating volume and ventilatory status is essential, with immediate resuscitation if required. If simple measures do not quickly restore hemodynamic stability, consider intensive care with invasive hemodynamic monitoring and aggressive cardiovascular support.[8,9,10]

Early institution of mechanical ventilation and sedation helps to reduce oxygen demand and improve oxygen delivery and extraction at the tissue level.[11] If possible, avoid prolonged neuromuscular blockade because of the risk of prolonged muscular weakness. However, brief administration (48 hours) of **cisatracurium** in general ICU patients with early, severe acute respiratory distress syndrome was associated with an improved adjusted 90-day mortality without increased muscle weakness.[12] This finding may not be generalized to other neuromuscular blocking agents (pancuronium, rocuronium, vercuronium). Sedation protocols should include a process of daily lightening of sedation with a careful clinical evaluation.

A seminal study demonstrated a marked improvement in 28-day mortality in patients for whom the following goals of resuscitation were accomplished within 6 hours of hospital admission:[9]

- central venous pressure (CVP): 8–12 mm Hg (in a mechanically ventilated patient, the target central venous pressure should be 12–15 mm Hg due to the increased intrathoracic pressure)
- mean arterial pressure (MAP) ≥65 mm Hg
- urine output ≥0.5 mL/kg/hour
- central venous (superior vena cava) or mixed venous oxygen saturation (SvO_2) ≥70%

Table 1: Classification of Sepsis, Severe Sepsis and Septic Shock

Clinical Staging[a]	Diagnostic Criteria
Sepsis	Clinical evidence suggestive of infection *plus*: Signs of a systemic inflammatory response to infection (≥2 of the following): • Tachypnea (>20 breaths/min or $PaCO_2$ <32 mm Hg [<4.3 kPa]) • Tachycardia (>90 beats/min) • Hyperthermia (>38°C) or hypothermia (<36°C) • WBC >12 × 10^9 cells/L, or <4 × 10^9 cells/L, or >10% immature (band) forms
Severe sepsis	Sepsis with hypotension (systolic blood pressure <90 mm Hg or a 40 mm Hg decrease from baseline in the absence of other causes), organ dysfunction and perfusion abnormalities such as: Oliguria: <0.5 mL/kg for at least 1 h in patients with urinary catheters Elevated plasma lactate (> normal upper limit) Altered mental status
Septic shock	Severe sepsis as defined above, despite adequate fluid resuscitation *Note:* patients who are on vasopressor agents may not be hypotensive

[a] Clinical staging and classification of sepsis is important but challenging. The above table reflects definitions from 1992 which have been expanded upon in subsequent works but not fundamentally changed.[1,2] Further, determination of severity of sepsis and organ dysfunction has been systematized into various scoring systems.[3,4] A detailed discussion of classification and scoring systems is beyond the scope of this chapter.

Figure 1: Early Management of Septic Shock[8]

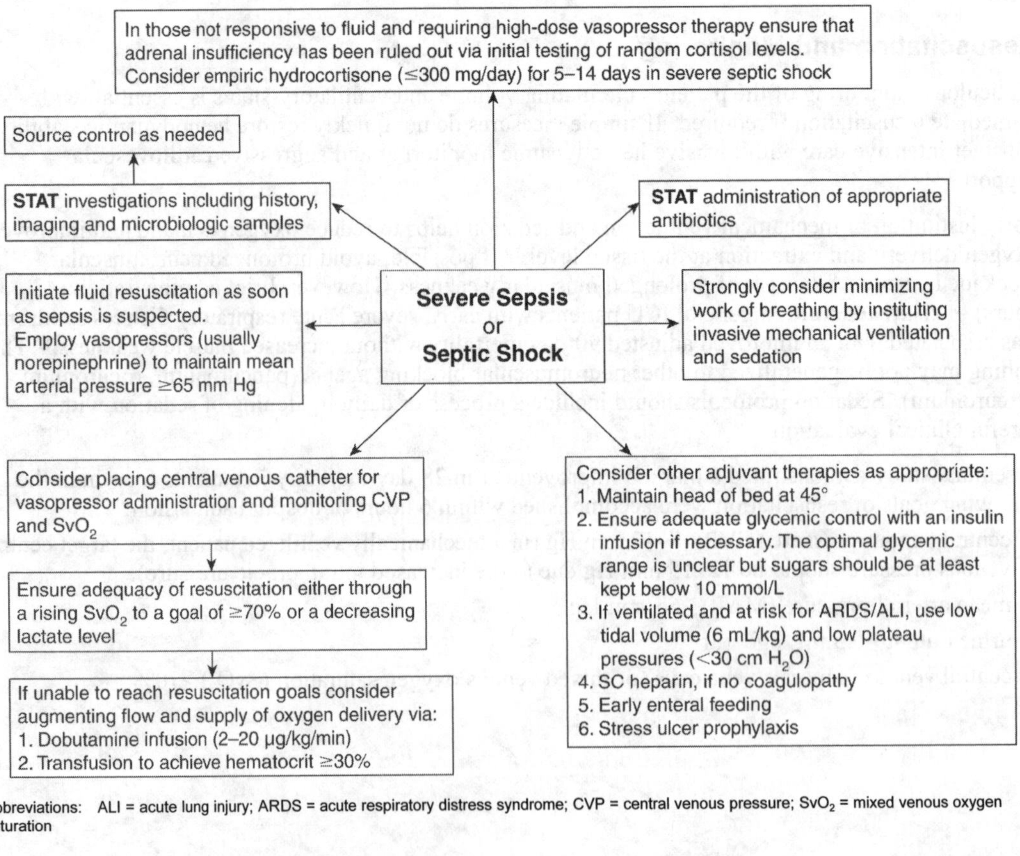
In those not responsive to fluid and requiring high-dose vasopressor therapy ensure that adrenal insufficiency has been ruled out via initial testing of random cortisol levels. Consider empiric hydrocortisone (≤300 mg/day) for 5–14 days in severe septic shock
Source control as needed
STAT investigations including history, imaging and microbiologic samples
STAT administration of appropriate antibiotics
Severe Sepsis or Septic Shock
Initiate fluid resuscitation as soon as sepsis is suspected. Employ vasopressors (usually norepinephrine) to maintain mean arterial pressure ≥65 mm Hg
Strongly consider minimizing work of breathing by instituting invasive mechanical ventilation and sedation
Consider placing central venous catheter for vasopressor administration and monitoring CVP and SvO_2
Ensure adequacy of resuscitation either through a rising SvO_2 to a goal of ≥70% or a decreasing lactate level
If unable to reach resuscitation goals consider augmenting flow and supply of oxygen delivery via:
1. Dobutamine infusion (2–20 μg/kg/min)
2. Transfusion to achieve hematocrit ≥30%
Consider other adjuvant therapies as appropriate:
1. Maintain head of bed at 45°
2. Ensure adequate glycemic control with an insulin infusion if necessary. The optimal glycemic range is unclear but sugars should be at least kept below 10 mmol/L
3. If ventilated and at risk for ARDS/ALI, use low tidal volume (6 mL/kg) and low plateau pressures (<30 cm H_2O)
4. SC heparin, if no coagulopathy
5. Early enteral feeding
6. Stress ulcer prophylaxis

Abbreviations: ALI = acute lung injury; ARDS = acute respiratory distress syndrome; CVP = central venous pressure; SvO_2 = mixed venous oxygen saturation

In the above study protocol, a packed red blood cell transfusion was given to achieve a hematocrit of ≥30% if fluid resuscitation did not result in an SvO_2 of ≥70% despite a CVP of 8–12 mm Hg (or 12–15 mm Hg in a mechanically ventilated patient). If the hematocrit was at or above this goal and the SvO_2 was not ≥70%, a **dobutamine** infusion was initiated to achieve the target saturation of ≥70%.

Although SvO_2 has typically been used to guide adequacy of resuscitation it is also reasonable to follow serial lactate values instead of measurements of SvO_2. In some contexts measuring lactate clearance may be easier (e.g., when the patient can have only a femoral central line) and has been shown to be noninferior to normalizing SvO_2.[13]

These are reasonable goals of initial resuscitation but strict adherence to absolute values is discouraged. As an example, the absolute value of CVP does not reflect the ability of administered fluid to increase cardiac output,[14] whereas the trend is more useful. Therefore CVP should be interpreted in the context of other indicators of volume status.

The exact nature of optimal resuscitation is not clear. In a recent large, multicentre RCT there was no difference in outcome between the specific resuscitation as outlined above,[9] a protocolized resuscitation algorithm which did not emphasize the optimization of SvO_2, and uncontrolled physician-directed resuscitation.[15] Despite this inconsistency it must be emphasized that early and aggressive resuscitation by an expert is paramount, and is more important than the specific aspects of the resuscitation algorithm.

Fluid Resuscitation

Crystalloids are recommended for initial resuscitation for severe sepsis and septic shock. A portion of resuscitation fluids may be given as **albumin**, although this fluid is more costly than crystalloids and has not shown a specific benefit.[16] Hydroxyethyl starches are not recommended as therapy for sepsis. Recent literature has shown an increased incidence of acute kidney injury and mortality associated with their use in critically ill patients.[17,18,19]

Fluid administration is best managed through a process of fluid challenges in the patient who is septic.[20] A minimum of 30 mL/kg of crystalloids is advised, however the total amount is patient specific and intravenous fluid can be continued as long as the patient is improving hemodynamically.[16,21] Fluid challenges should be administered in aliquots of 500–1000 mL over 30 minutes with defined safety and success endpoints. Positive responses to a fluid challenge include increased MAP, decreased vasopressor requirements and improved organ perfusion, most commonly demonstrated as increased urine output. It is important to note that aggressive fluid resuscitation should not continue indefinitely and that excessive fluid administration is associated with organ dysfunction and edema.

Transfusion Therapy

Maintaining hemoglobin above 70–80 g/L is a safe transfusion threshold for the general ICU population.[22] A higher concentration of 90–100 g/L may be required in patients with myocardial ischemia or to augment oxygen delivery in those with low mixed venous oxygen saturation.[23] Having not been formally studied in sepsis, erythropoietin and prophylactic fresh frozen plasma administration are not recommended.[24,25] Platelet transfusion guidelines in sepsis are largely from consensus opinion. For those at risk of bleeding and those who have active bleeding the recommended thresholds are 20 000/mm^3 and 50 000/mm^3 respectively.[26]

Glucose Control

Despite conflicting results in recent studies, it is prudent to maintain euglycemia in septic patients. Give iv regular human **insulin** by continuous infusion with a glycemic check every hour. Original data supported a glycemic goal of 4.4–6.1 mmol/L;[27] however, additional trials failed to demonstrate a benefit with an aggressive glucose control regimen.[28,29] Moreover, a significant increase in rate of hypoglycemia was observed. A large, multicentre, randomized trial showed that tight glucose control

(4.5–6 mmol/L) was associated with increased 90-day mortality compared to a less strict glucose parameter (≤10 mmol/L).[30,31] Although there are still unanswered questions in the debate over glucose control, in light of this large, well-designed trial and a meta-analysis[32] it is reasonable to aim for glucose levels of ≤10 mmol/L in the general ICU population.

Localization and Evacuation of Loculated Infections

Plain radiographs, ultrasonography and computed tomography are invaluable for localizing the nidus of infection. Drain abscesses whenever possible, and strongly consider removing infected foreign bodies.[33]

Consider the ability of a patient to tolerate transportation away from the ICU to facilitate imaging needs. Transportation imposes a small but very real risk of complications associated with moving a critically ill patient (extubation, hemodynamic collapse, dysrhythmia).

Persistent bacteremia, despite appropriate antimicrobial therapy, suggests a valvular or endovascular infection, or the emergence of a resistant microorganism. Intermittent bacteremias tend to be due to abscesses or localized infections which "shower" bacteria into the blood sporadically.

Anticipation and Prevention of Complications

- *Acute renal failure*: avoid nephrotoxic drugs; monitor and dialyze as needed. Intermittent hemodialysis and continuous venovenous hemofiltration are equally effective, although the latter may be better tolerated from a hemodynamic and fluid balance perspective.[34] The optimal dose of continuous renal replacement therapy (including continuous venovenous hemofiltration) in acute kidney injury in ICU patients has not been determined; studies have shown conflicting results.[35,36] A meta-analysis failed to show a difference in mortality between high-dose (>35 mL/kg/h) and low-dose (<25 mL/kg/h) continuous renal replacement therapy.[37] Early initiation of continuous venovenous hemofiltration appears to be associated with increased mortality in septic ICU patients without evidence of acute kidney injury.[38]
- *Acute respiratory distress syndrome (ARDS)*: anticipate and treat supportively (ventilatory support and judicious use of fluids). Lung-protective ventilation strategies should be used in patients with acute lung injury (ALI) or ARDS. This includes the use of low tidal volumes (6 mL/kg) and a goal of maintaining end-inspiratory pressures <30 cm of H_2O. Often, a moderate increase in arterial carbon dioxide tension ($PaCO_2$), i.e., permissive hypercapnia, is necessary to achieve these ventilator goals. Permissive hypercapnia may not be appropriate for patients with metabolic acidosis and is contraindicated in head injuries. Positive end-expiratory pressure (PEEP) should be used to minimize lung injury. The level of PEEP will vary from patient to patient but a reasonable starting point is 5–10 mm H_2O.[8] A meta-analysis demonstrated prone positioning to be associated with reduced mortality from ARDS in those maintained with low tidal volumes, and as such this strategy should be considered in appropriate patients.[39]
- *Aspiration*: whenever possible, raise the head of the patient's bed 45 degrees to minimize the risk of passive aspiration and ventilator-associated pneumonia.
- *Electrolyte and acid-base status*: correct metabolic derangements. Beware of refeeding syndrome in those with poor nutrition. This syndrome is characterized by metabolic disturbances upon re-initiation of feeding after a period of malnourishment. Advance feeds slowly in those at risk while monitoring electrolytes carefully. Metabolic acidosis should not be routinely corrected with **sodium bicarbonate** unless the pH is <7.15.[8] Some advocate using a pH threshold of 7 for initiation of bicarbonate.[40] Concern exists with sodium and fluid overload with sodium bicarbonate use. The primary focus in a severely acidotic patient should be to correct the underlying cause.
- *Edema, pericardial and pleural effusions*: maintain adequate intravascular volume before using **diuretics** to mobilize extravascular fluid. Generally, diuretics are not employed while patients are on vasopressors except in extenuating circumstances. Occasionally, diuretics are used when patients

are receiving positive inotropes. Drain empyemas as soon as possible with a large-bore chest tube. The majority of pleural effusions are transudative and can be drained with small-bore chest tubes, although it is not clear whether this adds additional benefit over diuresis but is often employed in selected patients. Be suspicious of a tamponade in a patient with a pericardial effusion.

- *Disseminated intravascular coagulation (DIC) and thrombocytopenia*: although **heparin** will theoretically prevent further consumption of clotting factors by reducing thrombin generation, its use in patients with bleeding is controversial. The first-line therapy for DIC is to manage the underlying illness and treat supportively. Fresh frozen plasma should only be given to a patient with an elevated INR if an invasive procedure is planned or if there is spontaneous bleeding.
- *Deep vein thrombosis (DVT)*: use **unfractionated heparin (UFH), low molecular weight heparins (LMWH)** or venous compression devices (see Chapter 48) to prevent deep vein thrombosis.[41,42] The PROTECT study demonstrated that **dalteparin**, a LMWH, was comparable to UFH in the prevention of proximal leg DVT.[43] Pharmacoeconomic analyses demonstrate LMWH are more cost-effective due to the decreased incidence of heparin-induced thrombocytopenia.[44]
- *Hepatic dysfunction*: be wary of toxic accumulation from medications that undergo biotransformation in the liver.
- *Stress ulcer prophylaxis*: if the patient is not being fed enterally, prophylaxis with **H_2-receptor blockers** or **proton pump inhibitors** (PPIs) reduces bleeding in those at risk.[45,46] It is particularly indicated in patients with prolonged mechanical ventilation, hypotension and coagulopathy.[41] H_2-receptor blockers and PPIs increase the incidence of ventilator-acquired pneumonia (VAP); assess the risk and benefits of their use in each patient.[47]
- *Impaired GI motility*: manage slow gastric emptying with prokinetic agents such as **metoclopramide** or **erythromycin**.[48] Additionally, a post-pyloric feeding tube may be placed. A prokinetic agent should not be given to a patient who has high gastric residuals secondary to a mechanical obstruction.
- *Adequate caloric intake* with **trace element and vitamin supplements**, preferably through the enteral route, is also important.[49] It is recommended to begin enteral feeds once the initial resuscitation is complete (or within 48 hours of presentation).[50] The use of enteral nutrition is preferred over total parenteral or partial parenteral nutrition in the first 7 days after diagnosis of severe sepsis/septic shock.[51]
- *CNS dysfunction*: be vigilant for the development of delirium. **Antipsychotics** are typically used to manage delirium although there is limited evidence supporting this practice.[52] Indeed the benefit may lie in the discontinuation of precipitating agents such as **benzodiazepines**. **Dexmedetomidine**, a novel alpha-2 agonist, may be useful as a sedative or for treatment of ICU delirium.[53,54] Evidence concerning duration of mechanical ventilation, length of ICU stay and mortality have been conflicting.[53,55] A large RCT (n=500) demonstrated a reduction in duration of mechanical ventilation by almost 2 days with dexmedetomidine compared to **midazolam**, but at the cost of more hypotension and bradycardia.[55] In a parallel study (n=498) there was no difference in duration of mechanical ventilation when dexmedetomidine was compared with **propofol**.[55] In addition, there was no difference in duration of ICU or hospital stay or mortality in either comparison. A previous meta-analysis of 24 heterogeneous trials concluded dexmedetomidine might reduce length of ICU stay in some critically ill patients but did not demonstrate reduced duration of mechanical ventilation.[53]

  Daily interruption of sedation has been shown to reduce the duration of mechanical ventilation and ICU and hospital length of stay,[56] although a well-designed randomized controlled trial demonstrated no benefit of daily sedation vacations with spontaneous breathing trials.[57] The most prudent course of action is to limit excessive sedation by utilizing sedation scores, sedation protocols and transitioning off of continuous infusions as soon as possible to achieve therapeutic goals.
- *Nosocomial infections*: strict adherence to handwashing, aseptic technique and other infection control principles is required to minimize the development of nosocomial infections.[58] Remove

central venous catheters, foley catheters and other invasive lines as soon as possible. Avoid nasogastric and nasotracheal intubation to prevent nosocomial sinusitis. Weaning protocols that utilize daily spontaneous breathing trials minimize the number of days on mechanical ventilation and lower the risk of ventilator-associated pneumonia.[59] Implementation of ventilator-associated pneumonia and central line infection bundles are requirements of modern ICU care.

- *Pneumothorax*: monitor airway pressure to prevent pneumothoraces in patients who are mechanically ventilated.

Empiric Antimicrobial Therapy

Antimicrobial therapy remains the cornerstone of treatment for sepsis and septic shock. However, the underlying disease, comorbid conditions and development of complications (e.g., ARDS, multi-organ dysfunction) often dictate the eventual outcome of therapy. Source control (see Goals of Therapy) if possible, is critical for the successful treatment of infections.

Broad-spectrum antibiotics should be administered immediately, with the first dose being ordered and administered STAT. There is good evidence that mortality increases dramatically with each hour that appropriate antibiotic administration is delayed in the septic patient.[60] If feasible, acquire all samples for microbial culture prior to the administration of antibiotics. Do *not* delay antibiotic administration in the critically ill patient for the sole purpose of maximizing the microbial yield or for initiation of imaging studies.

Initial antimicrobial therapy is empiric because gram-positive, gram-negative, mycobacterial, fungal and viral sepsis are often clinically indistinguishable. Antibiotic selection is based on the most likely source/site of infection and hence the most likely causative microorganisms and their anticipated susceptibility profiles (Table 2). The choice of antimicrobial agents, described in Table 3, may also be influenced by the presence of acute renal or hepatic failure, hypersensitivity reactions, need for fluid restriction, local antimicrobial susceptibility patterns, emergence of resistance and drug interactions. Another element that may factor into antibiotic selection is the local prevalence of severe *C. difficile*-associated diarrhea.[70]

Administer antibiotics iv in critically ill patients and reassess daily. Adjustments are guided by culture results, in vitro susceptibility patterns and clinical response. Occasionally, 2 effective antibiotics are continued to prevent the development of resistance. *Pseudomonas* is the classic example and it is standard of care to "double cover" to prevent the development of resistance but this is not based on strong evidence.[71] In specific cases some experts will use 2 effective antibiotics based on their mechanisms of action and potential synergy. Even in this scenario use should be limited to no longer than 3–5 days.[8]

There are several observational and retrospective studies of severe pneumococcal pneumonia (bacteremic) that support using combination antibiotic therapy with a **beta-lactam** and either a **macrolide** or a **fluoroquinolone**, although a macrolide is preferred.[72] Improvement in mortality was seen even after controlling for inadequate therapy in the mono-antibiotic group.[73,74,75] The use of 2 effective antibiotics with complementary mechanisms for other septic states is not routinely recommended as it does not improve outcomes.[76]

There is increasing evidence suggesting that serum procalcitonin (PCT)-guided algorithms may reduce antibiotic exposure in the ICU patient population without increasing mortality or length of ICU stay.[77] Although there is growing evidence of its role in safely stopping antibiotics, PCT should not be used as the primary means of diagnosing an infection in the critically ill.[78]

Candida is the fourth most common pathogen isolated in blood stream infections in the ICU, yet when to start antifungal therapy is not clear.[63,79] In special at-risk populations such as neutropenic patients, consider empiric antifungal therapy. Other patients need to be considered on a case-by-case basis. Risk factors for candidemia include multiple colonization sites, long-term broad-spectrum antibiotic therapy, hollow viscus rupture or abdominal surgery, intravenous catheters, prolonged ICU stay and use of total parenteral nutrition.[63,80]

Table 2: Empiric Antimicrobial Treatment of Sepsis and Septic Shock

Source of Infection	Common Pathogens	Initial Antimicrobial Regimen[a]
Community-acquired pneumonia[61]	*Streptococcus viridans*, *Streptococcus pyogenes*, *Streptococcus pneumoniae*, *Haemophilus influenzae*, *Legionella pneumophila*, *Staphylococcus aureus* (MRSA or MSSA), gram-negative bacilli (rarely *Pseudomonas aeruginosa* except in those with risk factors), *Mycoplasma pneumoniae*, *Chlamydia pneumoniae* Evaluate the potential of other pathogens based on risk factors	Extended-spectrum beta-lactam[b] (usually a 3rd generation cephalosporin is adequate) + extended-spectrum fluoroquinolone *or* macrolide ± vancomycin[c] *or* linezolid[c]
Intraperitoneal/ gastrointestinal tract[62]	Enteric gram-negative bacilli, *Bacteroides fragilis*, *Peptostreptococcus* spp., *Clostridia* spp., *Enterococcus* spp., less commonly *Candida* spp.	Meropenem or imipenem *or* piperacillin/tazobactam *or* ceftazidime + metronidazole Consider early empiric addition of an anticandidal agent (e.g., echinocandin, fluconazole) in severely ill patient with a hollow viscus rupture[63,64]
Urinary tract[65]	*Escherichia coli*, other enteric gram-negative bacilli, *Staphylococcus saprophyticus*, *Enterococcus* spp., less commonly, *Pseudomonas aeruginosa*	Ciprofloxacin + ceftazidime *or* meropenem or imipenem *or* piperacillin/tazobactam
	Extended-spectrum beta-lactamase (ESBL)-producing bacteria	Carbapenem
Meningitis[66]	*Neisseria meningitidis*, *H. influenzae*, *S. pneumoniae*, *Listeria monocytogenes*	Cefotaxime or ceftriaxone ± vancomycin (for penicillin-resistant pneumococcus) ± ampicillin (for elderly, alcoholic, immunocompromised or pregnant patients, in particular for *Listeria* coverage)
Necrotizing skin and soft tissues[67]	Group A streptococcus, *S. aureus*, *Clostridia* spp.	Extended-spectrum beta-lactam[b,d] + clindamycin ± vancomycin
	Gram-negative *Enterobacteriaceae* and anaerobes are prominent in perirectal/genital infections.	Extended-spectrum beta-lactam[b]
Intravascular device-associated[68]	*S. aureus*, coagulase-negative staphylococci Much less commonly, enteric gram-negative bacilli and *Candida* spp.	Vancomycin

(cont'd)

Table 2: **Empiric Antimicrobial Treatment of Sepsis and Septic Shock** *(cont'd)*

Source of Infection	Common Pathogens	Initial Antimicrobial Regimen[a]
Nosocomially-acquired infections	A broad range of gram-negative and gram-positive organisms are possible, particularly multidrug-resistant organisms	Carbapenem + ciprofloxacin + linezolid or vancomycin
Unknown source		Extended-spectrum penicillin with beta-lactamase inhibitor[e] or carbapenem ± vancomycin or linezolid ± ciprofloxacin

[a] Initial antibiotic selection is a suggestion only, all antibiotic choices should be based on local antibiograms. Antibiotics selected should cover as close to 100% of probable pathogens as is reasonable, yet as narrow in spectrum as possible. For example, in an institution with negligible carbapenem resistance, adding ciprofloxacin to a carbapenem for empiric treatment of nosocomially acquired infections is unnecessary.
[b] Extended-spectrum beta-lactam = 3rd or 4th generation cephalosporin, extended-spectrum penicillin with beta-lactamase inhibitor (piperacillin/tazobactam or ticarcillin/clavulanate) or carbapenem. Add metronidazole if a 3rd or 4th generation cephalosporin is selected to treat severe perirectal soft tissue infections or intraperitoneal/gastrointestinal tract infections.
[c] If increased risk of methicillin-resistant *S. aureus* (MRSA) such as local outbreaks, being a known carrier or close contact with a known carrier. Note that some patients may have community-associated MRSA with no risk factors.
[d] Penicillin is the antibiotic of choice for the most common pathogen, group A streptococcus, although it is impossible to be sure on initial evaluation the identity of the pathogen and therefore broad antibiotic coverage should be initiated.
[e] Institute a more focused antimicrobial choice once the nidus of infection and likely pathogens become more apparent.

Candidemia may be difficult to detect through blood cultures but is associated with increased mortality. In high-risk patients, consider sending blood samples for 1,3 beta-D-glucan assay and/or the mannan and anti-mannan antibody assays if results can be received in a timely manner. These can help with diagnosis of invasive candidal infections.[8] Consideration should also be given to early or prophylactic antifungal therapy in patients with hollow viscus rupture[64] or those who have developed unexplained fever or shock and have multiple risk factors for candidemia.[63,81] Bedside scoring systems aid in the difficult decision of when to initiate empiric antifungal therapy.[80] Although empiric antifungal therapy is recommended in guidelines for those at risk,[63,82] a trial randomizing high-risk patients to receive fluconazole or placebo showed no difference in outcomes.[83] Always maintain a high level of suspicion of occult fungal infections when evaluating critically ill immunocompromised patients.[63]

The most appropriate choice of empiric antifungal therapy is not clear but an **echinocandin** is generally preferred in those with more severe illness or recent azole exposure.[63,82,84] **Fluconazole** is a reasonable choice in less severe illness. Historically, **amphotericin B** has been the empiric antifungal of choice but has fallen out of favour due to its nephrotoxicity and metabolic derangements.

Vasoactive Agents for Cardiovascular Support

Although rapid fluid administration alone may be sufficient to restore hemodynamic stability, vasopressors are often necessary to restore an adequate mean arterial pressure (MAP) primarily by bolstering systemic vascular resistance.

Norepinephrine (0.03–1.5 μg/kg/min) is the pressor of choice in septic shock. It has peripheral vasoconstricting activity and may be superior to dopamine in septic shock by increasing peripheral resistance and improving splanchnic perfusion.[85,86] It is a potent vasoconstrictor and has lesser positive inotropic and chronotropic effects. **Dopamine** (5–20 μg/kg/min) has positive chronotropic, inotropic and vasoconstrictive effects. Use of dopamine is often limited by its strong positive chronotropic effects. A meta-analysis comparing dopamine and norepinephrine in patients with septic shock found a higher incidence of cardiac dysrhythmia and mortality with dopamine use.[87] Further, low-dose dopamine does not preserve renal function as previously thought.[88] **Epinephrine** is a second-line agent that possesses positive inotropic and vasopressor activity and is often utilized when norepinephrine alone is inadequate to maintain a target MAP. Epinephrine produces similar outcomes to norepinephrine plus dobutamine in septic shock.[89] Therefore, epinephrine may be a reasonable choice in septic shock, but a combination of norepinephrine and dobutamine allows greater control over relative degree of inotropy and vasopressor activity required. **Phenylephrine** (2–10 µg/kg/min) also has potent vasoconstricting properties and increases blood pressure. It acts only peripherally and its relative lack of chronotropy makes it useful in tachyarrhythmias. It is not a first- or second-line agent in septic shock because of its potential to reduce cardiac output by increasing afterload without increasing contractility.[8]

Occasionally, low-dose **vasopressin** (0.02–0.04 units/min) is used as an adjunctive or "rescue" vasopressor. The VASST trial randomized patients with septic shock to receive vasopressin and norepinephrine or norepinephrine alone.[90] No differences were noted between the 2 groups except significantly less renal failure in the "low norepinephrine" (<15 µg/min) plus vasopressin group. This study showed that vasopressin is safe and may be useful to "spare" high doses of norepinephrine in the septic patient who cannot tolerate tachycardia. However, it does not improve outcomes in the general ICU population. Vasopressin is not recommended as a single agent and should be used cautiously only in those with cardiac dysfunction.

Dobutamine (2–20 µg/kg/min) is a positive inotrope, but decreases systemic vascular resistance because of its vasodilatory properties. When added to norepinephrine, it may improve splanchnic blood flow[91] and it is often used in septic shock to improve oxygen delivery in a patient who has a mixed venous value of <70%, although studies have called into question the necessity of titrating resuscitation to mixed venous goals.[13,15]

Drotrecogin alfa

Drotrecogin alfa (activated protein C) was indicated for use in adult patients with severe sepsis and an Acute Physiology and Chronic Health Evaluation (APACHE II) score of ≥25 with multiple acute organ dysfunction. However in 2011, a large international study found no benefit for patients receiving drotrecogin alfa compared to those who did not. Subsequently the drug was withdrawn from the market worldwide.[92] There are currently no targeted anti-inflammatory medications for the treatment of sepsis, beyond the general anti-inflammatory class of corticosteroids.

Corticosteroids

Major clinical trials have yielded conflicting recommendations.[93,94,95] Many clinicians feel that corticosteroids can be an important therapeutic adjunct for a subset of patients who require them. Conversely, some studies suggest a higher risk of superinfections and new septic shock in those receiving them.[94,96,97] Identifying patients in whom the benefit is expected to outweigh risk is not straightforward. Consider administration of low-dose **hydrocortisone** (<300 mg/day) in patients whose hypotension does not adequately respond to fluids and vasopressors.[8,95] The practice of using an ACTH stimulation test to identify the cohort of patients who would benefit is no longer recommended.[8,97] However, it may be prudent to do a random cortisol level on all patients with shock initially unresponsive to fluid and low-dose vasopressors, to avoid missing those with profoundly low levels due to absolute adrenal insufficiency. Absolute adrenal deficiency is characterized by an absence of endogenous production of adrenal hormones and may be seen in bilateral adrenal infarcts, such as with Waterhouse-Fredrickson syndrome or thrombotic heparin-induced thrombocytopenia, or bilateral adrenal infiltration as seen in some disseminated malignancies or histoplasmosis. Hydrocortisone provides adequate mineralocorticoid activity, therefore adjunctive **fludrocortisone** (50 µg daily po) is recommended only if a corticosteroid without mineralocorticoid activity is used in place of hydrocortisone.

Immune Globulins

Immunotherapy to neutralize or remove specific exotoxins may be worthwhile if etiologic agents are identified (e.g., diphtheria, botulism, anthrax, clostridial septicotoxemia, toxic shock syndrome). However, as specific antisera are seldom available, immunoglobulins pooled from healthy donors are often used instead.

The use of polyclonal **iv immune globulins (IVIG)** is recommended in patients with hereditary or acquired immunodeficiency.[98,99] An observational study also suggested that IVIG at 2 g/kg × 1–2 doses could be useful in streptococcal toxic shock syndrome.[100] IVIG may improve outcome in cases of necrotizing fasciitis due to group A streptococcus (*Streptococcus pyogenes*) at a dose of 1 g/kg on day 1 and then 0.5 g/kg on days 2 and 3.[101] IVIG may also be useful in staphylococcal toxic shock syndrome.[102]

Currently there is clinical equipoise regarding the use of polyclonal IVIG in septic shock. There have been conflicting results in meta-analyses, and further well-designed, multicentre, randomized, placebo-controlled trials are needed.[103,104,105] Polyclonal IVIG is not recommended for use in septic shock outside of the specific indications cited above.

Therapeutic Tips

- Early recognition and treatment of sepsis are of paramount importance. Relevant antibiotics must be quickly available, ideally stored at the point of care to avoid delays in acquisition.
- When the CNS is the source of infection, consider covering with **acyclovir** until viral encephalitis (most commonly due to herpes simplex virus) is ruled out or another diagnosis is apparent (e.g., obvious bacterial meningitis). Strongly consider giving **dexamethasone** 0.15 mg/kg iv Q6H × 2–4 days as it improves outcomes in pneumococcal meningitis.[106,107,108] First dose should be administered before or concomitantly with antibiotics. Discontinue if culture results are negative for pneumococci.
- Culture-negative infections are particularly common among patients who have received partial antimicrobial therapy before cultures are obtained, and in immunocompromised patients undergoing bone marrow or solid organ transplants.
- Treat patients who have shock with no clear etiology for sepsis with appropriate antimicrobial therapy while investigating further. Distributive shock from sepsis may present concomitantly with other forms of shock such as cardiogenic shock, particularly in those patients who have pre-existing chronic disease.
- Biomarker assays such as procalcitonin are emerging as a useful adjunct in the evaluation of sepsis and may aid in determining the optimal duration of antimicrobial therapy.[109]
- Although sepsis typically involves low systemic vascular resistance, there is often some degree of myocardial depression. Bedside echocardiography facilitates the recognition and management of mixed shock states (low systemic vascular resistance and low cardiac output).
- Appropriate antimicrobial stewardship is challenging in the ICU. The balance between ensuring the best outcome for patients and avoiding the overuse of broad-spectrum agents can be difficult. Apply general principles of initial broad-spectrum therapy with re-evaluation and de-escalation of therapy based on microbiology results on a daily basis.[8] Occasionally, de-escalation is not prudent because of ongoing severe illness.

Table 3: Intravenous Antimicrobials Used in Sepsis and Septic Shock

Class[a]	Drug	Dose	Adverse Effects	Drug Interactions	Comments	Cost[b]
Aminoglycosides	*amikacin* generics	7.5 mg/kg Q12H iv or 15–20 mg/kg once daily iv	Nephrotoxicity, ototoxicity, neuromuscular blockade.	Penicillins may decrease serum levels.	Avoid as a first-line agent in septic shock because of nephrotoxicity and ototoxicity; monitor serum drug levels to guide dosing and avoid toxicity. Conventional dosing: desired serum peak level 40 µg/mL; desired trough <10 µg/mL. Once-daily dosing: desired trough is <1 µg/mL.	$$$
	gentamicin generics	1.5 mg/kg Q8H iv or 4–7 mg/kg once daily iv	See amikacin.	See amikacin.	See amikacin. Conventional dosing: desired peak 10 µg/mL; desired trough <2 µg/mL. Desired trough for once-daily dosing is <1 µg/mL.	$
	tobramycin generics	1.5 mg/kg Q8H iv or 4–7 mg/kg once daily iv	See amikacin.	See amikacin.	See amikacin. Conventional dosing: desired peak 10 µg/mL; desired trough <2 µg/mL. Desired trough for once-daily dosing is <1 µg/mL.	$
Carbapenems	*ertapenem* Invanz	1 g Q24H iv	Usually well tolerated. GI, hematologic reactions, rarely seizures.	Carbapenems may decrease valproic acid levels.	Low risk of cross-hypersensitivity with penicillins. May be used with caution in patients with penicillin allergy after a risk assessment and consideration of a graded challenge. Extended spectrum beta-lactam antibiotics have become the mainstay of treatment because of lack of nephrotoxicity and broad-spectrum activity vs. gram-negative organisms. No antipseudomonal activity. Once-daily dosing unique to carbapenem class.	$

(cont'd)

Table 3: **Intravenous Antimicrobials Used in Sepsis and Septic Shock** *(cont'd)*

Class[a]	Drug	Dose	Adverse Effects	Drug Interactions	Comments	Cost[b]
	imipenem/cilastatin Primaxin, generics	500 mg–1 g Q6H iv	Higher seizure risk than other carbapenems particularly with high doses and in presence of renal dysfunction.	See ertapenem. Avoid concurrent use with ganciclovir as seizures have been reported. Enhanced neurotoxic effects may occur with cyclosporine.	Low risk of cross-hypersensitivity with penicillins. May be used with caution in patients with penicillin allergy after a risk assessment and consideration of a graded challenge. Extended spectrum beta-lactam antibiotics have become the mainstay of treatment because of lack of nephrotoxicity and broad-spectrum activity vs. gram-negative organisms.	$$$
	meropenem Merrem, Meropenem for Injection	1 g Q8H iv (traditional dosing) *or* 500 mg Q6H iv (alternative dosing)[69]	See ertapenem.	See ertapenem.	Low risk of cross-hypersensitivity with penicillins. May be used with caution in patients with penicillin allergy after a risk assessment and consideration of a graded challenge. Extended spectrum beta-lactam antibiotics have become the mainstay of treatment because of lack of nephrotoxicity and broad-spectrum activity vs. gram-negative organisms.	$$$
Cephalosporins, third-generation	*cefotaxime* Claforan	2 g Q6–8H iv Meningitis: 2 g Q4–6H iv	Diarrhea, rash, hypersensitivity reactions, phlebitis, pseudomembranous colitis, hematologic reactions.	May increase INR with warfarin.	May be used with caution in patients with penicillin allergy after a risk assessment. If no alternative available and patient has history of immediate sensitivity reaction with penicillin consider a graded challenge or desensitization.	$$
	ceftazidime Fortaz, generics	2 g Q8H iv	See cefotaxime.	See cefotaxime.	See cefotaxime. Ceftazidime has good antipseudomonal activity, poor gram-positive coverage.	$$$$

Class[a]	Drug	Dose	Adverse Effects	Drug Interactions	Comments	Cost[b]
	ceftriaxone generics	1–2 g Q24H iv Meningitis: 2 g Q12H iv	See cefotaxime. Biliary sludge, particularly with high doses and rapid iv administration.	Do not reconstitute or mix with calcium-containing solutions. Do not administer simultaneously with calcium-containing iv solutions via a Y-site. Administration may be done sequentially provided the infusion lines are thoroughly flushed between infusions. See cefotaxime.	See cefotaxime.	$
Cephalosporins, fourth-generation	*cefepime* Maxipime, generics	2 g Q12H iv If neutropenic: 2 g Q8H iv	See cefotaxime. Risk of seizures particularly in those with renal dysfunction.	See cefotaxime.	See cefotaxime. Excellent activity against many resistant gram-negative pathogens including *Pseudomonas*. Good activity against most gram-positive organisms. Conflicting meta-analyses on the impact on mortality have been published.	$
Cyclic Lipopeptides	*daptomycin* Cubicin	Skin and soft tissue infections: 4 mg/kg daily iv Bacteremias: 6 mg/kg daily iv	Myalgias. Occasionally, rhabdomyolysis. Rarely, eosinophilic pneumonia.	No known significant drug interactions.	Effective against gram-positive organisms including MRSA and VRE. Should not be used in pneumonia because of deactivation by pulmonary surfactant in the lung.	$$$$
Fluoroquinolones	*ciprofloxacin* Cipro, generics	400 mg Q8–12H iv	Hypersensitivity reactions, lowers seizure threshold, prolongs QT_c interval.	Avoid using in conjunction with agents or conditions that prolong QT_c interval. As an inhibitor of CYP1A2, ciprofloxacin can increase serum concentrations of CYP1A2 substrates (e.g., theophylline).	Oral formulations available for step-down therapy; most appropriate fluoroquinolone for pseudomonal infections; emerging resistance worldwide.	$$
	levofloxacin Levaquin, generics	750 mg Q24H iv	See ciprofloxacin. Hypo- or hyperglycemia. Cases of severe liver injury including liver failure have been reported.	See ciprofloxacin. Not metabolized by CYP enzymes.	Oral formulations available for step-down therapy; effective against atypical pathogens of community-acquired pneumonia and many gram-positive cocci.	$

(cont'd)

Table 3: **Intravenous Antimicrobials Used in Sepsis and Septic Shock** *(cont'd)*

Class[a]	Drug	Dose	Adverse Effects	Drug Interactions	Comments	Cost[b]
	moxifloxacin Avelox	400 mg Q24H iv	See ciprofloxacin. Cases of severe liver injury including liver failure have been reported.	See ciprofloxacin. Not metabolized by CYP enzymes.	Oral formulations available for step-down therapy; improved activity against anaerobic bacteria as well as gram-positive cocci and enteric gram-negative bacilli; effective against atypical pathogens of community-acquired pneumonia.	$
Glycopeptides	*vancomycin* ❥ generics	15–20 mg/kg Q8–12H iv (monitor levels and adjust dose accordingly)	Nephrotoxicity, ototoxicity, phlebitis, "red man syndrome" (flushing/rash, hypotension) if infused too rapidly (<1 h).	Enhanced nephrotoxicity when used with aminoglycosides.	Desired serum levels: trough 15–20 μg/mL. Useful if serious infection with enterococci or coagulase-negative staphylococci, or for methicillin-resistant *S. aureus*.	$$$$
Glycylcyclines	*tigecycline* Tygacil	100 mg initially, then 50 mg Q12H iv	Nausea and vomiting relatively common, pancreatitis, injection site reactions, tooth discolouration.	Possible increased risk of pseudotumor cerebri in patients taking isotretinoin.	Broad spectrum; active against most gram-positive, gram-negative and anaerobic bacteria. No activity against *Pseudomonas*. Active against VRE and MRSA. Structurally similar to tetracyclines. Avoid in pregnant women. Tigecycline has been associated with an increased risk of mortality compared to other antibiotics when used for severe infections, particularly ventilator-associated pneumonia. Other antibiotics are preferred when susceptibilities permit their use.	$$$$
Lincosamides	*clindamycin* Dalacin C Phosphate Sterile Solution, generics	600–900 mg Q8H iv, can also be administered Q6H	Rash, thrombophlebitis, GI effects, pseudomembranous colitis, blood dyscrasias, elevated liver function tests.	May increase neuromuscular blocking action of other agents. Antagonism with erythromycin.	Used in necrotizing skin infections to reduce endotoxin production and for synergy with beta-lactams.	$
Macrolides	*azithromycin* Zithromax, generics	500 mg Q24H iv	Venous irritation/thrombophlebitis, prolongation of QT_c interval.	May increase serum concentrations of cardiac glycosides. Enhanced QT_c prolongation effect of amiodarone.	Used for coverage of atypical pathogens in community-acquired pneumonia (not necessary if patient is taking a fluoroquinolone).	$

Class[a]	Drug	Dose	Adverse Effects	Drug Interactions	Comments	Cost[b]
Nitroimidazoles	*metronidazole* generics	500 mg Q8–12H iv	Not common: thrombophlebitis, blood dyscrasias, neurological disturbances.	Increased lithium levels.	Excellent anaerobic coverage; caution if severe hepatic dysfunction.	$
Oxazolidinones	*linezolid* Zyvoxam	600 mg BID iv/po	Rarely lactic acidosis. Peripheral and optic neuropathy, myelosuppression.	May potentiate the pressor effect of adrenergic agents. Possible serotonin syndrome when used with SSRIs or MAOIs.	Effective against gram-positive organisms; 100% oral bioavailability but do not use orally in septic patients as bioavailability is unreliable; may have better outcomes than vancomycin in MRSA pneumonia.	$$$$$
Penicillins, extended-spectrum	*piperacillin/ tazobactam* Tazocin, Piperacillin/Tazobactam for Injection, other generics	3.375 g Q6H iv (4.5 g Q6H iv for *Pseudomonas*)	Usually well tolerated. Gastrointestinal, hematologic reactions.	Tetracyclines decrease effectiveness of penicillins. Increased methotrexate serum levels.	Extended spectrum beta-lactam antibiotics have become the mainstay of treatment because of lack of nephrotoxicity and broad-spectrum activity vs. gram-negative organisms.	$$
	ticarcillin/clavulanate Timentin	3.1 g Q4–6H iv	See piperacillin/tazobactam.	See piperacillin/tazobactam.	See piperacillin/tazobactam. Experts differ on whether ticarcillin/clavulanate is equivalent to piperacillin/tazobactam.	$
Azole Antifungals	*fluconazole* Diflucan,generics	400 mg Q24H iv	Gastrointestinal reactions, hepatic injury, exfoliative skin disorders.	Additive effect with other QT-prolonging agents. Increased levels of sulfonylureas, phenytoin. Rifampin decreases azole levels.		$
	voriconazole Vfend, generics	Loading dose of 6 mg/kg Q12H iv × 24 h, then 3–4 mg/kg Q12H iv Oral maintenance dose: <40 kg: 100 mg BID; maximum 150 mg BID ≥40 kg: 200 mg BID; maximum 300 mg BID	Gastrointestinal reactions, visual disturbances, rash, hepatic injury.	See fluconazole.	Avoid iv in moderate to severe renal impairment because of nephrotoxic vehicle. Effective against *Aspergillus*. Oral formulation available for step-down therapy and is safe in renal impairment.	$$$$$

(cont'd)

Table 3: **Intravenous Antimicrobials Used in Sepsis and Septic Shock** *(cont'd)*

Class[a]	Drug	Dose	Adverse Effects	Drug Interactions	Comments	Cost[b]
Echinocandin Antifungals	*anidulafungin* Eraxis	200 mg iv day 1, then 100 mg Q24H iv	Fever, rash, nausea, vomiting, phlebitis at injection site.	No clinically significant interactions.	Active against most candidal species and well tolerated.	$$$$$
	caspofungin Cancidas	70 mg iv day 1, then 50 mg Q24H iv	See anidulafungin.	Increased LFTs with cyclosporine. Dexamethasone, efavirenz, nevirapine, phenytoin, rifampin, carbamazepine decrease caspofungin levels.	See anidulafungin.	$$$$$
	micafungin Mycamine	100 mg Q24H iv	See anidulafungin.	Increased cyclosporine, nifedipine and sirolimus levels. Probably not clinically significant.	See anidulafungin.	$$$$$
Polyene Antifungals	*amphotericin B* Fungizone	0.6–1 mg/kg Q24H iv	Fever, electrolyte disturbances, nausea/vomiting, nephrotoxicity, anemia, hypotension, phlebitis.	Increased nephrotoxicity with other nephrotoxic drugs.	Use limited by renal failure or electrolyte disturbances.	$$
	amphotericin B lipid preparation Abelcet, AmBisome	3–5 mg/kg Q24H iv	Less nephrotoxicity than standard amphotericin B.	See amphotericin B.		$700

[a] In this table, antibacterial agents are presented first in alphabetical order followed by the antifungal agents.
[b] Cost of 1-day supply based on 70 kg body weight; includes drug cost only.
Dosage adjustment required in renal impairment; see Appendix I.
Abbreviations: LFT = liver function test; MAOI = monoamine oxidase inhibitor; MRSA = methicillin-resistant *S. aureus*; VRE = vancomycin-resistant enterococci
Legend: $ < $50 $$ $50–100 $$$ $100–150 $$$$ $150–200 $$$$$ $200–250

Suggested Readings

Angus DC, van der Poll T. Severe sepsis and septic shock. *N Engl J Med* 2013;369(9):840-51.

Dellinger RP, Levy MM, Rhodes A et al. Surviving Sepsis Campaign: international guidelines for management of severe sepsis and septic shock: 2012. *Crit Care Med* 2013;41(2):580-637.

Kumar A, Roberts D, Wood KE et al. Duration of hypotension before initiation of effective antimicrobial therapy is the critical determinant of survival in human septic shock. *Crit Care Med* 2006;34(6):1589-96.

Rivers E, Nguyen B, Havstad S et al. Early goal-directed therapy in the treatment of severe sepsis and septic shock. *N Engl J Med* 2001;345(19):1368-77.

Vincent JL, De Backer D. Circulatory shock. *N Engl J Med* 2013;369(18):1726-34.

References

1. American College of Chest Physicians/Society of Critical Care Medicine Consensus Conference: definitions for sepsis and organ failure and guidelines for the use of innovative therapies in sepsis. *Crit Care Med* 1992;20(6):864-74.
2. Levy MM, Fink MP, Marshall JC et al. 2001 SCCM/ESICM/ACCP/ATS/SIS International Sepsis Definitions Conference. *Crit Care Med* 2003;31(4):1250-6.
3. Ferreira FL Bota DP, Bross A et al. Serial evaluation of the SOFA score to predict outcome in critically ill patients. *JAMA* 2001;286(14):1754-8.
4. Vincent JL, Bruzzi de Carvalho F et al. Severity of illness. *Semin Respir Crit Care Med* 2010;31(1):31-8.
5. Beaulieu Y. Bedside echocardiography in the assessment of the critically ill. *Crit Care Med* 2007;35(5 Suppl):S235-49.
6. Harvey S, Harrison DA, Signer M et al. Assessment of the clinical effectiveness of pulmonary artery catheters in management of patients in intensive care (PAC-Man): a randomised controlled trial. *Lancet* 2005;366(9484):472-7.
7. Chittock DR, Dhingra VK, Ronco JJ et al. Severity of illness and risk of death associated with pulmonary artery catheter use. *Crit Care Med* 2004;32(4):911-5.
8. Dellinger RP, Levy MM, Rhodes A et al. Surviving Sepsis Campaign: international guidelines for management of severe sepsis and septic shock: 2012. *Crit Care Med* 2013;41(2):580-637.
9. Rivers E, Nguyen B, Havstad S et al. Early goal-directed therapy in the treatment of severe sepsis and septic shock. *N Engl J Med* 2001;345(19):1368-77.
10. Practice parameters for hemodynamic support of sepsis in adult patients in sepsis. Task Force of the American College of Critical Care Medicine, Society of Critical Care Medicine. *Crit Care Med* 1999;27(3):639-60.
11. Manthous CA, Hall JB, Olson D et al. Effect of cooling on oxygen consumption in febrile critically ill patients. *Am J Respir Crit Care Med* 1995;151(1):10-4.
12. Papazian L, Forel JM, Gacouin A et al. Neuromuscular blockers in early acute respiratory distress syndrome. *N Engl J Med* 2010;363(12):1107-16.
13. Jones AE, Shapiro NI, Trzeciak S et al. Lactate clearance vs central venous oxygen saturation as goals of early sepsis therapy: a randomized clinical trial. *JAMA* 2013;303(8):739-46.
14. Osman D, Ridel C, Ray P. Cardiac filling pressures are not appropriate to predict hemodynamic response to a volume challenge. *Crit Care Med* 2007;35(1):64-8.
15. ProCESS Investigators, Yealy DM, Kellum JA et al. A randomized trial of protocol-based care for early septic shock. *N Engl J Med* 2014;370(18):1683-93.
16. Finfer S, Bellomo R, Boyce N et al. A comparison of albumin and saline for fluid resuscitation in the intensive care unit. *N Engl J Med* 2004;350(22):2247-56.
17. Guidet B, Martinet O, Boulain T et al. Assessment of hemodynamic efficacy and safety of 6% hydroxyethylstarch 130/0.4 vs. 0.9% NaCl fluid replacement in patients with severe sepsis: the CRYSTMAS study. *Crit Care* 2012;16(3):R94.
18. Perner A, Haase N, Guttormsen AB et al. Hydroxyethyl starch 130/0.42 versus Ringer's acetate in severe sepsis. *N Engl J Med* 2012;367(2):124-34.
19. Zarychanski R, Abou-Setta AM, Turgeon AF et al. Association of hydroxyethyl starch administration with mortality and acute kidney injury in critically ill patients requiring volume resuscitation: a systematic review and meta-analysis. *JAMA* 2013;309(7):678-88.
20. Vincent JL, De Backer D. Circulatory shock. *N Engl J Med* 2013;369(18):1726-34.
21. Marik PE, Monnet X, Teboul JL. Hemodynamic parameters to guide fluid therapy. *Ann Intensive Care* 2011;1(1):1.
22. Hebert PC, Wells G, Blajchman MA et al. A multicenter, randomized, controlled clinical trial of transfusion requirements in critical care. Transfusion Requirements in Critical Care Investigators, Canadian Critical Care Trials Group. *N Engl J Med* 1999;340(6):409-17.
23. Vincent JL. Hemodynamic support in septic shock. *Intensive Care Med* 2001;27(Suppl 1):S80-92.
24. Corwin HL, Gettinger A, Rodriguez RM et al. Efficacy of recombinant human erythropoietin in the critically ill patient: a randomized, double-blind, placebo-controlled trial. *Crit Care Med* 1999;27(11):2346-50.
25. Stanworth SJ, Walsh TS, Prescott RJ et al. A national study of plasma use in critical care: clinical indications, dose and effect on prothrombin time. *Crit Care* 2011;15(2):R108.
26. Liumbruno G, Bennardello F, Lattanzio A et al. Recommendations for the transfusion of plasma and platelets. *Blood Transfus* 2009;7(2):132-50.
27. van den Berghe G, Wouters P, Weekers F et al. Intensive insulin therapy in critically ill patients. *N Engl J Med* 2001;345(19):1359-67.
28. Brunkhorst FM, Engel C, Bloos F et al. Intensive insulin therapy and pentastarch resuscitation in severe sepsis. *N Engl J Med* 2008;358(2):125-39.
29. De La Rosa Gdel C, Donado JH, Restrepo AH et al. Strict glycaemic control in patients hospitalised in a mixed medical and surgical intensive care unit: a randomised clinical trial. *Crit Care* 2008;12(5):R120.
30. The NICE-SUGAR Study Investigators et al. Intensive versus conventional glucose control in critically ill patients. *N Engl J Med* 2009;360(13):1283-97.
31. The NICE-SUGAR Study Investigators et al. Hypoglycemia and risk of death in critically ill patients. *N Engl J Med* 2012;367(12):1108-18.

32. Griesdale DE, de Souza RJ, van Dam, RM et al. Intensive insulin therapy and mortality among critically ill patients: a meta-analysis including NICE-SUGAR study data. *CMAJ* 2009;180(8):821-7.
33. Jimenez MF, Marshall JC; International Sepsis Forum. Source control in the management of sepsis. *Intensive Care Med* 2001;27(Suppl 1):S49-62.
34. Rabindranath K, Adams J, Macleod AM et al. Intermittent versus continuous renal replacement therapy for acute renal failure in adults. *Cochrane Database Syst Rev* 2007;(3):CD003773.
35. Vesconi S, Cruz DN, Fumagalli R et al. Delivered dose of renal replacement therapy and mortality in critically ill patients with acute kidney injury. *Crit Care* 2009;13(2):R57.
36. Van Wert R, Friedrich JO, Scales DC et al. High-dose renal replacement therapy for acute kidney injury: systematic review and meta-analysis. *Crit Care Med* 2010;38(5):1360-9.
37. Zhongheng Z, Xiao X, Hongyang Z. Intensive- vs less-intensive-dose continuous renal replacement therapy for the intensive care unit-related acute kidney injury: a meta-analysis and systematic review. *J Crit Care* 2010;25(4):595-600.
38. Payen D, Mateo J, Cavaillon JM et al. Impact of continuous venovenous hemofiltration on organ failure during the early phase of severe sepsis: a randomized controlled trial. *Crit Care Med* 2009;37(3):803-10.
39. Beitler JR, Shaefi S, Montesi SB et al. Prone positioning reduces mortality from acute respiratory distress syndrome in the low tidal volume era: a meta-analysis. *Intensive Care Med* 2014;40(3):332-41.
40. Boyd JH, Walley KR. Is there a role for sodium bicarbonate in treating lactic acidosis from shock? *Curr Opin Crit Care* 2008;14(4):379-83.
41. Perez J, Dellinger RP; International Sepsis Forum. Other supportive therapies in sepsis. *Intensive Care Med* 2001;27(Suppl 1):S116-27.
42. Davidson BL, Geerts WH, Lensing AW. Low-dose heparin for severe sepsis. *N Engl J Med* 2002;347(13):1036-7.
43. PROTECT Investigators for the Canadian Critical Care Trials Group and the Australian and New Zealand Intensive Care Society Clinical Trials Group, Cook D, Meade M et al. Dalteparin versus unfractionated heparin in critically ill patients. *N Engl J Med* 2011;364(14):1305-14.
44. Thirugnanam S, Pinto R, Cook DJ et al. Economic analyses of venous thromboembolism prevention strategies in hospitalized patients: a systematic review. *Crit Care* 2012;16(2):R43.
45. Steinberg KP. Stress-related mucosal disease in the critically ill patient: risk factors and strategies to prevent stress-related bleeding in the intensive care unit. *Crit Care Med* 2002;30(6 Suppl):S362-4.
46. Marik PE, Vasu T, Hirani A et al. Stress ulcer prophylaxis in the new millennium: a systematic review and meta-analysis. *Crit Care Med* 2010;38(11):2222-8.
47. Kahn JM, Doctor JN, Rubenfeld GD. Stress ulcer prophylaxis in mechanically ventilated patients: integrating evidence and judgement using a decision analysis. *Intensive Care Med* 2006;32(8):1151-8.
48. Camilleri M, Parkman HP, Shafi MA et al. Clinical guideline: management of gastroparesis. *Am J Gastroenterol* 2013;108(1):18-37.
49. Cerra FB, Benitez MR, Blackburn GL et al. Applied nutrition in ICU patients. A consensus statement of the American College of Chest Physicians. *Chest* 1997;111(3):769-78.
50. Marik PE, Zaloga GP. Early enteral nutrition in acutely ill patients: a systematic review. *Crit Care Med* 2001;29(12):2264-70.
51. Casaer MP, Mesotten D, Hermans G et al. Early versus late parenteral nutrition in critically ill adults. *N Engl J Med* 2011;365(6):506-17.
52. Girard TD, Pandharipande PP, Ely EW. Delirium in the intensive care unit. *Crit Care* 2008;12(Suppl 3):S3.
53. Tan JA, Ho KM. Use of dexmedetomidine as a sedative and analgesic agent in critically ill adult patients: a meta-analysis. *Intensive Care Med* 2010;36(6):926-39.
54. Reade MC, O'Sullivan K, Bates S et al. Dexmedetomidine vs. haloperidol in delirious, agitated, intubated patients: a randomised open-label trial. *Crit Care* 2009;13(3):R75.
55. Jakob SM, Ruokonen E, Grounds RM et al. Dexmedetomidine vs midazolam or propofol for sedation during prolonged mechanical ventilation: two randmized controlled trials. *JAMA* 2012;307(11):1151-60.
56. Girard TD, Kress JP, Fuchs BD et al. Efficacy and safety of a paired sedation and ventilator weaning protocol for mechanically ventilated patients in intensive care (Awakening and Breathing Controlled trial): a randomised controlled trial. *Lancet* 2008;371(9607):126-34.
57. Mehta S, Burry L, Cook D et al. Daily sedation interruption in mechanically ventilated critically ill patients cared for with a sedation protocol: a randomized controlled trial. *JAMA* 2012;308(19):1985-92.
58. Huskins WC. Interventions to prevent transmission of antimicrobial-resistant bacteria in the intensive care unit. *Curr Opin Crit Care* 2007;13(5):572-7.
59. Esteban A, Alia I, Tobin MJ et al. Effect of spontaneous breathing trial duration on outcome of attempts to discontinue mechanical ventilation. Spanish Lung Failure Collaborative Group. *Am J Respir Crit Care Med* 1999;159(2):512-8.
60. Kumar A, Roberts D, Wood KE et al. Duration of hypotension before initiation of effective antimicrobial therapy is the critical determinant of survival in human septic shock. *Crit Care Med* 2006;34(6):1589-96.
61. Mandell LA, Wunderink RG, Anzueto A et al. Infectious Diseases Society of America/American Thoracic Society consensus guidelines on the management of community-acquired pneumonia in adults. *Clin Infect Dis* 2007;44(Suppl 2):S27-72.
62. Solomkin JS, Mazuski JE, Baron EJ et al. Guidelines for the selection of anti-infective agents for complicated intra-abdominal infections. *Clin Infect Dis* 2003;37(8):997-1005.
63. Pappas PG, Kauffman CA, Andes D et al. Clinical practice guidelines for the management of candidiasis: 2009 update by the Infectious Diseases Society of America. *Clin Infect Dis* 2009;48(5):503-35.
64. Shan YS, Sy ED, Wang ST et al. Early presumptive therapy with fluconazole for occult Candida infection after gastrointestinal surgery. *World J Surg* 2006;30(1):119-26.
65. Wagenlehner FM, Weidner W, Naber KG. Pharmacokinetic characteristics of antimicrobials and optimal treatment of urosepsis. *Clin Pharmacokinet* 2007;46(4):291-305.
66. Tunkel AR, Hartman BJ, Kaplan SL et al. Practice guidelines for the management of bacterial meningitis. *Clin Infect Dis* 2004;39(9):1267-84.
67. Stevens DL, Bisno AL, Chambers HF et al. Practice guidelines for the diagnosis and management of skin and soft-tissue infections. *Clin Infect Dis* 2005;41(10):1373-406.
68. Raad I, Hanna H, Maki D. Intravascular catheter-related infections: advances in diagnosis, prevention, and management. *Lancet Infect Dis* 2007;7(10):645-57.
69. Patel GW, Duquaine SM, McKinnon PS. Clinical outcomes and cost minimization with an alternative dosing regimen for meropenem in a community hospital. *Pharmacotherapy* 2007;27(12):1637-43.
70. Gould CV, McDonald LC. Bench-to-bench bedside review: Clostridium difficile colitis. *Crit Care* 2008;12(1):203.
71. Hilf M, Yu VL, Sharp J et al. Antibiotic therapy for *Pseudomonas aeruginosa* bacteremia: outcome correlations in a prospective study of 200 patients. *Am J Med* 1989;87(5):540-6.

72. Sligl WI, Asadi L, Eurich DT et al. Macrolides and mortality in critically ill patients with community-acquired pneumonia: a systematic review and meta-analysis. *Crit Care Med* 2014;42(2):420-32.
73. Leroy O, Saux P, Bedos JP et al. Comparison of levofloxacin and cefotaxime combined with ofloxacin for ICU patients with community-acquired pneumonia who do not require vasopressors. *Chest* 2005;128(1):172-83.
74. Waterer GW. Monotherapy versus combination antimicrobial therapy for pneumococcal pneumonia. *Curr Opin Infect Dis* 2005;18(2):157-63.
75. Martin-Loeches I, Lisboa T, Rodriguez A et al. Combination antibiotic therapy with macrolides improves survival in intubated patients with community-acquired pneumonia. *Intensive Care Med* 2010;36(4):612-20.
76. Brunkhorst FM, Oppert M, Marx G et al. Effect of empirical treatment with moxifloxacin and meropenem vs meropenem on sepsis-related organ dysfunction in patients with severe sepsis: a randomized trial. *JAMA* 2012;307(22):2390-9.
77. Heyland DK, Johnson AP, Reynolds SC et al. Procalcitonin for reduced antibiotic exposure in the critical care setting: a systematic review and an economic evaluation. *Crit Care Med* 2011;39(7):1792-9.
78. Layios N, Lambermont B, Canivet JL et al. Procalcitonin usefulness for the initiation of antibiotic treatment in intensive care unit patients. *Crit Care Med* 2012;40(8):2304-9.
79. Sarosi GA. Fungal infections and their treatment in the intensive care unit. *Curr Opin Crit Care* 2006;12(5):464-9.
80. Leon C, Ruiz-Santana S, Saavedra P et al. A bedside scoring system ("Candida score") for early antifungal treatment in nonneutropenic critically ill patients with Candida colonization. *Crit Care Med* 2006;34(3):730-7.
81. Piarroux R, Grenouillet F, Balvay P et al. Assessment of preemptive treatment to prevent severe candidiasis in critically ill surgical patients. *Crit Care Med* 2004;32(12):2443-9.
82. Bow EJ, Evans G, Fuller J et al. Canadian clinic practice guidelines for invasive candidiasis in adults. *Can J Infect Dis Med Microbiol* 2010;21(4):e122-50.
83. Schuster MG, Edwards JE, Sobel JD et al. Empirical fluconazole versus placebo for intensive care unit patients: a randomized trial. *Ann Intern Med* 2008;149(2):83-90.
84. Kett DH, Shorr AF, Reboli AC et al. Anidulafungin compared with fluconazole therapy in critically ill patients. *Crit Care Med* 2010;14(Suppl 1):P72.
85. Martin C, Papazian L, Perrin G et al. Norepinephrine or dopamine for the treatment of hyperdynamic septic shock? *Chest* 1993;103(6):1826-31.
86. Marik PE, Mohedin M. The contrasting effects of dopamine and norepinephrine on systemic and splanchnic oxygen utilization in hyperdynamic sepsis. *JAMA* 1994;272(17):1354-7.
87. De Backer D, Aldecoa C, Njimi H et al. Dopamine versus norepinephrine in the treatment of septic shock: a meta-analysis. *Crit Care Med* 2012;40(3):725-30.
88. Bellomo R, Chapman M, Finfer S et al. Low-dose dopamine in patients with early renal dysfunction: a placebo-controlled randomised trial. Australian and New Zealand Intensive Care Society (ANZICS) Clinical Trials Group. *Lancet* 2000;356(9248):2139-43.
89. Annane D, Vignon P, Renault A et al. Norepinephrine plus dobutamine versus epinephrine alone for management of septic shock: a randomised trial. *Lancet* 2007;370(9588):676-84.
90. Russell JA, Walley KR, Singer J et al. Vasopressin versus norepinephrine infusion in patients with septic shock. *N Engl J Med* 2008;358(9):877-87.
91. Duranteau J, Sitbon P, Teboul JL et al. Effects of epinephrine, norepinephrine, or the combination of norepinephrine and dobutamine on gastric mucosa in septic shock. *Crit Care Med* 1999;27(5):893-900.
92. Health Canada. *Xigris (drotrecogin alfa) withdrawn worldwide*. Ottawa (ON): Health Canada; 2011. Available from: www.healthycanadians.gc.ca/recall-alert-rappel-avis/hc-sc/2011/13551a-eng.php.
93. Annane D, Sebille V, Charpentier C et al. Effect of treatment with low doses of hydrocortisone and fludrocortisone on mortality in patients with septic shock. *JAMA* 2002;288(7):862-71.
94. Sprung CL, Annane D, Keh D et al. Hydrocortisone therapy for patients with septic shock. *N Engl J Med* 2008;358(2):111-24.
95. Annane D, Bellissant E, Bollaert PE et al. Corticosteroids in the treatment of severe sepsis and septic shock. *JAMA* 2009;301(22):2362-75.
96. Minneci PC, Deans KJ, Banks SM et al. Meta-analysis: the effect of steroids on survival and shock during sepsis depends on the dose. *Ann Intern Med* 2004;141(1):47-56.
97. Marik PE, Pastores SM, Annane D et al. Recommendations for the diagnosis and management of corticosteroid insufficiency in critically ill adult patients: consensus statements from an international task force by the American College of Critical Care Medicine. *Crit Care Med* 2008;36(6):1937-49.
98. Schwartz SA. Intravenous immunoglobulin treatment of immunodeficiency disorders. *Pediatr Clin North Am* 2000;47(6):1355-69.
99. Spector SA, Gelber RD, McGrath N et al. A controlled trial of intravenous immune globulin for the prevention of serious bacterial infections in children receiving zidovudine for advanced human immunodeficiency virus infection. Pediatric AIDS Clinical Trials Group. *N Engl J Med* 1994;331(18):1181-7.
100. Kaul R, McGeer A, Norrby-Teglund A et al. Intravenous immunoglobulin therapy for streptococcal toxic shock syndrome—a comparative observational study. The Canadian Streptococcal Study Group. *Clin Infect Dis* 1999;28(4):800-7.
101. Darenberg J, Ihendyane N, Sjolin J et al. Intravenous immunoglobulin G therapy in streptococcal toxic shock syndrome: a European randomized, double-blind, placebo-controlled trial. *Clin Infect Dis* 2003;37(3):333-40.
102. Darenberg J, Soderquist B, Normark BH et al. Differences in potency of intravenous polyspecific immunoglobulin G against streptococcal and staphylococcal superantigens: implications for therapy of toxic shock syndrome. *Clin Infect Dis* 2004;38(6):836-42.
103. Turgeon AF, Hutton B, Fergusson DA et al. Meta-analysis: intravenous immunoglobulin in critically ill adult patients with sepsis. *Ann Intern Med* 2007;146(3):193-203.
104. Pildal J, Gotzsche PC. Polyclonal immunoglobulin for treatment of bacterial sepsis: a systematic review. *Clin Infect Dis* 2004;39(1):38-46.
105. Alejandria MM, Lansang MA, Dans LF et al. Intravenous immunoglobulin for treating sepsis, severe sepsis and septic shock. *Cochrane Database Syst Rev* 2013;9:CD001090.
106. de Gans J, van de Beek D; European Dexamethasone in Adulthood Bacterial Meningitis Study Investigators. Dexamethasone in adults with bacterial meningitis. *N Engl J Med* 2002;347(20):1549-56.
107. Brouwer MC, Heckenberg SG, de Gans J et al. Nationwide implementation of adjunctive dexamethasone therapy for pneumococcal meningitis. *Neurology* 2010;75(17):1533-9.
108. Brouwer MC, McIntyre P, de Gans J et al. Corticosteroids for acute bacterial meningitis. *Cochrane Database Syst Rev* 2010;(9):CD004405.
109. Becker KL, Snider R, Nylen ES. Procalcitonin assay in systemic inflammation infection and sepsis: clinical utility and limitataions. *Crit Care Med* 2008;36(3):941-52.

Chapter 120
Sexually Transmitted Infections

Richard Lester, MD, FRCPC

In this chapter, sexually transmitted infections (STIs) are presented according to whether the major initial manifestations are vaginal discharge, urethritis or cervicitis or genital lesions. Anogenital warts and pelvic inflammatory disease (an infection of the upper genital tract) are discussed as well.

Goals of Therapy

- Treat the infection
- Abolish symptoms
- Decrease spread to sexual partners
- Decrease vertical transmission from mother to newborn
- Reduce transmission of HIV
- Decrease probability of complications, such as infertility, chronic pain, sepsis

Investigations

- History:
  - duration of symptoms, if any
  - risk factors, e.g., sexual contact with person with known STI, recent new partner, >2 partners in past year, injection drug use, men having sex with men (MSM), commercial sex workers, nonbarrier contraception[1,2]
  - type and site of sexual exposure with or without barrier protection (e.g., oral, vaginal, anal, receptive and/or insertive)
  - risks for ascending infection such as recent childbirth or intrauterine contraceptive device insertion
  - past history of STIs, therapy and response
- Physical:
  - search for systemic signs of STIs, e.g., syphilis, disseminated gonococcus
  - inspect mucocutaneous regions including pharynx and anus
  - inspect external genitalia for lesions, inflammation, discharge
  - consider a digital rectal exam and anoscopy if perianal warts are present or if patient has rectal symptoms or has practised receptive anal intercourse
  - palpate for inguinal lymphadenopathy
  - in women: perform speculum examination to visualize cervix and vaginal walls and to evaluate endocervical and vaginal discharges; bimanual pelvic exam to detect uterine or adnexal masses or tenderness
  - in men: search for signs of urethral discharge, palpate testicles/epididymides
- Laboratory tests:
  - for women: clinician-collected tests include cervical or vaginal swabs. Patient-collected samples include first-void urine or vaginal self-collection; when collected properly, the patient-obtained

samples have similar sensitivity and specificity to the physician-collected specimens. Nucleic acid amplification tests (NAATs) are available for chlamydia, gonorrhea and, at some centres, trichomoniasis or mycoplasma.[3] NAATs will not give information on antibiotic susceptibility. Gonorrhea cultures should be obtained when antibiotic resistance is a concern. Vaginal swabs can be done to test for yeast or bacterial vaginosis by use of Gram stain and pH; wet preparations are useful for trichomoniasis or yeast. Antigen detection tests or culture improve sensitivity for trichomoniasis. Ultrasound if pelvic inflammatory disease (PID) is suspected; beta-hCG to rule out pregnancy; rectal specimens for chlamydia and lymphogranuloma venereum (LGV), as indicated

- for men: first-void urine for chlamydia and gonorrhea NAAT; urethral swab for gonorrhea culture if symptomatic and available; scrotal ultrasound if epididymo-orchitis or testicular torsion suspected, consider testing for LGV (culture, NAAT, serology); rectal specimens for chlamydia and LGV, as indicated (testing for LGV can be done by using a standard chlamydia NAAT and requesting genotyping if chlamydia positive)
- for external lesions: swabs for herpes (use viral media), bacteria, syphilis (send fluid from lesion for darkfield test, direct immunofluorescence antibody test or PCR) as indicated
- throat and rectal swabs for gonorrhea if indicated
- consider serology for syphilis, hepatitis B and hepatitis C (see Chapter 66), HIV (see Chapter 113) as indicated

Infections Characterized by Vaginal Discharge

Etiology

The 3 infections most frequently associated with vaginal discharge are *trichomoniasis* (caused by *Trichomonas vaginalis*), *bacterial vaginosis* (caused by a replacement of the normal vaginal flora by an overgrowth of anaerobic microorganisms, mycoplasmas and *Gardnerella vaginalis*) and *vulvovaginal candidiasis* (VVC; commonly caused by *Candida albicans*) (Table 1). There is an element of recurrence in these conditions. Recurrent vulvovaginal candidiasis (≥4 episodes/year) requires investigation and possibly referral. Address predisposing causes if present, e.g., use of systemic antibiotics, poorly controlled diabetes mellitus or HIV (consider testing).

Table 1: Differential Diagnosis of Vaginal Discharge[1,2]

Diagnostic Parameters		Candidiasis	Trichomoniasis	Bacterial Vaginosis
Signs/ symptoms	Pruritus	+	+	–
	Odour	–	+	+ (fishy)
	Discharge	white, clumpy & curdy	off-white or yellow, frothy	grey or milky, thin, copious
	Inflammation	+	+	–
Simple tests	Vaginal pH	<4.5 (normal)	>4.5	>4.5
	"Whiff" test[a]	–	–	+
Microscopic findings	Specific	budding yeast, pseudohyphae	motile trichomonads	clue cells,[b] predominant gram-negative curved bacilli and coccobacilli
	PMNs	++	+++	–
	Lactobacilli	+	–	–

[a] Malodour often intensified after addition of 10% potassium hydroxide (KOH).
[b] Clue cells are vaginal epithelial cells covered with numerous coccobacilli.
Abbreviations: PMN = polymorphonucleocyte

Nonsexually transmitted causes of vaginitis are numerous, e.g., atrophic vaginitis, trauma, malignancy, detergents, foreign bodies, contraceptive chemicals and allergy to latex condoms. Candidiasis and bacterial vaginosis are not usually considered sexually transmitted (Table 2).

Therapeutic Choices

Figure 1 depicts the management of vaginitis and cervicitis. Table 3, Table 4 and Table 5 detail the drugs used in the treatment of trichomoniasis, bacterial vaginosis and vulvovaginal candidiasis, respectively.

Pharmacologic Choices

Treatment of *trichomoniasis* is recommended for all patients except asymptomatic pregnant women. Treat sexual partner(s) irrespective of symptoms or test results.

Antibiotic treatment can be offered to all symptomatic women with bacterial vaginosis. Treatment is unnecessary in asymptomatic women except if undergoing IUD insertion, gynecologic surgery, therapeutic abortion, upper genital tract instrumentation or if the woman is at high-risk of preterm delivery.[5]

Uncomplicated VVC can be treated by a short course of topical antifungal formulations. Treatment is unnecessary in asymptomatic cases. Individualize therapy based on factors such as patient preference, cost, convenience, adherence, portability and history of response or side effects to prior treatments. Vaginal **nystatin** is less effective than vaginal **azoles**. Consider prophylactic oral **fluconazole** at start of antibiotic treatment in women prone to recurrent VVC secondary to antibiotic use.

Table 2: **Treatment of Sexual Contacts[1,2]**

Disease	Management of Partner
Anogenital warts (human papillomavirus)	Likelihood of transmission and duration of infectivity unknown, but condoms associated with decreased transmission of human papillomavirus
Bacterial vaginosis	No treatment
Chlamydia and gonorrhea	Refer all recent (<60 days) partners for testing and empiric treatment (Table 6, Table 7). No sexual contact for patient or partner until 1 wk after initiation of treatment
Genital herpes	Use condoms, be aware of asymptomatic shedding
Lymphogranuloma venereum	Refer all recent (<60 days) partners for testing and empiric treatment (Table 9)
Pelvic inflammatory disease	Refer all recent male partners (<60 days) for examination and treatment (Table 12, Table 13). Treat empirically for *C. trachomatis* and/or *N. gonorrhoeae*. No sexual contact for patient or partner until 1 wk after initiation of treatment
Syphilis, late latent	Test all long-term partners and any of their children who were possibly exposed during pregnancy
Syphilis, primary, secondary and early latent	Refer partners for empiric treatment (Table 8) even if seronegative. Trace-back period for primary, secondary and early latent syphilis is 3 months, 6 months and 1 year, respectively; refer all partners for testing and empiric treatment
Trichomoniasis	Treat current sexual partner. No sexual contact until patient and partner finished treatment and are asymptomatic
Vulvovaginal candidiasis	No treatment. Consider treatment of sex partner(s) in women with recurrent infections

Figure 1: **Management of Vaginitis and Cervicitis**

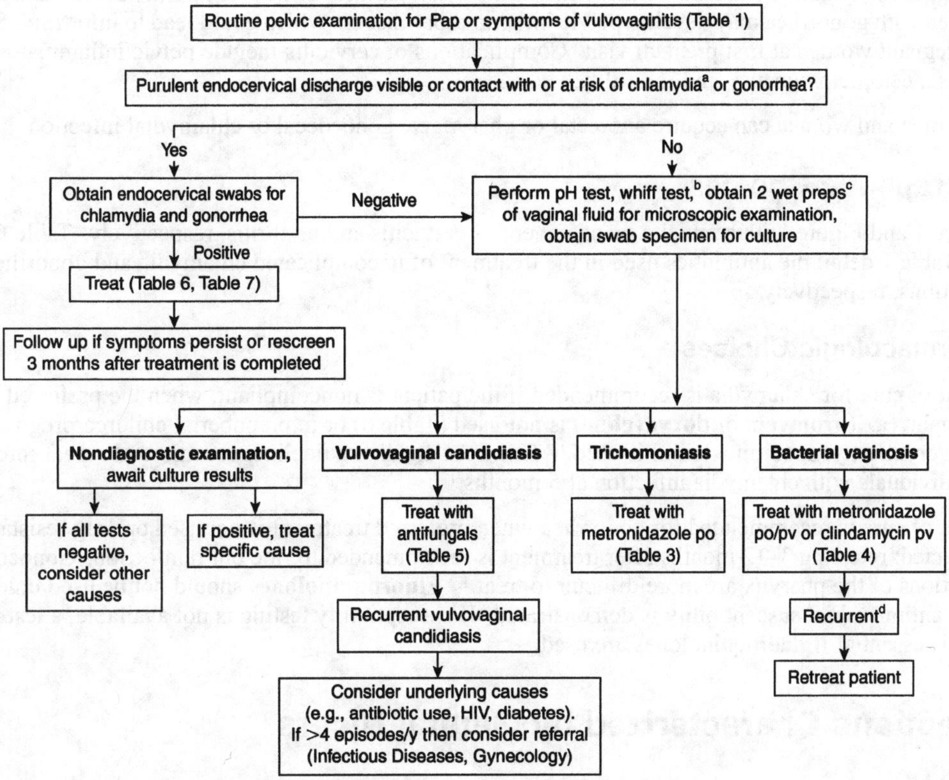

a Chlamydial nucleic acid amplification testing, e.g., PCR, of a first voided urine specimen is an option if vaginal examination is not possible.
b Malodour often intensified after addition of 10% potassium hydroxide (KOH).
c First sample mixed in a few drops of normal saline; second sample mixed with 10% KOH.
d Recurrent bacterial vaginosis may develop in ~15–30% of patients in the first 1–3 months of treatment.
Abbreviations: Pap = Papanicolaou test; po = orally; pv = intravaginally

Infections Characterized by Urethritis and Cervicitis

Etiology

The 2 main causes of urethritis and cervicitis are gonorrhea (caused by *Neisseria gonorrhoeae*) and chlamydia (caused by *Chlamydia trachomatis* serovars D to K). Nongonococcal, nonchlamydial causes of urethritis and cervicitis include *Mycoplasma genitalium*, *Ureaplasma urealyticum*, *T. vaginalis*, herpes simplex virus (HSV), herpes zoster (VZV), and adenovirus. Patients with gonorrhea are often infected with chlamydia and should receive presumptive treatment for both.[1,2] Test and treat sexual partners (Table 2). Symptoms may be absent and are not a prerequisite for screening individuals at risk of STIs. Screen for HIV and syphilis.

In men, symptoms include purulent discharge and severe dysuria ("drip and burn"). Complications of urethritis include epididymitis, seminal vesiculitis, prostatitis and disseminated infection (fever, skin and joint involvement). If epididymo-orchitis is due to sexual transmission, empiric therapy for both gonorrhea and chlamydia is required; continue the antichlamydial regimen for at least 10 days and until resolution occurs. Scrotal elevation, bedrest and analgesics are advisable. Epididymo-orchitis may require referral to rule out other diagnoses such as testicular torsion and abscess.

In women, symptoms include copious vaginal discharge, dysuria, intermenstrual uterine bleeding and menorrhagia. Chlamydia infection is often asymptomatic; therefore, screen high-risk women (e.g., young, sexually active women, women with multiple sex partners or new sex partners).[2] Up to 20% of women with gonorrhea may develop pelvic inflammatory disease which could lead to infertility. Screen all pregnant women at first prenatal visit. Complications of cervicitis include pelvic inflammatory disease, ectopic pregnancy and infertility.

Both men and women can acquire anorectal or pharyngeal gonococcal or chlamydial infection.

Therapeutic Choices

Figure 1 and Figure 2 illustrate the management of cervicitis and urethritis, respectively. Table 6 and Table 7 detail the antibiotics used in the treatment of uncomplicated chlamydia and gonorrhea infections, respectively.

Pharmacologic Choices

A test of cure for chlamydia is recommended if the patient is noncompliant, when the preferred treatment (**azithromycin** or **doxycycline**) is not used (Table 6) or in prepubertal children/pregnancy when erythromycin or amoxicillin is used.[1,2] Current Canadian guidelines recommend repeat screening of individuals with chlamydia infection at 6 months.[1]

A test of cure is recommended for gonorrhea when preferred treatment is not used or drug resistance is suspected; retesting 3–12 months after treatment is recommended to rule out reinfection. Gonococcal infections of the pharynx are more difficult to treat.[1,2] **Fluoroquinolones** should not be used unless prior antimicrobial susceptibility is demonstrated. If susceptibility testing is not available, a test of cure is essential if fluoroquinolones are used.

Infections Characterized by Genital Ulcers

Etiology

Several STIs are associated with genital ulcers including genital herpes, syphilis, lymphogranuloma venereum and chancroid. The two most common in North America are *genital herpes* (see Chapter 112) and syphilis. *Syphilis* is caused by *Treponema pallidum*, a bacterium that penetrates broken skin or mucous membranes, usually through sexual contact. Syphilis ulcers (chancres) are often single, large and painless while genital herpes ulcers are often multiple, small and painful. However, there is considerable overlap in clinical presentation of these conditions.

Lymphogranuloma venereum (LGV) is caused by the invasive *C. trachomatis* serovars L1, L2 and L3 which preferentially affect the lymph tissue.[1,2] LGV is transmitted through vaginal, anal or oral sexual contact. Suspect LGV if proctitis symptoms appear in men who have sex with men, particularly if accompanied by bloody anal discharge [Evidence: SORT C*].[1,2] Complications include colorectal fissures and secondary bacterial infections. Testing for LGV in suspicious cases is by special request to a reference laboratory. Test and treat sexual partners [Evidence: SORT C*].[1,2] See Table 2. Individuals with genital ulcers are at increased risk of acquiring and transmitting HIV.

* SORT (Strength of Recommendation Taxonomy) is a rating system (A, B or C) that addresses the quality of available evidence. For more information consult **How to Use *Compendium of Therapeutic Choices*** on page xxv.

Figure 2: **Management of Urethritis and Epididymo-orchitis in Males**

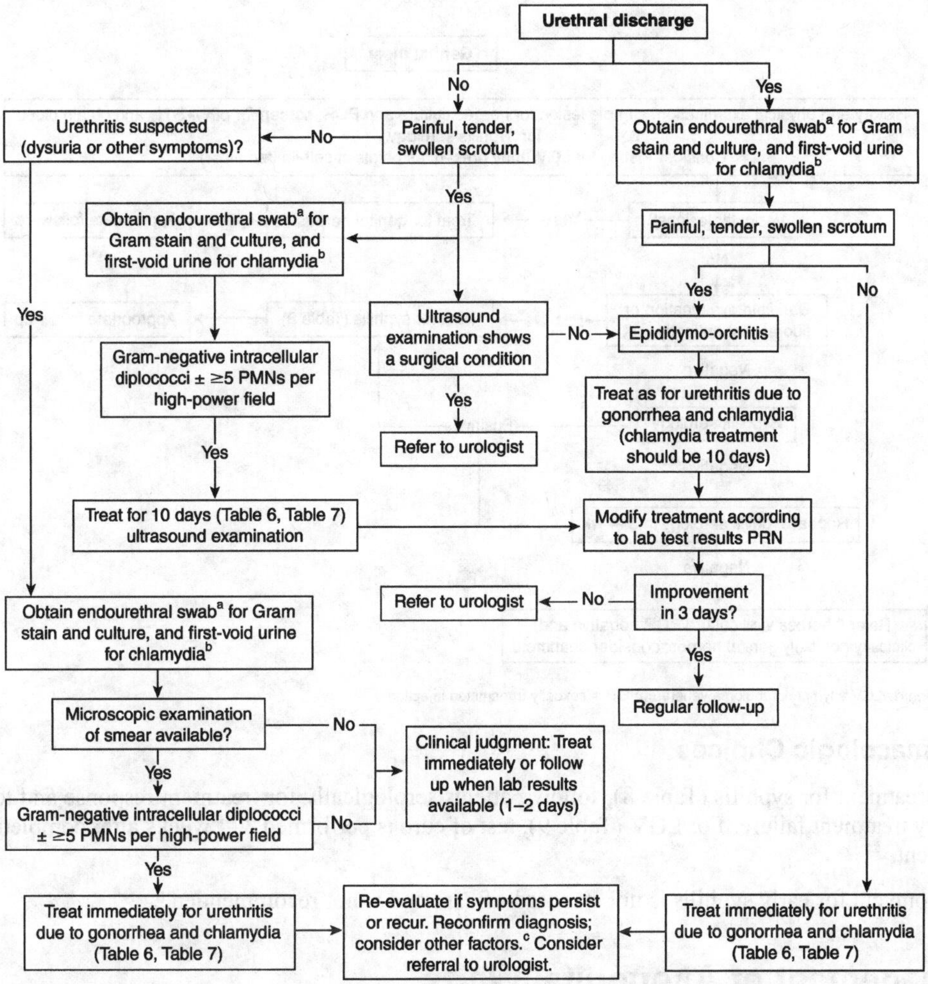

a Diagnosis of gonorrhea by culture, rather than nucleic acid amplification testing is preferred, in order to allow for antimicrobial susceptibility testing.
b Nucleic acid amplification testing, e.g., PCR, of a first-voided urine specimen is accurate for chlamydia detection.
c Re-exposure; nonadherence; antimicrobial resistance; other etiologies such as urinary tract infections, prostatitis; other microorganisms such as *T. vaginalis, U. urealyticum, M. genitalium*.
Abbreviations: PMN = polymorphonucleocyte; PRN = as needed

Chancroid, caused by *Haemophilus ducreyi*, is very rare in North America and requires special media to culture. Contact your laboratory if chancroid is suspected (one or more painful genital ulcers with a yellow-gray base and a surrounding erythematous ring, tender and sometimes suppurative inguinal lymphadenopathy, history of travel to an endemic area such as Africa, Asia or the Caribbean).

Refer individuals coinfected with HIV and syphilis and those with suspected or proven tertiary syphilis.

Therapeutic Choices

Figure 3 illustrates the management of genital ulcers (herpes, LGV and syphilis).

Figure 3: **Management of Genital Ulcers: Herpes, Lymphogranuloma Venereum and Syphilis**

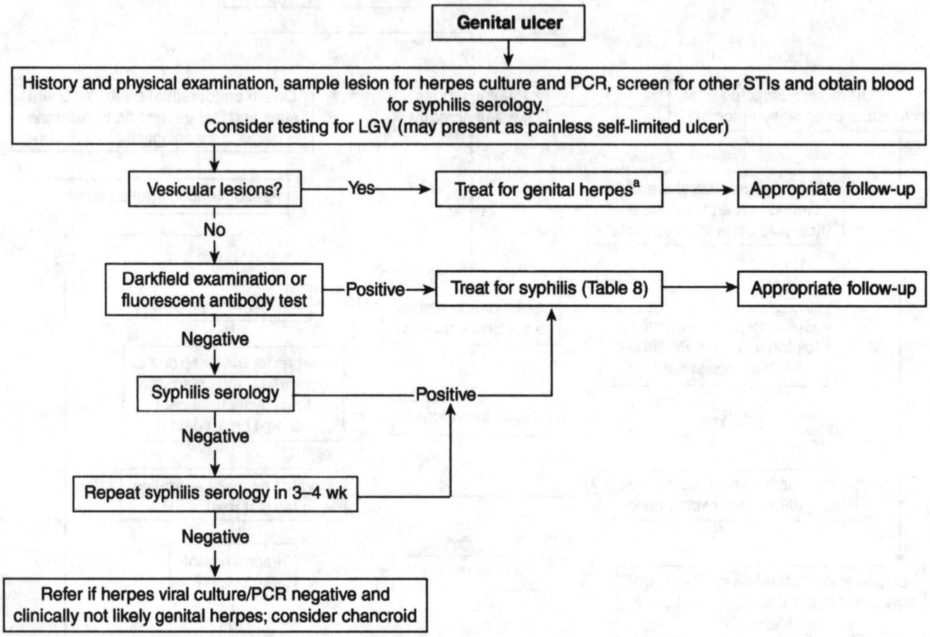

Abbreviations: LGV = lymphogranuloma venereum; STI = sexually transmitted infection

Pharmacologic Choices

After treatment for syphilis (Table 8), follow patients serologically for treatment response and to identify treatment failure. For LGV (Table 9), test of cure is performed 3–4 weeks after completion of treatment.

Azithromycin for early syphilis is not standard-of-care and is not recommended.[6]

Management of Anogenital Warts

Etiology

Anogenital warts are caused by the human papillomavirus (HPV). No definitive evidence suggests any of the available treatments is superior to the others, and no single treatment is ideal for all patients or all warts. Warts may resolve with or without treatment; however, there is a frustratingly high recurrence rate (approximately 33%) of genital warts 1 year after apparent cure. Refer patients with warts on their cervix or anal mucosa.

Therapeutic Choices

Figure 4 illustrates the management of anogenital warts.

Pharmacologic Choices

Imiquimod, **podophyllin** and **podophyllotoxin** (Table 10) are used to treat genital warts.

Figure 4: **Management of Anogenital Warts**

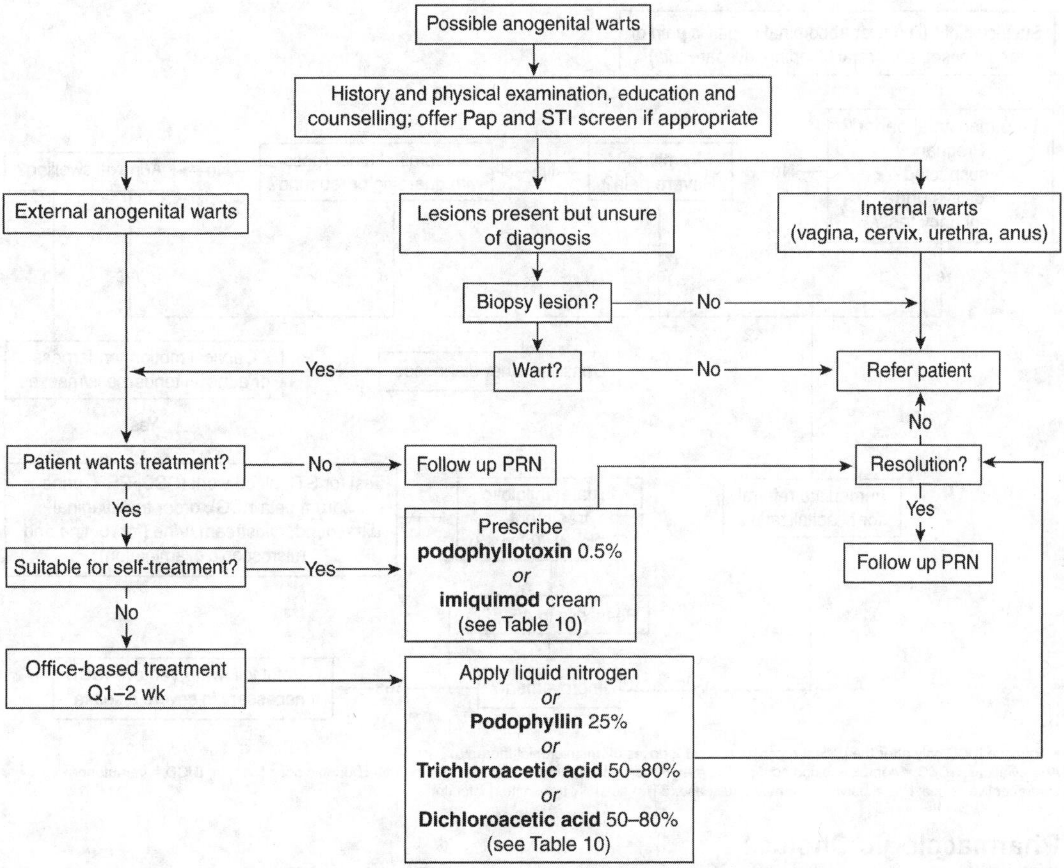

For *prevention* of genital warts, a quadrivalent **HPV vaccine** has been approved for females and males aged 9–26 years (Table 11). The vaccine does not prevent all strains of HPV. Annual cytology screening (Pap smear) is recommended until 2 consecutive tests are negative, then every 3 years until age 69.[7] A bivalent HPV vaccine that contains the 2 most common carcinogenic strains of HPV (types 16 and 18) is available but it does not prevent anogenital warts caused by HPV type 6 or 11.

Management of Pelvic Inflammatory Disease

Therapeutic Choices

Pelvic inflammatory disease (PID) includes infectious endometritis, salpingitis and peritonitis. Patients with PID should be hospitalized if they are pregnant, do not respond to or do not tolerate outpatient antibiotics, are nonadherent, have a tubo-ovarian abscess or are very ill (e.g., vomiting, high fever).[1,2] Test and treat sexual partners (Table 2). Figure 5 illustrates the management of PID. Table 12 and Table 13 detail the antibiotics used in the management of PID in outpatients and inpatients respectively.

Figure 5: **Management of Pelvic Inflammatory Disease**

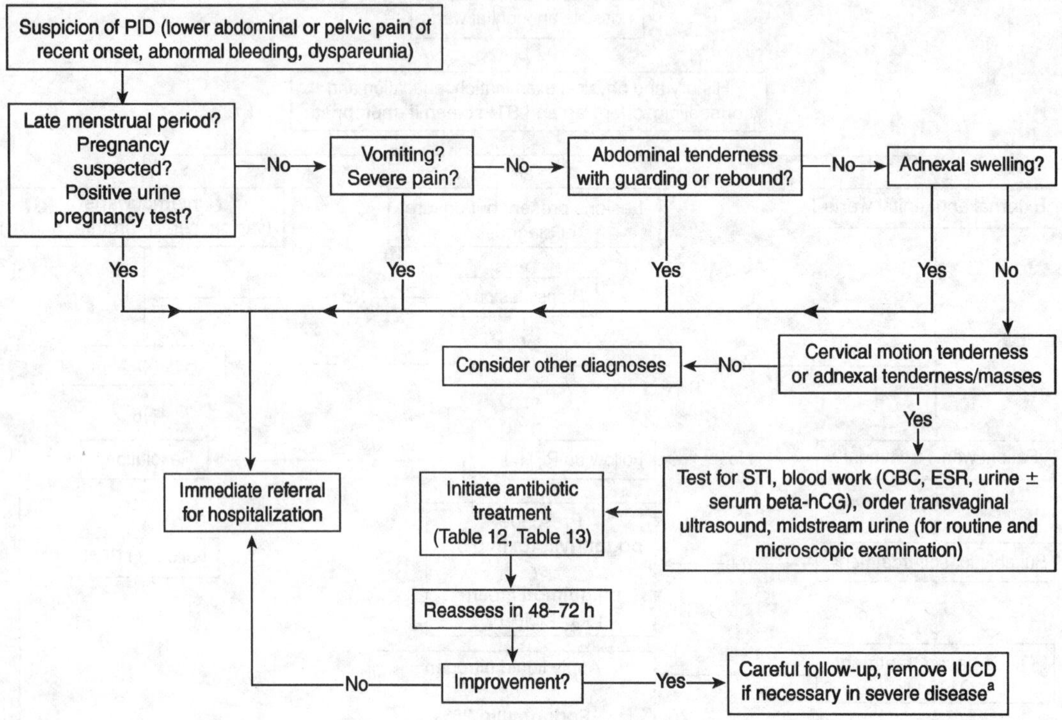

[a] Remove IUCD only after the patient receives at least 2 doses of antimicrobial therapy.
Abbreviations: CBC = complete blood count; ESR = erythrocyte sedimentation rate; hCG = human chorionic gonadotropin; IUCD = intrauterine contraceptive device; PID = pelvic inflammatory disease; STI = sexually transmitted infection

Pharmacologic Choices

Empiric antimicrobial therapy for PID should include coverage of the likely pathogens: *N. gonorrhoeae*, *C. trachomatis*, gram-negative facultative bacteria and streptococci. Consider anaerobic coverage since anaerobes are detected in the majority of PID cases. However, it is not known if elimination of anaerobes is necessary.

Choices during Pregnancy and Breastfeeding

Sexually transmitted infections (STIs) pose potential risk of complications for the expectant mother and the newborn. Therefore, screen pregnant women for chlamydia, gonorrhea, syphilis and hepatitis B virus and offer HIV testing in their first prenatal visit, and again in the third trimester if their risk of acquiring an STI is ongoing. Due to increased risks of complications and the potential for decreased efficacy of treatments during pregnancy, follow up is important to ensure therapeutic success. Consult experts and/or resources such as the Motherisk Program (www.motherisk.org or 416-813-6780) when appropriate. **Erythromycin estolate** salt, **fluoroquinolones**, **podophyllin**, **podophyllotoxin**, **imiquimod** and **tetracyclines** are relatively or absolutely contraindicated in pregnancy or breastfeeding. Several STIs may cause poor pregnancy outcomes and be vertically transmitted and cause congenital infections. Always seek up-to-date information.

Untreated *trichomoniasis* may lead to premature rupture of membranes, preterm delivery and low birth weight. Treat patient if symptomatic. Oral **metronidazole** is preferred either as a 2 g single dose or a 7-day course (Table 3) as two 2 g doses may increase the risk of preterm birth.[19] Treat sexual partners. Retest during pregnancy only if symptomatic. Screening for asymptomatic trichomoniasis is not recommended because a benefit of treatment has not been demonstrated.

Untreated *bacterial vaginosis* may cause premature rupture of membranes, preterm labour, preterm birth and postpartum endometritis. Screen if pregnancy is high-risk (previous preterm labour/delivery or premature rupture of membranes) or if patient is symptomatic. Otherwise, treatment has not been shown to improve outcomes. Systemic **metronidazole** or **clindamycin** are preferred over topical formulations (Table 4). Withhold breastfeeding during treatment with metronidazole and for 12–24 h after last dose. Avoid intravaginal clindamycin cream since it has been associated with adverse outcomes in newborns. Consider re-screening high-risk women.

Routine screening for *vulvovaginal candidiasis* is not necessary. Risks to pregnant mother are limited to the bothersome symptoms and irritation. Recurrences are common in pregnancy. If symptomatic, treat with *vaginal* "**azole**" antifungals (Table 5). Animal teratogenicity has been shown in the first trimester with continuous daily **fluconazole** doses of ≥400 mg. Data are lacking for single-dose use. Fluconazole may be used in recurrent VVC if benefit outweighs potential risk (see Appendix II). **Boric acid** vaginal suppositories are not currently recommended.

Untreated *chlamydial infections* may lead to preterm birth and premature rupture of membranes and may cause conjunctivitis and pneumonia in the newborn. Screen all pregnant women at first prenatal visit. **Amoxicillin, erythromycin** (not the estolate salt) or **azithromycin** are the preferred antibiotics (Table 6). Patients should abstain from sexual intercourse for 7 days after initiation of adequate treatment and until all sexual partners have been treated. Patients and ongoing sexual partners should have a follow-up test of cure 3–4 weeks after completing therapy. Co-treat for gonorrhea if this has not been ruled out.

Table 3: Antibiotics for the Treatment of Trichomoniasis[1,2]

Class	Drug	Dose	Adverse Effects	Drug Interactions	Comments	Cost[a]
Nitroimidazoles	*metronidazole, oral* Flagyl, generics	2 g po × single dose *or* 500 mg BID po × 7 days	GI upset, urethral burning, discolouration of urine (dark or reddish brown).	Disulfiram-like reaction with alcohol may occur during treatment.	Intravaginal metronidazole is ineffective in treatment of trichomoniasis. Treat current partner(s) irrespective of symptoms; efficacy increases if partner is also treated. No follow up necessary unless symptoms recur. Can be used in pregnancy or breastfeeding—benefit outweighs possible risks.	$

[a] Cost for specified duration of treatment; includes drug cost only.
Dosage adjustment required in renal impairment; see Appendix I.
Legend: $ <$10

Untreated *gonococcal infections* may lead to endometritis and pelvic sepsis in the mother and ophthalmia neonatorum and systemic infection in the newborn. Screen all pregnant women at first prenatal visit. **Ceftriaxone** is the preferred antibiotic (Table 7). Patients should abstain from sexual intercourse for 7 days after initiation of adequate treatment and until all sexual partners have been treated. Patients and ongoing sexual partners should have a follow-up test of cure 3–4 weeks after completing therapy. Co-treat for chlamydia if this has not been ruled out.

Untreated *syphilis infection* may lead to complications of systemic syphilis in the mother and congenital syphilis in the newborn. Fetal loss may also occur. Transmission during breastfeeding is theoretically possible during secondary syphilis. A **penicillin** regime is strongly preferred (Table 8). Consider desensitization if patient is allergic to penicillin and refer to a specialist. Risk of vertical transmission is reduced with maternal therapy but empiric therapy may be required for the newborn with appropriate follow up to rule out congenital syphilis.

External genital warts and *HPV infections* may proliferate during pregnancy and may be refractory to therapy. Respiratory papillomatosis may rarely occur in the newborn. Goal of treatment is to relieve symptoms only. Disease severity may increase in pregnancy and may spontaneously regress postpartum. **Di-** or **trichloroacetic acid** (Table 10), **cryotherapy**, **laser** or **surgical excision** are the preferred treatment options. Cytotoxic agents (podophyllin, podophyllotoxin and imiquimod) are contraindicated. Cesarean section is rarely indicated.

Pelvic inflammatory disease is uncommon in pregnancy but poses an increased risk of adverse outcomes for both the mother and the fetus. Suspected PID cases should be hospitalized for evaluation and treatment with parenteral therapy (Table 13). Outpatient regimens recommended for the treatment of PID are outlined in Table 12. **Fluoroquinolones** and **tetracyclines** are contraindicated in pregnancy and breastfeeding. Consult with an infectious disease expert.

A discussion of general principles on the use of medications in these special populations can be found in Appendix II and Appendix III. Other specialized reference sources are also provided in these appendices.

Therapeutic Tips

- Treat sexual partner(s) (Table 2).
- Discuss consistent and correct use of latex or polyurethane *condoms* for optimal risk reduction of STIs.[8,9,10,11,12]
- Recommend **Hepatitis B vaccine**, if not previously immunized.
- Discuss and counsel on risk of acquisition and transmission of HIV and STIs.[13]

Table 4: Antibiotics for the Treatment of Bacterial Vaginosis[1,2]

Class	Drug[a]	Dose	Adverse Effects	Comments	Cost[b]
Lincosamides	*clindamycin, oral* Dalacin C, Dalacin C Flavored Granules, generics	300 mg BID po × 7 days	GI upset, *C. difficile* colitis, diarrhea.	*Alternative treatment.* Can be used in pregnant and breastfeeding women; retest 1 month after completion to confirm efficacy of therapy. Coadministration of kaolin decreases clindamycin absorption.	$
	clindamycin, 2% vaginal cream Dalacin Vaginal Cream	1 applicatorful (5 g) daily pv × 7 days	Vulvovaginitis.	***Preferred treatment.*** Not recommended in high-risk pregnancy as it does not prevent preterm birth.[4] Topical clindamycin has been associated with adverse outcomes in the newborn when used in pregnancy. Delay treatment until completion of menstrual period. Contains mineral oil—may decrease effectiveness of condoms and diaphragms.	$$$
Nitroimidazoles	*metronidazole, oral* Flagyl, generics	Preferred dose: 500 mg BID po × 7 days Alternative dose: 2 g po × single dose Recurrent bacterial vaginosis (≥3 episodes per year): 500 mg BID po × 10–14 days	GI upset, urethral burning, dark or reddish brown discolouration of urine, metallic taste.	***Preferred treatment.*** Can be used in pregnancy or breastfeeding. Retest 1 month after completion of treatment to ensure therapeutic success. Single dose metronidazole is associated with higher failure rate. Disulfiram-like reaction with alcohol may occur during treatment.	$
	metronidazole, 0.75% vaginal gel NidaGel, generics	1 applicatorful (5 g) daily pv × 5 days Recurrent bacterial vaginosis (≥3 episodes per year): 1 applicatorful (5 g) daily pv × 10 days followed by 5 g pv twice weekly × 4–6 months	Vaginal discharge, yeast infection, vulva/vaginal irritative symptoms, pain and discomfort.	***Preferred treatment.*** Not recommended in high-risk pregnancy as it does not prevent preterm birth.[4] Topical treatment has similar cure rate as oral metronidazole.	$$

[a] Treatment of male sexual partners is not indicated and does not prevent recurrence. Treatment of asymptomatic patients is unnecessary except prior to IUD insertion, gynecologic surgery, therapeutic abortion, upper tract instrumentation or if high-risk pregnancy.

[b] Cost of preferred dose; includes drug cost only.

Dosage adjustment required in renal impairment; see Appendix I.

Legend: $ <$10 $$ $10–20 $$$ $20–30

Table 5: **Antifungals for the Treatment of Symptomatic Vulvovaginal Candidiasis**[1,2]

Class	Drug[a]	Dose	Adverse Effects	Comments	Cost[b]
Azole Antifungals, oral	*fluconazole* ❥ Diflucan-150, CanesOral, generics	Uncomplicated infection: 150 mg po × single dose Recurrent infection (≥4 episodes per year): 150 mg every 72 h × 3 doses then weekly for a minimum of 6 months; consider referral	Headache, nausea, abdominal pain, diarrhea, dyspepsia, dizziness.	Prescription not required. Contraindicated in pregnancy. Confirm diagnosis of recurrent VVC by vaginal culture and identification of species. If patient is prone to VVC and requires a course of antibiotics, consider prescribing prophylactic topical or oral antifungals (e.g., fluconazole 150 mg once weekly until antibiotic course is completed). Follow up required if symptoms persist despite treatment or recur within 2 months of onset.	$
	itraconazole Sporanox Capsules, Sporanox Oral Solution	Maintenance treatment: 200–400 mg monthly po × 6 months[1]	No significant side effects because of infrequent dosing.	Other antifungals (e.g., oral fluconazole, topical azoles) are preferred for maintenance.	$$/month
Azole Antifungals, topical[c]	*butoconazole 2% vaginal cream* Gynazole-1	Uncomplicated infection: 5 g pv × single dose	Local hypersensitivity.	Prescription required. Cream contains mineral oil; decreases effectiveness of condoms or diaphragms. Though a 1-day treatment, it takes a few days for symptoms to resolve. Follow up required if despite treatment symptoms persist or recur within 2 months of onset.	$$
	clotrimazole Canesten Vaginal, generics	Uncomplicated infection: 200 mg/vaginal tablet: 1 tablet daily pv × 3 days *or* 500 mg/vaginal tablet: 1 tablet pv × single dose *or* 1% vaginal cream: 1 applicatorful daily pv × 6 days *or* 2% vaginal cream: 1 applicatorful daily pv × 3 days *or* 10% vaginal cream: 1 applicatorful pv × single dose Recurrent infection (≥4 episodes/y): extend treatment period to 10–14 days then maintain with clotrimazole 500 mg vaginal tablets once monthly for at least 6 months	See butoconazole 2% vaginal cream.	Prescription not required. Also available in combination with external cream. Menstruation is not an indication to stop treatment. Safe for use in pregnancy; 7–14 days treatment period may be necessary. Follow up required if symptoms persist despite treatment or recur within 2 months of onset.	$

Class	Drug[a]	Dose	Adverse Effects	Comments	Cost[b]
	miconazole Monistat, generics	Uncomplicated infection: 400 mg/ovule: 1 ovule daily pv × 3 days *or* 1200 mg/ovule: 1 ovule pv × single dose *or* 2% vaginal cream: 1 applicatorful daily pv × 7 days *or* 4% vaginal cream: 1 applicatorful daily pv × 3 days	See butoconazole 2% vaginal cream.	Prescription not required. Also available in combination with external cream. Ovules contain hydrogenated vegetable oil and mineral oil which may decrease effectiveness of condoms or diaphragms. Treat for 7–14 days in pregnancy. Follow up required if symptoms persist despite treatment or recur within 2 months of onset.	$
	terconazole Terazol, generics	Uncomplicated infection: 0.4% vaginal cream: 1 applicatorful daily pv × 7 days *or* 80 mg vaginal ovule + 0.8% vaginal cream combination pack: 1 ovule daily pv × 3 days + external application of cream to vulva × 3 days	See butoconazole 2% vaginal cream.	Prescription required. Ovules contain hydrogenated vegetable oil; Decreased efficacy of latex condoms or diaphragms. Follow up required if symptoms persist despite treatment or recur within 2 months of onset.	$$
Polyenes	*nystatin* generics	Uncomplicated infection: Vaginal cream 25 000 units/g: 4 g once or twice daily pv × 14 days *or* Vaginal cream 100 000 units/g: 5 g daily pv × 14 days Severe infection: Vaginal cream 100 000 units/g: 5 g BID pv × 14 days	See butoconazole 2% vaginal cream.	Less effective than azole antifungals. Follow up required if symptoms persist despite treatment or recur within 2 months of onset.	$
Weak Acids	*boric acid vaginal capsules*[d]	Recurrent infection (≥4 episodes/y): 300–600 mg gelatin capsule daily pv × 14 days then maintain with 300 mg capsule pv × 5 days per month beginning the first day of menstrual cycle. Continue for at least 6 months	Local irritation, vaginal burning; more pronounced with higher dose.	Contraindicated in pregnancy. 300 mg capsules are less irritating than the 600 mg capsules. Usually reserved for treatment of recurrent or non-albicans VVC. Also useful in treatment of VVC in immunocompromised host.	$$

[a] Topical treatment is as effective as oral therapy.
[b] Cost for specified duration of treatment; includes drug cost only.
[c] Preferred treatment.
[d] Extemporaneously compounded preparation
Abbreviations: CCB = calcium channel blocker; H_2RA = H_2-receptor antagonist; PPI = proton pump inhibitor; VVC = vulvovaginal candidiasis
Legend: $ <$10 $$ $10–20

Table 6: **Antibiotics for the Treatment of Uncomplicated *Chlamydia* Infection**

Class	Drug[a]	Dose	Adverse Effects	Drug Interactions	Comments	Cost[b]
Fluoroquinolones	*levofloxacin* Levaquin, generics	500 mg daily po × 7 days	GI upset, headache.	Decreased levels with concurrent antacids or iron. Increases risk of tendon rupture with concomitant corticosteroid use. Avoid use with QT_c prolonging agents, e.g., Class 1A, III antiarrhythmics—may result in arrhythmias.	*Alternative treatment.* A test of cure is essential. Test and treat partners. Contraindicated in pregnant and breastfeeding women. Safety in children <18 y not established.	$
	ofloxacin generics	300 mg BID po × 7 days	See levofloxacin.	See levofloxacin.	See levofloxacin.	$$
Macrolides	*azithromycin* Zithromax, generics	Adults and children ≥45 kg: 1 g po × single dose	GI upset.	May increase digoxin levels.	***Preferred treatment.*** May be useful in situations when poor adherence is expected. Repeat dose if vomiting <1 h post-administration. Can be used in pregnant and breastfeeding women.	$
	erythromycin Eryc, generics	Adults: erythromycin base 500 mg QID po × 7 days If tolerance is a concern: erythromycin base 250 mg QID po × 14 days *Chlamydia trachomatis* in infants, ophthalmia neonatorum, infant pneumonia caused by *C. trachomatis*: erythromycin base 12.5 mg/kg QID po × 14 days; may need second course of treatment and follow up	GI upset.	May increase levels of carbamazepine, digoxin, HMG-CoA reductase inhibitors, e.g., simvastatin, protease inhibitors, sildenafil, theophylline, warfarin. Avoid use with pimozide, cisapride, disopyramide.	*Alternative treatment.* High incidence of GI side effects and QID dosing may discourage adherence. Can be used in pregnant and breastfeeding women. Do not use erythromycin estolate during pregnancy due to reports of cholestatic hepatitis. Conjunctivitis: use systemic therapy since topical treatment not adequate. Reports of infantile hypertrophic pyloric stenosis with erythromycin use in infants <6 wk; monitor signs and symptoms.	$

Class	Drug[a]	Dose	Adverse Effects	Drug Interactions	Comments	Cost[b]
Penicillins	*amoxicillin* (renal symbol) generics	500 mg TID po × 7 days	Rash, GI upset.	May decrease efficacy of oral contraceptives. Tetracyclines may decrease effectiveness of amoxicillin.	*Alternative treatment.* Main advantage is safety in pregnancy and breastfeeding.	$
Tetracyclines	*doxycycline* Vibramycin, generics	Adults and children ≥8 y: 100 mg BID po × 7 days	GI upset, rash, candidal vaginitis, photosensitivity.	Decreased levels with antacids, iron, barbiturates, bismuth, carbamazepine, phenytoin. Decreases effectiveness of penicillins and oral contraceptives.	***Preferred treatment.*** Similar high cure rates to azithromycin. Contraindicated in pregnant and breastfeeding women.	$

[a] Treat sexual partner(s). Repeat testing in all treated patients 6 months post-treatment since reinfection risk is high. Test of cure 3–4 weeks after completion of therapy if patient is pregnant, an alternative regimen is prescribed or nonadherence is suspected.

[b] Cost for specified duration of treatment; includes drug cost only.

(renal symbol) Dosage adjustment required in renal impairment; see Appendix I.

Legend: $ <$10 $$ $10–20

Table 7: **Antibiotics for the Treatment of Uncomplicated Gonorrhea Infections: Endocervical, Pharyngeal, Rectal, Urethral**[a,b,1,2,3]

Class	Drug[b]	Dose	Adverse Effects	Comments	Cost[c]
Aminoglycosides	*spectinomycin*	2 g im × single dose Children <9 y or <45 kg: 40 mg/kg im × single dose; maximum 2 g	Pain at injection site.	*Alternative treatment.* Used as last resort when resistance of *N. gonorrhea* to fluoroquinolones is too high and if cephalosporins are contraindicated. Not effective for pharyngeal infection; test of cure is recommended 3–5 days after treatment completion.	[d]
Cephalosporins, third-generation	*cefixime* Suprax	800 mg po × single dose Children <9 y: 8 mg/kg po × single dose; maximum 400 mg, follow-up culture required	GI upset, hypersensitivity reactions.	**Preferred** agent for heterosexual men and women. Although Canadian STI guidelines do not list cefixime as a preferred agent for the treatment of pharyngeal infections, recent studies show that it may be comparable to ceftriaxone for this indication when combined with azithromycin.[17,18] Repeat screening recommended.	$$
	cefotaxime Claforan generics	500 mg im × single dose[14] Ophthalmia neonatorum: 100 mg/kg im × single dose	GI upset, hypersensitivity reactions.	*Alternative treatment.* Ophthalmia neonatorum: use systemic therapy since topical antibiotic is ineffective.	$$
	ceftriaxone generics	Adults and children >9 y: 250 mg im × single dose Ophthalmia neonatorum: 25–50 mg/kg im/iv × single dose; maximum 125 mg	GI upset, hypersensitivity reactions.	***Preferred*** *agent for men who have sex with men or any patient with pharyngeal infection.* May be mixed with 1–2 mL of 1% lidocaine to reduce irritation. Do not reconstitute or mix with calcium-containing solutions. Do not administer simultaneously with calcium-containing iv solutions via a Y-site. Administration may be done sequentially provided the infusion lines are thoroughly flushed between infusions.	$$
Fluoroquinolones	*ciprofloxacin* Cipro, generics	500 mg po × single dose	GI upset, headache.	*Alternative treatment.* Use only if preferred treatments are not possible and susceptibility is demonstrated; test of cure is essential. Safety in children <18 y not established. Contraindicated in pregnant and breastfeeding women. Repeat screening recommended. Decreased levels with concurrent use of antacids or iron.	$

Class	Drug[b]	Dose	Adverse Effects	Comments	Cost[c]
	ofloxacin (renal) generics	400 mg po × single dose	See ciprofloxacin.	See ciprofloxacin.	$
Macrolides	*azithromycin* Zithromax, generics	2 g po × single dose	Diarrhea, nausea, vomiting; food may minimize adverse effects.	*Alternative treatment.* Bacterial resistance to azithromycin has emerged sporadically in Canada. Used if preferred treatments are not suitable. Prophylactic antiemetics may be needed. 2 g dose will also treat chlamydia infection.	$

[a] See Table 6 for cotreatment of chlamydia infection.
[b] Initiate empiric chlamydia therapy in all patients regardless of chlamydia test result as coinfection rates are high and chlamydia has a longer test window period. Azithromycin is preferred over doxycycline as cotreatment when gonorrhea is suspected as it provides adjunctive coverage for gonorrhea. Treat sexual partner(s).
[c] Cost for specified duration of treatment; includes drug cost only.
[d] Available through Health Canada, Special Access Programme, Therapeutic Products Directorate.
(renal) Dosage adjustment required in renal impairment; see Appendix I.
Legend: $ <$5 $$ $5–10

Table 8: Antibiotics for the Treatment of Syphilis[1,2]

Class	Drug	Dose	Adverse Effects	Comments	Cost[a]
Cephalosporins	*ceftriaxone* generics	All stages of syphilis (except neurosyphilis): 1 g daily iv/im × 10 days Neurosyphilis: 2 g daily iv/im × 10–14 days	GI upset, hypersensitivity reactions.	*Alternative treatment.* Use only in exceptional circumstances as a last resort. Not a satisfactory alternative to penicillin in pregnancy. Test and treat sexual contacts. Do not reconstitute or mix with calcium-containing solutions. Do not administer simultaneously with calcium-containing iv solutions via a Y-site. Administration may be done sequentially provided the infusion lines are thoroughly flushed between infusions.	$$–$$$
Penicillins	*benzathine penicillin G* Bicillin L-A	Primary, secondary and early latent (<1 y duration) syphilis: 2.4 million units im × single dose (consider a second dose 1 wk later if patient is pregnant) Late latent syphilis, syphilis of unknown duration, cardiovascular syphilis, tertiary syphilis not involving CNS: 2.4 million units weekly im × 3 doses	Jarisch-Herxheimer reaction: *not a drug allergy*; may occur at any stage but prevalent during early syphilis; fever, chills, rigors, sweating may occur; resolves within 24 h.	***Preferred treatment.*** Commonly confused with the short-acting benzylpenicillin (penicillin G). Can be used in pregnant and breastfeeding women; consider penicillin desensitization in pregnant women who are allergic to penicillin. Test and treat sexual contacts. Tetracyclines may decrease penicillin efficacy.	$$–$$$
	benzylpenicillin (penicillin G) generics	Neurosyphilis: 3–4 million units Q4H iv (16–24 million units daily) × 10–14 days	See benzathine penicillin G.	See benzathine penicillin G.	$$$
Tetracyclines	*doxycycline* Vibramycin, generics	Primary, secondary and early latent (<1 y duration) syphilis: 100 mg BID po × 14 days Late latent syphilis, syphilis of unknown duration, cardiovascular syphilis, tertiary syphilis not involving CNS: 100 mg BID po × 28 days; consider penicillin desensitization first even in penicillin-allergic patients	GI upset, rash, candidal vaginitis, photosensitivity.	*Alternative treatment.* Useful if patient is allergic to penicillins. Test and treat sexual contacts. Contraindicated in pregnant and breastfeeding women. Decreased levels with antacids, iron, barbiturates, bismuth, carbamazepine, phenytoin. Decreases efficacy of penicillins and oral contraceptives.	~$15

[a] Cost for specified duration of treatment; includes drug cost only.
Dosage adjustment required in renal impairment; see Appendix I.
Legend: $ <$100 $$ $100–200 $$-$$$ $100–300 $$$ $200–300

Table 9: Antibiotics for the Treatment of Lymphogranuloma Venereum[1,2]

Class	Drug	Dose	Adverse Effects	Drug Interactions	Comments	Cost[a]
Macrolides	*azithromycin* Zithromax, generics	1 g once weekly po × 3 wk; clinical efficacy data lacking Sexual partner: 1 g po × single dose; optimal duration of treatment unknown	GI upset.	May increase levels of digoxin.	*Last resort if doxycycline and erythromycin are contraindicated.* Test and treat sexual partner. Test of cure performed 3–4 wk after completion of therapy; follow up until chlamydial tests are negative. Can be used in pregnant and breastfeeding women. Repeat dose if vomiting <1 h post-administration.	$
	erythromycin base Eryc, generics	500 mg QID po × 3 wk	GI upset.	May increase levels of atorvastatin, carbamazepine, digoxin, lovastatin, protease inhibitors, sildenafil, simvastatin, theophylline. Avoid use with cisapride, clindamycin, disopyramide, pimozide.	*Alternative treatment.* Test and treat sexual partners. Test of cure performed 3–4 wk after completion of therapy; follow up until chlamydial tests are negative. Can be used in pregnant and breastfeeding women. Do not use erythromycin estolate during pregnancy due to reports of cholestatic hepatitis.	$$
Tetracyclines	*doxycycline* Vibramycin, generics	100 mg BID po × 3 wk Sexual partner: 100 mg BID po × 7 days	GI upset, rash, candidal vaginitis, photosensitivity.	Decreased levels with antacids, barbiturates, bismuth, carbamazepine, iron, phenytoin. Decreases efficacy of oral contraceptives and penicillins.	***Preferred treatment.*** Test and treat sexual partner. Test of cure performed 3–4 wk after completion of therapy; follow up until chlamydial tests are negative. Contraindicated in pregnant and breastfeeding women.	$$

[a] Cost for specified duration of treatment; includes drug cost only.
Legend: $ <$20 $$ $20–30

Table 10: Topical Drugs for the Treatment of External Anogenital Warts[a]

Class	Drug	Dose	Adverse Effects[b]	Comments	Cost[c]
Antimitotic Agents	*podophyllin 25% topical liquid* Podofilm	Office-based treatment Apply once per wk to warts only; may repeat 1–2 times Use a cotton applicator and allow to dry then remove with soap and water 1–4 h later. If no adverse local reaction, subsequent applications may be washed off after 6 h	Systemic: urticaria, fever, paresthesia, polyneuritis, paralytic ileus, blood dyscrasias, coma, death. Local: erythema, edema, pain, burning, itching, severe necrosis, scarring, paraphimosis, pseudoepitheliomatous hyperplasia.	Protect normal skin adjacent to lesion with petrolatum. Do not use in pregnancy. Do not use to treat cervical, meatal, vaginal or anal warts. Use only if other therapies are inappropriate.	$
	podophyllotoxin 0.5% topical solution Condyline, Wartec	Self-applied Apply to visible genital warts BID with a cotton swab × 3 days, followed by 4 days without therapy May repeat cycle ≤6 times. Total treated area should be <10 cm² and total daily volume should be <0.5 mL	Local irritation, pain, inflammation, erosion, burning, bleeding, pruritus, dizziness, insomnia.	Physicians: perform initial application to demonstrate proper application and to identify warts that require treatment. May require up to 3 months for response. Do not use in pregnancy. More effective than podophyllin with fewer side effects. Do not use to treat cervical, meatal, vaginal or anal warts.	$/3.5 mL bottle
Caustic Agents	*dichloroacetic acid (DCA) or trichloroacetic acid (TCA) 50–80% solution in 70% alcohol*	Office-based treatment Apply sparingly to warts weekly × 6–8 wk	Inflammation, erosion, pain, burning, ulceration, blistering.	Can be used in pregnant and breastfeeding women. Protect healthy skin with petroleum jelly. Does not need to be washed off.	$
Immune Response Modifiers	*imiquimod 5% cream* Aldara, generics	Self-applied Apply 3 times per wk on alternate days for up to 16 wk; rub cream in until no longer visible Wash hands before and after treatment application. Wash treatment area with soap and water 6–8 h after application	Local irritation, pain, mild to moderate erythema, burning.	Physicians: perform initial application to demonstrate proper application and to identify warts that require treatment. Treatment does not eliminate HPV infection; 10% recurrence rate. May require up to 3 months for response. Do not use in pregnancy.	$/packet
	imiquimod 3.75% cream Vyloma	Self-applied Apply QHS to external genital/perianal warts for up to 8 wk; rub cream in until no longer visible. Up to 1 packet may be used per day. Wash hands before and after application. Wash treatment area with mild soap and water 8 h after application	See imiquimod 5% cream.	Physicians: perform initial application to demonstrate proper application and to identify warts that should be treated. Treatment does not eliminate HPV infection. Do not use in pregnancy.	$/packet

[a] No therapy guarantees eradication of HPV. With or without treatment, most patients with genital warts experience complete clearance within 2 years.
[b] All treatments are associated with local skin reactions; decreasing intensity of treatment may help lessen these side effects.
[c] Cost of smallest available pack size unless specified otherwise; includes drug cost only.
Legend: $ <$15 $$ $15–30 $$$ $30–45

Table 11: Vaccines for the Prevention of External Anogenital Warts

Class	Drug	Dose	Adverse Effects	Comments	Cost
Vaccines	*quadrivalent human papillomavirus (types 6, 11, 16, 18) recombinant vaccine* Gardasil	Females: 9–45 y Males: 9–26 y 0.5 mL administered at 0, 2 and 6 months im Alternative schedule: 0, ≥1 month after first dose and ≥3 months after second dose	Pain, swelling, erythema and pruritus at injection site, headache, fatigue, syncope, lymphadenopathy,[15] anaphylaxis (rare).[16]	Prevention of external genital warts caused by human papillomavirus types 6 and 11. Not recommended in pregnancy. Can be used in breastfeeding mothers.	~$150/dose

Table 12: Antibiotic Combination Therapy for the Outpatient Management of Pelvic Inflammatory Disease[1,2]

Class	Drug[a]	Dose	Adverse Effects	Drug Interactions	Comments	Cost[b]
Cephalosporins + **Tetracyclines** ± **Nitroimidazoles**	*ceftriaxone* + *doxycycline* ± *metronidazole*	Ceftriaxone: 250 mg single dose im + Doxycycline: 100 mg BID po × 14 days ± Metronidazole: 500 mg BID po × 14 days	*Ceftriaxone:* GI upset, *C. difficile* colitis. *Doxycycline:* GI upset, rash, candidal vaginitis, photosensitivity. *Metronidazole:* GI upset, urethral burning, dark or reddish brown discolouration of urine.	*Ceftriaxone:* Increases anticoagulant effect of warfarin. Increased levels with probenecid. *Doxycycline:* Decreased levels with antacids, iron, barbiturates, bismuth, carbamazepine, phenytoin. Decreased efficacy of penicillins and oral contraceptives. *Metronidazole:* disulfiram-like reaction with alcohol may occur during treatment.	***Preferred treatment.*** Test and treat partners. Re-evaluate patients 2–3 days after initiation of therapy; if no improvement, parenteral therapy required. *Doxycycline:* contraindicated in pregnant and breastfeeding women. *Metronidazole:* provides anaerobic coverage.	$$$$$
Fluoroquinolones ± **Nitroimidazoles**	*levofloxacin* ± *metronidazole*	Levofloxacin: 500 mg daily po × 14 days ± Metronidazole: 500 mg BID po × 14 days	*Levofloxacin:* GI upset, headache. *Metronidazole:* GI upset, urethral burning, dark or reddish brown discolouration of urine.	*Levofloxacin:* Decreased levels with concurrent use of antacids or iron. Increased risk of tendon rupture with concomitant corticosteroid use. Caution with concomitant use of agents with QT_c prolongation, e.g., amiodarone; assess risks/benefits of therapy. *Metronidazole:* disulfiram-like reaction with alcohol may occur during treatment.	*Alternative treatment.* A test of cure is essential. Test and treat sexual partner(s). Levofloxacin is contraindicated in pregnant and breastfeeding women; safety in children <18 y not established. *Metronidazole:* provides anaerobic coverage.	$$
	ofloxacin ± *metronidazole*	Ofloxacin: 400 mg BID po × 14 days ± Metronidazole: 500 mg BID po × 14 days	*Ofloxacin:* GI upset, headache. *Metronidazole:* GI upset, urethral burning, dark or reddish brown discolouration of urine.	*Ofloxacin:* Decreased levels with concurrent use of antacids or iron. Increased risk of tendon rupture with concomitant corticosteroid use. Caution with concomitant use of agents with QT_c prolongation, e.g., amiodarone; assess risks/benefits of therapy. *Metronidazole:* disulfiram-like reaction with alcohol may occur during treatment.	*Alternative treatment.* A test of cure is essential. Test and treat sexual partner(s). Ofloxacin is contraindicated in pregnant and breastfeeding women; safety in children <18 y not established. *Metronidazole:* provides anaerobic coverage.	$

[a] Ensure antibacterials provide coverage for *N. gonorrhea*, *C. trachomatis*, gram-negative bacteria and streptococci. Also consider anaerobic coverage.
[b] Cost for duration of treatment; includes drug cost only.
Dosage adjustment required in renal impairment; see Appendix I.
Legend: $ <$25 $$ $25–50 $$$ $50–75 $$$$ $75-100 $$$$$ $100–125

Table 13: Antibiotic Combination Therapy for Inpatient Management of Pelvic Inflammatory Disease[1,2]

Class	Drug	Dose	Adverse Effects	Drug Interactions	Comments	Cost[a]
Aminoglycosides + **Lincosamides**	*gentamicin* ◗ + *clindamycin*	Gentamicin: loading dose 2 mg/kg im/iv, then maintenance dose 1.5 mg/kg Q8H or 5 mg/kg Q24H iv + Clindamycin: 900 mg Q8H iv Stop parenteral therapy 24 h after clinical improvement and continue with clindamycin 450 mg QID po or doxycycline 100 mg BID po for a total of 14 days	*Gentamicin:* ototoxicity, nephrotoxicity (monitor kidney function and gentamicin levels during treatment). *Clindamycin:* *C. difficile* colitis, diarrhea.	*Clindamycin:* monitor kidney function with concomitant aminoglycoside. May decrease therapeutic effect of live typhoid vaccine. Administer typhoid vaccine >24 h after last dose of clindamycin.	***Preferred treatment.*** Test and treat partners. Re-evaluate patients 2–3 days after initiation of therapy.	$$$$[b]
Fluoroquinolones + **Nitroimidazoles**	*levofloxacin* ◗ + *metronidazole*	Levofloxacin: 500 mg daily iv + Metronidazole: 500 mg Q8H iv Stop parenteral therapy 24 h after clinical improvement and continue with oral therapy	*Levofloxacin:* GI upset, headache. *Metronidazole:* GI upset, urethral burning, dark or reddish brown discolouration of urine.	*Levofloxacin:* Increased risk of tendon rupture with concomitant corticosteroid use. Caution with concomitant use of agents with QT_c prolongation properties, e.g., amiodarone; assess risks/benefits of therapy. *Metronidazole:* disulfiram-like reaction with alcohol may occur during treatment.	*Alternative treatment.* A test of cure is essential. Test and treat partner(s). *Levofloxacin:* contraindicated in pregnant and breastfeeding women; safety in children <18 y not established. *Metronidazole:* provides anaerobic coverage.	$$$
Fluoroquinolones + **Tetracyclines** + **Nitroimidazole**	*ciprofloxacin* ◗ + *doxycycline* + *metronidazole*	Ciprofloxacin: 200 mg Q12H iv + Doxycycline: 100 mg Q12H po/iv[c] + Metronidazole: 500 mg Q8H iv Stop parenteral therapy 24 h after clinical improvement and continue with oral therapy	*Ciprofloxacin:* GI upset, headache. *Doxycycline:* GI upset, rash, candidal vaginitis, photosensitivity. *Metronidazole:* GI upset, urethral burning, dark or reddish brown discolouration of urine.	*Ciprofloxacin:* Decreased absorption with concurrent use of antacids or iron. Increased risk of tendon rupture with concomitant corticosteroid use. *Doxycycline:* Decreased levels with antacids, iron, barbiturates, bismuth, carbamazepine, phenytoin. Reduces efficacy of penicillins and oral contraceptives. *Metronidazole:* disulfiram-like reaction with alcohol may occur during treatment.	*Alternative treatment.* Test of cure is essential. Doxycycline ensures coverage against *C. trachomatis* and metronidazole ensures anaerobic coverage. Oral doxycycline can be substituted for parenteral doxycycline because oral and iv bioavailability are similar.	$$

[a] Cost for 1-day supply; includes drug cost only.
[b] Cost based on dosage for 50 kg person.
[c] IV form is available through Health Canada, Special Access Programme, Therapeutic Products Directorate.
◗ Dosage adjustment required in renal impairment; see Appendix I.
Legend: $ <$25 $$ $25–50 $$$ $50–75 $$$$ $75–100

Suggested Readings

Hollier LM, Workowski KW. Treatment of sexually transmitted infections in pregnancy. *Clin Perinatol* 2005;32(3):629-56.

Public Health Agency of Canada. *Canadian guidelines on sexually transmitted infections*. Evergreen ed. Ottawa (ON): PHAC. Available from: www.phac-aspc.gc.ca/std-mts/sti-its/cgsti-ldcits/index-eng.php.

Sena AC, Miller WC, Hobbs MM et al. Trichomonas vaginalis infection in male sexual partners: implications for diagnosis, treatment, and prevention. *Clin Infect Dis* 2007;44(1):13-22.

Workowski KA, Berman S; Centers for Disease Control and Prevention (CDC). Sexually transmitted diseases treatment guidelines, 2010. *MMWR Recomm Rep* 2010;59(RR-12):1-110.

References

1. Public Health Agency of Canada. *Canadian guidelines on sexually transmitted infections*. Evergreen ed. Ottawa (ON): PHAC. Available from: www.phac-aspc.gc.ca/std-mts/sti-its/cgsti-ldcits/index-eng.php. Accessed December 15, 2013.
2. Workowski KA, Berman S; Centers for Disease Control and Prevention (CDC). Sexually transmitted diseases treatment guidelines, 2010. *MMWR Recomm Rep* 2010;59(RR-12):1-110.
3. College of Registered Nurses of British Columbia. Reproductive Health Certified Practice. *Sexually transmitted infections: gonorrhea*. Vancouver (BC): CRNBC; 2012. Available from: crnbc.ca/Standards/CertifiedPractice/Documents/ReproductiveHealth/721GonorrheaRe-portableSTIDST.pdf. Accessed November 6, 2012.
4. Yudin MH, Money DM; Infectious Diseases Committee. Screening and management of bacterial vaginosis in pregnancy. *J Obstet Gynaecol Can* 2008;30(8):702-16.
5. Public Health Agency of Canada. Section 4. Management and treatment of specific syndromes. Vaginal discharge (bacterial vaginosis, vulvovaginal candidiasis, trichomoniasis). In: *Canadian guidelines on sexually transmitted infections*. Ottawa (ON): PHAC; January 2008. Available from: www.phac-aspc.gc.ca/std-mts/sti-its/cgsti-ldcits/index-eng.php. Accessed December 15, 2013.
6. Riedner G, Rusizoka M, Todd J et al. Single-dose azithromycin versus penicillin G benzathine for the treatment of early syphilis. *N Engl J Med* 2005;353(12):1236-44.
7. National Advisory Committee on Immunization (NACI). Statement on human papillomavirus vaccine. An Advisory Committee Statement (ACS). *Can Commun Dis Rep* 2007;33(ACS-2):1-31.
8. Warner L, Stone KM, Macaluso M et al. Condom use and risk of gonorrhea and chlamydia: a systematic review of design and measurement factors assessed in epidemiologic studies. *Sex Transm Dis* 2006;33(1):36-51.
9. Winer RL, Hughes JP, Feng Q et al. Condom use and the risk of genital human papillomavirus infection in young women. *N Engl J Med* 2006;354(25):2645-54.
10. Wald A, Langenberg AG, Krantz E et al. The relationship between condom use and herpes simplex virus acquisition. *Ann Intern Med* 2005;143(10):707-13.
11. Hogewoning CJ, Bleeker MC, van den Brule AJ et al. Condom use promotes regression of cervical intraepithelial neoplasia and clearance of human papillomavirus: a randomized clinical trial. *Int J Cancer* 2003;107(5):811-6.
12. Bleeker MC, Hogewoning CJ, Voorhorst FJ et al. Condom use promotes regression of human papillomavirus-associated penile lesions in male sexual partners of women with cervical intraepithelial neoplasia. *Int J Cancer* 2003;107(5):804-10.
13. Kamb ML, Fishbein M, Douglas JM et al. Efficacy of risk-reduction counseling to prevent human immunodeficiency virus and sexually transmitted diseases: a randomized controlled trial. Project RESPECT Study Group. *JAMA* 1998;280(13):1161-7.
14. Centers for Disease Control and Prevention. *Updated recommended treatment regimens for gonococcal infections and associated conditions—United States, April 2007*. Available from: www.cdc.gov/STD/treatment/2006/GonUpdateApril2007.pdf. Accessed March 15, 2011.
15. Studdiford J, Lamb K, Horvath K et al. Development of unilateral cervical and supraclavicular lymphadenopathy after human papilloma virus vaccination. *Pharmacotherapy* 2008;28(9):1194-97.
16. Brotherton JML, Gold MS, Kemp AS et al. Anaphylaxis following quadrivalent human papillomavirus vaccination. *CMAJ* 2008;179(6):525-33.
17. Gratrix J, Bergman J, Egan C et al. Retrospective review of pharyngeal gonorrhea treatment failures in Alberta, Canada. *Sex Transm Dis* 2013;40(11):877-9.
18. Barbee LA, Kerani RP, Dombrowski JC et al. A retrospective comparative study of 2-drug oral and intramuscular cephalosporin treatment regimens for pharyngeal gonorrhea. *Clin Infect Dis* 2013;56(11):1539-45.
19. Klebanoff MA, Carey JC, Hauth JC et al. Failure of metronidazole to prevent preterm delivery among pregnant women with asymptomatic Trichomonas vaginalis infection. *N Engl J Med* 2001;345(7):487-93.

Chapter 121
Sinusitis

Susan R. Fryters, BScPharm, ACPR and
Edith M. Blondel-Hill, MD, FRCPC

Sinusitis is defined as inflammation and/or mucosal thickening of one or more of the paranasal sinus cavities, the cause of which may be allergic, viral, bacterial or fungal.[1] **Acute** sinusitis refers to cases lasting 4 weeks or less, while **recurrent** sinusitis is defined as 4 or more episodes of acute sinusitis per year, each lasting 10 days or more, with an absence of symptoms between episodes.[2,3,4,5] **Chronic sinusitis** refers to infections lasting 12 weeks or more with or without treatment.[1,3,4] Acute sinusitis can also be superimposed on chronic sinusitis.[2] Rhinitis and rhinosinusitis, most commonly associated with a viral or allergic etiology, are often misdiagnosed and treated as bacterial sinusitis.

Many similarities exist between sinusitis and otitis media, including histology, pathogenesis, etiologic agents and risk factors. In children, the 2 diseases frequently coexist.[2]

The paranasal sinuses are normally sterile. Acute sinusitis is most often secondary to viral respiratory infections. Viral upper respiratory tract infections (URTIs) are complicated by bacterial sinusitis in only 0.5–2% of adult cases and 6–13% of cases in children.[5,6,7,8,9,10]

This chapter addresses community-acquired bacterial sinusitis in children and adults. Bacteria commonly implicated in bacterial sinusitis in children and adults are listed in Table 2 and Table 3 respectively. The most common bacterial pathogens in acute sinusitis are *Streptococcus pneumoniae* and unencapsulated strains of *Haemophilus influenzae*. *Moraxella catarrhalis* is more common in children.[1] Up to 10% of cases of acute sinusitis in adults may be due to mixed anaerobic bacteria; these cases are often associated with concurrent dental disease. The microbiology of chronic sinusitis is less clear, although anaerobes, *Staphylococcus aureus* and *Enterobacteriaceae* are more common in chronic than in acute sinusitis.[11,12]

Goals of Therapy

- Optimize the symptomatic management of sinusitis, especially drainage of congested sinuses
- Eradicate infection
- Prevent recurrences and complications of sinusitis
- Reduce antibiotic use in ill-defined URTI to avoid the development of antibiotic resistance

Investigations

The diagnosis of acute bacterial sinusitis relies on history and physical examination. Differentiation of bacterial sinusitis from viral URTI is determined by the duration and severity of the symptoms described below.[9]

- Symptoms:
  - Adults: Persistent symptoms of URTI without improvement after 10–14 days, or worsening after 5 days, with both nasal congestion/purulent nasal discharge and facial pain, with or without fever, maxillary toothache or facial swelling. Nonspecific concurrent symptoms include headache, halitosis, hyposmia/anosmia, ear pain/pressure, fatigue and cough[1,2,3,13]

- Children: Symptoms of acute bacterial sinusitis are similar in children but often also include irritability, lethargy, prolonged cough and vomiting that occurs in association with gagging on mucus[1,2,3]
- Chronic: Patients with chronic sinusitis typically complain of purulent nasal discharge, postnasal drip and nasal obstruction accompanied by facial pain. Symptoms can mimic the pain of atypical and typical migraine, dental disease and tension headaches[14]

- Physical examination:
  - Of limited utility due to similarity of findings between viral URTI and acute bacterial sinusitis[12]
  - Physical findings of swelling and/or erythema over the symptomatic area, tenderness on palpation/percussion of paranasal sinuses, periorbital swelling, erythema/swelling of nasal mucosa, postnasal drip
  - The colour of nasal discharge/sputum should not be used to diagnose the sinusitis episode as bacterial since colour is related to the presence of neutrophils, not bacteria[5]
  - In addition:
    - assess patient for changes in extraocular movements and visual acuity to look for orbital complications
    - look for associated dental infection by checking the maxillary teeth for tenderness
- Objective measurements:
  - Transillumination of the sinuses has limited value in adults and no diagnostic value in children as findings are not specific to bacterial infection, and in children the sinuses are not yet fully formed
  - Nasal/nasopharyngeal cultures obtained from a direct swab through the nose are not recommended due to poor correlation with sinus pathogens
  - Plain sinus x-rays and CT scans are not routinely recommended in the diagnosis of sinusitis, as they will not distinguish between sinus abnormalities associated with viral URTI and bacterial sinusitis
  - CT scans may be useful for:
    - complications of sinusitis (*acute*—orbital cellulitis, cavernous vein thrombosis, brain abscess, meningitis, osteomyelitis, oral-antral fistula; *chronic*—mucocele, brain abscess, osteomyelitis, oral-antral fistula)[2]
    - chronic sinusitis unresponsive to treatment[3]
    - chronic progressive nasal obstruction without identified cause[2]
    - severe presentations in which diagnosis is suspected but not clear[2,3]
    - patients in whom surgery is being considered[2,15]
  - MRIs are not routinely recommended due to poor bone definition. May have a role in the diagnosis of fungal sinusitis or intracranial complications of sinusitis[12]
- Consider underlying risk factors, especially in recurrent and/or chronic sinusitis:
  - allergic rhinitis
  - asthma[16]
  - cystic fibrosis
  - eosinophilic nonallergic rhinitis[2]
  - gastroesophageal reflux disease
  - immunodeficiency
  - structural abnormalities, e.g., deviated septum, nasal polyps

Therapeutic Choices

Prevention of Sinusitis[2,3,16]

- Limit the spread of viral infections. Handwashing is an effective way to prevent the spread of infection.[17]
- Avoid exposure to environmental toxins, especially tobacco smoke.
- Reduce allergen exposure.

Nonpharmacologic Choices

- Local treatment with steam inhalation, cool mist humidifiers and/or saline nasal irrigation/sprays may be of benefit in both acute and chronic sinusitis to liquefy and soften crusting of nasal secretions and facilitate their removal, and to moisturize dry, inflamed nasal mucosae.[18,19]
- Although there are no scientific data on efficacy, the following comfort measures may be helpful in relieving symptoms in some patients:[2]
  - adequate rest and hydration
  - warm facial packs/compresses
  - sleeping with the head of the bed elevated
  - adding pine oil or menthol preparations to steam treatments.
- Surgical drainage for chronic sinusitis may be necessary, especially when it is unresponsive to maximal medical therapy.[20]

Pharmacologic Choices

Principles of Therapy in Sinusitis

The preferred initial strategy for managing symptoms in patients with nonsevere acute sinusitis (mild pain, temperature <38.3°C) is watchful waiting without initiation of antibiotic therapy and the use of analgesics/antipyretics and decongestants when needed.[5,21] Approximately 70% of cases of acute sinusitis will resolve within 2 weeks without antibiotic treatment.[22,23,24,25,26,27] However, if symptoms continue for longer than 7 days after diagnosis or worsen at any time, consider antibiotic therapy.[5] Overprescribing antibiotics has serious consequences including promotion of antibiotic resistance, increased costs and adverse drug effects, including *Clostridium difficile* infection.[16]

Symptomatic Management

Analgesics/antipyretics, such as **acetaminophen** or **ibuprofen**, can be used for control of pain and/or fever.

Nasal and oral **decongestants** may be beneficial in both acute and chronic infections.[18] Use oral decongestants with caution in patients with uncontrolled hypertension, cardiovascular disease, hyperthyroidism, diabetes, angle-closure glaucoma, urinary retention or in conjunction with MAO inhibitors. Limit use of topical decongestant sprays to 3–5 days as extended use may result in rhinitis medicamentosa (rebound congestion/hyperemia), which may be refractory to subsequent decongestant therapy.[2]

The efficacy and safety of nasal/oral decongestants have not been well studied in pediatric patients <12 years old.[15,28] Adverse events resulting in emergency room visits due to the use and/or misuse of oral cough and cold preparations are highest among children <6 years.[29] In addition, overdosage of oral cough and cold preparations, specifically **pseudoephedrine**, has been associated with deaths in several infants.[30] As a result, in December 2008 Health Canada issued an advisory instructing caregivers not to give certain nonprescription cough and cold medications to children younger than 6 years.[31] Some clinicians further advise against their use in children <12 years.[28] Carefully weigh the risks and benefits of these medications before prescribing and ask whether other cough and cold preparations are being used, to avoid overdose from multiple medications (including analgesic products) that contain the same ingredients.

Avoid antihistamines in acute sinusitis because of their tendency to cause excessive dryness, with thickening of secretions and crusting.[32] However **second-generation antihistamines** may have a role in chronic sinusitis when a clear allergic component is demonstrated.[18]

The use of intranasal **corticosteroid** sprays in acute sinusitis is controversial as placebo-controlled studies have shown conflicting results.[12,15] A meta-analysis of 3 well conducted, double-blind, randomized placebo-controlled studies found an overall rate of resolution or marked improvement of symptoms in 73% of corticosteroid-treated patients with acute sinusitis versus 66% in placebo-treated patients.[33] In other words, for every 100 patients treated with intranasal corticosteroids, 7 additional patients had complete or marked symptom relief. While some experts advocate routine use of intranasal corticosteroids,[34] others consider this benefit to be too modest to recommend them in all patients with acute sinusitis. Most experts agree that intranasal corticosteroids probably have a benefit in patients with recurrent and/or allergic rhinosinusitis.[1,5] Intranasal corticosteroids may also be beneficial in chronic sinusitis due to their ability to decrease nasal edema and inflammation and thus promote drainage.[2]

There is no evidence that **mucolytics** such as guaifenesin are useful adjuncts in acute sinusitis.[2]

Antibiotic Therapy

Information about antibiotic therapy can be found in Table 2, Table 3, Table 4 and Table 5.

Acute Upper Respiratory Tract Infection (URTI)

A Cochrane review of 6 randomized controlled trials comparing antibiotic therapy with placebo in acute URTI (the common cold) with <7 days of symptoms or <10 days of purulent rhinitis found that those receiving antibiotics did not have higher cure rates or greater improvement in symptoms than those receiving placebo.[35]

Acute Sinusitis

Multiple clinical trials and 2 meta-analyses have shown that ~70% of cases of acute sinusitis will resolve without antibiotic treatment.[22,23,24,25,26,27] Five meta-analyses of randomized, controlled trials comparing antibiotics to placebo in acute bacterial sinusitis have consistently found a benefit for antibiotic therapy over placebo but with a number needed to treat of 7–15 and in the majority of studies, a higher incidence of adverse events.[26,27,36,37,38] Antibiotic therapy should be reserved for those patients with bacterial sinusitis as defined by history, including duration of symptoms >10 days, and physical examination. There are no clinically significant differences in outcomes between first-line and second-line broader spectrum antibiotics, including fluoroquinolones.[25,26,27,39,40,41,42]

Amoxicillin remains the antibiotic of choice for acute bacterial sinusitis for the following reasons:[1,2,3,4,5,20]

- Provides adequate coverage for organisms involved in acute sinusitis
- Exhibits best activity of all oral beta-lactam agents against *S. pneumoniae*, including strains with intermediate susceptibility to penicillin (when high-dose amoxicillin is used)
- No other antibiotic has been proven superior to amoxicillin in clinical trials
- Lower potential to induce resistance compared to other antibiotic classes
- Relatively few adverse effects
- Relatively inexpensive

Although **macrolides** are frequently used in the treatment of sinusitis, their routine use cannot be recommended because:

- azithromycin and clarithromycin have inferior coverage of *H. influenzae* and *S. pneumoniae*, the 2 most common pathogens in acute bacterial sinusitis
- there is a higher rate of resistance, especially with *S. pneumoniae*, to macrolides than to amoxicillin or amoxicillin/clavulanate
- macrolides have been shown to be less efficacious than amoxicillin/clavulanate for treatment of acute otitis media

Macrolides, sulfamethoxazole/trimethoprim (SMX/TMP) and **oral cephalosporins** are no longer recommended for empiric therapy of sinusitis due to unpredictable/poor activity against *S. pneumoniae* and/or *H. influenzae*.

Failure of First-line Therapy

Amoxicillin/clavulanate offers the most appropriate spectrum of activity and is the agent of choice when first-line antibiotic therapy fails.[3,4,27]

Levofloxacin and **moxifloxacin** have good coverage of the pathogens involved. However, because of their broad spectrum, potential for increasing resistance and the risk of *C. difficile* infection, these fluoroquinolones should be reserved for patients who are allergic to beta-lactams or who have failed first-line antibiotic therapy.

Antibiotic therapy (especially with macrolides or fluoroquinolones) within the previous 3 months may be a risk factor for multi-drug–resistant *S. pneumoniae*. If this is the case, use an antibiotic from a different class.

Antibiotics *not* recommended for empiric treatment of acute bacterial sinusitis are listed in Table 1.

Table 1: Antibiotics *Not* Routinely Recommended as Empiric Therapy for Acute Bacterial Sinusitis[2,3,4]

Antibiotic	Comments
Cephalexin	No activity against penicillin intermediate/resistant *S. pneumoniae*. No activity against *Haemophilus* or *Moraxella* spp.
Cefaclor	No activity against penicillin intermediate/resistant *S. pneumoniae*. Poor activity against *H. influenzae* and *M. catarrhalis*.
Cefixime	No activity against penicillin intermediate/resistant *S. pneumoniae*. Excellent activity against *Haemophilus* spp. and *M. catarrhalis*. May be an option but only in combination with clindamycin.
Ceftriaxone	Routine use of this agent is not recommended in acute bacterial sinusitis due to potential for increased resistance to third-generation cephalosporins. May be an option in patients with severe acute bacterial sinusitis who have failed therapy. Three days of im/iv therapy is recommended, as a single dose is not as effective in eradicating penicillin-resistant *S. pneumoniae*.
Clindamycin	No activity against *Haemophilus* or *Moraxella* spp. Reasonable activity against *S. pneumoniae*. Clindamycin can be used in acute sinusitis but only in combination with cefixime or as an alternative to amoxicillin/clavulanate in chronic sinusitis.
Ciprofloxacin	Suboptimal coverage of *S. pneumoniae*.
Macrolides	Poor activity against *H. influenzae*. Significant macrolide resistance in *S. pneumoniae* and *Streptococcus pyogenes*.
SMX/TMP	Unpredictable/poor activity against *S. pneumoniae* and *H. influenzae*. No activity against *S. pyogenes*.

Abbreviations: SMX/TMP = sulfamethoxazole/trimethoprim

Duration of Therapy

Optimal duration of antibiotic therapy in acute bacterial sinusitis is not well defined. Traditionally, anywhere from a 7- to 14-day course of therapy has been recommended.[1,2,12,16] Some physicians continue antibiotic therapy until the patient is free of symptoms and then for an additional 7 days to ensure eradication of bacteria and to prevent relapse.[2,20] However, short-course optimal dose therapy has been shown to be effective in acute bacterial sinusitis (e.g., amoxicillin/clavulanate[43] or respiratory quinolones for 5 days[44,45,46]). A meta-analysis of 12 randomized controlled trials compared short-course (3–7 days) therapy to longer courses (6–10 days) with the same antibiotic at the same dose in acute uncomplicated sinusitis and found no differences in clinical success, microbiologic efficacy, relapses, adverse events or withdrawals.[48] In a subanalysis of 7 trials that compared 5-day vs. 10-day regimens, clinical success was similar but adverse events were fewer with the 5-day course of therapy. In adults with uncomplicated acute sinusitis, a shorter treatment duration of 5–7 days is recommended and has advantages in terms of lower potential for development of resistance, better adherence, fewer adverse events and lower costs [Evidence: SORT B*].[4,47,48,49] If first-line therapy has failed, choose a different antibiotic and treat for 5–10 days with the new agent (see Table 3).[4,49] For children, data on shorter durations of therapy are lacking, therefore it is still recommended to treat for 10 days.[4,49]

Chronic Sinusitis

Antibiotics should be used to treat chronic sinusitis if nasal purulence is present. A longer duration of therapy (at least 3 weeks) is required.

Choices during Pregnancy and Breastfeeding

Sinusitis and Pregnancy

Hormonal changes during pregnancy can cause temporary nasal congestion and symptoms of sinusitis due to vasodilation and increased blood volume.[16,21] Symptoms of this condition, pregnancy rhinitis de novo, usually disappear within 2 weeks after delivery.[21]

Infectious sinusitis has been reported to be as high as 1.5% in pregnancy, which represents a sixfold increase over that observed in a nonpregnant population.[50] The peak onset is in the second trimester. Classic signs and symptoms of sinusitis are absent in nearly half of women with documented purulent sinusitis during pregnancy.[50]

Uncontrolled sinusitis during pregnancy may aggravate coexisting asthma, which can have an adverse effect on pregnancy outcome and quality of life. Therefore, sinusitis during pregnancy should be actively evaluated and treated to optimize pregnancy outcome.[50]

Management of Sinusitis in Pregnancy

Nonpharmacologic measures such as humidification and nasal rinsing[50] should be tried first. **Acetaminophen** can be used if an analgesic or antipyretic is necessary. **NSAIDs** such as **ibuprofen** are an alternative but should be avoided in the third trimester because of the risk of premature closure of the ductus arteriosis.

Topical decongestants are preferred over **oral decongestants** to lessen fetal drug exposure. Since pregnant women have a tendency to develop rhinitis medicamentosa, likely due to hormonally-induced congestion, topical decongestants should be used minimally (e.g., before bedtime to help with sleep) for no more than 3–5 days, preferably after the first trimester and not during labour.[50] Avoid oral decongestants in the first trimester because of a possible risk of gastroschisis (a rare disorder involving failure of closure of the abdominal wall) in the newborn.[21,51] There is no specific information available

---

* SORT (Strength of Recommendation Taxonomy) is a rating system (A, B or C) that addresses the quality of available evidence. For more information consult **How to Use *Compendium of Therapeutic Choices*** on page xxv.

on the use of **intranasal corticosteroids** during pregnancy but because these drugs are poorly absorbed and undergo first-pass metabolism, very little drug (if any) would be expected to reach the fetus during maternal intranasal use.[50]

As in the general population, the antibiotic of choice to treat acute bacterial sinusitis in pregnancy is **amoxicillin**. When amoxicillin has failed, **amoxicillin/clavulanate** is safe to use in pregnancy. Respiratory fluoroquinolones (**levofloxacin** and **moxifloxacin**) should be avoided in pregnancy as safer alternatives exist. Impaired cartilage development has been reported in animal studies although there have been no reports suggesting an increased risk of major malformations, adverse effects in the fetal musculoskeletal system, spontaneous abortions, prematurity, intrauterine growth restriction or postnatal disorders.[52,53,54,55] **Doxycycline** is associated with tooth discolouration in the fetus and therefore should not be used. For the treatment of chronic sinusitis, **clindamycin** is considered safe to use in pregnancy.

Management of Sinusitis in Breastfeeding Women

As in pregnancy, nonpharmacologic measures such as humidification and nasal rinsing[50] are preferred first measures. **Acetaminophen** or **ibuprofen** can be used if an analgesic or antipyretic is necessary.

Topical decongestants such as **oxymetazoline**, **xylometazoline** and **phenylephrine** are considered safe in breastfeeding when used for no more than 3–5 days[56] and are preferred over **oral decongestants** to lessen drug exposure to the newborn. If oral decongestants are needed, only short-acting forms should be used and are best taken just after breastfeeding to minimize drug levels in breast milk. Breastfeeding mothers with poor or marginal milk production should be exceedingly cautious in using **pseudoephedrine** as reduced milk production has been reported in late-stage lactation.[56] With topical or oral decongestant use, watch for signs of toxicity in the infant such as irritability, nervousness, insomnia or excitation.[50,56] These products should not be used during breastfeeding of infants with hypertension or cardiac syndromes.[56]

Intranasal corticosteroids are considered safe for use in breastfeeding mothers as only very small doses are used, intranasal absorption is minimal and there is rapid first-pass metabolism by the liver.[56] Therefore, it is unlikely that these products pose any risk to the breastfed infant.[56]

The American Academy of Pediatrics lists **amoxicillin** as compatible with breastfeeding.[57] In addition, **amoxicillin/clavulanate** and **clindamycin** (for chronic sinusitis) may be used in nursing mothers. Caution is advised in using **levofloxacin**, **moxifloxacin** and **doxycycline**, and if used, avoid repeated or prolonged exposure.[56] With any antibiotic, observe infant for thrush, GI symptoms such as diarrhea, and rash.[56]

A discussion of general principles on the use of medications in these special populations can be found in Appendix II and Appendix III. Other specialized reference sources are also provided in these appendices.

Therapeutic Tips

- Most episodes of acute sinusitis resolve without antibiotic therapy.
- If patient shows no improvement after 72 hours of symptomatic therapy plus first-line antibiotic, change to a second-line antibiotic.[1,2,3,4,13]
- Inform patients that complete resolution of symptoms may take up to 14 days.[4]
- If the patient deteriorates at any time, reassess for acute complications, other diagnoses and/or adherence to treatment.
- Routine follow-up on completion of therapy in asymptomatic patients is not required.
- If a patient has received antibiotics (especially macrolides or fluoroquinolones) within the past 3 months, choose an antibiotic from a different class to treat acute bacterial sinusitis as there is a higher risk of multi-drug-resistant *S. pneumoniae*.

- The presence of tenacious, thick, brown nasal secretions should heighten the suspicion of a fungal infection.
- Refer to ear, nose and throat (ENT) specialist if a patient:[3]
  - fails second-line therapy[1]
  - experiences 4 or more episodes of bacterial sinusitis per year
  - has chronic sinusitis that is not responding to medical therapy (symptomatic and antibiotic)
  - has anatomic anomalies
  - develops complications

Table 2: Recommended Empiric Therapy for Bacterial Sinusitis in Children[3,4]

Infection	Usual Pathogens	Recommended Empiric Therapy	Comments
Acute Sinusitis (Symptoms <4 wk *and* ≤3 episodes per year)	*S. pneumoniae* *M. catarrhalis* *H. influenzae* Occasionally *S. aureus*, *S. pyogenes*, anaerobes	Standard-dose amoxicillin × 10 days *or* High-dose amoxicillin × 10 days Penicillin allergy:[a] ≤8 years: clindamycin + cefixime × 10 days; >8 years: doxycycline × 10 days **Severe infection[b] or immunocompromised:** amoxicillin + amoxicillin/clavulanate (7:1) × 10 days Nonsevere beta-lactam allergy: ceftriaxone × 10 days Severe beta-lactam allergy/anaphylaxis: levofloxacin[c] × 10 days	Refer to ENT specialist if ≥4 episodes per year High-dose amoxicillin should be used in children at high risk of penicillin-resistant *S. pneumoniae*: age <2 years, recent (<3 months) antibiotic exposure *and/or* daycare centre attendance (extrapolated from acute otitis media data).
Failure of First-line Agents: (No improvement or clinical deterioration after 72 h of antibiotic therapy *or* recurrence within 3 months)	*S. pneumoniae* *M. catarrhalis* *H. influenzae* Occasionally *S. aureus*, *S. pyogenes*, anaerobes	Amoxicillin/clavulanate (7:1) ± amoxicillin[d] × 10 days Penicillin allergy: clindamycin + cefixime × 10 days *or* ceftriaxone × 10 days Severe beta-lactam allergy: levofloxacin[c] × 10 days	Consider resistant organisms, especially penicillin-resistant *S. pneumoniae* and ampicillin-resistant *H. influenzae*.
Chronic Sinusitis (Symptoms ≥12 wk)	Anaerobes Occasionally *S. aureus*, *S. pneumoniae*, *H. influenzae*, *M. catarrhalis*, *S. pyogenes*, *Enterobacteriaceae*	Amoxicillin/clavulanate × 3 wk *or* Clindamycin × 3 wk	Longer duration of therapy may be required in exceptional circumstances.

[a] Sulfamethoxazole/trimethoprim is an alternative in penicillin allergy but resistance is significant. If used, close clinical monitoring is essential.
[b] Severe = high fever (≥39°C) and purulent nasal discharge or facial pain for 3–4 consecutive days.
[c] Levofloxacin use is justified in severe beta-lactam allergy/anaphylaxis as reliable therapeutic options are limited.
[d] If patient has failed high-dose amoxicillin therapy, amoxicillin/clavulanate alone is adequate to cover beta-lactamase-producing organisms.

Abbreviations: ENT = ear, nose and throat

Table 3: Recommended Empiric Therapy for Bacterial Sinusitis in Adults[3,4]

Infection	Usual Pathogens	Recommended Empiric Therapy	Comments
Acute Sinusitis (Symptoms <4 wk *and* ≤3 episodes per year)	*S. pneumoniae* *M. catarrhalis* *H. influenzae* Occasionally *S. aureus*, *S. pyogenes*, anaerobes	Amoxicillin × 5–7 days Beta-lactam allergy: doxycycline × 5–7 days **Severe infection[a] or immunocompromised:** amoxicillin + amoxicillin/clavulanate (7:1) × 5–7 days Nonsevere beta-lactam allergy: ceftriaxone × 5–7 days Severe beta-lactam allergy/anaphylaxis: levofloxacin × 5 days	Refer to ENT specialist if ≥4 episodes per year. Advise patients that symptoms are likely to last up to 14 days.
Failure of First-line Agents: (Clinical deterioration after 72 h of antibiotic therapy *or* no improvement post therapy *or* recurrence within 3 months)	*S. pneumoniae* *M. catarrhalis* *H. influenzae* Occasionally *S. aureus*, *S. pyogenes*, anaerobes	Amoxicillin/clavulanate ± amoxicillin[b] × 5–10 days Beta-lactam allergy: levofloxacin × 5–10 days[c] *or* moxifloxacin × 5–10 days[c]	Consider resistant organisms, especially penicillin-resistant *S. pneumoniae* and ampicillin-resistant *H. influenzae*. Quinolone use should be restricted (Table 5).
Chronic Sinusitis (Symptoms ≥12 wk)	Anaerobes Occasionally *S. aureus*, *S. pneumoniae*, *H. influenzae*, *M. catarrhalis*, *S. pyogenes*, *Enterobacteriaceae*	Amoxicillin/clavulanate × 3 wk Beta-lactam allergy: clindamycin × 3 wk	A single prolonged (3 wk) course of antibiotic may be of value in chronic sinusitis. Repeated courses of antibiotics are not recommended. Refer to ENT specialist if not responding. Investigations for allergy ± nasal polyps, underlying immunodeficiency and/or odontogenic disease may be indicated.

[a] Severe = high fever (≥39°C) and purulent nasal discharge or facial pain for 3–4 consecutive days.
[b] If patient has failed high-dose amoxicillin therapy, amoxicillin/clavulanate alone is adequate to cover beta-lactamase-producing organisms.
[c] Shorter durations of therapy have been shown to be effective in acute bacterial sinusitis but have not been well studied in patients who have failed first-line therapy. Use short-course therapy with caution in this patient population.[44]
Abbreviations: ENT = ear, nose and throat

Table 4: Antibiotics for Bacterial Sinusitis in Children

Class	Drug	Pediatric Dose	Adverse Effects	Drug Interactions	Comments	Cost[a]
Cephalosporins	*cefixime* Suprax	8 mg/kg/day divided BID po; maximum 400 mg/day	Nausea, vomiting, diarrhea,[b] hypersensitivity reactions (cross-reactivity with penicillins negligible).	May increase nephrotoxic effects of aminoglycosides; possible increased INR with warfarin.	Use in combination with clindamycin.	$$
	ceftriaxone generics	100 mg/kg daily iv	See cefixime.	Ceftriaxone may enhance the adverse/toxic effects of ethyl alcohol and the nephrotoxic effects of aminoglycosides. Ceftriaxone binds with iv calcium salts to form an insoluble precipitate.	Use if severe presentation of acute sinusitis.	~$250
Fluoroquinolones	*levofloxacin* Levaquin, generics	10–20 mg/kg/day divided daily or BID po	Usually well tolerated. Headache, dizziness may occur. QT_c prolongation. Rare: tendon rupture. Cases of severe liver injury including liver failure have been reported.	Antacids, sucralfate, metal cations, dairy products decrease levofloxacin absorption. Avoid use with other agents that prolong the QT_c interval. May increase warfarin effect. NSAIDs may increase risk of CNS stimulation/seizures.	Due to broad spectrum and potential for increased resistance, reserve quinolones for patients with beta-lactam allergy or those who have failed previous antibiotic therapy. Levofloxacin use is justified in children when reliable therapeutic options are limited (children with severe beta-lactam allergy and severe infection).	$
Lincosamides	*clindamycin* Dalacin C, Dalacin C Flavored Granules, generics	20–30 mg/kg/day divided TID or QID po; maximum 1.2–1.8 g/day	Diarrhea.[b]	Absorption of clindamycin decreased by kaolin, absorption of erythromycin decreased by clindamycin.	No activity against *H. influenzae* or *M. catarrhalis.* Alternative to amoxicillin/clavulanate in chronic sinusitis.	capsules: $ granules: $$$$
Penicillins	*amoxicillin* generics	Standard dose: 40 mg/kg/day divided TID po; maximum 1500 mg/day High dose: 90 mg/kg/day divided BID or TID po; maximum 2–3 g/day	Usually well tolerated. Nausea, vomiting, diarrhea,[b] hypersensitivity reactions.	Penicillins may increase serum concentration of methotrexate, and decrease serum concentration of the active metabolite of mycophenolate. Tetracyclines may decrease the therapeutic effect of penicillins.	First-line treatment for bacterial sinusitis in children. High-dose amoxicillin should be used in children at high risk of resistant *S. pneumoniae*: age <2 years; recent (<3 months) antibiotic exposure *and/or* daycare centre attendance.	$

(cont'd)

Table 4: **Antibiotics for Bacterial Sinusitis in Children** *(cont'd)*

Class	Drug	Pediatric Dose	Adverse Effects	Drug Interactions	Comments	Cost[a]
	amoxicillin/ clavulanate (7:1) ❥ ± *additional amoxicillin* Clavulin, generics	amoxicillin/clavulanate 45 mg/kg/day (amoxicillin component) divided BID–TID po + *additional* amoxicillin 45 mg/kg/day divided BID–TID po	Nausea, vomiting, hypersensitivity reactions. Diarrhea[b] more common with amoxicillin/clavulanate than with amoxicillin alone.	See amoxicillin.	If patient has failed standard-dose amoxicillin, combine amoxicillin/clavulanate with amoxicillin to increase the total dose of amoxicillin while minimizing diarrhea due to the clavulanate. If patient has failed high-dose amoxicillin therapy, amoxicillin/clavulanate alone is adequate to cover beta-lactamase-producing organisms.	$
Tetracyclines	*doxycycline* Vibramycin, generics	4 mg/kg/day divided BID po	Nausea, vomiting, diarrhea,[b] rash, photosensitivity.	May increase warfarin effect. May increase digoxin levels. Doxycycline seems to be minimally affected by food and dairy products as compared to demeclocycline and tetracycline. Aluminum, bismuth, iron and magnesium decreases absorption. Carbamazepine, phenytoin and phenobarbital may decrease doxycycline concentrations.	For children >8 years of age with penicillin allergy. Excellent activity against sinusitis pathogens, including beta-lactamase-producing *H. influenzae* and *M. catarrhalis*; *S. pneumoniae*, including penicillin-intermediate strains. Doxycycline resistance less than macrolide resistance in *S. pneumoniae*. Has not been associated with causing an increase in penicillin resistance among *S. pneumoniae* (macrolides have). Excellent pharmacokinetics/dynamics (high serum levels, concentration-dependent killing).	$

[a] Costs are given for a 10-day course of treatment based on 20 kg body weight, except for clindamycin (3 weeks); includes drug cost only.
[b] Antibiotic-associated diarrhea/colitis is commonly associated with clindamycin and beta-lactams, but any antibiotic can cause this condition.
❥ Dosage adjustment may be required in renal impairment; see Appendix I.
Legend: $ < $25 $$ $25–50 $$$ $50–75 $$$$ $75–100

Table 5: **Antibiotics for Bacterial Sinusitis in Adults**

Class	Drug	Dose	Adverse Effects	Drug Interactions	Comments	Cost[a]
Cephalosporins	*ceftriaxone* generics	1–2 g daily iv	Nausea, vomiting, diarrhea,[b] hypersensitivity reactions (cross-reactivity with penicillins negligible).	Ceftriaxone may enhance the adverse/toxic effects of ethyl alcohol and the nephrotoxic effects of aminoglycosides. Ceftriaxone binds with iv calcium salts to form an insoluble precipitate.	Use if severe presentation of acute sinusitis.	$60–$180
Fluoro-quinolones	*levofloxacin* ❥ Levaquin, generics	750 mg daily po × 5 days	Usually well tolerated. Headache, dizziness may occur. QT_c prolongation. Rare: tendon rupture. Cases of severe liver injury including liver failure have been reported.	Antacids, sucralfate, metal cations, dairy products decrease levofloxacin absorption. Avoid use with other agents that prolong the QT_c interval. May increase warfarin effect. NSAIDs may increase risk of CNS stimulation/seizures.	Due to broad spectrum and potential for increased resistance, reserve quinolones for patients with beta-lactam allergy or those who have failed previous antibiotic therapy.	$
	moxifloxacin Avelox	400 mg daily po	See levofloxacin.	See levofloxacin. No interaction with calcium.	See levofloxacin.	$$
Lincosamides	*clindamycin* Dalacin C, generics	300 mg QID po	Diarrhea.[b]	Absorption of clindamycin decreased by kaolin, absorption of erythromycin decreased by clindamycin.	No activity against *H. influenzae* or *M. catarrhalis*. Alternative to amoxicillin/clavulanate in chronic sinusitis.	$$
Penicillins	*amoxicillin* ❥ generics	500 mg–1 g TID po	Usually well tolerated. Nausea, vomiting, diarrhea,[b] hypersensitivity reactions.	Penicillins may increase serum concentration of methotrexate, and decrease serum concentration of the active metabolite of mycophenolate. Tetracyclines may decrease the therapeutic effect of penicillins.	First-line treatment for bacterial sinusitis in adults.	$

(cont'd)

Table 5: **Antibiotics for Bacterial Sinusitis in Adults** *(cont'd)*

Class	Drug	Dose	Adverse Effects	Drug Interactions	Comments	Cost[a]
	amoxicillin/ clavulanate ❥ Clavulin, generics	875 mg BID po	Nausea, vomiting, hypersensitivity reactions. Diarrhea[b] more common than with amoxicillin alone.	See amoxicillin.		$
Tetracyclines	*doxycycline* Vibramycin, generics	200 mg po once, then 100 mg BID po	Nausea, vomiting, diarrhea,[b] rash, photosensitivity.	May increase warfarin effect. May increase digoxin levels. Doxycycline seems to be minimally affected by food and dairy products as compared to demeclocycline and tetracycline. Aluminum, bismuth, iron and magnesium decrease absorption. Alcohol, carbamazepine, phenytoin and phenobarbital may decrease doxycycline concentrations.	Excellent activity against sinusitis pathogens, including beta-lactamase-producing *H. influenzae* and *M. catarrhalis*; *S. pneumoniae*, including penicillin-intermediate strains. Doxycycline resistance less than macrolide resistance in *S. pneumoniae*. Has not been associated with causing an increase in penicillin resistance among *S. pneumoniae* (macrolides have). Excellent pharmacokinetics/dynamics (high serum levels, concentration-dependent killing).	$

[a] Costs are given for a 5 to 7-day course of treatment except clindamycin (3 weeks); includes drug cost only.
[b] Antibiotic-associated diarrhea/colitis is commonly associated with clindamycin and beta-lactams, but any antibiotic can cause this condition.
❥ Dosage adjustment may be required in renal impairment; see Appendix I.
Abbreviations: DS = double strength; SR = sustained release
Legend: $ < $25 $$ $25–50 $$$ $50–75 $$$$ $75–100

Suggested Readings

Chow AW, Benninger MS, Brook I et al. IDSA clinical practice guideline for acute bacterial rhinosinusitis in children and adults. *Clin Infect Dis* 2012;54(8):e72-112.

De Muri GP, Wald ER. Sinusitis. In: Mandell GL, Bennett JE, Dolin R, eds. *Mandell, Douglas, and Bennett's principles and practice of infectious diseases*. 7th ed. Philadelphia (PA): Churchill Livingstone/Elsevier; 2009.

Desrosiers M, Evans GA, Keith PK et al. Canadian clinical practice guidelines for acute and chronic rhinosinusitis. *Allergy Asthma Clin Immunol* 2011;7(1):2.

Wilson JF. In the clinic. Acute sinusitis. *Ann Intern Med* 2010;153(5):ITC31-15.

References

1. Desrosiers M, Frenkiel S, Hamid QA et al. Acute bacterial sinusitis in adults: management in the primary care setting. *J Otolaryngol* 2002;31(Suppl 2):2S2-14.
2. Slavin RG, Spector SL, Bernstein IL et al. The diagnosis and management of sinusitis: a practice parameter update. *J Allergy Clin Immunol* 2005;116(6 Suppl):S13-47.
3. Alberta Medical Association. *Diagnosis and management of acute bacterial sinusitis*. Edmonton (AB): Toward Optimized Practice; 2008. Available from: www.topalbertadoctors.org/download/374/acute_bacterial_sinusitis_guideline.pdf. Accessed April 1, 2011.
4. Blondel-Hill E, Fryters S. *Bugs & drugs 2012*. Edmonton (AB): Alberta Health Services; 2012.
5. Rosenfeld RM, Andes D, Bhattacharyya N et al. Clinical practice guideline: adult sinusitis. *Otolaryngol Head Neck Surg* 2007;137(3 Suppl):S1-31.
6. Hickner JM, Bartlett JG, Besser RE et al. Principles of appropriate antibiotic use for acute rhinosinusitis in adults: background. *Ann Intern Med* 2001;134(6):498-505.
7. O'Brien KL, Dowell SF, Schwartz B et al. Acute sinusitis: principles of judicious use of antimicrobial agents. *Pediatrics* 1998;101(1 Suppl):174-7.
8. Wald ER, Chiponis D, Ledesma-Medina J. Comparative effectiveness of amoxicillin and amoxicillin-clavulanate potassium in acute paranasal sinus infections in children: a double-blind, placebo-controlled trial. *Pediatrics* 1986;77(6):795-800.
9. Druce HM. Diagnosis of sinusitis in adults: history, physical examination, nasal cytology, echo, and rhinoscope. *J Allergy Clin Immunol* 1992;90(3 Pt 2):436-41.
10. Fireman P. Diagnosis of sinusitis in children: emphasis on the history and physical examination. *J Allergy Clin Immunol* 1992;90(3 Pt 2):433-6.
11. Benninger MS, Anon J, Mabry RL. The medical management of rhinosinusitis. *Otolaryngol Head Neck Surg* 1997;117(3 Pt 2):S41-9.
12. De Muri GP, Wald ER. Sinusitis. In: Mandell GL, Bennett JE, Dolin R, eds. *Mandell, Douglas, and Bennett's principles and practice of infectious diseases*. 7th ed. Philadelphia (PA): Churchill Livingstone/Elsevier; 2009.
13. Anon JB, Jacobs MR, Poole MD et al. Antimicrobial treatment guidelines for acute bacterial rhinosinusitis. *Otolaryngol Head Neck Surg* 2004;130(1 Suppl):1-45.
14. Richards W, Roth RM, Church JA. Underdiagnosis and undertreatment of chronic sinusitis in children. *Clin Pediatr (Phila)* 1991;30(2):88-92.
15. American Academy of Pediatrics. Subcommittee on Management of Sinusitis and Committee on Quality Improvement. Clinical practice guideline: management of sinusitis. *Pediatrics* 2001;108(3):798-808.
16. Wilson JF. In the clinic. Acute sinusitis. *Ann Intern Med* 2010;153(5):ITC31-15.
17. Jefferson T, Del Mar C, Dooley L et al. Physical interventions to interrupt or reduce the spread of respiratory viruses: systematic review. *BMJ* 2009;339:b3675.
18. Poole MD. A focus on acute sinusitis in adults: changes in disease management. *Am J Med* 1999;106(5A):38S-47S.
19. Harvey R, Hannan SA, Badia L et al. Nasal saline irrigations for the symptoms of chronic rhinosinusitis. *Cochrane Database Syst Rev* 2007;(3):CD006394.
20. Brook I. Microbiology and antimicrobial management of sinusitis. *J Laryngol Otol* 2005;119(4):251-8.
21. Dykewicz MS, Hamilos DL. Rhinitis and sinusitis. *J Allergy Clin Immunol* 2010;125(2 Suppl 2):S103-15.
22. Gananca M, Trabulsi LR. The therapeutic effects of cyclacillin in acute sinusitis: in vitro and in vivo correlations in a placebo-controlled study. *Curr Med Res Opin* 1973;1(6):362-8.
23. Stalman W, van Essen GA, van der Graaf Y et al. The end of antibiotic treatment in adults with acute sinusitis-like complaints in general practice? A placebo-controlled double-blind randomized doxycycline trial. *Br J Gen Pract* 1997;47(425):794-9.
24. van Buchem FL, Knottnerus JA, Schrijnemaekers VJ et al. Primary-care-based randomised placebo-controlled trial of antibiotic treatment in acute maxillary sinusitis. *Lancet* 1997;349(9053):683-7.
25. Garbutt JM, Goldstein M, Gellman E et al. A randomized, placebo-controlled trial of antimicrobial treatment for children with clinically diagnosed acute sinusitis. *Pediatrics* 2001;107(4):619-25.
26. Ahovuo-Saloranta A, Rautakorpi UM, Borisenko OV et al. Antibiotics for acute maxillary sinusitis in adults. *Cochrane Database Syst Rev* 2014;2:CD000243.
27. Ip S, Fu L, Balk E et al. *Update on acute bacterial rhinosinusitis*. Evidence Report/Technology Assessment No. 124 AHRQ Publication No. 05-E020-1. Rockville (MD): Agency for Healthcare Research and Quality; 2005. Available from: www.ahrq.gov/downloads/pub/evidence/pdf/rhinoupdate/rhinoup.pdf. Accessed April 1, 2011.
28. Taverner D, Latte J. Nasal decongestants for the common cold. *Cochrane Database Syst Rev* 2007;(1):CD001953.
29. Schaefer MK, Shehab N, Cohen AL et al. Adverse events from cough and cold medications in children. *Pediatrics* 2008;121(4):783-7.
30. Centers for Disease Control and Prevention (CDC). Infant deaths associated with cough and cold medications--two states, 2005. *MMWR Morb Mortal Wkly Rep* 2007;56(1):1-4.
31. Health Canada. *Health Canada releases decision on the labelling of cough and cold products for children*. Available from: www.canadiensensante.gc.ca/recall-alert-rappel-avis/hc-sc/2008/13267a-eng.php. Accessed April 1, 2011.
32. Stafford CT. The clinician's view of sinusitis. *Otolaryngol Head Neck Surg* 1990;103(5 Pt 2):870-4.
33. Zalmanovici Trestioreanu A, Yaphe J. Intranasal steroids for acute sinusitis. *Cochrane Database Syst Rev* 2013;12:CD005149.

34. Desrosiers M, Evans GA, Keith PK et al. Canadian clinical practice guidelines for acute and chronic rhinosinusitis. *Allergy Asthma Clin Immunol* 2011;7(1):2.
35. Kenealy T, Arroll B. Antibiotics for the common cold and acute purulent rhinitis. *Cochrane Database Syst Rev* 2013;6:CD000247.
36. Rosenfeld RM, Singer M, Jones S. Systematic review of antimicrobial therapy in patients with acute rhinosinusitis. *Otolaryngol Head Neck Surg* 2007;137(3 Suppl):S32-45.
37. Falagas ME, Giannopoulou KP, Varkadas KZ et al. Comparison of antibiotics with placebo for treatment of acute sinusitis: a meta-analysis of randomised controlled trials. *Lancet Infect Dis* 2008;8(9):543-52.
38. Young J, De Sutter A, Merenstein D et al. Antibiotics for adults with clinically diagnosed acute rhinosinusitis: a meta-analysis of individual patient data. *Lancet* 2008;371(9616):908-14.
39. de Bock GH, Dekker FW, Stolk J et al. Antimicrobial treatment in acute maxillary sinusitis: a meta-analysis. *J Clin Epidemiol* 1997;50(8):881-90.
40. Piccirillo JF, Mager DE, Frisse ME et al. Impact of first-line vs second-line antibiotics for the treatment of acute uncomplicated sinusitis. *JAMA* 2001;286(15):1849-56.
41. de Ferranti SD, Ioannidis J, Lau J et al. Are amoxicillin and folate inhibitors as effective as other antibiotics for acute sinusitis? A meta-analysis. *BMJ* 1998;317(7159):632-7.
42. Karageorgopoulos DE, Giannopoulou KP, Grammatikos AP et al. Fluoroquinolones compared with beta-lactam antibiotics for the treatment of acute bacterial sinusitis: a meta-analysis of randomized controlled trials. *CMAJ* 2008;178(7):845-54.
43. Gehanno P, Beauvillain C, Bobin S et al. Short therapy with amoxicillin-clavulanate and corticosteroids in acute sinusitis: results of a multicentre study in adults. *Scand J Infect Dis* 2000;32(6):679-84.
44. Sher LD, McAdoo MA, Bettis RB et al. A multicenter, randomized, investigator-blinded study of 5- and 10-day gatifloxacin versus 10-day amoxicillin/clavulanate in patients with acute bacterial sinusitis. *Clin Ther* 2002;24(2):269-81.
45. Poole M, Anon J, Paglia M et al. A trial of high-dose, short-course levofloxacin for the treatment of acute bacterial sinusitis. *Otolaryngol Head Neck Surg* 2006;134(1):10-7.
46. Ferguson BJ, Anon J, Poole MD et al. Short treatment durations for acute bacterial rhinosinusitis: five days of gemifloxacin versus 7 days of gemifloxacin. *Otolaryngol Head Neck Surg* 2002;127(1):1-6.
47. Poole MD, Portugal LG. Treatment of rhinosinusitis in the outpatient setting. *Am J Med* 2005;118(Suppl 7A):45S-50S.
48. Falagas ME, Karageorgopoulos DE, Grammatikos AP et al. Effectiveness and safety of short vs. long duration of antibiotic therapy for acute bacterial sinusitis: a meta-analysis of randomized trials. *Br J Clin Pharmacol* 2009;67(2):161-71.
49. Chow AW, Benninger MS, Brook I et al. IDSA clinical practice guideline for acute bacterial rhinosinusitis in children and adults. *Clin Infect Dis* 2012;54(8):e72-112.
50. Incaudo GA. Diagnosis and treatment of allergic rhinitis and sinusitis during pregnancy and lactation. *Clin Rev Allergy Immunol* 2004;27(2):159-77.
51. Erebara A, Bozzo P, Einarson A et al. Treating the common cold during pregnancy. *Can Fam Physician* 2008;54(5):687-9.
52. Koren G. Use of the new quinolones during pregnancy. *Can Fam Physician* 1996;42:1097-9.
53. Berkovitch M, Pastuszak A, Gazarian M et al. Safety of the new quinolones in pregnancy. *Obstet Gynecol* 1994;84(4):535-8.
54. Loebstein R, Addis A, Ho E et al. Pregnancy outcome following gestational exposure to fluoroquinolones: a multicenter prospective controlled study. *Antimicrob Agents Chemother* 1998;42(6):1336-9.
55. Quinolones and pregnancy: worrying animal findings, few clinical data. *Prescrire Int* 1999;8(39):29-31.
56. Hale TW. *Medication and mothers' milk: a manual of lactational pharmacology*. 15th ed. Amarillo (TX): Hale Publishing; 2012.
57. American Academy of Pediatrics Committee on Drugs. Transfer of drugs and other chemicals into human milk. *Pediatrics* 2001;108(3):776-89.
58. Arrieta A, Arguedas A, Fernandez P et al. High-dose azithromycin versus high-dose amoxicillin-clavulanate for treatment of children with recurrent or persistent acute otitis media. *Antimicrob Agents Chemother* 2003;47(10):3179-86.
59. Arrieta A, Singh J. Management of recurrent and persistent acute otitis media: new options with familiar antibiotics. *Pediatr Infect Dis J* 2004;23(2 Suppl):S115-24.

Infectious Diseases

Chapter 122
Streptococcal Sore Throat

Andrew C. Steer, MBBS, BMedSc, MPH, FRACP, PhD

Goals of Therapy

- Provide symptomatic relief
- Shorten duration of symptoms
- Prevent suppurative complications, e.g., quinsy (peritonsillar abscess), mastoiditis, cervical lymphadenitis
- Prevent nonsuppurative complications, e.g., acute rheumatic fever (rare in Canada)
- Prevent spread of group A streptococci to contacts

Investigations

The probability of group A streptococci (*S. pyogenes*) as the cause of sore throat is greatest in a child with an acute sore throat who is >3 years old, lacks signs of a viral upper respiratory infection and has signs and symptoms as listed below.[1] However, seriously consider the diagnosis of streptococcal pharyngitis (strep throat) in any child presenting with an acute sore throat, with or without "classic" signs and symptoms because differentiating group A streptococcal pharyngitis from viral pharyngitis is very difficult clinically.

- Clinical diagnosis of streptococcal infection: a throat swab with positive rapid antigen detection test (RADT) and/or positive throat culture are the only true predictive features[2]
- Although not diagnostic, symptoms and signs suggestive of group A streptococcal sore throat include:
  - symptoms: sudden onset of sore throat, pain on swallowing, headache, abdominal pain, nausea, vomiting, fever (see Chapter 26)
  - signs: tender cervical adenopathy, erythematous pharynx and tonsils, pharyngeal exudate, scarlatiniform rash
  - note that the presence of features suggestive of a viral etiology (cough, rhinorrhea, hoarseness, oral ulcers) make the diagnosis of group A streptococcal sore throat much less likely
- Laboratory diagnosis:
  - RADT of throat swab: results available in 7–70 minutes. A positive RADT has a high specificity such that treatment can be commenced and a back-up throat culture is unnecessary. A negative RADT in adults allows withholding of antibiotics with no need for a back-up throat culture. However, the sensitivity of RADT can be too low (<90%) to rule out streptococcal infection in children or adolescents.[2] If the RADT is unavailable or is negative in children or adolescents, obtain a culture and withhold antibiotics for 24–48 hours until the results are available. If positive, recall and treat the patient for group A streptococci. This approach does not increase the risk of acute rheumatic fever[3] but avoids the unnecessary use of antibiotics
  - throat culture is "gold standard" (results available in 24–48 hours). A negative throat culture allows withholding of antibiotics from the majority of patients with sore throat

- viral throat culture rarely influences therapy (results available in days to weeks). A partial list of etiologic agents for acute sore throat is presented in Table 1
- repeat bacterial cultures are not necessary at the end of therapy or from asymptomatic family contacts (except in the case of household contacts of a patient with acute rheumatic fever)
- bacterial culture and RADT do not differentiate between carriage of and infection with group A streptococci
- streptococcal serology (antistreptolysin O or antideoxyribonuclease B titres): useful retrospectively in patients who have possible complications of streptococcal infection (e.g., rheumatic fever or post-streptococcal glomerulonephritis)[3] but are not useful in the diagnosis of acute streptococcal pharyngitis

Therapeutic Choices

Information about Therapeutic Choices can be found in Figure 1

Nonpharmacologic Choices

- Strict hand-washing to prevent spread of infection.
- Exclude from school or daycare for 24 hours after antimicrobial therapy is begun.

Pharmacologic Choices

Information about Pharmacologic Choices can be found in Table 2.

Analgesics

Acetaminophen or **ibuprofen** may be given for fever and pain. Lozenges and gargles may be indicated for symptomatic treatment of sore throat.

Adjunctive therapy with a **corticosteroid** appears to provide more rapid symptomatic relief in adults than antibiotics alone (likelihood of complete resolution of pain at 24 hours; RR 3.16 (95% CI 1.97–5.08); NNT = 3.7).[5] However, many questions remain such as the appropriate formulation and dose, complications and adverse effects, efficacy as monotherapy, efficacy in children and comparative efficacy versus other analgesics. Until more information is available, corticosteroids are not recommended as routine adjunctive treatment but may be considered on a case-by-case basis in adults [Evidence: SORT B*].[5]

Table 1: Selected Pathogens of Acute Pharyngitis

Viruses (adenoviruses, enteroviruses, cytomegalovirus, Epstein-Barr, influenza, herpes simplex virus and parainfluenza viruses)
Group A β-hemolytic streptococci (children: 15–30%; adults: 5–10%)[2]
Groups C and G β-hemolytic streptococci
Neisseria gonorrhoeae (consider sexual abuse if recovered from child's throat)
Mycoplasma pneumoniae[a]
Chlamydia trachomatis[a]
Chlamydophila pneumoniae[a,b]
Corynebacterium diphtheriae
Arcanobacterium hemolyticum[a]

[a] Role in acute pharyngitis is controversial.
[b] Previously *Chlamydia pneumoniae*.

* SORT (Strength of Recommendation Taxonomy) is a rating system (A, B or C) that addresses the quality of available evidence. For more information consult **How to Use *Compendium of Therapeutic Choices*** on page xxv.

Figure 1: **Management of Acute Sore Throat**

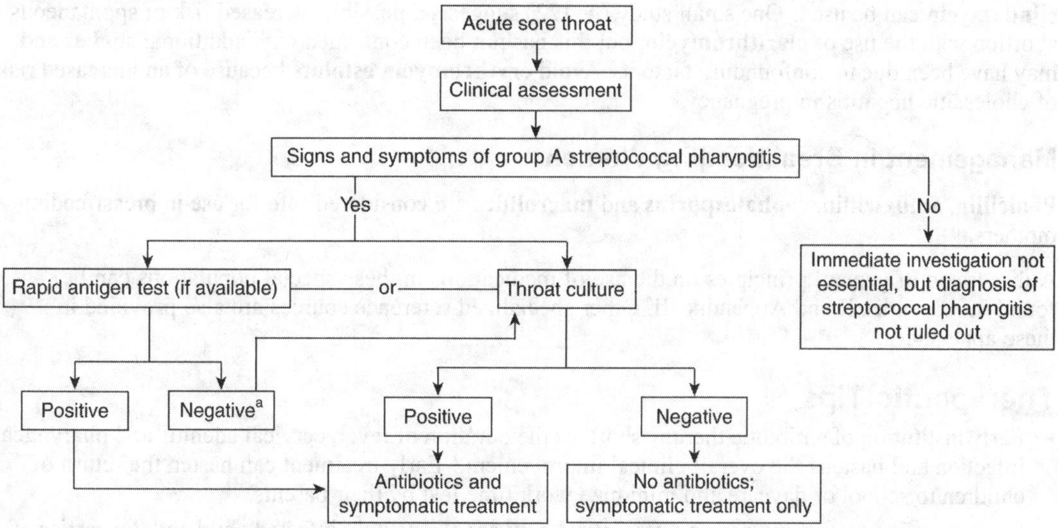

[a] Antibiotic therapy may be safely withheld from an adult based on a negative rapid antigen test.[4]

Antibiotics

Antibiotic therapy for group A streptococcal pharyngitis provides modest symptomatic benefit. It reduces throat soreness and fever by approximately one-half and shortens the course of the acute illness by an average of 16 hours.[6] Antibiotic therapy can prevent suppurative complications such as quinsy with the number needed to treat between 50 and 200.[7] Antibiotic therapy also prevents rheumatic fever if started within 10 days of illness onset, although rheumatic fever is exceedingly uncommon in Canada.[6,8]

Penicillin (or **amoxicillin**) is the drug of choice for streptococcal sore throat.[2] Although **cephalosporins** are effective, they should *not* replace penicillin or amoxicillin as the drug of choice because of their broader spectrum and consequent risk of promoting resistance. Amoxicillin is often used in children requiring liquid medication due to the poor palatability of penicillin V suspension.[2]

There are a number of treatment options for penicillin-allergic patients. For patients who do not have an immediate IgE-mediated hypersensitivity to penicillin, narrow spectrum cephalosporins, such as **cephalexin**, can be used.[2] For patients with an IgE-mediated anaphylactic hypersensitivity to penicillin, treatment with **clindamycin** or **clarithromycin** for 10 days or **azithromycin** for 5 days is recommended. **Erythromycin** is no longer preferred therapy for penicillin-allergic patients because of its high rate of gastrointestinal adverse events and availability of other more favourable agents.

Choices during Pregnancy and Breastfeeding

Streptococcal Sore Throat and Pregnancy

Streptococcal sore throat is more common in children aged 5–15 years than in adults, however, cases of streptococcal sore throat do occur in pregnancy. The management of streptococcal sore throat in pregnant women is the same as for children; if group A streptococci are identified on throat culture, treatment for 10 days is indicated.

Management during Pregnancy

Penicillin is considered safe in pregnancy. For penicillin-allergic patients, **azithromycin** and **clindamycin** can be used. One small study (n=122) suggests a possible increased risk of spontaneous abortion with the use of **clarithromycin**, but this has not been confirmed with additional studies and may have been due to confounding factors.[9] Avoid **erythromycin estolate** because of an increased risk of cholestatic hepatitis in pregnancy.

Management in Breastfeeding Women

Penicillin, **amoxicillin**, **cephalosporins** and **macrolides** are considered safe for use in breastfeeding mothers.[10]

A discussion of general principles on the use of medications in these special populations can be found in Appendix II and Appendix III. Other specialized reference sources are also provided in these appendices.

Therapeutic Tips

- Early institution of antibiotic therapy shortens the duration of fever, cervical adenitis and pharyngeal infection and hastens the overall clinical improvement.[6] Early treatment can hasten the return of children to school or daycare and minimize work time lost by their parents.
- Since there is no efficient way to differentiate between the acutely infected child and the carrier of group A streptococci, all symptomatic patients with a positive RADT or positive culture should receive antistreptococcal therapy. Note that acute rheumatic fever is rare in Canada but may develop after mild or subclinical streptococcal infections.[11]
- As discussed above, it is difficult to reliably differentiate between acute streptococcal infection and chronic carriage, however, chronic carriers of group A streptococci are not thought to play an important role in the spread of the bacteria to contacts. Therefore, as long as the patient is asymptomatic, repeated courses of antibiotics to eradicate carriage are generally not indicated.[2] If eradication therapy is desired, penicillin monotherapy is the least effective regimen in eradicating pharyngeal streptococcal carriage. Some advocate the use of **clindamycin** (20 mg/kg/day divided TID for 10 days; maximum 600 mg/day) or the addition of **rifampin** (20 mg/kg/day divided BID; maximum 600 mg/day) for the final 4 days of **penicillin** therapy to attempt to interrupt chronic pharyngeal carriage of group A streptococci.[12,13] For patients who have persistent symptoms and positive cultures at the end of initial treatment, one of the above regimens, a narrow-spectrum **cephalosporin** or **amoxicillin/clavulanate** may be considered.[2]

Table 2: **Drugs for Treatment of Group A Streptococcal Pharyngitis**

Class	Drug	Dose	Adverse Effects	Comments	Cost[a]
Cephalosporins	*cefadroxil* generics	Adults: 1 g daily po as a single dose or divided BID × 10 days	Hypersensitivity (some cross-reactivity with penicillins).	**Cephalosporins may be used if treatment failure with penicillin or in individuals with nonimmediate hypersensitivity to penicillins.**	$$
	cephalexin generics	Adults: 500 mg BID po × 10 days Children: 40 mg/kg/day divided BID po × 10 days; maximum 1 g/day	See cefadroxil.	See cefadroxil. Available as suspension.	$
Lincosamides	*clindamycin* Dalacin C, Dalacin C Flavored Granules, generics	Adults and children: 21 mg/kg/day divided TID po × 10 days; maximum 900 mg/day	*C. difficile* colitis, diarrhea (common).	An alternative for patients with erythromycin-resistant strain of group A Streptococcus and who cannot tolerate β-lactam antibiotics. May be used for treatment in symptomatic patients with multiple, recurrent episodes of pharyngitis. Available as suspension.	$$
Macrolides	*azithromycin* Z-Pak, Zithromax, generics	Adults: 500 mg once daily po × 5 days Children: 12 mg/kg once daily po × 5 days; maximum 500 mg/day	Lower frequency of GI effects than erythromycin.	**An alternative for penicillin-allergic patients.** A 5-day course is effective. Available as suspension. Less likely than other macrolides to interact with other drugs.	$
	clarithromycin Biaxin, generics	Adult: 250 mg BID po × 10 days Children: 15 mg/kg/day divided BID po × 10 days; maximum 500 mg/day	Lower frequency of GI effects than erythromycin.	**An alternative for penicillin-allergic patients.** Available as suspension. Increased levels of atorvastatin, carbamazepine, digoxin, lovastatin, prednisone, simvastatin, theophylline.	$
	erythromycin Eryc, generics	Adults: 1 g daily divided BID–QID po × 10 days Administer 1 hour before meals to prevent acid inactivation	Nausea, vomiting, epigastric distress, diarrhea, elevated liver enzymes, cholestatic jaundice.	**An alternative for penicillin-allergic patients.** Increased levels of atorvastatin, carbamazepine, digoxin, lovastatin, prednisone, simvastatin, theophylline.	$
	erythromycin estolate generics	Adults: 1 g daily divided BID–QID po × 10 days Children:[14] 40 mg/kg/day divided BID–TID po × 10 days; maximum 1 g/day	See erythromycin.	Contraindicated in pregnancy. Incidence of cholestatic hepatitis greater in pregnancy. **An alternative for penicillin-allergic patients.** Available as suspension. Increased levels of atorvastatin, carbamazepine, digoxin, lovastatin, prednisone, simvastatin, theophylline.	$

(cont'd)

Table 2: **Drugs for Treatment of Group A Streptococcal Pharyngitis** *(cont'd)*

Class	Drug	Dose	Adverse Effects	Comments	Cost[a]
	erythromycin ethylsuccinate generics	Adults: 1 g daily divided BID–QID po × 10 days Children: 40–50 mg/kg/day divided BID–QID po × 10 days; maximum 1 g/day	See erythromycin.	**An alternative for penicillin-allergic patients.** Available as suspension. Increased levels of atorvastatin, carbamazepine, digoxin, lovastatin, prednisone, simvastatin, theophylline.	$
Penicillins	*amoxicillin* ❥ generics	Adults and children: 50 mg/kg once daily or divided BID po × 10 days; maximum 1 g/day	Usually well tolerated. Rash, anaphylaxis (rare).	Available as chewable tablets and suspension.	$
	penicillin V potassium ❥ generics	Adults and children >27 kg:[14] 300 mg TID or 600 mg BID po × 10 days Children ≤27 kg:[14] 40 mg/kg/day divided BID–TID po × 10 days; maximum 750 mg/day	Anaphylaxis, gastrointestinal upset, diarrhea.	**Drug of choice.** Oral route for penicillin preferred.	$
Penicillinase-resistant Penicillins	*amoxicillin/ clavulanate* ❥ Clavulin, generics	Adults: 500 mg (amoxicillin component) BID po × 10 days Children: 40 mg/kg/day (amoxicillin component) divided TID po × 10 days; maximum dose of amoxicillin: 2 g/day	Diarrhea, gastrointestinal upset, anaphylaxis (rare).	May be used for treatment in symptomatic patients with multiple, recurrent episodes of pharyngitis. Available as suspension.	$$

[a] Cost of 10-day supply of tablets for adult dosage (except 5 days for azithromycin); includes drug cost only.

❥ Dosage adjustment may be required in renal impairment; see Appendix I.

Legend: $ < $10 $$ $10–20 $$$ $20–30

Suggested Readings

ESCMID Sore Throat Guideline Group, Pelucchi C, Grigoryan L et al. Guideline for the management of acute sore throat. *Clin Microbiol Infect* 2012;18(Suppl 1):1-28.

Gerber MA, Baltimore RS, Eaton CB et al. Prevention of rheumatic fever and diagnosis and treatment of acute Streptococcal pharyngitis: a scientific statement from the American Heart Association Rheumatic Fever, Endocarditis, and Kawasaki Disease Committee of the Council on Cardiovascular Disease in the Young, the Interdisciplinary Council on Functional Genomics and Translational Biology, and the Interdisciplinary Council on Quality of Care and Outcomes Research: endorsed by the American Academy of Pediatrics. *Circulation* 2009;119(11):1541-51.

Shulman ST, Bisno AL, Clegg HW et al. Clinical practice guideline for the diagnosis and management of group A streptococcal pharyngitis: 2012 update by the Infectious Diseases Society of America. *Clin Infect Dis* 2012;55(10):e86-102.

Spinks A, Glasziou PP, Del Mar CB. Antibiotics for sore throat. *Cochrane Database Syst Rev* 2013;11:CD000023.

Wessels MR. Clinical practice. Streptococcal pharyngitis. *N Engl J Med* 2011;364(7):648-55.

References

1. Wannamaker LW. Perplexity and precision in the diagnosis of streptococcal pharyngitis. *Am J Dis Child* 1972;124(3):352-8.
2. Gerber MA, Baltimore RS, Eaton CB et al. Prevention of rheumatic fever and diagnosis and treatment of acute Streptococcal pharyngitis: a scientific statement from the American Heart Association Rheumatic Fever, Endocarditis, and Kawasaki Disease Committee of the Council on Cardiovascular Disease in the Young, the Interdisciplinary Council on Functional Genomics and Translational Biology, and the Interdisciplinary Council on Quality of Care and Outcomes Research: endorsed by the American Academy of Pediatrics. *Circulation* 2009;119(11):1541-51.
3. Guidelines for the diagnosis of rheumatic fever. Jones Criteria, 1992 update. Special Writing Group of the Committee on Rheumatic Fever, Endocarditis, and Kawasaki Disease of the Council on Cardiovascular Disease in the Young of the American Heart Association. *JAMA* 1992;268(15):2069-73.
4. Shulman ST, Bisno AL, Clegg HW et al. Clinical practice guideline for the diagnosis and management of group A streptococcal pharyngitis: 2012 update by the Infectious Diseases Society of America. *Clin Infect Dis* 2012;55(10):e86-102.
5. Hayward G, Thompson MJ, Perera R et al. Corticosteroids as standalone or add-on treatment for sore throat. *Cochrane Database Syst Rev* 2012;10:CD008268.
6. Spinks A, Glasziou PP, Del Mar CB. Antibiotics for sore throat. *Cochrane Database Syst Rev* 2013;11:CD000023.
7. ESCMID Sore Throat Guideline Group, Pelucchi C, Grigoryan L et al. Guideline for the management of acute sore throat. *Clin Microbiol Infect* 2012;18(Suppl 1):1-28.
8. Catanzaro FJ, Stetson CA, Morris AJ et al. The role of the streptococcus in the pathogenesis of rheumatic fever. *Am J Med* 1954;17(6):749-56.
9. Einarson A, Phillips E, Mawji F et al. A prospective controlled multicentre study of clarithromycin in pregnancy. *Am J Perinatol* 1998;15(9):523-5.
10. Drugs and Lactation Database (LactMed). Bethesda (MD): U.S. National Library of Medicine. Available from: toxnet.nlm.nih.gov/cgi-bin/sis/htmlgen?LACT. Accessed August 15, 2013.
11. Carapetis JR, McDonald M, Wilson NJ. Acute rheumatic fever. *Lancet* 2005;366(9480):155-68.
12. Tanz RR, Poncher JR, Corydon KE et al. Clindamycin treatment of chronic pharyngeal carriage of group A streptococci. *J Pediatr* 1991;119(1 Pt 1):123-8.
13. Tanz RR, Shulman ST, Barthel MJ et al. Penicillin plus rifampin eradicates pharyngeal carriage of group A streptococci. *J Pediatr* 1985;106(6):876-80.
14. Anti-infective Review Panel. *Anti-infective guidelines for community-acquired infections*. Toronto (ON): MUMS Guideline Clearinghouse; 2012.

Chapter 123
Travellers' Diarrhea

Laurence Green, MD, FRCPC and
Michael Libman, MDCM, FRCPC

Travellers' diarrhea (TD) is defined as the passage of 3 or more unformed stools in a 24-hour period plus at least one other symptom of enteric disease such as abdominal pain or cramps, nausea, vomiting, fever, bloody diarrhea or tenesmus.[1] Diarrhea develops in an average of 15–40% of travellers depending on destination and season.[2] In 10% of cases, fever and/or bloody stools may occur.[2] Most cases in adults are caused by bacteria, predominantly enterotoxigenic *E. coli* (ETEC), enteroaggregative *E. coli* as well as *Campylobacter*, *Salmonella* and *Shigella*.[3,4] Other pathogens include viruses (norovirus, rotavirus) and protozoa, e.g., *Giardia intestinalis*. Incubation periods are short. Most TD cases occur within 2 weeks of arriving at a destination but could still occur within 2 weeks after returning home.[5,6] Because of the frequent unavailability of reliable medical care, travellers must be prepared to institute self-therapy. Fortunately, TD is self-limiting (usually lasting <7 days) and in most cases antibiotic treatment is not necessary for recovery.[7] An episode of TD does not confer protection against future attacks and more than one episode can be experienced in a single trip.

Goals of Therapy

- Reduce risk of infection in travellers
- Limit duration and severity of symptoms while travelling and during the immediate post-travel period

Investigations

- Counsel travellers about *self-diagnosis*:
  - distinguish mild symptoms (abdominal cramps, malaise, nausea and frequent bowel movements) from the high fever and bloody and mucoid stools of more severe infection requiring urgent antibiotic therapy
- Evaluate patients developing symptoms after returning home or presenting with symptoms persisting >2 weeks after their return:
  - history (e.g., destination and season of travel) and physical examination (signs of volume depletion, abdominal tenderness/guarding)
  - consider stool cultures especially in cases of dysentery, in food handlers, in health- and childcare workers, in immunocompromised patients and in those not improving with supportive care
  - consider stool parasitology exams for diarrhea persisting >2 weeks after return

Prevention of Travellers' Diarrhea

Therapeutic Choices

Nonpharmacologic Choices

- "Boil it, cook it, peel it or forget it" is a useful reminder but difficult to follow and actual protection is unproven.[8]

- Drink only boiled, bottled or carbonated beverages. Avoid bottled drinks if the cap is not sealed and intact. Alcoholic drinks do not sterilize water or ice.
- Bring clear water to a boil, or sterilize using chlorine (**sodium hypochlorite** 1.5% or in tablet form) or iodine (5 drops of 2% tincture of **iodine** per litre of clear water). Because of iodine's physiologic effects, do not use it for >3 weeks. *Iodine resin filters* have the advantage of filtering plus the iodine is not absorbed. *Ceramic microbial filters* are inexpensive, sturdy and highly effective, and may also protect against viruses. Filtration is particularly effective for protozoa, which are relatively resistant to regular doses of iodine and chlorine.[9]
- Avoid ice cubes unless made from safe water.
- Eat fruit (including tomatoes) only if it has been washed in safe water and peeled.
- Avoid salads and raw vegetables.
- Eat only thoroughly and recently cooked meats or fish.
- Avoid leftovers and condiments in open bottles.
- Avoid food from street vendors.
- Reassess the need for proton pump inhibitors and H_2-receptor antagonists in individuals travelling to areas with high rates of travellers' diarrhea since these agents increase the risk of acquiring intestinal pathogens.[10,11]
- Wash hands with soap and water before eating. Waterless alcohol-based hand sanitizers are also effective if hands are not visibly dirty.

Pharmacologic Choices

Table 1 lists medications used for the treatment and prevention of travellers' diarrhea.

Bismuth Subsalicylate

Bismuth subsalicylate (BSS) is effective in preventing and treating TD.[12,13] BSS may have antibacterial activity as well as antisecretory and anti-inflammatory properties. Side effects are minimal with short-term use (<3 weeks) at recommended doses. Black stools produced by BSS may create diagnostic confusion by simulating melena. Do not recommend BSS in travellers taking anticoagulants or salicylates or those who are allergic to salicylates. Chemoprophylaxis with BSS is also not recommended for young children due to concerns regarding excessive salicylate absorption and risk of bismuth encephalopathy at higher doses.[14] BSS is not recommended often for the prevention of TD.

Antibiotics

The benefits of *preventing* TD with antibiotics usually do not outweigh the risks, cost and inconvenience. Furthermore, antimicrobials are very effective in *treating* TD once it occurs. Most travellers should use antibiotics for treatment rather than prevention of TD. In the rare event where antibiotics are needed for prevention, prescribe them for short courses only (<3 weeks), and target those at greatest risk of TD or its complications (e.g., chronically ill or immunocompromised patients), or persons who undertake critical travel (e.g., diplomatic missions) or have diarrhea every time they travel.

Fluoroquinolones (**ciprofloxacin**, **levofloxacin**, **norfloxacin**, **ofloxacin**) effectively reduce attacks of TD by up to 90% and are relatively safe, although bacterial resistance severely limits their use in Thailand,[15,16] India,[17] Nepal[18] and Indonesia.[19] There is a risk of *Clostridium difficile*-associated diarrhea in travellers taking antibiotic prophylaxis or antibiotics for any purpose. **Sulfamethoxazole/trimethoprim** (SMX/TMP) and **doxycycline** are *no longer recommended* for prevention of TD due to significant bacterial resistance.[1]

Vaccines

An inactivated oral **cholera vaccine** contains the B subunit of cholera toxin, which has significant homology with the toxin of ETEC. There is insufficient evidence to support the use of this vaccine for protecting travellers against ETEC diarrhea.[20] Because of the vaccine's cost, uncertain/low efficacy, relatively short duration of protection, mild and self-limited nature of ETEC diarrhea and because TD responds rapidly to self-treatment, the inactivated oral cholera vaccine is not routinely recommended.[20,21] However, it is recommended for travellers at unusually high risk such as relief/aid workers or health care professionals working in cholera risk zones.[22] Updated *Immunization of Travellers* guidelines from the Public Health Agency of Canada is available at www.phac-aspc.gc.ca/publicat/cig-gci/p03-10-eng.php.

Probiotics

There is currently little evidence that probiotics such as *Lactobacillus* spp. or *Saccharomyces boulardii* are effective in the prevention of TD.[23,24]

Self-treatment of Travellers' Diarrhea

Therapeutic Choices

Figure 1 discusses the self-management of travellers' diarrhea in adults.

Nonpharmacologic Choices

Travellers with mild diarrhea may benefit from a simple diet that maintains hydration, contains a modest amount of sugars and electrolytes, and is devoid of fatty or oily foods and natural laxatives (e.g., caffeine, alcohol, excessive fruits). Bananas can provide a source of potassium. Dietary fibre may aggravate bloating and cramping.

Figure 1: Self-Management of Travellers' Diarrhea in Adults

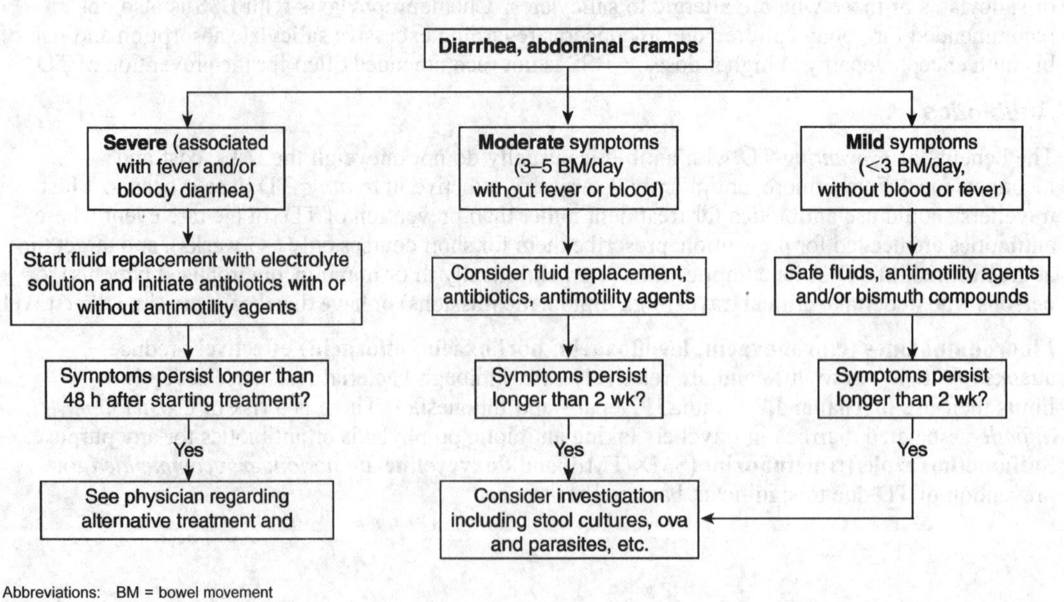

Abbreviations: BM = bowel movement

Pharmacologic Choices

Table 1 lists medications used for the treatment of travellers' diarrhea.

Oral Rehydration Salts (ORS)

Oral hydration, especially in infants, pregnant women and the frail elderly, is the cornerstone of all therapy. Commercially available sachets of **oral rehydration salts** (e.g., Gastrolyte, Pedialyte) are dissolved in safe water and the resulting liquid is consumed until thirst is quenched. The traveller should carry sufficient sachets to produce 2–4 litres of oral rehydration solution.

If ORS is unavailable, a less-ideal emergency substitute can be prepared by adding 1 level teaspoonful (5 mL) of table salt and 6 teaspoonfuls (30 mL) of sugar to 1 litre of safe water.[25] Alternatively, 1/4 teaspoonful (1 mL) of baking soda, 1/8 teaspoonful (0.5 mL) of salt and 1/2 teaspoonful (2.5 mL) of pasteurized honey can be added to 1 cup (240 mL) of fruit juice.[23] These ingredients may be harder to find.

Antimotility Agents

Loperamide provides relief for mild to moderate diarrhea (up to 5 loose stools per day and mild cramping pain) in adults and older children.[26] **Diphenoxylate with atropine** is not as effective as loperamide and has a less favourable side effect profile.[27] Do not use antimotility agents in children <3 years of age due to the risk of developing toxic megacolon and obscuring the severity of fluid loss. Do not use antimotility agents alone in patients with bloody diarrhea or fever (temperature >38.5°C) since the resulting inhibition of peristalsis could prolong the infection and could lead to complications such as ileus, megacolon and toxic megacolon.[28] However, the combination of loperamide and an antibiotic is safe and more effective than either alone in reducing the duration of diarrhea.[29,30]

Antibiotics

Travellers' diarrhea (commonly caused by ETEC) is usually a mild, self-limited disease that responds promptly to appropriate therapy. Advise patients to obtain a 1- to 3-day supply of antibiotics to take with them on their travels and to initiate therapy with the onset of symptoms, especially in the case of severe diarrhea with blood, cramps or high fever. Mild diarrhea can be managed with fluids and antimotility agents.

The **fluoroquinolones (ciprofloxacin**, **levofloxacin**, **norfloxacin**, **ofloxacin**) effectively reduce the duration of diarrhea by >50% relative to placebo.[31,32,33] In Thailand, the most common cause of dysentery (passage of grossly bloody stools) is *Campylobacter*, which is often fluoroquinolone-resistant. Because of this, **azithromycin** has become the antibiotic of choice for TD in Thailand[34] as well as in India, Indonesia and Nepal. Despite lack of data, it is reasonable to extend this recommendation to other Southeast Asian and Indian subcontinent countries.

SMX/TMP is rarely prescribed due to presumed bacterial resistance and is ineffective against *Campylobacter* (consider only for areas with low rates of this infection, e.g., inland Mexico during summer). SMX/TMP remains an alternative for those who cannot take a fluoroquinolone.

Several clinical trials have shown the effectiveness of a single dose of antibiotic in the treatment of TD (see Table 1 for recommended doses). The addition of loperamide to a single dose of antibiotic appears to be particularly effective.[23,29,35]

Travellers' Diarrhea in Children

The management of TD in children and infants is difficult because of the increased risk and rapid onset of severe and life-threatening dehydration, different infectious agents (e.g., rotavirus in children <3 years) and more limited antibiotic choices (e.g., fluoroquinolones are not recommended in children). Advise parents to travel with **oral rehydration salts** and educate them regarding their use. Recommend that they seek medical help early if their child is affected. Do not use **loperamide** in children under age 3. Use loperamide sparingly, if at all, in older children. **Bismuth subsalicylate** (BSS) is contraindicated in children <3 years of age and should be used cautiously in older children because of the risks of Reye's syndrome. Use of SMX/TMP in children is limited by the same resistance problems seen in adults. **Azithromycin** is safe in children and is the antibiotic of choice if antibiotics are deemed necessary. **Ciprofloxacin** has been avoided because of concern over its potential effects on cartilage development. However, studies in the past decade have not shown a problem with the short courses (1–3 days) that are used to treat TD.[36]

Choices during Pregnancy and Breastfeeding

Travellers' Diarrhea during Pregnancy

The pregnant traveller may be at increased risk of travellers' diarrhea and subsequent complications.[37] Decreased gastric acidity may increase the risk of diarrhea. Altered motility may worsen the outcome and significant volume depletion may precipitate premature labour, placental insufficiency or shock. Early fluid, energy and electrolyte replacement remains the cornerstone of management.[37]

Management

Chemoprophylaxis is not recommended.[37] Pregnant travellers should pay special attention to safe food and water preparation. This may include travelling with sufficient material to boil water.[37] Iodine preparations are not recommended because of the potential risk of causing thyroid disease in the fetus. It is prudent for the pregnant traveller to carry adequate supplies of **oral rehydration salts** and to learn how to use them. Fluoroquinolones are contraindicated because of the potential risk to the fetus although the short courses used in management of travellers' diarrhea have not been shown to increase teratogenicity. **Azithromycin** is considered safe in pregnancy and is the agent of choice if antibiotics are needed.[37] Sulfa-containing agents such as **sulfamethoxazole/trimethoprim** are safe in early pregnancy but carry the risk of kernicterus if given prepartum. **Bismuth subsalicylate** is not recommended because of the risk of bismuth encephalopathy. **Loperamide** is considered safe and can be used when necessary.

Travellers' Diarrhea during Breastfeeding

Breastfeeding should be continued during travel as it reduces the risk of contaminated food products infecting the infant. Women must be meticulous in hand-washing and breast hygiene to prevent infecting organisms being passed to the infant.

Management

Adequate management of diarrhea hinges on proper fluid, energy and electrolyte replacement.[38] **Azithromycin** and **loperamide** may be used in severe diarrhea.[38] Iodine for water sterilization, bismuth preparations and fluoroquinolones are best avoided in breastfeeding travellers.

A discussion of general principles on the use of medications in these special populations can be found in Appendix II and Appendix III. Other specialized reference sources are also provided in these appendices.

Therapeutic Tips

- Mild travellers' diarrhea usually resolves within 24 hours with antimotility agents and fluids.
- It is often best to wait and treat travellers' diarrhea when it occurs rather than use chemoprophylaxis since treatment options are effective and relatively quick in relieving symptoms.
- Discourage the use of nonprescription drugs purchased abroad as they are ineffective for both prophylaxis and treatment. Some foreign products contain chloramphenicol which may induce

aplastic anemia, or iodochlorhydroxyquin which can cause neurologic damage and optic atrophy with prolonged use.

- Investigate symptoms persisting >2 weeks after the return home (history, physical and stool parasitology as part of a first-line investigation). Irritable bowel syndrome is common. Also consider parasitic infection, antibiotic-associated colitis, disaccharidase deficiency and bowel carcinoma. Inflammatory bowel disease or celiac disease may be unmasked by an episode of travellers' diarrhea.
- Advise patients with fever or dysentery to seek medical attention if symptoms have not improved within 48 hours despite therapy.

Suggested Readings

DuPont HL, Ericsson CD, Farthing MJ et al. Expert review of the evidence base for prevention of travelers' diarrhea. *J Travel Med* 2009;16(3):149-60.

DuPont HL, Ericsson CD, Farthing MJ et al. Expert review of the evidence base for self-therapy of travelers' diarrhea. *J Travel Med* 2009;16(3):161-71.

Kollaritsch H, Paulke-Korinek M, Wiedermann U. Traveler's diarrhea. *Infect Dis Clin North Am* 2012;26(3):691-706.

Plourde PJ. Travellers' diarrhea in children. *Paediatr Child Health* 2003;8(2):99-103.

Table 1: Drugs Used for the Treatment and Prevention of Travellers' Diarrhea

Class	Drug	Dose	Adverse Effects	Comments	Cost[a]
Antiperistaltics	*loperamide* Imodium, Riva-Loperamide, other generics	**Adults:** 4 mg po initially, then 2 mg after each loose stool (maximum 16 mg/day) **Children:** 1–2 mg po initially, then 1–2 mg after each loose stool (maximum 3 mg daily for ages 3–5 y, 4 mg daily for ages 5–8 y and 6 mg daily for ages 8–12 y) Do not use for prophylaxis. Used for treatment only.	Abdominal cramping, rarely dizziness, dry mouth, skin rash.	Do not use in children <3 y. Use with an antibiotic only if experiencing fever or bloody stools. Prophylactic antimotility agents have no effect in preventing travellers' diarrhea.	$
Fluoroquinolones	*ciprofloxacin* Cipro, generics	**Adults:** Treatment: 500 mg BID po × 3 days or 750 mg po × 1 dose Prophylaxis:[b] 500 mg once daily po **Children:** Not recommended	Infrequent GI disturbance, CNS effects, skin rash.	Not recommended in southeast Asia and Indian subcontinent.	$
	levofloxacin Levaquin, generics	**Adults:** Treatment: 500 mg once daily po × 3 days or 1000 mg po × 1 dose Prophylaxis:[b] 500 mg once daily po **Children:** Not recommended	See ciprofloxacin.	See ciprofloxacin.	$
	norfloxacin generics	**Adults:** Treatment: 400 mg BID po × 3 days or 800 mg po × 1 dose Prophylaxis:[b] 400 mg once daily po **Children:** Not recommended	See ciprofloxacin.	See ciprofloxacin.	$
	ofloxacin generics	**Adults:** Treatment: 200–300 mg BID po × 3 days or 400 mg po × 1 dose Prophylaxis:[b] 300 mg once daily po **Children:** Not recommended	See ciprofloxacin.	See ciprofloxacin.	$
Intestinal Adsorbants	*bismuth subsalicylate* Pepto-Bismol, generics	**Adults:** Treatment: 524 mg (2 tablets) or 30 mL suspension Q30 min po (maximum 8 doses/day) Prophylaxis: 524 mg (2 tablets) or 30 mL suspension QID po **Children:** Not recommended	Blackening of stools and tongue, mild tinnitus.	Avoid in patients taking anticoagulants, therapeutic doses of salicylates or in whom salicylates are contraindicated (e.g., children and pregnant women). Decreases absorption of tetracyclines. May decrease the number of unformed stools passed but may not speed up illness recovery.	$

Class	Drug	Dose	Adverse Effects	Comments	Cost[a]
Macrolides	*azithromycin* Zithromax, generics	**Adults:** Treatment: 500 mg once daily po × 3 days or 1000 mg po × 1 dose **Children:** Treatment: 5–10 mg/kg (maximum 500 mg) once daily po × 3 days	GI disturbance infrequently.	Drug of choice for southeast Asia and Indian subcontinent. Can be used in children and in pregnancy. Available as suspension. Not recommended for prophylaxis.	$$
Sulfonamides	*sulfamethoxazole/ trimethoprim* generics	**Adults:** Treatment: 800/160 mg BID po × 3 days or 1600/320 mg po × 1 dose **Children ≤12 y:** Treatment: sulfamethoxazole 20–25 mg/kg + trimethoprim 4–5 mg/kg (as pediatric suspension) BID po × 3 days	GI disturbances, blood dyscrasias, skin reactions, Stevens-Johnson syndrome (rare).	Available as suspension. Due to the widespread emergence of resistance, consider SMX/TMP as second line when other antibiotics are contraindicated. Use only for regions where SMX/TMP resistance is uncommon (central Mexico in summer); not first choice in other geographic areas.	$
Vaccines	*Vibrio cholerae whole cell/B subunit vaccine* Dukoral	Prevention of enterotoxigenic *E. coli* diarrhea: Adults and children ≥2 y: Primary immunization: 2 doses po. 2nd dose administered within 7–42 days after the 1st dose and at least 1 wk before reaching destination Booster: 1 dose every 3 months if the risk is continuous Taken orally on an empty stomach (1 h before or 1 h after eating or drinking)	Abdominal pain (16%), diarrhea (12%), nausea (4%) and vomiting (3%).	Not enough evidence to routinely recommend this vaccine to all travellers. May consider for prevention of travellers' diarrhea in persons with chronic illnesses (e.g., heart failure, insulin-dependent diabetes mellitus, inflammatory bowel disease, chronic kidney disease) or in those with immune suppression.	$$$/1 dose

[a] Cost of 3-day treatment for adults unless otherwise specified; includes drug cost only.
[b] Start prophylactic treatment on the first day in the area of risk and continued for 1–2 days after return home, to a maximum of 3 weeks total.
Dosage adjustment may be required in renal impairment; see Appendix I.
Legend: $ <$10 $$ $10–20 $$$ $20–30

References

1. Hill DR, Ericsson CD, Pearson RD et al. The practice of travel medicine: guidelines by the Infectious Diseases Society of America. *Clin Infect Dis* 2006;43(12):1499-539.
2. DuPont HL. New insights and directions in traveler's diarrhea. *Gastroenterol Clin North Am* 2006;35(2):337-53.
3. Shah N, DuPont HL, Ramsey DJ. Global etiology of travelers' diarrhea: systematic review from 1973 to the present. *Am J Trop Med Hyg* 2009;80(4):609-14.
4. Adachi JA, Jiang ZD, Mathewson JJ et al. Enteroaggregative Escherichia coli as a major etiologic agent in traveler's diarrhea in 3 regions of the world. *Clin Infect Dis* 2001;32(12):1706-9.
5. Steffen R, van der Linde F, Gyr K et al. Epidemiology of diarrhea in travelers. *JAMA* 1983;249(9):1176-80.
6. Al-Abri SS, Beeching NJ, Nye FJ. Traveller's diarrhoea. *Lancet Infect Dis* 2005;5(6):349-60.
7. Leggat PA, Goldsmid JM. Travellers' diarrhoea: health advice for travellers. *Travel Med Infect Dis* 2004;2(1):17-22.
8. DuPont HL, Ericsson CD, Farthing MJ et al. Expert review of the evidence base for prevention of travelers' diarrhea. *J Travel Med* 2009;16(3):149-60.
9. U.S. Centers for Disease Control and Prevention. The Pre-travel consultation. Counseling & advice for travelers. In: *2014 Yellow book.* Available from: wwwnc.cdc.gov/travel/yellowbook/2014/chapter-2-the-pre-travel-consultation/water-disinfection-for-travelers.
10. Bavishi C, Dupont HL. Systematic review: the use of proton pump inhibitors and increased susceptibility to enteric infection. *Aliment Pharmacol Ther* 2011;34(11-12):1269-81.
11. Leonard J, Marshall JK, Moayyedi P. Systematic review of the risk of enteric infection in patients taking acid suppression. *Am J Gastroenterol* 2007;102(9):2047-56.
12. DuPont HL, Ericsson CD, Johnson PC et al. Prevention of travelers' diarrhea by the tablet formulation of bismuth subsalicylate. *JAMA* 1987;257(10):1347-50.
13. http://www.ncbi.nlm.nih.gov/pubmed/2406861
14. Pickering LK, Feldman S, Ericsson CD et al. Absorption of salicylate and bismuth from a bismuth subsalicylate-containing compound (Pepto-Bismol). *J Pediatr* 1981;99(4):654-6.
15. Rademaker CM, Hoepelman IM, Wolfhagen MJ et al. Results of a double-blind placebo-controlled study using ciprofloxacin for prevention of travelers' diarrhea. *Eur J Clin Microbiol Infect Dis* 1989;8(8):690-4.
16. Wistrom J, Norrby SR, Burman LG et al. Norfloxacin versus placebo for prophylaxis against travellers' diarrhoea. *J Antimicrob Chemother* 1987;20(4):563-74.
17. Jain D, Sinha S, Prasad KN et al. Campylobacter species and drug resistance in a north Indian rural community. *Trans R Soc Trop Med Hyg* 2005;99(3):207-14.
18. Shlim DR. Update in traveler's diarrhea. *Infect Dis Clin North Am* 2005;19(1):137-49.
19. Oyofo BA, Lesmana M, Subekti D et al. Surveillance of bacterial pathogens of diarrhea disease in Indonesia. *Diagn Microbiol Infect Dis* 2002;44(3):227-34.
20. Ahmed T, Bhuiyan TR, Zaman K et al. Vaccines for preventing enterotoxigenic Escherichia coli (ETEC) diarrhoea. *Cochrane Database Syst Rev* 2013;7:CD009029.
21. Committee to Advise on Tropical Medicine and Travel (CATMAT); National Advisory Committee on Immunization (NACI). Statement on new oral cholera and travellers' diarrhea vaccination. *Can Commun Dis Rep* 2005;31(ACS-7):1-11.
22. National Advisory Committee on Immunization. *Canadian immunization guide.* Evergreen ed. Ottawa (ON): Public Health Agency of Canada. Available from: www.phac-aspc.gc.ca/publicat/cig-gci/index-eng.php. Accessed February 11, 2014.
23. Committee to Advise on Tropical Medicine and Travel (CATMAT). An Advisory Committee Statement (ACS). Statement on travellers' diarrhea. *Can Commun Dis Rep* 2001;27:1-12.
24. Adachi JA, Ostrosky-Zeichner L, DuPont HL et al. Empirical antimicrobial therapy for traveler's diarrhea. *Clin Infect Dis* 2000;31(4):1079-83.
25. Government of Canada. Travel health and safety. *Oral rehydration solutions.* Available from: travel.gc.ca/travelling/health-safety/rehydration.
26. Johnson PC, Ericsson CD, DuPont HL et al. Comparison of loperamide with bismuth subsalicylate for the treatment of acute travelers' diarrhea. *JAMA* 1986;255(6):757-60.
27. Palmer KR, Corbett CL, Holdsworth CD. Double-blind cross-over study comparing loperamide, codeine and diphenoxylate in the treatment of chronic diarrhea. *Gastroenterology* 1980;79(6):1272-5.
28. DuPont HL, Hornick RB. Adverse effect of lomotil therapy in shigellosis. *JAMA* 1973;226(13):1525-8.
29. Ericsson CD, DuPont HL, Mathewson JJ et al. Treatment of traveler's diarrhea with sulfamethoxazole and trimethoprim and loperamide. *JAMA* 1990;263(2):257-61.
30. Taylor DN, Sanchez JL, Candler W et al. Treatment of travelers' diarrhea: ciprofloxacin plus loperamide compared with ciprofloxacin alone. A placebo-controlled, randomized trial. *Ann Intern Med* 1991;114(9):731-4.
31. DuPont HL, Ericsson CD, Mathewson JJ et al. Five versus three days of ofloxacin therapy for traveler's diarrhea: a placebo-controlled study. *Antimicrob Agents Chemother* 1992;36(1):87-91.
32. Salam I, Katelaris P, Leigh-Smith S, et al. Randomised trial of single-dose ciprofloxacin for travellers' diarrhoea. *Lancet* 1994;344(8936):1537-9.
33. Adachi JA, Ericsson CD, Jiang ZD et al. Azithromycin found to be comparable to levofloxacin for the treatment of US travelers with acute diarrhea acquired in Mexico. *Clin Infect Dis* 2003;37(9):1165-71.
34. Kuschner RA, Trofa AF, Thomas RJ et al. Use of azithromycin for the treatment of Campylobacter enteritis in travelers to Thailand, an area where ciprofloxacin resistance is prevalent. *Clin Infect Dis* 1995;21(3):536-41.
35. Ericsson CD, DuPont HL, Mathewson JJ. Single dose ofloxacin plus loperamide compared with single dose or three days of ofloxacin in the treatment of traveler's diarrhea. *J Travel Med* 1997;4(1):3-7.
36. Grady R. Safety profile of quinolone antibiotics in the pediatric population. *Pediatr Infect Dis J* 2003;22(12):1128-32.
37. Carroll ID, Williams DC. Pre-travel vaccination and medical prophylaxis in the pregnant traveler. *Travel Med Infect Dis* 2008;6(5):259-75.
38. Chen LH, Zeind C, Mackell S et al. Breastfeeding travelers: precautions and recommendations. *J Travel Med* 2010;17(1):32-47.

Chapter 124
Tuberculosis

Victoria J. Cook, MD, FRCPC and
James C. Johnston, MD, FRCPC

Goals of Therapy

- Prevent latent tuberculosis infection (LTBI) from progressing to clinically active disease
- Prevent person-to-person transmission, through early diagnosis, appropriate infection control and initiation of treatment
- Treat active disease by eradicating *Mycobacterium tuberculosis* (MTB) from the affected organ(s) and relieve symptoms
- Achieve cure without relapse, prevent complications, prevent development of drug resistance and death

Investigations[1,2,3,4,5,6,7]

- Thorough history with special attention to:
  - risk factors for infection with MTB, e.g., country of birth/origin, occupation, TB exposure, travel to endemic area, substandard housing (high household occupancy density, poor air quality, inadequate ventilation)[8]
  - risk factors for development of active tuberculosis (TB) once infected, e.g., recent TB infection, tuberculin skin test (TST) conversion within past 2 years, predisposing medical conditions such as HIV/AIDS, organ transplantation, end-stage renal disease, diabetes mellitus, hematologic malignancies, malnutrition, use of immunosuppressants (e.g., systemic corticosteroids, cancer chemotherapy), use of tumor necrosis-alpha (TNF-α) inhibitors, abnormal chest x-ray (fibronodular disease or calcified granulomas), current smoking (≥1 pack per day)
  - risk factors for drug resistance, e.g., previous treatment or previous drug-resistant disease, especially if not on directly observed therapy (DOT), nonadherence, HIV/AIDS, alcohol abuse, travel to or residence in countries with high prevalence of TB disease or high incidence of drug-resistant disease, contact with a patient with drug-resistant disease
  - previous TST results and details of previous LTBI or TB disease treatment
  - *Mycobacterium bovis* bacillus Calmette-Guérin (BCG) vaccination—including age at last BCG vaccination
- Physical examination:
  - nutritional status, fever, choroid tubercles, abnormal breath sounds, meningeal signs, erythema nodosum, adenopathy
  - concomitant diseases that may affect treatment, e.g., HIV/AIDS, liver disease, chronic renal insufficiency
  - prior to therapy: weight, visual acuity and colour vision testing
- Investigations:
  - chest x-ray (compare to old films if available)
  - obtain 3 sputum specimens (either spontaneous or induced at least 1 hour apart) for acid fast bacilli (AFB) smear *and* mycobacterial culture; negative sputum smears do not preclude a

diagnosis of active pulmonary TB (50% of the patients with active TB have negative sputum smears)
- first morning-voided midstream urine for smear (usually negative, not available at most labs but can aid in rapid diagnosis) and culture if renal TB suspected
- lumbar puncture with CSF samples sent for AFB smear (usually negative) and mycobacterial culture plus glucose, protein, white cell count and differential if meningitis is suspected
- baseline platelet count, ALT, AST, bilirubin and creatinine should be performed
- HbA_{1C} and hepatitis B and C serology should be performed in those with epidemiologic risk factors[9,10]
- counselling and testing for HIV should be performed for all patients with newly diagnosed active TB unless they refuse testing (an opt-out approach)[7]
- in HIV-infected persons, x-ray findings are more likely atypical; blood and stool cultures for mycobacteria may be positive for both tuberculous and nontuberculous mycobacteria in this population
- miliary disease is common and sputum smears are often negative in patients with HIV

- Special procedures:
  - serial or repeated sputum induction in an appropriately ventilated room has a similar yield to bronchoscopy, with less patient discomfort, fewer complications and less risk of nosocomial transmission
  - fibre optic bronchoscopy ± transbronchial biopsy is particularly useful when alternative diagnoses are suspected or if miliary TB is a concern; rapid diagnosis is possible if caseating granulomas or AFB are found on biopsy
  - gastric washings (fasting morning sample) may be positive in patients unable to produce sputum (7–20% sensitive)[11,12]
  - aspiration of pleural effusions for AFB smear (usually negative) and culture (positive in <25% of specimens), chemical and cytological analysis. Diagnosis often requires pleural biopsy for culture and histology via Abrams needle biopsy or video-assisted thoracic surgery; a combination of culture and pleural biopsy increases diagnostic yield of mycobacterial cultures to 90%
  - nucleic acid amplification tests (NAATs) are commercially available to identify mycobacteria directly from sputum specimens (95% sensitive, 90–100% specific if smear positive; 50–70% sensitive, 90–100% specific if smear negative, culture positive). Confirms the diagnosis of TB but does not replace the need for routine AFB smear and culture[13,14]
  - NAATs may be used for other body fluids or tissue samples under certain circumstances in experienced laboratories. Major advantage is rapid diagnosis and it is most useful in diagnosing meningeal TB
- *Mantoux test* (tuberculin skin test or TST) has 3 uses: the diagnosis of LTBI (Figure 1), to assist in the diagnosis of TB disease (Figure 2) and as an epidemiologic tool. It should not be performed on persons with previous, severe, blistering tuberculin reactions, documented active or prior history of TB, extensive burns or eczema, a major viral infection or a history of vaccination with a live virus vaccine (e.g., MMR) in the past month
  - 48–72 hours after intradermal inoculation, the widest transverse diameter of induration (not erythema) is measured; routine anergy screening is not recommended
  - false negative tests can occur in seriously ill patients and those with impaired cell-mediated immunity or with inappropriate technique/reading (e.g., drawing tuberculin material up into syringes more than 20 minutes before administration, significant exposure of tuberculin to sunlight). Patients' recall of test results is not reliable. Test results may vary by 15% between arms and between observers. A negative skin test should not preclude consideration of the diagnosis of TB. False negatives can also occur at the extremes of age

- false positive tests can occur in patients with a history of BCG vaccination, exposure to nontuberculous mycobacteria or with inappropriate technique/reading. BCG vaccination in infancy alone (<18 months) is associated with lower false positivity. BCG vaccination status should not preclude the diagnosis of latent TB infection in the event of contact
- reactivity to tuberculin antigen can diminish to nonreactivity with age
- repeated TST may boost reactivity. Thus, it is important in populations who are going to have serial TST (e.g., nursing home residents, health care workers) to perform an initial 2-step test to determine those whose response has waned over time. A second dose is administered 1–3 weeks after the first. Repeated skin testing will not induce a false-positive reaction but the initial test may stimulate the patient's ability to react to subsequent testing

- In vitro diagnostic tests, called interferon-gamma release assays (IGRAs), i.e., QuantiFERON-TB Gold (QFT-G), T-SPOT, are increasingly used to support the diagnosis of latent and active TB infection. Guidelines for their use are available.[15,16]
  - IGRAs should not be used to diagnose active TB in adults[11]
  - IGRAs may be used as supplementary evidence for active TB in children, when used in combination with clinical history and examination, TST results, microbiological and radiological investigations. This test should not replace other diagnostic modalities and a negative IGRA (or negative TST) does not rule out disease[17]
  - IGRAs are an acceptable alternative for LTBI diagnosis and may be used for LTBI screening in many situations where TST is indicated[15]
  - IGRAs may be used as a confirmatory LTBI test for adults with a positive TST and low risk for progression to active TB
  - IGRAs are not acceptable when repeat or serial testing is expected/indicated
  - IGRAs are the preferred test in people who received BCG more than once and/or after infancy
  - IGRAs are preferred in people with poor rates of return for TST reading
  - IGRAs may be used to supplement TST results when there is high risk of infection or progression to TB disease. Negative IGRA results do not rule out risk of active TB in this setting.

Therapeutic Choices

All patients with known or suspected pulmonary TB should be either hospitalized in a single negative pressure room and placed on respiratory precautions, or isolated at home if they can avoid high risk (e.g., young children) or unexposed contacts and respiratory precautions are followed as outlined by the health care team. Discontinue isolation when consecutive sputum smears are negative for AFB on 3 separate days *and* there is evidence of adherence to an appropriate treatment regimen for a minimum of 2 weeks with clinical response, in the absence of high risk for significant drug resistance. Continue isolation in patients with pulmonary or laryngeal multiple drug-resistant TB (MDR-TB) for duration of hospital stay or until cultures are negative on consecutive occasions.

Proper masks (which filter particles 1 micron in size, have a 95% filter efficiency when tested in the unloaded state and provide a tight facial seal) should be worn when caring for patients with known or suspected TB. Surgical masks do not prevent the inhalation of droplet nuclei but are appropriate for infectious TB patients. All patients with a chest x-ray consistent with TB should be isolated pending results of sputum smear for AFB. The radiographic appearance of TB is variable in patients with HIV infection and may be normal (12%).

Figure 1: Diagnosis and Management of Latent Tuberculosis Infection

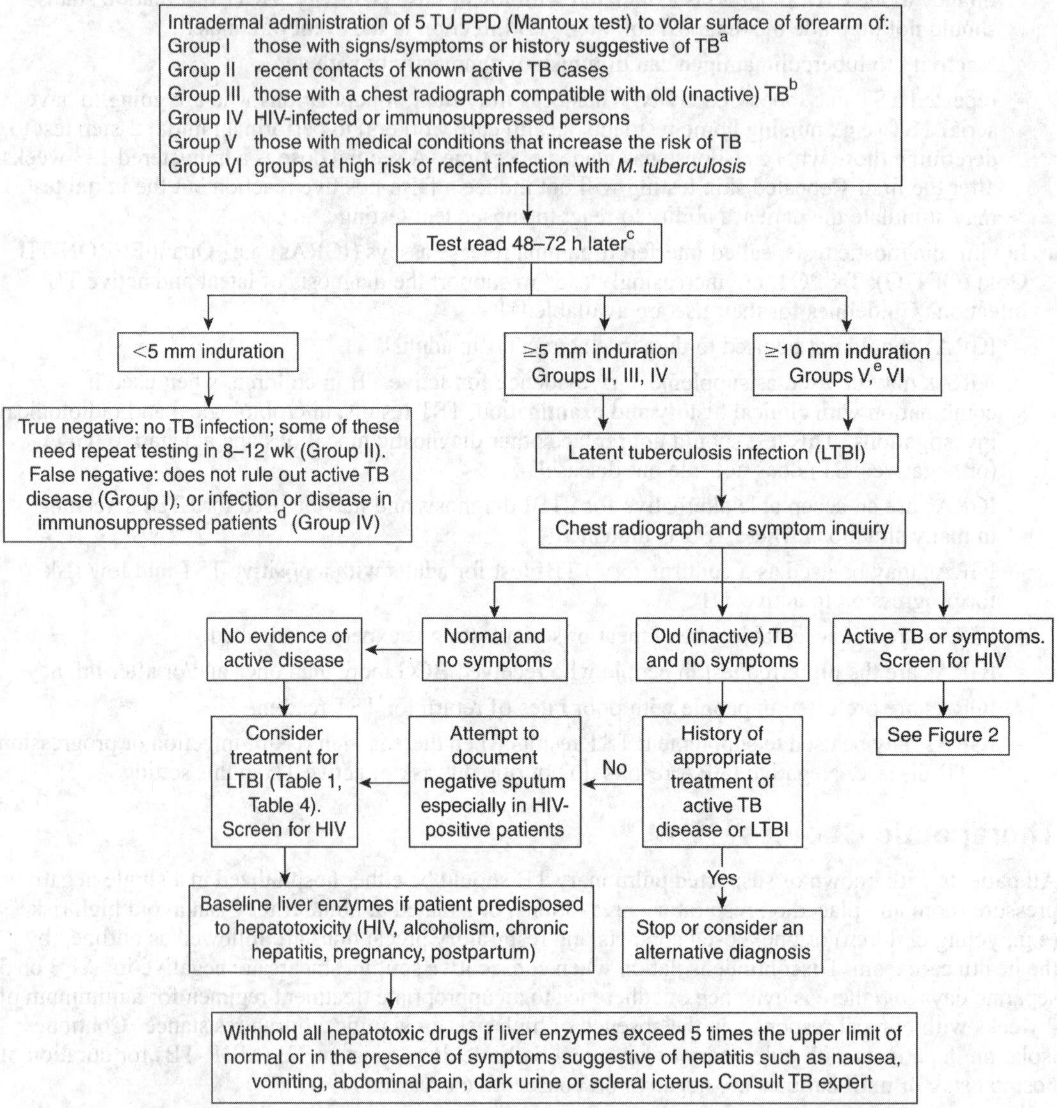

a In pediatric patients, active TB can be difficult to diagnose. The TST is often used to assist in the diagnosis of active TB in this population.
b If active TB disease is suspected, isolate the patient.
c A web-based tool is available to aid in the interpretation of a positive TST result (www.tstin3d.com/).
d Consider treatment for LTBI in HIV-positive patients or other severely immunocompromised patients (e.g., those on immunosuppressive drugs) with close contact with an active case of TB, a chest radiograph consistent with old (inactive) TB or a history of positive TST without a history of treatment for TB or LTBI. Consider primary preventive treatment in children ≤5 years who have had recent contact with an active case of TB, until repeat skin testing is available.
e For patients with end-stage renal disease consider a TST positive if induration ≥5 mm.
Abbreviations: LTBI = latent tuberculosis infection; PPD = purified protein derivative; TST = tuberculin skin test; TU = tuberculin units

Figure 2: **Diagnosis and Management of Active Pulmonary Tuberculosis Disease**

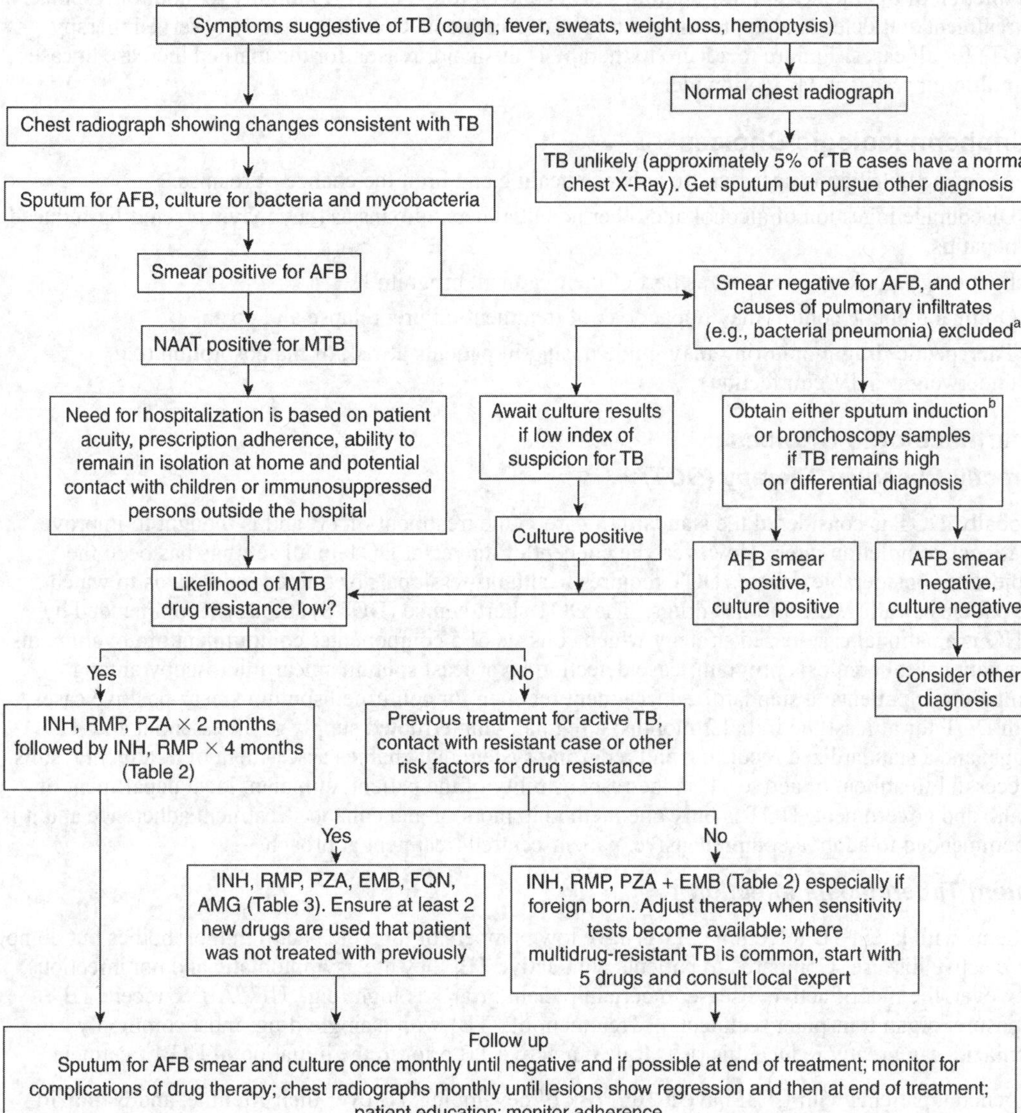

a 50% of pulmonary TB cases will be smear negative. Therefore, with suspicious chest radiograph and clinical scenario, consider initiating empiric anti-TB therapy.
b Induced sputum has higher yield, quicker turnaround and less risk to patients or health care workers than bronchoscopy.
c 15% of pulmonary TB cases will be culture negative but diagnosis is based on clinical and radiographic response to therapy in the appropriate clinical setting.

Abbreviations: AFB = acid fast bacilli; AMG = aminoglycoside; EMB = ethambutol; FQN = fluoroquinolone; INH = isoniazid; MTB = *Mycobacterium tuberculosis*; NAAT = nucleic acid amplification test; PZA = pyrazinamide; RMP = rifampin

Notify the local Department of Health for contact tracing. Close follow up of active TB cases is mandatory (initially, monthly visits and regular chest radiographs with a final chest x-ray at completion of treatment). Follow sputum smears and cultures for AFB monthly to monitor response to treatment and determine appropriate duration of treatment. Consider directly observed therapy (DOT) for all cases. Failure to adhere to therapy is the major reason for the marked increase in cases of multidrug-resistant TB worldwide.

Nonpharmacologic Choices[5,6,7]

- Adequate nutrition is necessary to enhance healing and limit the chance of relapse.[18]
- Discourage ingestion of alcohol and other potential hepatotoxins as they may worsen drug-induced hepatitis.
- Encourage smoking cessation as part of the treatment program.[19]
- Optimal diabetic control may impact risk of treatment failure, relapse and death.
- Therapeutic drug monitoring may guide dosing in patients at risk of malabsorption (e.g., underweight, HIV coinfection)

Pharmacologic Choices

Directly Observed Therapy (DOT)[20]

Globally, DOT is considered the standard of care in the treatment of TB and is thought to improve treatment completion rates. However, the concept of universal DOT in all settings has been the subject of considerable debate. DOT requires health professionals or trained individuals to watch the patients swallow the anti-TB drugs. The DOT short-course (DOTS) strategy recommended by WHO is a national case-based strategy which consists of 5 components: commitment of governments to a national tuberculosis program; case detection by at least sputum smear microscopy among symptomatic patients; a standardized treatment regimen for confirmed sputum smear-positive cases, with DOT for at least the initial 2 months; a regular, uninterrupted supply of all essential anti-TB drugs; and a standardized recording and reporting system that enables assessment of treatment results. Successful treatment of active TB is the responsibility of the patient, clinician, local department of health and government. DOT is only one method to monitor and enhance treatment adherence and it is recommended to adopt a comprehensive, patient-centred treatment approach.

Latent Tuberculosis Infection[21]

Patients with latent TB infection (LTBI) have low numbers of tubercle bacilli in their bodies but do not have active disease. Compared to patients with active TB, they are asymptomatic and noninfectious. However, the risk of active disease in certain patient groups is high (e.g., HIV/AIDS, recent TB exposure, organ transplant recipients). Treatment of LTBI with a single drug, most commonly isoniazid, can greatly reduce this risk. Rule out active TB prior to the initiation of LTBI treatment.

In general, patients with LTBI have a 10% risk of developing TB over their lifetime, and **isoniazid** can reduce this risk by over 90% in adherent patients. Offer treatment of LTBI to recent contacts, HIV-infected persons, organ transplant recipients, patients on immunosuppressive drugs (specifically corticosteroids and anti-TNF agents), those with end-stage renal disease and individuals with fibronodular disease on chest radiographs who have a tuberculin skin test of ≥5 mm.[7]

For those who have a TST ≥10 mm and are in a lower-risk group (Figure 1), the risk of adverse effects from isoniazid must be weighed against its benefit in reducing the risk of active disease. The risk of significant hepatitis increases with age and history of pre-existing liver disease; however, the risk of isoniazid-related hepatitis has been overestimated and is now reported as 1–3 per 1000 person-years.[9,22] Asymptomatic liver enzyme abnormalities (minor rises in aminotransferases 2–3 times normal) are common. For those with risk factors for reactivating dormant infection (e.g., diabetes, malnutrition, alcohol and cigarette use), age should not preclude offering LTBI treatment although the risk of hepatotoxicity must be considered in treatment decisions.

Isoniazid daily for 9 months (9INH) is the regimen of choice. If the source case is isoniazid-resistant or if the patient is unable to take isoniazid, **rifampin** for 4 months may be substituted (Table 1).[7,25] Short-course daily prophylaxis with rifampin and **pyrazinamide** for 8 weeks is no longer recommended due to high rates of hospitalization and death due to liver injury.[26,27,28,29,30] Short-course weekly isoniazid and **rifapentine** for 3 months is as effective as 9INH, with less hepatotoxicity but higher rates of poorly understood hypersensitivity reactions. Given this and the fact that rifapentine is available only through the Special Access Programme in Canada, its routine use is not recommended. Consultation with a TB expert is recommended in the event of contact with a drug-resistant source case or if an intermittent regimen is considered.

Baseline and monthly testing of aminotransferases is recommended for persons with risk factors for liver disease (e.g., alcohol use, post-partum, viral hepatitis).

Active Tuberculosis[7,24,31,32,33]

The standard approach to active TB treatment is to use multiple drugs for the appropriate duration and to ensure adherence by using a patient-centred approach (this can include the use of DOT). Treatment begins with an initial (bactericidal or intensive) phase over the first 2 months to rapidly eliminate the majority of organisms and prevent emergence of drug resistance. This is followed by a continuation (sterilizing) phase of 4–7 months to eradicate dormant organisms and prevent relapse by achieving long-lasting cure (Table 2). Knowledge of the local epidemiology of resistance is essential to ensure appropriate treatment. Adjust therapy (Table 3) when susceptibility results are available (usually 1–2 months into therapy). Dose adjustments may be required for some patients (e.g., low BMI, renal insufficiency) and can be guided by therapeutic drug monitoring. Single drug therapy must never be used for active TB, nor should a single drug ever be added to a failing regimen. **Rifampin**-based short-course treatment (Table 2) is the standard of care. Response to treatment is monitored by monthly smear and culture of sputum specimens, which are repeated until 2 consecutive samples are negative. Repeat susceptibility testing is recommended if cultures are persistently positive after 3 months.

Table 1: **Treatment Regimens for Latent TB Infection**[7]

Regimen[a,b]	Frequency[c] and Duration[d]	Comments
Isoniazid (INH)	Daily × 9 months	**Regimen of choice**; all others acceptable alternatives with variable levels of evidence.
INH	Daily × 6 months	Less effective than daily INH × 9 months.
INH	DOT: Twice weekly × 6–9 months	Level 2 evidence;[e] use in select circumstances.
Rifampin (RMP)	Daily × 4 months	For INH-resistant strains or in patients unable to tolerate INH.
INH + RMP	Daily × 3–4 months	Level 1 evidence.[e]
INH + RMP	DOT: Twice weekly × 3 months	Level 2 evidence;[e] use in select circumstances.
INH + rifapentine	DOT: Once weekly × 3 months	Rifapentine available in Canada only through the Special Access Programme.

[a] See Table 4 for appropriate doses.
[b] A regimen consisting of twice weekly isoniazid and rifampin directly-observed for 6 months was successful in a Canadian Aboriginal population.[23]
[c] DOT must be used throughout the duration of treatment with intermittent regimens.
[d] Completion of therapy is not determined by the duration of therapy but by the number of doses taken.[24]
[e] Level of evidence as defined in the *Canadian Tuberculosis Standards*:[7] Level 1 = multiple randomized trials; Level 2 = single randomized trial and/or multiple observational studies.

Abbreviations: DOT = directly observed therapy; INH = isoniazid; RMP = rifampin

Table 2: **Standard Treatment Regimens for Active Disease**

Regimen[a,b]	Frequency[c] and Duration[d]	Comments
Isoniazid (INH) + Rifampin (RMP) + Pyrazinamide (PZA) ± Ethambutol (EMB)	1) daily[e] × 2 months,[f] then INH + RMP daily × 4 months *or* 2) daily[e] × 2 months,[f] then INH + RMP 3 times weekly × 4 months *or* 3) daily for at least 2 weeks then 3 times weekly × 6 months Total duration of 6 months only if culture conversion at 2 months, noncavitary disease and fully sensitive organism. Extend continuation phase to 7 months (total duration 9 months) in patients with extensive disease, cavitation (at 2 months or end of treatment) and positive culture at 2 months as they are at a higher risk of relapse.[24]	Empiric treatment with EMB given prior to sensitivity results for areas with INH resistance ≥4%. In areas with INH resistance <4%, INH, RMP and PZA without EMB can be used pending sensitivity results. Consider intermittent therapy in the intensive phase of treatment only if HIV-negative, no cavitary disease present, smear-negative and excellent adherence with DOT. Twice-weekly regimens no longer recommended. Fixed-dose combinations are not recommended.
Isoniazid + Rifampin + Ethambutol	Daily[e] for 2 months then INH + RMP daily (or 3 times weekly) × 7 months	Empiric treatment given prior to sensitivity results in the elderly, those at high risk for liver toxicity and in pregnancy.

[a] See Table 4 for appropriate doses.
[b] Second-line drugs are available in the event of intolerance or multiple drug-resistant TB: cycloserine, ethionamide, p-aminosalicylic acid, streptomycin, amikacin and capreomycin.
[c] DOT is recommended for all regimens, but *must* be used throughout the treatment duration of intermittent regimens.
[d] Completion of therapy is not determined by the duration of therapy but by the number of doses taken.[24]
[e] Daily = 7 doses weekly or 5 doses weekly DOT.[24]
[f] Can switch to thrice-weekly DOT after an initial daily intensive phase or after 2 weeks of intensive treatment in HIV-negative patients.
Abbreviations: DOT = directly observed therapy; EMB = ethambutol; INH = isoniazid; PZA = pyrazinamide; RMP = rifampin

The standard short-course regimen for active TB can be used for empiric therapy in areas where there is minimal (<4%) or no isoniazid resistance. The regimen comprises a 2-month intensive phase of **isoniazid**, **rifampin** and **pyrazinamide** followed by a 4-month continuation phase of isoniazid and rifampin. **Ethambutol** is included in the initial regimen if isoniazid resistance exists or local susceptibilities are not known. If susceptibility results indicate full sensitivity, ethambutol may be discontinued assuming the patient is tolerating first-line therapy. Intermittent regimens are an option and thrice-weekly DOT with a rifampin-containing regimen can be given after an initial daily intensive phase or after at least 2 weeks of intensive treatment in HIV-negative patients with smear-negative, noncavitary disease. Thrice-weekly regimens are preferred over twice-weekly regimens in Canada based on the practical consideration that a single missed dose of a thrice-weekly regimen has less of an impact on treatment than 50% of a twice-weekly regimen. A longer period of treatment (minimum 9 months) is recommended for patients with drug-susceptible, extensive or cavitary pulmonary TB if sputum cultures remain positive after 2 months of treatment because of an increased risk of relapse and treatment failure.[24] This may reflect poor drug penetration at the site of disease or high bacillary burden at the time of diagnosis.[34] Short-course treatment (6 months) is only recommended with rifampin-based regimens that include isoniazid and pyrazinamide in the intensive phase of treatment.

No evidence is available to support recommendations in the case of *treatment interruptions*; however, it is a generally accepted practice to completely restart the 4-drug intensive phase regimen if treatment is interrupted for >14 days during the initial intensive phase of treatment or for >3 months during the continuation phase of treatment, due to concerns about resistance.[35] Consultation with a local TB expert is suggested when confronted with treatment interruptions, treatment failure or relapse, drug intolerance or adverse effects, or multiple drug resistance.

Drug-resistant Tuberculosis

Major risk factors for drug-resistant TB are a prior treatment for TB, exposure to a drug-resistant case and having been foreign born. Drug susceptibility testing (DST) can determine the extent of drug resistance. Research into alternative treatment includes investigation of respiratory quinolones (**moxifloxacin**, **levofloxacin**) and **ethambutol** as substitutes for isoniazid in the intensive phase of treatment and **linezolid** for the treatment of multidrug-resistant tuberculosis.[36,37] Despite widespread use of quinolones for nontuberculous infections, there is no indication at this time of widespread resistance in MTB isolates from patients exposed to these medications.[38] For isoniazid-resistant disease, the later generation **fluoroquinolones** are considered interchangeable with isoniazid.

Multidrug-resistant TB (MDR-TB) is resistant to both isoniazid and rifampin, and extensively drug-resistant TB (XDR-TB) is resistant to isoniazid, rifampin, quinolones and at least 1 of the 3 injectable second-line drugs (capreomycin, kanamycin, amikacin).[7] Both MDR-TB and XDR-TB are associated with high morbidity and mortality. Refer patients with MDR-TB and XDR-TB to a TB specialist for individualized treatment based on DST results. In general, for MDR-TB treatment should include at least 4 drugs that the isolate is sensitive to, including a fluoroquinolone and an injectable agent for at least 8 months followed by 3 or more drugs for another 12–18 months. All treatment should be directly observed and intermittent regimens should be avoided. Using an aggressive outpatient strategy in HIV-negative patients, the cure rate for patients with XDR-TB was comparable to those with MDR-TB.[39] A longer time to culture conversion and an extended duration of treatment was observed in those with XDR-TB.[39] Several new anti-TB drugs (e.g., bedaquiline, delamanid) may become available in the coming years for treatment of MDR-TB and XDR-TB. Surgery has been used as adjunctive therapy for drug-resistant TB.

Antituberculous Drug-induced Hepatotoxicity[40]

Drug-induced hepatotoxicity is defined as aspartate aminotransferase (AST) level >3 times the upper limit of normal in symptomatic patients (nausea, vomiting, abdominal pain, jaundice) or >5 times the upper limit of normal in asymptomatic patients. Withhold all hepatotoxic drugs and consult a local TB specialist. For active TB disease, consider promptly reinstituting a nonhepatotoxic regimen (e.g., ethambutol, streptomycin and a quinolone) when or as liver test results improve. Alcohol is the most important cofactor in isoniazid-induced hepatitis.[41]

Table 3: **Treatment Regimens for Drug-resistant Active Tuberculosis**[7]

Drug-resistant Active TB Disease[a]	Regimen[b]	Frequency[c] and Duration[d]
Isoniazid-resistant disease	Isoniazid (INH) + rifampin (RMP) + pyrazinamide (PZA) + ethambutol (EMB) ± a quinolone (FQN); consider addition of an aminoglycoside if severe disease	1) RMP + EMB + PZA daily[e] × 2 months then continue daily[e] or switch to 3 times weekly × 4–7 months *or* 2) RMP + EMB + PZA daily[e] × 2 months then RMP + EMB daily[e] or 3 times weekly × 10 months *or* 3) RMP + EMB + PZA + FQN daily[e] × 2 months then RMP + EMB + FQN daily[e] or 3 times weekly × 4–7 months
Rifampin-resistant disease	Isoniazid + pyrazinamide + ethambutol ± a quinolone or aminoglycoside	1) daily[e] INH + PZA + EMB + FQN × 2 months then INH + EMB + FQN daily[e] or 3 times weekly × 10–16 months *or* 2) daily[e] or 3 times weekly INH + PZA + aminoglycoside × 9 months *or* 3) daily[e] INH + PZA + EMB × 2 months then daily[e] or 3 times weekly INH + EMB × 16 months

[a] Always consult a TB expert in cases of drug-resistant active tuberculosis.
[b] Second-line drugs are available in the event of intolerance or multiple drug-resistant TB: cycloserine, ethionamide, p-aminosalicylic acid, amikacin and capreomycin. Amikacin is preferred over streptomycin due to ease of monitoring and lower toxicity.
[c] DOT is recommended for all regimens but must be used throughout the treatment duration of intermittent regimens.
[d] Completion of therapy is not determined by the duration of therapy but by the number of doses taken.[24]
[e] Daily = 7 doses weekly, or 5 doses weekly DOT.[24]
Abbreviations: DOT = directly observed therapy; EMB = ethambutol; FQN = fluoroquinolone; INH = isoniazid; PZA = pyrazinamide; RMP = rifampin

BCG Vaccine

Though used as a preventive measure against TB globally, BCG vaccine is not used generally in Canada except in some jurisdictions for First Nations infants to prevent more serious forms of TB and death.[7,42] The vaccine efficacy has been estimated to be 51% in preventing any TB disease.[43] BCG vaccine in infants has a protective effect in preventing TB meningitis and disseminated disease.[43] BCG vaccination is contraindicated in persons with or at risk of HIV infection.

Tuberculosis in Special Populations

Pediatric Tuberculosis

With rare exceptions (e.g., cavitary or laryngeal tuberculosis), children with TB are not considered contagious.[44,45] Untreated children <5 years are at increased risk of developing severe forms of TB such as miliary or meningeal TB; treatment should be initiated promptly upon suspicion of TB. Dose anti-TB medications by weight (mg/kg) in children. Regimens recommended in children are similar to those used in adults, including use of ethambutol which is now considered standard in empiric regimens although caution is advised with its use in young children who cannot be assessed effectively for visual toxicity. Children <5 years who are exposed to an infectious case of TB and are TST-negative are eligible for primary preventative therapy with isoniazid (or as guided by known drug sensitivities) until a repeat TST is performed in 8–12 weeks.[7] Consult a TB expert when exposures included children <6 months as TST results may be difficult to interpret.

Extrapulmonary Tuberculosis

The basic principles of management for extrapulmonary tuberculosis are similar to pulmonary TB. Prolonged treatment (≥12 months) is required for bone and joint, miliary and CNS tuberculosis. Prolonged treatment may also be required in patients slow to respond. In general, corticosteroids are indicated only for meningeal and pericardial TB as they have been shown to decrease mortality.[46,47] Corticosteroids may have a role in adrenal TB, life-threatening disseminated disease, obstructive endobronchial disease, pleural TB and drug reactions.

HIV Infection

Principles of treatment of active TB in HIV-infected adults are similar to treatment of individuals without HIV infection.[48,49,50] Daily or thrice-weekly DOT (continuation phase) is strongly recommended due to high risk of resistance and relapse of infection with less frequent administration.[24]A treatment duration of at least 8 months is suggested in patients with HIV infection who decline or are unable to take antiretrovirals (ARV).

Dose adjustments may be required for anti-TB and antiretroviral agents.[49] Rifamycins may substantially decrease the concentration of protease inhibitors (PIs) and non-nucleoside reverse transcriptase inhibitors (NNRTIs). Among the rifamycins, **rifabutin** is the least potent enzyme inducer and can be substituted for rifampin with similar efficacy though dose adjustments may still be required depending on the ARVs chosen.

The optimal time to initiate antiretroviral therapy in relation to anti-TB treatment has been uncertain due to various factors, including complex drug interactions and immune reconstitution inflammatory syndrome (IRIS). Recent evidence indicates that antiretroviral therapy should be initiated well before completion of the anti-TB regimen to reduce risk of mortality.[51] Initiate antiretroviral therapy within 2 weeks after the start of anti-TB therapy for patients with CD4 <50 cells/µL and within 8 weeks for all others.[7,52] For patients already receiving antiretrovirals, continue therapy during anti-TB treatment, especially if it has been successful. Monitor for signs and symptoms of IRIS (fever, malaise, local reactions in organs) particularly if anti-TB therapy and antiretroviral therapy are started at the same time.[7,53] If IRIS does occur, both antiretroviral and anti-TB treatments are continued while managing the inflammatory response.[52] Corticosteroids have been used to treat severe IRIS.

Management of HIV-infected patients with TB requires health care workers with expertise in these areas. Consultation with a respirologist, TB expert or HIV expert with experience managing HIV-related TB is strongly recommended due to possible drug interactions and the risk of the immune reconstitution syndrome.

For more information on the treatment of HIV, see Chapter 113.

Choices during Pregnancy and Breastfeeding

Active Tuberculosis and Pregnancy

There is no evidence to suggest that active TB is more common in pregnant women. Diagnosis of active TB may be more difficult as symptoms of fatigue or malaise may be attributed to pregnancy, and pregnant women with active TB are more often asymptomatic.[54,55] Clinical response to anti-TB therapy is similar to the general population, although pregnant and postpartum women may be at higher risk of hepatotoxicity.[56]

Infants born to mothers with active TB are at higher risk for low birth weight. Mothers with active TB may transmit congenital TB during pregnancy, or neonatal TB in the postpartum period. Both conditions carry a high mortality risk.[57] Given the risk to the fetus, pregnant women with suspected active TB should be investigated through standard diagnostic procedures, including a single posterior-anterior chest x-ray with double shielding (front and back) of the abdomen.[7] Active TB is not an indication for termination of pregnancy, but counselling should be provided for patients with drug-resistant disease regarding the potential risk of second-line therapy.[24]

Management of Active Tuberculosis in Pregnancy

Treatment of active TB should not be withheld during pregnancy or the postpartum period, as the risk of untreated active TB outweighs the risk of adverse events from anti-TB therapy.[7,24] The preferred initial treatment regimen includes **isoniazid**, **rifampin** and **ethambutol**.[7,24] These drugs cross the placenta, but teratogenic effects have not been demonstrated. The risk of teratogenicity with **pyrazinamide** has not been determined though it is unlikely to be teratogenic.[24] Its use could be considered if resistance to one of the initial drugs is suspected and susceptibility to pyrazinamide is likely, or in cases of extensive disease. **Aminoglycosides** have been associated with congenital deafness and should not be used.[24] Refer cases of drug resistant disease to a TB specialist, as commonly used second-line drugs have potential teratogenic effects and are not considered safe. **Pyridoxine** (Vitamin B6) is recommended in pregnant women prescribed isoniazid.

If a mother is suspected of having active TB during labour, the mother and infant should be separated after delivery and each should be investigated and treated as appropriate. A mother with active infectious TB should wear an appropriate mask during labour and respiratory precautions should be instituted.

Latent Tuberculosis in Pregnancy

Pregnancy is not an indication for latent TB testing. However, patients with very high risk for disease (e.g., HIV-positive, recent TB infection) may be tested, as positive test results may warrant treatment during pregnancy.[7] If possible, test for latent TB in high-risk patients before pregnancy. Chest x-ray remains part of the LTBI diagnostic procedure in pregnant women; a single posterior-anterior chest x-ray with double (front and back) shielding of the abdomen is recommended for women with positive TST and IGRA results.

Women who are receiving LTBI treatment should be advised to avoid pregnancy. If a patient becomes pregnant while on latent TB therapy, continuation of the regimen should be considered on a case-by-case basis.[58] In patients without high risk of disease, withhold latent therapy until

3 months postpartum to reduce the risk of hepatotoxicity. Daily **isoniazid** therapy for 9 months is the preferred regimen for high-risk patients with latent disease. Pregnant and postpartum women who are receiving isoniazid therapy should be monitored carefully for hepatotoxicity. Concomitant **pyridoxine** therapy is recommended.[24]

Management during Breastfeeding

Breastfeeding is not contraindicated in women receiving **isoniazid**, **rifampin** or **ethambutol** therapy.[24] The small concentrations of these drugs in the breast milk have not been shown to cause toxicity in infants. Breast milk does not provide adequate serum concentrations for treating an infant. **Pyridoxine** therapy is recommended for all infants under treatment or whose mothers are taking isoniazid therapy. Consultation with a TB expert is recommended before breastfeeding while taking second-line therapy.

A discussion of general principles on the use of medications in these special populations can be found in Appendix II and Appendix III. Other specialized reference sources are also provided in these appendices.

Therapeutic Tips

- Prescribe **pyridoxine** 25 mg/day (1 mg/kg/day for children) to prevent peripheral neuropathy in patients given **isoniazid** who have poor nutrition, alcoholism or other substance abuse disorders, diabetes, renal failure, HIV infection, seizure disorders or other disorders that might predispose to neuropathy.[7] Pregnant and breastfeeding women should also receive pyridoxine with isoniazid. Consider prescribing pyridoxine to all patients given isoniazid.[59]
- Recommend DOT in the treatment of TB, especially in patients with a history of treatment failure, drug resistance, disease relapse, HIV infection, substance abuse or psychiatric illness and in homeless patients.
- Before splitting a dose or switching to a second-line agent in patients who experience stomach upset, consider administering first-line anti-TB drugs with a small amount of food.[24] Evaluate patients with GI symptoms for drug-induced hepatitis.

Table 4: **Antibiotics for the Treatment of *M. tuberculosis***

Class	Drug	Dose	Adverse Effects	Drug Interactions	Comments	Cost[a]
Aminoglycosides	*amikacin* generics	**Active TB disease:** **Adults**: 15 mg/kg/day im/iv (up to 1 g/day) >59 y: 10 mg/kg/day im/iv (up to 750 mg/day) **Children**: 15–30 mg/kg/day im/iv (up to 1 g/day)	Vestibular/cochlear toxicity, ataxia (may be permanent), nystagmus, proteinuria, hypersensitivity reaction with fever, rash. Hematologic effects.[b]	Additive toxicity with other neurotoxic, ototoxic or nephrotoxic drugs.	Second-line agent in active TB disease. Avoid in children: risk of irreversible auditory nerve damage. Used in TB meningitis. Contraindicated in pregnancy; associated with congenital deafness. Target peak serum levels for this indication to 35–45 µg/mL.	~$100
	streptomycin generics	**Active TB disease:** **Adults**: 15 mg/kg/day (up to 1 g/day) im *or* 15 mg/kg (up to 1.5 g) 3 times weekly im >59 y: 10 mg/kg/day (up to 750 mg) im **Children**: 20–40 mg/kg/day (up to 1 g) im	See amikacin.	See amikacin.	See amikacin. Amikacin preferred over streptomycin due to ease of monitoring and lower toxicity.	$$$$$
Antimycobacterial Agents	*ethambutol* Etibi	**Active TB disease:** **Adults**: 15–20 mg/kg/day (up to 1.6 g) po *or* DOT: 25–40 mg/kg (up to 2.4 g) 3 times weekly po **Children**: 15–25 mg/kg/day (up to 1.6 g/day) po *or* DOT: 30–50 mg/kg (up to 2.4 g) 3 times weekly po	Ocular toxicity: decreased visual acuity, central scotomata, red-green colour blindness due to retrobulbar neuritis (dose-related; rare at 15 mg/kg/day). Skin rash: Stevens-Johnson syndrome, toxic epidermal necrolysis. Hematologic effects.[b] GI upset.[c] Neurologic effects: headache, dizziness, confusion, hallucinations.	Decreased levels with concomitant ingestion of aluminum hydroxide: separate doses by at least 4 h.	First-line agent in active TB disease. Assess colour vision and visual acuity at baseline and monitor monthly in patients receiving ethambutol for longer than 2 months (can use Ishihara-type diagrams[7] available online). Can be used in pregnancy.	$

(cont'd)

Table 4: **Antibiotics for the Treatment of *M. tuberculosis*** *(cont'd)*

Class	Drug	Dose	Adverse Effects	Drug Interactions	Comments	Cost[a]
	isoniazid generics	**Latent TB infection:** **Adults**: 5 mg/kg/day (up to 300 mg/day) po × 9 months *or* DOT: 900 mg twice weekly po × 6–9 months **Children**: 10–15 mg/kg/day (up to 300 mg) po × 9 months *or* DOT: 20–30 mg/kg (up to 900 mg) twice weekly po × 6–9 months **Active TB disease:** Daily therapy may be initially preferable to less frequent therapy. **Adults**: 5 mg/kg (up to 300 mg) daily po *or* 10 mg/kg (up to 600 mg) 3 times weekly po **Children**: 10–15 mg/kg/day (up to 300 mg daily) po *or* DOT: 20–30 mg/kg (up to 900 mg) 3 times weekly po Consult expert in patients with severe liver disease	Asymptomatic increase in hepatic aminotransferases and bilirubin (10–20%), clinical hepatitis (symptoms may occur within weeks to months), peripheral neuropathy (dose-related). Hematologic effects.[b] GI upset.[c] Gynecomastia, seizures, drowsiness, drug-induced lupus, toxic encephalopathy, fever, skin rash, mood changes, lymphadenopathy.	INH increases serum levels of carbamazepine, phenytoin, theophylline. Increased hepatotoxicity of INH with rifampin, ethanol, acetaminophen. Cross-hepatotoxicity may occur between drugs that are chemically related (e.g., INH and pyrazinamide). Both agents should be avoided if a reaction to one of them occurs.	First-line agent in active TB disease. Educate patients on symptoms of hepatitis (e.g., fatigue, flu-like symptoms, anorexia, nausea with or without vomiting). Can be used in pregnancy. Consider prescribing pyridoxine 25 mg/day or 1mg/kg/day for children to prevent peripheral neuropathy.[59]	$
	pyrazinamide generics	**Active TB disease:** **Adults**: 20–25 mg/kg/day (up to 2 g/day) po *or* DOT: 30–40 mg/kg (up to 4 g) 3 times weekly po **Children**: 30–40 mg/kg/day (up to 2 g/day) po *or* DOT: 60–80 mg/kg (up to 3 g) 3 times weekly po	Hepatotoxicity (rare with 2 months therapy), rash, arthralgia, increase in uric acid (acute gout rarely seen), drug fever, GI upset. Hematologic effects.[b]	Rifampin and pyrazinamide: liver injury in patients with latent TB infection.[28] Increased pyrazinamide levels: concomitant administration of allopurinol through inhibition of xanthine oxidase.	First-line agent in active TB disease.	$

Class	Drug	Dose	Adverse Effects	Drug Interactions	Comments	Cost[a]
Fluoroquinolones	*levofloxacin* Levaquin, generics	**Active TB disease:** Adults: 500–1000 mg daily po	Abdominal pain, nausea, vomiting, photosensitivity, dizziness, headache, drowsiness, insomnia, diarrhea, pseudomembranous colitis, eosinophilic meningitis, tendonitis and rupture. Cases of severe liver injury including liver failure have been reported.	Decreased absorption of fluoroquinolones with concomitant iron, calcium, magnesium, zinc, antacids, sucralfate. Separate doses by 2 h. Torsades de pointes is possible with concomitant use of other drugs that prolong QT_c interval.	Second-line agent in active TB disease and for drug-resistant disease.	$
	moxifloxacin Avelox	**Active TB disease:** Adults: 400 mg daily po	See levofloxacin. Cases of severe liver injury including liver failure have been reported.	See levofloxacin.	See levofloxacin.	$$
	ofloxacin generics	**Active TB disease:** Adults: 400 mg BID po	See levofloxacin.	See levofloxacin.	See levofloxacin.	$
Rifamycins	*rifabutin* Mycobutin	**Active TB disease:** Adults: 5 mg/kg/day (up to 300 mg/day) po DOT: 5 mg/kg (up to 300 mg) 3 times weekly po	Rash, orange discolouration of body fluids (contact lens staining), GI upset, liver toxicity, flu-like illness, neutropenia, leukopenia thrombocytopenia, myalgia, taste perversion.	Adjust rifabutin dose when combining with efavirenz or protease inhibitors.[52,60] Protease inhibitors decrease clearance of rifabutin while efavirenz increases clearance of rifabutin. Do not use with elvitegravir or rilpivirine. Avoid maraviroc. Consult TB/HIV expert; many interactions with HIV drugs. Decreased serum concentration of drugs due to hepatic enzyme induction, e.g., oral contraceptives, anticoagulants, antihyperglycemic agents, immunosuppressants, methadone. Adjust dose of affected drug when a rifamycin is initiated or discontinued.	First-line agent in active TB disease. Preferred rifamycin in HIV-infected patients treated with protease inhibitors.[52]	$$

(cont'd)

Table 4: **Antibiotics for the Treatment of *M. tuberculosis*** *(cont'd)*

Class	Drug	Dose	Adverse Effects	Drug Interactions	Comments	Cost[a]
	rifampin Rifadin, Rofact, generics	**Latent TB infection:** **Adults**: 10 mg/kg/day (up to 600 mg/day) po × 4 months **Children**: 10–20 mg/kg/day (up to 600 mg/day) po × 4 months **Active TB disease:** **Adults**: 10 mg/kg/day (up to 600 mg/day) po *or* DOT: 10 mg/kg (up to 600 mg/day) 3 times weekly po **Children**: 10–20 mg/kg/day (up to 600 mg/day) po *or* DOT: 10–20 mg/kg (up to 600 mg/day) 3 times weekly po Consult expert in patients with severe liver disease	Rash (petechial rash may suggest thrombocytopenia), orange discolouration of body fluids (contact lens staining), GI upset, liver toxicity, flu-like illness, subclinical disseminated intravascular coagulation, diarrhea, urticaria, ataxia, confusion, visual disturbances, acute interstitial nephritis. Hematologic effects.[b]	Avoid use with etravirine, elvitegravir, nevirapine, protease inhibitors and rilpivirine.[52,60] Increase dose of integrase inhibitors or maraviroc if used concomitantly with rifampin.[52,60] Consult TB/HIV expert; many interactions with HIV drugs. Decreased serum concentration of drugs due to hepatic enzyme induction, e.g., oral contraceptives, anticoagulants, antihyperglycemic agents, immunosuppressants, methadone. Adjust dose of affected drug when a rifamycin is initiated or discontinued.	First-line agent in active TB disease. Can be used in pregnancy.	$

[a] Cost based on 1-day supply for adult dose of active TB treatment; includes drug cost only.
[b] Hematologic effects may include any of eosinophilia, thrombocytopenia, transient leukopenia, hemolytic anemia, agranulocytosis, or sideroblastic or aplastic anemia.
[c] GI upset: nausea, vomiting, poor appetite, abdominal pain; common in the first few weeks of therapy—manage by administering with food or at bedtime; monitor AST to rule out hepatotoxicity.

Dosage adjustment may be required in renal impairment; see Appendix I.
Abbreviations: DOT = directly observed therapy; INH = isoniazid
Legend: $ < $5 $$ $5–15 $$$ $15–25 $$$$ $25–35 $$$$$ $35–45

Suggested Readings

American Thoracic Society; Centers for Disease Control and Prevention; Infectious Diseases Society of America. American Thoracic Society/Centers for Disease Control and Prevention/Infectious Diseases Society of America: controlling tuberculosis in the United States. *Am J Respir Crit Care Med* 2005;172(9):1169-227.

Blumberg HM, Burman WJ, Chaisson RE et al. American Thoracic Society/Centers for Disease Control and Prevention/Infectious Diseases Society of America: treatment of tuberculosis. *Am J Respir Crit Care Med* 2003;167(4):603-62.

Menzies D, ed. *Canadian tuberculosis standards*. 7th ed. Ottawa (ON): Canadian Thoracic Society; Public Health Agency of Canada; 2014. Available from: www.respiratoryguidelines.ca/tb-standards-2013.

World Health Organization. *Tuberculosis and air travel: guidelines for prevention and control*. 3rd ed. Geneva (CH): WHO; 2008. Available from: whqlibdoc.who.int/publications/2008/9789241547505_eng.pdf.

References

1. Targeted tuberculin testing and treatment of latent tuberculosis infection. This official statement of the American Thoracic Society was adopted by the ATS Board of Directors, July 1999. This is a Joint Statement of the American Thoracic Society (ATS) and the Centers for Disease Control and Prevention (CDC). This statement was endorsed by the Council of the Infectious Diseases Society of America. (IDSA), September 1999, and the sections of this statement. *Am J Respir Crit Care Med* 2000;161(4 Pt 2):S221-47.
2. Diagnostic Standards and Classification of Tuberculosis in Adults and Children. This official statement of the American Thoracic Society and the Centers for Disease Control and Prevention was adopted by the ATS Board of Directors, July 1999. This statement was endorsed by the Council of the Infectious Disease Society of America, September 1999. *Am J Respir Crit Care Med* 2000;161(4 Pt 1):1376-95.
3. Schluger NW. Changing approaches to the diagnosis of tuberculosis. *Am J Respir Crit Care Med* 2001;164(11):2020-4.
4. Greenaway C, Menzies D, Fanning A et al. Delay in diagnosis among hospitalized patients with active tuberculosis–predictors and outcomes. *Am J Respir Crit Care Med* 2002;165(7):927-33.
5. Menzies D, Fanning A, Yuan L et al. Hospital ventilation and risk for tuberculous infection in Canadian health care workers. Canadian Collaborative Group in Nosocomial Transmission of TB. *Ann Intern Med* 2000;133(10):779-89.
6. Menzies D, Fanning A, Yuan L et al. Factors associated with tuberculin conversion in Canadian microbiology and pathology workers. *Am J Respir Crit Care Med* 2003;167(4):599-602.
7. Menzies D, ed. *Canadian tuberculosis standards*. 7th ed. Ottawa (ON): Canadian Thoracic Society; Public Health Agency of Canada; 2014. Available from: www.respiratoryguidelines.ca/tb-standards-2013. Accessed May 17, 2014.
8. Advisory Committee Statement (ACS). Canadian Tuberculosis Committee. Housing conditions that serve as risk factors for tuberculosis infection and disease. *Can Commun Dis Rep* 2007;33(ACS-9):1-13. Available from: www.phac-aspc.gc.ca/publicat/ccdr-rmtc/07pdf/acs33-09.pdf. Accessed March 24, 2011.
9. Nolan CM, Goldberg SV, Buskin SE. Hepatotoxicity associated with isoniazid preventive therapy: a 7-year survey from a public health tuberculosis clinic. *JAMA* 1999;281(11):1014-8.
10. World Health Organization. *Collaborative framework for care and control of tuberculosis and diabetes*. Available from: whqlibdoc.who.int/publications/2011/9789241502252_eng.pdf. Accessed October 1, 2013.
11. Pai M, Minion J, Jamieson F et al. Chapter 3: Diagnosis of active tuberculosis and drug resistance. In: Menzies D, ed. *Canadian tuberculosis standards*. 7th ed. Ottawa (ON): Canadian Thoracic Society; Public Health Agency of Canada; 2014. Available from: www.respiratoryguidelines.ca/tb-standards-2013. Accessed May 17, 2014.
12. Singh M, Moosa NV, Kumar L et al. Role of gastric lavage and broncho-alveolar lavage in the bacteriological diagnosis of childhood pulmonary tuberculosis. *Indian Pediatr* 2000;37(9):947-51.
13. Coll P, Garrigo M, Moreno C et al. Routine use of Gen-Probe Amplified Mycobacterium Tuberculosis Direct (MTD) test for detection of Mycobacterium tuberculosis with smear-positive and smear-negative specimens. *Int J Tuberc Lung Dis* 2003;7(9):886-91.
14. Brodie D, Schluger NW. The diagnosis of tuberculosis. *Clin Chest Med* 2005;26(2):247-71.
15. Pai M, Kunimoto D, Jamieson F et al. Chapter 4: Diagnosis of latent tuberculosis infection. In: Menzies D, ed. *Canadian tuberculosis standards*. 7th ed. Ottawa (ON): Canadian Thoracic Society; Public Health Agency of Canada; 2014. Available from: www.respiratoryguidelines.ca/tb-standards-2013. Accessed May 17, 2014.
16. Mazurek GH, Jereb J, Vernon A et al. Updated guidelines for using interferon gamma release assays to detect Mycobacterium tuberculosis infection, United States, 2010. *MMWR Recomm Rep* 2010;59(RR-5):1-25.
17. Kitai I, Demers AM. Chapter 9: Pediatric tuberculosis. In: Menzies D, ed. *Canadian tuberculosis standards*. 7th ed. Ottawa (ON): Canadian Thoracic Society; Public Health Agency of Canada; 2014. Available from: www.respiratoryguidelines.ca/tb-standards-2013. Accessed May 17, 2014.
18. Khan A, Sterling TR, Reves R et al. Lack of weight gain and relapse risk in a large tuberculosis treatment trial. *Am J Respir Crit Care Med* 2006;174(3):344-8.
19. Slama K, Chiang CY, Enarson DA. Introducing brief advice in tuberculosis services. *Int J Tuberc Lung Dis* 2008;11(15):496-9.
20. Frieden TR, Munsiff SS. The DOTS strategy for controlling the global tuberculosis epidemic. *Clin Chest Med* 2005;26(2):197-205.
21. Blumberg HM, Leonard MK, Jasmer RM. Update on the treatment of tuberculosis and latent tuberculosis infection. *JAMA* 2005;293(22):2776-84.
22. LoBue PA, Moser KS. Use of isoniazid for latent tuberculosis infection in a public health clinic. *Am J Respir Crit Care Med* 2003;168(4):443-7.
23. McNab BD, Marciniuk DD, Alvi RA et al. Twice weekly isoniazid and rifampin treatment of latent tuberculosis infection in Canadian plains Aborigines. *Am J Respir Crit Care Med* 2000;162(3 Pt 1):989-93.

24. Blumberg HM, Burman WJ, Chaisson RE et al. American Thoracic Society/Centers for Disease Control and Prevention/Infectious Diseases Society of America: treatment of tuberculosis. *Am J Respir Crit Care Med* 2003;167(4):603-62.
25. Polesky A, Farber HW, Gottlieb DJ et al. Rifampin preventive therapy for tuberculosis in Boston's homeless. *Am J Respir Crit Care Med* 1996;154(5):1473-7.
26. Centers for Disease Control and Prevention (CDC). Fatal and severe hepatitis associated with rifampin and pyrazinamide for the treatment of latent tuberculosis infection--New York and Georgia, 2000. *MMWR Morb Mortal Wkly Rep* 2001;50(15):289-91.
27. Centers for Disease Control and Prevention (CDC). Update: fatal and severe liver injuries associated with rifampin and pyrazinamide for latent tuberculosis infection, and revisions in American Thoracic Society/CDC recommendations--United States, 2001. *MMWR Morb Mortal Wkly Rep* 2001;50(34):733-5.
28. Centers for Disease Control and Prevention (CDC). Update: fatal and severe liver injuries associated with rifampin and pyrazinamide treatment for latent tuberculosis infection. *MMWR Morb Mortal Wkly Rep* 2002;51(44):998-9.
29. Centers for Disease Control and Prevention (CDC); American Thoracic Society. Update: adverse event data and revised American Thoracic Society/CDC recommendations against the use of rifampin and pyrazinamide for treatment of latent tuberculosis infection–United States, 2003. *MMWR Morb Mortal Wkly Rep* 2003;52(31):735-9.
30. Ijaz K, Jereb JA, Lambert LA et al. Severe or fatal liver injury in 50 patients in the United States taking rifampin and pyrazinamide for latent tuberculosis infection. *Clin Infect Dis* 2006;42(3):346-55.
31. Hershfield E. Tuberculosis: 9. Treatment. *CMAJ* 1999;161(4):405-11.
32. Park SK, Kim CT, Song SD. Outcome of chemotherapy in 107 patients with pulmonary tuberculosis resistant to isoniazid and rifampin. *Int J Tuberc Lung Dis* 1998;2(11):877-84.
33. Small PM, Fujiwara PI. Management of tuberculosis in the United States. *N Engl J Med* 2001;345(3):189-200.
34. Benator D, Bhattacharya M, Bozeman L et al. Rifapentine and isoniazid once a week versus rifampicin and isoniazid twice a week for treatment of drug-susceptible pulmonary tuberculosis in HIV-negative patients: a randomised clinical trial. *Lancet* 2002;360(9332):528-34.
35. City of New York. Bureau of Tuberculosis Control. *Tuberculosis (TB): clinical policies and protocols*. 4th ed. New York (NY): New York City Department of Health and Mental Hygiene; 2008. Available from: www.nyc.gov/html/doh/downloads/pdf/tb/tb-protocol.pdf.
36. O'Brien RJ, Spigelman M. New drugs for tuberculosis: current status and future prospects. *Clin Chest Med* 2005;26(2):327-40.
37. Fortun J, Martin-Davila P, Navas E et al. Linezolid for the treatment of multidrug-resistant tuberculosis. *J Antimicrob Chemother* 2005;56(1):180-5.
38. Bozeman L, Burman W, Metchock B et al. Fluoroquinolone susceptibility among Mycobacterium tuberculosis isolates from the United States and Canada. *Clin Infect Dis* 2005;40(3):386-91.
39. Mitnick CD, Shin SS, Seung KJ et al. Comprehensive treatment of extensively drug-resistant tuberculosis. *N Engl J Med* 2008;359(6):563-74.
40. Saukkonen JJ, Cohn DL, Jasmer RM et al. An official ATS statement: hepatotoxicity of antituberculosis therapy. *Am J Respir Crit Care Med* 2006;174(8):935-52.
41. Kopanoff DE, Snider DE, Caras GJ. Isoniazid-related hepatitis: a U.S. Public Health Service cooperative surveillance study. *Am Rev Respir Dis* 1978;117(6):991-1001.
42. Wang L, Turner MO, Elwood RK et al. A meta-analysis of the effect of Bacille Calmette Guerin vaccination on tuberculin skin test measurements. *Thorax* 2002;57(9):804-9.
43. Public Health Agency of Canada. National Advisory Committee on Immunization (NACI). *Canadian immunization guide*. Evergreen ed. Available from: www.phac-aspc.gc.ca/publicat/cig-gci/index-eng.php. Accessed December 17, 2012.
44. Curtis AB, Ridzon R, Vogel R et al. Extensive transmission of Mycobacterium tuberculosis from a child. *N Engl J Med* 1999;341(20):1491-5.
45. Pineda PR, Leung A, Muller NL et al. Intrathoracic paediatric tuberculosis: a report of 202 cases. *Tuber Lung Dis* 1993;74(4):261-6.
46. Dooley DP, Carpenter JL, Rademacher S. Adjunctive corticosteroid therapy for tuberculosis: a critical reappraisal of the literature. *Clin Infect Dis* 1997;25(4):872-87.
47. Thwaites GE, Nguyen DB, Nguyen HD et al. Dexamethasone for the treatment of tuberculous meningitis in adolescents and adults. *N Engl J Med* 2004;351(17):1741-51.
48. Burman WJ, Jones BE. Treatment of HIV-related tuberculosis in the era of effective antiretroviral therapy. *Am J Respir Crit Care Med* 2001;164(1):7-12.
49. Dean GL, Edwards SG, Ives NJ et al. Treatment of tuberculosis in HIV-infected persons in the era of highly active antiretroviral therapy. *AIDS* 2002;16(1):75-83.
50. FitzGerald JM, Houston S. Tuberculosis: 8. The disease in association with HIV infection. *CMAJ* 1999;61(1):47-51.
51. Abdool Karim SS, Naidoo K, Grobler A et al. Timing of initiation of antiretroviral drugs during tuberculosis therapy. *N Engl J Med* 2010;362(8):697-706.
52. Panel on Antiretroviral Guidelines for Adults and Adolescents. *Guidelines for the use of antiretroviral agents in HIV-1 infected adults and adolescents*. Department of Health and Human Services; 2014. p. 1-284. Available from: www.aidsinfo.nih.gov/ContentFiles/AdultandAdolescentGL.pdf. Accessed May 3, 2014.
53. Narita M, Ashkin D, Hollender ES et al. Paradoxical worsening of tuberculosis following antiretroviral therapy in patients with AIDS. *Am J Respir Crit Care Med* 1998;158(1):157-61.
54. Knight M, Kurinczuk JJ, Nelson-Piercy C et al. Tuberculosis in pregnancy in the UK. *BJOG* 2009;116(4):584-8.
55. Kothari A, Mahadevan N, Girling J. Tuberculosis and pregnancy—Results of a study in a high prevalence area in London. *Eur J Obstet Gynecol Reprod Biol* 2006;126(1):48-55.
56. Davidson PT. Managing tuberculosis during pregnancy. *Lancet* 1995;346(8969):199-200.
57. Jana N, Vasishta K, Jindal SK et al. Perinatal outcome in pregnancies complicated by pulmonary tuberculosis. *Int J Gynaecol Obstet* 1994;44(2):119-24.
58. Bothamley G. Drug treatment for tuberculosis during pregnancy: safety considerations. *Drug Saf* 2001;24(7):553-65.
59. Snider DE. Pyridoxine supplementation during isoniazid therapy. *Tubercle* 1980;61(4):191-6.
60. U.S. Department of Health and Human Services. Centers for Disease Control and Prevention (CDC). *Managing drug interactions in the treatment of HIV-related tuberculosis*. Atlanta (GA): CDC; 2013. Available from: www.cdc.gov/tb/publications/guidelines/TB_HIV_Drugs/pdf/tbhiv.pdf. Accessed May 3, 2014.

Infectious Diseases

Chapter 125
Urinary Tract Infection

Lindsay Nicolle, MD, FRCPC

Goals of Therapy

- Relieve symptoms in acute infection
- Prevent complications of untreated acute infection
- Prevent recurrent infection
- Prevent pyelonephritis in pregnancy

Investigations

Table 1 details recommended investigations in a patient presenting with a urinary tract infection (UTI) as well as the most common infecting microorganisms. *Relapse* is a recurrence of UTI with the same organism due to persistence of the organism within the urinary tract, usually in the prostate or kidneys. Relapse usually occurs within a short period (e.g., within 4 weeks) after treatment completion. *Reinfection* is a recurrent UTI with a new species or strain of organism, usually occurring >2 weeks after treatment completion; it generally follows ascension of microorganisms from the periurethral area into the bladder.

Table 1: **Clinical Features and Diagnosis of UTIs**

Syndrome	Most Common Infecting Organisms[a]	Microbiologic Diagnosis	Urine Culture
Acute Uncomplicated UTI (Cystitis) Occurs in females with normal genitourinary tracts. Some women have a genetic predisposition for recurrent UTIs. Behavioural factors promoting infection include sexual intercourse and use of spermicides or diaphragm. Usual presenting symptoms include internal dysuria, frequency, suprapubic discomfort and urgency. Recurrences are common but of variable frequency.	*Escherichia coli* (80–90%), *Staphylococcus saprophyticus* (5–10%), *Klebsiella pneumoniae, Proteus mirabilis*	Presence of **any** quantitative count of a gram-negative organism or *S. saprophyticus* in a voided urine specimen with pyuria.	Generally not recommended. Culture if failure to respond to empiric therapy, early (<1 month) recurrence following therapy, diagnostic uncertainty or pregnant patient.
Acute Nonobstructive Pyelonephritis Occurs in women who also experience recurrent uncomplicated UTIs but at lower frequency than cystitis. Classic presentation includes fever and flank pain with or without associated irritative urinary symptoms. Nausea and vomiting may be present. Patients who present with UTIs with only lower tract symptoms or asymptomatic bacteriuria occasionally have associated occult renal infection. Bacteremic infection occurs most frequently in diabetic women or women >65 y.	*E. coli* (90%), *P. mirabilis* (5%), *K. pneumoniae* (5%)	$\geq 10^7$ cfu/L[b] in voided specimen.	Always indicated. Obtain before initiating antimicrobials. Consider blood cultures.

(cont'd)

Table 1: **Clinical Features and Diagnosis of UTIs** *(cont'd)*

Syndrome	Most Common Infecting Organisms[a]	Microbiologic Diagnosis	Urine Culture
Complicated UTI Occurs in individuals with an abnormal genitourinary tract due to structural or functional abnormalities, including indwelling catheter. Virtually all episodes of UTI in a male will be complicated. Patients may present with cystitis (lower tract) symptoms or fever/pyelonephritis. Management includes search for correctable anomalies; with persistent abnormalities, recurrent infection is common (50% by 6 wk post-therapy).	*E. coli* (50%), *P. mirabilis* (20%), *Enterococcus faecalis* (10%), *Pseudomonas aeruginosa*, *Providencia stuartii*, *Citrobacter* spp., *Enterobacter* spp., *Serratia* spp., group B streptococci	≥10^8 cfu/L[b] in voided specimen or any quantitative count for an "in and out" catheterized specimen.	Always, before antimicrobial therapy.
Bacterial Prostatitis **Acute:** Symptoms include acute onset chills, fever, perineal and low back pain, irritative and obstructive voiding. The prostate is tender, swollen, indurated and warm. Prostatic massage is not recommended because it may cause bacteremia.	*E. coli*, *Enterobacteriaceae*, *P. aeruginosa*, *Staphylococcus aureus*, others	Urine culture >10^8 cfu/L[b]; blood culture positive; aspirate prostate abscess if present (abnormalities are found in <5% of cases).	Voided urine specimen before empiric therapy.
Chronic: Common cause of recurrent UTIs in older men; increases with age. Intermittent urinary infection presenting as cystitis; history of recurrent UTIs. Symptoms of chronic prostatitis are not considered attributable to infection in the absence of microbiologic documentation (antimicrobial therapy does not improve these symptoms when compared to placebo).[1] Prostate examination is usually normal. Usually due to relapse.	*E. coli* (80%), *Klebsiella* spp, *P. aeruginosa*, *Proteus* spp, others	Post-prostatic massage urine culture positive with pyuria and negative midstream urine specimen.	Urine culture with acute symptoms.
Asymptomatic Bacteriuria Microbiologic evidence for a UTI in the absence of associated symptoms. Asymptomatic bacteriuria is more common in women; increases with age. In pregnancy, screen for asymptomatic bacteriuria at 12–16 wk.	*E. coli* (60–70%), *P. mirabilis*, group B streptococcus, coagulase-negative staphylococci, others	≥10^8 cfu/L[b] in 2 consecutive specimens in women or 1 specimen in men.	Screening for bacteriuria is not indicated for asymptomatic patients unless they are pregnant or about to undergo an invasive urologic procedure.

[a] *E. coli* is the most frequent organism causing UTIs. Individuals with a complicated UTI or recent exposure to antimicrobials are more likely to have organisms other than *E. coli* or organisms of increased antimicrobial resistance.
[b] 10^7 cfu/L = 10^4 cfu/mL; 10^8 cfu/L = 10^5 cfu/mL.
Abbreviations: cfu/L = colony-forming units/litre; UTI = urinary tract infection

Therapeutic Choices

Figure 1 details the management of recurrent acute, uncomplicated UTIs. Table 2 lists the various forms of UTIs and the recommended empiric antibiotic regimens for their treatment. Table 3 details the properties of common antibiotics used in the treatment of UTIs.

Figure 1: **Management of Recurrent Acute, Uncomplicated UTIs**

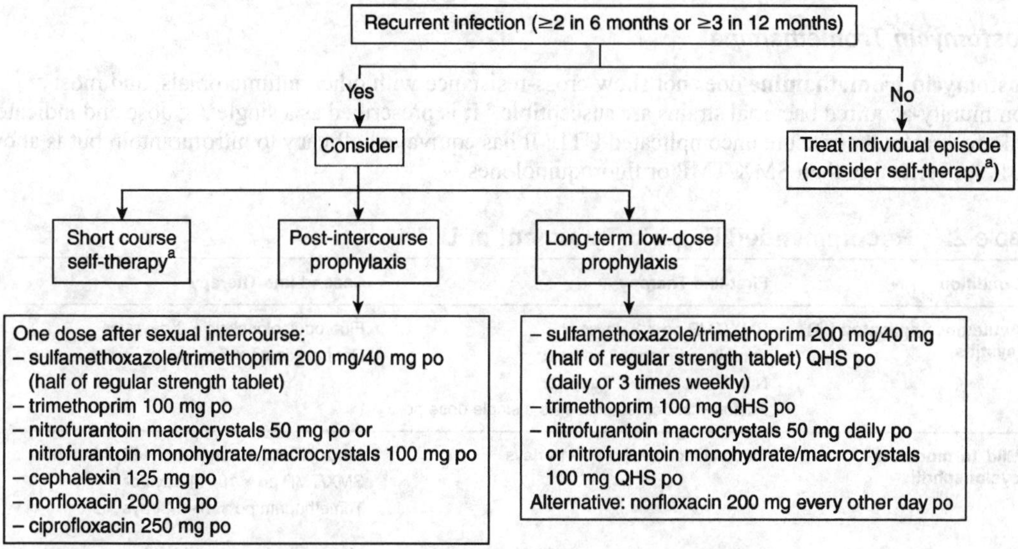

[a] Three-day course of treatment, self-administered on appearance of symptoms.

Pharmacologic Choices

Sulfamethoxazole/trimethoprim (SMX/TMP) and Trimethoprim (TMP)

SMX/TMP and **TMP** are the drugs of choice for most UTIs if local rates of resistance are <20% [Evidence: SORT C*].[2] Both may be used as 3-day therapy for acute uncomplicated UTIs. Resistance to SMX/TMP and TMP is increasing and must be considered in individuals who have failed empiric therapy or who have had recent prior therapy with these agents. Use of SMX/TMP is limited by sulfa allergy (TMP alone may be used in sulfa-allergic patients).

Nitrofurantoin

Nitrofurantoin, a urinary antiseptic, has been widely used to treat UTIs. It may not be as effective as SMX/TMP for 3-day therapy in the treatment of acute uncomplicated UTIs; however, a 5-day course is effective.[5] It is not recommended for treatment of pyelonephritis and is contraindicated in renal failure (ClCr <60 mL/min). Pulmonary and hepatic toxicity occur rarely but are more common with long-term use. Nitrofurantoin *monohydrate/macrocrystals* (MacroBID) is dosed twice daily and may be better tolerated than the standard *macrocrystal* formulation.

Amoxicillin and Amoxicillin/clavulanate

Resistance of *E. coli* to **amoxicillin** limits its current use; reserve for UTIs with streptococci or enterococci or when the infecting organism is known to be susceptible.

Amoxicillin is not recommended for empiric therapy of uncomplicated UTIs as it will be about 20% less effective than SMX/TMP.[2]

* SORT (Strength of Recommendation Taxonomy) is a rating system (A, B or C) that addresses the quality of available evidence. For more information consult **How to Use *Compendium of Therapeutic Choices*** on page xxv.

Amoxicillin/clavulanate may be considered when SMX/TMP, nitrofurantoin and fluoroquinolones cannot be used.[6] Amoxicillin with clavulanate is associated with substantial gastrointestinal (GI) side effects (10–25% incidence).

Fosfomycin Tromethamine

Fosfomycin tromethamine does not show cross-resistance with other antimicrobials, and most community-acquired bacterial strains are susceptible.[2] It is prescribed as a single 3 g dose and indicated only for treatment of acute uncomplicated UTI.[7] It has equivalent efficacy to nitrofurantoin but is about 10% less effective than SMX/TMP or fluoroquinolones.[2,7]

Table 2: **Recommended Empiric Treatment of UTIs**

Condition	First-line Therapy	Second-line Therapy
Acute uncomplicated UTI (cystitis)	SMX/TMP po × 3 days[a] *or* Trimethoprim po × 3 days[a] *or* Nitrofurantoin po × 5 days *or* Fosfomycin tromethamine as a single dose po	Fluoroquinolone[b] po × 3 days[a] *or* Cephalexin po × 7 days
Mild to moderate pyelonephritis[c,d]	Fluoroquinolone[b] po × 7–14 days	Amoxicillin/clavulanate po × 10–14 days *or* SMX/TMP po × 10–14 days *or* Trimethoprim po × 10–14 days
Severe pyelonephritis[c,e]	Aminoglycoside iv ± ampicillin[f] iv for initial therapy. If clinically appropriate, step down to oral therapy as in mild to moderate infections in order to complete 10–14 days	Fluoroquinolone[b] iv × 10–14 days *or* 3rd-generation cephalosporin iv ± aminoglycoside iv × 10–14 days *or* Carbapenem iv × 7–14 days (for extended-spectrum β-lactamase-producing organisms)
Mild to moderate complicated UTI[c,d]	Fluoroquinolone[b] po × 7–10 days *or* SMX/TMP po × 7–10 days *or* Trimethoprim po × 7–10 days *or* Nitrofurantoin po × 7–10 days	Amoxicillin/clavulanate po × 7–10 days *or* Cephalexin po × 7–10 days *or* Cefixime po × 7–10 days
Severe complicated UTI[c,e]	Aminoglycoside iv ± ampicillin[f] iv for initial therapy. If clinically appropriate, step down to oral therapy as in mild to moderate infections in order to complete 10–14 days	Fluoroquinolone[b] iv × 10–14 days *or* 3rd-generation cephalosporin iv × 10–14 days
Acute bacterial prostatitis[c]	Aminoglycoside iv ± cloxacillin iv ± ampicillin iv[f] Cloxacillin is useful only if *S. aureus* is known to be present.	Fluoroquinolone[b] iv or po × 4 wk *or* SMX/TMP po × 4 wk
Chronic bacterial prostatitis[c]	Fluoroquinolone[b] po × 4–6 wk	SMX/TMP po × 4–6 wk

[a] Treat for 7 days in women with symptoms lasting >1 wk or women with recurrent infections in <1 month.[2] Treat for 3 days in women ≥65 years.[3,4]
[b] Resistance to fluoroquinolones is increasing.
[c] Always obtain urine culture prior to initiating therapy. Use culture results to guide therapy after the first few days of treatment, particularly in step-down therapy.
[d] Hemodynamically stable, no vomiting.
[e] High fever, sepsis, vomiting.
[f] Include ampicillin if *Enterococcus* is a concern.
Abbreviations: SMX/TMP = sulfamethoxazole/trimethoprim; UTI = urinary tract infection

Fluoroquinolones

The renally excreted fluoroquinolones (**ciprofloxacin**, **levofloxacin**, **norfloxacin** and **ofloxacin**) are as effective as SMX/TMP for 3-day treatment of acute uncomplicated UTIs due to susceptible organisms, but are generally second-line therapy due to concerns about development of resistance. Fluoroquinolones could be considered when resistance to SMX/TMP is anticipated to be >20% in the population in which it is being prescribed.

Single-dose therapy with fluoroquinolones is not reliable for *Staphylococcus saprophyticus*.[8] In addition, single-dose therapy may have poor patient acceptance because symptoms persist for 48–72 hours. Fluoroquinolones are important agents in the treatment of *complicated* UTIs, particularly for patients infected with resistant organisms. Ciprofloxacin for 7 days is adequate therapy for less severe presentations of acute nonobstructive pyelonephritis.[9,10] Do not use fluoroquinolones to treat UTIs in children or pregnant women because of potential adverse effects on developing cartilage.

Cephalosporins

All cephalosporins, including **cefaclor**, **cefazolin**, **cefixime**, **cefuroxime** and **cephalexin**, are effective for treatment of UTIs. They are not as well studied as SMX/TMP or fluoroquinolones and are somewhat less effective for acute cystitis, especially with short courses of therapy. Cephalosporins may be associated with a greater likelihood of vulvovaginal candidiasis.[11] Third-generation cephalosporins such as **ceftriaxone** and **cefotaxime** are effective agents for parenteral treatment of pyelonephritis.

Carbapenems

Carbapenems (**ertapenem** and **meropenem**) are beta-lactam antibiotics useful in treating severe UTIs due to susceptible extended-spectrum beta-lactamase (ESBL)-producing *Enterobacteriaceae*.[12] Risk factors for infection or colonization with ESBL-producing organisms are recent hospitalization, residence in a long-term care facility, prolonged use of broad-spectrum antibiotics and travel to countries where these strains are endemic. Meropenem, but not ertapenem, is active against *P. aeruginosa*. Carbapenems are available for parenteral use only, and require dosage adjustment in patients with moderate or severe renal impairment since excretion of carbapenems is mainly renal.

Carbapenems may cause allergic reactions (anaphylaxis, angioedema and urticaria) in <3% of patients.[13] The reported incidence of cross-allergenicity between penicillins and carbapenems is about 1%.[14] More common adverse effects include nausea and vomiting, diarrhea, thrombophlebitis and rash. Reduce dose in patients with renal dysfunction to prevent drug accumulation.

Aminoglycosides

Aminoglycosides (**amikacin**, **gentamicin** and **tobramycin**) remain the therapy of choice for the treatment of acute pyelonephritis requiring parenteral therapy. Most gram-negative organisms, especially in patients with community-acquired infections, will remain susceptible to these agents. Initial parenteral therapy is switched to oral therapy as soon as symptoms and signs have settled (72–96 hours). With such short duration of therapy, ototoxicity and nephrotoxicity are unlikely. Aminoglycosides are usually interchangeable for the treatment of UTIs. Antimicrobial susceptibility and cost determine selection of an individual agent.

Natural Health Products

Cranberry

Evidence from clinical trials does not support the use of cranberry products (juice, powder or tablets) for the prevention of UTIs.[15] Consumption of large quantities of cranberry juice may result in an interaction with warfarin and raise INR.[16]

Choices during Pregnancy and Breastfeeding

UTIs during Pregnancy

Screen pregnant women for asymptomatic bacteriuria early in pregnancy.[17] Treat if asymptomatic bacteriuria is confirmed on 2 consecutive cultures. If left untreated, bacteriuria in pregnancy can progress to pyelonephritis and cause adverse effects to the fetus.[18] Antibiotic treatment has been shown to reduce the incidence of pyelonephritis, rate of preterm delivery and the risk of low-birth-weight babies.[17,19]

Management of UTIs during Pregnancy

Treat asymptomatic bacteriuria and symptomatic cystitis with a 3- to 7-day course of **amoxicillin** (if the organism is known to be susceptible), **amoxicillin/clavulanate**, **cephalexin** or **nitrofurantoin** with appropriate follow-up.[20] **Fosfomycin tromethamine** may also be used in pregnancy when the organism is susceptible.[21]

Nitrofurantoin is usually avoided near term because of the risk of inducing hemolytic anemia in the fetus or newborn, especially in those with glucose-6-phosphate dehydrogenase deficiency; however, this toxicity is rare.[22,23] Avoid **trimethoprim** and **SMX/TMP** in the first trimester of pregnancy as they are associated with antifolate teratogenicity.[24,25] Avoid **SMX** in the last 6 weeks of pregnancy as it may lead to neonatal hyperbilirubinemia. Avoid **fluoroquinolones** in pregnancy. Impaired cartilage development has been reported in animal studies, although there are no reports in humans suggesting an increased risk of major malformations, adverse effects in the fetal musculoskeletal system, spontaneous abortions, prematurity, intrauterine growth retardation or postnatal disorders.[26,27,28,29]

Ceftriaxone is the preferred empiric therapy for treating pyelonephritis in pregnancy. Step down to oral therapy once the patient is stabilized and urine culture results are available.[30,31,32,33]

Upon completion of therapy, follow up with a urine culture 1–2 weeks later, and then monthly until the baby is born.[24]

Management of UTIs during Breastfeeding

The American Academy of Pediatrics considers fluoroquinolones (**ciprofloxacin**, **ofloxacin**), **nitrofurantoin** and **SMX/TMP** to be compatible with breastfeeding.[34] **Amoxicillin** and **cephalosporins** are considered compatible with breastfeeding.

Prevention of UTIs during Pregnancy and Breastfeeding

Antimicrobial prophylaxis is effective to prevent recurrent symptomatic or asymptomatic UTI in pregnant women. **Nitrofurantoin** and **cephalexin** are preferred. The use of cranberry products is safe in pregnancy, but efficacy to prevent infection in this patient population is not known.[15,35]

A discussion of general principles on the use of medications in these special populations can be found in Appendix II and Appendix III. Other specialized reference sources are also provided in these appendices.

Therapeutic Tips

- Whenever possible, base initial selection of antimicrobial therapy on urine culture results.
- Antimicrobial susceptibility in populations is dynamic and the local prevalence of susceptibility must always be considered.
- Base selection of empiric therapy in symptomatic patients on anticipated local antimicrobial susceptibilities and an individual patient's recent antimicrobial exposure and tolerance.

- Asymptomatic bacteriuria is common in many populations but is benign. Asymptomatic bacteriuria should not be treated except in pregnancy or in patients undergoing invasive urologic procedures. Treatment of asymptomatic bacteriuria contributes to harmful outcomes including an increased frequency of symptomatic infections and reinfection with more resistant bacteria.[17]
- For women (including those ≥65 years) with uncomplicated acute bacterial cystitis, a 3-day course of antimicrobial therapy with **sulfamethoxazole/trimethoprim, trimethoprim** or a **fluoroquinolone** is preferred.[3,4]
- Use parenteral therapy for patients who are septic, unable to tolerate oral medications, pregnant with pyelonephritis or those with resistant organisms requiring parenteral therapy.
- Consider prophylaxis for women with frequent recurrent uncomplicated UTIs (see Figure 1).
- Without microbiologic confirmation of a bacterial infection, symptoms of chronic prostatitis are not an indication for antimicrobial therapy.[1]

Suggested Readings

Habermacher GM, Chason JT, Schaeffer AJ. Prostatitis/chronic pelvic pain syndrome. *Annu Rev Med* 2006;57:195-206.

Hooton TM. Clinical practice. Uncomplicated urinary tract infection. *N Engl J Med* 2012;366(11):1028-37.

Nicolle L; AMMI Canada Guidelines Committee. Complicated urinary tract infection in adults. *Can J Infect Dis Med Microbiol* 2005;16(6):349-60.

Nicolle LE. Uncomplicated urinary tract infection in adults, including uncomplicated pyelonephritis. *Urol Clin North Am* 2008;35(1):1-12.

Nicolle LE, Bradley S, Colgan R et al. Infectious Diseases Society of America guidelines for the diagnosis and treatment of asymptomatic bacteriuria in adults. *Clin Infect Dis* 2005;40(5):643-54.

Table 3: **Antimicrobials for the Treatment of UTIs**

Class	Drug	Dose	Adverse Effects	Drug Interactions	Cost[a]
Aminoglycosides	*amikacin* generics	15–20 mg/kg/day iv	Nephrotoxicity, usually reversible, increases with dose, dosing frequency greater than once daily and dosing duration lasting >7–10 days; ototoxicity, often irreversible.	Increases ototoxicity with loop diuretics, increases nephrotoxicity with other nephrotoxic drugs.	$$$$$
	gentamicin generics	3–5 mg/kg/day iv	See amikacin.	See amikacin.	$$$
	tobramycin generics	3–5 mg/kg/day iv	See amikacin.	See amikacin.	$$
Carbapenems	*ertapenem sodium* Invanz	1 g Q24H iv	Diarrhea, headache, infused vein complications, nausea, seizures.	Decreases serum concentration of valproic acid; concurrent use is not recommended. Probenecid decreases renal excretion of ertapenem; concurrent use is not recommended.	$$$$
	meropenem Merrem, Meropenem for Injection	0.5–1 g Q8H iv	See ertapenem sodium.	See ertapenem sodium.	$$$$$
Cephalosporins, first-generation	*cefazolin* generics	1 g Q8H iv	Hypersensitivity reactions, rash, nausea, vomiting, pseudomembranous colitis, renal and hepatic dysfunction.	Increased INR with warfarin.	$$
	cephalexin generics	500 mg QID po	See cefazolin.	See cefazolin.	$
Cephalosporins, second-generation	*cefuroxime axetil* Ceftin, generics	250 mg BID po	See cefazolin.	See cefazolin.	$
	cefuroxime sodium generics	750 mg Q8H iv	See cefazolin.	See cefazolin.	$$$$
Cephalosporins, third-generation	*cefixime* Suprax	400 mg once daily po	See cefazolin.	See cefazolin.	$
	cefotaxime Claforan	1 g Q8H iv	See cefazolin. Safe in hepatobiliary disease.	See cefazolin.	$$$

Class	Drug	Dose	Adverse Effects	Drug Interactions	Cost[a]
	ceftazidime Fortaz, generics	1 g Q8H iv	See cefazolin.	See cefazolin.	$$$$$
	ceftriaxone generics	1 g Q24H im or iv	See cefazolin.	See cefazolin. Do not reconstitute or mix with calcium-containing solutions. Do not administer simultaneously with calcium-containing iv solutions via a Y-site. Administration may be done sequentially, provided the infusion lines are thoroughly flushed between infusions.	$$
Fluoroquinolones	*ciprofloxacin* Cipro, Cipro XL, generics	**Oral:** Immediate-release: 250–500 mg BID Long-acting: 500–1000 mg once daily **Parenteral:** 200–400 mg BID iv	Abdominal pain, nausea, vomiting, photosensitivity, dizziness, headache, drowsiness, insomnia, diarrhea, pseudomembranous colitis. Potential adverse effects on developing cartilage; avoid in children and in pregnancy.	Concomitant iron, antacids, sucralfate reduce absorption of fluoroquinolones; increase INR with warfarin.	po: $ iv: $$$
	levofloxacin Levaquin, generics	250–750 mg once daily po or 500 mg once daily iv	See ciprofloxacin.	See ciprofloxacin.	po: $ iv: $$$$
	norfloxacin generics	400 mg BID po	See ciprofloxacin.	See ciprofloxacin.	$
	ofloxacin generics	300–400 mg BID po	See ciprofloxacin.	See ciprofloxacin.	$
Folate Antagonists	*trimethoprim* generics	100 mg BID po	Rash, pruritus.	Increases phenytoin levels; increased myelosuppression with methotrexate.	$
Nitrofuran Derivatives	*nitrofurantoin macrocrystals* generics	50–100 mg QID po	Headache, nausea, flatulence, loss of appetite; pulmonary and hepatic toxicity with long-term use; rare acute pulmonary toxicity.	Antacids may decrease absorption.	$
	nitrofurantoin monohydrate/macrocrystals MacroBID	100 mg BID po	See nitrofurantoin. The monohydrate/macrocrystal formulation is better tolerated than the macrocrystal formulation.	See nitrofurantoin.	$

(cont'd)

Table 3: **Antimicrobials for the Treatment of UTIs** *(cont'd)*

Class	Drug	Dose	Adverse Effects	Drug Interactions	Cost[a]
Penicillins	*amoxicillin* generics	500 mg TID po	Hypersensitivity reactions, rash, nausea, vomiting, pseudomembranous colitis, GI effects.	Decreases efficacy of oral contraceptives; increases methotrexate serum levels.	$
	amoxicillin/clavulanate Clavulin, generics	500 mg TID po ***or*** 875 mg BID po	See amoxicillin.	See amoxicillin.	$
	ampicillin generics	1 g Q6H iv	See amoxicillin.	See amoxicillin.	$$
	piperacillin generics	3 g Q6H iv	See amoxicillin.	See amoxicillin.	$$$$$
	piperacillin/ tazobactam Tazocin, Piperacillin/Tazobactam for Injection, other generics	3.375 g Q6H iv	See amoxicillin.	See amoxicillin.	$$$$$
	ticarcillin/clavulanate Timentin	3.1 g Q4–6H iv	See amoxicillin.	See amoxicillin.	$$$$
Phosphoric Acid Derivatives	*fosfomycin tromethamine* Monurol	One 3 g sachet (single dose)	Diarrhea, headache, nausea, vaginitis.	Metoclopropamide, probenicid decrease fosfomycin levels.	$$$
Sulfonamide Combinations	*sulfamethoxazole/ trimethoprim* (SMX/TMP) generics	800/160 mg (2 regular-strength tablets or 1 DS tablet) BID po	Hypersensitivity reactions, nausea, vomiting, diarrhea, rash, false increase in serum creatinine, renal impairment, neutropenia, thrombocytopenia, anemia, agranulocytosis.	Increases phenytoin levels, increases INR with warfarin, hypoglycemia with sulfonylureas, increased nephrotoxicity with cyclosporine.	$

[a] Cost of 1-day supply based on 70 kg body weight unless otherwise specified; includes drug cost only.
Dosage adjustment may be required in renal impairment; see Appendix I.
Abbreviations: INR = International Normalized Ratio
Legend: $ <$10 $$ $10–20 $$$ $20–40 $$$$ $40–60 $$$$$ $60–80

References

1. Alexander RB, Propert KJ, Schaeffer AJ et al. Ciprofloxacin or tamsulosin in men with chronic prostatitis/chronic pelvic pain syndrome: a randomized, double-blind trial. *Ann Intern Med* 2004;141(8):581-9.
2. Gupta K, Hooton TM, Naber KG et al. International clinical practice guidelines for the treatment of acute uncomplicated cystitis and pyelonephritis in women: a 2010 update by the Infectious Diseases Society of America and the European Society for Microbiology and Infectious Diseases. *Clin Infect Dis* 2011;52(5):e103-20.
3. Vogel T, Verreault R, Gourdeau M et al. Optimal duration of antibiotic therapy for uncomplicated urinary tract infection in older women: a double-blind randomized controlled trial. *CMAJ* 2004;170(4):469-73.
4. American College of Obstetricians and Gynecologists. ACOG Practice Bulletin No. 91: Treatment of urinary tract infections in nonpregnant women. *Obstet Gynecol* 2008;111(3):785-94.
5. Gupta K, Hooton TM, Roberts PL et al. Short-course nitrofurantoin for the treatment of acute uncomplicated cystitis in women. *Arch Intern Med* 2007;167(20):2207-12.
6. Hooton TM, Scholes D, Gupta K et al. Amoxicillin-clavulanate vs ciprofloxacin for the treatment of uncomplicated cystitis in women: a randomized trial. *JAMA* 2005;293(8):949-55.
7. Patel SS, Balfour JA, Bryson HM. Fosfomycin tromethamine. A review of its antibacterial activity, pharmacokinetic properties and therapeutic efficacy as a single-dose oral treatment for acute uncomplicated lower urinary tract infections. *Drugs* 1997;53(4):637-56.
8. Richard GA, Mathew CP, Kirstein JM et al. Single-dose fluoroquinolone therapy of acute uncomplicated urinary tract infection in women: results from a randomized, double-blind, multicenter trial comparing single-dose to 3-day fluoroquinolone regimens. *Urology* 2002;59(3):334-9.
9. Talan DA, Stamm WE, Hooton TM et al. Comparison of ciprofloxacin (7 days) and trimethoprim-sulfamethoxazole (14 days) for acute uncomplicated pyelonephritis pyelonephritis in women: a randomized trial. *JAMA* 2000;283(12):1583-90.
10. Sandberg T, Skoog G, Hermansson AB et al. Ciprofloxacin for 7 days versus 14 days in women with acute pyelonephritis: a randomised, open-label and double-blind, placebo-controlled, non-inferiority trial. *Lancet* 2012;380(9840):484-90.
11. MacDonald TM, Beardon PH, McGilchrist MM et al. The risks of symptomatic vaginal candidiasis after oral antibiotic therapy. *Q J Med* 1993;86(7):419-24.
12. Hawkey PM, Jones AM. The changing epidemiology of resistance. *J Antimicrob Chemother* 2009;64(Suppl 1):i3-10.
13. Prescott WA, Kusmierski KA. Clinical importance of carbapenem hypersensitivity in patients with self-reported and documented penicillin allergy. *Pharmacotherapy* 2007;27(1):137-42.
14. Frumin J, Gallagher JC. Allergic cross-sensitivity between penicillin, carbapenem, and monobactam antibiotics: what are the chances? *Ann Pharmacother* 2009;43(2):304-15.
15. Jepson RG, Williams G, Craig JC. Cranberries for preventing urinary tract infections. *Cochrane Database Syst Rev* 2012;(10):CD001321.
16. Rindone JP, Murphy TW. Warfarin-cranberry juice interaction resulting in profound hypoprothrombinemia and bleeding. *Am J Ther* 2006;13(3):283-4.
17. Nicolle LE, Bradley S, Colgan R et al. Infectious Diseases Society of America guidelines for the diagnosis and treatment of asymptomatic bacteriuria in adults. *Clin Infect Dis* 2005;40(5):643-54.
18. McDermott S, Daguise V, Mann H et al. Perinatal risk for mortality and mental retardation associated with maternal urinary-tract infections. *J Fam Pract* 2001;50(5):433-7.
19. Smaill F, Vazquez JC. Antibiotics for asymptomatic bacteriuria in pregnancy. *Cochrane Database Syst Rev* 2007;(2):CD000490.
20. Le J, Briggs GG, McKeown A et al. Urinary tract infections during pregnancy. *Ann Pharmacother* 2004;38(10):1692-701.
21. Stein GE. Single-dose treatment of acute cystitis with fosfomycin tromethamine. *Ann Pharmacother* 1998;32(2):215-9.
22. Pritchard JA, Scott DE, Mason RA. Severe anemia with hemolysis and megaloblastic erythropoiesis. A reaction to nitrofurantoin administered during pregnancy. *JAMA* 1965;194(4):457-9.
23. Bruel H, Guillemant V, Saladin-Thiron C et al. [Hemolytic anemia in a newborn after maternal treatment with nitrofurantoin at the end of pregnancy]. *Arch Pediatr* 2000;7(7):745-7. [French].
24. Anti-infective Review Panel. *Anti-infective guidelines for community-acquired infections*. Toronto (ON): MUMS Guideline Clearinghouse; 2010.
25. Sivojelezova A, Einarson A, Shuhaiber S et al. Trimethoprim-sulfonamide combination therapy in early pregnancy. *Can Fam Physician* 2003;49:1085-6.
26. Quinolones and pregnancy: worrying animal findings, few clinical data. *Prescrire Int* 1999;8(39):29-31.
27. Koren G. Use of the new quinolones during pregnancy. *Can Fam Physician* 1996;42:1097-9.
28. Berkovitch M, Pastuszak A, Gazarian M et al. Safety of the new quinolones in pregnancy. *Obstet Gynecol* 1994;84(4):535-8.
29. Loebstein R, Addis A, Ho E et al. Pregnancy outcome following gestational exposure to fluoroquinolones: a multicenter prospective controlled study. *Antimicrob Agents Chemother* 1998;42(6):1336-9.
30. Gilstrap LC, Ramin SM. Urinary tract infections during pregnancy. *Obstet Gynecol Clin North Am* 2001;28(3):581-91.
31. Wing DA, Hendershott CM, Debuque L et al. A randomized trial of three antibiotic regimens for the treatment of pyelonephritis in pregnancy. *Obstet Gynecol* 1998;92(2):249-53.
32. Millar LK, Wing DA, Paul RH et al. Outpatient treatment of pyelonephritis in pregnancy: a randomized controlled trial. *Obstet Gynecol* 1995;86(4 Pt 1):560-4.
33. Sanchez-Ramos L, McAlpine KJ, Adair CD et al. Pyelonephritis in pregnancy: once-a-day ceftriaxone versus multiple doses of cefazolin. A randomized, double-blind trial. *Am J Obstet Gynecol* 1995;172(1 Pt 1):129-33.
34. American Academy of Pediatrics Committee on Drugs. Transfer of drugs and other chemicals into human milk. *Pediatrics* 2001;108(3):776-89.
35. Dugoua JJ, Seely D, Perri D et al. Safety and efficacy of cranberry (vaccinium macrocarpon) during pregnancy and lactation. *Can J Clin Pharmacol* 2008;15(1):e80-6.

Cancer Chemotherapy Toxicity

Chapter 126
Chemotherapy-induced Nausea and Vomiting

Lynne Nakashima, BSc(Pharm), PharmD

Managing nausea and vomiting in patients receiving chemotherapy continues to be a challenge. Although data on relative emetogenicity are available for many iv chemotherapeutic agents, data are less available for oral chemotherapy regimens. However, managing nausea and vomiting in patients on oral chemotherapy is no less problematic.

Goals of Therapy

- Prevent or minimize *acute* (starting within 24 hours of chemotherapy), *delayed* (starting >24 hours after chemotherapy) and *anticipatory* (starting before chemotherapy as a conditioned response) nausea and vomiting to maintain quality of life, to help patient adherence with active treatment and to avoid treatment delays
- Decrease incidence and severity of nausea and vomiting (once it has occurred) and maintain patient comfort[1]
- Prevent complications, such as esophageal tears, dehydration, anorexia, malnutrition, weight loss, pathological bone fractures, metabolic alkalosis, chloride and potassium depletion[1]

Investigations

- A thorough history including:
  - onset and duration of symptoms
  - timing of nausea and/or retching and/or vomiting
  - impact on the patient, e.g., weight loss, asthenia
  - description of the vomiting episodes
  - medications
- Physical examination with particular attention to:
  - orthostatic hypotension
  - abdominal pain, distention, constipation, hemorrhage
  - neurologic assessment including cranial nerves, vestibular and pupillary functions, extrapyramidal signs
- Laboratory tests:
  - electrolytes: urea, creatinine, sodium, potassium, chloride (to assess hydration status); calcium, albumin (to assess for hypercalcemia)
  - drug screening, such as for digoxin if suspected as a cause of nausea and vomiting

Although medication is the most likely cause of nausea and vomiting in a patient receiving chemotherapy, rule out other potential causes (e.g., fluid/electrolyte abnormalities, bowel obstruction, CNS or hepatic metastases, infections and radiation therapy). Other drugs (e.g., opioids, digoxin, antibiotics) may cause or exacerbate nausea and vomiting; therefore, a thorough medication history is essential. Some chemotherapeutic agents are more likely to cause nausea and vomiting than others (Table 1). It is important to consider the emetogenic potential, the dose of the chemotherapy agents and the expected pattern of emesis of the chemotherapy regimen when choosing antiemetics.[2,3,4,5,6]

Table 1: **Emetogenic Potential of IV Chemotherapy Agents**[a]

Emetogenic Potential	Chemotherapy Agents		
High (>90%)	carmustine cisplatin	cyclophosphamide (>1500 mg/m^2) dacarbazine	mechlorethamine streptozocin
Moderate (30–90%)	carboplatin cyclophosphamide (<1500 mg/m^2) cytarabine (>1000 mg/m^2) daunorubicin	doxorubicin epirubicin ifosfamide irinotecan lomustine	methotrexate (dose-dependent) oxaliplatin procarbazine temozolomide
Low (10–30%)	altretamine (hexamethylmelamine) bortezomib capecitabine cetuximab cytarabine (<1000 mg/m^2) docetaxel etoposide 5-fluorouracil gemcitabine	hydroxyurea L-asparaginase lenalidomide melphalan mercaptopurine mitomycin mitoxantrone paclitaxel panitumomab pemetrexed	ralitrexed rituximab sunitinib 6-thioguanine teniposide thalidomide thiotepa topotecan trastuzumab
Minimal (<10%)	bevacizumab bleomycin busulfan chlorambucil	cladribine erlotinib fludarabine gefitinib	sorafenib vincristine vindesine vinorelbine

[a] Slowing infusion rate of certain chemotherapeutic agents (e.g., cisplatin) may decrease emesis.[7]

Patient-specific factors such as age <50 years, female gender and a history of motion sickness or chemotherapy-induced nausea and vomiting (CINV) may raise the risk of experiencing nausea and vomiting;[8] therefore, antiemetic regimens must be tailored to the individual patient.

Therapeutic Choices

Nonpharmacologic Choices[1,9,10,11]

- Dietary adjustments:
  - try small, light meals several times daily.
  - avoid foods high in fat or those with a heavy aroma.
  - try dry, starchy foods, such as crackers.
  - if unable to tolerate solid foods, try ice chips and small sips of clear liquids.
  - avoid food preparation because the smell of food cooking often worsens nausea.
- Behavioural methods:
  - relaxation techniques may help decrease physiologic arousal and anxiety.
  - individualized exercise programs may help decrease anxiety and depression.
  - systemic desensitization may be helpful for anticipatory nausea and vomiting.
- Other:
  - keep movement to a minimum; rest in bed or a chair to avoid vestibular stimulation.
  - acupuncture and acupressure may be effective in alleviating CINV.[12,13]
  - sleep has been shown to protect against CINV.[14]

Pharmacologic Choices

Nausea and vomiting are mediated through a number of receptors, however, the type 3 serotonin ($5\text{-}HT_3$) and neurokinin-1 (NK-1) receptors appear to be most important in CINV. Antiemetic agents targeting other neurotransmitters are important additional agents to help provide optimal prevention and treatment, but are not used as single agents for moderate or highly emetogenic chemotherapy regimens.

- Prevention of acute nausea and vomiting is the best way to prevent delayed nausea and vomiting.
- Successful prevention of acute and delayed CINV in a current chemotherapy cycle is the best way to prevent anticipatory nausea and vomiting in subsequent cycles.
- Use antiemetic therapy to *prevent* anticipatory nausea and vomiting, which usually worsens with each cycle; up to 30% of patients refuse further chemotherapy because of intolerable nausea and vomiting.[2,3]
- *Regularly scheduled and administered* antiemetics (not PRN) are more effective at preventing nausea and vomiting.

Figure 1 outlines the prevention of CINV and management of breakthrough nausea and vomiting for regimens with minimal, low, moderate and high emetogenic potential. Individual medications are detailed in Table 2.

Serotonin Antagonists

The first-generation $5\text{-}HT_3$ receptor antagonists ($5\text{-}HT_3RAs$) **granisetron** and **ondansetron** have equivalent efficacy and toxicity when used for the prevention of acute chemotherapy-induced nausea and vomiting.[15,16,17] Injectable **palonosetron**, a second-generation $5\text{-}HT_3RA$, is the only drug in this class effective in preventing acute *and* delayed nausea and vomiting associated with moderately emetogenic chemotherapy [Evidence: SORT A*].[18,19,20,21] Single-dose iv palonosetron prior to start of chemotherapy may be a more convenient option over the first-generation agents if multiple-day $5\text{-}HT_3RA$ dosing is anticipated. *Intravenous* dolasetron is no longer available due to increased risk of serious arrhythmias.[22] High-dose ondansetron may also increase the risk of serious cardiac arrhythmias. As a result the maximum recommended single iv ondansetron dose has been lowered to 16 mg.[23] Single-agent efficacy is reported, but when used in combination with a **corticosteroid** and **aprepitant** for highly emetogenic regimens, efficacy is improved. These drugs are generally well tolerated.

Neurokinin-1 Receptor Antagonists

The NK-1 receptor antagonists aprepitant and **fosaprepitant** bind to substance P, found in the brainstem and GI tract. Aprepitant is an oral NK-1 receptor antagonist while its prodrug fosaprepitant is used iv. When added to a $5\text{-}HT_3RA$ plus **dexamethasone** regimen for highly emetogenic chemotherapy, NK-1 receptor antagonists improve prevention of acute and delayed emesis.[24,25] Aprepitant is a moderate inhibitor of CYP3A4 and interacts with corticosteroids. Therefore, the dose of dexamethasone as an antiemetic is decreased with concomitant use of aprepitant. Aprepitant appears to be well tolerated, with asthenia/fatigue and hiccups being the most commonly reported side effects.[26]

Corticosteroids

Dexamethasone is the most commonly used corticosteroid, although several others including **methylprednisolone** have been studied.[27] The actual mechanism of action is unknown, but they appear to be effective as single agents or in combination with other antiemetics and are particularly effective in the prevention of delayed nausea and vomiting.[27,28] The combination of dexamethasone with a $5\text{-}HT_3RA$ and a NK-1 receptor antagonist is the most effective antiemetic regimen for acute nausea and vomiting.[29,30]

* SORT (Strength of Recommendation Taxonomy) is a rating system (A, B or C) that addresses the quality of available evidence. For more information consult **How to Use *Compendium of Therapeutic Choices*** on page xxv.

Dopamine Antagonists

Prochlorperazine and **metoclopramide** are the most commonly used dopamine antagonists in the management of nausea and vomiting in chemotherapy regimens with low emetogenicity or as rescue agents.[31] Both agents block the dopaminergic receptors in the chemoreceptor trigger zone. Prochlorperazine may also exhibit serotonin antagonistic activity at higher doses. The availability of a wide variety of dosage forms (tablet, suppository, injectable) facilitates prochlorperazine use, especially for outpatients. Low doses of metoclopramide (10–20 mg) are generally as effective as prochlorperazine; however, in high doses (1–3 mg/kg), metoclopramide provides significantly higher antiemetic activity.[32] A limitation to metoclopramide use is the development of extrapyramidal side effects.

Although insufficient evidence from randomized, controlled trials exists,[33] **haloperidol** may be useful in the management of refractory nausea and vomiting due to chemotherapy,[31,34,35] but may be less effective than metoclopramide.[36]

Olanzapine antagonizes several neurotransmitter receptors including dopamine and 5-HT receptors and has shown some activity in acute, delayed and breakthrough nausea and vomiting.[37,38,39]

Benzodiazepines

Benzodiazepines provide useful antianxiety, amnesic and sedating effects. **Lorazepam** and **alprazolam** are the most commonly used, and have been studied in cases of anticipatory nausea.[40,41] They are usually used in combination with other antiemetics.[31,42,43]

Cannabinoids

Nabilone is of limited use because it is available only as an oral formulation and is associated with several side effects including dry mouth, dizziness, drowsiness, mood alterations, hallucinations, delusions, tachycardia and hypotension.[2,44,45] Higher doses are associated with increased risk of side effects. It is generally used in refractory nausea and vomiting or in combination with other antiemetics.[2]

Antihistamines and Anticholinergics

The antihistamine **dimenhydrinate** and the antimuscarinic **scopolamine** are useful for treating vomiting due to motion sickness but they are considered no more effective than placebo against CINV.[46,47]

Therapeutic Tips

- If the patient can tolerate oral antiemetics, this is the recommended route of administration. However, *rectally* administered antiemetics such as prochlorperazine are especially useful in patients who are vomiting or unable to take oral medications and who are at home. For hospitalized patients, the *iv route* of administration is recommended in patients who are vomiting.

Figure 1: **Prevention and Management of Chemotherapy-induced Nausea and Vomiting**[31,42,43]

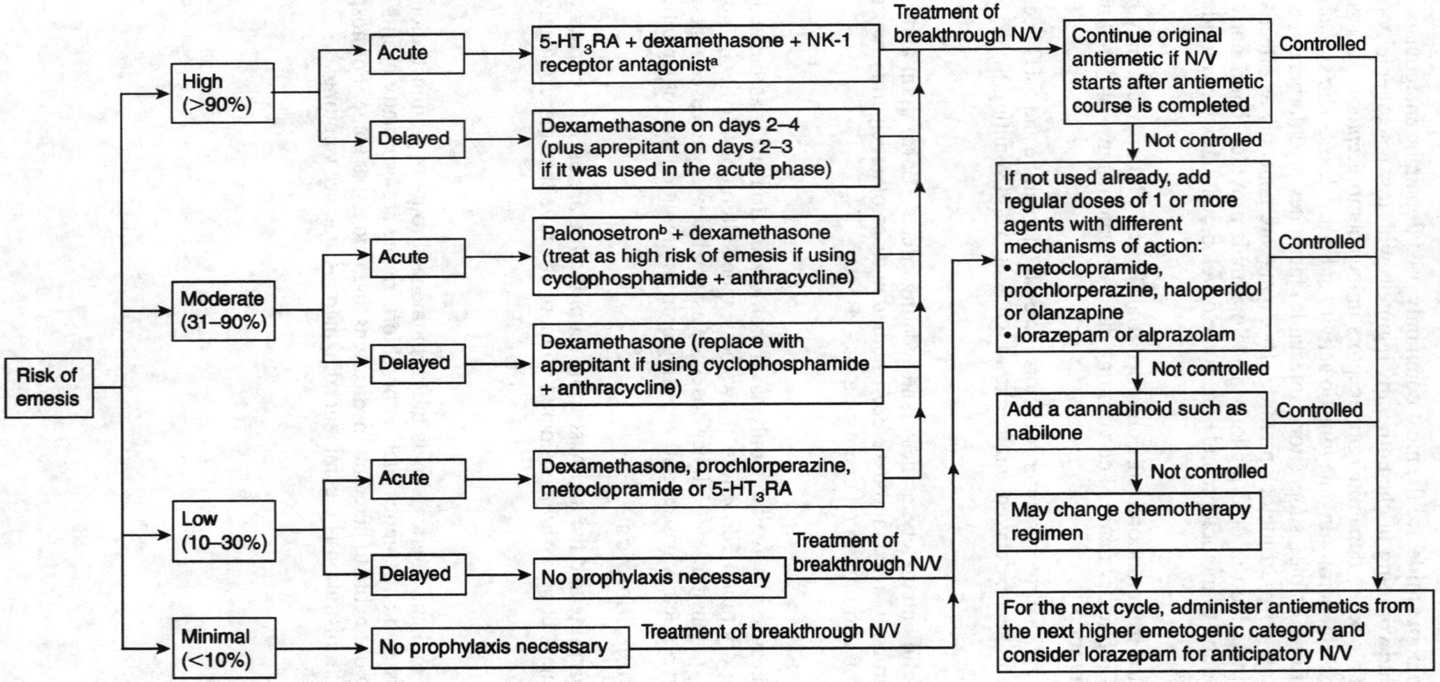

[a] Neurokinin-1 receptor antagonists are aprepitant and its injectable form fosaprepitant. Aprepitant is administered for 3 consecutive days starting 1 hour before start of chemotherapy cycle. A single dose of fosaprepitant injection on day one 30 minutes before start of chemotherapy may replace all 3 days of oral aprepitant dosing regimen.

[b] Palonosetron is the preferred 5-HT_3RA. If palonosetron is unavailable, use any other 5-HT_3RA.

Abbreviations: 5-HT_3RA = 5-HT_3 receptor antagonist; N/V = nausea and vomiting; NK-1 = neurokinin-1

Table 2: **Drugs Used for Chemotherapy-induced Nausea and Vomiting**[31,42,43]

Class	Drug	Dose	Adverse Effects	Drug Interactions	Cost[a]
Benzodiazepines	*lorazepam* Ativan, generics	0.5–2 mg Q4–6H po	Sedation.	Additive sedation occurs with other sedating medications such as opioid analgesics, hypnotics, alcohol; avoid or minimize concurrent use if possible.	$
Cannabinoids	*nabilone* Cesamet, generics	Starting dose is 0.5 mg BID po titrated up to 1–2 mg BID po as tolerated. Maximum 6 mg per day. First dose is given the night before start of chemotherapy and the second dose is usually administered 1–3 hours before chemotherapy.	Sedation, dizziness, ataxia, psychotropic effects ("high"), tachycardia, orthostatic hypotension, dry mouth.	See lorazepam.	$
Corticosteroids	*dexamethasone* Dexasone, generics	HEC, MEC or LEC: Acute: 12 mg single dose po/iv on day 1 Dose is increased to 20 mg in HEC or MEC if aprepitant or fosaprepitant is not also used HEC or MEC: Delayed: 8 mg once daily po on days 2–4	Mood changes, increased appetite, GI irritation, ulceration, fluid retention, weight gain, may mask signs of infection.	Dexamethasone is a CYP3A4 substrate. CYP3A4 inhibitors (e.g., ketoconazole, erythromycin, clarithromycin) may decrease its metabolism. Antacids and CYP3A4 inducers (e.g., carbamazepine, phenobarbital, phenytoin, rifampin) may increase its metabolism. Aprepitant and fosaprepitant may increase the serum concentration of dexamethasone. Dosing guidelines account for this by decreasing the recommended dose of dexamethasone (usually reduced from 20 mg to 8–12 mg) when aprepitant or fosaprepitant is coadministered.	$
Dopamine Antagonists	*haloperidol* generics	1–2 mg Q4–6H PRN po	Sedation, extrapyramidal effects.	See lorazepam.	$
	metoclopramide ❥ Metonia, other generics	10–40 mg Q4–6H PRN po/iv	Sedation, dose-related diarrhea, extrapyramidal effects.	See lorazepam. Anticholinergic agents antagonize effects of metoclopramide on GI motility.	po: $ iv: $$$$

(cont'd)

Table 2: **Drugs Used for Chemotherapy-induced Nausea and Vomiting**[31,42,43] *(cont'd)*

Class	Drug	Dose	Adverse Effects	Drug Interactions	Cost[a]
	olanzapine Zyprexa, generics	2.5–5 mg BID po	Dizziness, constipation, postural hypotension, akathisia, somnolence, dry mouth.	Concomitant use with benzodiazepines may cause cardiorespiratory depression and excessive sedation. Use with metoclopramide may raise risk of tardive dyskinesia. Strong CYP1A2 inhibitors (ciprofloxacin, fluvoxamine, ketoconazole, norfloxacin, ofloxacin) may decrease the metabolism of olanzapine. Olanzapine may decrease the therapeutic effect of antiparkinsonian agents.	$
	prochlorperazine ❥ generics	10 mg Q4–6H PRN po/iv or 25 mg Q12H pr	Sedation, anticholinergic effects (dry mouth, blurred vision, constipation, nasal congestion, urinary retention), extrapyramidal effects, hypotension, hypersensitivity, rare pancytopenia.	See lorazepam.	$
Neurokinin-1 Receptor Antagonists	*aprepitant* Emend	**Not used as monotherapy** Day 1: 125 mg 1 h before chemotherapy po Days 2 & 3: 80 mg once daily po	Asthenia/fatigue, diarrhea, dizziness, dyspepsia, hiccups.	Contraindicated with pimozide. Increases levels of drugs metabolized by CYP3A4 (e.g., dexamethasone, midazolam). Decreases levels of drugs metabolized by CYP2C9 (e.g., phenytoin, tolbutamide, warfarin). Increased levels of aprepitant with CYP3A4 inhibitors (e.g., erythromycin, clarithromycin, ketoconazole). Decreased levels of aprepitant with CYP3A4 inducers (carbamazepine, phenytoin, rifampin). Possible reduced effectiveness of oral contraceptives.	$$$$/ Tri-Pack
	fosaprepitant Emend IV	**Not used as monotherapy** Day 1 only: 150 mg infused iv over 20–30 min approximately 30 min prior to chemotherapy	See aprepitant.	Fosaprepitant is rapidly converted to aprepitant after injection. See aprepitant.	$$$$

Class	Drug	Dose	Adverse Effects	Drug Interactions	Cost[a]
Serotonin Antagonists	*granisetron* generics	po: 2 mg single dose or 1 mg BID iv: 0.01 mg/kg (maximum 1 mg) per day	Bradycardia, constipation, diarrhea, dizziness, headache, QT interval prolongation, sedation, transient increases in laboratory values of liver function tests.	No clinically significant drug interactions.	$$
	ondansetron Ondissolve ODF, Zofran, Zofran ODT, generics	po: 16–24 mg per day iv: up to 16 mg initially infused over no less than 15 min (do not exceed 8 mg if ≥75 years). Subsequent iv doses must not exceed 8 mg/dose and may be given 4 and 8 hours after the initial dose.	See granisetron.	No clinically significant drug interactions.	po: $ iv: $$
	palonosetron Aloxi	po: 0.5 mg single dose before start of chemotherapy iv: 0.25 mg single dose before start of chemotherapy	See granisetron.	No clinically significant drug interactions.	po: $$$ iv: $$$$

[a] Cost based on 50 kg body weight for a 1-day supply (unless otherwise specified); includes drug cost only.
Dosage adjustment may be required in renal impairment; see Appendix I.
Abbreviations: HEC = highly emetogenic chemotherapy; LEC = low emetogenic chemotherapy; MEC = moderately emetogenic chemotherapy
Legend: $ <25 $$ $25–50 $$$ $50–75 $$$$ $75–100

Suggested Readings

Basch E, Prestrud AA, Hesketh PJ et al. Antiemetics: American Society of Clinical Oncology clinical practice guideline update. *J Clin Oncol* 2011;29(31):4189-98.

Hesketh PJ. Chemotherapy-induced nausea and vomiting. *N Engl J Med* 2008;358(23):2482-94.

Multinational Association of Supportive Care in Cancer. *MASCC/ESMO antiemetic guideline 2013.* Available from: www.mascc.org/assets/documents/mascc_guidelines_english_2013.pdf.

National Comprehensive Cancer Network. *Clinical practice guidelines in oncology: antiemesis.* Version 2.2011. Available from: www.nccn.org/professionals/physician_gls/f_guidelines.asp. Registration required.

Navari RM. Management of chemotherapy-induced nausea and vomiting: focus on newer agents and new uses for older agents. *Drugs* 2013;73(3):249-62.

References

1. Roscoe JA, Morrow GR, Aapro MS et al. Anticipatory nausea and vomiting. *Support Care Cancer* 2011;19(10):1533-8.
2. Hesketh PJ. Chemotherapy-induced nausea and vomiting. *N Engl J Med* 2008;358(23):2482-94.
3. Lindley CM, Bernard S, Fields SM. Incidence and duration of chemotherapy-induced nausea and vomiting in the outpatient oncology population. *J Clin Oncol* 1989;7(8):1142-9.
4. Warr DG. Chemotherapy- and cancer-related nausea and vomiting. *Curr Oncol* 2008;15(Suppl 1):S4-9.
5. BC Cancer Agency. *Cancer management guidelines. Supportive care.* Available from: www.bccancer.bc.ca/HPI/CancerManagementGuidelines/SupportiveCare/default.htm. Accessed February 9, 2011.
6. Cancer Care Ontario. *Antiemetic Report.* October 2013. Accessed February 28, 2014.
7. Jordan NS, Schauer PK, Schauer A et al. The effect of administration rate on cisplatin-induced emesis. *J Clin Oncol* 1985;3(4):559-61.
8. Vidall C, Dielenseger P, Farrell C et al. Evidence-based management of chemotherapy-induced nausea and vomiting: a position statement from a European cancer nursing forum. *Ecancermedicalscience* 2011;5:211.
9. Jordan K, Sippel C, Schmoll HJ. Guidelines for antiemetic treatment of chemotherapy-induced nausea and vomiting: past, present, and future recommendations. *Oncologist* 2007;12(9):1143-50.
10. Wickham R. Best practice management of CINV in oncology patients: II. Antiemetic guidelines and rationale for use. *J Support Oncol* 2010;8(2 Suppl 1):10-5.
11. McMillan C, Dundee JW, Abram WP. Enhancement of the antiemetic action of ondansetron by transcutaneous electrical stimulation of the P6 antiemetic point, in patients having highly emetic cytotoxic drugs. *Br J Cancer* 1991;64(5):971-2.
12. Kaptchuk TJ. Acupuncture: theory, efficacy, and practice. *Ann Intern Med* 2002;136(5):374-83.
13. Garcia MK, McQuade J, Haddad R et al. Systematic review of acupuncture in cancer care: a synthesis of the evidence. *J Clin Oncol* 2013;31(7):952-60.
14. Dominguez-Ortega L, Cubedo-Cervera R, Cortes-Funes H et al. Sleep protects against chemotherapy induced emesis. *Cancer* 1996;77(8):1566-70.
15. Jordan K, Hinke A, Grothey A et al. A meta-analysis comparing the efficacy of four 5-HT3-receptor antagonists for acute chemotherapy-induced emesis. *Support Care Cancer* 2007;15(9):1023-33.
16. del Giglio A, Soares HP, Caparroz C et al. Granisetron is equivalent to ondansetron for prophylaxis of chemotherapy-induced nausea and vomiting: results of a meta-analysis of randomized controlled trials. *Cancer* 2000;89(11):2301-8.
17. Billio A, Morello E, Clarke MJ. Serotonin receptor antagonists for highly emetogenic chemotherapy in adults. *Cochrane Database Syst Rev* 2010;(1):CD006272.
18. Jin Y, Sun W, Gu D et al. Comparative efficacy and safety of palonosetron with the first 5-HT3 receptor antagonists for the chemotherapy-induced nausea and vomiting: a meta-analysis. *Eur J Cancer Care (Engl)* 2013;22(1):41-50.
19. Likun Z, Xiang J, Yi B et al. A systematic review and meta-analysis of intravenous palonosetron in the prevention of chemotherapy-induced nausea and vomiting in adults. *Oncologist* 2011;16(2):207-16.
20. Botrel TE, Clark OA, Clark L et al. Efficacy of palonosetron (PAL) compared to other serotonin inhibitors (5-HT3R) in preventing chemotherapy-induced nausea and vomiting (CINV) in patients receiving moderately or highly emetogenic (MoHE) treatment: systematic review and meta-analysis. *Support Care Cancer* 2011;19(6):823-32.
21. Celio L, Agustoni F, Testa I et al. Palonosetron: an evidence-based choice in prevention of nausea and vomiting induced by moderately emetogenic chemotherapy. *Tumori* 2012;98(3):279-86.
22. Health Canada. *ANZEMET (dolasetron mesylate): Withdrawal of 20 mg/mL intravenous injection due to potential risk of arrhythmias.* Available from: www.healthycanadians.gc.ca/recall-alert-rappel-avis/hc-sc/2011/14633a-eng.php.
23. GlaxoSmithKline. *Zofran (ondansetron hydrochloride dihydrate, ondansetron)—Important new safety information: Association of Zofran with changes in electrical activity in the heart.* 2012. Available from: www.gsk.ca/english/docs-pdf/Zofran_PC.pdf.
24. Hesketh PJ, Grunberg SM, Gralla RJ et al. The oral neurokinin-1 antagonist aprepitant for the prevention of chemotherapy-induced nausea and vomiting: a multinational, randomized, double-blind, placebo-controlled trial in patients receiving high-dose cisplatin-The Aprepitant Protocol 052 Study Group. *J Clin Oncol* 2003;21(22):4112-9.
25. Poli-Bigelli S, Rodrigues-Pereira J, Carides AD et al. Addition of the neurokinin 1 receptor antagonist aprepitant to standard antiemetic therapy improves control of chemotherapy-induced nausea and vomiting: results from a randomized, double-blind, placebo-controlled trial in Latin America. *Cancer* 2003;97(12):3090-8.
26. Dando TM, Perry CM. Aprepitant: a review of its use in the prevention of chemotherapy-induced nausea and vomiting. *Drugs* 2004;64(7):777-94.
27. Lindley C, Goodin S, McCune J et al. Prevention of delayed chemotherapy-induced nausea and vomiting after moderately high to highly emetogenic chemotherapy: comparison of ondansetron, prochlorperazine, and dexamethasone. *Am J Clin Oncol* 2005;28(3):270-6.
28. Ioannidis JP, Hesketh PJ, Lau J. Contribution of dexamethasone to control of chemotherapy-induced nausea and vomiting: a meta-analysis of randomized evidence. *J Clin Oncol* 2000;18(19):3409-22.

29. Nevidjon B, Chaudhary R. Controlling emesis: evolving challenges, novel strategies. *J Support Oncol* 2010;8(4 Suppl 2):1-10.
30. Roila F, Tonato M, Cognetti F et al. Prevention of cisplatin-induced emesis: a double-blind multicenter randomized crossover study comparing ondansetron and ondansetron plus dexamethasone. *J Clin Oncol* 1991;9(4):675-8.
31. National Comprehensive Cancer Network. *Clinical practice guidelines in oncology: antiemesis*. Version 2.2011. Available from: www.nccn.org/professionals/physician_gls/f_guidelines.asp. Accessed February 3, 2011. Registration required.
32. Gralla RJ. Metoclopramide. A review of antiemetic trials. *Drugs* 1983;25(Suppl 1):63-73.
33. Perkins P, Dorman S. Haloperidol for the treatment of nausea and vomiting in palliative care patients. *Cochrane Database Syst Rev* 2009;(2):CD006271.
34. Plotkin DA, Plotkin D, Okun R. Haloperidol in the treatment of nausea and vomiting due to cytotoxic drug administration. *Curr Ther Res Clin Exp* 1973;15(9):599-602.
35. Tornetta FJ. Double-blind evaluation of haloperidol for antiemetic activity. *Anesth Analg* 1972;51(6):964-7.
36. Grunberg SM, Gala KV, Lampenfeld M et al. Comparison of the antiemetic effect of high-dose intravenous metoclopramide and high-dose intravenous haloperidol in a randomized double-blind crossover study. *J Clin Oncol* 1984;2(7):782-7.
37. Navari RM, Einhorn LH, Passik SD et al. A phase II trial of olanzapine for the prevention of chemotherapy-induced nausea and vomiting: a Hoosier Oncology Group study. *Support Care Cancer* 2005;13(7):529-34.
38. Navari RM, Einhorn LH Loehrer PJ et al. A phase II trial of olanzapine, dexamethasone, and palonosetron for prevention of chemotherapy-induced nausea and vomiting: a Hoosier Oncology Group study. *Support Care Cancer* 2007;15(11):1285-91.
39. Navari RM, Nagy CK, Gray SE. The use of olanzapine versus metoclopramide for the treatment of breakthrough chemotherapy-induced nausea and vomiting in patients receiving highly emetogenic chemotherapy. *Support Care Cancer* 2013;21(6):1655-63.
40. Malik IA, Khan WA, Qazilbash M et al. Clinical efficacy of lorazepam in prophylaxis of anticipatory acute and delayed nausea and vomiting induced by high doses of cisplatin. A prospective randomized trial. *Am J Clin Oncol*1995;18(2):170-5.
41. Razavi D, Delvaux N, Farvacques C et al. Prevention of adjustment disorders and anticipatory nausea secondary to adjuvant chemotherapy: a double-blind, placebo-controlled study assessing the usefulness of alprazolam. *J Clin Oncol* 1993;11(7):1384-90.
42. American Society of Clinical Oncology, Kris MG, Hesketh PJ et al. American Society of Clinical Oncology guideline for antiemetics in oncology: update 2006. *J Clin Oncol* 2006;24(18):2932-47.
43. Roila F, Herrstedt J, Aapro M et al. Guideline update for MASCC and ESMO in the prevention of chemotherapy- and radiotherapy-induced nausea and vomiting: results of the Perugia consensus conference. *Ann Oncol* 2010;21(Suppl 5):v232-43.
44. Slatkin NE. Cannabinoids in the treatment of chemotherapy-induced nausea and vomiting: beyond prevention of acute emesis. *J Support Oncol* 2007;5(5 Suppl 3):1-9.
45. Sutton IR, Daeninck P. Cannabinoids in the management of intractable chemotherapy-induced nausea and vomiting and cancer-related pain. *J Support Oncol* 2006;4(10):531-5.
46. Wood CD. Antimotion sickness and antiemetic drugs. *Drugs* 1979;17(6):471-9.
47. Longo DL, Wesley M, Howser D et al. Results of a randomized double-blind crossover trial of scopolamine versus placebo administered by transdermal patch for the control of cisplatin-induced emesis. *Cancer Treat Rep* 1982;66(11):1975-6.

Chapter 127

Management of Side Effects of Chemotherapy and Radiation Therapy

Mova Leung, BScPhm, PharmD, BCOP

Radiation and chemotherapy (Table 1) are highly toxic therapies that confer side effects normally unacceptable in the treatment of other diseases. Furthermore, patients with cancer are living long enough for delayed side effects to manifest.

Cancer cells grow and divide faster than normal cells. Chemotherapeutic drugs exploit this difference by affecting fast-growing, highly proliferative cells during replication, killing more cancer cells than normal cells. Hematopoietic cells, the skin and its appendages and the epithelium of the intestine are also highly proliferative, thus they are susceptible to toxicity from chemotherapy.

Contrary to chemotherapy, where most side effects occur upon exposure and generally resolve over time once therapy is completed, any organ that is exposed to radiation can develop early (within days to months) toxicities or delayed (within months to years) toxicities. Radiation is delivered locally, thus toxicities usually occur locally. X-rays travel through the tissues from an entry point into, to an exit point out of, the body. Toxicities can occur throughout this area.

This chapter's focus is on select toxicities that are predictable and preventable in onset or severity. While pediatric management is generally the same, the focus is the adult patient.

Goals of Therapy

- Prevent toxicity if possible by treating risk factors and applying preventive measures
- Reduce the severity of toxicity and subsequent complications by early detection and management
- Improve or control symptoms of toxicity once they occur
- Improve or maintain quality of life and ability to perform activities of daily living
- Reduce hospitalization
- Prevent morbidity and mortality

Therapeutic Tips

- Patient education and involvement in preventive measures and detection are paramount
- Full disclosure of side effects to the patient will ensure better management of toxicity
- Contrary to some beliefs, discussion of side effects does not predispose patients to experiencing them[1,2]
- Frequency and severity of toxicity are dependent on the drug, dose, dosing schedule and route of administration.

Table 1: Common Chemotherapeutic Classes

Chemotherapy Class	Drugs
Alkylating agents	bendamustine, busulfan, carmustine (BCNU), chlorambucil, cyclophosphamide, ifosfamide, lomustine (CCNU), mechlorethamine, melphalan, streptozocin
Alkylating agents, nonclassic	dacarbazine (DTIC), procarbazine, temozolomide
Anthracyclines	daunorubicin, doxorubicin, epirubicin, idarubicin, liposomal doxorubicin
Anthracenediones	mitoxantrone
Antimetabolites	Antifolates: methotrexate, pemetrexed, raltitrexed Fluoropyrimidines: capecitabine, fluorouracil Cytidineanalogues: azacitidine, cytarabine (ara-C; cytosine arabinoside), gemcitabine Purine antimetabolites: azathioprine, cladribine, fludarabine, 6-mercaptopurine, 6-thioguanine
Antitumour antibiotics	bleomycin, dactinomycin, mitomycin C
Hormonal agents	Aromatase inhibitors: anastrozole, exemestane, letrozole Antiandrogens: abiraterone, bicalutamide, cyproterone, enzalutamide, flutamide, nilutamide Selective estrogen receptor modulators: raloxifene, tamoxifen Antiestrogen: fulvestrant GnRH analogues: buserelin, degarelix, goserelin, leuprolide
Immunomodulators	interferon, interleukin
Monoclonal antibodies	alemtuzumab, bevacizumab, cetuximab, panitumumab, pertuzumab, rituximab, tositumomab, trastuzumab, trastuzumab emtansine (T-DM1)
Mammalian target of rapamycin (mTOR) inhibitors	everolimus, temsirolimus
Platinums	carboplatin, cisplatin, oxaliplatin
Proteasome inhibitors	bortezomib
Small molecule kinase inhibitors	axitinib, crizotinib, dabrafenib, dasatinib, erlotinib, gefitinib, imatinib, lapatinib, pazopanib, regorafenib, ruxolitinib, sunitinib, sorafenib, trametinib, vandetanib, vemurafenib, vismodegib
Taxanes	cabazitaxel, docetaxel, nab-paclitaxel, paclitaxel
Thalidomide and analogues	lenalinomide, thalidomide
Topoisomerase I inhibitors	Camptothecin analogues: irinotecan (CPT-11), topotecan
Topoisomerase II inhibitors	Epipodophyllotoxins: etoposide (VP-16), teniposide
Vinca alkaloids	vinblastine, vincristine, vindesine, vinorelbine
Others	amsacrine, asparaginase, Bacillus Calmette Guerin (BCG)

Abbreviations: GnRH = gonadotropin-releasing hormone; nab-paclitaxel = nanoparticle albumin bound paclitaxel

Table 2: **Prevention and Management of Select Toxicities of Chemotherapies**

Toxicity/Organ Involved (Time frame to onset)	Classes/Drugs Commonly Implicated	Prevention	Management
Cardiac			
Coronary vasospasm and myocardial ischemia (within hours to days)	**Fluoropyrimidines** capecitabine, fluorouracil	Initiate cautiously in patients with coronary artery disease; avoid in patients with severe or unstable conditions. Prophylactic use of calcium channel blockers has shown some benefit for patients at risk.[3]	Usually reversible with cessation of the drug. Treat symptomatically with **nitrates** and **calcium channel blockers**. Discontinuation of fluoropyrimidine suggested.[4]
Heart failure (within months to years)	Lapatinib, trastuzumab	Cardiac monitoring for all patients receiving trastuzumab. More frequent monitoring if cardiac risk factors exist. Avoidance of simultaneous administration with other cytotoxic chemotherapies has dramatically reduced incidence of cardiotoxicity.[5,6]	Interruption of therapy for asymptomatic reductions in ejection fraction. Discontinuation usually recommended if clinically symptomatic or if interruptions are required multiple times.[5,7] Standard management of left ventricular dysfunction with ACE inhibitors, ARBs and/or beta-blockers. See Chapter 38.
	Anthracyclines daunorubicin, doxorubicin, epirubicin, idarubicin, liposomal doxorubicin	Limit cumulative doses. Consider discontinuing if serial ejection fraction drops 25% from baseline. **Dexrazoxane** used in the non-curative setting for patients whose lifetime cumulative anthracycline dose exceeds safe thresholds or who have underlying cardiac risk factors. Assess cardiac function periodically.[3,8]	Clinically indistinguishable from heart failure due to other causes. Treat symptomatically.[3,9] See Chapter 38.
Hypertension (within weeks to months)	Bevacizumab, many small molecule kinase inhibitors	Identify and manage risk factors for hypertension. Monitor blood pressure with every cycle of treatment with expectation of blood pressure elevations within the first few cycles of therapy.	Manage blood pressure aggressively but with consideration to the patient's clinical status and prognosis. See Chapter 39.
QT_c prolongation (within days to weeks)	Many small molecule kinase inhibitors	Initiate cautiously in patients with risk factors (e.g., congenital long QT syndrome, heart failure, electrolyte imbalances). Dose reductions based on QT_c are recommended for some drugs. Avoid concurrent use of drugs with additive risk of QT_c prolongation or high risk of cytochrome interactions (especially CYP3A4).[10]	If benefit of using the drug outweighs risk, monitor and resolve risk factors; perform baseline ECG and monitor frequently.
Venous thromboembolic events (within weeks to months)	Bevacizumab, sunitinib, thalidomide and analogues	Cancer is a major risk factor for venous thromboembolism and patients should receive prophylaxis accordingly. See Chapter 48. Routine prophylaxis for ambulatory patients receiving systemic chemotherapy is not recommended except for thalidomide and analogues.[11,12]	Vitamin K antagonists are used with caution as cancer patients are susceptible to wide fluctuations in INR. **Low molecular weight heparins** preferred for long-term anticoagulation.[11,12] See Chapter 48.

Toxicity/Organ Involved (Time frame to onset)	Classes/Drugs Commonly Implicated	Prevention	Management
Dermatologic			
Alopecia (within weeks to months)	Most conventional chemotherapies	To delay or minimize hair loss, treat hair gently by using mild shampoos, soft hairbrushes, and avoiding harsh chemicals and high heat settings on hair dryer. Scalp cooling remains controversial.[13]	Degree and location of hair loss can be partial or complete, depending on the chemotherapy regimen and the individual. Cosmetic intervention using wigs, hats or scarves.
Extravasation Leakage from iv line into surrounding tissues resulting in tissue inflammation and necrosis (during infusion to days)	Anthracyclines, antitumour antibiotics, mechlorethamine, platinums, taxanes, vinca alkaloids	Ensure good blood return from, and fluid flow into, the iv line. IV lines should not be placed in areas adjacent to tendons, nerves or arteries, or in areas affected by lymphedema or neurological weakness. The site should be monitored throughout chemotherapy treatment.[14,15,16]	Stop infusion. Aspirate any residual drug remaining in tissues. Apply cold compresses for 20 min 4 times daily for 1–2 days. Local heat application should be used for vinca alkaloids. Specific antidotes are **dimethylsulfoxide** (DMSO) for anthracyclines and antitumour antibiotics, and **sodium thiosulfate** for mechlorethamine. **Dexrazoxane** is a useful antidote for extravasation of anthracyclines.[17] Severe cases require plastic surgery.[14,16]
Hand-foot-skin reaction (within weeks to months)	Axitinib, regorafenib, sorafenib, sunitinib	Cool hands and feet frequently during treatment. Apply moisturizers and avoid extreme temperatures. Avoid irritation and friction from ill-fitting shoes and clothing. **Vitamin B_6** 150–200 mg/day sometimes prescribed (clinical evidence poor).[18,19]	Dose interruptions and reduction. Discontinue therapy if severe or recurs. Lanolin/petrolatum **emollients** (Bag Balm, Udderly Smooth) and wound care for desquamation and ulcerations.[20]
Hand-foot syndrome (within weeks to months)	Capecitabine, fluorouracil, liposomal doxorubicin		
Rash related to Epidermal Growth Factor Receptor (EGFR) inhibition (within weeks)	Cetuximab, erlotinib, gefitinib, lapatinib panitumumab	Moisturize liberally with hypoallergenic lotions. Limit UV exposure (apply sunscreen to exposed areas). Avoid harsh chemicals, soaps or detergents. Use cool or lukewarm water instead of hot water for showers. Avoid prolonged baths.[21] Proactive use of **topical corticosteroids** and oral **tetracyclines** can be considered.[22]	Mild reactions can be managed with **topical clindamycin** and corticosteroids. Oral tetracyclines in more severe rashes. Itch improves as rash improves. Severe itch may be alleviated with antihistamines. Avoid alcohol-containing products and acne treatments due to drying effect.[22]
Eyes, Ears, Nose and Throat (EENT)			
Conjunctivitis (within days)	Anthracyclines, cytarabine (doses >2 g/m^2), fluoropyramidines	Artificial tears may have a dilutional effect. For cytarabine, prednisolone 1% or dexamethasone 0.1% ophthalmic Q4–6H started before and continued >48 h post-cytarabine.[23] Ophthalmic diclofenac may also have a role.[24] No standard preventive measures for other chemotherapies.	Usually reversible upon discontinuation of offending agent. **Artificial tears** to provide local relief. **Corticosteroid ophthalmic preparations** to manage inflammation. Ocular pain may require analgesics.
Ototoxicity (within weeks to months)	Platinums	Audiograms every 3–4 cycles, especially in patients at risk (pre-existing hearing loss, chronic noise exposure, high cumulative doses of cisplatin).[25]	Can be irreversible. Reduce doses or avoid completely if possible.

(cont'd)

Table 2: **Prevention and Management of Select Toxicities of Chemotherapies** *(cont'd)*

Toxicity/Organ Involved (Time frame to onset)	Classes/Drugs Commonly Implicated	Prevention	Management
Gastrointestinal			
Cholinergic syndrome and acute diarrhea Abdominal cramps, flushing, miosis, lacrimation, rhinitis (during infusion to hours)	Irinotecan	Reduce the rate of infusion. Educate patient to report symptoms immediately so that treatment can be initiated.[26]	Symptoms managed with **atropine** 0.3–0.6 mg sc/iv PRN. Subsequent cycles of irinotecan may require prophylactic atropine.[27]
Constipation (within hours to days)	$5\text{-}HT_3$ antagonists, bortezomib, vinca alkaloids, thalidomides and analogues	Often unrecognized, constipation can occur 1 or 2 days after chemotherapy due to $5\text{-}HT_3$ antagonist antiemetics. See Chapter 126. Patient education and preventive measures, including laxatives and stool softeners, should be considered.	**Laxatives, stool softeners** and nonpharmacologic measures. Suppositories and enemas are used with prolonged, severe constipation, but they may introduce an infection risk in neutropenic patients. Educate patient to discontinue laxatives before the onset of chemotherapy-induced diarrhea.
Diarrhea (within days to weeks)	Alkylating agents, antimetabolites, irinotecan, platinums, taxanes, others	Educate patient on nonpharmacologic management, avoidance of potential triggers and careful monitoring. It is important to treat diarrhea before it progresses in severity. Patients starting chemotherapy at high risk for diarrhea should have antidiarrheal medications on hand. See Chapter 59.	Chemotherapy should be withheld until complete resolution of symptoms without the use of antidiarrheal therapy. Fluids and BRAT diet. **Loperamide** (high-dose regimen) or **diphenoxylate/atropine** PRN. Severe cases require **octreotide**, **antibiotics** and iv hydration.[28,29]
Mucositis (within days to weeks)	Most conventional chemotherapies, severity varies with agent and individual	Cryotherapy (ice chips) prevents mucositis or reduces its severity in patients receiving bolus treatments of fluorouracil or high-dose melphalan. **Palifermin** is used in patients receiving high-dose chemotherapy ± total body irradiation for autologous hematopoietic stem-cell transplant. Employ nonpharmacologic measures: basic oral hygiene and the use of a soft-bristle toothbrush that is replaced on a regular basis (includes brushing, flossing and the use of bland mouthwashes such as soda rinses, salt rinses or alcohol-free mouthwashes).[30]	Bland (saline or soda) rinses or combination **mouthwashes** for mild symptoms. Avoid alcohol-containing products. Combination mouthwashes usually are institution-specific and contain varying proportions of lidocaine, diphenhydramine, antacids, nystatin and dexamethasone. There is no optimal formulation. Systemic **analgesics** (e.g., opioids) for severe mucositis. Evidence supports the use of low-level laser therapy in transplant settings and in radiation therapy for head and neck cancer.[31,32]
Nausea and vomiting (during infusion to days)		See Chapter 126.	

Toxicity/Organ Involved (Time frame to onset)	Classes/Drugs Commonly Implicated	Prevention	Management
Hematologic			
Anemia (within weeks to months)	Most conventional chemotherapies, severity varies with agent and individual	No proven preventive measures. Erythropoietics should not be used prophylactically.	Packed red blood cells given to patients with severe or symptomatic anemia. Erythropoietics (**epoetin alfa** or **darbepoetin**) to reduce the need for transfusions in select patients with hemoglobin <100 g/L.[33] **Iron dextran** or **iron sucrose** iv for functional iron deficiency. Nonpharmacologic measures for fatigue: see Fatigue in Other toxicities below.
Neutropenia and febrile neutropenia (within days to weeks)	Most conventional chemotherapies, severity varies with agent and individual	Granulocyte colony stimulating factors (**pegfilgrastim** and **filgrastim**) in patients at high risk of febrile neutropenia where chemotherapy dosage reductions or delays should be avoided (i.e., patients who may expect a cure from their chemotherapy).[34,35] Antibiotics in select patients.[36,37] Employ nonpharmacologic measures: avoid infection (wash hands thoroughly and frequently, avoid large crowds and people with colds or flu, maintain good hygiene, monitor for symptoms of infection).[37,38]	Rapid recognition and response to potential infection required. Standard management of febrile neutropenia includes empiric broad-spectrum antibiotics, clinical assessment and supportive care. See Chapter 114.
Thrombocytopenia (within weeks)	Occurs rarely with many conventional chemotherapies; severity varies with agent and individual	No proven preventive measures.	Platelet transfusions are the mainstay of treatment for severe thrombocytopenia induced by chemotherapy.
Immunologic			
Hypersensitivity reactions Mediated by IgE, histamine, mast cells (during infusion to hours)	Asparaginase, bleomycin, cetuximab, epipodophyllotoxins, platinums, procarbazine	Preventive measures generally not initiated for most agents. For bleomycin, the use of a test dose is suggested but is not universally accepted.[39]	Stop chemotherapy infusion. Administer antihistamines, steroids, vasoconstrictors. Supportive care. Desensitization protocols if platinums must be continued.[40]
	Taxanes	Taxanes are premedicated with oral or iv corticosteroids (usually started at least 12 h prior to chemo) and antihistamines (H_1- and H_2-blockers given right before chemotherapy).	Stop chemotherapy infusion. Medical and supportive care with antihistamines, corticosteroids, vasoconstrictors, oxygen, bronchodilators. Reintroduction can be done cautiously, with slower infusions.
Infusion reactions Cytokine-mediated or result of interactions with molecular target (during infusion to hours)	Monoclonal antibodies	Premedication with corticosteroids and antihistamines generally required. Humanized monoclonal antibodies such as trastuzumab, bevacizumab and panitumumab can usually be administered without premedication.	Severe reactions require cessation of infusion and administration of vasopressors, corticosteroids, antihistamines and bronchodilators. Consider discontinuation of therapy in severe cases. Mild reactions can be managed by slowing the infusion rate[41] or administering antihistamines and/or corticosteroids before continuing infusion.

(cont'd)

Table 2: **Prevention and Management of Select Toxicities of Chemotherapies** *(cont'd)*

Toxicity/Organ Involved (Time frame to onset)	Classes/Drugs Commonly Implicated	Prevention	Management
Metabolic			
Hypokalemia, hypomagnesemia (within days to weeks)	Cetuximab, panitumumab, platinums	Treat deficiencies prior to chemotherapy. Monitor levels while on treatment. Mg^{++} and K^{+} given iv with some chemotherapy protocols.	Supplemental **magnesium** and **potassium** to replace deficits. Mild deficits often managed orally.
Tumour lysis syndrome Combination of hyperuricemia, hyperkalemia, hypocalcemia, hyperphosphatemia, renal failure, cardiac arrhythmias and seizure (within hours to days)	Seen in cancers with large tumor burden and high sensitivity to chemotherapy, e.g., leukemias, lymphomas	Prevention for patients at risk. Aggressive hydration ± diuretics to maintain adequate urine output, **allopurinol** or **rasburicase** to prevent and manage hyperuricemia. Close monitoring of serum electrolytes, with accordant adjustments of contents of iv fluids, and urine output.	Treatment of hyperkalemia, hyperphosphatemia and hypocalcemia if symptomatic or severe. Hyperuricemia is managed with allopurinol or rasburicase. Dialysis for severe electrolyte abnormalities or signs of acute renal failure.[42,43]
Musculoskeletal			
Arthralgias and myalgias (within hours to days)	Aromatase inhibitors, interferons, taxanes, others	Increased hydration prior to and during therapy may benefit myalgias associated with interferon.[44] No proven preventive measures for taxanes or aromatase inhibitors although gabapentin and antihistamines have been tried.[45]	Systemic analgesics and rest. Introduce mild exercise, behavioural (e.g., relaxation techniques) and physical therapies (e.g., massage).[46] May be related to abrupt cessation of corticosteroids in premedications or antiemetic regimens (for taxanes) and should be ruled out. NSAIDs may be cautiously considered only after other modalities have failed.
Osteoporosis (within months to years)	Aromatase inhibitors, antiandrogens	Calcium and vitamin D intake should be assessed prior to therapy and maintained at 1200 mg/day (or more) of elemental calcium and 800 IU/day of vitamin D.[47]	See Chapter 83.
Neurologic			
Central or autonomic neurotoxicity (within weeks to months)	Vinca alkaloids	For constipation, use stool softeners or stimulant laxatives if necessary.	Dose reduction may be necessary with severe toxicity, or the drugs may have to be avoided altogether. Rule out other causes such as CNS metastases or leptomeningeal disease.

Toxicity/Organ Involved (Time frame to onset)	Classes/Drugs Commonly Implicated	Prevention	Management
Cognitive changes "Chemo fog" or "chemo brain" (within weeks to months)	All therapies	See Suggested Readings for patient education and nonpharmacologic measures.	"Chemo fog" usually resolves once treatment is complete but can be persistent in a subset of patients. Rule out contributing conditions (e.g., anemia, metabolic disorders). Because pharmacologic (e.g., methylphenidate, modafinil) and nonpharmacologic (e.g., cognitive training) measures for severe deficits have demonstrated mixed results, they are not routinely recommended [Evidence: SORT B*].[48,49]
Peripheral nerve toxicity	Bortezomib, platinums, taxanes, vinca alkaloids (within weeks to months)	Usually cumulative dose-related. Education and increased monitoring in patients at risk (e.g., diabetic neuropathy) so that dose adjustments can be made prior to severe damage. Avoid extremes of temperature. No established preventive measures.	Dose reductions or longer intervals between cycles. With severe toxicity, the drugs may have to be avoided altogether. **Gabapentin**, **pregabalin**, **duloxetine** and **venlafaxine** may be used for persistent neuropathy but the evidence is poor.[50]
	Oxaliplatin—peripheral sensory, pharyngeal and laryngeal neuropathies; precipitated by cold temperatures (within hours to days)	Pharyngeal/laryngeal symptoms occur within hours of exposure, are cold-triggered and may worsen in severity and duration with repeated administration. Nonpharmacologic measures: avoid cold exposure (e.g., from the wind, refrigerator, cold water) while receiving oxaliplatin.[51]	Acute onset symptoms can be managed with bronchodilators and antihistamines but usually resolve spontaneously. Persistent symptoms may be alleviated by slowing the rate of infusion of oxaliplatin and/or withholding oxaliplatin from the chemotherapy regimen.[52] Persistent pain may be alleviated with **duloxetine**.[53] **Venlafaxine**, **gabapentin** and **pregabalin** can be considered for persistent pain if other options are ineffective, but there is limited supporting evidence.[50,54]
Renal			
Hemorrhagic cystitis (within weeks to months)	Cyclophosphamide, ifosfamide	**Mesna**, diuresis and hydration administered while on chemotherapy. Administer chemotherapy as early in the day as possible to minimize the amount of damaging metabolites in prolonged contact with the bladder at night. Educate patient to drink plenty of fluids to urinate frequently.	Mild cases can be managed with bladder irrigation or the use of intravesical astringents (e.g., alum) or systemic antifibrinolytics (e.g., **tranexamic acid**). Cystoscopy and/or surgery may be required for more severe cases.[55]
Nephrotoxicity (within days to weeks)	Carmustine, ifosfamide, methotrexate, mitomycin, platinums, streptozocin	Prevention varies with the chemotherapy. Vigorous hydration and alkalinization of the urine with **sodium bicarbonate** is required (45–50 mEq/L of iv fluid) to prevent nephrotoxicity before, during and after administration of high doses of methotrexate. Saline-based hydration and forced diuresis with mannitol reduces cisplatin nephrotoxicity.[56]	Correct electrolyte and metabolic abnormalities. Maintain intravascular volume and urine output. Dose reductions and aggressive hydration with subsequent chemotherapy treatment. Dialysis in severe cases.

(cont'd)

* SORT (Strength of Recommendation Taxonomy) is a rating system (A, B or C) that addresses the quality of available evidence. For more information consult **How to Use *Compendium of Therapeutic Choices*** on page xxv.

Table 2: **Prevention and Management of Select Toxicities of Chemotherapies** *(cont'd)*

Toxicity/Organ Involved (Time frame to onset)	Classes/Drugs Commonly Implicated	Prevention	Management
Reproductive			
Gonadal toxicity (within months to years)	Alkylating agents, other regimens	Sperm, oocyte or embryo banking. The decision to use fertility preservation must be made relatively quickly, ideally before chemotherapy begins. Use chemotherapies with the least effect on spermatogenesis or ovarian function. Gonadotropin-releasing hormones are not indicated but may be considered when proven options are not available.[57]	Discuss assisted reproduction techniques with patients. Assess for psychosocial concerns that may have developed due to infertility.[57]
Sexuality changes Altered functioning, reduced libido (within weeks to months)	All therapies	Prevalent in both men and women during and after chemotherapy (can be months or years). Education and communication prior to its development may facilitate management.	Ensure any changes in sexual functioning are addressed, rather than ignored or suppressed.
Other			
Carcinogenesis (within years)	Alkylating agents, cladribine, fludarabine, non-classic alkylating agents, topoisomerase II inhibitors	Use the least amount of chemotherapy possible to control the disease.	Case specific.
Fatigue (within days to months)	Most therapies	Prevent and manage contributing factors (pain, emotional distress, sleep issues, anemia, nutrition deficits, medications).	Treat contributing factors (e.g., anemia, pain). Exercise may be beneficial for some patients with moderate to severe fatigue, but must be undertaken with caution. Use energy conservation techniques and behavioural therapies.[58]
Flu-like syndrome Fever, myalgias, chills (within hours to days)	Dacarbazine, interferon, gemcitabine, monoclonal antibodies, procarbazine	Premedication with acetaminophen or NSAIDs and adequate hydration.	Control fever and aches/pains with **acetaminophen** or **NSAIDs** (unless patient has thrombocytopenia). Supportive care.
Hot flashes (within days to weeks)	Hormonal therapies	Identify and avoid triggers (e.g., caffeine, alcohol, stress). Employ environmental modification.[59]	Behavioural and relaxation techniques. Exercise may help. **Venlafaxine**, **SSRIs** (e.g., citalopram), **clonidine** or **gabapentin**. Little data to distinguish management in men compared to women.[59]
Teratogenicity	Most therapies	Avoid chemotherapy in the first trimester. Avoid chemotherapies with high risk of teratogenicity (e.g., antifolates, imatinib).[60]	Contraception necessary while patient receives chemotherapy.

Abbreviations: ACE = angiotensin converting enzyme; ARB = angiotensin II receptor blocker; BRAT = Bananas, Rice, Applesauce, Toast; SSRI = selective serotonin reuptake inhibitor

Table 3: Prevention and Management of Side Effects of Radiation Therapy

Toxicity (Time frame to onset)	Location of Radiation	Prevention	Management
Cardiac			
Heart disease (years)	Breast, head and neck, lung, mediastinum	Manage and control risk factors for coronary artery disease.[61]	Routine cardiac testing if asymptomatic changes are present.
Pericardial disease (weeks for acute, or months to years for chronic)	Breast, head and neck, lung, mediastinum	Use of shielding methods and lower doses of radiation have reduced the risk of pericarditis.[61]	Supportive care with **NSAIDs** during the acute period. Chronic pericarditis may require pericardiectomy.[9]
CNS			
Edema (weeks to years)	Brain	No proven preventive measures.	Typically **dexamethasone** 4 mg QID po for moderate to severe symptoms with a slow taper after radiation completed. IV dexamethasone and mannitol may be required for life-threatening edema.[62]
Headache (weeks to months)	Brain	Low-dose steroids (dexamethasone or prednisone) may help prevent the occurrence of headaches.[64]	May indicate brain edema. **Corticosteroids**, **antiepileptics** are usually indicated.
Somnolence syndrome and fatigue (weeks to months, or chronic)	Brain, head and neck, lung	No proven preventive measures although various agents are under investigation and exploration.[62]	**Corticosteroids** may decrease the duration of somnolence syndrome in children.[63] Also see Table 2, Fatigue.
Dermatologic			
Alopecia (during treatment to weeks)	Brain		See Table 2, Alopecia.
Erythema and pruritus (during treatment to weeks)	In radiated area (and exit point)	Wash with mild soaps, shampoos or water alone, using hands rather than abrasive washcloths. Avoid frequent bathing or showering to prevent drying. Avoid friction by wearing loose-fitting clothes. Moisturize radiated area with plain, unscented, preferably lanolin-free hydrophilic moisturizers (e.g., Glaxal Base, Lubriderm). Avoid hot or cold packs, extreme temperatures, harsh chemicals and deodorants in the radiation treatment field. Use an electric razor if shaving is required. Protect from sun. Improve skin elasticity with moisturizers (and sunscreen).[65]	May apply a thin film of moisturizer. Low potency topical **corticosteroids** for short periods (up to 8 wk) for relief of itchiness.[64]

(cont'd)

Table 3: **Prevention and Management of Side Effects of Radiation Therapy** *(cont'd)*

Toxicity (Time frame to onset)	**Location of Radiation**	**Prevention**	**Management**
Desquamation (during treatment to weeks)	In radiated area	Wash with mild soaps, shampoos or water alone, using hands rather than abrasive washcloths. Avoid frequent bathing or showering to prevent drying. Avoid friction by wearing loose-fitting clothes. Moisturize radiated area with plain, unscented, preferably lanolin-free hydrophilic moisturizers (e.g., Glaxal Base, Lubriderm). Avoid hot or cold packs, extreme temperatures, harsh chemicals and deodorants in the radiation treatment field. Use an electric razor if shaving is required. Protect from sun. Improve skin elasticity with moisturizers (and sunscreen).[65]	If dry desquamation, use saline compresses and moisturize with plain, unscented, lanolin-free moisturizers (e.g., Glaxal Base, Lubriderm) or vitamin E preparations. If moist desquamation, apply principles of moist wound healing using nonadherent dressings. Add absorbent dressings on top if necessary. Hydrogel and hydrocolloid products may also be considered. Systemic analgesics may be required until recovery.[66,67,68]
Fibrosis, skin discolouration, photosensitivity, ulceration or atrophy (months to years)	In radiated area		Avoid trauma to area. Wound care for severe symptoms. Physical therapy with gentle massage and myofascial release.[64,65]
Eyes, Ears, Nose and Throat (EENT)			
Dental caries (months to years)	Head and neck	Frequent dental check-ups. Maintain oral hygiene, use of fluoride toothpastes and topical fluoride. Manage dry mouth. Avoid sugary foods and drinks.	Progression of caries can be rapid and destructive. Prevention and early dental management is key to preventing tooth loss.[69]
Gastrointestinal			
Bowel adhesions and obstruction (months)	Abdomen	Early recognition and intervention to prevent morbidity. Educate patient about potential symptoms.	Surgical intervention is required (e.g., bypass or resection).
Candidiasis (oral) (weeks to months)	Head and neck	Maintain good oral hygiene. Early recognition and treatment is important to prevent systemic dissemination.[70]	**Nystatin** suspension in mild cases. Oral **fluconazole** in moderate to severe cases or if refractory to nystatin. **Itraconazole** used in refractory cases.
Diarrhea (during treatment to months)	Abdomen, pelvis	See Table 2, Diarrhea. **Probiotics** containing lactobacilli may have preventative effects but dosing is unclear.[71]	**Loperamide** and **diphenoxylate/atropine**.[28] **Octreotide** if other therapies fail.[71]
Esophagitis (during treatment to weeks or chronic)	Chest or mediastinum, head and neck	Acid-reducing agents to reduce acidity and possibly ulceration of mucosa.	Systemic **analgesics**, **topical lidocaine**, **sucralfate** and **nystatin** are commonly used. Acid-reducing agents may be helpful in those with a component of reflux. Treatment interruptions may be required. Chronic esophagitis (fibrosis) may require systemic analgesics and endoscopic dilatation.[72,73]
Mucositis (during treatment to weeks)	Head and neck, abdomen	**Benzydamine** oral rinse may prevent radiation-induced mucositis in patients receiving treatment for head and neck cancer.[30]	SeeTable 2, Mucositis.

Toxicity (Time frame to onset)	Location of Radiation	Prevention	Management
Nausea and vomiting (during treatment to days)	From highest to lowest risk: total body > upper abdomen > cranial, head and neck > breast	**5-HT3 receptor antagonists ± dexamethasone** are used in accordance with the emetogenicity of radiation therapy.[74]	See Chapter 126 for antiemetic options.
Proctitis (weeks to months, or chronic)	Abdomen, pelvis	**Sulfasalazine** will help reduce the incidence and severity of acute symptoms.[75]	Use sitz baths and topical anti-inflammatory preparations for anal irritation. **Topical corticosteroids** (e.g., Proctofoam) by enema or suppository. Symptomatic management of urgency, tenesmus or loose movements with antispasmodics and antidiarrheals. **Sucralfate enemas** for chronic proctitis with rectal bleeding.[76]
Taste alterations (weeks to months, or chronic)	Head and neck	There are no proven preventive measures. Avoidance of radiation to parotid glands.[77]	Experiment with foods; monitor nutritional intake. Alleviate dry mouth to improve taste.
Xerostomia Dry mouth (during treatment to weeks, or chronic)	Head and neck	Avoid unnecessary irradiation of salivary glands. Use oral lubricants or artificial saliva, sugarless gum or popsicles, ice cubes and water intake to moisten mouth.	Oral lubricants or artificial saliva preparations. **Pilocarpine** stimulates saliva production if there is residual salivary function. Stringent oral hygiene is paramount to prevent dental caries and oral infection. Sugary foods and drinks should be avoided.[72,78]
Hematologic			
Myelosuppression (weeks to months)	Pelvis, total body		See Table 2, Neutropenia and febrile neutropenia, Anemia and Thrombocytopenia.
Musculoskeletal			
Osteoradionecrosis (months to years)	Head and neck	Full dental checkup with extraction of problematic teeth. Avoid use of ill-fitting dentures. Control xerostomia and maintain good oral hygiene.	Débridement and irrigation. Topical and oral **antibiotics** may be required. Resection of affected areas. Hyperbaric oxygen for resistant cases.[69,80]
Trismus Inability to open mouth completely due to tonic contraction of muscles of mastication (weeks to months)	Head and neck	Early detection and treatment to prevent consequences of condition (poor intake or hygiene). Physical therapy to perform mechanical stretching of the muscles of mastication.[69]	Mechanical devices to stretch muscles around mouth.[79]

(cont'd)

Table 3: **Prevention and Management of Side Effects of Radiation Therapy** *(cont'd)*

Toxicity (Time frame to onset)	Location of Radiation	Prevention	Management
Renal			
Urinary frequency or dysuria (weeks or chronic)	Pelvis		Treat symptomatically with anticholinergics (e.g., **oxybutynin**, **tolterodine**) or alpha$_1$- adrenergic antagonists (e.g., **tamsulosin**, **doxazosin**). See Chapter 67 and Chapter 68. Rule out infection.
Hemorrhagic cystitis (months to years)	Pelvis	Limit amount of radiation exposure to the bladder if possible.	See Table 2, Hemorrhagic cystitis.
Reproductive			
Erectile dysfunction and reduced sexual function (months or chronic)	Pelvis	Prevalent in both men and women during and after radiation therapy (can be months or years). Education and communication prior to its development may facilitate management.	Penile implants, **phosphodiesterase inhibitors** (e.g., sildenafil), mechanical devices for men. Vaginal dilators and lubricants for women.[81,82] See Table 2, Sexual changes.
Gonadal toxicity	Pelvis, craniospinal		See Table 2, Gonadal toxicity.
Vaginal irritation (weeks or chronic)	Pelvis	Educate patients on the importance of vaginal dilatation methods. See Chapter 73.	Water-soluble lubricant, vaginal dilators.
Respiratory			
Pneumonitis (months to years)	Chest	Minimize risk and severity by limiting the area of the lung that is irradiated.[83] **Pentoxifylline** has demonstrated benefit in preventing early and late toxicities.[84]	**Prednisone** (starting dose of 1 mg/kg/day po, taper over weeks) or **dexamethasone** (16–20 mg/day) po. Identify and manage any concurrent infection.
Other			
Carcinogenesis (years)	Cervix, chest, oral cavity, pharynx, testes and others	Reduce risk by using modern radiation techniques to limit radiation doses and the volume of normal tissue exposed; regular screening where indicated (e.g., mammography for breast cancer in patients receiving high-dose radiation to the chest)	Cancer specific.

Table 4: **Pharmacologic Therapy for Prevention and Management of Side Effects of Chemotherapy and Radiation Therapy**

Toxicity	Drug	Dose	Adverse Effects	Comments
Anemia	*darbepoetin alfa* Aranesp	Usual: 500 µg Q3 wk sc	Edema, nausea, arthralgias, injection site reactions, uncontrolled hypertension, thrombotic and vascular events, seizures. Hemoglobin targets of >120 g/L and use outside of chemotherapy treatment period associated with increased morbidity and mortality.	Rule out other etiologies. Consider iron supplementation for functional iron deficiency (impairment of iron mobilization despite iron parameters in normal ranges).
	epoetin alfa Eprex	40 000 U Q1 wk sc Titrate to 60 000 U after 4 wk if still clinically symptomatic		
	iron dextran Infufer, generics	Total dose calculated according to weight and hemoglobin target. Usually given in 100 mg increments iv over several weeks	Hypersensitivity reactions, blood pressure changes, arrhythmias, fever, chills, nausea, delayed infusion reactions.	Test dose required. Hypersensitivity reactions may occur even if the test dose was tolerated.
	iron sucrose Venofer	100–200 mg iv over 1 h Usual total dose: 1000 mg	Hypersensitivity reactions, hypotension, headache, nausea.	Test dose should be considered if patient suspected to be at risk for hypersensitivity reactions.
Diarrhea	*diphenoxylate/ atropine* Lomotil	1 tablet (2.5 mg diphenoxylate) TID–QID PRN po	Sedation.	
	loperamide Imodium, Riva-Loperamide, other generics	Standard-dose: 4 mg STAT po, then 2 mg after every loose bowel movement until 12 h after diarrhea resolves (maximum dose 16 mg/day) High-dose: 4 mg STAT po then 2 mg Q2H until 12 h after diarrhea resolves[85]	Dizziness.	High-dose regimen is required for irinotecan-based chemotherapy protocols and for other chemotherapy regimens where diarrhea nonresponsive to standard regimen.
	octreotide Sandostatin, generics	100–150 µg TID sc with dose escalation up to 500 µg TID PRN	Fatigue, fever, arthralgias, myalgias, hyperglycemia, gallstones, abdominal cramps.	Can also be given as a continuous infusion.
Erectile dysfunction	*sildenafil* Viagra	25–100 mg po 30–60 min prior to sexual activity	Headache, flushing, dyspepsia, epistaxis, visual disturbances.	Use caution in patients with cardiovascular disorders. Contraindicated in patients taking nitrates.
	tadalafil Cialis	2.5–20 mg po at least 60 min prior to sexual activity	See sildenafil.	See sildenafil.
	vardenafil Levitra, Staxyn	5–20 mg po 30–60 min prior to sexual activity	See sildenafil.	See sildenafil.

(cont'd)

Table 4: **Pharmacologic Therapy for Prevention and Management of Side Effects of Chemotherapy and Radiation Therapy** *(cont'd)*

Toxicity	Drug	Dose	Adverse Effects	Comments
Extravasation	*dimethylsulfoxide* Rimso-50, generics	Apply in a thin layer topically to extravasated area. Repeat Q8H for 1 wk[14]	Skin irritation.	For extravasation due to antitumour antibiotics and anthracyclines. If a nonocclusive dressing is required, allow dimethylsulfoxide to air dry first.
	sodium thiosulfate generics	4 mL of sodium thiosulfate 25% is diluted with 6 mL of sterile water. Inject 2 mL of the resulting solution sc throughout the extravasation area[14]	Local irritation.	For extravasation due to mechlorethamine. Although used, evidence for efficacy is poor.
Heart failure	*dexrazoxane* Zinecard	Given iv at a dose of 10 times that of doxorubicin or epirubicin within 30 min of their administration[88]	Myelosuppression, injection site reaction, phlebitis, nausea.	Because of its mechanism of action and role as a "protectant," reduction in antitumour efficacy has not been ruled out.[3,89]
Hemorrhagic cystitis	*mesna* Uromitexan, generics	Bolus iv: calculated to equal 60% of the total daily dose of ifosfamide in 3 doses (15 min before and 4 and 8 h after ifosfamide) Oral: calculated to equal 100% of the total daily dose of ifosfamide in 3 equal doses (20% as an iv bolus, then 40% given po at 2 h and 40% at 6 h after ifosfamide completed)	Headache, flushing, dizziness, constipation, nausea and vomiting, fatigue, fever.	Mesna is given on each day that ifosfamide is given. Other dosing protocols exist. Mesna is used in all ifosfamide treatments and in regimens using high-dose cyclophosphamide (for transplant).
	tranexamic acid Cyklokapron, generics	10 mg/kg TID–QID iv or 1–1.5 g TID–QID po	Nausea, vomiting, diarrhea.	
Hot flashes	*clonidine* Dixarit, generics	0.025–0.05 mg daily to BID po	Sedation, hypotension, xerostomia, constipation.	Avoid abrupt cessation. Treatment should be tapered.
	gabapentin Neurontin, generics	100 mg BID po titrated to effect and increased as tolerated to 600 mg TID (do not increase dose more often than every 3 days)	Dizziness, fatigue, edema, ataxia.	Not a Health Canada-approved indication.
	SSRIs	See Chapter 75		In patients taking tamoxifen, avoid initiating SSRIs that strongly inhibit CYP2D6 activity (e.g., paroxetine, fluoxetine).
	venlafaxine Effexor XR, generics	37.5 mg QHS po (extended-release tablet), increased every 5–7 days to 150 mg/day	Nausea, sleep disturbance, drowsiness, nervousness, dizziness, dry mouth.	Avoid abrupt cessation. Treatment should be tapered.

Toxicity	Drug	Dose	Adverse Effects	Comments
Mucositis and oral candidiasis	*benzydamine*, Pharixia, other generics	Gargle 15 mL for 30 sec to 2 min Q2H PRN	Numbness, local irritation, nausea and vomiting.	Can be diluted with water to reduce irritation.
	fluconazole Diflucan, generics	100–200 mg daily po × 7–14 days Esophageal mucositis: increase to 200–400 mg daily po	Headache, dizziness, nausea and vomiting, hypercholesterolemia, altered liver function tests.	
	itraconazole solution Sporanox Oral Solution	200 mg daily po × 7–14 days	Nausea, edema, diarrhea, rash, pruritus, chest pain, abnormal liver function.	Itraconazole capsules are less effective due to variable absorption.
	nystatin generics	5–10 mL TID po Rinse, then spit or swallow (if extends to throat or esophagus)	Diarrhea, nausea, stomach pain.	Chilling nystatin may improve palatability, but avoid in patients receiving oxaliplatin (pharyngeal neuropathies can be triggered by cold).
	palifermin Kepivance	Autologous hematopoietic stem cell transplant: 60 µg/kg daily for the 3 days preceding conditioning chemotherapy for transplant, then 60 µg/kg daily for 3 days starting the day of stem cell infusion	Edema, hypertension, dysesthesias, rash, taste alteration, mouth/tongue discolouration or thickness, proteinuria, cough, rhinitis, arthralgias.	Should not be administered within 24 h before or after conditioning chemotherapy regimen (may worsen mucositis).
Neutropenia	*filgrastim* Neupogen	5 µg/kg daily sc for 7–10 days starting at least 24 h after chemotherapy (round to nearest vial size)	Fever, arthralgias, splenomegaly, injection site reactions.	Avoid administration within 24 h of chemotherapy (can worsen neutropenia).
	pegfilgrastim Neulasta	6 mg × 1 dose sc at least 24 h after chemotherapy	See filgrastim.	See filgrastim.
Peripheral nerve toxicity	*duloxetine* Cymbalta	30 mg/day, increase as tolerated every 7 days to 60 mg/day	Nausea, dizziness, fatigue, insomnia.	Better tolerated if given with food. Do not discontinue abruptly.
	gabapentin Neurontin, generics	200–300 mg/day, increase as tolerated every 1–7 days by 50–100% of dose	Dizziness, dry mouth, blurred vision, drowsiness, water retention.	Usual maintenance dose 300–1200 mg daily in divided doses.
	pregabalin Lyrica, generics	75–150 mg/day, increase as tolerated every 5–7 days by 50–100% of dose	See gabapentin.	Usual maintenance dose 75–300 mg/day in divided doses.
	venlafaxine Effexor XR, generics	37.5 mg QHS po (extended-release tablet), increased every 5–7 days to 150 mg/day	Nausea, sleep disturbance, drowsiness, nervousness, dizziness, dry mouth.	Avoid abrupt cessation. Treatment should be tapered.

(cont'd)

Table 4: **Pharmacologic Therapy for Prevention and Management of Side Effects of Chemotherapy and Radiation Therapy** *(cont'd)*

Toxicity	Drug	Dose	Adverse Effects	Comments
Pneumonitis	*pentoxifylline* Trental, generics	400 mg TID po during radiation	Nausea, vomiting, renal impairment.	
Proctitis	*hydrocortisone/ pramoxine* Proctofoam-HC	1 applicatorful pr BID–TID and after bowel evacuation	Local irritation, itching and pain.	
	sucralfate enema Sulcrate	3 g (15 mL of oral suspension) rectally once to twice daily	Minimal adverse effects.	Can also be specially compounded from tablets into 15–20 mL volumes.[90]
	sulfasalazine Salazopyrin, generics	500–1000 mg BID po during radiation	Headaches, rash, GI disturbances, abnormal liver function tests, blood dyscrasias.	
Rash related to EGFR inhibition	*clindamycin topical* Clindets (pledgets), Dalacin T Solution, generics	Apply to affected area BID until resolution	Dryness, burning, itchiness, erythema, peeling of skin.	Avoid alcohol-containing solutions to minimize irritation and drying. Can also be prescribed as an extemporaneous compound.
Tumour lysis syndrome	*allopurinol* ❥ generics	Prevention of hyperuricemia in low risk (solid tumours): 300–600 mg/day po usually started 1–2 days prior to chemotherapy and continued for 3–7 days Prevention for high risk or for treatment: 100 mg/m^2 TID (maximum 800 mg/day)[42,43]	Precipitation of hypoxanthine can cause obstructive uropathy. Hypersensitivity reactions, skin rash.	Reduce 6-mercaptopurine and/or azathioprine doses by 65–75% with concomitant allopurinol. Reduce allopurinol in renal insufficiency. Doses greater than 300 mg should be divided.
	rasburicase Fasturtec	0.1–0.2 mg/kg/day iv over 30 min for up to 7 days in the treatment and prophylaxis of hyperuricemia	Fever, peripheral edema, bronchospasm.	When administered to patients with G6PD deficiency it can cause severe hemolysis.
Xerostomia (dry mouth)	*pilocarpine* Salagen, generics	2.5–5 mg TID–QID po. Titrate slowly to minimize side effects. Maximum 30 mg/day	Sweating, urinary frequency, nausea, vomiting, lacrimation, rhinitis, dizziness, diarrhea.	Avoid in patients with asthma, glaucoma. Use with caution in patients with COPD or cardiovascular disease.

❥ Dosage adjustment may be required in renal impairment; see Appendix I.

Suggested Readings

BC Cancer Agency. *Cancer drug manual*. Available from: www.bccancer.bc.ca/HPI/DrugDatabase/default.htm.

Berkey FJ. Managing the adverse effects of radiation therapy. *Am Fam Physician* 2010;82(4):381-8, 394.

Canadian Cancer Society. *Cognitive changes and chemotherapy*. Available from: www.cancer.ca/en/cancer-information/diagnosis-and-treatment/chemotherapy-and-other-drug-therapies/chemotherapy/side-effects-of-chemotherapy/cognitive-changes-and-chemotherapy/.

Cancer Care Ontario. CCO Toolbox. *Drug formulary*. Available from: www.cancercare.on.ca/toolbox/drugformulary/.

References

1. Nair K, Dolovich L, Cassels A et al. What patients want to know about their medications. Focus group study of patient and clinician perspectives. *Can Fam Physician* 2002;48:104-10.
2. Howland JS, Baker MG, Poe T. Does patient education cause side effects? A controlled trial. *J Fam Pract* 1990;31(1):62-4.
3. Floyd JD, Nguyen DT, Lobins RL et al. Cardiotoxicity of cancer therapy. *J Clin Oncol* 2005;23(30):7685-96.
4. Youssef G, Links M. The prevention and management of cardiovascular complications of chemotherapy in patients with cancer. *Am J Cardiovasc Drugs* 2005;5(4):233-43.
5. Mackey JR, Clemons M, Cote MA et al. Cardiac management during adjuvant trastuzumab therapy: recommendations of the Canadian Trastuzumab Working Group. *Curr Oncol* 2008;15(1):24-35.
6. Yeh ET, Tong AT, Lenihan DJ et al. Cardiovascular complications of cancer therapy: diagnosis, pathogenesis, and management. *Circulation* 2004;109(25):3122-31.
7. Moy B, Goss PE. Lapatinib-associated toxicity and practical management recommendations. *Oncologist* 2007;12(7):756-65.
8. van Dalen EC, Caron HN, Dickinson HO et al. Cardioprotective interventions for cancer patients receiving anthracyclines. *Cochrane Database Syst Rev* 2008;(2):CD003917.
9. Carver JR, Shapiro CL, Ng A et al. American Society of Clinical Oncology clinical evidence review on the ongoing care of adult cancer survivors: cardiac and pulmonary late effects. *J Clin Oncol* 2007;25(25):3991-4008.
10. van Noord C, Eijgelsheim M, Stricker BH. Drug- and non-drug-associated QT interval prolongation. *Br J Clin Pharmacol* 2010;70(1):16-23.
11. Mandala M, Falanga A, Roila F et al. Venous thromboembolism in cancer patients: ESMO Clinical Practice Guidelines for the management. *Ann Oncol* 2010;21(Suppl 5):v274-6.
12. Lyman GH, Khorana AA, Kuderer NM et al. Venous thromboembolism prophylaxis and treatment in patients with cancer: American Society of Clinical Oncology clinical practice guideline update. *J Clin Oncol* 2013;31(7):2189-204.
13. Grevelman EG, Breed WP. Prevention of chemotherapy-induced hair loss by scalp cooling. *Ann Oncol* 2005;16(3):352-8.
14. Wengstrom Y, Margulies A; European Oncology Nursing Society Task Force. European Oncology Nursing Society extravasation guidelines. *Eur J Onc Nurs* 2008;12(4):357-61.
15. Schrijvers DL. Extravasation: a dreaded complication of chemotherapy. *Ann Oncol* 2003;14(Suppl 3):iii26-30.
16. Doellman D, Hadaway L, Bowe-Geddes LA et al. Infiltration and extravasation: update on prevention and management. *J Infus Nurs* 2009;32(4):203-11.
17. Mouridsen HT, Langer SW, Buter J et al. Treatment of anthracycline extravasation with Savene (dexrazoxane): results from two prospective clinical multicentre trials. *Ann Oncol* 2007;18(3):546-50.
18. Lorusso D, Stefano A, Carone V et al. Pegylated liposomal doxorubin-related palmar-plantar erythrodysesthesia ('hand-foot' syndrome). *Ann Oncol* 2007;18(7):1159-64.
19. Lassere Y, Hoff P. Management of hand-foot syndrome in patients treated with capecitabine (Xeloda). *Eur J Oncol Nurs* 2004;8(Suppl 1):S31-40.
20. Manchen E, Robert C, Porta C. Management of tyrosine kinase inhibitor-induced hand-foot skin reaction: viewpoints from the medical oncologist, dermatologist, and oncology nurse. *J Support Oncol* 2011;9(1):13-23.
21. Melosky B, Burkes R, Rayson D et al. Management of skin rash during EGFR-targeted monoclonal antibody treatment for gastrointestinal malignancies: Canadian recommendations. *Curr Oncol* 2009;16(1):16-26.
22. Lacouture ME, Anadkat MJ, Bensadoun RJ et al. Clinical practice guidelines for the prevention and treatment of EGFR inhibitor-associated dermatologic toxicities. *Support Care Cancer* 2011;19(8):1079-95.
23. Cancer Care Ontario Formulary. *Cytarabine*. Available from: www.cancercare.on.ca/cms/one.aspx?pageId=11752. Accessed March 6, 2014.
24. Matteuci P, Carlo-Stella C, Di Nicola M et al. Topical prophylaxis of conjunctivitis induced by high-dose cytosine arabinoside. *Haematologica* 2006;91(2):255-7.
25. Bokemeyer C, Berger CC, Hartmann JT et al. Analysis of risk factors for cisplatin-induced ototoxicity in patients with testicular cancer. *Br J Cancer* 1998;77(8):1355-62.
26. AHFS Drug Information. *Irinotecan*. Bethesda (MD): American Society of Health-System Pharmacists. Available from: www.ahfsdruginformation.com. Subscription required.
27. Cancer Care Ontario Formulary. *Irinotecan*. Available from: www.cancercare.on.ca/cms/one.aspx?pageId=11752. Accessed March 6, 2014.
28. Benson AB, Ajani JA, Catalano RB et al. Recommended guidelines for the treatment of cancer treatment-induced diarrhea. *J Clin Oncol* 2004;22(14):2918-26.
29. Barbounis V, Koumakis G, Vassilomanolakis M et al. Control of irinotecan-induced diarrhea by octreotide after loperamide failure. *Support Care Cancer* 2001;9(4):258-60.
30. Peterson DE, Bensadoun RJ, Roila F et al. Management of oral and gastrointestinal mucositis: ESMO clinical practice guidelines. *Ann Oncol* 2011;22(Suppl 6):vi78-84.
31. Bensinger W, Schubert M, Ang KK et al. NCCN Task Force Report: prevention and management of mucositis in cancer care. *J Natl Compr Canc Netw* 2008;6(Suppl 1):S1-21.

32. Clarkson JE, Worthington HV, Furness S et al. Interventions for treating oral mucositis for patients with cancer receiving chemotherapy. *Cochrane Database Syst Rev* 2010;(8):CD001973.
33. Rizzo JD, Brouwers M, Hurley P et al. American Society of Clinical Oncology/American Society of Hematology clinical practice guideline update on the use of epoetin and darbepoetin in adult patients with cancer. *J Clin Oncol* 2010;28(33):4996-5010.
34. Kouroukis CT, Chia S, Verma S et al. Canadian supportive care recommendations for the management of neutropenia in patients with cancer. *Curr Oncol* 2008;15(1):9-23.
35. National Comprehensive Cancer Network. NCCN clinical practice guidelines in oncology. *Myeloid growth factors*. V.I.2010. Available from: subscriptions.nccn.org. Registration required.
36. Herbst C, Naumann F, Kruse EB et al. Prophylactic antibiotics or G-CSF for the prevention of infections and improvement of survival in cancer patients undergoing chemotherapy. *Cochrane Database Syst Rev* 2009;(1):CD007107.
37. Flowers CR, Seidenfeld J, Bow EJ et al. Antimicrobial prophylaxis and outpatient management of fever and neutropenia in adults treated for malignancy: American Society of Clinical Oncology clinical practice guideline. *J Clin Oncol* 2013;31(6):794-810.
38. American Cancer Society. *Infections in people with cancer*. Available from: www.cancer.org/treatment/treatmentsandsideeffects/physicalside-effects/infectionsinpeoplewithcancer/index. Accessed March 5, 2014.
39. Cancer Care Ontario Formulary. *Bleomycin*. Available from: www.cancercare.on.ca/cms/one.aspx?pageId=11752. Accessed March 6, 2014.
40. Zanotti KM, Markman M. Prevention and management of antineoplastic-induced hypersensitivity reactions. *Drug Saf* 2001;24(10):767-79.
41. Chung CH. Managing premedications and the risk for reactions to infusional monoclonal antibody therapy. *Oncologist* 2008;13(6):725-32.
42. Coiffier B, Altman A, Pui CH et al. Guidelines for the management of pediatric and adult tumor lysis syndrome: an evidence-based review. *J Clin Oncol* 2008;26(16):2767-78.
43. Tosi P, Barosi G, Lazzaro C et al. Consensus conference on the management of tumor lysis syndrome. *Haematologica* 2008;93(12):1877-85.
44. Hauschild A, Gogas H, Tarhini A et al. Practical guidelines for the management of interferon-alpha-2b side effects in patients receiving adjuvant treatment for melanoma: expert opinion. *Cancer* 2008;112(5):982-94.
45. Martoni A, Zamagni C, Gheka A et al. Antihistamines in the treatment of taxol-induced paroxystic pain syndrome. *J Natl Cancer Inst* 1993;85(8):676.
46. Thorne C. Management of arthralgias associated with aromatase inhibitor therapy. *Curr Oncol* 2007;14(Suppl 1):S11-19.
47. Papaioannou A, Morin S, Cheung AM et al. 2010 clinical practice guidelines for the diagnosis and management of osteoporosis in Canada: summary. *CMAJ* 2010;182(17):1864-73.
48. Von Ah D, Jansen C, Allen DH. Putting evidence into practice: evidence-based interventions for cancer and cancer treatment-related cognitive impairment. *Clin J Oncol Nurs* 2011;15(6):607-15.
49. Fardell JE, Vardy J, Johnston IN et al. Chemotherapy and cognitive impairment: treatment options. *Clin Pharmacol Ther* 2011;90(3):366-76.
50. Piccolo J. Kolesar JM. Prevention and treatment of chemotherapy-induced peripheral neuropathy. *Am J Health Syst Pharm* 2014;71(1):19-25.
51. Pasetto LM, D'Andrea MR, Rossi E et al. Oxaliplatin-related neurotoxicity: how and why? *Crit Rev Oncol Hematol* 2006;59(2):159-68.
52. Benson AB, Bekaii-Saab T, Chan E et al. Metastatic colon cancer, version 3.2013: featured updates to the NCCN Guidelines. *J Natl Compr Canc Netw* 2013;11(2):141-52.
53. Smith EM, Pang H, Cirrincione C et al. Effect of duloxetine on pain, function, and quality of life among patients with chemotherapy-induced painful peripheral neuropathy: a randomized clinical trial. *JAMA* 2013;309(13):1359-67.
54. Weickhardt A, Wells K, Messersmith W. Oxaliplatin-induced neuropathy in colorectal cancer. *J Oncol* 2011;2011:201593.
55. Cancer Care Ontario Formulary. *Cyclophosphamide*. Available from: www.cancercare.on.ca/cms/one.aspx?pageId=11752. Accessed March 6, 2014.
56. Kintzel PE. Anticancer drug-induced kidney disorders. *Drug Saf* 2001;24(1):19-38.
57. Loren AW, Mangu PB, Beck LN et al. Fertility preservation for patients with cancer: American Society of Clinical Oncology clinical practice guideline update. *J Clin Oncol* 2013;31(19);2500-10.
58. National Comprehensive Cancer Network. NCCN clinical practice guidelines in oncology. *Cancer-related fatigue*. V.I.2010. Accessed from: subscriptions.nccn.org. Registration required.
59. Kligman L, Younus J. Management of hot flashes in women with breast cancer. *Curr Oncol* 2010;17(1):81-6.
60. Koren G, Carey N, Gagnon R et al. *Cancer chemotherapy and pregnancy*. SOGC Clinical Practice Guideline 2013;no. 288. Available from: www.sogc.org/wp-content/uploads/2013/04/gui288CPG1303E.pdf. Accessed October 14, 2013.
61. Lancellotti P, Nkomo VT, Badano LP et al. Expert consensus for multi-modality imaging evaluation of cardiovascular complications of radiotherapy in adults: a report from the European Association of Cardiovascular Imaging and the American Society of Echocardiography. *J Am Soc Echocardiogr* 2013;26(9):1013-32.
62. Shaw EG, Robbins ME. The management of radiation-induced brain injury. In: Small W, Woloschak GE, eds. *Radiation toxicity: a practical guide*. New York (NY): Springer; 2006.
63. Butler JM, Rapp SR, Shaw EG. Managing the cognitive effects of brain tumor radiation therapy. *Curr Treat Options Oncol* 2006;7(6):517-23.
64. Robbins MA, Gosselin TK. Symptom management in radiation oncology: acute and long-term side effects. *Am J Nurs* 2002;102(Suppl 4):32-6.
65. Wood G, Casey L, Triotti A. Skin changes. In: Small W, Woloschak GE, eds. *Radiation toxicity: a practical guide*. New York (NY): Springer; 2006.
66. Kumar S, Juresic E, Barton M et al. Management of skin toxicity during radiation therapy: a review of the evidence. *J Med Imaging Radiat Oncol* 2010;54(3):264-79.
67. BC Cancer Agency. *Care of radiation skin reactions*. Revised July 18, 2012. Available from: www.bccancer.bc.ca/NR/rdonlyres/79E81484-6809-41CF-8CC2-0646DA6003F8/64011/CareofRadiationSkinReactions.pdf. Accessed May 29, 2013.
68. Bolderston A, Lloyd NS, Wong RK et al. The prevention and management of acute skin reactions related to radiation therapy: a systematic review and practice guideline. *Support Care Cancer* 2006;14(8):802-17.
69. Whitmyer CC, Waskowski JC, Iffland HA. Radiotherapy and oral sequelae: preventive and management protocols. *J Dent Hyg* 1997;71(1):23-9.
70. Pappas PG, Kauffman CA, Andes D et al. Clinical practice guidelines for the management of candidiasis: 2009 update by the Infectious Diseases Society of America. *Clin Infect Dis* 2009;48(5):503-35.
71. Gibson RJ, Keefe DM, Lalla RV et al. Systematic review of agents for the management of gastrointestinal mucositis in cancer patients. *Support Care Cancer* 2013;21(1):313-26.
72. Constine LS, Milano MT, Friedman D et al. Late effects of cancer treatment on normal tissues. In: Halperin EC, Perez CA, Brady LW, eds. *Perez and Brady's principles and practice of radiation oncology*. 5th ed. Philadelphia (PA): Wolters Kluwer/Lippincott Williams & Wilkins; 2008.

73. Bendell J, Willett C. Upper gastrointestinal tract. In: Small W, Woloschak GE, eds. *Radiation toxicity: a practical guide*. New York (NY): Springer; 2006.
74. Multinational Association of Supportive Care in Cancer. *MASCC/ESMO antiemetic guideline 2011*. Available from: www.mascc.org/assets/documents/MASCC_Guidelines_English_2011.pdf.
75. Keefe DM, Schubert MM, Elting LS et al. Updated clinical practice guidelines for the prevention and treatment of mucositis. *Cancer* 2007;109(5):820-31.
76. Mendenhall WM, McKibben BT, Hoppe BS et al. Management of radiation proctitis. *Am J Clin Oncol* 2013 Mar 11. [Epub ahead of print].
77. Jensen SB, Pedersen AM, Vissink A et al. A systematic review of salivary gland hypofunction and xerostomia induced by cancer therapies: management strategies and economic impact. *Support Care Cancer* 2010;18(8):1061-79.
78. Dirix P, Nuyts S, Van den Bogaert W. Radiation-induced xerostomia in patients with head-and-neck cancer: a literature review. *Cancer* 2006;107(11):2525-34.
79. Bensadoun RJ, Riesenbeck D, Lockhart PB et al. A systematic review of trismus induced by cancer therapies in head and neck cancer patients. *Support Care Cancer* 2010;18(8):1033-8.
80. Hancock PJ, Epstein JB, Sadler GR. Oral and dental management related to radiation therapy for head and neck cancer. *J Can Dent Assoc* 2003;69(9):585-90.
81. Mcconnell Greven K, Paunesku T. Radiation complications of the pelvis. In: Small W, Woloschak GE, eds. *Radiation toxicity: a practical guide*. New York (NY): Springer; 2006.
82. Miles CL, Candy B, Jones L et al. Interventions for sexual dysfunction following treatments for cancer. *Cochrane Database Syst Rev* 2007;(4):CD005540.
83. Marks LB, Yu X, Vujaskovic Z et al. Radiation-induced lung injury. *Semin Radiat Oncol* 2003;13(3):333-45.
84. Berkey FJ. Managing the adverse effects of radiation therapy. *Am Fam Physician* 2010;82(4):381-8, 394.
85. Maroun JA, Anthony LB, Blais N et al. Prevention and management of chemotherapy-induced diarrhea in patients with colorectal cancer: a consensus statement by the Canadian Working Group on Chemotherapy-Induced Diarrhea. *Curr Oncol* 2007;14(1):13-20.
86. Mar Fan HG, Clemons M, Xu W et al. A randomised, placebo-controlled, double-blind trial of the effects of d-methylphenidate on fatigue and cognitive dysfunction in women undergoing adjuvant chemotherapy for breast cancer. *Support Care Cancer* 2008;16(6):577-83.
87. Minton O, Richardson A, Sharpe M et al. Psychostimulants for the management of cancer-related fatigue: a systematic review and meta-analysis. *J Pain Symptom Manage* 2011;41(4):761-7.
88. Cancer Care Ontario. Seymour L, Bramwell V and members of the Systemic Treatment Disease Site Group. *Use of dexrazoxane as a cardioprotectant in patients receiving doxorubicin or epirubicin chemotherapy for the treatment of cancer*. Practice Guideline Report #12-5. (Archived). Available from: www.cancercare.on.ca/cms/one.aspx?objectId=10425&contextId=1377. Accessed December 19, 2011.
89. Swain SM, Whaley FS, Gerber MC et al. Cardioprotection with dexrazoxane for doxorubicin-containing therapy in advanced breast cancer. *J Clin Oncol* 1997;15(4):1318-32.
90. Erickson MA. *Compounding hotline*. Available from: www.pharmacytimes.com/publications/issue/2006/2006-11/2006-11-6069. Accessed March 6, 2014.

Palliative Care

Chapter 128
End-of-Life Care

David Dupéré, MD, FRCPC

Patients at the end of life are confronted with many troubling symptoms (Table 1) requiring a team approach to care. This chapter provides management strategies for common end-of-life symptoms. The therapies presented are recommended by experienced palliative care teams and can be used in the home setting.

Table 1: Symptoms at the End of Life[a,1]

Symptom	Incidence (%)
Noisy and moist breathing	56
Urinary dysfunction	53
Pain	51
Restlessness and agitation	42
Dyspnea	22
Nausea and vomiting	14
Sweating	14
Jerking, twitching	12

[a] End of life refers to the final 48 hours of life.

Goals of Therapy

- Limit physical and emotional suffering by adequately managing pain and other symptoms
- Support the ability to enjoy remaining life while avoiding inappropriate prolongation of death

Investigations

- History and physical exam to determine the nature and severity of symptoms
- Detailed medication history including nonprescription medications, herbal remedies, vitamins and other natural therapies—having knowledge of the benefit of, or intolerance to, prior treatments can save time
- Minimal diagnostic testing helps to preserve quality of life—avoid invasive investigations whenever possible

Therapeutic Choices

Four rules are essential for optimal symptom management in the palliative setting:

- Any symptom is as distressing as a patient claims it to be.
- Treatment risks, benefits and alternatives need to be discussed in the context of the dying patient's values, culture, goals and fears.
- Individualize medication choice and doses—preset recipes are not adequate.
- Cause of symptoms is irrelevant and investigation is pointless when disease is advanced and death very near, unless detection would direct a useful change in symptomatic treatment.

Dyspnea

- Patients' awareness of their own breathing is completely subjective, potentially distressing and easily misinterpreted; patient comfort is a priority and an observer's opinion or objective measurements are irrelevant.
- Manage effectively by choosing therapies that treat symptoms with the greatest impact on activities of daily living. Treat reversible causes or components when appropriate.
- Associated anxiety requires special management.

Nonpharmacologic Choices

- Oxygen is a potent symbol of medical care that clearly has a role in the hypoxic patient.[2] Carefully consider oxygen use in the hypoxic patient who thinks they will not benefit or the nonhypoxic patient who thinks they will; try on a continuous or as-needed basis and ask the patient if it helps. Similarly, let the patient choose the flow rate. Sometimes a mask with compressed air flow provides a sense of security.
- Provide reassurance, information and support to the patient and family.
- Suggest relaxation therapies or breathing exercises.
- Suggest physical therapies, e.g., exercise program to avoid deconditioning.
- Offer an electric fan for cool air flow to face.
- Open a window; for bedbound patients, allow clear line of sight to the outside.

Pharmacologic Choices

Table 4 lists drugs used in the treatment of dyspnea.

Respiratory Sedatives

Opioids

Oral and parenteral **opioids** are effective and recommended in the management of breathlessness in end-of-life care [Evidence: SORT A*].[3,4] The acute situation may require frequent parenteral dosing (e.g., morphine 5–10 mg sc or iv Q30 minutes until settled). Otherwise, the usual dosing regimen involves Q4H dosing with Q1H breakthrough doses. There is no clear evidence for the role of nebulized opioids.[3,4]

Sublingual **fentanyl** has been shown to be effective for breathlessness.[5,6] Onset is quick but duration of effect is only about 40–60 minutes.[7] Sublingual fentanyl tablets are available in Canada, but the lowest available dose is higher than the usual starting dose of fentanyl for this indication. Some palliative care protocols use the parenteral formulation sublingually at a starting dose of 25–50 µg. This option can be beneficial in the home setting when parenteral access may be limited.[8] Patients need access to a home care nurse or a pharmacy willing to prepare doses in advance.

Intermittent dyspnea can be treated with intermittent opioids. If titrated to control dyspnea, opioids will not hasten death.[9]

Nonopioids

Benzodiazepines such as clonazepam, diazepam, lorazepam and midazolam have been widely used to manage dyspnea in the palliative care setting, despite a lack of strong evidence of efficacy.[10,11] Though their use is not validated, benzodiazepines may provide improved control of dyspnea compared to

* SORT (Strength of Recommendation Taxonomy) is a rating system (A, B or C) that addresses the quality of available evidence. For more information consult **How to Use *Compendium of Therapeutic Choices*** on page xxv.

opioids in terms of duration of action, potency and reduced adverse effects, especially in the absence of pain or when there is a clear component of anxiety.

Phenothiazines (e.g., promethazine, chlorpromazine) can effectively relieve refractory cases of dyspnea without causing respiratory depression.[12]

Corticosteroids have a specific role in the management of dyspnea resulting from obstructive lesions, lymphangitic carcinomatosis or COPD. CNS adverse effects may limit their utility.

Pain

- Determine the cause. Differentiate nociceptive (somatic, visceral) from neuropathic (dysesthetic, neuralgic) pain to guide the choice of treatment (see Chapter 21).
- Measure the pain intensity. Numeric rating scales that ask patients to grade their pain on a scale of 0 (no pain) to 10 (worst pain) are easy to use, reproducible and validated.[13,14]
- Review multidimensional aspects of pain. Assess response to, and adverse effects of, previously used analgesics as well as coping skills, past drug/alcohol abuse, concerns about addiction, metabolic abnormalities, cognitive impairment and finances.

Pharmacologic Choices

Table 4 lists drugs used in the treatment of pain.

A step-wise approach to pain management is mandated in all cases (see Chapter 14 and Chapter 21 for discussions of acute pain and neuropathic pain). For mild pain, **nonopioid analgesics** can be tried (e.g., acetaminophen, ASA, other NSAIDs) with or without an opioid. In the acute palliative care setting, **opioids** (e.g., morphine and hydromorphone) are usually the mainstay of therapy.

- Titrate opioid doses gradually to achieve adequate pain control without opioid toxicity.
- Use Q4H dosing (po/sc/iv/pr) for dose titration. The acute situation may require more frequent parenteral dosing (e.g., morphine 5–10 mg sc or iv Q30 min until settled).
- A breakthrough dose (estimated as 10% of the total 24-hour dose) ordered as Q1H PRN allows for control of interdose pain and provides essential dosing information to help with opioid titration.
- Regularly review and adjust doses to a new Q4H dose = (all Q4H + all PRN doses in previous 24 hours)/6.
- There is no ceiling effect or maximum safe dose for opioids. Patients' response to opioids can vary greatly and doses in the hundreds of milligrams Q4H may be required. Side effects may be the limiting factor.
- Educate patients and caregivers about anticipated side effects of opioid use (Table 2).
- Opioid toxicity can result from altered opioid metabolism (e.g., dehydration, renal failure) and may respond to a dose reduction or, when possible, a correction of the altered metabolism. Significant toxicity requires a switch to another opioid at 50–75% of the equianalgesic dose. Avoid **meperidine** as its neurotoxic metabolite can accumulate in patients with reduced renal function, possibly causing seizures.
- Adjuvant drugs (Table 3) may be useful in specific pain syndromes (e.g., corticosteroids in bone pain or hepatic capsular pain).

Terminal Delirium and Agitation

Patients often exhibit increasing confusion, drowsiness and/or restlessness and moaning with progressive multi-organ failure.

- Identify and eliminate reversible causes (e.g., dehydration, visual or hearing impairment)[16] although this is rarely successful.
- Palliative sedation: Consider heavy sedation to render the patient unaware of a severe symptom (e.g., pain, dyspnea, restlessness, hemorrhage) when a usual intervention has not provided an acceptable level of comfort.[17] **Midazolam** and **methotrimeprazine** are commonly used. Review the option with the patient and/or caregivers and explain that this usually involves cessation of nutrition and hydration.
- Never give opioids as sedatives.

Table 2: Management of Adverse Effects of Opioids

Category	Effects	Comments	Management
General	Nausea	Very common, tolerance develops in 2–3 days	Dimenhydrinate or metoclopramide PRN (see Chapter 64)
	Constipation	Ongoing treatment is mandatory	Daily laxatives (e.g., softener + stimulant, polyethylene glycol + stimulant) (see Chapter 58)
	Somnolence	Very common, tolerance develops in 2–3 days	Reassure patient
	Pruritus	Less common	Antihistamines; may require a change of opioid
	Dry mouth	Less common	Chew gum; suck on hard candy or ice chips; use saliva substitutes
Neurotoxic	Myoclonus	Uncommon in early titrated opioid use	May require change of opioid
	Delirium	See myoclonus	See myoclonus
	Visual hallucinations	See myoclonus	See myoclonus

Table 3: Adjuvant Analgesics

Type/Description of Pain	Suggested Drug Treatment
Bone pain	**NSAID** with cytoprotection (e.g., **naproxen**[a] 500 mg BID po/pr with **misoprostol** 200 μg BID po or **omeprazole** 20 mg daily po[15]) Severe cases: **dexamethasone** 4–8 mg QAM po/sc/iv
Closed space pain	**Dexamethasone** as for bone pain
Pleuritic pain	**NSAID** as for bone pain
Neuropathic pain	See Chapter 21
Burning/dysesthetic	Add tricyclic antidepressant (TCA),[b] e.g., **amitriptyline**, **desipramine** or **nortriptyline** 25 mg BID–TID po; increase gradually up to 150 mg/day if necessary
Shock-like/lancinating	Add **gabapentin**[a] 300 mg QHS po; increase gradually up to 1200 mg TID if necessary *or* **pregabalin**[a] 50–150 mg BID po; titrate weekly by 50–150 mg/day up to a maximum of 600 mg/day Severe cases: **dexamethasone** as above for severe bone pain

[a] Dosage adjustment may be required in renal impairment; see Appendix I.
[b] Decrease doses of TCAs by 50% in the presence of hepatic or renal impairment or in the frail elderly.

Nonpharmacologic Choices

- Reassure and educate the caregivers about the possibility of delirium and agitation.

Pharmacologic Choices

Table 4 lists drugs used in the treatment of delirium and agitation.

- Optimize doses or discontinue current medication (e.g., sedatives).
- **Haloperidol** is the mainstay of treatment for delirium. If doses >20 mg/day are ineffective, consider more sedating agents such as **methotrimeprazine** or **midazolam** in regular doses or as a continuous infusion if necessary.

Respiratory Secretions

Pooling of secretions is common with decreased levels of consciousness. This symptom (unfortunately named "death rattle") is usually of no consequence to the patient but can be quite distressing to the caregivers.

Nonpharmacologic Choices

- Educate the caregivers that the patient is unaware of the distressful breathing sounds and it is not a source of suffering.
- Position patient semi-prone if possible.
- If possible and not too distressing for the patient, use mouth swabs to remove secretions directly.

Pharmacologic Choices

Table 4 lists drugs used in the treatment of respiratory secretions.

- Regular use of anticholinergics at the onset of this symptom decreases secretions; there is no effect on built-up secretions.
- **Scopolamine** is the usual choice but is sedating. To avoid sedation, **glycopyrrolate** may be given.[18]

Therapeutic Tips

- At the end of life, goals of care focus on achieving patient comfort. Discontinue interventions that do not play a role in supporting comfort (e.g., blood work, vital signs, blood glucose monitoring). Often the routine medical approach (e.g., iv fluid rehydration[19]) is best replaced by what truly keeps the patient comfortable (e.g., good mouth care to control thirst).
- Choose medications with the goal of providing comfort. Most medications used to treat chronic diseases (e.g., antianginal agents) rarely have a role at end of life and should be discontinued. Opioids and medications with sedating properties are frequently required and their use should be guided solely by any ongoing need to control symptoms.
- Successful end-of-life care in the home requires 24-hour access to a supportive multidisciplinary team ready to deal rapidly with issues as they arise.

Table 4: **Drugs for End-of-Life Symptoms**

Class	Drug	Indication	Starting Doses	Adverse Effects	Comments	Cost[a]
Analgesics	*morphine* M.O.S., Morphine HP Injection, MS-IR, Statex, generics	Pain, dyspnea	PO, immediate-release: 5–10 mg Q4–6H po + appropriate PRN use IV/SC: 2.5–5 mg Q4–6H + appropriate PRN use	Nausea, vomiting, constipation, sedation, drowsiness, confusion, respiratory depression, urinary retention, dry mouth, myoclonus.	Highly individual dosing requirements. Dose escalation based on pain relief and adverse effects.	$
	hydromorphone Dilaudid, generics	Pain, dyspnea	PO, immediate-release: 2–4 mg Q4–6H + appropriate PRN use IV/SC: 1–2 mg Q4–6H + appropriate PRN use	See morphine.	See morphine.	$
	fentanyl generics	Dyspnea	SL: 25–50 µg (0.5–1 mL parenteral solution 50 µg/mL) Q1H PRN Ask patient to hold liquid under tongue for about 10 min without swallowing if possible	See morphine.	See morphine.	$$$$
Antiemetics	*dimenhydrinate*[b] Gravol Preparations, generics	Nausea, vomiting	PO/IM/PR: 25–50 mg Q4–6H PRN	Sedation, anticholinergic effects, confusion. The elderly may be particularly susceptible.	Additive sedation with other sedating medications.	po/pr: $ im: $$
	metoclopramide Metonia, other generics	Nausea, vomiting	PO/SC: 5–10 mg Q4–6H PRN	Diarrhea, abdominal cramps and distention, headache, hyperprolactinemia, drowsiness, fatigue, extrapyramidal effects.	See dimenhydrinate.	po: $ sc: $$
	prochlorperazine, generics	Nausea, vomiting	PO/IM/PR: 5–10 mg Q4–6H PRN	Sedation, anticholinergic effects (dry mouth, blurred vision, constipation, nasal congestion, urinary retention), extrapyramidal effects, hypotension, hypersensitivity; pancytopenia (rare).	See dimenhydrinate.	po/pr: $ im: $$

(cont'd)

Table 4: **Drugs for End-of-Life Symptoms** *(cont'd)*

Class	Drug	Indication	Starting Doses	Adverse Effects	Comments	Cost[a]
Antimuscarinics	*glycopyrrolate* generics	Respiratory secretions	SC: 0.2–0.6 mg Q2–4H PRN	Dizziness, blurred vision, dry mouth, urinary retention.	Rarely causes sedation or delirium.	$$$$/ 4 doses
	scopolamine (hyoscine hydrobromide)[b] generics	Respiratory secretions	SC: 0.3–0.8 mg Q2–4H PRN	Sedation, dizziness, blurred vision, dry mouth, urinary retention.		$$$/ 4 doses
Antipsychotics	*haloperidol* generics	Agitation, nausea	PO/SC: 0.5–2 mg Q4–8H PRN	Sedation, extrapyramidal effects.	Usual drug of choice.	$
	methotrimeprazine Nozinan, generics	Agitation, nausea, adjuvant analgesia	PO/SC: 5–10 mg Q4–6H PRN	See haloperidol.		po: $ sc: $$
	chlorpromazine generics	Dyspnea, nausea	PO/SC: 10 mg Q6H	See haloperidol. Hypotension with im/iv administration.		$
Benzodiazepines	*midazolam* generics	Agitation, dyspnea	SC: 1–2 mg Q30 min to Q1H PRN	Sedation, hypotension, transient apnea.		$$$
	lorazepam Ativan, generics	Agitation, dyspnea	PO/SL: 1–2 mg Q6–8H PRN	Sedation (up to 80%), dizziness.		$
	clonazepam Rivotril, generics	Agitation, dyspnea	PO: 0.25–0.5 mg Q8–12H PRN	Sedation, dizziness.		$
Corticosteroids	*dexamethasone* Dexasone, generics	Nausea, dyspnea, adjuvant analgesia	PO/SC: 4–8 mg daily	Mood changes, increased appetite, GI irritation, ulceration, fluid retention, weight gain, may mask signs of infection.		$

[a] Cost of 1-day supply, unless otherwise specified; includes drug cost only.
[b] Available without a prescription.
Dosage adjustment may be required in renal impairment; see Appendix I.
Legend: $ <$5 $$ $5–25 $$$ $25–45 $$$$ $45–65

Suggested Readings

LeGrand SB. Delirium in palliative medicine: a review. *J Pain Symptom Manage* 2012;44(4):583-94.

Lo B, Rubenfeld G. Palliative sedation in dying patients: "we turn to it when everything else hasn't worked". *JAMA* 2005;294(14):1810-6.

Morrison RS, Meier DE. Clinical practice. Palliative care. *N Engl J Med* 2004;350(25):2582-90.

Quigley C. The role of opioids in cancer pain. *BMJ* 2005;331(7520):825-9.

Stevenson J, Abernethy AP, Miller C et al. Managing comorbidities in patients at the end of life. *BMJ* 2004;329(7471):909-12.

University of Toronto, Faculty of Medicine, Continuing Education. *Ian Anderson continuing education program in end-of-life care*. Toronto (ON): University of Toronto. Available from: www.cme.utoronto.ca/endoflife/.

References

1. Lichter I, Hunt E. The last 48 hours of life. *J Palliat Care* 1990;6(4):7-15.
2. Bruera E, de Stoutz N, Velasco-Leiva A et al. Effects of oxygen on dyspnoea in hypoxaemic terminal-cancer patients. *Lancet* 1993;342(8862):13-4.
3. Jennings AL, Davies AN, Higgins JP et al. Opioids for the palliation of breathlessness in terminal illness. *Cochrane Database Sys Rev* 2001;(4):CD002066.
4. Viola R, Kiteley C, Lloyd NS et al. The management of dyspnea in cancer patients: a systematic review. *Support Care Cancer* 2008;16(4):329-37.
5. Benitez-Rosario MA, Martin AS, Feria M. Oral transmucosal fentanyl citrate in the management of dyspnea crises in cancer patients. *J Pain Symptom Manage* 2005;30(5):395-7.
6. Gauna AA, Kang SK, Triano ML et al. Oral transmucosal fentanyl citrate for dyspnea in terminally ill patients: an observational case series. *J Palliat Med* 2008;11(4):643-8.
7. Zhang H, Zhang J, Streisand JB. Oral mucosal delivery: clinical pharmacokinetics and therapeutic applications. *Clin Pharmacokinet* 2002;41(9):661-80.
8. Harlos M. *Palliative care incident pain and incident dyspnea protocol.* Winnipeg (MB): Palliative Medicine, University of Manitoba; 2002. Available from: www.palliative.info/incidentpain.htm.
9. Gallagher R. Killing the symptom without killing the patient. *Can Fam Physician* 2010;56:544-6.
10. Simon ST, Higginson IJ, Booth S et al. Benzodiazepines for the relief of breathlessness in advanced malignant and non-malignant diseases in adults. *Cochrane Database Syst Rev* 2010;20(1):CD007354.
11. Wedzicha JA, Wallis PJ, Ingram DA et al. Effect of diazepam on sleep in patients with chronic airflow obstruction. *Thorax* 1988;43(9):729-30.
12. O'Neill PA, Morton PB, Stark RD. Chlorpromazine--a specific effect on breathlessness? *Br J Clin Pharmacol* 1985;19(6):793-7.
13. McCaffery M, Pasero C. 0-10 numeric pain rating scale. In: *Pain: clinical manual.* St. Louis (MO): Mosby; 1999. p. 16.
14. Hawker GA, Mian S, Kendzerska T et al. Measures of adult pain: Visual Analog Scale for Pain (VAS Pain), Numeric Rating Scale for Pain (NRS Pain), McGill Pain Questionnaire (MPQ), Short-Form McGill Pain Questionnaire (SF-MPQ), Chronic Pain Grade Scale (CPGS), Short Form-36 Bodily Pain Scale (SF-36 BPS), and Measure of Intermittent and Constant Osteoarthritis Pain (ICOAP). *Arthritis Care Res (Hoboken)* 2011;63(Suppl 11):S240-52.
15. Singh G, Triadafilopoulos G. Appropriate choice of proton pump inhibitor therapy in the prevention and management of NSAID-related gastrointestinal damage. *Int J Clin Pract* 2005;59(10):1210-7.
16. Casarett DJ, Inouye SK et al. Diagnosis and management of delirium near the end of life. *Ann Intern Med* 2001;135(1):32-40.
17. Cherny NI, Radbruch L. European Association for Palliative Care (EAPC) recommended framework for the use of sedation in palliative care. *Palliat Med* 2009;23(7):581-93.
18. Wildiers H, Menten J. Death rattle: prevalence, prevention and treatment. *J Pain Symptom Manage* 2002;23(4):310-7.
19. Bruera E, Hui D, Dalal S et al. Parenteral hydration in patients with advanced cancer: a multicenter, double-blind, placebo-controlled randomized trial. *J Clin Oncol* 2013;31(1):111-8.

Appendix I
Dosage Adjustment in Renal Impairment

James McCormack, BSc(Pharm), PharmD
Bruce Carleton, BPharm, PharmD and
Piera Calissi, BSc(Pharm), PharmD, FCSHP

Careful dosage adjustment may reduce the risk of drug toxicity in patients with impaired renal function. The following is an approach to empiric dosage adjustments (dose and/or interval) in adult patients based on an estimate of renal function (Figure 1, Table 1). This approach does not apply to patients on dialysis (consult specialized references).

Patient/Drug Considerations

The following questions should be answered prior to making empiric dosage adjustments. Table 2 provides drug-specific information.

Is the patient's renal function impaired?

Use the following formula[1] to estimate the *weight-corrected creatinine clearance* (ClCr) and to guide empiric dosage adjustments:

$$\text{Males: ClCr (mL/s/70 kg)} = \frac{(140 - \text{age}) \times 1.5}{\text{serum creatinine } (\mu\text{mol/L})}$$

Females: ClCr (mL/s/70 kg) = 0.85 × above equation

Many clinicians may be more familiar with a ClCr formula that includes weight. When using formulas to estimate ClCr, first identify the reason for the ClCr determination. If an estimate of the patient's true ClCr (in mL/second) is needed, then use a ClCr formula that includes weight. However, if the estimate of the degree of renal impairment is to guide dosage adjustments, use a weight-corrected estimate of ClCr rather than the patient's actual ClCr. This weight-corrected estimate is then compared to a "normal" ClCr for a 70 kg male (1.8–2 mL/s) to approximate the degree of renal dysfunction. Charts that suggest empiric dosage adjustments are usually based on the assumption that the baseline or normal ClCr is 1.8–2 mL/s. In addition, a weight-corrected ClCr is easier to calculate.

Elderly (>65 years) or malnourished patients may have relatively low muscle mass and therefore produce less creatinine. If the actual serum creatinine for such patients is used, the formula can often overestimate renal function. A rule of thumb in such patients is not to use a serum creatinine <100 µmol/L in the above formula.

Over the last few years, a new equation (Modification of Diet in Renal Disease—MDRD) to estimate the glomerular filtration rate (GFR) has found its way into clinical use. The MDRD is recommended for staging chronic kidney disease because it has improved predictive performance over the Cockcroft-Gault equation in estimating the GFR. Some clinicians also use the MDRD to estimate the GFR in order to adjust medication doses in patients with renal impairment. However, in adjusting drug doses in patients with renal impairment, the improved accuracy of the MDRD equation to predict the

GFR will not, in most cases, result in measurably improved outcomes such as enhanced medication safety or efficacy. This is because most recommendations for drug dosing in patients with renal impairment are not based on specific pharmacokinetic or pharmacodynamic outcome data. Instead, the dosage recommendations are based on somewhat broad and arbitrary GFR cut-off points. Given this, both the Cockcroft, Gault and MDRD equations provide sufficiently accurate estimates of renal function for use in drug dosage adjustment. Clinicians should likely choose the equation that is easiest to use or the one with which they are most familiar. Most importantly, clinicians need to determine rational starting doses using not only these equations, but also based on the urgency of the need for a response to drug therapy. All these issues make the current debate about which formula to use to estimate renal function somewhat irrelevant. However, regardless of the method used, there is a critical next step: titrate the dose whenever possible, and determine the correct dose by monitoring a patient's response to the dose chosen.

In general, if ClCr estimates are >1 mL/s/70 kg, empiric dosage adjustments are not required because changes in ClCr from 2 to 1 mL/s/70 kg are associated with relatively small changes in the half-life of a drug or its active metabolite. However, as ClCr falls below 1 mL/s/70 kg, empiric dosage adjustments should be based on the following questions.

Figure 1: Empiric Dosage Adjustment Based on Renal Function (Adults)

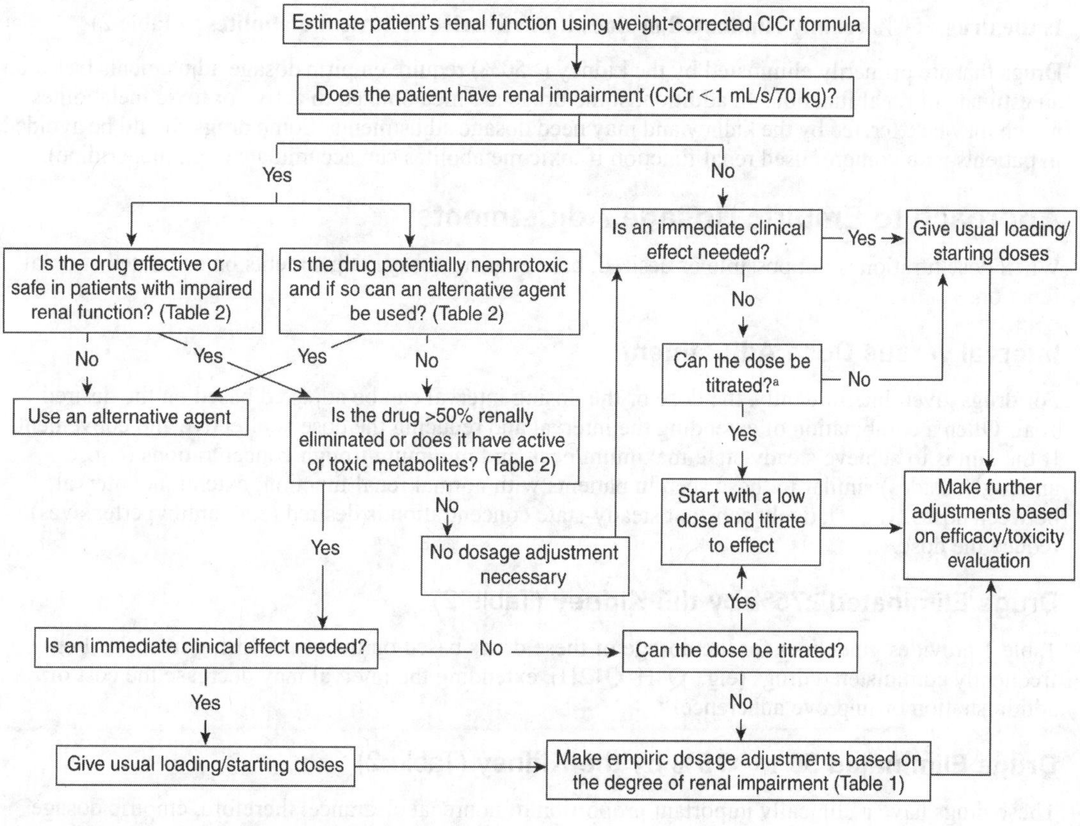

[a] For example, antihypertensives, antihyperglycemics, antidepressants.
Abbreviations: ClCr = creatinine clearance

Is the drug effective/safe in patients with renal impairment? (Table 2, Comments column)

Some drugs are ineffective or potentially toxic in patients with clinically important renal dysfunction (ClCr <0.5 mL/s/70 kg) and should be avoided.

Is the drug nephrotoxic? (Table 2, Comments column)

A number of drugs have the potential to worsen renal function and an alternative non-nephrotoxic agent should be used if possible.

Is an immediate clinical effect required?

When failure to elicit an immediate response (e.g., life-threatening conditions or severe pain) poses a clinically important risk of mortality or morbidity, drug dosing should be aimed at obtaining a therapeutic response within minutes or hours irrespective of renal function. In an attempt to achieve a rapid response, usual initial doses should be used, followed by empiric dosage adjustments once the patient has responded.

If an immediate effect is not required, can the dose be titrated?

Many conditions do not require an immediate or maximal effect, and dose titration can often be used to determine the lowest effective dose. To identify the correct dose for any patient, but particularly in patients with renal impairment, start with a low dose (e.g., one-quarter or one-half of the typically recommended dose), and titrate up to a clinical effect.

Is the drug >50% renally eliminated or does it have active or toxic metabolites? (Table 2)

Drugs that are primarily eliminated by the kidney (>50%) require empiric dosage adjustments based on an estimate of renal function. In addition, some drugs are metabolized to active or toxic metabolites which may be excreted by the kidney and may need dosage adjustments. Some drugs should be avoided in patients with compromised renal function if toxic metabolites can accumulate (e.g., meperidine).

Approach to Empiric Dosage Adjustments

When dose titration is not possible or desired, base empiric dosage adjustments on estimates of renal function.

Interval versus Dose Adjustment

For drugs given intermittently, the dose or the dosing interval can be adjusted based on the desired goal. Often a combination of extending the interval and reducing the dose is effective and convenient. If the aim is to achieve steady-state maximum/peak and minimum/trough concentrations (e.g., aminoglycosides) similar to those seen in patients with normal renal function, extend the interval between doses. If a relatively constant steady-state concentration is desired (e.g., antihypertensives), reduce the dose.

Drugs Eliminated ≥75% by the Kidney (Table 2)

Table 1 provides guidelines for the dosage of these drugs based on the usual dosing interval. For frequently administered drugs (e.g., Q4H–Q12H), extending the interval may decrease the cost of administration or improve adherence.

Drugs Eliminated 50 to <75% by the Kidney (Table 2)

These drugs have a clinically important proportion of nonrenal clearance, therefore, empiric dosage adjustments are generally not required until renal function estimates are <0.75 mL/s/70 kg (Table 1).

Drugs Eliminated <50% by the Kidney (Table 2)

For drugs eliminated <50% by the kidney, empiric dosage adjustments are generally not required, assuming the drug has no active or toxic metabolites. However, these drugs may require dosage adjustment in patients with clinically important liver dysfunction.

Drugs with Active or Toxic Metabolites (Table 2, Comments column)

Empiric dosage adjustments for drugs with active or toxic metabolites which are dependent on renal elimination should be made as though the drug were 75–100% renally eliminated.

Further Dosage Adjustments Based on Clinical Response

All of the above recommendations are for empiric dosage adjustments, and further dosage changes must always be made based on a patient-specific assessment of efficacy and toxicity. Serum drug concentration monitoring may guide dosage adjustments for certain drugs (Table 2, Comments column).

Table 1: **Suggested Empiric Dosage Adjustments in Adults for Drugs Primarily Renally Eliminated** based on percentage renal elimination and estimated creatinine clearance (normal ClCr = 2 mL/s/70 kg)

How to Use Table 1:

1. Estimate renal function (weight-corrected ClCr), *e.g., a patient with an estimated ClCr of 0.42 mL/s/70 kg is receiving iv ampicillin.*
2. Determine percentage renal elimination of drug (Table 2), *e.g., ampicillin is 75–100% renally eliminated, according to Table 2.*
3. Determine normal dosing interval, *e.g., usual dosing interval for ampicillin is Q6H.*
4. Using above information, determine empiric dosage adjustment, *e.g., the patient's ClCr is between 0.25 and 0.5 mL/s/70 kg. Therefore, the empiric dosing adjustment is to administer the ampicillin Q12H.*

			Normal Dosing Interval				
% Renal Elimination of Drug:	**75–100%**	**50–74%**	**Q4H**	**Q6H**	**Q8H**	**Q12H**	**Q24H**
	>1	>0.75	No adjustment required	No adjustment required	No adjustment required	No adjustment required	No adjustment required
Estimated ClCr (mL/s/70 kg)	0.5–1	0.33–0.75	Q6H	Q8H	Q12H	Q24H	Reduce dose by 25%[a]
	0.25–0.5	0.16–0.33	Q8H	Q12H	Q24H	Q24H and reduce dose by 25%[a]	Reduce dose by 50%[a]
	<0.25	<0.16	Q12H	Q24H	Q24H and reduce dose by 25%[a]	Q24H and reduce dose by 50%[a]	Reduce dose by 75%[a]

[a] For certain drugs, decreasing the dose is not appropriate, or one may need to extend interval >Q24H if available dosage forms do not permit specific dose reductions.

Table 2: Dosage Adjustment in Renal Impairment—Adults[a]

Drug	% Renal Elimination <50	50–74	≥75	Comments
5-aminosalicylic acid	•			
abacavir	•			
abatacept	•			
acarbose	•			
acebutolol		•		Active metabolite; assume ≥75% renal elimination for dosage adjustment
acetaminophen	•			
acetazolamide			•	Avoid; ineffective in severe renal impairment
acitretin	•			
acyclovir			•	
adalimumab	•			
adefovir dipivoxil	•			Nephrotoxic. Active metabolite; assume ≥75% renal elimination for dosage adjustment
adenosine	•			
alemtuzumab	•			
alendronate	•			Avoid in severe renal impairment
alfacalcidol	•			
alfuzosin	•			
aliskiren	•			
allopurinol	•			Active metabolite; assume ≥75% renal elimination for dosage adjustment
almotriptan			•	
alprazolam	•			
alprostadil	•			
alteplase	•			
aluminum salts	•			Avoid in severe renal impairment as may accumulate
amantadine			•	
amikacin			•	Nephrotoxic; monitor serum drug concentrations
amiloride		•		Avoid in severe renal impairment
aminophylline	•			
amiodarone	•			Active metabolite but no dosage adjustment required
amitriptyline	•			Active metabolite but no dosage adjustment required
amlodipine	•			
amoxicillin		•		
amoxicillin/clavulanate		•		

[a] *Omission of a drug from this table does not imply that dosage adjustment is NOT required in renal impairment. Refer to specific references for dosing in dialysis.*

Table 2: **Dosage Adjustment in Renal Impairment—Adults**[a] *(cont'd)*

	% Renal Elimination			
Drug	**<50**	**50–74**	**≥75**	**Comments**
amphetamine, mixed salts		•		Active metabolite but no dosage adjustment required
amphotericin	•			Nephrotoxic
ampicillin			•	
anakinra			•	
anidulafungin	•			
apixaban	•			
aprepitant	•			
aripiprazole	•			
ASA	•			Nephrotoxic
asenapine	•			
atazanavir	•			
atenolol			•	
atomoxetine	•			
atorvastatin	•			Active metabolite but no dosage adjustment required
atovaquone	•			
atropine	•			
auranofin			•	Avoid; nephrotoxic
azathioprine	•			Active metabolite; assume ≥75% renal elimination for dosage adjustment
azilsartan	•			
azithromycin	•			
baclofen			•	
belimumab	•			
benazepril	•			
benztropine	•			
bezafibrate		•		Avoid in renal impairment
bisacodyl	•			Active metabolite but no dosage adjustment required
bismuth subsalicylate	•			
bisoprolol		•		
bivalirudin	•			Reduce dose in severe renal impairment
boceprevir	•			
bromocriptine	•			
brompheniramine	•			
budesonide	•			
bumetanide	•			Larger doses may be required in severe renal impairment

[a]*Omission of a drug from this table does not imply that dosage adjustment is NOT required in renal impairment. Refer to specific references for dosing in dialysis.*

Table 2: **Dosage Adjustment in Renal Impairment—Adults**[a] *(cont'd)*

Drug	% Renal Elimination <50	50–74	≥75	Comments
buprenorphine	•			
bupropion	•			Active metabolite; assume ≥75% renal elimination for dosage adjustment
buserelin	•			
buspirone	•			
butalbital	•			Active metabolite; assume ≥75% renal elimination for dosage adjustment
caffeine	•			Active metabolite; assume ≥75% renal elimination for dosage adjustment
calcitonin	•			
calcitriol	•			
calcium salts	•			
canagliflozin	•			Less effective in moderate and ineffective in severe renal impairment
candesartan	•			
captopril		•		
carbamazepine	•			Active metabolite but no dosage adjustment required
carvedilol	•			Active metabolite but no dosage adjustment required
cascara				Route of elimination unknown
caspofungin	•			
cefaclor		•		
cefadroxil			•	
cefazolin			•	
cefepime			•	
cefixime		•		
cefotaxime		•		Active metabolite; assume ≥75% renal elimination for dosage adjustment
cefoxitin			•	
cefprozil		•		
ceftazidime			•	
ceftriaxone	•			
cefuroxime			•	
celecoxib	•			Nephrotoxic
cephalexin			•	
certolizumab pegol	•			Polyethylene glycol component renally eliminated
cetirizine		•		
chloral hydrate	•			Avoid. Active metabolite; assume ≥75% renal elimination for dosage adjustment
chlordiazepoxide	•			Active metabolite; assume ≥75% renal elimination for dosage adjustment

[a] *Omission of a drug from this table does not imply that dosage adjustment is NOT required in renal impairment. Refer to specific references for dosing in dialysis.*

Table 2: **Dosage Adjustment in Renal Impairment—Adults**[a] *(cont'd)*

Drug	% Renal Elimination <50	50–74	≥75	Comments
chloroquine		•		
chlorpheniramine	•			
chlorpromazine	•			Active metabolite but no dosage adjustment required
chlorpropamide	•			Avoid. Active metabolite; assume ≥75% renal elimination for dosage adjustment
chlorthalidone		•		Avoid; ineffective at low ClCr
chlorzoxazone	•			
cidofovir			•	Avoid; nephrotoxic. Active metabolite; assume ≥75% renal elimination for dosage adjustment
cilazapril	•			Active metabolite; assume ≥75% renal elimination for dosage adjustment
cimetidine		•		
cinacalcet	•			
ciprofloxacin		•		
citalopram	•			
clarithromycin	•			Active metabolite; assume ≥75% renal elimination for dosage adjustment
clindamycin	•			
clobazam	•			
clodronate			•	Avoid; nephrotoxic
clomiphene	•			
clomipramine	•			Active metabolite but no dosage adjustment required
clonazepam	•			
clonidine	•			
clopidogrel	•			
cloxacillin	•			
clozapine	•			Active metabolite but no dosage adjustment required
codeine	•			Active metabolite; assume ≥75% renal elimination for dosage adjustment
colchicine	•			Avoid in renal impairment
colestipol	•			
cyclobenzaprine	•			
cyclophosphamide	•			Active metabolites. Dosage adjustment recommended in severe renal impairment
cyclosporine	•			Nephrotoxic; monitor serum drug concentrations
cyproheptadine	•			
cyproterone acetate	•			
dabigatran			•	Contraindicated in severe renal impairment

[a]*Omission of a drug from this table does not imply that dosage adjustment is NOT required in renal impairment. Refer to specific references for dosing in dialysis.*

Table 2: **Dosage Adjustment in Renal Impairment—Adults**[a] *(cont'd)*

Drug	% Renal Elimination <50	50–74	≥75	Comments
dalteparin			•	
danazol	•			
dantrolene	•			
dapsone	•			
daptomycin			•	
darbepoetin alfa	•			
darifenacin	•			
darunavir	•			
deferoxamine			•	
delavirdine	•			
delta-9-tetrahydro-cannabinol/cannabidiol	•			
denosumab	•			
desipramine	•			Active metabolite but no dosage adjustment required
desloratadine	•			Active metabolite; assume ≥75% renal elimination for dosage adjustment
desmopressin			•	
desvenlafaxine	•			Manufacturer recommends dosage adjustment if ClCr <0.5 mL/s, although <50% renal elimination
dexamethasone	•			
dexbrompheniramine	•			
dexlansoprazole	•			
dexrazoxane	•			Reduce dose by 50% in patients with moderate to severe renal impairment
dextroamphetamine		•		Active metabolite but no dosage adjustment required
dextromethorphan	•			Active metabolite; assume ≥75% renal elimination for dosage adjustment
diazepam	•			Active metabolite but no dosage adjustment required
diclofenac	•			Nephrotoxic
dicyclomine			•	
didanosine	•			Active metabolite; assume ≥75% renal elimination for dosage adjustment
diflunisal	•			Nephrotoxic
digoxin			•	Monitor serum concentrations
dihydroergotamine	•			Active metabolite
diltiazem	•			Active metabolite but no dosage adjustment required
dimenhydrinate	•			
dimethyl fumarate	•			
diphenhydramine	•			

[a] *Omission of a drug from this table does not imply that dosage adjustment is NOT required in renal impairment. Refer to specific references for dosing in dialysis.*

Table 2: **Dosage Adjustment in Renal Impairment—Adults**[a] *(cont'd)*

Drug	**% Renal Elimination** <50	50–74	≥75	**Comments**
diphenoxylate	•			Active metabolite
dipyridamole	•			
divalproex	•			
dobutamine	•			
docusate	•			
dofetilide			•	
dolasetron	•			Active metabolite but no dosage adjustment required. Avoid in severe renal impairment
dolutegravir	•			
domperidone	•			
donepezil	•			Active metabolite but no dosage adjustment required
doxazosin	•			
doxepin	•			Active metabolite but no dosage adjustment required
doxycycline	•			
doxylamine	•			
dronabinol	•			
dronedarone	•			
droperidol	•			
duloxetine	•			
dutasteride	•			
efavirenz	•			
eletriptan	•			
emtricitabine			•	
enalapril	•			Active metabolite; assume ≥75% renal elimination for dosage adjustment
enfuvirtide	•			
enoxaparin			•	
entacapone	•			
entecavir		•		
eplerenone	•			Use contraindicated by manufacturer if ClCr <0.8 mL/s
epoetin alfa	•			
eprosartan	•			
eptifibatide	•			Dosage adjustment recommended for patients with renal impairment
ergotamine	•			Avoid in renal impairment
ertapenem			•	

[a]*Omission of a drug from this table does not imply that dosage adjustment is NOT required in renal impairment. Refer to specific references for dosing in dialysis.*

Table 2: **Dosage Adjustment in Renal Impairment—Adults**[a] *(cont'd)*

Drug	% Renal Elimination <50	50–74	≥75	Comments
erythromycin	•			
escitalopram	•			Active metabolite but no dosage adjustment required
esmolol	•			
esomeprazole	•			
estrogens	•			
etanercept	•			
ethacrynic acid	•			Avoid in severe renal impairment
ethambutol		•		
ethopropazine				Route of elimination unknown
ethosuximide	•			
etidronate		•		Nephrotoxic
etodolac	•			Nephrotoxic
etravirine	•			
exenatide			•	Avoid in severe renal impairment
ezetimibe	•			
famciclovir	•			Active metabolite; assume ≥75% renal elimination for dosage adjustment
famotidine			•	
fampridine			•	Use contraindicated by manufacturer if ClCr <1 mL/s
febuxostat	•			
felodipine	•			
fenofibrate	•			Active metabolite; assume ≥75% renal elimination for dosage adjustment
fentanyl	•			
ferumoxytol	•			
fesoterodine		•		Active metabolite
fexofenadine	•			Active metabolite; assume ≥75% renal elimination for dosage adjustment
fidaxomicin	•			
filgrastim	•			
finasteride	•			
fingolimod	•			
flecainide	•			Active metabolite; assume ≥75% renal elimination for dosage adjustment
fluconazole		•		
flucytosine			•	
fludrocortisone	•			
flunarizine	•			

[a]*Omission of a drug from this table does not imply that dosage adjustment is NOT required in renal impairment. Refer to specific references for dosing in dialysis.*

Table 2: Dosage Adjustment in Renal Impairment—Adults[a] *(cont'd)*

Drug	% Renal Elimination			Comments
	<50	50–74	≥75	
fluoxetine	•			Active metabolite but no dosage adjustment required
flupentixol	•			
fluphenazine	•			
flurazepam	•			Active metabolite but no dosage adjustment required
flurbiprofen	•			Nephrotoxic
fluvastatin	•			
fluvoxamine	•			
folic acid	•			% renal elimination increased with large doses
fondaparinux			•	
fosamprenavir	•			
fosaprepitant	•			
foscarnet			•	Avoid; nephrotoxic
fosfomycin	•			
fosinopril	•			Active metabolite but no dosage adjustment required
frovatriptan	•			
furosemide		•		Larger doses may be required in severe renal impairment
gabapentin			•	
galantamine	•			
ganciclovir			•	
gemfibrozil	•			Active metabolite; assume ≥75% renal elimination for dosage adjustment
gentamicin			•	Nephrotoxic; monitor serum drug concentrations
glatiramer	•			
gliclazide	•			
glimepiride	•			Active metabolite; assume ≥75% renal elimination for dosage adjustment
glucosamine	•			
glyburide	•			Avoid. Active metabolite but no dosage adjustment required
glycopyrrolate	•			
goserelin	•			
granisetron	•			
guaifenesin				Route of elimination unknown
guanfacine		•		
haloperidol	•			
heparin	•			
hydralazine	•			

[a]*Omission of a drug from this table does not imply that dosage adjustment is NOT required in renal impairment. Refer to specific references for dosing in dialysis.*

Table 2: **Dosage Adjustment in Renal Impairment—Adults**[a] *(cont'd)*

Drug	% Renal Elimination <50	50–74	≥75	Comments
hydrochlorothiazide			•	Avoid; ineffective at low ClCr
hydrocodone	•			Active metabolite; assume ≥75% renal elimination for dosage adjustment
hydrocortisone	•			
hydromorphone	•			
hydroxychloroquine	•			
hydroxyzine		•		
hyoscine	•			
ibuprofen	•			Nephrotoxic
ibutilide	•			Active metabolite but no dosage adjustment required
imipenem/cilastatin		•		
imipramine	•			Active metabolite but no dosage adjustment required
indapamide	•			Avoid; ineffective at low ClCr
indinavir	•			
indomethacin	•			Nephrotoxic
infliximab	•			
insulin	•			
interferon alfa	•			
interferon beta	•			
irbesartan	•			
iron salts	•			
isoniazid	•			
isosorbide dinitrate or 5-mononitrate	•			Active metabolite but no dosage adjustment required
isotretinoin	•			Avoid in renal impairment
itraconazole	•			
ketoconazole	•			
ketoprofen	•			Nephrotoxic
ketorolac			•	Nephrotoxic
ketotifen		•		
labetalol	•			
lacosamide			•	Manufacturer recommends a maximum daily dose of 300 mg in patients with end stage renal disease
lamivudine		•		Active metabolite; assume ≥75% renal elimination for dosage adjustment
lamotrigine	•			
lanreotide	•			

[a]*Omission of a drug from this table does not imply that dosage adjustment is NOT required in renal impairment. Refer to specific references for dosing in dialysis.*

Table 2: **Dosage Adjustment in Renal Impairment—Adults**[a] *(cont'd)*

	% Renal Elimination			
Drug	**<50**	**50–74**	**≥75**	**Comments**
lansoprazole	•			
leflunomide	•			Active metabolite; assume ≥75% renal elimination for dosage adjustment
leuprolide	•			
levetiracetam		•		
levodopa	•			Active metabolite but no dosage adjustment required
levofloxacin			•	
levonorgestrel	•			
levothyroxine	•			
lidocaine	•			Active metabolite but no dosage adjustment required
linagliptin	•			
linezolid	•			
liothyronine				No data on renal elimination
liraglutide	•			
lisdexamfetamine	•			
lisinopril			•	
lithium			•	Nephrotoxic; monitor serum drug concentrations
loperamide	•			
lopinavir/ritonavir	•			
loratadine	•			Active metabolite. Consider dosage adjustment in severe renal impairment
lorazepam	•			
losartan	•			Active metabolite but no dosage adjustment required
lovastatin	•			
loxapine	•			
lurasidone	•			Active metabolite; assume ≥75% renal elimination for dosage adjustment
magnesium salts	•			Avoid in severe renal impairment as may accumulate
maprotiline	•			Active metabolite but no dosage adjustment required
maraviroc	•			Modify dose when taking concurrent potent CYP3A4 inhibitors
medroxyprogesterone	•			
mefenamic acid	•			Nephrotoxic
mefloquine	•			
megestrol	•			
meloxicam	•			Nephrotoxic
memantine			•	
meperidine	•			Active metabolite; assume ≥75% renal elimination for dosage adjustment

[a]*Omission of a drug from this table does not imply that dosage adjustment is NOT required in renal impairment. Refer to specific references for dosing in dialysis.*

Table 2: Dosage Adjustment in Renal Impairment—Adults[a] *(cont'd)*

Drug	% Renal Elimination <50	50–74	≥75	Comments
mercaptopurine	•			Active metabolite; assume ≥75% renal elimination for dosage adjustment
meropenem		•		
mesna			•	
metformin			•	Avoid in severe renal impairment
methadone	•			
methazolamide	•			Avoid; ineffective in severe renal impairment
methimazole	•			
methocarbamol	•			
methotrexate			•	Avoid; nephrotoxic
methotrimeprazine	•			Active metabolite but no dosage adjustment required
methoxsalen	•			
methyldopa	•			Active metabolite; assume ≥75% renal elimination for dosage adjustment
methylnaltrexone		•		
methylphenidate	•			
methylprednisolone	•			
metoclopramide			•	Active metabolites; assume ≥75% renal elimination for dosage adjustment
metolazone		•		Dosage reduction not necessary in renal impairment
metoprolol	•			
metronidazole	•			Active metabolite but no dosage adjustment required
mexiletine	•			Active metabolite but no dosage adjustment required
micafungin	•			
miconazole	•			
midazolam	•			
midodrine	•			Active metabolite; assume ≥75% renal elimination for dosage adjustment
milrinone			•	
minocycline	•			
mirabegron	•			Manufacturer recommends a maximum daily dose of 25 mg in patients with severe renal impairment
mirtazapine			•	
misoprostol	•			
mitoxantrone	•			
moclobemide	•			
montelukast	•			
morphine	•			Active metabolite; assume ≥75% renal elimination for dosage adjustment

[a] *Omission of a drug from this table does not imply that dosage adjustment is NOT required in renal impairment. Refer to specific references for dosing in dialysis.*

Table 2: **Dosage Adjustment in Renal Impairment—Adults**[a] *(cont'd)*

Drug	% Renal Elimination			Comments
	<50	50–74	≥75	
moxifloxacin	•			
mycophenolate	•			
nabilone	•			
nabumetone	•			Nephrotoxic. Active metabolite; assume ≥75% renal elimination for dosage adjustment
nadolol			•	
nadroparin			•	
nafarelin	•			
naloxone	•			
naltrexone	•			Active metabolite but no dosage adjustment required
naproxen	•			Nephrotoxic
naratriptan		•		
natalizumab	•			
nateglinide	•			
nebivolol	•			Active metabolites; assume ≥75% renal elimination for dosage adjustment
nelfinavir	•			Active metabolite but no dosage adjustment required
nevirapine	•			
niacin	•			
nicotine	•			
nicoumalone	•			
nifedipine	•			
nimodipine	•			
nitrofurantoin	•			Avoid in renal impairment
nitroglycerin	•			
nitroprusside	•			
nizatidine		•		
norethindrone	•			
norfloxacin			•	
nortriptyline	•			Active metabolite but no dosage adjustment required
octreotide	•			Reduce dose in severe renal impairment
ofloxacin			•	
olanzapine	•			
olmesartan	•			Not recommended in severe renal impairment
olsalazine	•			

[a]*Omission of a drug from this table does not imply that dosage adjustment is NOT required in renal impairment. Refer to specific references for dosing in dialysis.*

Table 2: **Dosage Adjustment in Renal Impairment—Adults**[a] *(cont'd)*

Drug	% Renal Elimination <50	50–74	≥75	Comments
omalizumab	•			
omega-3 fatty acids	•			
omeprazole	•			
ondansetron	•			
orlistat	•			
orphenadrine	•			Active metabolites; assume ≥75% renal elimination for dosage adjustment
oseltamivir	•			Active metabolite. Dosage adjustment recommended in severe renal impairment
oxaprozin	•			Nephrotoxic
oxazepam	•			
oxcarbazepine	•			Active metabolite; assume ≥75% renal elimination for dosage adjustment
oxtriphylline	•			
oxybutynin	•			Active metabolite but no dosage adjustment required
oxycodone	•			
oxymetazoline				Route of elimination unknown
palifermin	•			
paliperidone		•		Manufacturer recommends dosage adjustment in renal impairment
palonosetron			•	Active metabolite but no dosage adjustment required
pamidronate		•		Nephrotoxic
pantoprazole	•			
paroxetine	•			
pegfilgrastim	•			Polyethylene glycol component renally eliminated
peginterferon alfa	•			Polyethylene glycol component renally eliminated
penicillamine	•			Avoid; nephrotoxic
penicillin G/V		•		
pentamidine	•			Nephrotoxic when given iv
pentazocine	•			
pentoxifylline	•			
perampanel	•			
perindopril	•			Active metabolite; assume ≥75% renal elimination for dosage adjustment
perphenazine	•			
phenazopyridine		•		
phenelzine	•			
pheniramine			•	

[a]*Omission of a drug from this table does not imply that dosage adjustment is NOT required in renal impairment. Refer to specific references for dosing in dialysis.*

Table 2: Dosage Adjustment in Renal Impairment—Adults[a] *(cont'd)*

Drug	% Renal Elimination <50	50–74	≥75	Comments
phenobarbital	•			Active metabolite but no dosage adjustment required
phenylephrine	•			
phenytoin	•			
pimozide	•			
pinaverium bromide	•			
pindolol	•			
pioglitazone	•			
piperacillin			•	
piperacillin/tazobactam			•	
pipotiazine	•			Avoid in renal impairment due to risk of hypotension
piroxicam	•			Nephrotoxic
pizotifen	•			
posaconazole	•			
potassium salts			•	May accumulate in renal impairment
pramipexole			•	
prasugrel	•			Active metabolite but no dosage adjustment required
pravastatin	•			
prazosin	•			
prednisone	•			
pregabalin			•	
primaquine	•			
primidone	•			Active metabolite but no dosage adjustment required
procainamide		•		Active metabolite; assume ≥75% renal elimination for dosage adjustment
prochlorperazine	•			Active metabolite; assume ≥75% renal elimination for dosage adjustment
procyclidine	•			Active metabolite; assume ≥75% renal elimination for dosage adjustment
progesterone	•			
proguanil	•			Active metabolite but no dosage adjustment required
promethazine	•			
propafenone	•			
propranolol	•			
propylthiouracil	•			
prucalopride		•		
pseudoephedrine			•	
pyrazinamide	•			Avoid in severe renal impairment

[a]*Omission of a drug from this table does not imply that dosage adjustment is NOT required in renal impairment. Refer to specific references for dosing in dialysis.*

Table 2: **Dosage Adjustment in Renal Impairment—Adults**[a] *(cont'd)*

Drug	% Renal Elimination <50	50–74	≥75	Comments
pyridoxine		•		% renal elimination increased with large doses
pyrimethamine	•			
quetiapine	•			
quinapril	•			Active metabolite; assume ≥75% renal elimination for dosage adjustment
quinidine	•			Active metabolite but no dosage adjustment required
quinine	•			
quinupristin/dalfopristin	•			
rabeprazole	•			
raloxifene	•			
raltegravir	•			
ramipril	•			Active metabolite; assume ≥75% renal elimination for dosage adjustment
ranitidine		•		
rasagiline	•			Conclusive data not available for renally impaired patients
rasburicase	•			
repaglinide	•			
ribavirin	•			Avoid in renal impairment
rifabutin	•			Active metabolite but no dosage adjustment required
rifampin	•			Active metabolite but no dosage adjustment required
rilpivirine	•			
risedronate			•	Avoid in severe renal impairment
risperidone	•			Active metabolite; assume ≥75% renal elimination for dosage adjustment
ritonavir	•			Active metabolite but no dosage adjustment required
rituximab	•			Nephrotoxic
rivaroxaban	•			Avoid in severe renal impairment
rivastigmine	•			
rizatriptan	•			Active metabolite but no dosage adjustment required
roflumilast	•			
ropinirole	•			
rosiglitazone	•			
rosuvastatin	•			
rotigotine	•			
rufinamide	•			
saquinavir	•			
saxagliptin	•			Active metabolite; assume ≥75% renal elimination for dosage adjustment

[a] *Omission of a drug from this table does not imply that dosage adjustment is NOT required in renal impairment. Refer to specific references for dosing in dialysis.*

Table 2: **Dosage Adjustment in Renal Impairment—Adults**[a] *(cont'd)*

	% Renal Elimination			
Drug	**<50**	**50–74**	**≥75**	**Comments**
scopolamine	•			
selegiline	•			Active metabolite but no dosage adjustment required
senna				% renally eliminated unknown
sertraline	•			
sildenafil	•			
silodosin	•			
simeprevir	•			
simvastatin	•			
sitagliptin			•	
sodium aurothiomalate			•	Avoid; nephrotoxic
sodium phosphates				% eliminated not established; may accumulate in renal impairment
sofosbuvir			•	No dose adjustment recommended in mild and moderate renal impairment
solifenacin		•		Active metabolite
sotalol		•		
spectinomycin			•	Dosage adjustment unnecessary
spironolactone	•			Avoid. Active metabolite; assume ≥75% renal elimination for dosage adjustment
stavudine	•			Active metabolite; assume ≥75% renal elimination for dosage adjustment
stiripentol	•			
streptomycin			•	Nephrotoxic; monitor serum drug concentrations
sucralfate	•			Al^{++} may accumulate
sulfadiazine		•		Nephrotoxic
sulfamethoxazole/ trimethoprim		•		
sulfasalazine	•			Active metabolite but no dosage adjustment required
sulfinpyrazone	•			Avoid; nephrotoxic
sulindac	•			Nephrotoxic. Active metabolite but no dosage adjustment required
sumatriptan	•			
tacrolimus	•			
tadalafil	•			Active metabolite; assume ≥75% renal elimination for dosage adjustment
tamsulosin	•			
telaprevir	•			
telbivudine			•	
telmisartan	•			
temazepam	•			

[a]*Omission of a drug from this table does not imply that dosage adjustment is NOT required in renal impairment. Refer to specific references for dosing in dialysis.*

Table 2: **Dosage Adjustment in Renal Impairment—Adults**[a] *(cont'd)*

	% Renal Elimination			
Drug	**<50**	**50–74**	**≥75**	**Comments**
tenecteplase	•			
tenofovir			•	Nephrotoxic
tenoxicam	•			Nephrotoxic
terazosin	•			
terbinafine		•		
teriflunomide	•			
teriparatide	•			Do not use if ClCr <0.5 mL/s
tetracycline		•		Nephrotoxic
theophylline	•			
thiamine	•			
thiothixene	•			
tiaprofenic acid			•	Nephrotoxic
ticagrelor	•			
ticarcillin			•	
ticarcillin/clavulanate		•		
ticlopidine	•			
tigecycline	•			
timolol	•			
tinzaparin			•	
tipranavir	•			
tirofiban		•		
tizanidine	•			
tobramycin			•	Nephrotoxic; monitor serum drug concentrations
tocilizumab	•			
tolbutamide	•			
tolcapone	•			
tolterodine	•			
topiramate			•	
tramadol	•			Active metabolite; assume ≥75% renal elimination for dosage adjustment
trandolapril	•			Active metabolite; assume ≥75% renal elimination for dosage adjustment
tranexamic acid			•	
tranylcypromine	•			Active metabolite; assume ≥75% renal elimination for dosage adjustment
trazodone	•			
triamterene	•			Avoid. Nephrotoxic. Active metabolite but no dosage adjustment required

[a]*Omission of a drug from this table does not imply that dosage adjustment is NOT required in renal impairment. Refer to specific references for dosing in dialysis.*

Table 2: Dosage Adjustment in Renal Impairment—Adults[a] *(cont'd)*

Drug	% Renal Elimination <50	50–74	≥75	Comments
triazolam	•			
trifluoperazine	•			
trihexyphenidyl			•	
trimeprazine	•			
trimethoprim			•	
trimipramine	•			
triprolidine	•			
triptorelin	•			Conclusive data not available for renally impaired patients but dosage adjustment may be required
trospium	•			Conclusive data not available for renally impaired patients but dosage adjustment may be required
L-tryptophan	•			
ulipristal	•			
ursodiol	•			
ustekinumab	•			
valacyclovir	•			Active metabolite; assume ≥75% renal elimination for dosage adjustment
valganciclovir		•		Nephrotoxic. Active metabolite; assume ≥75% renal elimination for dosage adjustment
valproic acid	•			
valsartan	•			
vancomycin			•	Nephrotoxic; monitor serum drug concentrations
vardenafil	•			
varenicline			•	
vasopressin	•			
venlafaxine	•			Active metabolite; assume ≥75% renal elimination for dosage adjustment
verapamil	•			Active metabolite but no dosage adjustment required
verteporfin	•			
vigabatrin			•	
vitamin B_{12}		•		% renal elimination increased with large doses
vitamin C			•	
vitamin D	•			
vitamin E	•			
voriconazole	•			Avoid iv formulation in renal impairment; nephrotoxic vehicle
warfarin	•			
xylometazoline				Route of elimination unknown

[a]*Omission of a drug from this table does not imply that dosage adjustment is NOT required in renal impairment. Refer to specific references for dosing in dialysis.*

Table 2: **Dosage Adjustment in Renal Impairment—Adults[a]** *(cont'd)*

Drug	**% Renal Elimination <50**	**50–74**	**≥75**	**Comments**
yohimbine				Avoid. Route of elimination unknown
zafirlukast	•			
zanamivir	•			
zidovudine	•			Reduce dose in severe renal impairment
ziprasidone	•			
zoledronic acid			•	
zolmitriptan	•			Active metabolite but no dosage adjustment required
zolpidem	•			
zopiclone	•			
zuclopenthixol	•			

[a] Omission of a drug from this table does not imply that dosage adjustment is NOT required in renal impairment. Refer to specific references for dosing in dialysis.

Abbreviations: ASA = acetylsalicylic acid; ClCr = creatinine clearance; CYP3A4 = cytochrome P450 3A4

Suggested Readings

Dersch D, McCormack J. Estimating renal function for drug dosing: rewriting the gospel? *Can J Hosp Pharm* 2008;61(2):138-43. Available from: www.cjhp-online.ca/index.php/cjhp/article/view/31.

Vidal L, Shavit M, Fraser A et al. Systematic comparison of four sources of drug information regarding adjustment of dose for renal function. *BMJ* 2005;331(7511):263.

References

1. McCormack JP Cooper J, Carleton B. Simple approach to dosage adjustment in patients with renal impairment. *Am J Health Syst Pharm* 1997;54(21):2505-9.

[a]*Omission of a drug from this table does not imply that dosage adjustment is NOT required in renal impairment. Refer to specific references for dosing in dialysis.*

Appendix II
Drug Use during Pregnancy

Orna Diav-Citrin, MD and
Gideon Koren, MD, FRCPC

The following is an overview of drug use during pregnancy. This information is not intended to be a comprehensive review; the reader is therefore encouraged to seek additional and confirmatory information.

Principles of Prescribing in Pregnancy

Many pregnant women are exposed to a variety of medications that may exert therapeutic, toxic or teratogenic effects on the fetus. Since the thalidomide disaster, many physicians and pregnant women tend to withhold any medication during pregnancy, although the risk of teratogenic effect from most drugs in therapeutic doses is nonexistent. Major congenital defects occur in 1–3% of the general population at birth.[1] Of the major defects, about 25% are of genetic origin (genetically inherited diseases, new mutations and chromosomal abnormalities) and 65% are of unknown etiology (multifactorial, polygenic, spontaneous errors of development and synergistic interactions of teratogens). Only 2–3% of malformations are thought to be associated with drug treatment. The remaining defects are related to other environmental exposures including infectious agents, maternal disease states, mechanical problems and irradiation.[2,3]

Optimal prescribing in pregnancy is a challenge and should provide maximal safety to the fetus as well as therapeutic benefit to the mother. To date, very few drugs are proven teratogens in humans. However, drug-induced malformations are important because they are potentially preventable.

Maternal physiologic changes during pregnancy may alter the pharmacokinetics of drugs. Clearance rates of many drugs increase during late pregnancy due to increases in both renal and hepatic elimination (e.g., digoxin, phenytoin), while for other drugs the clearance rate decreases (e.g., theophylline). Generally, little is known about the relationship between maternal serum drug concentration and risk of teratogenicity.

The importance of **timing of drug exposure** is better understood; the effect produced by a teratogenic agent depends upon the developmental stage in which the conceptus is exposed. Several important phases in human development are recognized:[3]

- The **"all or none" period**, the time from conception until somite formation, corresponds to the first 17 days after conception. Insults to the embryo in this phase are likely to result in either death and miscarriage or intact survival. The embryo is undifferentiated, and repair and recovery are possible through multiplication of the still totipotential cells. Consider that exposure to teratogens during the presomitic stage usually does not cause congenital malformations unless the agent persists in the body beyond this period.[3,4]
- The **embryonic period**, from 18–60 days after conception when the basic steps in organogenesis occur. This is the period of maximum sensitivity to teratogenicity since tissues are differentiating rapidly and damage becomes irreparable. Exposure to teratogenic agents during this period has the greatest likelihood of causing a structural anomaly. The pattern of anomalies produced depends on which systems are differentiating at the time of teratogenic exposure.

- The **fetal phase**, from the end of the embryonic stage to term, when growth and functional maturation of formed organs and systems occurs. Teratogen exposure in this period will affect fetal growth (e.g., intrauterine growth restriction) and the size or function of an organ, rather than cause gross structural anomalies. The term **fetal toxicity** is commonly used to describe such an effect.

The potential effect of psychoactive agents (e.g., antidepressants, antiepileptics, alcohol and other drugs of abuse) on the developing central nervous system has led to the new field of behavioural teratology.

Many organ systems continue structural and functional maturation long after birth. Most of the adenocarcinomas associated with 1st trimester exposure to diethylstilbestrol occurred many years later.

Teratogens must reach the developing conceptus in sufficient amounts to cause their effects. Large molecules with a molecular weight greater than 1000 (e.g., heparin) do not easily cross the placenta into the embryonic-fetal bloodstream. Other factors influencing the rate and extent of placental transfer of drugs include polarity, lipid solubility and the existence of a specific carrier protein (e.g., P-glycoprotein).

In an attempt to provide the practitioner with a better assessment of fetal risk, the US Food and Drug Administration (FDA) developed a classification of fetal risk in 1979.[5] These categories initially appeared logical but are not helpful in counselling individual patients. Drug manufacturers may have legal rather than scientific reasons for assigning particular designations. The classification frequently results in ambiguity and even false alarm. For example, oral contraceptives are denoted as X (contraindicated in pregnancy), despite failure of 2 meta-analyses to show increased teratogenic risk. In 1994 the Teratology Society stated that the FDA ratings are inappropriate and should be replaced by narrative statements that summarize and interpret available data regarding hazards of developmental toxicity and provide estimates of teratogenic risk.[6] During the last few years the FDA has begun a process to change the present system.

Teratology Counselling[7]

- Ascertain the clinical facts regarding the nature of the exposure: the length, dosage and timing during pregnancy, as well as other exposures of concern (e.g., alcohol, cigarette smoking, herbal remedies).
- Collect all available current data regarding the agent and the risk of exposure.
- Counselling should include background human baseline risk for major malformations, whether the fetus is at increased risk, which anomaly has been associated with the agent in question, a risk assessment, methods of prenatal detection when available, limitations in our knowledge and limitations of prenatal diagnostic capabilities.
- Additional considerations include the potential risk of the medical condition for which a drug is prescribed, known interactions between the disease state and the pregnancy, and preventive measures when applicable (e.g., folic acid supplementation in carbamazepine exposure).
- Because more than 50% of pregnancies are unplanned, teratogenic risk assessment should be started prior to pregnancy.

Table 1 lists drugs with sufficient evidence to prove their teratogenic effect in humans. Use an alternative in pregnancy when possible. Table 2 lists possible teratogenic drugs with insufficient evidence as yet for teratogenicity in humans.

Drugs of Choice during Pregnancy

Table 3 presents drugs of choice during gestation for common maternal conditions.

Note: Antenatal drug/chemical risk counselling or information on safety of drug use during breastfeeding is available from the Motherisk Program, Hospital for Sick Children, Toronto, Ontario. Tel.: 416-813-6780; email: momrisk@sickkids.ca; Web site: www.motherisk.org.

Table 1: Proven Teratogenic Drugs in Humans[7]

Drug	Adverse Effects
Angiotensin-onverting Enzyme inhibitors (ACEIs) and Angiotensin II antagonists	Adverse effects relate to hemodynamic effects of ACEIs and angiotensin II antagonists on the fetus. In late pregnancy, ACEI fetopathy: intrauterine renal insufficiency, neonatal hypotension, oliguria with renal failure, hyperkalemia, complications of oligohydramnios (fetal limb contractures, lung hypoplasia and craniofacial anomalies), prematurity, intrauterine growth restriction and fetal death. 1st trimester exposure: questionable teratogenic risk of cardiovascular and CNS malformations.[8] Several cohort studies and meta-analyses suggest the observed risk is associated with the underlying maternal conditions.[9,10,11,12,13,14]
Antineoplastic agents	A significant increase in the incidence of various fetal malformations and early miscarriages following 1st trimester exposure.[15]
Carbamazepine	1st trimester exposure: 1% risk of neural tube defects (10 × baseline risk) and an increased risk of cardiovascular malformations. A pattern of malformations similar to the fetal hydantoin syndrome has also been associated.[16]
Cocaine	Abruptio placenta, prematurity, fetal loss, decreased birth weight, microcephaly, limb defects, urinary tract malformations and poorer neurodevelopmental performance. Methodological problems make the findings difficult to interpret. Cocaine abuse is often associated with poly-drug abuse, alcohol consumption, smoking, malnutrition and poor prenatal care. Human epidemiology indicates the risk of major malformation from cocaine is probably low, but the anomalies may be severe.[17]
Corticosteroids (systemic)	1st trimester exposure: <1% increased risk of oral clefts.[18]
Coumarin anticoagulants (e.g., nicoumalone, warfarin)	1st trimester exposure (6–9 wk gestation): fetal warfarin syndrome (nasal hypoplasia and calcific stippling of the epiphyses). Intrauterine growth restriction and developmental delay (CNS damage), eye defects and hearing loss. Warfarin embryopathy is found in up to ⅓ of the cases where a coumarin derivative was given throughout pregnancy. Associated with high rate of miscarriage. Risk of CNS damage due to hemorrhage after the 1st trimester.[19,20]
Diethylstilbestrol	Vaginal clear cell adenocarcinoma in offspring exposed in utero before 18th wk (>90% of the cancers occurred after 14 y of age). High incidence of benign vaginal adenosis. Increased miscarriage rate and preterm delivery. In males exposed in utero: no signs of malignancy but genital lesions in 27% and pathologic changes in spermatozoa in 29%. The drug is not currently available in Canada.[21]
Ethanol	Fetal alcohol spectrum disorders include 4 diagnostic categories: fetal alcohol syndrome (FAS); partial FAS; alcohol-related neurodevelopmental disorders; alcohol-related birth defects. FAS presents as growth impairment, developmental delay and dysmorphic facies. Cleft palate and cardiac anomalies may occur. Full expression of the syndrome occurs with chronic daily ingestion of 2 g alcohol per kg (8 drinks/day) in about one-third of offspring and partial effects in three-quarters of offspring.[22,23,24,25,26] Alcohol-related neurodevelopmental disorders are much more common than FAS.[27]
Folic acid antagonists: aminopterin and methotrexate	Fetal aminopterin-methotrexate syndrome: CNS defects, craniofacial anomalies, abnormal cranial ossification, abnormalities in first branchial arch derivatives, intrauterine growth restriction and mental retardation after 1st trimester exposure. Maternal dose of methotrexate needed to induce defects is probably above 10 mg/wk.[28]
Hydantoins (phenytoin)	Fetal hydantoin syndrome: craniofacial dysmorphology, anomalies and hypoplasia of distal phalanges and nails, growth restriction, mental deficiency and cardiac defects.[29]
Lithium	Small increase in risk for cardiac teratogenesis in early gestation (1%). The risk of Ebstein's anomaly (a congenital heart defect, characterized by anterior displacement of the tricuspid valve, enlarged right chambers, often with atrial septal defect and arrhythmias) exceeds spontaneous rate of occurrence. Fetal echocardiography if exposed in 1st trimester.[30,31]
Misoprostol	1st trimester exposure: limb defects. Moebius sequence (a congenital facial palsy with impairment of ocular abduction, as a result of dysfunction of cranial nerves VI and VII) and CNS injuries. Absolute teratogenic risk: 1–2%. Uterine contraction inducing activity causing vascular disruption defects.[32,33,34]

(cont'd)

Table 1: Proven Teratogenic Drugs in Humans[7] *(cont'd)*

Drug	Adverse Effects
Mycophenolate mofetil	1st trimester exposure: ear, eye and craniofacial malformations, oral clefts, cardiac, finger, urogenital, gastrointestinal, CNS and skeletal malformations.[35,36,37]
Retinoids (acitretin, isotretinoin) and megadoses of Vitamin A	Systemic exposure: potent human general and behavioural teratogens. Risk of retinoic acid embryopathy: craniofacial anomalies, cardiac defects, abnormalities in thymic development and alterations in CNS development (congenital anomalies in 28% of prospectively ascertained pregnancies that resulted in births). Risk for associated miscarriage: 40%.[38,39]
Tetracyclines	Discolouration of the teeth after 17 wk gestation when deciduous teeth begin to calcify. Close to term: crowns of permanent teeth may be stained. Oxytetracycline and doxycycline associated with a lower incidence of enamel staining.[40,41]
Thalidomide	Malformations limited to tissues of mesodermal origin, primarily limbs (reduction defects), ears, cardiovascular system and gut musculature. Critical period: 34–50th day after the beginning of the last menstrual period. A single dose of <1 mg/kg has produced the syndrome. Embryopathy found in about 20% of pregnancies exposed in the critical period.[42]
Valproic Acid	1st trimester exposure: neural tube defects with 1–2% risk of meningomyelocele, primarily lumbar or lumbosacral, cardiovascular malformations and hypospadias. Fetal valproate syndrome: craniofacial dysmorphology, cardiovascular defects, long fingers and toes, hyperconvex fingernails and cleft lip, has been delineated by some investigations. Neurobehavioural teratogen.[43,44,45,46,47,48]

Table 2: Possible Teratogenic Drugs in Humans[a,49]

Drug	Adverse Effects
Diazepam	A questionable small increase in the incidence of cleft lip and palate (small studies). Larger studies did not confirm the association.[50]
Fluconazole	High-dose treatment: multiple synostosis, congenital heart defects, skeletal anomalies and recognizable dysmorphic facial features (case reports).[51]
HMG-CoA reductase Inhibitors (statins)	A questionable increase in the risk of CNS and limb anomalies (retrospective data), not confirmed by several prospective cohort studies.[52,53]
Methimazole	Scalp defects such as aplasia cutis congenita suggested through case reports and an epidemiological study in which methimazole had been added to animal feeds as a weight enhancer; methimazole embryopathy (choanal and esophageal atresia, scalp defects, minor facial anomalies and psychomotor delay).[54,55]
Paroxetine	A questionable increase in the risk of cardiac malformations, which may be associated with the underlying psychiatric disorder.[56]
Penicillamine	High-dose treatment: connective tissue disorders (cutis laxa) (case reports).[57]
Sulfamethoxazole/trimethoprim	Possible increased risk of neural tube and cardiovascular defects and oral clefts with 1st trimester exposure. Folic acid supplementation may reduce these risks.[58,59,60]

[a] This list is not exhaustive.

Table 3: Drugs of Choice for Select Conditions during Pregnancy[7]

Condition	Drugs of Choice	Alternative	Comments
Allergy[61,62]	Antihistamines: chlorpheniramine, desloratadine, diphenhydramine, dimenhydrinate, loratadine	Intranasal preparations of sodium cromoglycate, beclomethasone, budesonide, fluticasone; cetirizine, fexofenadine	
Anticoagulation	Heparin and low molecular weight heparins[63,64]		
Anxiety	Short-term treatment: benzodiazepines[50] Long-term treatment: citalopram, fluoxetine, sertraline[56,65,66,67]		Watch for possible transient neonatal effects when benzodiazepines or SSRIs used close to term. Short- or intermediate-acting benzodiazepines (e.g., lorazepam, oxazepam) may be preferred if needed for regular use near term. For diazepam, there is a questionable small increase in the incidence of cleft lip and palate (small studies). Larger studies did not confirm the association.
Asthma[68]	Inhaled bronchodilators (ipratropium bromide, salbutamol or terbutaline) and inhaled corticosteroids (beclomethasone, budesonide, fluticasone)	Systemic corticosteroids and theophylline	
Bacterial infections[5]	Cephalosporins, clindamycin, erythromycin, penicillins	Aminoglycosides (amikacin, gentamicin, tobramycin), azithromycin, clarithromycin, quinolones	
Bipolar disorder	Lithium[31,69]	Carbamazepine, lamotrigine	With lithium, monitor using fetal echocardiography. Avoid valproic acid when possible, especially in the 1st trimester (if not possible to avoid, limit dose to <600–1000 mg/day). With carbamazepine and valproic acid, prescribe periconceptional folate supplementation: 5 mg po daily, ideally starting 3 months before trying to conceive and continuing at least until the end of the 1st trimester. Monitor using level II ultrasound for prevention of neural tube defects.
Constipation[70]	Bulk-forming agents (e.g., methylcellulose, psyllium hydrophilic mucilloid)	Docusate sodium, glycerin suppository, lactulose, mineral oil	Long-term use of mineral oil can decrease absorption of lipid soluble vitamins A, D, E and K.
Cough[71]	Antihistamines (in the case of cough due to rhinitis or allergy), codeine (when indicated)	Dextromethorphan	Avoid high doses of codeine close to term (risk of neonatal opioid withdrawal).

(cont'd)

Table 3: **Drugs of Choice for Select Conditions during Pregnancy[7]** *(cont'd)*

Condition	Drugs of Choice	Alternative	Comments
Depression	Citalopram, fluoxetine, sertraline,[56,66,67,72] tricyclic antidepressants	Other selective serotonin reuptake inhibitors, bupropion, venlafaxine	Neonatal withdrawal may occur when used in 3rd trimester. There is a questionable association between paroxetine exposure in pregnancy and cardiac malformations.
Diabetes mellitus	Human insulin[73]	Metformin[74] in gestational diabetes in 3rd trimester, glyburide[75]	Important to achieve strict glycemic control before conception and during the 1st trimester.
Diarrhea	Bulk-forming agents (e.g., methylcellulose, psyllium hydrophilic mucilloid), kaolin pectin[76]	Loperamide	
Dyspepsia	Alginic acid compound, antacids (various combinations of aluminum, calcium, magnesium salts), omeprazole,[77] ranitidine	Famotidine	
Epilepsy[78,79,80]	Carbamazepine, lamotrigine	Benzodiazepines (e.g., clonazepam) (see "Anxiety"), phenobarbital, phenytoin, valproic acid (see Comments).	The drug of choice for epilepsy in pregnancy should be the drug that best controls the seizures; monotherapy should be favoured. Use the lowest effective dose. Avoid valproic acid when possible, especially in the 1st trimester (if not possible to avoid, limit dose to <600–1000 mg/day). With carbamazepine and valproic acid, prescribe periconceptional folate supplementation: 5 mg po daily, ideally starting 3 months before trying to conceive and continuing at least until the end of the 1st trimester. Monitor using level II ultrasound for prevention of neural tube defects.
Fever and pain	Acetaminophen[81]	ASA, NSAIDs[82]	Avoid full anti-inflammatory doses of NSAIDs in 3rd trimester due to the risk of oligohydramnios and premature closure of ductus arteriosus.
Hemorrhoids (3rd trimester)	Topical hydrocortisone/pramoxine,[83] topical lidocaine, topical zinc oxide		
Herpetic infections	Acyclovir, valacyclovir[84,85]		
Hypertension[86]	Hydralazine, methyldopa	Beta-blockers, calcium channel blockers	With beta-blockers, reduced birth weight and persistent beta-blockade possible in newborn. Monitor growth using serial ultrasounds in the 3rd trimester. Monitor newborn for hypoglycemia, bradycardia, hypotension and respiratory problems during the first 24–48 h.
Hyperthyroidism[87]	Propylthiouracil		Perform fetal ultrasound near term for goitre detection.

Condition	Drugs of Choice	Alternative	Comments
Migraine (abortive therapy)	Acetaminophen	ASA, NSAIDs, sumatriptan[88,89,90]	Avoid full anti-inflammatory dose of NSAIDs in 3rd trimester due to the risk of oligohydramnios and premature closure of ductus arteriosus.
Nausea/Vomiting	Doxylamine/pyridoxine (Diclectin)[91,92]	Dimenhydrinate, metoclopramide,[93,94] ondansetron[95]	
Schizophrenia[96]	Phenothiazines	Haloperidol, risperidone	Watch neonate for possible adverse effects if taken close to term. Continue present antipsychotic if the woman is stable and unplanned pregnancy occurs. Monitor the woman for metabolic complications (weight gain, hyperglycemia, hyperlipidemia), especially with second-generation antipsychotics.
Vaginal candidiasis	Vaginal: clotrimazole, miconazole, nystatin Topical azoles are preferred[97,98]	Fluconazole: single systemic dose of 150 mg[99]	

References

1. Heinonen OP, Slone D, Shapiro S. *Birth defects and drugs in pregnancy*. Littleton (MA): Publishing Sciences Group; 1977.
2. Koren G, Pastuszak A, Ito S. Drugs in pregnancy. *N Engl J Med* 1998;338(16):1128-37.
3. Brent RL, Beckman DA. Environmental teratogens. *Bull NY Acad Med* 1990;66(2):123-63.
4. Adam MP. The all-or-none phenomenon revisited. *Birth Defects Res A Clin Mol Teratol* 2012;94(8):664-9.
5. Briggs GG, Freeman RK, Yaffe SJ. *Drugs in pregnancy and lactation: a reference guide to fetal and neonatal risk*. 9th ed. Philadelphia (PA): Lippincott Williams & Wilkins; 2011.
6. FDA classification of drugs for teratogenic risk. Teratology Society Public Affairs Committee. *Teratology* 1994;49(6):446-7.
7. Koren G. *Medication safety in pregnancy and breastfeeding*. New York (NY): McGraw-Hill; 2007.
8. Cooper WO, Hernandez-Diaz S, Arbogast PG et al. Major congenital malformations after first-trimester exposure to ACE inhibitors. *N Engl J Med* 2006;354(23):2443-51.
9. Malm H, Artama M, Gissler M et al. First trimester use of ACE-inhibitors and risk of major malformations. *Reprod Toxicol* 2008;26(1):67.
10. Lennestal R, Otterblad Olausson P, Kallen B. Maternal use of antihypertensive drugs in early pregnancy and delivery outcome, notably the presence of congenital heart defects in the infants. *Eur J Clin Pharmacol* 2009;65(6):615-25.
11. Diav-Citrin O, Shechtman S, Halberstadt Y et al. Pregnancy outcome after in utero exposure to angiotensin converting enzyme inhibitors or angiotensin receptor blockers. *Reprod Toxicol* 2011;31(4):540-5.
12. Li D, Yang C, Andrade S et al. Maternal exposure to angiotensin converting enzyme inhibitors in the first trimester and risk of malformations in offspring: a retrospective cohort study. *BMJ* 2011;343:d5931.
13. Moretti ME, Caprara D, Drehuta I et al. The fetal safety of angiotensin converting enzyme inhibitors and angiotensin II receptor blockers. *Obstet Gynecol Int* 2012;2012:658310.
14. Polifka JE. Is there an embryopathy associated with first-trimester exposure to angiotensin-converting enzyme inhibitors and angiotensin receptor antagonists? A critical review of the evidence. *Birth Defects Res A Clin Mol Teratol* 2012;94(8):576-98.
15. Selig BP, Furr JR, Huey RW et al. Cancer chemotherapeutic agents as human teratogens. *Birth Defects Res A Clin Mol Teratol* 2012;94(8):626-50.
16. Jones KL, Lacro RV, Johnson KA et al. Pattern of malformations in the children of women treated with carbamazepine during pregnancy. *N Engl J Med* 1989;320(25):1661-6.
17. Addis A, Moretti ME, Ahmed-Syed F et al. Fetal effects of cocaine: an updated meta-analysis. *Reprod Toxicol* 2001;15(4):341-69.
18. Park-Wyllie L, Mazzotta P, Pastuszak A et al. Birth defects after maternal exposure to corticosteroids: prospective cohort study and meta-analysis of epidemiological studies. *Teratology* 2000;62(6):384-92.
19. Hall JG, Pauli RM, Wilson KM. Maternal and fetal sequelae of anticoagulation during pregnancy. *Am J Med* 1980;68(1):122-40.
20. Schaefer C, Hannemann D, Meister R et al. Vitamin K antagonists and pregnancy outcome. A multi-centre prospective study. *Thromb Haemost* 2006;95(6):949-57.
21. Mittendorf R. Teratogen update: carcinogenesis and teratogenesis associated with exposure to diethylstilbestrol (DES) in utero. *Teratology* 1995;51(6):435-45.
22. Lemoine P, Harousseau H, Borteyru JP et al. [Les enfants des parents alcoholiques: anomalies observées a propos de 127 cas]. *Ouest Med* 1968;21:476-82. [French].
23. Ulleland CN. The offspring of alcoholic mothers. *Ann N Y Acad Sci* 1972;197:167-9.
24. Jones KL, Smith DW, Ulleland CN et al. Pattern of malformation in offspring of chronic alcoholic mothers. *Lancet* 1973;1(7815):1267-71.
25. Jones KL, Smith DW. Recognition of the fetal alcohol syndrome in early infancy. *Lancet* 1973;2(7836):999-1001.
26. Rosett HL, Ouellette EM, Weiner L et al. Therapy of heavy drinking during pregnancy. *Obstet Gynecol* 1978;51(1):41-6.
27. Breiner P, Nulman I, Koren G. Identifying the neurobehavioral phenotype of fetal alcohol spectrum disorder in young children. *J Popul Ther Clin Pharmacol* 2013;20(3):e334-9.
28. Hyoun SC, Obican SG, Scialli AR. Teratogen update: methotrexate. *Birth Defects Res A Clin Mol Teratol* 2012;94(4):187-207.
29. Mercier-Parot L, Tuchmann-Duplessis H. The dysmorphogenic potential of phenytoin: experimental observations. *Drugs* 1974;8(5):340-53.
30. Congenital malformations. *N Engl J Med* 1983;309(5):311-2.
31. Jacobson SJ, Jones K, Johnson K et al. Prospective multicenter study of pregnancy outcome after lithium exposure during the first trimester. *Lancet* 1992;339(8792):530-3.
32. Pastuszak AL, Schuler L, Speck-Martins CE et al. Use of misoprostol during pregnancy and Möbius' syndrome in infants. *N Engl J Med* 1998;338(26):1881-5.
33. Koren G, Schuler L. Taking drugs during pregnancy. How safe are the unsafe? *Can Fam Physician* 2001;47:951-3.
34. Vauzelle C, Beghin D, Cournot MP et al. Birth defects after exposure to misoprostol in the first trimester of pregnancy: prospective follow-up study. *Reprod Toxicol* 2013;36:98-103.
35. Le Ray C, Coulomb A, Elefant E et al. Mycophenolate mofetil in pregnancy after renal transplantation: a case of major fetal malformations. *Obstet Gynecol* 2004;103(5 Pt 2):1091-4.
36. Anderka MT, Lin AE, Abuelo DN et al. Reviewing the evidence for mycophenolate mofetil as a new teratogen: case report and review of the literature. *Am J Med Genet A* 2009;149A(6):1241-8.
37. Hoeltzenbein M, Elefant E, Vial T et al. Teratogenicity of mycophenolate confirmed in a prospective study of the European Network of Teratology Information Services. *Am J Med Genet A* 2012;158A(3):588-96.
38. Lammer EJ, Chen DT, Hoar RM et al. Retinoic acid embryopathy. *N Engl J Med* 1985;313(14):837-41.
39. Dai WS, LaBraico JM, Stern RS. Epidemiology of isotretinoin exposure during pregnancy. *J Am Acad Dermatol* 1992;26(4):599-606.
40. Forti G, Benincori C. Doxycycline and the teeth. *Lancet* 1969;1(7598):782.
41. Sanchez AR, Rogers RS, Sheridan PJ. Tetracycline and other tetracycline-derivative staining of the teeth and oral cavity. *Int J Dermatol* 2004;43(10):709-15.
42. Newman CG. Teratogen update: clinical aspects of thalidomide embryopathy—a continuing preoccupation. *Teratology* 1985;32(1):133-44.
43. Bjerkedal T, Czeizel A, Goujard J et al. Valproic acid and spina bifida. *Lancet* 1982;2(8307):1096.
44. Robert E, Guibaud P. Maternal valproic acid and congenital neural tube defects. *Lancet* 1982;2(8304):937.
45. Centres for Disease Control (CDC).Valproate: a new cause of birth defects—report from Italy and follow-up from France. *MMWR Morb Mortal Wkly Rep* 1983;32(33):438-9.
46. Christianson AL, Chesler N, Kromberg JG. Fetal valproate syndrome: clinical and neurodevelopmental features in two sibling pairs. *Dev Med Child Neurol* 1994;36(4):361-9.

47. Moore SJ, Turnpenny P, Quinn A et al. A clinical study of 57 children with fetal anticonvulsant syndromes. *J Med Genet* 2000;37(7):489-97.
48. Jentink J, Loane MA, Dolk H et al. Valproic acid monotherapy in pregnancy and major congenital malformations. *N Engl J Med* 2010;362(23):2185-93.
49. Motherisk. Toronto (ON): Hospital for Sick Children. Available from: www.motherisk.orgwomen/index.jsp. Accessed November 2013.
50. Enato E, Moretti M, Koren G. The fetal safety of benzodiazepines: an updated meta-analysis. *J Obstet Gynaecol Can* 2011;33(1):46-8.
51. Lopez-Rangel E, Van Allen MI. Prenatal exposure to fluconazole: an identifiable dysmorphic phenotype. *Birth Defects Res A Clin Mol Teratol* 2005;73(11):919-23.
52. Godfrey LM, Erramouspe J, Cleveland KW. Teratogenic risk of statins in pregnancy. *Ann Pharmacother* 2012;46(10):1419-24.
53. Winterfeld U, Allignol A, Panchaud A et al. Pregnancy outcome following maternal exposure to statins: a multicentre prospective study. *BJOG* 2013;120(4):463-71.
54. Diav-Citrin O, Ornoy A. Teratogen update: antithyroid drugs-methimazole, carbimazole, and propylthiouracil. *Teratology* 2002;65(1):38-44.
55. Cassina M, Dona M, Di Gianantonio E et al. Pharmacologic treatment of hyperthyroidism during pregnancy. *Birth Defects Res A Clin Mol Teratol* 2012;94(8):612-9.
56. Diav-Citrin O, Ornoy A. Selective serotonin reuptake inhibitors in human pregnancy; to treat or not to treat? *Obstet Gynecol Int* 2012;2012:698947.
57. Rosa FW. Teratogen update: penicillamine. *Teratology* 1986;33(1):127-31.
58. Hernandez-Diaz S, Werler MM, Walker AM et al. Folic acid antagonists during pregnancy and the risk of birth defects. *N Engl J Med* 2000;343(22):1608-14.
59. Hernandez-Diaz S, Werler MM, Walker AM et al. Neural tube defects in relation to use of folic acid antagonists during pregnancy. *Am J Epidemiol* 2001;153(10):961-8.
60. Matok I, Gorodischer R, Koren G et al. Exposure to folic acid antagonists during the first trimester of pregnancy and the risk of major malformations. *Br J Clin Pharmacol* 2009;68(6):956-62.
61. Seto A, Einarson T, Koren G. Pregnancy outcome following first trimester exposure to antihistamines: meta-analysis. *Am J Perinatol* 1997;14(3):119-24.
62. Källén B. Use of antihistamine drugs in early pregnancy and delivery outcome. *J Matern Fetal Neonatal Med* 2002;11(3):146-52.
63. Fouda UM, Sayed AM, Ramadan DI et al. Efficacy and safety of two doses of low molecular weight heparin (enoxaparin) in pregnant women with a history of recurrent abortion secondary to antiphospholipid syndrome. *J Obstet Gynaecol* 2010;30(8):842-6.
64. Romualdi E, Dentali F, Rancan E et al. Anticoagulant therapy for venous thromboembolism during pregnancy: a systematic review and a meta-analysis of the literature. *J Thromb Haemost* 2013;11(2):270-81.
65. Ferreira E, Martin B, Morin C. *Grossesse et allaitement: guide thérapeutique*. 2nd ed. Montréal (QC): CHU Sainte-Justine; 2013.
66. Koren G, Nordeng HM. Selective serotonin reuptake inhibitors and malformations: case closed? *Semin Fetal Neonatal Med* 2013;18(1):19-22.
67. Reis M, Källén B. Combined use of selective serotonin reuptake inhibitors and sedatives/hypnotics during pregnancy: risk of relatively severe congenital malformations or cardiac defects. A register study. *BMJ Open* 2013;3(2). pii:e002166.
68. Lim A, Stewart K, König K et al. Systematic review of the safety of regular preventive asthma medications during pregnancy. *Ann Pharmacother* 2011;45(7-8):931-45.
69. Gentile S. Lithium in pregnancy: the need to treat, the duty to ensure safety. *Expert Opin Drug Saf* 2012;11(3):425-37.
70. Trottier M, Erebara A, Bozzo P. Treating constipation during pregnancy. *Can Fam Physician* 2012;58(8):836-8.
71. Gilbert C, Mazzotta P, Loebstein R, Koren G. Fetal safety of drugs used in the treatment of allergic rhinitis: a critical review. *Drug Saf* 2005;28(8):707-19.
72. Källén B. The safety of antidepressant drugs during pregnancy. *Expert Opin Drug Saf* 2007;6(4):357-70.
73. Lepercq J, Lin J, Hall GC et al. Meta-analysis of maternal and neonatal outcomes associated with the use of insulin glargine versus NPH insulin during pregnancy. *Obstet Gynecol Int* 2012;2012:649070.
74. Gui J, Liu Q, Feng L. Metformin vs insulin in the management of gestational diabetes: a meta-analysis. *PLoS One* 2013;8(5):e64585.
75. Berggren EK, Boggess KA. Oral agents for the management of gestational diabetes. *Clin Obstet Gynecol* 2013;56(4):827-36.
76. Black RA, Hill DA. Over-the-counter medications in pregnancy. *Am Fam Physician* 2003;67(12):2517-24.
77. Pasternak B, Hviid A. Use of proton-pump inhibitors in early pregnancy and the risk of birth defects. *N Engl J Med* 2010;363(22):2114-23.
78. Battino D, Tomson T. Management of epilepsy during pregnancy. *Drugs* 2007;67(18):2727-46.
79. Harden CL, Meador KJ, Pennell PB et al. Management issues for women with epilepsy—Focus on pregnancy (an evidence-based review): II. Teratogenesis and perinatal outcomes: Report of the Quality Standards Subcommittee and Therapeutics and Technology Subcommittee of the American Academy of Neurology and the American Epilepsy Society. *Epilepsia* 2009;50(5):1237-46.
80. Holmes LB, Hernandez-Diaz S. Newer anticonvulsants: lamotrigine, topiramate and gabapentin. *Birth Defects Res A Clin Mol Teratol* 2012;94(8):599-606.
81. Niederhoff H, Zahradnik HP. Analgesics during pregnancy. *Am J Med* 1983;75(5A):117-20.
82. Daniel S, Matok I, Gorodischer R et al. Major malformations following exposure to nonsteroidal antiinflammatory drugs during the first trimester of pregnancy. *J Rheumatol* 2012;39(11):2163-9.
83. Ebrahimi N, Vohra S, Gedeon C et al. The fetal safety of hydrocortisone-pramoxine (Proctofoam-HC) for the treatment of hemorrhoids in late pregnancy. *J Obstet Gynaecol Can* 2011;33(2):153-8.
84. Stone KM, Reiff-Eldridge R, White AD et al. Pregnancy outcomes following systemic prenatal acyclovir exposure: conclusions from the international acyclovir pregnancy registry, 1984-1999. *Birth Defects Res A Clin Mol Teratol* 2004;70(4):201-7.
85. Pasternak B, Hviid A. Use of acyclovir, valacyclovir, and famciclovir in the first trimester of pregnancy and the risk of birth defects. *JAMA* 2010;304(8):859-66.
86. Society of Obstetricians and Gynaecologists of Canada. Diagnosis, evaluation and management of the hypertensive disorders of pregnancy. *J Obstet Gynaecol Can* 2008;30(3 Suppl 1):1-49. Available from: www.sogc.org/guidelines/documents/gui206CPG0803_001.pdf. Accessed November 13, 2013.
87. De Groot L, Abalovich M, Alexander EK et al. Management of thyroid dysfunction during pregnancy and postpartum: an Endocrine Society clinical practice guideline. *J Clin Endocrinol Metab* 2012;97(8):2543-65.
88. Källén B, Nilsson E, Otterblad Olausson P. Delivery outcome after maternal use of drugs for migraine: a register study in Sweden. *Drug Saf* 2011;34(8):691-703.
89. Hilaire ML, Cross LB, Eichner SF. Treatment of migraine headaches with sumatriptan in pregnancy. *Ann Pharmacother* 2004;38(10):1726-30.
90. ezvalová-Henriksen K, Spigset O, Nordeng H. Triptan safety during pregnancy: a Norwegian population registry study. *Eur J Epidemiol* 2013;28(9):759-69.

91. cKeigue PM, Lamm SH, Linn S et al. Bendectin and birth defects: I. A meta-analysis of the epidemiologic studies. *Teratology* 1994;50(1):27-37.
92. shkenazi-Hoffnung L, Merlob P, Stahl B et al. Evaluation of the efficacy and safety of bi-daily combination therapy with pyridoxine and doxylamine for nausea and vomiting of pregnancy. *Isr Med Assoc J* 2013;15(1):23-6.
93. Matok I, Gorodischer R, Koren G et al. The safety of metoclopramide use in the first trimester of pregnancy. *N Engl J Med* 2009;360(24):2528-35.
94. asternak B, Svanström H, Mølgaard-Nielsen D et al. Metoclopramide in pregnancy and risk of major congenital malformations and fetal death. *JAMA* 2013;310(15):1601-11.
95. Pasternak B, Svanström H, Hviid A. Ondansetron in pregnancy and risk of adverse fetal outcomes. *N Engl J Med* 2013;368(9):814-23.
96. Gentile S. Antipsychotic therapy during early and late pregnancy. A systematic review. *Schizophr Bull* 2010;36(3):518-44.
97. Public Health Agency of Canada. *Canadian guidelines on sexually transmitted infections*. Evergreen ed. Ottawa (ON): PHAC; updated January 2010. Available from: www.phac-aspc.gc.ca/std-mts/sti-its/cgsti-ldcits/section-6-4-eng.php. Accessed November 13, 2013.
98. Young GL, Jewell D. Topical treatment for vaginal candidiasis (thrush) in pregnancy. *Cochrane Database Syst Rev* 2001;(4):CD000225.
99. Mølgaard-Nielsen D, Pasternak B, Hviid A. Use of oral fluconazole during pregnancy and the risk of birth defects. *N Engl J Med* 2013;369(9):830-9.

Appendix III
Drug Use during Breastfeeding

M.S. Brochet, BPharm, MSc and
S. Ito, MD, FRCPC

The following is an overview of drug use during breastfeeding. This information is not intended to be a comprehensive review; the reader is therefore encouraged to seek additional and confirmatory information.

Principles of Drug Use during Breastfeeding

Clinicians can use the following general principles to manage cases where drug exposure in a breastfed infant is questioned:

- Almost all drugs are excreted to some degree in breast milk.
- Breast milk/feeding has tangible medical and other benefits compared to formula.[1,2,3]
- Even when the breast milk:maternal plasma concentration ratio approaches or exceeds 1, the amount of drug ingested by the infant rarely attains therapeutic levels.
- Brief exposure to a drug, as might be expected in the case of analgesics given to relieve postpartum pain, is usually of less concern than a drug given for long periods of time. The amount of drug ingested by the infant can, on occasion, be minimized by feeding the infant just before or at the time of maternal dosing.
- In the case of chronic drug therapy, the infant is usually exposed to lower concentrations of the drug while breastfeeding than while the fetus is in utero. Nevertheless, in most cases the long-term consequences of chronic exposure to subtherapeutic levels of medications are not known.
- Recommendations about breastfeeding during drug therapy depend on knowing if small amounts of the drug (subtherapeutic amounts) taken for even short periods of time may be associated with the following:
  - idiosyncratic reactions, e.g., chloramphenicol
  - interference with genetically abnormal metabolic pathways, e.g., nitrofurantoin in patients with G6PD deficiencies
  - synergistic effects with drugs the infant receives therapeutically, e.g., caffeine in coffee and tea may enhance effects of therapeutic caffeine or aminophylline in the neonate

Clinicians require a reasonable knowledge of pharmacology and therapeutics in the newborn as well as a knowledge of the amount of drug excreted in breast milk.

The Drugs and Lactation database (LactMed) is a reliable and authoritative web-based resource about drug excretion in breast milk and recommendations for breastfeeding during maternal therapy.[5] It is free of charge and run by the US National Library of Medicine. LactMed is housed within the TOXNET Web site.

Consider several important questions when a breastfeeding mother starts drug therapy:[4]

- Is the drug absorbed from the GI tract?
- Is the drug ever given directly to infants for therapeutic reasons?
- Does the estimated dose delivered through breast milk approach a therapeutic quantity?

- Are the effects of the drug easily recognized in the infant?
- Are there idiosyncratic or allergic reactions to the drug that are not dose-related?
- Are there less toxic alternatives for maternal therapy?
- Is there a potential for drug accumulation during prolonged therapy?
- Could subtherapeutic doses of the drug mask early signs of medical conditions in the infant?
- Is the risk posed by the drug substantial enough to outweigh the significant proven benefits of breastfeeding?

Drugs Compatible with Breastfeeding

Drugs considered compatible with breastfeeding far outnumber those considered contraindicated during breastfeeding. Table 1 discusses some examples of drugs considered to be compatible with breastfeeding.

Table 1: Drugs Compatible with Breastfeeding[a]

Therapeutic Class	Drugs/Drug Classes Compatible with Breastfeeding	Comments
Analgesics	Acetaminophen, morphine	• For most **opioid analgesics**, the amount of drug excreted in breast milk is small, and short-term use should be of no major concern. If used for longer than 3 days monitor closely for drowsiness/sedation, difficulty breathing, difficulty breastfeeding, decreased tone, particularly in premature infants and neonates.[6] **Meperidine** is an exception; in neonates, the long half-lives of meperidine (13 h) and normeperidine (63 h) may result in accumulation in plasma, possibly leading to neurobehavioural depression.[7,8] • In addition, use **codeine** with caution at the lowest effective dose for the shortest period of time. Mothers with ultra-rapid metabolizer CYP2D6 genotype (Chinese, Japanese, Hispanic 0.5–1%; Caucasian 1–10%; African American 3%; North African, Ethiopian, Saudi Arabian 16–28%) may experience intensified effects from a regular dosing regimen of codeine due to increased conversion of codeine to morphine, causing morphine toxicity. Resultant high levels of morphine in maternal serum could cause relatively high morphine levels in breast milk.[4] Mothers experiencing morphine toxicity, whether due to this genotype or morphine overdose, should not breastfeed. Codeine use should be limited to less than 3–4 days in a breastfeeding mother. • **Oxycodone** and **hydrocodone** are also metabolized by CYP2D6 to a potent active metabolite; see codeine for information regarding the ultra-rapid metabolizer CYP2D6 genotype.[4] Maternal oxycodone use has been associated with a similar incidence of neonatal CNS depression as codeine[9] and levels in breast milk strongly correlated with plasma levels in one study.[10] Use of oxycodone or hydrocodone while breastfeeding should be considered only in patients who cannot take other opioids and should be limited to less than 3–4 days. • The amount of **morphine** excreted in breast milk could reach 7.5% of the pediatric dose.[11] Despite widespread use of morphine by breastfeeding mothers, there is only one case report of a nursing infant with therapeutic plasma concentrations.[12] • Limited data indicates that **hydromorphone** is excreted into breast milk in small amounts.[4] • Data for **tramadol** are lacking. Short-term use may be a concern due to its long half-life (7 h for tramadol and 8.5 h for the active metabolite in newborns) especially in premature infants: monitor for increased sleepiness. Excretion into breast milk is low, therefore it is unlikely to affect healthy babies. An exclusively breastfed infant would receive about 10% of the therapeutic dose for a child.[13] • **Methadone** levels in human milk are low. An exclusively breastfed infant would receive <5% of the weight-adjusted maternal dose.[b] **Buprenorphine** levels in milk could reach 2.5% of the weight-adjusted maternal dose[b] in an exclusively breastfed infant. It has poor oral bioavailability and low drug concentrations in breastfed infant's serum and urine have been documented.

(cont'd)

Table 1: **Drugs Compatible with Breastfeeding**[a] *(cont'd)*

Therapeutic Class	Drugs/Drug Classes Compatible with Breastfeeding	Comments
		One study suggested that extradural buprenorphine administration in the mother suppressed infant breastfeeding but 3 others were inconclusive.[14] Levels of methadone or buprenorphine in breast milk are insufficient to prevent symptoms of neonatal abstinence syndrome.[4] • Data for **naltrexone** are lacking.[14]
Antibiotics	Aminoglycosides, cephalosporins, clindamycin, fluoroquinolones, macrolides, metronidazole, nitrofurantoin, penicillins, sulfonamides	• For many antibiotics, the amounts ingested by a breastfed infant will be below therapeutic levels (e.g., **penicillins**, **cephalosporins**), but might be sufficient to result in idiosyncratic reactions (e.g., **chloramphenicol**) or cause anemia in an infant with G6PD deficiency (e.g., **nitrofurantoin**, **sulfonamides**). Other potential problems are modifications to the normal GI flora leading to thrush and diarrhea. However, clinical significance of these risks is usually not high enough to justify discontinuation of breastfeeding. • **Aminoglycosides** are excreted in breast milk when administered im or iv to the mother; because the drugs are poorly absorbed from the GI tract, it is unlikely that renal toxicity or ototoxicity would occur in the infant. • Only small amounts of oral **clindamycin** are excreted in breast milk (2–6% of the recommended pediatric dosage). It is unlikely that these quantities would be clinically relevant but at least one case of bloody stools has been reported in the breastfed infant of a mother receiving clindamycin. Topical clindamycin (not used in the nipple area) is generally associated with lower maternal systemic drug levels and lower breast milk excretion compared to systemic use.[14] • **Erythromycin** is excreted in breast milk in low amounts and is compatible with breastfeeding. Limited data regarding **clarithromycin** and **azithromycin** demonstrate that these drugs are excreted in breast milk in small amounts, but the amount of drug ingested by a breastfed infant is likely below therapeutic pediatric levels.[15,16] No data are available regarding the excretion of **telithromycin** in breast milk. • **Metronidazole** use during breastfeeding has raised some concerns based on reports that it is mutagenic in bacteria and carcinogenic in rodents during life-long ingestion. Specific untoward effects in a nursing infant as a result of metronidazole ingestion have not been reported. Without more direct evidence of the harmful effects of short-term use in humans, it seems overly conservative to withhold the drug or discontinue breastfeeding in patients with symptomatic infections. For the treatment of trichomoniasis with a single oral dose of metronidazole 2 g, some clinicians now recommend an interruption of breastfeeding for 12–24 h, especially with young babies.[7] Topical metronidazole (as long as it is not used in the nipple area) is considered compatible with breastfeeding since blood levels and excretion into breast milk are lower than with maternal systemic metronidazole use. • Fluoroquinolones have traditionally not been used in infants because of concerns regarding adverse effects on joint development. Studies indicate little risk. Short-term use of **ciprofloxacin**, **levofloxacin**, **norfloxacin** or **ofloxacin** is acceptable in nursing mothers. These quinolones are excreted in breast milk in small amounts which do not result in significant serum concentrations in breastfed infants. The calcium in breast milk may also decrease quinolone absorption in the infant.[14] There are no data available for **moxifloxacin**. Maternal use of **gatifloxacin** eye drops presents negligible risk for the nursing infant.[14] • The **sulfonamides** are excreted in breast milk in small amounts. **Nitrofurantoin** excretion is also small. In each case, there are concerns about these drugs causing anemia in an infant with G6PD deficiency which is more common in those of African, Greek, middle-eastern and south-east Asian origin. Use with caution in mothers breastfeeding premature infants or neonates with hyperbilirubinemia.[7] Use alternatives unless the infection is not responding to other therapy. • Some reviews classify **tetracyclines** as contraindicated in breastfeeding based on concerns of staining of dental enamel or bone deposition. Available data indicate that harm is unlikely with short-term use of tetracyclines. Milk levels are low and calcium in breast milk limits absorption of tetracyclines. However, as a precaution based on the theoretical risk, prolonged or repeated courses should be avoided during breastfeeding.[14]

(cont'd)

Table 1: Drugs Compatible with Breastfeeding[a] *(cont'd)*

Therapeutic Class	Drugs/Drug Classes Compatible with Breastfeeding	Comments
Anticoagulants	Heparin (unfractionated and low molecular weight), warfarin	• **Heparin**, administered parenterally for acute short-term therapy of thrombophlebitis, has not been shown to be excreted in breast milk. Heparin is a large polysaccharide molecule that is inactivated in the GI tract when taken orally. Its transfer into breast milk and risk to a breastfed infant are considered negligible.[7] • The amount of **benzyl alcohol** used as preservative in multidose vials of unfractionated heparin or low molecular weight heparin is too low to pose any risk to a breastfeeding baby.[11] • Few data are available regarding the effects of **low molecular weight heparins** during breastfeeding. There is a case report of 12 full-term neonates being breastfed by mothers treated with 20 or 40 mg of **enoxaparin** injected subcutaneously daily.[17] No anticoagulant effects, as measured by anti-Xa activity levels, were detected in the babies. It is thought that with the relatively high molecular weight of enoxaparin and its inactivation in the GI tract if orally ingested, its transfer into breast milk and risk to a breastfed infant should be considered negligible.[7] No drug was found in breast milk of 2 patients who received 5000–10 000 IU of **dalteparin**.[18] In a study of 15 lactating mothers after once daily routine dalteparin 2500 IU sc no quantitative correlation was noted between anti-Xa activities in plasma and milk.[19] There are no data available on excretion into milk of **nadroparin** or **tinzaparin**; however based on their molecular weight and inactivation by the GI tract, excretion into breast milk is expected to be negligible. • There are 3 case reports of **danaparoid** use by breastfeeding mothers. One report described the use of **lepirudin** during lactation. The amount of these large molecules excreted into breast milk is expected to be very small. Additionally, their deactivation in the GI tract after oral ingestion makes risk to a breastfeeding infant via ingestion from breast milk negligible.[20,21] • The use of **fondaparinux** during breastfeeding has not been described in humans. Although animal data suggest the drug is excreted into milk, the effect on a nursing infant is probably not clinically significant because it is not absorbed after oral ingestion.[11,21] • Among breastfed infants whose mothers were taking **warfarin**, the drug was undetectable in plasma and the bleeding time was not affected.[21]
Antidepressants	Desvenlafaxine, SSRIs, tricyclic antidepressants, venlafaxine	• Except for **doxepin** there are no reports of untoward effects of any of the **tricyclic antidepressants** in breastfed infants.[22] • **Sertraline** is transferred into breast milk resulting in an estimated infant dose of between 0.5% and 5% of the weight-adjusted maternal dose[b,23,24,25,26] There is a case report of serotonergic symptoms in a premature infant exposed in utero and via breast milk, but a causative link is uncertain.[27] There are also reports of uneventful breastfeeding during maternal sertraline use.[28] • **Paroxetine** is transferred into breast milk resulting in an estimated infant dose of between 0.1% and 4.3% of the weight-adjusted maternal dose[b]. In these studies, paroxetine was not detected in the serum of the majority of infants (in whom it was measured) and no adverse effects were reported.[28,29,30,31,32] • The amount of **fluoxetine** excreted in breast milk is 2–18% of the weight-adjusted maternal dose.[b,23,24,25,26,28,29,30,31,32,33] Nearly therapeutic serum concentrations were reported in some symptomatic infants.[34,35,36,37,38,39,40,41,42] Also, infants breastfed by mothers on fluoxetine had poorer weight gain, although the significance is unclear.[38] A few cases of colic have been associated with fluoxetine.[35,39] Because of the long half-lives of fluoxetine and its active metabolites, caution is advised, particularly when breastfeeding a preterm infant or neonate.[14] • Excretion of **fluvoxamine** seems to be low and no adverse effects were reported in the few available cases.[28,43] • The amount of **citalopram** excreted in breast milk is approximately 0.7–9% of the weight-adjusted maternal dose[b]. In one study, a single infant presented an "uneasy" sleep pattern which improved when maternal dose was decreased.[44,45,46,47] The amount of **escitalopram** excreted in breast milk is less than 8% of the weight-adjusted maternal dose[b] and no adverse effects were reported in the available cases.[14]

(cont'd)

Table 1: **Drugs Compatible with Breastfeeding**[a] *(cont'd)*

Therapeutic Class	Drugs/Drug Classes Compatible with Breastfeeding	Comments
		• **Venlafaxine** and its metabolites are excreted in breast milk in approximately 5–9% of the weight-adjusted maternal dose.[b,48,49] In one study of 7 infants the active metabolite O-desmethylvenlafaxine was detected in the plasma of 4 infants. No adverse effects were reported in the infants.[50] Excretion of **desvenlafaxine** (O-desmethylvenlafaxine) into breast milk is less than 7% of the maternal weight-adjusted dose[b] and serum drug levels of breastfed infants are less than 6% of simultaneous maternal levels.[51] • Although **bupropion**, **moclobemide** and **mirtazapine** have not been studied extensively, for each of these drugs the amount excreted in breast milk is less than 2% of the weight-adjusted maternal dose.[b] No adverse effects were reported[14,52,53,54,55,56,57] except for bupropion (two case reports of possible seizure) although the significance is unclear.[58,59] Limited data indicate that excretion of **trazodone** into breast milk is low but data on its active metabolites are lacking.[60,61,62,63] The amount of **duloxetine** excreted into breast milk seems to be low, less than 1% of the weight-adjusted maternal dose[b] is excreted into breast milk.[64,65] • Overall, no significant short-term effect has been reported for the commonly used antidepressants such as tricyclics and SSRIs. Clinical significance of reported adverse events remains unclear. Base the choice of antidepressants on the maternal condition and response. No matter what drug is used, use caution until more experience is gained.
Antiepileptics	Carbamazepine, clonazepam, phenytoin, valproic acid	• The excretion into milk is low: approximately 5% and 2% of the weight-adjusted maternal dose[b] for **carbamazepine** and its epoxide metabolite, less than 4% for **valproic acid**, and less than 8% for **phenytoin**. Limited data for **clonazepam** indicate that the weight adjusted maternal dose is <3% therefore risk for toxicity is expected to be low.[14] However the long half-life and lipophilicity of clonazepam could be a concern. Despite sporadic case reports of adverse effects, these antiepileptics are believed to be compatible with breastfeeding.[7,66] • **Phenobarbital**, **ethosuximide** and **primidone** may warrant more caution because the infant's exposure may reach therapeutic levels. The infant exposure levels for phenobarbital, ethosuximide and primidone are estimated at 100%, 50% and >10%, respectively, of the levels expected when the drug is given directly to an infant in a therapeutic dose.[66] Whether this high-level exposure precludes breastfeeding or not depends on various factors in each individual case. In selected cases, regular monitoring of clinical signs (e.g., lethargy, poor feeding, sedation) and of drug concentrations in breast milk and/or in infant's plasma may guide breastfeeding.
Antifungals	Amphotericin B, caspofungin, fluconazole, ketoconazole, topical antifungals	• Data on **amphotericin B** are lacking. However, it is virtually unabsorbed orally and is commonly used in pediatrics.[70,71] • Although data are lacking on topical fungicidal agents like **clotrimazole**, **miconazole**, **terconazole** and **nystatin** in breastfeeding, systemic absorption in the mother is very poor. Milk levels are probably too low to be clinically relevant. Most of these topical antifungals are used in pediatrics. • Data on **caspofungin** in breastfeeding are lacking but it has poor oral bioavailability. • **Lamotrigine** plasma levels as high as 50% of maternal serum levels were found in breastfed infants whose mothers were taking lamotrigine. Many infants have been breastfed without adverse reactions but this drug may be of concern.[14] • **Gabapentin** excretion into breast milk is 1.3–3.8% of the weight-adjusted maternal dose[b] and serum drug levels of breastfed infants are <12% of simultaneous maternal levels.[67,68,69] • Data on **topiramate** are lacking. The long elimination half-life and inadequately studied possible long-term effects on neurobehaviour and cognitive development may be of concern. • **Clobazam**, **levetiracetam**, **oxcarbazepine**, **pregabalin** and **vigabatrin** have not been extensively studied and their use during breastfeeding should be evaluated on an individual basis.

(cont'd)

Table 1: **Drugs Compatible with Breastfeeding**[a] *(cont'd)*

Therapeutic Class	Drugs/Drug Classes Compatible with Breastfeeding	Comments
Antihistamines	Cetirizine, desloratadine, fexofenadine, loratadine	• **Loratadine** and **fexofenadine** (based on terfenadine data) result in infant exposure levels of <1% of the weight-adjusted maternal dose.[b,73,74] • **Desloratadine** is the active metabolite of loratadine. The calculated maximum expected dose of desloratadine in milk is 0.46% of the maternal weight-adjusted dose[b] of loratadine.[73] • Although data on **cetirizine** are lacking, use during breastfeeding is considered acceptable since the drug is safely used in infants >6 months.[11] • Other antihistamines may be given, but data on the concentrations of these drugs in breast milk are lacking. Infants should be monitored for irritability or drowsiness.[75] • Antihistamines are not usually contraindicated during breastfeeding. Alternatives to oral antihistamines that may be considered during breastfeeding include nasally administered **corticosteroids** or **cromolyn**. **Cromolyn** and **nedocromil** eye drops are considered acceptable during breastfeeding because of their low bioavailability.[7]
Antihypertensives	Labetalol, metoprolol, propranolol Benazepril, captopril, enalapril, quinapril, ramipril Methyldopa Nifedipine Hydrochlorothiazide, furosemide	• Beta-blockers that are safe to use even in the neonatal period are **labetalol**, **metoprolol** and **propranolol**.[66,76,77] • **Acebutolol**, **atenolol** and **sotalol** (although the latter is not indicated as an antihypertensive agent) may cause relatively high exposure levels, 10%, 25% and 20%, respectively, of those expected when the drug is given directly to an infant in a therapeutic dose. This may not be a problem in post-neonatal infants. However, exercise caution in the early neonatal period because newborns may have low clearance of atenolol and sotalol as a result of immature renal function (low GFR). Signs of beta-blockade have been reported in a breastfed infant of a woman taking atenolol (bradycardia, cyanosis, hypotension, hypothermia) and acebutolol (hypotension, bradycardia, tachypnea, drowsiness).[78,79,80] • **Methyldopa** and some **ACE inhibitors** (**benazepril**, **captopril**, **enalapril**, **quinapril** and **ramipril**) are not excreted into breast milk in clinically significant amounts and are considered compatible with breastfeeding.[11,14,81,82] Data concerning the use of **angiotensin II receptor antagonists** during lactation are lacking. Use with caution in breastfeeding mothers.[7] • **Nifedipine** is excreted into breast milk in low amounts and no adverse effects have been reported in infants. It is considered compatible with breastfeeding. Very limited data indicates amounts of **diltiazem** and **verapamil** in breast milk are low and would not be expected to have any adverse effects in breastfed infants.[14] • Data on **diuretics** are lacking. Intense diuresis may decrease breast milk production. **Hydrochlorothiazide** <50 mg daily is considered acceptable during breastfeeding based on a case report where an exclusively breastfed infant received <1% of the usual neonatal dose.[14] Although there is little data available regarding the amount of **furosemide** in breast milk, its short half-life, high protein binding and extensive use in neonates and pediatrics indicate that small maternal doses may be acceptable.[11]
Antimalarial agents (prophylactic)	Chloroquine, mefloquine, proguanil	• The very small amount of **chloroquine**, **mefloquine** and **proguanil** excreted in breast milk is not thought to be harmful to a nursing infant.[7] • There is no information on the amount of **primaquine** that enters into human breast milk but the drug may cause severe hemolysis in G6PD-deficient individuals. Because data are not yet available on the safety and efficacy of **atovaquone/proguanil** in infants weighing <11 kg, the medication should not be given to a woman who is breastfeeding an infant less than this weight unless the potential benefit to the woman outweighs the potential risk to the infant. Consider mefloquine. • Quantity of antimalarial medication transferred in breast milk is insufficient to provide adequate protection against malaria. Infants who require chemoprophylaxis should receive the recommended dosages of appropriate antimalarial drugs.[83,84]

(cont'd)

Table 1: **Drugs Compatible with Breastfeeding**[a] *(cont'd)*

Therapeutic Class	**Drugs/Drug Classes Compatible with Breastfeeding**	**Comments**
Antimanic agents		• **Lithium** should be used with caution in breastfeeding mothers. Lithium is excreted in breast milk, occasionally in quantities sufficient to produce infant serum levels ranging from 10–50% of maternal serum levels. In an infant exposed to lithium in utero and through breastfeeding, cyanosis, T-wave abnormalities and decreased muscle tone were reported. Other studies have reported no adverse effects.[7,85] • Monitoring of drug concentrations in milk and/or infant's serum may be justified.[86] Consider periodic thyroid evaluation of the infant as lithium can reduce thyroxine production. Monitor changes in infant hydration carefully as hydration status can greatly alter lithium serum levels.[7]
Antipsychotics	Chlorpromazine, haloperidol, olanzapine, quetiapine, risperidone	• The amount of **olanzapine** excreted into breast milk is less than 4% of the weight-adjusted maternal dose.[b] Few adverse effects have been reported among breastfed infants but monitoring for sedation (especially in those <2 months of age) is recommended.[14,87,88,89] • Less than 0.5% of the weight-adjusted maternal dose[b] of **quetiapine** is excreted into breast milk. Monitor infants (particularly those <2 months old) for sedation. No developmental problems or adverse events have been noted in infants breastfed during maternal use.[14,90,91,92] • The amount of **risperidone** excreted into breast milk is <5 % of the weight-adjusted maternal dose[b]. Although no adverse effects in infants have been reported, monitor for sedation, especially in infants <2 months old.[14,93] • **Chlorpromazine** is excreted into breast milk in low amounts (4% of the recommended pediatric dose) but milk levels do not appear to correlate well with the maternal dose or serum level. Monitor the infant for excessive drowsiness during breastfeeding.[14,94] • **Clozapine** appears to be excreted into breast milk in low amounts (1.2% of the weight-adjusted maternal dose[b]). Use during breastfeeding may be of concern due to its serious adverse effect profile (agranulocytosis and CNS depression). Monitor infant for excessive sedation. Periodic monitoring of the infant's white blood cell count is advisable.[14,94,95] • The use of **haloperidol** may be of concern due to lack of data. Doses <40 mg/day are excreted in low amounts in breast milk. Infants should be monitored for sedation and extrapyramidal effects.[94] • Case reports for **aripiprazole**, **flupentixol**, **methotrimeprazine**, **paliperidone**, **perphenazine**, **trifluoperazine**, **ziprasidone** and **zuclopenthixol** indicate that these medications are excreted into breast milk in low amounts (<1% of the weight-adjusted maternal dose[b]).[11] Data are lacking for **loxapine** and **pimozide**.
Antivirals	Acyclovir, valacyclovir	• **Acyclovir** and **valacyclovir** (which is almost entirely transformed to acyclovir) excretion into milk are low (less than 1% of the maximal daily pediatric dosage). No adverse effects were reported in breastfed infants.[96] • No studies have been reported on the excretion of **amantadine** in human milk. However, amantadine is a dopamine agonist. Clinical studies using amantadine concurrently with neuroleptic medications have demonstrated a decrease of prolactin and galactorrhea induced by neuroleptic drugs. The maternal prolactin level in a mother with established lactation may not affect her ability to breastfeed.[97,98] • Data on **famciclovir** in breastfeeding and pediatrics are lacking. Acyclovir and valacyclovir are preferred.[14]
	Oseltamivir	• Even though the amount of **oseltamivir** excreted in breast milk seems to be low (less than 1% of the usual pediatric dosage and 0.5% of the weight-adjusted maternal dose[b] after 75 mg twice daily for 5 days in a 9 months postpartum nursing mother), it would not be expected to cause any adverse effects in breastfed infants, especially if the infant is older than 2 months.[99,100] • No data are available regarding the excretion of **zanamivir** in breast milk, but due to the poor inhaled absorption and very low plasma levels, it would not be expected to cause any adverse effects in breastfed infants.[100]

(cont'd)

Table 1: **Drugs Compatible with Breastfeeding**[a] *(cont'd)*

Therapeutic Class	Drugs/Drug Classes Compatible with Breastfeeding	Comments
Anxiolytics and sedatives	Lorazepam, oxazepam	• If used occasionally as a sedative, **benzodiazepines** are not contraindicated during breastfeeding.[101] Benzodiazepines with shorter half-lives, lower lipophilicity and no active metabolites are preferred in breastfeeding mothers (e.g., oxazepam, lorazepam). • Benzodiazepines taken over a longer period of time to treat chronic maternal conditions may be of concern. The benzodiazepines and their metabolites are excreted in breast milk, are poorly metabolized by the neonate, and have been associated with drowsiness in nursing infants. Consequently, discourage the chronic use of a benzodiazepine in breastfeeding mothers unless the infant's condition is closely monitored.
Asthma therapy	Inhaled bronchodilators, inhaled corticosteroids	• **Inhaled bronchodilators** and **inhaled corticosteroids** are acceptable during breastfeeding as bioavailability and maternal serum levels are low.[102] • The average amount of **terbutaline** an exclusively breastfed infant would receive ranges from 0.2–0.7% of the weight-adjusted maternal dose.[b] Serum levels were undetectable in the infant in one case.[103,104] • The amount of **budesonide** in breast milk is low (0.3% of the weight-adjusted maternal dose[b]).[105] • No data are available regarding the excretion of **omalizumab** into breast milk. • Data on excretion of the leukotriene receptor inhibitor **montelukast** into milk are lacking. However, it does not penetrate the CNS or many other tissues and is highly protein-bound, making the probability of the baby being exposed via breast milk likely very low.[7] The manufacturer of **zafirlukast** indicates that it is excreted into milk in low concentrations (0.5% of the weight-adjusted maternal dose[b]).[106] It has been used in children as young as 12 months.[107]
Contraceptives	Progestin-only formulations	• **Progestin-only contraceptives** should be considered for post-partum women and may be introduced immediately after delivery (or 4–6 weeks postpartum in the case of levonorgestrel intrauterine device to allow time for uterine involution). **Estrogen-containing contraceptives** (including pills, patch, vaginal ring) should not be started until breastfeeding is fully established (approximately 6 weeks) as even low-dose formulations can decrease milk yield.[108]
Corticosteroids	Prednisolone, prednisone	• **Prednisone** and **prednisolone** are excreted in breast milk in low amounts and are not expected to cause adverse effects in the baby. Depending on maternal dose administered, baby will be exposed to 1–10% of a neonatal dose.[11,109]
Decongestants, oral	Pseudoephedrine	• 5.5% of the weight-adjusted maternal dosage[b] is excreted in breast milk after a single oral dose of 60 mg of **pseudoephedrine**. Decreased milk production was reported at the same dosage. Irritability was reported in infants exposed to pseudoephedrine in one study of breastfeeding mothers.[75,110] Use should be limited to a few days and discontinued if a decrease in milk production is observed. No data are available on the use of **phenylephrine** during breastfeeding, therefore an alternate drug may be preferred, especially while nursing a newborn or preterm infant. • Intranasal isotonic **saline solutions** or **topical decongestants** (**oxymetazoline, xylometazoline**) are preferred over oral decongestants.
Diabetes therapy	Insulin, metformin	• Human **insulin** is normally found in breast milk. Amount of synthetic insulin secreted into breast milk is unknown but, if secreted, this peptide would be destroyed in the infant's GI tract with no significant absorption.[7] • **Metformin** levels in milk are low and infants would receive less than 0.5% of their mother's weight-adjusted dosage. It is sometimes detectable in low levels in the serum of breastfed infants but no adverse effects in breastfed infants were reported in one study. Metformin should be used with caution while nursing newborn and premature infants and those with renal impairment.[14] • The amount of **glyburide** excreted in breast milk seems to be low (less than 1% of the weight-adjusted maternal dose[b]): no adverse effects on breastfed infant's blood glucose have been reported but data are limited.[111]

(cont'd)

Table 1: **Drugs Compatible with Breastfeeding**[a] *(cont'd)*

Therapeutic Class	Drugs/Drug Classes Compatible with Breastfeeding	Comments
		• No data are available regarding the excretion of **acarbose** into breast milk. However less than 2% of a dose of acarbose is absorbed from the mother's gastrointestinal tract making it unlikely that any drug reaches the infant through breast milk.[112] • No data are available regarding the excretion of **gliclazide**, **glimepiride**, **nateglinide**, **pioglitazone**, **repaglinide** and **rosiglitazone** in breast milk. An alternate drug may be preferred, especially while nursing a newborn or preterm infant. Some experts recommend monitoring the breastfed infant's blood glucose during maternal therapy with hypoglycemic agents.[112]
Gastrointestinal drugs	Antacids, sucralfate	• **Aluminum**, **calcium** and **magnesium antacids** and **sucralfate** are partially or poorly absorbed orally and are considered safe to use.[7]
	Antidiarrheals	• Use of **loperamide** during breastfeeding is unlikely to affect the infant as it is minimally absorbed orally. Based on its chemical and pharmacological similarity to narcotics, occasional small doses of **diphenoxylate** may be acceptable while breastfeeding an older infant, but alternatives are preferred, especially while nursing a newborn.[7,14]
	GI motility agents	• The excretion into milk of **domperidone** and **metoclopramide** are less than 0.05% and 6% respectively of a daily pediatric dose. No adverse events are reported for domperidone but intestinal discomfort was reported in 2 breastfed infants of mothers taking metoclopramide.[113,114,115] Domperidone is used to increase milk production in some women who do not respond to a nonpharmacologic approach.
	H_2 antagonists	• Though considered safe for use by breastfeeding mothers, **cimetidine** and **ranitidine** may concentrate in milk whereas **famotidine** and **nizatidine** have the lowest concentrations, making them preferable choices.[7,21] Ranitidine has been widely used in pediatrics primarily for gastroesophageal reflux. Adverse effects have not been reported in nursing infants.
	Laxatives	• **Psyllium** is acceptable to use during breastfeeding because it is not absorbed from the gastrointestinal tract. There have been no cases of loose stools reported in breastfed infants.[14] • **Docusate**, **bisacodyl** and **magnesium hydroxide** are not appreciably absorbed from the gastrointestinal tract and therefore these drugs are unlikely to be found in the maternal serum or breast milk.[7,14] One postpartum patient receiving a laxative containing docusate in a dose of 120 mg daily in addition to danthron 100 mg daily stated that diarrhea occurred in her breastfed infant.[14] • Usual doses of **senna** are acceptable to use during breastfeeding. However, a laxative effect was observed in a few case reports. **Cascara** is not a first-line choice due to case reports of a laxative effect in breastfed infants and unknown oral absorption.[7,14] • No data are available regarding the excretion of **lactulose** into breast milk; however less than 3% of a dose of lactulose is absorbed from the mother's GI tract, making it unlikely that any drug reaches the infant through breast milk.[11] • Oral **polyethylene glycol** (e.g., PEG-3350) and rectal **glycerin** are negligibly absorbed from the GI tract and unlikely to have significant levels in breastmilk.[11]
	Misoprostol	• **Misoprostol** levels in breast milk are low; amount ingested by the nursing infant would not be expected to cause adverse effects.[14]
	Proton pump inhibitors	• **Proton pump inhibitors** are unstable in an acid milieu and, when ingested via milk, would probably be destroyed in the infant's stomach prior to absorption.[7] **Pantoprazole** and **omeprazole** are excreted in milk in small quantities.[116,117] Lansoprazole and omeprazole are used for the treatment of gastroesophageal reflux in neonates and pediatrics. **Esomeprazole** is the s-enantiomer of omeprazole and therefore would also not be expected to cause any adverse effects in breastfed infants.[117]

(cont'd)

Table 1: **Drugs Compatible with Breastfeeding**[a] *(cont'd)*

Therapeutic Class	Drugs/Drug Classes Compatible with Breastfeeding	Comments
Migraine therapy	Eletriptan, sumatriptan	• Occasional use of **sumatriptan** and **eletriptan** seems to be acceptable because the amount of these drugs excreted into milk is low (3.5% and 0.02% of the weight-adjusted maternal dosage,[b] respectively). Data on **almotriptan**, **frovatriptan**, **naratriptan**, **rizatriptan** and **zolmitriptan** are lacking.[7] • Because there is limited published experience with **ergotamine**, **dihydroergotamine** and **methysergide** during breastfeeding, and adverse effects in the infant cannot be ruled out, most authorities consider these drugs to be undesirable to use while nursing.[7,14]
Muscle relaxants	Cyclobenzaprine, methocarbamol	• The excretion of **cyclobenzaprine**, **methocarbamol** and **orphenadrine** into milk has not been reported. However, occasional cyclobenzaprine and methocarbamol exposures are acceptable because of cyclobenzaprine's structural similarities to amitriptyline (see "Antidepressants") and the very short half-life of methocarbamol. No adverse events have been published, but infants (especially those that are newborn or premature) should be monitored for sedation while nursing.[7]
NSAIDs	Diclofenac, flurbiprofen, ibuprofen, indomethacin, naproxen	• Most NSAIDs have been shown to be present in breast milk in small amounts and are considered safe to use. The use of short-acting drugs, such as **ibuprofen** and **flurbiprofen**, may be preferred over those with a longer half-life such as **naproxen**.[7] • Less than 1% of the pediatric dose of **diclofenac** is excreted into breast milk. Diclofenac also has a short half-life.[14,120] • The amount of **indomethacin** excreted in breast milk is less than 4% of a typical neonatal dose and it is considered safe to use while breastfeeding. However, other agents with more published information on use during breastfeeding may be preferable especially while nursing a newborn or preterm infant.[11] • Data on **celecoxib** are limited to a few infants but milk levels were low and adverse effects were not noted when taken short term.[7] More data are needed to determine risk since the drug has a long half-life and high oral absorption.
Scabicides, pediculicides	Permethrin	• **Permethrin** 5% cream is the treatment of choice for scabies. **Permethrin** 1% or **pyrethrins/piperonyl butoxide** may be used for the treatment of head lice while breastfeeding.[118] Topical absorption of permethrin and pyrethrins is low. Permethrin is rapidly metabolized to inactive metabolites and excreted in urine. Overt toxicity is unlikely. Avoid application on nipples. Percutaneous absorption of piperonyl butoxide is unknown.[7,119] • **Lindane** is not recommended because it is absorbed through the mother's skin and excreted into milk fat. Direct contact of lindane with neonatal skin results in significant absorption. Direct exposure is potentially toxic in infants with reports of elevated liver enzymes, seizure disorders and hypersensitivity. It may also have estrogenic effects that could inhibit lactation.[14,119] Lindane is not currently available in Canada.
Smoking cessation	Nicotine replacement therapy	• Data on **nicotine patches** are limited but the amount of nicotine and cotinine excreted in breast milk seem to be less than 8% of the weight-adjusted maternal dose[b]. With a 21 mg transdermal patch, nicotine passes into breast milk in amounts equivalent to smoking 17 cigarettes daily. Lower patch strengths of 7 and 14 mg provide proportionately lower amounts of nicotine to the breastfed infant. No studies on nicotine spray or nicotine gum use in nursing mothers have been reported. Nicotine gum may produce large variations in peak levels when gum is chewed rapidly: fluctuations similar to smoking itself. Some clinicians recommend to wait 2–3 h after using the gum before breastfeeding.[121] • Data on **varenicline** are lacking but transfer is possible and effect on CNS is a concern.[7] • For information on the use of **bupropion** during breastfeeding, see Antidepressants.

(cont'd)

Table 1: **Drugs Compatible with Breastfeeding**[a] *(cont'd)*

Therapeutic Class	Drugs/Drug Classes Compatible with Breastfeeding	Comments
Thyroid agents	Antithyroid agents	• The estimated level of exposure to **propylthiouracil** in breastfeeding infants is less than 1% of the therapeutic dose standardized by weight, and the thyroid function of the infant is not affected.[122] **Methimazole** in doses up to 20 mg/day has been documented not to affect the infant's thyroid function.[123,124,125] For either drug, no adverse effects in breastfed infants have been reported so far and monitoring of infants' thyroid function is not necessary if development is progressing normally.[125]
	Thyroid hormones	• **Levothyroxine** is compatible with breastfeeding. Thyroid hormones cross into breast milk in low amounts. Their presence is not likely to affect the infant's thyroid.[21]
Vaccines		• Women who are breastfeeding can be vaccinated with Td, Tdap, pneumococcal, meningococcal, hepatitis A, hepatitis B, HPV, rabies, typhoid, MMR, varicella, HPV and cholera vaccines if indicated. Safety of the Japanese encephalitis vaccine in breastfeeding is unknown and it should be administered only if the risk of disease outweighs the unknown risk of vaccination. Yellow fever vaccine is not recommended for breastfeeding women and BCG vaccine should be used with caution. Women who receive smallpox vaccine as postexposure prophylaxis should avoid breastfeeding and other close contact with their baby until the scab has separated from the vaccination site.[126]

[a] This list is not exhaustive or definitive. Drugs not listed in the table are not necessarily contraindicated. Individualized risk assessment is required when prescribing any medication to a breastfeeding woman.

[b] Weight-adjusted maternal dose is a mother's dose based on body weight (e.g., mg/kg). Experts recommend that an amount of drug received by the infant via breast milk which is >10% of the weight-adjusted maternal dose should be a theoretical level of concern when considering the acceptability of drug exposure. The estimated amount of drug received by the infant via breast milk is calculated by multiplying the standard milk intake (150 mL/kg/day) by the drug concentration in breast milk.

Abbreviations: GFR = glomerular filtration rate.

Drugs for Nonmedical Use (Table 2)

Tobacco smoking and alcohol ingestion are the most common sources of nonmedicinal drug exposure in breastfed infants in Canada. Because they so often occur in the same individual, it is difficult to study their independent effects. Increasingly, these drugs are used together with illicit drugs such as marijuana and cocaine.

Table 2: **Breastfeeding and Nonmedical Use of Drugs**

Drug	Comments on Breastfeeding
Alcohol	• Not compatible with breastfeeding. The alcohol metabolizing capacity (alcohol and aldehyde dehydrogenase) is premature throughout the neonatal and infantile period. Overall, motor development is slightly slower in infants breastfed by mothers who regularly drink alcohol. Chronic or heavy consumers of alcohol should not breastfeed.[7] • Short-term alcohol consumption by nursing mothers reportedly has an immediate effect on the odour characteristics of the milk and the feeding behaviour of their infants, resulting in less consumption of milk.[127] To avoid exposure of the infant to alcohol, breastfeeding mothers should not consume alcohol or should consume no more than one drink 2–3 h before breastfeeding.[7]
Caffeine	• Hypothetically, a nursing infant ingests 0.11% of the maternal dose after the mother drinks 1–2 cups of coffee. This is an insignificant amount of the drug, but it must be remembered that the half-life of caffeine is 80 h in the term newborn and 97.5 h in a premature infant (20–30 times that of an adult). Therefore, repeated ingestion might lead to accumulation of caffeine in the infant during the first 2 weeks of postnatal life. This has yet to be studied.

(cont'd)

Table 2: **Breastfeeding and Nonmedical Use of Drugs** *(cont'd)*

Drug	Comments on Breastfeeding
Recreational or street drugs	• No systematic studies of recreational or street drug (or drug metabolite) excretion exist.
Tobacco	• Discourage during breastfeeding because there are well-documented health risks to the mother and infant from second-hand smoke. Infant exposure to nicotine is largely through inhalation of second-hand smoke. In mothers unwilling to stop smoking during breastfeeding, it should be noted that breastfed babies of mothers who continue to smoke have better immunity and less respiratory infections than bottle-fed babies of mothers who continue to smoke.[128] • Nicotine is concentrated in human breast milk.[129,130] One study suggests that cigarette smoking significantly reduces breast milk production.[131] • Encourage nursing mothers to speak to their health care providers regarding options for smoking cessation.

References

1. Kramer MS, Aboud F, Mironova E et al. Breastfeeding and child cognitive development: new evidence from a large randomized trial. *Arch Gen Psychiatry* 2008;65(5):578-84.
2. Verhasselt V, Milcent V, Cazareth J et al. Breast milk-mediated transfer of an antigen induces tolerance and protection from allergic asthma. *Nat Med* 2008;14(2):170-5.
3. Section on Breastfeeding. Breastfeeding and the use of human milk. *Pediatrics* 2012;129(3):e827-41.
4. Sachs HC; Committee on Drugs. The transfer of drugs and therapeutics into human breast milk: an update on selected topics. *Pediatrics* 2013;132(3):e796-809.
5. Akus M, Bartick M. Lactation safety recommendations and reliability compared in 10 medication resources. *Ann Pharmacother* 2007;41(9):1352-60.
6. Health Canada; Janssen-Ortho. *Important safety information about use of Tylenol with Codeine No. 2, 3, 4 and elixir in nursing mothers and ultra-rapid metabolizers of codeine*; October 6, 2008. Available from: healthycanadians.gc.ca/recall-alert-rappel-avis/hc-sc/2008/14526a-eng.php. Accessed October 1, 2013.
7. Hale TW. *Medications and mothers' milk: a manual of lactational pharmacology.* 15th ed. Amarillo (TX): Hale Publishing; 2012.
8. Wittels B, Scott DT, Sinatra RS. Exogenous opioids in human breast milk and acute neonatal neurobehavior: a preliminary study. *Anesthesiology* 1990;73(5):864-9.
9. Lam J, Kelly L. Ciszkowski C et al. Central nervous system depression of neonates breastfed by mothers receiving oxycodone for postpartum analgesia. *J Pediatr* 2012;160(1):33-7.
10. Seaton S, Reeves M, McLean S. Oxycodone as a component of multimodal analgesia for lactating mothers after Caesarean section: relationships between maternal plasma breast milk and neonatal plasma levels. *Aust N Z J Obstet Gynaecol* 2007;47(3):181-5.
11. Ferreira E, Martin B, Morin C. *Grossesse et allaitement: guide thérapeutique.* 2nd ed. Montréal (QC): CHU Sainte Justine; 2013.
12. Robieux I, Koren G, Vandenbergh H et al. Morphine excretion in breast milk and resultant exposure of a nursing infant. *Clin Toxicol* 1990;28(3):365-70.
13. Ilett KF, Paech MJ, Page-Sharp M et al. Use of a sparse sampling study design to assess transfer of tramadol and its O-desmethyl metabolite into transitional breast milk. *Br J Clin Pharmacol* 2008;65(5):661-6.
14. Drugs and Lactation Database (LactMed). Bethesda (MD): U.S. National Library of Medicine. Available from: toxnet.nlm.nih.gov/cgi-bin/sis/htmlgen?LACT. Accessed October 2, 2013.
15. Sedlmayr T, Peters F, Raasch W et al. [Clarithromycin, a new macrolide antibiotic. Effectiveness in puerperal infections and pharmacokinetics in breast milk]. *Geburtshilfe Frauenheilkd* 1993;53(7):488-91. [German].
16. Kelsey JJ, Moser LR, Jennings JC et al. Presence of azithromycin breast milk concentrations: a case report. *Am J Obstet Gynecol* 1994;170(5 Pt 1):1375-6.
17. Guillonneau M, de Crepy A, Aufrant C et al. [Breast-feeding is possible in case of maternal treatment with enoxaparin]. *Arch Pediatr* 1996;3(5):513-4. [French].
18. Harenberg J, Leber G, Zimmermann R et al. [Prevention of thromboembolism with low-molecular weight heparin in pregnancy]. *Geburtshilfe Frauenheilkd* 1987;47(1):15-8. [German].
19. Richter C, Sitzmann J, Lang P et al. Excretion of low molecular weight heparin in human milk. *Br J Clin Pharmacol* 2001;52(6):708-10.
20. Lindhoff-Last E, Bauersachs R. Heparin-induced thrombocytopenia-alternative anticoagulation in pregnancy and lactation. *Semin Thromb Hemost* 2002;28(5):439-46.
21. Briggs GG, Freeman RK, Yaffe SJ. *Drugs in pregnancy and lactation: a reference guide to fetal and neonatal risk.* 9th ed. Philadelphia (PA): Lippincott Williams & Wilkins; 2011.
22. Frey OR, Scheidt P, von Brenndorff AI. Adverse effects in a newborn infant breast-fed by a mother treated with doxepin. *Ann Pharmacother* 1999;33(6):690-3.
23. Birnbaum CS, Cohen LS, Bailey JW et al. Serum concentrations of antidepressants and benzodiazepines in nursing infants: a case series. *Pediatrics* 1999;104(1):e11.
24. Stowe ZN, Hostetter AL, Owens MJ et al. The pharmacokinetics of sertraline excretion into human breast milk: determinants of infant serum concentrations. *J Clin Psychiatry* 2003;64(1):73-80.
25. Dodd S, Stocky A, Buist A et al. Sertraline in paired blood plasma and breast-milk samples from nursing mothers. *Hum Psychopharmacol* 2000;15(4):161-264.
26. Epperson N, Czarkowski KA, Ward-O'Brien D et al. Maternal sertraline treatment and serotonin transport in breast-feeding mother-infant pairs. *Am J Psychiatry* 2001;158(10):1631-7.
27. Müller MJ, Preuß C, Paul T et al. Serotonergic overstimulation in a preterm infant after sertraline intake via breastmilk. *Breastfeed Med* 2013;8(3):327-9.

28. Hendrick V, Fukuchi A, Altshuler L et al. Use of sertraline, paroxetine and fluvoxamine by nursing women. *Br J Psychiatry* 2001;179:163-6.
29. Begg EJ, Duffull SB, Saunders DA et al. Paroxetine in human milk. *Br J Clin Pharmacol* 1999;48(2):142-7.
30. Ohman R, Hagg S, Carleborg L et al. Excretion of paroxetine into breast milk. *J Clin Psychiatry* 1999;60(8):519-23.
31. Stowe ZN, Cohen LS, Hostetter A et al. Paroxetine in human breast milk and nursing infants. *Am J Psychiatry* 2000;157(2):185-9.
32. Misri S, Kim J, Riggs KW et al. Paroxetine levels in postpartum depressed women, breast milk, and infant serum. *J Clin Psychiatry* 2000;61(11):828-32.
33. Epperson CN, Jatlow P, Czarkowski K et al. Maternal fluoxetine treatment in the postpartum period: effects on platelet serotonin and plasma drug levels in breastfeeding mother-infant pairs. *Pediatrics* 2003;112(5):e425-9.
34. Moretti ME, Sharma A, Bar-Oz B et al. Fluoxetine and its effects on the nursing infant: a prospective cohort study. *Clin Pharmacol Ther* 1999;65(2):141.
35. Kristensen JH, Ilett KF, Hackett LP et al. Distribution and excretion of fluoxetine and norfluoxetine in human milk. *Br J Clin Pharmacol* 1999;48(4):521-7.
36. Taddio A, Ito S, Koren G. Excretion of fluoxetine and its metabolite, norfluoxetine, in human breast milk. *J Clin Pharmacol* 1996;36(1):42-7.
37. Yoshida K, Smith B, Craggs M et al. Fluoxetine in breast-milk and developmental outcome of breast-fed infants. *Br J Psychiatry* 1998;172:175-8.
38. Chambers CD, Anderson PO, Thomas RG et al. Weight gain in infants breast-fed by mothers who take fluoxetine. *Pediatrics* 1999;104(5):e61.
39. Lester BM, Cucca J, Andreozzi L et al. Possible association between fluoxetine hydrochloride and colic in an infant. *J Am Acad Child Adolesc Psychiatry* 1993;32(6):1253-5.
40. Hale TW, Shum S, Grossberg M. Fluoxetine toxicity in a breast-fed infant. *Clin Pediatr (Phila)* 2001;40(12):681-4.
41. Suri R, Stowe ZN, Hendrick V et al. Estimates of nursing infant daily dose of fluoxetine through breast milk. *Biol Psychiatry* 2002;52(5):446-51.
42. Piontek CM, Wisner KL, Perel JM. Serum fluvoxamine levels in breastfed infants. *J Clin Psychiatry* 2001;62(2):111-3.
43. Kristensen JH, Hackett LP, Kohan R et al. The amount of fluvoxamine in milk is unlikely to be a cause of adverse effects in breastfed infants. *J Hum Lact* 2002;18(2):139-43.
44. Rampono J, Kristensen JH, Hackett LP et al. Citalopram and demethylcitalopram in human milk; distribution, excretion and effects in breast fed infants. *Br J Clin Pharmacol* 2000;50(3):263-8.
45. Schmidt K, Olesen OV, Jensen PN. Citalopram and breast-feeding: serum concentration and side effects in the infant. *Biol Psychiatry* 2000;47(2):164-5.
46. Spigset O, Carieborg L, Ohman R et al. Excretion of citalopram in breast milk. *Br J Clin Pharmacol* 1997;44(3):295-8.
47. Heikkinen T, Ekblad U, Kero P et al. Citalopram in pregnancy and lactation. *Clin Pharmacol Ther* 2002;72(2):184-91.
48. Hendrick V, Altshuler L, Wertheimer A et al. Venlafaxine and breast-feeding. *Am J Psychiatry* 2001;158(12):2089-90.
49. Ilett KF, Hackett LP, Dusci LJ et al. Distribution and excretion of venlafaxine and O-desmethylvenlafaxine in human milk. *Br J Clin Pharmacol* 1998;45(5):459-62.
50. Ilett KF, Kristensen JH, Hackett LP et al. Distribution of venlafaxine and its O-desmethyl metabolite in human milk and their effects in breastfed infants. *Br J Clin Pharmacol* 2002;53(1):17-22.
51. Rampono J, Teoh S, Hackett LP et al. Estimation of desvenlafaxine transfer into milk and infant exposure during its use in lactating women with postnatal depression. *Arch Womens Ment Health* 2011;14(1):49-53.
52. Briggs GG, Samson JH, Ambrose PJ et al. Excretion of bupropion in breast milk. *Ann Pharmacother* 1993;27(4):431-3.
53. Baab SW, Peindl KS, Piontek CM et al. Serum bupropion levels in 2 breastfeeding mother-infant pairs. *J Clin Psychiatry* 2002;63(10):910-1.
54. Haas JS, Kaplan CP, Barenboim D et al. Bupropion in breast milk: an exposure assessment for potential treatment to prevent post-partum tobacco use. *Tob Control* 2004;13(1):52-6.
55. Aichhorn W, Whitworth AB, Weiss U et al. Mirtazapine and breast-feeding. *Am J Psychiatry* 2004;161(12):2325.
56. Kristensen JH, Ilett KF, Rampono J et al. Transfer of antidepressant mirtazapine into breast milk. *Br J Clin Pharmacol* 2007;63(3):322-7.
57. Buist A, Dennerstein L, Maguire KP et al. Plasma and human milk concentrations of moclobemide in nursing mothers. *Human Psychopharmacol Clin Exp* 1998;13(8):579-82.
58. Chaudron LH, Schoenecker CJ. Bupropion and breastfeeding: a case of a possible infant seizure. *J Clin Psychiatry* 2004;65(6):881-2.
59. Corriveau D. *Utilisation de Wellbutrin SR chez la femme enceinte et chez la femme allaitant.* In: GlaxoSmithKline, Personal Communication; 2001.
60. Verbeek RK, Ross SG, McKenna EA. Excretion of trazodone in breastmilk. *Br J Clin Pharmacol* 1986;22(3);367-70.
61. Misri S, Corral M, Wardrop AA et al. Quetiapine augmentation in lactation: a series of case reports. *J Clin Psychopharmacol* 2006;26(5):508-11.
62. Misri S, Sivertz K. Tricyclic drugs in pregnancy and lactation: a preliminary report. *Int J Psychiatry Med* 1991;21(2):157-71.
63. Newport DJ, Ritchie JC, Knight BT et al. Venlafaxine in human breast milk and nursing infant plasma: determination of exposure. *J Clin Psychiatry* 2009;70(9):1304-10.
64. Lobo ED, Loghin C, Knadler MP et al. Pharmacokinetics of duloxetine in breast milk and plasma of healthy postpartum women. *Clin Pharmacokinet* 2008;47(2):103-9.
65. Boyce PM, Hackett LP, Ilett KF. Duloxetine transfer across the placenta during pregnancy and into milk during lactation. *Arch Womens Ment Health* 2011;14(2):169-72.
66. Ito S. Drug therapy for breast-feeding women. *N Engl J Med* 2000;343(2):118-26.
67. Ohman I, Vitols S, Tomson T. Pharmacokinetics of gabapentin during delivery, in the neonatal period, and lactation: does a fetal accumulation occur during pregnancy? *Epilepsia* 2005;46(10):1621-4.
68. Ohman I, Tomson T. Gabapentin kinetics during delivery, in the neonatal period, and during lactation. *Epilepsia* 2009;50(Suppl 10):108.
69. Kristensen JH , Ilett KF, Hackett LP et al. Gabapentin and breastfeeding: a case report. *J Hum Lact* 2006;22(4):426-8.
70. Mactal-Haaf C, Hoffman M, Kuchta A. Use of anti-infective agents during lactation, Part 3: Antivirals, antifungals, and urinary antiseptics. *J Hum Lact* 2001;17(2):160-6.
71. Ilett KF, Kristensen JH. Drug use and breastfeeding. *Expert Opin Drug Saf* 2005;4(4):745-68.
72. Reed BR. Dermatologic drug use during pregnancy and lactation. *Dermatol Clin* 1997;15(1):197-206.
73. Hilbert J, Radwanski E, Affrime MB et al. Excretion of loratadine in human breast milk. *J Clin Pharmacol* 1988;28(3):234-9.
74. Lucas BD, Purdy CY, Scarim SK et al. Terfenadine pharmacokinetics in breast milk in lactating women. *Clin Pharmacol Ther* 1995;57(4):398-402.
75. Ito S, Blajchman A, Stephenson M et al. Prospective follow-up of adverse reactions in breast-fed infants exposed to maternal medication. *Am J Obstet Gynecol* 1993;168(5):1393-9.

76. Sandstrom B, Regardh CG. Metoprolol excretion into breast milk. *Br J Clin Pharmacol* 1980;9(5):518-9.
77. Ho TK, Moretti ME, Schaeffer IJ et al. Maternal beta-blocker usage and breast feeding in the neonate. *Pediatr Res* 1999;45(4):67A.
78. Schimmel MS, Eidelman AI, Wilschanski MA et al. Toxic effects of atenolol consumed during breast feeding. *J Pediatr* 1989;114(3):476-8.
79. Dumez Y, Tchobroutsky C, Hornych H et al. Neonatal effects of maternal administration of acebutolol. *Br Med J (Clin Res Ed)* 1981;283(6299):1077-9.
80. Boutroy MJ, Bianchetti G, Dubruc C et al. To nurse when receiving acebutolol: is it dangerous for the neonate? *Eur J Clin Pharmacol* 1986;30(6):737-9.
81. Jones HM, Cummings AJ. A study of the transfer of alpha-methyldopa to the human foetus and newborn infant. *Br J Clin Pharmacol* 1978;6(5):432-4.
82. White WB, Andreoli JW, Cohn RD. Alpha-methyldopa disposition in mothers with hypertension and in their breast-fed infants. *Clin Pharmacol Ther* 1985;37(4):387-90.
83. Committee to Advise on Tropical Medicine and Travel (CATMAT). Canadian recommendations for the prevention and treatment of malaria among international travellers. *Can Commun Dis Rep* 2004;30(Suppl 1):1-62. Available from: www.phac-aspc.gc.ca/publicat/ccdr-rmtc/09vol35/35s1/page5-eng.php. Accessed October 2, 2013.
84. Recommendations for the prevention of malaria among travelers. *MMWR Recomm Rep* 1990;39(RR-3):1-10. Available from: www.cdc.gov/mmwr/preview/mmwrhtml/00001584.htm. Accessed October 2, 2013.
85. Viguera AC, Newport DJ, Ritchie J et al. Lithium in breast milk and nursing infants: clinical implications. *Am J Psychiatry* 2007;164(2):342-5.
86. Tunnessen WW, Hertz CG. Toxic effects of lithium in newborn infants: a commentary. *J Pediatr* 1972;81(4):804-7.
87. Kirk M. *Zyprexa—Emploi chez les femmes enceintes ou allaitantes*. In: Touzin J, ed. Toronto (ON): Eli Lilly Canada, Inc.; 2008:15.
88. Gilad O, Merlob P, Stahl B et al. Outcome of infants exposed to olanzapine during breastfeeding. *Breastfeed Med* 2011;6(2):55-8.
89. Gardiner SJ, Kristensen JH, Begg EJ et al. Transfer of olanzapine into breast milk, calculation of infant drug dose, and effect on breast-fed infants. *Am J Psychiatry* 2003;160(8):1428-31.
90. Lee A, Giesbrecht E, Dunn E et al. Excretion of quetiapine in breast milk. *Am J Psychiatry* 2004;161(9):1715-6.
91. Rampono J, Kristensen JH, Ilett KF et al. Quetiapine and breast feeding. *Ann Pharmacother* 2007;41(4):711-4.
92. Yazdani-Brojeni P, Taguchi N, Garcia-Bournissen F et al. Quetiapine in human milk and simulation-based assessment of infant exposure. *Clin Pharmacol Ther* 2010;87(Suppl 1):S3-4.
93. Weggelaar NM, Keijer WJ, Janssen PK. A case report of risperidone distribution and excretion into human milk: how to give good advice if you have not enough data available. *J Clin Psychopharmacol* 2011;31(1):129-31.
94. Yoshida K, Smith B, Craggs M et al. Neuroleptic drugs in breast-milk: a study of pharmacokinetics and of possible adverse effects in breast-fed infants. *Psychol Med* 1998; 28(1):81-91.
95. Dev VJ, Krupp P. Adverse event profile and safety of clozapine. *Rev Contemp Pharmacother* 1995;6:197-208.
96. Sheffield JS, Fish DN, Hollier LM et al. Acyclovir concentrations in human breast milk after valaciclovir administration. *Am J Obstet Gynecol* 2002;186(1):100-2.
97. Siever LJ. The effect of amantadine on prolactin levels and galactorrhea on neuroleptic-treated patients. *J Clin Psychopharmacol* 1981;1(1):2-7.
98. Correa N, Opler LA, Kay SR et al. Amantadine in the treatment of neuroendocrine side effects of neuroleptics. *J Clin Psychoharmacol* 1987;7(2):91-5.
99. Wentges-van Holthe N, van Eijkeren M, van der Laan JW. Oseltamivir and breastfeeding. *Int J Infect Dis* 2008;12(4):451.
100. Tanaka T, Nakajima K, Murashima A et al. Safety of neuraminidase inhibitors against novel influenza A (H1N1) in pregnant and breastfeeding women. *CMAJ* 2009;181(1-2):55-8.
101. Kelly LE, Poon S, Madadi P et al. Neonatal benzodiazepines exposure during breastfeeding. *J Pediatr* 2012;161(3):448-51.
102. NAEPP expert panel report. Managing asthma during pregnancy: recommendations for pharmacologic treatment-2004 update. *J Allergy Clin Immunol* 2005;115(1):34-46.
103. Lindberg C, Boreus LO, de Chateau P et al. Transfer of terbutaline into breast milk. *Eur J Resp Dis* 1984;134:87-91.
104. Lonnerholm G, Lindstrom B. Terbutaline excretion into breast milk. *Br J Clin Pharmacol* 1982;13(5):729-30.
105. Falt A, Bengtsson T, Kennedy BM et al. Exposure of infants to budesonide through breast milk of asthmatic mothers. *J Allergy Clin Immunol* 2007;120(4):798-802.
106. e-CPS. Ottawa (ON): Canadian Pharmacists Association; 2013. Accolate [product monograph]. Available from: www.e-therapeutics.ca. Subscription required.
107. Berlin CM, Briggs GG. Drugs and chemicals in human milk. *Semin Fetal Neonatal Med* 2005;10(2):149-59.
108. Black A, Francoeur D, Rowe T et al. Canadian contraception consensus. *J Obstet Gynaecol Can* 2004;26(4):347-87, 389-436.
109. Ost L, Wettrell G, Bjorkhem I et al. Prednisolone excretion in human milk. *J Pediatr* 1985;106(6):1008-11.
110. Aljazaf K, Hale TW, Ilett KF et al. Pseudoephedrine: effects on milk production in women and estimation of infant exposure via breastmilk. *Br J Clin Pharmacol* 2003;56(1):18-24.
111. Feig DS, Briggs GG, Kraemer JM et al. Transfer of glyburide and glipizide into breast milk. *Diabetes Care* 2005;28(8):1851-5.
112. Everett JA. Use of oral antidiabetic agents during breastfeeding. *J Hum Lact* 1997;13(4):319-21.
113. Kauppila A, Arvela P, Koivisto M et al. Metoclopramide and breast feeding: transfer into milk and the newborn. *Eur J Clin Pharmacol* 1983;25(6):819-23.
114. Kauppila A, Anunti P, Kivinen S et al. Metoclopramide and breast feeding: efficacy and anterior pituitary responses of the mother and the child. *Eur J Obstet Gynecol Reprod Biol* 1985;19(1):19-22.
115. Lewis PJ, Devenish C, Kahn C. Controlled trial of metoclopramide in the initiation of breast feeding. *Br J Clin Pharmacol* 1980;9(2):217-9.
116. Plante L, Ferron GM, Unruh M et al. Excretion of pantoprazole in human breast. *J Reprod Med* 2004;49(10):825-7.
117. Marshall JK, Thompson AB, Armstrong D. Omeprazole for refractory gastroesophageal reflux disease during pregnancy and lactation. *Can J Gastroenterol* 1998;12(3):225-7.
118. Centers for Disease Control and Prevention, Workowski KA, Berman SM. Sexually transmitted diseases treatment guidelines, 2006. *MMWR Recomm Rep* 2006;55 (RR-11):1-94.
119. Porto I. Antiparasitic drugs and lactation: focus on anthelmintics, scabicides, and pediculicides. *J Hum Lact* 2003;19(4):421-5.
120. Taketomo CK, Hodding JH, Kraus DM. *Pediatric & neonatal dosage handbook: a comprehensive resource for all clinicians treating pediatric and neonatal patients*. 18th ed. Hudson (OH): Lexicomp; 2011.
121. Ilett KF, Hale TW, Page-Sharp M et al. Use of nicotine patches in breast-feeding mothers: transfer of nicotine and cotinine into human milk. *Clin Pharmacol Ther* 2003;74(6):516-24.
122. Kampmann JP, Johansen K, Hansen JM et al. Propylthiouracil in human milk. Revision of a dogma. *Lancet* 1980;1(8171):736-7.

123. Azizi F. Effect of methimazole treatment of maternal thyrotoxicosis on thyroid function in breast-feeding infants. *J Pediatr* 1996;128(6):855-8.
124. Azizi F, Khoshniat M, Bahrainian M et al. Thyroid function and intellectual development of infants nursed by mothers taking methimazole. *J Clin Endocrinol Metab* 2000;85(9):3233-8.
125. Mandel SJ, Cooper DS. The use of antithyroid drugs in pregnancy and lactation. *J Clin Endocrinol Metab* 2001;86(6):2354-9.
126. Part 3: Vaccination of specific populations. Immunization in pregnancy and breastfeeding. In: Public Health Agency of Canada. Canadian immunization guide. Available from: www.phac-aspc.gc.ca/publicat/cig-gci/p03-04-eng.php#a8. Accessed November 19, 2013.
127. Mennella JA, Beauchamp GK. The transfer of alcohol to human milk. Effects on flavor and the infant's behavior. *N Engl J Med* 1991;325(14):981-5.
128. Dorea JG. Maternal smoking and infant feeding: breastfeeding is better and safer. *Matern Child Health J* 2007;11(3):287-91.
129. Luck W, Nau H. Nicotine and cotinine concentrations in serum and milk of nursing smokers. *Br J Clin Pharmacol* 1984;18(1):9-15.
130. Hardee GE, Stewart T, Capomacchia AC. Tobacco smoke xenobiotic compound appearance in mothers' milk after involuntary smoke exposures. I. Nicotine and cotinine. *Toxicol Lett* 1983;15(2-3):109-12.
131. Hopkinson JM, Schanler RJ, Fraley JK et al. Milk production by mothers of premature infants: influence of cigarette smoking. *Pediatrics* 1992;90(6):934-8.

Appendix IV
Nutritional Supplements

L. Maria Gutschi, BScPhm, PharmD

Vitamins and **minerals** cannot usually be synthesized in the body but occur naturally in certain foods. They are essential in small quantities for normal body metabolism, functioning as cofactors within enzyme systems required for the function of life. Some vitamins such as A and D serve in hormonal or epigenetic pathways. If steady intakes are not met, deficiency diseases occur, which can sometimes lead to death. However, excess intake can result in toxicities, even at doses which were generally thought to be safe. Most individuals in North America ingest sufficient vitamins and minerals in their diets to prevent deficiency diseases; a small number may be at risk and require supplementation of particular nutrients for identified deficiencies. Insufficient vitamin D levels may be common in Canadians due to our northern climate since it is derived primarily from exposure to sunlight.

Nutritional supplements are defined as substances occurring naturally in food which are required for normal functioning of the body. Nutrient supplementation can contribute to overall health and vitality, providing sufficient vitamins, minerals and other nutrients for prevention of deficiency diseases.

Although preliminary studies may suggest that nutrient supplementation prevents or reduces risk of chronic disease, a benefit is yet to be proven by large trials in most cases. Additionally, long-term nutrient supplementation may be harmful.

Chronic intake of some drugs can affect or interact with vitamins and minerals. Depending on the nature of interaction, it may be necessary to avoid combination therapy, or drug therapy may necessitate supplementation.

Dietary Reference Intakes for Nutrients

The *Dietary Reference Intakes (DRIs)* are a comprehensive set of nutrient reference values for healthy populations that can be used for assessing and planning diets.[1,2] Established cooperatively by Canada and the United States, DRIs are derived from scientific data and provide a range of values from optimal to maximum based on indicators of good health, prevention of chronic disease and evaluation of the possible adverse effects of excess intake.

The *Recommended Dietary Allowance (RDA)* is defined as the average daily dietary intake level thought to be sufficient to meet the nutrient requirement of nearly all (97–98%) healthy individuals in a particular life stage and gender group.

The *Adequate Intake (AI)* is a recommended average daily nutrient intake level based on observed/experimentally determined estimates of nutrient intake by a group (or groups) of apparently healthy people who are assumed to be maintaining an adequate nutritional state. The AI is used when there are insufficient data to establish the estimated average requirement on which to base the RDA of a nutrient. It is expected to meet or exceed the needs of most people in the age, gender or life-stage group.

Selected DRIs for common nutrients are presented in Table 1.

Table 2 provides information on the roles, food sources and toxicity related to excess intake of the **fat-soluble vitamins** (A, D, E and K).

Table 3 provides information on the roles, food sources and toxicity related to excess intake of the **water-soluble vitamins**: thiamine (B_1), riboflavin (B_2), niacin (B_3), pantothenic acid (B_5), biotin (B_7), folic acid (B_9), cyanocobalamin (B_{12}) and ascorbic acid (C). Choline, while not a vitamin, is an essential nutrient usually grouped with the B-complex vitamins.

Table 4 provides information on selected **essential minerals**. Macrominerals (with requirements measured in mg to g per day) include calcium, magnesium, phosphorous, potassium and sodium while microminerals (with requirements measured in µg to mg per day) include copper, chromium, fluoride, iodine, iron, manganese, molybdenum, selenium, vanadium and zinc.

Goals of Therapy

- Identify and correct any identified nutritional deficiencies (Table 5)
- Tailor supplementation to individual and specific diets
- Ensure excess is not consumed and limit antioxidant supplementation
- Ensure no significant drug-nutrient interactions (Table 6)
- Assess benefit versus risk in individual patients for prevention or treatment of disease (Table 7)

Treatment of a disease or condition with micronutrient supplementation should be supported by good evidence and monitored for adverse events.

Indications for General Preventive Supplementation

A benefit from micronutrient supplementation is unlikely for most of the general adult population;[3] encourage consumption of whole foods such as fruits, vegetables, whole grains, legumes, nuts and fish as these may contain other important nutrients required for optimal health (e.g., phytochemicals such as flavonoids, isothiocyanates, isoflavones, saponins) and have been shown to decrease risk of chronic disease and overall mortality.[4,5] The benefit on overall mortality of supplementation with specific nutrients (e.g., vitamin D and omega-3 fatty acids/fish oils) awaits more evidence from prospective randomized controlled trials.[6] Most Canadians have adequate intake of micronutrients although deficiencies in vitamins A, C, D, calcium, magnesium, zinc and folate have been identified in high-risk groups (e.g., those at the lowest level of income and/or educational attainment).[7] See Table 5 for a discussion of common deficiencies.

Certain groups of individuals may require specific preventive supplementation.

Populations with increased requirements:

- Pregnancy and breastfeeding
  - **multivitamin** with **folic acid**[8] (0.4–1 mg/day; 5 mg/day periconceptionally if at high risk)
  - **calcium** (intake from dietary sources recommended but many people do not ingest enough): age 14–18 years = 1300 mg/day; age 19+ = 1000 mg/day[1]
  - **vitamin D**: consider 2000 IU/day for pregnant women during winter months[9]
  - **iron** supplementation, if required (total = 27 mg/day).[1,10] Routine iron supplementation during pregnancy in nonanemic women (hemoglobin >130 g/L) may not be without adverse effects[11] and 16 mg/day total supplementation is proposed.[12] Intermittent iron supplementation (± folic acid) may be an alternative for preventing gestational anemia in nonanemic women with adequate antenatal care. Intermittent supplementation is less likely to result in adverse events such as nausea and GI disturbances compared with a daily regimen, and results in similar maternal and infant outcomes.[13] Additionally, the risk of high hemoglobin concentrations may be reduced. The most commonly used intermittent dosing schedule is 120 mg total weekly elemental iron, given on 1 day of the week in 2 divided doses. This regimen is not recommended for women who are anemic at the start of their pregnancy[13]

- Drug-nutrient interactions (see Table 6)

Populations at risk of inadequate intake:

- Very low calorie diet (<800 kcal/day), either voluntary or involuntary (overall insufficient intake)
- Exclusion diets—lack intake of certain foods, e.g., whole grains, deeply coloured vegetables and fruits, fortified cereals, animal-source foods:
  - vegan diets:[1,14] vitamin B_{12}, vitamin D, calcium and omega-3 fatty acids (from microalgae), iron, zinc
  - lacto-ovo-vegetarians:[1,14] vitamin B_{12}, zinc
- Chronic substance abuse: vitamin C, vitamin B_1, folic acid, vitamin B_6 and vitamin B_2 (riboflavin) in particular for alcohol abuse[1]
- Poverty, social isolation, institutionalization:[15] vitamin A, vitamin C, magnesium, calcium, folic acid, vitamin B_{12}, vitamin D
- At-risk elderly (possibly due to polypharmacy, poor oral health, functional limitations, depression, dementia, social isolation): encourage increased oral intake to manage insufficient micronutrient intake.[16,17] Vitamin B_{12} deficiency (primarily due to chronic food-cobalamin malabsorption and to a lesser extent pernicious anemia)[18] and vitamin D deficiency are common in this group and may require supplementation
  - routine vitamin and mineral supplementation may be associated with increased mortality in elderly women, particularly supplemental iron.[19] Supplementation is not associated with a decreased risk of infections in elderly persons living at home[20]

Populations at risk of malabsorption:

- After bariatric surgery: vitamins A, D, K, B_1, B_{12}, C and folic acid; calcium, copper, iron, selenium, and zinc. Patients require routine supplementation with vitamins and minerals for 2 years or more, with doses higher than those provided by nonprescription supplements[21,22]
- GI diseases known to cause malabsorption or maldigestion (e.g., lactose intolerance, gluten-sensitive enteropathy, food allergies): fat-soluble vitamins, vitamin B_{12}, vitamin K, zinc, iron, calcium
- Swallowing, chewing or dental problems

Table 1: **Daily Dietary Reference Intakes for Vitamins and Selected Minerals**[1,2]

	Vitamins													Minerals				
Age, Gender or Life Stage	**A (IU)**	**B_1 (mg)**	**B_2 (mg)**	**B_3 (mg)**	**Pan-tothenic Acid[a] (B_5) (mg)**	**B_6 (mg)**	**Biotin[a] (B_7) (µg)**	**Folate[b] (B_9) (µg)**	**B_{12} (µg)**	**C (mg)**	**D (IU)**	**E (mg)**	**K[a] (µg)**	**Ca[a] (mg)**	**Fe (mg)**	**F[a] (mg)**	**Se (µg)**	**Zn (mg)**
0–6 months[a]	1333	0.2	0.3	2	1.7	0.1	5	65	0.4	40	400	4	2	200	0.27	0.01	15	2
7–12 months[a]	1667	0.3	0.4	4	1.8	0.3	6	80	0.5	50	400	5	2.5	260	11[c]	0.5	20	3[c]
1–3 y	1000	0.5	0.5	6	2	0.5	8	150	0.9	15	600	6	30	700	7	0.7	20	3
4–8 y	1333	0.6	0.6	8	3	0.6	12	200	1.2	25	600	7	55	1000	10	1	30	5
9–13 y	2000	0.9	0.9	12	4	1.0	20	300	1.8	45	600	11	60	1300	8	2	40	8
14–18 y Male	3000	1.2	1.3	16	5	1.3	25	400	2.4	75	600	15	75	1300	11	3	55	11
14–18 y Female	2333	1.0	1.0	14	5	1.2	25	400[d]	2.4	65	600	15	75	1300	15	3	55	9
14–18 y Pregnancy	2500	1.4	1.4	18	6	1.9	30	600[d]	2.6	80	600	15	75	1300	27	3	60	12
14–18 y Breastfeeding	4000	1.4	1.6	17	7	2.0	35	500	2.8	115	600	19	75	1300	10	3	70	13
19–50 y Male	3000	1.2	1.3	16	5	1.3	30	400	2.4	90	600	15	120	1000	8	4	55	11
19–50 y Female	2333	1.1	1.1	14	5	1.3	30	400[d]	2.4	75	600	15	90	1000	18	3	55	8
19–50 y Pregnancy	2567	1.4	1.4	18	6	1.9	30	600[d]	2.6	85	600	15	90	1000	27	3	60	11
19–50 y Breastfeeding	4333	1.4	1.6	17	7	2	35	500	2.8	120	600	19	90	1000	9	3	70	12
51–70 y Male	3000	1.2	1.3	16	5	1.7	30	400	2.4	90	600	15	120	1000	8	4	55	11
51–70 y Female	2333	1.1	1.1	14	5	1.5	30	400	2.4	75	600	15	90	1200	8	3	55	8
≥71 y Male	3000	1.2	1.3	16	5	1.7	30	400	2.4	90	800	15	120	1200	8	4	55	11
≥71 y Female	2333	1.1	1.1	14	5	1.5	30	400	2.4	75	800	15	90	1200	8	3	55	8

[a] RDA unknown; values represent AI.
[b] As dietary folate equivalents DFE (1 DFE = 1 µg folate from food = 0.5 µg folic acid supplement taken on an empty stomach = 0.6 µg from a fortified food or a supplement consumed with food).
[c] Value represents RDA.
[d] All women capable of becoming pregnant should take a supplement of 400 µg of folic acid daily, in addition to the amount of folate found in a healthy diet; this supplement should continue until a pregnancy is confirmed and prenatal care begins. The critical time for neural tube formation is shortly after conception.
Abbreviations: AI = adequate intake; Ca = calcium; F = fluoride; Fe = iron; RDA = recommended dietary allowance; Se = selenium; Zn = zinc

Table 2: Fat-soluble Vitamins[1,2,23]

Nutrient	Role and Sources	Toxicity	Prevention of Toxicity
vitamin A (retinol)	Required for vision, bone growth, reproduction, cell division, cell differentiation. Regulates immune system and gene transcription. Food sources (preformed vitamin A): liver, whole milk, fortified food products, cod liver oil.	TUL: 10 000 IU/day. Teratogenic at doses >10 000 IU/day. Hepatotoxic. High intake of preformed vitamin A through diet or supplementation is associated with osteoporosis and fracture risk;[24] can occur subclinically without signs or symptoms of hypervitaminosis at total doses of 5000 IU/day; risk may be highest in those with low vitamin D intake.[25]	Avoid supplementation of preformed vitamin A (retinol). Encourage dietary intake from vegetables and fruits as there is no evidence of increased osteoporosis risk from dietary intake.
beta-carotene	Food sources (carotenoids): coloured fruits and vegetables.	No TUL established for dietary beta-carotene.[26] However, oral beta-carotene supplements increase risk of first-time nonfatal MI, increase risk of CV mortality[27,28] in adult male smokers; increase risk of lung cancer diagnosis and death in patients at high risk.[28] Vitamin A and beta-carotene supplementation, singly or combined, increase risk of overall mortality.[26]	No RDA established, but 3–6 mg/day recommended. Supplementation with beta-carotene not generally required but may be used for patients/populations at risk of vitamin A deficiency[1] (recent immigrants or refugees from developing countries with high incidence of vitamin A deficiency or measles; patients with Crohn's disease, celiac disease, pancreatic diseases). High serum concentrations of alpha-carotene (also found in yellow-orange and dark green vegetables) are associated with decreased risk of mortality.[29] Lycopene, lutein and zeaxanthin are carotenoids which do not have vitamin A activity but have health promoting activity.
vitamin D (D_3: cholecalciferol D_2: ergocalciferol)	Modulates transcription of >50 genes in cell differentiation, immunity, insulin secretion, hypertension. Required for calcium metabolism. Food sources: salmon, sardines, tuna and fish oils, fortified milk/orange juice, some mushrooms.	TUL: 4000 IU/day. Hypercalcemia, hypercalciuria, reversible renal impairment, GI symptoms. Single yearly high doses (500 000 IU orally or 300 000 IU IM) have been associated with increased risk of falls and fracture rates especially in the first months post-dose.[30] 400 IU/day plus 2 g/day of calcium was associated with small increased risk of nephrolithiasis.[31] Persons with primary hyperparathyroidism, sarcoidosis, tuberculosis and lymphoma may have increase risk of hypercalcemia with supplementation.	Cholecalciferol (vitamin D_3) most useful in primary care. Avoid large single doses (10 000 IU or more). Doses >2000 IU/day for >4 months unlikely to be beneficial unless patient assessed as a high risk of deficiency. Total amounts of vitamin D ingestion from various supplements should be recorded/monitored.

Nutrient	Role and Sources	Toxicity	Prevention of Toxicity
vitamin E (α-tocopherol)	Required as an antioxidant for protection from damaging effects of free radicals. Food sources: nuts, seeds, vegetable oils.	TUL: 1000 mg (1500 IU)/day. GI upset at doses of 200–800 mg/day, antiplatelet effects and bleeding at 800–1200 mg/day. Other toxicity can occur at 1200 mg/day (emotional disturbances, thrombophlebitis, lipid and thyroid effects, gonadal dysfunction).[32] Intervention trials have not supported the hypothesis that vitamin E decreases CV risk[33,34] or prevents cancer.[33,35] Vitamin E supplementation: • showed a small increased risk of heart failure in people at high risk of CVD[35] • may increase risk of death from any cause at doses >400 IU/day[36] • has no significant effect on the incidence or number of days of respiratory infections or antibiotic use[37] • may increase risk of prostate cancer[38]	Little or no supplementation in patients with a history of stroke, CABG surgery, MI or those at risk of prostate cancer. Limit vitamin E supplementation for others to <400 IU/day. Ensure no significant drug-nutrient interactions which can increase bleeding risk (see Table 6).
vitamin K	Required for blood clotting and bone formation. Food sources: green leafy vegetables, vegetable oils.	TUL has not been determined.	Single ingredient oral supplements are not available in Canada. Excess intake of vitamin K from food sources may interfere with the effect of vitamin K antagonist anticoagulants, e.g., warfarin.

Abbreviations: AI = adequate intake, established when evidence is insufficient to develop an RDA; is set at a level assumed to ensure nutritional adequacy; AREDS = Age-Related Eye Disease Study; CABG = coronary artery bypass graft; CV = cardiovascular; GI = gastrointestinal; HDL = high-density lipoprotein; MI = myocardial infarction; RDA = recommended dietary allowance, i.e., average daily level of intake sufficient to meet the nutrient requirements of nearly all (97–98%) healthy individuals; TUL = tolerable upper limit, i.e., maximum average daily intake likely to cause no risk of adverse health effects

Table 3: Water-soluble Vitamins[1,2,23]

Nutrient	Role and Sources	Toxicity	Prevention of Toxicity
vitamin B_1 (thiamine)	Required coenzyme for mitochondrial enzymes involved in critical roles in the production of energy from food. Food sources: wide variety of foods including cereals (rice, wheat), legumes, nuts, pork.	TUL has not been determined.	
vitamin B_2 (riboflavin)	Integral component of flavoenzymes required for redox reactions and metabolism of carbohydrates, fats and proteins. Food sources: wide variety of foods including fortified cereals, milk and milk products, meat, eggs, nuts.	TUL has not been determined.	
vitamin B_3 (niacin, nicotinic acid, niacinamide)	Required to produce hemoglobin and to increase its oxygen-carrying capacity. Helps maintain blood glucose levels in normal range. Food sources: wide variety of foods including beans, meats, cereals, vegetables.	TUL: 35 mg/day Prostaglandin-mediated flushing occurs in doses >30 mg/day (itching, increased intracranial blood flow, headache). Use of large doses (>3 g/day) may cause elevated liver enzyme levels and is a risk factor for jaundice and hepatotoxicity (more common with sustained-release formulations), GI symptoms, impaired glucose tolerance.	Limit routine supplementation to <30 mg/day. Treatment of lipid disorders requires larger doses and should be monitored by a clinician.
vitamin B_5 (pantothenic acid)	Component of coenzyme A which is required to produce energy from food. Food sources: liver and kidney, yeast, egg yolk, and broccoli.	TUL has not been determined.	
vitamin B_6 (pyridoxine)	Has role in production of >100 enzymes required for chemical reactions, e.g., glycogen phosphorylation. Food sources: fortified cereals, poultry, potatoes, spinach, bananas.	TUL: 100 mg/day Sensory neuropathy can occur with high-dose supplementation (100–500 mg/day); reversible upon discontinuation.	Avoid high-dose supplementation.
vitamin B_7 (biotin)	Required for mammalian carboxylase enzymes. Food sources: egg yolks, liver, yeast.	TUL has not been determined.	

Nutrient	Role and Sources	Toxicity	Prevention of Toxicity
folic acid (folate)[a]	Required for new cell growth formation and maintenance, especially during periods of rapid growth. Food sources: legumes (cooked kidney, pinto, fava beans), green leafy vegetables (spinach), liver, fortified flour (mandatory in Canada), fortified breakfast cereals, oranges.	TUL: 1000 µg/day Doses >1500 µg/day can cause irritability, confusion, exacerbation of seizure frequency, precipitate or exacerbate vitamin B_{12} deficiency. Potential increase in CV risk and colon cancer[39,40] and chronic high doses may increase risk of solid cancers.[41] Increased rate of cognitive decline in elderly who take large doses is possibly related to low vitamin B_{12} levels.[42]	Studies demonstrate mixed results regarding unmetabolized folic acid or intracellular folate and increased cancer and CV risk;[39,43] more study is required to delineate risk/benefit profile. Avoid supplements unless higher folate need is identified (e.g., pregnancy, breastfeeding, methotrexate use). Limit total supplement intake to ≤0.4 mg/day. Emphasize foods high in folate (e.g., green leafy vegetables, fruits) as intake from foods is not associated with adverse effects.
vitamin B_{12} (cyanocobalamin)	Required for red blood cell formation, DNA synthesis and neurological function. Food sources: meat, fish, shellfish, eggs, poultry, fortified cereals.	TUL has not been determined.	
choline	Although not a vitamin, choline is an essential nutrient for structural integrity of cell membranes, cholinergic neurotransmission, and lipid and cholesterol transport and metabolism. Accelerates synthesis and release of acetylcholine. Food sources: milk, liver, eggs, peanuts; small amounts are synthesized in humans from phospholipids. Dietary sources provide approximately 730–1040 mg/day of choline, mostly as lecithin (phosphatidylcholine).[44]	TUL: 3.5 g/day Ingestion of 7.5 g/day may cause hypotension. Cholinergic signs (sweating and diarrhea) and a fishy body odour may occur with doses of 10–16 g/day.[44]	
vitamin C (ascorbic acid)	Required for collagen formation, *l*-carnitine and protein synthesis. Vitamin C is an important physiological antioxidant and regenerates other antioxidants including vitamin E. Food sources: fruits (especially citrus), vegetables (peppers).	TUL: 2 g/day Several grams taken at once can cause nausea, vomiting, esophagitis and heartburn, flushing and diarrhea. Sleep disturbances and fatigue have also been reported. Long-term ingestion of 2 g/day may precipitate urate or oxalate stones in the urinary tract and increase risk of nephrolithiasis.[45]	Limit supplementation to <2 g/day.

[a] Folate refers to the form found naturally in foods; folic acid is the synthetic form used in fortified foods and supplements.
Abbreviations: AI = adequate intake, established when evidence is insufficient to develop an RDA; is set at a level assumed to ensure nutritional adequacy; CV = cardiovascular; GI = gastrointestinal; RDA = recommended dietary allowance, i.e., average daily level of intake sufficient to meet the nutrient requirements of nearly all (97–98%) healthy individuals; TUL = tolerable upper limit, i.e., maximum average daily intake likely to cause no risk of adverse health effects

Table 4: Selected Macro- and Microminerals[1]

Nutrient	Sources	Toxicity	Management
calcium	Food sources: dairy products, calcium-set tofu, fortified foods, kale and related greens (broccoli, bok choy, cabbage).	TUL: 2500 mg/day Studies demonstrated mixed results concerning increased risk of cardiac events, particularly MI, if excess calcium supplementation is used with or without vitamin D.[46,47,48,49,50] More trials required to determine if there is a risk of calcium supplementation, especially in persons with adequate dietary calcium intake.	Typical diet provides 500–1000 mg elemental calcium/day; avoid total amounts (from diet and oral supplements) >1.2 g/day. Ensure adequate vitamin D intake.
iron[a]	Food sources (heme iron from hemoglobin): meat, poultry, fish.	TUL: 45 mg/day Excess iron is stored in tissues and organs, e.g., liver, heart and may lead to cirrhosis, heart failure. Iron is extremely toxic in overdose; accidental poisoning/death has occurred in children with ingestion of as little as 200 mg.[51]	Avoid supplementation unless prescribed for known or suspected iron deficiency or for increased need. Absorption of nonheme iron, e.g., from plant sources, may be influenced by enhancers (ascorbic or malic acid) or inhibitors (polyphenols, phytates, soy protein).
magnesium	Food sources: green leafy vegetables; nuts, seeds, whole grains, foods high in fibre.	TUL: 350 mg/day Acute: doses of >5 g are associated with hypotension, nausea, vomiting, facial flushing leading to muscle weakness, breathing difficulties, cardiac arrythmias (plasma levels >1.74–2.61 mmol/L). Chronic: high doses from supplementation/medications may cause diarrhea, nausea, cramping.	Average intake is generally less than recommended, however low dietary intake does not generally result in symptomatic magnesium deficiency. Toxicity risks increased with impaired renal function.
potassium	Food sources: fruits and vegetables, especially tropical fruits, baked potatoes with skin.	TUL has not been determined for healthy adults. Doses >11 g as a single dose may lead to hyperkalemia in persons who are not accustomed to high intakes even if there is normal kidney function. Acute or chronic renal failure, excessive aldosterone secretion and medications (e.g., potassium-sparing diuretics, ACEIs, ARBs, SMX/TMP) increase risk of hyperkalemia.	Routine supplementation of potassium is not recommended.

Nutrient	Sources	Toxicity	Management
selenium	Food sources: organ meats, seafood; plant sources dependent on selenium content of soil. Average diet provides approximately 100 μg/day.	TUL: 400 μg/day Selenosis (hair and nail brittleness and loss, gastrointestinal upset, garlic breath odour, fatigue, irritability and mild neuropathy) is rare.[1] Cases were reported in 13 subjects taking supplements which, due to a manufacturing error, contained 27.3 mg (27 300 μg) per tablet.[52]	
zinc	Food sources: shellfish, red meat, nuts, legumes.	TUL: 40 mg/day Acute: nausea, vomiting, anorexia, abdominal cramps. Chronic: doses 150–450 mg/day affect copper status, alter iron function, decrease immune function, decrease HDL. Doses >80 mg/day as used in the AREDS study have been associated with significant increase in genitourinary hospitalizations.[53]	Avoid high-dose supplementation. Monitor persons on high doses of zinc for treatment of macular degeneration for genitourinary effects (urinary retention, UTI, urinary lithiasis). See Chapter 28.

[a] RDAs are given as doses of elemental iron. Requirements are 1.8 times higher in vegetarians due to the lower bioavailability of iron from a vegetarian diet.

Abbreviations: ACEI = angiotensin-converting enzyme inhibitor; AI = adequate intake, established when evidence is insufficient to develop an RDA; is set at a level assumed to ensure nutritional adequacy; ARB = angiotensin II receptor blocker; AREDS = Age-Related Eye Disease Study; HDL = high-density lipoprotein; MI = myocardial infarction; RDA = recommended dietary allowance, i.e., average daily level of intake sufficient to meet the nutrient requirements of nearly all (97–98%) healthy individuals; SMX/TMP = sulfamethoxazole/trimethoprim; TUL = tolerable upper limit, i.e., maximum average daily intake likely to cause no risk of adverse health effects; UTI = urinary tract infection

Table 5: Supplementation to Prevent or Treat Common Known Deficiency States

Deficiency	Patient Groups Affected	Recommendations
***vitamin D* (cholecalciferol)** *Adequate* levels:[a] >50 nmol/L *Deficiency* (<25 nmol/L) may be associated with muscle pain, bone pain *Suboptimal* levels (25–75 nmol/L) may be associated with:[54,55] • Bone health, osteoporosis • Increased CV risk • Muscle weakness and falls • Increased risk of cognitive decline in the elderly,[56] schizophrenia,[57] type I diabetes, depression, cancer (colon, possibly breast and prostate), cancer mortality, multiple sclerosis Observational data only[58]—awaiting randomized controlled trial evidence Measurement of vitamin D levels is not routinely required unless high risk of deficiency or concerns regarding toxicity[59]	Approximately 10% of Canadians have inadequate levels for bone health and are at risk for rickets or osteomalacia; 60% have levels <75 nmol/L,[60] the suggested level needed for overall health and disease prevention. Patient groups at increased risk of deficiency/suboptimal levels include:[54] • Dark skinned individuals • Sunscreen use (SPF >8) • Lack of sunlight due to northern latitude, use of occlusive clothing, staying indoors (e.g., elderly, obese or institutionalized persons) • Medication-induced (see Table 6) Modest decrease in overall mortality, primarily seen in elderly women who are institutionalized or in dependent care.[61]	Health Canada RDA (Table 1) differs from those of other groups: Osteoporosis Canada[62] • Adults <50 y at low risk of deficiency: 400–1000 IU daily • Adults ≥50 y and those at moderate-high risk: 800–2000 IU daily International Osteoporosis Foundation[63] • Older adults: 800–1000 IU/day • Obese, limited skin exposure, non-European populations: 2000 IU/day Canadian Cancer Society[64] • Adults during fall and winter: 1000 IU/day • Older adults, dark skin or little sun exposure: 1000 IU/day all year Canadian Pediatric Society[65] • Pregnancy and breastfeeding: consider vitamin D_3 2000 IU/day during winter months Maintenance range: 400–2000 IU/day Evidence and safety supports use of 800–1000 IU/day in Canadians. For severe deficiency (levels <25 nmol/L), consider bolus dosing followed by maintenance: • 2000–4000 IU of D_3 daily for 8–20 weeks **or** • 600 000 IU of D_2 over 8 weeks (e.g., 50 000 IU weekly for 8–12 weeks)[54] Optimal form of vitamin D and regimen for bolus dosing for severe deficiency have not been established. Appropriate vitamin D levels may improve dietary absorption of calcium.[54,66]
vitamin B_{12} Pernicious anemia occurs in 2–4% of US population; overall rates of vitamin B_{12} insufficiency is estimated at 1.5–15%[67]	Persons with macrocytosis or neurologic symptoms. Persons >60 y (marginal depletion reported to be >20%).[68] Persons with gastric, ileal, pancreatic, Crohn's, or celiac disease. Chronic use of PPIs, metformin or H_2 receptor antagonists. Exclusion diets.[69]	Encourage persons at risk of vitamin B_{12} deficiency to consume foods high in vitamin B_{12}. Malabsorption of vitamin B_{12} from food is the main cause of deficiency in the elderly. Consider 1000 µg/day orally for persons taking drugs known to deplete vitamin B_{12} stores.

Deficiency	Patient Groups Affected	Recommendations
calcium	Postmenopausal women.[70] Vegans or those who limit dairy product intake (e.g., due to lactose intolerance). Persons with anorexia or excess exercise leading to amenorrhea.[71]	In postmenopausal women, ≤400 IU vitamin D and ≤1000 mg of calcium supplements provided no benefit for the primary prevention of fractures;[72] high quality evidence for the benefit of higher doses of vitamin D is lacking but 800–2000 IU/day is often recommended.[70] Excess calcium supplementation should be avoided (limit to ≤1200 mg/day from all sources).[70] Calcium carbonate should be taken with food to improve absorption; calcium citrate can be taken without food and is more readily absorbable. Avoid doses >500 mg elemental calcium at one time. Constipation, gas or bloating may be managed with smaller, more frequent dosing, or differing formulations or salts.
iron	Female adolescents, women with heavy menstrual losses. Those at high risk of malabsorption (e.g., Crohn's or celiac disease). Patients with renal failure, especially those on dialysis. Persons who engage in intense aerobic exercise; female and vegetarian athletes, distance runners may also be at risk.[51]	Adult men and postmenopausal women should not take a supplement unless evaluated, as deficiency is rare and supplementation may be harmful.[19] Vegetarians/vegans should consider consuming nonheme sources of iron together with foods high in vitamin C (e.g., citrus fruits) to improve absorption.

[a] Evidence of the relationship between disease due to vitamin D insufficiency and 25-hydroxyvitamin D levels is evolving.
Abbreviations: CV = cardiovascular; IU = international unit; PPI = proton pump inhibitor; RDA = recommended dietary allowance; SPF = sun protection factor

Table 6: **Clinically Significant Drug-Nutritional Supplement Interactions**[32,73]

Supplement	Drug	Interaction	Management
beta-carotene, vitamin A	Hepatotoxic drugs (acetaminophen, carbamazepine, isoniazid, methotrexate)	May increase risk of liver disease.	Avoid combination.
	Retinoids (isotretinoin, acitretin, etretinate, tazarotene)	Additive toxic effects.	Avoid combination.
	Warfarin	Increased risk of vitamin A toxicity and bleeding.	Avoid combination.
calcium	Diuretics	Possible hypocalcemia (with loop diuretics) or hypercalcemia (with thiazides).	May require calcium supplementation with loop diuretics.
	Fluoroquinolones, tetracyclines, bisphosphonates, glucocorticoids	Decreased absorption, possible decreased efficacy, risk of treatment failure.	Separate calcium doses at least 4 h apart from bisphosphonates; consider temporarily discontinuing supplementation while receiving fluoroquinolones or tetracyclines. Normal dairy intake is unlikely to decrease efficacy.
folic acid	Methotrexate (low-dose)	Increased folate requirements to prevent GI and liver toxicity.	Supplement with 1–5 mg/day; avoid on days when methotrexate ingested.
	Phenytoin	Folic acid may be a cofactor in phenytoin metabolism, decrease serum phenytoin levels with large doses of folic acid and potential increase in seizure frequency.	Avoid folic acid supplements >1 mg/day.
iron	Allopurinol	Increased iron storage in liver.	Avoid combination.
	Bisphosphonates, fluoroquinolones, levothyroxine, levodopa, tetracyclines	Form insoluble complexes with iron.	Separate doses at least 2 h apart. Avoid iron and levodopa combination.
	PPIs,[74] H_2 blockers	Impaired iron absorption.	Separate doses at least 2 h apart.
magnesium	Bisphosphonates, tetracyclines	Forms insoluble complexes; results in reduced absorption.	Separate doses by at least 2 h.
	Diuretics	Loop/thiazide diuretics: possible magnesium depletion. Potassium-sparing diuretics: reduced magnesium excretion.	Regular monitoring of magnesium levels required.
	PPIs[75]	Chronic long-term use of PPIs may cause hypomagnesemia. Possibly accompanied by hypocalcemia and hypokalemia.	Periodic monitoring suggested. Supplements may be required.
niacin	Antidiabetic drugs	Impairs glucose tolerance in a dose-dependent manner.	Doses >4 g/day may increase plasma glucose by an average of 16% and HbA_{1c} by 21%; increased requirements for antidiabetic drugs may be necessary.

Supplement	Drug	Interaction	Management
	Carbamazepine	Niacin 60–80 mg/day may increase carbamazepine levels.	Monitor carbamazepine levels, avoid niacin supplementation.
	HMG-CoA reductase inhibitors	Increased risk of myopathies.	Monitor signs and symptoms, use lowest dose possible.
pyridoxine (vitamin B_6)	Antiepileptic drugs (phenytoin, phenobarbital)	Can decrease phenytoin and phenobarbital serum levels by increasing metabolism.	Discontinue pyridoxine or increase dose of antiepileptic drug.
	Isoniazid	Acts as an antagonist and can induce peripheral neuropathy.	Supplementation recommended but limit pyridoxine to 10–50 mg/day.
	Levodopa	Decreased anti-parkinson effect.	Avoid supplementation; consider treatment with levodopa/carbidopa combination.
vitamin B_{12}	H_2 blockers	Possible decreased vitamin B_{12} levels but evidence is conflicting.	
	Metformin	10–30% of patients who take metformin may have decreased vitamin B_{12} absorption.	Supplementation of crystalline vitamin B_{12} may be required.
	PPIs[74]	Decreased absorption of nonheme iron, retards clinical response to iron supplementation.	May require change to heme iron formulation if iron-deficiency anemia occurs on chronic PPI therapy. Supplementation of crystalline vitamin B_{12} may be required, especially in the elderly or if on PPI >10 y.
vitamin D	Antiepileptic drugs (carbamazepine, phenytoin, phenobarbital)	Increased vitamin D metabolism to inactive compounds and decreased calcium absorption.	Supplementation may be required.
	Cholestyramine, colestipol, orlistat	Decreased absorption.	Supplementation may be required.
	Corticosteroids	Can impair vitamin D metabolism; long-term use can contribute to development of osteoporosis as corticosteroids also inhibit calcium absorption.	Supplementation may be required.
	Rifampin	Increased vitamin D metabolism.	Supplementation may be required.
vitamin E	Warfarin, ASA, NSAIDs	May increase risk of bleeding.	Limit vitamin E dose ≤200 IU/day and monitor INR.

Abbreviations: HbA_{1c} = hemoglobin A_{1c}; INR = International Normalized Ratio; PPI = proton pump inhibitor

Table 7: Evidence-based Supplementation to Prevent or Treat Disease

Disease/Condition	Supplement	Evidence of Benefit/Risk	Recommendations
Age-related macular degeneration	*antioxidants plus copper and zinc*	May be beneficial; data primarily from AREDS[76] in patients with age-related macular degeneration (AMD). The addition of lutein and zeaxanthin or omega-3 fatty acids to the original AREDS formula did not demonstrate reduced risk of progression of AMD.[77]	Discuss supplementation with specialist/family physician since data are not available for other patient groups. Beta-carotene–containing formulations are no longer recommended for prevention of AMD progression because of an increased risk of lung cancer.[77] Lutein and zeaxanthin may be a suitable replacement for beta-carotene in the original AREDS formulation.
Cardiovascular disease, primary prevention	*omega-3 fatty acids*	Benefits of fatty fish/omega-3 fatty acid supplementation have been questioned.[78,79] Definitive benefits to be determined in upcoming trials.	2 servings weekly of low-mercury fish (tuna, sardines, salmon) recommended. May consider supplementation to provide 1 g/day of EPA+DHA[a] in those who do not consume fish. Persons with sensitivity to finned fish appear to tolerate fish oil supplements;[80] alternatively a DHA supplement derived from algae may be used for vegetarians or those with severe allergies.
	vitamin D	Supplementation in older patients (>70 y) with isolated systolic hypertension did not improve blood pressure, despite baseline low 25-hydroxyvitamin D levels.[81] Dosing of 100 000 IU/3 months may be a study limitation.	Vitamin D supplementation is unlikely beneficial for primary prevention of cardiovascular disease.
Cardiovascular disease, secondary prevention	*B vitamins (folic acid, vitamin B_6, vitamin B_{12}) and antioxidants*	No benefit seen on CV events with B vitamins and potential harm from antioxidants.[82,83,84,85]	Avoid routine use.
	omega-3 fatty acids	Decreased risk of CV death, sudden cardiac death and nonfatal CV events and overall mortality (primarily in high risk patients).[86] Benefit seen primarily in those at high risk. No benefit seen if post MI patients optimally treated[87] or given low doses.[88] Lack of benefit seen when initiated after acute phase of CV event.[82] Lack of benefit for prevention of recurrent AF.[89]	1 g/day of EPA+DHA[a,90] **or** ≥ 2 servings of fish weekly as part of a Mediterranean diet.[91] Formulation of omega-3 acid ethyl esters used in trials (Omacor/Lovanza) is not yet available in Canada. Given within 3 months of an MI. Monitor INR if on warfarin.

Disease/Condition	Supplement	Evidence of Benefit/Risk	Recommendations
Cancer prevention, colon	*folic acid*	1 mg/day in high-risk patients with polyps not effective in reducing colon cancer[92] and may increase risk. Supplementation in the general population does not appear to be beneficial.[93]	Avoid supplementation for cancer prevention especially in those at high risk; Increasing folate from dietary sources may be beneficial.
	calcium, vitamin D	Additional studies are needed on use of calcium, vitamin D before these can be routinely recommended.	
	antioxidants		Avoid antioxidant supplementation.[26,94]
Cancer prevention, other	*vitamin E*	Long-term vitamin E supplementation does not prevent cancer.[95] Supplementation increases risk of prostate cancer by 17%; effect is apparent by the 3rd year of supplementation.[38]	Limit or avoid vitamin E supplementation, especially in those at high risk (e.g., smokers). Avoid in males, especially those >60 y.
	selenium	Selenium supplementation does not prevent cancer.[38]	Limit supplementation for primary prevention of cancer.
	B vitamins (folic acid, vitamin B_6, vitamin B_{12})	Vitamin B supplementation does not decrease overall risk of breast cancer.[96]	Limit supplementation for primary prevention of breast cancer.
	beta-carotene	Beta-carotene supplements increase risk of gastric and lung cancer at doses of 20–30 mg/day and at any dose in patients at high risk (smokers, asbestos exposure).[85,97]	Avoid beta-carotene, retinol especially in those at high risk (smokers); supplement with foods high in alpha-carotenes.[29]
	vitamin D	Benefit of vitamin D for cancer prevention awaiting clarification from definitive trials as data are conflicting (possible increased risk of pancreatic cancer with high vitamin D levels).[98]	Canadian Cancer Society recommends 800–1000 IU/day during winter months in patients at moderate to high risk of insufficiency.[64]
Childhood development (cognitive and visual)	*omega-3 fatty acids*	Maternal supplementation with omega-3 fatty acids during pregnancy did not result in significant differences in cognitive or visual development.[99,100]	More study required.
Cognitive decline	*B vitamins (folic acid, vitamin B_6, vitamin B_{12}) and antioxidants*	Supplementation does not prevent cognitive decline, nor does antioxidant supplementation (vitamin C, vitamin E, beta-carotene).[101]	Avoid high-dose vitamin B and antioxidant supplementation.
	omega-3 fatty acids/fish oil	Recommendation regarding omega-3 fatty acid supplementation to prevent cognitive decline is awaiting current trial results.	A possible decreased risk with fish consumption has been seen in observational trials.[101]

(cont'd)

Table 7: Evidence-based Supplementation to Prevent or Treat Disease *(cont'd)*

Disease/Condition	Supplement	Evidence of Benefit/Risk	Recommendations
Diabetes	*omega-3 fatty acids*	Omega-3 fatty acids lower triglycerides and VLDL but have no effect on glycemic control; LDL levels may increase insignificantly. Insufficient data to make recommendations for diabetes prevention.[102]	Awaiting controlled clinical trial data to support observational data.
	vitamin D	Risk of type 1 diabetes may be decreased in children who were supplemented—may prevent type 1 diabetes.[103]	No change to current recommendations until RCT evidence is available. Data are insufficient to recommend vitamin D for primary prevention of type 2 diabetes or for glycemic control.
	B vitamins (folic acid, vitamin B_6, vitamin B_{12})	High dose vitamin B therapy (folic acid, vitamin B_{12} and vitamin B_6) did not slow progression of diabetic nephropathy and increased risk of vascular events.[104]	Avoid supplementation.
Gout	*vitamin C*	Vitamin C supplementation (median dose of 500 mg per day) modestly decrease serum uric acid levels in healthy patients.[105] but a small RCT did not show any urate-lowering effects in patients with gout.[106]	Limit doses to <2 g/day. More study required to determine optimal dose and effect on clinical outcomes (number of gouty attacks).
Heart failure	*omega-3 fatty acids*	May be considered in those with mild to moderate heart failure.[107] Those with preserved ejection fraction >40% may not benefit.	1 g daily of EPA+DHA.[a] The formulation of omega-3 acid ethyl esters used in trials (Omacor/Lovanza) is not yet available in Canada. Monitor for increased bleeding if on warfarin. Doses >3 g/day may be associated with bleeding.
	coenzyme Q_{10}	Supplementation has no effect on exercise capacity or LV function in patients with heart failure despite increased blood levels.[108]	Higher quality studies required to determine if there are benefits on morbidity or mortality when added to current standard of care.
Headache	*omega-3 fatty acids*	Dietary intervention of increased n-3 EPA and DHA and decreased n-6 LA intake decreased the number and intensity of headaches and increased quality of life.[109]	Unknown if supplementation will result in similar outcomes. Larger confirmatory trials needed before recommendation can be made.

Disease/Condition	Supplement	Evidence of Benefit/Risk	Recommendations
Mood disorders (major depressive disorder)	*B vitamins (folic acid, vitamin B_6, and vitamin B_{12})*	Limited data suggest potential benefit, especially in women when used as adjunctive therapy.[110] Supplemental vitamin B_6, B_{12} and folic acid decrease risk of depression after stroke or TIA.[111] Folate 0.5 mg/day decrease depressive and somatic symptoms in patients partially responsive or nonresponsive to SSRIs.[112] Improves cognitive function and decrease depressive symptoms in elderly with dementia and known folate deficiency.[112]	No evidence for efficacy as monotherapy. Balance potential benefit of folic acid supplementation with long-term risk. Uncertain whether benefit occurs in those with or without folate deficiency. Supplementation of vitamin B_6 25 mg, vitamin B_{12} 500 µg and folic acid 2 mg daily may be considered for stroke patients at risk of depression, but awaiting confirmatory data.
	omega-3 fatty acids/fish oil	Data primarily as adjunctive therapy at doses of 1–4 g/day; EPA alone or with DHA appears to show greater benefits.[a,110] Fish oil supplementation during pregnancy does not reduce risk of postpartum depression and has not been shown to improve neurodevelopment in offspring.[100,113,114]	More study required.
	selenium	Insufficient evidence for the use of selenium to prevent postpartum depression.[114]	More study required.
Pain, chronic or neuropathic	*vitamin D*	One trial has shown a beneficial effect of supplementation with vitamin D in chronic pain conditions.[115]	Recommendation regarding use of vitamin D to decrease incidence of chronic pain awaits high quality trial evidence.[116]
Pregnancy-related conditions	*calcium*	Oral calcium may prevent pre-eclampsia and decrease risk of death or complications related to hypertension.[117]	1 g daily in divided doses may be beneficial, especially those with low baseline calcium intake or at high risk of pre-eclampsia.
Psychotic disorders/ schizophrenia	*omega-3 fatty acids/fish oil*	May be beneficial for early prevention in persons at ultra-high risk of psychosis.[118] May allow decreased antipsychotic doses, but its use for treatment of schizophrenia remains experimental.[119] Little evidence for benefit for manic symptoms of bipolar disorder.[120]	Requires confirmatory trials.
	folic acid	Supplementation improved negative symptoms in patients with specific gene variants (*FOLH1*).[121]	Folic acid 2 mg and vitamin B_{12} 400 µg may be beneficial in those with *FOLH1* gene variants.

(cont'd)

Table 7: Evidence-based Supplementation to Prevent or Treat Disease *(cont'd)*

Disease/Condition	Supplement	Evidence of Benefit/Risk	Recommendations
Respiratory conditions	*vitamin C*	Limited evidence that vitamin C may decrease pneumonia incidence and decrease respiratory symptoms; benefits seen in those at high risk of or known to have malnutrition/insufficient intake.[122] Vitamin C supplementation halves the risk of a common cold in persons who are under extreme physical stress for short periods of time (e.g., marathon runners, skiers, soldiers in subarctic conditions). No benefit seen for duration or severity of cold.[123] Vitamin C prophylaxis is not beneficial in reducing incidence of the common cold in the general population.[123]	Vitamin C prophylaxis may have a small, but consistent effect on the duration of symptoms of the common cold. Children particularly, may benefit.[123]
	zinc	Zinc lozenges may reduce the duration of the common cold when administered within 24 hours of onset of symptoms.[124]	Zinc lozenges ≥75 mg/day for the duration of the cold is the recommended dose.
Systemic lupus erythematosus	*vitamin D*	Supplementation with vitamin D 2000 IU improved inflammatory and hemostatic markers as well as disease activity in patients with SLE and vitamin D insufficiency.[125]	Vitamin D supplementation may be beneficial, but larger trials required before routine supplementation can be recommended.
Triglyceridemia	*omega-3 fatty acids*	Efficacy appears similar to fibrates.[90]	2–4 g/day of EPA+DHA[a] supplements in capsule form under medical supervision. Adverse events include GI disturbances, burping, potential increased risk of bleeding.

[a] EPA and DHA are essential fatty acids found in cold water fish.
Abbreviations: ALA = alpha-linolenic acid; AREDS = Age-Related Eye Disease Study; CVD = cardiovascular disease; DHA = docosahexaenoic acid; DM = diabetes mellitus; EPA = eicosapentaenoic acid; FOLH1 = folate hydrolase 1; LA = linoleic acid; LV = left ventricular; RCT = randomized controlled trial; SSRI = selective serotonin reuptake inhibitor; TIA = transient ischemic attack

References

1. Institutes of Medicine of the National Academies. *Dietary Reference Intakes (DRIs): Recommended dietary allowances and adequate intakes, vitamins and elements*. Available from: www.iom.edu/Activities/Nutrition/SummaryDRIs/~/media/Files/Activity%20Files/Nutrition/DRIs/RDA%20and%20AIs_Vitamin%20and%20Elements.pdf. Accessed February 4, 2011.
2. Health Canada. *Dietary reference intakes tables*. Available from: www.hc-sc.gc.ca/fn-an/nutrition/reference/table/index-eng.php. Accessed March 23, 2011.
3. McCormick DB. Vitamin/mineral supplements: of questionable benefit for the general population. *Nutr Rev* 2010;68(4):207-13.
4. Sofi F, Cesari F, Abbate A et al. Adherence to Mediterranean diet and health status: meta-analysis. *BMJ* 2008;337:a1344.
5. Ford ES, Bergmann MM, Kroger J et al. Healthy living is the best revenge: findings from the European Prospective Investigation into Cancer and Nutrition-Potsdam Study. *Arch Intern Med* 2009;169(15):1355-62.
6. VITAL Study. *The vitamin D and OMEGA-3 Trial (VITAL)*. Available from: www.vitalstudy.org/. Accessed March 30, 2011.
7. Tarasuk V, Fitzpatrick S, Ward H. Nutrition inequities in Canada. *Appl Physiol Nutr Metab* 2010;35(2):172-9.
8. Wilson RD, Johnson JA, Wyatt P et al. Pre-conceptional vitamin/folic acid supplementation 2007: the use of folic acid in combination with a multivitamin supplement for the prevention of neural tube defects and other congenital anomalies. *J Obstet Gynaecol Can* 2007;29(12):1003-26.
9. Vitamin D supplementation: recommendations for Canadian mothers and infants. *Paediatr Child Health* 2007;12(7):583-98.
10. Pena-Rosas JP, De-Regil LM, Dowswell T et al. Daily oral iron supplementation during pregnancy. *Cochrane Database Syst Rev* 2012;12:CD004736.
11. Ziaei S, Norrozi M, Faghihzadeh S et al. A randomized placebo-controlled trial to determine the effect of iron supplementation on pregnancy outcome in pregnant women with hemoglobin > or = 13.2 g/dl. *BJOG* 2007;114(6):684-8.
12. Cockell KA, Miller DC, Lowell H. Application of the Dietary Reference Intakes in developing a recommendation for pregnancy iron supplements in Canada. *Am J Clin Nutr* 2009;90(4):1023-8.
13. Pena-Rosas JP, De-Regil LM, Dowswell T et al. Intermittent oral iron supplementation during pregnancy. *Cochrane Database Syst Rev* 2012;7:CD009997.
14. American Dietetic Association; Dietitians of Canada. Position of the American Dietetic Association and Dietitians of Canada: vegetarian diets. *J Am Diet Assoc* 2003;103(6):748-65.
15. Kirkpatrick SI, Tarasuk V. Food insecurity is associated with nutrient inadequacies among Canadian adults and adolescents. *J Nutr* 2008;138(3):604-12.
16. Marian M, Sacks G. Micronutrients and older adults. *Nutr Clin Pract* 2009;24(2):179-95.
17. Mucci E, Jackson SH. Nutritional supplementation in community-dwelling elderly people. *Ann Nutr Metab* 2008;52(Suppl 1):33-7.
18. Andres E, Loukili NH, Noel E et al. Vitamin B12 (cobalamin) deficiency in elderly patients. *CMAJ* 2004;171(3):251-9.
19. Mursu J, Robien K, Harnack LJ et al. Dietary supplements and mortality rate in older women: the Iowa Women's Health Study. *Arch Intern Med* 2011;171(18):1625-33.
20. Avenell A, Campbell MK, Cook JA et al. Effect of multivitamin and multimineral supplements on morbidity from infections in older people (MAVIS trial): pragmatic, randomised, double blind, placebo controlled trial. *BMJ* 2005;331(7512):324-9.
21. Shankar P, Boylan M, Sriram K. Micronutrient deficiencies after bariatric surgery. *Nutrition* 2010;26(11-12):1031-7.
22. Schweitzer DH, Posthuma EF. Prevention of vitamin and mineral deficiencies after bariatric surgery: evidence and algorithms. *Obes Surg* 2008;18(11):1485-8.
23. Linus Pauling Institute. Oregon State University. Micronutrient Research for Optimal Health. Micronutrient Information Center. Available from: lpi.oregonstate.edu/infocenter/. Accessed March 23, 2011.
24. Feskanich D, Singh V, Willett WC et al. Vitamin A intake and hip fractures among postmenopausal women. *JAMA* 2002;287(1):47-54.
25. Caire-Juvera G, Ritenbaugh C, Wactawski-Wende J et al. Vitamin A and retinol intakes and the risk of fractures among participants of the Women's Health Initiative Observational Study. *Am J Clin Nutr* 2009;89(1):323-30.
26. Bjelakovic G, Nikolava D, Gluud LL et al. Mortality in randomized trials of antioxidant supplements for primary and secondary prevention: systematic review and meta-analysis. *JAMA* 2007;297(8):842-57.
27. Tornwall ME, Virtamo J, Korhonen PA et al. Effect of alpha-tocopherol and beta-carotene supplementation on coronary heart disease during the 6-year post-trial follow-up in the ATBC study. *Eur Heart J* 2004;25(13):1171-8.
28. Omenn GS, Goodman GE, Thornquist MD et al. Effects of a combination of beta carotene and vitamin A on lung cancer and cardiovascular disease. *N Engl J Med* 1996;334(18):1150-5.
29. Li C, Ford ES, Zhao G et al. Serum {alpha}-carotene concentrations and risk of death among US adults: the third National Health and Nutrition Examination Survey Follow-up Study. *Arch Intern Med* 2011;171(6):507-15.
30. Sanders KM, Stuart AL, Williamson EJ et al. Annual high-dose oral vitamin D and falls and fractures in older women: a randomized controlled trial. *JAMA* 2010;303(18):1815-22.
31. Jackson RD, LaCroix AZ, Gass M et al. Calcium plus vitamin D supplementation and the risk of fractures. *N Engl J Med* 2006;354(7):669-83.
32. Rogovik AL, Vohra S, Goldman RD. Safety considerations and potential interactions of vitamins: should vitamins be considered drugs? *Ann Pharmacother* 2010;44(2):311-24.
33. Lee IM, Cook NR, Gaziano JM et al. Vitamin E in the primary prevention of cardiovascular disease and cancer: the Women's Health Study: a randomized controlled trial. *JAMA* 2005;294(1):56-65.
34. Sesso HD, Buring JE, Christen WG et al. Vitamins E and C in the prevention of cardiovascular disease in men: the Physicians' Health Study II randomized controlled trial. *JAMA* 2008;300(18):2123-33.
35. Lonn E, Bosch Y, Yusuf S et al. Effects of long-term vitamin E supplementation on cardiovascular events and cancer: a randomized controlled trial. *JAMA* 2005;293(11):1338-47.
36. Miller ER, Pastor-Barriuso R, Dalal D et al. Meta-analysis: high-dosage vitamin E supplementation may increase all-cause mortality. *Ann Intern Med* 2005;142(1):37-46.
37. Meydani SN, Leka LS, Fine BC et al. Vitamin E and respiratory tract infections in elderly nursing home residents: a randomized controlled trial. *JAMA* 2004;292(7):828-36.
38. Klein EA, Thompson IM, Tangen CM et al. Vitamin E and the risk of prostate cancer: the Selenium and Vitamin E Cancer Prevention Trial (SELECT). *JAMA* 2011;306(14):1549-56.
39. Sauer J, Mason JB, Choi SW. Too much folate: a risk factor for cancer and cardiovascular disease? *Curr Opin Clin Nutr Metab Care* 2009;12(1):30-6.
40. Cole BF, Baron JA, Sandler RS et al. Folic acid for the prevention of colorectal adenomas: a randomized clinical trial. *JAMA* 2007;297(21):2351-9.

41. Ebbing M, Bonaa KH, Nygard O et al. Cancer incidence and mortality after treatment with folic acid and vitamin B12. *JAMA* 2009;302(19):2119-26.
42. Morris MC, Evans DA, Bienias JL et al. Dietary folate and vitamin B12 intake and cognitive decline among community-dwelling older persons. *Arch Neurol* 2005;62(4):641-5.
43. Vollset SE, Clarke R, Lewington S et al. Effects of folic acid supplementation on overall and site-specific cancer incidence during the randomised trials: meta-analyses of data on 50 000 individuals. *Lancet* 2013;381(9871):1029-36.
44. Linus Pauling Institute. Oregon State University. Micronutrient Information Center. *Choline*. Available from: lpi.oregonstate.edu/infocenter/othernuts/choline/. Accessed March 8, 2012.
45. Taylor EN, Stampfer MJ, Curhan GC. Dietary factors and the risk of incident kidney stones in men: new insights after 14 years of follow-up. *J Am Soc Nephrol* 2004;15(12):3225-32.
46. Bolland MJ, Grey A, Avenell A et al. Calcium supplements, with or without vitamin D and risk of cardiovascular events: reanalysis of the Women's Health Initiative limited access data set and meta-analysis. *BMJ* 2011;342:d2040.
47. Lewis JR, Calver J, Zhu K et al. Calcium supplementation and the risks of atherosclerotic vascular disease in older women: results of a 5-year RCT and a 4.5-year follow up. *J Bone Miner Res* 2011;26(1):35-41.
48. Michaelsson K, Melhus H, Warensjo Lemming E et al. Long term calcium intake and rates of all cause and cardiovascular mortality: community based prospective longitudinal cohort study. *BMJ* 2013;346:f228.
49. Xiao Q, Murphy RA, Houston DK et al. Dietary and supplemental calcium intake and cardiovascular disease mortality: the National Institutes of Health-AARP diet and health study. *JAMA Intern Med* 2013;173(8):639-46.
50. Langsetmo L, Berger C, Kreiger N et al. Calcium and vitamin D intake and mortality: results from the Canadian Multicentre Osteoporosis Study (CaMos). *J Clin Endocrinol Metab* 2013;98(7):3010-8.
51. Office of Dietary Supplements, National Institutes of Health. *Dietary supplement fact sheet: Iron.* Available from: ods.od.nih.gov/factsheets/Iron-HealthProfessional/. Accessed January 13, 2011.
52. Centers for Disease Control and Prevention. *CDC alert on adverse effects associated with consuming "Total Body Formula" and "Total Body Mega Formula".* Available from: dhhs.ne.gov/publichealth/han%20Documents/advisory041408.pdf. Accessed January 3, 2011.
53. Johnson AR, Munoz A, Gottlieb JL et al. High dose zinc increases hospital admissions due to genitourinary complications. *J Urol* 2007;177(2):639-43.
54. Holick MF. Vitamin D deficiency. *N Engl J Med* 2007;357(3):266-81.
55. Stone S, Regier L, Jensen B. *Vitamin D: therapeutic overview & evaluation of evidence for current claims.* Saskatoon Health Region: RxFiles; Dec 2010. Available from: www.rxfiles.ca. Subscription required.
56. Llewellyn DJ, Lang IA, Langa LM et al. Vitamin D and risk of cognitive decline in elderly persons. *Arch Intern Med* 2010;170(13):1135-41.
57. McGrath JJ, Burne TH, Feron F et al. Developmental vitamin D deficiency and risk of schizophrenia: a 10-year update. *Schizophr Bull* 2010;36(6):1073-8.
58. Chung M, Balk EM, Brendel M et al. Vitamin D and calcium: a systematic review of health outcomes. *Evid Rep Technol Assess (Full Rep)* 2009;(183):1-420.
59. Ontario Health Technology Advisory Committee. OHTAC recommendation. *Clinical utility of vitamin D testing.* Available from: www.health.gov.on.ca/english/providers/program/ohtac/tech/recommend/rec_vitamin%20d_201002.pdf. Accessed January 13, 2011.
60. Langlois K, Green-Finestone L, Little J et al. Vitamin D status of Canadians as measured in the 2007 to 2009 Canadian Health Measures Survey. *Health Rep* 2010;21(1):47-55.
61. Bjelakovic G, Gluud LL, Nikolova D et al. Vitamin D supplementation for prevention of mortality in adults. *Cochrane Database Syst Rev* 2011;(7):CD007470.
62. Hanley DA, Cranney A, Jones G et al. Vitamin D in adult health and disease: a review and guideline statement from Osteoporosis Canada (summary). *CMAJ* 2010;182(12):1315-9.
63. Dawson-Hughes B, Mithal A, Bonjour JP et al. IOF position statement: vitamin D recommendations for older adults. *Osteoporos Int* 2010;21(7):1151-4.
64. Canadian Cancer Society. *Vitamin D.* Available from: www.cancer.ca. Accessed January 13, 2011.
65. Vitamin D supplementation: recommendations for Canadian mothers and infants. *Paediatr Child Health* 2007;12(7):583-9.
66. Heaney RP. Vitamin D and calcium interactions: functional outcomes. *Am J Clin Nutr* 2008;88(2):541S-544S.
67. Office of Dietary Supplements, National Institutes of Health. *Dietary Supplement Fact Sheet: Vitamin B12.* Available from: ods.od.nih.gov/factsheets/VitaminB12-HealthProfessional/#h5. Accessed January 13, 2011.
68. Allen LH. How common is vitamin B-12 deficiency? *Am J Clin Nutr* 2009;89(2):693S-6S.
69. Hudson B. Vitamin B-12 deficiency. *BMJ* 2010;340:c2305.
70. Papaioannou A, Morin S, Cheung AM et al. 2010 clinical practice guidelines for the diagnosis and management of osteoporosis in Canada: summary. *CMAJ* 2010;182(17):1864-73.
71. Health Canada. *Vitamin D and calcium: updated Dietary Reference Intakes.* Available from: www.hc-sc.gc.ca/fn-an/nutrition/vitamin/vita-d-eng.php. Accessed January 13, 2011.
72. Moyer VA; U.S. Preventive Services Task Force. Vitamin D and calcium supplementation to prevent fractures in adults: U.S. Preventive Services Task Force recommendation statement. *Ann Intern Med* 2013;158(9):691-6.
73. Sulli MM, Ezzo DC. Drug interactions with vitamins and minerals. *US Pharm* 2007;1:42-55.
74. McColl KE. Effect of proton pump inhibitors on vitamins and iron. *Am J Gastroenterol* 2009;104(Suppl 2):S5-9.
75. Mouchantaf R. Proton pump inhibitors: hypomagnesemia accompanied by hypocalcemia and hypokalemia. *Can Adverse React Newsl* 2011;21(3):1-2. Available from: www.hc-sc.gc.ca/dhp-mps/medeff/bulletin/carn-bcei_v21n3-eng.php#_Proton_pump_inhibitors.
76. Age-Related Eye Disease Study Research Group. A randomized, placebo-controlled, clinical trial of high-dose supplementation with vitamins C and E, b-carotene, and zinc for age-related macular degeneration and vision loss: AREDS report no. 8. *Arch Ophthalmol* 2001;119(10):1417-36.
77. Age-Related Eye Disease Study 2 Research Group. Lutein + zeaxanthin and omega-3 fatty acids for age-related macular degeneration: the Age-Related Eye Disease Study 2 (AREDS2) randomized clinical trial. *JAMA* 2013;309(19):2005-15.
78. Hooper L, Thompson RL, Harrison RA et al. Omega 3 fatty acids for prevention and treatment of cardiovascular disease. *Cochrane Database Syst Rev* 2004;(4):CD003177.
79. Risk and Prevention Study Collaborative Group, Roncaglioni MC, Tombesi M et al. n-3 fatty acids in patients with multiple cardiovascular risk factors. *N Engl J Med* 2013;368(19):1800-8.
80. Mark BJ, Beaty AD, Slavin RG. Are fish oil supplements safe in finned fish-allergic patients? *Allergy Asthma Proc* 2008;29(5):528-9.

81. Witham MD, Price RJ, Struthers AD et al. Cholecalciferol treatment to reduce blood pressure in older patients with isolated systolic hypertension: the VitDISH randomized controlled trial. *JAMA Intern Med* 2013;173(18):1672-9.
82. Galan P, Kesse-Guyot E, Czernichow S et al. Effects of B vitamins and omega 3 fatty acids on cardiovascular diseases: a randomised placebo controlled trial. *BMJ* 2010;341:c6273.
83. Kris-Etherton PM, Lichtenstein AH, Howard BV et al. Antioxidant vitamin supplements and cardiovascular disease. *Circulation* 2004;110(5):637-41.
84. Myung SK, Ju W, Cho B et al. Efficacy of vitamin and antioxidant supplements in prevention of cardiovascular disease: systematic review and meta-analysis of randomised controlled trials. *BMJ* 2013;346:f10.
85. Fortmann SP, Burda BU, Senger CA et al. Vitamin and mineral supplements in the primary prevention of cardiovascular disease and cancer: an updated systematic evidence review for the U.S. Preventive Services Task Force. *Ann Intern Med* 2013 Nov 12. [Epub ahead of print].
86. Marik PE, Varon J. Omega-3 dietary supplements and the risk of cardiovascular events: a systematic review. *Clin Cardiol* 2009;32(7):365-72.
87. Rauch B, Schiele R, Schneider S et al. OMEGA, a randomized, placebo-controlled trial to test the effect of highly purified omega-3 fatty acids on top of modern guideline-adjusted therapy after myocardial infarction. *Circulation* 2010;122(21):2152-9.
88. Kromhout D, Giltay EJ, Geleijnse JM et al. n-3 fatty acids and cardiovascular events after myocardial infarction. *N Engl J Med* 2010;363(21):2015-26.
89. Macchia A, Grancelli H, Varini S et al. Omega-3 fatty acids for the prevention of recurrent symptomatic atrial fibrillation: results of the FORWARD (randomized trial to assess efficacy of PUFA for the maintenance of sinus rhythm in persistent atrial fibrillation). *J Am Coll Cardiol* 2013;61(4):463-8.
90. Kris-Etherton PM, Harris S, Apel LJ et al. Fish consumption, fish oil, omega-3 fatty acids, and cardiovascular disease. *Circulation* 2002;106(21):2747-57.
91. National Institute for Health and Clinical Excellence. *MI: secondary prevention: secondary prevention in primary and secondary care for patients following a myocardial infarction*. Available from: www.nice.org.uk/nicemedia/live/14302/65691/65691.pdf. Accessed November 19, 2013.
92. Cole BF, Baron JA, Sandler RS et al. Folic acid for the prevention of colorectal adenomas: a randomized clinical trial. *JAMA* 2007;297(21):2351-9.
93. Cooper K, Squires H, Carroll C et al. Chemoprevention of colorectal cancer: systematic review and economic evaluation. *Health Technol Assess* 2010;14(32):1-206.
94. Wilkins T, Reynolds PL. Colorectal cancer: a summary of the evidence for screening and prevention. *Am Fam Physician* 2008;78(12):1385-92.
95. Lonn E, Bosch J, Yusuf S et al. Effects of long-term vitamin E supplementation on cardiovascular events and cancer: a randomized controlled trial. *JAMA* 2005;293(11):1338-47.
96. Zhang SM, Cook NR, Albert CM et al. Effect of combined folic acid, vitamin B6, and vitamin B12 on cancer risk in women: a randomized trial. *JAMA* 2008;300(17):2012-21.
97. Druesne-Pecollo N, Latino-Martel P, Norat T et al. Beta-carotene supplementation and cancer risk: a systematic review and metaanalysis of randomized controlled trials. *Int J Cancer* 2010;127(1):172-84.
98. World Health Organization. International Agency for Research on Cancer. *Vitamin D and cancer*. Available from: www.iarc.fr/en/publications/pdfs-online/wrk/wrk5/Report_VitD.pdf. Accessed April 5, 2011.
99. Gould JF, Smithers LG, Makrides M. The effect of maternal omega-3 (n-3) LCPUFA supplementation during pregnancy on early childhood cognitive and visual development: a systematic review and meta-analysis of randomized controlled trials. *Am J Clin Nutr* 2013;97(3):531-44.
100. Makrides M, Gibson RA, McPhee AJ et al. Effect of DHA supplementation during pregnancy on maternal depression and neurodevelopment of young children: a randomized controlled trial. *JAMA* 2010;304(15):1675-83.
101. Plassman BL, Williams JW, Burke JR et al. Systematic review: factors associated with risk for and possible prevention of cognitive decline in later life. *Ann Intern Med* 2010;153(3):182-93.
102. Hartweg J, Perera R, Montori V et al. Omega-3 polyunsaturated fatty acids (PUFA) for type 2 diabetes mellitus. *Cochrane Database Syst Rev* 2008;(1):CD003205.
103. Zipitis CS, Akobeng AK. Vitamin D supplementation in early childhood and risk of type 1 diabetes: a systematic review and meta-analysis. *Arch Dis Child* 2008;93(6):512-7.
104. House AA, Eliasziw M, Cattran DC et al. Effect of B-vitamin therapy on progression of diabetic nephropathy: a randomized controlled trial. *JAMA* 2010;303(16):1603-9.
105. Juraschek SP, Miller ER, Gelber AC. Effect of oral vitamin C on uric acid: a meta-analysis of randomized clinical trials. *Arthritis Care Res (Hoboken)* 2011;63(9):1295-306.
106. Stamp LK, O'Donnell JL, Frampton C et al. Clinically insignificant effect of supplemental vitamin C on serum urate in patients with gout: a pilot randomized controlled trial. *Arthritis Rheum* 2013;65(6):1636-42.
107. Howlett JG, McKelvie RS, Arnold JM et al. Canadian Cardiovascular Society Consensus Conference guidelines on heart failure, update 2009: diagnosis and management of right-sided heart failure, myocarditis, device therapy and recent important clinical trials. *Can J Cardiol* 2009;25(2):85-105.
108. Madmani ME, Solaiman AY, Tamr Agha K et al. Coenzyme Q10 for heart failure. *Cochrane Database Syst Rev* 2013;9:CD008684.
109. Ramsden CE, Faurot KR, Zamora D et al. Targeted alteration of dietary n-3 and n-6 fatty acids for the treatment of chronic headaches: a randomized trial. *Pain* 2013;154(11):2441-51.
110. Freeman MP, Fava M, Lake J et al. Complementary and alternative medicine in major depressive disorder: the American Psychiatric Association Task Force Report. *J Clin Psychiatry* 2010;71(6):669-81.
111. Almeida OP, Marsh K, Alfonso H et al. B-vitamins reduce the long-term risk of depression after stroke: the VITATOPS-DEP trial. *Ann Neurol* 2010;68(4):503-10.
112. Fava M, Mischoulon D. Folate in depression: efficacy, safety, differences in formulations, and clinical issues. *J Clin Psychiatry* 2009;70(Suppl 5):12-7.
113. Mozurkewich EL, Clinton CM, Chilimigras JL et al. The Mothers, Omega-3, and Mental Health Study: a double-blind, randomized controlled trial. *Am J Obstet Gynecol* 2013;208(4):313.e1-9.
114. Miller BJ, Murray L, Beckmann ML et al. Dietary supplements for preventing postnatal depression. *Cochrane Database Syst Rev* 2013;10:CD009104.
115. Knutsen KV, Brekke M, Gjelstad S et al. Vitamin D status in patients with musculoskeletal pain, fatigue and headache: a cross-sectional descriptive study in a multi-ethnic general practice in Norway. *Scand J Prim Health Care* 2010;28(3):166-71.

116. Straube S, Derry S, Moore RA et al. Vitamin D for the treatment of chronic painful conditions in adults. *Cochrane Database Syst Rev* 2010;(2):CD007771.
117. Hofmeyr GJ, Lawrie TA, Atallah AN et al. Calcium supplementation during pregnancy for preventing hypertensive disorders and related problems. *Cochrane Database Syst Rev* 2010;(8):CD001059.
118. Amminger GP, Schafer MR, Papageorgiou K et al. Long-chain omega-3 fatty acids for indicated prevention of psychotic disorders: a randomized, placebo-controlled trial. *Arch Gen Psychiatry* 2010;67(2):146-54.
119. Joy CB, Mumby-Croft R, Joy LA. Polyunsaturated fatty acid supplementation for schizophrenia. *Cochrane Database Syst Rev* 2006;(3):CD001257.
120. Montgomery P, Richardson AJ. Omega-3 fatty acids for bipolar disorder. *Cochrane Database Syst Rev* 2008;(2):CD005169.
121. Roffman JL, Lamberti JS, Achtyes E et al. Randomized multicenter investigation of folate plus vitamin B12 supplementation in schizophrenia. *JAMA Psychiatry* 2013;70(5):481-9.
122. Hemila H, Louhiala P. Vitamin C for preventing and treating pneumonia. *Cochrane Database Syst Rev* 2013;8:CD005532.
123. Hemila H, Chalker E. Vitamin C for preventing and treating the common cold. *Cochrane Database Syst Rev* 2013;1:CD000980.
124. Singh M, Das RR. Zinc for the common cold. *Cochrane Database Syst Rev* 2013;6:CD001364.
125. Abou-Raya An About-Raya S, Helmii M. The effect of vitamin D supplementation on inflammatory and hemostatic markers and disease activity in patients with systemic lupus erythematosus: a randomized placebo-controlled trial. *J Rheumatol* 2013;40(3):265-72.

Glossary of Abbreviated Terms

5-ASA	5-aminosalicylic acid
AC	before meals
ACE	angiotensin-converting enzyme
ACEI	angiotensin-converting enzyme inhibitor
ADHD	attention-deficit hyperactivity disorder
AIDS	acquired immunodeficiency syndrome
AMD	age-related macular degeneration
aPTT	activated partial thromboplastin time
ARB	angiotensin receptor blocker
ASA	acetylsalicylic acid
AST	aspartate aminotransferase
AUC	area under the concentration curve
BCG	bacillus Calmette-Guérin
BID	twice daily
BMD	bone mineral density
BMI	body mass index
BMR	basal metabolic rate
BP	blood pressure
BPH	benign prostatic hyperplasia
bpm	beats per minute
BSA	body surface area
BUN	blood urea nitrogen
C&S	culture and sensitivity
CABG	coronary artery bypass graft
cAMP	cyclic adenosine monophosphate
cART	combination antiretroviral therapy
CBC	complete blood count
CBT	cognitive behavioural therapy
CCB	calcium channel blocker
CDC	Centers for Disease Control (US)
cfu/L	colony-forming units/litre
cGMP	cyclic guanosine monophosphate
CI	confidence interval
CK	creatine kinase
ClCr	creatinine clearance
CNS	central nervous system
COPD	chronic obstructive pulmonary disease
CPK	creatine phosphokinase
CPR	cardiopulmonary resuscitation
CRP	C-reactive protein
CSF	cerebrospinal fluid
CT	computed tomography
DEET	diethyltoluamide
DHA	dihydroxyacetone; docosahexaenoic acid
DHEA	dehydroepiandrosterone
DMARD	disease-modifying antirheumatic drug
DNA	deoxyribonucleic acid
DOT	directly observed therapy
DOTS	directly observed therapy – short course
DPI	dry powder inhaler
DVT	deep vein thrombosis
DXA	dual energy x-ray absorptiometry
ECG	electrocardiogram
ECT	electroconvulsive therapy
EDTA	ethylenediaminetetraacetic acid
EEG	electroencephalogram
EMLA	eutectic mixture of local anesthetics
ENT	ear, nose and throat
EPA	eicosapentaenoic acid
EPS	extrapyramidal symptoms
ESR	erythrocyte sedimentation rate
FDA	Food and Drug Administration (USA)
FEV	forced expiratory volume
FEV_1	forced expiratory volume in one second
FiO_2	fraction of inspired oxygen
FSH	follicle-stimulating hormone
fT3	free triiodothyronine
fT4	free thyroxine
G6PD	glucose-6-phosphate dehydrogenase
GERD	gastroesophageal reflux disease
GFR	glomerular filtration rate
GGT	gamma glutamyl transpeptidase
GI	gastrointestinal

GnRH gonadotropin-releasing hormone
GnRH-a gonadotropin-releasing hormone analogue
h hour(s)
H_2RA H2-receptor antagonist
Hb hemoglobin
HbA_{1c} glycosylated hemoglobin
HCG human chorionic gonadotropin
HDL-C high-density lipoprotein cholesterol
HEPA high efficiency particulate air
HFA hydrofluoroalkane
HIV human immunodeficiency virus
HLA human leukocyte antigen
HPO hypothalamic-pituitary-ovarian
HPV human papillomavirus
HS bedtime
IBW ideal body weight
ICU intensive care unit
im, IM intramuscular
INR International Normalized Ratio
IOP intraocular pressure
IU international unit
IUD intrauterine device
IUS intrauterine system
iv, IV intravenous
J joule
LCD liquor carbonis detergens
LDL-C low-density lipoprotein cholesterol
LH luteinizing hormone
LMWH low-molecular-weight heparin
MAO monoamine oxidase
MAOI monoamine oxidase inhibitor
MDI metered-dose inhaler
MI myocardial infarction
MIC minimum inhibitory concentration
min minute(s)
MRI magnetic resonance imaging
MRSA methicillin-resistant *S. aureus*
ms millisecond
MSSA methicillin-sensitive *S. aureus*
NG nasogastric
NNT number needed to treat
NSAID nonsteroidal anti-inflammatory drug
NSTEMI non-ST segment elevation myocardial infarction
NYHA New York Heart Association
OCD obsessive-compulsive disorder
OR odds ratio
OTC over-the-counter (nonprescription)
PABA para-aminobenzoic acid
PC after meals
PCR polymerase chain reaction
PDE5 phosphodiesterase type 5
po, PO by mouth
PPI proton pump inhibitor
pr, PR rectally
PRN when necessary
PSA prostate specific antigen
PT prothrombin time
PTH parathyroid hormone
PTSD post-traumatic stress disorder
PTT partial thromboplastin time
pv, PV vaginally
QHS each bedtime
QID four times per day
RA rheumatoid arthritis
RBC red blood cell
RCT randomized controlled trial
REM rapid eye movement
RICE rest, ice, compression, elevation
RR relative risk
SAM-e S-adenosyl-methionine
SaO_2 oxygen saturation
sc, SC subcutaneous
s second(s)
SIADH syndrome of inappropriate antidiuretic hormone
sl, SL sublingual
SMX/TMP sulfamethoxazole/trimethoprim
SNRI serotonin-norepinephrine reuptake inhibitor
SOGC Society of Obstetricians and Gynaecologists of Canada
SPF sun protection factor
SSRI selective serotonin reuptake inhibitor
STI sexually transmitted infection
STEMI ST segment elevation myocardial infarction
TID three times per day
TNFα tumor necrosis factor-alpha
TSH thyroid-stimulating hormone

USP	United States Pharmacopoeia
UTI	urinary tract infection
UVA	ultraviolet-A
UVB	ultraviolet-B
UVC	ultraviolet-C
WBC	white blood cell
WHI	Women's Health Initiative
WHO	World Health Organization
wk	week(s)
y	year(s)

Index

B

D

E

F

G

H

I

J

K

L

M

N

O

Q

R

S

W

X

Y

Z